AF530769

Textbook of Radiology & Imaging

Textbook of Radiology & Imaging

Edition 8

David Sutton

Rodney Reznek, Janet Murfitt

Volume 2

Adaptation Editor

Bharat Aggarwal

Director, Radiology Services, Max Healthcare, New Delhi, India

Adjunct Professor, Koita Centre for Digital Health (KCDH) of Indian Institute of Technology, Bombay

Associate Editors

Amit Kumar Sahu
Consultant
Department of Radiology
Max Superspeciality Hospital, Saket
New Delhi, India

Akshay D. Baheti
Professor
Department of Radiodiagnosis
Tata Memorial Center and Homi Bhabha National University
Mumbai, Maharashtra, India

Varsha Joshi
Senior Consultant Radiologist
Vijaya Diagnostic Centers
Hyderabad, Telangana, India

Section Editors

Girish Gandikota
Professor and Vice Chair of Radiology
University of Chapel Hill, North Carolina
Adjunct Professor, Radiology and Rheumatology
University of Michigan
Ann Arbor, MI, United States

Mukesh Harisinghani
Professor of Radiology
Harvard Medical School,
Massachusetts General Hospital
Boston, MA, United States

Puneet Bhargava
Professor, Director
Gastrointestinal Imaging
Abdominal Imaging Radiologist, University of Washington School of Medicine Hospitals,
Seattle, WA, United States

Sandeep S. Hedgire
Assistant Clinical Director
Cardiovascular Division, Director, Vascular Imaging
Department of Radiology, Massachusetts General Hospital, Harvard Medical School,
Boston, MA, United States

Subba R. Digumarthy
Associate Professor of Radiology
Harvard Medical School
Boston, MA, United States
Head of Thoracic Oncology Imaging
Division of Thoracic Imaging and Intervention
Massachusetts General Hospital Boston, MA, United States

Sujit Vaidya
Consultant Radiologist
The Royal London Hospital, Barts Health NHS Trust
Queen Mary University of London,
London, United Kingdom

Suresh K. Mukerji
Professor of Radiology & Radiation Oncology
University of Louisville & University of Illinois, Robert Wood Johnson Medical School, Rutgers University, New Brunswick, NJ, United States.
Faculty, Otolaryngology Head Neck Surgery, Michigan State University
National Director of Head & Neck Radiology; ProScan Imaging
Bruce Bradley Fellow; The Leapfrog Group

Suyash Mohan
Associate Professor of Radiology & Neurosurgery, Perelman School of Medicine at the University of Pennsylvania
Philadelphia, PA, United States
Formerly, Clinical Lecturer-II University of Michigan, Ann Arbor, MI, United States

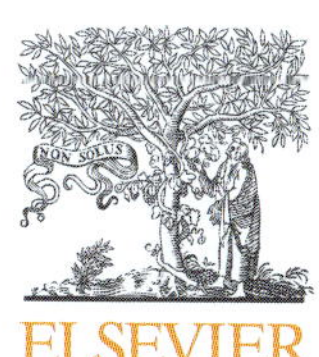

ELSEVIER

Elsevier
RELX India Pvt. Ltd.
Registered Office: 818, 8th floor, Indraprakash Building, 21, Barakhamba Road, New Delhi-110 001
Corporate Office: 14th Floor, Building No. 10B, DLF Cyber City, Phase II, Gurgaon-122 002, Haryana, India

Textbook of Radiology & Imaging, 2 Volume Set, 7e, David Sutton, Rodney Reznek, Janet Murfitt.

Publisher's note: Elsevier takes a neutral position with respect to territorial disputes or jurisdictional claims in its published content, including in maps and institutional affiliations.

ISBN: 978-0-443-07109-6

This adaptation of **Textbook of Radiology & Imaging, 2 Volume Set, 7e, by David Sutton, Rodney Reznek, Janet Murfitt** was undertaken by RELX India Private Limited and is published by arrangement with Elsevier Ltd.

Textbook of Radiology & Imaging, 2 Volume Set, 8e by David Sutton, Rodney Reznek, Janet Murfitt.
Adaptation Editor: Bharat Aggarwal

Adaptation ISBN: 978-81-312-5961-0
Adaptation e-ISBN: 978-81-312-5964-1

Set ISBN: 978-81-312-5959-7
Set e-ISBN: 978-81-312-5962-7

First Printed in India 2024, Reprinted 2025

Notice

The adaptation has been undertaken by RELX India Pvt. Ltd and its sole responsibility. Medical Students, radiology residents, practitioners and researchers must always rely on their own experience and knowledge in evaluating and using any information, methods, compounds or experiments described herein. Because of rapid advances in the medical sciences, in particular, independent verification of diagnoses and drug dosages should be made. To the fullest extent of the law, no responsibility is assumed by Elsevier, authors, editors or contributors in relation to the adaptation or for any injury and/or damage to persons or property as a matter of products liability, negligence or otherwise, or from any use or operation of any methods, products, instructions, or ideas contained in the material herein.

Although all advertising material is expected to conform to ethical (medical) standards, inclusion in this publication does not constitute a guarantee or endorsement of the quality or value of such product or of the claims made of it by its manufacturer.

Authorised Territory for Print form only is India, Pakistan, Bangladesh, Nepal, Srilanka, Bhutan, Maldives, Singapore, Malaysia, Brunei, Indonesia, Philippines, Thailand, Vietnam, Cambodia, Laos and Myanmar.

Publisher's `e-book' shall have `World' rights for selling globally through 3PP websites as approved by Proprietor.

Content Strategist: Mrinalini Bakshi
Content project Manager: Shivani Pal
Senior Production Executive: Dhan Singh
Senior Graphic Artist: Gopalakrishnan Venkatraman

Typeset by Aptara

Printed in India by Sanat Printers

Foreword

When I was a resident in the late 1980s, the only general radiology textbook we referred to was Dr. David Sutton's Textbook of Radiology. My copy was heavily underlined and annotated and dog-eared and had multiple short, "xeroxed" pages of newer information from journals stuck to the original pages by tape or gum, increasing the weight of the textbook significantly.

Even though in the later years, other textbooks became popular, Sutton was always the first book that would come to mind when we wanted residents to read up on a specific topic. In those days, with no Internet, no Pubmed, no Radiopaedia, and no other online resources, our only avenues to learn were general radiology and specialty textbooks and the popular grey and yellow journals, which in India, we would receive only about 6-9 months after publication.

Dr. Sutton died in 2002. The last (7th) edition of his book was also published in 2002. Given its immense popularity, it is no wonder that Elsevier has decided to resurrect an 8th edition of this book, in a new avatar, especially for a South Asian audience. This is no mean task. Radiology has advanced by leaps and bounds since the time Dr. Sutton updated his book. Residents, fellows, and consultants now have access to a large number of online teaching resources, some very good, many free, and some behind paywalls, but all available at the click of a mouse or the touch of a thumb. The large language models such as Chat-GPT4 are also increasing access to textual knowledge, especially for specifically structured questions. Textbooks therefore now face significant competition for eyeballs and money.

Elsevier was wise and I would say lucky to find and choose my friend Dr. Bharat Aggarwal to helm this project to bring to life this 8th edition. A third-generation radiologist, Bharat is one of the finest radiologists I have known over the last 30 years. He understands the nuances of the subject, is widely read and traveled, and hence has been able to put together an enviable roster of renowned radiologists of Indian origin, both in India and from the US and the UK, as Associate and Section Editors. His Associate Editors, Drs. Amit Sahu, Akshay Baheti, and Varsha Joshi are radiologists I have known for the last many years, all of them passionate teachers and educators. His Section Editors are all internationally renowned experts in their field. Drs. Suyash Mohan, Suresh Mukherji, Sandeep Hedgire, Mukesh Harisinghani, Sujit Vaidya, Subba Digamurthy, Girish Gandikota, and Puneet Bhargava have all put tremendous effort into their individual sections to bring the book to fruition.

It has taken about 4 years, two of which were during the challenging COVID-19 times, to make sure that each chapter in the book is as good, if not better than any online resource, with new images, algorithms, flowcharts, and tables. Some new sections have been added including Women's, Pediatric Imaging, and Interventional Radiology. It is a complete textbook that would give residents most of the information they need during their residency days and clear their examinations.

It has taken a lot of effort to maintain the flavor, language, and flow of the original book, while still ensuring that every statement of fact has been vetted and that all information is current up to the date of publication.

I congratulate Dr. Bharat Aggarwal and his team for this effort and I am sure that the book will serve as a popular and invaluable resource, not only for residents, but even for consultants, who can use this as a quick reference resource when stuck on a specific subject.

Dr Bhavin Jankharia

Preface

Radiology is a continuously evolving field. With each passing year, advancements in technology enable greater precision and improved safety. The adoption of digital tools, artificial intelligence and machine learning, coupled with a better understanding of the molecular basis of disease, has enabled the introduction of new therapies and altered decision pathways for patient care. The role of the radiologist is now central to treatment planning and disease monitoring, therefore making it vital for radiologists to not only provide diagnoses but also actively contribute to decision-making in patient care. The modern radiologist now, more than ever before, must have a strong foundational knowledge while adapting to the evolving technological advances. It is with this premise that we have adapted this new edition of Sutton's Textbook of Radiology.

It has been an honor to be invited by Elsevier to edit and update Sutton's Textbook of Radiology, the gold standard and a key reference book for practicing radiologists over multiple generations. I have attempted to share my experiences as a radiologist, a journey that began when I learned radiology from my father, Dr. Sudarshan K. Aggarwal, perhaps one of the greatest visionaries of Indian Radiology. The Diwan Chand Aggarwal Imaging Center, started by my grandfather in 1924 and taken forward by my uncle Dr. Satyapal Aggarwal, was scaled to an institution under the stewardship of my father, and managed under one core tenet—**patient first.** This created an academic environment and pushed the institute to be a teaching center from where over 100 radiology residents completed their training and are now leading radiologists across the globe. I continue to follow this philosophy of combining high-quality clinical care and academic pursuit in my ongoing tenure at Max Healthcare, one of the largest healthcare providers in India.

Despite the fact that the last revision of this book was in 2002, it has continued to be a favorite textbook among radiology residents, mainly because of the comprehensive coverage of each topic and the presentation style. We have preserved the unique style of the textbook and retained material that continues to be relevant even two decades later. This edition of Sutton is aimed at recreating an exhaustive resource and reference text for radiologists to solve diverse clinical scenarios using the latest and most appropriate technology, and develop a sound process-driven approach.

New sections on radiology physics and techniques, pediatric radiology, interventional radiology, and emergency radiology have been added to make the book comprehensive. The first section includes chapters on quality assurance, structured reporting, information technology in radiology, and a primer in artificial intelligence—knowledge of which is now extremely important to practicing radiologists. The remaining sections have been reorganized to emphasize the need for sub-specialty radiology. Chapters on nuclear medicine and dental radiology provide the practicing radiologist with an understanding of all imaging-based diagnostic techniques available today. The evolving radiology lexicons that radiologists should use in their daily practice to communicate their findings for consistent care have also been incorporated into the book.

This book was put together through the COVID-19 pandemic, the biggest medical calamity faced by our generation. I want to extend my heartfelt gratitude to all the contributors who, despite being personally and professionally impacted by COVID-19 at the frontlines during the pandemic, stood true to their commitment and contributed high-quality material that will lay the foundation for the careers of the radiologists of the future.

I acknowledge the proactivity, guidance, and support extended by the section editors, all of whom are leaders in their fields—a big thanks to Dr. Suresh Mukherji, Dr. Suyash Mohan, Dr. Girish Gandikota, Dr. Sandeep Hedgire, Dr. Mukesh Harisinghani, Dr. Sujit Vaidya, Dr. Puneet Bhargava, and Dr. Subba Digumarthy. I would also like to thank Dr. Rajesh Gothi and Dr. Shivani Khanna for editorial support, and the management of Max Healthcare for their support.

I would have been unable to complete this project without the commitment shown by my associate editors, Dr. Amit Sahu and Dr. Akshay Baheti, right from the acceptance of this challenge to its planning and smooth execution, along with Dr. Varsha Joshi.

Most importantly I thank the patient community that my family has served over almost a century, for shaping my professional career and encouraging me to be a better doctor.

There are absolutely no words to describe the encouragement and support I have received from my wife, Suman, and children, Samir and Divya, in this extended, almost four-year journey of editing Sutton and the endless personal time ungrudgingly shared.

This book is my contribution to the legacy of my family and to the specialty of Radiology.

Dr Bharat Aggarwal

Contributors

Amogh N. Hegde
Senior Consultant Radiologist
Raffles Hospital, Singapore

Abhay Kumar Kapoor
Senior Consultant & Head
Department of Interventional Oncology, RGCI & RC
Delhi, India

Aditi Chandra
Senior Consultant, Tata Medical Center
Kolkata, India

Aditya S. Pandey
Professor and Chair, Department of Neurosurgery
Professor, Neurological Surgery, Radiology, Otolaryngology – Head and Neck Surgery
Surgical Director, Comprehensive Stroke Center
Director, Strategic Vision and Outside Collaborations – Neurosurgery
Ann Arbor, MI, United States

Ali Rashidi
Department of Radiology, Molecular Imaging Program at Stanford (MIPS)
Stanford University School of Medicine
Stanford, CA, United States

Alistair D. Calder
Radiology Department, Great Ormond Street Hospital
London, United Kingdom

Late Allan Midyet
Imaging Institute for Neuroradiology

Anagha Rajeev Joshi
Professor and Head of Department
Department of Radiology
Lokmanya Tilak Municipal Medical College and General Hospital
Sion, Mumbai, Maharashtra, India

Anand Kirwadi
Consultant Musculoskeletal Radiologist
Manchester University Hospitals Foundation Trust
Manchester, United Kingdom

Anbarasu Arangasamy
Consultant Radiologist & Director
Aran Diagnostic Imaging
Coimbatore, Tamil Nadu, India

Anisha Gehani
Junior Consultant
Tata Medical Center
Kolkata, West Bengal, India

Ankit Balani
Consultant Radiologist
Vijaya Diagnostic Center Pvt. Ltd
Hyderabad, Telangana, India

Anu Eapen
Professor, Department of Radiodiagnosis
Christian Medical College
Vellore, Tamil Nadu, India

Anuj Jain
Locum Consultant Radiologist, Department of Radiology & Nuclear Medicine
North Cumbria Integrated Care
Carlisle, United Kingdom

Argha Chatterjee
PDCC Gastro-Radiology, SGPGIMS
Lucknow, Uttar Pradesh, India
Associate Consultant
Tata Medical Center
Kolkata, West Bengal, India

Arman Parsai
Consultant Radiologist at Barts Health
London, United Kingdom

Ashok Adams
Consultant Radiologist at Barts Health
London, United Kingdom

Betty Simon
Professor, Department of Clinical Radiology
Christian Medical College
Vellore, Tamil Nadu, India

Bhawan Paunipagar
Partner and Consultant Radiologist, Sai Scans (3T MRI), Akshay PET-CT, Akshay CT
Sangli and Kolhapur, Maharashtra, India

Bojan Kovacina
Radiologist
Jewish General Hospital
Assistant Professor
McGill University
Montreal, QC, Canada

52 Arthritis

STEPHEN JUDGE, MICHAEL BROOKS, LAUREN GOLDMAN, GIRISH GANDIKOTE

Radiographic examinations for joint and back pain are ubiquitous in both general and subspecialty radiology practices and become essential for the interpreting radiologist to differentiate inflammatory from degenerative causes of joint disease, having implications for patient management. Degenerative, or osteoarthritis (OA), is characterized by asymmetric chondral wear resulting in nonuniform joint space narrowing. As the joint space narrows, abnormal motion across the joint surfaces causes bony productive change in the form of subchondral sclerosis and osteophyte formation, as well as subchondral cysts or geodes.

In contrast, there are imaging findings and concepts that are shared among the inflammatory arthritides. Recognizing the radiographic hallmarks of inflammatory arthritis, including marginal bone erosions, uniform joint space narrowing, and regional soft-tissue swelling, will allow the radiologist to offer more definitive radiological diagnoses. Focal discontinuity of subchondral bone indicates osseous erosion, which indicates underlying joint inflammation. Specifically, understanding the concept of periarticular or marginal erosions is considered one of the most important imaging features in being able to distinguish an inflammatory arthropathy from OA. Joint inflammation will initially produce erosions at the margins or periphery of joints, known as the "bare area," representing the portion of the joint that is intra-articular, but not covered or essentially not protected by hyaline cartilage (Fig. 52.1). Eventually, destruction of the articular cartilage is uniform throughout the joint space, which leads to symmetric joint space narrowing, rather than asymmetric patterns seen in degenerative arthritis [1].

Additionally, and of equal importance, understanding the classic distribution tendencies will lead the radiologist down different diagnostic pathways. In monoarticular arthropathy, excluding infection is imperative before suggesting inflammatory arthropathy from a separate etiology. Successful diagnosis of a suspected inflammatory arthropathy that involves multiple joints should be tackled utilizing a distribution approach. *For example, proximal distribution process of the hands or feet without bony proliferative changes suggests rheumatoid arthritis; however a distal distribution process of the hands or feet with associated bone proliferation suggests a seronegative arthropathy.* Imaging and distribution characteristics of both degenerative OA and inflammatory arthritides will be addressed throughout this chapter, while offering a framework or an approach to be utilized during image interpretation to increase diagnostic accuracy (Fig. 52.2).

Degenerative and Erosive OA

Overview

OA, also known as degenerative joint disease, is considered the most prevalent chronic joint disease. The overall disease prevalence of OA is thought to be on the rise, in part due to an aging population, but also due to the increasing prevalence of obesity [2]. The condition is most notably a noninflammatory arthropathy characterized by progressive cartilage degeneration with resultant hypertrophic bony proliferation, osteophyte formation, which far outpaces the body's intrinsic ability for cartilage repair.

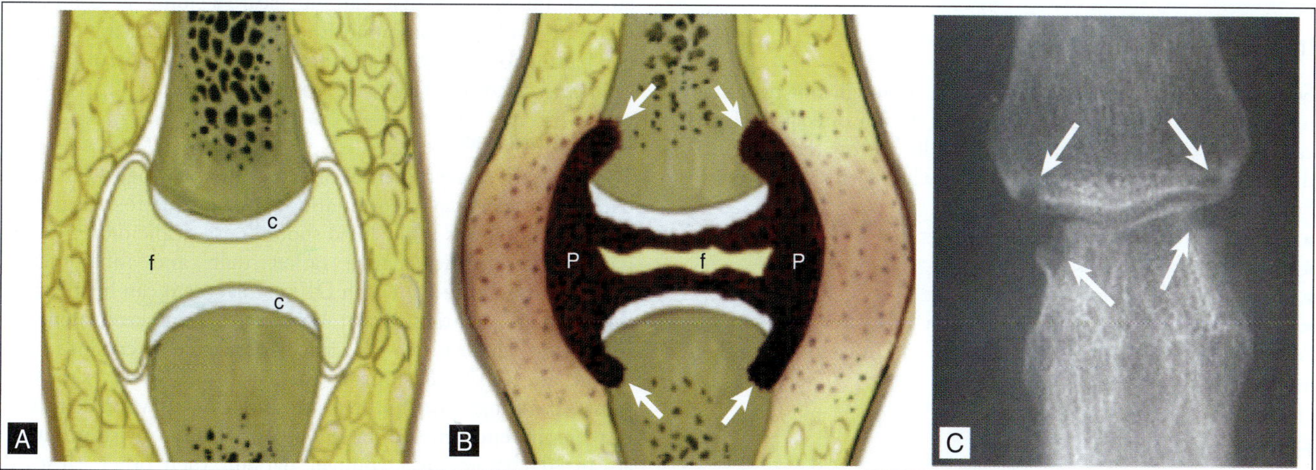

Figure 52.1 (A) Illustration of synovial joint shows joint fluid (*f*) and articular cartilage (c). (B) Illustration and (C) radiograph show inflammatory arthritis, synovitis, and pannus (*P*) causing cartilage destruction. Marginal erosions (*arrows*) are seen where subchondral bone plate is exposed to intraarticular synovitis.

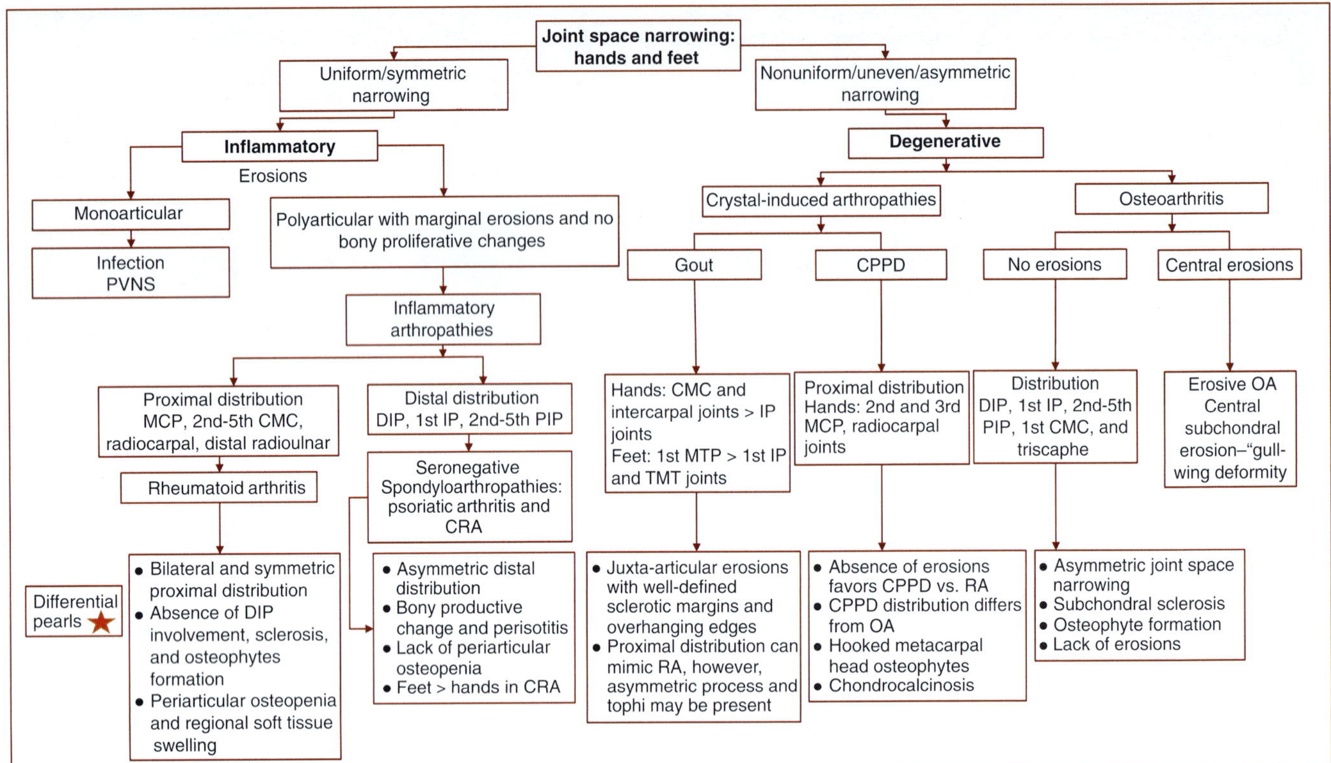

Figure 52.2 Approach to the radiographic evaluation of arthropathies, using the distal extremities as a model. *CMC*, carpometacarpal; *CPPD*, calcium pyrophosphate dihydrate crystal deposition disease; *CRA*, chronic reactive arthritis; *DIP*, distal interphalangeal; *IP*, interphalangeal; *MCP*, metacarpophalangeal; *MTP*, metatarsophalangeal; *OA*, osteoarthritis; *PIP*, proximal interphalangeal; *PVNS*, pigmented villonodular synovitis; *RA*, rheumatoid arthritis; *TMT*, tarsometatarsal.

Pathology

Although the pathophysiology underlying OA is not completely understood, it is thought to be fundamentally attributable to multiple intrinsic and extrinsic factors, including but not limited to repetitive mechanical stresses, history of trauma and/or instability, normal aging processes within articular cartilage, genetic factors predisposing to premature cartilage destruction, and in some cases even to hormonal factors such as low estrogen levels [3]. Even as part of the normal aging process, chondrocytes decrease in number resulting in increased fragility of the cartilage matrix due to decreasing proteoglycan production. Increased degradative enzymes may result from this process and contribute to the rapidity of onset.

Imaging Appearance

Several imaging manifestations of OA, although not necessarily unique to this entity, are so widespread within osteoarthritic disease processes that they serve to markedly narrow the differential diagnosis of joint pathology, especially when seen simultaneously. Such findings include:

- Asymmetric joint space narrowing
- Subchondral sclerosis
- Subchondral cyst formation
- Periarticular osteophyte proliferation

Additional imaging manifestations seen in OA can most easily be assessed based on anatomic location.

Hands/Wrists

First, identifying the distribution of joint involvement in the hands and wrists is essential in narrowing the differential diagnosis for various arthritides. OA is known to affect the interphalangeal joints of the hand (Fig. 52.3), *with special predilection for the distal interphalangeal (DIP) joint. Additionally, primary OA targets the first carpometacarpal joint and scapho-trapezial-trapezoid articulations.* Nodular deformities from osteophytes and soft-tissue swelling at the distal *(Heberden nodes)* and proximal *(Bouchard nodes)* interphalangeal joints are common clinical findings [4].

Erosive OA—It is an inflammatory variant of OA. It has marked female predilection. Typically presenting in the peri- and postmenopausal patient. Distribution pattern in the hands and feet is essentially the same as encountered in primary OA, manifesting as mixed erosive and productive changes of the interphalangeal joints. The first carpometacarpal joint is commonly involved, and less commonly the scapho-trapezial-trapezoid. It has pathognomonic central subchondral erosions resulting in a "*gullwing deformity*" (Fig. 52.4) [5].

Differential Pearls

The hallmark of asymmetric joint space narrowing, resulting in hypertrophic osteophyte formation, and lack of erosions involving the small joints of the hand should raise suspicion for underlying osteoarthritic change rather than and inflammatory arthropathy. Erosive OA with DIP involvement can be mistaken for psoriatic arthritis (PsA); however, careful assessment for "gull-wing" deformity with lack of periarticular erosions leans toward erosive OA. Rheumatoid arthritis rarely involves the DIP joints. If radiographic findings are similar in appearance to OA, but are in encountered in an atypical joint distribution, or advanced changes in a younger patient, then other causes of atypical or secondary OA (post-traumatic arthrosis, crystal-induced arthritis, hemophilic and neuropathic arthropathy) should be entertained.

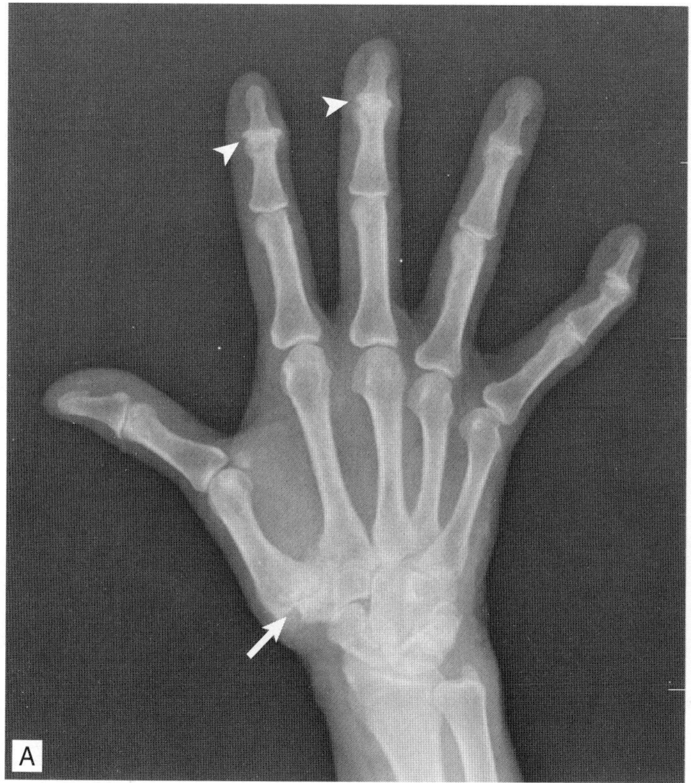

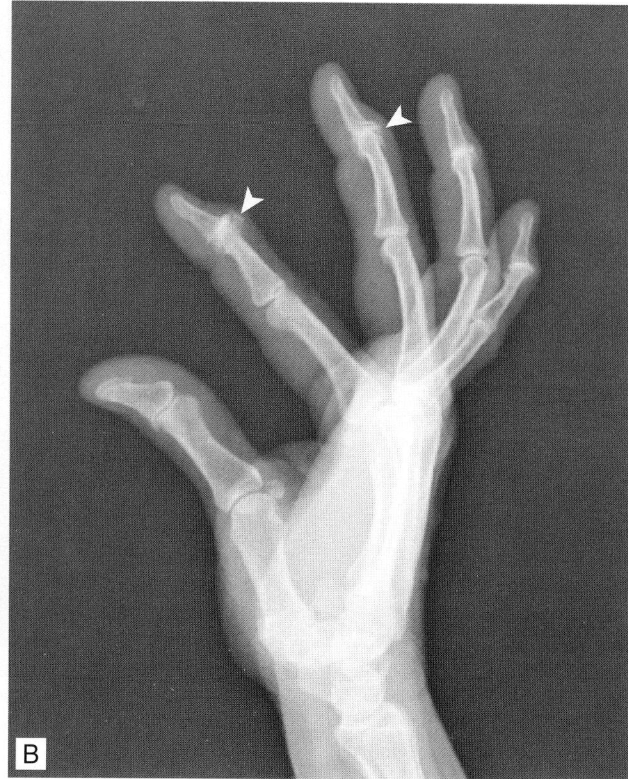

Figure 52.3 Classic osteoarthritis of the hands. PA (A) and lateral (B) radiographs demonstrate 2nd-5th DIP joint space narrowing with prominent marginal osteophytes (*arrowheads*), as well as severe narrowing at the 1st CMC joint (*arrow*) with subchondral sclerosis and osteophyte formation.

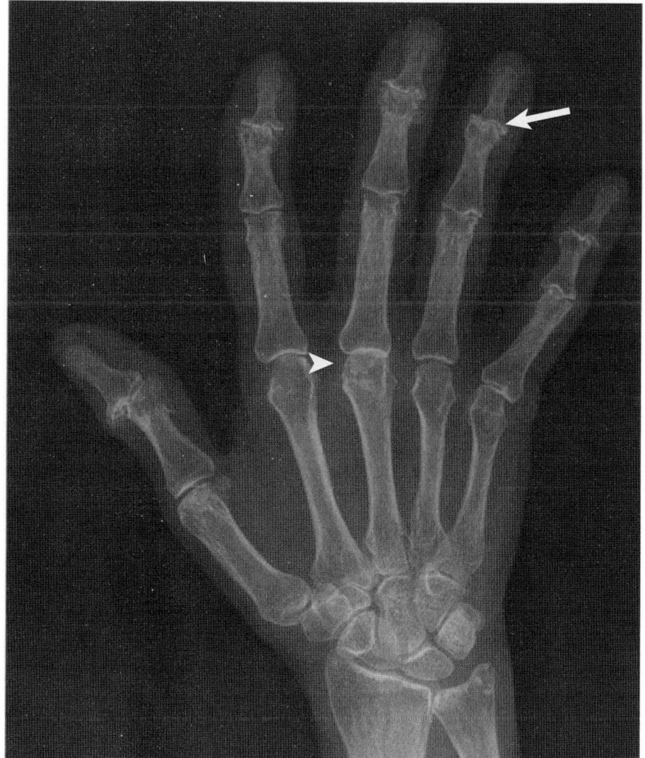

Figure 52.4 Erosive osteoarthritis. Frontal radiograph of the hands in a 76-year-old female demonstrating central subchondral erosions of the 2nd–5th DIP joints resulting in the classic gullwing deformity (*white arrow*) seen in erosive osteoarthritis. Also, note the atypical distribution of 2nd and 3rd MCP narrowing with subchondral cystic change and chondrocalcinosis (*arrowhead*), suggestive of coexistent CPPD arthropathy.

Shoulders

- Primary OA—No specific cause. Related to age, gender, and genetic factors. Most commonly seen in patients over the age of 50, with women being affected more often than men
- Secondary OA—Has a known cause (i.e., previous injury or shoulder dislocations, infection, or rotator cuff tear)

Superomedial aspect of the humeral head is frequently the earliest site of osteoarthritic cartilage loss in the glenohumeral joint (Fig. 52.5). Marginal osteophyte formation is seen at the inferior humeral head-neck junction (Fig. 52.5).

- Large size of inferomedial humeral head osteophytes may even result in neurologic symptoms if they impinge on the axillary nerve as it courses through the quadrilateral space
- Small fragments of osteophytes may additionally fracture and result in intra-articular bodies

Joint degeneration can be accelerated in the presence of accompanying soft-tissue abnormality, including but not limited to rotator cuff pathology and/or shoulder instability. Glenohumeral OA superimposed upon severe rotator cuff disease can result in rotator cuff arthropathy, a specific form of OA that results in superior displacement of the humeral head with respect to the glenoid. Abnormal articulation of the humerus with the acromion leads to rounding of the greater tuberosity (*femoralization*) with associated concave erosion of the undersurface of the acromion (*acetabularization*).

The acromioclavicular (AC) joint is also a common site of OA, with typical findings of joint space narrowing, subchondral sclerosis and cystic change, and osteophyte formation.

Hips

Classic OA of the hip results from progressive cartilage degeneration with following typical radiographic imaging manifestations (Fig. 52.6) [6]:

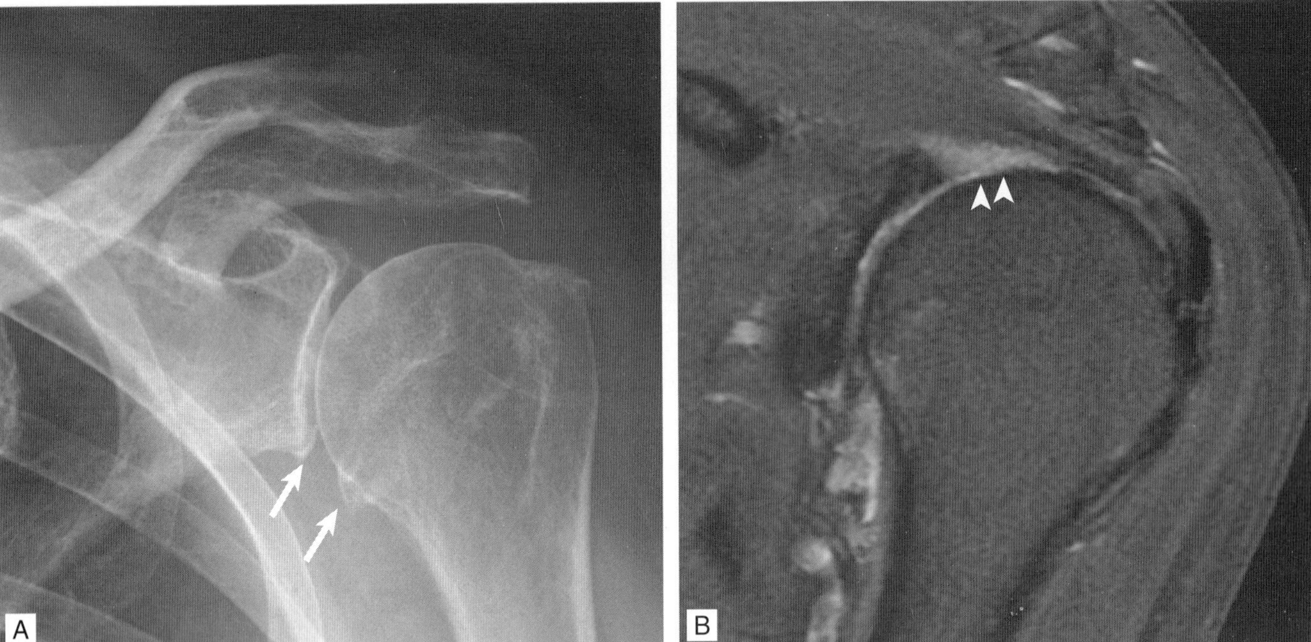

Figure 52.5 Classic glenohumeral arthritis. Frontal radiograph (A) of the shoulder demonstrates joints space narrowing, glenoid subchondral sclerosis, inferior glenoid rim, and inferomedial humeral head–anatomic neck osteophyte formation (*arrows*). Coronal proton density fat-saturated MR image (B) in the same patient showing focal high-grade chondral wear along the superomedial aspect of the humeral head (*arrowheads*), as well as inferomedial humeral head osteophyte formation.

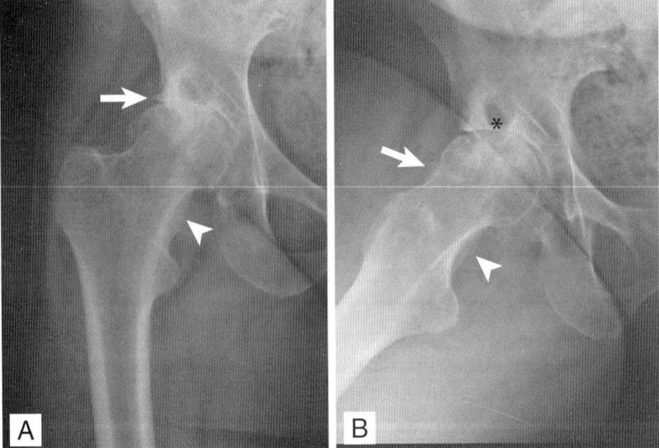

Figure 52.6 Classic OA of the hip. AP (A) and frog leg lateral (B) radiographs demonstrate severe superolateral joint space narrowing of the right hip joint with bone-on-bone articulation, subchondral sclerosis, subchondral cyst (*), calcar buttressing (*arrowheads*), prominent acetabular spurring (*arrow* in A), and femoral head–neck junction ring osteophytes.

- Superolateral femoral head subluxation and joint space narrowing along the weight-bearing portion of the joint is seen in 80% of cases, whereas medial subluxation/narrowing (protrusio) is seen in 20% of hip OA cases
- Subchondral sclerosis and cyst formation
- Osseous productive change
  - Femoral head–neck junction ring osteophytes
  - Acetabular osteophytes
  - Femoral neck (calcar) buttressing

OA in young adults is often associated with underlying morphologic abnormalities:

- Femoroacetabular impingement
- Developmental dysplasia of the hip

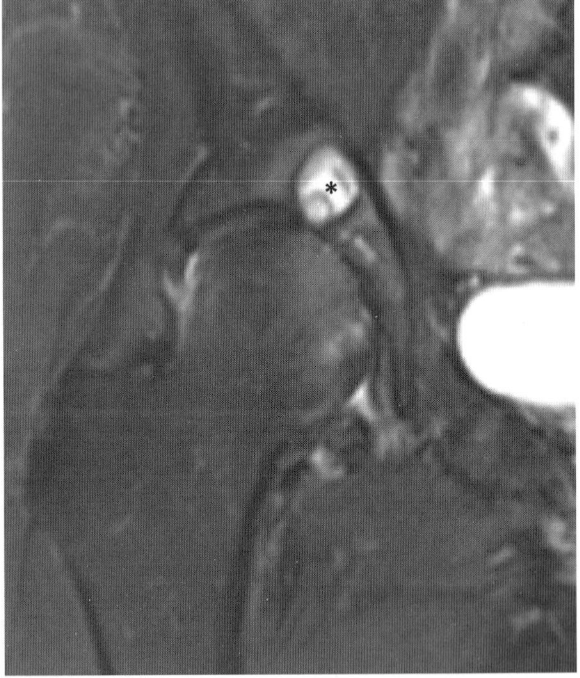

Figure 52.7 Egger cyst. Coronal STIR MR image of the right hip demonstrating a large singular acetabular subchondral cyst known as an Egger cyst (*), an early hallmark of hip osteoarthritis.

One of the earliest imaging manifestations of OA of the hip is frequently a singular acetabular cyst, or Egger cyst, resulting from bone contusion ultimately giving rise to microfractures and intrusion of synovial fluid within the superior acetabulum (Fig. 52.7). More advanced OA may include superolateral femoral head subluxation which is found to occur in 80% of cases (though protrusion is also

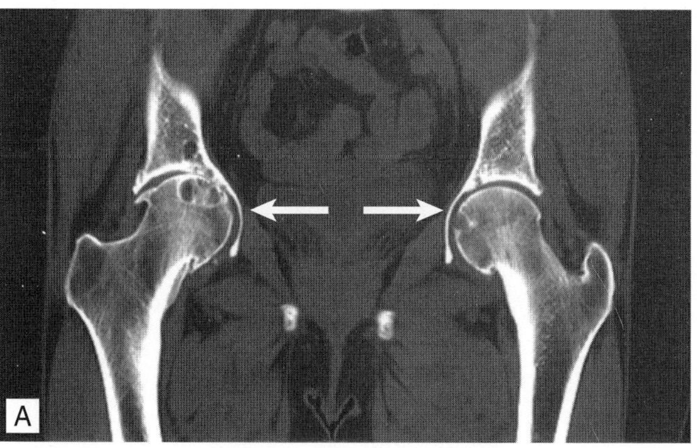

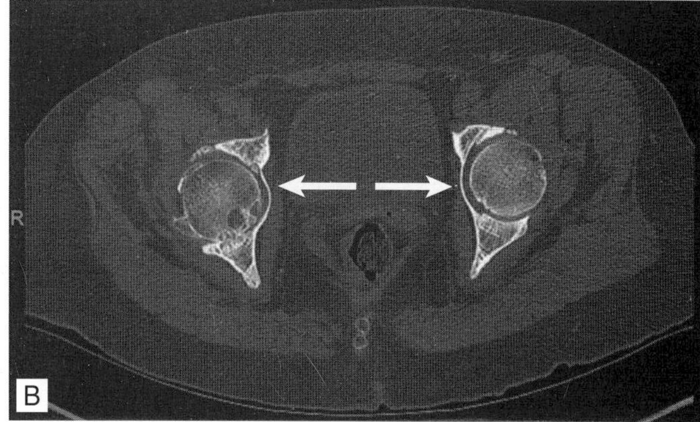

Figure 52.8 Bilateral acetabular protrusio due to Otto disease. Coronal (A) and axial (B) CT images demonstrate medial intrapelvic convexity of the medial acetabular wall, with concentric joint space loss, subchondral cystic change, and osteophyte formation.

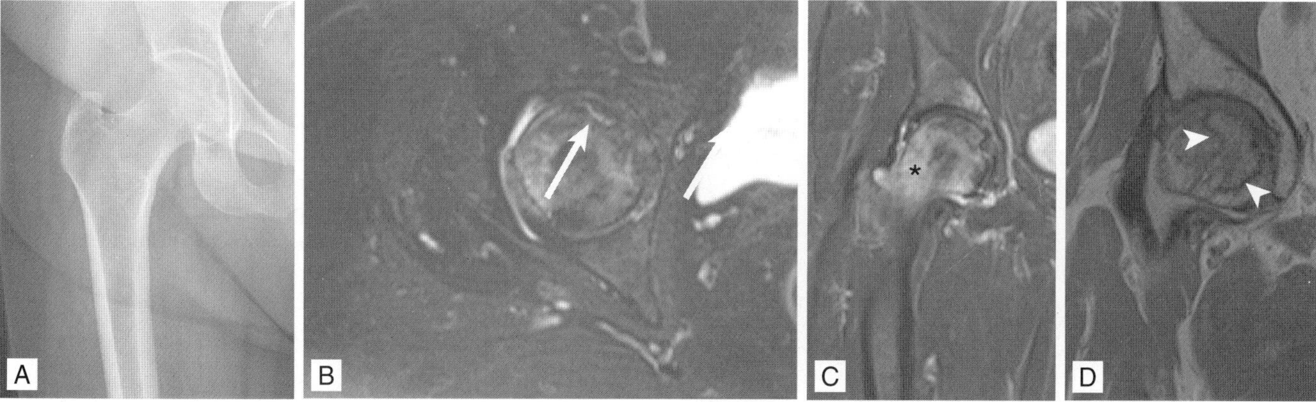

Figure 52.9 Subchondral fracture with underlying avascular necrosis. Normal appearing frontal AP radiograph (A) of the right hip in a 67-year-old female presenting with acute hip pain. Axial T2-fat suppression image (B) demonstrates curvilinear hyperintense T2 signal undercutting the subarticular surface of the femoral head (*white arrow*) with associated intense subchondral bone marrow edema extending into the femoral neck on the coronal IR image (C) (*), compatible with an acute subchondral insufficiency fracture. Coronal PD image (D) demonstrates femoral head avascular necrosis with classic double-line sign (*arrowheads*).

noted in a minority of OA cases, occasionally attributed to a variant of OA of the hip known as Otto disease) (Fig. 52.8).

The differential diagnosis of hip pain is broad, which can present diagnostic challenges; however, MRI has become an invaluable tool in assessing patients with hip pain who have normal or inconclusive radiographs [7] including subchondral insufficiency fractures (Fig. 52.9), early chondral wear, labral tear and degeneration (Fig. 52.10), occult fractures, transient migratory osteoporosis, septic arthritis, and bone lesions.

Rapidly progressing OA of the hip should prompt a search for underlying pathology, most commonly an insufficiency fracture of the superior subchondral femoral head surface (Fig. 52.11).

Knees

The knees are the most commonly affected joint in clinical practice and consists of three separate compartments—medial tibiofemoral, lateral tibiofemoral, and patellofemoral. Radiographs are the first-line imaging modality for evaluation; typical findings include:

- Joint space narrowing (typically demonstrated on notch views with the knee in approximately 40 degrees of flexion)
- Prominent periarticular osteophyte formation
- Subchondral cysts
- Joint malalignment; most commonly varus (Fig. 52.12) [8]

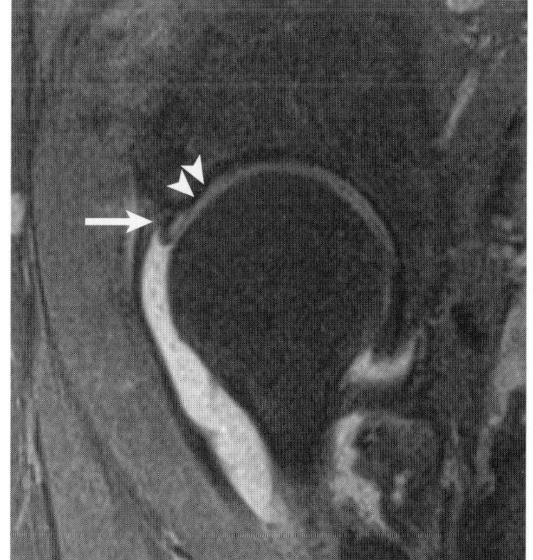

Figure 52.10 Acetabular labral tear and chondral degeneration. Sagittal proton density fat-suppressed MR image in a 58-year-old female with left hip pain demonstrating degenerative tearing of the anterosuperior acetabular labrum (*arrow*) and high-grade thinning of the acetabular (*arrowheads*) and femoral head cartilage, compatible with osteoarthritis. Radiographs of the left hip were normal.

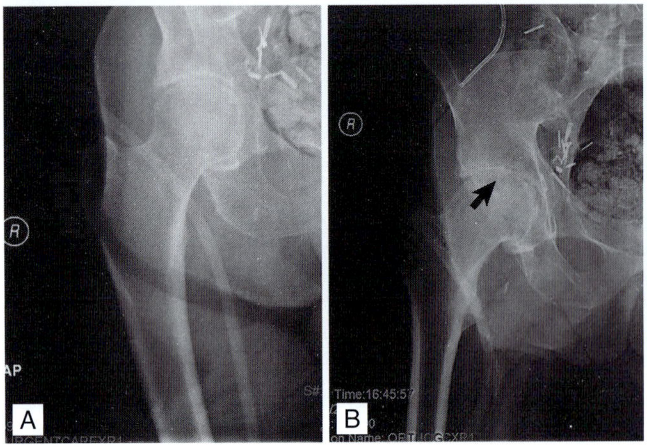

Figure 52.11 Rapidly destructive osteoarthritis of the hip. Initial AP radiograph (A) of the right hip demonstrated mild superolateral joint space narrowing. AP radiograph of the right hip obtained 6 months later (B) demonstrated interval bone-on-bone articulation, subchondral cystic change, and collapse of the femoral head (*arrow*), compatible with rapidly progressive osteoarthritis.

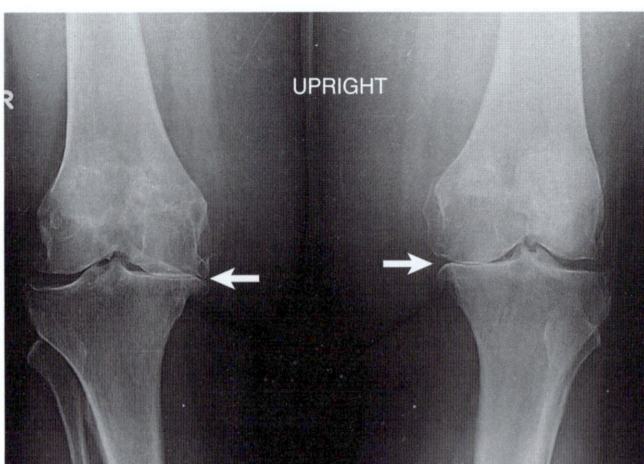

Figure 52.12 Classic case of OA of the knees. Frontal radiographs demonstrating bone-on-bone articulation of the medial tibiofemoral compartments with subchondral sclerosis and osteophyte formation (*arrows*) resulting in genu varus alignment.

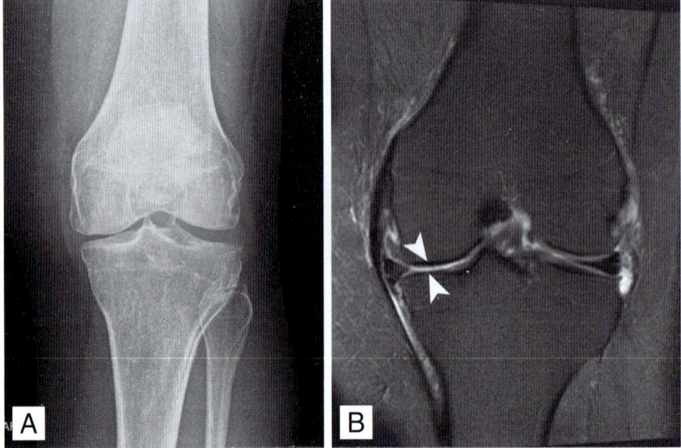

Figure 52.13 Early osteoarthritic change on MRI. AP radiograph (A) demonstrated mild narrowing of the medial tibiofemoral compartment with small osteophytes. Coronal PD fat-suppression image (B) demonstrates diffuse chondral thinning overlying the central surfaces of the medial femoral condyle and medial tibial plateau (*arrowheads*).

The patellofemoral joint can be assessed radiographically utilizing a dedicated sunrise view, which involves flexion of the knee to 45 degrees and imaging with placement of the x-ray beam aiming inferiorly to superiorly from the patient's feet. Magnetic resonance imaging (MRI) can play an important role both in determining early cartilage degeneration (Fig. 52.13), and in assessing for mitigating factors in the development or progression of knee OA, such as subchondral insufficiency fractures (Fig. 52.14) and/or meniscal degeneration (Fig. 52.15).

Ankles/Feet

The subtalar joint is most involved; *posterior subtalar compartment oftentimes being the most severely affected* (Fig. 52.16). Involvement of the tibiotalar joint can also be seen especially in the setting of previous trauma and/or recurrent ankle instability. Disease may be more widespread, involving many or all joints of the midfoot, including the tarsometatarsal joints (Fig. 52.17). OA of the forefoot typically presents with involvement of the first metatarsophalangeal (MTP) joint and can lead to malalignment and severe motion restriction, known as hallux rigidus (Fig. 52.18). The presence of alignment deformities of this joint (e.g., hallux valgus) should prompt a search for associated early or advanced degenerative changes, especially on more advanced cross-sectional imaging.

Spine

Degenerative processes of the spine are exceedingly common and frequently visualized on radiographic imaging. More commonly, manifestations of OA of the lumbar spine include intervertebral disc space narrowing, subchondral endplate sclerosis, horizontal osteophyte formation, and facet degenerative changes, which may ultimately give rise to associated spinal canal and neuroforaminal narrowing (Fig. 52.19). Specific entities associated with OA of the spine include Baastrup's disease, a condition in which the spinous processes are in closer approximation resulting in enlargement, flattening, and sclerosis of apposing interspinous surfaces [9]. Uncovertebral joint (apophyseal) osteophytes and facet joint OA in the cervical spine contribute to neuroforaminal narrowing. MRI is particularly useful in the setting of degenerative disc disease both to quantify the extent of degeneration, and to further clarify associated pathology such as disc herniation and/or annular tears, ligamentum flavum hypertrophy, or facet cyst formation, all of which may ultimately contribute to severity of patient symptoms including pain and/or radiculopathy.

Inflammatory Arthropathies

Rheumatoid Arthritis

Overview

Rheumatoid arthritis is an autoimmune systemic inflammatory arthropathy that predominantly affects the musculoskeletal system, with imaging findings reflecting the underlying pathophysiology of the disease process. RA is seen in all age groups, but is most likely to present between ages 20 and 55, with women more commonly affected than men at a ratio of 3:1. Prevalence is quite high at approximately 1% of the worldwide population, and is

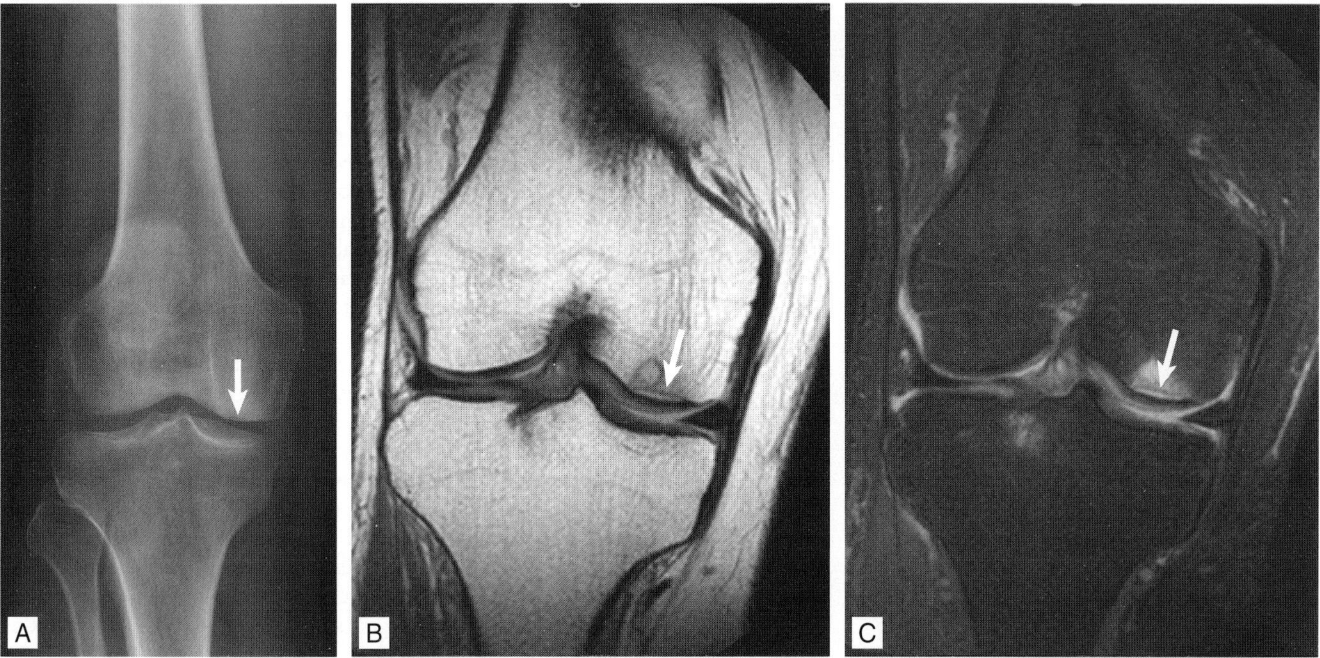

Figure 52.14 Subchondral insufficiency fracture. AP radiograph (A) demonstrates a linear subchondral lucency along the medical femoral condyle (*arrow*), compatible with a subchondral insufficiency fracture. Coronal T1 (B) and T2 fat-suppression (C) images demonstrate subchondral linear hypointense T1 and T2 signal corresponding to the radiographic lucency (*arrows*), outlined by intense bone marrow edema, compatible with an acute subchondral insufficiency fracture. Note the normal appearing underlying articular cartilage.

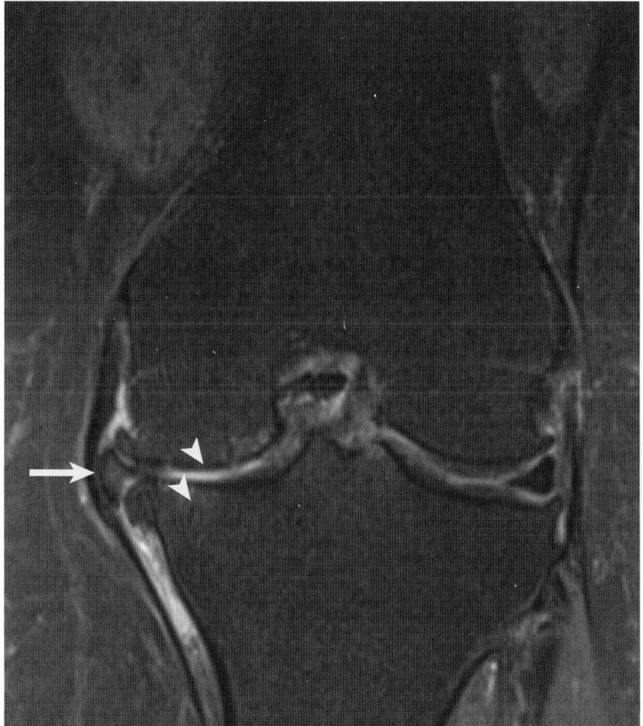

Figure 52.15 Advanced OA on MRI. Coronal proton density fat-saturated MR image demonstrating degeneration and extrusion of the medial meniscal body (*arrow*), with associated complete, diffuse full thickness medial tibiofemoral compartment cartilage loss, marginal osteophytes, cystic change, and reactive subchondral bone marrow edema (*arrowhead*).

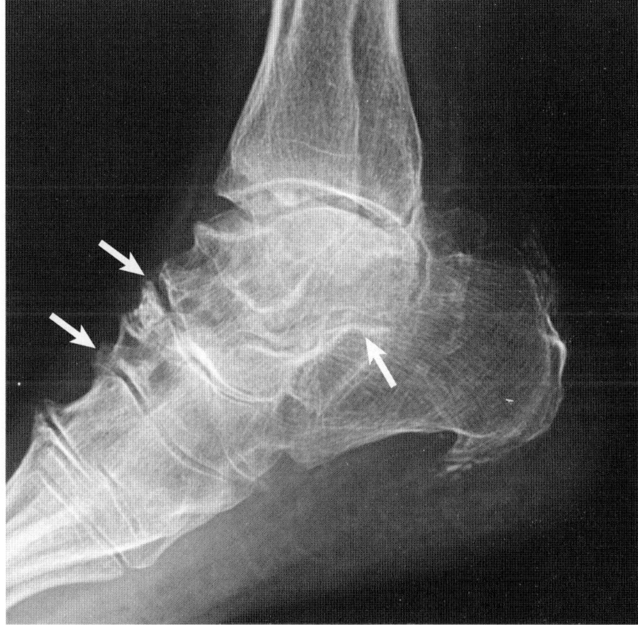

Figure 52.16 OA of the subtalar joint. Lateral radiograph of the ankle/hindfoot demonstrating severe degenerative changes of the subtalar joint, as well as the visualized joints of the midfoot and hindfoot.

particularly prevalent among some Native American populations. Although there is some debate regarding the pathogenesis of rheumatoid arthritis, it is generally felt that genetic predisposition accounts for nearly half of the risk of development of the disease [10], with 70% of patients being HLA-DR4 positive [11]. Additionally, presumed environmental triggers have been reported, including smoking, periodontal disease, and alterations in gut microbiome [1,12].

Pathology

Synovitis or inflammation of the synovium lining joint surfaces, tendon sheaths, and bursae, can be seen in infection, noninfectious inflammatory processes, and degenerative conditions, is thought to

Figure 52.17 Midfoot OA. AP radiograph of the left foot demonstrates severe narrowing across the 2nd and 3rd tarsometatarsal joints (*arrows*) with subchondral sclerosis, cystic change, and prominent dorsal osteophyte formation.

be the primary underlying pathologic process in RA. Hypertrophied synovial proliferation, known as pannus, can be characterized as either hypervascular due active hyperemia, or hypovascular due to chronic inactive proliferation. Synovitis and pannus formation can ultimately result in periarticular marginal erosions, as the outer margins of synovial joints, known as "bare areas," because they are not covered or protected by hyaline cartilage (Fig. 52.1). Hypertrophied synovium, which may involve joints, tendon sheaths, or bursae, is invasive inflammatory tissue, leading to eventual erosion of contiguous bone and cartilage surfaces, fibrous/osseous ankylosis, and ligamentous laxity/rupture [13]. Similarly, synovial proliferation within the tendon sheath results in tenosynovitis, and if severe, can lead to tendon failure and/or rupture.

Imaging Findings

Along with a thorough clinical examination and laboratory markers, imaging evaluation can offer invaluable clues to the early diagnosis of RA, as well as monitoring of disease remission or progression depending on the imaging modality utilized for the assessment. Radiography remains the initial imaging modality in the evaluation of RA; however MRI and ultrasonography (USG) have emerged as critical tools in the assessment of early disease and monitoring of therapy. Throughout this section, multiple examples will illustrate early changes related to RA, including synovitis, tenosynovitis, joint effusions, bone marrow edema, and early erosions all of which are largely imperceptible upon radiographic examination [11]. Given that early pathological changes are related to the synovium, both USG and MRI have emerged as superior imaging modalities for the detection of early changes related to RA and other inflammatory arthridities compared with CT and radiography. When performed by an adept sonographer or trained musculoskeletal radiologist, USG has proved to be highly accurate in identifying both osseous and soft-tissue inflammatory changes, and is highly sensitive in detecting osseous erosions compared with radiography. USG and MRI are comparable in their ability to detect early osseous erosions [13].

In addition, USG is incredibly useful in detecting intra-articular synovitis (and tenosynovitis) manifest by noncompressible hypoechogenic synovial hypertrophy with or without power Doppler activity. Increased power Doppler activity indicates hyperemia and is a marker of acute inflammation.

Similarly, MRI also demonstrates synovitis with high sensitivity compared with USG, as evidence by synovial thickening that can be detected as relative hypointense proliferative material outlined by hyperintense joint fluid. However, synovium and joint fluid can have similar appearing signal intensities on unenhanced MR images. The addition of IV gadolinium-based contrast agents adds specificity, as inflamed synovium will demonstrate enhancement, while bland joint fluid will not. Furthermore, when compared with radiography, CT, and USG, MRI provides a unique look at underlying subchondral inflammation, as evidenced by bone marrow edema changes and enhancement of subchondral bone, which if identified has been shown to be an indicator of erosion formation.

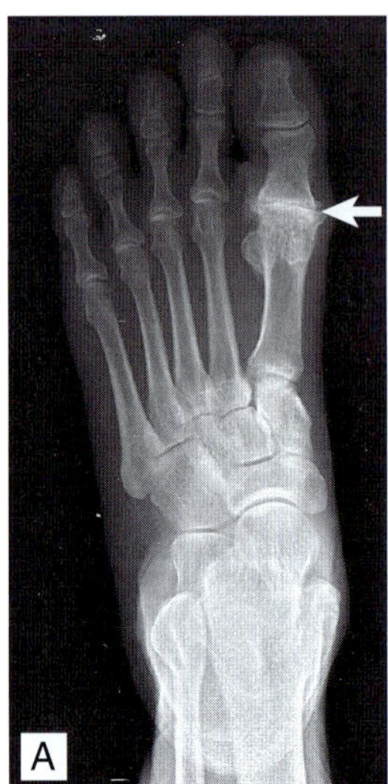

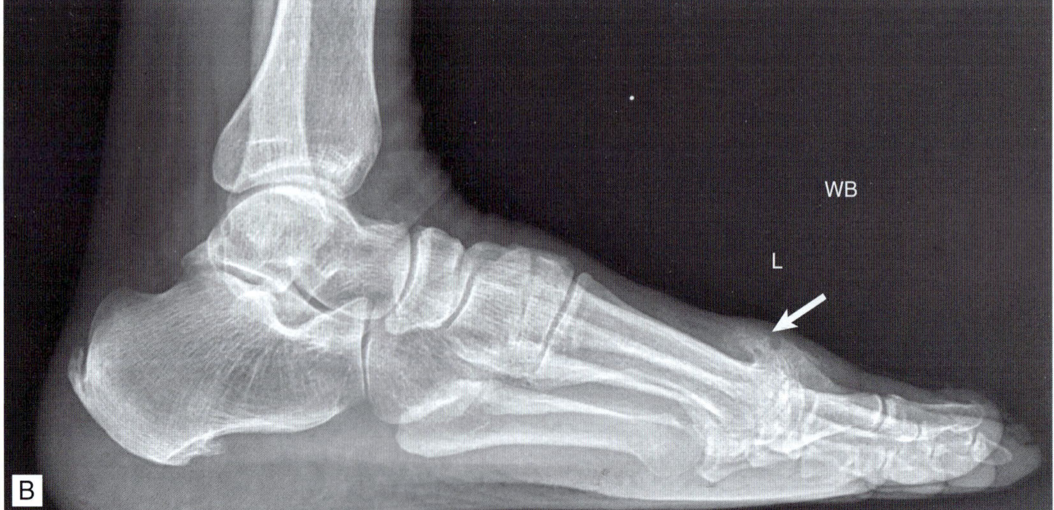

Figure 52.18 1st MTP OA. AP (A) and lateral (B) radiographs of the left foot demonstrate severe osteoarthritis of the 1st MTP joint with prominent dorsal osteophytes (*arrows*), compatible with radiographic evidence of hallux rigidus.

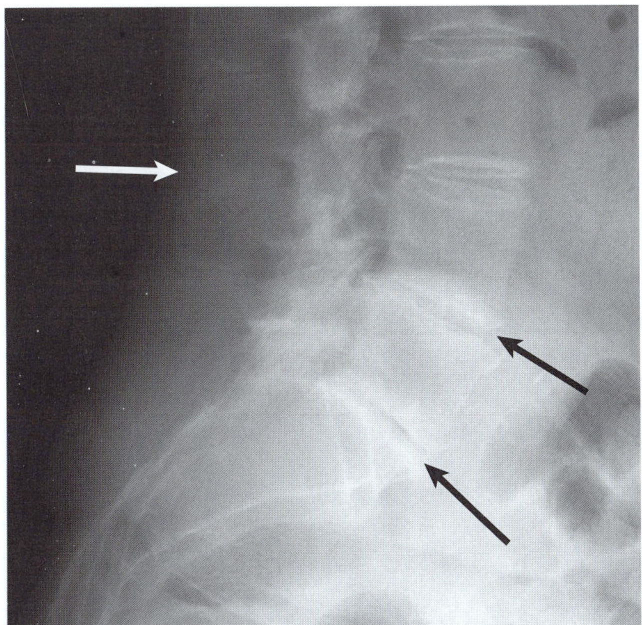

Figure 52.19 Degenerative disc disease. Lateral radiograph of the lumbar spine in an 82-year-old female with back pain demonstrating moderate-to-severe narrowing at L4-5 and L5-S1 (*black arrows*) with subchondral endplate sclerosis, as well as anterior marginal and posterolateral osteophytes, which in combination with facet arthrosis likely contributes to neuroforaminal narrowing. There is also squaring of the spinous processes with narrowing of the interspinous spaces demonstrating subchondral irregularity and sclerosis, compatible with Baastrup's disease (*white arrow*).

The wide spectrum of imaging findings encountered in patents with RA will be described based upon location and pathophysiology with corresponding imaging manifestations across multiple imaging modalities. Classic feature of RA is a bilateral symmetric inflammatory arthritis involving more than three joints with the absence of bony proliferation, helping to differentiate from OA and seronegative spondyloarthropathies. Additionally, over 60% of patients present with symmetric arthritis of the small joints of the hand. Erosive changes with predominant proximal distribution and the absence of periarticular bony productive changes are findings indicative of rheumatoid arthritis.

Typical Patterns and Distribution of RA

Upper Extremity

Hands and Wrists

- Bilateral, symmetric, and polyarticular process
- Commonly affected joints include the metacarpophalangeal (MCP) joints with erosions of the second and third, as well as the third proximal interphalangeal (PIP) joint
- All wrist joints, ulnar and radial styloid
- DIP joints are rarely involved

Earliest, but subtle radiographic findings include soft-tissue swelling and periarticular osteopenia and thought to be the result of subchondral osteoclast activation secondary to regional synovitis and inflammation, which can easily identified by MR imaging or USG. Synovitis leads to subtle radiographic findings of initial joint space widening due joint effusions, as well as periarticular cortical thinning, indistinctness, and bone loss, known as the dot-dash appearance, and eventually contributing to erosions (Fig. 52.20).

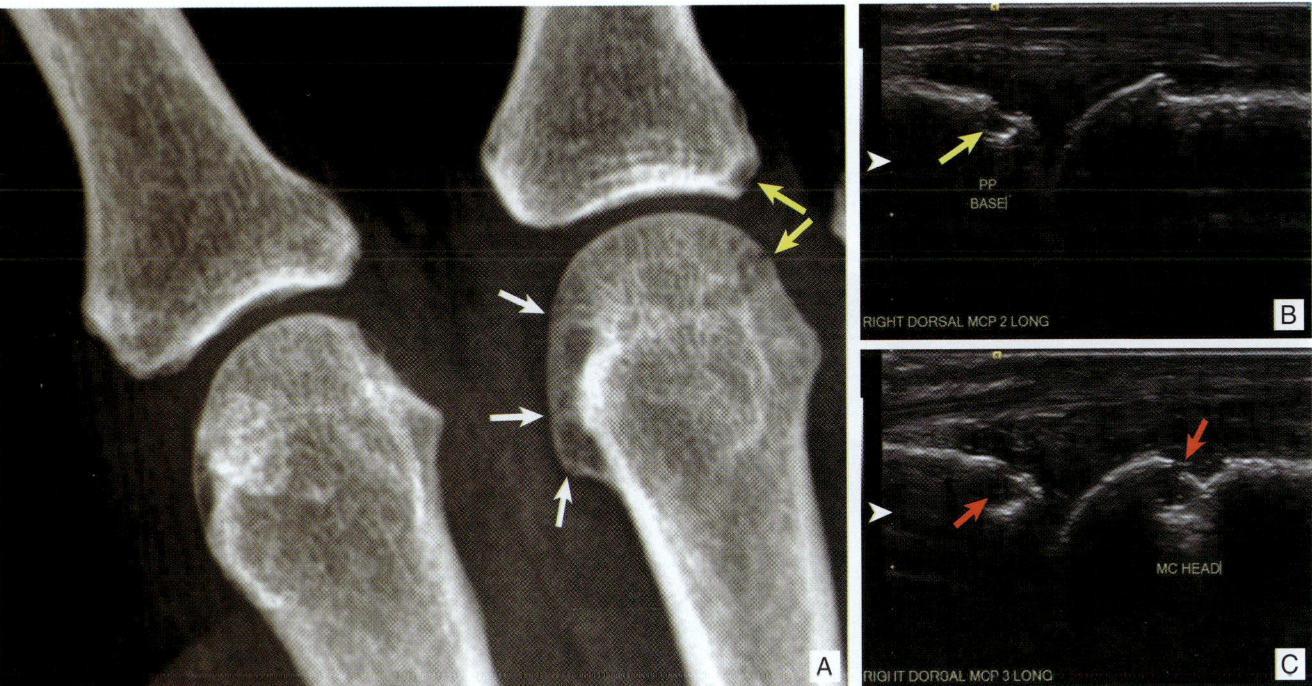

Figure 52.20 Early radiographic findings in a patient with RA with USG confirmation. PA coned down view (A) of the right 2nd and 3rd MCP joints demonstrates subtle widening of the 2nd MCP joint indicating joint capsule distension with fluid and synovitis. Localized osteopenia of the 2nd and 3rd metacarpal heads with subtle irregularity and discontinuity of the cortex (*white arrows*), described as the "dot-dash" appearance of early erosive change. Also note the early erosions at the base of the 3rd proximal phalanx and head of the 3rd metacarpal (*yellow arrows*). Corresponding USG images in the same patient demonstrate 2nd and 3rd MCP joint capsular distension with synovitis, erosion at the base of the 2nd proximal phalanx (B—*yellow arrow*) which is not appreciated on the radiographs, and confirmation of the 3rd MCP joint erosions (C—*red arrows*) as seen on the radiographs.

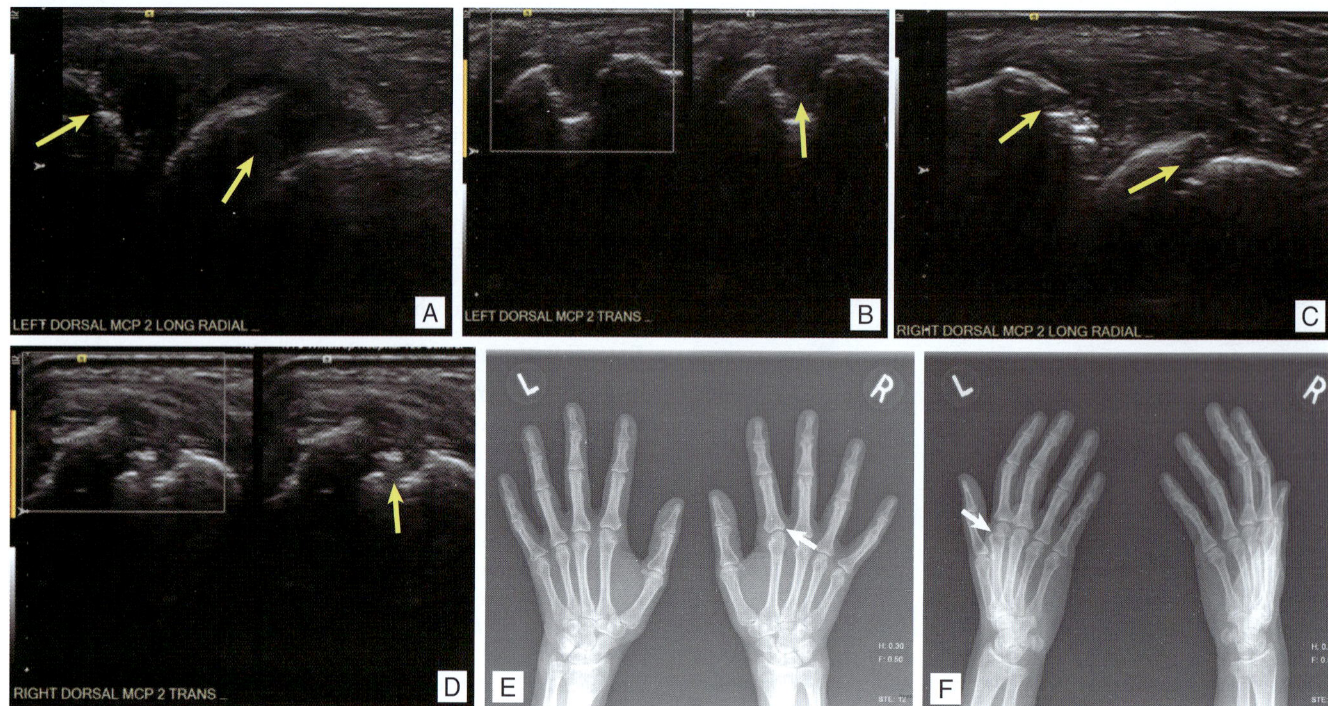

Figure 52.21 Erosions in patient with RA. USG images clearly demonstrate osseous erosions of the left (A and B) and right (C and D) 2nd metacarpal heads (*yellow arrows*) which are less conspicuous on AP (E) and lateral (F) radiographs (*white arrows*).

Early in the disease process, the most involved joints include the second and third MCP and the third PIP joints of the hand (Fig. 52.20), which may be inconspicuous at radiography, but clear on USG (Figs. 52.20 and 52.21) and MR imaging (Fig. 52.22).

MRI findings of early rheumatoid arthritis in the hand and wrist include the following:

- Periarticular and/or marginal erosions, as well as ulnar styloid erosions and pannus formation are typical (Figs. 52.22 and 52.23)
- Pannus formation outlined by joint effusions (Fig. 52.23)
- Tenosynovitis of flexor or extensor tendons
- Subchondral bone marrow edema, which may reflect an early manifestation of erosive disease (Fig. 52.23)
- Enhancement of synovium and tendon sheaths on postcontrast imaging

USG is complimentary to radiography and MRI, playing a critical role in the evaluation of early rheumatoid arthritis. There is excellent ability to detect early effusions and erosions of small joints (Figs. 52.20 and 52.21).

- *Erosions* in USG are defined as periarticular cortical discontinuity of the bone surface visible in two perpendicular planes [14]. Acute erosions demonstrate irregular margin, poorly defined osseous base, and associated active synovitis. The absence of synovitis may reflect chronic erosion [15]. Power Doppler imaging can be used to detect hyperemia and synovitis (Fig. 52.24)

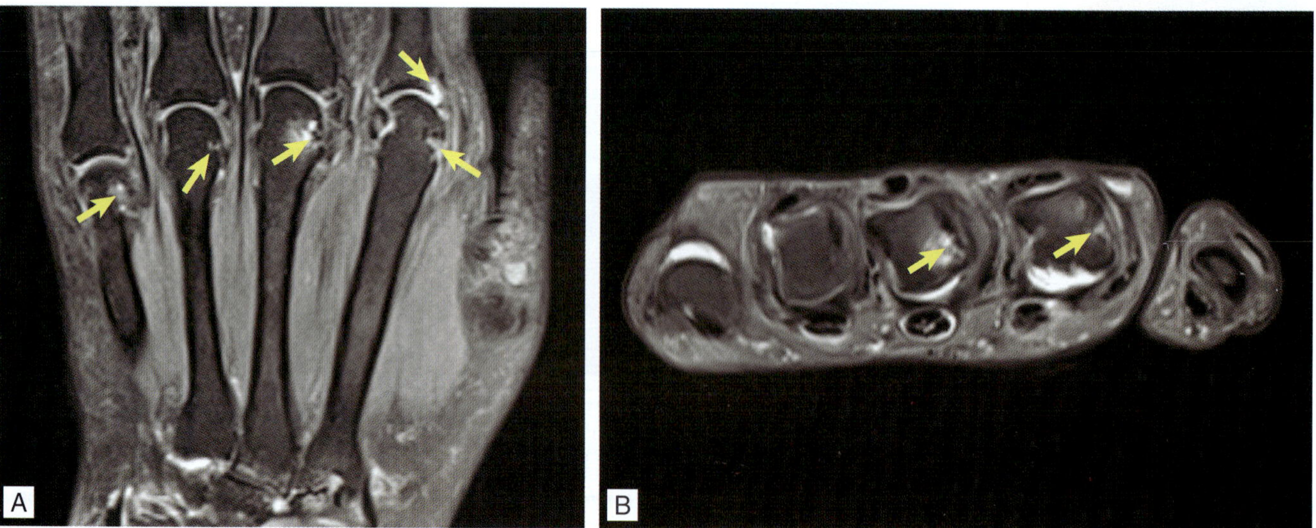

Figure 52.22 Synovitis and erosions in a woman with rheumatoid arthritis. Coronal PD fat-suppression (A) and axial T2 fat-suppression (B) images demonstrate periarticular erosions (*arrows*) at the 2nd–5th metacarpal heads, radial base of the 2nd proximal phalanx, and at the base of the 2nd metacarpal.

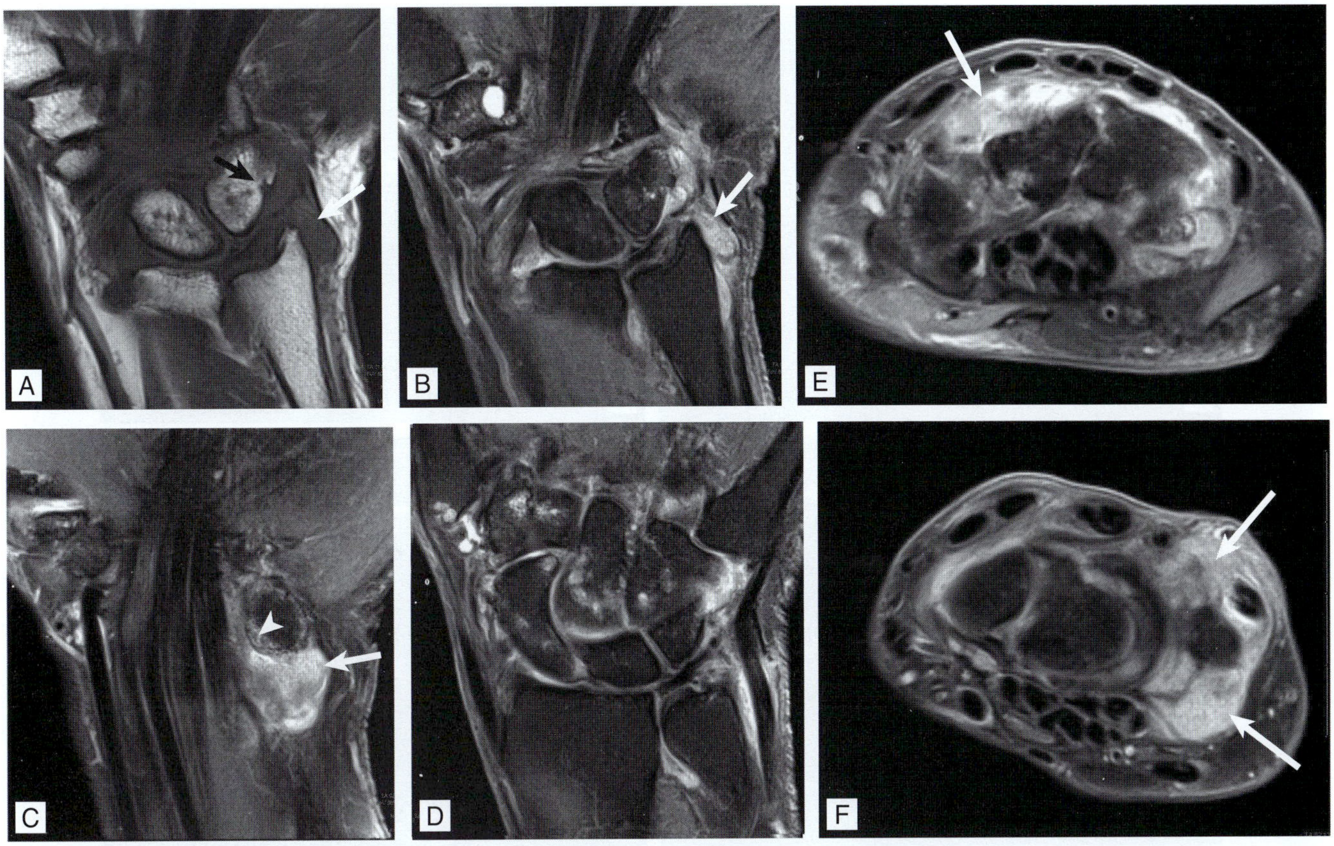

Figure 52.23 MR imaging findings in early RA. Coronal PD (A) and coronal (B, C, D) and axial (E and F) PD-weighted fat-suppressed images demonstrate a triquetral erosion (*black arrow*), with extensive dorsal carpal, ulnocarpal, radiocarpal, and pisotriquetral recess synovitis (*white arrows*) manifest as intermediate-signal intensity outlined by high-signal joint fluid. Additionally, patchy areas of bone marrow edema and scattered erosions are seen throughout the carpal bones (*arrowhead*).

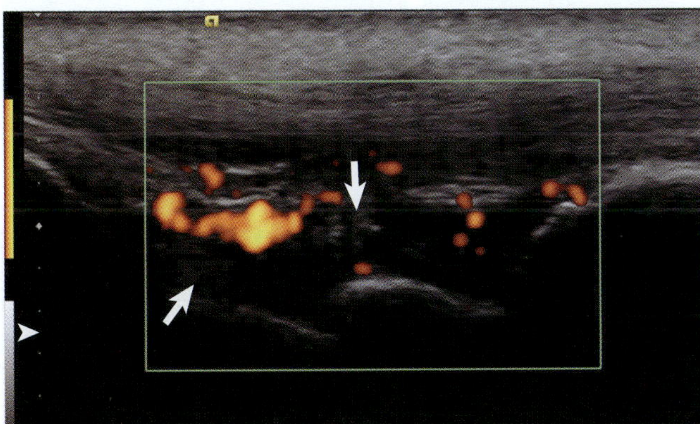

Figure 52.24 Hyperemia and active synovitis on USG. A 66-year-old male patient presenting with wrist pain and normal radiographs. Longitudinal USG image acquired of the dorsal carpal recesses of the left wrist demonstrates abnormal, noncompressible intra-articular tissue surrounded by joint fluid, compatible with synovial hypertrophy (*arrows*), exhibiting increased power Doppler signal, consistent with active synovitis.

- *Joint effusion* is identified as abnormal hypoechoic or anechoic intra-articular fluid that is displaceable and compressible, without demonstration of Doppler signal
- *Synovitis* is abnormal hypoechoic intra-articular tissue that is nondisplaceable, poorly compressible, with possible Doppler signal. It can be detected early in the disease course and is considered a strong predictor of bone erosion development

Following features allow USG to be used as a screening tool for the diagnosis of early inflammatory arthritis:

- Ease of detection of tenosynovitis and tendon rupture (Fig. 52.25). Tenosynovitis is abnormal anechoic/hypoechoic tendon sheath thickening or distention, related to the presence of abnormal tenosynovial fluid and/or synovial hypertrophy
- Superiority in the evaluation of rheumatoid nodules, which may be below the resolution of other forms of cross-sectional imaging

Later disease manifestations include uniform joint space narrowing and destruction, ulnar capping and translocation (with carpal bones subluxing ulnarly such that the lunate articulates with the ulna), as well as volar subluxation of the carpal bones upon the radius (Fig. 52.26). Ulnar capping refers to productive bone changes seen at the ulnar styloid sometimes seen with long-term rheumatoid arthritis. Scapholunate dissociation leads to volar intercalated segmental instability or dorsal intercalated segmental instability. Ulnar drift and volar subluxation is often present involving the metacarpal joints. "Hitchhiker's thumb" results in flexion deformity at the thumb MCP joint with extension at the interphalangeal joint (Fig. 52.27). Swan-neck deformity refers to PIP joint hyperextension and DIP joint hyperflexion (Fig. 52.28).

Late severe destruction of osseous structures may give pencil-in-cup appearance in phalanges and may destroy distal ulna or proximal carpal row (Fig. 52.29).

Differential Pearls

1. *Systemic lupus erythematosus (SLE)* differs from RA in that associated arthropathy is nonerosive and joint subluxations are reducible.

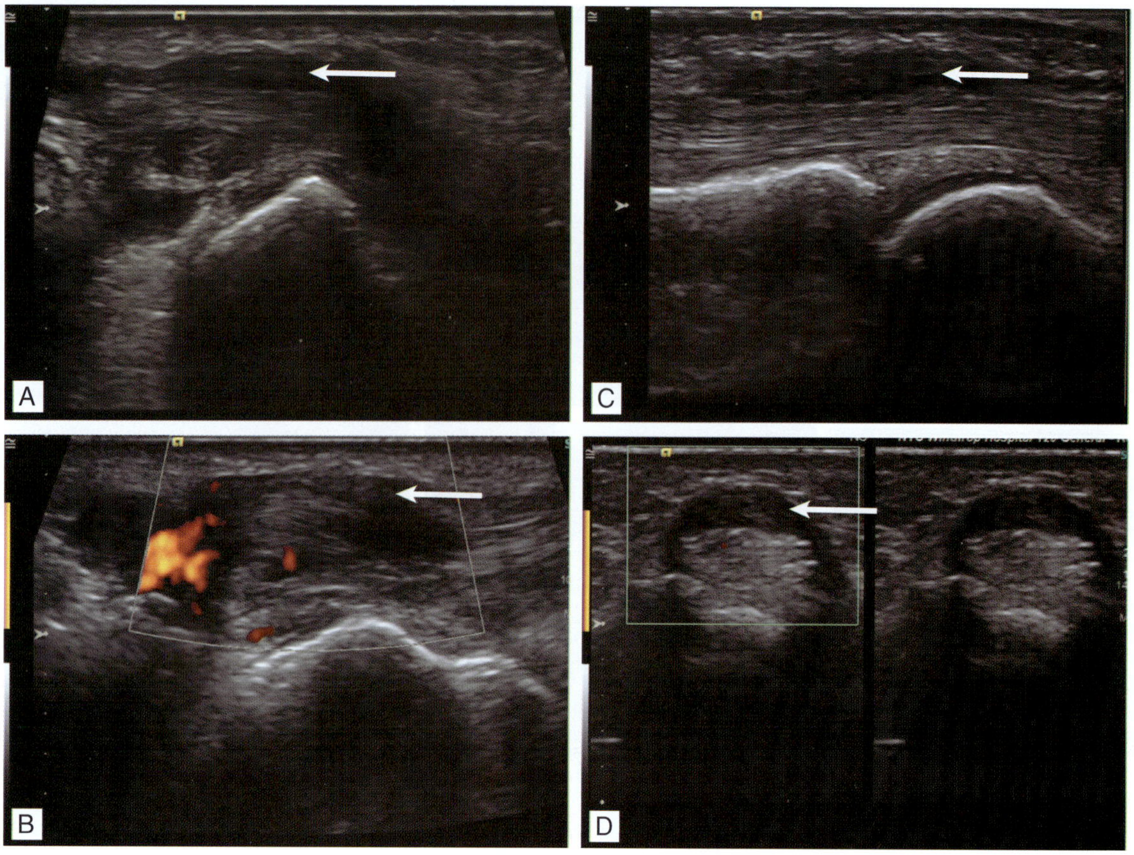

Figure 52.25 USG findings in early presentation of RA. Longitudinal USG images (A and B) acquired of the left wrist demonstrate abnormal tenosynovial thickening of the extensor carpi ulnaris tendon (*arrows*) with increased power Doppler signal, compatible with tenosynovitis. Longitudinal (C) and transverse (D) USG images demonstrate tenosynovitis of the 3rd flexor tendon (*arrows*).

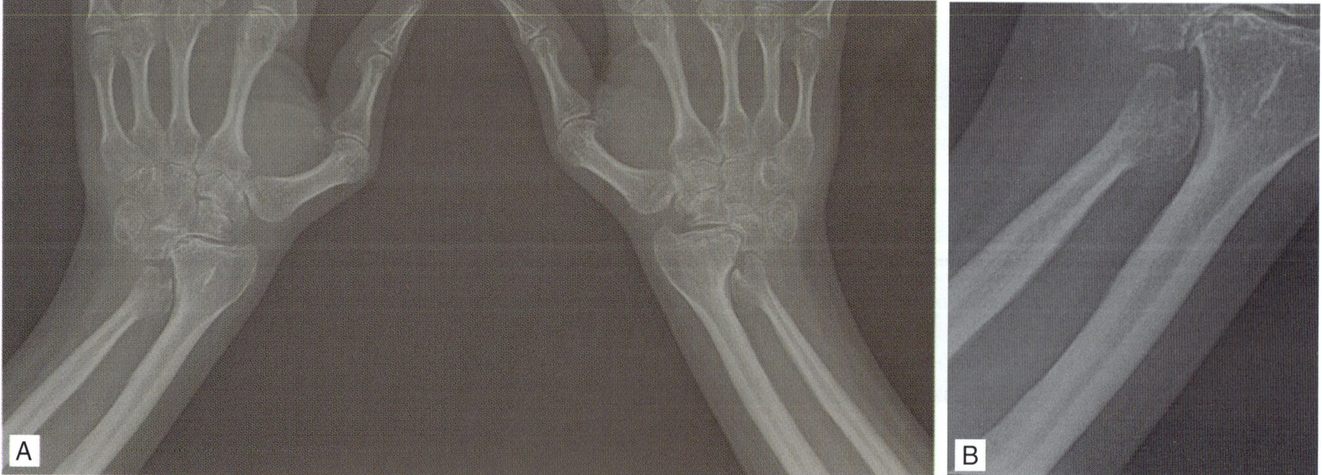

Figure 52.26 Later stage findings in RA. AP radiographs of the wrists (A) show ulnar capping and ulnar translocation. Zoomed in AP radiograph of the left ulnar styloid (B) highlights the ulnar capping, which refers to productive bone changes seen at the ulnar styloid sometimes seen with long-term rheumatoid arthritis. Ulnar translocation involves volar subluxation of the carpal bones upon the radius.

2. *Erosive OA* may be differentiated as it typically follows the distribution of OA, with predominantly DIP involvement as well as involvement of the first carpometacarpal and scapho-trapezium-trapezoid joints.
3. *Psoriatic arthropathy* is more apt to have associated periostitis, with a distribution favoring the DIP joints.
4. The absence of DIP involvement, subchondral sclerosis, and osteophyte formation excludes *OA*.

Shoulder and Elbow. The AC joint may demonstrate erosions on both sides of the joint, with end-stage penciling of the clavicle as well as resorption at the coracoclavicular ligament insertions. Glenohumeral joint involvement typically begins with erosions at

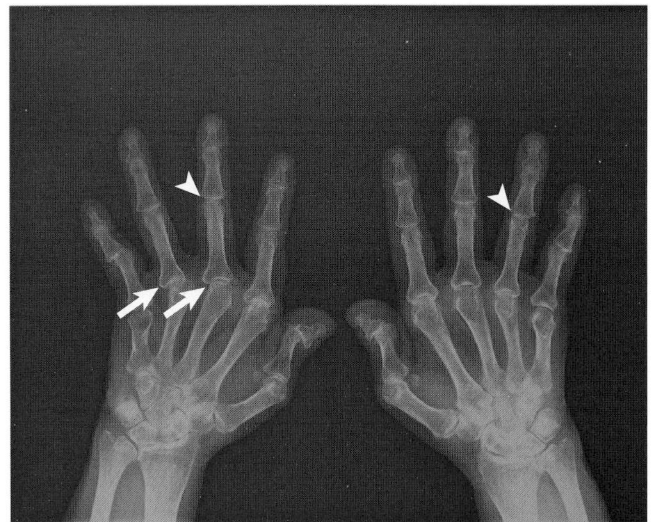

Figure 52.27 Late-stage changes in RA. Radiographs demonstrate uniform joint space narrowing of the MCP joints with ulnar subluxation (*arrows*), periarticular erosions at the base of the left 3rd middle phalanx and base of the right 4th middle phalanx (*arrowheads*). Hitchhiker thumb is also demonstrated.

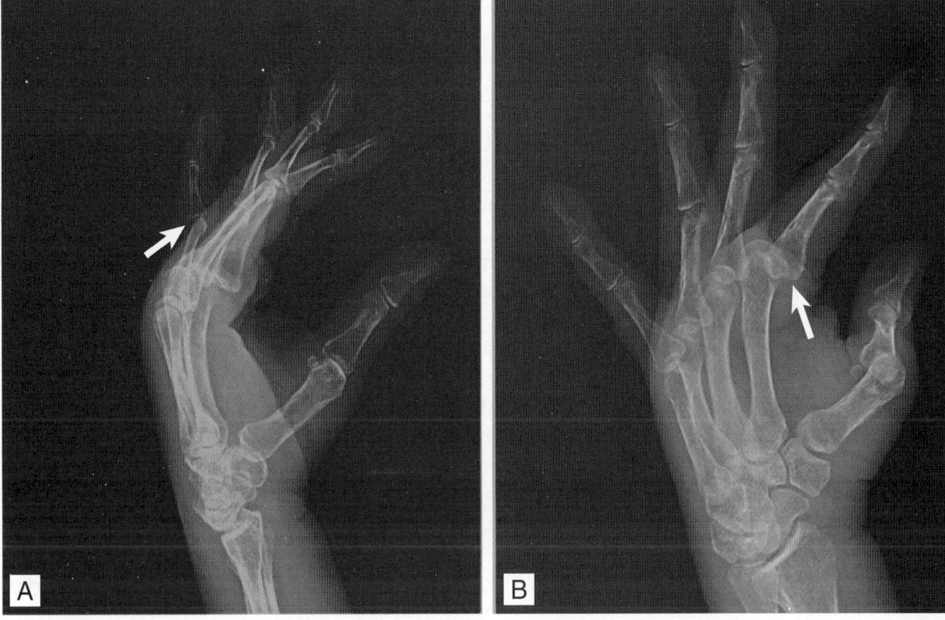

Figure 52.28 Late-stage changes in RA. AP (A) and lateral (B) radiographs demonstrate swan-neck deformity of the 5th finger (*arrow* in A). Also note volar subluxations (*arrow* in B) and periarticular osteopenia of the MCP joints.

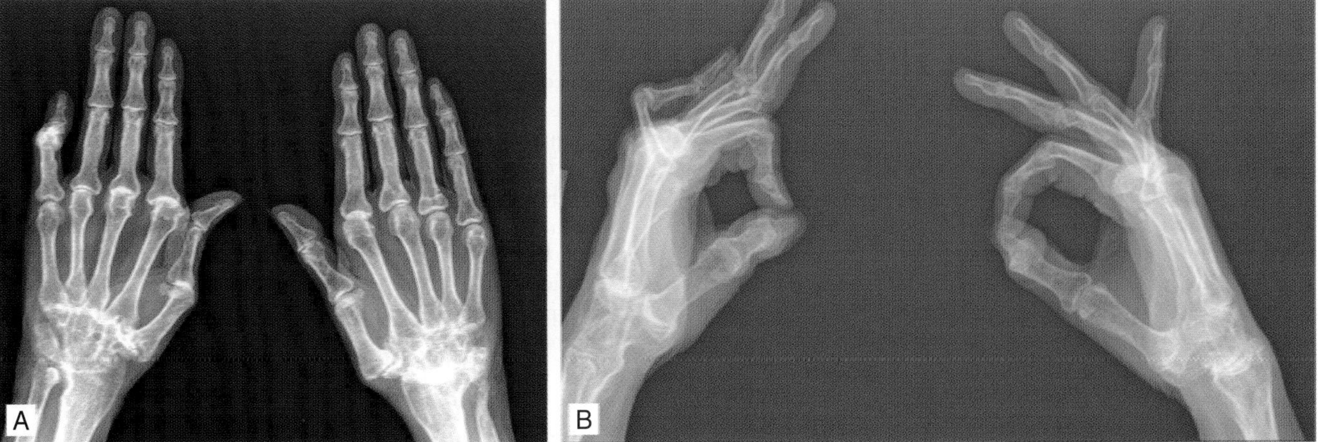

Figure 52.29 Advanced RA changes. Radiographs demonstrate severe uniform, bilateral symmetric joint space narrowing of the 2nd MCP joints with ulnar deviation and volar subluxation, erosion of the left ulnar head and styloid, distal radioulnar joint erosions with scalloping along the ulnar aspect of the distal radius, and extensive carpal ankyloses.

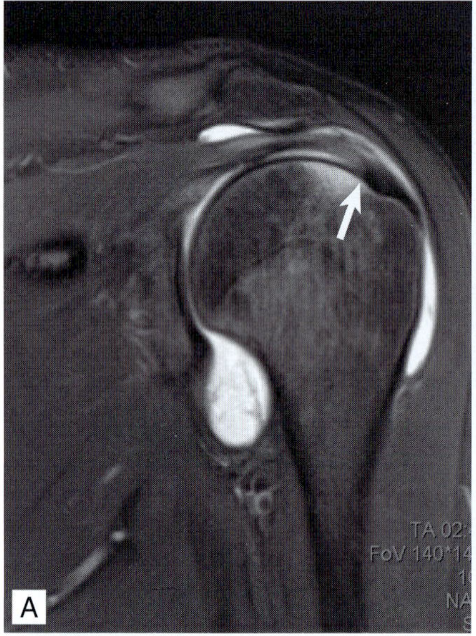

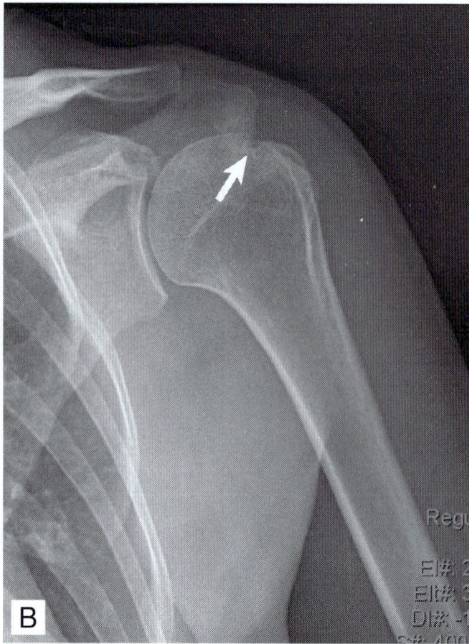

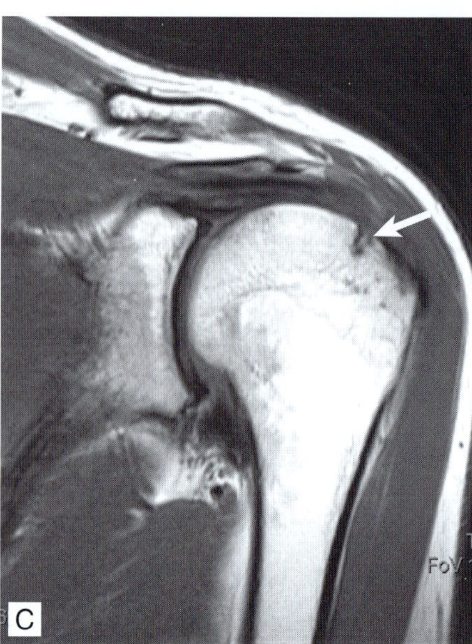

Figure 52.30 Glenohumeral RA. (A) Focal bone marrow edema (*arrow*) along the superior humeral head subjacent to the rotator cuff insertion, suggestive of early erosive change. Subsequent radiographs (B) and MRI (C) acquired 2 years later demonstrate osseous erosions of the superior humeral head in the previous sites of osteitis (*arrows*).

the junction of the cartilage-covered humeral head and the greater tuberosity (Fig. 52.30).

- Later stages result in uniform disruption of the glenohumeral joint
- Hatchet-like mechanical erosions at the medial surgical neck due to impaction against the inferior glenoid may result
- Concomitant rotator cuff pathology may result in synovitis extending into the subacromial/subdeltoid bursa

Elbow involvement may demonstrate joint effusions, olecranon bursitis, and/or diffuse erosive changes. Decompression of synovial fluid through weak joint capsules of large joints is common, and presumably related to the associated higher pressure of the inflammatory arthropathy (Fig. 52.31).

Lower Extremity

Hip and Knee: Typical imaging findings for hip and knee involvement include bilateral, symmetric, and uniform cartilage space narrowing, acetabular protrusio deformity (Fig. 52.32), periarticular osteopenia, and possible associated insufficiency fractures.

Ankle and Foot

- Tibiotalar and MTP joint effusions are relatively common
- Retrocalcaneal bursitis may be seen
- Earliest erosive changes are typically demonstrated at the fifth MTP joint and posterior calcaneal tubercle (Fig. 52.32)

Axial Skeleton

Erosive changes are most commonly seen at the C1–C2 level and are typically centered around the dens (Fig. 52.33). Atlantoaxial subluxation may result from disruption of the transverse ligament by inflammatory pannus formation, with normal atlantodens interval measuring less than 4 mm.

- Flexion views will demonstrate maximal atlantoaxial subluxation, which is seen in up to 30% of patients with chronic rheumatoid arthritis
- Note that subluxation may also be present in other seronegative spondyloarthropathies, but in this setting would likely be accompanied by syndesmophytes and/or vertebral body fusion

Atlantoaxial impaction results from erosions and collapse of the C1–C2 facets, which may result in protrusion of the dens through the foramen magnum. This may ultimately result in clinical symptoms of spinal cord compression. Other imaging manifestations of RA in the spine may include facet joint erosive change and thinning of the spinous processes.

Sacroiliac joint changes are less common and severe than those in seronegative spondyloarthropathies but may be seen in up to 30% of those with long-standing disease. Such changes are more commonly seen in women and rarely result in fusion.

Seronegative Spondyloarthropathies

The term seronegative spondyloarthropathy refers to a group of inflammatory arthritides that were initially characterized as rheumatoid arthritis, but which lacked serum rheumatoid factors [16]. Ankylosing spondylitis (AS) is the prototypical disease described in the spectrum of seronegative spondyloarthopathies, but other disorders in this category include PsA, arthritis-related inflammatory bowel disease (IBD), reactive arthritis, uveitis-related to HLA-B27, and other undifferentiated or indistinguishable forms of these diseases. As this initial description, additional diagnostic criteria for this category of arthritides include axial and peripheral articular involvement, and an association with human leukocyte antigen HLA-B27. The overall prevalence is estimated at 1%, making this group of inflammatory arthritides more common than rheumatoid arthritis [17]. The predominant imaging approach to recognizing a seronegative inflammatory process includes polyarticular joint space narrowing, with predominant distal distribution of the hands and feet, and the addition of bony proliferation. Additionally, this group of diseases is characterized by enthesitis, or inflammation of enthesis, which are osseous attachment sites for ligaments and tendons. Diagnostic classification criteria set

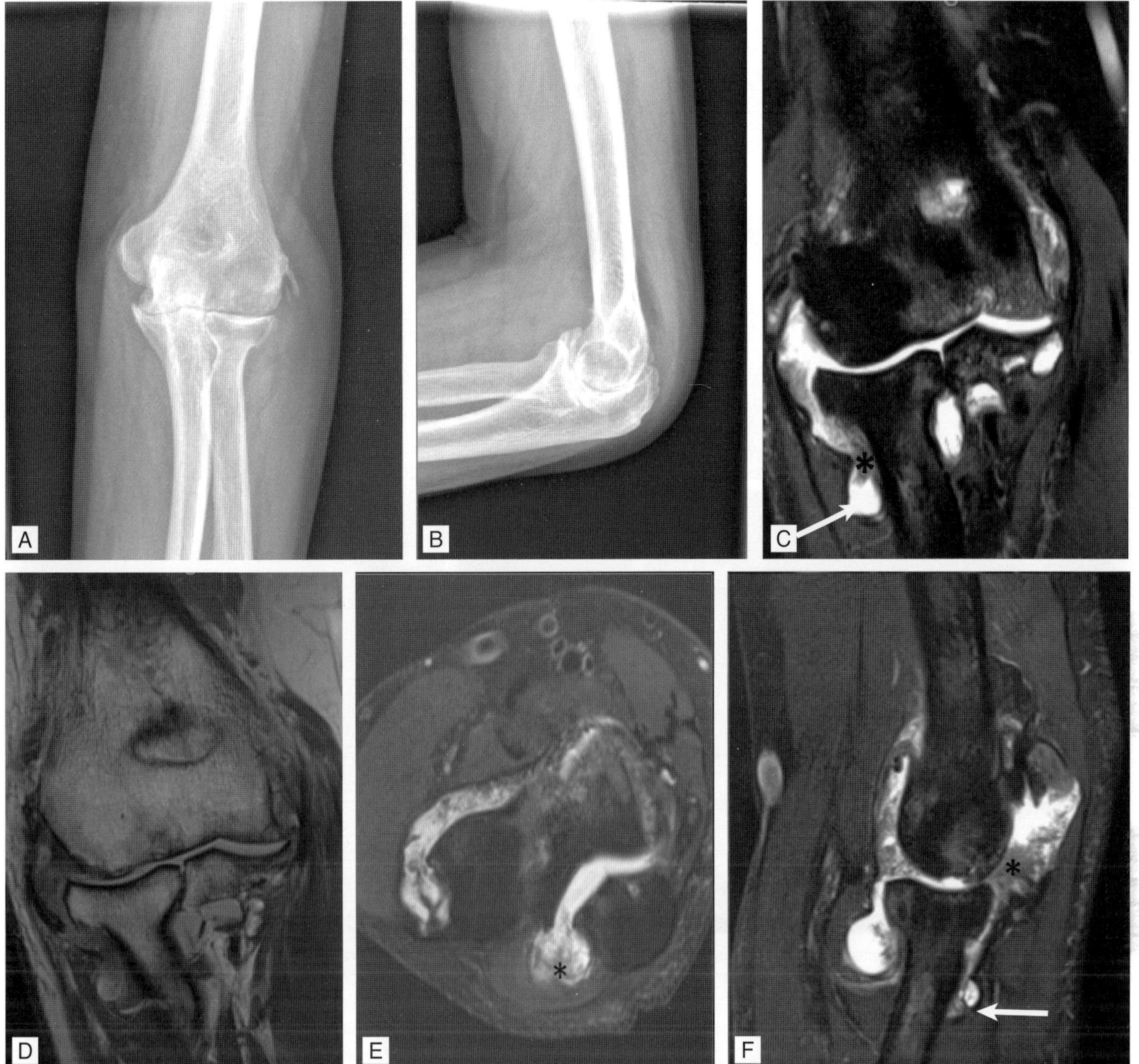

Figure 52.31 Elbow RA. AP (A) and lateral (B) radiographs show severe uniform joint space narrowing of the radiocapitellar and ulnotrochelar articulations with subchondral erosions of the capitellum, trochlea, radial head, and olecranon without bony productive change. Images also demonstrate diffuse osteopenia and large joint effusion, the findings of which are typical of RA. Coronal T2-weighted fat-suppressed (C) and PD fat-suppressed (D) images in the same patient demonstrate complete uniform cartilage loss of the radiocapitellar and ulnotrochelar joints, with osseous erosions. Axial (E) and sagittal (F) T2-weighted fat-suppressed images also show a large effusion surrounding exuberant lobulated low-signal hyperplastic synovial tissue, pannus (*), significantly distending the joint capsule and bicipital-radial bursa, as well as synovitis and joint fluid decompressing through weakened joint capsule (*white arrows*).

forth by the Assessment of SpondyloArthritis international Society for patients younger than 45 presenting with low back pain includes the following:

1. Either MRI or radiographic evidence of sacroiliitis and at least one clinical finding (mucosal ulcerations involving the mouth, intestines, or genitals, infections, erythema nodosum, inflammatory back pain, arthritis, Achilles enthesitis, dactylitis, uveitis, psoriasis, Crohn's disease/ulcerative colitis, good response to nonsteroidal anti-inflammatory medications, family history of spondyloarthropathy, positive HLA-B27, and elevated C-reactive protein); OR
2. HLA-B27 positive and at least two clinical findings

MRI is an essential tool in the diagnostic algorithm and is included in the criteria because both the sensitivity and specificity for the diagnosis of axial spondyloarthropathy is greater than 90% when there is MRI evidence of sacroiliitis combined with one specific clinical feature.

Ankylosing Spondylitis

Overview

AS is an inflammatory condition predominantly affecting the spine and sacroiliac joints. The peak onset typically occurs between 15 and 30 years of age, with males being more

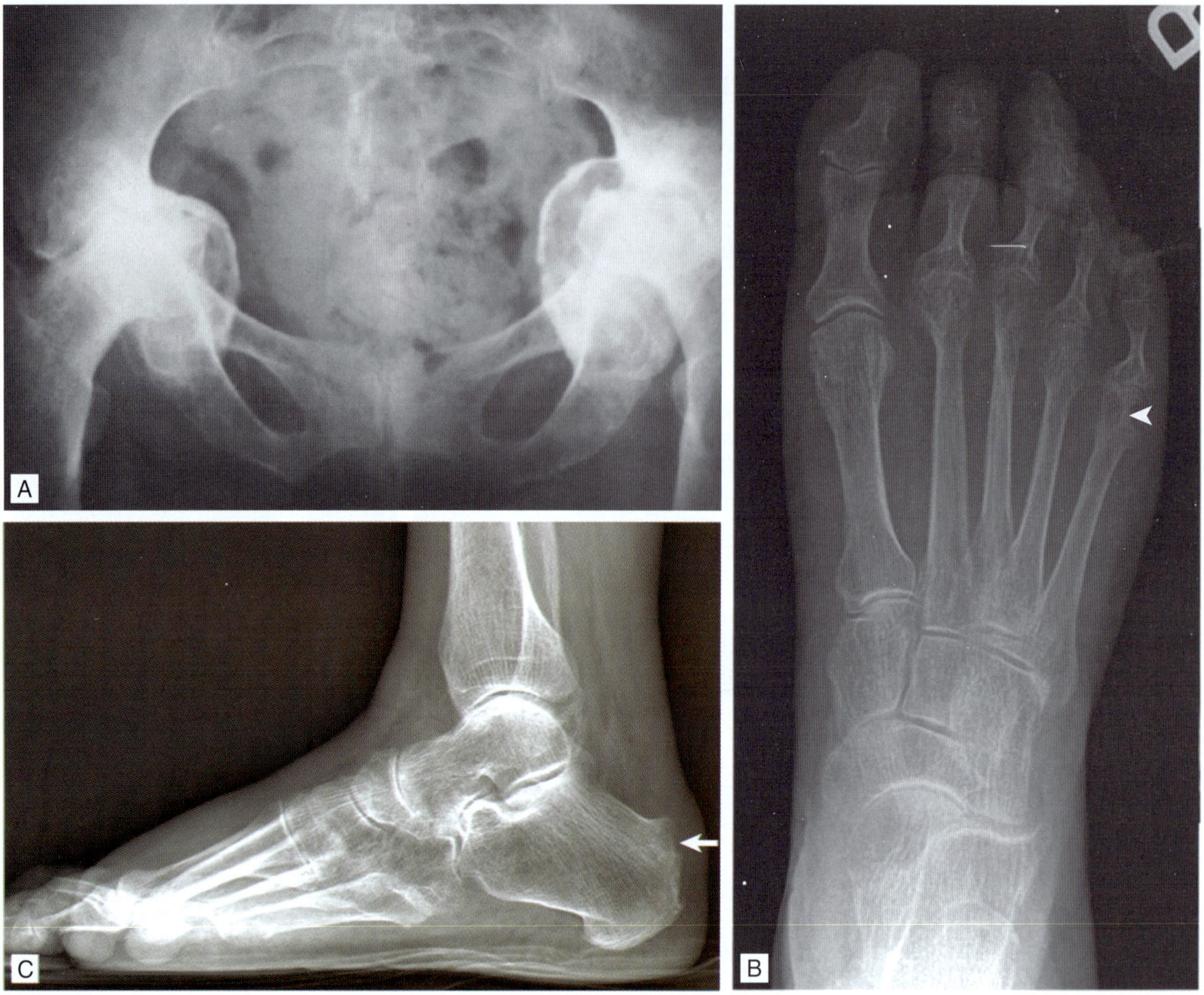

Figure 52.32 (A) Rheumatoid arthritis—extreme protrusio with medial migration and erosion of the femoral heads (B and C). Foot RA. AP (A) and lateral (B) views of the foot demonstrate calcaneal tubercle (*arrow*) and 5th metatarsal head periarticular erosions (*arrowhead*).

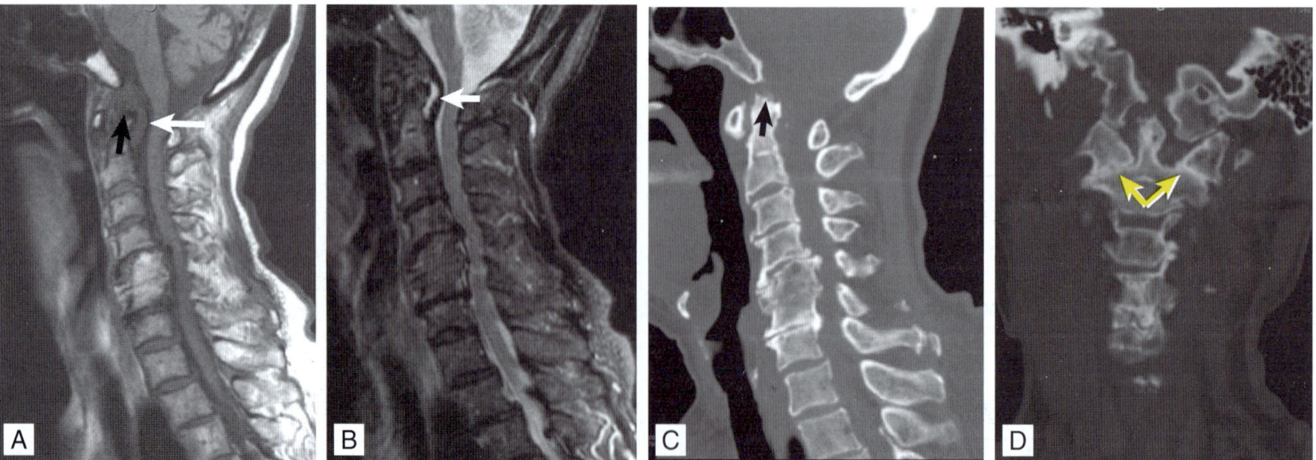

Figure 52.33 Cervical spine RA. Sagittal T1 (A) and T2 (B) MR images show extensive pannus formation surrounding the odontoid (*white arrows*) with effacement of the thecal sac and posterior displacement of the spinal cord, as well as erosion of the dens (*black arrow*). Corresponding CT image (C) demonstrates confirms odontoid erosions, as well as advanced erosive change across the C1–C2 facets (D—*yellow arrows*).

commonly affected than females at a 4:1 ratio. The prevalence in the general population is relatively low at 0.1%. Serum HLA-B27 positivity is detected in over 90% of patients afflicted with this condition.

Pathology

Pathophysiology of AS involves both synovial changes and entheseal inflammation, with fibrous ankylosis reflecting a relatively late manifestation.

Imaging

Radiographic findings of AS typically consist of bilateral, symmetric sacroiliitis (though asymmetric involvement is a common manifestation early in the disease process) (Fig. 52.34). Erosive changes are initially identified along the inferior one-third of the SI joints, which is the synovial portion of the joint, as well demonstrating an iliac-sided predominance due to the thinner hyaline cartilage layer in comparison to the sacrum, eventually leading to subchondral sclerosis and fusion across the SI joints later in the disease process.

Characteristic radiographic findings of the axial skeleton include the following:

- *Romanus lesions or corner entheseal erosions* (active inflammatory spondylitis) at the anterior-superior and anterior-inferior aspects of the vertebral body endplates, at the attachment sites of the annulus fibrosus (Fig. 52.35), which appear as focal edema/enthesitis on MRI
- *Osteitis or "shiny corner" sign* reflecting reactive sclerotic repair or healing secondary to inflammatory Romanus erosions at the anterior-superior and anterior-inferior aspects of the vertebral body endplates (Fig. 52.36)
- Healing new bone formation at the annulus fibrosus enthesis results in vertical syndesmophyte formation, which is ossification of the outer margin of the annulus (Fig. 52.37)
- Thin syndesmophytes bridging the outer layer of the annulus fibrosis and ossification of the posterior interspinous ligaments produces a dense linear line known as the dagger sign, which in combination with fused facets results in what is known as the trolley track sign (Fig. 52.38)
- Eventually leads to long column fusion which creates the "bamboo spine" appearance

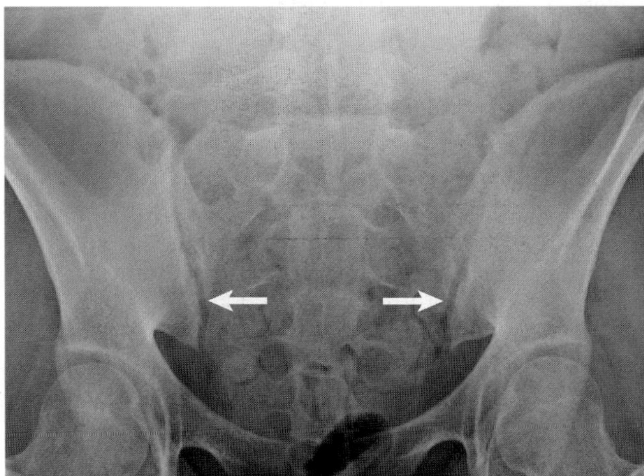

Figure 52.34 Bilateral sacroiliitis in patient with ankylosing spondylitis. Frontal radiograph of the pelvis demonstrating bilateral symmetric sacroiliac joint widening and cortical indistinctness compatible with sacroiliitis in a patient with ankylosing spondylitis.

- Careful attention should be directed toward the evaluation of the posttraumatic AS patient [18], even in the setting of minimal or low-grade trauma, as the fused spine acts as a lever arm placing great stress on the spine, which can result in a transverse "carrot-stick" fracture (Fig. 52.39) across disco-vertebral

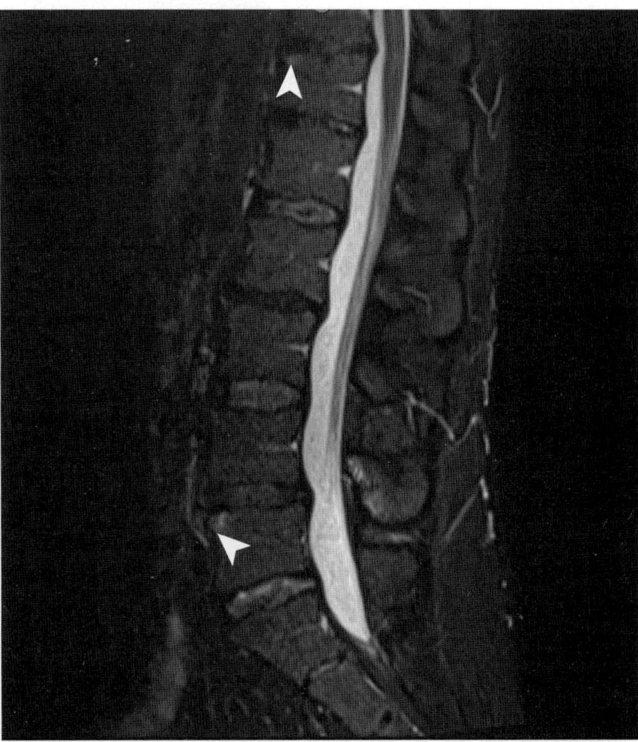

Figure 52.35 Spondylitis in a patient with AS. Corner entheseal erosions (active inflammatory spondylitis) at the anterior-superior and anterior-inferior aspects of the T12 and L5 vertebral body endplates (*arrowheads*), at the attachment sites of the annulus fibrosus, which appear as focal edema/enthesitis on MRI.

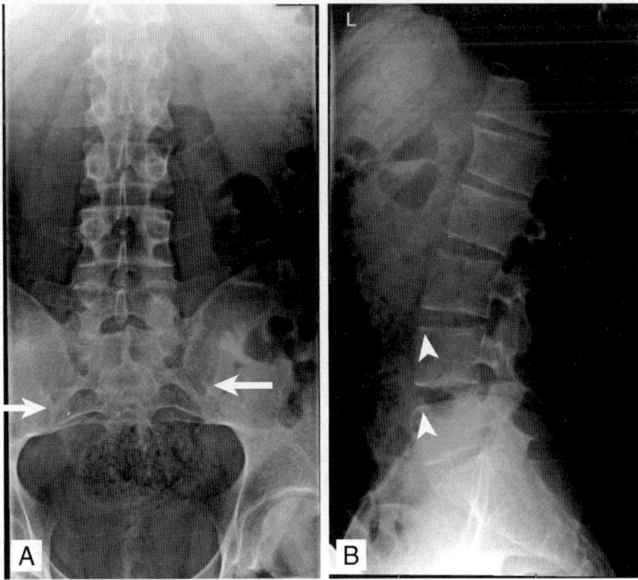

Figure 52.36 Shiny corners in a patient with AS. AP radiograph of the lumbar spine (A) in a 25-year-old male demonstrates fusion of the sacroiliac joints (*arrows*). Lateral view (B) demonstrating osteitis or "shiny corners" appearing as increased sclerosis (*arrowheads*) of the anterosuperior endplates of the L4 and L5 vertebral bodies.

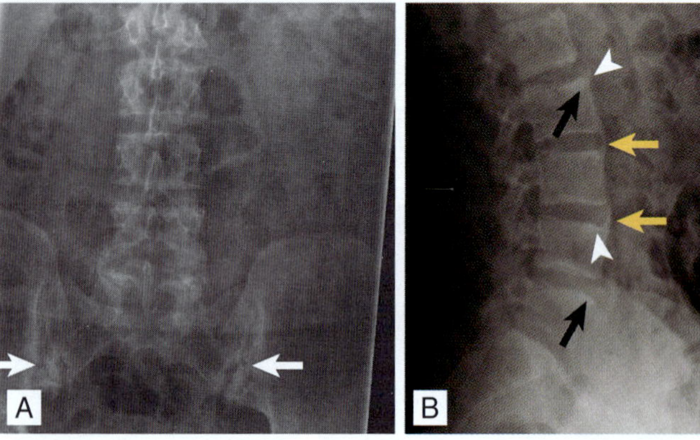

Figure 52.37 Ankylosing spondylitis. AP radiograph (A) demonstrates bilateral and symmetric sacroiliitis (*white arrows*). Lateral radiograph (B) demonstrates corner erosions of the anterior superior endplate of L2 and L4 (*white arrowheads*) which occur exactly at the site of attachment of the annulus fibrosus to the vertebral endplate, indicating a Romanus erosion, while there are corner foci of sclerotic repair at L2 and L5 (*black arrows*), compatible with osteitis or shiny corners. There is also healing new bone formation at the annulus fibrosus enthesis that results in vertical syndesmophyte formation (*yellow arrows*), which is ossification of the outer margin of the annulus.

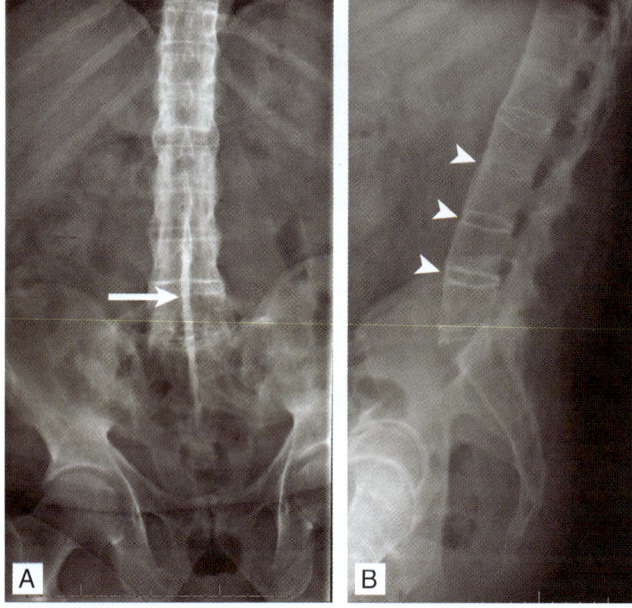

Figure 52.38 Syndesmophytes in AS. AP and lateral radiographs demonstrate fusion across the SI joints, thin syndesmophytes bridging the outer layer of the annulus fibrosis (*white arrowheads*) resulting in the classic bamboo spine appearance, and ossification of the posterior interspinous ligaments (*white arrow*) produces a dense linear line known as the dagger sign, which in combination with fused facets results in what is known as the trolley track sign.

junctions. Carrot-stick fractures can cause significant comorbidity if coupled with an unstable fracture pattern or epidural hematoma

Inflammatory spondylodiscitis, known as Andersson lesions, is a noninfectious disco-vertebral process seen in patients with AS. MR imaging can detect early changes of spondylodiscitis, typically revealing hemispherical increased signal intensity along adjacent subchondral endplates, as well as increased intradiscal signal, which can mimic discitis-osteomyelitis (Fig. 52.40). Both Romanus and Anderson lesions may demonstrate post-contrast enhancement, presumably related to the resulting associated local inflammatory hyperemia. More distal peripheral disease is less common and often seen with inadequate treatment. Unlike sacroiliac joint involvement, AS of peripheral joints is typically asymmetric.

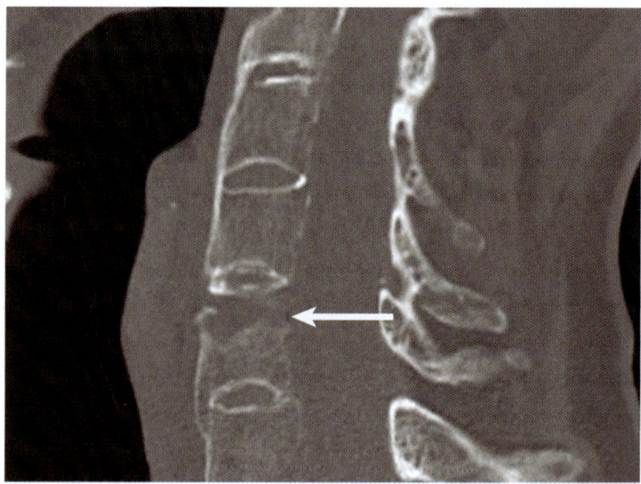

Figure 52.39 "Carrot-stick" facture in patient with AS. Sagittal CT image in a patient with known ankylosing spondylitis and subsequent transverse ("carrot stick") fracture through the superior C6 vertebral body (*arrow*) and posterior elements.

Differential Pearls

Bilateral and symmetric sacroiliitis.

Inflammatory Bowel Disease

Overview

IBD is well known to be associated with peripheral arthritis and spondyloarthropathy, among other causes of musculoskeletal system-related pain, which occur in up to 53% of patients [19]. IBD-related spondyloarthropathy, which can be categorized as axial versus peripheral arthropathy, is considered one of the most common extraintestinal manifestations of IBD, occurring in up to 30% of patients with IBD [20].

Pathology

Serum HLA-B27 positivity is detected in over 50% of patients with enteropathic arthropathy, most commonly in those with axial skeletal involvement. It is felt that predisposing genetic factors may also play a role in disease and symptom onset. IBD-related spondyloarthropathy consists of both axial arthropathy (sacroiliitis, inflammatory back pain, and ankylosing spondylitis) and peripheral arthropathy (nondeforming arthritis that waxes and wanes with bowel activity and flares) [21].

Imaging

Axial arthropathy includes sacroiliitis and spondylitis is common and indistinguishable from AS, appearing as bilateral and symmetric, as well as Romanus lesions and shiny corners, noninfectious spondylodiscitis, and thin bridging vertical syndesmophytes (Fig. 52.41). Additional synovial inflammatory changes can be seen along the facet joints, costosternal, costovertebral, and costotransverse joints.

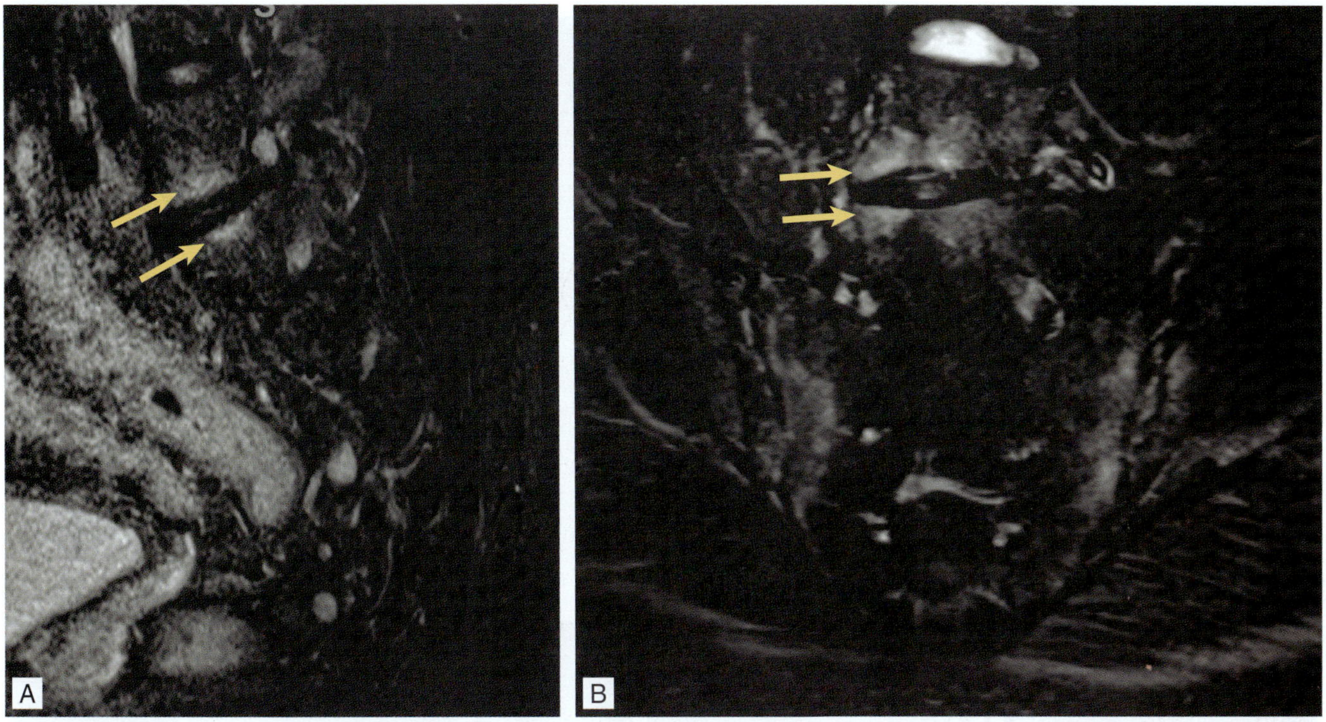

Figure 52.40 Inflammatory spondylodiscitis. Sagittal (A) and coronal oblique (B) T2-weighted fat-suppressed images through the sacrum demonstrate hemispherical increased signal intensity along adjacent L5 and S1 subchondral endplates (*yellow arrows*), as well as increased intradiscal signal, compatible with inflammatory spondylodiscitis (Anderson lesion). Additionally, there is bilateral subchondral bone marrow edema along the SI joints compatible with sacroiliitis.

MR imaging can detect acute inflammatory spondylitis and sacroiliitis earlier than radiographs, allowing for potential treatments before progressive structural damage.

MR findings of acute inflammatory sacroiliitis include the following (Fig. 52.42):

- Subchondral bone marrow edema seen as a hyperintense signal on STIR or T2-weighted fat-suppressed images along the subchondral surface of the SI joints, as well as subchondral enhancement, which be seen in association with erosions (Fig. 52.42)
- Synovitis of the SI joints manifested by intra-articular enhancement
- Enthesitis of the interosseous SI joint ligaments as evidenced by hyperintense signal seen on STIR or T2-weighted fat-suppressed
- Later findings and structural changes related chronic sacroiliitis, which can be appreciated on radiographs and MRI include subchondral sclerosis, erosions, periarticular fat deposition due to chronic inflammation, and bony bridging (ankylosis)

Peripheral IBD-related arthropathy manifestation included dactylitis and enthesitis.

- Radiographic findings are usually nonspecific and normal, but can show periarticular osteopenia, soft-tissue swelling, and rarely erosions of the MCP joints, as well as arthropathy of large weight-bearing joints
- Enthesitis, focal inflammation at a tendon, ligament, or joint capsule osseous attachment site, are common findings in all patients with seronegative spondyloarthropathies (6–50% of patients), manifested as bone marrow edema on MR imaging at enthesis sites (Fig. 52.42)

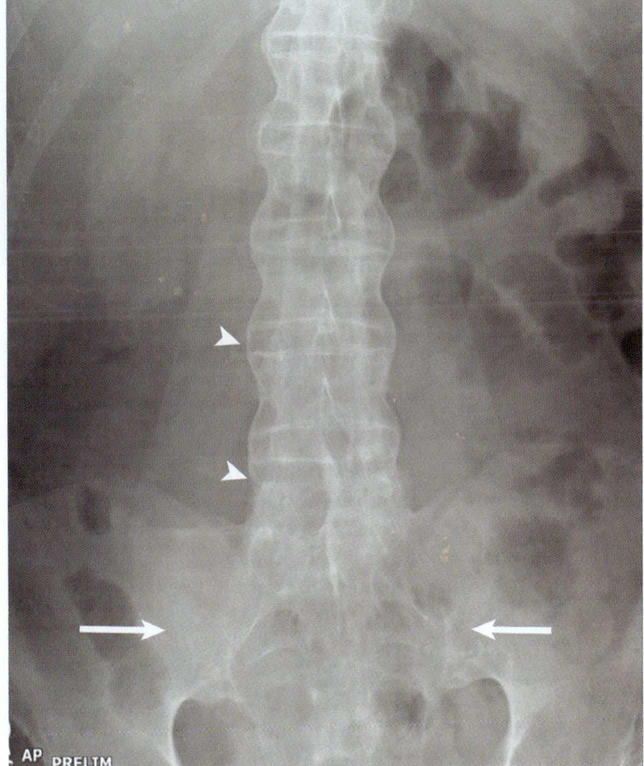

Figure 52.41 IBD-related spondyloarthropathy. AP preliminary radiograph in a 65-year-old male with Crohn's disease obtained for small bowel series demonstrates classic thin bridging vertical syndesmophytes (*arrowheads*) and fused SI joints, (*arrows*), indistinguishable from AS.

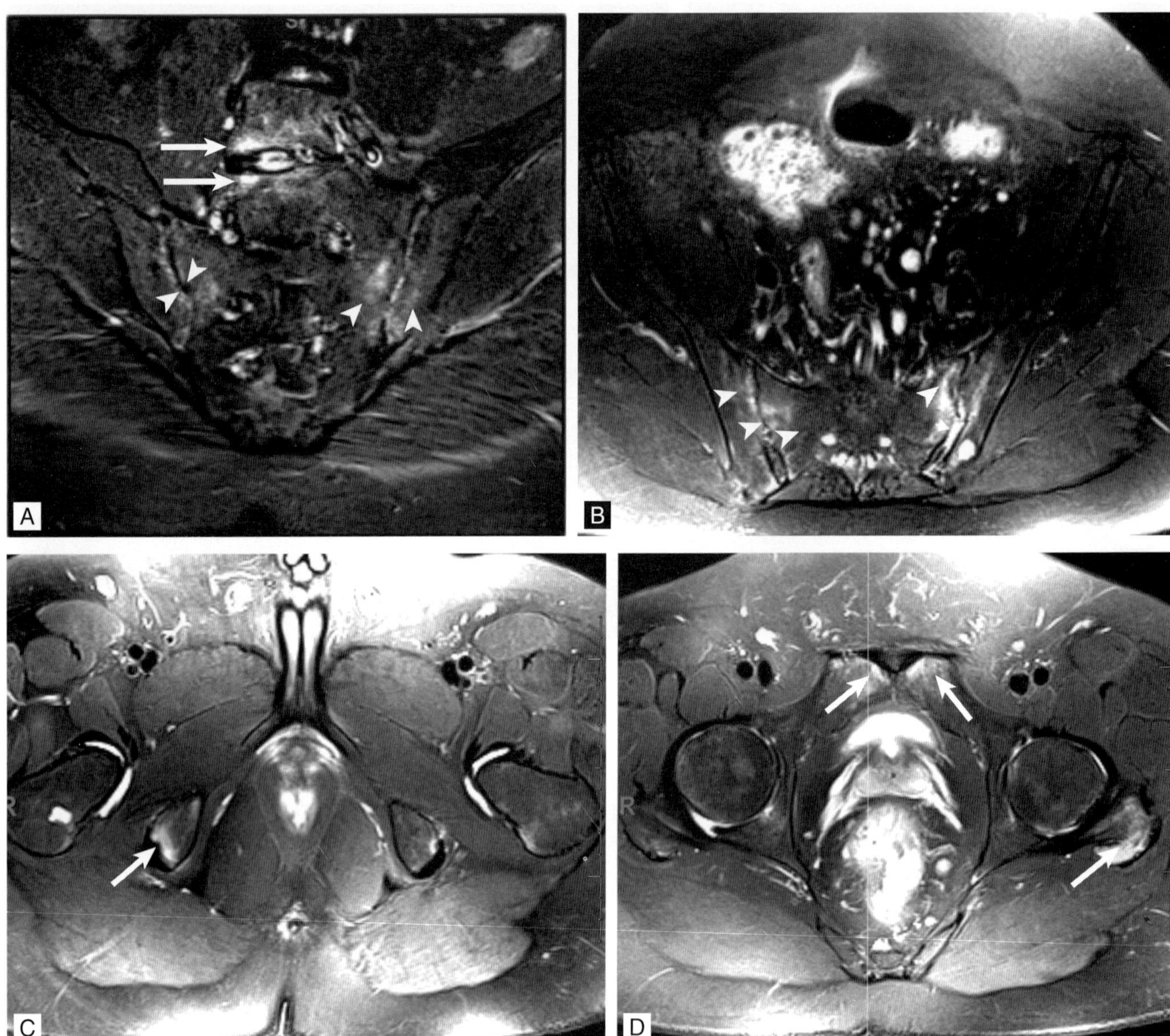

Figure 52.42 IBD-related spondyloarthropathy. Coronal (A) and axial oblique IR (B) images demonstrate bilateral sacroiliac joint bone marrow edema, erosions, and fluid accumulation with SI joints, left greater than right, as well as inferior predominance involving the synovial portions of the SI joints (*arrowheads*). Axial PD fat-suppressed images (C and D) demonstrate multifocal entheseal bone marrow edema (*white arrows*), compatible with enthesitis at the hamstring tendon origins, adductor insertions, gluteal tendon insertions, and the L4–L5 endplates at the attachment sites of the annulus fibrosus.

Other musculoskeletal manifestations of IBD-related spondyloarthropathy include osteonecrosis, which may be encountered more frequently due to high incidence of steroid use in this population, and osteomyelitis of the pelvic bones and spine due to direct extension from intra-abdominal abscess and fistulas.

Psoriatic Arthropathy

Overview

Psoriatic arthropathy (PsA) is considered under the category of seronegative spondyloarthropathy, presenting with peripheral joint involvement and affecting the axial skeleton including the sacroiliac joint and spine. Most patients, approximately 70%, develop psoriatic skin lesions several years before experiencing musculoskeletal symptoms, while 15% of patients develop arthritis before skin changes, and the remaining patients report arthritis and skin changes developing simultaneously. Patient symptoms clinically overlap with rheumatoid arthritis, including joint stiffness, pain, and swelling, limited range of motion, morning stiffness, and fatigue; however, patients with psoriatic arthropathy present with nail psoriasis and dactylitis and usually test negative for rheumatoid factor. Additionally, contrary to RA, patients with PsA, exhibit an asymmetric and distal distribution pattern in the extremities. In 2005, Moll and Wright classified PsA into five subtypes:

1. *Classic PsA or predominant DIP joint arthritis of the hands and feet*: It manifests as distinct periarticular erosive changes of the DIP joints with bony proliferative changes, often associated with nail dystrophy
2. *Arthritis mutilans*: A destructive form of PsA with extensive osteolysis of the DIP and PIP joints of the hands and feet resulting is severe digital abnormalities including "pencil-in-cup" and "opera glass" deformities

3. *Symmetrical peripheral polyarthritis resembling RA*: It affects more than five joints of the fingers, wrists, and toes with erosions and ankyloses of the interphalangeal joints. 15–20% of cases cannot be distinguished from RA (although patients are RF negative)
4. *Asymmetrical mono or oligarthritis usually involving the knees or peripheral small joints*: It is the most common form of PsA (70% of cases), affecting less than five joints, exhibiting an asymmetric distribution of both small and large joints, including the classic finding of "sausage digit"
5. *Axial spondyloarthropathy*: These findings are similar to AS, including spondylitis, bulky asymmetric syndesmophytes, and asymmetric sacroiliitis

Pathology

Although the precise pathophysiology of psoriatic arthropathy has yet to be delineated, the development of psoriatic arthropathy is likely due to combination of hereditary and environmental factors. It has been postulated that this process may represent a reactive arthropathy from psoriatic plaque flora. Serum HLA-B27 positivity is detected in approximately 60% of patients who demonstrate peripheral and axial involvement.

Imaging

A plethora of radiographic findings are associated with psoriatic arthropathy and can be subdivided based on peripheral and axial distributions of inflammatory changes.

Peripheral Joints

Hand/Wrists (Involved in 25%)

- *Row pattern*: Classic DIP prevalence with asymmetric distribution
  - Begins as periarticular or marginal erosions of the DIP joints with peripheral bony productive change at the joint borders, coined the "mouse-ear" deformity (Fig. 52.43)
  - More advanced changes include distal phalangeal tuft erosions, acro-osteolysis (Box 52.1), as well as DIP and PIP joint ankyloses (Fig. 52.44)
- Progressive osseous erosions lead to other advanced findings seen in PsA including:
  - *"Pencil-in-cup" deformity*: It is described as marked thinning/erosion of the distal aspect of the proximal phalanx exhibiting a pointed end and accompanied bone resorption at the base of the distal phalanx creating a concave appearance (Fig. 52.45) [22]. Typical radiographic finding in PsA, but not specific as it can be seen in other inflammatory arthropathies
  - Five percent of patients may develop arthritis mutilans resulting from osteolysis and articular collapse of the phalanges. This can be associated with the clinical manifestation of "telescoping fingers"

BOX 52.1 Differential Diagnosis of Acro-Osteolysis

- Scleroderma
- Dermatomyositis
- PsA
- Reactive arthritis
- Sarcoidosis
- Juvenile chronic arthritis
- Extreme temperature; frostbite/burns
- Trauma
- Hyperparathyroidism
- Porphyria
- Drug toxicity (i.e., phenytoin)
- Vascular insult/occlusion
- Raynaud disease

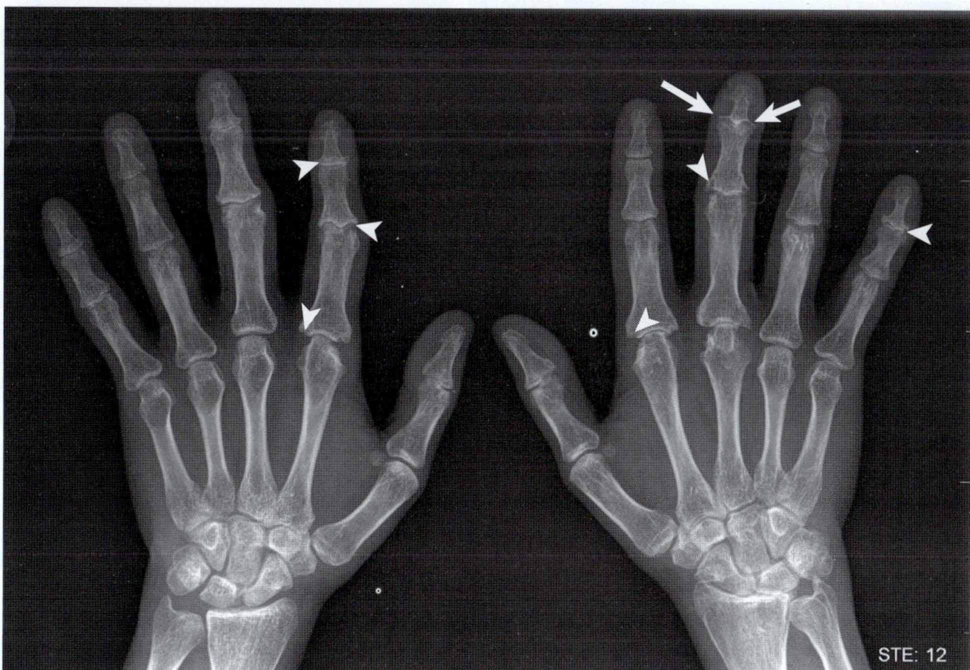

Figure 52.43 Psoriatic arthritis. AP radiographs of the hands demonstrated asymmetric distribution of periarticular erosions with bony productive change at the right 3rd DIP joint, known as "mouse-ear" deformity (*arrows*). Periarticular erosions are identified at the right 5th DIP, 3rd PIP, joint and 2nd and 3rd MCP joints. Early periarticular erosions at the left 2nd DIP joint, 2nd PIP joint, and 2nd MCP joint.

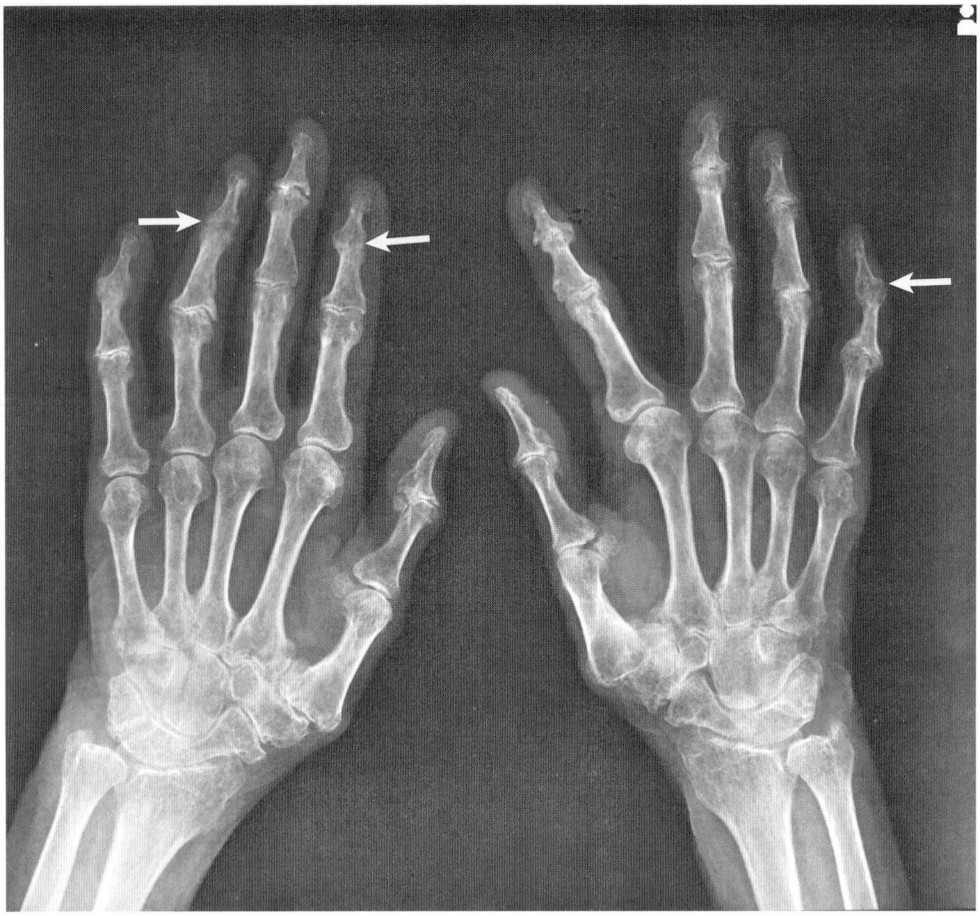

Figure 52.44 Psoriatic arthritis. AP radiographs of the hands demonstrate asymmetric erosive changes with bony productive change as well as ankyloses across multiple DIP joints (*arrows*).

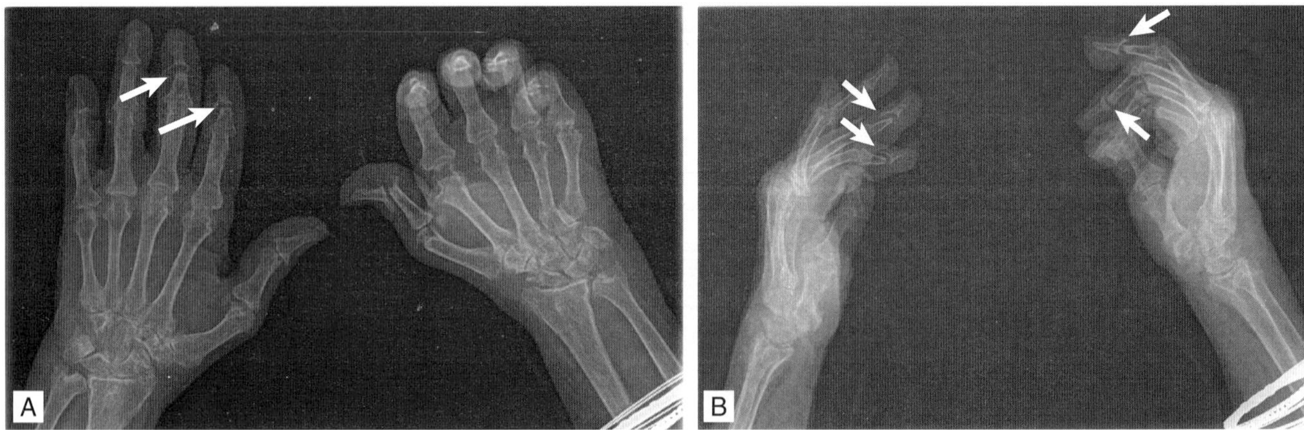

Figure 52.45 Advanced changes in psoriatic arthritis. AP (A) and oblique (B) radiographs of the hands demonstrate marked erosive changes of the left 2nd and 3rd DIP and right 3rd and 4th DIP joints, resulting in the appearance of the pencil-in-cup deformity (*arrows*) and shortening of the middle phalanges with subluxation of the right 1st IP joint resulting in telescoping fingers, as well as flexion deformities of the right hand. Additionally periarticular erosions are also identified about the 1st MCP joints, and metacarpal heads.

- *Ray pattern*: Early PsA of the hands and feet can result in *dactylitis*, known as a "sausage digit," manifest as soft-tissue swelling of an entire digit and periostitis due to inflammation and synovitis about the DIP and PIP joints, as well as flexor tenosynovitis (Fig. 52.46)
  - The MCP joints are typically spared early in the disease process, although can be eventually involved if untreated
  - A combination of endosteal and periosteal bone proliferation can lead to an "ivory" phalanx [22], which results in increased radiodensity of an entire phalanx (Fig. 52.47)
  - Any compartment of the wrist may be involved; fairly nonspecific

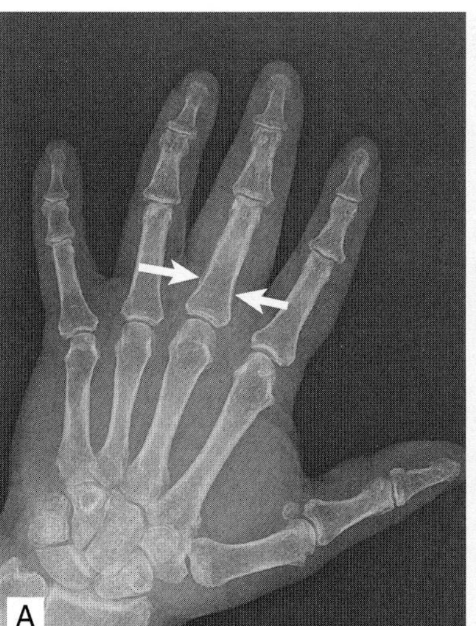

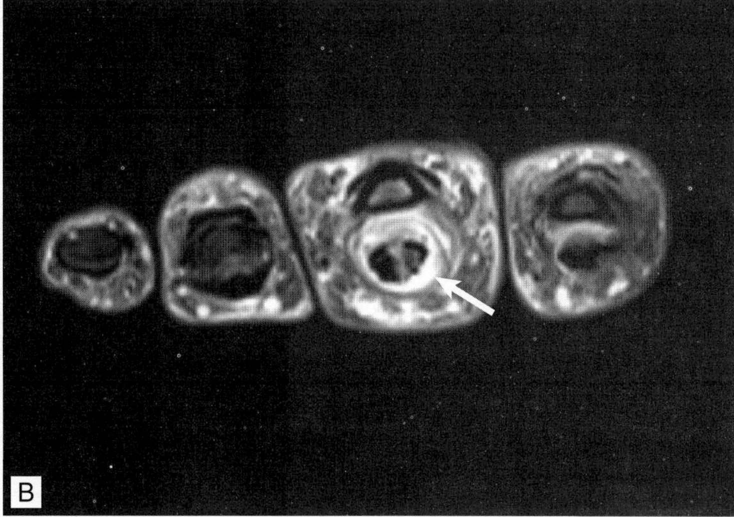

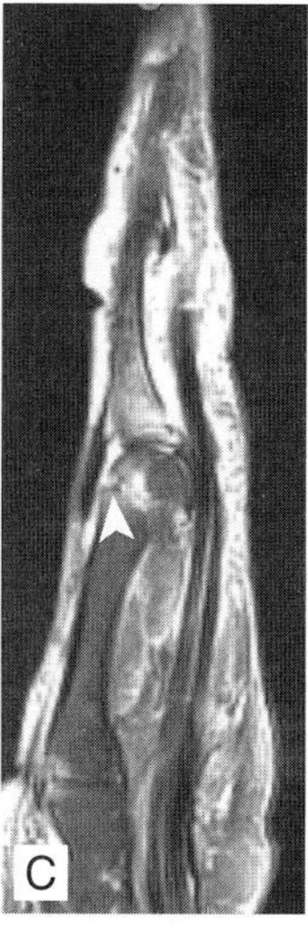

Figure 52.46 Dactylitis in a psoriatic arthritis. AP radiograph (A) of the left hand in a 58-year-old male with history of psoriasis, demonstrating fusiform swelling of the 3rd digit (sausage digit) with periosteal proliferation along the 3rd proximal phalanx (*arrows*). Corresponding axial (B) and sagittal T2-fat-suppression (C) MR sequences demonstrate tenosynovitis of the 3rd flexor tendon (*arrow*) with regional soft-tissue edema, intense bone marrow edema within the 3rd proximal phalanx, 3rd MCP joint effusion, and erosion dorsal aspect of the 3rd metacarpal head (*arrowhead*).

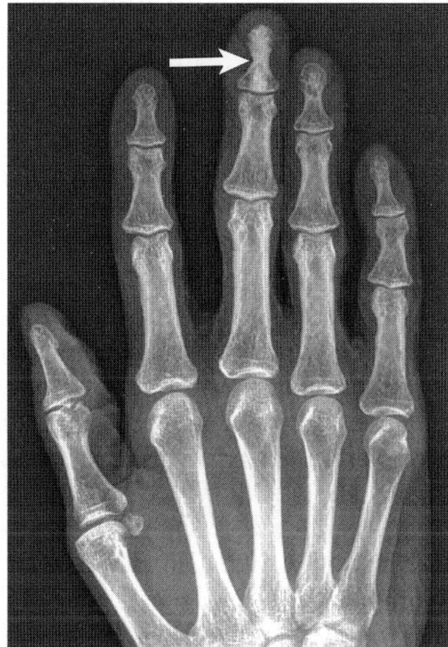

Figure 52.47 Ivory phalanx. Frontal radiograph of the hand in an 80-year-old female with history of psoriasis demonstrating diffusely increased density within the 3rd digit distal phalanx (*arrow*) compatible with an "ivory phalanx."

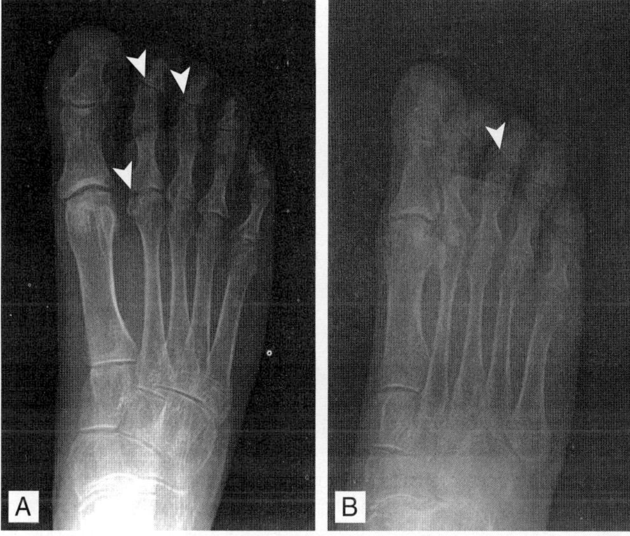

Figure 52.48 Psoriatic arthritis. AP (A) and oblique (B) radiographs of the right foot demonstrate 2nd, 3rd, and 4th DIP joint periarticular erosions (*arrowheads*), as well as at the bases of the 2nd and 3rd proximal phalanges.

Feet/Ankles

Overall, the features and distribution are same as seen in the hands (Fig. 52.48). Typically manifests as interphalangeal joint involvement, with ivory phalanx commonly observed in the distal phalanx of the great toe. Commonly observed erosive changes are seen at the posterior tubercle of the calcaneus, but is nonspecific as it can also be a typical finding in patients with chronic reactive arthritis. Enthesitis is a commonly observed imaging finding at the malleoli, Achilles tendon insertion, and plantar aponeurosis.

Axial Manifestations

- Sacroiliitis
  - Common finding in patients with PsA
  - Initially appears as bilateral and asymmetric, but progresses to symmetric involvement later in the disease process (Figs. 52.49 and 52.50)
  - Late manifestations include bilateral ankylosis, although this is less common than in AS
- Spondylitis
  - Syndesmophytes present as bulky vertical/nonmarginal paravertebral ossifications that may be asymmetric with "skipped bodies"
- Enthesitis
  - Considered a hallmark clinical and imaging finding in seronegative spondyloarthropathies, including PsA
  - Most commonly identified at the Achilles tendon insertion, origin of the plantar aponeurosis, and tendinous attachment sites about the pelvis

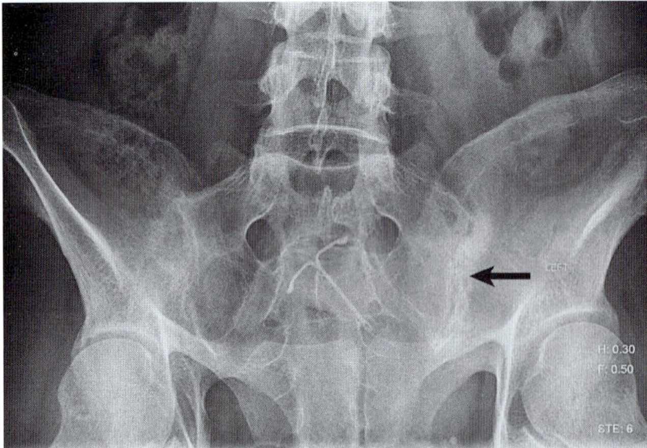

Figure 52.49 Asymmetric sacroilitis in patient with psoriatic arthropathy. AP view of the sacrum demonstrates asymmetric left-sided sacroiliac joint subchondral irregularity, erosions, sclerosis, and partial fusion (*black arrow*), compatible with asymmetric sacroiliitis.

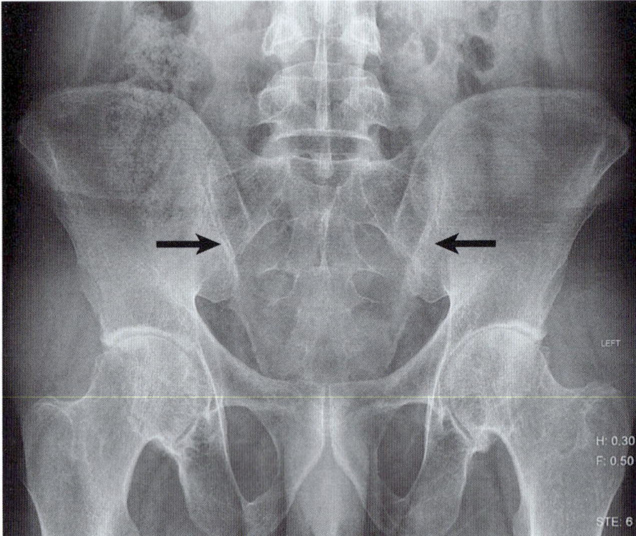

Figure 52.50 Psoriatic arthritis. AP radiograph of the pelvis demonstrating asymmetric sacroilitis, left greater than right as evidenced by subchondral sclerosis and indistinctness of the subchondral margins (*arrows*) due to underlying erosions with an iliac-sided predominance, as well as partial ankyloses. Additionally, note the concentric bilateral hip joint space narrowing, more commonly seen in inflammatory arthropathies compared with superolateral and inferomedial joint space narrowing commonly seen in osteoarthritis.

Diagnostic Pearls

- Distal, asymmetric distribution in the hands and feet with bony productive change and the absence of periarticular osteopenia can help to differentiate between psoriatic and rheumatoid arthritis
- PsA may be distinguished radiographically from chronic reactive arthritis (CRA) due to the propensity of CRA to involve a single articulation of the foot
- Bilateral and asymmetric sacroiliitis seen in PsA versus AS

Chronic Reactive Arthropathy

Overview

The term chronic reactive arthropathy (CRA) refers to the triad of arthritis, urethritis, and conjunctivitis [23]. From a musculoskeletal standpoint this condition often presents with heel pain as an initial manifestation, following an enteric or urogenital infection.

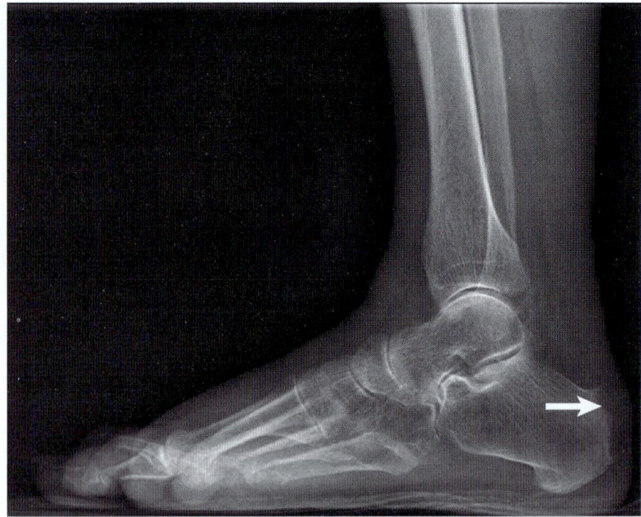

Figure 52.51 Chronic reactive arthritis. Erosions of the posterior calcaneal tubercle (*arrow*).

Pathology

There is a strong association of CRA with HLA-B27 positivity. There has also been a demonstrable association between this condition and HIV-positive status, and is thought to be triggered by a preceding gastrointestinal or genitourinary infection, which may have a subclinical presentation. Additionally, joint fluid and synovial cultures are sterile, hence the term "reactive."

Imaging

Radiographic findings are nonspecific, but are similar to other forms of seronegative spondyloarthropathies, such as PsA, including irregular erosions, enthesitis, bone proliferation, periostitis, and digital soft-tissue swelling, either presenting as unilateral or bilateral, as well as asymmetric distributions. However, compared with PsA, CRA more often targets the joint of the feet rather than the hands.
Imaging features include:

- Erosions of the posterior tubercle of the calcaneus at the Achilles tendon insertion (Fig. 52.51) in conjunction with erosions of the MTP joints and interphalangeal joint of the great toe
  - *Lower extremity predominance*: MTP joints, first interphalangeal joint, and the calcaneus are the most frequent targeted sites in the foot
- Enthesitis
- Sausage digit with associated periostitis
- Bulky paravertebral osteophytes syndesmophytes, indistinguishable from PsA
- Asymmetric sacroiliitis

Differential Pearls

Radiographic changes are identical to *PsA*; however, the predominant distal distribution and feet greater than hands in *CRA*, as well as clinical history allows for a more accurate diagnosis of *CRA* versus *PsA*.

Connective Tissue Diseases of Joints

Systemic Lupus Erythematosus

Overview

SLE is an autoimmune disorder characterized by inflammation, immune complex deposition, vasculitis, and vasculopathy [24]. It affects 1 in 700 white females and roughly 1 in 245 Black females.

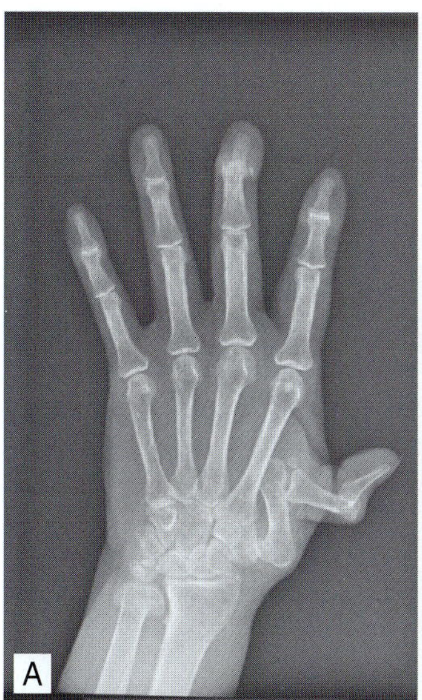

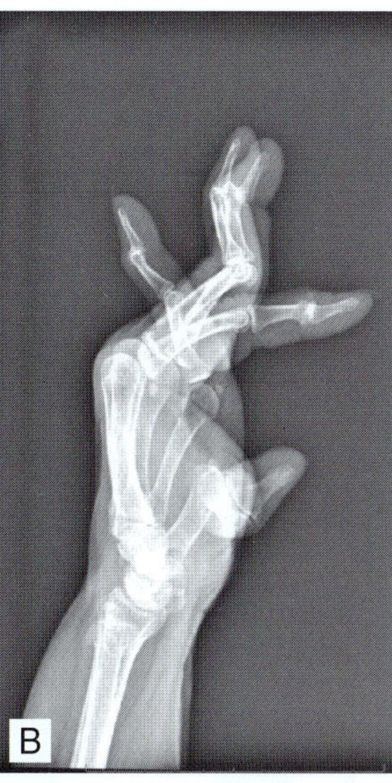

Figure 52.52 SLE-related arthropathy. AP (A) and lateral (B) radiographs demonstrate hyperextension deformity involving the 2nd through 5th proximal interphalangeal joints with associated compensatory flexion deformity at the distal interphalangeal joints, compatible with swan-neck deformity, as well as 1st CMC joint subluxation.

The condition may affect individuals of all ages, although the peak onset is typically between 10 and 40 years of age [25,26].

Pathology

The underlying pathophysiology of SLE is thought to be related to autoantibodies reacting with components of various cell nuclei, ultimately resulting in deposition of immune complexes within end organs. Cells affected by the disorder are often present within synovial fluid, which likely gives rise to the majority of musculoskeletal manifestations of lupus.

Imaging Findings

It is mostly considered a symmetric, polyarticular disease. The most frequent findings in the hands and wrists consist of reducible, deforming, but nonerosive arthropathy due to ligamentous laxity and muscle contracture, distinguishing SLE from RA (Fig. 52.52).

- *Swan-neck deformity*: Hyperextension deformity of the PIP joint with compensatory flexion deformity at the DIP joint
- *Boutonniere deformity*: Flexion contracture of the PIP joint with compensatory extension deformity at the DIP joint
- MCP joint subluxation with ulnar deviation
- Subluxation of the first carpometacarpal (CMC) joint
- Tenosynovitis is a common presenting sign, typically involving the flexor tendons of the hand. Tendon ruptures may occur later in the disease process
- Increased incidence of septic arthritis may be seen in this population, thought to be due increased steroid treatments
- Avascular necrosis and insufficiency fractures are common, usually involving the hips, knees, and shoulders. It may result from steroid therapy and/or osteopenia, but given the high incidence (10%), there is likely an underlying component related directly to the disease itself. Widespread osteonecrosis in unusual locations should suggest SLE as a possible etiology

Jaccoud's arthropathy is a disease entity characterized by a deforming, nonerosive arthritis that occurs in approximately 10–35% of SLE patients [27]. This condition does not involve the synovium but causes capsular fibrosis.

Imaging Findings

- Lateral deviation of the hands and feet may be seen when examined without weight-bearing; with pressure, these deformities vanish
- Joint spaces are mainly preserved
- "Hook" erosions of the metacarpal heads may possibly be due to local capsular pressure; true erosions are not typically found

Scleroderma/Progressive Systemic Sclerosis

Overview

Scleroderma is a multisystem disorder characterized by skin thickening and vasculitis. It mostly affects younger patients, with roughly 50% of patients presenting before the age of 40. It has a strong female predominance of roughly 80%.

Pathology

Though the underlying etiology is unknown, characteristic antibodies associated with the disease (ANA, anticentromere) suggest an underlying immunologic abnormality. Vascular damage is considered to be the primary event in disease onset, with endothelial cell activation, intimal thickening, and vascular narrowing ultimately giving rise to an impaired angiogenic response.

Imaging Findings

- Best diagnostic clue is acro-osteolysis (Figs. 52.53 and 52.54) in conjunction with soft-tissue calcification (Fig. 52.54)
- Early skin changes usually appear as soft-tissue swelling. Mid-disease skin changes include tapering of the skin at the ends of digits. Late-disease skin changes include marked contractures
- Calcinosis appears as punctate, globular, or sheet-like areas of mineralization, most commonly affecting the hands [28]
- Tenosynovitis, occasionally with the presence of fibrotic nodules, is considered an early finding
- Muscular fibrosis and atrophy may occur later in the disease; early myopathy may also occur but is virtually indistinguishable from other etiologies
- Arthritis is uncommon early in the disease; erosions may develop later in the disease process, as may other signs of end-stage joint involvement including:
    - DIP joint ankylosis
    - Subluxation and erosion of the trapezium/base of first metacarpal
    - Radial and proximal migration of the first carpometacarpal joint is thought to be a hallmark of progressive systemic sclerosis
- Hyperparathyroidism, thermal injury/burns, and PsA can all have similar appearances on imaging and should be maintained in the differential diagnosis

Crystal-Induced Arthropathies

Gout

Overview

This disease entity is due to a biochemical derangement in which hyperuricemia results in monosodium urate or uric acid crystal deposition within periarticular soft tissues, cartilage, and bone.

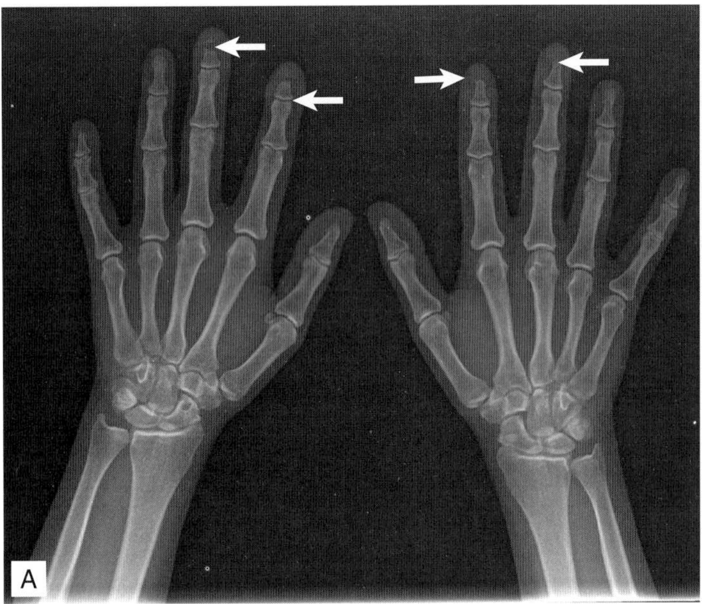
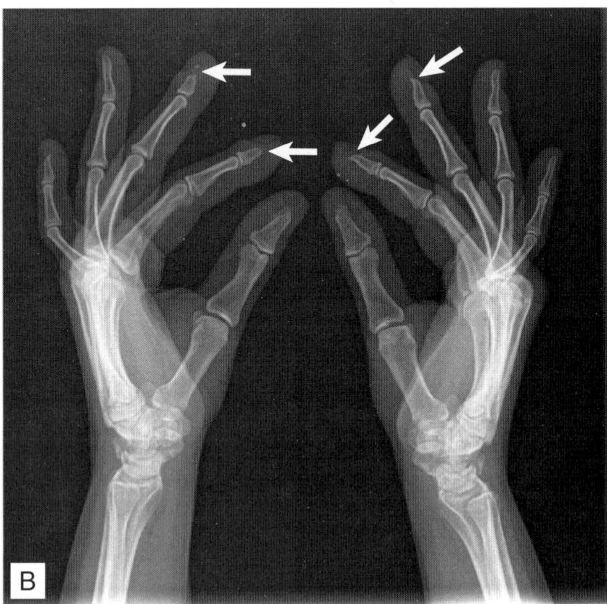

Figure 52.53 Acro-osteolysis in scleroderma. AP (A) and lateral (B) radiographs demonstrate distal phalangeal acro-osteolysis (*arrows*).

Although most cases are idiopathic, there may be a familial component and in some cases a relation to chronic disease (typically renal pathology or conditions creating high rates of cellular turnover, such as widespread tumor).

Pathology

Hyperuricemia ultimately gives rise to sodium urate crystal deposition in soft tissues and joints. The underlying cause of the primary gout is thought to be abnormal purine metabolism, whereas the secondary gout is believed to be attributable to increased serum uric acid levels.

Imaging Findings

Initial clinical presentation is usually of monoarticular joint involvement, commonly the foot. Although any joint can be affected, the first MTP joint is most commonly affected with gout, followed by the first interphalangeal and tarsometatarsal joints. Erosive changes as will be described can be mono- or polyarticular, and usually exhibit an asymmetric distribution. Similarly, any of the joints of the hand and wrist can be involved; the carpometacarpal and intercarpal joints are most frequently affected. Various imaging findings seen in gout can be subdivided based on modality.

Radiographic Findings

- Pain, erythema, and regional periarticular soft-tissue swelling may be the first and only radiographic finding encountered in an acute gouty attack
- Known as "podagra" if affecting the first MTP joint
- Juxta-articular erosions, away from the joint, characterized as well-defined sharp sclerotic margins and overhanging edges (rat-bite erosions) are the typical appearance of gouty erosions (Fig. 52.55)
- Urate crystal deposits within the soft tissues, often seen with chronic gout, result in dense nodules due to crystal deposition,

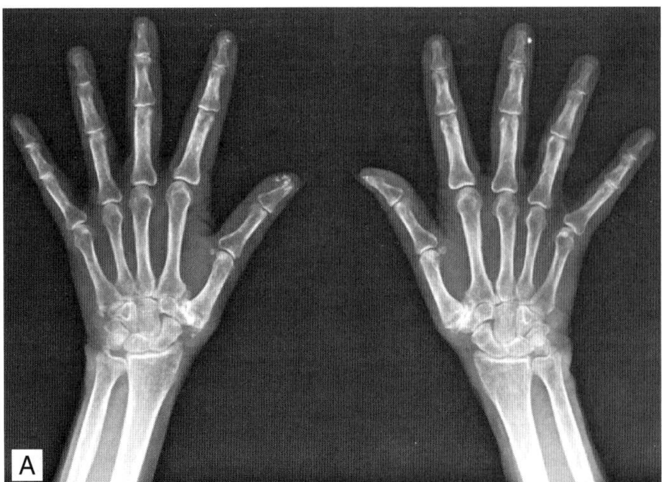
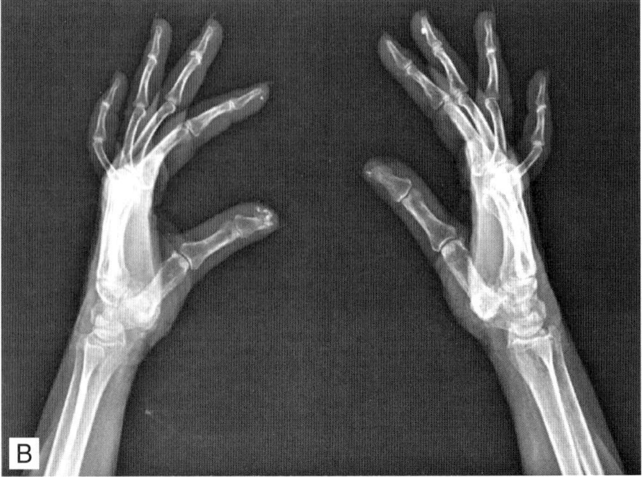

Figure 52.54 Acro-osteolysis + soft-tissue calcifications in scleroderma. AP (A) and lateral (B) radiographs demonstrate acro-osteolysis of the right 1st and 2nd distal phalanx, left 2nd and 3rd distal phalanges, distal phalangeal soft-tissue calcification, as well as advanced 1st CMC arthrosis with radial migration of the 1st metacarpal.

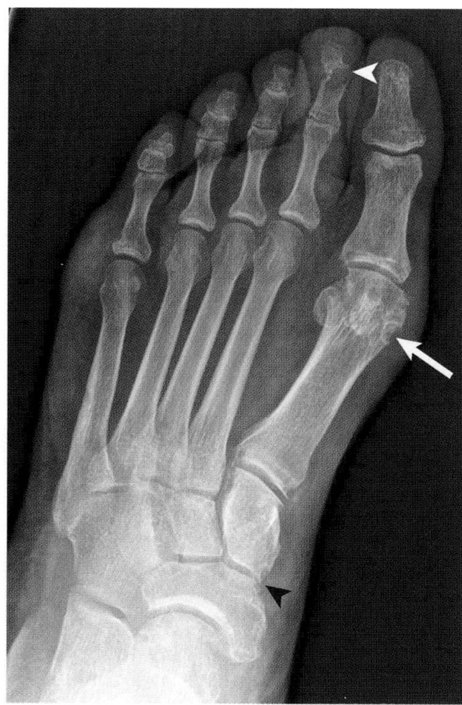

Figure 52.55 Gout. AP radiograph of the foot demonstrating the hallmark findings of gout including classic juxta-articular erosions of the 1st metatarsal head with overhanging edges (*arrow*), normal bone density, and preservation of the 1st MTP joint space. Additionally, there are punched out erosions across the 2nd DIP joint (*white arrowhead*), as well as erosions along the medial aspect of the naviculocuneiform articulation (*black arrowhead*).

sometimes with internal calcifications and/or cloudy amorphous density, known as tophus. Tophus and adjacent joint erosion may exist synchronously (Figs. 52.56–52.59)

- Preservation of the joint space until late in the disease process

USG Finding

- Typically demonstrate joint effusions, tophi, and periarticular erosions [29]. Erosions in gout are usually deeper and more destructive compared with RA erosions
- Tophi appear as inhomogeneous hypoechoic to hyperechoic surrounded by thin anechoic rim, may exhibit a nodular or infiltrative appearance, and can cause posterior acoustic enhancement due to attenuation of the sound beam and calcifications (Figs. 52.60 and 52.61)
- Tendon involvement is usually peritendinous or around the tendon, but can be seen as intratendinous deposit. Common tendons include the Achilles and peroneal tendons in the foot, as well as the popliteus tendon insertion and along the intercondylar groove associated with cruciate ligaments are common intra-articular sites within the knee. Additionally, the patellar tendon and infrapatellar fat pad are site of tophus formation
- Double contour sign refers to the sonographic appearance of hyperechoic linear crystal deposits with the underlying hyperechoic line of subchondral bone (Fig. 52.62)
- Hyperechoic aggregates may also be visualized within joint fluid

CT Findings

- Dual-energy CT can be highly valuable in distinguishing urate crystal deposition from calcium depositions, which may otherwise have very similar appearances on other imaging modalities (Fig. 52.61) [30]

MRI Findings: Can identify intraosseous tophus deposits; however, although MRI is very sensitive in the detection of soft tissue and bone pathology, the findings may not be specific as the erosive changes can mimic septic joint-osteomyelitis. The site of involvement, distribution, radiographic, and clinical correlation are often necessary to conclude the correct diagnosis.

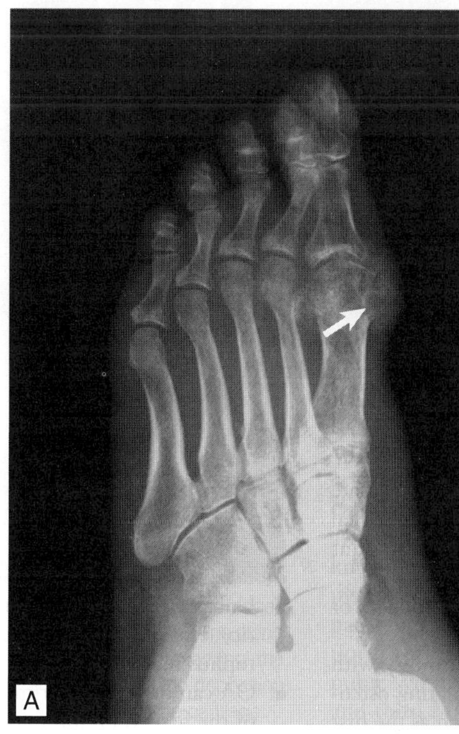

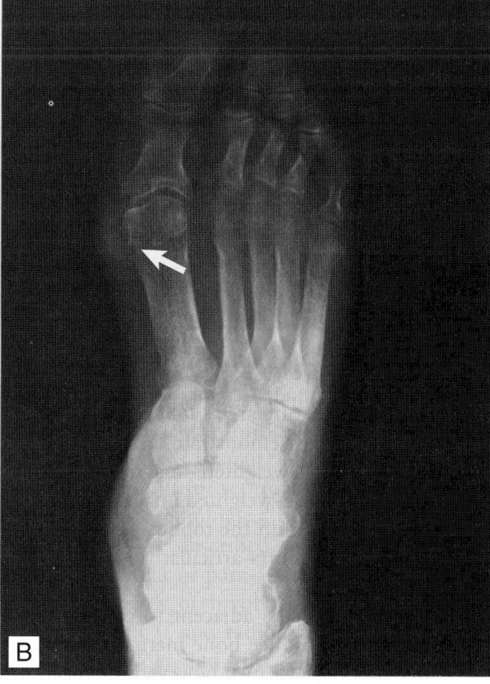

Figure 52.56 *Tophaceous gout.* Oblique radiograph of the left foot (A) and AP radiograph of the right foot (B) demonstrates tophus formation with the soft tissues adjacent to the 1st MTP joints, associated with typical juxta-articular erosions of the 1st metatarsal heads (*arrows*).

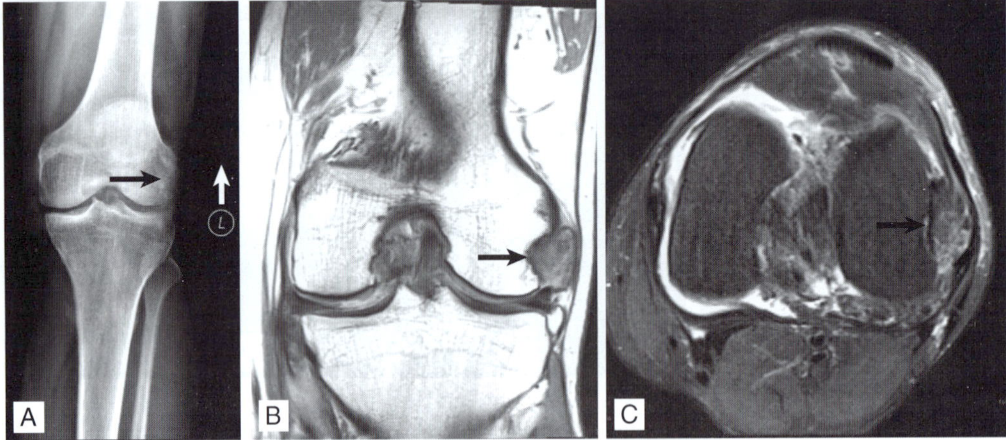

Figure 52.63 Gout AP radiograph (A) demonstrates increased calcified soft density adjacent to popliteus tendon origin and erosion in popliteal groove (*black arrow*). Corresponding coronal PD (B) and axial T2-weighted fat-suppressed (C) images demonstrate intermediate signal tophus at the origin of the popliteus tendon with erosion of the popliteal groove (*black arrows*).

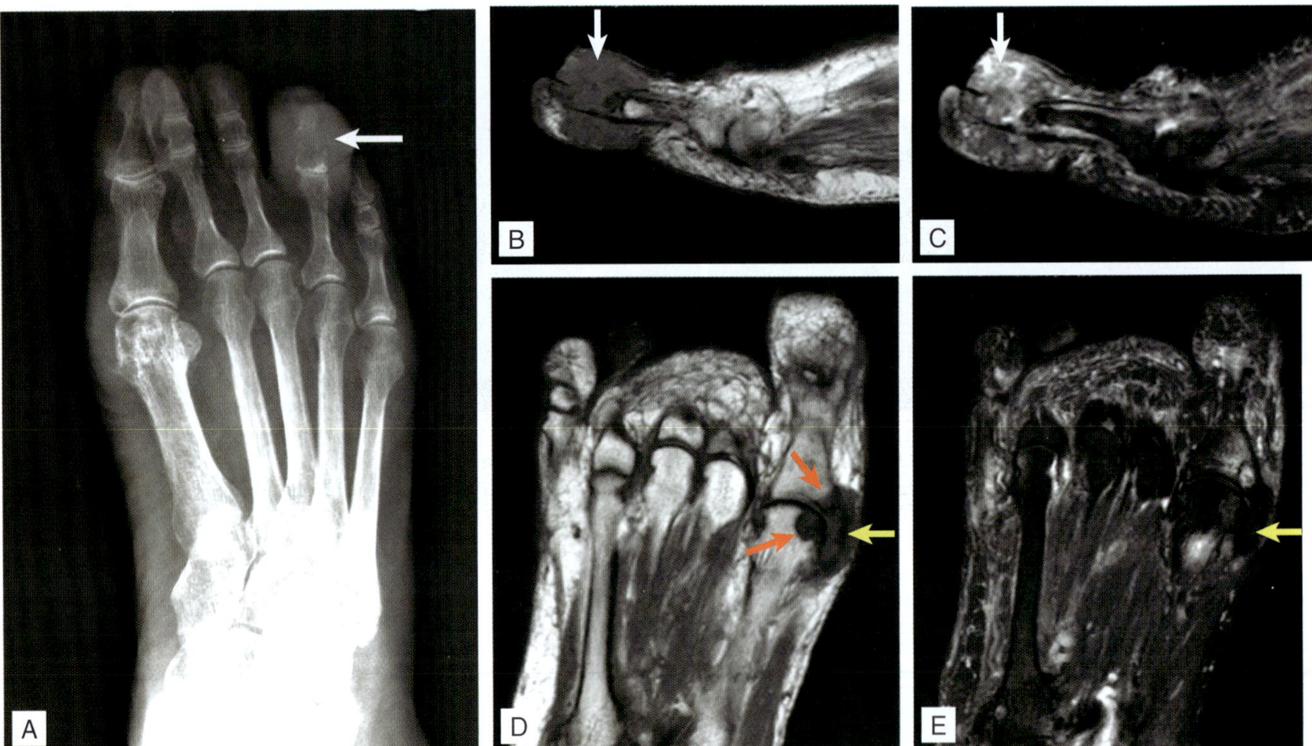

Figure 52.64 Gout versus osteomyelitis. AP radiograph of the right foot (A) demonstrates punched out erosion of the 4th DIP joint with associated amorphous partially calcified soft-tissue mass (*white arrow*). Patient had a history of gout and diabetes but no draining soft-tissue wound or ulcer. Sagittal T1 and IR (B and C) sequences demonstrate a gouty tophus infiltrating and eroding the 4th DIP joint (*white arrows*), with resultant bone marrow edema. Long-axis T1 and T2 fat-suppressed image (D and E) demonstrate corresponding juxta-articular erosion seen on the radiographs with tophus exhibiting intermediate signal on both sequences eroding the adjacent bone. Surgical pathology confirmed gouty tophus status post amputation. Additionally, note the 1st MTP joint erosions (*red arrows*) and adjacent low-to-intermediate signal tophus (*yellow arrows*).

Pathology

The underlying pathology of pseudogout is felt to be mostly idiopathic, although hereditary and even secondary causes such as hemochromatosis, hyperparathyroidism, hypothyroidism, and ochronosis have been theorized, which have been shown to have increased association with CPPD. The pseudogout crystals may be pathologically distinguished from other disease processes and crystal deposition diseases through the characteristic rhomboid positive birefringence CPPD crystals observed on polarized light microscopy.

Imaging Findings

Chondrocalcinosis is a pathognomonic radiographic finding that corresponds to crystal deposition into hyaline or fibrocartilaginous structures, appearing as punctate and linear calcifications.

- Typical locations of chondrocalcinosis include:
  - TFCC
  - Hyaline cartilage and fibrocartilage (menisci) of the knee
  - Pubic symphysis
  - Glenohumeral joint

the shoulder being the most frequent site of involvement in up to 69% of cases [33]. Interestingly, most cases of HADD are asymptomatic and frequently encountered on radiographs as an incidental finding; however, is a common cause of nontraumatic joint pain.

Distribution and Location

HADD presents as a monoarticular process, with the shoulder and hip known to be the most common site of involvement. However, when patients present with a painful monoarticular process in an atypical location, treating physicians must rely on radiological interpretation and clinical presentation to avoid misdiagnosing HADD as another possibly more ominous process.

Shoulder

- *Common locations*: Rotator cuff tendons are most common site of HADD (supraspinatus > infraspinatus > subscapularis > teres minor)
- *Uncommon locations*: Biceps tendon, pectoralis major tendon insertion, and subacromial–subdeltoid bursa

Hip

- *Common locations*: Gluteal tendon insertion
  - *Greater trochanter*: Gluteus medius and minimus tendon insertions
  - *Gluteal tuberosity*: Gluteus maximus tendon insertion
- Uncommon locations around the hip:
  - Rectus femoris origin
  - Iliopsoas insertion
  - Common hamstring tendon origins
  - Labrum and/or hip capsule (rare)

Elbow

- *Common locations*: Flexor and extensor tendon complex origins
- *Uncommon locations*:
  - Ulnar and radial collateral ligaments
  - Biceps and triceps tendon insertions

Wrist/Hand

- *Common locations*:
  - Flexor carpi ulnaris tendon insertion upon the pisiform is the most common site in the wrist
  - Periarticular regions of the MCP and interphalangeal joints

Knee

- Usually an uncommon or atypical site for HADD
  - Occur adjacent to the femoral condyles, fibular head, prepatellar region, popliteus tendon, and collateral ligaments

Foot/Ankle

- Usually an uncommon or atypical site for HADD
  - Seen in the flexor hallucis longus and brevis tendons, as well as the peroneus muscles
  - Adjacent to the MTP joints known as acute calcific periarthritis/hydroxyapatite pseudopodagra
    - Often mistaken for acute tophaceous gout

Neck

- Usually an uncommon or atypical site for HADD
  - Longus coli muscle and tendon with calcific deposition anterior to C2

- Pr
  ph
- M

Pathop

The und
trauma
rise to re
ing alon
four pat
1. Preca
   lagin
2. Calci
   proce
   into
   homo
3. Resor
   intrat
   and p
   sues,
   a. M
   b. Fl
      gr
   c. C
      lea
   d. Ty
      de
      an
      mi
   e. Un
      H
4. Repar
   collag

Imaging

Radiogr homogen
tendon o
erosions
involvem
cern for
Milwa
arthropat
vated col
thinning
destructi
predilecti
resembles
dence of
CT Findi insertions.
cortical e
ation of l
tween cal
appearan
preciated.
MRI Find malities a
hypointe
on gradie
of HAD

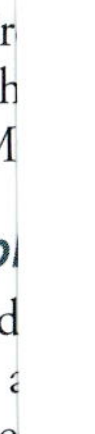

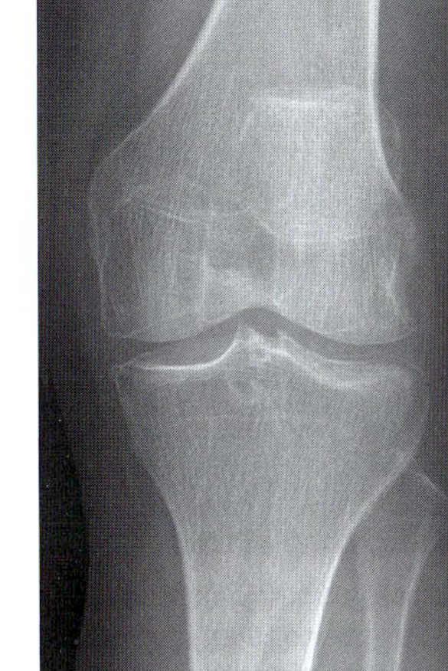

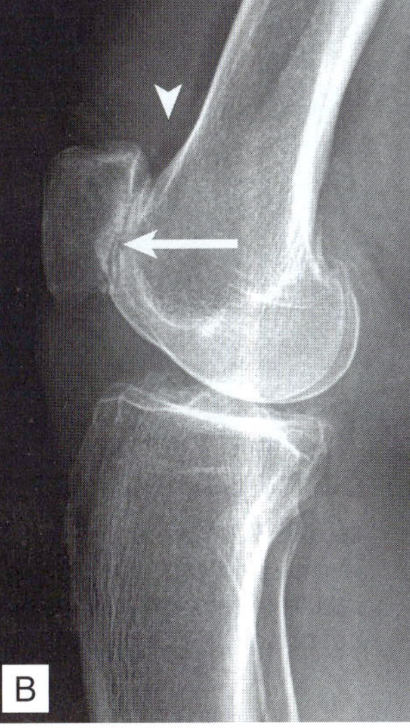

Figure 52.65 *Isolated patellofemoral arthrosis CPPD.* AP (A) and lateral (B) views of the knee demonstrate tricompartmental chondrocalcinosis (*arrowhead*) with advanced arthrosis of the patellofemoral joint (*arrow*).

- Typical locations of tendon chondrocalcinosis include:
  - Gastrocnemius, quadriceps, and Achilles tendons (the most common)
  - Triceps, rotator cuff, and cruciate ligaments (less common)
- Distribution of arthropathy:
  - *Knee*: Patellofemoral compartment may manifest as isolated disease, or out of proportion compared with the tibiofemoral compartments (Fig. 52.65)
  - *Wrist*: Radiocarpal articulation
  - *Hands*: Second and third MCP joints
  - *Spine*: Usually surrounding the dens and anterior arch of C1, discogenic calcifications

Radiographic appearance (Fig. 52.66):

- Chondrocalcinosis
- Joint space narrowing, subchondral sclerosis, subchondral cysts, and geode formation
- Hooked-like osteophytes emanating from the metacarpal heads
- Cause of scapholunate advanced collapse (SLAC wrist)

USG appearance: The pseudogout may demonstrate a thin echogenic band, which is often interrupted, within the mid-zone of the articular cartilage (Figs. 52.66 and 52.67) [32].

- In contrast to gout, calcium pyrophosphate crystals aggregate in the middle layer of cartilage, appearing as hyperechoic irregular foci of a variable length embedded within anechoic appearing hyaline cartilage
- Punctate, round echogenic foci may also be demonstrated within fibrocartilaginous structures (e.g., TFCC or menisci)
- May demonstrate echogenic intra-articular aggregates as can be seen in gout, but unlike gout these aggregates are uniformly round with sharply defined outer margins (Fig. 52.67)

Crowned dens syndrome is a typical manifestation of the pseudogout involvement of the spine (Fig. 52.68).

Differential Pearls

1. Septic arthritis
   a. Clinical presentation and imaging findings can often be indistinguishable from CPPD arthritis, thus joint aspiration may be necessary in those clinical situations
2. CPPD versus RA
   a. The absence of MCP erosions would favor CPPD versus RA
   b. Erosions of the dens and mass-like deposition around the C1–C2 articulations can mimic pannus formation in RA; however, CT imaging can be used to identify calcifications that would be present in CPPD but not associated with pannus in a patient with RA

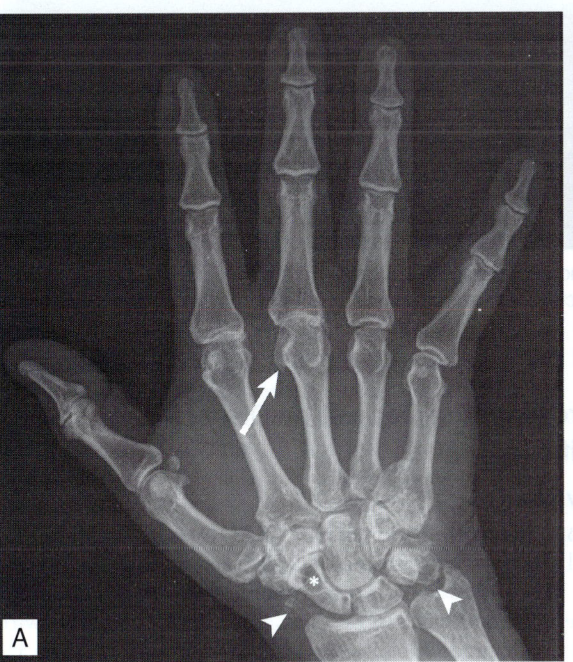

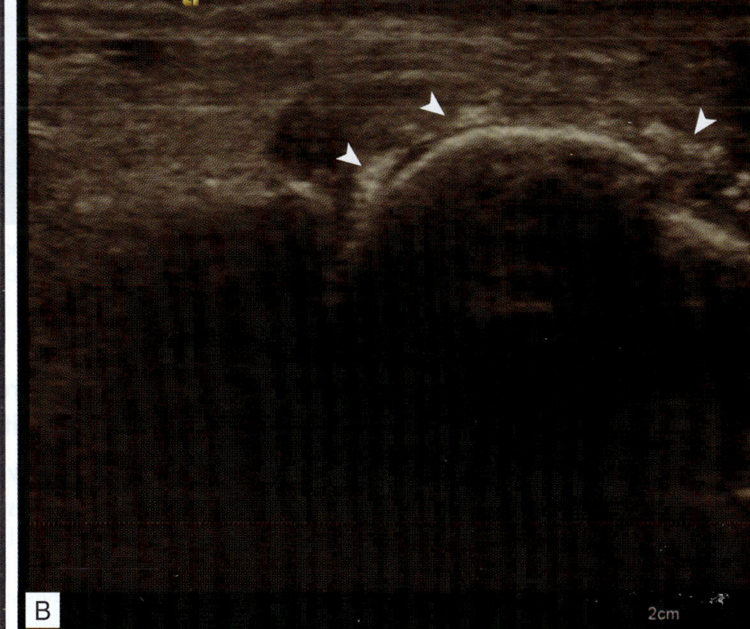

Figure 52.66 CPPD arthropathy. PA radiograph (A) of the right hand demonstrates radiocarpal and TFCC chondrocalcinosis (*arrowheads*) with carpal geodes (*). There is also narrowing of the 2nd and 3rd MCP joint with subchondral sclerosis and hooked osteophyte emanating from the 3rd metacarpal head (*arrow*). Corresponding USG of the 3rd MCP joint (B) demonstrated an irregular pattern of calcium deposition along the 3rd metacarpal head (*arrowheads*).

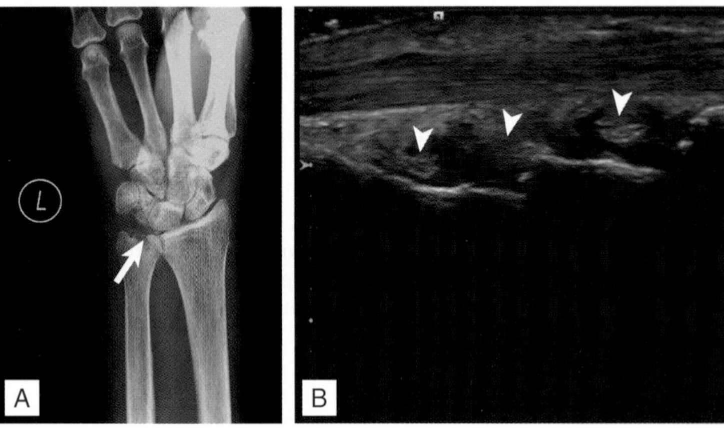

Figure 52.67 CPPD arthropathy. Oblique radiograph of the left wrist (A) demonstra
images (B and C) show rounded echogenic foci with the dorsal carpal recesses, outli
radiographs (*arrowheads*), demonstrating increased power Doppler signal, indicating
left wrist pain and cellulitis, the findings of which likely reflect the clinical presentatior

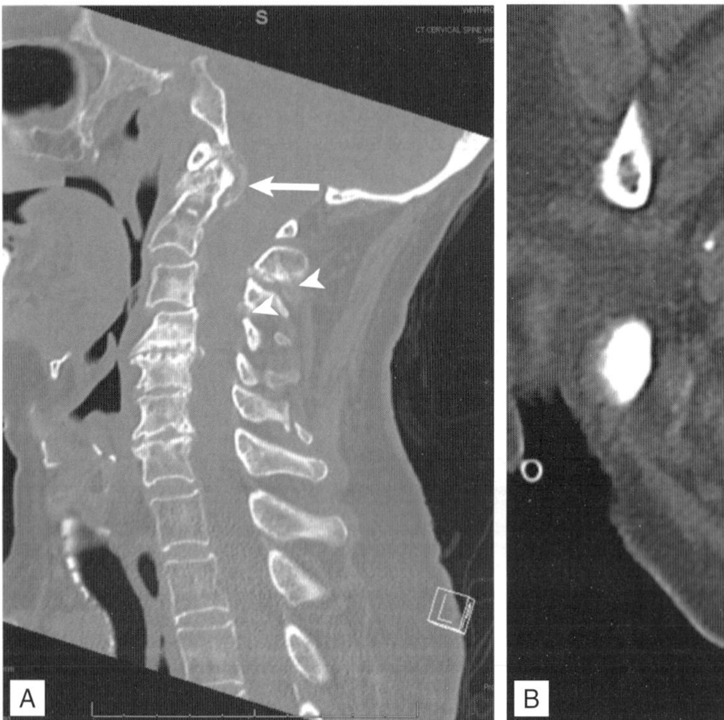

Figure 52.68 CPPD crowned dens syndrome. Sagittal (A) and axial (B) CT images s
cogenic and interspinous calcifications (*arrowheads*), the findings of which are chara
arthritis pannus is excluded by the presence of calcifications.

3. CPPD results in chondral destruction, producing an imaging appearance similar to OA
   a. CPPD distribution is different compared with OA
   b. Radiocarpal, glenohumeral, and, the second and third MCP joints are more commonly affected in CPPD
   c. Geodes and joint destruction encountered in CPPD is often more severe compared with OA
   d. Metacarpal head hooked osteophytes are commonly seen in CPPD, and may be more prominent in cases of hemochromatosis

Hyd
Calc

Over

Hydı
logic
dons
The ı
a slig
of th

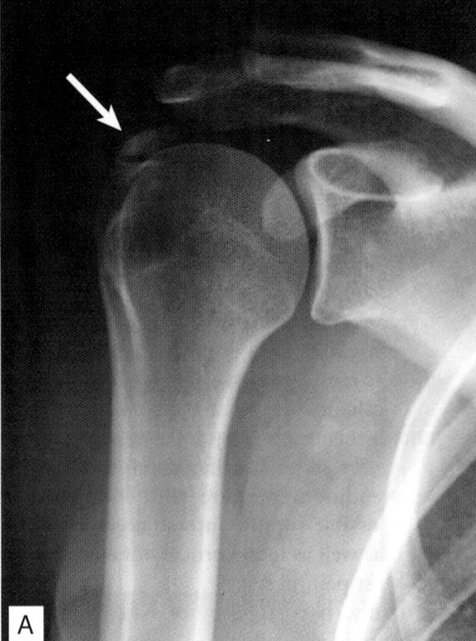

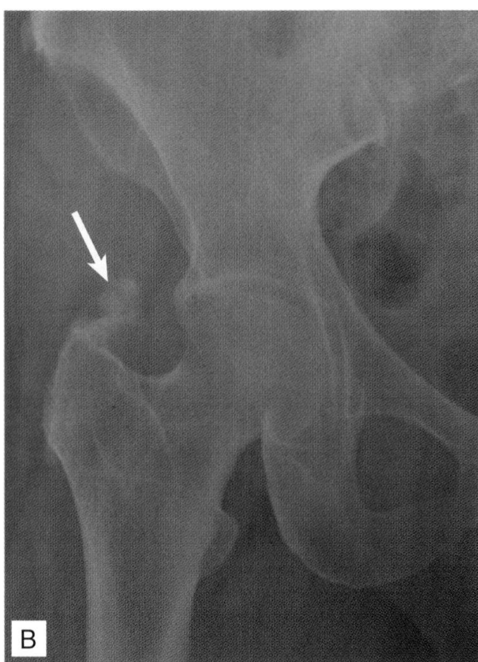

Figure 52.69 Calcific tendinosis. AP radiographs of the shoulder and hip demonstrate globular homogenous calcific deposits along the course of the rotator cuff (*arrow* in A) and the gluteal tendon insertions (*arrow* in B).

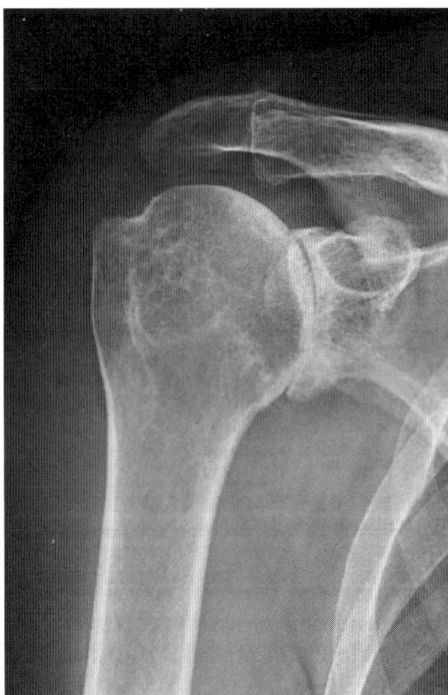

Figure 52.70 Milwaukee shoulder. AP radiograph of the right shoulder demonstrates uniform narrowing of the glenohumeral joint space, diffuse subchondral sclerosis, and intra-articular calcifications. Differential consideration would include chondrocalcinosis from calcium pyrophosphate deposition. Joint aspiration confirmed diagnosis of calcium hydroxyapatite crystals.

in hyperintense T2 signal representing reactive edema and inflammatory response within the tendon proper, peritendinous tissues, or adjacent bursa (Fig. 52.71) [37]. Aggressive picture at MR imaging with extensive localized inflammatory response, enhancement, and osseous involvement can mimic tumor.

- Edema may be extensive and can mimic infection or focal mass
- Soft-tissue calcification with cortical erosion and intraosseous migration resulting in bone marrow edema and periostitis may raise concern for neoplasm, particularly surface chondroid lesions (Figs. 52.72 and 52.73)

Correlation with radiographs and/or CT is crucial in rendering the correct diagnosis in the setting of neoplasm versus HADD.

USG Findings: Appears as echogenic foci within the tendon, with or without posterior acoustic shadowing (Fig. 52.74). USG can be utilized to perform diagnostic exams and therapeutic procedures (*barbotage*) [34]. Barbotage refers to a percutaneous intervention that allows for fragmentation and aspiration of calcific material within a joint or bursa.

Differential Pearls

Potential pitfalls and mimics in the acute setting

1. Infection
   a. Clinical manifestation of localized pain and in some cases fever
   b. Patients presenting with HADD will typically have normal WBC counts, but can elevated inflammatory markers
   c. MR imaging of calcium extrusion into the peribursal soft tissues/bursa aids in the diagnosis
   d. Acute onset of neck with stiffness and odynophagia (Fig. 52.75)
      i. Longus coli calcific tendinosis can mimic retropharangeal abscess [35]
2. Tumor
   a. Bone marrow edema associated with adjacent soft-tissue calcification and cortical destruction may raise concern for neoplasm, particularly surface chondroid lesions
3. Crystalline arthropathy (i.e., gout)
   a. Gouty tophi typically are more faintly calcified
   b. Elevated urate levels are seen in gout and not HADD
   c. MRI appearance of a tophus maybe indistinguishable from HADD

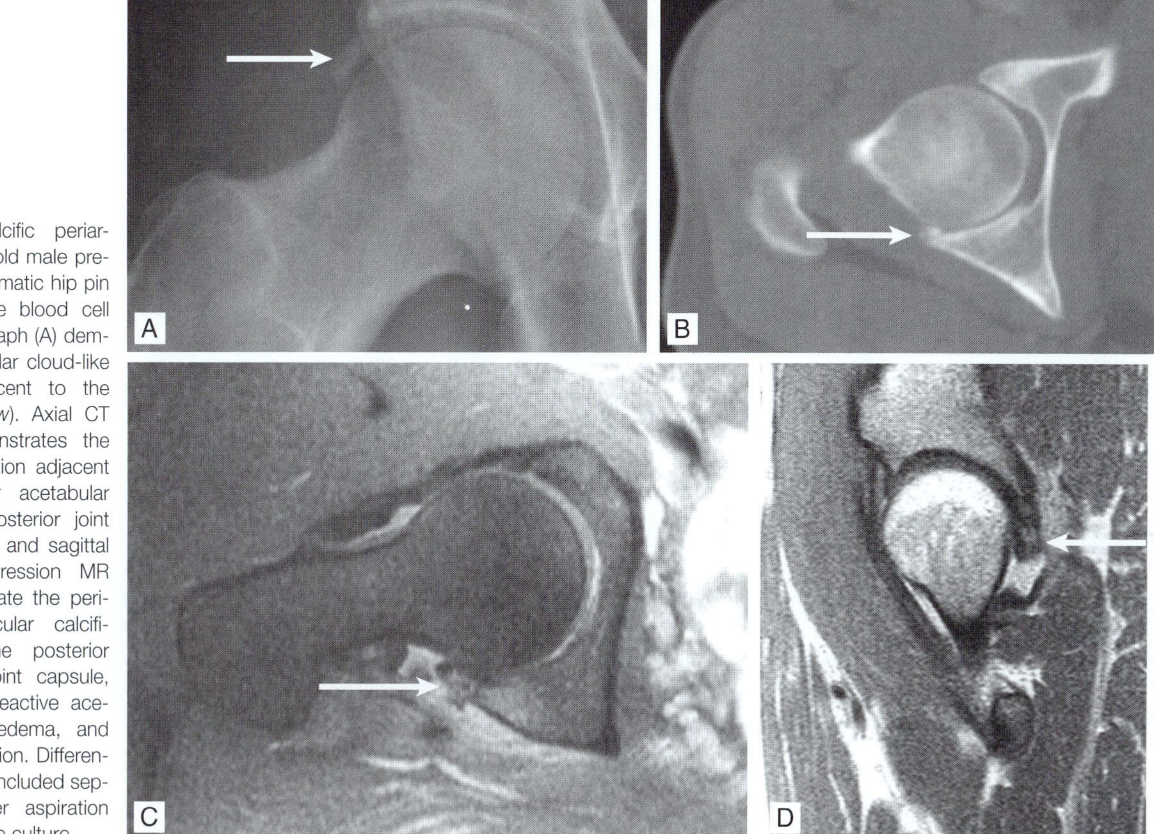

Figure 52.71 Calcific periarthritis. A 35-year-old male presenting with atraumatic hip pin and normal white blood cell count. AP radiograph (A) demonstrates a globular cloud-like calcification adjacent to the acetabulum (*arrow*). Axial CT image (B) demonstrates the focus of calcification adjacent to the posterior acetabular rim along the posterior joint capsule. Axial (C) and sagittal (D) PD fat-suppression MR images demonstrate the pericapsular/intra-articular calcification along the posterior aspect of the joint capsule, with associated reactive acetabular marrow edema, and reactive joint effusion. Differential consideration included septic joint, however aspiration confirmed negative culture.

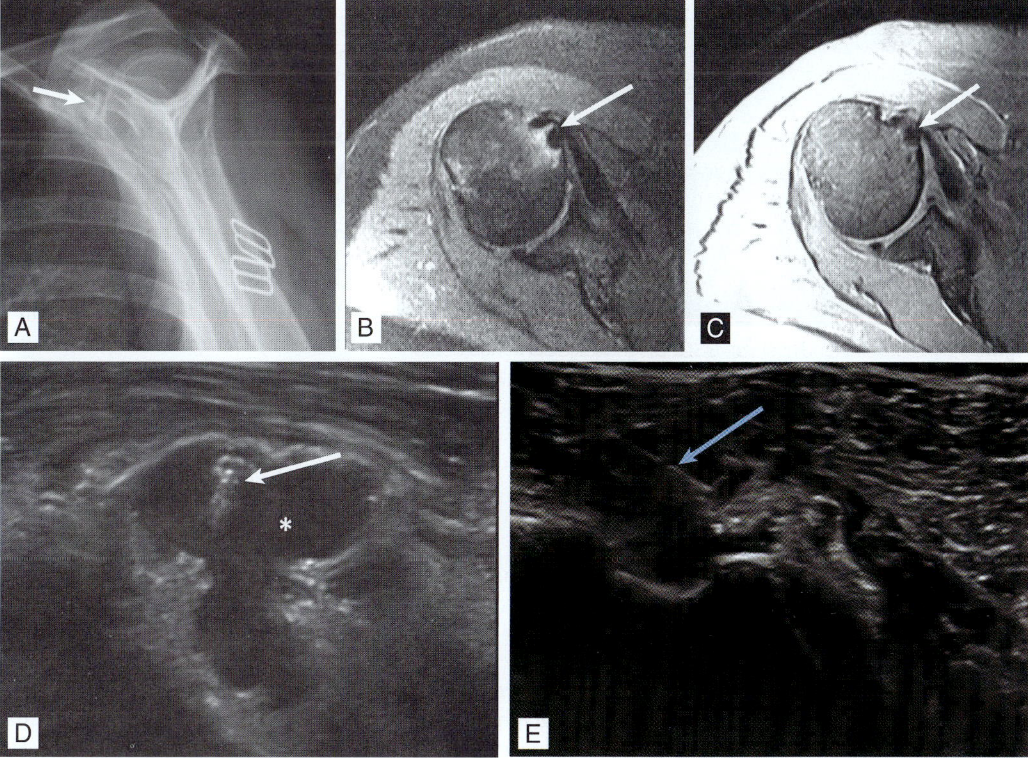

Figure 52.72 Calcific tendinosis with cortical erosion. A 55-year-old male with shoulder pain and limited range of motion. Scapular Y-view of the right shoulder (A) showing focal area of calcification along the course of the subscapularis. Axial PD fat suppression MR image (B) and gradient echo image (C) of the right shoulder in the same patient shows a focus of low signal with blooming artifact within the superior fibers of the subscapularis tendon with subjacent cortical erosion and bone marrow edema (*arrows*), compatible with calcific tendinosis with subcortical erosion rather than chondroid surface lesion. Diagnostic ultrasound (D) shows the corresponding hyperechoic calcification (*arrow*) surrounding by bursal fluid (*). Mechanical barbotage (E) with mechanical disruption (*blue arrow* indicating needle) of the calcification with numerous passes after aspiration and then followed with steroid injection.

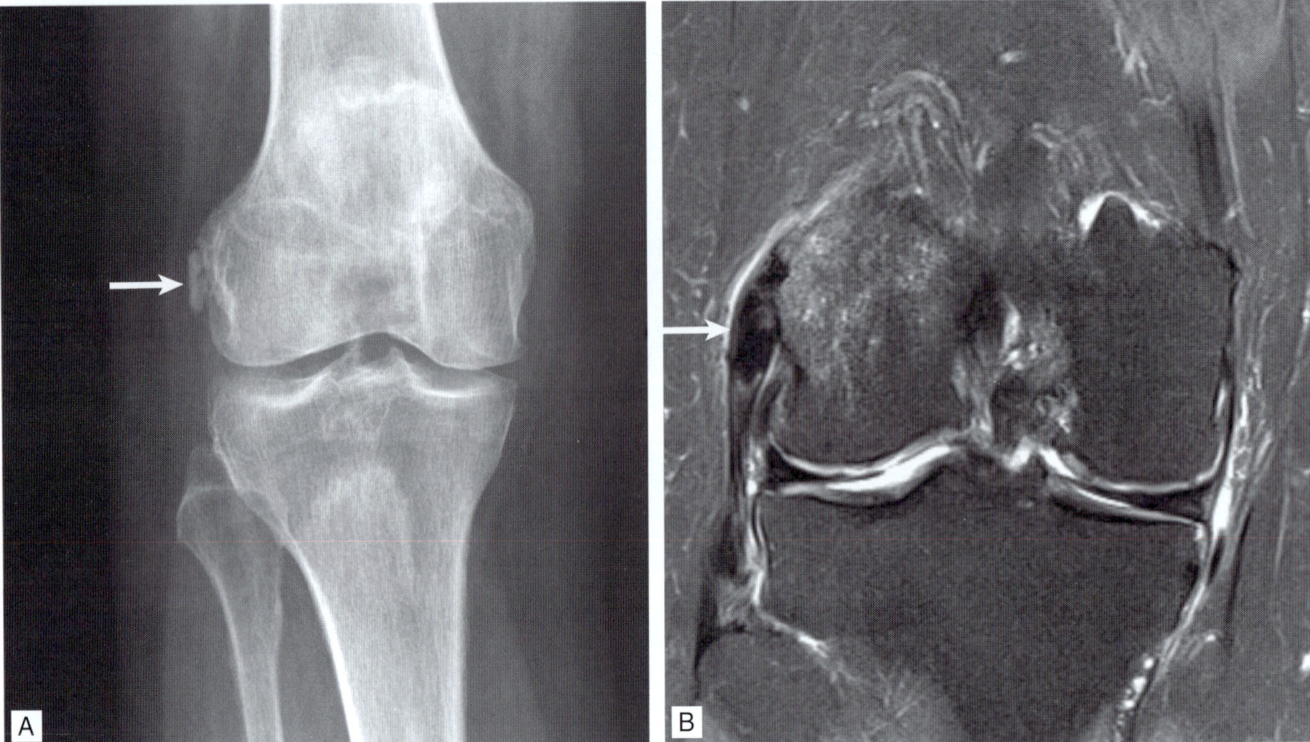

Figure 52.73 Atypical calcific tendinosis. A 55-year-old female with right knee pain and tenderness to palpation over the lateral joint space. Initial radiograph (A) demonstrates globular calcification adjacent to the lateral femoral condyle (*arrow*). Coronal proton density fat-saturated MR image (B) demonstrating marked edema of the lateral femoral condyle with low-signal intensity deposit/mineralization of the proximal lateral collateral ligament (*arrow*) compatible with acute calcific periarthritis.

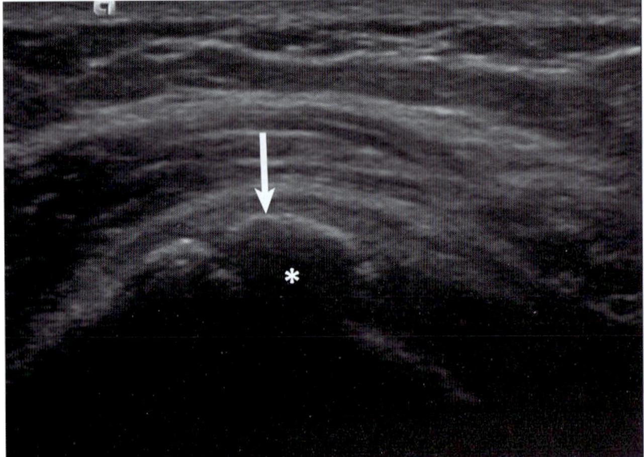

Figure 52.74 Calcific tendinosis on USG. Diagnostic USG image demonstrated hyperechoic calcium deposit with the supraspinatus tendon (*arrow*) with posterior acoustic shadowing (*).

4. Other osseous mimics
   a. *Avulsion fractures*: Usually history of trauma or sports-related injury
   b. *Post-traumatic ossification*: Pellegrini-Stieda and myositis ossificans
   c. Accessory ossicles
   d. Juxtacortical chondromas

Radiographic correlation is essential when encountered with a potential case of HADD. CT is superior to radiographs to depict continuity between the tendinous, cortical, and medullary processes. MRI offers superior resolution to assess the degree of tendon, bursal, and osseous involvement.

Factors that can aid in making the diagnosis of calcific tendinosis/HADD include:

1. Location within or adjacent to tendon or ligament
2. The absence of joint fluid or soft-tissue mass
3. Relatively acute clinical presentation

Metabolic, Hematologic, and Other Miscellaneous Causes of Arthritis

Hemochromatosis

Overview

Primary hemochromatosis is an autosomal recessive disorder caused by a single-site mutation on HFE gene, which allows cellular uptake of iron-based transferrin.

Secondary hemochromatosis has a variety of causes but usually results from hemosiderosis from multiple blood transfusions.

Pathology

Increased GI uptake of iron and cellular uptake manifests as a progressive increase in total body iron stores, ultimately resulting in abnormal iron deposition in multiple organs.

Imaging Findings

The best diagnostic clue on imaging is typically the large hooked osteophytes involving the second and third metacarpal heads/MCP joints with associated joint space narrowing, subchondral sclerosis, and subchondral cyst formation (Fig. 52.76).

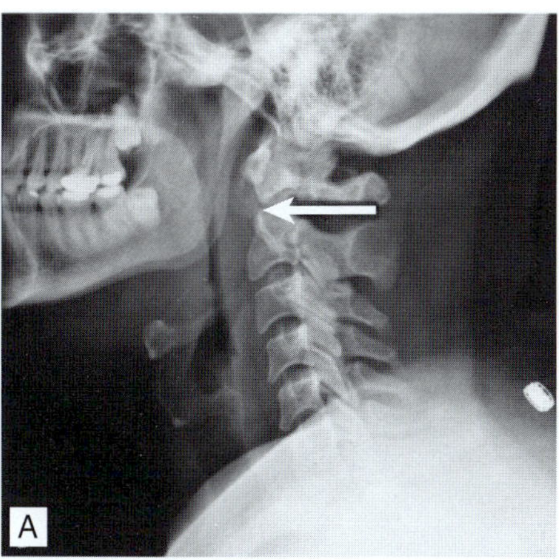
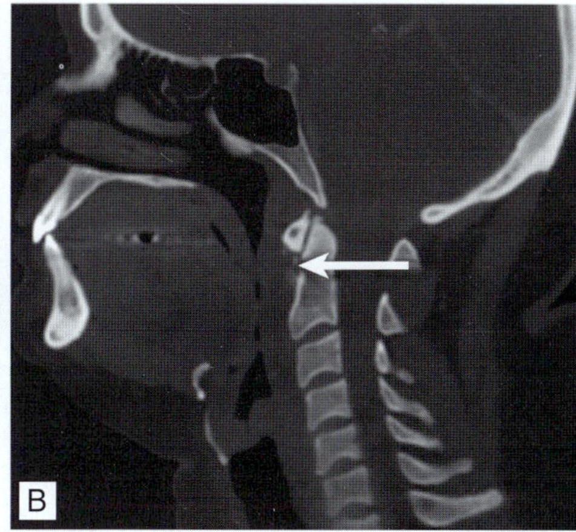
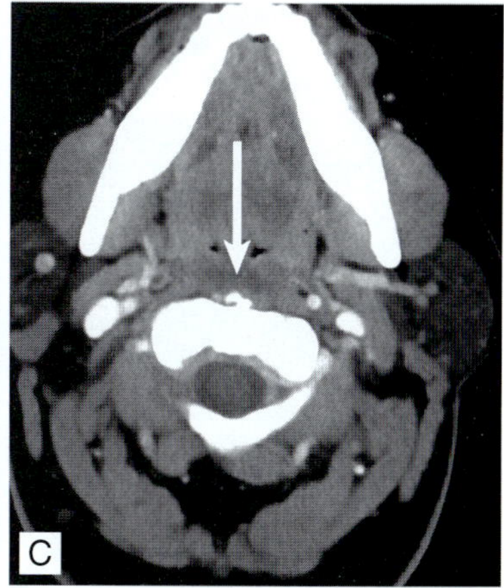

Figure 52.75 Longus colli calcific tendinosis. A 42-year-old female with neck pain and difficulty swallowing. Lateral radiograph (A) and sagittal reformatted CT image (B) of the cervical spine showing amorphous calcification (*arrows*) anterior to the C2 vertebral body. Corresponding postcontrast axial CT image (C) showing reactive fluid anterior to the calcification (*arrow*) without rim enhancement or abnormal adenopathy, the findings of which are compatible with longus colli calcific tendinosis.

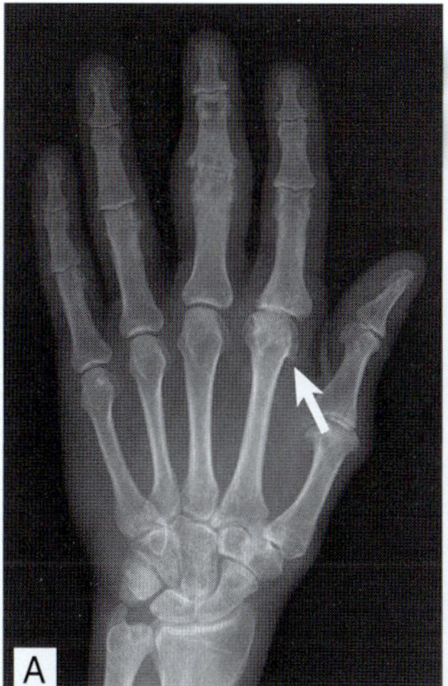
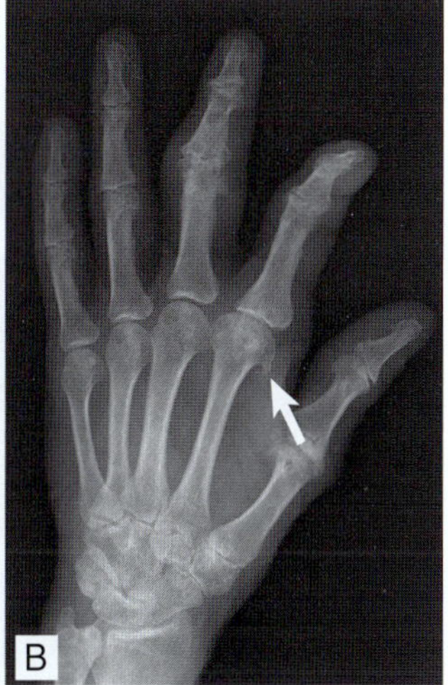

Figure 52.76 *Hemochromatosis.* AP (A) and oblique (B) demonstrate narrowing of the 2nd MCP joint with sclerosis, cystic change, and hooked/beaked-like osteophytes emanating from the 2nd metacarpal head (*arrows*). Additionally, are advanced arthritic changes in the 3rd PIP joint, geode formation with the head of the 3rd distal phalanx, and erosions of the ulna.

Differential Pearls

- Hooked osteophytes in hemochromatosis are typically larger than those present in CPPD
- If an arthritic pattern suggestive of CPPD develops in a young adult (especially a male), hemochromatosis should be considered as a potential cause
- MCP involvement can also be difficult to distinguish from RA; however, hooked osteophytes would not be expected in a patient with RA
- Distal sites in the hands are more commonly seen with OA changes rather than the more proximal distribution of hemochromatosis [38]

Hemodialysis-Associated Amyloid Arthropathy

Overview

Amyloidosis is a multisystem disorder caused by deposition of amyloid fibrillary protein aggregates in patients on long-term hemodialysis (HD) targeting the musculoskeletal system, manifested by erosive peripheral arthropathy, spondyloarthropathy, and carpal tunnel syndrome.

Pathology

HD-related amyloid arthropathy is thought to be due insufficient elimination of $\beta 2$ microglobulin, resulting in amyloid fibril deposition into bone, joints, muscle, tendons, and bursae, thus contributing to arthritis and tendon pathologies. However, the pathogenesis is likely multifactorial, including chronicity of renal failure, as well as the duration of HD.

Distribution

The most commonly affected locations include the shoulders, hips, and wrists, with imaging findings resembling that of inflammatory arthropathies, while spinal involvement may masquerade as discitis-osteomyelitis.

Imaging Findings

Erosive and destructive peripheral arthropathy.

Radiographic Appearance

- Juxta-articular erosions and subchondral cysts/geodes of variable sizes, usually demonstrating well-defined sclerotic margins at the sites of tendon and ligament attachments
- Eventually can lead to a destructive arthropathy with subluxations and joint contractures
- Most commonly seen around the hips, shoulders, and carpal bones

USG Appearance

- Amyloid deposits appear as intra-articular, intrabursal, periarticular lobulated echogenic masses with associated joint effusions, synovitis, and bursitis (Fig. 52.77)
- Tenosynovial amyloid deposition with the flexor and extensor tendons of the wrist

MRI Appearance

- Amyloid deposition can be identified along intra-articular, bursal, and tendon synovial surfaces, eroding and communicating with osseous cysts, and extension into periarticular soft tissues

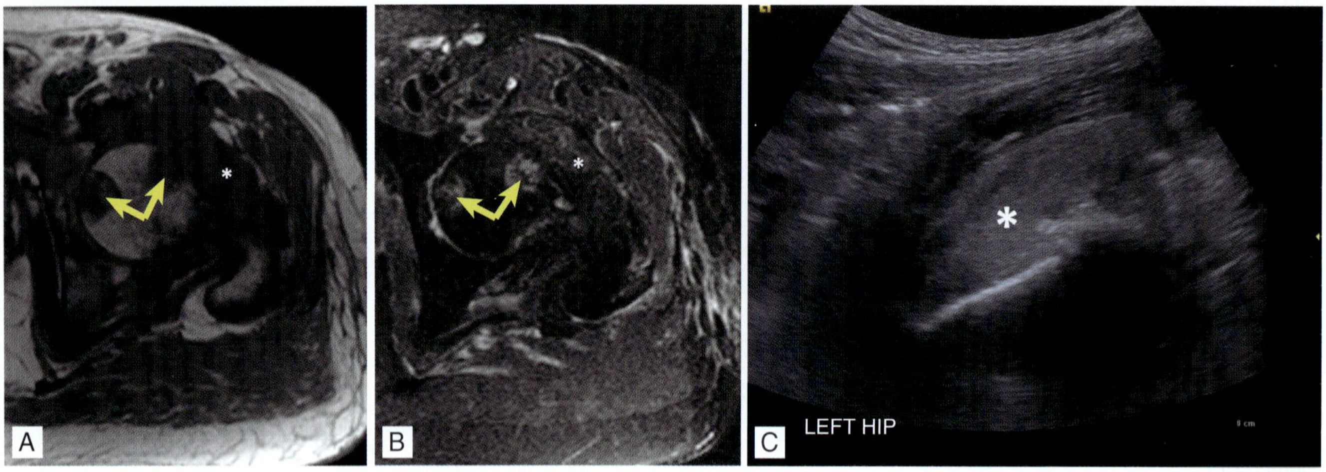

Figure 52.77 HD-related amyloidosis in a patient with ESRD on long-term HD. Axial T1 (A) and T2 (B) fat-suppressed images extensive lobulated intra-articular synovial mass throughout the left hip joint (*white* *), demonstrating hypointense T1 and predominantly low-to-intermediate signal on T2-weighted sequences, the imaging characteristics of which are suggestive of intra-articular amyloid deposition/dialysis-related amyloidosis. There is an osseous erosion along the fovea capitis and anteromedial aspect (*yellow arrows*) of the femoral head–neck junction, with amyloid deposition infiltrating in continuity within the osseous erosions, demonstrating associated perierosional edema adjacent to the femoral neck erosion. Corresponding USG (C) in the same patient demonstrates with intra-articular mass (*) as lobulated and echogenic.

- Intra-articular amyloid deposition appears as an abnormal intra-articular lobulated mass with capsular distension and joint effusion, demonstrating a hypointense signal on T1-weighted images, with variable but usually hypointense-to-intermediate signal on T2-weighted sequences (Fig. 52.77)
- Erosions, cysts, and intraosseous lesions demonstrate amyloid deposits that are in continuity with intra-articular deposits, exhibiting signal characteristics of low-signal intensity on all pulse sequences
  - No paramagnetic effect on gradient echo imaging (no blooming)
- MRI findings usually demonstrate periarticular tendon thickening with low-signal intensity infiltration of the tendons, particularly at the shoulder and flexor tendons of the wrist
  - Infiltration of the carpal tunnel is commonly associated with carpal tunnel syndrome

Spondyloarthropathy: Amyloid deposits have been identified as soft-tissue masses within the intervertebral discs or within the facet joints, as well as the ligamentum flavum, atlanto-occipital, and atlantoaxial joints of the cervical spine [39].

Subchondral endplate erosions with intervertebral disc space narrowing and lack of prominent osteophytes can mimic discitis-osteomyelitis; however, the process will usually be identified at multiple disc levels. Subchondral edema along the endplates with persistent intradiscal low signal suggest HD-related process, rather than infection. Biopsy may still be required in ambiguous clinical scenarios. Amyloid deposits and erosions can be identified in expected locations, usually demonstrating the amyloid tissue to be low signal on all sequences. Amyloid-induced atlantoaxial synovial hypertrophy can produce a soft tissue, partially calcified mass encasing and eroding the dens (Fig. 52.78), that may indistinguishable from rheumatoid arthritis pannus formation or crowned-dens findings in CPPD. However, calcifications in RA pannus formation are absent.

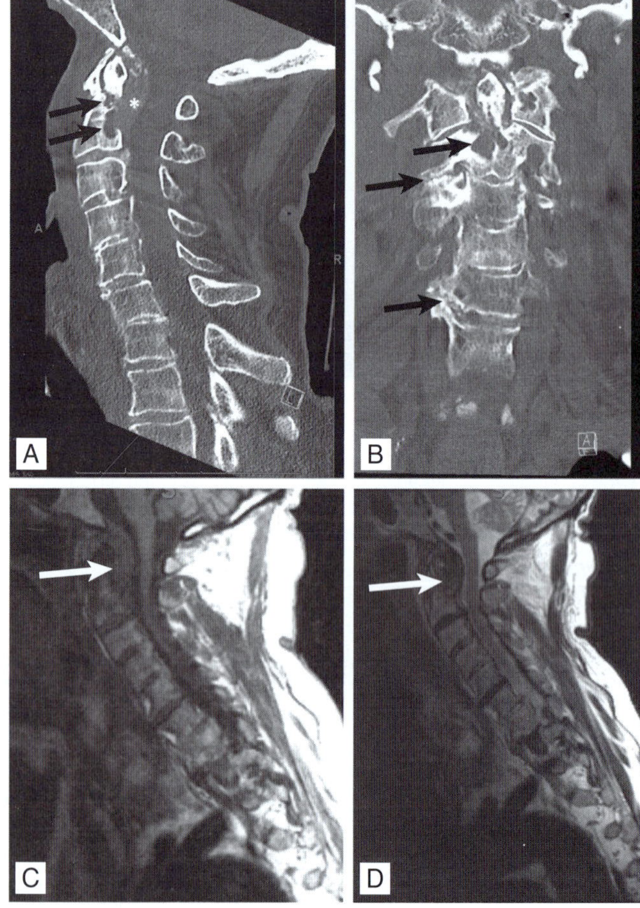

Figure 52.78 *HD-related spondyloarthropathy.* Amyloid and crystal deposition in patient with ESRD on long-term HD. Sagittal (A) and coronal (B) CT images demonstrate a partially calcified soft-tissue mass encasing the odontoid and displacing the spinal cord (*white* *), with well-defined punched out erosions involving the C1–C2 articulation, base of the odontoid, and facet joints (*black arrows*). Sagittal T1 (C) and T2 (D) MR images demonstrate the C1–C2 mass to be of low T1 and T2 signal (*white arrows*).

Differential Pearls

1. Differential considerations for this condition on an imaging basis should include multiple myeloma, metastatic disease, gouty erosions, brown tumors, hemophilic arthropathy, or pigmented villonodular synovitis (PVNS)
   - Biopsy may be required for definitive diagnosis

2. Imaging finding in combination with clinical history can help rendering an accurate diagnosis of HD-related arthropathy
   - Be aware of HD-related complications including pathological factures and *compressive myelopathy*
3. Tendon and joint capsule thickening in the setting of low-signal intensity erosions in a patient on long-term HD may also suggest *amyloidosis*

Ochronosis (Alkaptonuria)

Overview

Alkaptonuria is a genetic autosomal recessive metabolic disorder that results in pathologic blue–black pigmentation of connective tissues in patients due to an underlying enzymatic deficiency of homogentisic acid oxidase [41]. Musculoskeletal manifestations of alkaptonuria may be referred to as ochronosis due the yellow (ocher) histological appearance of connective tissues.

Pathology

The absence of homogentisic acid oxidase enzyme leads excessive homogentisic acid, which binds to collagen in connective tissues, leading to inflammation, degeneration, and progressive arthropathy.

Imaging Findings

Spine

- The most common imaging manifestation is multilevel thoracic and lumbar discogenic calcification, disc space narrowing with endplate sclerosis, bridging osteophytes, and osteoporosis [40] (Fig. 52.79A)
- SI joints and pubic symphysis are also commonly affected
- The differential diagnosis for discogenic calcifications included
  - OA, CPPD, AS, ochronosis, hemochromatosis, hyperparathyroidism, and amyloidosis

Peripheral Joints

- Large joints may also be involved with demonstration of cartilage space narrowing, subchondral sclerosis, and possible intra-articular osteochondral fragments
- Knee is the most commonly involved peripheral joint, followed by hip and shoulder

Differential Pearls

Lack of osteophyte formation as well as advanced degenerative changes in a younger patient can help differentiate from OA; however, in some cases still may indistinguishable from OA.

Multicentric Reticulohistiocytosis (Also Known as Lipoid Dermatoarthritis)

Overview

This rare condition results from infiltration of lipid-laden histiocytes into various tissues including skin, bone, cartilage, and synovium.

Pathology

Abnormal accumulation results in soft-tissue nodules, acro-osteolysis, and chronic destructive polyarthritis.

Imaging Findings

- Symmetric well-defined marginal erosions involving the DIP joints of the hand are typically seen (Fig. 52.79B) [42]
- MCP joints and carpal bones, as well as larger peripheral joints are also affected, but less frequent than the DIP joints
- Noncalcified soft-tissue nodules

Differential Pearls

- DIP distribution less likely to be seen with *RA*
- Erosions encountered in *gout* and *PsA* are usually asymmetric
- Erosions with overhanging edges and calcified soft-tissue nodules (tophi) are seen with *gout*

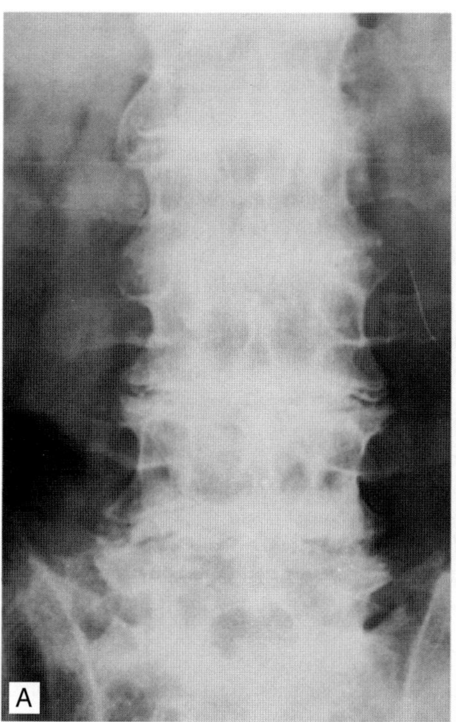

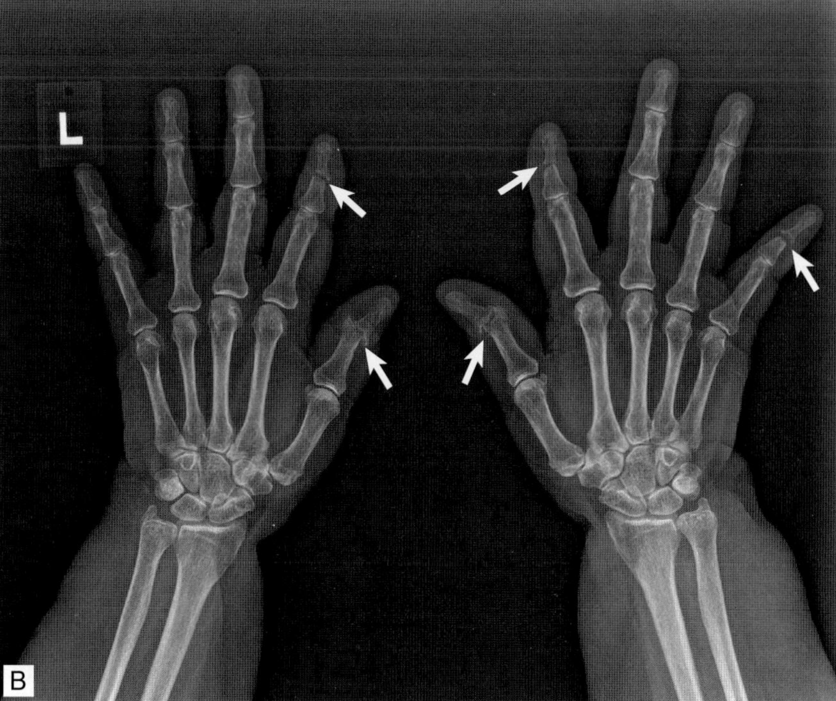

Figure 52.79 (A) Ochronosis. The intervertebral disc spaces are narrowed and calcified. (B) Multicentric reticulohistiocytosis. Erosive changes with radial subluxation of the 1st distal phalanges, erosive changes at the 2nd DIP joints bilaterally, and the right 5th DIP joint (*arrows*).

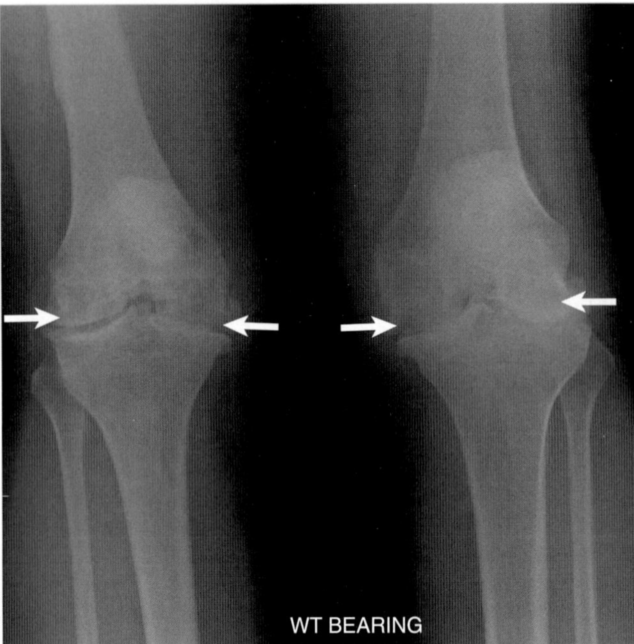

Figure 52.80 Hemophilia arthropathy. A 20-year-old male patient with AP radiographs of the knees demonstrate epiphyseal overgrowth, squaring/flattening of the condyles (*arrows*), widening of the intercondylar notch, and advanced secondary osteoarthritic changes.

Hemophilic Arthropathy

Overview

Hemophilic arthropathy is a destructive arthropathy triggered by acute on chronic hemarthrosis and chronic synovitis that can lead to chronic pain, limited range of motion, and decreased quality of life. Approximately 50–80% of patients the hemophilia will develop a severe arthropathy.

Pathology

Hemophilia A (the absence of clotting factor VIII) and hemophilia B (the absence of clotting factor IX) are both X-linked recessive bleeding disorders with intra-articular spontaneous bleeding and recurrent hemarthroses contributing to synovitis, chronic inflammation, and fibrosis, leading to chondral degeneration and subchondral bone destruction. Abnormal bleeding and clotting within joint spaces preferentially affects large joints including the knee, elbow, ankle, and hip.

Imaging Findings

Radiographic Appearance

- Large effusions are often noted, typically with increased density due to a predominantly hemorrhagic component and/or hemosiderin deposits within the synovium in the case of chronic bleeding
- Knee
  - Epiphyseal overgrowth (ballooning) due to hyperemia, flat condylar surfaces, and widening of the intercondylar notch (Fig. 52.80) [43]
- Elbow
  - Enlarged radial head and widening of the trochlea notch
- Secondary osteoarthritic changes as evidenced by symmetrical joint space loss, erosions, subchondral sclerosis, cysts, and osteophytes
- Typical gracile appearance of long bone diaphyses

MRI

- Shown to demonstrate heterogeneous signal intensity within joint effusions and/or fluid–fluid levels due to blood products, as well low-signal intensity and susceptibility artifact lining the synovium due to hemosiderin deposition

Differential Pearls

- Radiographic features may be indistinguishable from *juvenile idiopathic arthritis*; however, hemosiderin deposits can be demonstrated MR imaging
- *Pigmented villonodular synovitis* and *hemophilia* will both exhibit persistently hypointense signal of the synovium on all sequences and blooming on gradient echo images; however, *PVNS* tends to manifest as a more focal nodular pattern, rather than a diffuse intra-articular process, and the radiographic findings encountered with *hemophilia* will be absent in a patient with *PVNS*

Sarcoidosis

Overview

Sarcoidosis is a systemic chronic granulomatous disease characterized by noncaseating granulomas in multiple organs, including the heart and lungs, abdominal organs, central nervous system, and the musculoskeletal system including bone, joints, and soft tissues. Joint involvement is a commonly encountered clinical presentation, classified as either acute arthritis or chronic/recurrent arthritis. Acute sarcoidosis, known as Lofgren syndrome, is a syndrome characterized by erythema nodosum, hilar adenopathy, constitutional symptoms, and polyarthritis involving the ankles, wrist, PIP and MCP joint, and the elbows.

Pathology

Sarcoidosis is an immune-mediated disease resulting from an antigenic stimulation that triggers inflammatory response. An inflammatory response is caused by CD4(+) T cells that interact with antigen-presenting cells to initiate formation and maintenance of granulomas. The synovial granuloma formation incites an intra-articular inflammatory response, synovitis, and osseous erosions.

Distribution

Musculoskeletal sarcoidosis with osseous involvement is found in approximately 5% of patients with sarcoid. Although sarcoid can involve any site of the axial or appendicular skeleton, the most commonly encountered sites are the distal and middle phalanges of the second and third digits. Long bone and vertebral body involvement are less common, but must be differentiated from a metastatic or bone marrow hematological process.

Imaging Findings

Radiographic Findings

- Lacy trabecular configuration considered pathognomonic (Fig. 52.81) [44]
- Characteristically no periosteal reaction
- Granulomas extend into the soft tissues, causing diffuse swelling (sausage dactylitis)

Differential Pearls

The abnormal lace-like trabecular pattern of phalangeal osteolysis and destruction is considered pathognomonic. If acro-osteolysis is observed, scleroderma may be considered in the differential, but patients with scleroderma will exhibit soft-tissue calcifications.

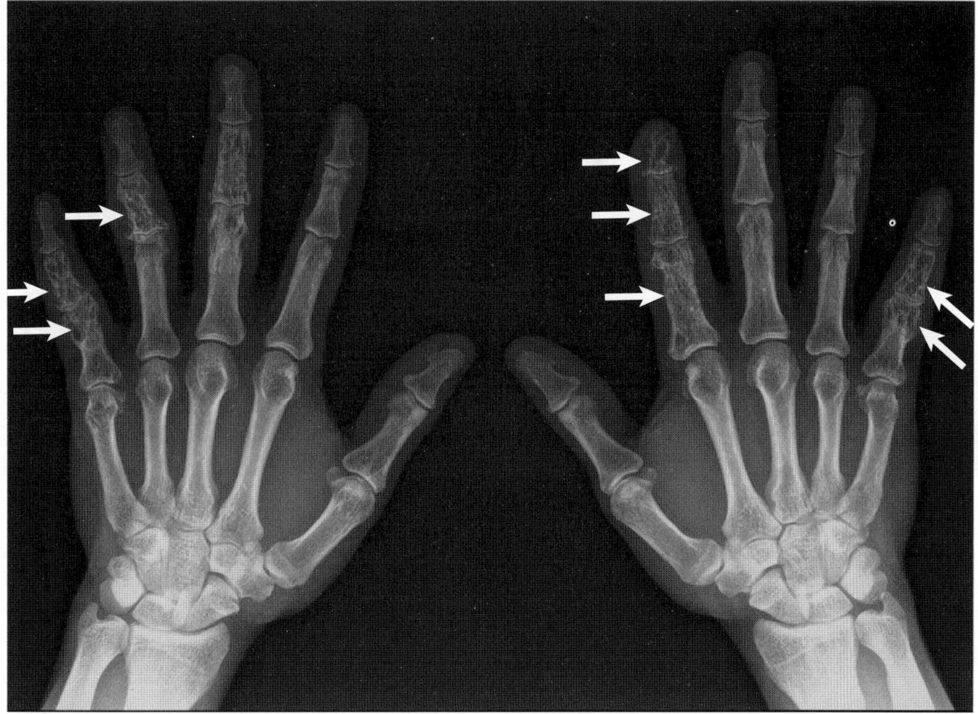

Figure 52.81 Musculoskeletal sarcoidosis. Radiographs demonstrate phalangeal expansion, trabecular thickening, and lucencies resulting in a lace-like pattern of osseous destruction (*arrows*).

Pigmented Villonodular Synovitis

Overview

PVNS is considered a benign neoplastic process of synovial hyperplasia, which can be villous, nodular, or villonodular demonstrating synovial hemosiderin deposition [45]. Given the synovial etiology, not only can PVNS involve intra-articular synovial lining, but can also be extra-articular, seen along tendon sheaths and bursae.

Pathology

The etiology of PVNS is of neoplastic synovial proliferation. Repeated hemorrhagic effusions and intra-articular inflammation result in synovial iron deposition in synovium and nodules. With continued proliferation of abnormal synovium, focal erosions and subchondral cysts develop.

Distribution

PVNS presents as a monoarticular arthropathy, most commonly involves the knee joint (80% of cases), either the localized intra-articular nodular variant or the diffuse intra-articular form, followed by the hip joint. Ankle, shoulder, and elbow are also sites of potential PVNS, as is virtually any synovial joint. When encountered along a tendon sheath, the lesion is referred to as tenosynovial giant cell tumor and pigmented villonodular bursitis when identified within a bursa.

Imaging Findings

Radiographic Appearance

- Joint effusion, soft-tissue swelling, extrinsic erosions, subchondral cysts, and preserved joint space
- The absence of calcification [45]

MRI Appearance

- Focal nodular mass or diffuse villonodular proliferation (Fig. 52.82)
- Lesion predominantly demonstrates low-to-intermediate signal on T1- and T2-weighted images (Fig. 52.82). Increased signal on T2-weighted images is likely due to intralesional joint fluid or regional synovitis (Fig. 52.82)
- The associated hemosiderin-laden nodules produce characteristic blooming artifact on gradient MRI sequences
- The typical MRI appearance consists of a large joint effusion with synovial-based masses exhibiting blooming effect on gradient echo sequences
- Postcontrast images demonstrate, variable inhomogeneous enhancement

Differential Pearls

Differential consideration of intra-articular soft-tissue masses:

1. Intra-articular nodular synovitis
   a. Similar MR appearance to PVNS, but generally less hemosiderin deposition and smaller joint effusions
2. Gout
   a. Can appear similar to PVNS with extrinsic erosions; however, calcified gouty tophus on radiographs should exclude PVNS
3. Amyloid
   a. Can appear similar to PVNS, but blooming artifact not identified
4. Hemophilic arthropathy
   a. Diffuse hypointense synovial proliferation on T1- and T2-weighted sequences, as well as blooming artifact can be indistinguishable from diffuse intra-articular PVNS; however radiographic appearance and clinical history help to decipher the two conditions
5. Synovial chondromatosis
   a. Low-signal masses can be confused with PVNS, but if calcified on radiographic evaluation, excludes PVNS
   b. Chondral bodies will not exhibit blooming on gradient echo images

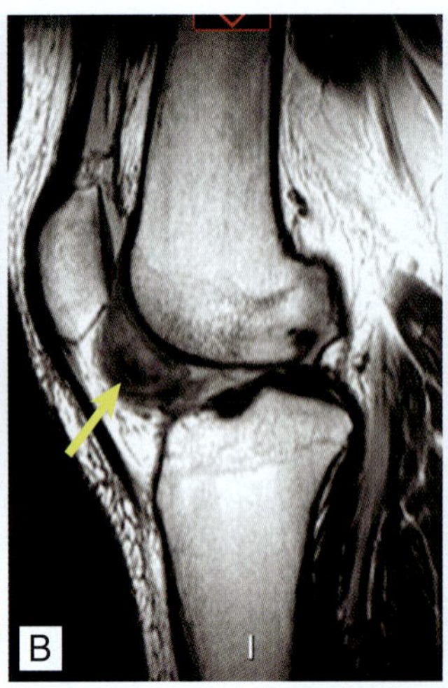

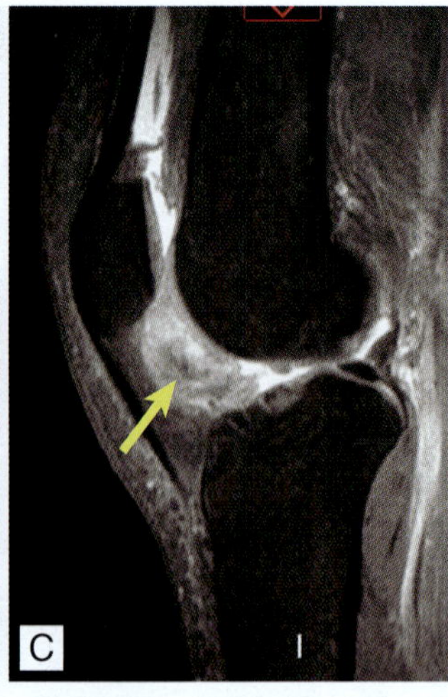

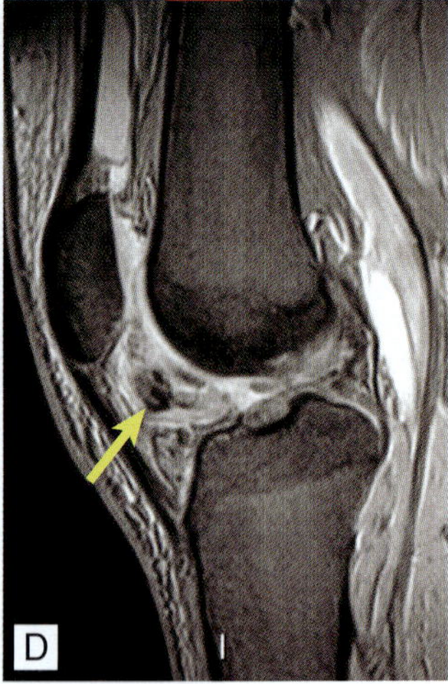

Figure 52.82 Localized intra-articular PVNS of the knee. Lateral radiograph (A) shows a noncalcified soft-tissue density within Hoffa fat pad (*white arrow*). Sagittal PD (B) and T2-weighted fat-suppressed sequences (C) reveal a focal nodular soft-tissue mass within Hoffa's fat pad (*yellow arrows*) demonstrating hypointense-to-intermediate signal on the PD image and heterogeneous increased signal and perilesional synovitis on the T2-weighted image, while the sagittal gradient echo image (D) clearly exhibits hypointense signal compatible with blooming artifact of hemosiderin.

Synovial Chondromatosis

Overview

Synovial chondromatosis is a benign neoplasm that causes synovial membrane proliferation and the formation of cartilaginous or osseous bodies within a joint, bursa, or tenosynovial structure. It is classified into two subtypes: *primary* is usually monoarticular and is of unknown etiology, whereas *secondary* is usually a result of degeneration, trauma, or neuropathic arthropathy.

Pathology

Genetic features suggest synovial chondromatosis is of benign neoplastic etiology.

Synovial membranes over proliferate creating nodular densities (which range from millimeters to greater than 2 cm) which may remain attached to synovium and develop blood supply and may become osseous, or become loose within a joint and become cartilaginous. In the ladder, the cartilage is provided nutrients through the synovial fluid. The underlying articular cartilage destruction is most likely mechanical in origin; not inflammatory.

Distribution

The distribution is commonly monoarticular and predominantly intra-articular, particularly in large joints. From most to least commonly involved joints: knee (50–65%) > hip > shoulder > elbow. The most common bursal locations are subdeltoid and popliteal. Tenosynovial chondromatosis most commonly involves the hands and feet.

Extracapsular spread is a potential risk through the usual sites of joint decompression; across rotator cuff tear into subacromial/subdeltoid bursa, from hip into iliopsoas bursa, and rare extension into adjacent muscle and fascial tissue. The round bodies of synovial chondromatosis are generally similar in size and may appear lamellated, with concentric rings of calcification. Occasionally will form conglomerate mass within joint or extend into extracapsular tissue.

Imaging Findings

Radiographic Findings

- Multiple round bodies (Fig. 52.83) of similar size which may range from small foci of speckled calcifications to large round, lamellated cartilage or ossified bodies
- These may conglomerate or be free floating [46]
- May or may not have associated osseous erosions, which are likely mechanical/degenerative in etiology
- May be difficult to visualize on radiograph (20–50%)

MRI Findings

- Eighty percent of patients have degenerative erosions detectable by MR
- Large effusion (hyperintense on fluid-sensitive sequences, low signal on T1)
- Bodies are of variable MR signal, depending on proportion of calcium, chondroid, and mature ossific tissue
  - The majority (77%) have low-to-intermediate T1 signal, with hyperintense T2 signal intensity (Fig. 52.83)
- T1WI FS with contrast shows enhancing hyperplastic synovium, surrounding low-signal effusion and bodies
- Malignant transformation to chondrosarcoma is unusual (5% of cases) and, although difficult to distinguish from benign disease, is suggested by multiple recurrences and marrow invasion [47]

Lipoma Arborescens

Overview

Lipoma arborescens involves infiltration of fat tissue in synovium forming frond-like masses.

Pathology

Chronic synovial irritation leads to inappropriate proliferation of fat. Can be seen from both degenerative and inflammatory arthropathies, as well as with previous trauma. Mature adipocytes proliferate within subsynovium generating enlarged synovial fronds [47, 48]. Additionally, may see osseous or chondroid metaplasia in some cases.

Imaging

Radiographic Findings

- Limited
- Joint distension ± visible fat density

CT Findings

- Fat density synovial masses

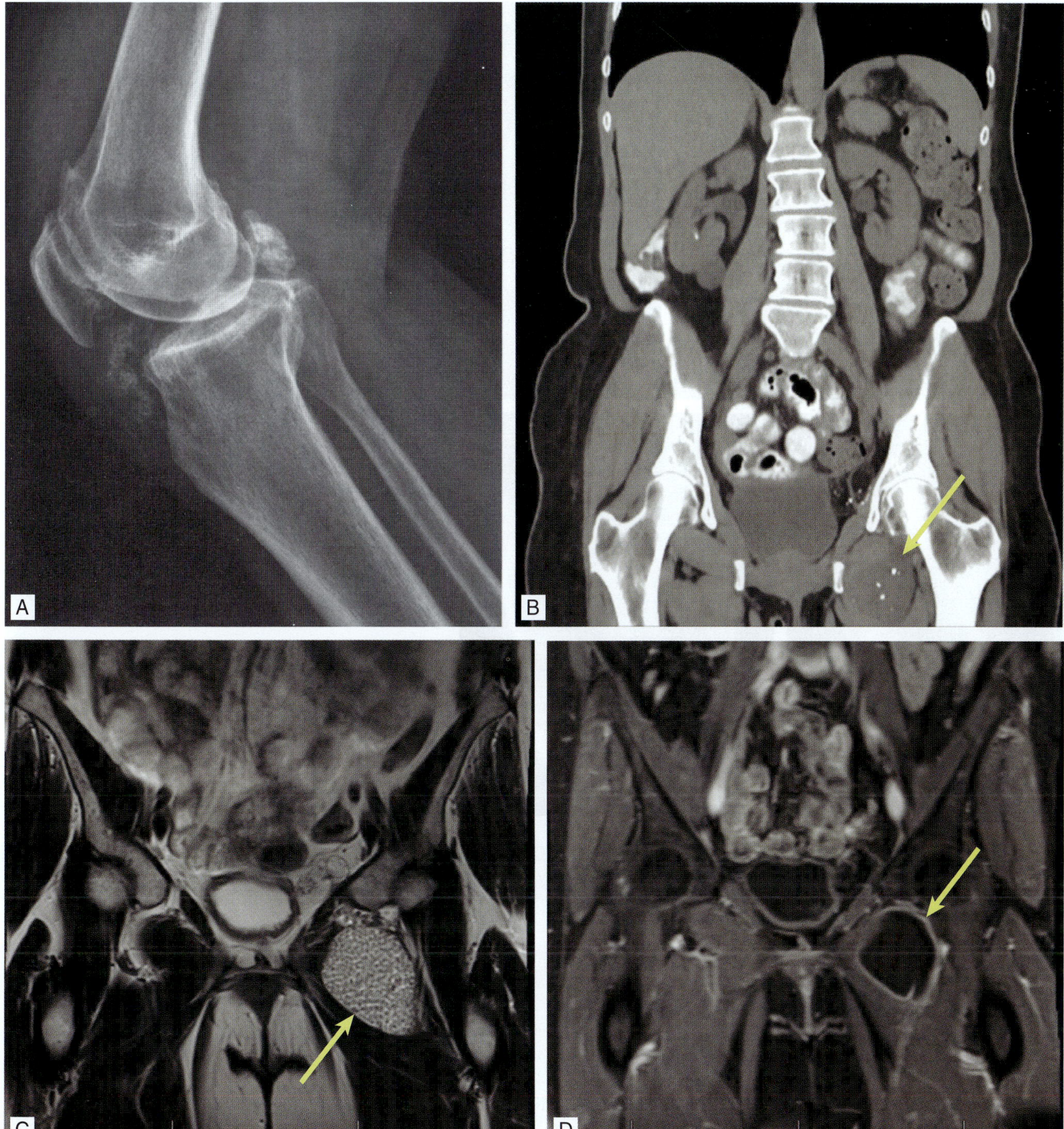

Figure 52.83 Synovial chondromatosis. Lateral radiograph of knee (A) shows multiple round bodies in anterior and posterior joint space. Coronal CT image (B) of a different patient shows an enlarged obturator bursa with multiple calcified intrabursal bodies. Corresponding coronal T2 (C) demonstrates high-signal fluid distending the bursa, outlining innumerable foci of uniform shape and size low signal within the bursa corresponding to the areas of mineralization. The coronal T1 postcontrast image (D) demonstrates peripheral enhancement of the bursa without any internal enhancement.

MR Findings

- High-signal intensity synovial masses on T1 that match intensity of subcutaneous fat. These enhance on T1 contrast-enhanced images (Fig. 52.84)
- Low-signal intensity on STIR/any fat-suppressed sequence

Hypertrophic Osteoarthropathy

Overview/Pathology

Syndrome characterized by proliferation of skin (1°) and bone (1° and 2°) in distal extremities of an indeterminate cause.

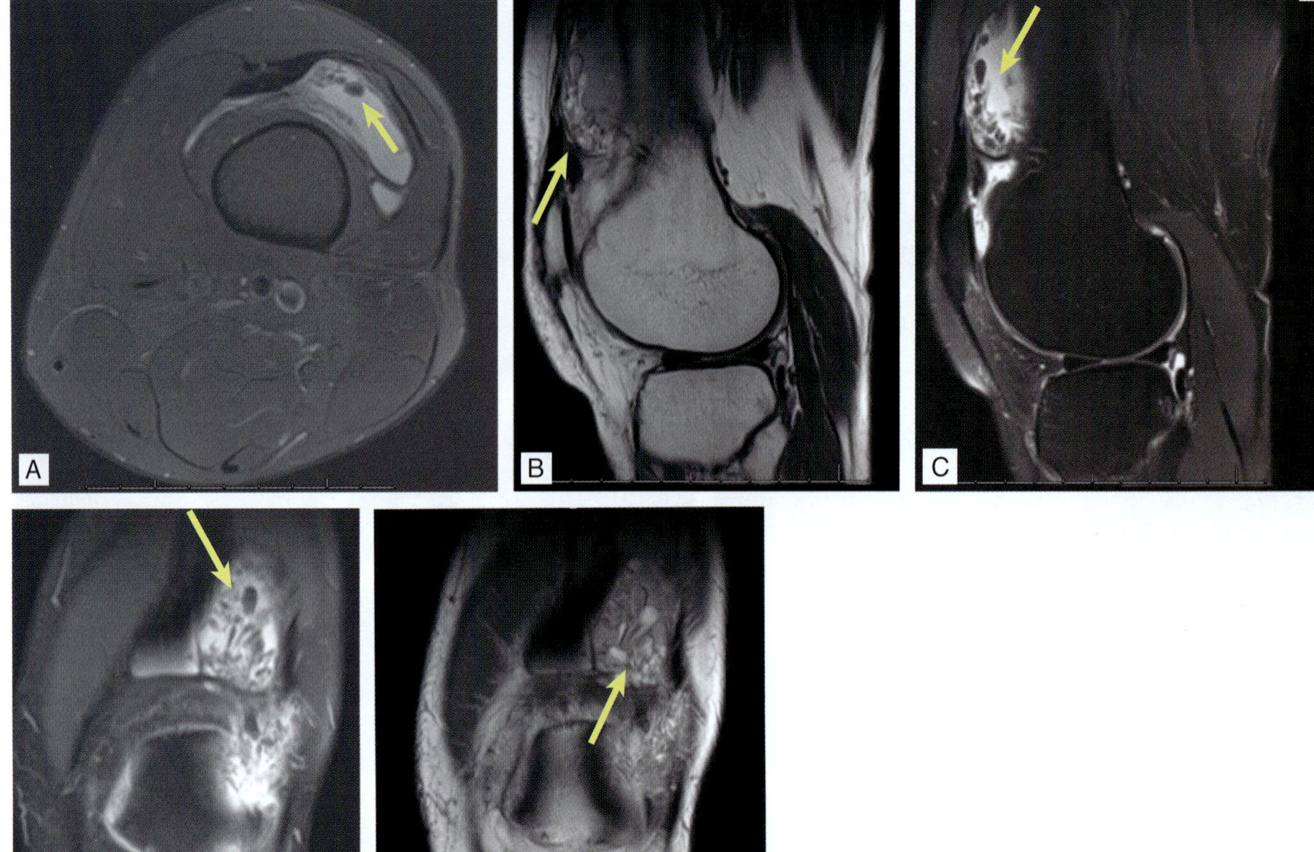

Figure 52.84 *Lipoma arborescens.* Axial T2FS (A) shows a low intensity frond-like structures (*yellow arrow*) in the suprapatellar recess outlined by joint fluid. Sagittal T1 (B) and T2FS (C) confirm the signal to be equivalent to adipose fat.

Genetic inheritance is classified as primary HOA. *Pachydermoperiostosis* is a rare disorder with autosomal recessive inheritance, which involves primary HOA, thickening of the skin of the face (pachyderma), excessive sweating (hyperhidrosis), and rheumatological symptoms (joint effusion, arthritis, acro-osteolysis, periosteal ossification). The secondary HOA has multiple mechanisms that can be broken down by organ system as follows:

- *Pulmonary*: Cancer (including primary pleural), fibrosis, or infection
- *Cardiac*: Cyanotic congenital heart disease, PDA, endocarditis
- *Gastrointestinal*: Cancer, IBD, cirrhosis
- *Systemic*: Lymphoma, POEMS

Imaging

Radiographs

- Periosteal reaction without underlying osseous lesion or injury
  - Commonly symmetric [49] (Fig. 52.85)
  - Thickness/extent dependent on disease duration
    - Shorter duration of disease → diaphyseal; later extends to metaphyses and epiphyses [50]
- Acro-osteolysis more commonly seen in patients with primary HOA and cyanotic heart disease
- Joints
  - Findings limited to soft-tissue swelling → clubbing of digits
  - No joint space narrowing or osseous erosions

MR Findings

- Normal marrow signal
- T1 hypointense periosteal reaction
- Fluid-sensitive sequences show linear high signal that may be seen on either side of low-signal periosteal reaction

Diffuse Idiopathic Skeletal Hyperostosis

Overview/Pathology

Disease entity defines by flowing/uninterrupted coarse osteophytes bridging four adjacent vertebral bodies without severe loss of intervertebral disc height and without degeneration of apophyseal and sacroiliac (SI) joints. The cause for this exaggerated response is unknown, although has possible associations with diabetes mellitus, dyslipidemia, hyperuricemia, alcohol intake, and poor dietary habits. This is a disease of middle-aged to older adults and is very uncommon before age 50.

Imaging

Radiography

- Uninterrupted anterior vertebral ossification (Fig. 52.86)
  - New bone formation begins adjacent to midvertebral body [51]
- Preservation of disc spaces and facets (relative) [52]

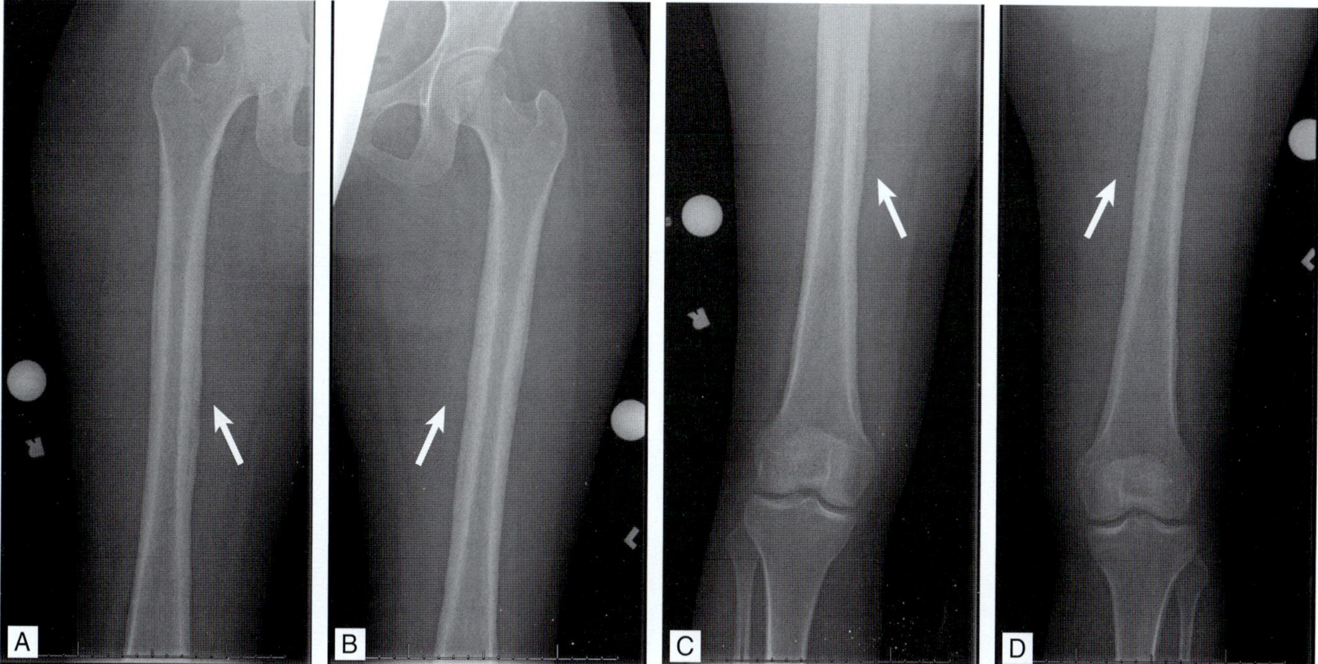

Figure 52.85 Hypertrophic osteoarthropathy. AP radiographs of the bilateral hips (A and B) and bilateral femurs (C and D) demonstrate smooth, benign-appearing thick periosteal reaction along both femoral diaphyses, which is bilaterally symmetric and consistent with hypertrophic pulmonary osteoarthropathy (HPOA). Specifically, this reflects HPOA in this patient with reported history of chronic pulmonary hypertension/interstitial lung disease.

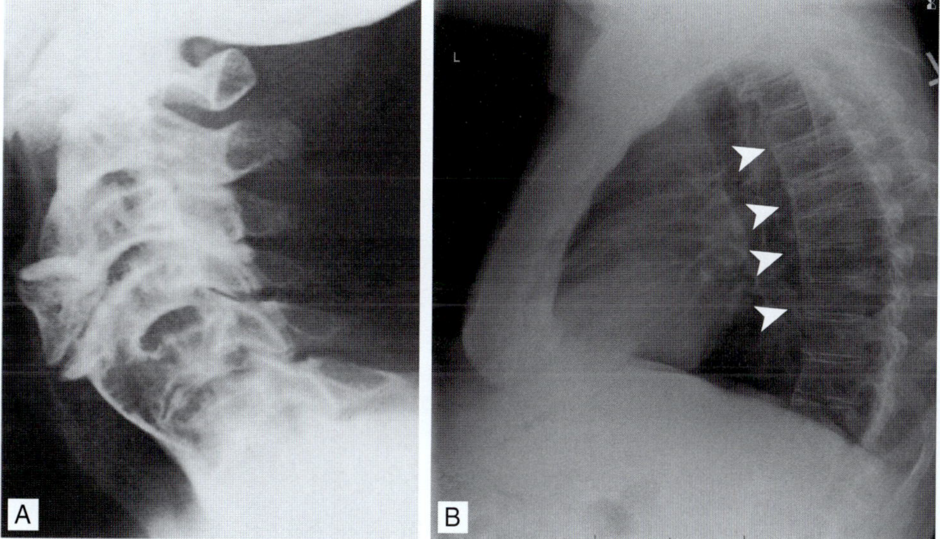

Figure 52.86 Diffuse idiopathic skeletal hyperostosis. Lateral radiographs of cervical (A) and dorsal (B) spine of two different patients show diffuse, flowing ossification of the anterior longitudinal ligaments compatible with diffuse idiopathic skeletal hyperostosis.

MR Findings

- T1WI will show flowing ossification of the anterior longitudinal ligament that may be difficult to distinguish from the anterior vertebral body
  - Hypointense if predominantly calcified
  - Isointense or hyperintense if marrow fat present
  - May show minimal enhancement (similar to vertebral marrow) on contrast-enhanced images
- T2WI
  - Anterior longitudinal ligament ossification may be hypointense unless substantial fatty marrow content

Summary

Differentiating inflammatory from degenerative causes of joint disease significantly impacts patient management (Fig. 52.87). Assessing for symmetric (inflammatory vs infectious) versus asymmetric (degenerative) joint space narrowing and identifying the distribution of joints involved are the first steps in leading a radiologist down the correct diagnostic pathway. Additionally, examining for periarticular or marginal erosions is essential to correctly distinguishing an inflammatory arthropathy from OA. Successfully implementing the systematic

Arthropathy	Appendicular Distribution	Axial Distribution	Radiographic Pearls	Differential Diagnosis and Pitfalls
OA	DIP, 1st IP, 2nd-5th PIP, 1st CMC, and scapho-trapezio-trapezoid (triscaphe) joint.	Intervertebral disc space narrowing, subchondral endplate sclerosis, horizontal osteophyte formation, and facet degenerative changes	Asymmetric joint space narrowing Subchondral sclerosis Osteophyte formation Lack of erosions	RA - rarely involves DIP joints. If radiographic findings are similar in appearance to OA, but are in encountered in an atypical joint distribution, or advanced changes in a younger patient, then other causes of atypical or secondary osteoarthritis should be considered.
Erosive OA	DIP, PIP, 1st CMC, and scapho-trapezio-trapezoid joints.		Pathognomonic central subchondral erosions resulting in a "gullwing deformity"	Erosive OA with DIP involvement can be mistaken for psoriatic arthritis, however careful assessment for "gull-wing" deformity with lack of peri-articular erosions leans toward erosive OA.
RA	Proximal Distribution 2nd and 3rd MCP, 3rd PIP, 2nd-5th CMC, Radiocarpal, Distal Radioulnar	Erosive changes with pannus at the C1-2 articulation Atlantoaxial subluxation and impaction Facet joint erosions	Peri-articular erosions Bilateral and symmetric proximal distribution Peri-articular osteopenia and regional soft tissue swelling Alignment abnormalities (Boutonniere and Swan-neck deformities, MCP ulnar deviation and volar subluxations, hitchhiker thumb)	SLE differs from RA in that associated arthropathy is non-erosive and joint subluxations are reducible EOA differs from RA in that it follows the distribution of OA, with predominant DIP, 1st CMC, and scapho-trapezio-trapezoid joints. PsA favors a distal distribution with bony proliferation and periostitis. Absence of DIP, subchondral sclerosis, and osteophyte formation.
PsA	Distal Distribution DIP, 1st IP, 2nd-5th PIP Enthesitis (Achilles tendon insertion, origin of the plantar aponeurosis, and tendinous attachment sites about the pelvis)	Bilateral and asymmetric sacroiliitis Syndesmophytes present as bulky vertical/non-marginal paravertebral ossifications that may be asymmetric	Asymmetric distal distribution Bony productive change and perisotitis Lack of peri-articular osteopenia Pencil-in-cup deformity Sausage digit/Dactylitis	Distal asymmetric distribution in the hands and feet with bony productive change and absence of periarticular osteopenia can help to differentiate between psoriatic and rheumatoid arthritis PsA asymmetric distal compared to symmetry seen in OA Bilateral and asymmetric sacroiliitis seen in PsA versus AS Radiographic changes are identical to PsA, however the predominant distal distribution with feet greater than hands in CRA, as well as clinical history allows for a more accurate diagnosis of PsA vs. CRA
AS	Hips show uniform joint space narrowing with axial migration and protrusio	Bilateral and symmetric sacroiliitis Thin, flowing bridging vertical syndesmophytes Enthesitis	Enthesial corner erosions (Romanus lesion) and healing osteitis (shiny corners) Bamboo spine Carrot stick fractures Inflammatory spondylodiscitis	May be indistinguishable from IBD-related spondyloarthropathy
Gout	Hands: CMC and intercarpal joints > IP joints Feet: 1st MTP > 1st IP and TMT joints		Juxta-articular erosions with well-defined sclerotic margins and overhanging edges "rat-bite" Preservation of joint space until late in the disease process	Proximal distribution can mimic RA, however unlike RA, gout is an asymmetric process with well-defined erosions, and tophi may be present OA can be seen superimposed upon gouty changes, especially of the 1st MTP joint and tarsometatarsal joints Septic arthritis can mimic gout, but location, history, and lack of soft tissue ulcer should render a correct imaging diagnosis
CPPD	Proximal Distribution Hands: 2nd and 3rd MCP, radiocarpal, and glenohumeral joints	Crowned dens syndrome (erosions of C1-2 can mimic RA pannus, chondrocalcinosis in CPPD not seen in pannus of RA)	Hooked metacarpal head osteophytes Chondrocalcinosis	Proximal distribution can mimic RA, however, absence of erosions favors CPPD vs. RA CPPD distribution differs from OA Geodes and joint destruction in CPP often more severe in CPPD vs. OA Septic arthritis clinical and imaging presentation may be indistinguishable from CPPD arthritis, thus joint aspiration may be necessary

Figure 52.87 Summary of systematic approach to arthritis.

approach that has been outlined to recognize the radiographic hallmarks allows a prompt and confident diagnosis by the interpreter and subsequently appropriate management for the patient.

Suggested Readings

- EY Chang, KC Chen, BK Huang, A Kavanaugh, Adult inflammatory arthritides: what the radiologist should know, Radiographics 36 (6) (2016) 1849–1870.
- JW Bijlsma, F Berenbaum, FP Lafeber, Osteoarthritis: an update with relevance for clinical practice, Lancet 377 (9783) (2011 Jun 18) 2115–2126, doi:10.1016/S0140-6736(11)60243-2. PMID: 21684382.
- MS Taljanovic, DM Melville, LH Gimber, LR Scalcione, MD Miller, CK Kwoh, et al., High-resolution US of rheumatologic diseases, Radiographics 35 (7) (2015 Nov-Dec) 2026–2048, doi:10.1148/rg.2015140250. PMID: 26562235.
- JM Moll, I Haslock, IF Macrae, V Wright, Associations between ankylosing spondylitis, psoriatic arthritis, Reiter's disease, the intestinal arthropathies, and Behcet's syndrome, Medicine (Baltimore) 53 (5) (1974 Sep) 343–364, doi:10.1097/00005792-197409000-00002. PMID: 4604133.
- G Girish, KN Glazebrook, JA Jacobson, Advanced imaging in gout, AJR Am J Roentgenol 201 (3) (2013 Sep) 515–525, doi:10.2214/AJR.13.10776. PMID: 23971443.

53

Endocrine and Metabolic Bone Diseases

SCOTT D. WUERTZER, LEON LENCHIK

Homeostasis of Bone

In general, metabolic bone diseases affect the skeleton in one of two ways: there is either too much or too little bone (Fig. 53.1). The latter, which comprises most of the metabolic bone diseases, is due to some combination of a decrease in the amount of bone formed and an increase in the amount of bone resorbed. This shift typically occurs from abnormal vitamin D and calcium metabolism, resulting from abnormal diet, renal or endocrine dysfunction, or drug therapy.

Role of Imaging

Conventional radiographs are used to evaluate metabolic bone disorders due to their wide availability and low cost (Fig. 53.2). Depending on the ratio of bone formation to resorption, the bone may appear normal, radiodense (osteosclerosis), or radiolucent (osteopenia). Because metabolic processes usually involve the entire skeleton, the radiographic findings are usually diffuse or multifocal. On occasion, focal lesions may be found, such as brown tumors in hyperparathyroidism (Fig. 53.3). In osteopenic patients, radiographs help establish a differential diagnosis and serve an important role in the diagnosis and management of fractures [1].

More advanced imaging, including computed tomography (CT), magnetic resonance imaging (MRI), and bone scintigraphy, are often used for the early diagnosis of specific disorders [2]. In particular, CT is more sensitive than radiographs for the diagnosis of nondisplaced fractures, bony erosions, and soft-tissue findings. MRI is more sensitive than radiographs for the diagnosis of occult fractures, bone and soft-tissue neoplasms, infection, and osteonecrosis. MRI is also more sensitive and specific for the evaluation of ligament, tendon, and muscle injuries. Bone scintigraphy, which uses a physiologic marker (methylene diphosphonate), is more sensitive to bone turnover than radiographs or CT. Because it can screen the entire body, bone scintigraphy is often used for determining the location and distribution of disease.

For the evaluation of osteoporosis, clinical management often necessitates quantitative imaging. Conventional radiographs can be subject to technical errors and interpreter subjectivity. For example, an osteoporotic patient may appear normal if an improper technique has been used during image acquisition. Likewise, the same radiographs on a patient may be interpreted as normal by one radiologist and osteopenic by another. For this reason, various quantitative methods for measuring bone mass have been developed, with dual x-ray absorptiometry (DXA) and quantitative CT (QCT) being the most widely used. QCT is a volumetric technique that expresses bone mineral density (BMD)

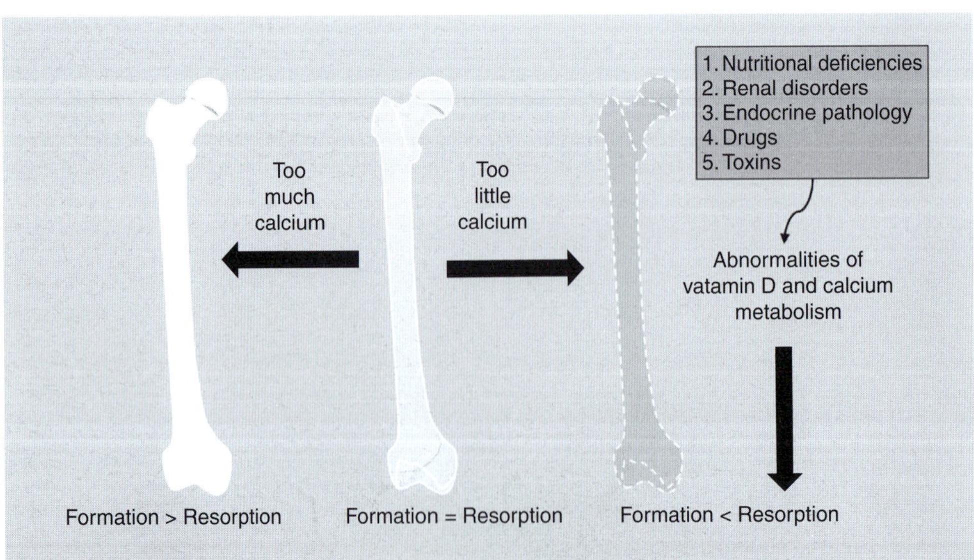

Figure 53.1 Homeostasis of bone. Metabolic and endocrine disorders of the skeleton are the result of too much or too little calcium. There is a critical balance between formation of bone and the resorption of bone. Most disease involves resorption of bone from abnormalities of vitamin D and calcium metabolism.

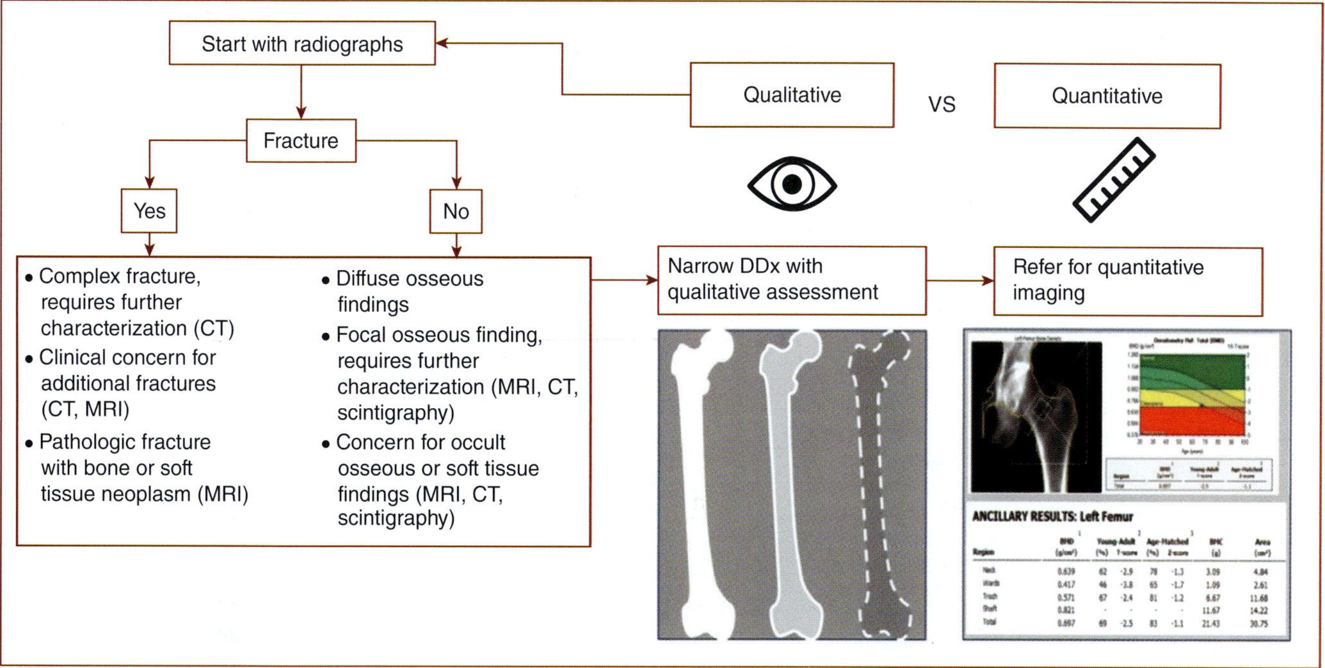

Figure 53.2 Role of imaging. The imaging of patients with metabolic and endocrine disorders should begin with radiographs, which provide a qualitative assessment, and progress to more advanced imaging (CT, MRI, or scintigraphy). In osteoporotic patients, clinical management often requires quantitative assessment (DXA, QCT). *CT*, computed tomography; *DXA*, dual x-ray absorptiometry; *MRI*, magnetic resonance imaging; *QCT*, quantitative computed tomography.

in mg/cm^3. In contrast, DXA is an area-based two-dimensional technique that expresses BMD in g/cm^2. Over the last decade, DXA has gained a higher acceptance rate over QCT, due to lower radiation dose, higher precision, and ease of use [3].

Dual X-ray Absorptiometry

DXA is routinely used for the diagnosis of osteoporosis, assessment of fracture risk, and monitoring of drug therapy [4]. A DXA scanner produces x-rays with two energy peaks, allowing

Figure 53.3 Brown tumors. Patient with a parathyroid adenoma. A lateral radiograph of the tibia and fibula shows a well-defined, mildly expansile lesion in the mid tibia consistent with a brown tumor. Smaller brown tumors are noted in the proximal and distal tibia.

a differential absorption of radiation by bone and soft tissue, from which the BMD is calculated. A typical DXA scan consists of a BMD measurement in the lumbar spine and the proximal femur, which are the most common sites of osteoporotic fractures. When the patient exceeds the weight limit of the table, or the hip and spine measurements are invalid, BMD can be measured in the nondominant forearm (Table 53.1).

In pediatric patients, a hip scan is usually not appropriate, and instead, a whole-body scan is obtained. Because the skull contains mostly cortical bone, the head is typically excluded from the final analysis, when whole-body scans are reported.

For point-of-care diagnosis of vertebral fractures, lateral evaluation of the thoracic and lumbar spine can be obtained, known as vertebral fracture assessment (VFA). VFA should be performed in patients with height loss, history of vertebral fracture, or chronic steroid therapy (>5 mg, >3 months).

BMD measurements are expressed as the number of standard deviations from the young-adult mean (T-score) or the age-matched mean (Z-score). The World Health Organization

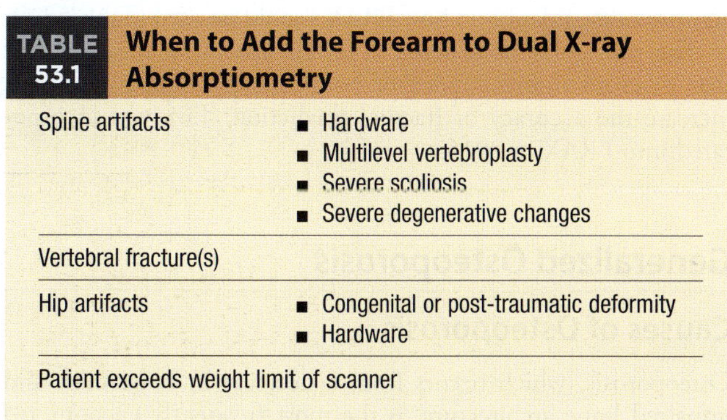

TABLE 53.1 When to Add the Forearm to Dual X-ray Absorptiometry

Spine artifacts	■ Hardware ■ Multilevel vertebroplasty ■ Severe scoliosis ■ Severe degenerative changes
Vertebral fracture(s)	
Hip artifacts	■ Congenital or post-traumatic deformity ■ Hardware
Patient exceeds weight limit of scanner	

TABLE 53.2 WHO Criteria for Osteoporosis

Diagnosis	T-Score
Normal	≥−1
Osteopenia	Between −1 and −2.5
Osteoporosis	≤−2.5, without fractures
Severe (established) osteoporosis	≤−2.5, with fractures

TABLE 53.3 Potential Artifacts on Dual X-ray Absorptiometry

Increase bone mineral density	■ Degenerative disease ■ Fracture ■ Vertebroplasty ■ Sclerotic metastases ■ Paget disease of bone ■ Vascular calcifications ■ Overlying objects ■ Contrast in bowel ■ Patient motion
Decrease bone mineral density	■ Laminectomy defects ■ Lytic metastases ■ Contrast in bowel ■ Patient motion

(WHO) defines osteoporosis as a T-score, which is 2.5 standard deviations or more below the young–adult mean (Table 53.2).

The printout from a DXA scan includes images of the spine, hip, or forearm, which should be inspected for proper patient positioning, proper scan analysis, and artifacts. Artifacts may falsely increase or decrease BMD. When possible, the spine, hip, or forearm artifacts should be removed from the region of interest. Other artifacts may be external to the patient, which should be removed before scanning (Table 53.3).

Although low BMD is the single best predictor for future fracture in postmenopausal women and older men, fractures are multifactorial in origin. In fact, in the study of osteoporotic fractures, 54% of the patients were not osteoporotic by BMD. These patients, however, could benefit from treatment, and the WHO introduced the Fracture Risk Assessment Tool (FRAX) in 2008 [5]. FRAX is a tool that calculates the 10-year probability of osteoporotic fractures based on widely validated clinical risk factors, including BMD as an input. FRAX has models for more than 50 countries and is considered the gold standard for fracture risk assessment. In the United States, the National Osteoporosis Foundation and the International Society for Clinical Densitometry provide guidance on how FRAX should be used (Table 53.4).

The trabecular bone score (TBS) is a textural measurement that gives an indirect index of bone microarchitecture [6]. To increase the accuracy of fracture prediction, TBS was incorporated into FRAX in 2015.

Generalized Osteoporosis

Causes of Osteoporosis

Osteoporosis, which occurs from a decrease in bone mass and impaired bone architecture, is the most frequently encountered

TABLE 53.4 National Osteoporosis Foundation and International Society for Clinical Densitometry Guidelines for FRAX

- Should only be used in patients with osteopenia by dual x-ray absorptiometry
- Should NOT be used in patients on therapy
- Should NOT be used in patients <50 years old
- Should NOT be used if previous hip or vertebral fracture

TABLE 53.5 Causes of Osteoporosis

Generalized	■ Postmenopausal ■ Age-related ■ Idiopathic juvenile osteoporosis ■ Drugs—steroids, heparin ■ Endocrine-related ■ Deficiency states—malnutrition, scurvy, calcium deficiency, alcoholism, liver disease ■ Congenital—osteogenesis imperfecta, ochronosis, homocystinuria, Gaucher disease, chronic anemia
Regional	■ Disuse osteoporosis ■ Complex regional pain syndrome (reflex sympathetic dystrophy) ■ Transient osteoporosis of the hip ■ Regional migratory osteoporosis ■ Periarticular osteoporosis with arthritis

metabolic bone disease [7]. On radiographs, the decreased density of bones is best described as osteopenia because generalized osteopenia is not specific to osteoporosis and can be seen in a variety of conditions, including osteoporosis, osteomalacia, hyperparathyroidism, and certain neoplasms.

There are many causes of osteoporosis, which can be categorized as generalized or regional, depending on the extent of skeletal involvement (Table 53.5).

Findings of Osteoporosis

The findings of osteoporosis are most pronounced in the axial skeleton [1]. Typically, vertebral endplates and vertical trabeculae are accentuated (Fig. 53.4A). *This pattern is different from osteomalacia, which has a more indistinct, fuzzy trabecular pattern due to deficient mineralization. The pattern is also different from renal osteodystrophy, which has endplate sclerosis (e.g., rugger-jersey appearance).* In the hip, tensile and compressive trabeculae are typically more prominent (Fig. 53.4B). In advanced disease, endosteal and intracortical resorption of bone becomes prominent, producing cortical thinning most evident in the long bones (Fig. 53.4C).

With a loss of bone mass, there is an increase in fracture risk, particularly in the femoral neck, thoracolumbar spine, distal radius, proximal humerus, and pelvis.

Atypical Femoral Fractures (Bisphosphonate-Related Proximal Femur Fracture)

Atypical femoral fractures (AFFs) are transversely oriented fractures in the lateral cortex of the femur, which are most frequently seen in

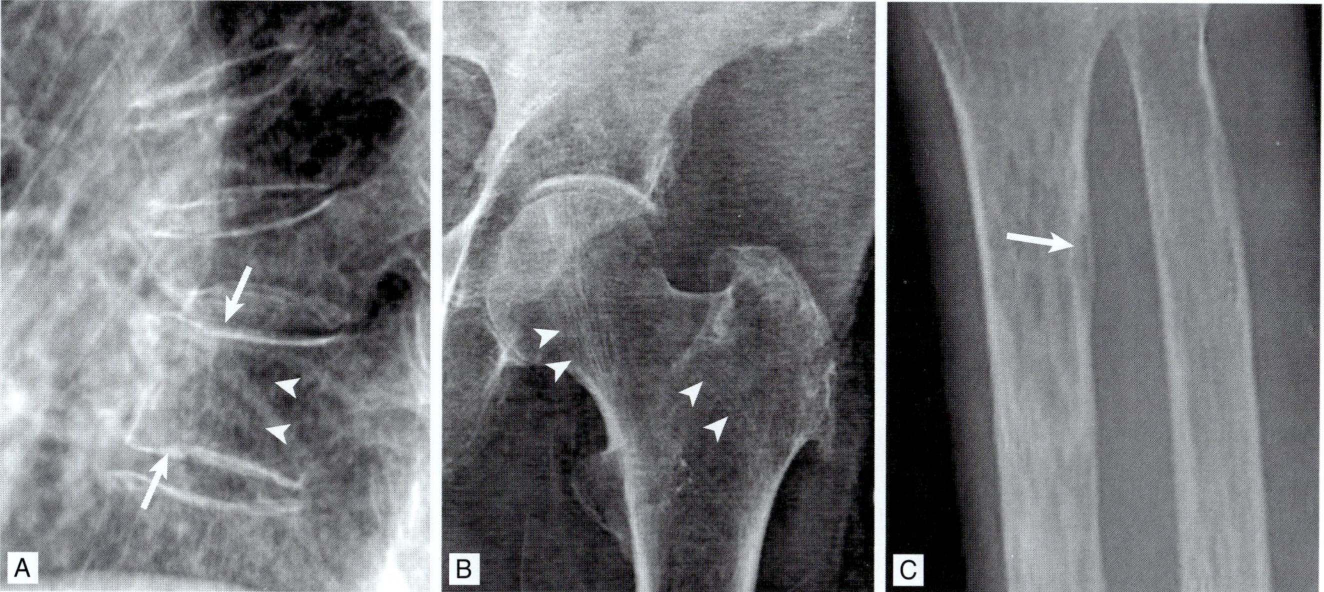

Figure 53.4 Findings of osteoporosis. (A) Vertebral endplates (*arrows*) and vertical trabeculae (*arrowheads*) are accentuated. (B) Tensile and compressive trabeculae are accentuated (*arrowheads*). (C) Endosteal and intracortical (*arrow*) resorption of bone, producing cortical thinning in the radius and ulna.

TABLE 53.6 Atypical Femoral Fractures. ASBMR Revised Definition (2013)

Located in the femoral diaphysis anywhere between the lesser trochanter and the supracondylar flare

Major features (four of five required)	▪ No trauma or minimal trauma ▪ Mainly transverse but may have short, medial oblique component ▪ Must involve the lateral cortex and can have a "medial spike" ▪ No comminution or minimal comminution ▪ Endosteal or periosteal thickening
Minor features (associated with AFFs but not required for diagnosis)	▪ Generalized diaphyseal thickening ▪ Bilaterality ▪ Prodromal symptoms, such as groin pain ▪ Delayed healing
Exclusion criteria	▪ Not spiral or comminuted ▪ Not femoral neck or intertrochanteric ▪ No malignant bone tumor (primary or metastatic) or other bone diseases (e.g., Paget disease, fibrous dysplasia)

patients taking long-term bisphosphonates for osteoporosis (Fig. 53.5A) [8]. The fractures, however, have also been reported in patients taking other osteoporosis medications and in patients with no exposure to these drugs. AFFs are considered a form of insufficiency fracture. The major features, minor features, and exclusion criteria have been well defined by the American Society for Bone and Mineral Research (ASBMR) (Table 53.6).

If the initial radiographs show endosteal or periosteal thickening without a fracture, MRI or CT can be performed for further characterization. A fluid-sensitive MRI sequence usually shows edema around the fracture site (Fig. 53.5B) and a CT usually shows a discrete fracture line.

When an AFF is identified, radiographs of the contralateral hip and entire femur should be performed because up to 44% of patients will have a contralateral fracture [9]. Antiresorptive treatment should be stopped. When surgery is indicated, intramedullary nailing is the preferred treatment (Fig. 53.5C).

Primary Osteoporosis

Generalized osteoporosis can occur from primary (idiopathic) or secondary etiologies [7]. The primary form is more common and can be subdivided into type 1 (postmenopausal) or type 2 (age-related). Postmenopausal osteoporosis occurs in women typically aged 50–65. There is a disproportionate loss of trabecular bone, giving rise to rapid bone loss and an increase in fractures, particularly of the vertebrae and distal radius. Vertebral fractures may lead to a marked kyphotic deformity (Fig. 53.6A and B).

Age-related osteoporosis differs from postmenopausal osteoporosis in that there is a proportionate loss of cortical and trabecular bone. Fractures occur most commonly in the femoral neck, proximal humerus, tibia, and pelvis (Fig. 53.7). Patients tend to be older, and the ratio of affected women to men is approximately 2:1.

Idiopathic juvenile osteoporosis is a rare self-limiting disease that affects both genders and occurs typically before puberty [10]. Patients present with bone pain, backache, or limp related to fractures, characteristically of the metaphysis of the long bones from minimal trauma. The diagnosis is one of exclusion, particularly from leukemia, lymphoma, and hypercorticosteroid states. Another diagnostic consideration is osteogenesis imperfecta (OI), which also presents with generalized osteopenia and multiple fractures.

Secondary Osteoporosis

Secondary osteoporosis has many causes, including those related to drugs, endocrine disorders, congenital factors, and nutrition [7].

Steroid-Induced Osteoporosis

With hypersteroidism, whether endogenous or exogenous, the main skeletal finding is osteopenia. Histological studies show the decreased bone formation and increased resorption. Biochemically,

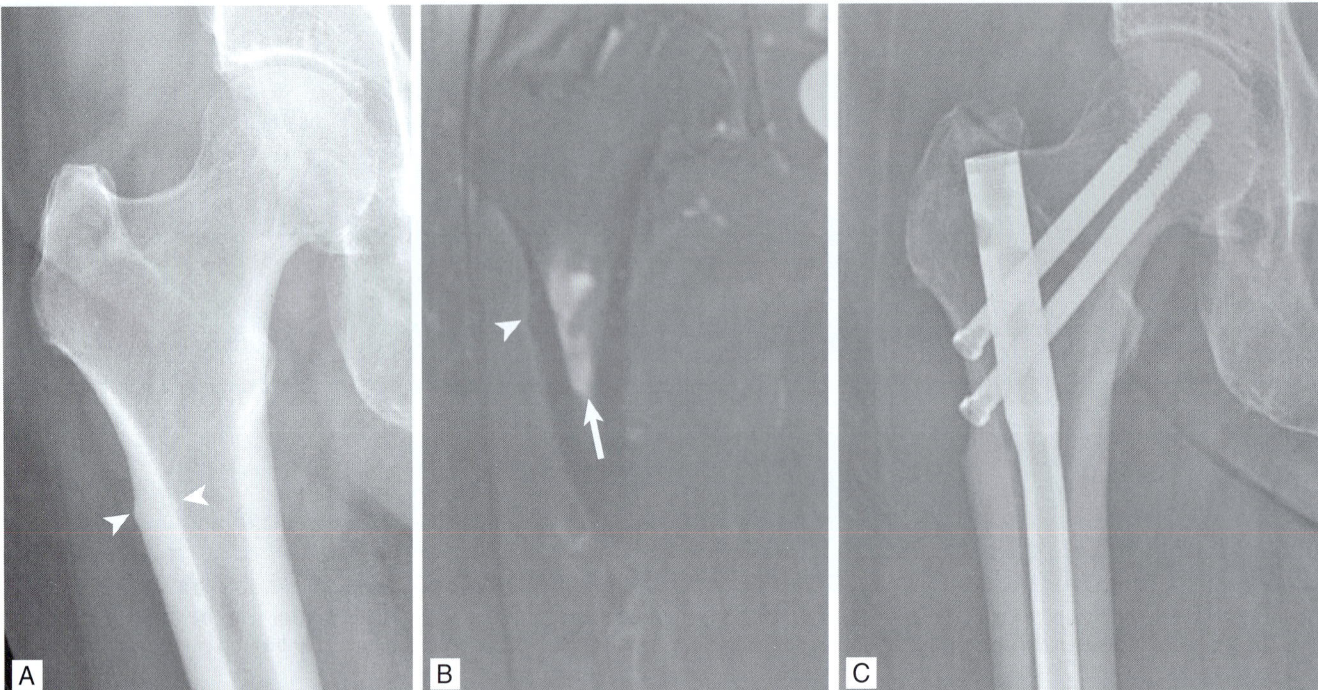

Figure 53.5 Atypical femoral fracture (bisphosphonate-related proximal femur fracture). A 78-year-old woman with right thigh pain on chronic bisphosphate treatment for the last 6 years. (A) Radiograph of the right proximal femur shows mild subtrochanteric periosteal and endosteal thickening (*arrowheads*) along the lateral femur. (B) Fluid-sensitive MRI shows the cortical thickening (*arrowhead*) and surrounding edema-like signal (*arrow*). (C) Follow-up radiographs show the placement of an intramedullary rod for prophylactic treatment to prevent propagation to a complete fracture. *MRI*, magnetic resonance imaging.

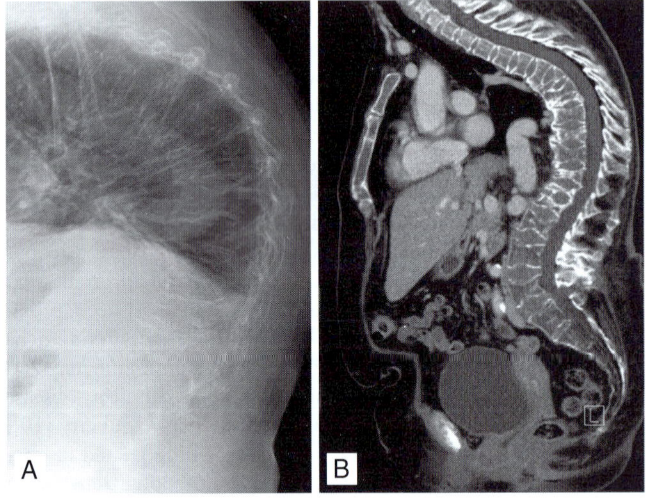

Figure 53.6 Postmenopausal osteoporosis in a 61-year-old woman (A) Lateral radiograph of the thoracic spine shows kyphotic deformity with multiple compression fractures. (B) Sagittal CT delineates the extent of fractures and shows accentuated vertebral body endplates with prominent vertical trabeculae.

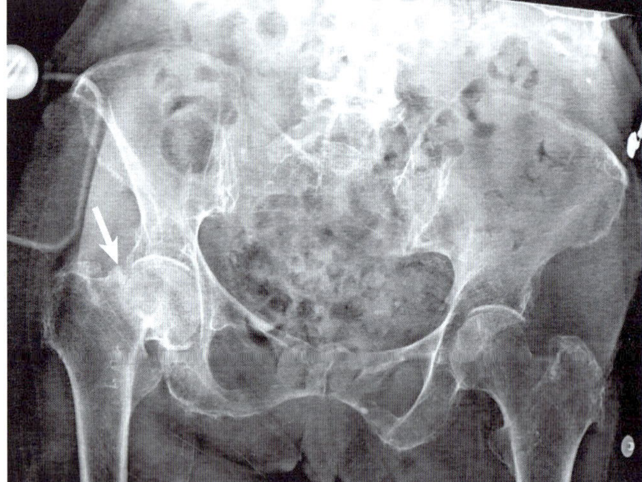

Figure 53.7 Age-related osteoporosis. A 92-year-old woman with right hip pain. Radiograph of the pelvis shows an acute right subcapital femur fracture (*arrow*). The pelvis and left proximal femur show prominent primary tensile and compressive trabeculae.

there is a negative calcium balance with hypercalciuria. Exuberant callus formation at fractures occurs, particularly in long bones, ribs (Fig. 53.8A), and vertebral bodies. With vertebral bodies, a characteristic increased density of the endplates occurs (Fig. 53.8B). Steroid-induced osteonecrosis can occur anywhere in the skeleton from vascular compression due to the accumulation of fat in the marrow. *The most common sites include the femoral head, humeral head, distal femur (Fig. 53.9A and B), and proximal tibia.* Early diagnosis often requires MRI.

Hypogonadism

Besides osteoporosis, hypogonadism in boys causes delayed closure of the epiphyseal plates, which results in long limbs compared with the trunk. A similar hypogonadal disorder in girls (Turner's syndrome) results in short stature, an increased carrying angle at the elbow (cubitus valgus), and a short fourth metacarpal (Fig. 53.10A). Premature closure of the medial aspect of the physis in the radius can lead to bowing of the radius (Fig. 53.10B) and a decrease in the carpal angle, which

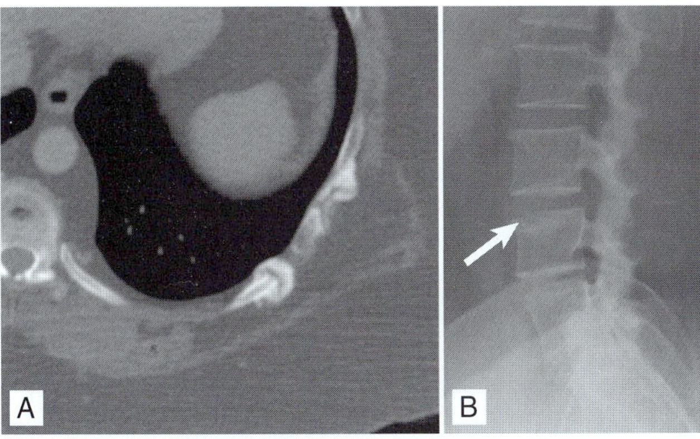

Figure 53.8 Steroid-induced osteoporosis. A 39-year-old woman on chronic steroids for juvenile rheumatoid arthritis. (A) Multiple left-sided rib fractures with exuberant callus. (B) Sclerotic endplate (*arrow*) at the site of acute L4 compression fracture.

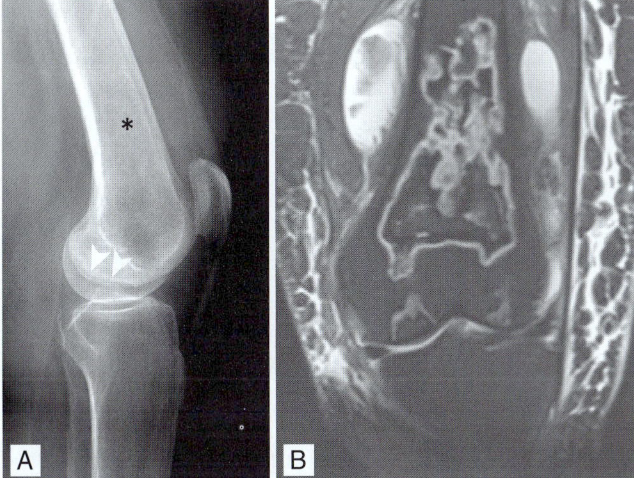

Figure 53.9 Steroid-induced osteonecrosis. A 67-year-old woman on chronic steroids for rheumatoid arthritis. (A) Lateral radiograph of the knee shows patchy areas of sclerosis (*asterisk*) in the femur suggestive of osteonecrosis. Subchondral collapse within the lateral femoral condyle from osteonecrosis (*arrowheads*). (B) Coronal T2-weighted MRI with fat saturation confirms the diagnosis of extensive osteonecrosis throughout the distal femur with the classic, serpentine-like outline of lesions in the metadiaphysis and femoral condyles.

is formed by a line through the proximal margins of the scaphoid and lunate and a second line through the proximal margins of the triquetrum and lunate. The findings resemble a Madelung deformity with a carpal angle less than 130° (Fig. 53.10C). Similar findings occur in the lower leg with premature closure of the medial physis in the tibia that leads to tibia varum (Blount disease) (Fig. 53.10D).

Thyroid Disorders

In hyperthyroidism, generalized osteoporosis may occur. There is an increase in both bone formation and resorption. Increased cortical striations in the long bones can be seen. In the spine, vertebral compression fractures and kyphosis are common. In children, hyperthyroidism can lead to accelerated skeletal maturation. Thyroid acropachy is a rare condition, which usually follows therapy for previous hyperthyroidism. There is characteristic periosteal thickening in the extremities with a predilection for the hand, specifically the thumb (Fig. 53.11A and B). It must be distinguished from hypertrophic osteoarthropathy (HPO), which is also found in the extremities. *In HPO, there is more frequently symmetric involvement of the tibia and fibula* (Fig. 53.12A and B). Isolated hand or feet findings are rare in HPO. Exophthalmos, pretibial myxedema, and clubbing are frequently present in thyroid acropachy.

Hypothyroidism may occasionally affect the skeletal system. In children, maturation is delayed, and growth is retarded. The sequence of epiphyseal formation is normal but delayed (Fig. 53.13A). Wormian bones occur in the skull, and the paranasal sinuses are underdeveloped. The sella is either small and bowl-shaped in young children or a larger round configuration in older children (cherry sella). In the spine, vertebral bodies can be bullet-shaped, especially at the thoracolumbar junction. The epiphyses are fragmented and can simulate Perthes' disease in the hip. The long bones are short and the pelvis is often narrow with coxa vara deformities (Fig. 53.13B).

Hyperpituitarism (Acromegaly)

Although generalized osteoporosis can occur with hyperpituitarism, some of the more characteristic skeletal findings allow for a more accurate diagnosis. Gigantism in the immature skeleton, and acromegaly in the adult, result from excessive growth hormone production by an eosinophilic adenoma. Most of the radiographic findings of hyperpituitarism occur due to increased soft-tissue thickness and bony overgrowth. In the skull, there are enlarged mastoid air cells and sinuses, frontal bossing, and prognathism. Pituitary fossa enlargement may be identified

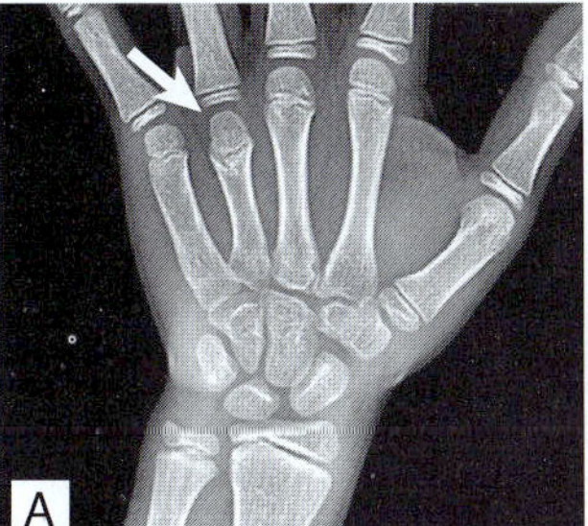

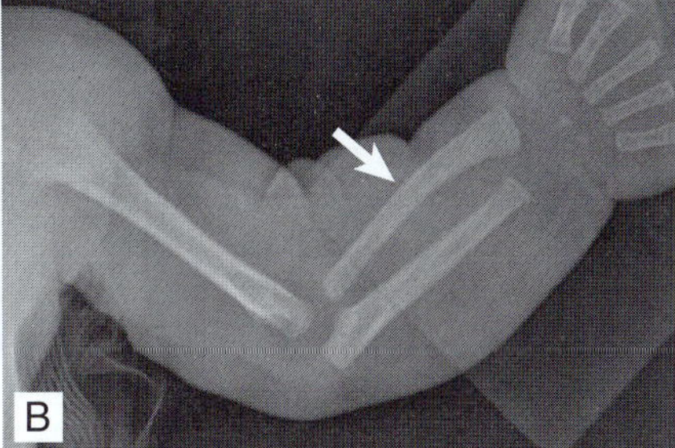

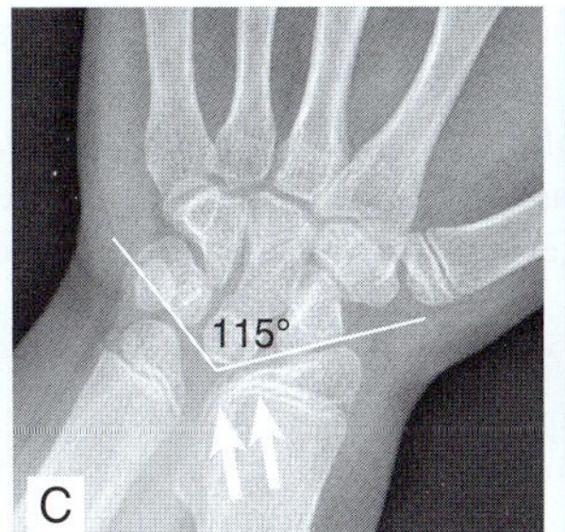

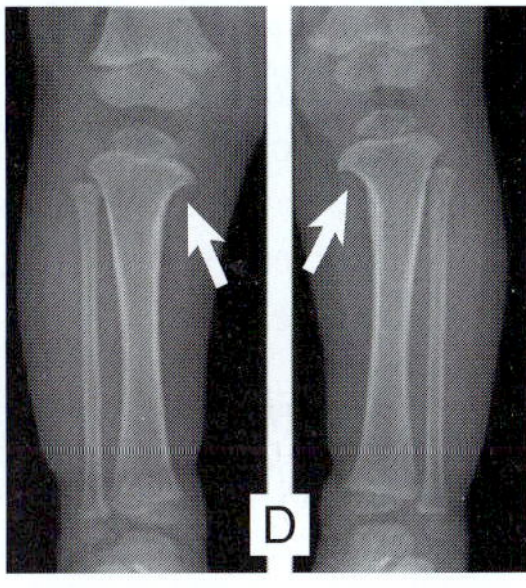

Figure 53.10 Turner syndrome (*TS*). (A) A 9-year-old girl with TS shows shortening of the fourth metacarpal (*arrow*). This finding is not unique to TS and can occur with pseudohypoparathyroidism and pseudopseudohypoparathyroidism. (B) A 1-month-old girl with TS has short forearms with bowing of the radius (*arrow*). (C) A 10-year-old girl with TS has a decreased carpal angle (less than 130 degrees, as depicted by the two intersecting lines). This finding is caused by premature closure of the medial aspect of the radial physis (*arrows*). (D) A 26-month-old girl with TS has bilateral tibia varum (Blount disease) from premature closure of the medial aspect of the physis (*arrows*).

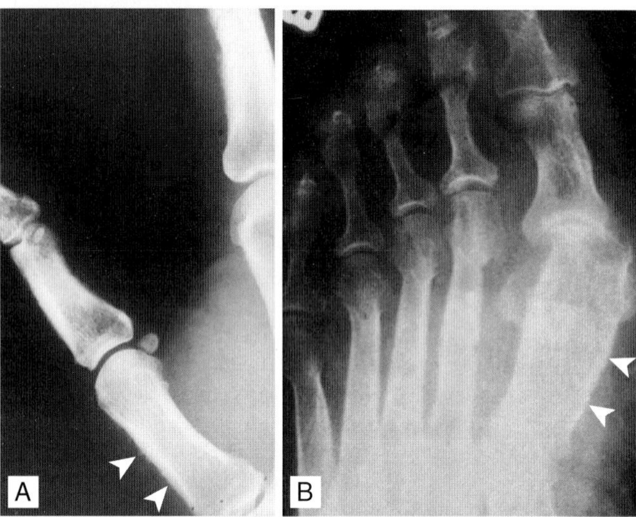

Figure 53.11 Thyroid acropachy. (A) Periostitis along the lateral aspect of the first metacarpal (*arrowheads*). (B) Dense periostitis along the medial margin of the first metatarsal in a different patient (*arrowheads*). Although this finding can occur in any of the digits, the first digit is a characteristic site.

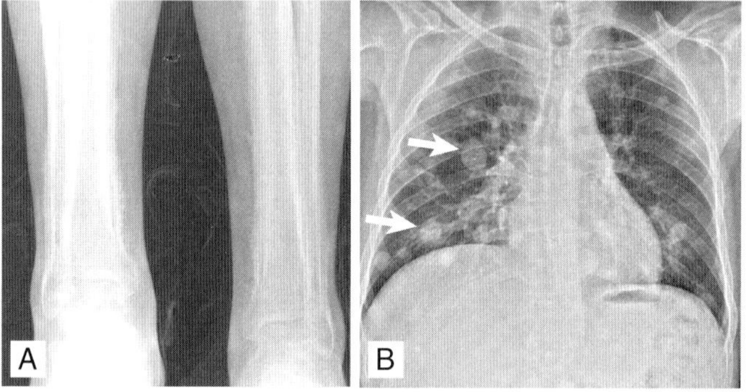

Figure 53.12 Hypertrophic pulmonary osteoarthropathy (HPO). A 48-year-old man with metastatic renal cell carcinoma (RCC) and HPO. (A) HPO has a symmetric distribution in the tibia and fibula compared with thyroid acropachy. HPO occurs less frequently in an isolated hand or foot distribution. (B) Chest radiograph shows metastatic RCC (*arrows*) to the lungs. In this case, the lower extremity series was obtained first, which prompted the radiologist to recommend a chest radiograph.

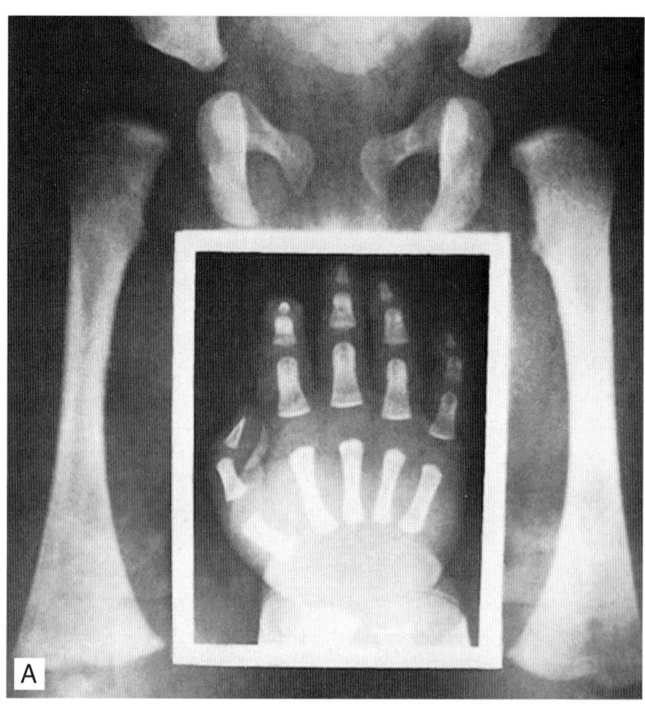

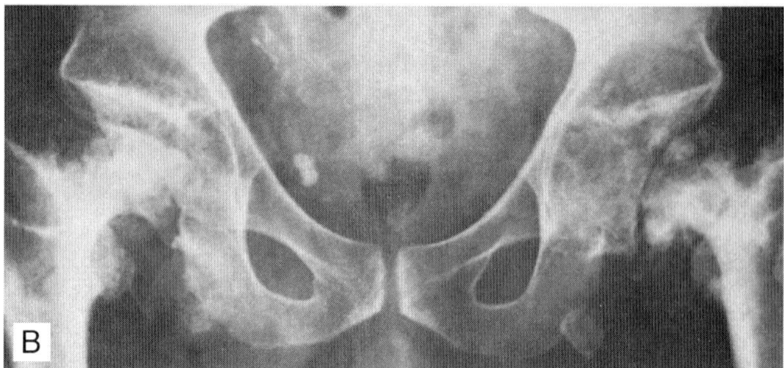

Figure 53.13 Congenital hypothyroidism. (A) A 12-month-old child with congenital hypothyroidism. Radiograph shows delayed ossification of the carpals and the proximal femoral epiphyses. (B) A 39-year-old man with congenital hypothyroidism, left untreated until the age of 35 years. Radiograph shows bilateral coxa vara and incompletely ossified, deformed femoral heads.

radiographically, but MRI is needed for pituitary adenoma evaluation. In the spine, enlargement of the vertebral bodies with posterior scalloping can occur. *The hands have characteristic enlargement of the bones with spade-like terminal tufts or arrowhead distal phalanges* (Fig. 53.14). Widening of the joint spaces due to overgrowth of articular cartilage can occur. In the feet, there can be an increase in the thickness of the heel pads. There is often bony proliferation at attachment sites for ligaments and tendons.

Hyperparathyroidism

As a result of bone resorption, generalized osteopenia is the most common finding of hyperparathyroidism. Brown tumors can also contribute to the osteopenic appearance. Brown tumors are cyst-like lesions that are characteristic of hyperparathyroidism (Fig. 53.15A and B). They consist of fibrous tissue, giant cells, and osteoclasts. Hyperparathyroidism will be discussed in more detail in the metabolic section.

Pregnancy

Generalized osteoporosis can occur with pregnancy. The exact cause is unknown but presumably relates to changes in mineral metabolism with increased calcium resorption. Pregnant patients may present with fragility fractures [11]. Localized osteoporosis, specifically transient osteoporosis of the hip (TOH), can occur in pregnant patients. *TOH typically occurs in the third trimester*. The exact etiology is unknown but likely relates to local factors at the hip, possibly from altered biomechanics of pregnancy or an alteration in the neural reflex pathway, similar to reflex sympathetic dystrophy. Patients typically present with a limp from hip pain or a fracture.

Increased weight of pregnancy from the growing fetus combined with an expansion of the pelvis for vaginal delivery places increased stress on the sacroiliac joints and pubic symphysis. Radiographically, this stress may manifest as osteitis condensans ilii at the sacroiliac joints and osteitis pubis at the pubic symphysis (Fig. 53.16). With osteitis condensans ilii, a well-defined triangular-shaped focus

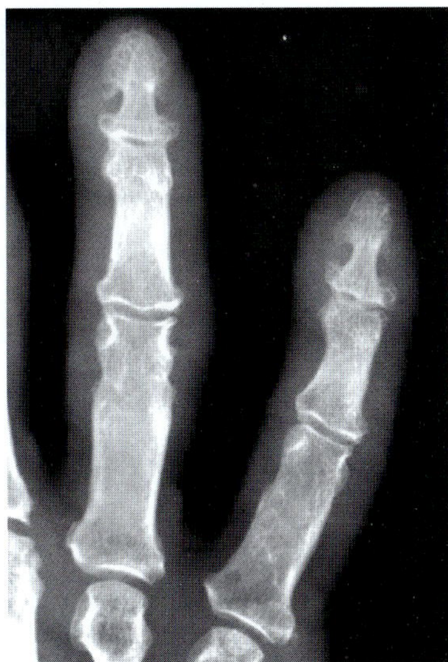

Figure 53.14 Acromegaly. Diffuse enlargement of the soft tissues of the fourth and fifth fingers widened joint spaces at the metacarpophalangeal joints and proximal interphalangeal joints, and spade-like appearance of the distal phalanges.

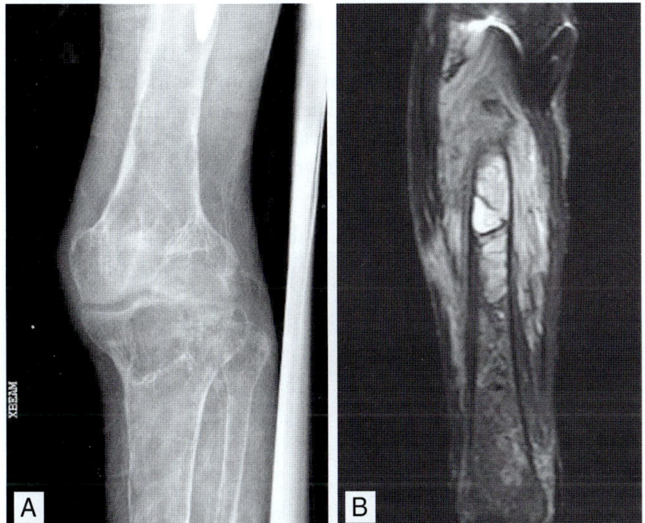

Figure 53.15 Osteopenia from brown tumors. A 43-year-old man with end-stage renal disease. (A) Frontal radiograph of the knee shows osteopenia from extensive brown tumor involvement. Large cyst-like lesions throughout all of the imaged bones of the knee with areas of endosteal scalloping and cortical thinning. (B) MR STIR image of the femur shows diffuse marrow involvement with cystic areas of increased signal intensity. The signal characteristics of brown tumors may vary on MRI, depending on the amount of solid or cystic components.

of sclerosis occurs along the iliac side of the sacroiliac joint. Typically, the findings are bilateral and symmetric with the preservation of the sacroiliac joint. With osteitis pubis, there are subchondral erosions with surrounding sclerosis. The findings are usually bilateral and symmetric. With time, sclerosis can resolve and ankylosis can occur.

Diabetes

Many musculoskeletal findings, including generalized osteoporosis, can occur in diabetes mellitus (DM) (Table 53.7) [12,13].

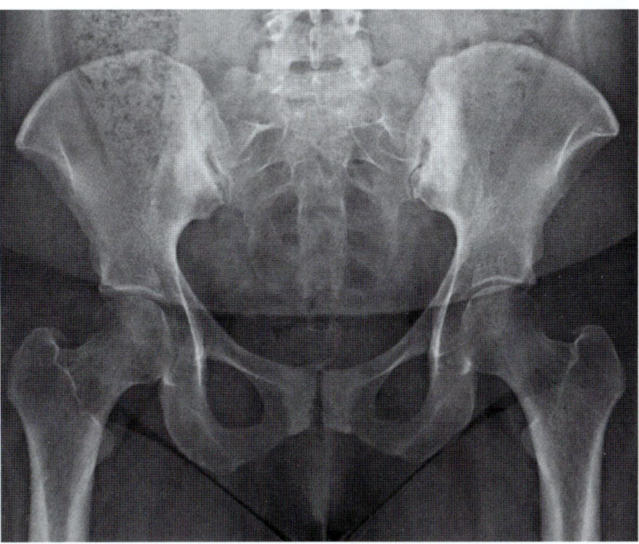

Figure 53.16 Osteitis condensans ilii and osteitis pubis. A 35-year-old woman with three vaginal deliveries in the last 5 years. Characteristic findings of osteitis condensans ilii, including bilateral triangular-shaped areas of sclerosis in the ilium. The sacroiliac joints and sacrum are unremarkable. Osteitis pubis is also present with sclerosis and mild subchondral erosions on both sides of the pubic symphysis.

TABLE 53.7 Musculoskeletal Complications of Diabetes Mellitus

Bone	▪ Osteoporosis ▪ Osteoporosis-related fractures ▪ Delayed fracture healing ▪ Osteomyelitis ▪ DISH
Joints	▪ Neuropathic osteoarthropathy ▪ Septic arthritis ▪ Association with gout, osteoarthritis
Soft tissues	▪ Fibroproliferative disorders ▪ Muscle infarction ▪ Vascular calcifications

The exact mechanism of osteoporosis in DM is unknown, but low bone turnover and decreased bone formation from osteoblast dysfunction likely contribute a role. Both types 1 and 2 DM are associated with increased fracture risk, and fracture healing may be prolonged.

Osteomyelitis is common in diabetic feet with the direct spread from soft-tissue ulceration, which typically occurs at pressure points over the first and fifth toes and posterior calcaneus (Fig. 53.17A–D). As the infection spreads through dependent tissues, septic arthritis can occur. Due to poor blood supply, the degree of osteopenia and periostitis from infection in DM may be decreased compared with osteomyelitis in nondiabetic patients. MRI can help delineate soft-tissue edema, abscesses, and marrow changes.

Diffuse idiopathic skeletal hyperostosis (DISH) is more common in patients with DM compared with age-matched controls (Fig. 53.18). Chronic elevation of serum insulin and insulin-like growth factor 1 (IGF-1) likely contribute to DISH in DM.

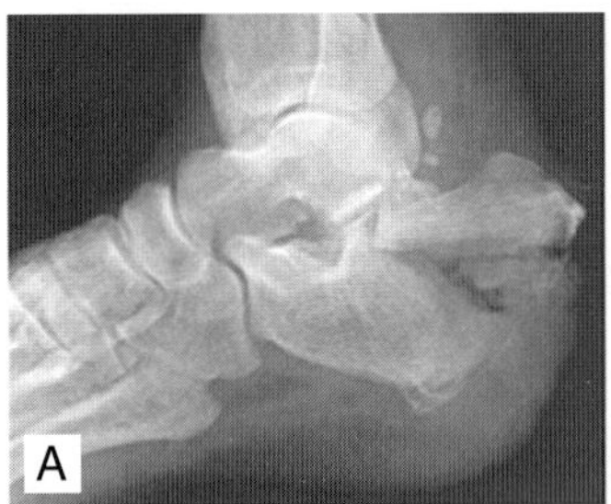
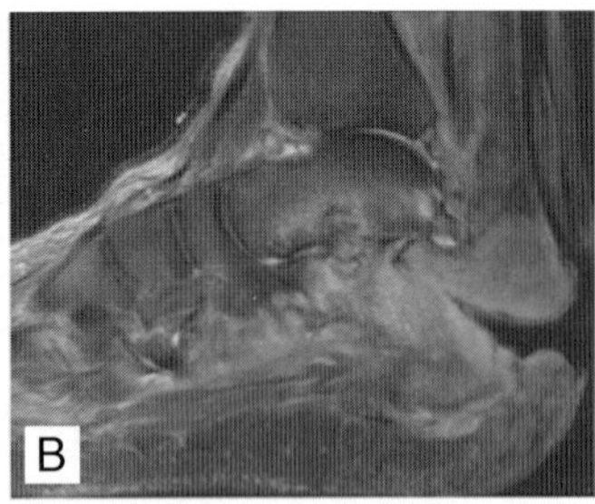
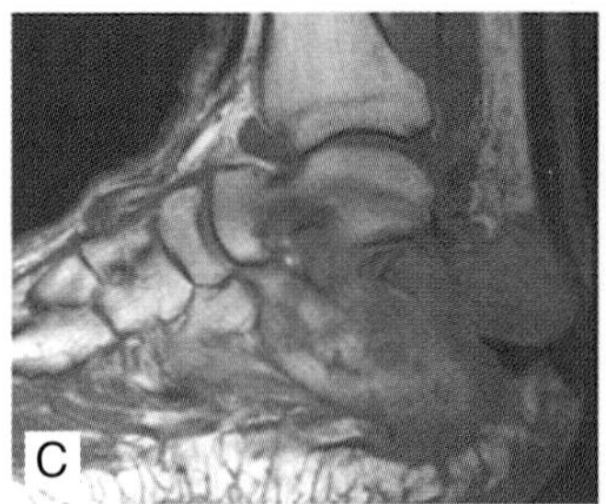
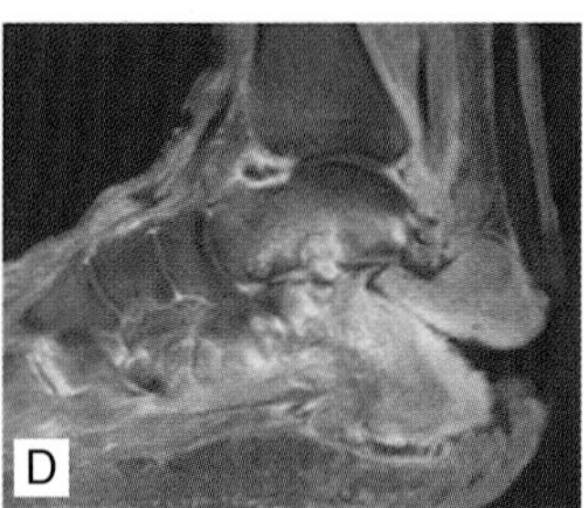

Figure 53.17 Acute osteomyelitis. A 51-year-old man with diabetes mellitus. (A) Pathologic fracture of the calcaneus. This type of avulsion fracture is common in diabetic patients where the Achilles is stronger than the underlying, infected bone. (B) Sagittal T2-weighted MR image shows increased, edema-like signal throughout the posterior half of the calcaneus due to a combination of osteomyelitis and the fracture. (C) Sagittal T1-weighted MR image shows confluent areas of low signal intensity in the same location. The posterior ulcer tracks directly into the bone. (D) Sagittal T1-weighted MR image with contrast shows enhancement of the infected bone.

Although neuropathic osteoarthropathy (Charcot joint) can be seen with other diseases, DM is by far the leading cause. Due to a decrease in sensory feedback, an initial injury and the associated inflammation may not be recognized by the patient. Subsequently, a cycle of degenerative and destructive change will ensue, which manifests itself as joint space loss, sclerosis, osteophytosis, fragmentation, fracture, and joint dislocation (Fig. 53.19A–C). Neuropathic osteoarthropathy associated with DM typically affects the feet, specifically the tarsometatarsal joints and intertarsal joints. Patients with DM frequently present with findings of a chronic Lisfranc fracture dislocation as a result of peripheral neuropathy (Fig. 53.20A and B). An association between DM and other arthropathies, including gout and osteoarthritis, has been suggested. This association, however, more likely relates to an increased frequency of obesity in patients with DM.

Many fibroproliferative disorders, including adhesive capsulitis, Dupuytren's contracture, diabetic cheiroarthropathy, flexor tenosynovitis (trigger finger) (Fig. 53.21A and B), and carpal tunnel syndrome, occur with a higher frequency in diabetic patients. The pathogenesis and association with DM are not well understood, but they are likely multifactorial, with chronic hyperglycemia contributing to glycosylation of collagen, decreased collagen degradation, and diabetic microangiopathy.

Muscle infarction (myonecrosis) tends to occur from microangiopathy in patients with poorly controlled diabetes. Myonecrosis presents as acute pain and swelling, typically in the thigh and calf (Fig. 53.22A and B). There may be a palpable mass, and symptoms can be unilateral or bilateral, involving noncontiguous muscle groups. Clinically, the main differential consideration is myositis and/or an abscess. With myonecrosis, there should not

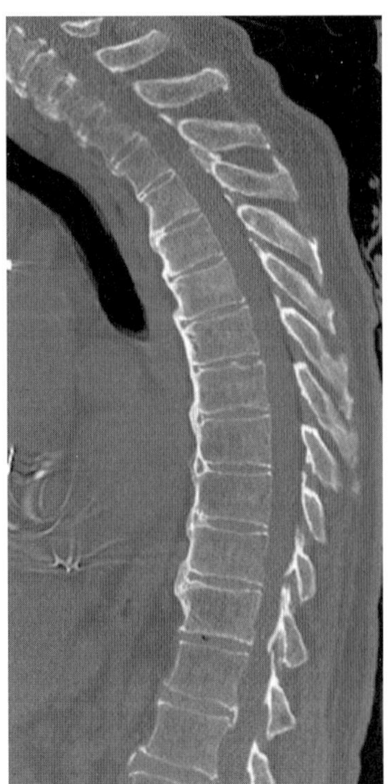

Figure 53.18 Diffuse idiopathic skeletal hyperostosis (DISH). A 79-year-old man with diabetes mellitus. Sagittal CT image shows flowing ossification along the anterior longitudinal ligament of multiple contiguous thoracic vertebral bodies, which is common in patients with diabetes mellitus. *CT*, computed tomography.

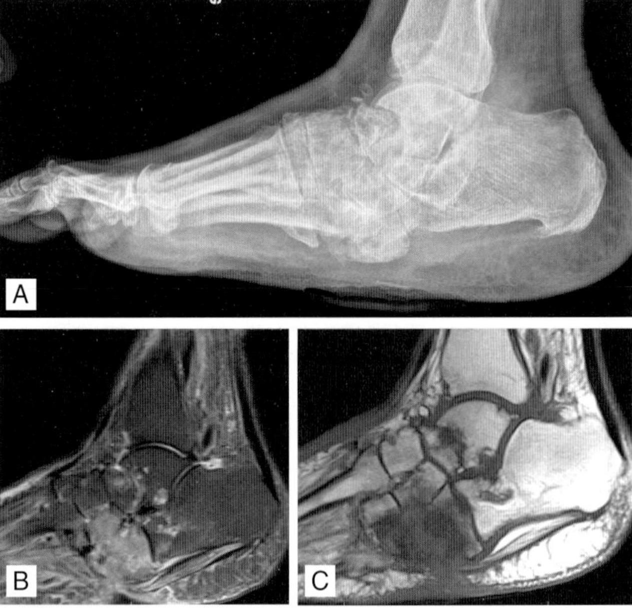

Figure 53.19 Charcot joint with acute osteomyelitis. A 71-year-old man with diabetes mellitus. (A) Lateral radiograph of the foot and ankle shows neuropathic osteoarthropathy (Charcot joint) in the midfoot. A combination of chronic degenerative and destructive change is centered at the Chopart joint. (B) Sagittal T2-weighted image shows edema-like signal throughout the cuboid, suspicious for osteomyelitis. (C) Sagittal T1-weighted MR image of the same area shows a plantar ulcer with a track that extends into the cuboid. There is diffuse low signal intensity throughout the cuboid. This combination of findings confirms the diagnosis of acute osteomyelitis.

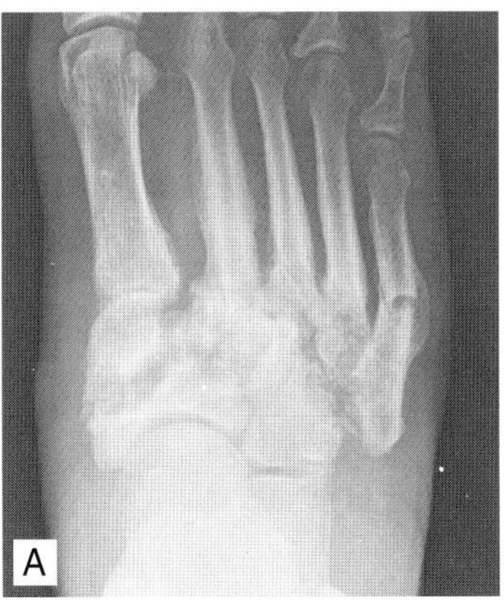

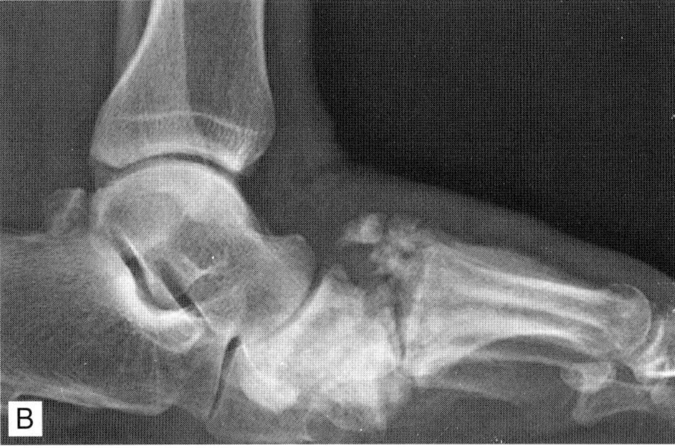

Figure 53.20 Chronic Lisfranc fracture dislocation. A 63-year-old man with DM and Charcot arthropathy. Frontal and lateral radiographs of the right foot show classic findings of neuropathic osteoarthropathy including severe degenerative and destructive changes across the Lisfranc joint. (A) Frontal radiograph shows multiple proximal metatarsal fractures and lateral dislocation of the second to fifth metatarsals. (B) Lateral radiograph also shows multiple chronic metatarsal base fractures with dorsal dislocation at the Lisfranc joint. These findings are typical in a patient with diabetes mellitus. *DM*, diabetes mellitus.

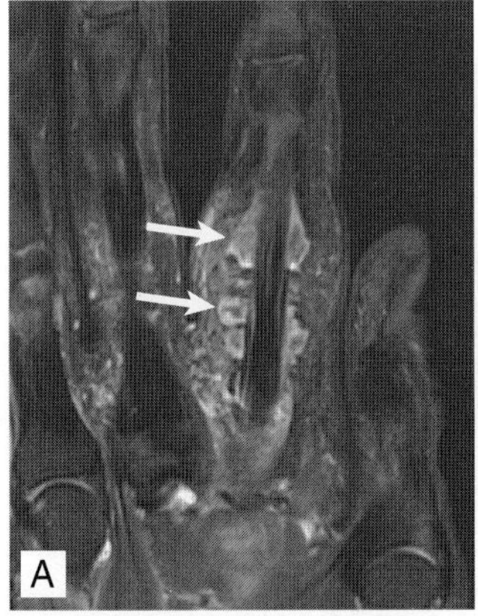

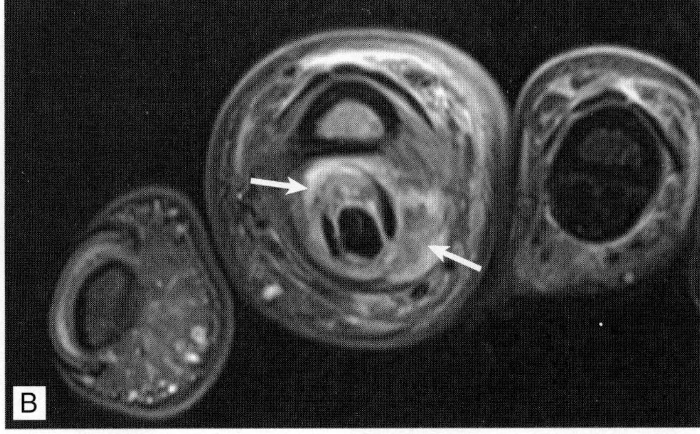

Figure 53.21 Stenosing flexor tenosynovitis (trigger finger). A 62-year-old man with DM presents with index finger pain and no trauma history. Surgically confirmed with trigger finger with superimposed infection. (A) Coronal T2-weighted MR image shows complex fluid (*arrows*) in the tendon sheath surrounding the flexor tendons. (B) Axial T2-weighted MR image shows similar findings of a complex tenosynovitis (*arrows*). *DM*, diabetes mellitus.

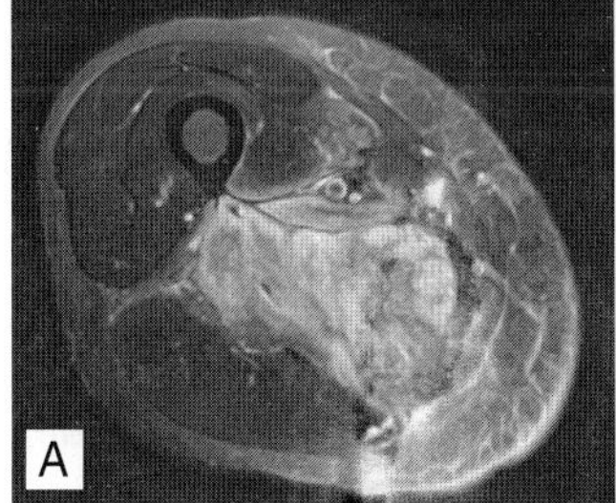

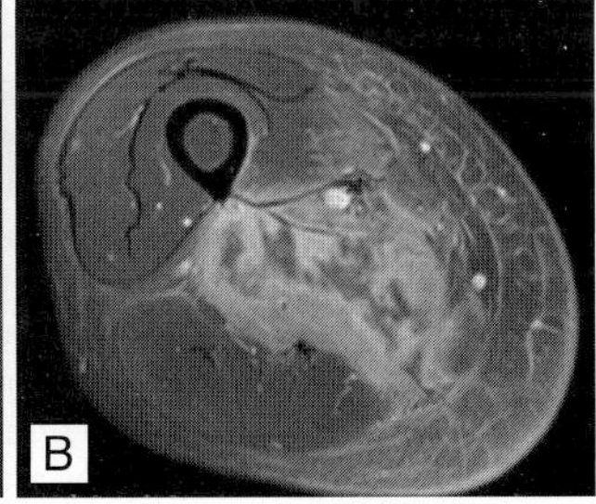

Figure 53.22 Myonecrosis. A 24-year-old woman with poorly controlled DM presents with pain in right thigh. (A) T2-weighted axial MR image of thigh shows diffuse edema-like signal throughout an enlarged, adductor magnus. (B) T1-weighted, fat-saturated MR image with contrast shows patchy areas of enhancement in a serpentine-like configuration around areas of necrotic muscle. The enhancement pattern combined with preserved central muscle fibers helps distinguish myonecrosis from an intramuscular abscess. *DM*, diabetes mellitus.

be a fever or leukocytosis. On MRI, myonecrosis typically shows muscle enlargement. On fluid-sensitive sequences, there is intramuscular edema and subfascial fluid. Contrast images show heterogeneous areas of muscle that do not enhance interposed with enhancing muscle. On MRI, intramuscular abscesses typically show a homogenous fluid collection with only peripheral enhancement (Fig. 53.23A and B).

Scurvy

Scurvy is rare before 6 months of age since the storage of vitamin C in the neonate is generally adequate. Normal osteoblastic activity depends on vitamin C. Without it, the organic matrix of bone cannot be laid down properly. Clinically, children present with limb pain and irritability. Swelling of the gums is also characteristic. Radiographically, four characteristic signs are seen: (1) the epiphysis is small with a well-defined sclerotic margin (Wimberger ring sign); (2) the zone of provisional calcification at the growing metaphysis is dense, giving a white line (Frankel line); (3) beneath this is a lucent zone, due to lack of mineralization of osteoid (*Trummerfeld zone*); (4) finally, as this area is weakened, it is prone to fractures which occur at the cortical margin, resulting in (*Pelkan*) spurs (Fig. 53.24) [7].

In addition, due to capillary fragility, subperiosteal hemorrhages occur, which may give rise to periosteal elevation and subsequent new bone formation, particularly following treatment (Fig. 53.25). After treatment, dense bands of bone persist, resembling growth arrest lines.

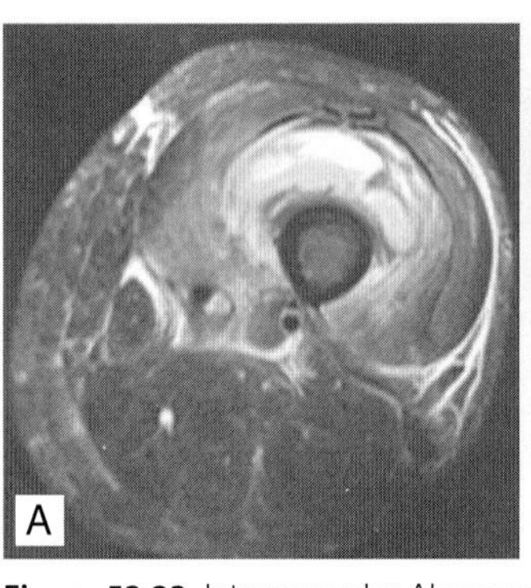
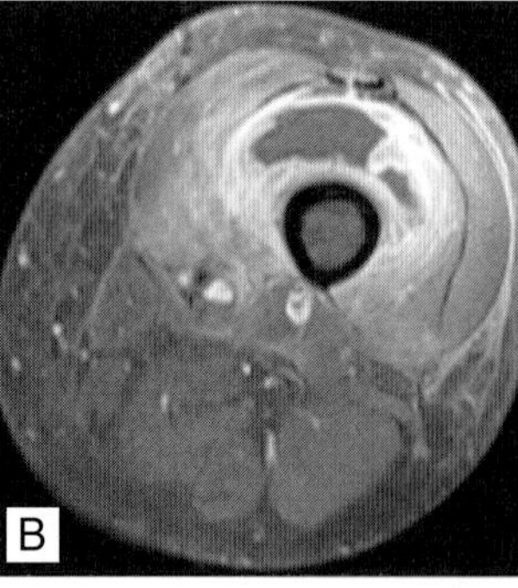

Figure 53.23 Intramuscular Abscess. A 37-year-old man with history of intravenous drug abuse presents with leg pain, fever, and elevated white blood cell count. A large amount of purulent fluid was evacuated from the deep compartment of the leg at surgery. (A) Axial T2-weighted MR image confirms the presence of a large, complex intramuscular abscess in the vastus musculature. (B) Axial T1-weighted, fat-saturated MR image with contrast shows peripheral enhancement of the fluid collection. The enhancement pattern combined with no internal muscle fibers confirms the diagnosis of abscess as opposed to myonecrosis.

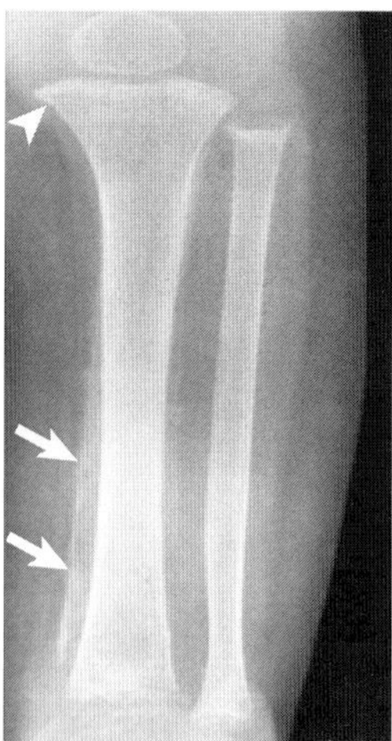

Figure 53.25 Scurvy with subperiosteal hemorrhage. Along the medial aspect of the distal tibia, there is elevation of the periosteum from subperiosteal hemorrhage (*arrows*). Additionally, there is spur (Pelkan) formation in the proximal tibia (*arrowhead*).

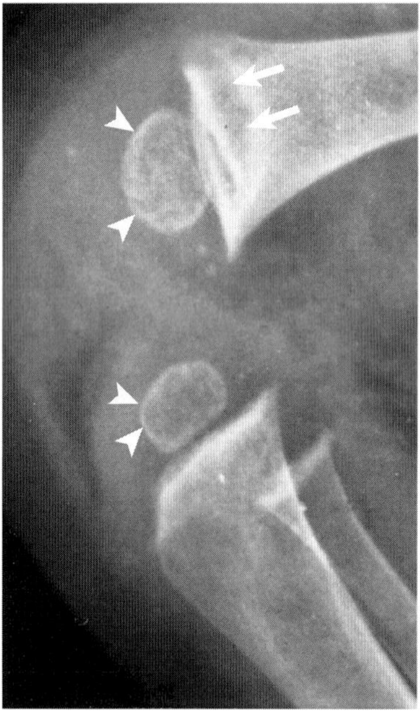

Figure 53.24 Scurvy. Lateral radiograph of knee. The margins of the epiphyses are sclerotic, which is the Wimberger ring sign (*arrowheads*). There is a dense zone of provisional calcification, giving a white line of Frankel. Deep to this line, there is a lucent zone known as the Trummerfeld zone, which is seen best in the distal femur (*arrows*).

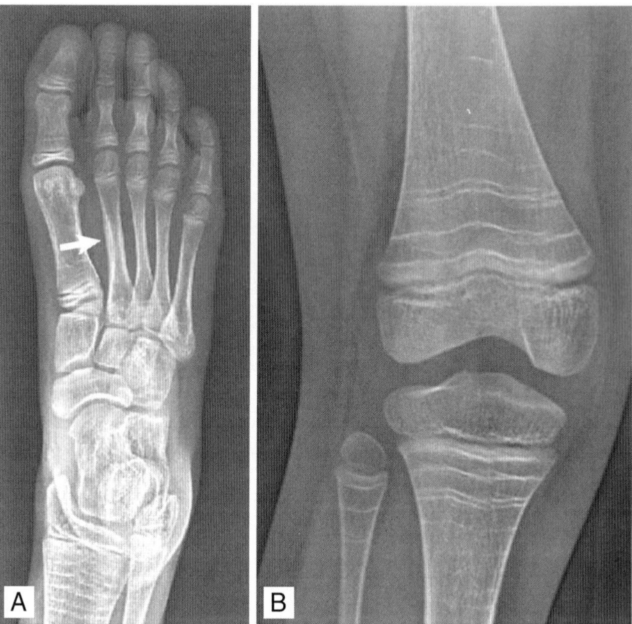

Figure 53.26 Osteogenesis imperfecta (OI). A 9-year-old girl with OI presents for Zoledronate infusion. (A) Frontal radiograph of the foot shows diffuse osteopenia, a healing second metatarsal fracture (*arrow*), and sclerotic metaphyseal bands in the tibia. (B) Frontal knee radiograph shows characteristic sclerotic metaphyseal bands (zebra stripes) in the distal femur, proximal tibia, and proximal fibula as the result of cyclical bisphosphonate therapy.

Congenital

Numerous congenital disorders can lead to generalized osteoporosis, including OI, ochronosis, and homocystinuria.

OI is an inherited disorder of connective tissue that exhibits osteoporosis, wormian bones, and fractures that heal with marked callus formation. Blue sclera, premature otosclerosis, and dentinogenesis imperfecta may be present. Cyclical treatment with bisphosphonates can lead to characteristic sclerotic metaphyseal bands on radiographs, "zebra stripes" (Fig. 53.26A and B) [14]. *The number of bands closely corresponds to the cycles of treatment received.*

Alkaptonuria is a rare hereditary disorder of tyrosine metabolism. Homogentisic acid accumulates in the tissues, particularly connective tissue. Ochronosis refers to the black pigment that is deposited in the tissues, producing the radiographic findings. Generalized osteoporosis can occur, but the most characteristic finding is disc calcification in the spine (Fig. 53.27A and B). Kyphoscoliosis and an advanced disease resembling ankylosing spondylitis may also develop. In extraspinal sites, severe joint space narrowing with minimal osteophyte formation or sclerosis may occur.

Homocystinuria is a rare hereditary disorder with deficient cystathiamine synthetase, which converts homocysteine to cystathionine and cysteine. In one form of the disease (pyridoxine-resistant), changes in the skeleton include osteoporosis, arachnodactyly, epiphyseal enlargement, scoliosis, sternal deformity, and

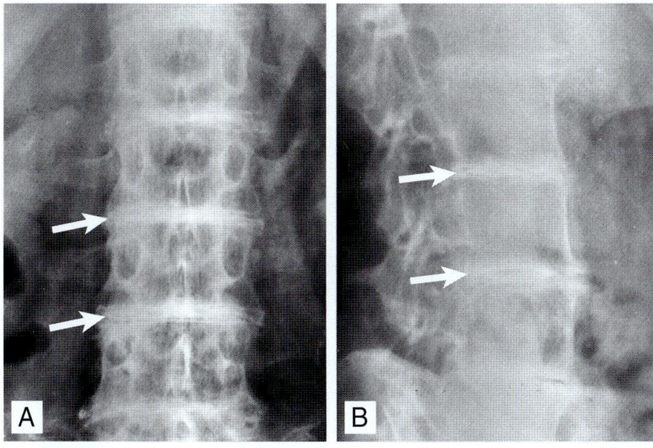

Figure 53.27 Ochronosis. A 56-year-old woman with ochronosis. Frontal (A) and lateral (B) radiographs of the lumbar spine show intervertebral disc calcification (*arrows*), which is a hallmark of ochronosis.

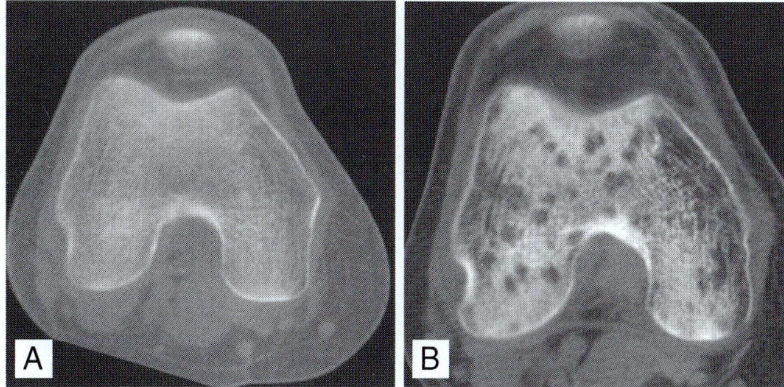

Figure 53.28 Disuse osteoporosis with medullary involvement on CT. A 34-year-old man with giant cell tumor (GCT) in the tibia (not shown in image). (A) Pretreatment CT through the distal femur shows normal trabecular bone. (B) Follow-up CT approximately 7 months after curettage and packing of the GCT in the tibia shows a speckled pattern of osteoporosis in the distal femur. This pattern is frequently seen on CT and should not be confused for a neoplastic process.

valgus deformity of the knees and hips. The radiographic findings, however, are not unique to homocystinuria, and the diagnosis is typically made through laboratory and genetic testing.

Regional Osteoporosis

Osteoporosis can occur in any region of the body. Regional osteoporosis usually involves the appendicular skeleton due to disuse, complex regional pain syndrome, TOH, or regional migratory osteoporosis (RMO). Additionally, periarticular osteoporosis can occur in association with arthritis.

Disuse Osteoporosis

Disuse osteoporosis is acute osteopenia that develops when the limb is immobilized. The findings usually occur after a fracture but can occur with any etiology that limits the use of the extremity, including paralysis or infection. Typically, resorption of cortical and trabecular bone occurs at the fracture site. All the bones distal to the fracture site are usually involved. These changes occur approximately 5 weeks after immobilization and reverse after activity resumes.

Besides generalized osteoporosis, a more speckled pattern of medullary involvement can involve any bone from the articular surface to the diaphysis (Fig. 53.28A and B) [15]. Varying degrees of demineralization may affect the subperiosteal, intracortical, or endosteal layers of the cortex. Cortical tunneling caused by prominent Haversian canals may be present (Fig. 53.29A and B). Periarticular changes include a characteristic radiolucent line deep to the articular cortex from endosteal resorption and a broadband of resorption at the physeal scar in adults. On fluid-sensitive MRI sequences, disuse osteoporosis presents as areas of increased signal intensity that may vary in morphology from dot like in the early stage, linear in the intermediate stage, and patchy or confluent in later stages (Fig. 53.30A and B) [16].

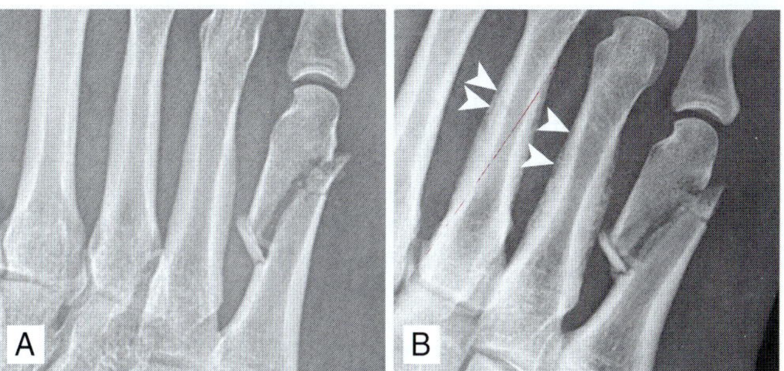

Figure 53.29 Disuse osteoporosis with cortical involvement. A 49-year-old woman with a fifth metatarsal fracture. (A) Oblique radiograph of the foot shows an acute oblique fracture through the fifth metatarsal shaft. There is normal cortical and medullary mineralization. (B) Oblique radiograph of the foot obtained 5 weeks later shows some healing at the fracture site with disuse osteopenia throughout the foot. The third and fourth metatarsal shafts show cortical demineralization with cortical tunneling (*arrowheads*).

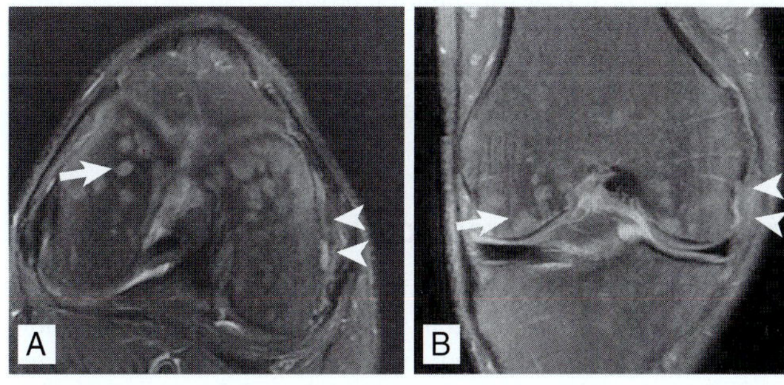

Figure 53.30 Disuse osteoporosis with medullary involvement on MRI. (A and B) Axial and coronal T2-weighted, fat-saturated images of the knee show patchy areas of increased signal intensity from disuse osteoporosis (*arrows*). The patient had a previous sprain of medial collateral ligament, which is thickened with intermediate signal intensity (*arrowheads*).

Complex Regional Pain Syndrome

The current terminology of complex regional pain syndrome (CRPS) comes from a special task force of the International Association of the Study of Pain in 1994. Previous names for this entity include reflex sympathetic dystrophy, Sudeck atrophy, and algodystrophy [17].

Although the pathogenesis is not fully understood, the most widely accepted theory involves an abnormal neural reflex pathway, which leads to muscle atrophy and increased vascularity. The main clinical findings include pain, which may be severe, and

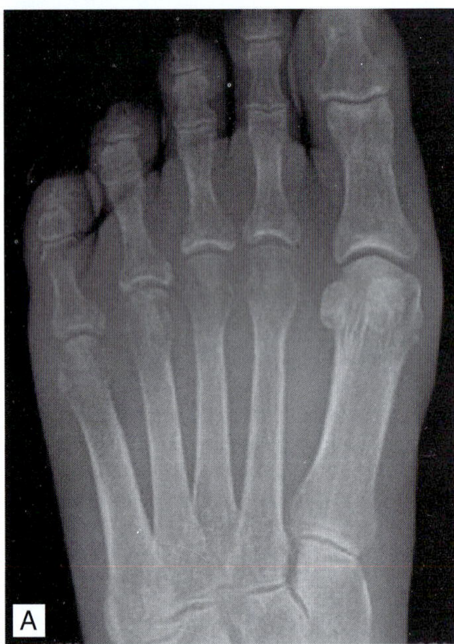

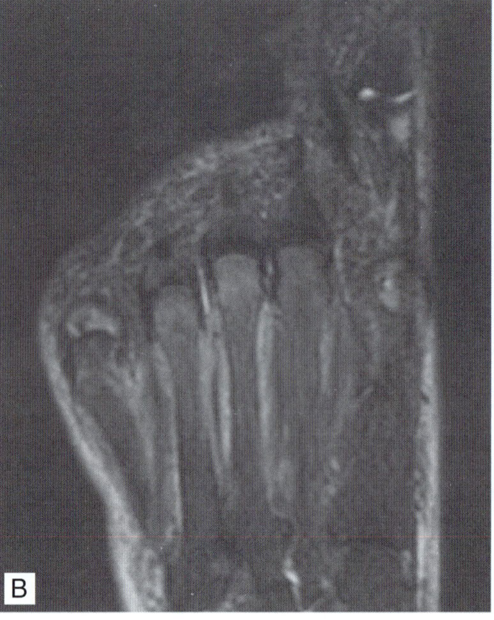

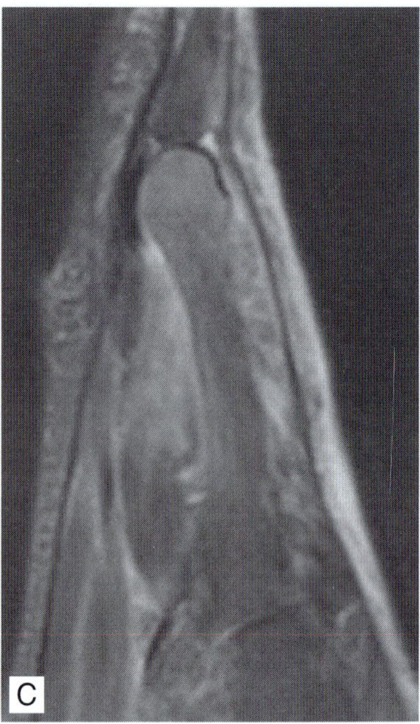

Figure 53.31 Complex regional pain syndrome (CRPS). A 70-year-old woman presents to podiatrist with dorsal foot pain. She reports "stubbing" her fifth toe previously. (A) Frontal radiograph of the foot shows osteopenia, which is most pronounced in the second to fifth metatarsal heads and necks. (B) Long-axis short-tau inversion recovery (STIR) MR image shows varying degrees of edema-like signal throughout the second to fifth metatarsal heads and necks. The intrinsic musculature of the foot has increased signal intensity within it. (C) Sagittal T2-weighted, fat-saturated MR image shows similar osseous findings. There is a small metatarsophalangeal joint effusion, and the skin is thickened and edematous. Although the MR images are nonspecific, they exclude a stress fracture and help confirm the clinical suspicion of CRPS.

atrophic skin changes. CRPS tends to occur after trauma, with or without a fracture, but may also follow infection, degenerative disease of the cervical spine, central nervous system abnormality, or peripheral neuropathy.

Diffuse osteopenia is the most characteristic radiographic finding, which is often most pronounced in a periarticular distribution (Fig. 53.31A). There is often thinning of the cortices with subperiosteal, intracortical, and endosteal bone resorption. A metaphyseal band of resorption can occur. The findings overlap with disuse osteoporosis, but osteopenia occurs more rapidly with CRPS. Juxtacortical or subchondral erosions may be present with CRPS. In the early stages, MR imaging findings include periarticular marrow edema, soft-tissue edema, joint effusion, skin enhancement (Fig. 53.31B and C). In more advanced stages, muscle atrophy may be present.

Transient Osteoporosis of the Hip

TOH is a type of transient regional osteoporosis, which was first described in pregnant women in their third trimester. TOH is now more frequently encountered in middle-aged men. Pain occurs spontaneously and can be unilateral or bilateral. In women, the left hip is more frequently involved. Pain tends to progress over a few weeks and is aggravated by weight-bearing. The clinical findings usually regress over months. By 2–6 months, the limp resolves, and joint motion is restored. The pathogenesis is not completely understood. In many cases, a subchondral insufficiency fracture can be identified on MRI, which suggests fracture as the etiology. TOH, however, can be bilateral or migrate to other joints, suggesting additional factors, such as self-limiting ischemia or disruption in the neural reflex pathway may contribute to the etiology.

On radiographs, there is marked osteoporosis of the femoral head but no subchondral collapse. Joint space is usually preserved. On occasion, patients present with the symptoms of TOH but show no radiographic findings. *On MRI, if there is edema-like signal throughout the femoral head without a subchondral insufficiency fracture, then a diagnosis of transient bone marrow edema is more appropriate* (Fig. 53.32A–F) [18].

Regional Migratory Osteoporosis

RMO is a type of transient regional osteoporosis that migrates between joints, typically the knee, ankle, or foot. Middle-aged men are affected the most. The symptoms develop rapidly with severe pain and swelling of the affected joint. Similar to TOH, the pain usually decreases over time and completely resolves by 6–9 months. *RMO differs from TOH because the symptoms migrate and affect a different joint in the same extremity or contralateral side.* With the migration, contiguous joints are usually involved, and more than one joint can be symptomatic at any given time. Although not fully understood, the pathogenesis for RMO is likely related to CRPS and TOH [18].

The radiographic findings develop several weeks after the onset of symptoms with the hallmark finding of severe regional osteopenia. The joint spaces are maintained. On MRI, the affected joint has an edema-like signal throughout the marrow and a reactive effusion is often present (Fig. 53.33A–C). Similar to TOH, patients can have MRI findings without any radiographic findings. In these cases, transient marrow edema syndrome is the preferred terminology.

Periarticular Osteoporosis With Arthritis

Periarticular osteoporosis occurs in the early stages of rheumatoid arthritis and can advance into the adjacent diaphysis over time (Fig. 53.34A and B). *Although this type of osteoporosis is most frequently described in rheumatoid arthritis, it can be seen with other types of inflammatory arthritides* [19]. The osteoporosis occurs from osteoclast resorption of the subchondral trabecular

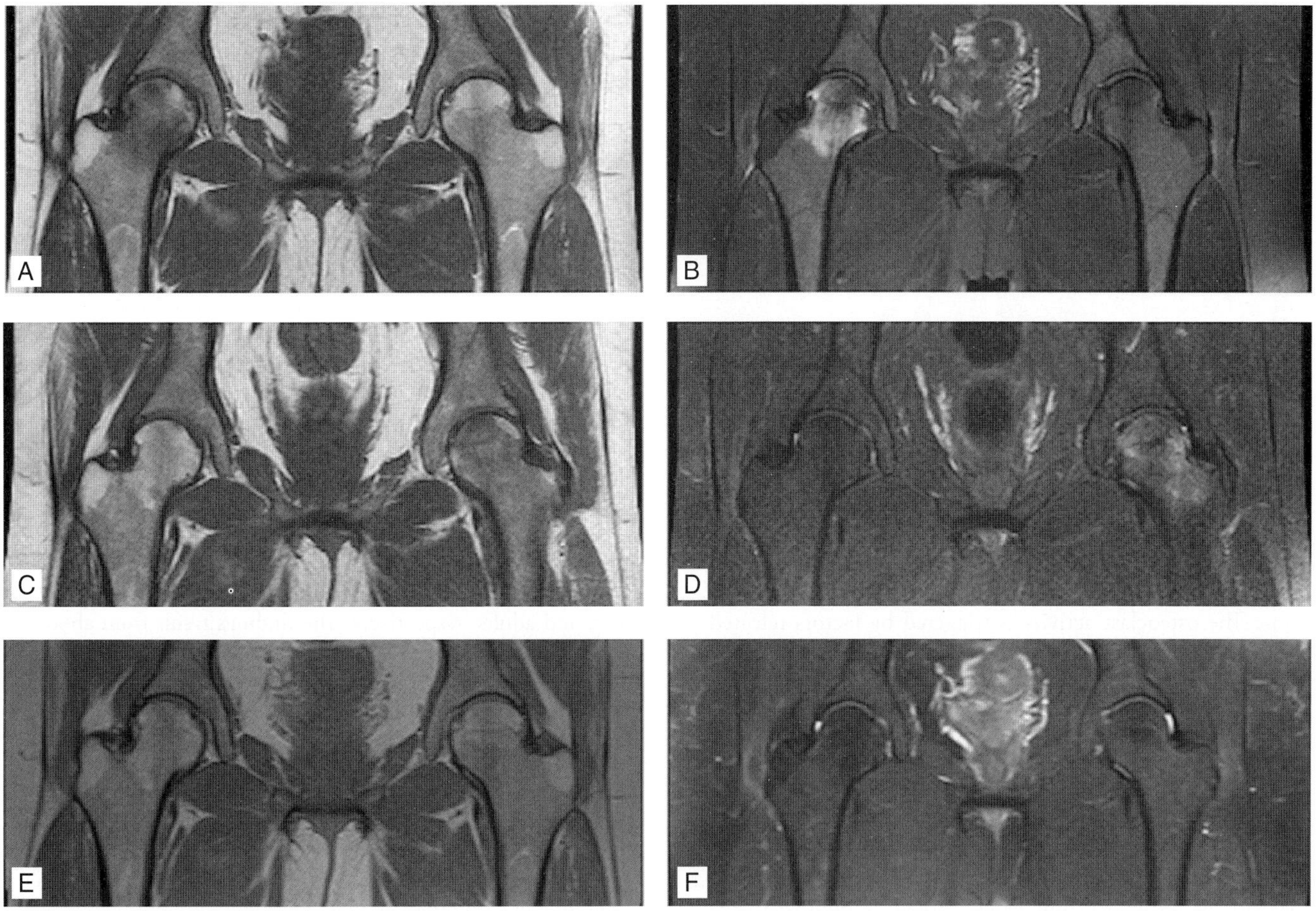

Figure 53.32 Transient bone marrow edema syndrome. A 41-year-old woman presents with right hip pain. Initial radiographs were normal. No trauma, signs of infection, or risk factors for osteonecrosis. (A and B) Coronal large field-of-view T1- and T2-weighted images of the pelvis show diffuse low signal intensity in the right femoral head and neck on the T1-weighted image and diffuse increased signal intensity in the right femoral head and neck on the T2-weighted, fat-saturated image. Patient is treated conservatively. Her pain resolves in the right hip, but it migrates to the left side. (C and D) Follow-up MRI in 8 months is normal on the right side with low T1, high T2 signal in the left femoral head and neck. Again, the patient is treated conservatively, and the pain improves. (E and F) Follow-up MRI in 4 months (12 months after the original) is normal. On each study, a small field-of-view was obtained for each symptomatic hip to exclude a subchondral insufficiency fracture.

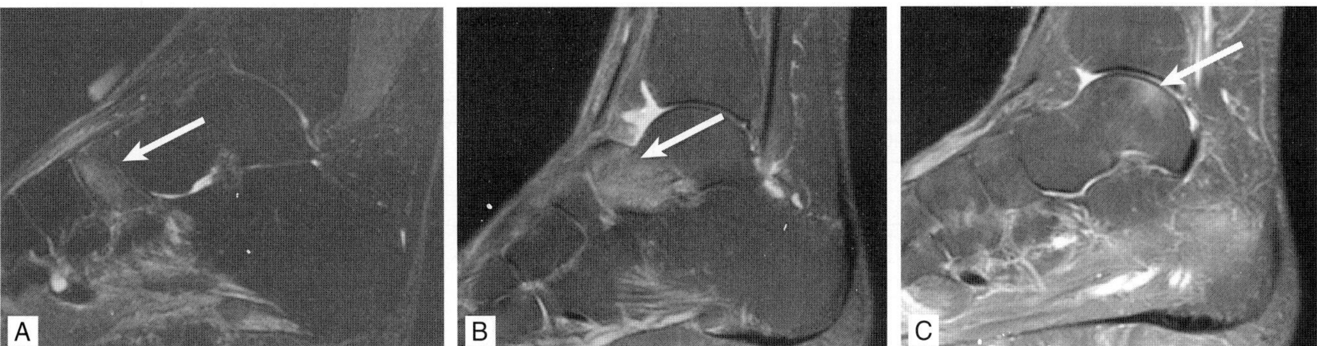

Figure 53.33 Regional migratory osteoporosis (RMO). A 48-year-old woman presents initially with left ankle pain. No trauma. (A) Sagittal STIR MR image of the left foot shows diffuse increased signal intensity in the navicular (*arrow*), concerning for a stress reaction. She was treated conservatively, and the pain resolved. She returned several months later with pain in the contralateral right ankle. (B) Sagittal T2-weighted, fat-saturated image of the right ankle shows edema within the talar head and neck (*arrow*) without a fracture. A moderate-sized tibiotalar joint effusion is present. Again, she was treated conservatively and returns for a final MR of her right ankle to reassess the talar head. (C) Sagittal T2-weighted, fat-saturated image of the ankle shows resolution of the edema in the talar head but new, patchy areas of edema-like signal in the talar dome (*arrow*) and the posterior calcaneus (not shown). A small reactive joint effusion is present. Each finding is nonspecific in isolation, but the migratory pattern combined with the clinical picture suggests RMO.

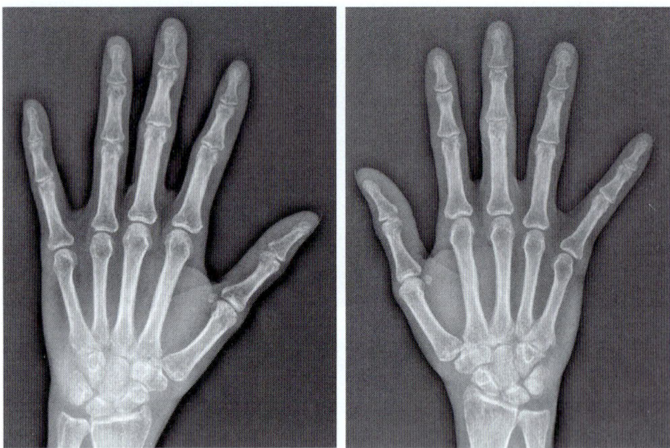

Figure 53.34 Periarticular osteoporosis. A 43-year-old man with recently diagnosed rheumatoid arthritis. Bilateral radiographs of the hands show diffuse periarticular osteopenia, which is most pronounced at the metacarpophalangeal joints. There are no erosions.

bone. The osteoclast activity is triggered by factors released by the inflamed synovium around the joint. Disuse of the joint may also be a contributing factor to the regional osteoporosis.

Biochemistry of Bone Metabolism

Serum calcium homeostasis is regulated by feedback pathways that involve the kidneys, intestines, and bones (Fig. 53.35). The bones, which contain 99% of the calcium in the human body, serve as a calcium and phosphorous reservoir that regulates the majority of serum calcium levels. Stored as hydroxyapatite in bone, calcium is exchanged with the extracellular space to maintain homeostasis. Hypocalcemia triggers the secretion of parathyroid hormone (PTH), which works to elevate serum calcium levels. Vitamin D is also an integral part of calcium homeostasis. Vitamin D has a prohormone form (cholecalciferol), which is derived from the diet and the action of ultraviolet light on the skin. Cholecalciferol is first hydroxylated in the liver to 25-hyroxycholecalciferol (25-HCC) and then hydroxylated in the kidney to the active form of 1,25-dihydroxcholecalciferol (1,25-DHCC). In the kidney, PTH stimulates the synthesis of 1-α-hydroxylase, required to produce 1,25-DHCC.

Bone homeostasis is maintained by two effects of 1,25-DHCC: (1) mobilization of calcium and phosphorous and (2) promotion of mineralization and maturation of organic matrix. The former increases osteoclastic activity and requires the presence of both 1,25-DHCC and PTH. In the intestine, 1,25-DHCC is the primary mediator of calcium and phosphorous absorption. In the kidneys, 1,25-DHCC and PTH enhance calcium reabsorption in the distal convoluted tubules. 1,25-DHCC self regulates by suppressing PTH secretion and suppressing the conversion of 25-HCC to 1,25-DHCC in the kidney. Finally, there are receptors in other organs, particularly the pituitary, placenta, and breast, which help regulate the increased demand for calcium during growth, pregnancy, and lactation.

Rickets and Osteomalacia

Rickets and osteomalacia are the same disorder, occurring in children and adults, respectively. The findings result from abnormal mineralization of the growth plate in the developing skeleton or abnormal mineralization of osteoid in the mature skeleton [7]. Based on bone homeostasis, the etiologies can be classified into two broad categories: low calcium (calcipenic) state or low phosphorous (phosphopenic) state.

Vitamin D deficiency or resistance may lead to a calcipenic state. It can occur for multiple reasons, including nutritional deficiency, malabsorption, hydroxylation defects in the liver or kidney, and various drugs. A nutritional deficiency occurs when a poor diet is combined with low exposure to ultraviolet light. When there is adequate ultraviolet light, the body can typically generate sufficient vitamin D.

Malabsorption states, including Crohn's disease and celiac disease, can result in rickets and osteomalacia. In celiac disease, the small bowel is less responsive to the action of vitamin D in calcium transport. Liver disease (ductal or hepatocellular) and renal disorders can result in rickets and osteomalacia through defective

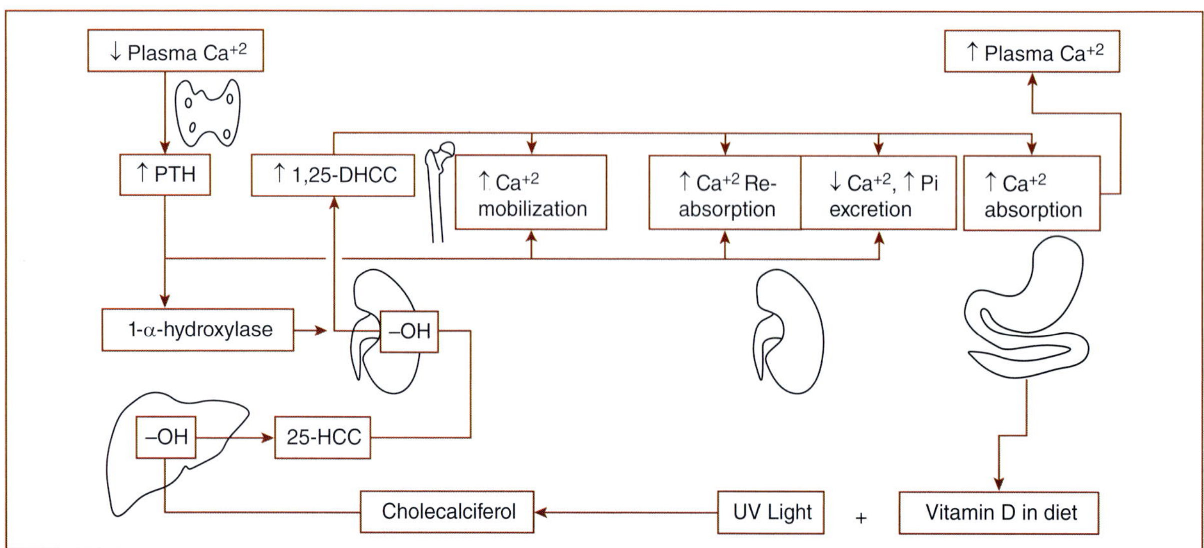

Figure 53.35 Biochemistry of bone metabolism. The diagram shows the pathways between the parathyroid glands, kidneys, intestines, and bones to maintain calcium homeostasis and vitamin D metabolism. The role of the liver and intestines are also shown. *Ca*$^{+2}$, calcium; *DHCC*, dihydroxycholecalciferol; *HCC*, hydroxycholecalciferol; *–OH*, hydroxylation; *Pi*, phosphate; *PTH*, parathyroid hormone.

vitamin D metabolism. With biliary disease, there will be malabsorption of vitamin D in the intestine. Hepatocellular disease interferes with the hydroxylation of cholecalciferol, and renal disease disrupts the hydroxylation of 25-hydroxycholecalficerol.

Drug therapy may produce rickets and osteomalacia, particularly long-term anticonvulsant therapy (phenytoin), by interfering with vitamin D hydroxylation. Many toxins have been found to cause rickets and osteomalacia by causing tubular damage and phosphate deficiency. These include aluminum hydroxide, magnesium sulfate, and cadmium, the latter being associated with alkaline battery manufacture.

Phosphopenic rickets or osteomalacia typically occur with renal tubular disorders, including X-linked hypophosphatemia and Fanconi's syndrome. X-linked hypophosphatemia, which is also known as familial vitamin D-resistant rickets, is the most common heritable cause of rickets and osteomalacia [20].

Rarely, hypophosphatemia results from phosphaturic mesenchymal tumors also referred to as "oncogenic osteomalacia." The tumors may be found in bone or soft tissues. Oncogenic osteomalacia has also been reported in association with prostatic carcinoma, lung carcinoma, neurofibromatosis, and fibrous dysplasia.

Rickets

Regardless of the etiology of rickets, the radiological features are similar, although varying in severity and location. The skeletal effects are due to a lack of mineralization of osteoid. Consequently, the most noticeable changes are at the metaphysis, where the most rapid growth is occurring [7]. The initial abnormality is a loss of the normal zone of provisional calcification adjacent to the metaphysis. The metaphyseal margin is indistinct, progressing to a frayed appearance with a widening of the growth plate due to a lack of calcification of the metaphyseal bone (Fig. 53.36A). Weight-bearing and stress on the uncalcified bone give rise to splaying, followed by cupping of the metaphysis (Fig. 53.36B). A similar but less marked finding occurs in the subperiosteal layer, which leads to an indistinct cortical margin. In particular, there is often haziness of the cortical margins in the epiphysis. Eventually, a generalized decrease in bone density is seen. *Looser zones, which typically occur with osteomalacia, are less frequent in rickets.*

With treatment, increased mineralization results in a dense white line at the zone of provisional calcification that eventually becomes contiguous with the metaphysis. In cases of intermittent dietary vitamin deficiency, or inadequate treatment, the metaphysis may show multiple regions of sclerosis.

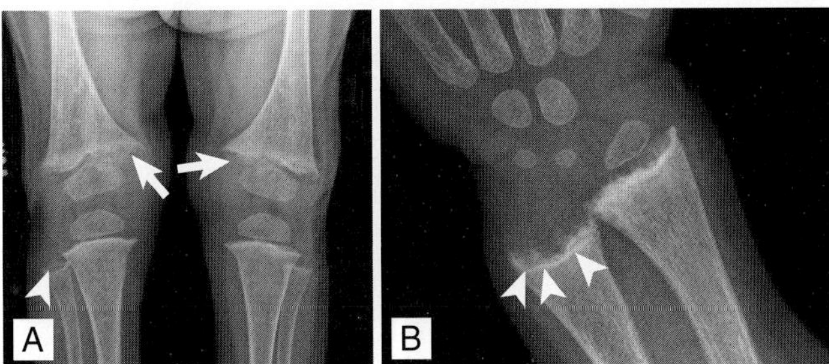

Figure 53.36 Rickets. A 16-month-old girl with rickets. (A) Frontal radiographs of the bilateral knees show widened, frayed metaphyses (*arrows*) in the distal femora. The proximal tibia and fibula show metaphyseal splaying with early cupping in the fibula (*arrowhead*). (B) Frontal radiograph of the wrist shows frayed metaphyses in the distal radius and ulna with cupping of the distal ulna (*arrowheads*).

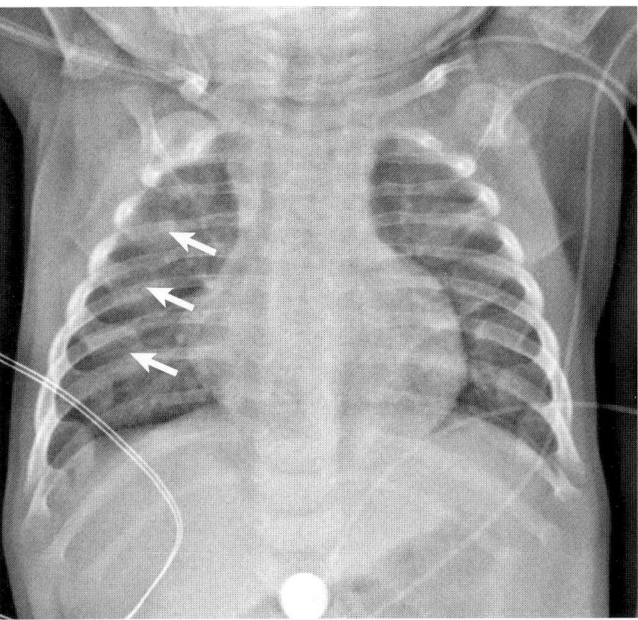

Figure 53.37 Rachitic rosary. A 5-month-old boy with rickets. Frontal radiograph of the chest shows expansion of the anterior rib ends at the costochondral junctions (*arrows*). On physical exam, this finding leads to an appearance of a row of beads, hence the term "rachitic rosary."

In severe cases of rickets, bone deformities are common: bowing of the long bones, especially the lower limbs, thoracic kyphosis with a pigeon chest, enlargement of the anterior ribs, causing the rachitic rosary (Fig. 53.37), and bossing of the skull. Complications of fractures and slipped capital femoral epiphyses may be present.

The differential diagnosis for rickets includes hypophosphatasia and Schmid metaphyseal chondroplasia (SMCD). *With hypophosphatasia, serum alkaline phosphatase levels will be low, whereas with other causes of rickets the levels will be elevated. With SMCD, the findings will resemble rickets but result from an inborn error in endochondral ossification.*

Osteomalacia

In adults, the most common finding of osteomalacia is generalized osteopenia with a coarse, indistinct trabecular pattern. These findings highlight the characteristic histopathology of under mineralized, excessive osteoid. Bone pain and fatigue are frequent symptoms. Serum alkaline phosphatase is elevated, and serum phosphorus is low.

The hallmark of osteomalacia is the pseudofracture (Looser zone), which is usually perpendicular or nearly perpendicular to the cortical bone (Fig. 53.38A and B) [7]. With time, these zones become progressively more prominent, with sclerotic margins. They represent sites of subclinical stress fractures that are repaired by unossified osteoid. They are frequently bilateral and symmetrical, occurring at regular stress sites. Common sites of involvement are pubic rami, medial margin of the proximal femur, scapula, lower ribs, and proximal ulna.

Radiographic findings commonly encountered with osteomalacia include compression fractures of the vertebral bodies, endplate deformities, and "codfish" vertebra appearance. Bowing and fractures of the long bones (Fig. 53.38A and B) and basilar invagination can occur.

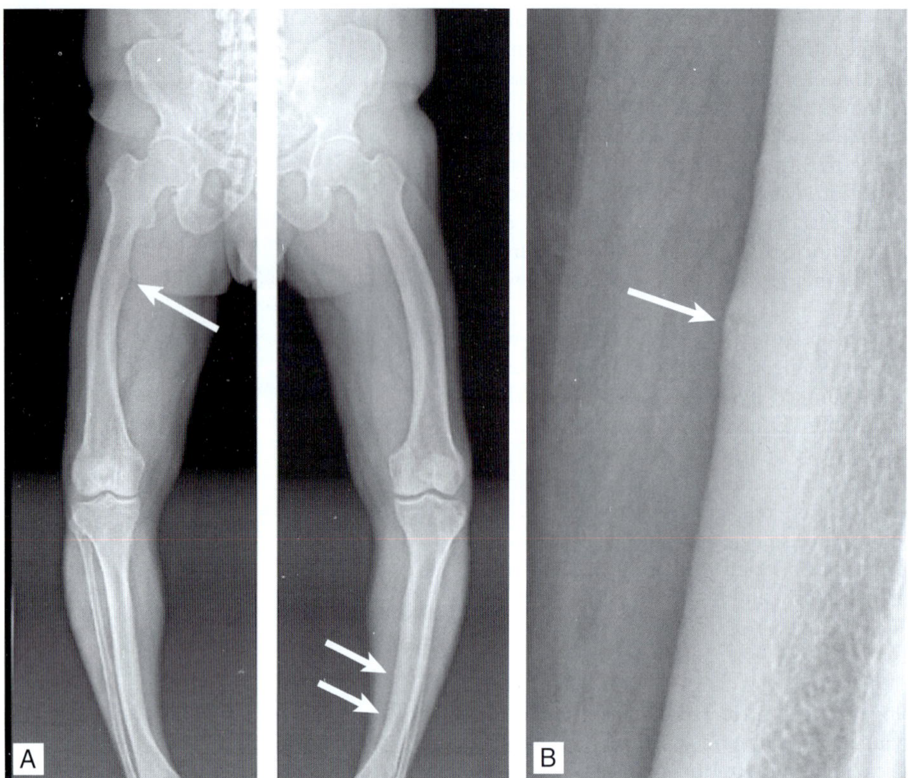

Figure 53.38 Osteomalacia and looser zones. A 39-year-old man with X-linked hypophosphatemia. (A) Genu varum from bowing of the long bones bilaterally. Pseudofractures (looser zones) of the medial right femur (*arrow*) and the medial left tibia (*arrows*). (B) Magnified view of the left tibia shows the perpendicularly oriented pseudofracture (*arrow*) with surrounding sclerosis.

Parathyroid Disorders

Hyperparathyroidism

Hyperparathyroidism has primary, secondary, and tertiary forms. In the primary form, increased hormone production occurs as a result of parathyroid adenomas (75%), hyperplasia, or carcinoma. It occurs most commonly in middle-aged and older adults and is more common in women (2:1). Symptoms may include weakness, lassitude, constipation, polydipsia, polyuria, peptic ulceration, renal calculi, or psychiatric problems.

Radiographically, the most characteristic finding is bone resorption, which can be classified as subperiosteal, subchondral, intracortical, trabecular, subligamentous, or subtendinous.

Subperiosteal erosion of bone along the radial aspect of the middle phalanx of the middle and index fingers is pathognomonic (Fig. 53.39) [7]. Other sites of subperiosteal erosion include the medial aspect of the proximal tibia (Fig. 53.40A), femur, and humerus, as well as ribs. Subchondral bone resorption is also common, typically involving the distal end of the clavicle, symphysis pubis, and sacroiliac joints (Fig. 53.40B). This type of resorption may also occur at the vertebral endplates, leading to Schmorl's nodes (Fig. 53.40C).

Intracortical bone resorption is another feature of hyperparathyroidism, resulting from osteoclastic activity within the Haversian canals. Radiographs show multiple small (2–5 mm) rounded or linear lucencies within the cortex (Fig. 53.41). The finding is not unique to hyperparathyroidism and can be seen in other conditions with rapid bone turnover, such as disuse osteoporosis, glucocorticoid-induced osteoporosis, hyperthyroidism, and osteomalacia.

Trabecular resorption presents as a granular or mottled appearance (salt-and-pepper), which is most frequently seen in the diploic space of the skull (Fig. 53.42A and B). Subligamentous and subtendinous resorption occurs at sites of ligament or tendon insertions and is most commonly seen at the ischial tuberosities, greater and lesser trochanters, inferior calcaneus, and inferior surface of the distal clavicle.

Brown tumors are focal areas of intense osteoclastic activity. They typically present as a lytic lesion, which may be expansile and lead to a pathologic fracture. The lesions are typically well

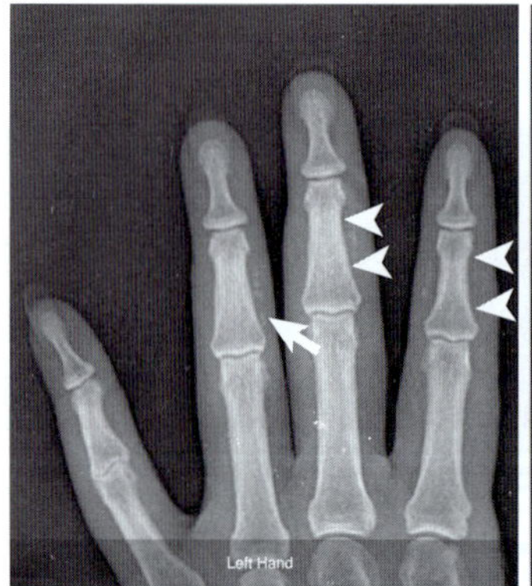

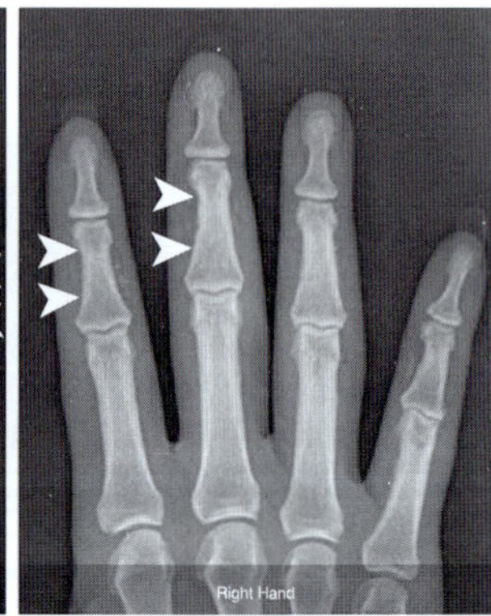

Figure 53.39 Subperiosteal resorption. A 51-year-old man with end-stage renal disease and secondary hyperparathyroidism. Bilateral subperiosteal resorption along the radial side of the middle phalanges of the index and middle fingers (*arrowheads*). Small vessel calcifications were also noted (*arrow*).

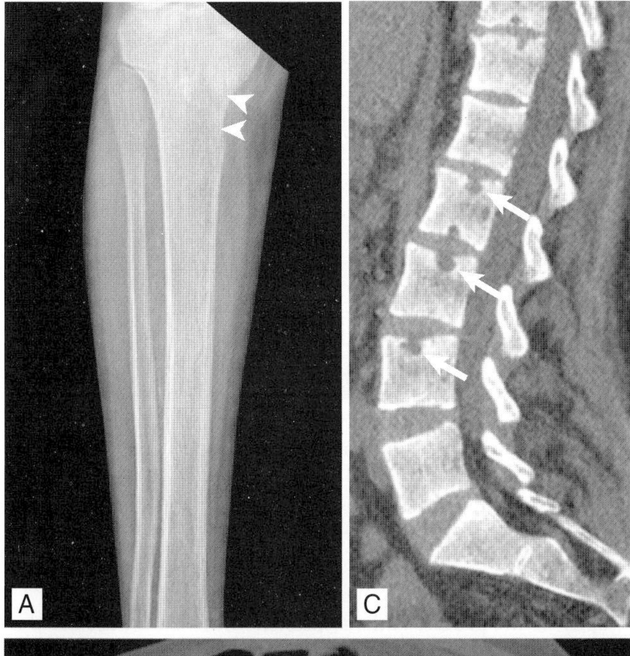
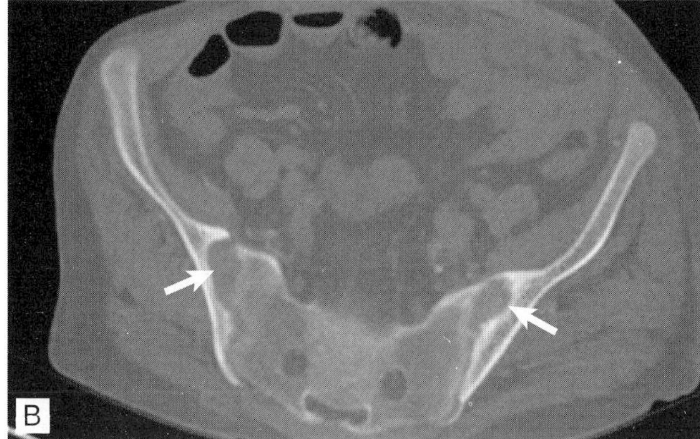

Figure 53.40 Subperiosteal and subchondral resorption. A 24-year-old woman with end-stage renal disease and secondary hyperparathyroidism due to granulomatosis with polyangiitis (Wegener's). (A) Subperiosteal resorption along the medial side of the proximal tibia (arrowheads). (B) Axial CT of pelvis shows widening and erosions of the bilateral sacro-iliac joints from subchondral resorption (arrows). (C) Sagittal CT of lumbar spine shows multiple Schmorl's nodes (arrows) from subchondral resorption at the endplates.

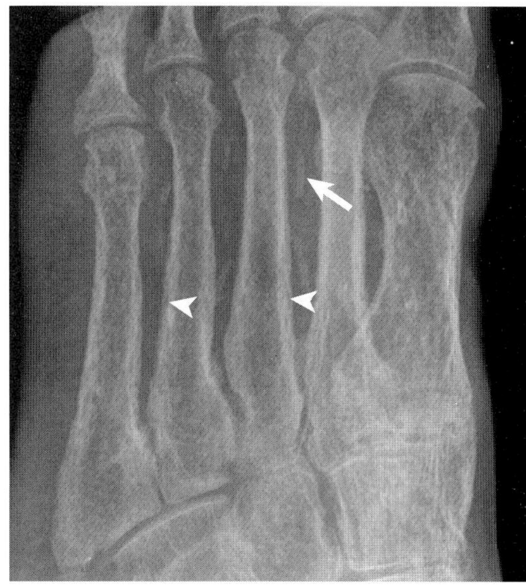

Figure 53.41 Intracortical resorption. A 44-year-old man with end-stage renal disease and secondary hyperparathyroidism. Severe osteopenia with intracortical resorption in all of the metatarsal shafts (*arrowheads*). Small vessel calcifications also noted (*arrow*).

marginated and can be multilocular (Fig. 53.43A and B). They may become more sclerotic or resolve following treatment.

Rarely, hyperparathyroidism may result in erosive arthropathy in the hands, wrists, and shoulders, which can mimic rheumatoid arthritis. Unlike rheumatoid arthritis, hyperparathyroidism usually involves the distal interphalangeal joints and often has subperiosteal resorption. Renal calculi have been reported in as many as 50% of patients with hyperparathyroidism. Most calculi are calcium oxalate, although a minority are uric acid stones. Nephrocalcinosis also occurs, but it is less common.

The term secondary hyperparathyroidism (2° HPT) is used in patients with parathyroid hyperplasia in response to persistent hypocalcemia. This response can be seen in rickets, osteomalacia, and chronic renal failure. The skeletal changes are similar to those of primary hyperparathyroidism, with brown tumors occurring less frequently. Nevertheless, because secondary hyperparathyroidism is so much more common than primary hyperparathyroidism, brown tumors are often associated with secondary hyperparathyroidism. Osteosclerosis is one of the hallmark findings of

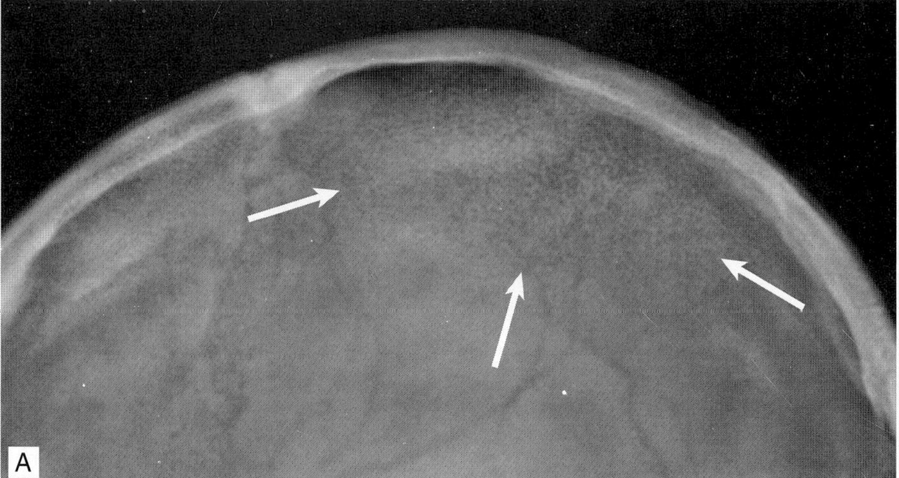
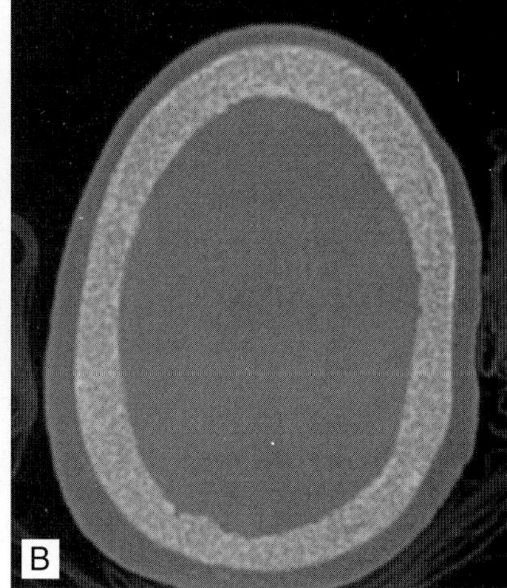

Figure 53.42 Salt-and-pepper calvarium. Two different elderly patients with end-stage renal disease. (A) The radiograph (*arrows*) and (B) the CT show a mottled diploic space, which is the characteristic salt-and-pepper pattern of hyperparathyroidism.

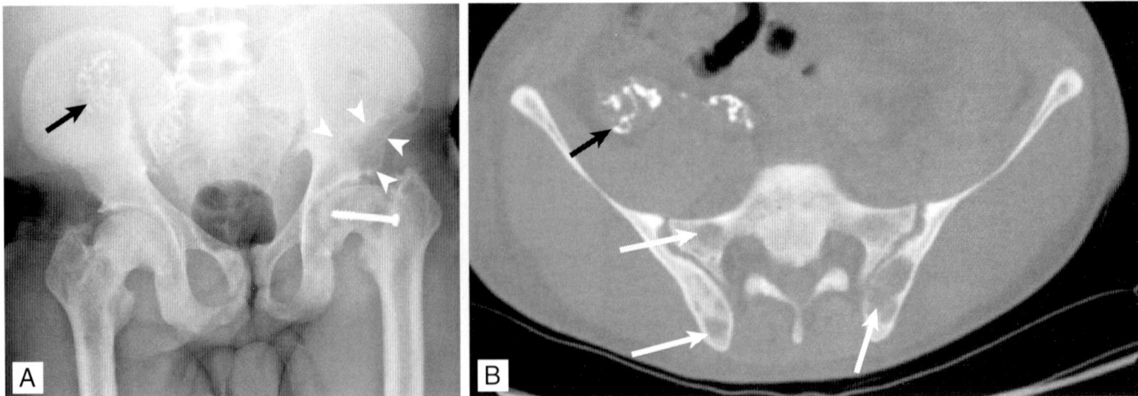

Figure 53.43 Brown tumors. A 26-year-old man with end-stage renal disease. (A) Frontal radiograph of the pelvis with multiple well-defined lytic lesions with the largest in the left ilium (*arrowheads*). These are consistent with brown tumors given the patient's history and the other radiographic findings. The bones are diffusely sclerotic with osseous resorption at the bilateral sacroiliac joints, pubic symphysis, and ischial tuberosities. Calcifications (*black arrow*) in a failed transplant kidney in the right lower quadrant and postsurgical changes from a left slipped capital femoral epiphysis are noted. (B) Axial CT of the pelvis shows diffuse sclerosis with multiple well-defined brown tumors (*arrows*). Subchondral osseous resorption at the bilateral sacroiliac joints and the calcified transplant kidney (*black arrow*) are again noted.

secondary hyperparathyroidism, which is characteristically seen in the superior and inferior margins of the vertebral bodies. These ill-defined broad bands of sclerosis produce a "rugger-jersey" appearance in the spine (Fig. 53.44). Calcification of arteries and soft tissues can occur and are typically seen with secondary hyperparathyroidism of renal osteodystrophy.

Tertiary hyperparathyroidism applies to cases where secondary hyperparathyroidism gives rise to autonomous hyperparathyroidism. Treatment of the underlying disorder fails to control the hyperparathyroidism. Surgical removal of the autonomous parathyroid tissue is necessary.

Hypoparathyroidism

Hypoparathyroidism typically occurs from the excision of or trauma to the gland during thyroidectomy. Idiopathic hypoparathyroidism, either autoimmune or familial, can occur without atrophy of the glands. Patients present with neuromuscular dysfunction from hypocalcemia. The typical radiographic findings of hypoparathyroidism include osteosclerosis, subcutaneous and basal ganglia calcification, and spinal abnormalities that resemble DISH [21].

Pseudohypoparathyroidism (PHP) is inherited in a dominant fashion and is characterized by normal parathyroid glands with end-organ resistance to PTH. Characteristic clinical features include short stature, obesity, abnormal dentition, and mental retardation. Similar to idiopathic hypoparathyroidism, PHP results in hypocalcemia and hyperphosphatemia. *Characteristic radiographic features include short metacarpals, especially the fourth and fifth, cone-shaped epiphyses, and bowing deformities* (Fig. 53.45A and B). Soft-tissue calcifications and basal ganglia calcifications may be present. In some cases, changes of secondary hyperparathyroidism may occur.

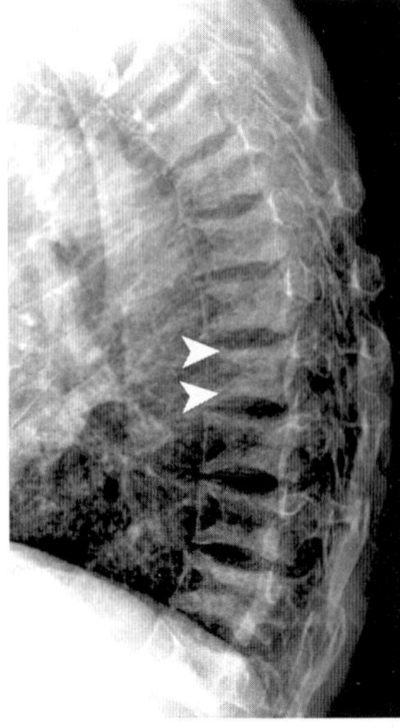

Figure 53.44 Rugger-jersey spine. A 42-year-old man with end-stage renal disease secondary to genitourinary tuberculosis. Lateral radiograph of dorsal spine shows typical end-plate sclerosis (*arrowheads*) with alternating lucent bands produces the classic rugger-jersey spine appearance.

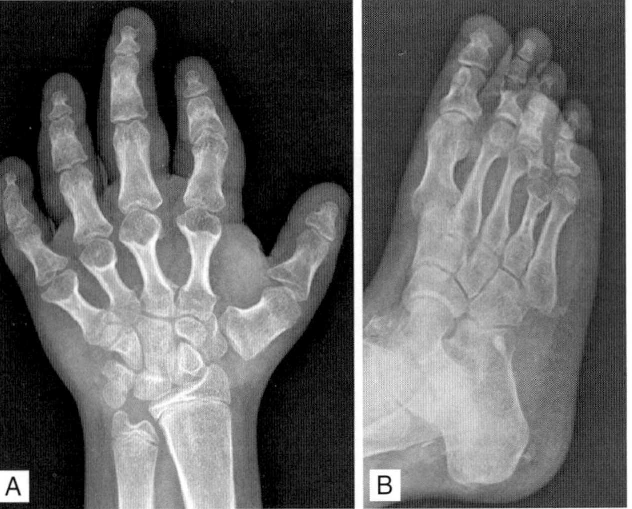

Figure 53.45 Pseudohypoparathyroidism. A 14-year-old boy with short stature and developmental delay followed by pediatric endocrinologist for pseudohypoparathyroidism. (A) Frontal radiograph of the hand shows brachydactyly. The phalanges are broad, and the epiphyses coned. (B) Oblique radiograph of the foot shows a shortened fourth metatarsal and multiple soft-tissue calcifications scattered around the ankle.

Pseudo pseudohypoparathyroidism (PPHP) presents with the same clinical and radiographic appearances as PHP, but with normal blood chemistry.

Renal Osteodystrophy

Chronic renal failure can have a significant effect on the skeletal system [22]. In children, renal failure typically occurs from a congenital abnormality. In adults, the most common cause of renal failure is glomerulonephritis. The radiographic findings are a combination of secondary hyperparathyroidism and rickets (children) or osteomalacia (adults).

The most common finding of secondary hyperparathyroidism in renal osteodystrophy is subperiosteal resorption. The prevalence of osseous resorption has been shown to increase from 10% of patients in the early stages of the disease to 50–70% of patients after 3–9 years of dialysis. Rickets is characterized by irregular, widened growth plates, and poorly defined epiphyses. The presence of Looser zones indicates osteomalacia.

Osteopenia has been reported in up to 85% of patients, likely a combination of osteomalacia, osteoporosis, and hyperparathyroidism. Osteosclerosis, which occurs in 9–34% of patients, may be the only manifestation of renal osteodystrophy. Osteosclerosis has a predilection for the axial skeleton (rugger-jersey spine), the pelvis, ribs, and clavicles. It can also affect the metaphyses of long bones and the skull.

Calcification of arteries, articular cartilage, and periarticular tissues occurs frequently in renal osteodystrophy. In fact, chronic renal failure is the most common cause of periarticular calcified masses (Fig. 53.46). The deposits of calcification can be massive, bilateral, and tend to occur around the hips, elbows, shoulders, and wrists. In the setting of renal failure, these calcified masses are best described as uremic tumoral calcinosis or secondary tumoral calcinosis. The imaging and histologic findings are identical to the familial form of tumoral calcinosis (primary).

Calciphylaxis, also known as calcific uremic arteriolopathy, is a rare condition of subcutaneous vascular calcification, which can lead to thrombotic occlusion and ischemic skin necrosis (Fig. 53.47). In the proper clinical setting, imaging can suggest calciphylaxis, leading to an earlier clinical diagnosis [23].

Tumoral Calcinosis

Tumoral calcinosis is a hereditary disease, leading to dysfunction of phosphate regulation. It is typically a diagnosis of exclusion seen in patients of African descent in the second and third decades of life. Patients present with large tumor-like lesions around the joints, which may affect mobility. Radiographs usually show large, lobulated calcified masses, fibrous septations, and fluid-calcium levels (milk of calcium) (Fig. 53.48A–C) [24]. Extensor surfaces of the hips, elbow, shoulder, foot, and wrist are frequently involved. Laboratory values will be normal, with the exception of hyperphosphatemia.

Metal and Drug Toxicity

Lead

Lead poisoning occurs in children who ingest lead-containing paint or water from lead-containing pipes. Lead deposition is most common in the growing metaphyseal regions (lead lines) (Fig. 53.49A) [25]. The width of lead lines typically varies based on the amount of lead ingested and the length of exposure time. Because lead impedes osteoclasts, there is unopposed osteoblastic activity. As a result, most of the dense bone from lead toxicity occurs from calcium deposition as opposed to actual lead deposition. *A serious complication of lead toxicity is lead encephalopathy* (Fig. 53.49B). If encephalopathy is suspected, radiographs of the knees should be obtained to look for lead lines, which are typically present.

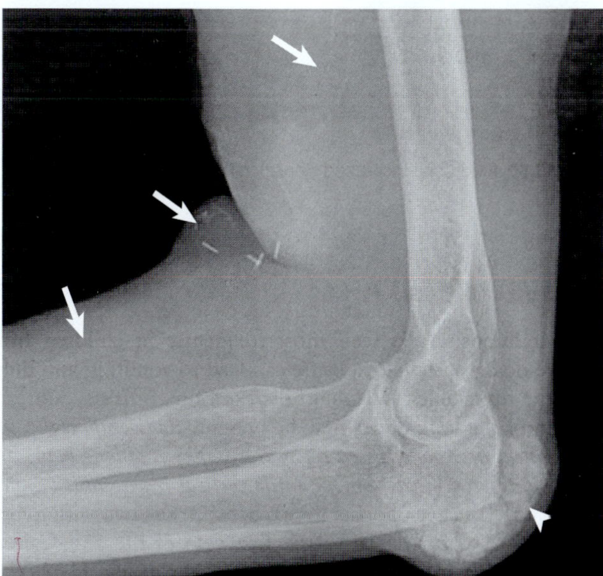

Figure 53.46 Soft-tissue calcifications in renal osteodystrophy. Periarticular calcified mass along the extensor surface of the elbow (*arrowhead*) in a middle-aged woman with end-stage renal disease. Extensive vascular calcifications and AV fistula calcification (*arrows*).

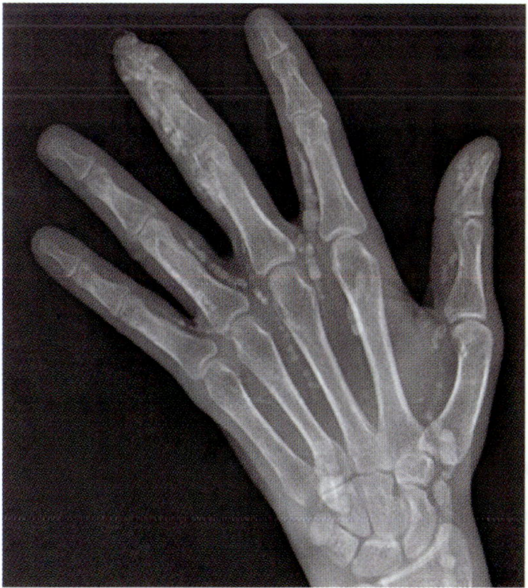

Figure 53.47 Calciphylaxis. A 34-year-old man with end-stage renal disease on hemodialysis presented with a painful, middle finger. Evaluated by dermatology for soft-tissue necrosis in the distal long finger, leading to biopsy-proved calciphylaxis. Extensive soft tissue and vascular calcification on imaging help confirm the diagnosis.

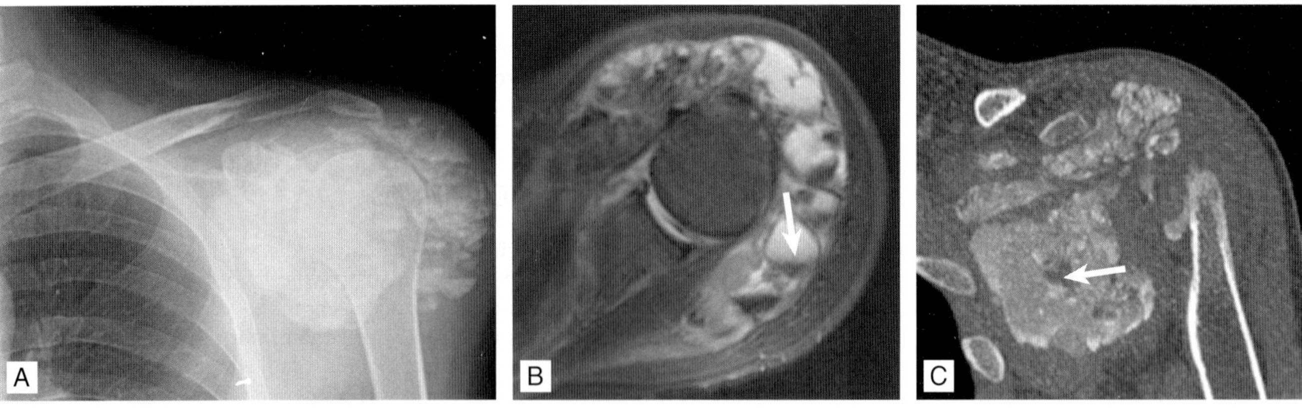

Figure 53.48 Tumoral calcinosis. A 33-year-old man referred to orthopedic oncology service for a left shoulder mass. (A) Large, lobulated periarticular calcified mass with numerous septations. (B and C) MRI and CT of the same mass show numerous septations and fluid-calcium levels (*arrows*). *MRI*, magnetic resonance imaging.

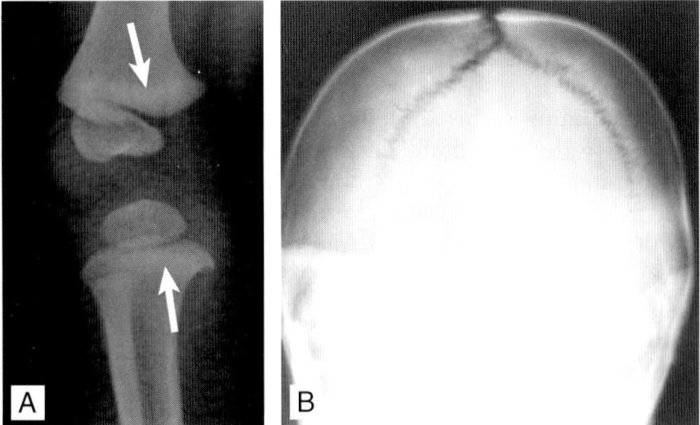

Figure 53.49 Lead toxicity. (A) Dense metaphyseal bands in the femur and tibia (*arrows*). (B) Suture widening in a patient with lead encephalopathy and increased intracranial pressure.

Fluorosis

Fluorosis, which occurs from chronic fluoride poisoning, is endemic in some parts of the Middle and Far East. It may also occur from occupational exposure in the aluminum smelting industry or from drinking water with high concentrations of fluorine. Radiographs show a generalized increase in density (Fig. 53.50), which is due to a diminished osteoclastic response caused by the fluorine rather than actual fluorine deposition. Cortical thickening, coarsened trabeculae, and calcification of ligamentous and musculotendinous attachments are key findings of fluorosis [26]. Unless the levels of fluorine are exceptionally high, fluorosis is rare in children.

Hypervitaminosis D

Excessive intake of vitamin D, which typically occurs with large treatment doses, leads to hypercalcemia and hypercalciuria. Radiographic findings of soft-tissue calcification, cortical thickening, and coarsened trabeculae may be present in children or adults [25]. In children, dense metaphyseal bands similar to lead poisoning may be present. In adults, a generalized osteopenia is more common, and amorphous, periarticular soft-tissue calcification may be present.

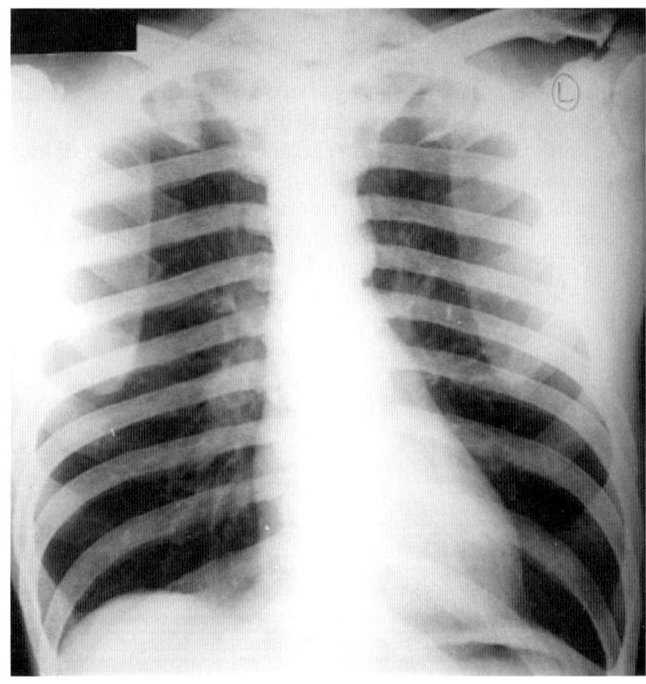

Figure 53.50 Fluorosis. Increased density of all the visualized bones.

Hypervitaminosis A

Hypervitaminosis A is seen most frequently in children from excessive dosages. Acute exposure can lead to vomiting and bulging of the fontanelles. With chronic exposure, pruritis, anorexia, and pain of the long bones may be present. *Radiographically, linear periosteal new bone is seen along the diaphyses of long bones and should be differentiated from infantile cortical hyperostosis (Caffey's disease)* [25]. The age of onset differs between the two with hypervitaminosis A occurring after the first year of life and Caffey's disease affecting infants in the first 6 months of life. Hypervitaminosis A rarely affects the mandible, which is almost always affected in Caffey's disease. Hypervitaminosis A may show additional osseous findings not present in Caffey's disease, including splaying and cupping of the metaphyses and invagination of the epiphyses (Fig. 53.51A–C).

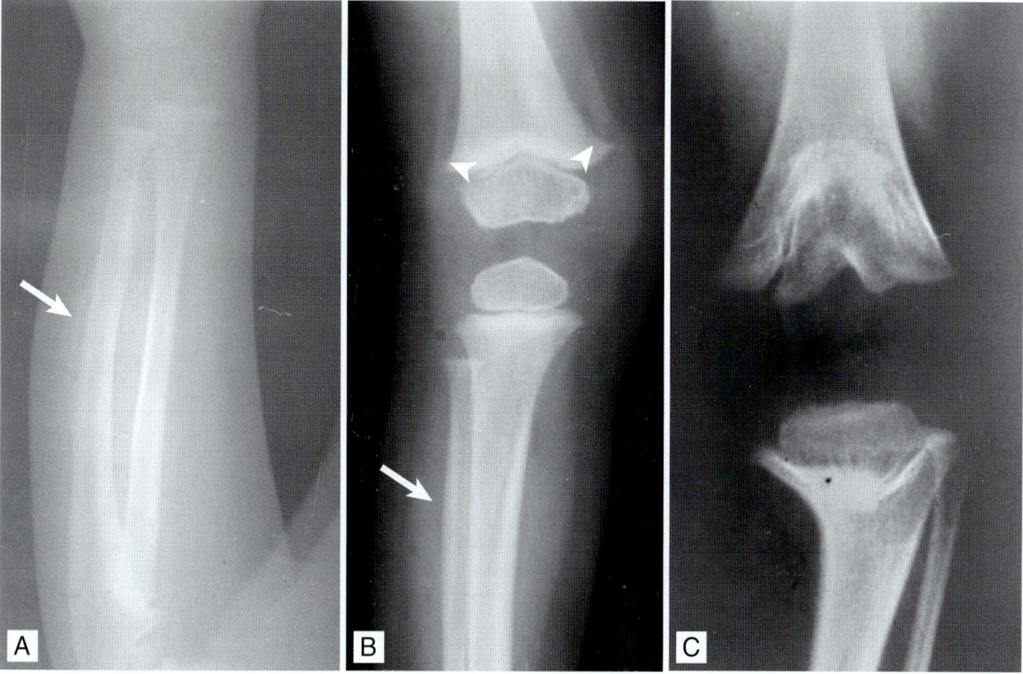

Figure 53.51 Hypervitaminosis A. (A) Linear periostitis (*arrow*) along the diaphysis of the ulna. (B) The same patient shows more subtle periostitis along the lateral fibula (*arrow*), splaying of the femoral metaphysis (*arrowheads*), and early epiphyseal invagination. (C) Different patient shows more advanced findings of coned-shaped epiphyses with invagination into the metaphysis at both the distal femur and proximal tibia.

Approach to Qualitative Imaging

The evaluation of patients with metabolic and endocrine disorders often requires an assessment with both qualitative and quantitative imaging. Qualitative imaging is critical for managing fractures and establishing a differential diagnosis. Because of their low cost and availability, radiographs should be the first study in the evaluation. Typically, the findings can be categorized as diffuse osteopenia (Table 53.8) or diffuse osteosclerosis (Table 53.9). If the findings are more focal, advanced imaging with CT, MRI, or scintigraphy can be performed to further characterize these lesions. In cases of a focal finding, infection, tumor, or fracture would be a more likely diagnosis. Because different diseases produce osteopenia or osteosclerosis through different effects on bone homeostasis, there are some key radiographic findings, which can help establish a diagnosis (Fig. 53.52).

Approach to Quantitative Imaging

The evaluation of patients with metabolic and endocrine disorders often requires an assessment with both qualitative and quantitative imaging. Quantitative imaging, which is an invaluable tool for clinical management, can help diagnose osteoporosis, assess the risk of fracture, identify patients for drug therapy, and monitor therapy. To produce an accurate report with clinically relevant information, a checklist approach can be applied to DXA interpretation (Fig. 53.53). The results should then be reported with a structured template (Fig. 53.54).

TABLE 53.8 Diffuse Osteopenia

Cause of Osteopenia	Effects on Bone	Key Findings
Osteoporosis	↓ Bone mass, normal matrix–mineralization ratio	Accentuation of vertical trabeculae in spine, compressive and tensile trabeculae in hip, and cortical thinning in long bones
Osteomalacia (adults)	↓ Mineralization, normal matrix	Looser zones, long bone bowing
Rickets (children)	↓ Mineralization, normal matrix	Metaphyseal fraying, wide physes, long bone bowing, large rib ends
Hyperparathyroidism	↑ Resorption, normal matrix, normal mineralization	Subperiosteal resorption
Neoplasm	Osteolysis from multiple myeloma or metastases, oncogenic osteomalacia	Focal lytic lesions

TABLE 53.9 Diffuse Osteosclerosis

Cause of Osteosclerosis	Effects on Bone	Key Findings
Renal osteodystrophy	Adults: Effects of 2° HPT > osteomalacia, Children: Effects of rickets >2° HPT	Rugger-jersey spine, periostitis, soft tissue and vascular calcification, osteopenia
Metal and drug toxicity	Fluorosis, hypervitaminosis A and D toxicity, heavy metal toxicity	Ligamentous calcification, periostitis
Miscellaneous	Congenital—osteopetrosis, pyknodysostosis	
	Metastatic—breast, prostate	
	Hematopoietic—sickle cell disease, mastocytosis, myelofibrosis	

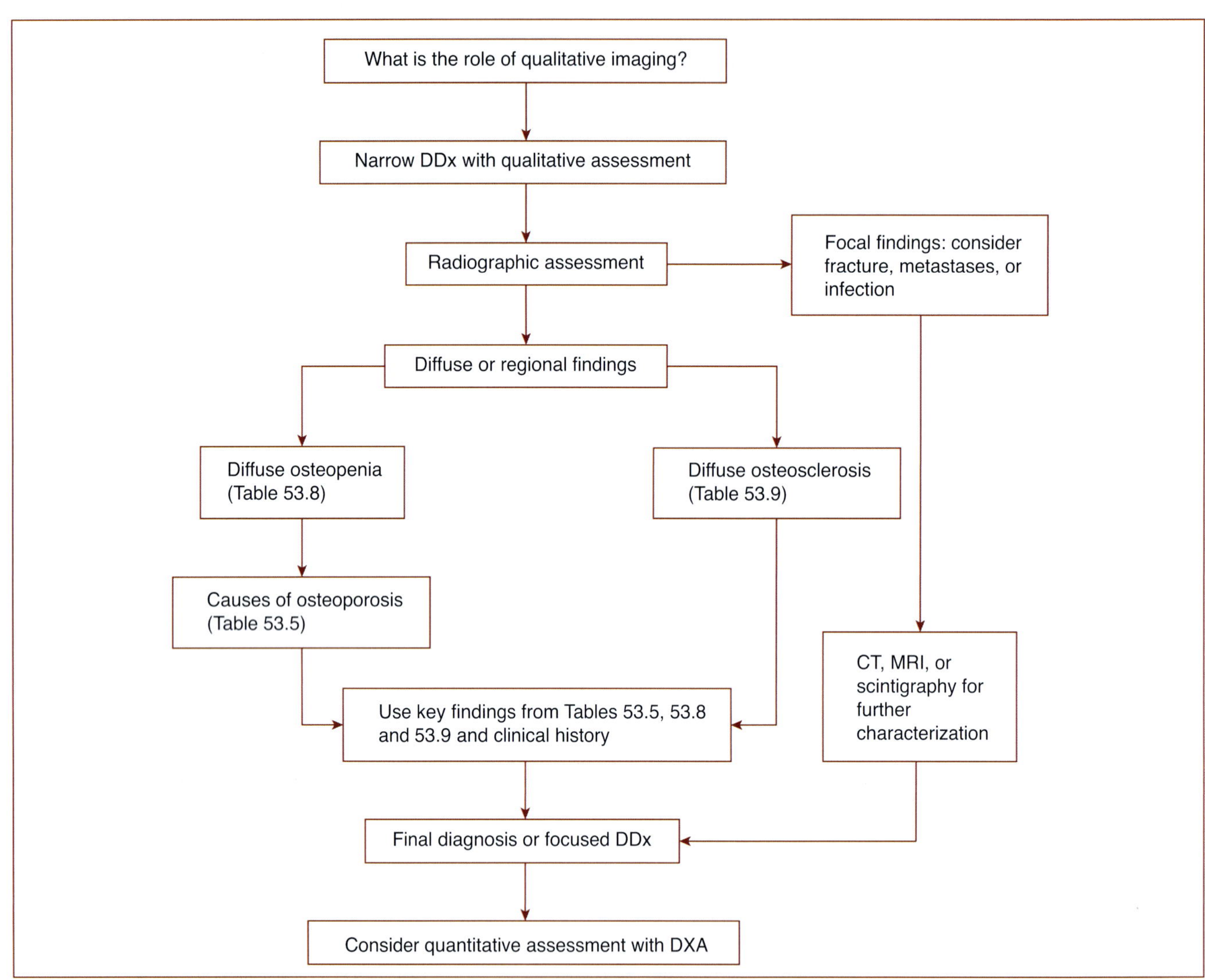

Figure 53.52 Approach to qualitative imaging.

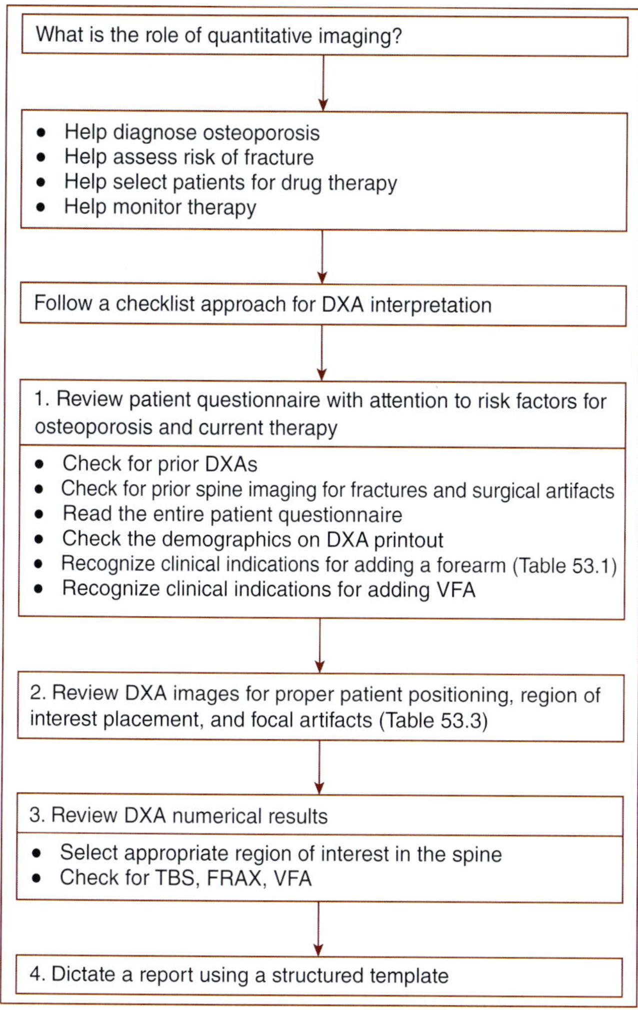

Figure 53.53 Approach to quantitative imaging.

Suggested Readings

- Y Fan, W Peh, Radiology of osteoporosis: old and new findings, Semin Musculoskelet Radiol 20 (03) (2016 Oct 14) 235–245.
- CY Chang, DI Rosenthal, DM Mitchell, A Handa, SV Kattapuram, AJ Huang, Imaging findings of metabolic bone disease, RadioGraphics 36 (6) (2016 Oct) 1871–1887.
- M Proisy, A Rouil, H Raoult, C Rozel, P Guggenbuhl, D Jacob, et al., Imaging of musculoskeletal disorders related to pregnancy, Am J Roentgenol 202 (4) (2014 Apr) 828–838.
- R Chanchlani, P Nemer, R Sinha, L Nemer, V Krishnappa, E Sochett, et al., An overview of rickets in children, Kidney Int Rep 5 (7) (2020 Jul) 980–990.
- M Sellami, H Riahi, K Maatallah, H Ferjani, MC Bouaziz, MF Ladeb, Skeletal fluorosis: don't miss the diagnosis! Skeletal Radiol 49 (3) (2020 Mar) 345–357.

BONE DENSITOMETRY (DXA)
INDICATION: Screening for osteoporosis
TECHNICAL QUALITY: Spine scan is not aligned with the scanner table.

CLINICAL HISTORY:
Age: 67.1 years
Race: White
Gender: Female
Menopausal Status: Post-menopausal
Risk Factors: Corticosteroid use for greater than 3 months.
Osteoporosis Therapy: None

TECHNIQUE: The study was performed using a [Device Trade Name] bone densitometer.

RESULTS:
Lumber Spine:
BMD measured in L1-L4 region of interest is 0.942 g/cm^2.
T-score: - 2.0
Z-score: - 0.3
Comments: Suboptimal spine positioning. Mild degenerative changes that may overestimate BMD.

FEMORAL NECK:
BMD measured in left femoral neck region of interest is 0.639 g/cm^2.
T-score: - 2.9
Z-score: - 1.3
Comments: None

TOTAL HIP:
BMD measured is left total hip region of interest is 0.697 g/cm^2.
T-score: - 2.5
Z-score: - 1.1
Comments: None

FOREARM:
BMD measured in the left mid radius (33%) region of interest is 0.697 g/cm^2.
T-score: - 2.5
Z-score: - 1.1
Comments: None

CONCLUSION:
1. Diagnosis: Osteoporosis.
2. Fracture Risk: Increased risk. FRAX is not applicable in the setting of osteoporosis.
3. Monitoring: No prior studies are available for comparison.
4. Consider repeat DXA in 1 year if the patient continues steroid treatment.

Figure 53.54 Structured template for reporting DXA results. *DXA*, dual x-ray absorptiometry.

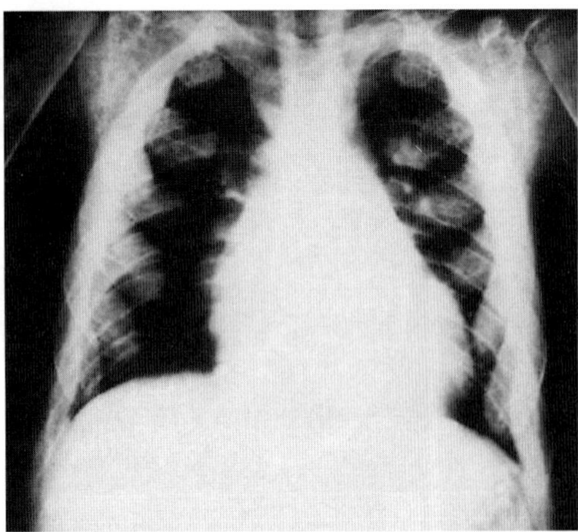

Figure 54.3 Thalassemia (boy aged 15). A chest film shows gross expansion of bone structures due to marrow hyperplasia. Note particularly involvement of the ribs and scapulae.

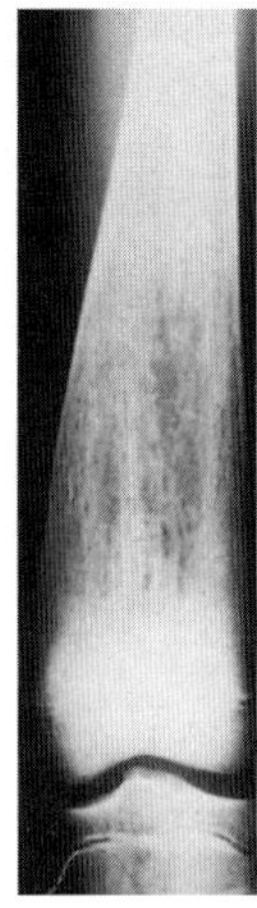

Figure 54.5 Thalassemia. Considerable marrow expansion has produced a flask shape of the distal femur. The coarsened trabecular pattern and cortical thinning are obvious.

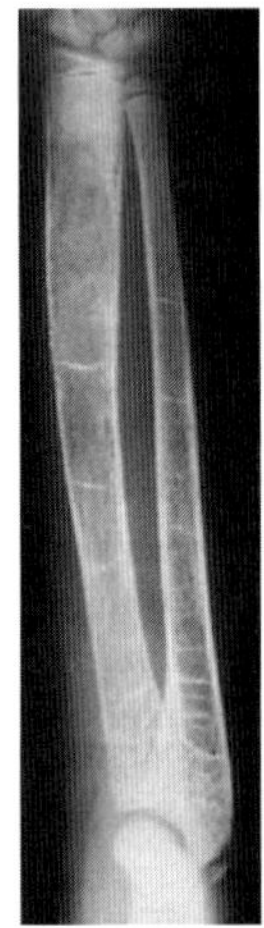

Figure 54.4 Thalassemia. Considerable bone expansion, cortical thinning, and simplification of trabecular pattern are demonstrated in the forearm of a 15-year-old boy.

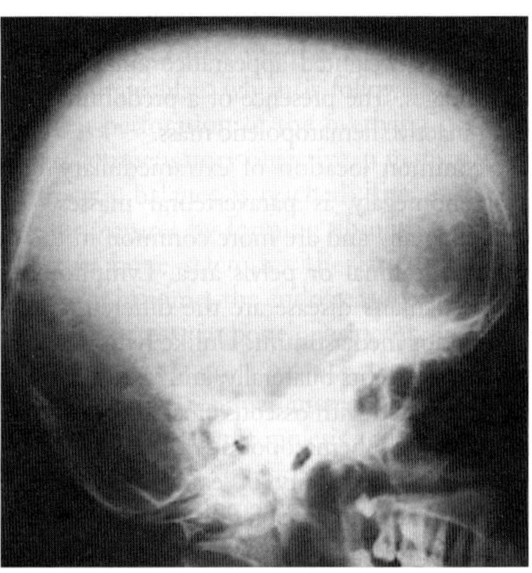

Figure 54.6 Thalassemia. Thickening of the outer table of the skull in the frontal area with perpendicular striation—"hairbrush sign."

changes result in the "classical" appearance of the "hair-on-end" in the skull imaging, distinguished by cortical erosions (Fig. 54.7). In the skull radiograph, gross thinning of the cortical bone, coarse trabeculation, and widening of marrow space are prominent features that are better visualized on CT images. On MR images, bone marrow expansion with T1-weighted signal hypointensity is a secondary finding to red marrow hyperplasia [2].

Development of the skull's air spaces, especially the maxillary and the mastoids, is impaired because of hyperplasia of the marrow, accounting for the clinical manifestation of "rodent" facies, with malocclusion.

The spine shows only diffuse demineralization with the same generalized coarsened trabecular pattern observed in the appendicular skeleton.

Although osteoporosis and osteopenia are common causes of morbidity in thalassemia major [3], vertebral collapse is uncommon. Osseous abnormalities of this type may also be observed in fewer forms of thalassemia and its variants, including those associated with other abnormal hemoglobins and the sickle cell trait. However, in all these conditions, the changes tend to be much less prominent than in thalassemia major.

Sickle Cell Disease

This chronic hemolytic anemia is congenital and hereditary in origin and results from a single gene mutation. The erythrocytes, when hypoxic, become abnormal in shape, being unusually long and slender. The abnormal hemoglobin that they contain has a reduced oxygen-carrying capacity. The disease occurs almost exclusively in black-skinned races, especially those in Central Africa or their descendants, who are homozygous for the sickling trait. This trait may be crossed with normal or abnormal hemoglobins, including thalassemia. In these crossed types, the patient is less severely affected, both clinically and radiologically.

Differentiation of the true homozygous state from the variants (combined with hemoglobin C is the most common) is of some importance. The former group's median survival age is 42 and 48 for men and women, respectively, whereas the latter may have a normal lifespan.

The homozygous sickle cell disease is characterized clinically by early onset of the severe anemic picture, with frequent skeletal and abdominal crises. These acutely painful episodes, lasting for several days, are due essentially to infarction, attributed to vascular blockage by collections of erythrocytes that have undergone sickling in areas

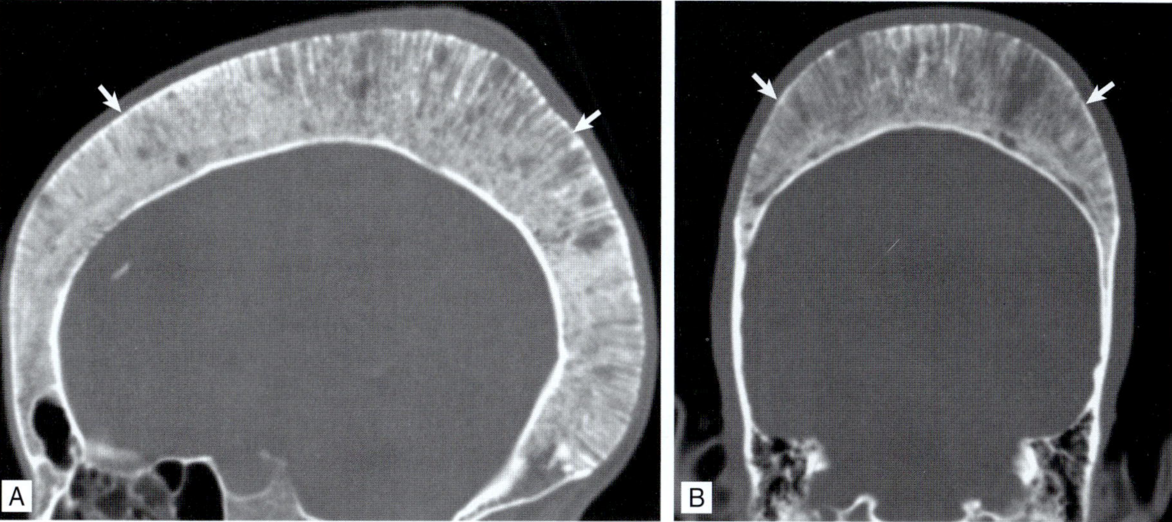

Figure 54.7 Classical "hair-on-end" appearance. Sagittal (A) and coronal (B) CT images of the skull in a patient with thalassemia major (Cooley's anemia) show thinning of the outer and inner cortical bones, coarse linear trabeculation of cancellous bone, and widening of marrow space. *CT*, computed tomography.

of capillary stasis, with resultant hypoxia. Infarcts may affect many systems. The fundamental skeletal abnormalities consist of marrow hyperplasia with superimposition of bone necrosis areas due to infarction and subsequent growth disparities. A further clinical complication is the development of infection within these infarcts, particularly in lesions developing in children's long bones.

Radiological Changes

The chronic hemolytic state is reflected by the development of characteristic and diagnostic radiological abnormalities, affecting primarily the erythropoietic skeleton and the soft tissues involved by extramedullary hematopoiesis. The frequency with which abnormalities are discovered increases with age. All variants of sickle cell disease produce essentially similar radiological abnormalities.

1. *Marrow hyperplasia* is fundamental. However, in this disease, the effects on the skeleton, which are so prominent in thalassemia major, occur in modified form, even in its worst clinical manifestations being less severe. A generalized osteoporotic appearance is evident throughout the hematopoietic areas of the skeleton, but even in infants and children, it is recognized more easily in the axial than in the peripheral skeleton. Decreased T1 signal intensity equal to or less than intervertebral disc can be diagnosed in MRI [4]. This feature is not diagnostic, but in a black-skinned child should arouse suspicion. Unlike severe thalassemia, significant modeling abnormalities are uncommon so that the air spaces of the paranasal sinuses are rarely affected. The diploic space of the skull may be widened, with consequent bossing. If a state of erythrocytic balance is achieved, diffuse trabecular thickening is likely to develop. Such an appearance may be seen incidentally in an asymptomatic adult sickle cell trait carrier. A coarse medullary pattern is associated with enlarged vascular channels in bone, especially in proximal or middle phalanges in more advanced cases
2. *Endosteal apposition of bone:* Inward cortical thickening is separated occasionally by a thin zone of translucency to result in the appearance in the long bones of "a bone within a bone" (Fig. 54.8). This sign may be observed in other conditions, including Gaucher's disease. In severe cases, the medullary

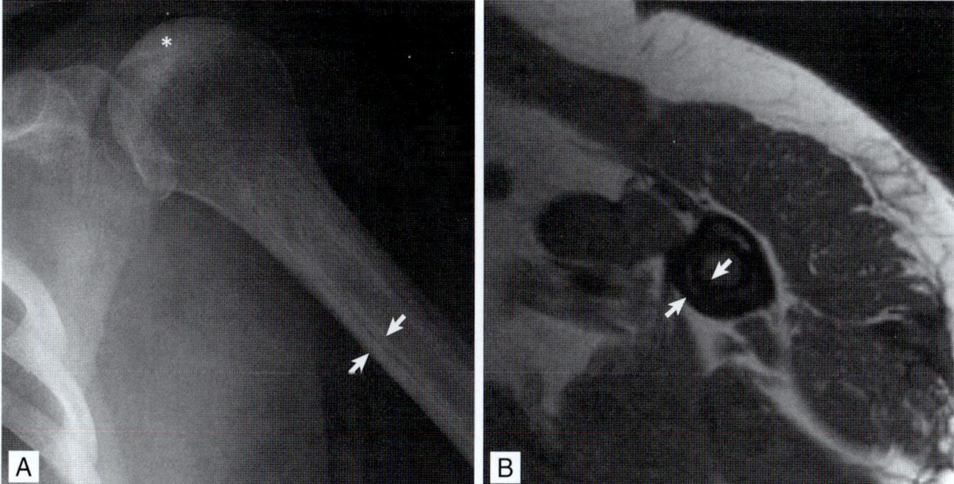

Figure 54.8 "Bone-within-a-bone" appearance of a patient with sickle cell disease. Left humerus anteroposterior radiograph (A) and axial T1-weighted MR image demonstrate separation and thickening of the cortical bone, resembling a dual layering of cortex with interposition of a thin zone without mineralization (*arrows*). Note the presence of a "snow cap" sign of the humeral head (*asterisk*), indicating avascular necrosis.

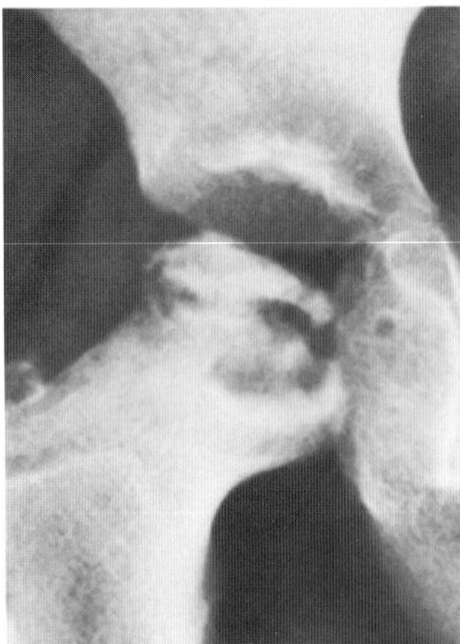

Figure 54.9 Sickle cell disease. Infarction in the proximal femoral metaphysis has produced a large defect with avascular necrosis of the femoral head. These features are similar to those of Perthes disease.

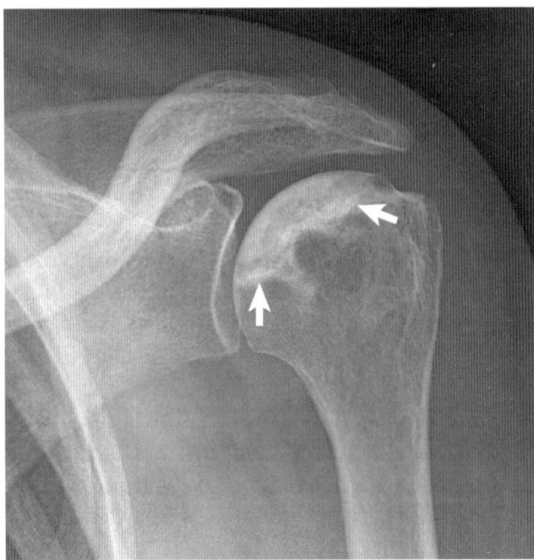

Figure 54.10 Avascular necrosis and "snow cap" sign of the shoulder in a patient with sickle cell disease. Left shoulder anteroposterior radiograph shows subarticular areas of increased density (*arrows*) indicating sclerotic bone due to recurring episodes of ischemia and infarction in the proximal left humerus.

cavities may ultimately be grossly narrowed and almost obliterated so that a diffuse and generalized increase in bone density results. This does not occur in the axial skeleton, which is a persistent red marrow area, and this provides an important diagnostic feature even in the absence of other signs

3. *Avascular necrosis/infarction of bone* provides the diagnostic hallmark of this disease. Infarction of various tissues, which results from vaso-occlusion, is considered the cause of the classic clinical episodes of sickle cell crises. Unlike thalassemia, in which infarction is virtually unknown, this type of skeleton involvement is common. The consequent radiological abnormalities are comparable to those observed in other systemic disorders such as dysbaric osteonecrosis (Caisson disease) and Gaucher's disease. Such infarcts are usually multiple and most commonly affect the humeral and femoral heads (Fig. 54.9) and medullary bone. Medullary infarcts may be of two varieties, with either sharply defined margins or producing diffuse sclerosis. In their mildest form, they may be recognized in an asymptomatic patient. The classic "snow cap" sign refers to the subarticular area of increased density, particularly in humeral and femoral heads, reflecting the revascularization of an area of bone that has been necrotic (Figs. 54.10 and 54.11). At this phase of development, bone scans are usually abnormal with increased activity. On the radiographs and CT imaging, osteopenia and progressive microfractures are the most common findings which result in abnormal sclerosis and fragmentation. On MRI, a linear signal hypointensity on T1-weighted images demonstrates avascular necrosis. On T2-weighted MRI, in addition to the linear hypointensity, an inner line of signal hyperintensity makes a "double line sign" as a clue for avascular necrosis [4]. Nevertheless, in acute infarction, a photon deficiency is often present within 24 hours of the insult. However, repairing bone is brittle and fractures easily—varying from "osteochondritis dissecans" to complete collapse

Femoral heads affected in childhood present an appearance exactly comparable to Perthes disease. In young black children, the areas with a preference for infarctions are the small tubular bones of the hands and feet, causing destructive changes accompanied by massive and painful soft-tissue swellings and periosteal reactions, which may be florid and reflect associated infarction of cortical bone (sickle cell dactylitis or "hand–foot" syndrome). These findings may indicate the correct diagnosis, but other causes of infantile periosteal reactions, such as cortical hyperostosis of the infantile or traumatic types, tuberculous dactylitis, or possibly hypervitaminosis A, may require consideration. The formation of

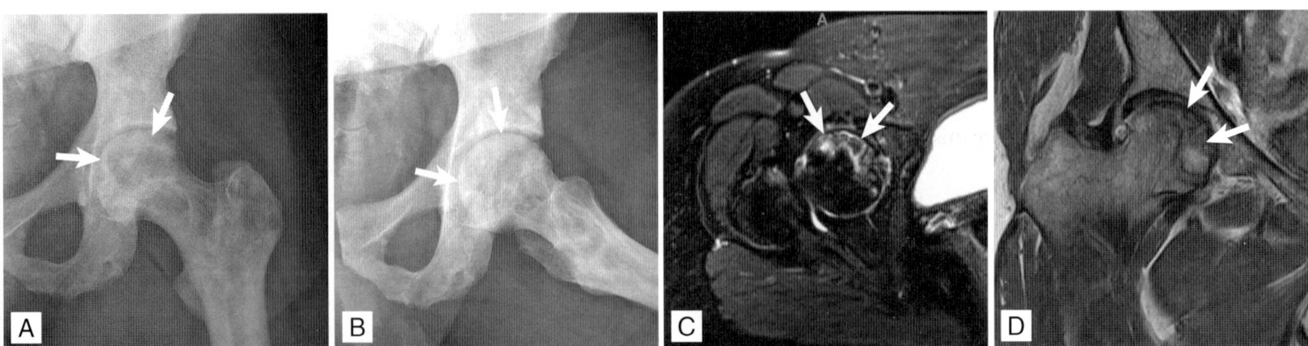

Figure 54.11 Avascular necrosis and "snow cap" sign of the hip in a patient with sickle cell disease. Left hip anteroposterior (A) and lateral (B) radiographs show subarticular areas of increased density (*arrows*), indicating sclerotic bone due to recurring episodes of ischemia and infarction in the femoral head, which is referred to as a "snow cap" sign. Right coronal hip proton-density-weighted (C) and axial fat-suppressed T2-weighted (D) MR images show the subarticular areas of bone infarction (*arrows*), which are characterized by areas of edema pattern indicating osseous ischemia and necrosis, as well as a geographic demarcation zone that has the characteristic double line with adjacent healthy cancellous bone and normal MRI signal of bone marrow.

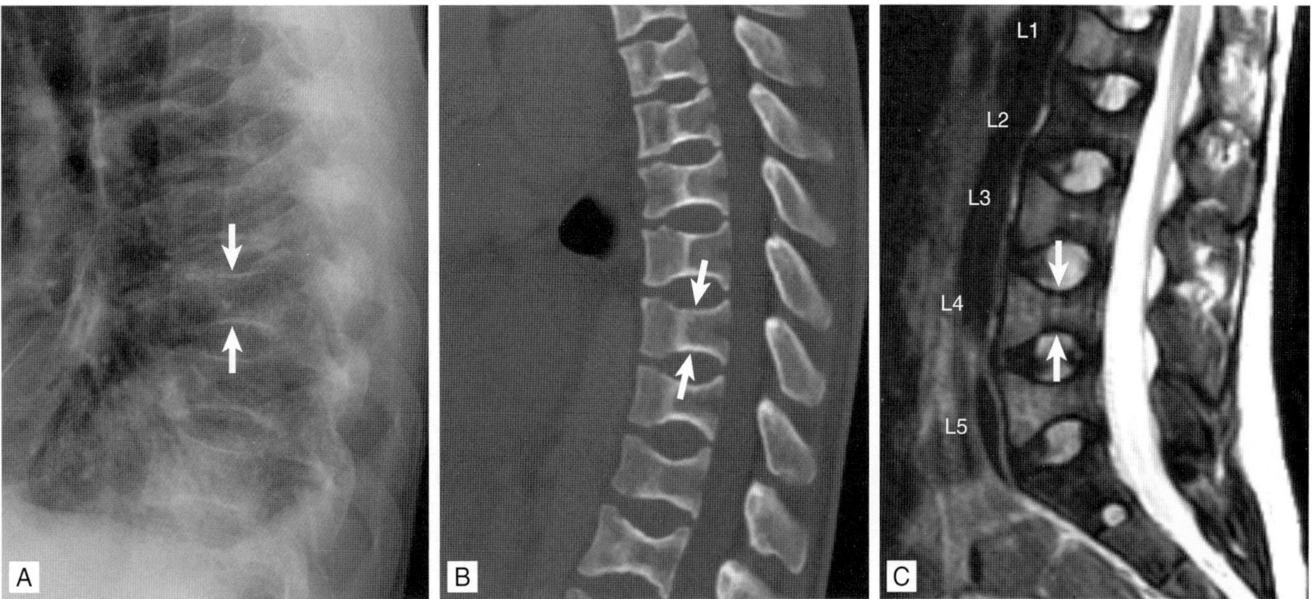

Figure 54.12 Classic "H-shaped" or "Lincoln log" appearance of the vertebrae with sickle cell disease. Lateral radiograph (A), sagittal CT image (B), and sagittal MR image (C) of the thoracolumbar spine in a patient with sickle cell disease demonstrate effects of vertebral endplate bone infarctions during development, manifesting as focal depressions of the center of the upper and lower endplates (*arrows*), resembling the shape of the letter H or a "Lincoln log," which are square-notched miniature toy logs used to build small buildings and blockhouses. *CT*, computed tomography.

perpendicular bony spicules on the skull, uncommon even in thalassemia, is distinctly unusual. More important is the possibility of a superadded infection, which is discussed later.

Infarcts of vertebral bodies are another characteristic of radiological stigma. Generalized depressions of the central portions of the vertebral end-plates are common and may be demonstrated in an asymptomatic patient. The depressions are often concave and rounded, initially simulating an ordinary nucleus pulposus impression on an already porotic bone. Infarction may be diagnosed when the center of the depression is flat and the sides slope obliquely, producing characteristic H-shaped vertebrae (Fig. 54.12). The diaphysis of the long bones, especially in the older child and the adolescent, are predilection sites for infarction. Typically, they involve the zones between the mid diaphysis and the metaphysis, the so-called "intermediate fifths." When the metaphysis is involved, significant deformities may occur due to growth arrest.

Central metaphyseal defects and lucencies are typical. These, in turn, may produce fragmentation and deformity of the epiphyses. They may also be the sites of pathological fractures. Infarcts may be massive, causing bone destruction, sequestration, reactive sclerosis, and even involucrum formation. The pattern may suggest acute pyogenic osteomyelitis.

Superimposed infection/secondary osteomyelitis: The areas of bone necrosis caused by infarction are especially susceptible to infection, classically by salmonella organisms of the paratyphoid B group. Differentiation between the pure infarct and those infected in this way may be extremely difficult both radiologically and pathologically since cultures are often sterile. Such lesions are liable to occur, especially in the tubular bones of the hands (Fig. 54.13) and feet in infants and the long bones (Fig. 54.14) and the spine of older children.

In the adult, septic arthritis may be superimposed on an adjacent infarct. Radiographs are mostly normal, and CT shows a different marrow density between the normal bone marrow and the infection. However, MRI has high sensitivity and specificity for the diagnosis of osteomyelitis. Bone marrow hypointensity on T1-weighted and hyperintensity on T2-weighted images are in

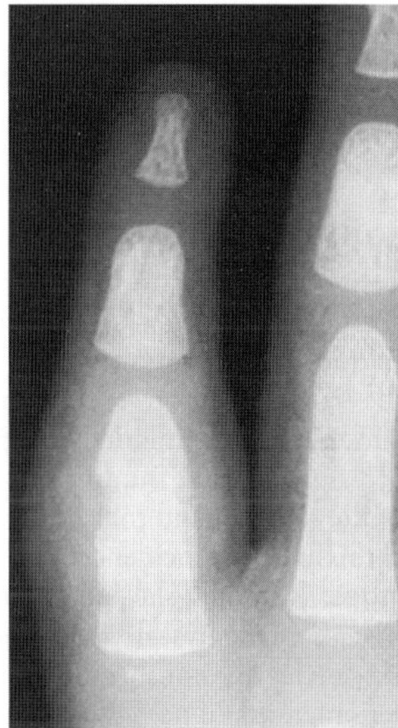

Figure 54.13 Sickle cell disease. Soft-tissue swelling surrounds an expanded proximal phalanx. Medullary expansion is present with simplification of trabecular pattern and penetration of the cortex. The distinction between these changes and osteomyelitis is extremely difficult.

favor of the diagnosis of osteomyelitis. With appropriate treatment, either by conservative antibiotic therapy or by active surgical measures, including sequestrectomy, healing usually occurs with remarkable rapidity.

Soft-tissue involvement may be seen in other chronic hemolytic anemias and such disorders of the marrow as Gaucher's disease. These may consist of heterotopic masses of hematopoietic tissue in the dorsal paravertebral areas and hepatosplenomegaly, renal papillary necrosis, or bowel infarction. Heterotopic masses of hematopoietic tissue may develop in the dorsal paravertebral areas. The release of iron pigments by accelerated destruction of erythrocytes may accelerate the formation of biliary calculi.

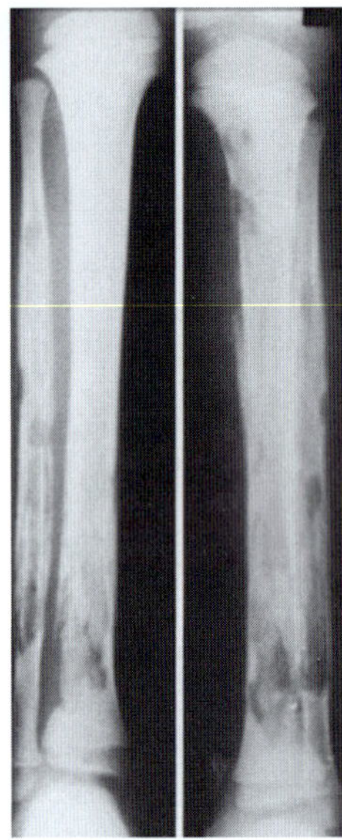

Figure 54.14 Sickle cell disease with salmonella osteomyelitis (Nigerian boy aged 4). Extreme destructive changes in the long bones have been caused by infection superimposed upon infarction. Numerous sequestra are present. (Courtesy: Mr. Geoffrey Walker.)

Erythroblastosis Fetalis (Hemolytic Disease of the Newborn)

Hemolytic anemia occurring in the fetus and newborn results from an immunological incompatibility between the mother and fetus's blood, most commonly due to the Rh factor, although other hematological errors of this type are known. The severity may vary widely, from mild anemia to icterus neonatorum and fetal hydrops. The Rh-positive erythrocytes of the fetus, crossing the placental barrier in a mother without Rh antigen, stimulate the maternal formation of anti-Rh antibodies that traverse the placenta to enter the fetal circulation, there to hemolysis the fetal red blood cells. The danger of infants being affected by this incompatibility increases with the number of conceptions, but early recognition of the disorder and the adoption of prophylactic measures has greatly reduced its incidence.

Radiological Changes: The only skeletal abnormality is the development of transverse metaphyseal translucencies in the long bones. These translucencies are nonspecific, as they may also occur with other severe maternal illnesses during pregnancy and in congenital syphilis. With successful treatment, the translucent areas ossify with residual growth lines. In the spine, such growth lines often cause "ghost shadows" within the vertebral bodies. Fetal hydrops may be diagnosed sonographically by the detection of growth retardation, effusions, and subcutaneous edema. The enlargement of the placenta displaces the fetus.

Other Chronic Anemias

Iron Deficiency Anemia

The anemia of infants suffering from iron deficiency may produces radiological changes in the skull due to marrow hyperplasia similar to those of the less severe congenital anemias. An inadequate diet is a usual cause, but malabsorption or abnormal loss of iron may be important factors. The widening of the diploic space and the subsequent bossing of the skull vault is again characteristic, but the disease has never been reported to cause changes sufficiently severe to involve the long bones and facial bones.

Hereditary Spherocytosis

This is an inherited defect in which the red blood cells are of an abnormal round shape. The anemia in which results may produce mild changes comparable to the other congenital anemias. Removal of the spleen permits the bone structures to revert to a normal appearance.

Fanconi's Anemia

This syndrome of congenital aplastic anemia with multiple congenital anomalies (not to be confused with the other syndrome described by the same author and concerned with osteomalacia and an abnormal renal tubular mechanism) is of interest in that the hematological changes are unlikely to appear before the age of 2 years. These consist of hypoplastic anemia, marrow hypoplasia, and skin pigmentation. The defect is inherited, and congenital abnormalities of the skeleton are associated, such as the deficient formation of the thumb bones, first metacarpal, and radius; other abnormalities, including congenital dislocation of the hip and club foot, short stature, and microcephaly, have also been observed. These are evident long before the hematological abnormalities become apparent, and the latter is not responsible for any skeletal abnormalities. Some cases have been terminated in leukemia.

Polycythemia

This condition is due to an increased level of erythropoietin and the overproduction of red blood cells. Although occasionally responsible for bone infarction, it produces no characteristic radiological changes in the skeleton. Transition to myeloid metaplasia is common. Pulmonary abnormalities in polycythemia may occur in the form of increased reticulation or fine mottling.

Diseases Primarily Involving White Blood Cells

Leukemia

Children are most commonly affected, almost invariably by an acute form of leukemia. In adults, the disease may also be acute, but it is more commonly chronic. Hematopoietic tissue is widely distributed throughout the skeleton of a child but is confined in the adult to the "red marrow" areas of the axial skeleton and the proximal ends of the humeri and femur. Thus, radiological changes in the bones are common in the younger age groups. More than half of the children affected show skeletal abnormalities, while in adults, these are found in fewer than 10% of cases. Although the diagnosis is usually confirmed by examining the blood and sternal marrow, bone changes may precede the development of a grossly pathological blood picture, especially in the so-called *aleukemic* type. Differentiation between myeloid and lymphatic types of leukemia cannot be made by radiological examination.

Radiological Changes

These are observed mainly in *children* and consist of the following (Table 54.2):

1. *Metaphyseal translucencies.* In children, the most characteristic sign occurring in up to 90% of cases is the presence of bands of translucency running transversely across the metaphysis (Fig. 54.15). Such bands may be narrow and incomplete in the early stages of the disease, but they may be found to traverse the metaphysis completely and be as much as 5 mm in width in a few weeks. The most rapidly growing areas—knees, wrists, and ankles—are commonly affected first, but later the metaphysis of the shoulders,

TABLE 54.2 Radiological Findings of Diseases Involving the White Blood Cells

Disease	Radiologic Findings
Leukemia	▪ Bands of translucency running transversely across the metaphysis ▪ Cortical erosion of metaphysis (leukemic lines) ▪ Diffusely scattered osteolytic lesions; mostly common in the shafts of the long bones ▪ Periosteal reaction with sunburst pattern associated with underlying bony lesions
Myeloid metaplasia	▪ Patchy or diffuse bone density increase with areas of relative translucency due to fibrosis ▪ Irregular periosteal reactions, particularly near the ends of long bones

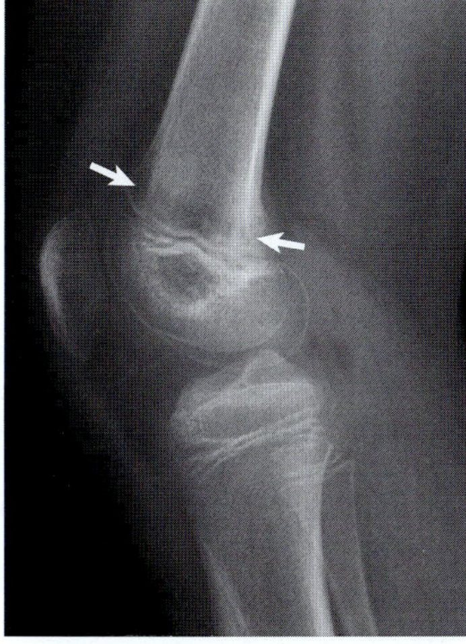

Figure 54.15 Metaphyseal translucent band in a child with leukemia. Lateral radiograph of the left knee shows a translucent band transversing the metaphysis of the distal left femur metaphysis (*arrows*).

hips, and vertebral bodies also may be involved. With treatment, remission may occur, and the bands of translucency resolve

2. *Metaphyseal cortical erosions (leukemic lines)* on the medial side of the proximal ends of the humeral (Fig. 54.16) and tibial shafts sometimes occur as an early feature. They are usually bilateral
3. *Osteolytic lesions* develop in over half of the cases. Usually, they are punctuating and diffusely scattered, although solitary and larger lesions may occur. Although such leukemic deposits may involve any portion of the skeleton, they are commonest in the shafts of the long bones. When the vertebral bodies are involved, collapse often occurs before specific areas of rarefaction can be identified. Prominent convolution marking and sutural widening can demonstrate skull involvement
4. *Periosteal reactions* are usually associated with underlying bony lesions and are distinguished by a sunburst pattern of periosteal reaction
5. *Osteosclerosis of the metaphysis* is a rare but well-recognized primary manifestation. It may develop during treatment

In *metastatic neuroblastoma,* skeletal changes take place, which may be indistinguishable from leukemia. Separation of the sutures of the skull in the former condition is a helpful differentiating sign.

In *adults,* skeletal lesions are rare. As has been stressed before, the deposits occur essentially in red marrow areas. Changes include *osteoporosis, translucent areas* of leukemic bone destruction (which tend to be oval with the long axis parallel to the shaft), and *vertebral destruction* and *collapse*. Periosteal reactions are unusual. Occasionally, generalized *osteosclerosis* of the marrow area is evident. This is likely to be caused by trabecular thickening during remission periods and may be patchy in type. However, in some instances, the leukemic changes may be a secondary and terminal process in myeloid metaplasia. On MRI, signal hypointensity in T1-weighted and hyperintensity in T2-weighted and short-tau inversion recovery (STIR) sequences, compared with normal bone marrow, are expected findings.

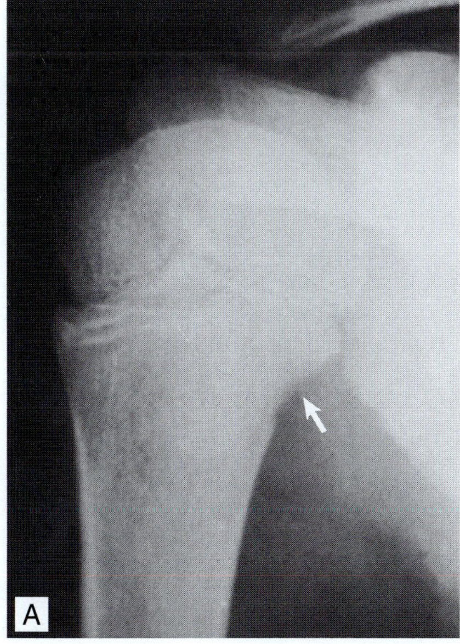

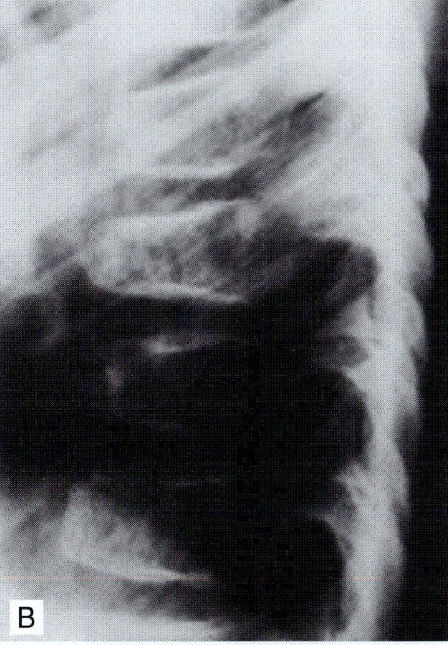

Figure 54.16 Lymphatic leukemia. (A) Erosions of the medial side of the proximal metaphyses (*arrow*) of both humeri were present in this 8-year-old child. The disease was in an aleukemic phase, not an uncommon finding even when skeletal changes are present. (B) The same child complained of back pain. Multiple vertebral collapses are shown with the preservation of disc-space height. Overall, bone density is reduced with a simplified trabecular pattern.

Myeloid Metaplasia (Myelofibrosis/Myelosclerosis)

This syndrome occurs by replacing bone marrow tissue with fibrous tissue due to an unknown etiology and is characterized by the triad of myelofibrosis, myeloid metaplasia, and features in the peripheral blood film, which simulate leukemia. The relation between myeloid metaplasia, myelosclerosis, and other diseases, including polycythemia vera and chronic myeloid leukemia, is intimate. The typical patient is a middle-aged or elderly adult, the primary disorder being metaplasia of the marrow cells to fibrous tissue. The usual presenting complaints are fatigue and abdominal fullness due to hepatosplenomegaly. Obliteration of the hematopoietic tissue results in progressive anemia, the appearance of immature red and white cells in the peripheral blood, and compensatory splenomegaly. In the later stages of the disease, the fibrous tissue becomes converted to bone, and endosteal cortical thickening develops. Polycythemia may be followed by myeloid metaplasia, and it appears probable that nearly half of the developed cases of myeloid metaplasia previously had some form of this blood disorder. Purine hypermetabolism may manifest itself as secondary gout.

Radiological Changes

In the sclerotic stage of the disease, the increased density of the bones may be diffuse or patchy (Table 54.2). Areas of relative translucency due to fibrosis may persist (Fig. 54.17). The increased density is due to new bone deposition on the trabeculae and the endosteal cortical thickening with the loss of the normal cortico medullary distinction. Narrowing of the medullary space becomes visible and resembles the later bones of sickle cell anemia in the long bones. Irregular periosteal reactions may occur, particularly near the ends of long bones. These may be well organized and continuous with the cortex or separated from it by a translucency zone. Although the red marrow areas (particularly the pelvis) are especially subject to these pathological changes, the entire skeleton may be affected. The density of the skull is associated with obliteration of the diploic space, although some persistent areas of fibrosis may remain translucent. Splenomegaly is almost invariably evident (Fig. 54.18). On MRI, T1- and T2-weighted sequences demonstrate hypointense marrow.

Differentiation must be made from other conditions causing a generalized increase of bone density. The congenital sclerosing dysplasias, including osteopetrosis, are likely to be encountered in adult life only as an incidental finding or associated with a pathological fracture. Fluorosis is likely to occur in an endemic area. Mastocytosis may cause some confusion, but the lesions are usually less diffuse and are accompanied by urticaria pigmentosa. Sclerosing and widespread metastasis, particularly prostatic, should not be forgotten.

Myelodysplastic Syndrome

Myelodysplastic syndrome (MDS) [5] is a clonal disorder of hematopoietic, specifically myeloid, stem cells, which leads to a group of hematologic neoplasms. The chance of transformation to acute myeloid leukemia increased in some of the patients. MDS frequently affects patients over 65 years' age and is more common in males. Although mostly asymptomatic, clinical manifestations resulting from pancytopenia, including fatigue, shortness of breath, petechiae or bleeding, and infection. Following the exclusion of other cytopenia causes, a bone marrow aspirate and biopsy are utilized for diagnosis. Low-dose whole-body multidetector computed tomography [6] and MRI [7] providing valuable information and are used as prognostic predictors in patients with MDS. Prognosis ultimately depends on multiple factors such as the severity of cytopenias and the percentage of blasts in the bone marrow.

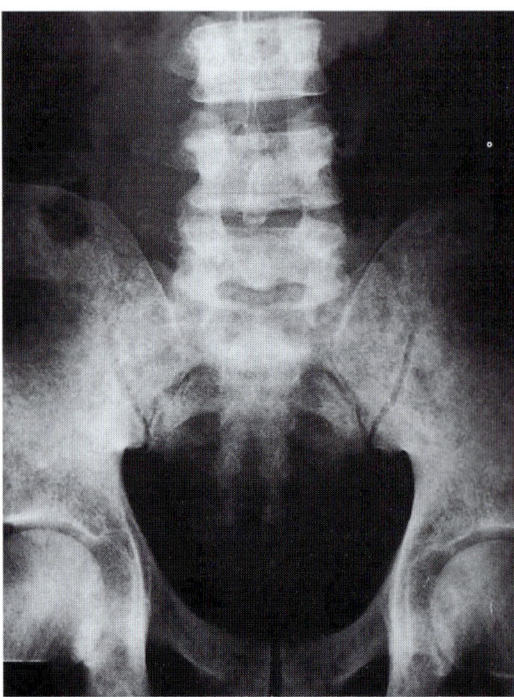

Figure 54.17 Myeloid metaplasia. Widespread but patchy areas of sclerosis are shown throughout the pelvis and lumbar spine.

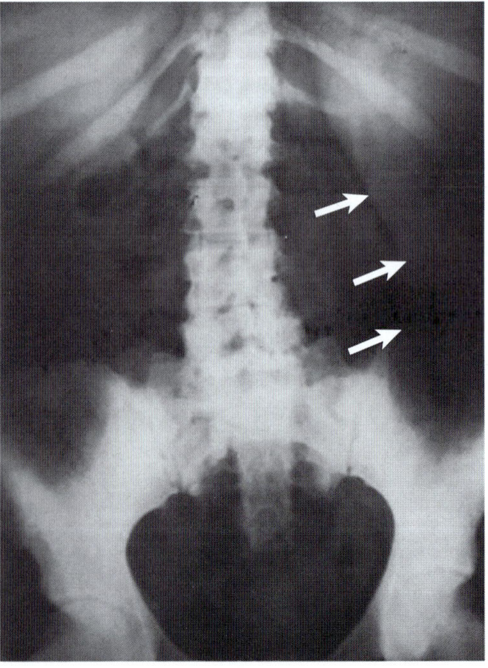

Figure 54.18 Myeloid metaplasia (woman aged 63). All the bones are diffusely dense, with lack of distinction between cortical and medullary bone. The spleen is grossly enlarged (*arrows*).

Diseases of the Lymphoreticular System

Four main groups of the disorder will be considered, divided for convenience as follows:

1. Lymphomas: Hodgkin's, non-Hodgkin's lymphomas, mastocytosis
2. Plasma-cell disease: Plasmacytoma, multiple myeloma, Waldenström macroglobulinemia (WM), POEMS syndrome
3. Histiocytosis: Langerhans cell histiocytosis, Erdheim–Chester disease, Rosai–Dorfman disease, Juvenile Xanthogranuloma
4. Storage disorders: Gaucher's disease, Niemann–Pick disease, Tay–Sachs disease, Fabry disease

Lymphomas

Lymphomas are a common type of blood cancer that primarily affects B-cell, T-cell, and natural killer cells. The most common subtypes of lymphoma and their main radiologic findings are summarized in Table 54.3.

Hodgkin's Disease

This defined tumor has an agreed classification on histological grounds, named after Rye. This comprises nodular sclerosis Hodgkin's disease, a complaint of young women involving intrathoracic lymph nodes, and three categories, lymphocyte-predominant Hodgkin's disease, mixed cellularity Hodgkin's disease, and lymphocyte-depleted Hodgkin's disease. The last three comprise a spectrum with, in the order listed, a worsening outlook.

Bone involvement always implies a less favorable prognosis. It is a feature of widespread disease and has been found at postmortem in more than half of the cases. Skeletal lesions at presentation are far less common. Primary Hodgkin's disease of bone probably does not occur. There is no correlation between the variety of Hodgkin's disease and the nature of the individual bony lesions it produces. The age of onset varies widely from childhood to old age, but the diagnosis is most commonly made in young adults. The red marrow areas are the most frequent presentation sites, the majority of lesions being found in the spine, thoracic cage, and pelvis. Bone pain may precede, by several months, the development of these lesions, and the importance of serial radiological examination, either radiographic or scintigraphic, must be stressed.

Radiological Changes: In the skeleton, most early bone lesions are destructive and often large when they are first observed, either from direct involvement from affected soft tissues, particularly

TABLE 54.3 Radiological Findings of Lymphomas

Lymphomas		Commonly Involved Skeleton Areas	Radiologic Findings
Hodgkin's disease		▪ Thoracolumbar spine (most common) ▪ Long bones ▪ Ribs and sternum ▪ Skull, clavicle, and scapulae	▪ Osteolytic, sclerotic, or mixed-type bone involvement ▪ Thoracolumbar spine (most frequently involved area): ○ Anterior scalloping of a vertebral body (rare and specific) ○ Ivory vertebral body (sclerotic type): a solitary dense vertebra ○ The intervertebral discs are usually spared ▪ Long bones: ○ The osteolytic type identifies as the predilection sites that are the red marrow areas in the proximal portions of the femora and humerus ○ Small oval translucencies in the long axis of the bone, extended throughout the marrow cavity associated with endosteal scalloping of the cortex ▪ Ribs and sternum: ○ Usually osteolytic and expanding in type
Non-Hodgkin's lymphoma	Low-grade non-Hodgkin's lymphoma	▪ Knee (with associated synovial effusion) ▪ Proximal end of the humerus	▪ The earliest finding: diffuse patchy medullary destruction or sclerosis with very poorly defined margins
	High-grade non-Hodgkin's lymphoma	▪ Primary skeletal involvement is probably extremely rare ▪ Can be solitary or multiple	▪ Resemble very closely to osteolytic type of Hodgkin's disease ▪ Large and diffuse irregular margins with scalloping of the inner aspects of the cortex ▪ Pathologic fractures in the femoral and humeral necks, and vertebral bodies ▪ Cortex erosions followed by the formation of large associated soft-tissue masses with relatively little periosteal reaction
	Burkitt lymphoma	▪ Mandible and maxilla (most common) ▪ Spine and long bones	▪ Large destructive, purely osteolytic, and rapidly growing lesions ▪ In long bones, the permeative lytic nature of the tumor, particularly with cortical erosions, may resemble an Ewing's sarcoma
Mastocytosis		▪ Spine, ribs, pelvis, skull, and tubular bones	▪ The initial finding: osteopenia and osteoporosis ▪ Diffuse areas of lytic and sclerotic lesions

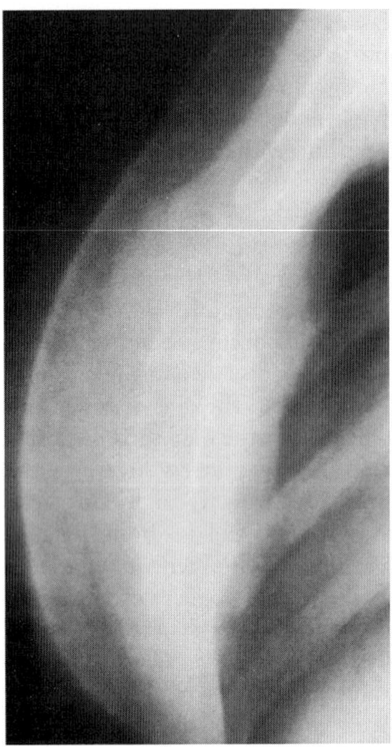

Figure 54.19 Hodgkin's disease. An expanding, destructive lesion involves the body of the sternum, with anterior and posterior soft-tissue masses. Bizarre changes in this bone should always arouse suspicion of lymphoma.

lymph nodes, or infiltration of bone marrow. About a third are essentially osteolytic in type (Fig. 54.19). The majority is, however, of mixed type with patchy sclerosis and destruction. Diffuse trabecular thickening causes sclerotic lesions in the remainder. Such an appearance may develop in a few months, being preceded by bone pain, and may well show no preliminary bone destruction. It may also follow the treatment of a formerly osteolytic lesion. Conversely, some sclerotic lesions may be observed to become osteolytic or normal following treatment. Whereas the osteolytic lesions may thin, displace, and erode the overlying cortex and develop associated soft-tissue masses, the primary sclerotic lesion does not cause enlargement of the affected bone.

Positron emission tomography (PET)/CT is a sensitive means of detecting the presence of bony lesions, particularly when sclerotic deposits have developed. With this method, bone marrow biopsy is no longer performed for adults in most trials, and instead, three positive foci detected by PET are considered bone involvement. PET/CT scans also increase disease staging sensitivity and improve the clinical outcomes in children [8].

MRI is extremely sensitive in the diagnosis of Hodgkin's disease. Whole-body MRI (WB-MRI) and PET/CT are valuable diagnostic techniques in assessing bone marrow involvement in patients with lymphoma [9]. When CT and PET scans do not yield a definite diagnosis, MRI is often helpful to diagnose bone involvement [8]. A T1 hypointensity and T2 hyperintensity suggest bone involvement on MRI [10].

- *The thoracolumbar spine* is the most frequently involved area. A rare but more specific diagnostic feature is anterior scalloping of a vertebral body, attributed to the long-standing mass effect of adjacent paravertebral lymph nodes. Several vertebrae may be affected. The sclerotic type shows a diffuse increase of density, possibly also with some anterior vertebral scalloping. A solitary dense vertebra, the so-called ivory vertebral body, is suggestive of this disease (Fig. 54.20). In all these types, the intervertebral discs are usually spared, aiding differentiation from an infection. Even in the rare cases where a disc space does become narrowed, preservation of density of the vertebral end-plates usually permits differentiation from an infective discitis where the loss of this density is an early diagnostic sign
- *The ribs* lesions may be observed on chest radiographs, which are usually osteolytic and expanding in type

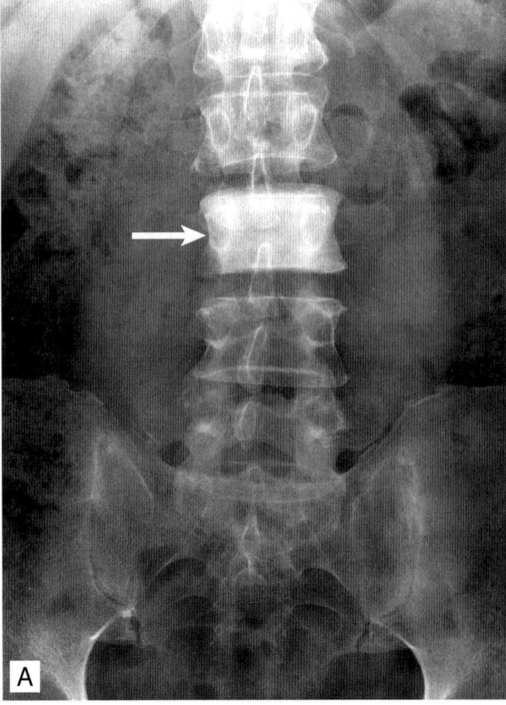

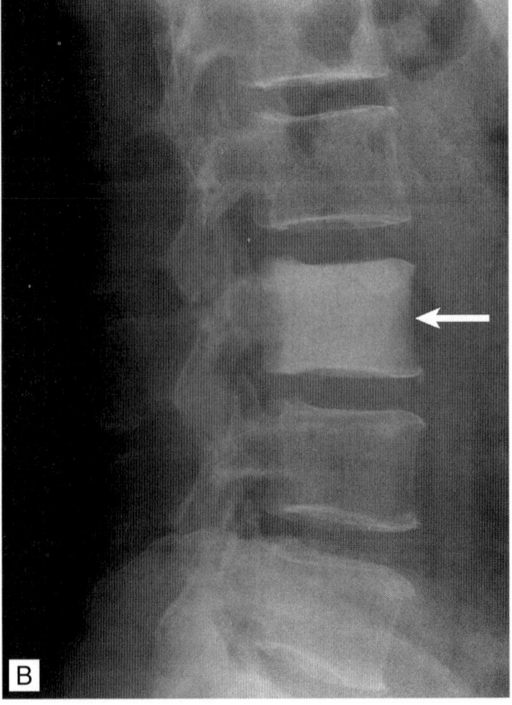

Figure 54.20 Ivory vertebral body in lymphoma. Anteroposterior radiograph (A) and lateral radiograph (B) of the lumbar spine show a markedly sclerotic, dense vertebral body (*arrows*), which is called an "ivory" vertebral body indicating neoplastic disease.

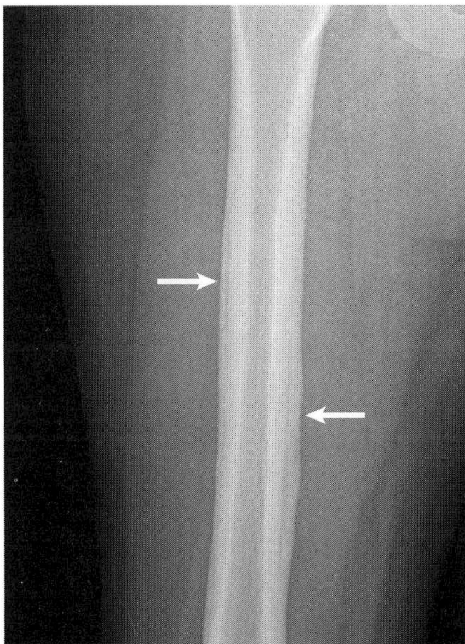

Figure 54.21 Hypertrophic osteoarthropathy in a patient with thoracic Hodgkin's disease. Right femur anteroposterior radiograph shows hypertrophic osteoarthropathy (*arrows*) of femur diaphysis characterized by mineralized periosteal thickening, which can be a sign of neoplastic pulmonary disease.

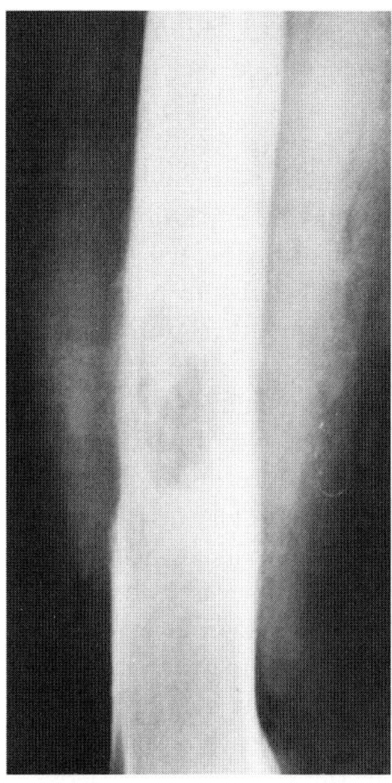

Figure 54.22 Non-Hodgkin's lymphoma. A purely destructive lesion is present in the distal femur of a woman patient. The margins are ill-defined with cortical destruction. Periosteal new bone formation is present adjacent to this destruction. These appearances resemble metastasis and osteosarcoma.

- *The sternum* is also a not-infrequent site for a lesion to appear, again usually osteolytic, but sometimes mixed in type with perpendicular spicules of new bone
- *In the pelvis*, mixed or sclerosing types tend to predominate. Osteolytic lesions, rather nonspecific in appearance, are not uncommon in the ischia, and change from either type to the mixed pattern may be observed in serial examinations
- *In the long bones,* the predilection sites are the red marrow areas in the proximal portions of the femora and humerus. These are usually of the osteolytic type and many small translucencies, oval in the long axis of the bone, extend throughout the marrow cavity associated with endosteal scalloping of the cortex. Although such an appearance is a feature of this disease, it may also be seen in non-Hodgkin's lymphoma, leukemia, and Gaucher's disease. The fusion of such areas may produce a "honeycomb pattern," with coarse residual trabeculation, like the medullary changes of Gaucher's disease. Organized periosteal reactions are not infrequent. Such a feature is rare in Gaucher's disease
- *The skull, clavicles, and scapulae* are sometimes affected. Pathological fractures are uncommon. With sclerosing lesions in elderly individuals, confusion with Paget's disease may easily arise, but the characteristic enlargement of the affected bone in that disease will probably be absent. Differentiation in all these lesions must be made from metastasis. Intrathoracic disease may present with hypertrophic osteoarthropathy (Fig. 54.21)

Non-Hodgkin's Lymphoma

This forms a much more difficult spectrum of disease with a continually evolving classification. That commonly used is based on lymph node histology and cytoimmuno chemistry. As a simplification, non-Hodgkin's lymphomas (NHLs) are categorized according to the histological architecture of the tumor into follicular or diffuse forms and according to their cell type into B-cell and T-cell tumors. As a working formulation, the tumor is then classified as low, medium, or high grade. In general, low-grade tumors tend to be follicular B-cell lymphomas, and high-grade tumors tend to be diffuse T-cell lymphomas.

It is difficult to assess how many patients present with primary skeletal non-Hodgkin's lymphoma; the proportion is probably less than one-third. The majority of patients have diffuse disease at diagnosis. Experience suggests that low-grade NHL may present as a primary bone tumor, although it can be multifocal and systemic in older patients. It is unlikely that high-grade NHL ever presents primarily in the skeleton.

Low-Grade Non-Hodgkin's Lymphoma: Skeletal involvement by low-grade NHL may be with localized pain and swelling, often over a protracted period. The tumor may be asymptomatic or presenting with pathological fracture. Males are affected twice as commonly as females. The majority is observed in the third and fourth decades, although presentation during later years is not unusual. The lesions may be multifocal in the older age group.

These tumors may be confused with other malignancies, including *osteosarcoma, metastasis,* and *malignant round cell tumors.* Differentiation between these tumors in a young adult may be extremely difficult, not only on clinical and radiological grounds but also histologically.

The lesion may arise as a primary tumor within the bone marrow and tend to remain confined to the skeleton, although it may spread to other bones and only at a later stage to lymph nodes and viscera.

The condition is localized to a single bone with a marked predilection for the long bones in their primary form. Nearly half of the cases occur near the knee (Fig. 54.22), often with an associated synovial effusion. The proximal end of the humerus is another common site, and about a third of cases are found in the flat bones of the axial skeleton. Spinal, rib, and pelvic involvement tend to occur with the extra skeletal form and the older age group.

The tumor may be extremely radiosensitive, and radiotherapy alone or in combination with surgery has resulted in many long survivals. Although a primary lesion may have regressed entirely with radiotherapy, generalized skeletal dissemination is likely to occur eventually.

The earliest evidence of the tumor is diffuse medullary destruction or sclerosis of a patchy nature with very poorly defined margins. At this stage, it may be impossible to differentiate the lesion radiologically from any other aggressive neoplasm. In particular, an osteolytic metastasis is likely to present the greatest difficulty. The lesion may resemble other primary malignant neoplasms stimulating little or no reactive bone formation, such as Ewing's tumor, fibrosarcoma, or malignant fibrous histiocytoma.

Radiological confusion with osteomyelitis may also arise, particularly as the overlying periosteal reaction is present in half of the cases (Fig. 54.22). The periosteal reaction may be present before medullary changes become evident. Scintigraphically, the features are unremarkable. Usually, increased activity is detected, or multifocal lesions may be found. Radiologically, the area of destruction spreads widely through the marrow cavity and remains patchy. Much of the adjacent cortex undergoes resorption with the development of well-defined soft-tissue swelling from soft-tissue tumor extension. Cortical thickening and reactive sclerosis are not prominent features, although they may occur exceptionally.

In the generalized form of the disease, lesions may be detected throughout the skeleton, and each presents the same characteristics as a solitary focus.

High-Grade Non-Hodgkin's Lymphoma: This malignant tumor is rarer than Hodgkin's disease and mainly affects older patients in the fifth and sixth decades. Nonetheless, several cases have been observed in children, and a male sex preponderance has been found. A proportion of these patients develop frank *lymphocytic leukemia.*

The incidence of bone lesions is 10–20%, although more are detected at postmortem. Prognostically, bone lesions imply a poor outcome. Primary skeletal involvement is probably extremely rare.

In the skeleton, these resemble very closely to those of Hodgkin's disease; other lesions grow more rapidly and are almost always osteolytic in type. Areas of destruction, commonly in red marrow areas, may be large with diffuse and irregular margins and with scalloping of the inner aspects of the cortex. They may be solitary or multiple and, because of their osteolytic nature, pathological fractures are common. The latter affects especially the femoral and humeral necks and may cause the collapse of vertebral bodies. When the lesions are multiple, they all tend to be of the same osteolytic type, unlike Hodgkin's disease, when all the different bone change types may be present. Erosion of the cortex is likely to be followed by the formation of large associated soft-tissue masses with relatively little periosteal reaction. Such erosions usually occur through an area of the cortex that has already been thinned and expanded by the underlying pathological process, emphasizing the radiological similarity of the individual lesions to Ewing's sarcoma.

Burkitt Lymphoma: *Burkitt's tumor* is an exceptional and particularly aggressive form of non-Hodgkin's lymphoma common in African children. The disease is associated with Epstein–Barr virus and is especially prevalent in endemic malarial areas.

Large, destructive lesions develop, especially in the mandible and maxilla (Fig. 54.23). Radiologically, these lesions are purely osteolytic and grow rapidly. The jaw lesions are characterized by the resorption of the lamina dura with multiple lytic foci that eventually merge with radiating spicules of bone. Spinal lesions are characterized by lytic, ill-defined destructive foci with paravertebral masses. In long bones, the permeative lytic nature of the tumor, particularly with cortical erosions, may resemble an Ewing's sarcoma. Foci develop in soft tissues, particularly the kidneys, ovaries, and abdominal lymph nodes. Regression can occur following the use of cytotoxic drugs.

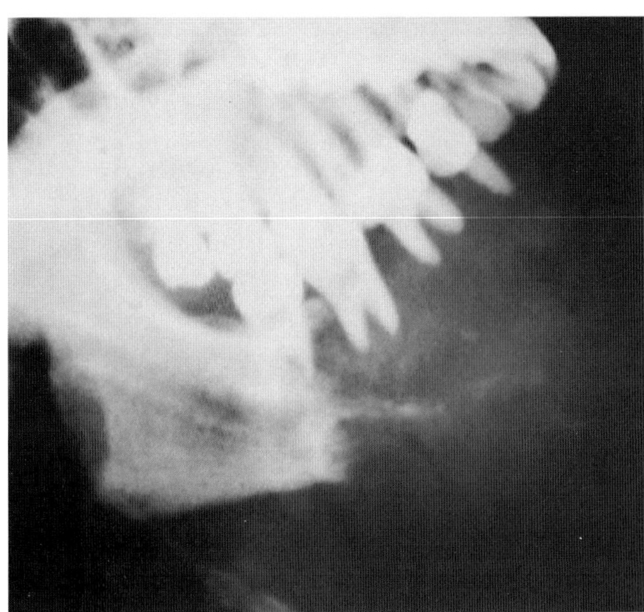

Figure 54.23 Burkitt's tumor. A large destructive lesion in the mandible of this African child is typical of this form of lymphoma.

Mastocytosis

The rare condition of urticaria pigmentosa is associated with enlargement of the liver, spleen, and lymph nodes due to the proliferation of mast cells. The disease is relatively benign, but a few instances of leukemic termination have been recorded. Bone changes are usually identified in early adult life.

Radiological Changes: In 70% of cases, skeletal changes, which are mostly generalized, are present. The most common presentations in the initial steps are osteopenia and osteoporosis [11]. There are diffuse areas of lytic and sclerotic lesions throughout the axial and appendicular skeleton (Fig. 54.24). Any bone may be affected; however, spine, ribs, pelvis, skull, and tubular bones are more to have lytic lesions [12]. The expansion of some trabeculae and the thickening of others may cause the osseous structures to have a coarse pattern. The appearance may closely resemble *sickle cell anemia*, the *sclerosing types of leukemia*, *Gaucher's disease,* and *osteopetrosis*. Occasionally the dense areas are sharply defined, of considerable size, and localized to a few areas. Particularly in young adults, differentiation from Hodgkin's disease must be made.

Plasma Cell Diseases

Plasma cells represent the end product of B-lymphocyte maturation. Pathological proliferation produces either a local tumor (plasmacytoma) or disseminated disease (myelomatosis). Table 54.4 summarizes the main radiologic findings of plasma cell diseases.

Plasmacytoma

This condition is unifocal, causing a localized destructive lesion in a red marrow area of the skeleton. Many other descriptive terms (such as solitary myeloma) for this localized lesion have been used. Although it may remain localized for many years and without health disturbance, it ultimately transitions to generalized

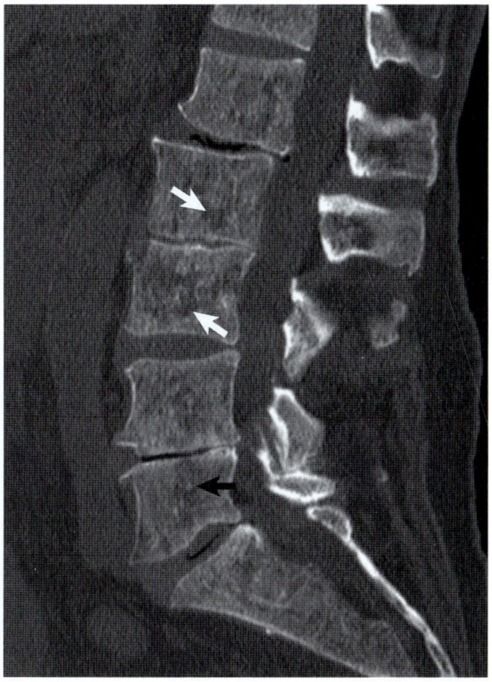

Figure 54.24 Mastocytosis of the spine. Sagittal CT image of the lumbosacral spine shows an abnormal pattern of cancellous bone, characterized by areas of lytic (*white arrows*) and sclerotic (*black arrow*) lesions in all vertebral bodies. *CT*, computed tomography.

myelomatosis. A latent interval of 5–10 years is usual; consequently, the outlook is better than multiple myeloma. Compared with the latter, these lesions are uncommon, but the exact incidence is difficult to assess as they are frequently asymptomatic. For example, a plasmacytoma in a rib may be noted incidentally on a routine examination of the chest (Fig. 54.25).

When symptoms occur, they are commonly those of bone pain, particularly backache. The vertebral bodies, especially in the thoracolumbar and lumbar regions, are the most common sites for these lesions and are likely to undergo partial collapse. The pelvis, especially the ilium, ribs, femur, and humerus, is the next most commonly involved sites. The vast majority of affected individuals are between the fifth and seventh decade of age. The differential diagnosis always includes a solitary osteolytic metastasis.

Differential diagnosis of these tumors may be difficult. Given the age group, *osteolytic metastasis* is the most common differential diagnosis. In vertebrae, such metastases are likely to involve the pedicles more commonly. Metastatic disease apart, the development of a solitary osteolytic lesion in a vertebral body in a late middle age patient should always be considered a plasmacytoma (Fig. 54.26). *Chordoma* may also produce similar features. Other differential diagnoses to be considered, especially with an expanding lytic focus in a rib, are *fibrous dysplasia*, a "brown" tumor of hyperparathyroidism, and, particularly when the lesion is adjacent to an articular surface, a *giant cell tumor*. The resemblance to a giant cell tumor may be close; however, these lesions are found in early adult life and have a different distribution, commonly affecting the appendicular skeleton, whereas plasmacytoma is more likely to be axial.

TABLE 54.4 Radiological Findings of Plasma-Cell Diseases

Plasma-Cell Disease	Commonly Involved Skeleton Areas	Radiologic Findings
Plasmacytoma	▪ Vertebral bodies, especially in the thoracolumbar and lumbar regions(most common) ▪ Pelvis, especially the ilium, ribs, femur, and humerus, is the next most commonly involved sites	▪ These lesions arise in areas of red marrow function ▪ Bone expansion: may be considered thinning of the overlying cortex ▪ Vertebral body collapse ▪ Well defined and sharply demarcated margins, characteristically without a sclerotic reaction ▪ Network appearance in the area of destruction due to coarse trabecular strands of increased density
Multiple myeloma	▪ The axial skeleton is affected predominantly ▪ Shafts of long bones and the skull	▪ Generalized reduction in bone density ▪ Localized radiolucency areas in red marrow areas ▪ The rounded and oval defects characteristically have sharply defined edges ▪ Classic lesion: punched-out "raindrop" lesions, circular defects varying in diameter from a few millimeters to 2 or 3 cm ▪ Myelomatous lesions may erode the cortex and extend into the adjacent soft tissues. (The resulting soft-tissue masses help differentiate the advanced forms of the disease from metastatic carcinoma lesions, which much less commonly produce extension into the soft tissues.) ▪ Vertebral body collapse which resulted in paravertebral soft-tissue shadows ▪ Pathologic fractures with remarkably quick healing and massive callus and new bone formation without any evidence of reactive sclerosis
Waldenström macroglobulinemia	▪ Spine	▪ Diffuse demineralization and compression fracture of the spine due to bone marrow infiltration

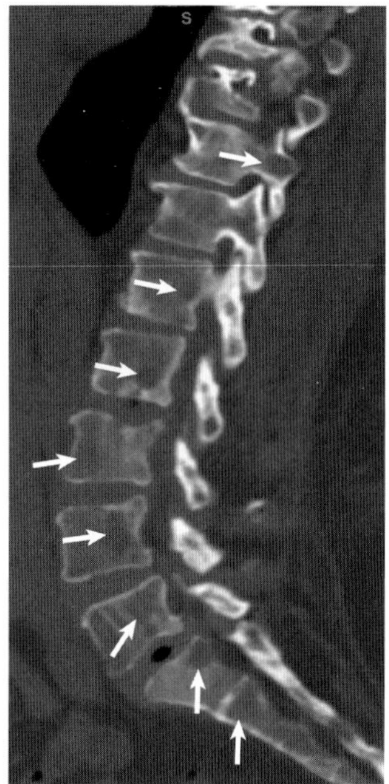

Figure 54.29 Multiple myeloma of the spine. Sagittal CT image of the lumbosacral spine shows multiple areas of lytic vertebral bone lesions (*arrows*). *CT*, computed tomography.

In some advanced cases, lytic defects may be due also to secondary amyloidosis, which can complicate many chronic disorders such as rheumatoid disease and long-standing infections.

Pathological fractures are very often the initiating factor in the diagnosis of the disease. These fractures heal remarkably quickly and soundly with massive callus and new bone formation. This response is somewhat surprising given the numerous cystic lesions and widespread osteoporosis, which are likely to be present without any evidence of reactive sclerosis.

Whole-body radiography and *traditional bone scintigraphy* are techniques with low accuracy in evaluating skeletal involvement in multiple myeloma.

Whole-body low-dose (WBLD) CT is more sensitive than whole-body radiography and is recommended as the initial diagnostic procedure for diagnosing lytic bone lesions in multiple myeloma patients (Fig. 54.29).

Whole-body MRI is the best technique for the assessment of bone marrow involvement in patients with multiple myeloma. Moreover, whole-body MRI is more sensitive than PET/CT to reveal focal or diffuse bone involvement. Multiple myeloma bone lesions have T1-weighted hypointensity and T2-weighted intermediate to hyperintensity in the MRI [14].

Waldenström Macroglobulinemia

Waldenström macroglobulinemia (WM) is a rare malignant subtype of the lymphoplasmacytic lymphoma with immunoglobulinM (IgM) monoclonal gammopathy infiltrating bone marrow. It mostly affects older patients. The median age of patients is usually between 63 and 68, and males are more prone to get the disease [15]. Although serum hyperviscosity, due to the circulating IgM, is the most distinguishing presentation of WM and can lead to high-output cardiac failure, the most common disease manifestation is anemia, resulting from bone marrow infiltration. Infiltration and deposition of IgM in organs distinguished by lymphadenopathy and hepatosplenomegaly in the physical examination [16]. A rare complication of WM is Bing–Neel syndrome, which is characterized by infiltration of CNS and presenting with headache, ataxia, vertigo, diplopia, and nystagmus.

Bone marrow infiltration may cause diffuse demineralization and a compression fracture of the spine. Although rare, the lytic bone disease may be visible on the bone surveys. On MRI, iso-/hypo-intensity to muscle and abnormal marrow enhancement can be noticed on T1-weighted images.

POEMS Syndrome

An uncommon condition with the acronym POEMS is characterized by chronic progressive polyneuropathy, organomegaly (hepatosplenomegaly), endocrinopathy (commonly diabetes mellitus), M-proteins (plasma-cell dyscrasia), and skin changes (hirsutism, pigmentation, edema). The pick incidence of the disease is in the fifth and sixth decades of life. Bone pain and fractures are rare [17] and radiologically presents with multiple sclerotic lesions, most commonly in the spine and pelvis.

Histiocytosis

The basic pathological abnormality in this group of diseases is a proliferation of histiocytic cells occurring particularly in the bone marrow, spleen, liver, lymphatic glands, and lungs. In the more chronic forms, these cells become swollen with lipid deposits, essentially cholesterol (although the blood cholesterol level remains normal), and they present the pathological appearances of "foam cells." Some of these become necrotic and are replaced by fibrous tissue.

Various forms of the condition have been regarded as separate entities in the past, which are outlined in Table 54.6.

Langerhans Cell Histiocytosis

Langerhans cell histiocytosis (LCH) is an idiopathic condition with unknown pathophysiology that involves dendritic antigen-presenting cells, although a neoplastic or an abnormal reactive process was defined as possible etiologies. The disease may involve bone marrow, lungs, liver, spleen, lymph nodes, gastrointestinal (GI) tract, pituitary gland, and a widespread disease increase mortality. LCH is a rare disease that mostly occurs in children <15 years of age and affects both sex equally.

The mildest and most common expression of histiocytosis is *eosinophilic granuloma*. Pathological changes are predominantly bony, although occasionally pulmonary involvement may occur. Children, especially boys between 3 and 12, are most commonly affected, although these lesions may be observed in adolescents, young adults, and the middle-aged. Any bone may be affected. The skull, pelvis, and femora between them account for nearly two-thirds of all cases. Clinically, pain and swelling may be accompanied by mild fever. Histologically, the eosinophilic infiltration is found around collections of histiocytes. In this relatively mild form, necrosis and fibrosis are rare, and the appearance of foam cells suggests a more serious variety.

Hand–Schüller–Christian disease is a more chronic form of the LCH disease, with the dissemination of lesions in the lungs, lymph nodes, liver, and spleen, in addition to virtually constant and early involvement of the skeleton. Moreover, exophthalmos, due to the mass effect on the orbital bone, and diabetes insipidus, due to direct infiltration of the posterior pituitary gland. Children below the age of 5 years are most frequently affected, although sporadic cases occur at later ages up to middle life. The course of the disease is chronic, often extending over 10 or more years. It is characterized by soreness of the mouth and loose teeth due to deposits in the gums and jaws, and skin lesions. Abnormalities in

TABLE 54.6 Radiological Findings of Histiocytosis

Disease		Commonly Involved Skeleton Areas	Radiologic Findings
Langerhans cell histiocytosis	Eosinophilic granuloma	▪ Thoracic spine ▪ Diaphysis or metaphysis of long bones	▪ Mostly presents as a solitary lesion ▪ Characteristic finding: translucent bone destruction areas, with sharply defined margins and considerable size ▪ Partial or complete collapse of spine presents as a classic fining: vertebra plana. (Consider DDX: Ewing's tumor, neuroblastoma metastasis, benign osteoblastoma, atypical tuberculous focus) ▪ No sclerotic margin in the active phase, peripheral sclerosis around the lesion in the healing phase
	Hand–Schüller–Christian disease	▪ Skull, mandible, and maxilla ▪ Vertebrae and pelvis ▪ Long bones (less common)	▪ Similar finding as those of eosinophilic granulomas with far more numerous lesions ▪ "Geographical skull": Merging of numerous bone lesions to produce widespread irregular defects usually likened to a map ▪ "Float in air" appearance: lesions in the mandible and maxilla around the tooth roots with dense and unaffected teeth
	Letterer–Siwe disease	▪ Widely spread in the flat bones	▪ Purely lytic lesions, indistinguishable from Hand–Schüller–Christian disease
Erdheim–Chester disease		▪ Distal ends of the femurs and proximal and distal tibia (The most characteristic in differentiating from Langerhans cell histiocytosis)	▪ Pathognomonic bilateral, symmetric cortical osteosclerosis of the diaphyseal and metaphyseal regions of the distal ends of lower—and sometimes upper limbs (epiphyses classically spare) ▪ Osteosclerosis of long bones differentiate it from Langerhans cell histiocytosis, which mostly presents with sharply defined lytic lesions in the axial skeleton ▪ Extensive fatty marrow replacement by signal hypointensity on T1-weighted images, and the heterogeneous signal on T2-weighted images/STIR
Rosai–Dorfman disease		▪ Long bones (metaphysis, diaphysis, or epiphysis), skull, and spine	▪ Osteolytic and intramedullary lesions

the temporal bone are common, with an associated otitis media. The eventual prognosis is good since spontaneous remission, possibly initiated or accelerated by radiotherapy, occurs in most cases. Over 10%, however, terminate fatally.

The least common form of LCH is *Letterer–Siwe disease*. This is an acute or subacute disseminated form of the disease, occurring very rarely in infants below 2 years and presenting a more severe clinical picture. It is characterized by pyrexia, with a rash and mouth sores, bleeding gums, respiratory symptoms, and failure to thrive. Particular involvement of the extra skeletal tissues occurs with enlargement of the liver, spleen, and lymph nodes. The disease usually ends fatally, often in a few months and at the most in 2 years. In those cases with a rapidly fatal outcome, skeletal lesions are unlikely to be demonstrated radiologically, having insufficient time to develop. Nevertheless, histological change may be present in the bone marrow, with widespread masses of histiocytes and eosinophilic infiltration, comparable with the early histological picture of the benign eosinophilic granuloma. Only in the rare cases that survive, fibrosis and cholesterol-containing foam cells become apparent.

In summary, histiocytosis is a disease primarily of childhood, although exceptionally, its more benign manifestations may be observed in early adult life. The older the child and the more the lesions are confined to the skeleton rather than other tissues, the better the prognosis. It must be appreciated that the benign eosinophilic granuloma may deteriorate to a chronic, multifocal form of the spectrum, and rarely vice versa.

Radiological Changes: In *eosinophilic granuloma,* translucent bone destruction areas, with sharply defined margins and often of considerable size, are characteristic (Fig. 54.30). The round or oval defects may have scalloped margins (Fig. 54.31). Although they provoke no sclerotic margin in the active phase, the healing phase, which usually develops by spontaneous regression, is marked by peripheral sclerosis around the lesion and slow reconstitution of the bony structure (Fig. 54.32). This healing phase may be accelerated by biopsy, radiotherapy, or steroid injection. True expansion is uncommon except in ribs and vertebral bodies. Apparent expansion may result from thickening of the overlying periosteum, especially if the cortex has been partially eroded (Fig. 54.33) or infarction has occurred. In approximately, two-thirds of patients, the lesions are *solitary.* The *differential diagnosis* of a solitary lesion of this type may be extremely difficult and is from either osteomyelitis or Ewing's tumor, which has a similar age incidence. Skeletal surveys,

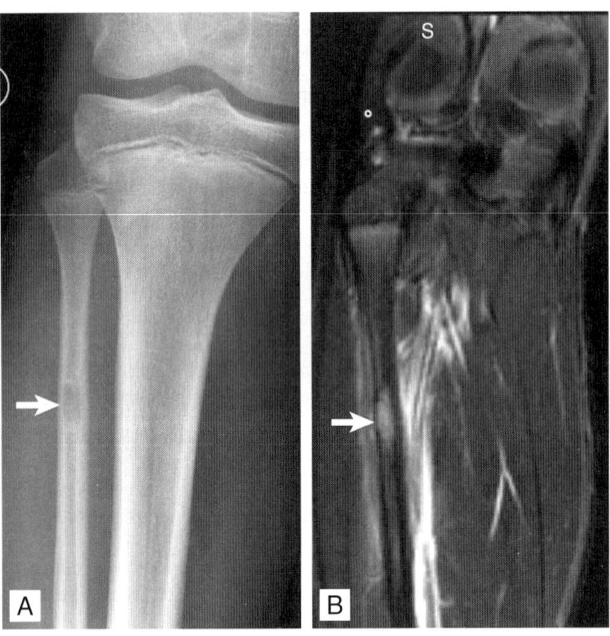

Figure 54.30 Eosinophilic granuloma of the fibula. Anteroposterior radiograph (A) demonstrates an area of centrally located osteolysis with sharply demarcated and partially sclerotic margins in the proximal fibula diaphysis (*arrow*). Fluid-sensitive fat-suppressed coronal (B) MR images redemonstrate the lytic bone lesion and additional characteristic surrounding edema pattern and periosteal reaction.

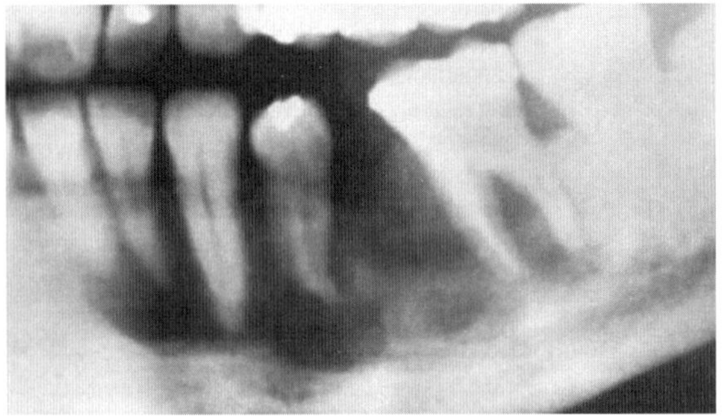

Figure 54.31 Histiocytosis. A purely osteolytic lesion is present in the mandible, with well-defined, slightly scalloped margins. The lamina dura has been destroyed. The teeth seem to 'float in air'.

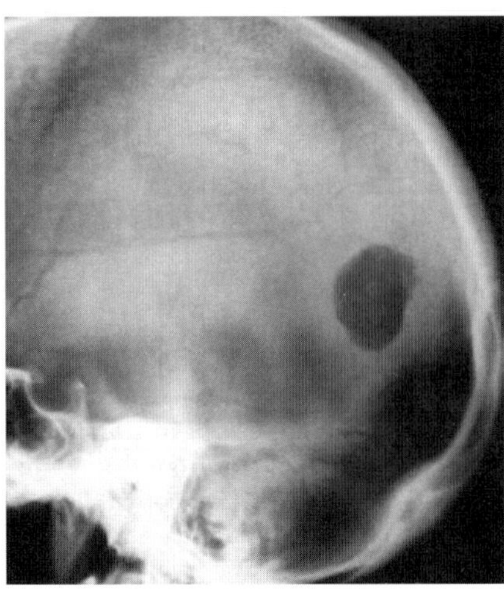

Figure 54.32 Histiocytosis. Lateral skull radiograph showing a well-defined osteolytic lesion with a narrow zone of transition and no sclerosis in the posterior parietal region.

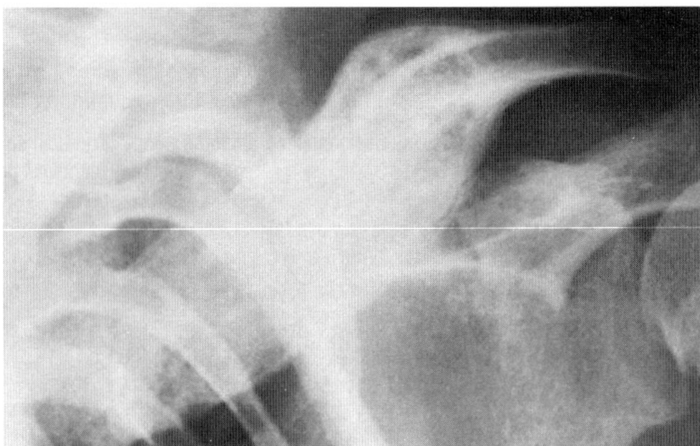

Figure 54.33 Histiocytosis. Extensive involvement of a bone, here the clavicle, is often associated with layered periosteal new bone causing bony expansion. Ill-defined areas of resorption may be visualized in the lesion. This was the only abnormality found in a young girl over several years of follow-up.

scintigraphic or radiographic, may disclose the presence of other asymptomatic lesions, facilitating the diagnosis. *Multiple* eosinophilic granulomas are usually found to be in different phases of evolution. As one lesion resolves, another may appear in a different part of the skeleton. In the skull particularly, new lesions several centimeters in diameter may appear in as many weeks. Button sequestra may be observed.

Solitary lesions in the spine may collapse, partially or completely, the latter presenting the classic appearance of *vertebra plana* (Figs. 54.34 and 54.35). The most commonly affected site is the thoracic spine. At one time, the lesions were considered to represent an "osteochondritis" and were named *Calvé's disease*. During the phase of collapse, the walls of the affected vertebral body tend to bulge laterally, and paravertebral soft-tissue shadows may be evident. The disc spaces on either side remain intact and may appear widened. As healing occurs, a remarkably good reconstitution of these vertebral bodies may occur if sufficient

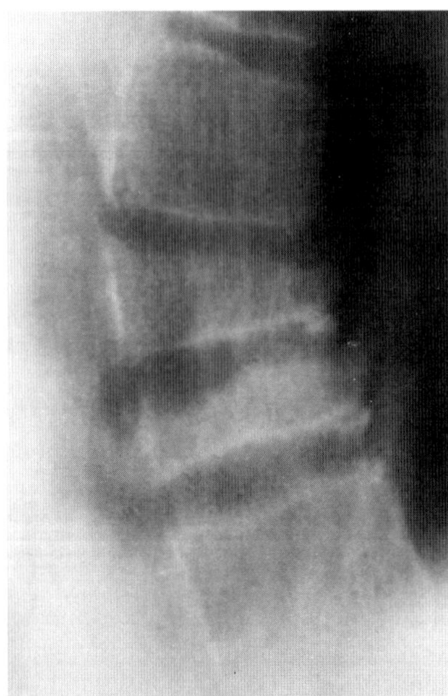

Figure 54.34 Histiocytosis. Vertebral lesions in the thoracic spine are shown on a lateral tomogram. The bodies of T7 and T8 have collapsed with a slight increase in bone density. Note the relative preservation of the disc spaces.

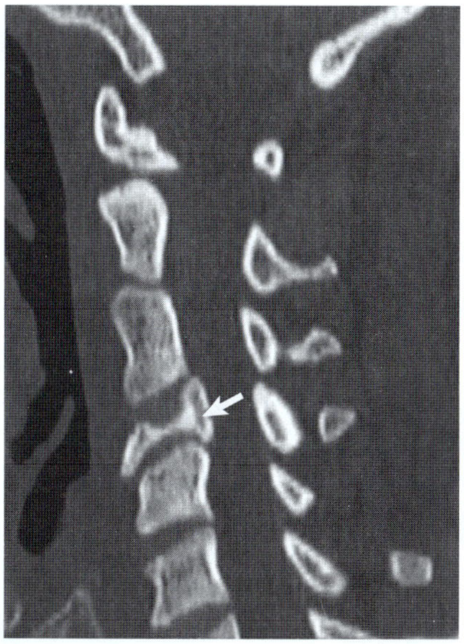

Figure 54.35 Vertebra plana of the cervical spine in a patient with eosinophilic granuloma. Sagittal cervical spine CT image shows a collapse of the fourth cervical vertebral body (*arrow*) due to eosinophilic granuloma. *CT*, computed tomography.

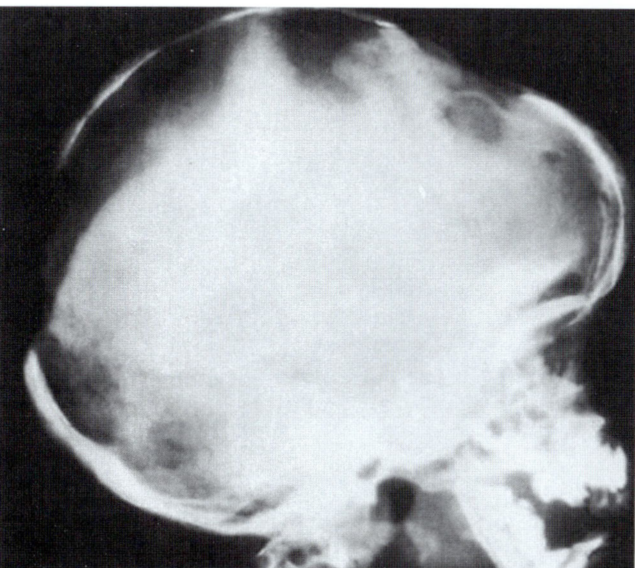

Figure 54.36 Histiocytosis. Extensive skull involvement in a child with the Hand–Schüller–Christian type of lesion. The areas of destruction in the flat bones of the skull have a map-like configuration.

years of growth remain. The vast majority of vertebral plana lesions, especially in a relatively healthy child, are caused by an eosinophilic granuloma, and confirmatory biopsy is usually unnecessary. The *differential diagnosis* of the collapse of a single vertebral body includes the relative rarities of Ewing's tumor, metastasis from neuroblastoma, benign osteoblastoma, atypical tuberculous focus, and chronic recurrent multifocal osteomyelitis (Table 54.7) [18].

This benign form of histiocytosis occasionally affects long bones and initially has a preference for the diaphysis. However, metaphyseal involvement may occur again, confusing with a pyogenic infection. A rare entity, *chronic granulomatous* (*Landing–Shirkey*) *disease*, tends to cause skeletal lesions, including those in the metaphysis, which simulate the radiological appearance of multiple eosinophilic granulomas closely. This condition is usually due to inherited and inadequate responses of leucocytes to infection.

The bone defects in *Hand–Schüller–Christian disease* are essentially the same as those of eosinophilic granulomas. They are far more numerous and particularly affect the flat bones. In the skull, they often merge to produce widespread irregular defects usually likened to a map and described as the "geographical skull," and both tables often being involved (Fig. 54.36). Lesions in the mandible and maxilla begin around the tooth roots so that the teeth, which are never affected, remain dense and appear to "float in air" (Fig. 54.31). Several vertebrae may be completely or partially collapsed, and extensive lesions may develop in the scapulae, ribs, and pelvis. Osteolytic pelvic lesions or vertebral collapse in a child are suggestive of this disease. Long bone involvement is less common (Fig. 54.37). In a relatively early stage, sclerotic reaction around the sharply defined margins of these lesions is absent. When healing occurs, the lesions fill in by sclerosis in the same way as eosinophilic granulomas. New lesions may appear after the original ones have begun to heal, emphasizing the wide spectrum of radiological changes in histiocytosis again. The lungs usually show a fine nodular infiltration in the acute phase. With healing, these infiltrations get fibrotic and persist as linear strands of increased density, but the presence

TABLE 54.7 Differential Diagnosis of the Collapse of a Single Vertebral Body (Vertebral Plana)

- Langerhans cell histiocytosis (eosinophilic granuloma)
- Ewing's tumor
- Metastasis from neuroblastoma
- Benign osteoblastoma
- Atypical tuberculous focus
- Chronic recurrent multifocal osteomyelitis

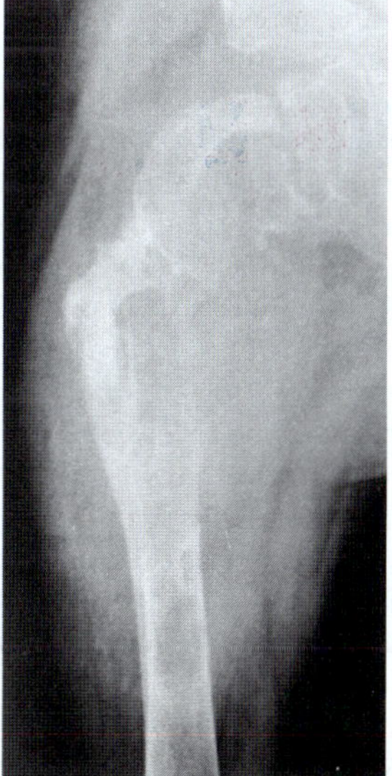

Figure 54.37 Hand–Schüller–Christian. Very extensive radiolucencies are present both in the metaphysis and diaphysis of this child's femur. A healed pathological fracture is present. Histiocytosis should always be considered in the differential diagnosis of bizarre bone lesions.

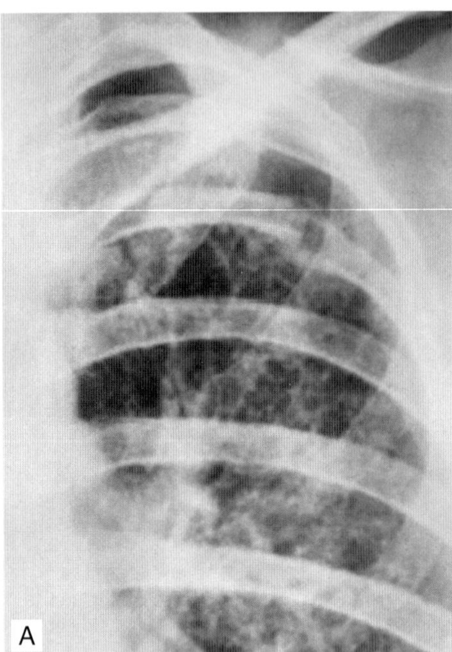

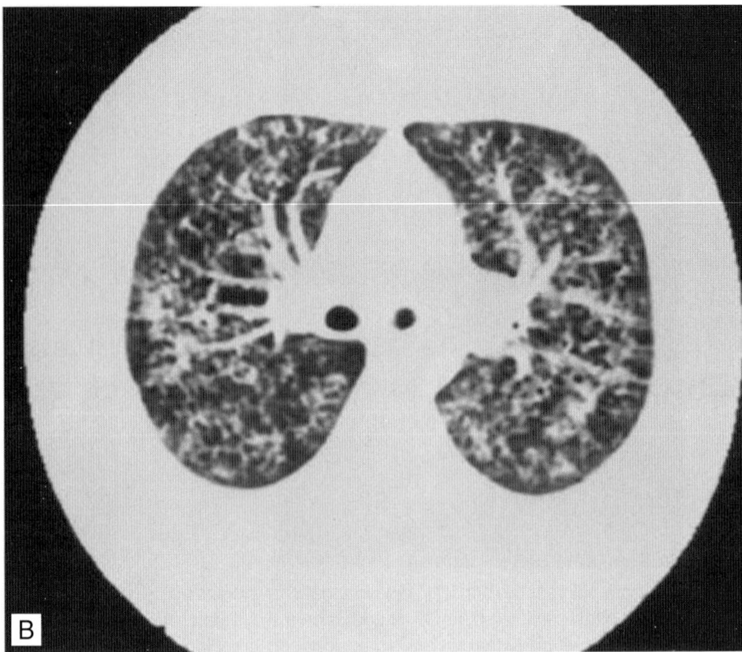

Figure 54.38 Histiocytosis. Adult pulmonary involvement (man aged 20). (A) A localized view from a chest radiograph demonstrates a coarse interstitial pulmonary fibrosis. Note also a pathological fracture of the left fourth rib due to a bony deposit. (B) A CT scan demonstrates peripheral interstitial pulmonary fibrosis with thickened interlobular septa and irregular honeycombing.

of pulmonary changes in histiocytosis indicates a worse prognosis (Fig. 54.38).

Bone lesions in *Letterer–Siwe disease* are indistinguishable from Hand–Schüller–Christian disease and are purely lytic. However, they tend to be even more widely spread in the flat bones, especially in the metadiaphyseal areas of the long bones (Fig. 54.39). Diffuse pulmonary infiltration is common. This may closely resemble miliary tuberculosis and is a variety of honeycomb lung.

Erdheim–Chester Disease

Erdheim–Chester disease [19,20] is a rare inflammatory disorder of unknown etiology, in which non-Langerhans foamy histiocytes infiltrate multiple organs. Erdheim–Chester disease clinical spectrum depends on the extent and distribution of the lesions. Although the disease primarily affects bone, it may involve every organ and causes a range of clinical manifestations from asymptomatic bone involvement to multisystemic, life-threatening forms. The most common clinical manifestations at the time of onset are bone pain, diabetes insipidus, and neurological and constitutional symptoms. Although therapeutic approaches with biologic agents and BRAF-inhibitors are developed and used in recent years, the overall prognosis is poor. Pediatrics are rarely affected, and males are slightly more prone to disease involvement.

Radiological Changes: Bone involvement is the most common presenting clinical feature and present in all patients with Erdheim–Chester disease. Distal ends of the femurs and proximal and distal tibia are the most characteristic involved sites (Fig. 54.40) that help differentiate from Langerhans cell histiocytosis in which craniofacial bones, pelvis, scapula, and proximal limbs are commonly involved.

On *radiographs*, a bilateral, symmetric cortical osteosclerosis of the diaphyseal and metaphyseal regions of the distal ends of lower—and sometimes upper—limbs are pathognomonic; epiphyses classically spared, and the axial skeleton is rarely affected. Mixed sclerotic and lytic lesions may rarely be observed. Osteosclerosis helps differentiate from Langerhans cell histiocytosis, which mostly presents with sharply defined lytic lesions in the axial skeleton, including the spine, skull, mandible, and Paget's disease, presenting with the axial skeleton and asymmetric appendicular skeleton involvement.

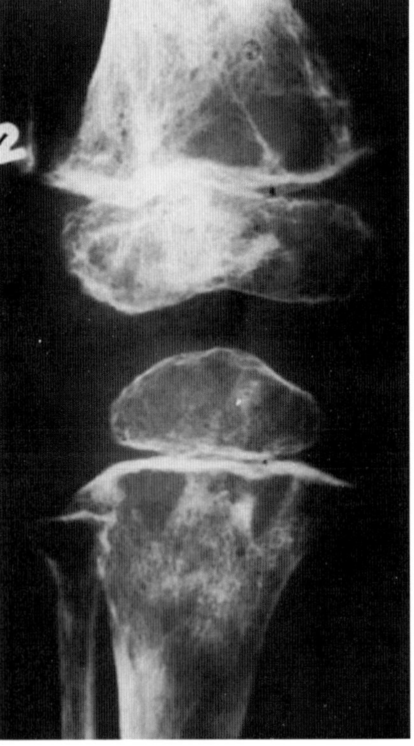

Figure 54.39 Letterer–Siwe type. Massive destructive lesions are present throughout the skeleton but particularly affect the metadiaphyseal areas of the long bones. Metastases could produce a similar appearance from neuroblastoma or the advanced stages of leukemia.

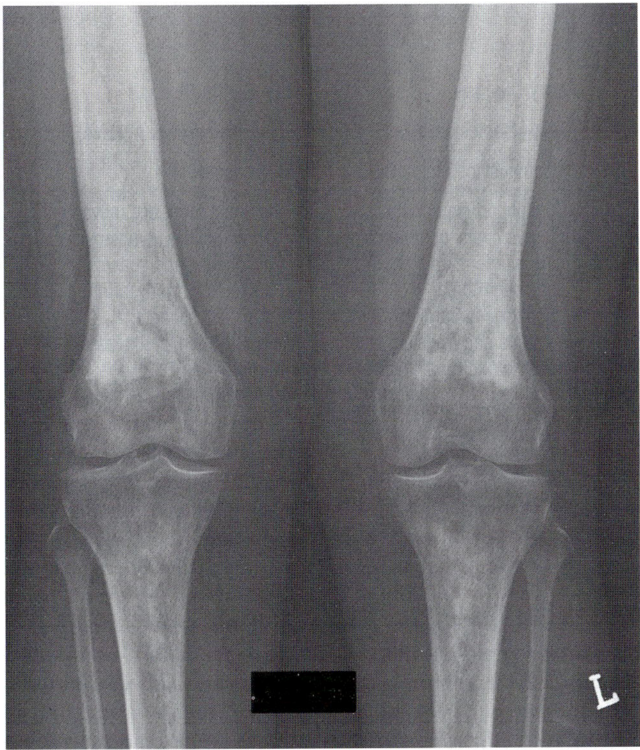

Figure 54.40 Erdheim–Chester disease. Bilateral, symmetric cortical osteosclerosis of the diaphyseal, and metaphyseal regions of the distal ends of femur and proximal ends of tibia. Epiphyses are classically spared.

On *technetium-99m bone scintigraphy*, the intense symmetric activity of the appendicular skeleton without reaching the epiphyseal regions is the pathognomonic finding.

The *FDG PET/CT scan*, like radiographs and Tc-99m bone scintigraphy, reveals a bilateral and symmetric uptake of FDG in the long bones. The advantage of this imaging technique is giving an accurate evaluation of both the skeletal and extra skeletal extent of the disease.

On *MRI*, an extensive replacement of the fatty marrow by signal hypointensity on T1-weighted images, the heterogeneous signal on T2-weighted images/STIR, and enhancement after gadolinium injection attributed to skeletal involvement. Moreover, MRI is a useful technique to evaluate the extent of medullary bone disease and the presence of associated osteonecrosis.

Considering the sclerotic bone changes and the age group, renal osteodystrophy, myelofibrosis, osteoblastic metastases, and chronic focal osteomyelitis are acquired syndromes that may mimic Erdheim–Chester disease radiographically.

Rosai–Dorfman Disease

Rosai–Dorfman disease [21,22] is an idiopathic and rare non-Langerhans cell histiocytosis disorder characterized by painless, peripheral, and massive cervical lymphadenopathy. Other lymph nodes and extranodal sites such as bone, skin, upper respiratory tract, gastrointestinal tract, and central nervous system may also be involved. Skeletal involvement mostly occurs secondarily to other extraosseous manifestations. Children and young adults are mostly affected, and males are slightly more prone to disease. Cervical lymphadenopathy is the most common presenting symptom, mostly accompanied by fever, malaise, and night sweat. The overall prognosis of the disease is good with spontaneous regression unless the vital organs get involved and require treatment.

Radiological Changes: Bone involvement in Rosai–Dorfman disease presents with gradual swelling, pain, and tenderness. Long bones, skull, and spine are the most commonly affected regions, although any bone may be affected. The metaphyses, diaphysis, or epiphyses of long bones may be involved.

On *radiographs*, skeletal involvement of Rosai–Dorfman disease represents osteolytic and intramedullary lesions.

On *MRI*, a hypointensity on T1-weighted or hyperintensity on a postcontrast T2-weighted image represent the typical appearance of marrow replacement in Rosai-Dorfman disease.

In patients with systemic Rosai-Dorfman disease, the FDG-PET scan is a sensitive indicator for early prediction of treatment response.

Juvenile Xanthogranuloma

Juvenile xanthogranuloma (JXG) [23] is a benign and rare form of non-Langerhans cell histiocytosis disease, which causes proliferative skin disorder. JXG usually occurs in infancy or early childhood, and up to 20% of cases have lesions at birth. The most common presentation is a solitary well-defined yellowish cutaneous papule found on the head, neck, extremities, or upper torso. Extracutaneous JXG mostly affects the eye, although the systemic disease may involve all other organs. In most cases, the disease has a course of spontaneous involution.

Storage Disorders of the Lymphoreticular System

Several conditions have been described in which the lymphoreticular system is the site of abnormal deposition of lipoproteins, usually due to inborn errors of metabolism. Table 54.8 summarizes the storage disorder features.

Gaucher's Disease

Young Jewish females are particularly susceptible to this hereditary condition caused by the deficiency of ß-glucosidase resulting in glucocerebroside accumulation. It is not confined to this ethnic group or sex. Although manifestations of the condition commonly become apparent in the later years of childhood and early adult life, the disease may be so chronic and of such insidious onset that it may be recognized for the first time only in middle age or even later life. In infancy, the rapidly fatal course of this systemic disease is characterized by gross neurological changes and pulmonary infiltration.

In the juvenile and young adult variety, the principal complaint is weakness and fatigue with progressive dementia. On clinical examination, splenic enlargement is detected in 95% of cases. Bone pain may be present, sometimes severe. In the chronic form of the disease, characteristic and diagnostic bone changes may be expected. Histological examination reveals numerous large histiocytes within which an abnormal lipoprotein, kerasin, is present. These cells are disseminated throughout the marrow of the hematopoietic skeleton, in addition to the spleen and liver. Yellowish-brown pigmentation is a common presentation of skin involvement.

Radiological Changes: *Diffuse infiltration* of the bone marrow causes widespread and irregular medullary radiolucency. Bone marrow infiltration in adults can be seen by MRI. The areas of signal hypointensity in T1-weighted images, known as dark marrow, represent the extent of marrow infiltration. In children, alternatively, bone scintigraphy is a useful method for the evaluation of bone marrow infiltration [24].

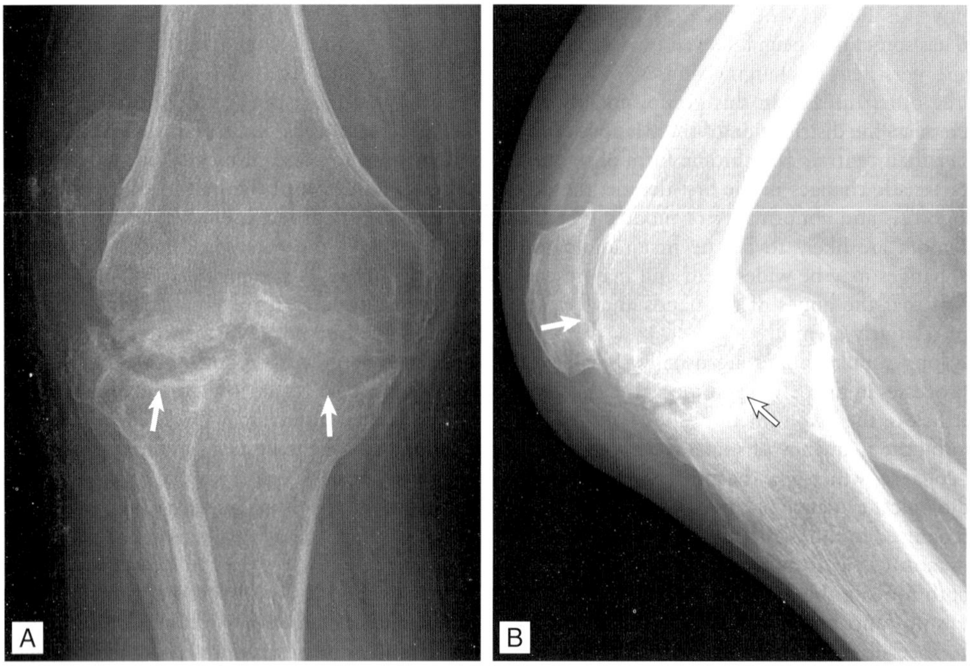

Figure 54.43 Hemophilia of the knee. Anteroposterior (A) and lateral (B) left knee radiographs in a hemophilic patient demonstrate partial joint space loss of the distal left femur due to recurring inflammation due to episodes of intra-articular hemorrhages.

of childhood and adolescence. Milder forms of the disease may cause the formation of large, soft-tissue hematoma without significant joint involvement. This is true of *Von Willebrand's disease*, which affects both sexes equally and is transmitted in an autosomal dominant manner. However, if the factor VIII level is low, bleeding into joints can occur in this condition. The most common affected joints are the knee, ankle, elbow, and shoulder.

Radiological Changes: These are caused by bleeding into joints, within bony structures, and beneath the periosteum in the skeleton. Frequent repetition of such episodes, particularly at an early age, increases their severity.

Intra-articular hemorrhage: In the early stages of the disease, the soft-tissue distension of a joint due to a hemarthrosis cannot be distinguished radiologically from a frank traumatic or inflammatory synovial effusion. Frequent repetition of hemorrhagic incidents results in synovial thickening and articular erosions. Initially, these erosions tend to be marginal in distribution (Fig. 54.43). Simultaneously, the bony structures near an affected joint are likely to become porotic, partly through disuse, but particularly through persistent hyperemia associated with the organization of the hemarthrosis. As with hyperemia of any other cause, this latter factor commonly causes enlargement of the growing epiphyses. Such epiphyses may become abnormal in shape and often fuse prematurely. Differentiation from chronic inflammatory synovitis, particularly tuberculous, may present radiological difficulty. The trabecular pattern of the bone becomes coarse and often has a lattice appearance. Secondary degenerative changes develop prematurely (Fig. 54.44). The knee is affected almost invariably; involvement is frequently bilateral. The intercondylar notch becomes wide and deep. The patella may develop an unusually rectangular shape, and its proximal articular surface is a common site of erosion. The elbows and ankles also are commonly affected. A characteristic abnormality in the former joint is an enlarged and deformed radial head. The shoulders and wrists are less frequently involved. Bleeding into the hip is unusual, but avascular necrosis of the femoral head causes an appearance comparable to Perthes disease when this does occur. Distended joint capsules, particularly those of the elbows, may become radiologically dense by deposition within them of hemosiderin. This, too, produces a low signal on MR images of diseased synovium.

Intraosseous hemorrhage: Juxta-articular cystic lesions may be observed in the later stages of the disease, with a peculiar predilection for the proximal humeral epiphyses olecranon processes. Although many are comparable to the post-traumatic subarticular cysts of degenerative joint disease, some of these cysts are remote from the articular surfaces and have led to the belief that they may be caused by hemorrhage within the bone itself.

Subperiosteal hemorrhage: Large osteolytic lesions, hemophiliac pseudotumors, occur in about 1% or 2% of severely affected patients. They arise especially in the iliac wings and in the shafts of the long bones of the lower limb (Fig. 54.45), although other bones, including the calcaneum, have been involved. These destructive lesions have been attributed to bleeding below the periosteum or muscle attachments and often are accompanied by large swellings, sometimes relatively painless, of the soft tissues. Relation to a former traumatic incident may occasionally be established. Absorption of the underlying cortex and medulla with the elevation of the periosteal margins results in an appearance that may be highly suggestive of a malignant bone tumor. Calcification is not uncommon within the space-occupying lesions. However, a diagnostic clue may be provided by evidence in an adjacent joint of a hemophiliac arthropathy. Failure to appreciate the nature of this entity, nevertheless, has resulted in iatrogenic disasters by inappropriate treatment.

The diagnosis of hemophilia is likely to be made clinically, but the radiologist must be aware of its skeletal manifestations, including not only the typical arthropathies and bone cysts, but also and importantly, the rare hemophiliac pseudotumors. Although *radiographs* can diagnose hemophilic arthropathies in

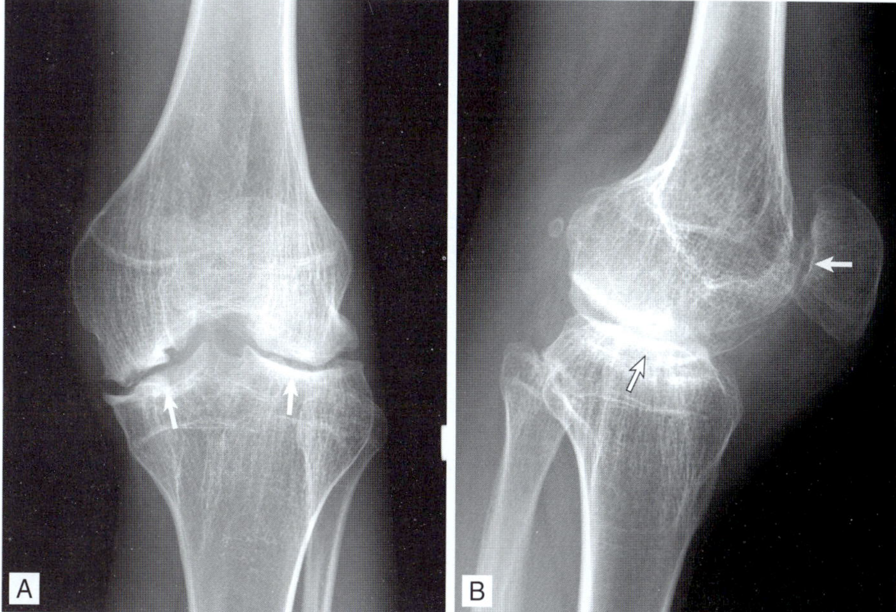

Figure 54.44 Hemophilia of the knee with secondary degeneration. Anteroposterior (A) and lateral (B) right knee radiographs show complete joint space loss with erosions of the articular surfaces (*arrows*) due to many recurring episodes of inflammation from intra-articular hemorrhage.

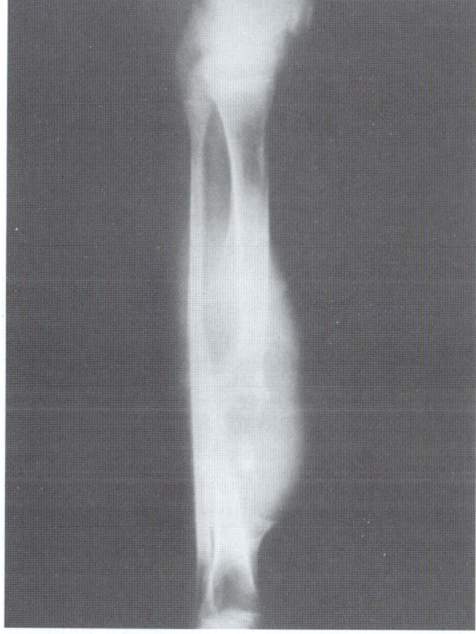

Figure 54.45 Hemophiliac pseudotumor. A huge destructive lesion in the tibia, with relatively well-defined margins, is associated with some periosteal reaction. Although an initial impression may be of a malignant tumor, changes in hemophilic arthropathy can be seen in the knee and ankle.

the later stage, *ultrasonography* has the potential to diagnose hemophilic arthropathy earlier before articular distraction occurs [29]. Also, the CT scan has comparable diagnostic performance with MRI in diagnosing cenobite is before osseous destruction occurs. However, MRI is still considered the gold standard diagnostic tool for assessing hemophiliac arthropathy [30].

Bone Marrow Changes

Bone marrow, with the main function of hematopoiesis, consists of cellular components, including hematopoietic and fat cells and supporting structures. Physiologically, bone marrow has two forms of red and yellow marrow. Red marrow has many erythropoietic cells and is hematopoietically active, whereas yellow marrow mostly consists of fat cells and is hematopoietically inactive.

The best imaging method of evaluating bone marrow is MRI using T1-weighted pulse sequences, which are exquisitely fat sensitive and thus most accurate for evaluating bone marrow changes. On T1-weighted images, red marrow demonstrates lower signal intensity than yellow marrow, which characteristically percent with high signal intensity on T1-weighted images [31].

Bone Marrow Conversion and Reconversion

Bone marrow conversion is a physiologic process starting from childhood and lasting by the age of 25. During this process, red bone marrow, which fills the entire skeleton, converts to yellow marrow. Conversion starts from the distal of the limbs and continues proximally to the axial skeleton. Within the long bones, epiphysis, diaphysis, and metaphysis get involved, respectively. In the vertebrae, the conversion starts from the center and continues to progress peripherally. As a result of the conversion, normal bone marrow in adults has a high signal intensity on T1-weighted and a low signal intensity on fat-suppressed T2-weighted MR images [32].

Bone marrow reconversion is a reversing process in which yellow marrow is replaced by red marrow. This process usually occurs as a physiologic response to the needs of the body to the medical or nonmedical conditions, including:

- Medical conditions:
  - Diabetes mellitus
  - Hemoglobinopathies
  - Obesity and related respiratory disorders
  - Treatment with hematopoietic growth factors
- Nonmedical conditions:
  - Smoking
  - Strenuous sports (e.g., marathon running)

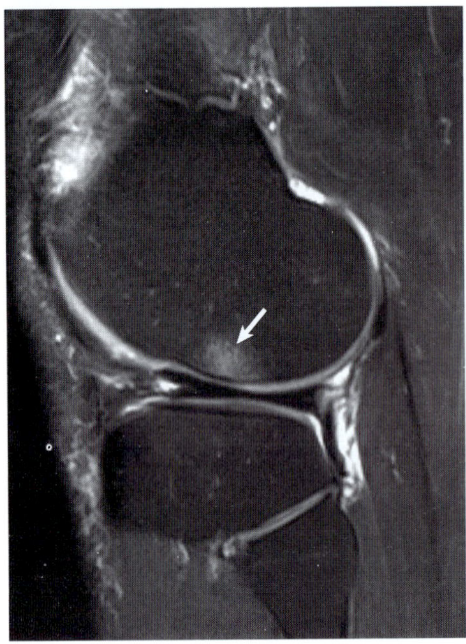

Figure 54.46 Bone bruise of the knee in a patient with a recent anterior cruciate ligament injury. Sagittal fat-suppressed MR image of the left knee in a patient with recent anterior cruciate ligament injury (not shown) demonstrates a characteristic bone bruise (*arrow*), also known as a bone contusion, at the lateral condylopatellar sulcus, which resulted from a collision with the posterior lateral tibia during pivot shift subluxation.

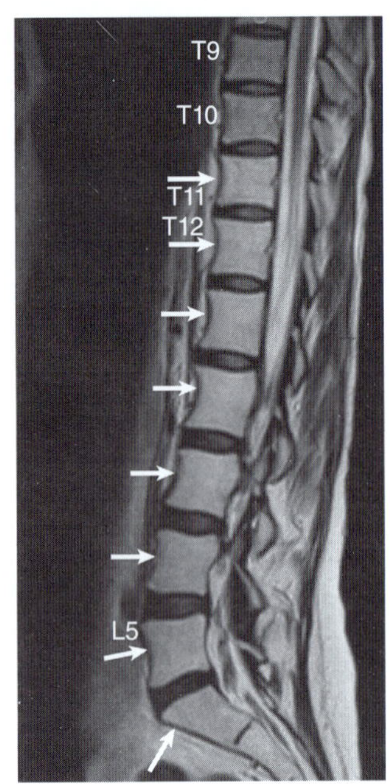

Figure 54.47 Fatty replacement of the vertebral body bone marrow. Sagittal T1-weighted thoracolumbosacral MR image shows replacement of the normal bone marrow with fatty marrow extending from T11 to S1 (*arrows*) following radiation. Note the red marrow contents in the T9 and T10 vertebral bodies.

On T1-weighted images, symmetric bone marrow distribution with increasing red marrow amounts is characteristic for reconversion [31].

Bone Marrow Edema

Bone marrow edema results from increased interstitial fluids in the marrow space. The most common underlying cause of bone marrow edema is trauma, which results in trabecular disruption and hemorrhage to the extracellular space. On MRI, areas of signal hyperintensity on fat-suppressed T2-weighted images are typical for bone marrow edema. The appearances are similar on STIR MR images.

The imaging patterns of bone marrow edema can vary depending on the mechanisms of trauma. A shearing- and avulsion-type injury can demonstrate a linear pattern, whereas an impaction injury results in a globular bone bruise (Fig. 54.46) [33].

Radiation-Induced Marrow Changes

Depending on time and dose, bone marrow may show different MR signals and imaging appearance during and after radiation therapy (Table 54.10). The acute phase mostly occurs within days 1–3 of radiation and represents bone marrow edema with a signal hypointensity on T1-weighted and signal hyperintensity on fat-saturated T2-weighted and STIR sequences images. Following that and in the days 4–10, hemorrhagic areas may be visualized on the MR images as a focal hyperintensity on T1-weighted and hypointensity on the STIR or T2-weighted images. Ultimately, and mostly on days 10–14, a fatty marrow replaces the normal bone marrow and gives a bright appearance on T1-weighted and dark appearance on fat-suppressed MR images (Fig. 54.47). Nonetheless, depending on the dose of radiation, these imaging findings may differ from weeks to months.

Radiation therapy may cause short-term complications in adults, including "irradiation osteitis," which presents on MRI as a signal hypointensity on T1-weighted or signal hyperintensity on the STIR or T2-weighted images in the radiation field, and *insufficiency fractures* on weight-bearing bones due to diminished elastic resistance. In addition, local radiation causes arteritis and fibrosis, which results in *avascular necrosis*. However, in children, radiation may cause impairment to the growth plate and skeletal maturation cessation. Nevertheless, the severity of impairment varies based on the administered dose and the age that the patient receives radiation treatment [32].

TABLE 54.10 Radiation-Induced Marrow Changes

	Days 1–3	Days 4–10	After Day 10
Mechanism	Bone marrow edema	Hemorrhage	Replacement of normal marrow by fatty marrow
T1-weighted MRI findings	Signal hypointensity	Focal signal hyperintensity	Bright appearance
Fat-suppressed fluid-sensitive MRI findings	Signal hyperintensity	Focal signal hypointensity	Dark appearance

Postmarrow Transplant Changes

Autologous or allogeneic stem cell transplantation is a commonly used therapy for hematologic malignancies. The evaluation of bone marrow before and after the transplantation is mostly performed by MRI. After transplantation and during the first days, a treatment-induced bone marrow edema is a common finding characterized by hypointense areas of marrow on T1-weighted and hyperintense areas of marrow on T2-weighted sequences images. Within 3 months following the transplantation, a band pattern may develop in the spine, which can be seen on T1-weighted images. The banding pattern gradually transforms into a homogeneous bone marrow appearance. After years, fatty bone marrow conversion, as typically seen in adults, is a common imaging finding following a bone marrow transplantation [32].

Suggested Readings

- AS Roberts, AS Shetty, VM Mellnick, PJ Pickhardt, S Bhalla, CO Menias, Extramedullary haematopoiesis: radiological imaging features, Clin Radiol 71 (9) (2016) 807–814.
- R Haidar, KM Musallam, AT Taher, Bone disease and skeletal complications in patients with β thalassemia major, Bone 48 (3) (2011) 425–432.
- AG Ormond Filho, BC Carneiro, D Pastore, IP Silva, SR Yamashita, FD Consolo, et al., Whole-body imaging of multiple myeloma: diagnostic criteria, Radiographics 39 (4) (2019) 1077–1097.
- YX Zhang, MX Li, SF Wei, L Zhang, TM Cheng, YH Ge, Multislice spiral computed tomography imaging in evaluating hemophilic arthropathy, Chin Med J (Engl) 133 (14) (2020) 1669–1675.
- A Małkiewicz, M Dziedzic, Bone marrow reconversion – imaging of physiological changes in bone marrow, Pol J Radiol 77 (4) (2012) 45–50.

55 Musculoskeletal Infections

RAJ CHARI, RAMY MANSOUR

Introduction

Musculoskeletal infections have traditionally been associated with mainly osteomyelitis, septic arthritis, and cellulitis. *Bone and soft-tissue infection (BSTI)* is an inclusive terminology that is rather broader and not just limited to bone and joints and is a common disease and the clinical presentation can be varied depending on the type of infection. The BSTI depending upon the anatomical plane is included in Table 55.1.

The etiology of *osteomyelitis* is different in children and adults. *In children, the etiology is typically hematogenous.* The nature of blood supply to the diaphysis, metaphysis, and epiphysis depends on the age of the patient. In infants, as a result of the diaphyseal vessels extending through the cartilaginous growth plate to reach the epiphysis, there is an increased frequency of epiphyseal and joint infections. In early childhood, these diaphyseal vessels terminate in the metaphysis-forming venous sinusoidal lakes with a slow, turbulent flow which allows blood-borne organisms to seed, proliferate, and cause metaphyseal osteomyelitis [1–4]. *In adults*, the hematogenous spread is less common and the bacterial access is *usually due to direct inoculation* from penetrating trauma, surgery, or adjacent contaminated soft tissue. Other etiologies are vascular insufficiency causing contiguous infection in the case of diabetic foot and osteomyelitis in immunocompromised patients [5].

The *soft tissue infection* etiology can be variable depending upon the anatomical site and include mechanism-related (bite, trauma, etc.) and patient-related (critical illness, elderly age, immunocompromised state, liver and kidney disease, and vascular insufficiency, etc.) risk factors [6].

Imaging of BSTI depends on the affected structure and tissue plane. Different imaging techniques include radiographs, ultrasonography (USG), computed tomography (CT), magnetic resonance imaging (MRI), and nuclear medicine studies.

- Radiographs are generally the first imaging technique to be considered when BSTI is suspected, even when the presentation is of soft-tissue infection, the radiographs are useful to determine the underlying bone and joint integrity [2]
- USG can be used either as the primary imaging technique or as an adjunct to other techniques, it is a relatively cheap, dynamic, and effective investigation aiding in the diagnosis and potential intervention of soft tissue and joint infections [1]
- Cross-sectional imaging techniques, such as CT and MRI, are useful to study the extent of BSTI in three dimension, bone architecture, and tissue plane [7]
- Functional imaging, such as three-phase bone scintigraphy, positron emission tomography using fluorodeoxyglucose, gallium scintigraphy, labeled leukocytes, and labeled antibodies against leukocyte surface antigens, antigranulocyte antibodies, etc. have a role in troubleshooting and surveillance [8]. Flow chart showing approach to diagnosis and intervention of soft tissue and bone infection is shown in (Fig. 55.1)

Soft-Tissue Infection

Cellulitis

Human skin serves as the principal barrier and the first line of defense against microbial infection and infection commonly follows a breach of the skin layer [8]. *Cellulitis is the most common form of musculoskeletal infection*, it is a spreading inflammatory reaction of infectious origin occurring along the skin, subcutaneous, and fascial planes with edema and skin changes. The common pathogens associated with cellulitis are *Streptococcus pyogenes* or *Staphylococcus aureus*. Predisposing factors include stasis, poor general health, skin laceration or ulceration, venepuncture, eczema, and immunosuppression [9].

USG is an ideal technique of investigation and cross-sectional imaging is rarely necessary. The appearances range from diffuse swelling, hyperechogenicity of the skin, and subcutaneous tissues to a variable cobblestone appearance depending on the anatomical site, the orientation of the interlobular fat septa, and degree of subcutaneous edema. USG appearances (Fig. 55.2) are similar to that of subcutaneous edema of systemic cause such as cardiac failure; *however, the presence of hyperemia on Doppler imaging is the diagnostic of cellulitis.*

On MRI there is T2/STIR hyperintensity of the affected area with diffuse linear or ill-defined soft-tissue thickening with corresponding T1 hypointensity and postcontrast enhancement. Subcutaneous

TABLE 55.1 Bone and Soft-Tissue Infection (BSTI) Terminology

Anatomic Plane	Terminology
Skin	Cellulitis
Fascia	Infective fasciitis/necrotizing fasciitis
Muscle	Pyomyositis
Tendon sheath	Infective tenosynovitis
Bursa	Septic bursitis
Joint	Septic arthritis
Periosteum	Infective periostitis
Bone	Osteomyelitis
Prosthesis	Prosthetic infection

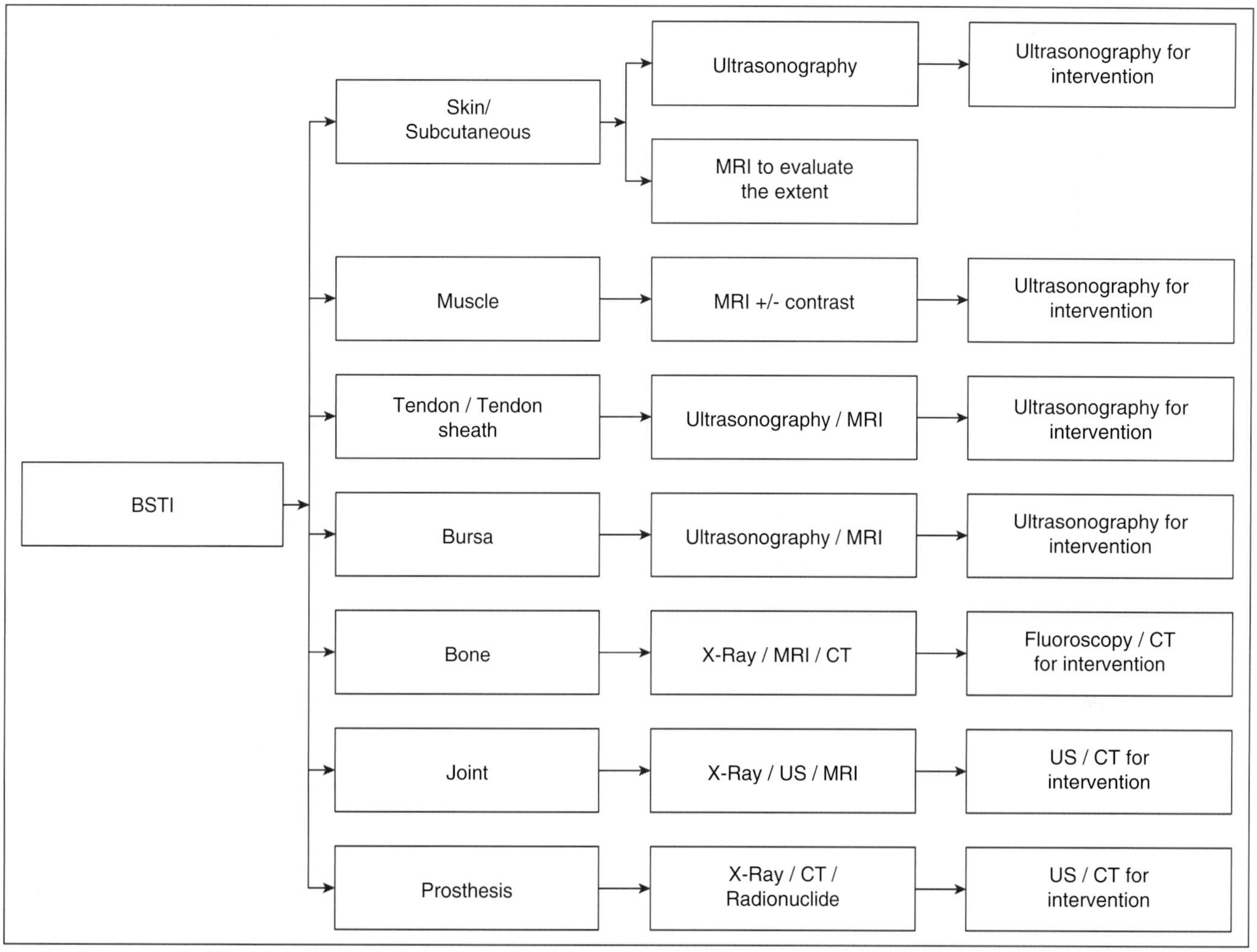

Site	Diagnosis	Intervention
BSTI → Skin/Subcutaneous	Ultrasonography	Ultrasonography for intervention
	MRI to evaluate the extent	
BSTI → Muscle	MRI +/- contrast	Ultrasonography for intervention
BSTI → Tendon / Tendon sheath	Ultrasonography / MRI	Ultrasonography for intervention
BSTI → Bursa	Ultrasonography / MRI	Ultrasonography for intervention
BSTI → Bone	X-Ray / MRI / CT	Fluoroscopy / CT for intervention
BSTI → Joint	X-Ray / US / MRI	US / CT for intervention
BSTI → Prosthesis	X-Ray / CT / Radionuclide	US / CT for intervention

Figure 55.1 A flow chart of the approach of diagnosis and intervention of soft tissue and bone infection.

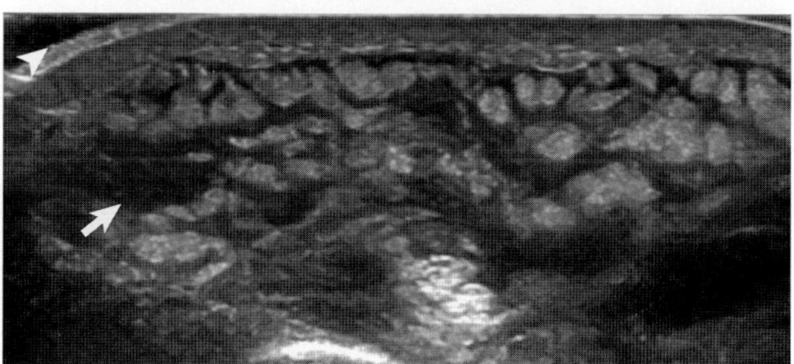

Figure 55.2 Transverse plane USG images showing extensive subcutaneous edema (*arrow*) of the dorsum of the wrist with thickened overlying skin (*arrowhead*), the appearances are typical of cellulitis.

edema of a local or systemic cause may mimic cellulitis on MRI, but without postcontrast enhancement.

CT of cellulitis shows subcutaneous fat stranding with thickening of overlying skin. Cellulitis is usually managed medically by antibiotics and treatment of underlying cause where necessary; however, image-guided intervention or surgical drainage is necessary if an abscess is formed [10,11]. *Phlegmonous change* refers to unbounded, nonspecific inflammation of soft tissue and can be of infectious origin. It is less focal and indistinct in nature compared with a walled-off abscess. It is often difficult to differentiate small or early abscess from phlegmon on USG. They both appear as ill-defined hypoechoic lesions without identifiable wall and the presence of internal color signals on color Doppler. Larger abscesses can be readily distinguished as a hypoechoic fluid collection on USG and presence of Doppler signals only in the periphery.

Necrotizing Fasciitis

Necrotizing fasciitis is an aggressive infection of the skin and soft tissue with *necrosis of the muscle, fascia, and subcutaneous tissues*. This infection typically spreads rapidly along the fascial plane, which has a poor blood supply. The reported mortality rate is as high as 29% even with treatment [12]. Direct inoculation of bacteria through a breach in the skin is seen in the majority of cases, gram-positive cocci such as *S. aureus* and Streptococci are seen in single site infection. Polymicrobial infections, however, occur with a combination of gram-negative and anaerobic bacteria, which aid rapid spread and difficulty in treatment. Gas-producing organisms (gram negative) lead to subcutaneous gas formation, whereas toxin-producing organisms (gram positive) cause toxic shock-like symptoms [13]. Although the term necrotizing fasciitis encompasses all soft-tissue infections deep to the hypodermis, depending upon the anatomical site, *Fournier gangrene* for the perineum or *Ludwig angina* for the submandibular region are recognized as subtypes [14]. Although there are no recognized risk factors, there is an association with pre-existing comorbidities, such as diabetes, vascular disease, immunosuppression, obesity, and drug abuse [15].

Figure 55.3 (A) Coronal STIR. (B) Axial STIR image of the thigh showing an ill-defined fluid collection (*arrow*) within the adductor magnus muscle with significant surrounding soft tissue edema in keeping with pyomyositis. (C) Axial T1 image showing isointense fluid collection with slightly hyperintense capsule (*arrow*).

Clinical presentation is usually out of proportion of pain, fever, and sepsis.

At MRI, the key finding is high T2/STIR signal intensity with corresponding low T1 signal intensity and variable contrast enhancement (depending on the degree of necrosis) along the deep fascia and deep intermuscular fascia involving multiple muscular compartments. If the signal changes are limited to superficial fascia or peripheral portions of the deep fascia, it is unlikely to represent necrotizing fasciitis. The presence of characteristic low signal foci in all sequences and blooming artifact on the gradient-echo sequence in the soft tissue is suggestive of free air and diagnostic of necrotizing fasciitis, however, the absence of the same does not exclude necrotizing fasciitis [16–18].

USG features include diffuse thickening of the subcutaneous tissue, subcutaneous hyperemia, perifascial fluid, distorted appearance of the visual field when there is the presence of soft-tissue air. CT studies show focal subcutaneous fat infiltration, asymmetric fascial thickening, and increased circumference of the affected limb with or without soft-tissue gas [19].

Pyomyositis

Skeletal muscles have ample blood supply and healthy muscles are generally resistant to infection, however, the hematogenous spread of predominantly *S. aureus* in individuals with predisposing conditions such as diabetes, malnutrition, human immunodeficiency virus (HIV) infection, immunodeficiency, drug abuse, malignancy, or trauma can cause primary pyomyositis.

Pyomyositis or infective myositis goes through three stages:

- The first invasive stage is characterized by nonspecific muscle edema similar to myositis

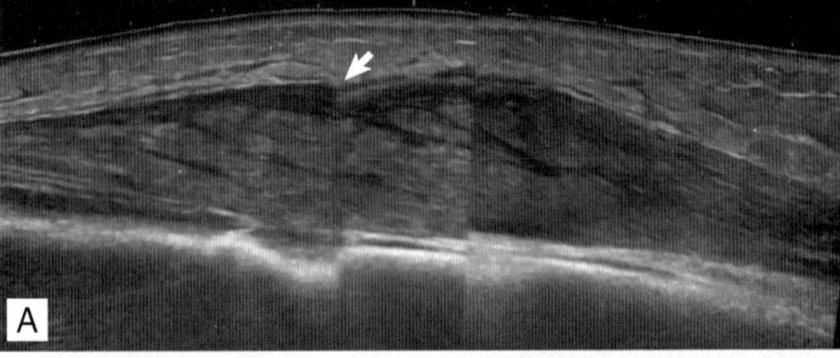

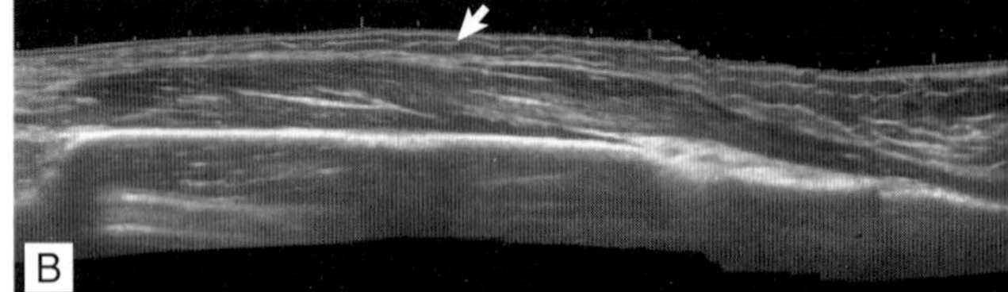

Figure 55.4 (A) Ultrasonography image of the triceps muscle, showing edema, fusiform enlargement (*arrow*), and ill-defined fluid collection interspersed between the muscle fibers in keeping with pyomyositis, the blood cultures of the patient grew *Staphylococcus aureus*. (B) Ultrasonography image 2 weeks later after antibiotic therapy shows complete resolution.

- The second suppurative stage is characterized by intramuscular abscess formation (Figs. 55.3 and 55.4)
- The third late stage is characterized by septicemia and multiorgan failure with a significantly high mortality rate [20]

Multiple muscle involvement is seen in up to 40% of cases due to bacterial seeding, the majority of cases, however, involve a single muscle. Lower limb muscles are affected more often with a predilection to the quadriceps compartment.

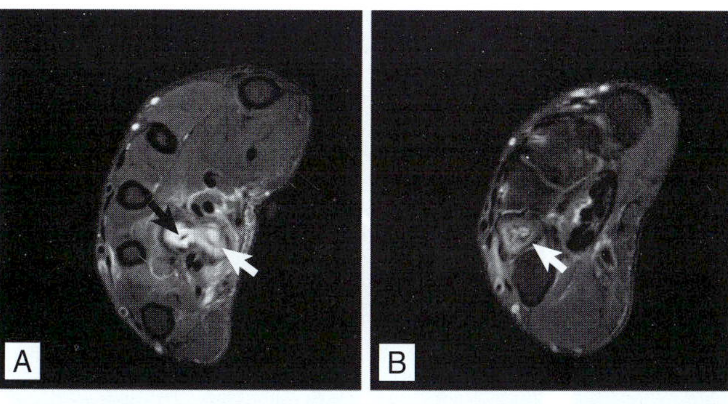

Figure 55.5 (A) MRI axial STIR images of the wrist. Foreign body within the flexor tendon sheath (*black arrow*) causing septic flexor tenosynovitis (*white arrow*) and (B) osteomyelitis of the fourth metacarpal (*arrow*).

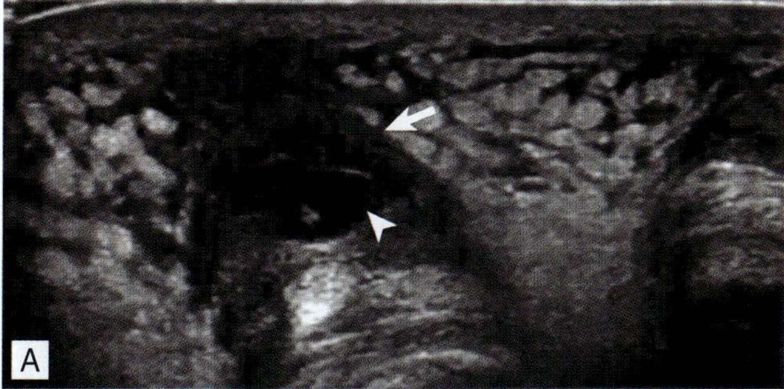

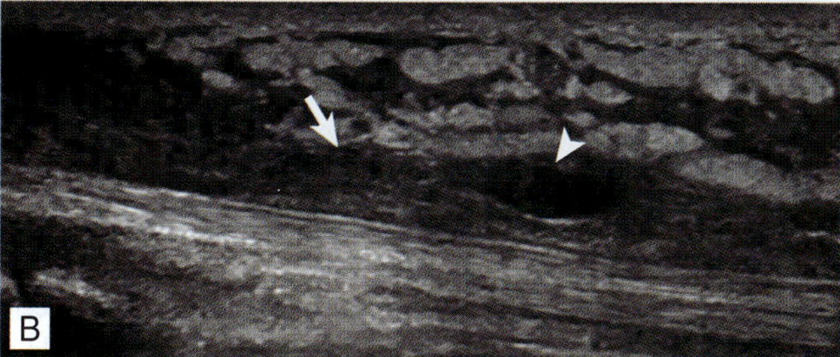

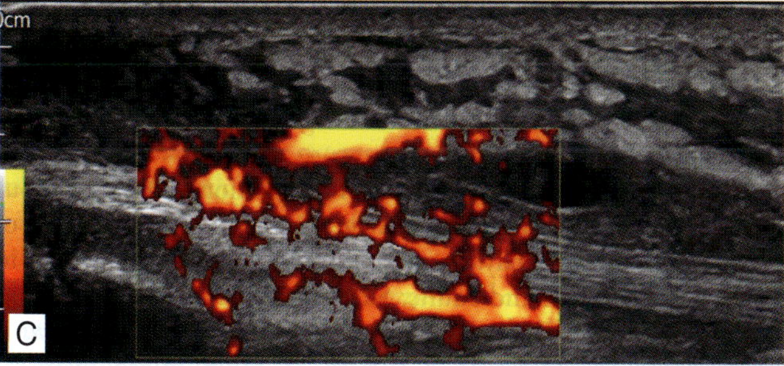

Figure 55.6 (A) Transverse USG image. (B) Longitudinal USG image of the dorsum of the hand showing significantly thickened extensor tendon sheath (*arrow*) with an associated abscess formation along the tendon sheath (*arrowhead*). (C) Longitudinal USG image with Doppler, showing significant hyperemia. The appearances are representative of infective tenosynovitis.

MRI may show only nonspecific muscle edema with high T2/STIR and isointense T1 signal change in the early stages and indistinguishable from other conditions causing myositis. In the initial stages, infectious myositis should be differentiated from inflammatory myositis by clinical features such as duration of onset of symptoms, muscle weakness, serum markers as the imaging may not be of help. However, a muscle biopsy remains the gold standard for the diagnosis [21].

As the disease progresses, *the hallmark intramuscular abscess is formed with surrounding inflammatory changes* disproportionate and more extensive compared with the size of the abscess itself. Depending upon the age and content of the abscess, the signal characteristics are low to intermediate at T1 and high T2 signal change (Fig. 55.3). Peripheral contrast enhancement and lack of central enhancement is pathognomonic and differentiates from solid sinister lesions, which show central enhancement [22].

Careful evaluation should be performed along with clinical correlation to differentiate myonecrosis from an abscess. Myonecrosis commonly occurs with a background of ischemia, sickle cell crisis, compartment syndrome, and crush injury. On MRI, T2 hyperintensity and T1 iso/hypointensity with associated perifascial, perimuscular, subcutaneous edema and dot-like, streaky, or curvilinear enhancing foci within a region of muscle separated from normal muscle by an enhancing rim [23]. On CT, the affected muscle shows relatively low attenuation changes and increased circumference of the affected limb in the early phase and intramuscular fluid collection with peripheral contrast enhancement in the late phase [24]. On USG, the affected muscle shows low attenuation changes and the collection may have heterogeneous contents with postacoustic enhancement (Fig. 55.4).

Infectious Tenosynovitis

Infectious tenosynovitis refers to the infection of the space between the inner visceral layer adherent to the tendon and an outer parietal layer with inflammatory reaction and pus within the tendon sheath. The most common pathogen is *S. aureus*, less commonly and the mechanism of bacterial inoculation into the tendon sheath is by penetrating trauma or rarely, spread from infected adjacent soft tissues. Less commonly, fungi, *Mycobacterium tuberculosis*, and nontuberculous mycobacterial infections are seen, particularly in immunocompromised individuals. *It commonly affects the flexor tendons of the hands and wrist.* Compared with the extensor tendons around the wrist, the flexor tendon sheaths communicate with adjacent bursae and hence the direct spread of infection is more common with flexor tendons (Fig. 55.5).

USG has an edge over MRI since it is dynamic and has a higher resolution in the periphery. USG can demonstrate thickening of the tendon and tendon sheath with hyperemia on Doppler imaging (Fig. 55.6), it can also be used for guided aspiration of fluid for microbial analysis.

MRI is also able to show tendon and tendon sheath thickening and the presence or absence of fluid. It is particularly useful to depict the extent and anatomical relations of the tenosynovitis (Fig. 55.5). Often it is difficult to differentiate from inflammatory tenosynovitis, apart from when there is a presence of preceding history of penetrating trauma. In the late phases, suppurative tenosynovitis shows the presence of pus within the tendon sheath and clinically presents with *Kanavel sign* (sausage-like fingers, proximal interphalangeal joint flexion, pain on passive extension, and tenderness over the flexor tendon sheath), which is more specific for infective tenosynovitis when compared with inflammatory tenosynovitis [1,10,25].

Septic Bursitis

Inflammation of various bursae is a common clinical problem due to chronic repetitive strain or mechanical reasons and presents as sterile inflammation of the bursal wall with free fluid in the bursa. *Septic bursitis is caused by bacterial inoculation of the synovial bursae and S. aureus is the most common pathogen involved.* Superficial bursae are more commonly involved due to the chance of direct inoculation due to trauma, for example, Olecranon bursa, prepatellar

BOX 55.1 Causes for Periosteal Reaction

Infection	Acute osteomyelitis
	Chronic osteomyelitis
Tumors	Osteogenic tumors
	Chondroid tumors
	Ewing's sarcoma
	Lymphoma
	Leukemia
Trauma	Fracture
	Stress fracture
	Insufficiency fracture
Auto inflammatory conditions	CRMO
	SAPHO
	Majeed syndrome
Drugs induced	Vitamin A
	Fluorides
	Prostaglandins
	Variconozole
Metabolic	Hypertrophic pulmonary osteoarthropathy
	Thyroid acropathy
	Rickets
Congenital / Genetic	Pachydermoperiostosis
	Periosteal reaction of newborn
	Caffey's disease
Vascular	Venous insufficiency

Periosteal reaction may be focal or multifocal

- Focal forms include those related to infection, trauma, stress, and neoplasm
- Multifocal involvement can be seen with multiple areas of one disease such as chronic multifocal osteomyelitis (CRMO) or, especially when diffuse, heralds a systemic process such as hypertrophic osteoarthropathy, which may be primary (pachydermoperiostitis) or secondary such as from underlying pulmonary pathology in the setting of hypertrophic pulmonary osteoarthropathy, chronic venous stasis/insufficiency, thyroid acropachy, hypervitaminosis A, fluorosis, and infantile cortical hyperostosis (Caffey disease) [27,46,47]

Although drug-related periostitis including prostaglandin, vitamin A, and fluoride have long been known, the association of voriconazole with periostitis is a relatively recent observation. The pathogenesis of drug-induced periostitis is still unknown. Postulated theories suggest a role for neural reflex, neuroendocrine mechanisms, involvement of megakaryocytes, or large clump of platelets [48].

Subperiosteal Abscess

A subperiosteal abscess is most commonly found in pediatric forms of osteomyelitis, as these patients are known to have looser adherence of the periosteum to the underlying cortex. In addition to MRI, USG has also been found to be a useful technique to establish the diagnosis and to follow patients with known subperiosteal abscess (Fig. 55.7), with the benefits of decreased exam time and precluding the need for sedation or anesthesia [33,47].

Intraosseous "Brodie's" Abscess

First described by Brodie, intraosseous abscesses occur most often in children, have a predilection for the metaphysis of long bones, and are observed in the subacute or chronic stage of osteomyelitis when the organism has reduced virulence. An intraosseous abscess is an intraosseous cavity filled with pus, with a rim of granulation tissue.

On MRI, intraosseous abscesses demonstrate high T2 and low to intermediate T1-weighted signal, rim enhancement after contrast administration (Fig. 55.9), and occasionally have a rim of medullary sclerosis or associated periosteal new bone formation. In pediatric patients, occasionally the abscess will traverse the physis and extend into the epiphysis (Fig. 55.10), although with effective antibiotic treatment, growth disturbance is rare. The penumbra sign, a discrete peripheral rim of mildly hyperintense signal about the low signal central abscess cavity on T1-weighted images, seen in 75% of intraosseous abscesses and histologically representing a rim of hypervascular granulation tissue. The penumbra sign has high specificity for the identification of bone or soft-tissue abscess [49,50]. The rim sign has also been described as a useful indicator of an intraosseous abscess on MRI, appearing as well-defined T1 and T2/STIR hypointense rim about the periphery of the abscess cavity (Fig. 55.9). The term cloaca is used to indicate an opening or rupture of the bony cortex overlying an area of osteomyelitis that allows granulation tissue and/or intramedullary pus to be discharged out of the bone. Inherently, the term implies either active or chronic infection of the bone, and a cloaca is often continuous with an intraosseous abscess (Brodie's abscess) [38–40].

Chronic Osteomyelitis

Chronic osteomyelitis can be associated with a sinus tract, draining granulation tissue and/or pus from the bone to the skin. Chronic osteomyelitis demonstrates inhomogeneous marrow signal, with areas of active disease demonstrating high T2, low T1 signal, interposed with areas of fibrosis which will demonstrate low signal on both T1- and T2-weighted images features of chronic osteomyelitis also include cortical remodeling and sequestra (Figs. 55.11 and 55.12) [43,51]. A sinus tract is an abnormal channel that originates or ends in one opening. A soft-tissue ulcer can show a sinus tract leading to a deeper soft-tissue collection or abscess. An extra-articular soft-tissue process can follow a sinus tract into a joint. MRI findings of the sinus tract include linear fluid-filled structure extending from bone to the skin surface with a hypointense signal on T1-weighted images and a hyperintense signal on T2-weighted images (Figs. 55.11 and 55.12). On contrast-enhanced images, in the setting of infection, sinus tracts display a "tram track" pattern of peripheral enhancement. Longstanding sinus tracts from chronic osteomyelitis may lead to malignant transformation, with squamous cell carcinoma being the most frequent malignancy developing from the epithelial lining of the tract.

A *bony sequestrum* is defined as a piece of devitalized bone that has become separated from the surrounding bone during the process of necrosis (Fig. 55.11) [51,52]. The presence of a sequestrum is definitive for chronic osteomyelitis. The presence of dead bone usually with fistulous tracts secondary to infection confirms the presence of chronic osteomyelitis. This devitalized bone becomes distinct from or "sequestered" from the adjacent more viable bone. Such nonviable, necrotic, and distinct bone contains

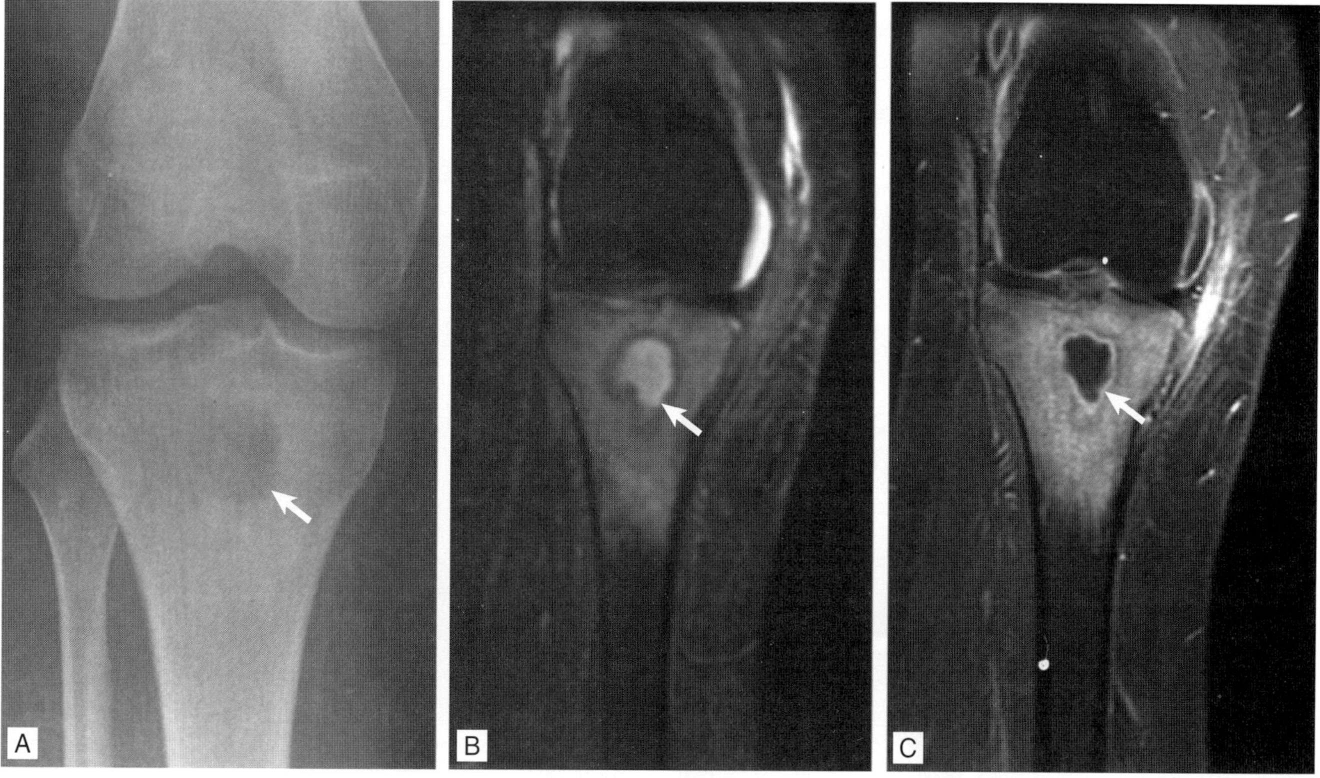

Figure 55.9 (A) Anteroposterior radiograph view of the knee showing a well-defined lucency in the proximal tibia (*white arrow*), representing an abscess. (B) Coronal STIR image showing an interosseous collection (*arrow*) with surrounding bone marrow edema, (C) corresponding coronal T1FS with contrast, showing rim enhancement.

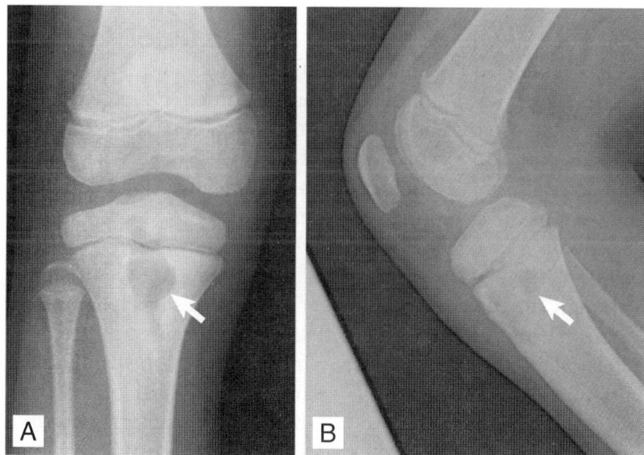

Figure 55.10 (A) Anteroposterior and (B) lateral radiograph views of the knee in a child showing well-defined lucency involving the tibial metaphysis in keeping with a Brodie's abscess. The key recognizing feature is extension of the lucency across the growth plate.

bacteria that are protected from circulating antibiotics and is called sequestrum.

Sequestrum is adequately depicted with radiographs and best identified with CT (Figs. 55.11 and 55.12). On CT a sequestrum will appear as a focal area of mineralization surrounded by relative lucency (Fig. 55.11). The appearance of sequestrum on MRI is not well described but is likely seen as poorly visualized areas of a decreased signal. Importantly, the sequestrum, if identified as such, often in conjunction with CT imaging, should not enhance, especially if cortically based. However, peripheral enhancement due to granulation tissue surrounding the sequestrum may be possible [53–56].

An *involucrum* describes the formation of a spherical capsule of viable new bone around an area of sequestered and necrotic bone. The involucrum can be viewed as a response to wall-off the necrotic, infected sequestrum. It often involves periosteal new bone formation. The involucrum consists of different layers.

- The inner lining of the involucrum faces the sequestrum and consists of granulation tissue
- The outer layer of the involucrum consists of expansile, coarse, woven bone, which is typically sclerotic in the mature stage

Eventually, the outer margin of the involucrum merges with the surrounding bone.

On MR images, the inner granulation tissue lining of the involucrum may demonstrate signal hyperintensity on T1-weighted MR images, like the penumbra sign described in subacute chronic osteomyelitis (Fig. 55.11). The signal intensities of the osseous component of the involucrum vary and include edema pattern on STIR and T2-weighted images, and hypo- or hyperintensity on T1-weighted MR images depending on the amounts of marrow fat contents and sclerotic bone.

Differential diagnostic consideration of an involucrum consist of cortical thickening secondary to an osseous stress reaction, benign bone lesions (osteoid osteoma, osteoblastoma, fibrous dysplasia), malignant bone lesions (osteosarcoma, Ewing sarcoma, lymphoma, and chondrosarcoma), Paget's disease, avascular necrosis, and healing or healed trauma.

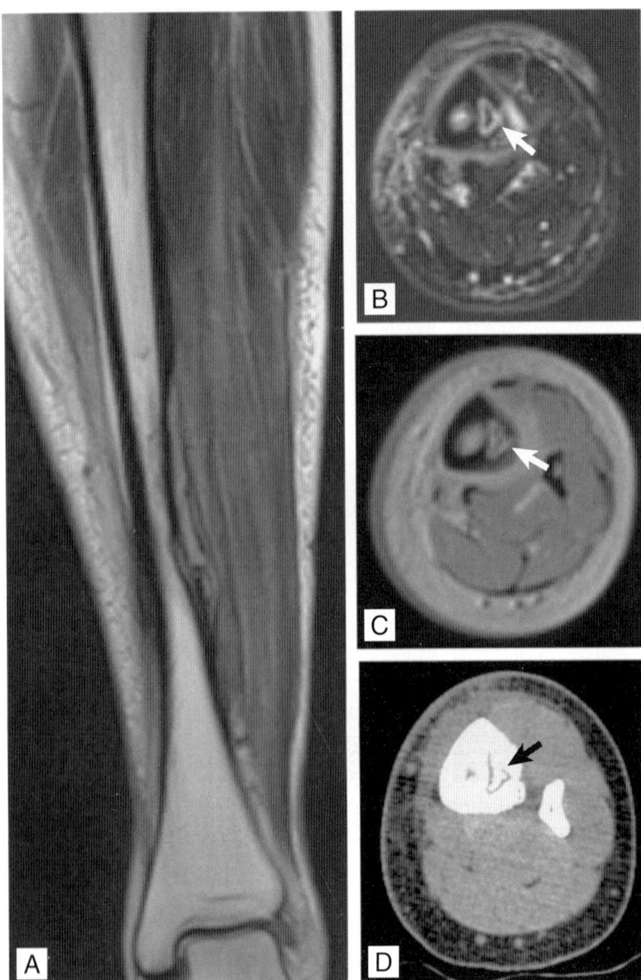

Figure 55.11 A patient with chronic osteomyelitis of the tibia. (A) Coronal T1, (B) axial STIR, and (C) axial postcontrast-enhanced T1 image showing cortical bone defect with enhancement of the granulation tissue (*white arrow*). (D) Axial unenhanced CT image showing hyperdense sequestrum (*black arrow*).

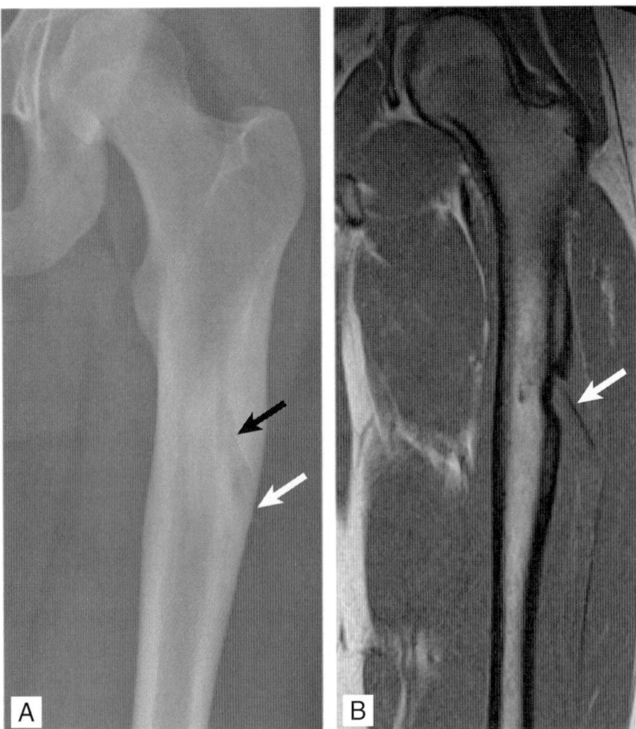

Figure 55.12 A patient with chronic osteomyelitis of the femur. (A) Frontal radiograph of the femur showing cortical thickening and a linear cortical lucency in keeping with cloaca (*black arrow*), a subtle linear hyperdensity along the cloaca is in keeping with the dead bone (sequestrum) (*white arrow*). (B) Coronal T1 image showing the cortical defect and a linear low signal sequestrum (*arrow*).

The term *cloaca* is used to indicate an opening or rupture of the bony cortex overlying an area of osteomyelitis that allows granulation tissue and/or intramedullary pus to be discharged out of the bone. A cloaca presents as focal partial-thickness defect (incomplete) or full-thickness (complete) perforation within the involucrum. Inherently, the term implies either active or chronic infection of the bone, and a cloaca is often continuous with an intraosseous abscess (Brodie's abscess).

On radiographs, the visibility of a cloaca depends on the location relative to the direction of the x-ray beam, whereas even small and incomplete cloacae are well visible on high-resolution CT images. CT can demonstrate focal thickening of the cortex with a lucent tract extending from the soft tissues into the bone. MRI can demonstrate and characterize a cloaca to better advantage, although the mineralized contents are less well visualized than on CT image. On MRI, cloaca demonstrates hypointense signal on T1-weighted images and hyperintense signal on T2-weighted images through the most superficial osseous cortex that can extend only intracortical or can extend to the medullary cavity.

After an osseous infection is cleared, the remnants of a cloaca often remain at the cortex of the bone. This is essentially reparative callus, but there can be a relative lucency at the site of the previous opening. Thus, it can be difficult to determine when a cloaca is closed on imaging [57–60].

CRMO is an autoinflammatory disorder characterized by metaphyseal osteitis and the periosteal reaction of the skeleton of children and adolescents [65]. CRMO is also termed chronic nonbacterial osteomyelitis and is a noninfective bone condition discussed in the appropriate chapter of this book.

Tuberculous Osteomyelitis

Although the incidence of skeletal tuberculosis has fallen markedly in recent years, the disease has not yet been eradicated and is relatively common in developing countries and individuals with immunocompromise. Hematogenous spread of infection to the skeleton is assumed to be from the lung and may occur at the time of primary infection or later from postprimary foci. Chest radiography, however, shows active disease in less than 50% of cases, the organism presumably having laid dormant and become active later. The bacillus lodges in the spongiosa of the metaphysis of a long bone.

The tuberculous reaction is destructive and accompanied by pus which may later become calcified. Calcification of abscesses is rarely seen currently if antibiotic treatment is adequate. In contradistinction to pyogenic osteomyelitis, neither sequestration nor periostitis is a prominent feature. Abscesses often point to the skin and a sinus tract may be demonstrated after injection of contrast medium.

Tuberculous osteomyelitis can remain localized to bone or involve adjacent joints and soft tissue (Fig. 55.13). In general, tuberculosis confined to the bone is relatively infrequent.

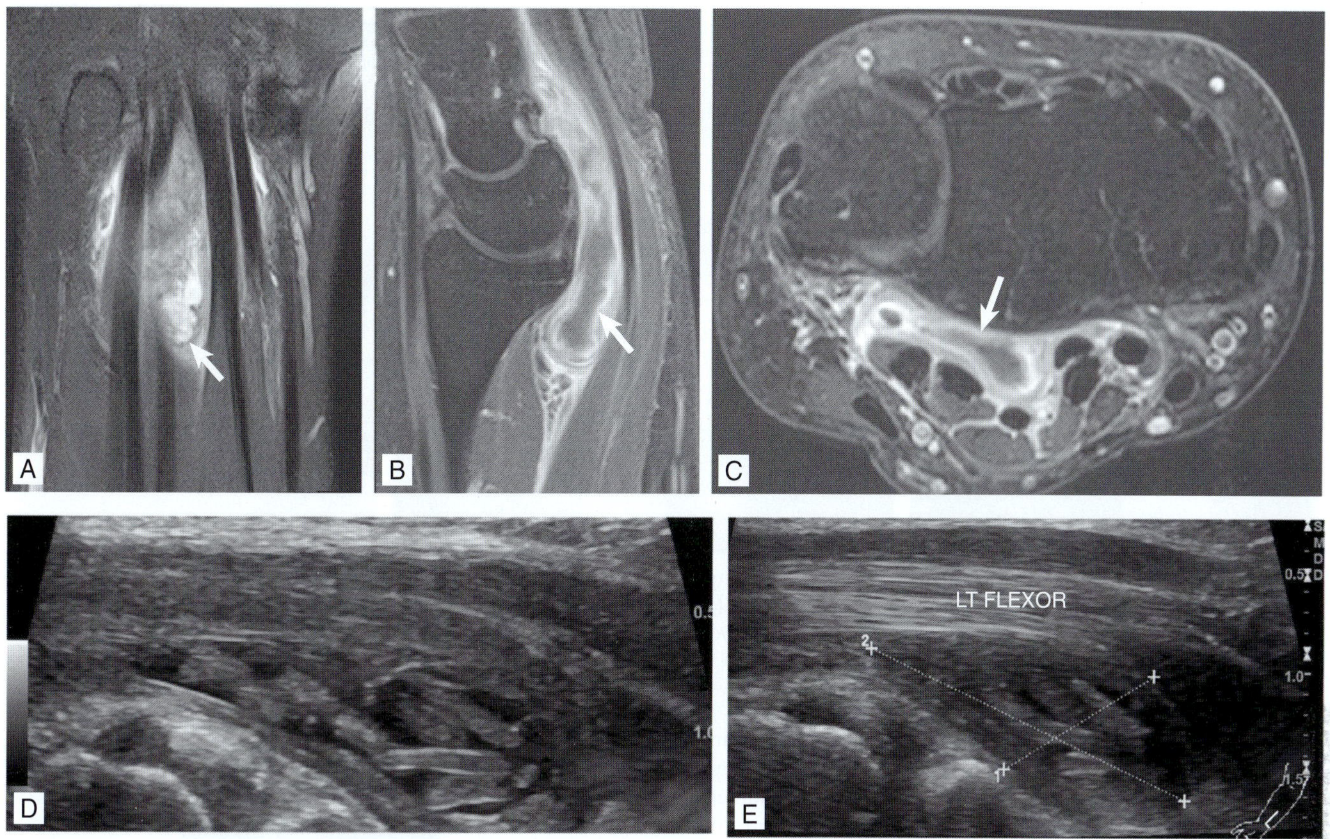

Figure 55.13 (A) MRI coronal STIR image of wrist showing severe flexor tenosynovitis. (B and C) Sagittal and axial contrast-enhanced T1FS images showing significant contrast enhancement of the thickened tendon sheath (*arrows*). Histopathology confirmed tubercular tenosynovitis. (D and E) Corresponding USG images of the same patient as in image A: transverse (D) and longitudinal (E) images showing severe tenosynovitis. (Courtesy: Dr. Graeme Thompson, Oxford University Hospital.)

Virtually any bone can be affected, including the pelvis, phalanges and metacarpals, long bones, ribs, sternum, skull, patella, carpal, and tarsal bones, although tuberculous osteomyelitis has a predilection for the spine (thoracic and lumbar segments) and weight-bearing joints (i.e., hip and knee joints). The metaphysis is the site of election; an oval or rounded focus will be found which soon crosses the epiphyseal line. No surrounding sclerosis is to be expected. The greater trochanter is a common site, particularly in adolescents and young adults (Fig. 55.14).

Tuberculous dactylitis is an uncommon form of extrapulmonary tuberculosis involving the small bones of the hand or the foot usually affecting children of less than 6 years of age, before growth plate fusion. It commonly involves the metacarpals and proximal phalanges of the hands manifested as soft-tissue swelling and periostitis. Children aged 6 years and below account for 85% of cases (1–3). The hematopoietic marrow of the involved bones is favorable for the hematogenous spread of tuberculosis causing fusiform bone expansion, thinned cortex, and granulation tissue formation. The plain radiographic features include fusiform soft-tissue swelling and periostitis. "Spina ventosa" refers to a cyst-like cavity due to the destruction and expansion of the involved bone giving it a "wind-filled sail" appearance (Fig. 55.14). *The presence of diffuse osteopenia and absence of sequestration distinguish tuberculous osteomyelitis from pyogenic osteomyelitis.* The CT scan features include bony sclerosis and destruction. On MRI the lesion demonstrates low signal on T1 and heterogeneous increased signal on T2-weighted sequences with bone expansion [61,62].

Diabetic Foot

Charcot joint or neuropathic osteoarthropathy frequently demonstrates marrow abnormality in the absence of infection and it is a commonly encountered diagnostic dilemma [45]. Neuropathic osteoarthropathy and infection however often coexist. Plain radiograph of the foot has a good sensitivity in identifying osteomyelitis of the digits (Fig. 55.15). The diagnostic difficulty in the MRI diagnosis of osteomyelitis in a patient with Charcot or neuropathic osteoarthropathy is largely because the marrow signal is discordant, the marrow shows high signal intensity on T2-weighted images without a matching confluent medullary pattern of marrow replacement on T1-weighted images (Fig. 55.16). Vascular insufficiency and tissue necrosis pose additional difficulty in the MRI diagnosis of osteomyelitis in the diabetic population. Vascularity is necessary for fat metabolism required to produce confluent, medullary T1 marrow replacement, as well as measurable contrast enhancement. Nonenhancing necrotic bone medullary tissue lacks T1 marrow replacement and bone marrow enhancement which is a potential source of false-negative MRI in a diabetic patient [44–46].

Postoperative Joint Infection

Joint infection after joint surgery (open or minimal access) is rather rare but a serious complication since it can lead to irreparable joint damage, early diagnosis, and treatment are hence essential. Different types of joint surgeries include arthroscopy,

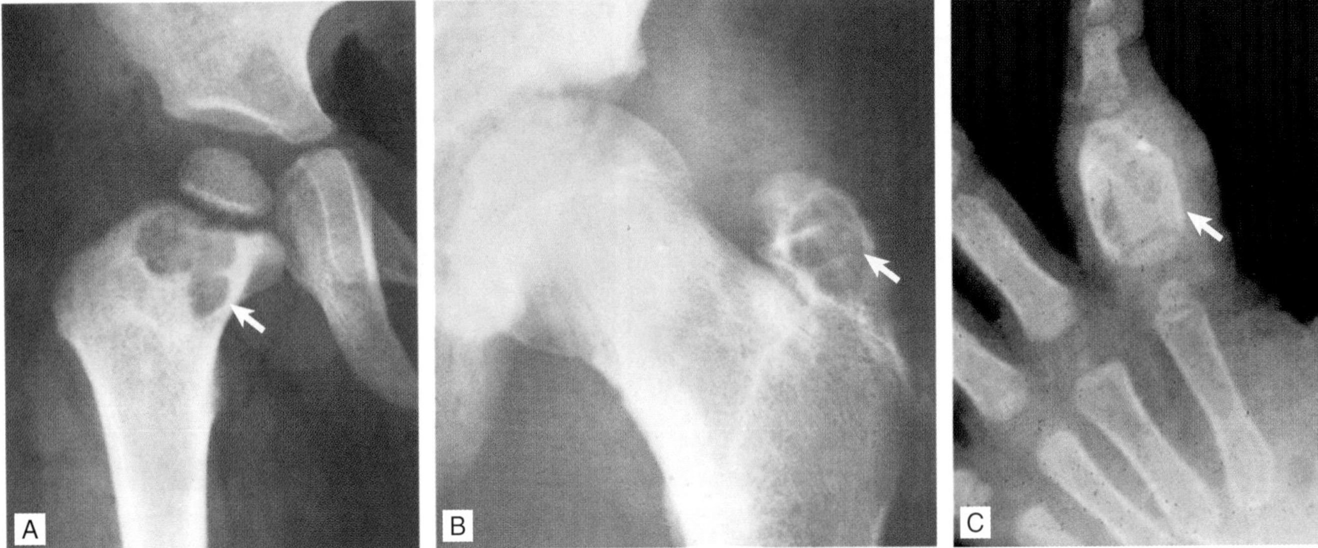

Figure 55.14 Plain radiographs showing examples of tuberculosis. (A) Anteroposterior view of the hip in a child showing well-defined lucency with sclerotic margin, extending to the growth plate. (B) Anteroposterior view of the hip in an adolescent showing well-defined expansile lesion involving the greater trochanter which is a common site, particularly in adolescents and young adults. The lesion may start in the bone or in the overlying bursa, extending into the bone. (C) Anteroposterior view of the hand showing proximal phalanx with characteristic medullary expansion (spina ventosa).

arthrotomy, synovectomy, arthrodesis, and arthroplasty. The incidence of infection in the minimal access surgeries (arthroscopic) is significantly less (0.42%), compared with open surgeries involving prostheses (1–2%). The incidence of the infection increases even further in cases of revision joint surgeries (4–5%) [63,64].

Incidence of infection within 90 days of surgery is considered acute infection and the commonest cause of infection is direct inoculation, however, there can be influence from patient-specific (e.g., immunosuppression) and procedure-specific (e.g., sterilization, duration) factors. The bacteria when conveyed through arthroscopy instruments into the joint deposit in the synovial membrane causing an acute inflammatory response. As the synovium has no barrier mechanism against the bacteria, they easily infiltrate the synovial fluid and cause purulent infection.

Incidence of infection after 90 days of surgery is considered chronic infection and the cause is usually hematogenous. The longer the prosthesis indwelling time, the higher the cumulative risk for hematogenous infections during the entire implant lifetime. The development of modern detection methods for microbial

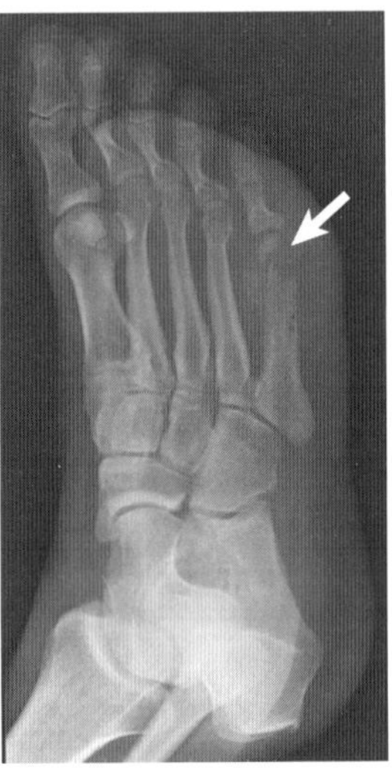

Figure 55.15 Plain radiograph of the foot showing destruction of the head of the fifth metatarsal (*arrow*) in a patient with diabetes mellitus, in keeping with diabetic foot.

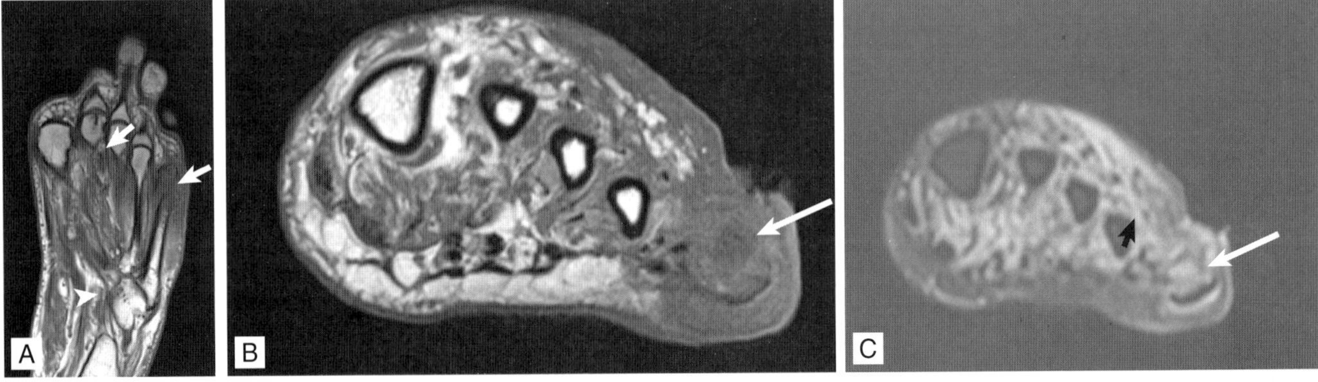

Figure 55.16 (A) Long-axis T1 and (B) short-axis T1 images of the foot showing destruction of the head of the fifth metatarsal (*arrow*). (C) Corresponding short-axis STIR image showing bone marrow edema with marrow fat replacement (*white arrow*) and surrounding soft tissue edema (*black arrow*) in a patient with diabetes mellitus, the appearances are consistent with diabetic foot.

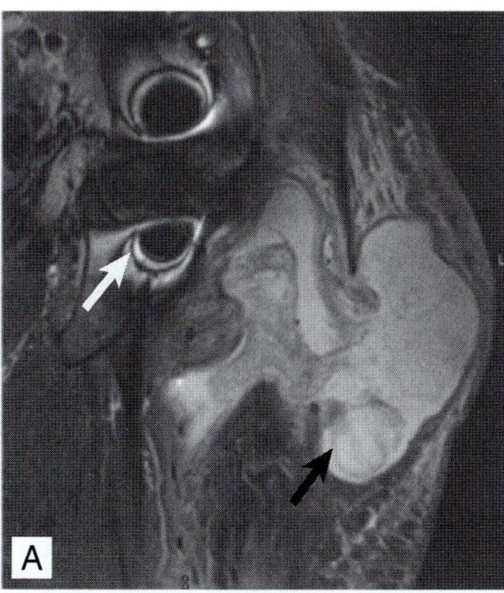

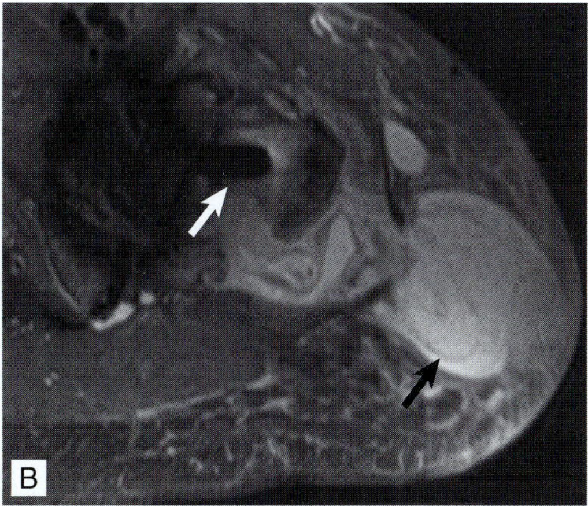

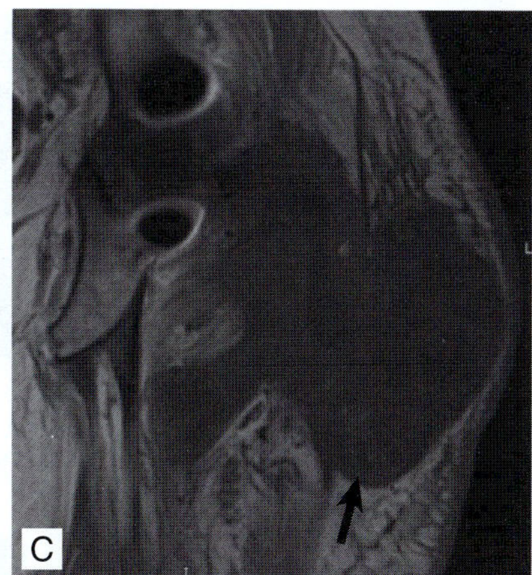

Figure 55.17 (A) Coronal T2FS, (B) axial STIR, and (C) coronal T1 showing a large complex collection (*black arrow*) surrounding a hip resurfacing prosthesis (*white arrow*), representing postoperative infection.

biofilms helps to recognize even chronic infections that would previously have been missed. Early infection is commonly caused by *S. aureus*, streptococci, enterococci, and delayed infection by coagulase-negative staphylococci or *Cutibacterium* species.

Plain radiographs provide important information in the late phase of the disease, and tend to be normal in acute infection; however, may serve as a baseline radiograph for follow-up. Patients with suspicion for concomitant septic spread should undergo an MRI or USG to look for features of joint infection, such as effusion, synovitis, etc. (Fig. 55.17).

When evaluating joint prosthesis infection, the plain radiograph forms the most important technique of imaging. Series of x-rays can be compared against each other to look for signs of prosthetic loosening. The CT scan may also assist in distinguishing between septic and aseptic loosening. MRI is usually of little help in evaluating prosthetic infection due to the presence of susceptibility artifacts from the metalwork. Three-phase bone scintigraphy using technetium has high sensitivity, but low specificity in detecting prosthetic infection. Positron emission tomography using fluorodeoxyglucose presents very divergent results in the literature. A definitive diagnosis of infection should be made by isolating the microorganism through cultures on material obtained from joint fluid, surgical wound secretions, or surgical debridement material.

Brucellosis

This disease is more prevalent in the United Kingdom than was once thought. Transmission is from unpasteurized milk or by direct contact with affected animals. *Brucellusmelitensis* infects sheep, *Br. abortus* infects cattle, and *Br. suis* pigs.

The bones are affected in 10% of cases, most often the spine and especially the lumbar region. Widespread granulomatous lesions may be present:

1. *Spinal lesions.* These bear a marked resemblance to other forms of osteomyelitis. Focal sclerosis develops to a marked degree around the end-plate (Fig. 55.18).The disk is rapidly destroyed and adjacent vertebrae are rapidly affected. Healing is by the production of extremely large, coarse, and shaggy bridging osteophytes
2. *Changes in other bones.* The radiographic appearances resemble those of subacute osteomyelitis
3. *Changes in joints.* These resemble the changes of *synovial tuberculosis.* In advanced cases, erosive lesions may be seen

In obscure and atypical bone infections, it is always advisable to test samples of the blood and the synovial fluid of affected joints for agglutination reaction for brucellosis, and also for typhoid and paratyphoid group of bacilli [65].

Actinomycosis

Bony lesions due to this disease are rarely seen. They usually result from direct extension of soft-tissue lesions. Manifestations may be seen in the following sites:

1. *Mandible.* Chronic osteomyelitis arises by direct spread from oral infections and infected cervical glands. The lesion appears to be irregularly destructive
2. *Ribs and thoracic spine.* Destructive foci and periosteal reaction in these bones arise from pleuropulmonary lesions
3. *Right side of the pelvis and lumbar spine.* The infection spreads to these bones from ileocecal foci. Spinal lesions are usually accompanied by paravertebral abscesses. The disc is usually spared
4. *Lower extremity.* Infection of the lower extremity is very uncommon because of the endogenous habitat of the organism. It can cause destructive changes to the skin, underlying soft tissue and progress deeper to involve bone and called mycetoma (Fig. 55.19). Very rarely, destructive metastatic foci are found in other bones [66]

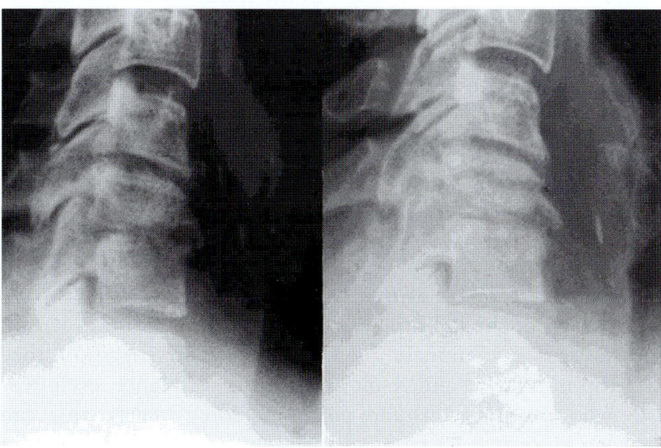

Figure 55.18 Brucellosis. Vertebro-discal destruction with florid new bone formation are characteristic features of this disease.

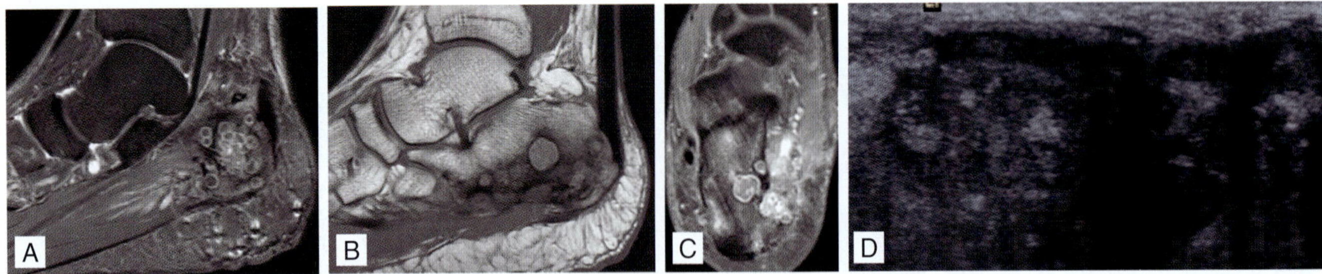

Figure 55.19 Sagittal STIR(A), T1(B), and axial STIR (C) MRI images of the ankle showing several punched out bone lesions involving the calcaneum bone with lesions of similar signal intensity in the soft tissue of the medial aspect of the ankle. Corresponding USG image (D) showing hypoechogenic soft-tissue abnormality in keeping with mycetoma. (Courtesy: Dr. Graeme Thompson, Oxford University Hospital.)

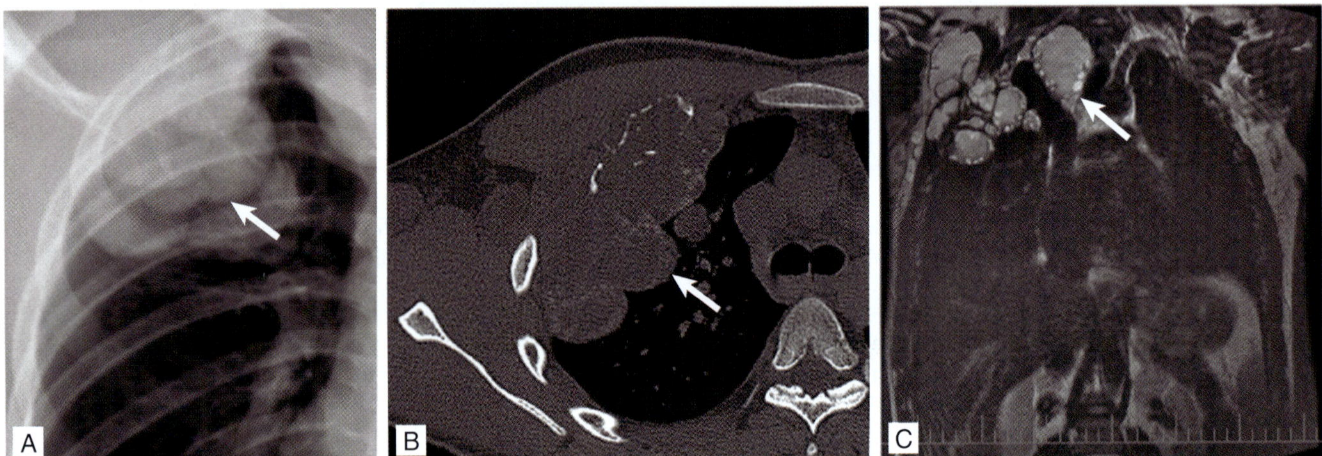

Figure 55.20 A 22-year-old man. (A) Plain radiograph of the chest shows right lung apical opacity (*arrow*) with rib destruction. (B) CT axial image shows osteolytic expansile *lesion* of the second anterior rib with endosteal scalloping, cortical disruption, and extensive multilobular extra osseous component (*arrow*). (C) MRI coronal T2 image shows heterogeneous multicystic expansile lesion in the anterior second rib and superior mediastinum. Small cysts represent daughter cysts inside a mucinous matrix (*arrow*).

Hydatid Disease (*Echinococcus*)

The bone is involved in less than 2% of affected patients with hydatid disease. The pelvis, spine, and proximal long bones are usually involved. The disease is found in sheep-farming areas. The enlarging cysts in bone absorb trabeculae and spread along the medulla, thinning the cortex and expanding the bone (Fig. 55.20). Later, the cystic lesions become well defined, so that fibrous dysplasia may be simulated in long bones. Around the hip joint, both the acetabulum and femoral head and neck are destroyed by large cystic lesions. Fusion may result. In the spine, the cysts break out of the cortex, forming large paraspinal masses that do not calcify, but do cause paraplegia. The appearance may resemble dumb-bell tumors in neurofibromatosis [67].

Cysticercosis

Cysticercosis is a common parasitic infection in humans, it is caused by consumption of contaminated food or water with viable eggs of *Taenia solium* or regurgitation of eggs into the stomach from the intestine of people harboring a gravid worm. If the eggs contaminate food sources, upon ingestion they develop into larvae and result in cysticercosis. Hence, even people who do not consume pork, including vegetarians, can develop cysticercosis. Humans carrying the adult tapeworm in the intestines are the definitive hosts and pigs are the intermediate hosts in the natural life cycle and are infected with the larval form most commonly in the muscles. If the *T. solium* eggs are accidentally ingested, the larval stage develops in various tissues like the brain, muscles, subcutaneous tissues and results in human cysticercosis (Fig. 55.21).

USG is the preferred technique of imaging. The USG findings evaluated were cyst size, shape, and margin; the presence of scolex; the presence of abscess/surrounding inflammation; and the location of the lesion. The most common USG appearance of soft-tissue cysticercosis is the formation of an intramuscular abscess with an eccentrically situated typical hypoechogenic cyst with a focal hyperechogenic scolex within (Fig. 55.22) clinically present as myalgia or mass. Subcutaneous cysticercosis may cause painless or painful subcutaneous nodules with similar imaging appearance.

On MRI, the cysticercosis is seen as a cystic lesion oriented in the direction of the muscle fibers with hyperintense T2W and hypointense on T1W signal intensity. Peripheral rim enhancement of the cyst wall is also known.

Cat-scratch Disease

Cat-scratch disease affects an estimated 22,000 people in the United States each year, more than half of whom are children or adolescents. The method of inoculation of the causative organism *Bartonella henselae*, a gram-negative bacillus is thought to be by the scratch of a cat [68]. Painful lymphadenopathy is the hallmark of cat-scratch disease proximal to the site of inoculation, usually upper limb, axilla, or neck. Nodes typically range in size from 1 to

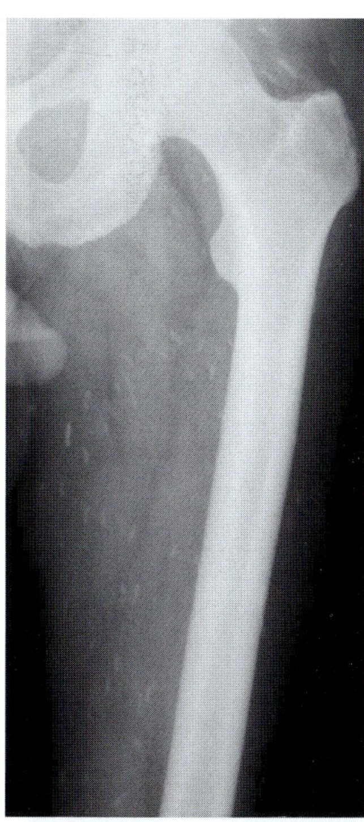

Figure 55.21 Frontal radiograph of the left thigh showing multiple elongated calcified bodies in the soft tissue of thigh in keeping with a sequelae of cysticercosis. (Courtesy: Dr. John Curtis, Aintree University Hospital.)

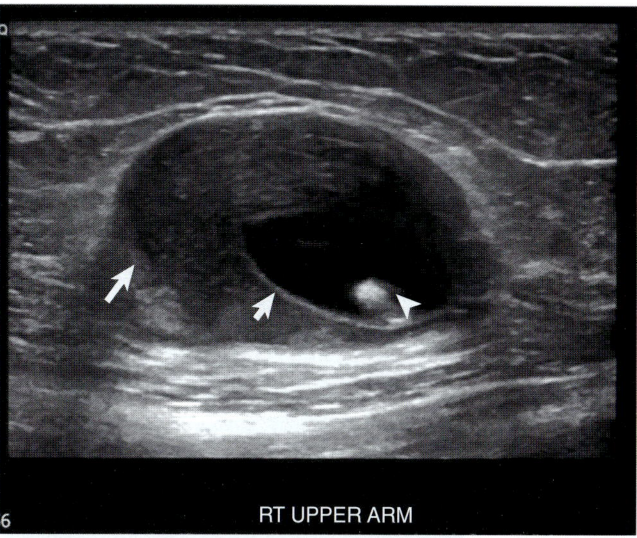

Figure 55.22. A 30-year-old lady with recent history of traveling to India, presented with swelling in the right upper arm. The ultrasonography showed a well-defined soft-tissue lesion within the brachialis muscle containing a hyperechogenic scolex (*arrowhead*), surrounded by a cyst (*small arrow*), and peripheral abscess (*big arrow*) compatible with cysticercosis.

5 cm. Recognition of the disease is sometimes difficult because the illness takes many forms, from regional lymphadenitis to generalized nonspecific lymphadenopathy. Disseminated infection occurs in 5–10% of cases, along with generalized lymphadenopathy, multiple granulomas of the liver and spleen are seen; bone lesions may also develop in both the axial skeleton and extremities [69].

USG is the preferred technique of evaluation of the regional lymphadenopathy, as well as systemic granulomas, which are typically initially hypoechogenic and show calcification in the late phase. CT is useful for the systemic assessment and visceral granulomas are typically hypoattenuating on nonenhanced CT and become isodense to the surrounding tissues, or demonstrate rim enhancement with contrast administration. MRI can be used for further evaluation of the local and systemic form of the disease, the affected lymph nodes, as well as the granulomas, which show T2 hyperintensity with contrast enhancement (Fig. 55.23) [69].

Syphilis

Very few cases of syphilis of bone are now seen, yet up to the time of the Second World War it was a condition that merited serious consideration in the differential diagnosis of most conditions of bone.

Congenital Syphilis

Lesions may be found in infants whose serological reactions are negative, especially when the mother is receiving treatment. They may appear early, that is, from birth to 4 years or later, that is, between the ages of 5 and 15 years.

Radiographic Appearances

The lesions may be widespread and usually symmetrical. Generally, they are best shown in the lower ends of the radius and ulna and around the knee. Changes are:

1. *Periostitis*. This is the commonest feature and is seen either as a thin layer or as more marked laminated layers. Marked thickening on the convexity of a diaphysis may be seen in later cases as, for example, in the so-called "sabre tibia"
2. *Metaphysitis*. There may be irregularity of metaphyses, and metaphyseal fractures may occur (Fig. 55.24)
3. *Osteitis* or *osteomyelitis*. Erosions on the upper medial surfaces of the tibiae are very characteristic of congenital syphilis. Sometimes more diffuse osteomyelitis of single bones is seen. Syphilis is a productive lesion, so sclerosis will be found frequently in such lesions
4. *Syphilitic dactylitis* is rare; it resembles *Tuberculous dactylitis*
5. *Skull lesions* may be purely sclerotic or may present as a combination of sclerosis and osteolysis. In purely sclerotic lesions, new bone may be laid down in the frontal and parietal regions, so producing the "hot cross bun" skull

Acquired Syphilis

Any bone may be affected by this condition. Radiological manifestations comprise periostitis and osteomyelitis.

- Periostitis

This sign may be seen as a simple laminated periosteal reaction or as a more exuberant lace-like appearance. Bony spiculation at right angles to the shaft is rare, but when it occurs, it may mimic a neoplastic lesion.

- Osteomyelitis

This may occur as a localized or as a diffuse lesion. The localized lesion is termed a gumma (Fig. 55.25), but a more diffuse lesion is often referred to as "gummatous osteitis" (Figs. 55.26 and 55.27). Sclerosis is generally found; irregularity of bone trabeculation is often apparent. Syphilis causes a combination of destruction and proliferation of bone.

It is important to remember the possibility of syphilis when presented with an atypical bone lesion.

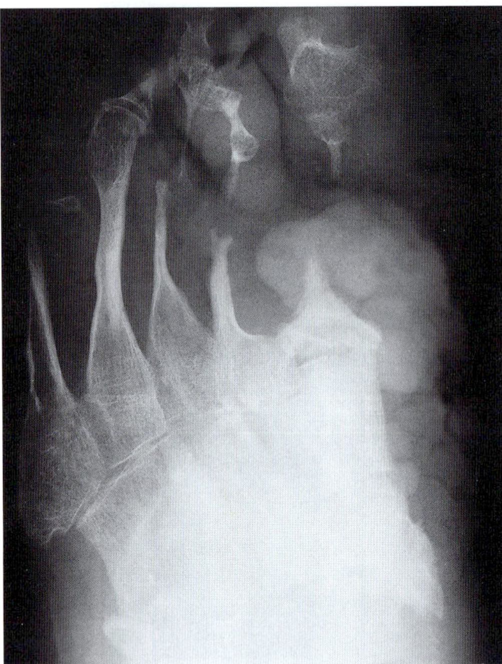

Figure 55.30 Leprosy. 'Cup and pencil' or 'licked candy stick' appearances demonstrated associated with thickening and irregularity of the soft tissues, presumably the result of chronic infection in the soft tissues.

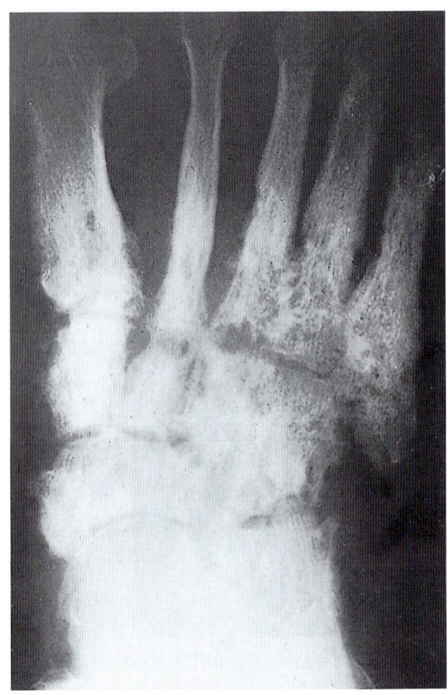

Figure 55.31 Mycetoma (Madura foot). Diffuse infiltrating destruction affecting the whole tarsus and proximal ends of the metatarsals.

gives a "licked candy stick" appearance with bone loss both longitudinally and circumferentially (Fig. 55.30). In addition, Charcot-like changes take place in the tarsus. These patients have abnormal, thickened nerves, and arterial occlusions. An abnormal stance potentiates this bone resorption in the denervated weight-bearing foot

With anesthesia, plantar ulceration and BSTIs are superimposed, so that pyogenic osteomyelitis is common in these patients. These changes are superimposed upon those of the neuropathic osteopathy.

3. A *diffuse osteoporosis* is seen, which is nonspecific. Nerve calcification is occasionally seen

Coccidioidomycosis

This is a chronic granulomatous condition caused by a fungus and found in the south-western parts of the United States. The lesions are multiple and are most commonly found in the spine, pelvis, hands, and feet. The bone lesions have the appearances of acute and chronic osteomyelitis; the joint lesions are similar to those found in tuberculous arthritis.

Mycetoma

Mycetoma implantation occurs mainly in the (bare) feet in semi-desert regions throughout the tropics. The skull and knees may also be implanted, usually by thorns. Different organisms are found in different regions—*M. mycetoma* in the Middle East, Africa, and India, and *Streptomyces somaliensis* and *pelletieri* in the Sudan. Lesions due to *M. mycetoma* are usually localized as large, well-defined black fungus balls, which can be seen on soft-tissue radiographs. These erode the cortices and cause cystic defects in the medulla. Madura foot results (the lesions were first described in that region of India). With superadded infection through the implantation track, gross bone destruction results (Fig. 55.31). Reactive sclerosis and a shaggy periostitis with bone resorption give an appearance likened to "melting snow." With *S. pelletieri*, diffuse infection occurs earlier but the end-stage appearances after secondary infection are usually similar.

Suggested Readings

- NA Kothari, DJ Pelchovitz, JS Meyer, Imaging of musculoskeletal infections, Radiol Clin N Am 39 (4) (2001) 653–671.
- MF Termaat, PG Raijmakers, HJ Scholten, The accuracy of diagnostic imaging for the assessment of chronic osteomyelitis: a systematic review and meta-analysis, J Bone Joint Surg Am 87 (11) (2005) 2464–2471.
- MR Hayeri, P Ziai, ML Shehata, OM Teytelboym, BK Huang, Soft-tissue infections and their imaging mimics: from cellulitis to necrotizing fasciitis, Radiographics 36 (6) (2016) 1888–1910, doi:10.1148/rg.2016160068.
- SJ Theodorou, DJ Theodorou, D Resnick, Imaging findings of complications affecting the upper extremity in intravenous drug users: featured cases, Emerg Radiol 15 (4) (2008) 227–239.
- MB McCarville, JY Chen, JL Coleman, et al., Distinguishing osteomyelitis from Ewing Sarcoma on radiography and MRI, AJR Am J Roentgenol 205 (2015) 640–650.

56 Shoulder

VIJAY PAPINENI, ANAND KIRWADI

Introduction

The shoulder joint is a ball and socket joint that favors a great degree of complex movements over stability because of the relatively large articular surface of the humeral head articulating with a shallow glenoid fossa. Hence, the shoulder is one of the most unstable joints. The labral cartilage, joint capsule, and surrounding soft tissues play important roles in providing stability by deepening the glenoid fossa.

For the initial assessment of patients presenting with shoulder trauma, conventional radiography and computed tomography (CT) are preferred screening investigations of choice. Ultrasonography (USG) and magnetic resonance imaging (MRI) are preferred choices for rotator cuff (RC) assessment, especially in patients older than 40 years of age. For patients younger than 40 years of age with suspected intraarticular derangement or recurrent shoulder instability, CT or MR arthrography or plain MRI are the preferred initial screening examinations.

Functional Anatomy

Bony Anatomy

Humerus: The articular surface of the humeral head is covered with hyaline cartilage. Important bony landmarks of the proximal humerus are the greater tuberosity, lesser tuberosity, and bicipital groove, which act as attachment sites for RC tendons.

The greater tuberosity has three facets, superior, middle, and inferior. The anatomic neck of the humerus is the transition of the proximal humerus to the humeral head. The surgical neck is few centimeters below the anatomic neck and is a frequent fracture site (Fig. 56.1).

The *scapula* is a flat bone that glides over the thoracic surface to facilitate rotating arm movement. The glenoid fossa is perpendicular to the body of the scapula. The osseous glenoid fossa is markedly smaller than the humeral head.

There are three bony projections from the body of the scapula—the coracoid process anteriorly, scapular spine posteriorly, and acromion process superiorly.

Different structures that form the superior border of the supraspinatus outlet are known as the coracoacromial arch (CAA). Anatomic variations of CAA can predispose to supraspinatus impingement. The two components of CAA are

1. Bony component: the acromion and acromioclavicular (AC) joint
2. Ligamentous component: the coracoacromial ligament

The shape of the acromion can contribute to impingement. There are four acromial types as per Bigliani classification as summarized and shown in Figs. 56.2 and 56.3. *Type 2 morphology is the commonest type*. Type 3 and 4 acromion are more likely to predispose to supraspinatus impingement.

Os acromiale: The four ossification centers of the acromion (preacromion, mesoacromion, metaacromion, and basiacromion) fuse at varying ages up to 25 years. Failure of fusion of these ossification centers results in os acromiale. There are seven types of os acromiale; the commonest is type A, which occurs at the junction of meso- and metaacromion (Fig. 56.4).

The *clavicle* medially articulates with the sternum at the sternoclavicular (SC) joint. Laterally it connects to the scapula with the AC joint.

Muscles and Labrum

The *RC* is also referred to as the SITS muscle, with reference to the first letter of their names (Supraspinatus, Infraspinatus, Teres minor, and Subscapularis, respectively). The muscles arise from the scapula and connect to the head of the humerus, forming a cuff around the glenohumeral (GH) joint (Table 56.1; Figs. 56.5 and 56.6). The supraspinatus and infraspinatus tendons fuse

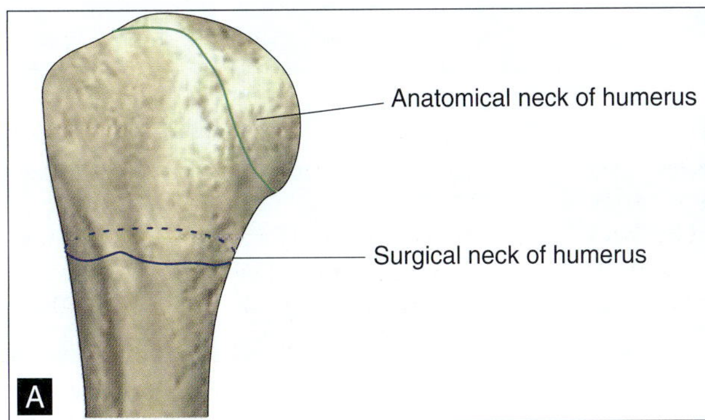

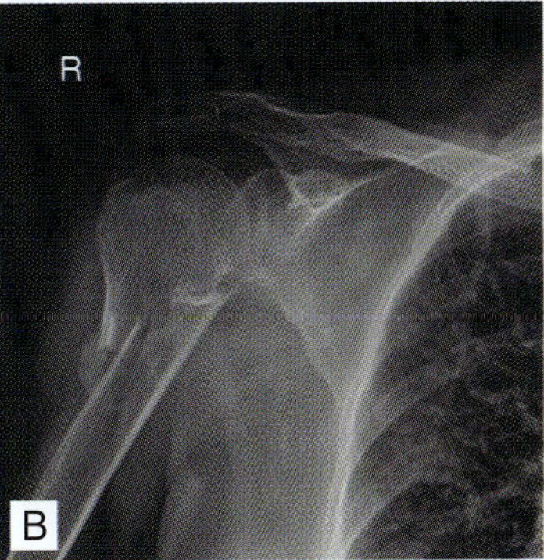

Figure 56.1 (A) The anatomic and surgical neck of the humerus. (B) Radiograph shows fracture of the surgical neck of the humerus.

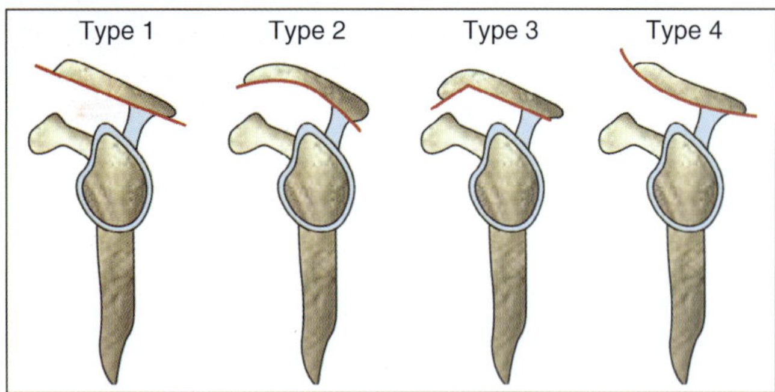

Figure 56.2 Types of acromion. Type 1, flat or slightly convex undersurface. Type 2, concave undersurface. Type 3, hooked undersurface. Type 4, convex undersurface.

laterally before inserting onto the superior and middle facets of the greater tuberosity of the humerus. Common tendon formed by the fusion of the supraspinatus and infraspinatus tendons with infraspinatus fibers remaining in a superficial position [1]. The subscapularis inserts into the lesser tuberosity and is separated from the free edge of the supraspinatus tendon by the rotator interval (RI) and intraarticular part of the long head of the biceps tendon (LHBT). Apart from the long head of the biceps, the rest of the tendons remain completely extraarticular.

Other shoulder girdle muscles include the biceps, teres major, coracobrachialis, triceps, and deltoid musculature (Table 56.2).

The LHBT runs caudally inside the bicipital groove and eventually leaves the groove to end in the proximal musculotendinous junction. Along its intraarticular course, the long head of biceps (LHB) is suspended by the coracohumeral ligament (CHL), the superior GH ligament, and the pulley fibers.

Labral anatomy: The glenoid labrum is a tough triangular fibrocartilaginous tissue that is attached along the bony margins of the glenoid fossa. This increases the surface area and the depth of the glenoid fossa, aiding in GH joint stability. This is in continuity with the glenoid articular cartilage and the capsule externally. For the purpose of imaging, the glenoid is divided into four quadrants or described as a clock face with 12'o clock located superiorly and 3'o clock anteriorly [1] (see Fig. 56.6).

Three types of superior labral attachments have been described at the 12 o'clock position where the biceps tendon inserts.

- Type 1: There is no recess between the labrum and glenoid cartilage
- Type 2: There is a small recess
- Type 3: There is a large sublabral recess between the 11 and 1 o'clock positions

A sublabral foramen is an unattached anterosuperior labrum at the 1 to 3 o'clock position. This sublabral recess and foramen can

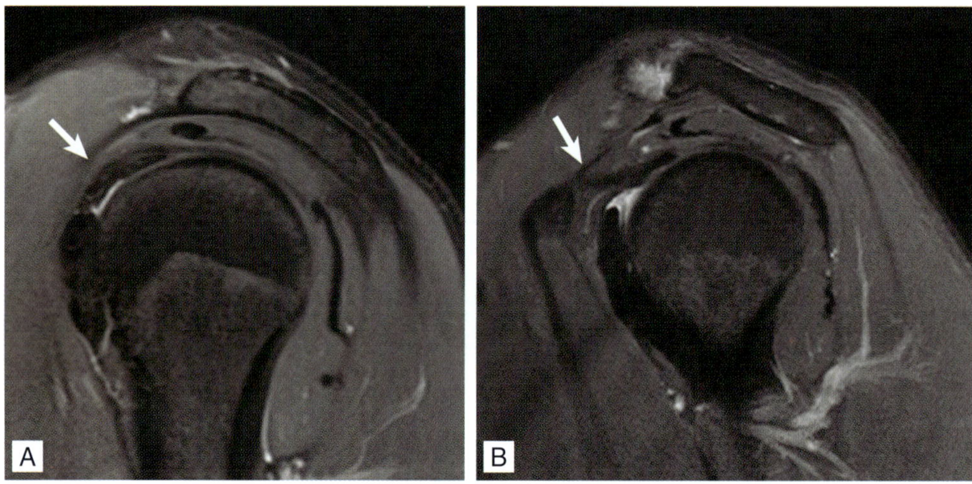

Figure 56.3 Bigliani classification. (A) Type 2 acromion. (B) Type 3 acromion and coracoacromial ligament (*arrow*).

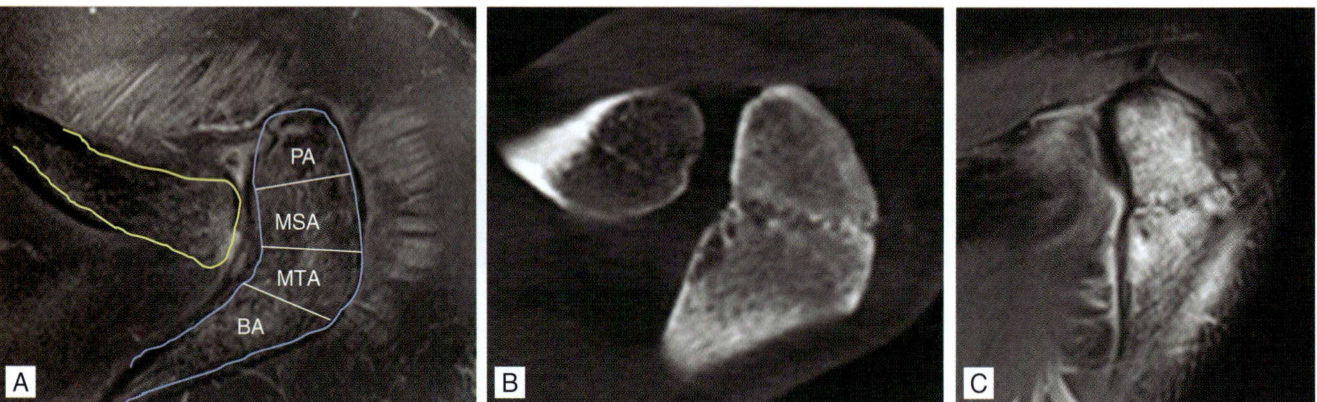

Figure 56.4 (A) Preacromion (PA), mesoacromion (MSA), metaacromion (MTA), and basiacromion (BA) drawn on a normal axial magnetic resonance image (MRI). The *blue outline* indicates the acromion, and the *yellow outline* indicates the clavicle. (B) Os acromiale on computed tomography. (C) Symptomatic os acromiale MRI with bone marrow edema on both sides of the synchondrosis.

TABLE 56.1 Rotator Cuff Anatomy

	Origin	Insertion	Action
Supraspinatus	Supraspinous fossa	Superior facet of the greater tuberosity	Initiation of abduction of arm to 15 degrees at the glenohumeral joint; stabilization of humeral head in the glenoid cavity; then the deltoid and trapezius muscles take over
Infraspinatus	Infraspinous fossa	Middle facet of the greater tuberosity	External rotation of the arm at the glenohumeral joint; stabilization of the humeral head in the glenoid cavity
Subscapularis	Subscapularis fossa	Lesser tuberosity	Internal rotation of the arm; stabilization of the humeral head in the glenoid cavity
Teres minor	Lateral border of the scapula	Inferior facet of the greater tuberosity	Internal rotation of the arm; stabilization of the humeral head in the glenoid cavity

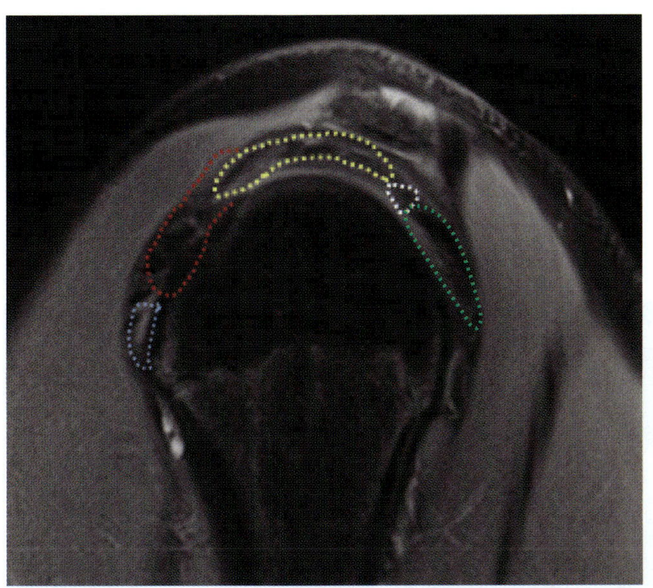

Figure 56.5 Proton Density (PD) fat-saturated sagittal oblique magnetic resonance imaging shows the rotator cuff tendon insertions. The subscapularis is in *green*, the long head of the biceps is in *white*, the supraspinatus is in *yellow*, the infraspinatus is in *red*, and the teres minor is in *blue*.

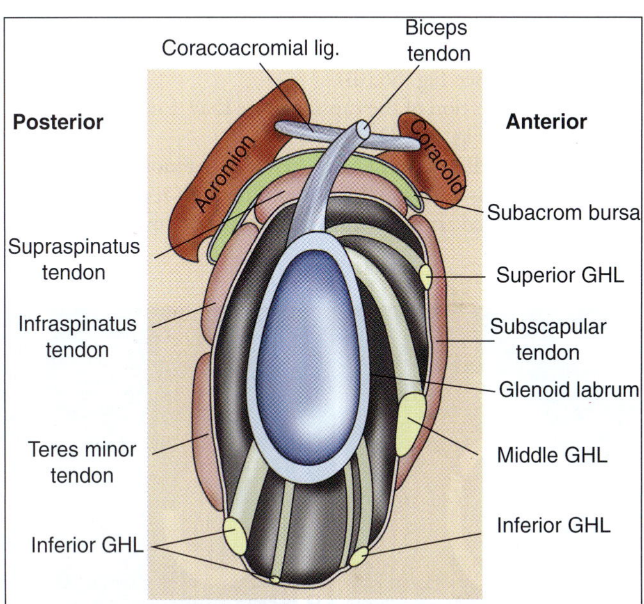

Figure 56.6 Diagram shows the muscles, tendons, and ligaments around the shoulder joint. *BT,* biceps tendon; *GHL,* glenohumeral ligament; *IGHLC,* inferior glenohumeral ligament complex; *MGHL,* middle glenohumeral ligament; *SGHL,* superior glenohumeral ligament.

TABLE 56.2 Other Shoulder Girdle Muscles

	Origin	Insertion	Action
Biceps	Long head: superior glenoid tubercle Short head: coracoid process	Radial tubercle	Weak arm flexor at the shoulder
Deltoid	Lateral clavicle, acromion, and scapular spine	Deltoid tubercle in the humerus shaft	Clavicular part: flexion and internal rotation of the arm Acromial part: abduction of the arm beyond the initial 15 degrees Spinal part: extension and external rotation of the arm
Triceps	Long head: infraglenoid tubercle and inferior labrum	Olecranon process	Elbow joint: extension of the forearm Shoulder joint: extension and adduction of the arm (long head)
Coracobrachialis	Coracoid process	Anteromedial aspect of the humerus shaft	Adduction and flexion of the arm at the shoulder joint
Teres major	Posterior surface of the inferior angle of the scapula	Medial aspect of the intertubercular groove	Extension and internal rotation of the humerus

be confused with a superior labral anterior posterior (SLAP) tear (Fig. 56.7).

A *Buford complex* is a developmental labral variant. At the 1 to 3 o'clock position, the anterosuperior labrum is absent, and the middle GH ligament is usually thickened and cordlike (see Fig. 56.7). It is seen in approximately 1.5% of individuals.

Ligaments and Capsule

Capsule

Glenohumeral joint stability is provided by the joint capsule and the labrum. The insertion of the anterior joint capsule can be slightly variable, inserting from the base of the glenoid labrum and more medially into the scapula.

According to Moseley and Övergaard [2], there are three capsular insertions that can be distinguished in the axial plane (Fig. 56.8):

- Type I: insertion at the tip or basis of the anterior labrum
- Type II: insertion of the capsule not more than 1 cm medial to the labrum (see Fig. 56.8B)
- Type III: insertion of the capsule more than 1 cm medial to the labrum (see Fig. 56.7D)

Type III can predispose to or be the result of anterior dislocation.

Some patients with shoulder instability with recurrent dislocations are offered surgery for correction of multi-directional instability, which is aimed at tightening the ligaments and decreasing the overall size of the shoulder capsule.

Glenohumeral Ligaments

These are capsular ligaments that fuse with RC musculature or attach to the glenoid labrum (see Figs. 56.6 and 56.9).

- The superior glenohumeral ligament (SGHL) arises from the supraglenoid tubercle and merges with the CHL before inserting into the lesser tuberosity
- The middle glenohumeral ligament (MGHL) arises most commonly from the labrum and inserts into the lesser tuberosity and fuses with subscapularis fascia
- The inferior glenohumeral ligament (IGHL) is the largest and most important component of the GH labroligamentous complex and is composed of the anterior band, posterior band, and axillary pouch. It extends between the labrum to the humeral neck

Coracohumeral Ligament

The CHL is a strong ligament of the shoulder joint and is a part of the RC interval. It originates from the lateral aspect of the base of the coracoid process, runs laterally, and envelops the LHBT tendon superiorly (Fig. 56.10). It attaches to the margin of the greater and lesser tubercles of the humerus.

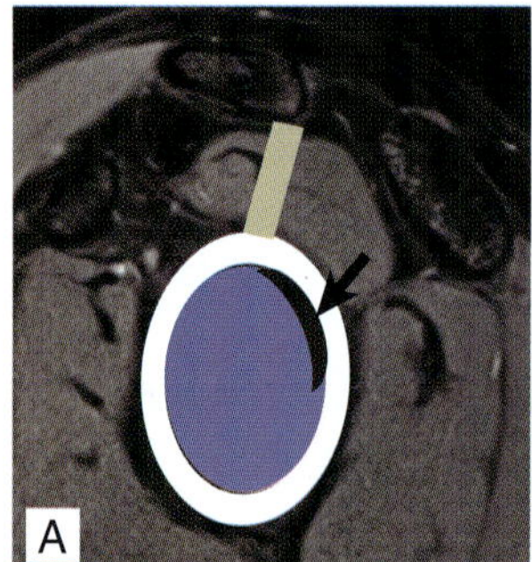

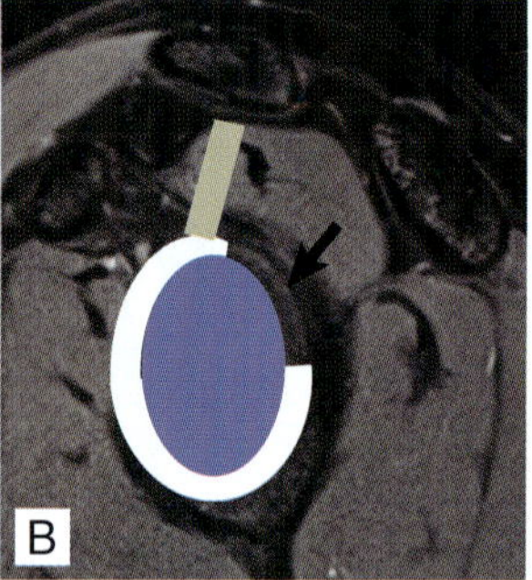

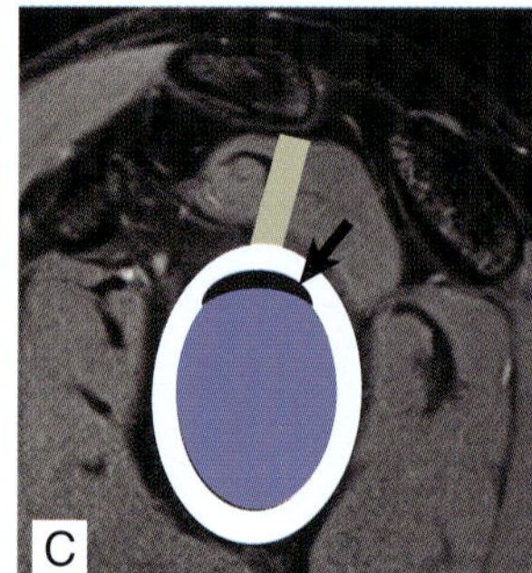

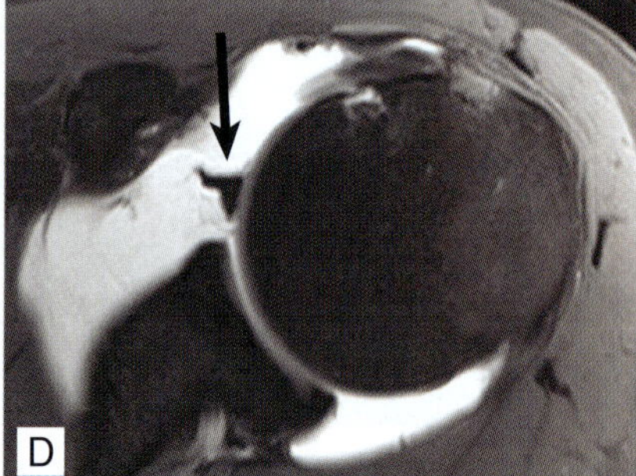

Figure 56.7 (A) Diagram shows the sublabral foramen from the 1 to 3 o'clock positions. (B) The Buford complex with deficient labrum from the 1 to 3 o'clock positions. (C) Sublabral recess from the 11 to 1 o'clock positions. (D) Axial T2-weighted fat-saturated saline magnetic resonance arthrography image demonstrates the presence of the Buford complex (*arrow*). The image also shows type 3 capsular insertion.

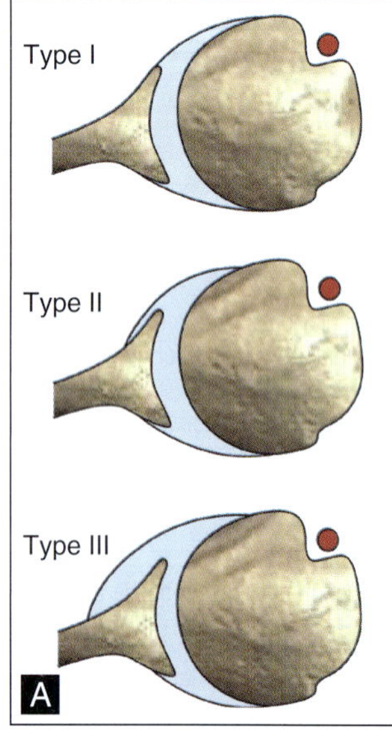

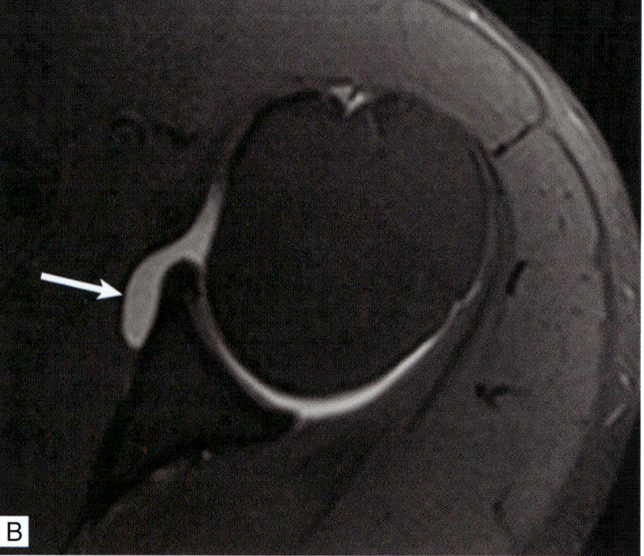

Figure 56.8 (A) Diagram shows the types of capsular insertion. (B) Axial T1-weighted fat-saturated magnetic resonance angiography image shows type II capsular insertion (*white arrow*).

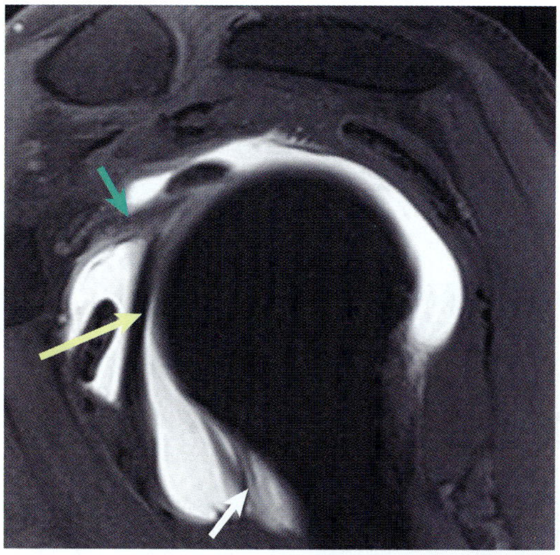

Figure 56.9 Sagittal oblique magnetic resonance arthrography shows the glenohumeral ligaments (GHLs). The *green arrow* indicates the superior GHL, the *yellow arrow* indicates the middle glenohumeral ligament, and the *white arrow* indicates the anterior band inferior GHL.

Rotator Interval

The RI is a triangular space between the tendons of the subscapularis and supraspinatus; and the base of the coracoid process. The LHBT and SGHL form the content of the RI (see Fig. 56.10). The CHL and SGHL act as stabilizers, preventing subluxation and anterior dislocation of the LHBT.

The RI may show abnormal soft tissue on USG or MRI, which may suggest frozen shoulder.

Acromioclavicular Joint

The AC joint is a diarthrodial synovial joint between the medial facet of the acromion and lateral end of the clavicle. Articular surfaces are covered by fibrocartilage with an intraarticular disk that has similar morphology to the meniscus. The joint is innervated by various branches of suprascapular, lateral pectoral, and axillary nerves. The anterior, posterior, superior, and inferior AC and coracoclavicular ligaments are the major stabilizers of the joint.

Nerves

Suprascapular Nerve

The suprascapular nerve is a branch from the upper trunk of the brachial plexus. It innervates the supraspinatus and infraspinatus muscles (Fig. 56.11). Compression of the suprascapular nerve may lead to nonspecific muscle edema and later to muscular atrophy.

Whereas nerve compression at the suprascapular notch affects both the supra- and infraspinatus muscles, compression at the spinoglenoid notch only affects the infraspinatus muscle.

Axillary Nerve

The axillary nerve is located posterior to the axillary artery and anterior to the subscapularis muscle (see Fig. 56.11B). Compression of the axillary nerve in the quadrilateral space (formed between the humerus laterally, the triceps medially, the teres minor muscles superiorly, and the teres major muscle inferiorly) may lead to atrophy of the teres minor muscle and possibly parts of the deltoid muscle.

Alignment

Glenohumeral alignment can be assessed by plain radiographs or cross-sectional modalities such as CT or MRI examination. The

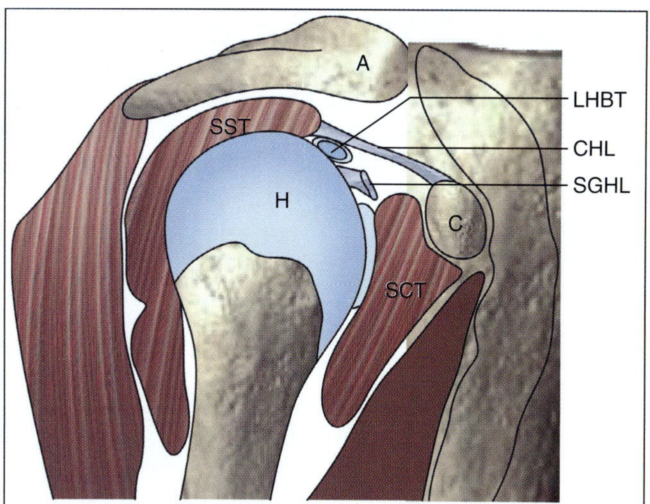

Figure 56.10 Diagram shows the location of the long head of biceps tendon (LHBT) in relation to the coracohumeral ligament (CHL) and superior glenohumeral ligament (SGHL). *A,* Acromion; *C,* Coracoid process; *H,* humerus; *SCT,* subscapularis; *SST,* supraspinatus.

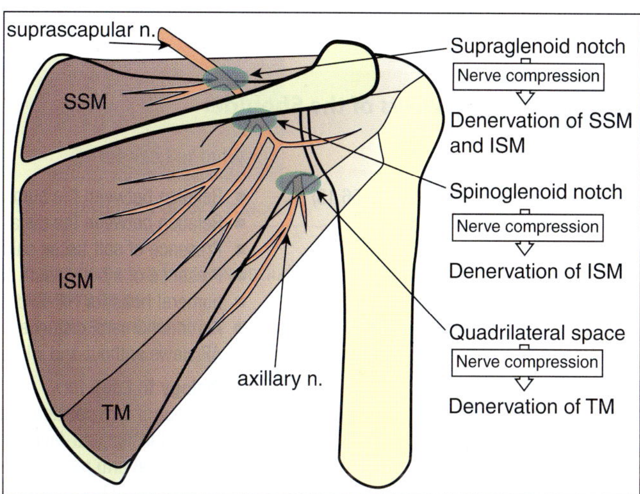

Figure 56.11 The course of the suprascapular nerve along the superior and posterior scapula and the course of the axillary nerve in the quadrilateral space. *ISM,* Infraspinatus mucle; *SSM,* supraspinatus mucle; *TM,* teres minor muscle.

acromiohumeral space measures 8 to 12 mm and is significantly reduced in a full-thickness RC tears (Fig. 56.12). Reduced acromiohumeral space leads to other reactive osseous changes along the undersurface of the acromion and humeral head.

Imaging Modalities

Plain Radiographs

Plain radiography is the first-line imaging method to be used for shoulder pathology.

As a basic principle, the plain radiographs should be obtained in at least two perpendicular planes.

Standard series of shoulder radiography are described in Table 56.3. Plain films are inadequate in diagnoses of bone marrow edema, occult fractures, and pathologic conditions of the RC muscles and tendons and the glenoid labrum [3,4].

Anteroposterior (AP) and axillary views are by far the most common views in the initial assessment of shoulder evaluation.

TABLE 56.3 Routine Views of the Shoulder—cont'd

View	What to Look for
Y view (Fig. 56.16)	■ Relation between the humeral head and the glenoid fossa ■ Good to distinguish between anterior and posterior dislocation of the shoulder **Pathology to Look for:** ■ Fractures of the scapular body, acromion, coracoid process, proximal humerus ■ Relationship of the humeral head to the glenoid fossa

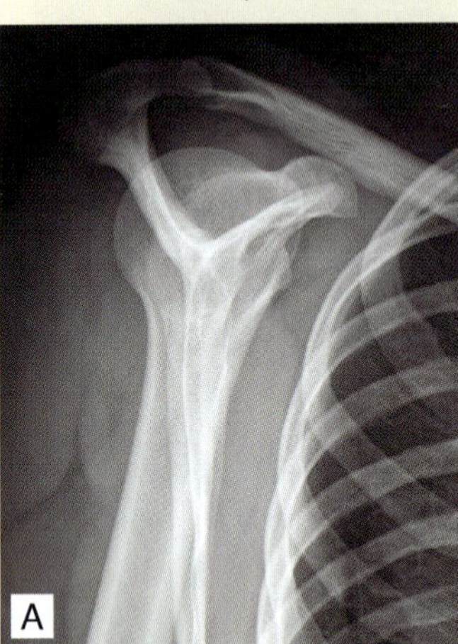

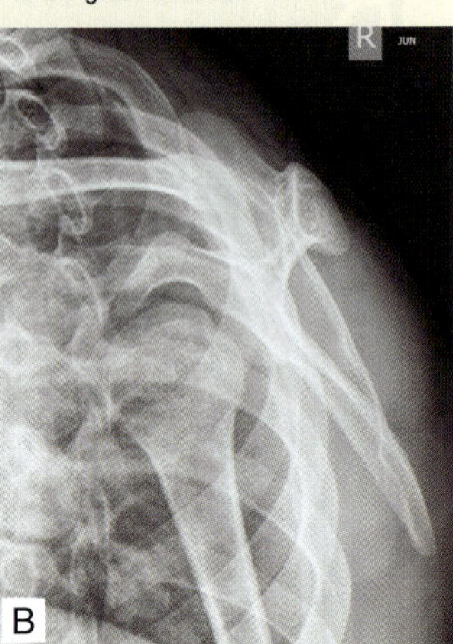

Figure 56.16 Shoulder Y view shows a normal appearance (A) and anterior dislocation (B).

AC, acromioclavicular; *GH*, glenohumeral; *OA*, osteoarthritis.

Special Views

Detail description of the specialized views is beyond the scope of the current textbook. However, Table 56.4 lists some special views, their indications, and what to look for on each of them [3,4].

TABLE 56.4 Anatomy and Pathology to Look for on Special Views

Special View	Anatomy and Pathology to Look for
Bernageau view	Glenoid rim lesions and Hill-Sachs lesions in cases of anterior instability
Stryker view or notch view	Used to detect humeral head fractures associated with anterior dislocation of the shoulder
West point view	Anteroinferior glenoid rim fractures, bony Bankart lesions from prior glenohumeral dislocations
Bicipital groove view	To demonstrate the bicipital sulcus, GT, and LT; erosions of the groove as well as spurs are imaged
Leclercq test	Diagnose tear in the RC of the shoulder; radiographic demonstration of reduction in the subacromial space in opposing abduction of the shoulder
AC joint views (Zanca view)	Better demonstration of the AC joint free from superimposition and aid in the assessment of distal osteophytes
PA sternoclavicular view	Sternoclavicular articulation/dislocation/arthritis
Anterior oblique SC view	Sternoclavicular articulation/dislocation/arthritis

AC, acromioclavicular; *GT*, greater tuberosity; *LT*, lesser tuberosity; *PA*, posteroanterior; *RC*, rotator cuff; *SC*, sternoclavicular.

- The **light bulb sign** refers to the abnormal AP radiograph appearance of the humeral head in posterior shoulder dislocation (Fig. 56.17A). When the humerus dislocates, it also internally rotates such that the head contour projects like a lightbulb when viewed from the front.
- The **trough line sign** is a sign of posterior shoulder dislocation on AP shoulder radiograph (Fig. 56.17A). Frontal radiographs reveal two nearly parallel lines in the superomedial aspect of the humeral head secondary to impaction fracture.

Pseudo cyst of the humerus or **humeral head pseudolesion**: Plain radiograph may sometimes show a lucent lesion in the region of the humeral greater tuberosity. This is an anatomical variant due to increased cancellous bone in the region of the greater tuberosity. Pseudocysts have a typical radiological appearance and they should not be misdiagnosed. The key is to look other views which appear normal and rarely requires further imaging (Fig. 56.17B).

Computed Tomography

Indications: Computed tomography is the investigation of choice to assess the bony anatomy and pathology after trauma. CT is used in the diagnosis of occult and complex fractures of the GH joint or the scapula and in the evaluation of fracture-dislocations and shoulder prostheses. It has a pivotal role in assisting planning operative management in complex fractures. Its multiplanar and three-dimensional reconstruction capabilities facilitate both interpretation and preoperative planning (Fig. 56.18).

Other important indications for CT scan include pathologies such as osteoid osteoma, heterotrophic ossification, bone-forming

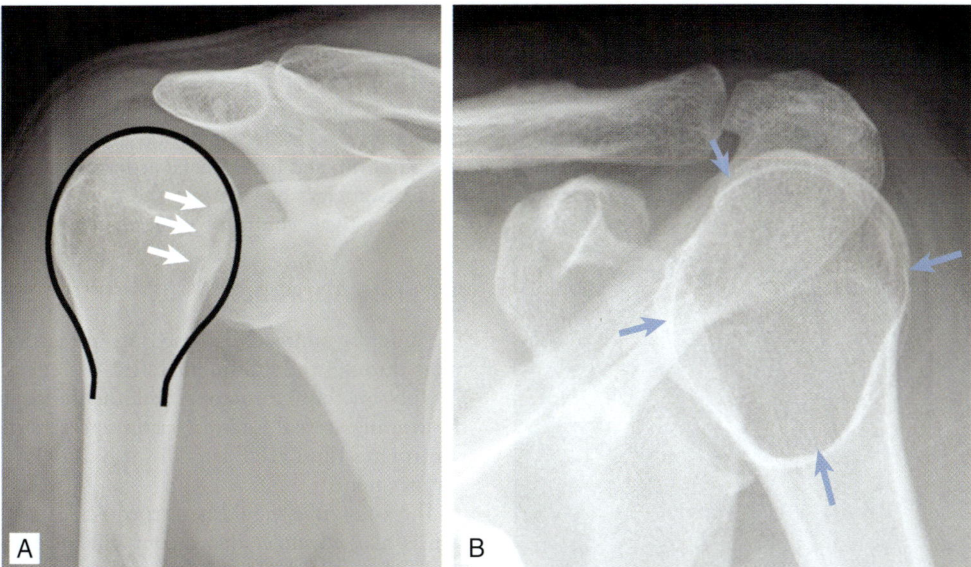

Figure 56.17 (A) Plain film shows the lightbulb sign and trough line sign (*white arrows*) in posterior dislocation of the glenohumeral joint. (B) Plain radiograph shows a lucent lesion (*blue arrows*) in the region of the humeral greater tuberosity. This is a normal anatomic variant called *pseudocyst of the humerus* or *humeral head pseudolesion*. (Courtesy: Rajesh Botchu.)

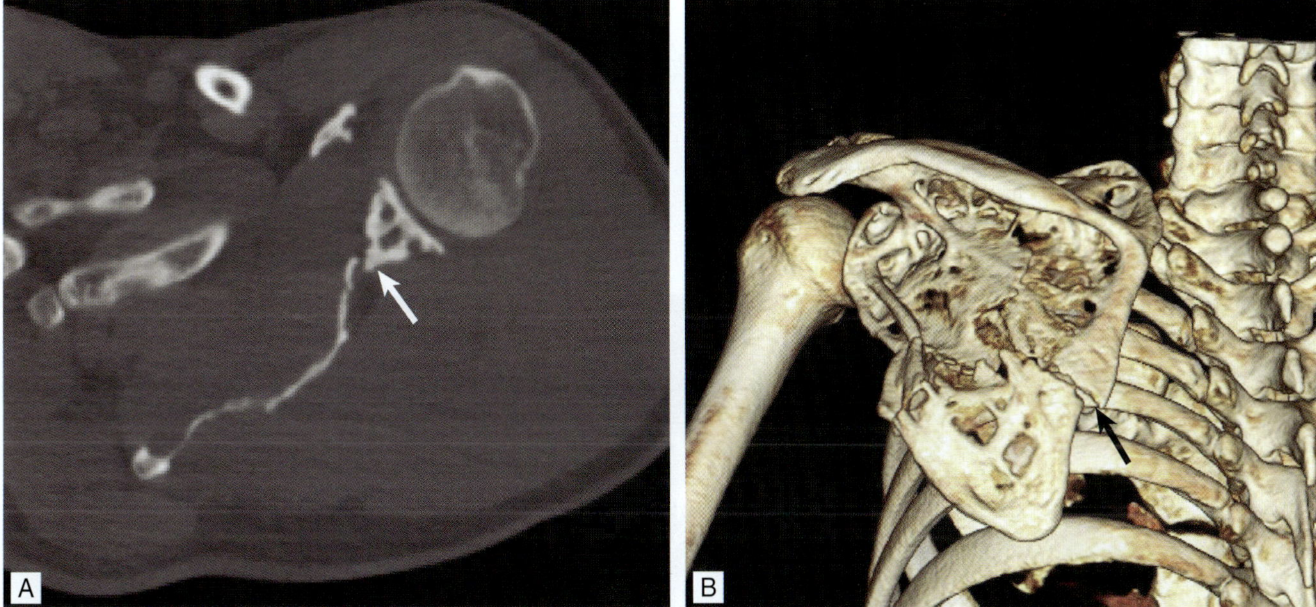

Figure 56.18 Computed tomography of the shoulder with multiplanar axial (A) and three-dimensional (B) reformats show an infiltrative lytic scapular lesion secondary to plasmacytoma with a pathological fracture (*arrows*).

tumors, crystal deposition disease, and conditions in which MRI is contraindicated.

The Walch classification is commonly used to describe GH pathology in primary osteoarthritis (OA) [5]. It is used in assisting preoperative planning and stratifies the outcomes of shoulder arthroplasty for different types of glenoid.

- Type A glenoids have centered humeral heads with either minor (type A1) or major (type A2) glenoid erosion (Fig. 56.19)
- Type B glenoids consist of posterior subluxation of the humeral head. Type B1 glenoids contain posterior subluxation with no erosion. Type B2 involves posterior erosion with a biconcave glenoid
- Type C glenoids show severe erosion of greater than 25 degrees and are considered hypoplastic [5,6]

Friedman and coworkers [7] introduced a method to calculate the *glenoid version* using a line drawn along the axis of the scapula. This line is from the medial tip of the scapula to the center of the glenoid fossa (Fig. 56.20). The version is defined as the angular difference in a perpendicular to the scapular axis line and a line along the edges of the glenoid fossa [5,6]. Glenoid retroversion can be associated with recurrent posterior GH instability.

Humeral torsion can be measured with CT by comparing an image obtained just below the coracoid process with an image obtained about 2.5 cm proximal to the interepicondylar line (Fig. 56.21). Increased humeral torsion may predispose to recurrent GH joint dislocation.

Dual-Energy Computed Tomography

Dual-energy CT scan is useful in distinguishing between urate mineralization and calcification and can be used for cases in which the clinical or biochemical presentation not typical.

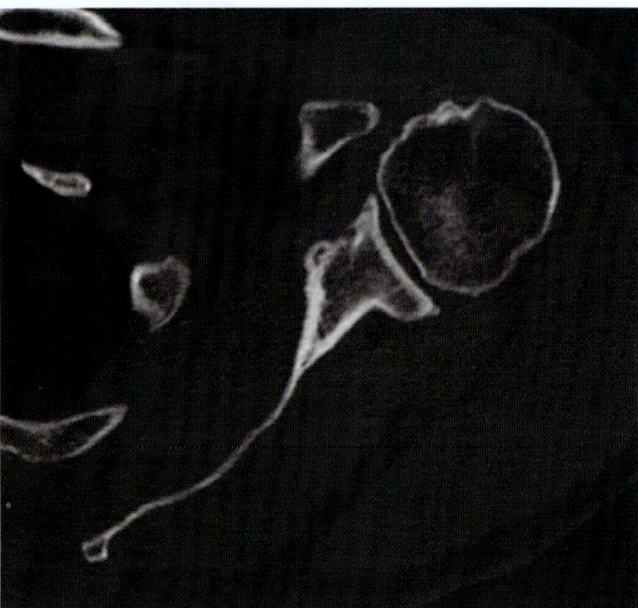

Figure 56.19 Axial computed tomography shows a type A1 glenoid with decreased joint space and a centered humeral head.

CT Arthrography

Computed tomography arthrography (CTA) is being increasingly performed to evaluate bony Bankart lesions and Hill Sachs lesions in traumatic cases. Evaluation of the RC and labrum are limited [8].

Indications and advantages of CTA include

- In claustrophobic patients or if MRI is contraindicated
- Recent studies using CTA have demonstrated equivalency or supremacy over MRI in diagnosing various pathologies, including articular surface RC tears, labral lesions, osseous or cartilaginous defects, and calcified structures such as Bennett lesions (mineralization of the posterior band of the inferior GH ligament in throwers) or chondrocalcinosis [9]
- Because of recent advances in helical scanning and multirow detectors, it has lesser motion artifacts, submillimeter spatial resolution, and better metal artifacts reduction algorithms
- Disadvantages of CTA are the use of ionizing radiation and inferior tissue contrast resolution compared with MRI

Anterior Approach

The anterior approach is based on intraarticular needle placement through the RC interval. The patient is positioned comfortably on the fluoroscopy table in the supine position with the arm in external rotation (palm up). External rotation of the arm rotates the LHBT laterally, avoiding injury during needle advancement.

The x-ray tube should be perpendicular to the GH joint. The skin is marked under fluoroscopy guidance at the superior and medial aspect of the humeral head, lateral to the medial articular cortex of the humerus. After local anaesthesia infiltration to the skin and subcutaneous tissues, a 21-gauge needle is inserted perpendicular to the shoulder down to the humeral head. When the needle is in contact with the bone, a small amount of local anesthetic is injected. This should be without any undue resistance if the needle is in an intraarticular position. With intermittent screening, the positive contrast is slowly injected; it should flow freely away from the needle tip with no resistance during the injection. There should not be any pooling of contrast around the needle tip. The contrast will outline the GH joint (Fig. 56.22). Approximately 12 to 15 mL of contrast is injected. Contrast can be seen along the LHBT, which is normal because it has an intraarticular course.

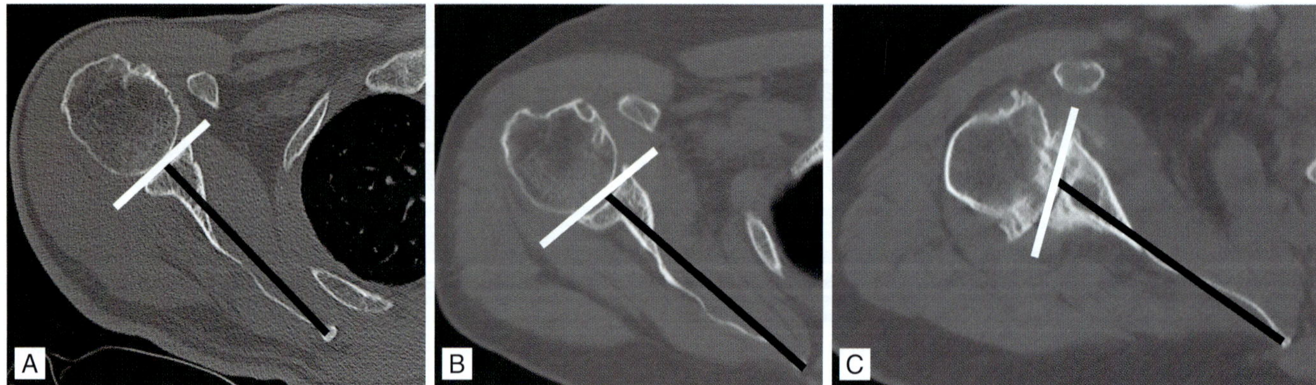

Figure 56.20 Measurement of the glenoid version using Friedman line landmarks on computed tomography. (A) Friedman line (*black line*) drawn from the tip of the scapular body to the center of the articular surface. The angle between this and a line parallel to the glenoid surface (*white line*) determine native version, which is normally 90 degrees. The normal range of glenoid version is 90 to 97 degrees. (B) Glenoid anteversion: increased angle. (C) Glenoid retroversion: decreased angle.

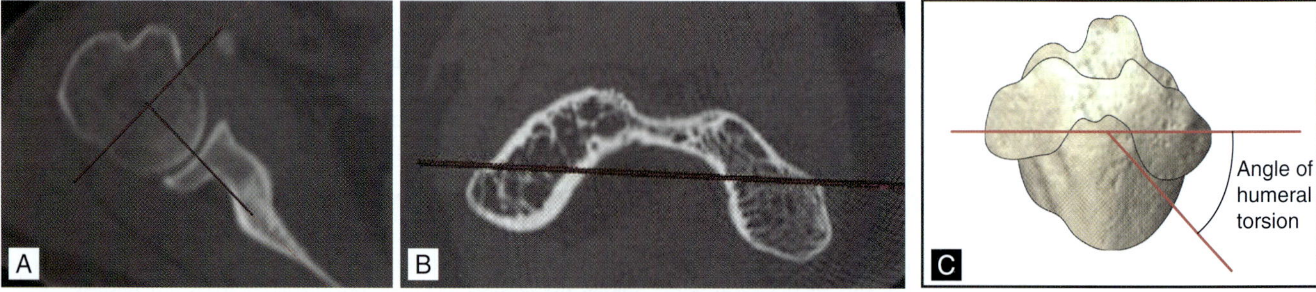

Figure 56.21 Computed tomography scan shows humeral torsion measurement. The proximal reference line is perpendicular to the humeral articular surface (A), and the distal reference line is along the distal transepicondylar line (B). (C) The angle between these two lines (angle of humeral torsion).

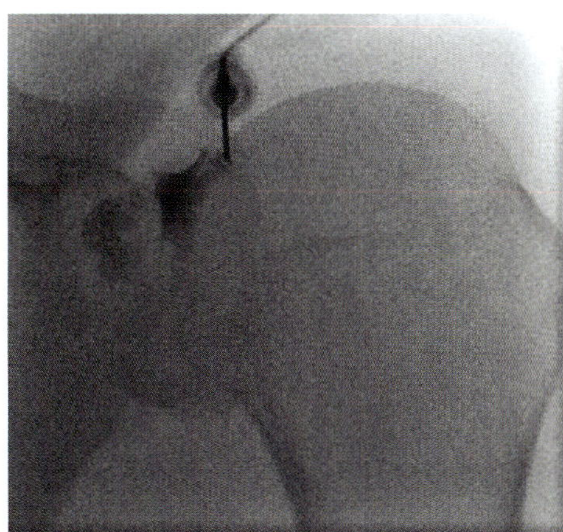

Figure 56.22 Fluoroscopic image shows an anteroposterior view of the shoulder during the rotator interval approach for arthrogram injection.

Some pathologies can be inferred during the arthrogram. If there is extravasation of contrast into the subacromial-subdeltoid (SASD) space, a full-thickness RC tendon tear is inferred. Hill-Sachs lesions can also be identified.

Posterior Approach

When anterior instability is suspected, a posterior approach may be used to preserve the anterior stabilizing structures.

Computed tomography scanning is performed with the patient's arm in the neutral position. Axial images reconstructed at 0.625-mm-thick at 0.3-mm intervals, and multiplanar reformats are created oblique parallel and perpendicular to the plane of the supraspinatus muscle belly.

Ultrasonography

Ultrasonography (USG) has become an important imaging tool in the evaluation of superficial soft tissue structures such as the SASD bursa, RC, and biceps tendon. The advantages include low cost, accessibility, and capability for real-time imaging that enables dynamic assessment and needle guidance.

USG and MRI have shown to have comparable diagnostic accuracy in the evaluation of RC disease, which is the most common cause of shoulder pain. As per a metaanalysis [10,11], the overall diagnostic accuracy of USG in the characterization of full-thickness and partial-thickness tears is as high as MRI and magnetic resonance arthrography (MRA) with a specificity 0.90 or greater. Performing shoulder USG involves sticking to some basic rules, which include

1. It should be performed in a logical and systematic fashion that is reproducible and easy to implement in daily practice.
2. It should be performed with gentle toggling (i.e., rocking and angling) of the transducer to eliminate the anisotropy artifact that may mimic tendinopathy or a tear.
3. Power Doppler, dynamic examination to assess impingement, and comparison with the opposite side are very handy and helpful adjuvants. The authors prefer to use the following technical guidance listed in Table 56.5 in their routine practice.

Anisotropy is the most common pitfall where the normal hyperechoic tendon appears artifactually hypoechoic when the tendon fibers are not perpendicular to the sound beam. A small angulation of 2°–3° will produce this artifact as the ultrasound beam is reflected away from the transducer. This can falsely mimic tendinopathy or tears, especially in an inexperienced hand.

TABLE 56.5 Ultrasound Examination of the Shoulder

Structure to Examine	Patient Position	Technique	Normal Finding	Pathology
Anterior				
Long head of the biceps (Fig. 56.23A and B)	Elbow flexed to 90 degrees, arm in neutral position, forearm supinated (palm up)	Find the bicipital groove over the anterior humerus in the short axis with the long head of the biceps tendon (LHBT) sitting with in it. Follow the LHBT proximally (intraarticular course) and distally down to the myotendinous junction (level of the pectoralis major tendon) in both the short and long axes.	The LHBT shows homogenous bright fibrillar echo texture with no thickening, tears or heterogeneity, or subluxation. Minimal fluid around it is normal as it communicates with the shoulder joint. Beware of anisotropy.	Tendon dislocation or subluxation, tendon tear, tendinopathy, fluid distension of the tendon sheath
Subscapularis (Fig. 56.23C)	Rotate the arm externally fixing the elbow on the iliac crest to show the subscapularis tendon and its insertion on the lesser tuberosity.	Examine the tendon both in the long and short axes during both internal and extern rotations. The full width of the tendon should be examined. Subcoracoid impingement can be assessed on dynamic examination as demonstrated by bunching of the tendon against the coracoid during internal rotation.	The flat subscapularis tendon can be seen inserting onto the lesser tubercle. Demonstrate the multipinnate structure of the tendon: superior, middle, and inferior fibers.	Tendinopathies and tears more commonly involve the most cranial portion of the tendon, which can be hard to visualize. Look for the biceps tendon dislocation, which may lie anterior to the subscapularis tendon. Look for subcoracoid impingement.

Continued

TABLE 56.5 Ultrasound Examination of the Shoulder—cont'd

Structure to Examine	Patient Position	Technique	Normal Finding	Pathology
Superior				
Supraspinatus (Fig. 56.24A and B)	Place the patient's arm posteriorly, placing the palmar side of the hand on the superior aspect of the iliac wing with the elbow flexed and directed posteriorly ("reaching to get a wallet from the back pocket").	Examine the tendon both in long and short axes. Pay extra attention to examine the free edge of the tendon (right next to the intraarticular biceps tendon), where most tears occur.	The tendon has a curved contour following the convex humeral head inserting onto the greater tuberosity. It has a bright homogenous fibrillary pattern. The SASD bursa should be seen as a single thin hyperechoic line paralleling the tendon.	Look for tendinopathy, tendon tear, cartilage interface sign, sagging of the bursa, rotator cuff calcific tendinitis, SASD bursitis. Thickening of the bursa or presence of fluid in the bursa (separation of the hyperechoic line by hypoechoic fluid) is abnormal.
Acromioclavicular (AC) joint (Fig. 56.24C)	Elbow flexed to 90 degrees, arm in neutral position, forearm supinated (palm up)	Place the transducer in the coronal plane over the shoulder to examine the AC joint. Sweep the transducer anteriorly and posteriorly over this joint to assess the presence of an os acromiale.	The undersurface of the AC joint, which can have spurs or osteophytes causing impingement, is unfortunately not visible.	Degenerative change of the joint: osteophytes; subchondral cyst formation, os acromiale, joint instability AC joint cyst or Geyser phenomenon
Posterior				
Infraspinatus (Fig. 56.25A)	Elbow flexion with then palm of the hand positioned over the opposite shoulder with forearm across the chest. Imaging planes: both longitudinal and transverse	Place the probe just below the scapular spine over the posterior shoulder in a slightly oblique axial plane that parallels the orientation of the scapular spine. Examine the long-axis view of the infraspinatus tendon. Move the probe more distally to examine the longitudinal axis of the teres minor. Examine both tendons in the short axis.	There is an overlap of supraspinatus and infraspinatus tendons, so it is difficult to separate them. From the free edge, the initial 1.5 cm of the rotator cuff is considered the supraspinatus, and the next 1.5 cm is the infraspinatus tendon. The thickness of the posterior rotator cuff can be significantly less than that of the anterior part (3.6 mm vs 6 mm), so thinning should not be interpreted as partial tears.	Look for tendinopathy, tears, and calcific tendinopathy.
Glenohumeral joint (Fig. 56.25B)	Same as for the infraspinatus	Move the probe medially along the long axis of the infraspinatus until you see the glenoid margin and the glenohumeral joint	Normal labrum a sharp hyperechoic triangle continuous with the underlying glenoid. It is a good idea to increase the depth of the field for better visualization. Examine the posterior recess for joint effusion. In thin patients, the posterior labrum can be clearly seen. Move the transducer medial to the labrum on transverse plane to visualize the spinoglenoid notch to look for a paralabral cyst.	Joint effusion, movement of the labrum during dynamic examination, paralabral cyst associated with SLAP lesions, suprascapular notch ganglion
Dynamic examination (Fig. 56.26)	Depends on which tendon is being interrogated. "Chicken flapping" (abduction and adduction) can demonstrate the supraspinatus tendon sliding under the AC joint.	Typically, longitudinally along the supraspinatus tendon	The SASD should be seen sliding effortlessly between the AC joint and the supraspinatus tendon with no bunching.	Subacromion impingement is demonstrated as bunching of the bursa against the acromion during dynamic examination.

AC, acromioclavicular; *SASD*, subacromial-subdeltoid; *SLAP*, superior labral anterior posterior.

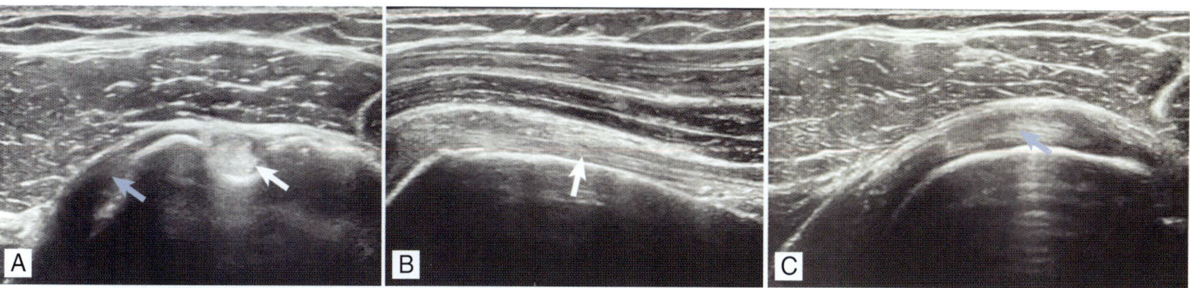

Figure 56.23 Ultrasound images show the short- (A) and long-axis (B) views of the long head of the biceps in the bicipital grove. (C) Ultrasound image shows the subscapularis in a long-axis view.

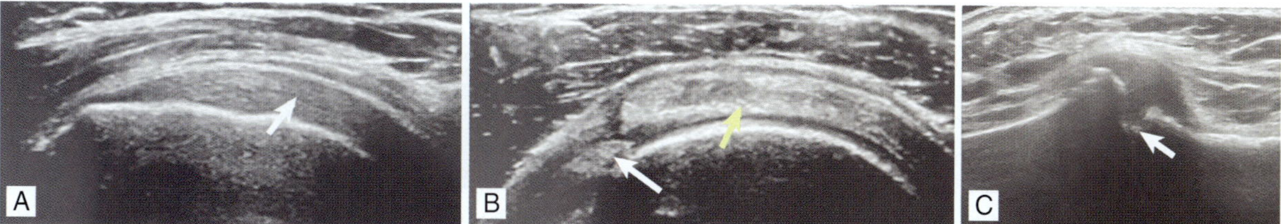

Figure 56.24 Ultrasound images shows the long- (A, *white arrow*) and short-axis (B, *yellow arrow*) views of the supraspinatus. The long head of the biceps (B, *white arrow*) is anterior to the free edge of the supraspinatus. (C) Ultrasound image shows the acromioclavicular joint (*white arrow*).

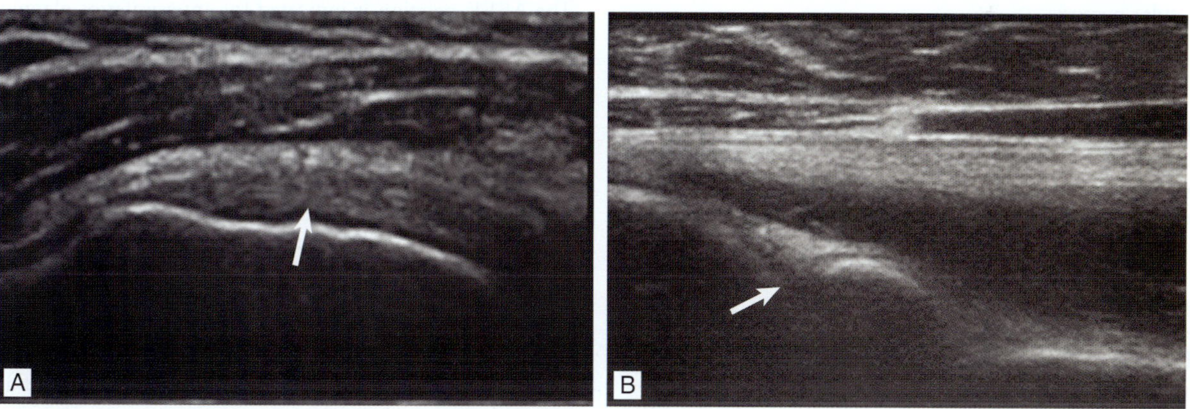

Figure 56.25 Ultrasound images shows long-axis view of the infraspinatus (A, *white arrow*) and a view of the glenohumeral joint (B, *white arrow*).

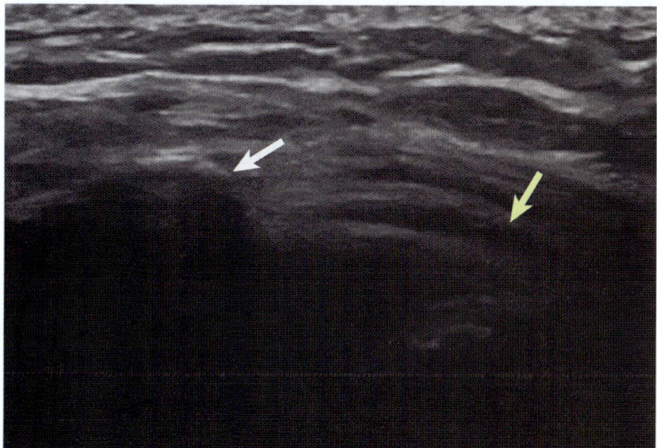

Figure 56.26 Ultrasound image show bunching of the subacromion subdeltoid bursa (*yellow arrow*) against the acromion (*white arrow*).

Magnetic Resonance Imaging

Soft tissue injures involving the RC, ligaments, articular cartilage, and labrum are better assessed by MRI examination. If there is a contraindication for MRI scan, other modalities such as USG and CT examination can be considered depending on the clinical information.

Indications

- Trauma (including dislocation)
- Occult fractures, dislocation, myotendinous injuries
- Internal derangement
- RC tendinosis, tears, and muscle bulk
- Glenoid labral tears
- LHB pathology
- Impingement with or without bursitis
- Infection (septic arthritis)
- Inflammatory processes

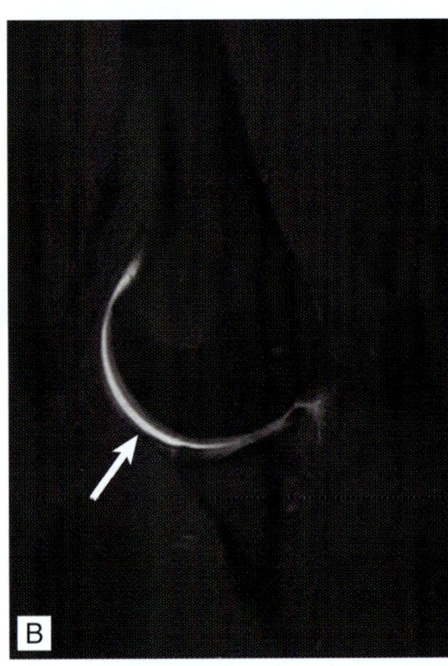

Figure 56.27 (A) The planning plane used to obtain the images. (B) Magnetic resonance image obtained with abduction external rotation (ABER) position shows the stretched out inferior capsule (*white arrow*).

- Nerve-related pathology
- Avascular necrosis
- Local staging of bone and soft tissue tumors

Patient Positioning and Coils

- Supine position with handheld in palm-facing-up position
- Dedicated shoulder coil with or without sandbag is normally used
- Images are obtained in all three planes (axial, sagittal, and coronal)
- A saturation band may be placed along the medial boundary of the imaging volume to decrease effects of motion from the thoracic cavity
- Use fluid-sensitive sequences such as T2 fat saturated and STIR (short tau inversion recovery (STIR) in soft tissue and bone tumors
- Use the abduction external rotation (ABER) position for MRA (Fig. 56.27)

Standard Protocol

Although the imaging protocols for shoulder vary substantially across institutions, the objectives remain the same. A representative protocol may include some combination of the following sequences (this is only a guide because protocols depend on institutional preferences and local practices) (Table 56.6).

TABLE 56.6 Magnetic Resonance Imaging Protocol for the Shoulder

	Field of View (mm)	Slice Thickness (mm)
Axial PDFS	140	3
Coronal oblique PDFS	140	3
Coronal oblique T2 weighted	140	3
Sagittal oblique T1 weighted	140	3

PDFS, Proton density fat saturated.

Special Sequences

The ABER position is indicated for anteroinferior glenoid labral assessment (see Fig. 56.27). The ABER position has an added value in demonstrating Perthes lesions more clearly, especially when the patient is properly positioned [12].

Need for Intravenous Contrast

- Not routinely used
- Mainly used in bone and soft tissue tumors to enable biopsy of the enhancing solid components and to assess post chemotherapy response before surgery

Magnetic Resonance Arthrography

- Indications: GH instability, labral tear, assessment of articular cartilage
- Protocols are listed in Table 56.7

Injection Procedure

This can be done under ultrasound or fluoroscopy guidance with the patient positioned in the lateral decubitus or supine position,

TABLE 56.7 Magnetic Resonance Imaging Protocol for Magnetic Resonance Arthrography

	Field of View (mm)	Slice Thickness (mm)
Coronal T1-weighted FS	140	3
Sagittal oblique T1-weighted FS	140	3
Axial T1-weighted FS	140	3
Coronal T2-weighted FS or PDFS	140	3
Sagittal oblique T1	140	3
ABER	140	3

ABER, abduction external rotation; *FS*, fat saturated; *PDFS*, Proton density fat saturated.

respectively. The procedure is detailed earlier in the CT arthrography section. After contrast has been injected into the GH joint patient is escorted to the MR scanner. The dilution of gadolinium is usually 1:200, so 0.1 mL in a 20-mL syringe [13]. In recent years, MRA using normal saline is gaining popularity to avoid complications associated with direct gadolinium injection and long-term effects of gadolinium deposition. If saline is used, T2-weighted sequences are used instead of the T1-weighted fat-saturated sequences.

Air bubbles are frequently encountered and are well-known artifacts commonly seen at MR arthrography of the shoulder (Fig. 56.28) which can be misinterpreted as intra-articular bodies, metal, chondrocalcinosis, or possible labral tear when they are in close apposition to fibrocartilaginous structures. Attention to detail while injecting the contrast often prevents noticeable accumulation of intraarticular gas.

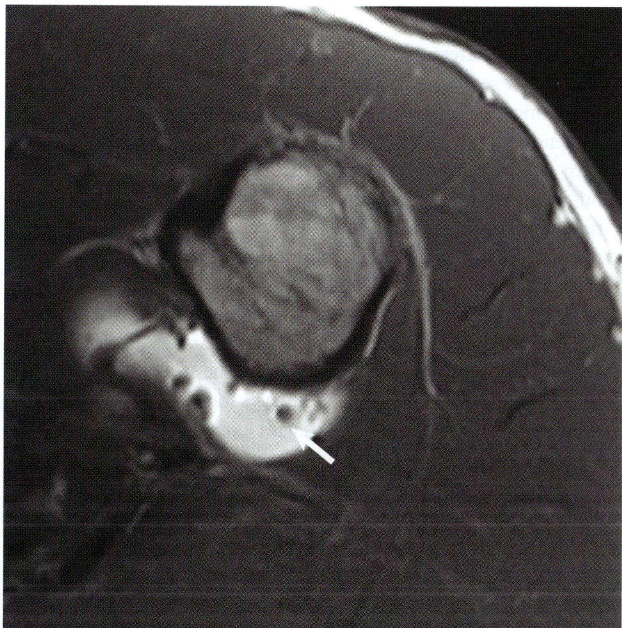

Figure 56.28 Inadvertent introduction of Air bubbles (*white arrow*) during injection, seen as artifacts on a magnetic resonance arthrography image.

Metal Artifact Reduction Sequences

Metal artifact reduction sequences are used to reduce the magnetic field distortion caused by metalwork. It is intended to reduce the size and intensity of susceptibility artifacts. There are several techniques used for reducing metal artifacts during MRI. These include

- Lowering magnetic field strength: 1.5 T instead of 3 T
- Increasing bandwidth, matrix: 512 pixel and number of excitations to maintain a good signal-to-noise ratio
- Using spin-echo and avoid gradient-echo when possible
- STIR for fat suppression instead of selective fat suppression
- Using shorter echo spacing and thinner slices

Shoulder pathology

Rotator Cuff Pathology

Subacromial Impingement

This occurs because of chronic impingement of the subacromial bursa and supraspinatus tendon between the humeral head and the CAA. Patients normally present with pain on overhead abduction of the upper arm. Etiologic factors can be developmental and acquired.

- Developmental factors tend to be type 3 acromial morphology, laterally downsloping acromion, and os acromiale
- Acquired causes tend to be prominent osteophytes along the inferior aspect of the AC joint, subacromial spur formation, or thickened CAA (Fig. 56.29)

It is usually a clinical diagnosis; however, dynamic USG can demonstrate the impingement. USG and MR scans demonstrate thickening and fluid distention of the subacromial subdeltoid bursa. Subsequently, if not treated appropriately, this leads to tendinopathy and tear of the supraspinatus. These features are best evaluated in coronal and sagittal oblique images on MR examination (see Fig. 56.29).

Subcoracoid Impingement

This is caused by a reduction in the space between the coracoid process and the lesser tuberosity of the humeral head. This leads to chronic compression of the subscapularis, and if severe narrowing, the LHBT can also be involved. Patients usually present with anterior shoulder pain exacerbated by internal rotation.

The normal coracohumeral distance is 10 mm or higher. Large RC tears can lead to anterior subluxation of the humeral head, subsequently reducing the coracohumeral distance and predisposing the patient to subcoracoid impingement. This is best evaluated on axial oblique images on MRI examination (Fig. 56.30). Significant tendinopathic changes will be seen in the subscapularis

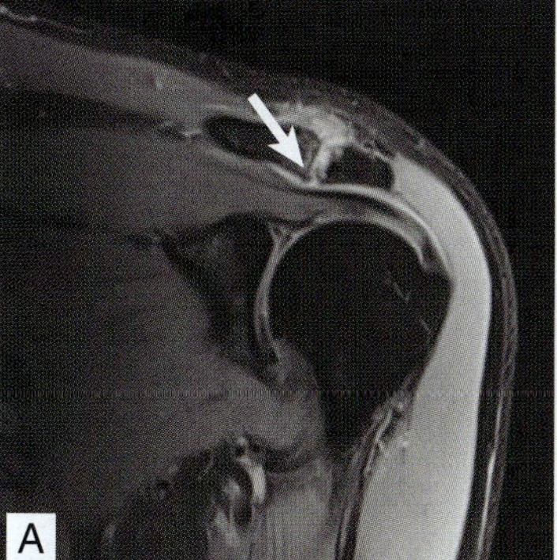

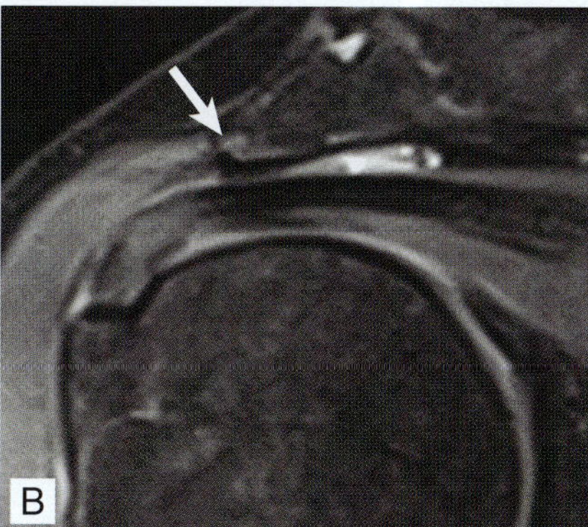

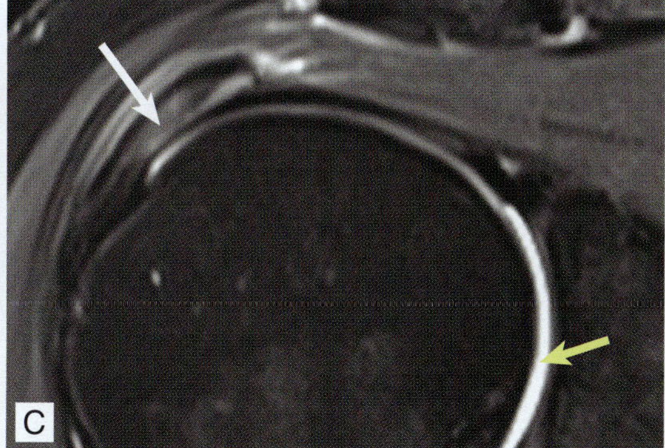

Figure 56.29 Coronal T2-weighted fat-saturated MRI images show rotator cuff impingement caused by acromioclavicular joint osteophyte (*arrow* in A); laterally downsloping acromion (*arrow* in B). (C) The high T2 signal of supraspinatus tendinopathy (*white arrow*) is usually less bright than fluid signal (*yellow arrow*) in the glenohumeral joint.

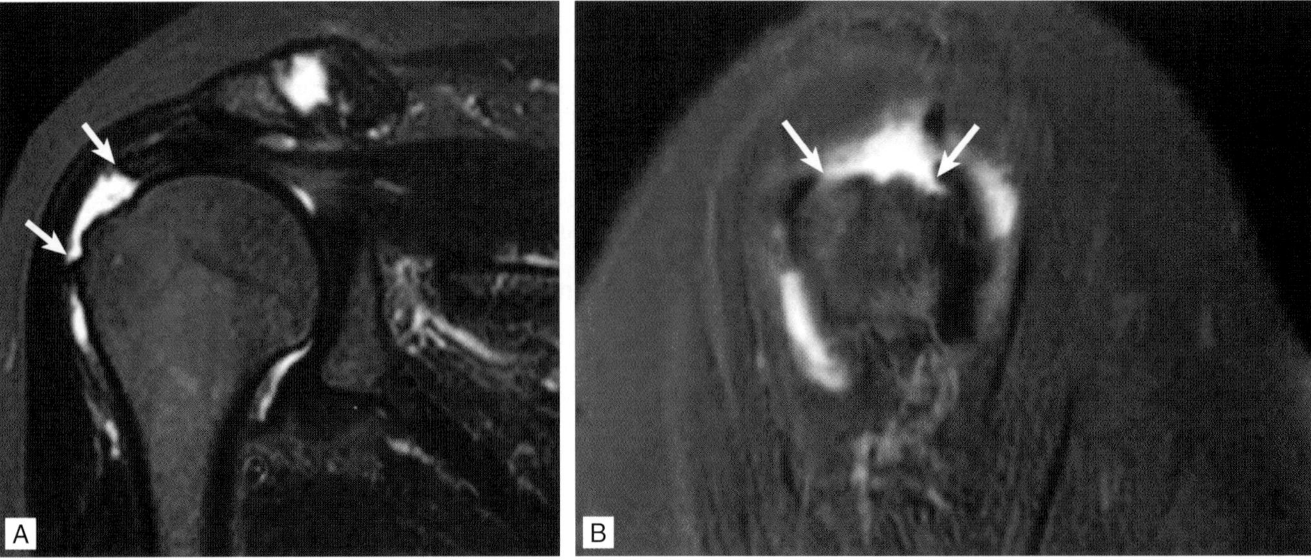

Figure 56.40 T2-weighted fat-saturated magnetic resonance imaging shows a full-thickness tear of the supraspinatus in coronal (A) and sagittal planes (B) marked by *white arrows.*

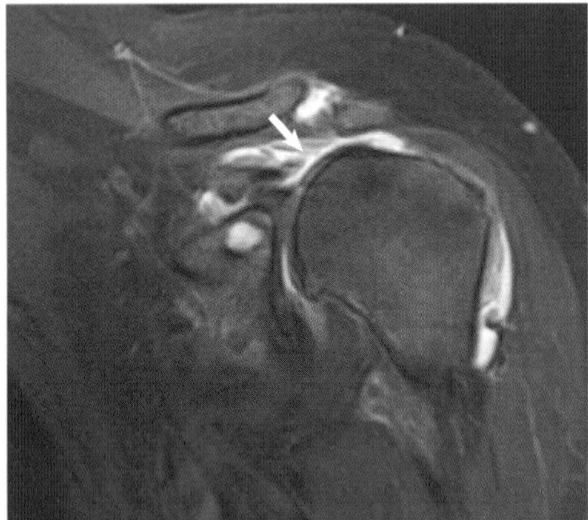

Figure 56.41 Coronal T2-weighted fat-saturated image shows grade 3 retraction of a completely torn supraspinatus tendon (*white arrow*).

- Grade 1: proximal stump near the bony insertion
- Grade 2: proximal stump is at the level of the humeral head (see Fig. 56.40A).
- Grade 3: proximal stump at the level of glenoid or more proximal (Fig. 56.41)

The higher the grade of retraction, the more challenging to repair and the poorer the surgical outcome.

Muscle Atrophy Grading

Fatty replacement and muscle atrophy is seen in chronic cases and can be graded using the *Goutallier classification.*

It is assessed on a sagittal MRI scan image (Fig. 56.42). Higher grades correlate with poorer functional outcomes after RC tear repair [13].

- Grade 0: normal muscle
- Grade 1: some fatty streaks
- Grade 2: less than 50% fatty muscle atrophy
- Grade 3: 50% fatty muscle atrophy
- Grade 4: greater than 50% fatty muscle atrophy

Subscapularis Tendon Tear

Subscapularis tendon tears are relatively uncommon compared with tears in the supraspinatus and infraspinatus tendons. Most often, these develop after a large RC tear involving the supraspinatus tear propagating anteriorly to involve the cranial fibers. Isolated tears tend to be caused by trauma. MRI demonstrates

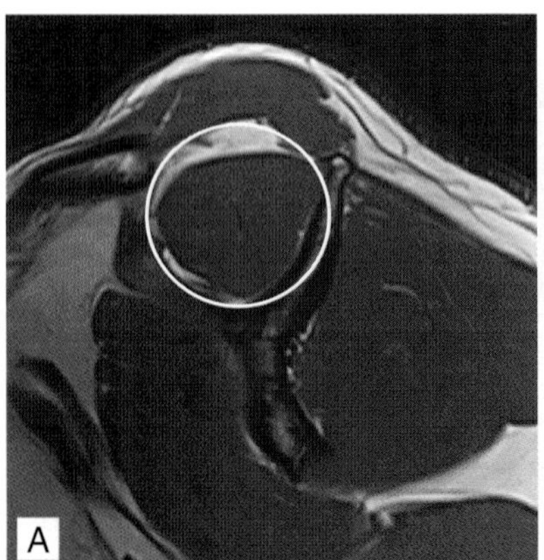

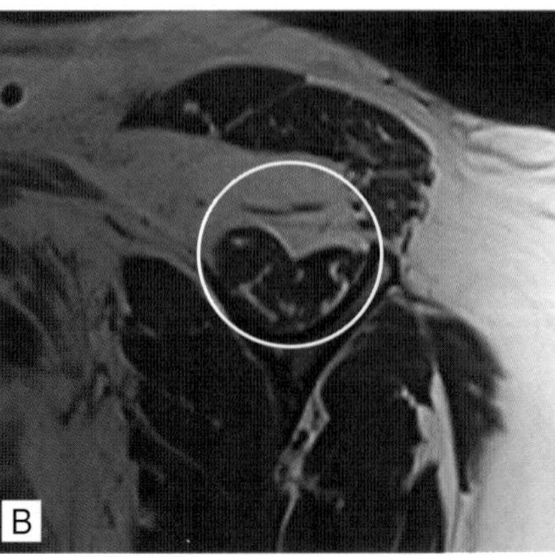

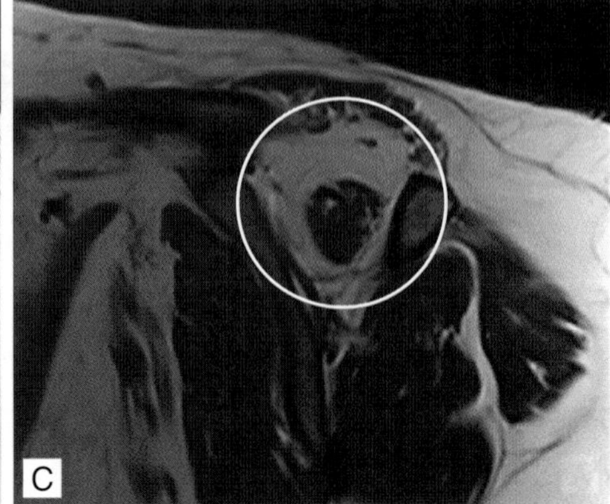

Figure 56.42 Sagittal T1-weighted magnetic resonance imaging shows grades 0 (A), 2 (B), and 4 (C) supraspinatus muscle atrophy outlined in *white.*

tendinopathic changes in the subscapularis tendon with or without tears. There might be fluid distension of the subscapularis bursa. The changes on MRI scan are best evaluated on axial oblique and sagittal images (Fig. 56.43).

Long Head of the Biceps Tendon: Tears, Tendinopathy, and Tenosynovitis

The LHBT has intracapsular and extracapsular portions. A small amount of fluid is seen in the tendon sheath because it is intracapsular in location. A significant amount of fluid must be present in the sheath to objectively diagnose tenosynovitis of the LHBT.

The tendon will appear thickened and heterogeneous in signal intensity because of tendinopathic changes. Most commonly, tears develop after long-standing tendinopathy. Acute tears tend to be traumatic in nature. Tears of the subscapularis and pulley structures result in LHBT subluxation and dislocation. The changes on MRI are best evaluated on axial oblique images (see Fig. 56.44). It should be noted that the biceps tendon is also prone to magic-angle artifact on coronal oblique PD fat sat images.

Misdiagnosis of Biceps Tendon Tears: Complete tears of the biceps tendon are more common in the proximal part within the bicipital groove (Fig. 56.45). The tendon retracts distally, usually to the level of the pectoralis major tendon insertion or beyond. The tendon sheath, along with mesotenon, is still intact and can thicken and may be partially filled with hematoma. This can be misinterpreted as an intact bicep tendon. This pitfall can be avoided by (1) proximally identifying the collapsed synovial sheath within the bicipital groove and (2) by scanning distally in a transverse plane to the midarm where the retracted swollen biceps tendon can be appreciated [16,17].

Rotator Interval and Biceps Pulley

The joint capsule in the RI is reinforced by SGHL and CHL, which form part of the biceps pulley. The LHBT is located within

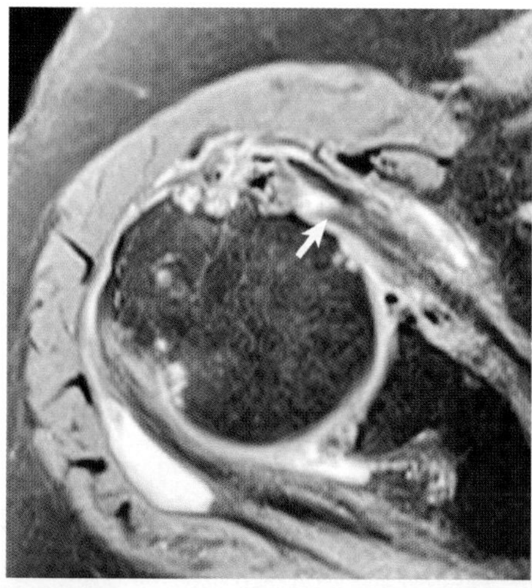

Figure 56.43 Subscapularis tendinopathy, articular surface tear (*white arrow*), and intrasubstance delamination.

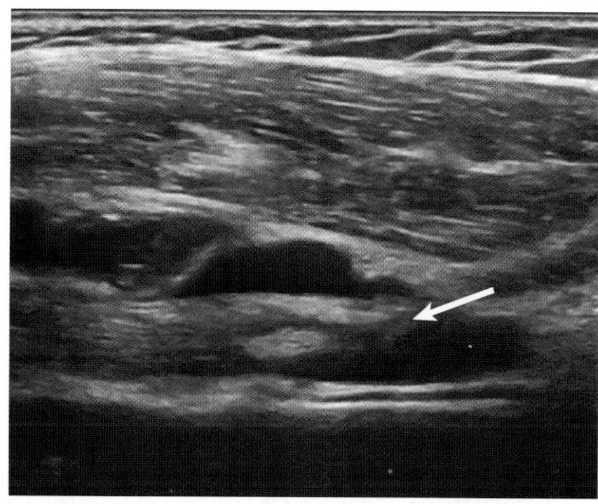

Figure 56.45 Longitudinal ultrasound scan shows biceps tendon rupture (*white arrow*) at the level of the midarm.

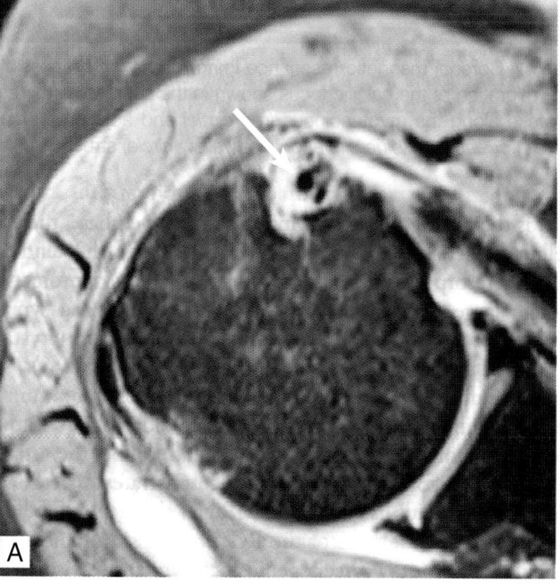

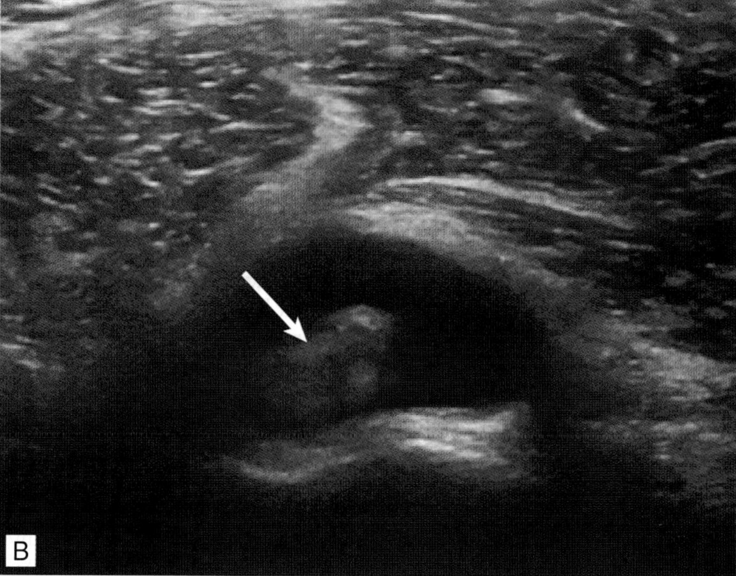

Figure 56.44 Axial T2-weighted magnetic resonance imaging (A) and ultrasound scan (B) show longitudinal split tears of the biceps tendon with fluid distension of the tendon sheath (*white arrows*).

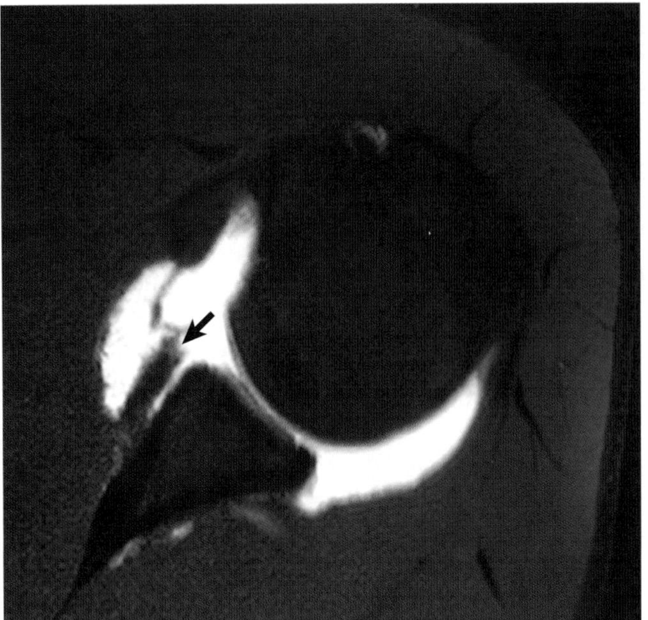

Figure 56.54 Axial Magnetic resonance arthrogram shows an anterior labral periosteal sleeve avulsion lesion (*black arrow*).

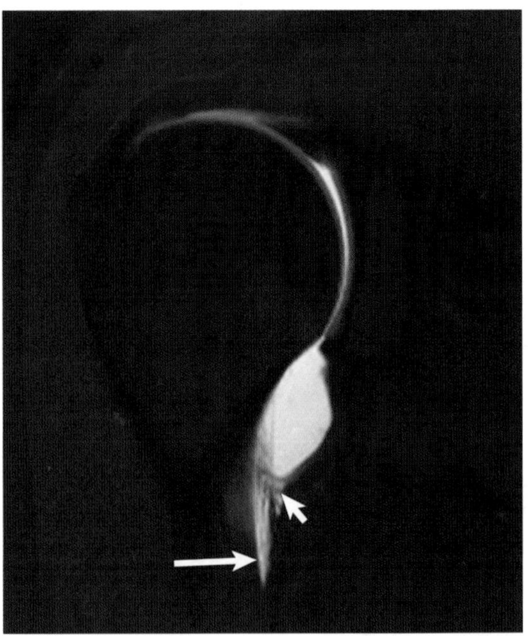

Figure 56.56 Coronal Magnetic resonance arthrogram shows contrast extension along the humeral shaft (*long white arrow*) caused by a tear in the inferior glenohumeral ligament (*short white arrow*) attachment onto the humerus in keeping with a humeral avulsion of the glenohumeral ligament lesion.

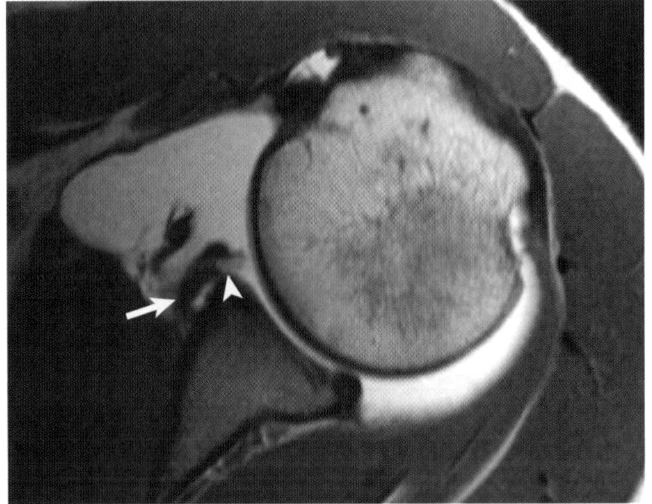

Figure 56.55 Axial Magnetic resonance arthrogram shows undisplaced tear of the anteroinferior labrum (*white arrow*) with an intact periosteal sleeve (*arrowhead*) – (Perthes Lesion).

Anterior Labral Periosteal Sleeve Avulsion: Anterior labral periosteal sleeve avulsion (ALPSA) involves an avulsion of the anteroinferior scapular periosteum along with the glenoid labrum, which is medially displaced (Fig. 56.54). Recurrent dislocations can lead to development of chronic ALPSA lesions with medialized periosteum.

Perthes Lesion: This is an undisplaced tear of the anteroinferior labrum with intact adjacent glenoid periosteum. Because this is undisplaced, it can be challenging to identify this lesion on an axial image or even at arthroscopy. ABER views make this type of lesion more obvious because of stretching of the anteroinferior labrum (Fig. 56.55).

Humeral Avulsion of the Glenohumeral Ligament: Humeral avulsion of the glenohumeral ligament (HAGL) represents the tear of the anterior aspect of the IGHL from its humeral attachment caused by soft tissue stretching during anterior dislocation. Sometimes there may be associated injuries or tear of the subscapularis and LHBT. Occasionally, the tear can extend posteriorly to involve axillary pouch and the posterior band as well. This is best evaluated on coronal images, with loss of normal "U-shaped" configuration of the IGHL to a "J shape" (Fig. 56.56).

Bone Lesions Associated With TUBS

Soft tissue Bankart lesions can be associated with bony avulsion injury resulting in *Bony Bankart lesions* (Figs. 56.57 and 56.58).

Glenoid Bone Loss: Young (<25–30 years) and highly athletic patients (especially overhead or contact athletes) with multiple recurrent dislocations warrant surgical intervention. Patients with greater than 25% to 30% of the glenoid surface bone loss or acute Bankart fracture benefit from early operative intervention [15].

Hill-Sachs lesion is secondary to impaction of the posterolateral aspect of the humeral head against the anteroinferior glenoid. It is best evaluated on axial images; depth and total percentage of humeral head circumference should be calculated (see Fig. 56.58). This should be done at or above the level of the coracoid. More inferiorly, the posterior aspect of the humeral head flattens naturally and should not be confused with a Hill-Sachs lesion. Larges lesions are prone to recurrent dislocations/subluxation and may need bone augmentation. Hill-Sachs lesions with 20% to 30% articular involvement are treated with anterior stabilization and bone grafting of the defect [15,23].

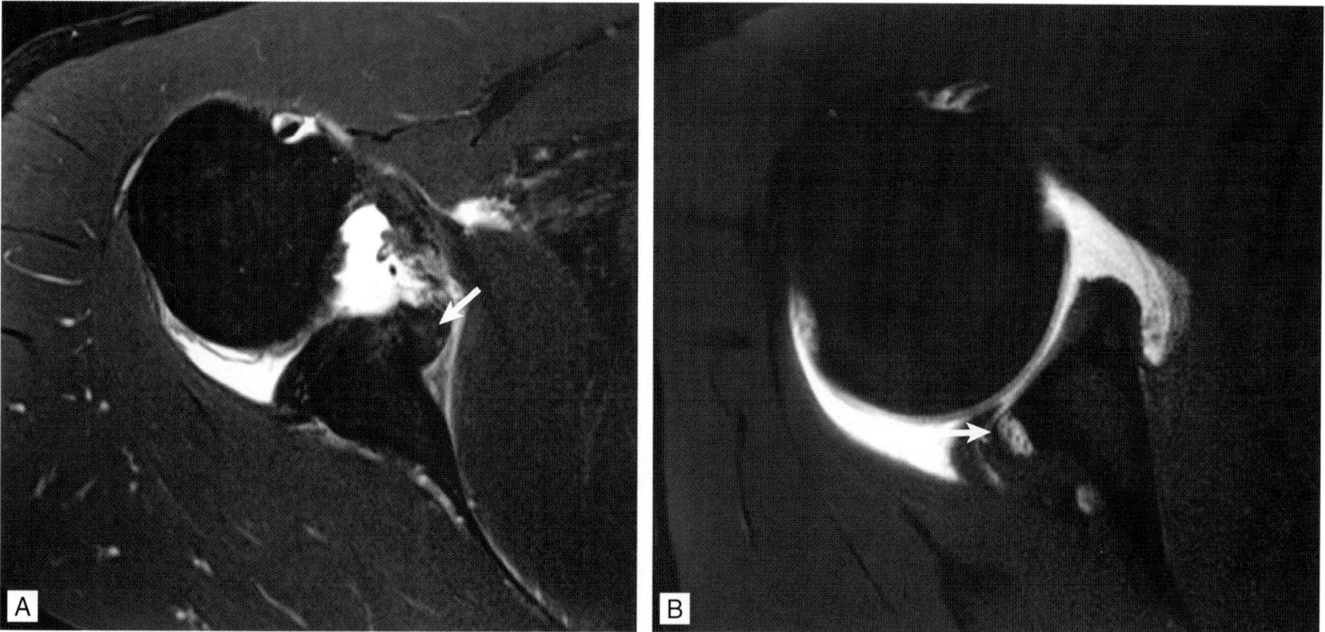

Figure 56.57 Axial magnetic resonance arthrogram images shows osseous Bankart (A, *white arrow*) and reverse Bankart (B, *white arrow*) lesions.

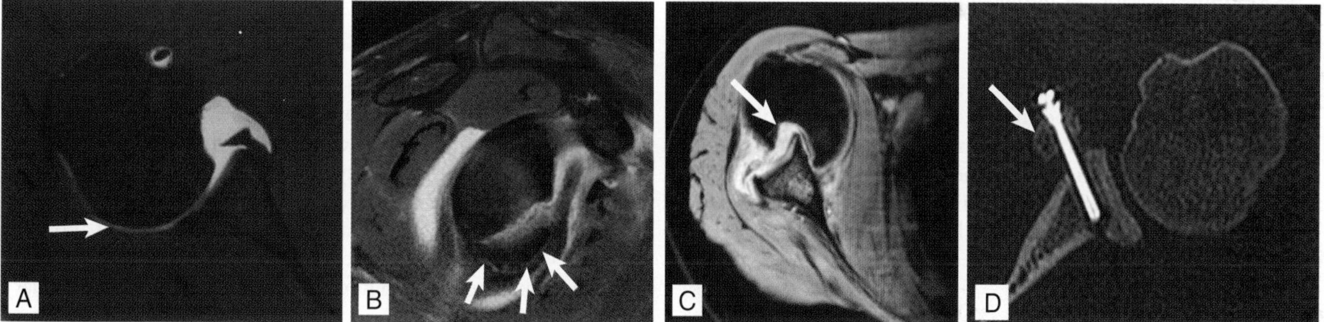

Figure 56.58 (A) Posterior subluxation of the humeral head (*white arrow*) caused by capsular laxity. (B) Large bony Bankart lesion (*white arrows*). (C) Large Hill-Sachs lesion (*white arrow*) with an impacted humeral head. (D) Nonunion of the bone block (*white arrow*) used for the Latarjet procedure.

Posterior Instability

This develops after posterior dislocation, which is much less common (<5%) than anterior dislocation. Posterior dislocation often results from violent muscle contraction caused by an epileptic fit or electric shock. It is often difficult to diagnose correctly on an AP radiograph. Reverse Bankart lesions can be seen in the posteroinferior quadrant. Similarly, reverse Hill-Sachs lesions are present in the anterior aspect of the humeral head caused by impaction onto the posterior osseous glenoid. Again, like the anterior labral lesions, these are best evaluated on axial images.

Variants of posterior glenoid pathology (soft tissue and bony) include:

Soft tissue: reverse Bankart lesion (see Fig. 56.57B), Bennett, posterior labrocapsular periosteal sleeve avulsion (POLPSA), reverse HAGL, Kim lesion.

POLPSA: similar to the ALPSA lesion but is located in the posteroinferior quadrant. The labrum may be intact but degenerate (Fig. 56.59).

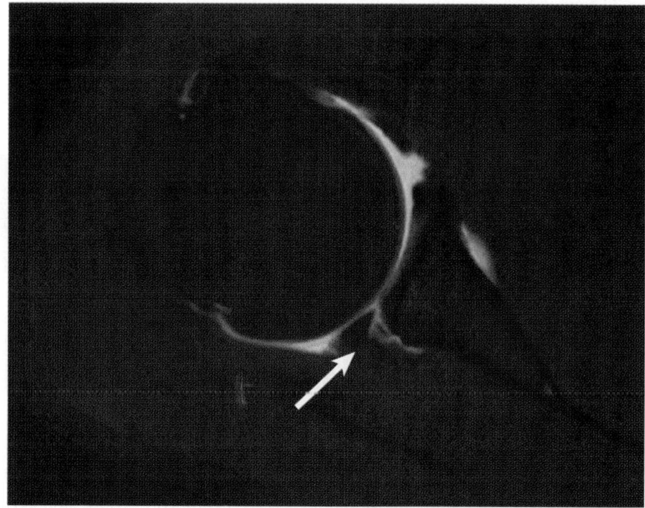

Figure 56.59 Axial Magnetic resonance arthrogram image with reverse posterior labrocapsular periosteal sleeve avulsion (*white arrow*).

Bennett lesion: extraarticular avulsion injury of the posterior band of the IGHL. This manifests as ossification in a crescent shape along the posteroinferior glenoid rim along the posterior band of IGHL attachment. In chronic cases, this is better appreciated on CT than on MRI.

POLPSA and Bennett lesions may be considered as acute and chronic manifestations of the same spectrum of underlying pathology.

Bony: reverse Hill-Sachs, posterior IGHL avulsion.

Atraumatic Instability

This usually tends to be caused by congenital capsular laxity or glenoid hypoplasia. Overhead throwing athletes may also develop this involving the throwing arm. It goes with a pneumonic *AMBRI: a*traumatic, *m*ultidirectional instability, *b*ilateral, *r*ehabilitation (the treatment of choice), *i*nferior capsular shift surgery (required if conservative treatment fails).

On axial MRI, the subscapularis and posterior joint recesses may seem capacious. The glenoid labrum may be hypoplastic with some chronic changes.

Microinstability usually results from chronic repetitive microtrauma to the capsular structures. It is commonly seen in overhead throwing athletes and tends to be unilateral, affecting the dominant arm. Capsular recesses tend to be capacious. In chronic cases, patients can develop labral degeneration, a frying, tear, or even RC injury because of impingement.

Labral Tears

The glenoid labrum can be injured during an acute episode of trauma to the shoulder or in a chronic setting of overuse as well. Like menisci, minor variations in the labral contour can be seen frequently. Subtle intrasubstance signal intensity changes are also relatively common in the labrum with advancing age. Labral tears can be seen as fluid-filled clefts on standard MRI. However, these are best evaluated on MRA.

Superior labral anteroposterior (SLAP) tears (Fig. 56.60): These are commonly seen in throwing athletes because of repetitive traction and torsion injury. Occasionally, they can develop after an isolated episode of trauma. The labral tissue between the 11 and 3'o clock positions is involved. It was initially described by the Snyder classification consisting of four types. More than 10 types have been described in the current literature. A type 2 tear is by far the commonest one to be identified. The description of the tear is more important to the referring clinician. The patient often presents with catching sensation with or without instability.

Important features to differentiate a tear from the normal variants are irregular margins of a tear, lateral extension, width of the lesion, and presence of more than one high signal intensity line in the labrum. The SLAP tears are best evaluated on coronal images.

Pseudo-SLAP Lesion: There is a sulcus between the long head of the biceps origin and superior labrum. When this sulcus is deep, it can fill with contrast material on MRA (best observed on oblique coronal images) and mimic a SLAP tear [23].

Paralabral cysts can develop secondary to a glenoid labral tear, resulting in leakage of the joint fluid. Extension of the cysts into the suprascapular and spinoglenoid notch may cause compression of the suprascapular nerve, leading to denervation changes in the muscles supplied by the suprascapular nerve and its branches. The cysts appear hypointense on T1-weighted images and hyperintense on T2 weighted images. On MRA, the contrast does not fill these paralabral cysts and hence can be missed on T1 fat-saturated images.

Adhesive Capsulitis

Adhesive capsulitis is a clinical condition of unknown etiology that usually presents as gradual onset shoulder pain and a severely reduced range of movements, especially external rotation. It has an incidence of 3% to 5% and typically affects women in their 50s. The incidence in patients with diabetes is reported to be two to four times higher than in the general population, where it can also present at a younger age. Adhesive capsulitis results in synovitis in the RI and thickening of the joint capsule predominantly in the axillary pouch.

Plain films are usually normal, and USG has limited value. Subtle nonspecific signs that may be encountered on USG scan are a thickened CHL and echogenic soft tissue around the LHB at the RI.

Magnetic resonance imaging is more reliable in the diagnosis or raising the suspicion of adhesive capsulitis: MRI features may include any of the following (Fig. 56.61):

- Fibrovascular soft tissue thickening in the RI
- Subcoracoid fat pad effacement

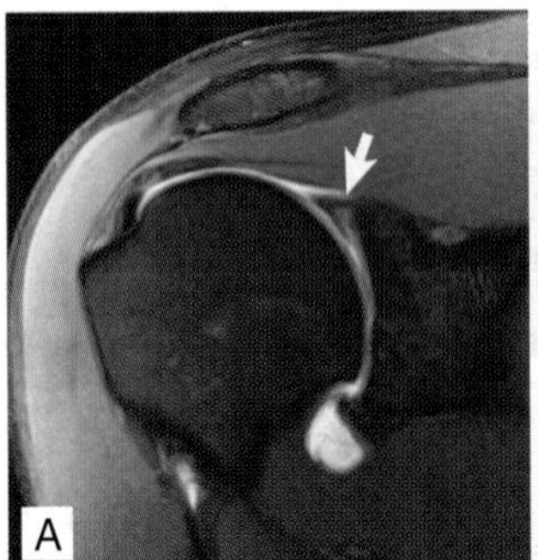

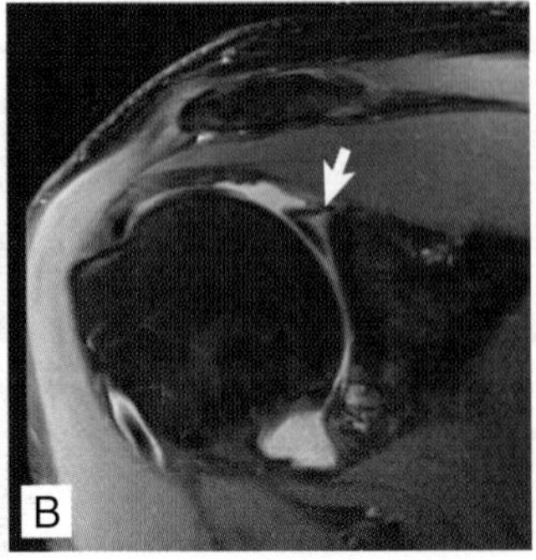

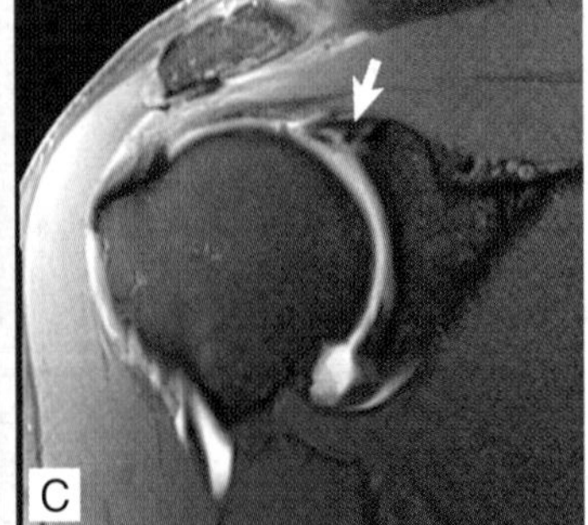

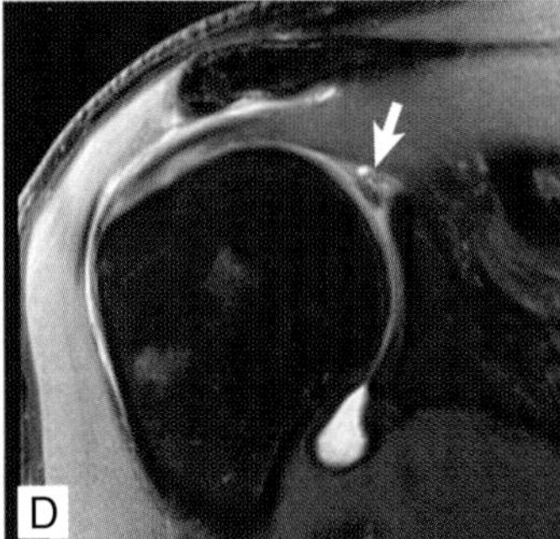

Figure 56.60 Magnetic resonance arthrogram with saline Proton density fat saturated (PDFS) images shows the most common types of superior labral anterior posterior tears. (A) Type 1 shows fraying of the labrum (*white arrow*). (B) Type 2 shows the detachment of the superior labrum and biceps anchor (*white arrow*). (C) Type 3 shows a bucket-handle tear of the superior labrum without extension into the long head of biceps tendon (*white arrow*). (D) Type 4 shows bucket handle tear of the superior labrum with extension into the long head of biceps (*white arrow*).

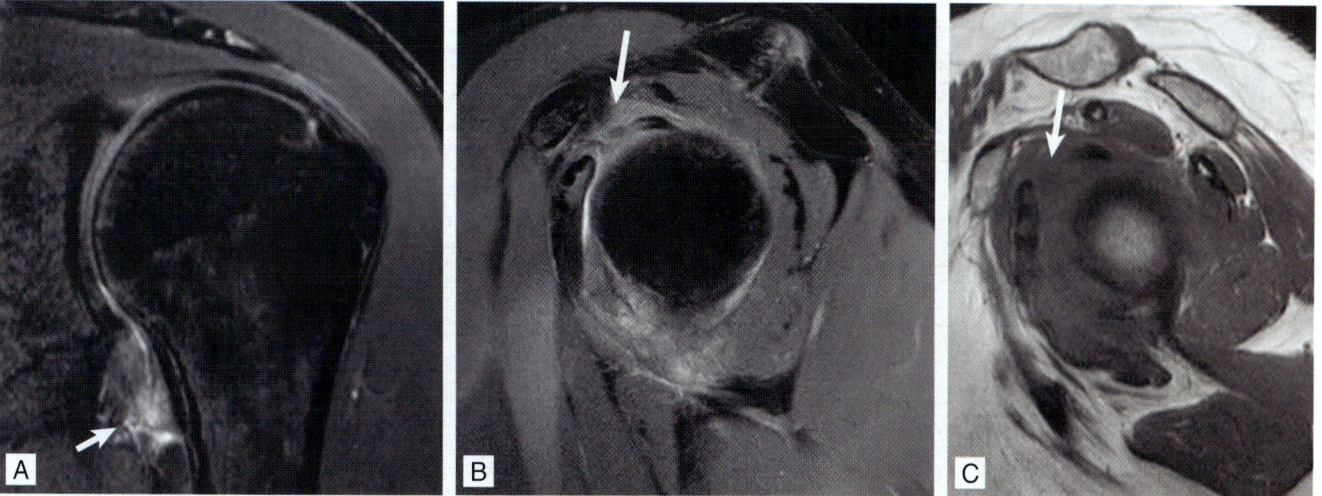

Figure 56.61 Coronal (A) and sagittal (B) Proton density fat saturated (PDFS) images show thickening of the axillary pouch (*white arrow* in A) and edema in the rotator interval (*white arrow* in B), respectively. (C) Sagittal T1 image of a different patient shows loss of fat signal in the rotator interval (*white arrow*).

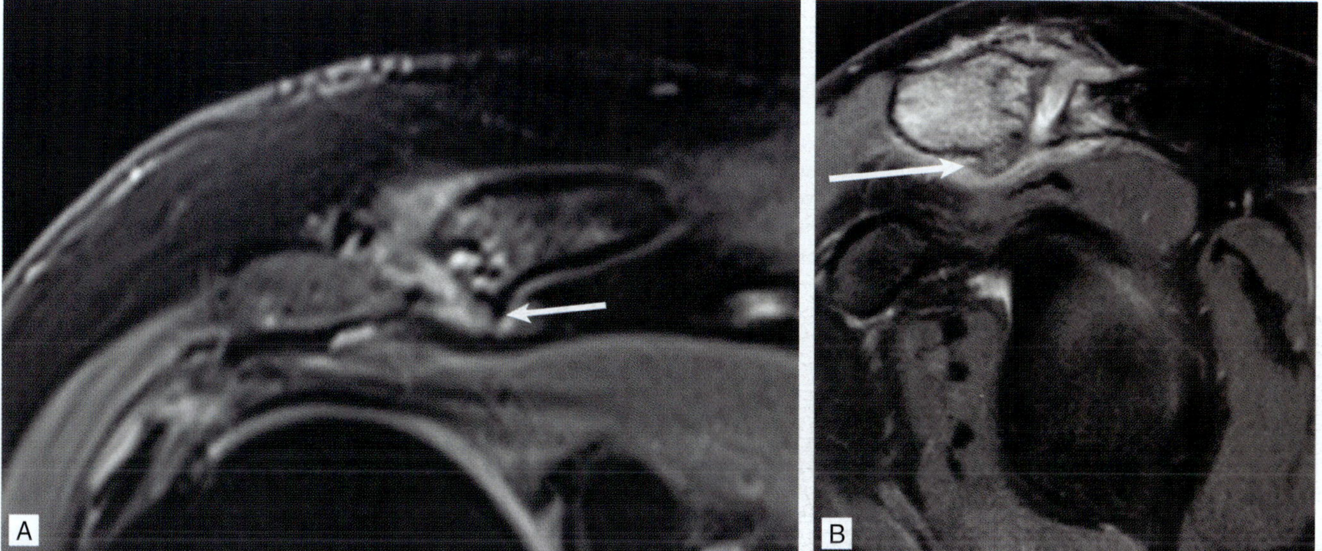

Figure 56.62 Coronal (A) and sagittal (B) Proton density fat saturated (PDFS) images show prominent osteophyte formation (*white arrows*) along the undersurface of the lateral end of clavicle resulting in supraspinatus impingement.

- Thickening of inferior GH ligaments or joint capsule with obliteration of axillary recess best seen on coronal oblique images at the midglenoid level
- More recent evidence suggests that postgadolinium MRI provides greater specificity in the diagnosis.

Acromioclavicular Joint Pathology

Osteoarthritis

Acromioclavicular joint OA most commonly presents in the fourth decade of life. An incomplete fibrocartilaginous disk and a small joint surface area of the AC joint, which under high loads during everyday activities, are thought to lead to early OA.

Magnetic resonance imaging is much more sensitive in identifying the early changes than plain radiographs. Common hallmarks of OA such as joint space reduction, capsular thickening, osteophyte formation, subchondral marrow edema, and cystic changes can be seen (Fig. 56.62). Prominent osteophytes along the undersurface of the lateral end of the clavicle and severe capsular thickening can predispose to RC impingement. Patients with symptomatic ACJ OA also have some form of internal derangement finding on MRI examinations, especially RC abnormalities.

Acromioclavicular Joint Cyst (Geyser Phenomenon)

Acromioclavicular joint fluid is common with OA. When there is a full-thickness RC tear, fluid from the GH joint can escape into

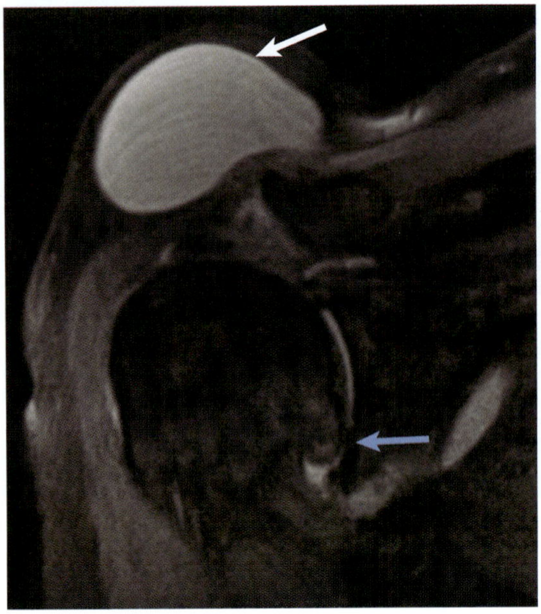

Figure 56.63 Proton density fat saturated (PDFS) magnetic resonance imaging shows a large fluid-filled cystic mass (*white arrow*) superficial to the acromioclavicular joint. Note the advanced degenerative changes of the glenohumeral joint (*blue arrow*).

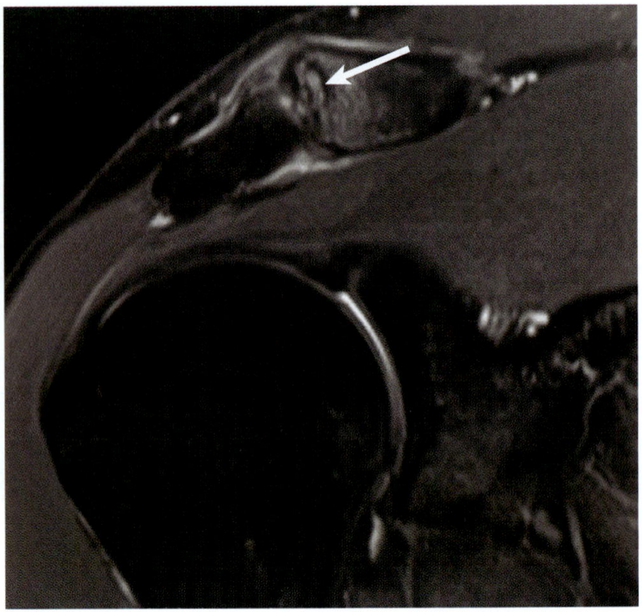

Figure 56.64 PDFS magnetic resonance imaging shows early posttraumatic distal clavicular osteolysis (*white arrow*).

the SASD bursa and track into the AC joint. If there is considerable pressure, a large fluid-filled cystic mass can develop superficial to the AC joint and mimic a soft tissue mass lesion. This development of a fluid-filled mass is also known as the Geyser sign (Fig. 56.63).

Distal Clavicular Osteolysis

This may be posttraumatic or stress related secondary to repetitive microtrauma.

On MRI, there will be subchondral marrow edema, cystic change, cortical irregularity involving the lateral clavicle. The acromion is relatively not affected. Joint space widening, capsular thickening, and effusion can be seen. In chronic stages, there will be osteolysis of the lateral end of the clavicle. Axial and coronal images are the best planes to evaluate these changes (Fig. 56.64).

Other important causes of distal clavicle erosions/resorption are hyperparathyroidism, rheumatoid arthritis, psoriasis & scleroderma. These etiologies should be considered, especially if the abnormality is bilateral.

Nerve Pathology

Parsonage-Turner Syndrome (Acute Brachial Neuritis)

This is usually, a self-limiting condition that is idiopathic, although viral neuritis, recent immunization, autoimmune mechanisms, trauma, strenuous exercise, and surgery have been proposed.

Most often, it is associated with a recent viral infection, suggesting inflammation or autoimmune response of brachial plexus and normally presents as sudden onset of severe shoulder pain and weakness. It can be bilateral in up to one-third of cases and can take up to 1 to 3 weeks to resolve completely. Although the suprascapular nerve is most often involved, the axillary nerve is affected in up to half of cases. In the acute stage, MRI demonstrates edema within the muscles involved (Fig. 56.65). Chronic stages demonstrate muscle atrophy and fatty replacement.

Nerve entrapments around the shoulder joint are summarized in Table 56.8.

Suprascapular Nerve Entrapment

Suprascapular nerve entrapment is a relatively uncommon condition. Narrow fibro-osseous tunnels at the suprascapular notch and spinoglenoid notch with their overlying ligaments predispose to suprascapular nerve entrapment.

Causes include trauma (e.g., scapular and humeral fractures, anterior shoulder dislocation); anomalous, thickened, or calcific scapular ligaments; iatrogenic injury; repetitive overhead activities; and forceful rotational movements performed during sports. Extrinsic compression by space-occupying lesions such as ganglion or paralabral cysts, hematomas, varices, lipomas, and malignant neoplasms have been reported.

Whereas acute denervation shows edema and T2 hyperintensity of the involved muscles, chronic compression shows fatty infiltration and a decrease in muscle bulk of the involved muscles (Fig. 56.66; see also Fig. 56.11).

Quadrilateral space syndrome is a rare disorder caused by axillary nerve and posterior humeral circumflex artery compression within the quadrilateral space. The compression is most

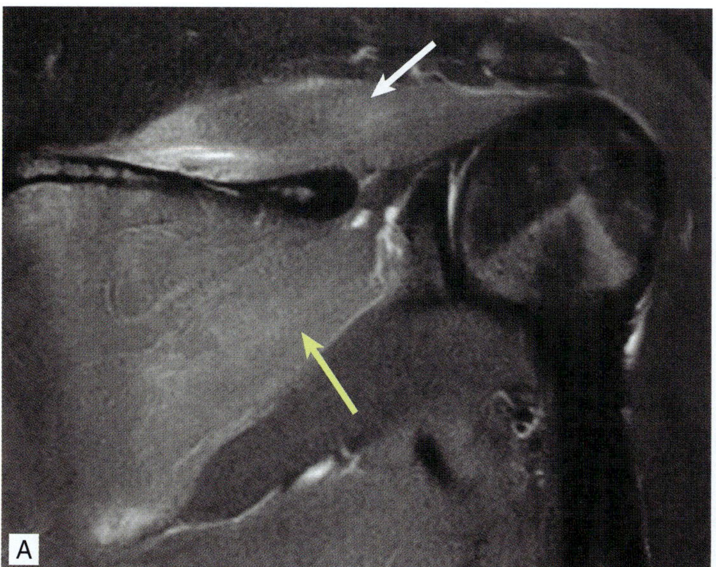

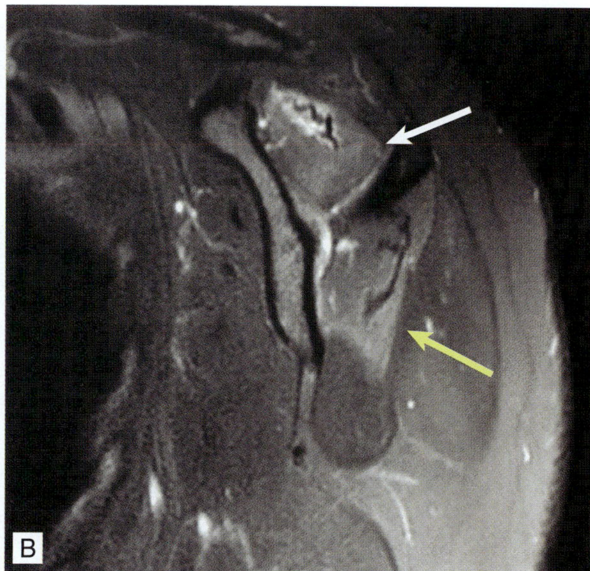

Figure 56.65 T2-weighted fat-saturated coronal (A) and sagittal (B) images show edema in the supraspinatus (*white arrows*) and infraspinatus (*yellow arrows*) in a patient with Parsonage-Turner syndrome.

TABLE 56.8 Summary of Nerve Involvement Around the Shoulder

Nerve Involvement	Causes/Etiology	Findings
Suprascapular nerve entrapment at the suprascapular notch	Acute or repetitive trauma, hematoma, paralabral cysts, mass lesions	Denervation edema or atrophy of the SST and INS muscles
Suprascapular nerve entrapment at the spinoglenoid notch	Acute or repetitive trauma, hematoma, paralabral cysts, mass lesions	Denervation edema or atrophy of the INS muscle
Axillary nerve entrapment in the quadrilateral space (quadrilateral space syndrome)	Trauma, fibrous bands, hypertrophy of the muscular border	Denervation edema or atrophy of teres minor with or without the deltoid muscle
Parsonage-Turner syndrome	Inflammation of brachial plexus	Denervation edema or atrophy of the muscles involved

INS, infraspinatus; *SST*, supraspinatus.

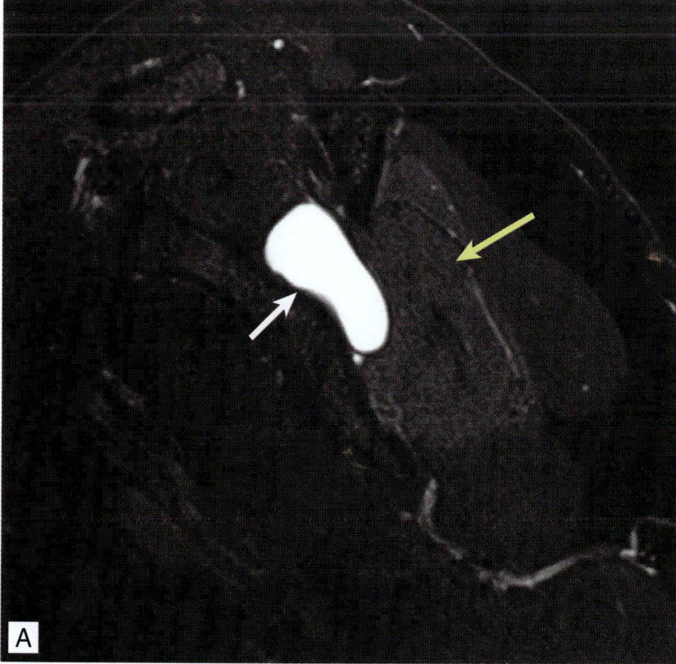

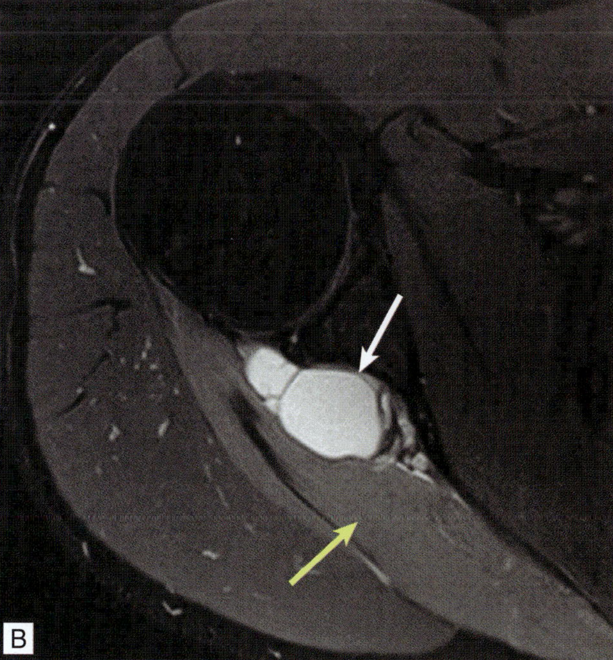

Figure 56.66 Sites of nerve entrapment. Sagittal (A) and (B) axial images show paralabral cyst (*white arrows*) formation with edema in the infraspinatus (*yellow arrows*) caused by suprascapular nerve compression.

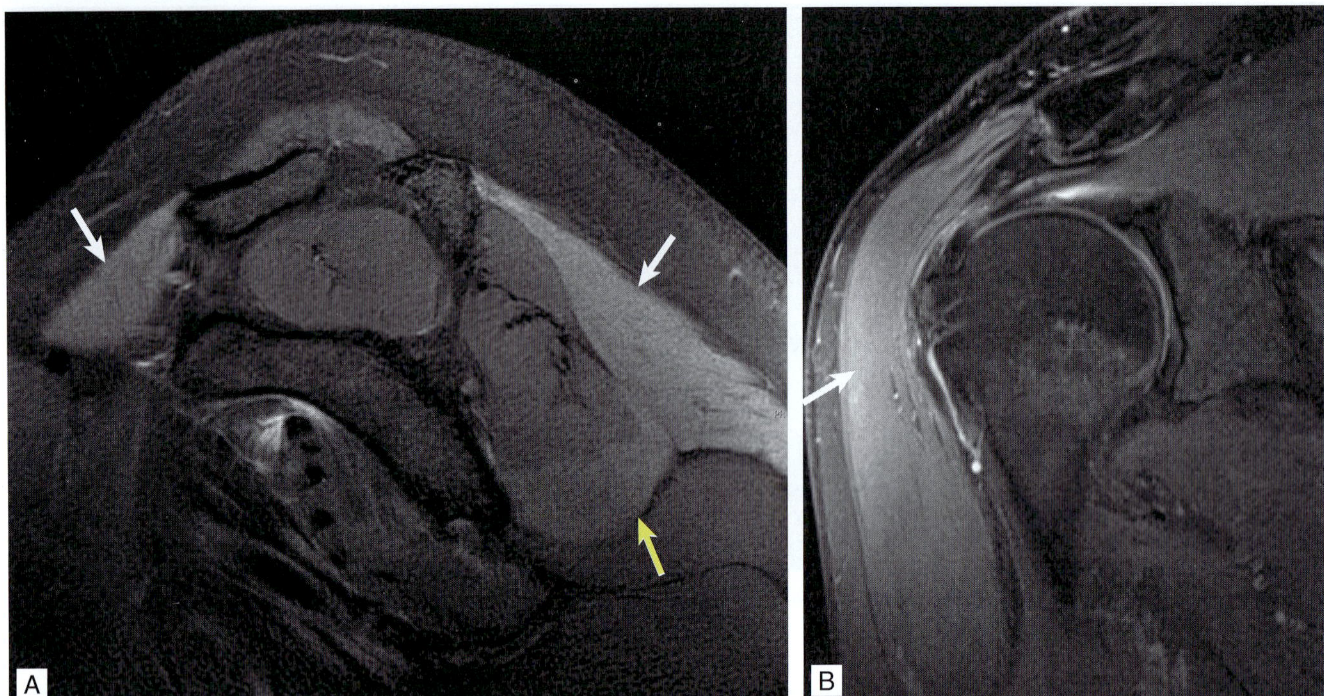

Figure 56.67 Saggital (A) and Coronal (B) T2-weighted fat-saturated images show diffuse edema in the deltoid (*white arrows*) and teres minor (*yellow arrow*) caused by quadrilateral space syndrome.

frequently caused by trauma, fibrous bands, or hypertrophy of one of the muscular borders leading to denervation of the teres minor or deltoid musculature (Fig. 56.67).

Suggested Readings

- E Llopis, P Montesinos, MT Guedez, L Aguilella, L Cerezal, Normal shoulder MRI and MR arthrography: anatomy and technique, Semin Musculoskelet Radiol 19 (2015) 212–230.
- M Jarraya, FW Roemer, MR-arthrography and CT-arthrography in sports-related glenolabral injuries: a matched descriptive illustration, Insights Imaging (2) (2016 Apr 7) 167–177.
- J-S Roy, C Braën, J Leblond, Diagnostic accuracy of ultrasonography, MRI and MR arthrography in the characterisation of rotator cuff disorders: a systematic review and meta-analysis, Br J Sports Med 49 (20) (2015 Oct) 1316–1328, doi:10.1136/bjsports-2014-094148.
- MH Lee, SE Sheehan, JF Orwin, KS Lee, Comprehensive shoulder US examination: a standardized approach with multimodality correlation for common shoulder disease, Radiographics 36 (2016) 1606–1627.
- T De Coninck, SS Ngai, Imaging the glenoid labrum and labral tears, Radiographics 36 (2016) 1628–1647.

57 The Elbow

MONICA KALUME-BRIGIDO, GIRISH GANDIKOTE

Anatomy

Bones and Joints

The elbow joint is a synovial joint comprised of three bones (the distal humerus, proximal radius, and ulna) and three articulations (ulnotrochlear, radiocapitellar, and proximal radioulnar joints), all covered by the same joint capsule. There are three joint recesses: two anteriorly, at the coronoid and radial fossae, and one posteriorly, at the olecranon fossa. Each of these recesses has a fat pad, which are intracapsular but extrasynovial (Fig. 57.1A and B) and are displaced in the presence of joint effusion (Fig. 57.1C) [1]. Intraarticular bodies can be seen on these recesses, particularly the coronoid and olecranon. *A meniscus-like structure can also be seen in the lateral aspect of the radiocapitellar joint, which can be associated with painful snapping* [2].

The articular surfaces of the bones are covered with hyaline cartilage. Anatomic variations, such as the pseudodefect of the capitellum, can be misinterpreted as osteochondral lesions (Fig. 57.2). This is a normal groove seen in the posterior junction of the capitellum and humerus. The posterior location helps to distinguish this normal variant from a true osteochondral defect, which tends to be located anteriorly [3,4]. An additional pseudodefect is seen along the trochlear grove at the junction of the olecranon and coronoid process, which lacks hyaline cartilage and where intraarticular bodies can also be found. An osseous ridge is also seen here, known as transverse trochlear ridge, and can simulate a central osteophyte [3,4].

A normal variant in the bone, the supracondylar process of the humerus, is a cortical osseous spur seen in 0.1 to 2.7% of the population and located in the anteromedial distal humerus, pointing distally and medially (Fig. 57.3). It is located about 4 to 8 cm proximal to the medial epicondyle and has a variable size ranging from 0.2 to 2 cm [5,6]. *It should not be misinterpreted as osteochondroma.* The ligament of Struthers is a fibrous band that joins the bone spur to the medial epicondyle and can cause median nerve and brachial artery compression [6]. A pseudo-osseous lesion can also be misinterpreted as a lytic lesion on radiographs and corresponds to the radial tuberosity viewed en face (Fig. 57.4). Table 57.1 summarizes anatomic variations and pseudolesions in the elbow.

Ligaments

The collateral ligaments of the elbow are thickening of the joint capsule and provide stabilization of the joint.

Medial Ligaments

The ulnar collateral ligament (UCL) complex has three bundles: anterior, transverse, and posterior (Fig. 57.5A). The anterior bundle is the strongest and most crucial stabilizer against valgus stress. It is also the most frequently injured bundle [3,7,8]. It originates from the inferior surface of the medial epicondyle and inserts distally in the sublime tubercle of the ulna or up to 3 to 4 mm distal to the joint line [7]. The posterior bundle forms the floor of the cubital tunnel. It originates from the undersurface of the medial epicondyle and inserts in the medial aspect of the olecranon (at the trochlear notch of the ulna). The transverse bundle is variably present and plays no role in the stabilization of the elbow [8].

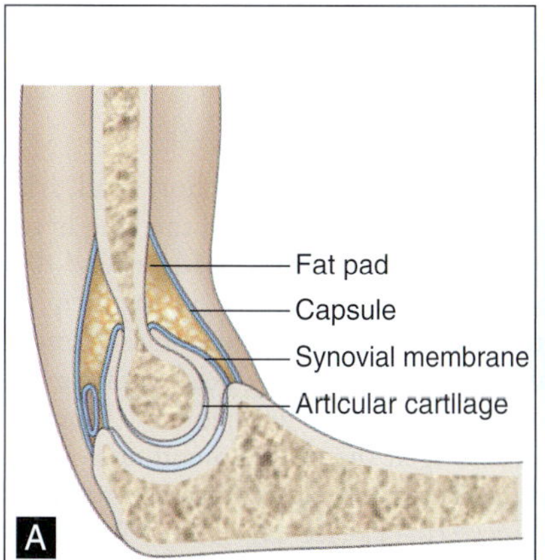

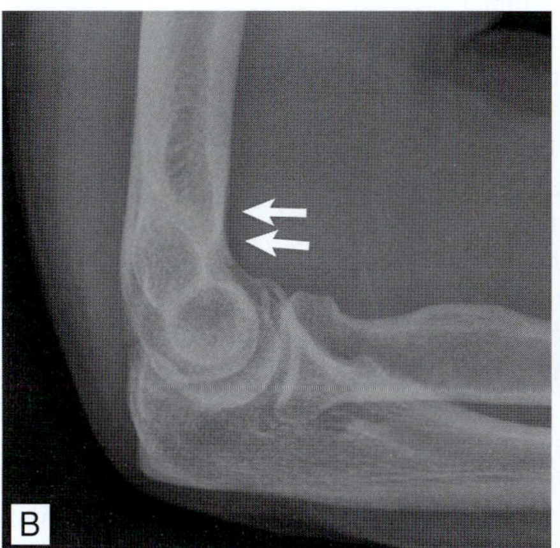

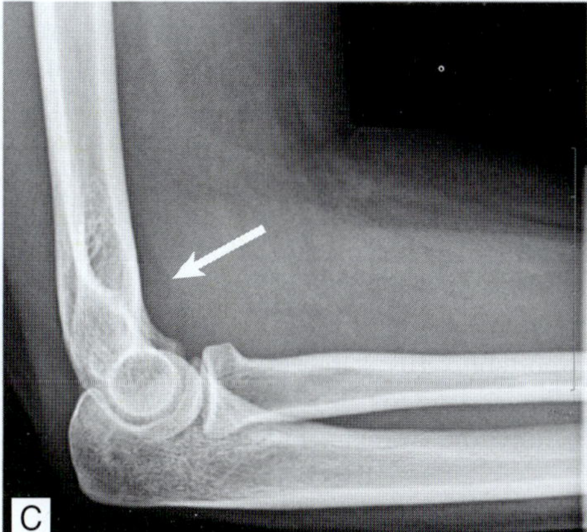

Figure 57.1 (A) Lateral illustration shows the elbow joint with the anterior and posterior intracapsular but extrasynovial fat pads. Lateral radiograph (B) shows the normal lucent fat pad just anterior to the distal humerus (*arrows*) and the displaced fat pad (C) in the presence of joint effusion (sail sign) (*arrow*).

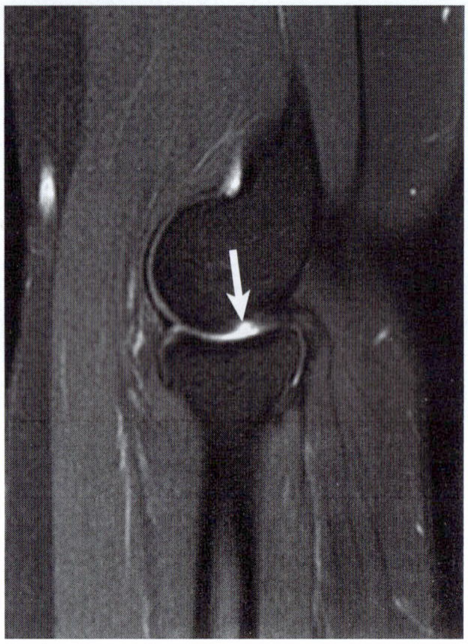

Figure 57.2 Pseudodefect of the capitellum: sagittal PD-weighted magnetic resonance image with fat saturation shows the normal groove in the posterior capitellum (*arrow*). The location, smooth margins, and lack of bone marrow edema distinguish it from a true osteochondral defect.

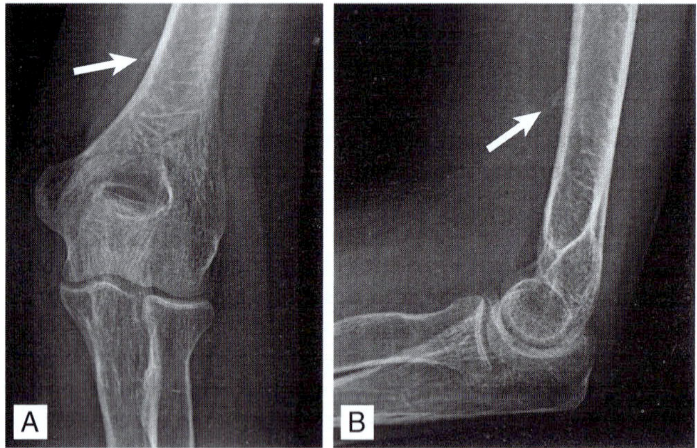

Figure 57.3 Supracondylar process of the humerus: radiograph frontal (A) and lateral (B) views show the anteromedial distal humerus osseous spur, pointing distally and medially (*arrows*).

Lateral Ligaments

The radial collateral ligament (RCL) complex has four components: lateral ulnar collateral ligament (LUCL), RCL, annular ligament (AL), and accessory collateral ligament (variably present) (Fig. 57.5B). The LUCL is the most critical and primary stabilizer against posterolateral rotatory instability (PLRI) [8,9]. Both the LUCL and RCL originate from the inferior surface of the lateral epicondyle and can be indistinguishable here. The LUCL originates just posterior to the RCL and extends distally to insert into the supinator crest of the ulna [8]. The RCL is intimately associated with the common extensor muscles superficially and extends distally to blend with the AL and supinator muscle fascia. It is an important varus stabilizer. The AL wraps around the proximal radius and inserts in the sigmoid notch of the ulna. It provides stability to the proximal radioulnar joint [8].

Muscles and Tendons

Anterior Compartment

The biceps brachii and brachialis muscles are the main flexors of the elbow.

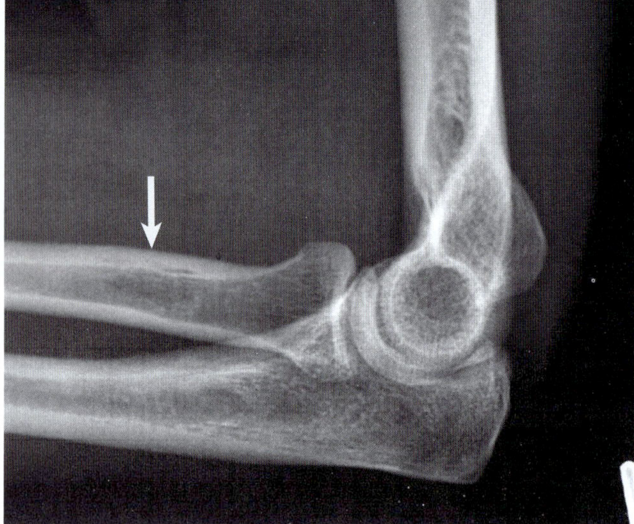

Figure 57.4 Radial tuberosity pseudolesion. Lateral radiograph shows the radial tuberosity viewed en face, simulating a lytic lesion (*arrow*).

TABLE 57.1 Imaging Pitfalls and Anatomic Variations

Variation	Description
Pseudodefect of the capitellum	Posterior capitellum; simulates OCD on MRI; no associated bone marrow edema; a true OCD is more often anterior
Pseudodefect of the trochlear grove	Junction of coronoid and olecranon process; not covered by articular cartilage; simulates OCD on MRI
Transverse trochlear ridge	Junction of the coronoid and olecranon process at the trochlear groove; simulates central osteophyte
Supracondylar process of the humerus	Anteromedial distal humerus, points to the medial epicondyle; can compress the median nerve; simulates osteochondroma
Proximal radius pseudo lytic lesion	Radial tuberosity seen on radiographs en face; simulates lytic lesion on radiographs
Anconeus epitrochlearis muscle	Anatomic variant; located between the medial epicondyle and olecranon process; can cause ulnar nerve compression

MRI, magnetic resonance imaging; *OCD*, osteochondral defect.

The biceps brachii muscle has two heads: the short head, arising from the coracoid process of the scapula, and the long head, arising from the supraglenoid tubercle. Both heads extend distally, cross the elbow joint, and insert separately in the bicipital radial tuberosity; the tendon of the short head inserts more distally and anteriorly and tendon of the long head inserts more proximally [10] (Fig. 57.6). The bicipital aponeurosis (Lacertus fibrosis) is a fibrous band arising at the musculotendinous junction of the distal biceps brachii and extending medially to blend with the antebrachial fascia [10,11] (see Fig. 57.6). An intact bicipital aponeurosis prevents a greater degree of retraction of a completely torn tendon, mainly when the tear involves the short head of the biceps. Therefore, the classic clinical presentation of a visible distal arm mass (Popeye sign) will not be present. This

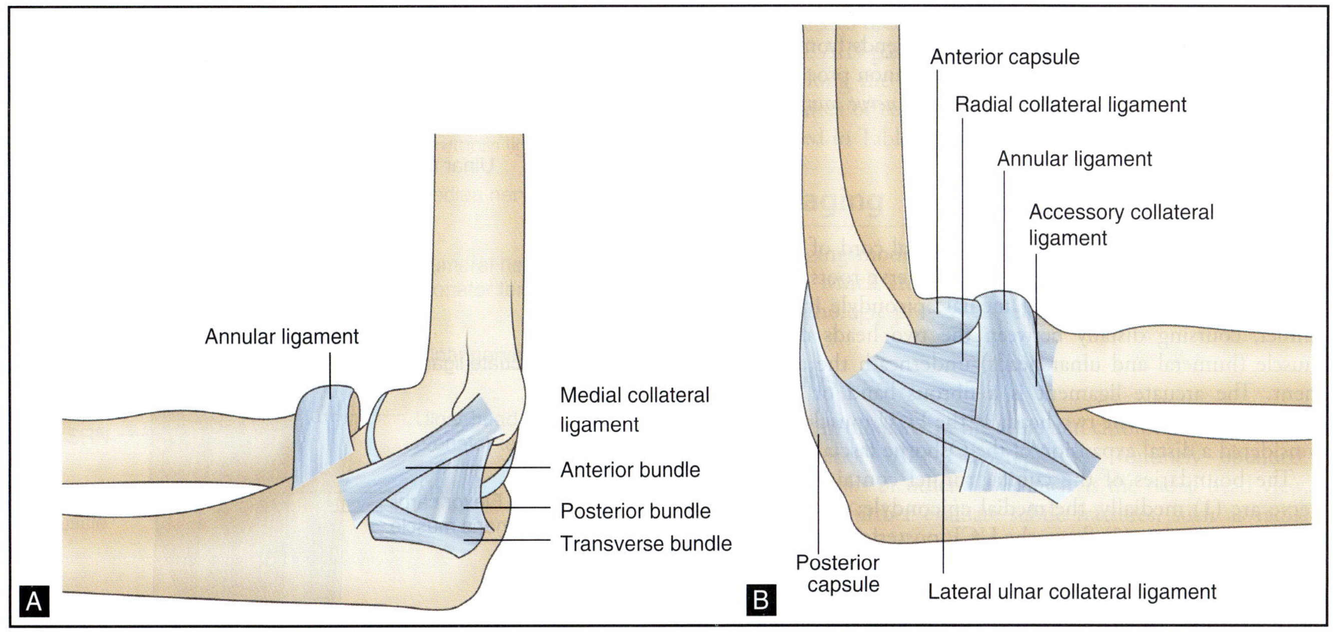

Figure 57.5 Lateral elbow illustration shows the ulnar collateral ligament (A) and the radial collateral ligament (B) complex with their components.

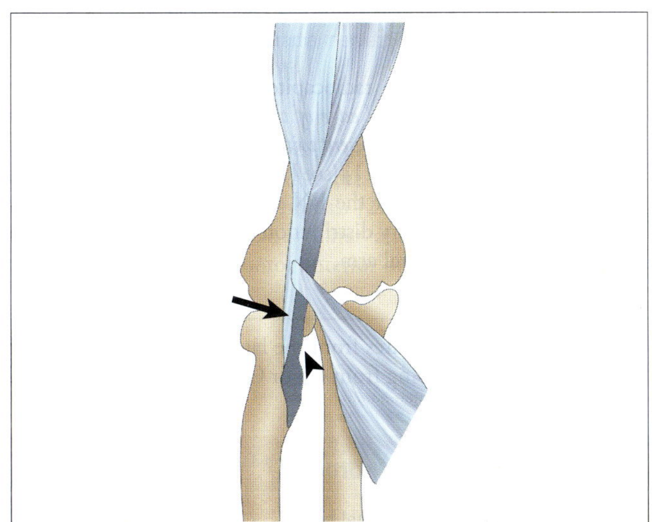

Figure 57.6 Frontal illustration shows the two heads of the biceps brachii tendon (*short head*, *arrowhead and long head*, *arrow*) inserting separately in the radial tuberosity. Note the bicipital aponeurosis (lacertus fibrosis) extending medially from the biceps musculotendinous junction to blend with the antebrachial fascia bicipital aponeurosis.

may lead the clinicians to underestimate the extent of the tendon tear [10,11]. *The distal tendon has no tendon sheath. The presence of fluid in this location should not be diagnosed as tenosynovitis.* Instead, there is a bursa called bicipitoradial bursa, which is located between the radial tuberosity and the distal biceps tendon [12].

The brachialis muscle arises from the anterior surface of the humerus and inserts in the coronoid process of the ulna. This muscle is located deep to the biceps brachii.

Medial Compartment

Several muscles of the forearm arise from the medial and lateral elbow. The medial muscle compartment includes the medial flexor-pronator group.

A common flexor tendon (CFT) originates in the medial epicondyle and gives rise to the superficial forearm flexor muscles. These muscles include pronator teres (PT), flexor carpi radialis, flexor carpi ulnaris (FCU), palmaris longus, and flexor digitorum superficialis (FDS) [13]. The CFT lies superficial to the medial collateral ligament (MCL).

Lateral Compartment

The lateral compartment includes the extensor-supinator muscle group.

A common extensor tendon (CET) originates in the lateral epicondyle and gives rise to several extensor muscles of the forearm. These muscles include the extensor carpi radialis brevis, extensor digitorum, extensor digiti minimi, and extensor carpi ulnaris [13]. The brachioradialis and extensor carpi radialis longus arise from the lateral supracondylar ridge. The supinator muscle has different origins in the lateral epicondyle and lateral capsular structures (humeral head) and in the ulna (ulnar head). The muscle wraps around the proximal radial shaft, where it inserts laterally. The CET lies superficial to the RCL and is intimately related to it.

Posterior Compartment

The posterior elbow contains the extensors, which includes the triceps, anconeus, and anconeus epitrochlearis.

The triceps brachii muscle is composed of three heads. It originates from the infraglenoid tubercle of the scapula (long head), the upper posterior humerus (lateral head), and the lower posterior humerus (medial head). The tendon primarily inserts on the olecranon process of the ulna [13,14]. The medial head has a separate insertion from the long and lateral heads, located anterior and deep on the olecranon process. The superficial tendon at the insertion is composed of the long and lateral heads. The deep tendon seen beneath is composed of the medial head [14]. The medial head is in close proximity to the ulnar nerve. The olecranon bursa is located in the superficial soft tissues overlying the olecranon process, between the skin and bone [12].

The anconeus muscle extends from the lateral epicondyle to the lateral aspect of the olecranon process [13].

intersect the capitellum are important landmarks evaluated on the lateral view to identify elbow malalignment [24]

- Radial head view: This is a variant of the lateral view. It includes 90% flexion with the x-ray beam angled 45 degrees toward the radial head and neck. It provides a better evaluation of subtle fractures of the radial head and coronoid process [25] because it decreases the overlap of other bones

Computed Tomography

Computed tomography (CT) is the imaging modality of choice for trauma with complex fractures and elbow dislocation, detecting occult or additional fractures, evaluating degree of articular surface step-off, and detecting the presence of intraarticular fracture fragments. Three-dimensional CT reconstructions are helpful for preoperative planning. Intravenous contrast is given if vascular injury is suspected.

In the chronic setting, CT can be used to evaluate soft tissue ossifications, including myositis ossificans, heterotopic ossifications and their relation to adjacent nerves, fracture healing process, and intraarticular osseous bodies. Additional usefulness of CT includes evaluation of hardware and possible complications with the use of metal-suppression protocol, evaluation of musculoskeletal tumors, and guidance of percutaneous biopsies.

Dual-energy CT is an accurate imaging modality used to diagnose gout with high sensitivity and specificity [26]. It detects urate deposits at and around the joints and can be a problem-solving tool in complex cases with unusual clinical presentation of gout.

Computed tomography arthrography is useful to evaluate osteochondral bodies in the joint. It can be used to evaluate the osteochondral defect, capsular and ligament disruption, particularly in patients with contraindication for MRI.

Ultrasonography

Both USG and magnetic resonance imaging (MRI) are the preferred imaging modalities to evaluate the soft tissues, including the muscles, tendons, ligaments, and nerves.

Ultrasonography is performed using a high-frequency linear transducer, at least 10 MHz. It is commonly requested to evaluate for medial and lateral epicondylitis but also tendon and ligament tears and nerve pathology. Normal tendons and ligaments appear hyperechoic on USG; tendons have a fibrillar appearance, and ligaments have a striated, more compact appearance (Fig. 57.10)

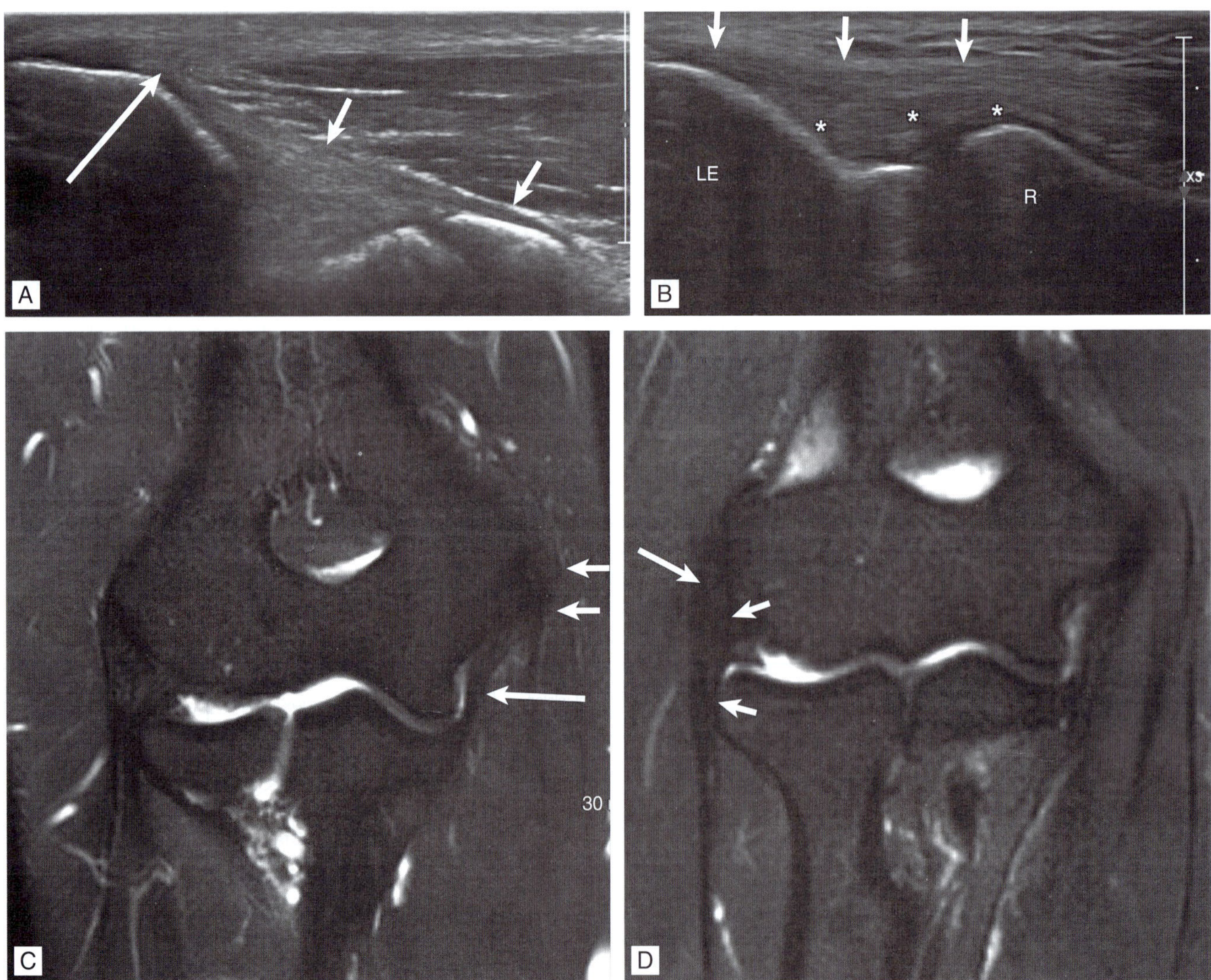

Figure 57.10 Longitudinal ultrasound image show the normal hyperechoic (A) ulnar collateral ligament (*short arrows*) and common flexor tendon (CFT; *long arrow*) (B), the radial collateral ligament (*asterisks*), and the common extensor tendon (CET; *arrows*). The corresponding coronal T2-weighted magnetic resonance image with fat saturation shows the normal low signal intensity of the ulnar collateral ligament (*long arrow* in C) and CFT (*short arrows* in C), the radial collateral ligament (*short arrows* in D), and the CET (*long arrow* in D).

[17,27]. If these structures are not imaged perpendicular to the ultrasound beam, their normal hyperechogenicity is lost, simulating pathology (anisotropy artifact). Normal nerve has a honeycomb appearance in the short-axis view and fascicular appearance in the long-axis view with hypoechoic nerve fascicles and hyperechoic connective tissue [17,27].

Advantages of USG include its low cost, quick and easy accessibility, and ability to correlate with site of pain and compare with the asymptomatic opposite side. It can perform dynamic imaging, which is helpful to distinguish partial versus complete tear of tendons and ligaments and to evaluate the source of snapping, clicking, and impingement.

High-frequency linear transducer allows great visibility of the nerves and sites of nerve compressions, although early muscle denervation changes are better evaluated with MRI.

An additional role of US is to guide therapeutic interventions, such as aspirations, injections, and tendon fenestrations [17,27]. Ultrasound elastography is also a promising technique, which is designed to distinguish tissues with different stiffness, and has a potential to improve assessment of tendon disorders [28].

Magnetic Resonance and Magnetic Resonance Arthrography

These modalities have higher sensitivity and specificity in the evaluation of the ligamentous structures. Conventional MRI is preferred to detect occult bone injuries. Magnetic resonance arthrography (MRA) is more accurate than conventional MRI in the evaluation of ligament and tendon tears [29].

Studies are best performed on a high-field strength magnet using surface coils, with images obtained in the coronal, axial, and sagittal planes. Sequences include T1 weighted, T2 weighted with fat saturation, proton-density weighted with fat saturation, and STIR (short tau inversion recovery). In MRA, the protocol consists of T1-weighted imaging with fat saturation in all planes plus a T2-weighted imaging with fat saturation.

Magnetic resonance arthrography examination is performed after intraarticular injection of diluted gadolinium, which is most commonly performed guided by fluoroscopy. The solution can be injected using a lateral approach through the radiocapitellar joint or a posterior approach through the triceps.

Magnetic arthrography images are obtained with the patient in the supine position with the arm held at the side, in anatomic position, or in prone position with the arm over the head ("superman position") for larger patients. *FABS position (flexed elbow, abducted shoulder, forearm supinated) improves visualization of the distal biceps tendon* [30].

- Normal tendons and ligaments should have homogeneous, low signal intensity relative to skeletal muscle in all sequences [3,4] (see Fig. 57.10). The humeral attachment of the UCL has a broad insertion. It is normal to have some mild signal change there because of fat interdigitation, which should not be misdiagnosed as pathologic [3,4]. The insertion of the ligament on the sublime tubercle is tight, although there is some variability [3]. There should be little or no fluid or contrast between the ligament and the sublime tubercle. Normal nerves on MRI demonstrate intermediate signal on T1-weighted images, nearly isointense to muscle, and slightly increased signal on T2-weighted images [4]. The characteristic honeycomb appearance with a high T1 fat signal surrounding the nerve and low signal central dots related to the fascicles is appreciated
- Partial-thickness ligament tears are best evaluated with distended joints, which are best accomplished with MRA [31]. An example of this is a partial tear of the anterior bundle of the UCL at the attachment on the sublime tubercle of the ulna [32]. MRA is also preferred to improve diagnosis of stability of osteochondral lesion and in the evaluation of intraarticular bodies, which is better assessed with the joint distended [33]

Elbow Pathology

Traumatic Events: Acute and Chronic Overuse Injuries

The stability of the elbow joint is accomplished by the integrity of the primary and secondary stabilizers, with the primary stabilizers playing the major role [8,32].

- Primary stabilizers: the anterior bundle of the MCL, the LUCL, and the ulnotrochlear joint
- Secondary stabilizers: the CET, the common flexor/pronator tendon, and the radiocapitellar joint

Disruption of these structures can occur acutely or associated with chronic repetitive overuse injuries. Ligament tears, fractures, and elbow dislocations with or without associated fractures can lead to elbow instability. Traumatic events, including elbow fractures and dislocations, as well as osteochondral lesions are addressed in other chapter.

Ulnar Collateral Ligament Injury

Injuries of the UCL are most common secondary to chronic repetitive valgus stress during athletic activities associated with throwing or overhead motion, as seen with baseball pitchers [8,32]. A fall onto an outstretched hand can also be a cause of injury in older and nonathletic individuals. The most common mechanism associated with overhead motion activity involves medial tension overload, lateral compression, and extension overload [8,32]:

- Medial tension overload: leads to injury of the anterior bundle of the UCL. Other possible injuries include ulnar nerve traction and CFT injury
- Lateral compression: leads to capitellum and radial head bone contusion and osteochondral injuries
- Extension overload (shear force): leads to posteromedial osteophyte formation of the olecranon process and trochlea

Disruption of the anterior bundle of the UCL leads to valgus instability. Tears occur more often in the midsubstance and at the sublime tubercle insertion. They can be partial or complete [8,32].

- **Imaging diagnosis**
    - Radiographs: These can be normal or demonstrate joint effusion, associated fractures, such as avulsion of the sublime tubercle of the ulna or elbow dislocation if complex injury, and findings associated with the capitellar osteochondral defect. Ligament calcifications and posteromedial osteophytes can be seen in a chronic injury
    - USG: This is focused on the anterior bundle of the UCL. It is best evaluated on the longitudinal plane. Findings include [17,27]
        - Sprain: hypoechogenicity and heterogeneity without fiber discontinuity
        - Partial tear: hypoechoic swelling and heterogeneity with partial fiber discontinuity (Fig. 57.11A)
        - Complete tear: complete fiber discontinuity with variable echogenicity related to fluid and hemorrhage. Dynamic imaging with gentle valgus stress helps distinguish a partial versus complete tear by assessing asymmetric

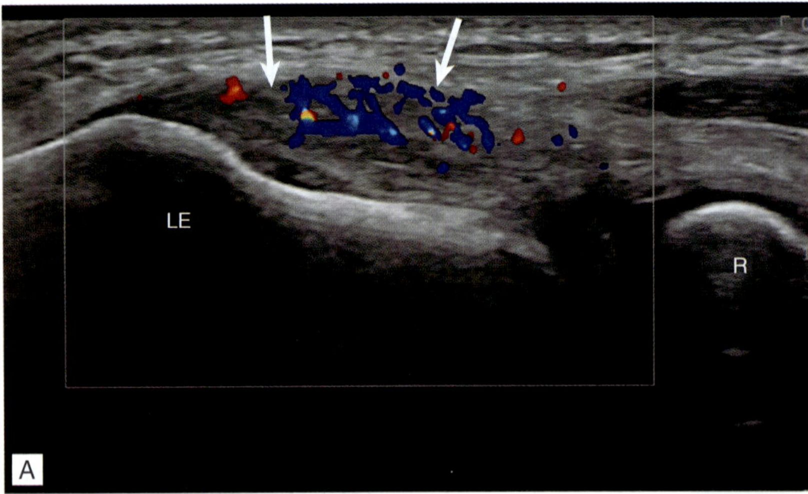

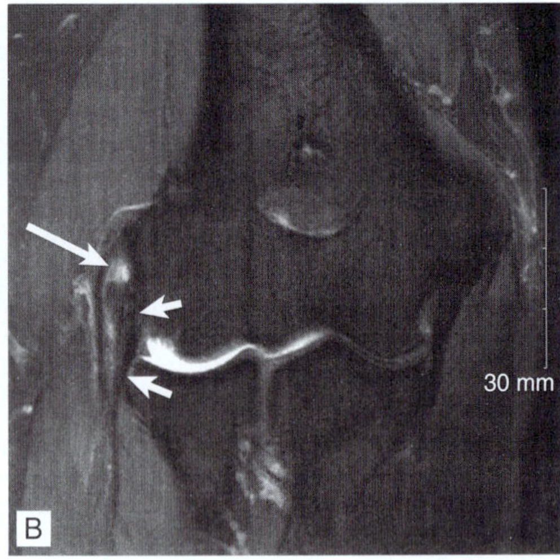

Figure 57.13 Lateral epicondylitis. (A) Longitudinal ultrasound image shows hypoechoic thickening of the common extensor tendon (CET) at the lateral epicondyle (LE) with increased vascularity on color Doppler (*arrows*). (B) Coronal T2-weighted magnetic resonance image with fat saturation of a companion case shows thickening with increased signal in the CET and partial fiber discontinuity (*long arrow*) consistent with a partial tear. The radial collateral ligament is intact (*short arrows*). *R*, radius.

  - MRI: This is best seen on coronal and axial planes. Findings include [31,41] increased T1 and T2 signal abnormality in the common tendon origin (Fig. 57.13B), fluid-filled or contrast-filled clefts (if MRA) if associated partial tendon tears (see Fig. 57.13B), complete tendon fibers discontinuity if a complete tear, peritendinous edema, cortical irregularity and reactive bone marrow edema in the epicondyle, and intratendinous ossifications, most commonly in chronic cases, after bone marrow signal in all sequences
- **Treatment:** There are different treatment options for epicondylitis, ranging from activity restrictions and conservative treatment to second-line treatments such as tendon fenestration, extracorporeal shockwave therapy, botulinum toxin injection, steroid injection (only short-term relief), and autologous blood or platelet-rich plasma injection, which are reported with variable outcomes [35]. Surgery is reserved for severe cases unresponsive to conservative treatment [40]

Biceps Brachii Tendon Injury

Distal biceps tendon tear is less common than proximal tendon tear [42]. *The most common site is near the insertion on the radial tuberosity, related to a zone of hypovascularity, as well as associated with mechanical impingement at the radial tuberosity* [42]. Other less common sites include the muscle belly and musculotendinous junction. The mechanism of injury usually involves a forced extension against active elbow flexion [42].

Tears can be related to acute trauma (occurring at any age) or related to chronic tendinopathy (fourth to sixth decades of life). It can coexist with tendinosis and bicipitoradial bursitis [42,43].

Tendon tears can be partial or complete (more common) and can involve one or both tendon heads with variable degree of retraction [10]. *An intact lacertus fibrosis can prevent tendon retraction, making the clinical diagnosis more challenging (lack of Popeye sign)* [10,11,42].

The clinical presentation consists of anterior elbow pain and swelling with history of a "popping sensation" in the anterior elbow at the time of injury; it can present with bruising and a visible lump in the arm (Popeye sign) related to the retracted torn tendon.

- **Imaging diagnosis:** Radiographs are used to exclude other possibilities. The diagnosis can be made with both USG and MRI
  - USG: Both axial and longitudinal planes are essential. Anisotropy can be an issue because of the oblique course of the tendon [27]. Different sonographic approaches are used to improve visualization of the distal tendon, including anterior, lateral, medial, and posterior [43]. Dynamic imaging with pronation and supination of the forearm are very helpful to distinguish partial versus complete tears; visualization of tendon motion indicates partial rather than complete tear. This can be identified using the lateral and medial sonographic approaches. USG findings include [27,43]
    - Tendinosis: hypoechoic swelling without fibers discontinuity. It can involve one or both tendon heads
    - Partial tear: thinning or thickening of the tendon with focal areas of fibers discontinuity. Hypoechogenicity also seen with associated tendinosis. Adjacent fluid can be present, related to bicipitoradial bursal fluid
    - Complete tear: complete tendon discontinuity with waviness and variable degree of proximal tendon retraction, which should be reported (Fig. 57.14A). Fluid and hematoma with variable echogenicity are seen filling the tendon gap. Posterior acoustic shadowing is also present and associated to refraction artifact secondary to the wavy torn and retracted tendon
  - MRI: best seen on sagittal and axial planes
    - Tendinosis: intermediate signal on T1 and intermediate to high signal on T2-weighted images without fibers discontinuity
    - Partial tear: high signal on T2-weighted images with partial fibers discontinuity. Intact fibers are seen. It can involve one or both tendon heads. High T2 fluid signal can also be seen within the bicipitoradial bursa [31,44]. Surrounding soft tissue edema is also seen
    - Complete tear: complete tendon discontinuity with waviness, involving one or both tendon heads, and proximal tendon retraction, if disrupted lacertus fibrosus is present [45]; soft tissue swelling and fluid with mixed low and high signal on T1 and T2-weighted

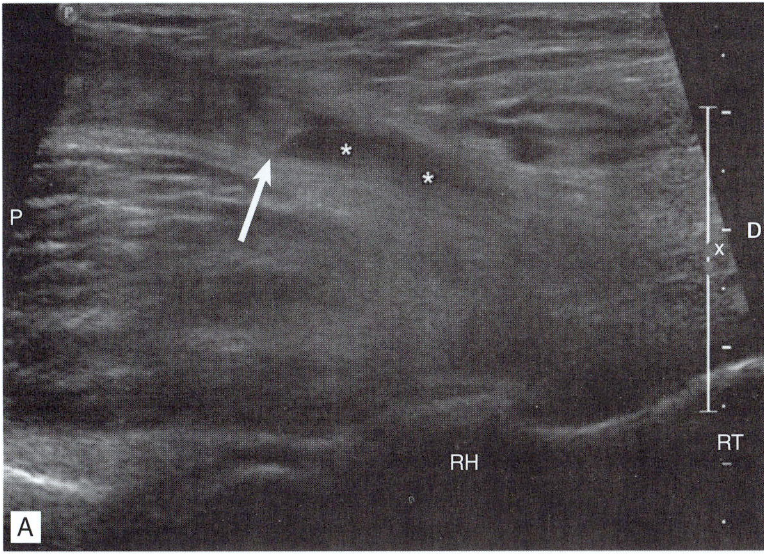

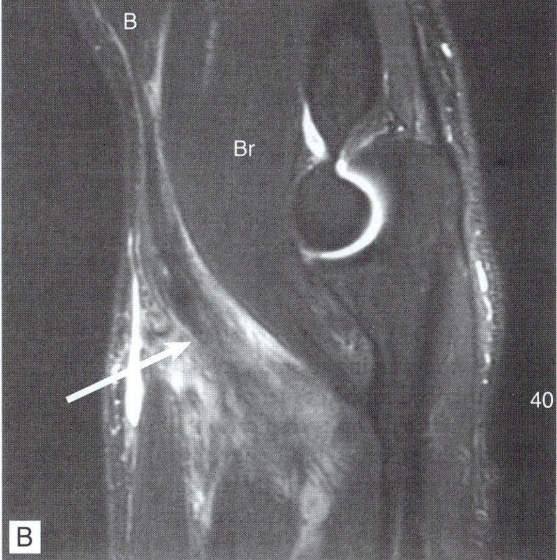

Figure 57.14 Complete tear of long head of biceps brachii tendon. (A) Longitudinal ultrasound image and (B) sagittal T2-weighted image with fat saturation show complete fibers discontinuity with proximal tendon retraction (*arrow*), hematoma filling the tendon gap (*asterisks*), and diffuse soft tissue swelling. *B,* Biceps; *Br,* brachialis; *RH,* radial head; *RT,* radial tuberosity.

images related to hemorrhage and hematoma seen at the tendon gap (Fig. 57.14B)

- **Treatment:** Patients with partial low-grade tears are treated conservatively. Those with complete tears are most commonly treated surgically with reattachment of the torn tendon to the bicipital tuberosity, particularly in acute tears in active individuals of all ages [42,45]

Triceps Tendon Injury

Triceps tendon injury is uncommon, with a prevalence of 3.8% [46]. Tears can be associated with (1) acute traumatic event, such as a direct blow, including deceleration force applied to the arm with the triceps muscle contracted, as seen on football players, or (2) repetitive overseas seen with weightlifters.

Contributing factors leading to underlying tendinopathy and predisposing to tear with a less significant trauma include diabetes, rheumatoid arthritis, history of chronic renal failure, gout, connective tissue disease, and the use of steroids systemically or locally to treat olecranon bursitis [46]. Age can range from childhood to older adult, with a mean of 46 years old. It is most common in males [46]. The clinical presentation includes acute pain and swelling in the posterior elbow with limited extension [31].

- Tears can be partial (most frequent) or complete. The most common tear is an avulsion from the osseous tendon insertion [46]. Musculotendinous junction injury is much less common. Partial tears most frequently involve the superficial layer (combined lateral and long heads), preserving the deep layer (medial head) [47]. Associated small bone avulsion from the olecranon process can be present with partial and complete tears, with variable degrees of retraction. Tendon calcifications can also be seen in chronic tears [47]
- **Imaging diagnosis:** Both USG and MRI are used
  - Radiographs: These can be normal or may demonstrate small olecranon avulsed osseous fragment (Fig. 57.15), triceps traction spur, or displaced olecranon fracture [32]. Tendon calcifications can be visualized as a result of chronic tear
  - USG: Findings of tendinosis, partial tear, and complete tear with varying degrees of retraction are similar to those described for biceps tendon injuries [27,47]

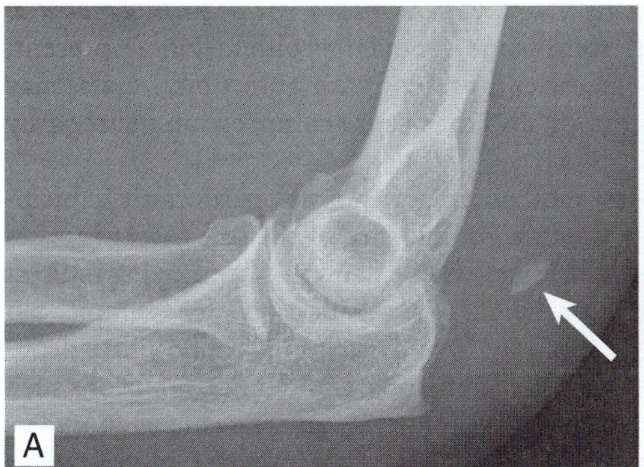

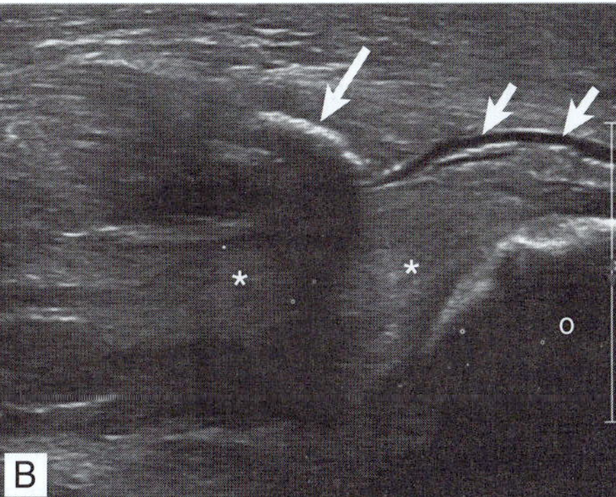

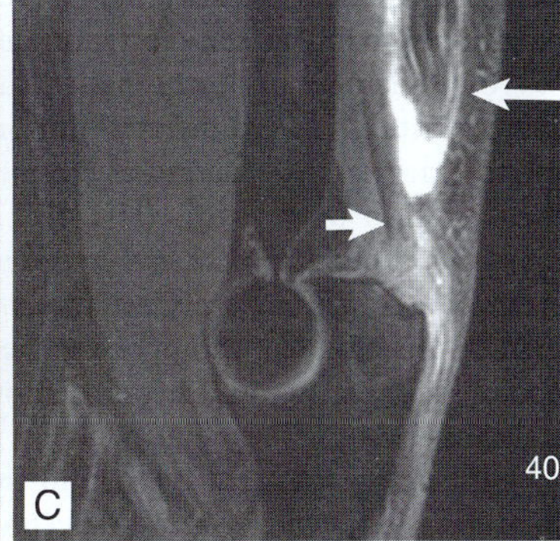

Figure 57.15 Triceps tendon tear. (A) Lateral radiograph shows olecranon osseous avulsion (*arrow*). (B) Longitudinal ultrasound image shows a partial tear with complete fiber discontinuity and retraction of the superficial tendon (long and lateral heads, *arrow*) with intact deep medial head fibers (*asterisks*). Note the hyperechoic osseous fragment attached to the retracted tendon (*arrow*). (C) Sagittal T2-weighted magnetic resonance image with fat saturation of a companion case shows the retracted tendon stump of the superficial fibers (*long arrow*) and the intact deep fibers (*short arrow*).

  - Intratendinous hyperechoic focus with posterior acoustic shadowing can be seen at the tendon stump if olecranon avulsed bone fragment is present (see Fig. 57.15) or in chronic tears with resultant ossifications
  - Dynamic imaging with gentle flexion and extension distinguishes partial tear (showing tendon motion) from complete tears (no motion)
  - Disruption of the superficial fibers with fluid filling the tendon gap and the normal hyperechoic intact fibers of the deep tendon are most commonly seen with partial tears (see Fig. 57.15) [47]
- MRI: Best seen on sagittal and axial planes. MRI findings of the varying degrees of injury are similar to those described for biceps tendon tear [31,46] (see Fig. 57.14)
  - Intratendinous ossifications after bone marrow signal in all sequences and bone morrow edema in the olecranon process are seen if there is an associated fracture. Fluid distending the olecranon bursa and soft tissue as well as muscle edema can also be encountered

- **Treatment:** Treatment is conservative if low-grade partial tear, not associated with tendon retraction or extension weakness. Patients with complete tears are treated surgically with tendon repair by direct reattachment in the olecranon. If chronic tears with retraction and scarring, tendon graft reconstruction is required [48]. If associated olecranon fracture with a large fragment, open reduction and internal fixation of the bone is performed

Elbow Arthritis

Elbow arthritis is most commonly secondary to prior trauma but can also result from rheumatoid arthritis, crystal-induced arthropathy, prior septic arthritis, hemophilia, and primary osteoarthritis (OA) [49]. The diagnosis is based on the patient's history, clinical presentation, laboratory tests, and imaging findings. Symptoms include pain, stiffness and limited range of motion, instability, and joint "catching" (which can be related to lose bodies) [49].

Plain radiographs are the first-line imaging modality in evaluating elbow arthritis, including AP, lateral, and oblique views. The imaging findings are variable, according to the underlying process, and are similar in appearance to those seen in any other synovial joint involved by the same disease. Primary OA is characterized by asymmetric joint space narrowing, subchondral sclerosis, subchondral cysts, osteophyte formation, variable joint effusion, and possible intraarticular bodies (Fig. 57.16). Intraarticular bodies are commonly found in the olecranon and coronoid fossae (see Fig. 57.16). Inflammatory arthropathy, such as rheumatoid arthritis, characteristically demonstrates uniform joint space narrowing, variable degree of subchondral erosions, joint laxity, and variable joint effusion or synovitis (Fig. 57.17). *If multiple small, nearly equal in size intraarticular osseous bodies are present, in the absence of other features of OA, synovial osteochondromatosis should be considered.* In this case, CT shows better the small intraarticular osseous bodies, and MRI would better demonstrate the unossified cartilaginous bodies.

Ultrasonography can be helpful to distinguish synovitis from joint effusion, which is not anechoic and easily compressible because simple fluid and may demonstrate central hyperemia on color Doppler [27]. The presence of bursitis and associated tendon or ligament pathology can also be addressed, such as

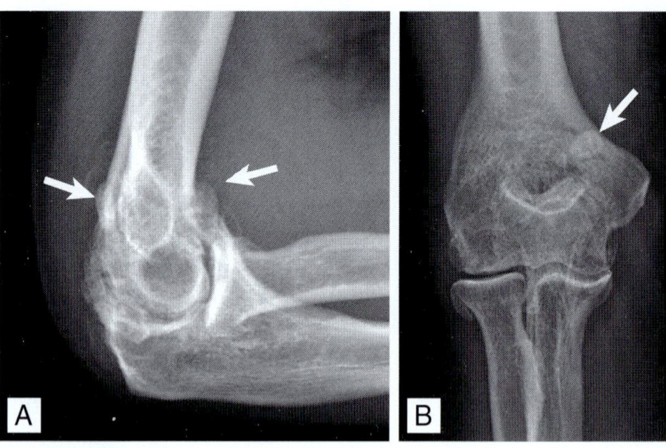

Figure 57.16 Elbow osteoarthritis. Lateral (A) and frontal (B) radiographs show joint space narrowing, osteophyte formation, and intraarticular bodies (*arrows*) in the coronoid and olecranon fossae.

tendinosis, tenosynovitis, and the presence of gouty tophus. USG is also used to guide aspiration, synovial biopsy, and injections (e.g., steroids in the joint or bursa).

Dual-energy CT can be used for the diagnosis of gout with the detection of urate deposits at and around the joints [26].

Magnetic resonance imaging is also used to evaluate synovial hypertrophy; the extent of hyaline cartilage loss; associated bone marrow changes, including cysts and erosions; the presence of intraarticular bodies bursitis; and associated tendon or ligament pathology. Hemosiderin deposition can be identified, particularly using specific MR sequences such as gradient echo, as small foci of low signal intensity related to blooming artifact [50]. This is seen with pigmented villonodular synovitis and hemophilic arthropathy, which is also associated with synovial hypertrophy, cartilage loss, and erosions.

Bursitis

Olecranon bursitis and bicipitoradial bursitis are the most common types of bursitis in the elbow. A native bursa, different from an adventitious bursa, has a synovial lining and when normal is collapsed and difficult to be visualized by imaging [12]. Potential causes of bursal enlargement include traumatic, inflammatory, and infectious processes. The diagnosis is made by clinical presentation and imaging findings. The location is the key. *The distal biceps tendon has no tendon sheath* [12]. *Therefore, fluid here should not be misdiagnosed as tenosynovitis.* If significant synovial proliferation is present, bicipitoradial bursitis can present with antecubital mass, may be mistaken as tumor, and may cause compression neuropathy symptoms [12].

Radiographs are most commonly normal, particularly in bicipitoradial bursitis, or show prominence of the soft tissues in cases of olecranon bursitis. It can also be helpful in identifying indirect signs of the nature of the bursitis: calcifications, for example, can be seen with gout (Fig. 57.18) and calcium pyrophosphate deposition, synovial osteochondromatosis, and chronic infections such as tuberculosis; erosions and joint effusion are a clue of an underlying inflammatory arthropathy, and the presence of gas can be seen with infection. USG and MRI are the best imaging modalities for the evaluation of bursitis. The bursa can be distended with fluid or synovial proliferation (or both) and demonstrates variable

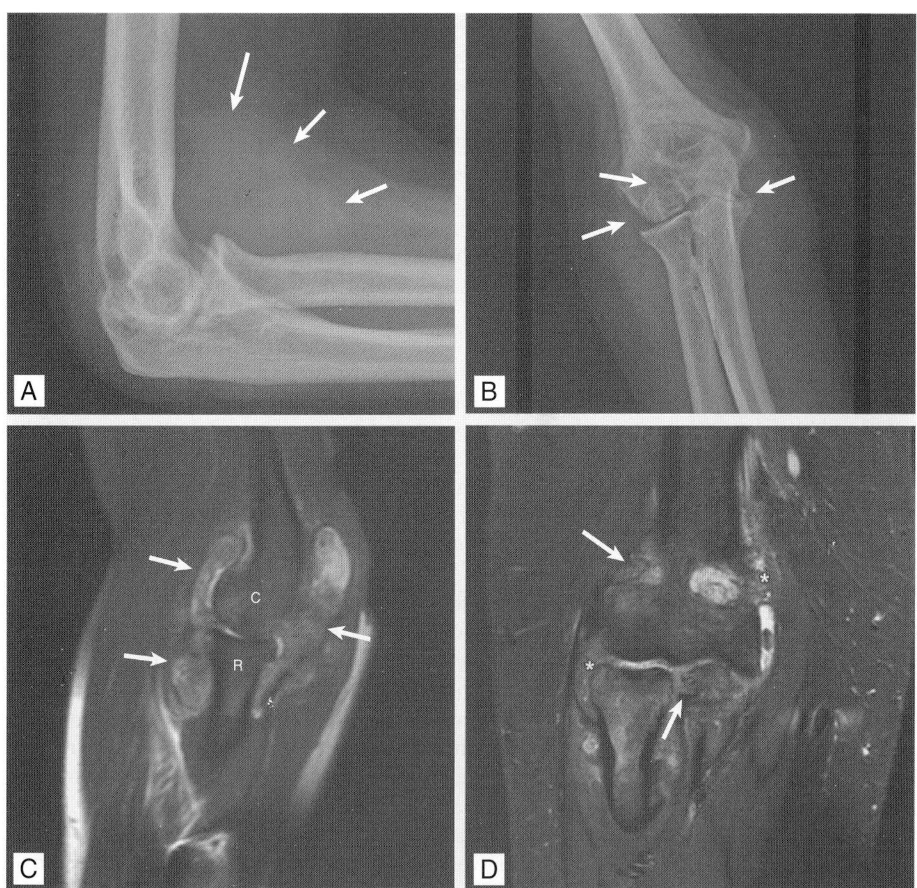

Figure 57.17 Elbow rheumatoid arthritis. (A) Lateral radiograph shows distended joint recess (*arrows*). (B) Frontal radiograph shows joint space narrowing and erosive changes (*arrows*). Sagittal (C) and coronal (D) T2-weighted magnetic resonance images with fat saturation show the extensive synovial proliferation and erosive change (*arrows* and *asterisks*). *C,* capitellum; *R,* radius.

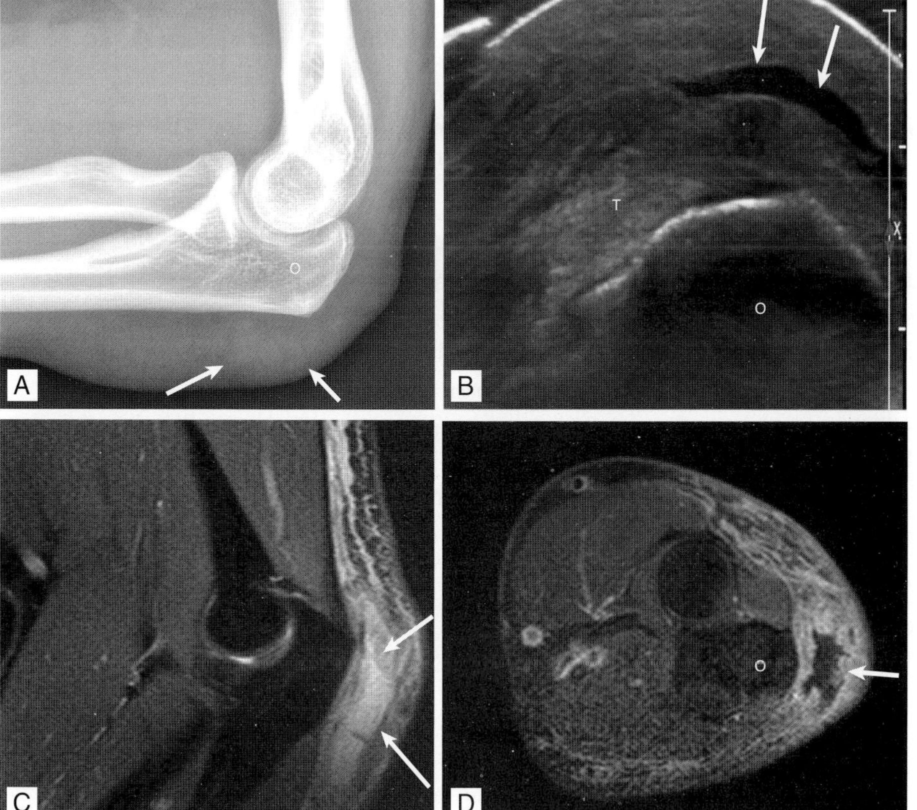

Figure 57.18 Olecranon bursitis. (A) Lateral radiograph shows the distended bursa posterior to the olecranon process (O) with internal calcifications (*arrows*) consistent with gout. (B) Longitudinal USG image shows an example of simple anechoic fluid (*arrows*) in the olecranon bursa. Sagittal T2-weighted magnetic resonance image with fat saturation (C) and axial T1-weighted magnetic resonance image after intravenous contrast injection (D) show an example of infected bursitis with distended bursa; diffuse soft tissue swelling; and thickened, irregular peripheral postcontrast enhancement (*arrows*).

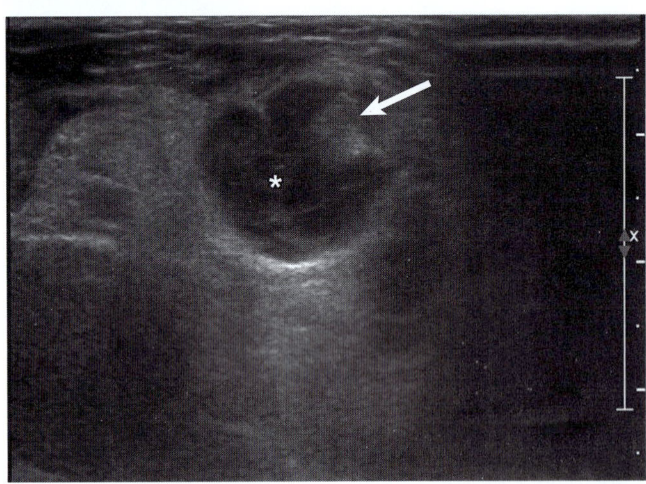

Figure 57.19 Bicipitoradial bursitis. Transverse ultrasound image shows complex hypoechoic fluid (*asterisk*) surrounding the hyperechoic biceps tendon (*arrow*).

echogenicity on USG (Fig. 57.19) and signal intensity on MRI, depending on the nature of fluid and presence of synovial proliferation. Table 57.4 summarizes the features of both elbow bursitis. Bone marrow signal change on MRI can be reactive or associated with erosions if inflammatory or infectious bursitis, with surrounding soft tissue swelling (see Fig. 57.18).

The treatment is most commonly conservative with antiinflammatory drugs, steroid injection (if no suspicion for infection), and surgical treatment if conservative treatment has failed or there is recurrence or compression neuropathy in the case of bicipitoradial bursitis.

Neuropathies

The clinical presentation of neuropathies varies according to the affected nerve and the level of compromise. The most commonly involved is the ulnar nerve at the elbow. The diagnosis is based on clinical neurologic examination and electrodiagnostic studies, in addition to USG, MRI, or MR neurography. Radiographs and CT can identify fractures or other processes that could be causing nerve compression. Both USG and MRI can identify the site of the nerve abnormality and possible causes associated with it. In some cases, the location of impingement may not be seen; in these cases, the diagnosis is made by indirect findings, such as muscle denervation or atrophy. Table 57.2 summarizes the compression neuropathies at and just above the elbow.

Ulnar Nerve

Although the pathology of the ulnar nerve in the elbow can be associated with acute trauma, most cases are related to a chronic process involving external compression, traction, or friction of the nerve. This compromises the blood supply and Schwann cells of the nerve, damaging the axons [51].

- *The most common site of compression of the ulnar nerve is at the elbow, within the cubital tunnel, or the epitrochlear groove* [52]
- Several factors are associated with ulnar compression neuropathy in the elbow, including ulnar nerve subluxation/dislocation, hypertrophy of the medial head of the triceps muscle, snapping triceps syndrome, presence of an anconeus epitrochlearis muscle, thickening of the Osborne ligament, extrinsic compression, and chronic nerve irritation by osseous abnormalities (e.g., prominent osteophytes, fracture deformities, heterotopic ossification, postsurgical changes, including orthopedic hardware, or compression by space-occupying masses) [15]
  - Ulnar nerve subluxation/dislocation is seen in approximately 16% of asymptomatic healthy individuals [53]. *It can be associated with laxity or the absence of the cubital tunnel retinaculum* (Osborne ligament) [53]
  - Snapping triceps syndrome has an unknown cause. It is escribed in weightlifters and may be related to an increase in the bulk of the triceps muscle [53]
  - The anconeus epitrochlearis muscle can cause ulnar neuropathy by compressing the nerve against the medial epicondyle, but it can be present in asymptomatic individuals [15]

TABLE 57.4 Elbow Bursitis

	Olecranon (Miner's or Student Elbow)	Bicipitoradial
Location	Superficial to the olecranon process	Between distal BT and RT
Incidence	Very common	Uncommon
Causes	Trauma (acute or chronic overuse)[a] Systemic conditions: RA, gout, CPPD	Repetitive overuse,[a] RA, synovial chondromatosis, PVNS, chronic infection, such as TB
Associated conditions	Tendinosis or tear	Tendinosis or tear (partial > complete)
Clinical symptoms	Swelling with or without pain, fever, warmth and erythema/cellulitis if infection	Pain, limited range of motion, with or without antecubital mass and radial nerve or PIN compression neuropathy symptoms
Imaging	USG: bursal fluid: anechoic (simple fluid), hypo-[a] or hyperechoic (complex fluid) with or without synovial proliferation and hyperemia on color Doppler MRI: bursal fluid ↓T1/↑T2 (simple fluid) or variable T1/T2 (complex fluid) with or without synovial proliferation and postcontrast enhancement	

[a]Most common.

BT, biceps tendon; *CPPD*, calcium pyrophosphate deposition; *MRI*, magnetic resonance imaging; *PIN*, posterior interosseous nerve; *PVNS*, pigmented villonodular synovitis; *RA*, rheumatoid arthritis; *RT*, radial tuberosity; *TB*, tuberculosis; *USG*, ultrasonography.

- **Clinical presentation:** It can sensory only or with progressive motor deficit in severe cases. It includes medial elbow pain; paresthesia in the ulnar aspect of the fourth and fifth digits and medial side of the forearm; and weakness of the intrinsic muscles of the hand, FCU, and ulnar fibers of the flexor digitorum profundus (FDP) muscle, leading to the clawlike hand deformity [19]
- **Imaging diagnosis**
  - Radiographs: These can identify OA with medial elbow osteophytes, heterotopic ossification, or other possible causes of nerve compression
  - USG:
    - Hypoechoic swelling of the nerve with loss of the normal speckled or fascicular appearance [52] (Fig. 57.20A and B); cross-sectional area greater than 10 mm^2 at the level of the medial epicondyle supports the diagnosis of cubital tunnel syndrome [20]
    - USG can identify the presence of anconeus epitrochlearis muscle extending between the medial epicondyle and the olecranon process. A space-occupying mass or other causes of nerve compression can also be visualized
    - Dynamic imaging with flexion and extension of the elbow identifies ulnar nerve dislocation or snapping triceps [53]:
      - In isolated nerve dislocation, the nerve dislocates anterior and medially over the medial epicondyle with flexion and reduces with the extension of the elbow (Fig. 57.20C and D)
      - In snapping triceps, the nerve and the medial head of the triceps dislocate over the medial epicondyle with flexion of the elbow, reducing with extension
    - In advanced cases, increased muscle echogenicity and volume loss can be seen with muscle atrophy

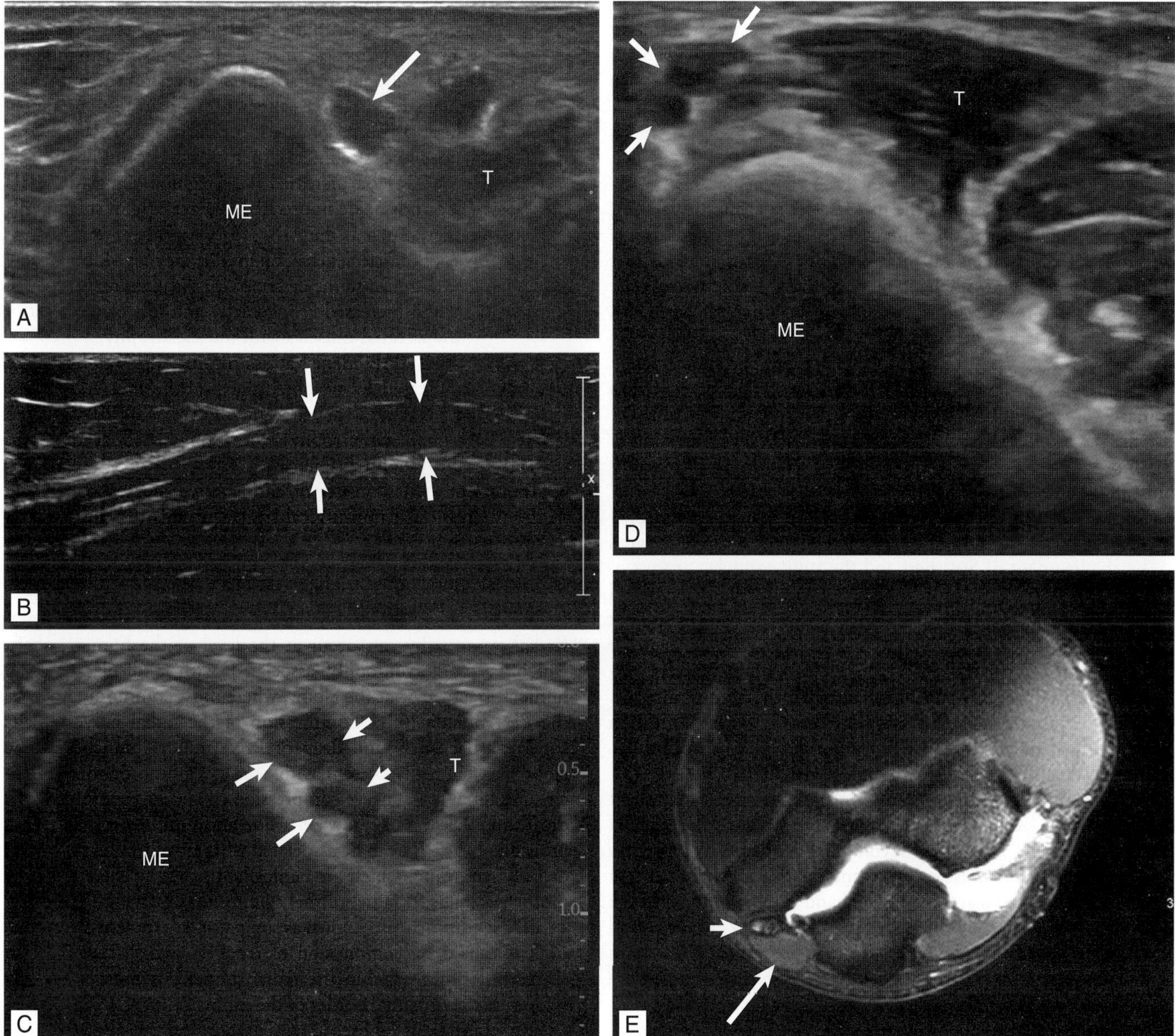

Figure 57.20 Cubital tunnel syndrome. Axial (A) and longitudinal (B) ultrasound images show hypoechoic swelling of the nerve with loss of the normal fascicular pattern (*arrows*) at the level of the medial epicondyle (ME). Axial ultrasound image (C) with the elbow in extension shows the hypoechoic prominent nerve behind the ME (*arrows*) and dislocated anterior to the ME with elbow flexion (D). (E) Axial T2-weighted magnetic resonance image with fat saturation shows an example of anconeus epitrochlearis muscle (*long arrow*) and the prominent ulnar nerve with increased T2 signal (*short arrow*). *T,* medial head of the triceps muscle.

- MRI
  - Nerve thickening with loss of normal fascicular appearance and increased T2-weighted signal [19] (see Fig. 57.20E)
  - Early muscle denervation changes are better evaluated with MRI. Findings include swelling with high T2-weighted signal in the affected musculature [19] (see Table 57.2) without fatty replacement or abnormal signal on the T1-weighted image
  - In advanced cases, the affected muscles show increased T1-weighted signal and residual increased or decreased T2-weighted signal related to muscle atrophy [19]
  - MRI can also identify abnormal contents in the cubital tunnel or other causes of nerve compression, such as accessory muscle, thickened and irregular cubital retinaculum, or soft tissue masses (see Fig. 57.20E)
  - If a nerve sheath tumor is suspected, MRI with intravenous gadolinium injection can show postcontrast enhancement
- **Treatment:** Treatment is conservative or surgical with nerve decompression if there is failure of conservative treatment, progression of symptoms, or sensory and motor deficit with muscle atrophy [19,51]

Median Nerve

Compression neuropathy of the median nerve around the elbow is uncommon and is a major differential diagnosis of carpal tunnel syndrome. Compression can occur by the lacertus fibrosus, the PT muscle (PT syndrome), or the presence of a supracondylar process of the humerus. Compression can also involve the AIN, a branch of the median nerve. Clinical symptoms include paresthesias in the palmar aspect of the first three fingers and motor deficit involving the muscles innervated by the median nerve, with a common complaint including weakness in grip and clenching the fist, and later thenar muscle atrophy [54]. Isolated compression of the motor branch AIN presents clinically with motor symptoms only, involving the muscles related to it (see Table 57.2).

- **Supracondylar process syndrome:** This is a rare syndrome related to compression of the median nerve in a tunnel created by the ligament of Struthers and the supracondylar process of the humerus (bone spur). Although the median nerve and brachial artery can both be compressed by the osseous spur or the ligament when passing deep to it, isolated median nerve compression is most commonly seen [6]. Supracondylar process fracture can also result in neurovascular compromise [6]. Patients present clinically with median nerve compression symptoms, exacerbated by elbow extension and pronation [6]. The bone spur can also be palpable above the elbow
- **PT syndrome:** The compression of the median nerve may occur deep to the lacertus fibrosus, between the ulnar and humeral heads of the PT muscle (most common), or beneath the fibrous arch of the FDS muscle. It presents clinically with pain and numbness in the volar forearm and hand with parenthesis in the median nerve distribution in the digits and thenar eminence and minimal motor findings with grip weakness. There is also pain to palpation of the PT [55]. *It can be misdiagnosed as carpal tunnel syndrome but is clinically distinguished by the presence of thenar eminence numbness in the distribution of the palmar cutaneous branch (a distal branch of the median nerve proximal to the carpal tunnel) and absence of nocturnal paresthesia symptoms* [55,56]
- **AIN syndrome:** Also called Kiloh-Nevin syndrome, it results from compression of the AIN, which can be caused by fibrous bands originating from the ulnar head of the PT muscle and the FDS muscle, by the presence of accessory muscles, aberrant or thrombosed adjacent vessels, or extrinsic compression by space-occupying masses or distended bicipitoradial bursa [23]. Supracondylar fractures or posterior elbow dislocation can damage the nerve by damaging the posterior neurofibers of the median nerve, making up the AIN [22]. Because the AIN is a motor branch and innervates the FDP of the second and third fingers and flexor pollicis longus (FPL), clinical manifestations include weakness to flex the interphalangeal joint of the thumb or the distal interphalangeal joint of the index and long fingers, with difficulty to handwrite and inability to make the OK sign with the thumb and index fingers [22,23]. No numbness
- **Imaging diagnosis**
  - Radiographs can help identify the presence of a supracondylar process, fractures, or other possible causes of median nerve compression
  - USG and MRI: These may not demonstrate the cause of the nerve compression, particularly when associated to small fibrous bands or scar, but can exclude other causes of compression, such as masses, enlarged bursa, enlarged asymmetrical muscle belly, and supracondylar process of the humerus
    - Focal change in nerve caliper, nerve distortion, or abnormal nerve course may be identified (Fig. 57.21)
    - Hypoechoic swelling of nerve fascicles on USG (see Fig. 57.21) or increased T2-weighted signal on MRI may or not be demonstrated, particularly in small nerve branches such as the AIN [18]
    - Signs of muscle denervation may be the only visible finding and are similar to the described for the ulnar nerve:
      - USG: increased echogenicity and loss of the bulk of the affected muscles with muscle atrophy
      - MRI early denervation: normal T1-weighted and increased T2-weighted signal of the affected muscles
      - MRI late denervation: increased T1-weighted signal (fat atrophy) with some residual increased T2-weighted signal
- **Treatment:** This consists of conservative therapy or surgical decompression if nonsurgical treatment fails to relieve symptoms [23,54,55]

Radial Nerve

Radial neuropathy can occur at the level of the humeral shaft, which is most commonly associated with a displaced spiral humeral fracture or at the elbow, where most commonly involves the PIN branch [57]. Compression of the radial nerve and its superficial (sensory) and deep or PIN (motor) branches at the elbow can clinically present with sensory, motor, or mixed deficits. Proximal radial nerve compression can lead to complete wrist drop and weakness of elbow extension and supination [58]. Compression of the PIN can be associated with radial tunnel syndrome or PIN syndrome, which are clinically distinct by the absence of motor weakness in radial tunnel syndrome [21].

- PIN syndrome: Also known as supinator entrapment syndrome. It is caused by compression of the PIN, which can occur in many locations within the radial tunnel but most frequently seen at the proximal border of the supinator muscle at the nerve entry (arcade of Frohse) [21]. Compression can also be associated with a thickened leading edge of the extensor carpi radialis brevis muscle and prominent radial recurrent vessels around the nerve [21]. Ganglion cysts or other soft tissues masses, radiocapitellar joint synovitis, and fractures are other causes of PIN compression [59]. Activities associated with repetitive pronation

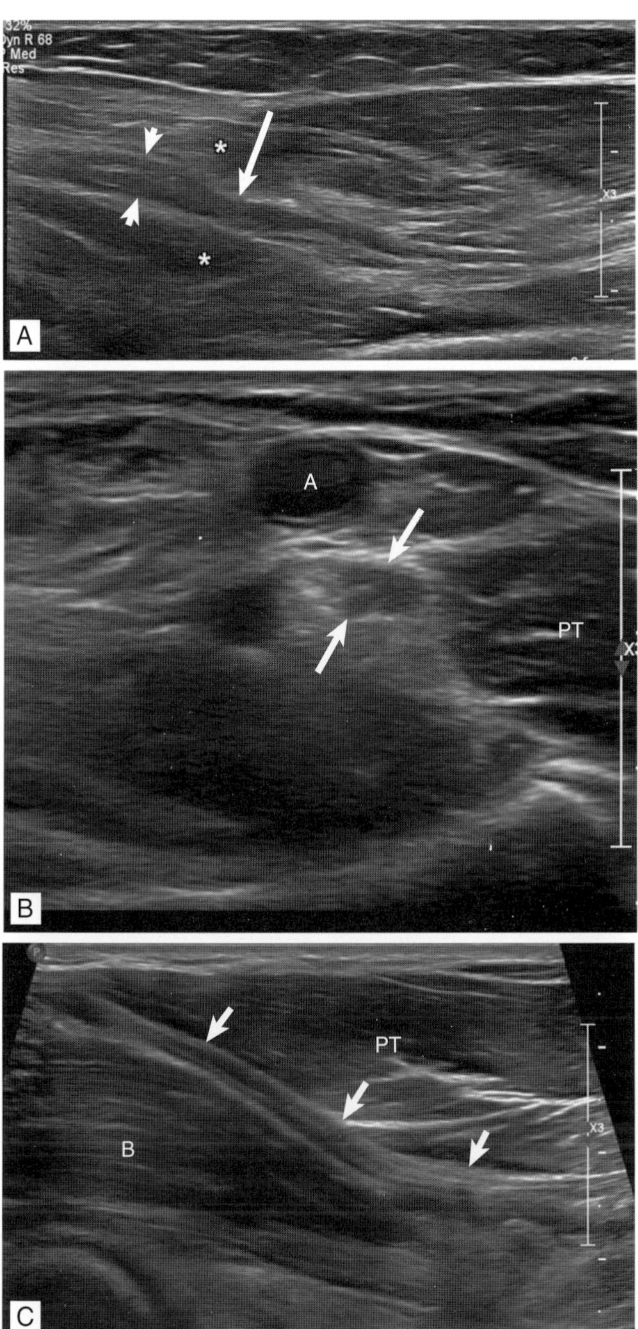

Figure 57.21 Pronator teres syndrome. Longitudinal (A) and transverse (B) ultrasound images show the focal narrowing of the median nerve (*long arrow*) between the two heads of the pronator teres muscle (PT, *asterisks*) and hypoechoic swelling of the nerve proximal to it (*short arrows*). (C) Longitudinal ultrasound image shows the normal appearance of the median nerve as it dives between the two heads of the PT muscle (*arrows*). *B,* brachialis.

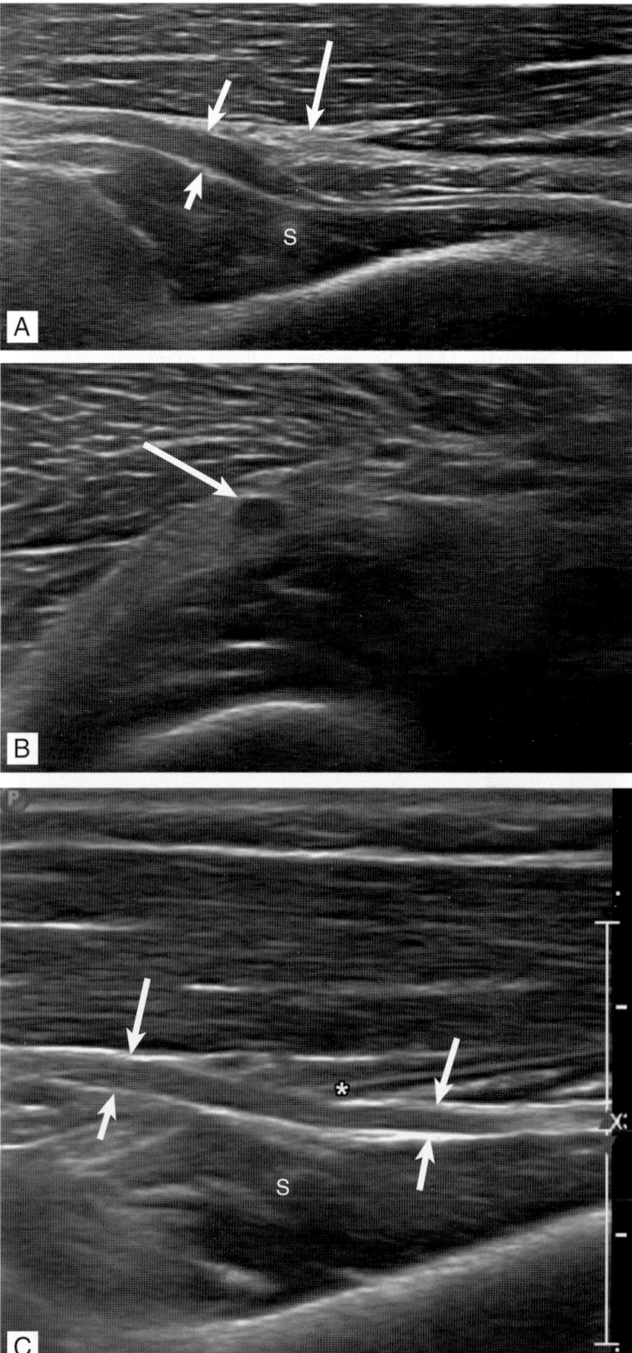

Figure 57.22 Posterior interosseous nerve syndrome. Longitudinal (A) and transverse (B) ultrasound images show focal narrowing of the nerve at the entrance in the supinator muscle (S, *long arrow*) with hypoechoic nerve swelling proximally (*arrows*). (C) Longitudinal ultrasound image shows a normal posterior interosseous nerve with normal mild narrowing as it enters the supinator muscle (*asterisk*).

and supination motion are at increased risk, such as in tennis players, swimmers, and violinists [59]. Patients present with insidious pain along the lateral elbow or proximal forearm and pain elicited by resisted forearm supination [21,60]. Motor deficit of the innervated muscles with ulnar wrist drop and limited finger extension or finger drop is characteristic [58]

- **Imaging diagnosis:** Both USG and MRI can identify a focal change in nerve caliper and morphology; change in the course of the nerve; intrinsic nerve abnormalities such as nerve sheath tumor; and other extrinsic causes of nerve compression, including enlarged bursa, synovitis, ganglion cysts, or other soft tissue masses [21,59]. Findings of lateral epicondylitis can be demonstrated on both imaging modalities, which can share similar symptoms of pain in the lateral elbow or proximal forearm and can coexist with PIN compression [21]. Imaging findings are similar to other neuropathies and include
  - USG: This shows hypoechoic swelling proximal to the compression site (Fig. 57.22) and evidence of muscle

denervation, which is better demonstrated on later stages, when increased echogenicity and decreased muscle bulk are seen, related to muscle atrophy
    - MRI: This is focal nerve swelling with increased T2 signal and muscle denervation edema or atrophy in the innervated muscles, including the supinator and proximal forearm extensor muscles [21]
- **Treatment:** This consists of conservative therapy or surgical treatment if persistent symptoms [60]

Suggested Readings

- ML Sampaio, ME Schweitzer, Elbow magnetic resonance imaging variants and pitfalls, Magn Reson Imaging Clin N Am 18 (2010) 633–642.
- LS Beltran, JT Bencardino, J Beltran, Imaging of sports ligamentous injuries of the elbow, Semin Musculoskelet Radiol 17 (2013) 455–465.
- C Martinoli, S Bianchi, F Pugliese, L Bacigalupo, C Gauglio, M Valle, L Derchi, Sonography of entrapment neuropathies in the upper limb (wrist excluded), J Clin Ultrasound 32 (2004) 438–450.
- DE Grayson, The elbow: Radiographic imaging pearls and pitfalls, Semi Roentgenol 40 (3) (2005) 223–224.
- JA Batlle, L Cerezal, MDL Parra, B Alba, S Resano, JB Sanchez, The elbow review of anatomy and common collateral ligament complex pathology using MRI, Insights Imaging 10 (2019) 43.

58

Imaging of the Wrist and Hand

MATTHEW D. KAY, MIHRA S. TALJANOVIC

Introduction

The broad functionality and dexterity of the wrist and hand are products of their complex anatomy. This chapter presents an overview of wrist and hand functional anatomy and their relationship to common conditions that radiologists and referring clinicians should be familiar with.

Functional Anatomy

Wrist—Bones

Wrist bony anatomy includes the distal radius and ulna, carpal bones, and proximal metacarpals.

The eight carpal bones of the wrist are arranged in two carpal rows, proximal and distal (Fig. 58.1). From radial to ulnar, the proximal carpal row consists of the *scaphoid, lunate,* and *triquetrum*. The *pisiform* is positioned palmar to the triquetrum and included in the proximal carpal row. The distal carpal row, from radial to ulnar, consists of the trapezium, trapezoid, capitate, and hamate.

Carpal ossification commences after birth, occurring sequentially from the capitate (1–3 months), hamate (2–4 months), triquetrum (2–3 years), lunate (2–4 years), scaphoid (4–6 years), trapezium (4–6 years), trapezoid (4–6 years), and finally pisiform (8–12 years) (see Fig. 58.1).

Although less common than tarsal coalitions, carpal coalitions (osseous or nonosseous fusion) do exist, and almost all combinations of carpal coalitions have been described. The most common is the *lunotriquetral coalition* followed by the capitohamate, scapho-trapezium, and scapholunate coalitions. Carpal coalitions that cross carpal rows and involve multiple carpal bones are rare and more commonly associated with syndromes such as arthrogryposis multiplex congenita, diastrophic dwarfism, dyschondrosteosis, Ellis-van Creveld syndrome, fetal alcohol syndrome, hand–foot–genital syndrome, Holt-Oram syndrome, Nievergelt syndrome, otopalato-digital syndrome, symphalangism, and Turner syndrome.

Wrist—Joints

The *wrist* is a complex of joints formed between

- the distal radius and ulna (*distal radioulnar joint [DRUJ]*);
- the distal radius and proximal carpal row (*radiocarpal joint*);
- the multiple intercarpal joints (*midcarpal joint* and *pisotriquetral joint*);
- the distal carpal row and metacarpals (*common carpometacarpal joints* and *first carpometacarpal joint*).

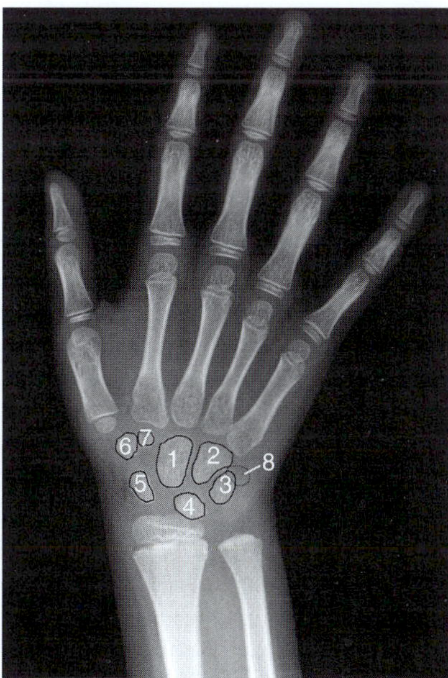

Figure 58.1 Posteroanterior radiograph of the hand demonstrates the sequence of carpal ossification starting with the (*1*) capitate, (*2*) hamate, (*3*) triquetrum, (*4*) lunate, (*5*) scaphoid, (*6*) trapezium, (*7*) trapezoid, and (*8*) pisiform.

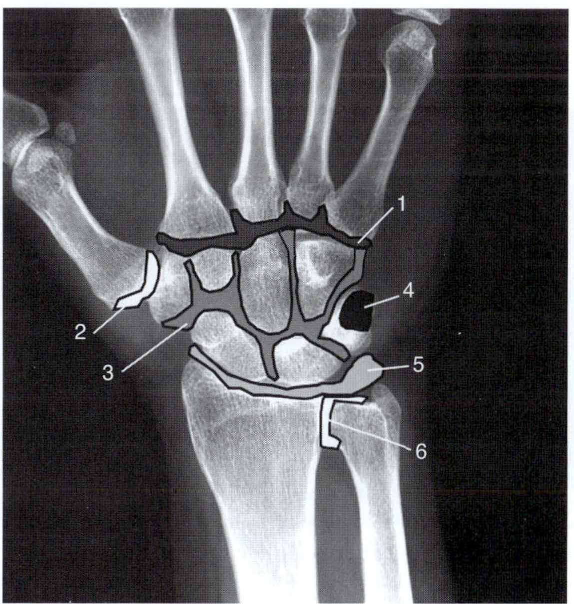

Figure 58.2 The six compartments of the wrist are the (*1*) common carpometacarpal, (*2*) first carpometacarpal joint, (*3*) midcarpal, (*4*) pisotriquetral, (*5*) radiocarpal, and (*6*) distal radioulnar.

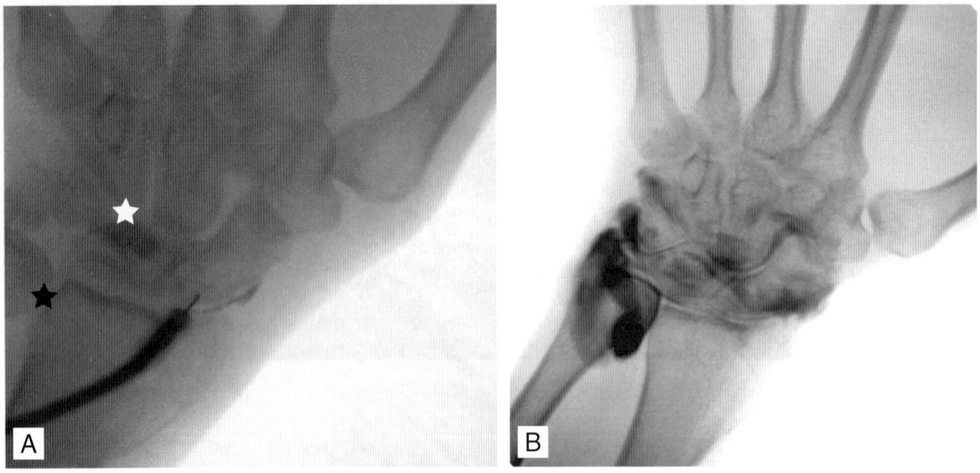

Figure 58.3 (A) Fluoroscopic image demonstrates the standard dorsal approach to arthrography of the radiocarpal joint at the level of the radioscaphoid joint. This patient was being injected with approximately 3 mL from a contrast solution of 10 mL of sterile normal saline, 10 mL of iodinated contrast and 0.1 mL of gadolinium-based contrast as they went on to magnetic resonance arthrography (MRA). The *white star* and the *black star* show the locations for dorsal approach to injecting the midcarpal and distal radioulnar joints, respectively. (B) Fluoroscopic image with contrast that was initially injected via the radiocarpal articulation demonstrates extension and communication from the radiocarpal compartment into the distal radioulnar and midcarpal compartments. This was caused by a central triangular fibrocartilage disk and lunotriquetral ligament tear that were demonstrated on the subsequent MRA.

The wrist is divided into six compartments (Fig. 58.2) by the intervening ligaments, and communication between these compartments during arthrography may imply capsular or ligamentous injury in young patients (Fig. 58.3). Communication normally exists between the midcarpal and carpometacarpal joints and in older people between different compartments.

The *DRUJ* functions as a pivot joint and lies between the convex articular surface of the ulnar head and the ulnar notch of the distal radius. Thin capsular ligaments protect the joint with redundant synovium proximally *(sacciform recess)*. Supination and pronation are functions of both the proximal radioulnar joint and DRUJ; the range of motion can be extended by internal shoulder rotation.

The distal ulna does not articulate directly with the proximal carpal row given the intervening triangular fibrocartilage. Located along the ulnar side of the wrist, the *triangular fibrocartilage complex (TFCC)* consists of (Fig. 58.4)

1. Articular disk
2. Ulnocarpal meniscus homolog
3. Dorsal radioulnar ligament
4. Volar radioulnar ligament
5. Ulnar collateral ligament of the wrist
6. Extensor carpi ulnaris tendon sheath
7. Ulnocarpal ligamentous complex (palmar ulnolunate, lunocapitate, and palmar ulnotriquetral extrinsic ligaments) [1]

The TFCC separates the DRUJ from the radiocarpal joint. The articular disk is contiguous with the distal radius articular cartilage extending from the ulnar notch of the radius to the ulnar styloid. The TFCC stabilizes the DRUJ and the ulnar side of the proximal carpal row. The radius accepts most of the axial force transferred from the proximal carpal row, and the TFCC transfers the residual to the distal ulna.

Altered ulnar length, with respect to the radius, significantly affects axial load transfer.

- When the distal ulna is shorter than the distal radius, it is referred to as *negative ulnar variance* and increases radial load.

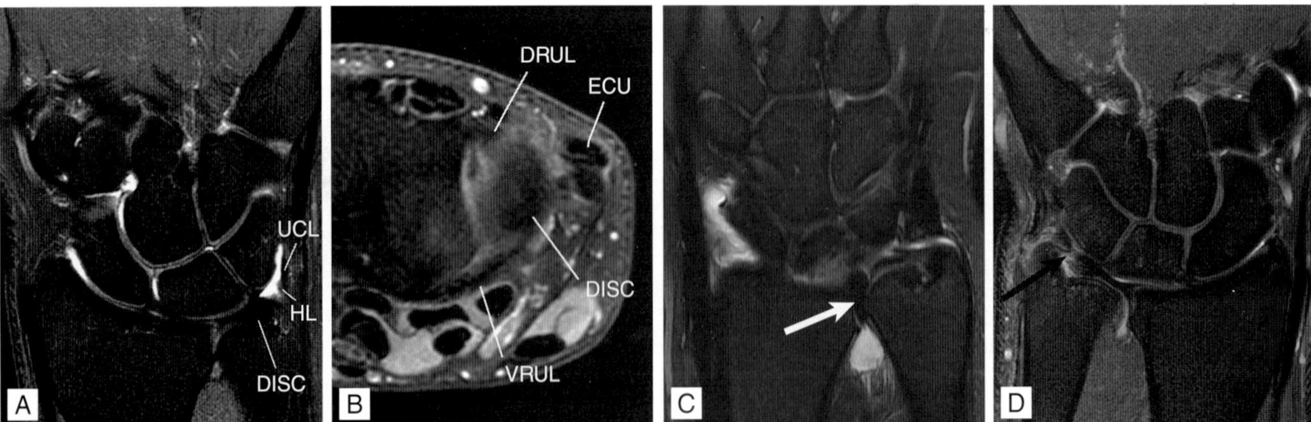

Figure 58.4 Coronal (A) and axial (B) T2-weighted fat-saturated MRI of the wrist demonstrate normal components of the triangular fibrocartilage complex (TFCC): articular disk (DISC), ulnocarpal meniscal homolog (HL), ulnar collateral ligament of the wrist (UCL), dorsal radioulnar ligament (DRUL), and volar radioulnar ligament (VRUL). The TFCC also receives support from the extensor carpi ulnaris tendon (ECU) sheath and the ulnocarpal ligamentous complex (not shown). (C) Coronal T2-weighted fat-saturated image from a wrist magnetic resonance arthrography in a different patient demonstrates the triangular fibrocartilage disk is torn and flipped into the distal radioulnar articulation (*white arrow*). (D) Coronal T2-weighted fat-saturated MRI, from another patient demonstrates peripheral tears of the ulnar styloid and foveal attachments of the triangular fibrocartilage disk (*black arrow*).

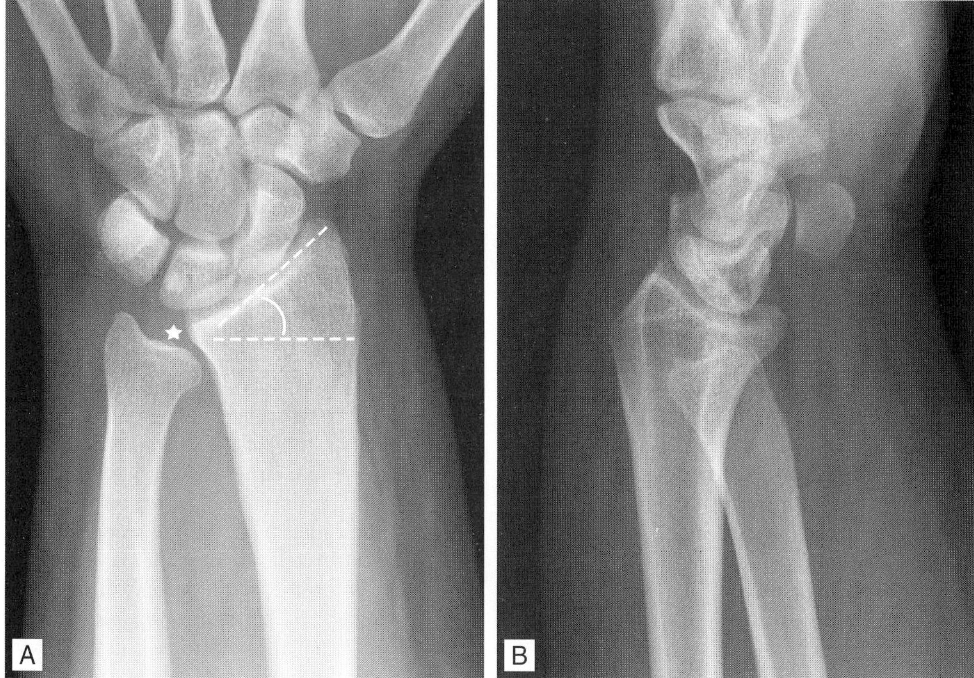

Figure 58.5 Posteroanterior (A) and lateral (B) radiographs demonstrate Madelung deformity with steepening of the radial styloid inclination, a result of premature fusion at the ulnar margin of the distal radius epiphysis. This case demonstrates negative ulnar variance (*star*) caused by prior ulnar osteotomy or epiphysiodesis.

- Similarly, when the distal ulna is longer than the distal radius, it is referred to as *positive ulnar variance*, resulting in increased ulnar load. Variations to neutral distal ulna and radius alignment could be congenital, posttraumatic, or postsurgical and lead to ulnar impingement and ulnar abutment
- *Madelung deformities* (Fig. 58.5) occur when the ulnar margin of the distal radius epiphysis fuses prematurely but the radial margin growth continues. The growth imbalance results in positive ulnar variance and bowing of the radius with steepening of the radial styloid inclination, predisposing to dorsal subluxation of the ulna (at the DRUJ) and palmar subluxation of the proximal carpal row

The radiocarpal joint is an ellipsoid joint. The *scapholunate* (Fig. 58.6) and *lunotriquetral ligaments* complete the proximal carpal row's convexity to articulate with the concavity formed by

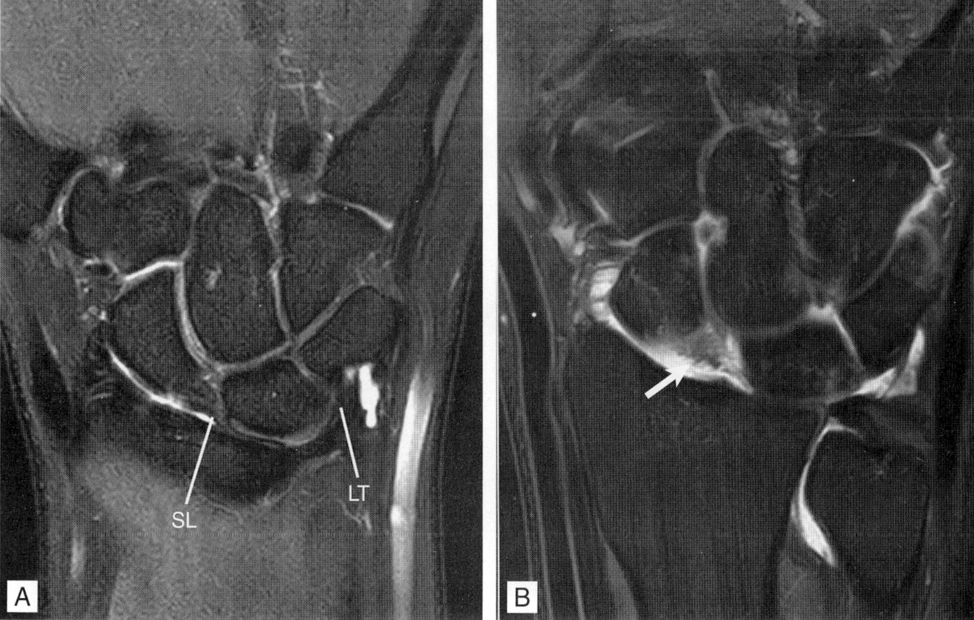

Figure 58.6 (A) Coronal T2-weighted fat-saturated MRI with normal scapholunate (SL) and lunotriquetral (LT) ligaments at the near junction of the volar and proximal components (small focus of T2 high signal degenerative cystic change is present in the capitate). (B) Coronal T2-weighted fat-saturated MRI in a different patient demonstrates complete tear of the scapholunate ligament with remnant dorsal fibers present interposed between the scaphoid and lunate (*arrow*).

the distal radius and the TFC articular disk. The pisiform is a sesamoid of the *flexor carpi ulnaris* tendon and articulates only with the triquetrum at the *pisotriquetral joint*. The *pisiform ligament complex* (flexor carpi ulnaris insertion, abductor digiti minimi origin, pisohamate ligament, pisotriquetral ulnar ligament, and pisometacarpal ligament) stabilizes the pisotriquetral joint and likely assists abductor digiti minimi function and ulnar deviation.

The midcarpal joint is undulating and irregular. On the radial side, the *triscaphoid joint* is formed by the distal scaphoid pole that articulates with the concavity of the trapezium and trapezoid. The convexity of the proximal capitate and hamate articulates with the concavity formed by the ulnar border of the scaphoid, distal lunate, and triquetrum.

Wrist—Ligaments

The intercarpal joints capsule and intrinsic wrist ligaments limit the distal wrist mobility [2]. The ligaments of the wrist are divided into extrinsic and intrinsic ligaments. The *extrinsic ligaments* secure the carpal bones to the distal radius, distal ulna, and metacarpal bases (except the *dorsal intercarpal ligament*) [3]. The *intrinsic ligaments* interconnect the carpal bones, such as the scapholunate and lunotriquetral, previously introduced.

The palmar extrinsic ligaments (Fig. 58.7) arising from the distal radius are

- Radioscaphocapitate
- Long radiolunate (also referred to as the radiotriquetral or radiolunotriquetral)
- Short radiolunate
- Radioscapholunate (ligament of Testut and Kuenz) ligaments

The palmar extrinsic ligaments arising from the distal ulnar (also the ulnocarpal ligamentous complex) are

- Palmar ulnolunate
- Palmar ulnotriquetral
- Palmar ulnocapitate ligaments (see TFCC)

The dorsal extrinsic ligaments (Fig. 58.8) are

- Dorsal radiocarpal (also referred to as the dorsal radiotriquetral or radiolunotriquetral)
- Dorsal ulnotriquetral
- Dorsal intercarpal ligaments (also referred to as the dorsal scaphotriquetral ligament with two bands, the triquetroscaphoid and triquetrotrapezoidal bands)

Dorsal intercarpal ligament; extends from the triquetrum to the scaphoid, often attaching to both lunate and trapezium along its course.

Two extrinsic collateral ligaments of the wrist exist, the 1) radial and 2) ulnar collateral ligaments. Like the dorsal ulnotriquetral ligament, the collateral ligaments are sometimes considered thickened capsule rather than actual ligaments [3].

The multiple dorsal and palmar carpometacarpal ligaments connecting the carpal bones to the second through fifth metacarpal bases are extrinsic ligaments. The common carpometacarpal compartment is formed by the second through fifth carpometacarpal joints (see Fig. 58.2). The *first carpometacarpal joint* is isolated by a complex of ligaments with three dorsal (dorsoradial, dorsal central and posterior oblique), two palmar (anterior oblique or beak, and ulnar collateral or volar trapeziometacarpal), and two ulnar (dorsal trapeziometacarpal and intermetacarpal) ligaments (Fig. 58.9).

The proximal carpal row intrinsic ligaments are the scapholunate and lunotriquetral ligaments (Fig. 58.10). Both have palmar/volar, proximal, and dorsal components. The intrinsic ligaments between carpal rows include the scaphotrapezium-trapezoid, scaphocapitate, triquetrocapitate, and triquetrohamate ligaments. The distal carpal row intrinsic ligaments are the trapeziotrapezoid, trapeziocapitate,

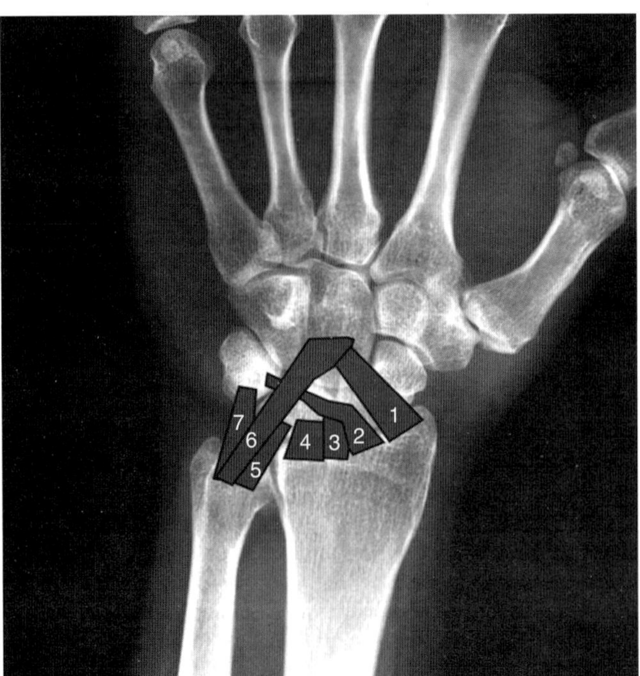

Figure 58.7 Posteroanterior radiograph of the wrist demonstrating the palmar extrinsic ligaments of the wrist (excluding the carpometacarpal ligaments): (*1*) radioscaphocapitate, (*2*) long radiolunate, (*3*) radioscapholunate (ligament of Testut and Kuenz), (*4*) short radiolunate (*5*) palmar ulnolunate, (*6*) lunocapitate, and (*7*) palmar ulnotriquetral ligaments.

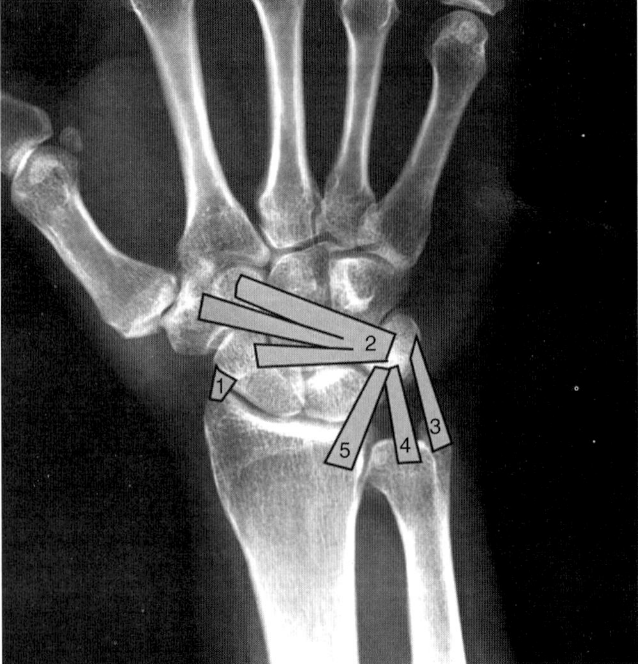

Figure 58.8 Posteroanterior radiograph of the wrist demonstrating the dorsal and collateral extrinsic ligaments of the wrist (excluding the carpometacarpal ligaments): (*1*) radial collateral, (*2*) intercarpal, (*3*) ulnar collateral, (*4*) dorsal ulnotriquetral, and (*5*) dorsal radiocarpal ligaments.

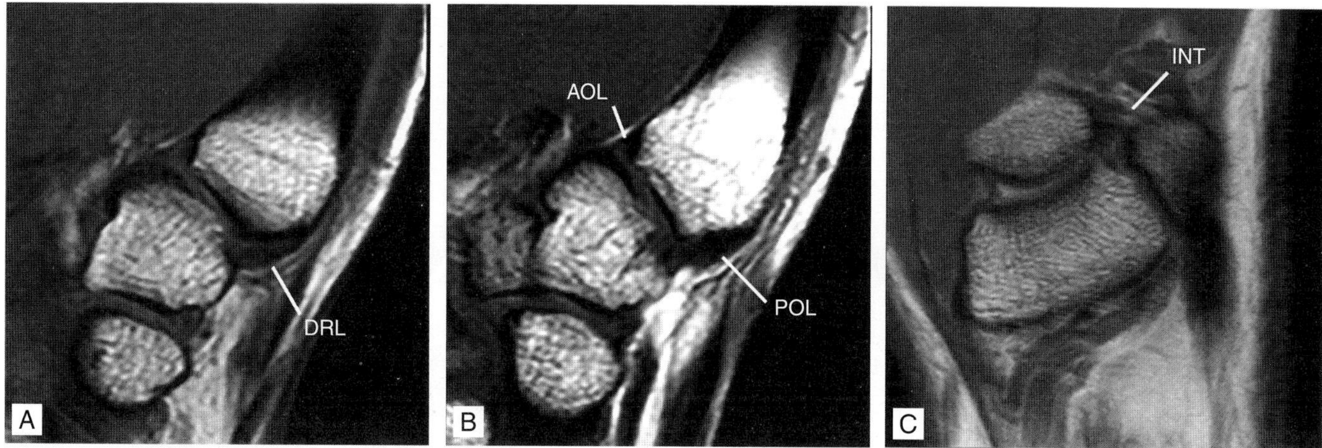

Figure 58.9 Coronal T1-weighted MRI with intact (A) dorsoradial (DRL), anterior oblique (AOL) (B), and posterior oblique ligaments (POL) of the first carpometacarpal joint. Sagittal proton density–weighted MRI (C) from a different patient demonstrates an intact intermetacarpal (INT) ligament, extending from the ulnar base of the first metacarpal.

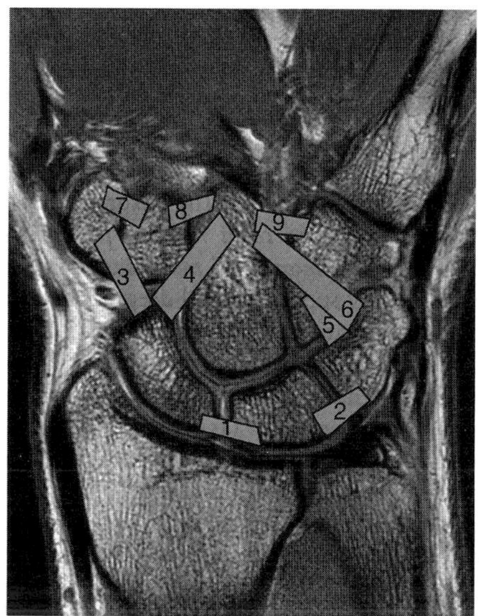

Figure 58.10 Coronal proton density–weighted MRI demonstrating the intrinsic ligaments of the wrist: (*1*) scapholunate (volar band), (*2*) lunotriquetral (volar band), (*3*) scaphotrapezium-trapezoid, (*4*) scaphocapitate, (*5*) triquetrohamate, (*6*) triquetrocapitate (or triquetro-hamate-capitate), (*7*) trapeziotrapezoid, (*8*) trapeziocapitate, and (*9*) capitohamate.

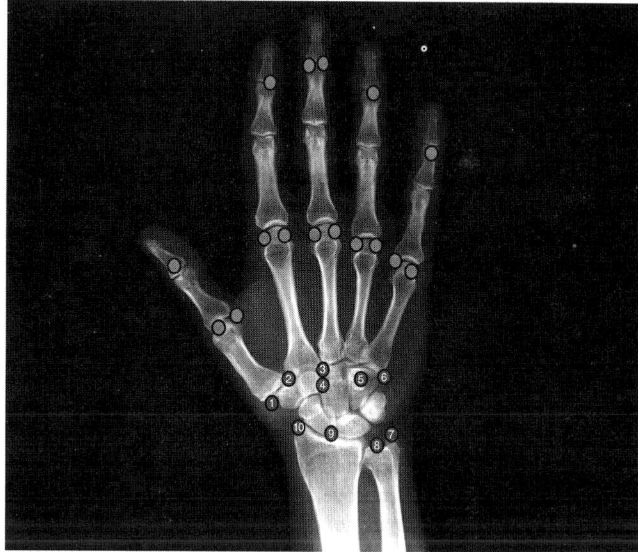

Figure 58.11 Posteroanterior radiograph of the hand and wrist demonstrates the various sites of possible sesamoids and the more common accessory ossicles, including the (*1*) os paratrapezium, (*2*) trapezium secundarium, (*3*) os styloideum, (*4*) os centrale, (*5*) os hamuliproprium, (*6*) os vesalianum carpi, (*7*) lunula (*8*) os triangulare, (*9*) os epilunate, and (*10*) os radiostyloideum.

and capitohamate ligaments. *The most critical intrinsic ligaments and most common wrist ligament injuries involve the scapholunate ligament and those associated with the TFCC.*

Hand—Bones

The hand contains five *metacarpals*, five *proximal phalanges*, four *middle phalanges*, and five *distal phalanges*. The thumb does not have a middle phalanx. The metacarpals and phalanges each have two ossification centers. The primary ossification center is the diaphysis. The secondary ossification center or epiphysis location varies. For all phalanges and the first metacarpal, the epiphysis is at the base, but for the second through fifth metacarpals, it is the head.

The metacarpal and phalangeal primary ossification centers begin in utero between the 8th and 10th weeks of gestation.

The secondary ossification centers first ossify at

- The metacarpals (3 years)
- The proximal phalanges (3–4 years)
- The middle phalanges (4–5 years)
- The distal phalanges (4–5 years)

The primary and secondary ossification centers fuse later during the second decade of life (13–20 years). *Bone age assessment* using standardized templates and methods, commonly the Gruelich-Pyle or Tanner-Whitehouse methods or more recently automated software, is useful in pediatric radiology to diagnose and manage conditions that may alter skeletal maturation.

Multiple (>20) accessory ossicles of the wrist and hand have been documented. Ossicles are a result of failure of ossification center fusion (Fig. 58.11). Sesamoids are embedded within a tendon adjacent to the joint or joint capsule and help with load bearing, stability, and shock absorption (see Fig. 58.11). There are

TABLE 58.2 Pulleys of the Index, Middle, Ring and Little Fingers

Pulleys, From Proximal to Distal	Location
Annular pulley 1 (A1 pulley)	Volar to the metacarpophalangeal joint
A2 pulley	Volar to the proximal phalanx shaft
Cruciate pulley (C1 pulley)	Volar and just proximal to the proximal interphalangeal joint
A3 pulley	Volar to the proximal interphalangeal joint
C2 pulley	Volar and just distal to the proximal interphalangeal joint
A4 pulley	Volar to the middle phalanx shaft
C3 pulley	Volar and just proximal to the distal interphalangeal joint
A5 pulley	Volar to the distal interphalangeal joint

insert at the *ulnar* margin of the extensor expansions of the first and second MCP joints and the thumb and index finger proximal phalanges, respectively. The palmar interossei originating from the fourth and fifth metacarpals insert at the *radial* margin of the extensor expansions of the fourth and fifth MCP joints and the ring and little finger proximal phalanges, respectively.

TABLE 58.3 Pulleys of the Thumb

Pulleys, From Proximal to Distal	Location
Annular pulley (A1 pulley)	Volar to the metacarpophalangeal joint
Annular variable pulley or ligament	Between the A1 and oblique pulleys
Oblique pulley	Volar to the proximal phalanx
A2 pulley	Volar to the interphalangeal joint

Flexor Pulley System

The flexor tendon pulleys are fibrous sheaths oriented to stabilize and prevent bowstringing of the flexor tendons. The index through little fingers (Table 58.2) each have eight pulleys, five annular, and three cruciate. In comparison, the thumb (Table 58.3) has three or four pulleys, two annular and an oblique (the annular variable pulley is sometimes included as part of the oblique pulley). The most important pulleys, biomechanically for the prevention of bowstringing, are the A2 and A4 pulleys (Figs. 58.16 and 58.17), with the A1 pulley implicated in *trigger finger* and *stenosing tenosynovitis*.

Flexor Tendons

The *flexor digitorum superficialis* tendons are superficial to the *flexor digitorum profundus* tendons until they split at the

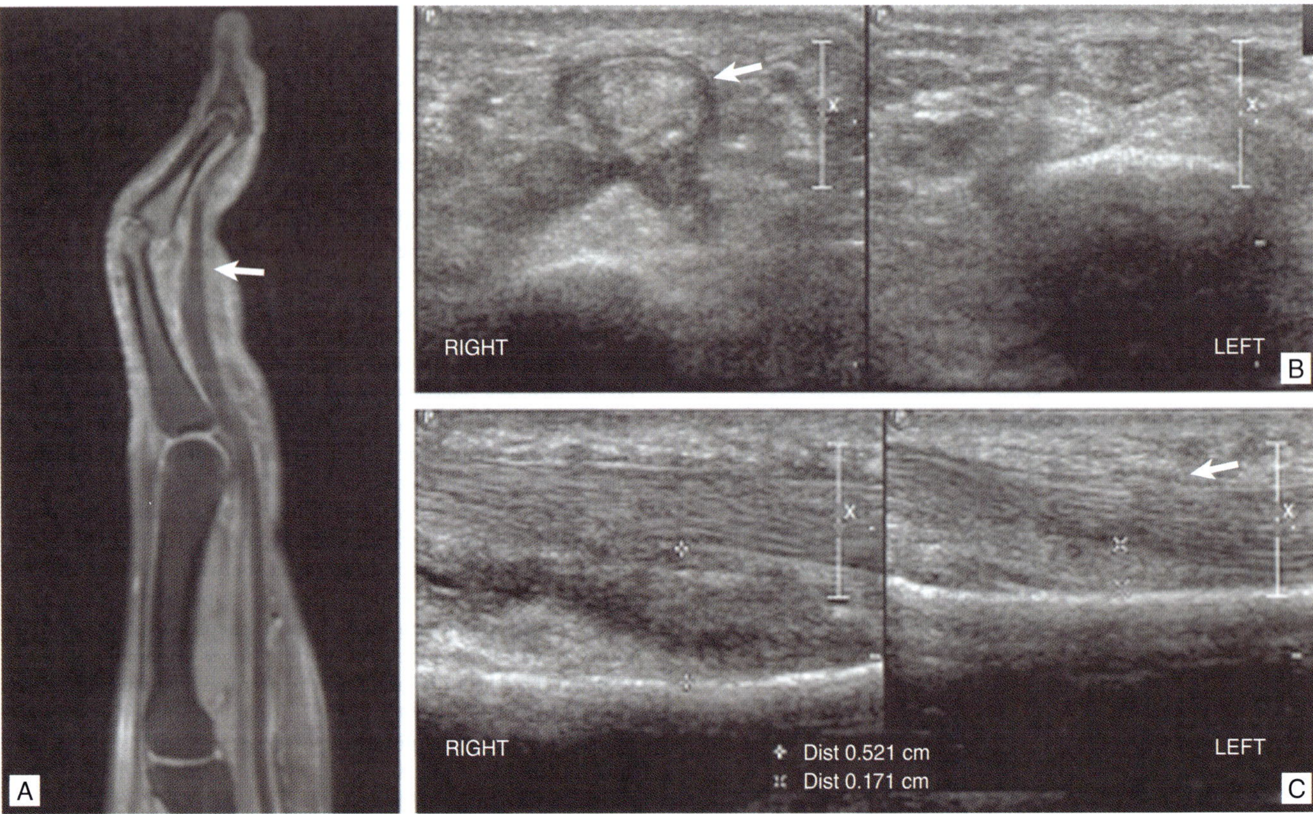

Figure 58.16 Sagittal proton density–weighted fat-saturated MRI (A) demonstrates bowstringing of the middle finger flexor tendons (*arrow*) caused by A2, A3, and C1 pulley tears. Mild bone edema is also demonstrated on either side of the proximal interphalangeal joint without fracture. Transverse (B) and longitudinal (C) real-time ultrasonography at the level of the right middle finger proximal phalanx demonstrates thickening of the flexor digitorum profundus and superficialis tendons with trace fluid in the tendon sheath (*arrow*). The right middle finger A2 pulley is indistinct in comparison with the left middle finger A2 pulley (*arrow*) at a similar level, and there is increased distance between the flexor tendons and volar cortex of the underlying proximal phalanx cortex (as demonstrated by the calipers), consistent with an A2 pulley rupture and resultant bowstringing.

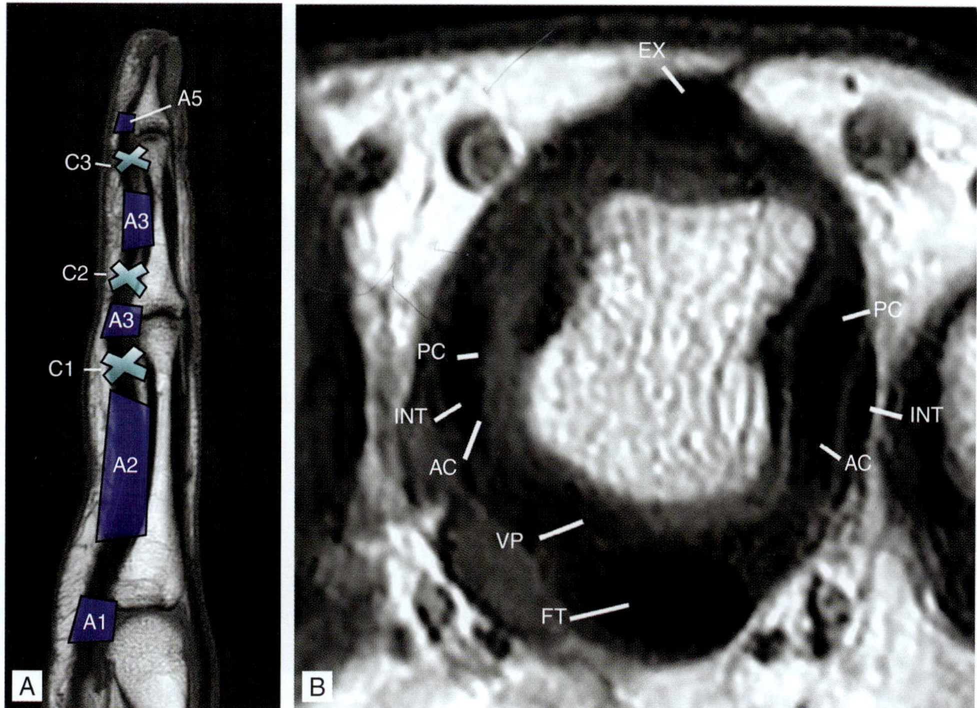

Figure 58.17 (A) Sagittal T1-weighted MRI overlaid with locations of the annular (A1, A2, A3, A4, and A5) and cruciate (C1, C2 and C3) pulleys of the fingers. (B) Axial T1-weighted MRI at the level of the middle finger metacarpophalangeal joint demonstrates location of the volar plate (VP), flexor digitorum profundus and superficialis (FT), interosseous tendon (INT), accessory collateral ligament (AC), proper collateral ligament (PC), and extensor digitorum tendon (EX). Note the interface between AC, PC, and INT can be difficult to define, with the AC palmar to the PC and INT superficial to both the AC and PC.

proximal phalanx of the index through to the little fingers. The flexor digitus superficialis splits into ulnar and radial slips, allowing passage of flexor digitorum profundus tendon. These two slips insert at the palmar base of the middle phalanx of the respective finger. The flexor digitorum profundus continues distally to insert at the palmar base of the distal phalanx. The thumb only has an interphalangeal joint, and flexion is facilitated by *flexor pollicis longus*, the tendon inserts, like the flexor digitorum profundus tendons, to the palmar base of the distal phalanx. The *vincula* are vascular connective bands anchoring the flexor digitorum profundus and superficialis tendons to the phalanges. Each tendon has a vincula longus and brevis.

Extensor Mechanism

The *extensor mechanism* [4] (Fig. 58.18) of the fingers is a complex of interconnections between the *extensor digitorum tendon* and a fibrous sheath, reinforced by the lumbricals and interossei. The dorsal MCP joint is covered by a fibrous sheath or the *extensor hood*, supported by *sagittal bands* (Figs. 58.18 and 58.19), and more distally, immediately dorsal to the proximal phalanx, by transverse and oblique fibers of a fibrous sheath that receives contributions from the lumbricals and interossei. The extensor digitorum tendon continues along the midline to the middle phalanx's dorsal base as the *central slip* with *lateral* and *medial slips* that merge with intrinsic tendons from either the lumbricals or interossei, becoming the *medial* and *lateral conjoined* tendons. The central slip also receives some reinforcement from these intrinsic tendons. More distally, the *triangular ligament* joins the lateral and medial conjoined tendons at the midline before they merge to form the *terminal extensor tendon* that

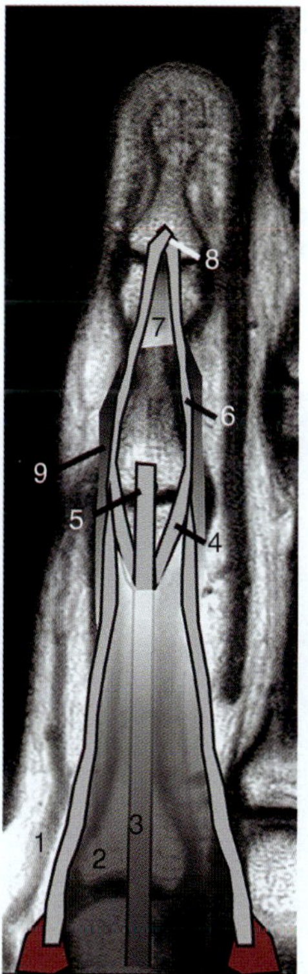

Figure 58.18 Coronal T1-weighted MRI overlaid with the extensor mechanism of the fingers: (*1*) lumbrical or interossei and tendon, (*2*) extensor hood and sagittal slips or bands, (*3*) extensor digitorum tendon, (*4*) lateral and medial slips, (*5*) central slip, (*6*) lateral and medial conjoined tendons, (*7*) triangular ligament, (*8*) terminal extensor tendon, and (*9*) transverse and oblique retinacular ligaments.

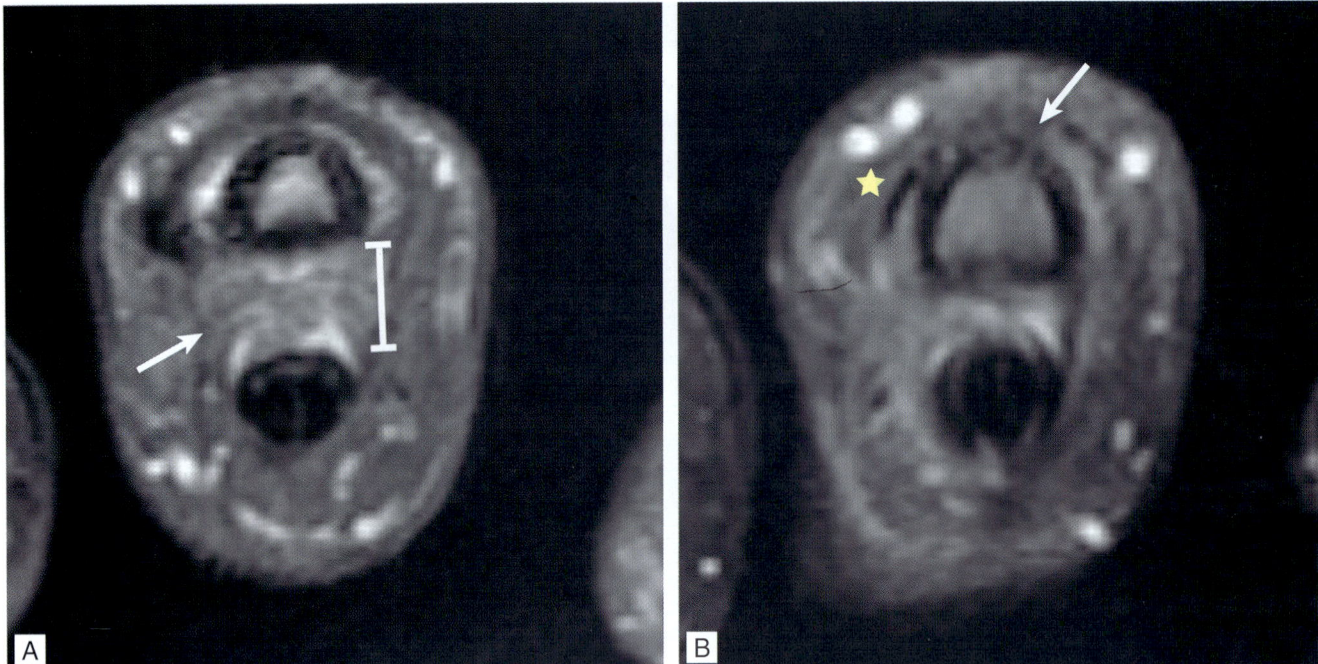

Figure 58.19 (A) Axial T2-weighted fat-saturated MRI demonstrates indistinctness of the middle finger A2 pulley (*arrow*), consistent with rupture. The increased separation of the flexor digitorum profundus and superficialis tendons from the underlying proximal phalanx cortex (interval line) reflects bowstringing. There is also bone edema involving the proximal phalanx with surrounding subcutaneous edema. (B) Axial T2-weighted fat-saturated MRI, from a different patient demonstrates rupture of the radial sagittal band (*arrow*) at the level of the proximal phalanx of the middle finger with ulnar deviation of the extensor tendon or central slip (*star*).

inserts to the dorsal base of the distal phalanx. The conjoined fibers receive additional support by *transverse* and *oblique retinacular ligaments* at the proximal and distal interphalangeal joints levels, respectively. Both of these ligaments have palmar origins, the transverse retinacular ligament from the volar plate of the proximal interphalangeal joint and the oblique retinacular ligament, with a longer course, from the proximal phalanx and flexor tendon sheath.

Nerves of the Hand and Wrist

Median Nerve

The *median nerve* extends through the carpal tunnel (Fig. 58.20) and divides into thenar or *recurrent muscular* and *digital cutaneous* branches distal to the carpal tunnel. However, in some, it bifurcates more proximally, giving rise to a *bifid median nerve*, commonly associated with

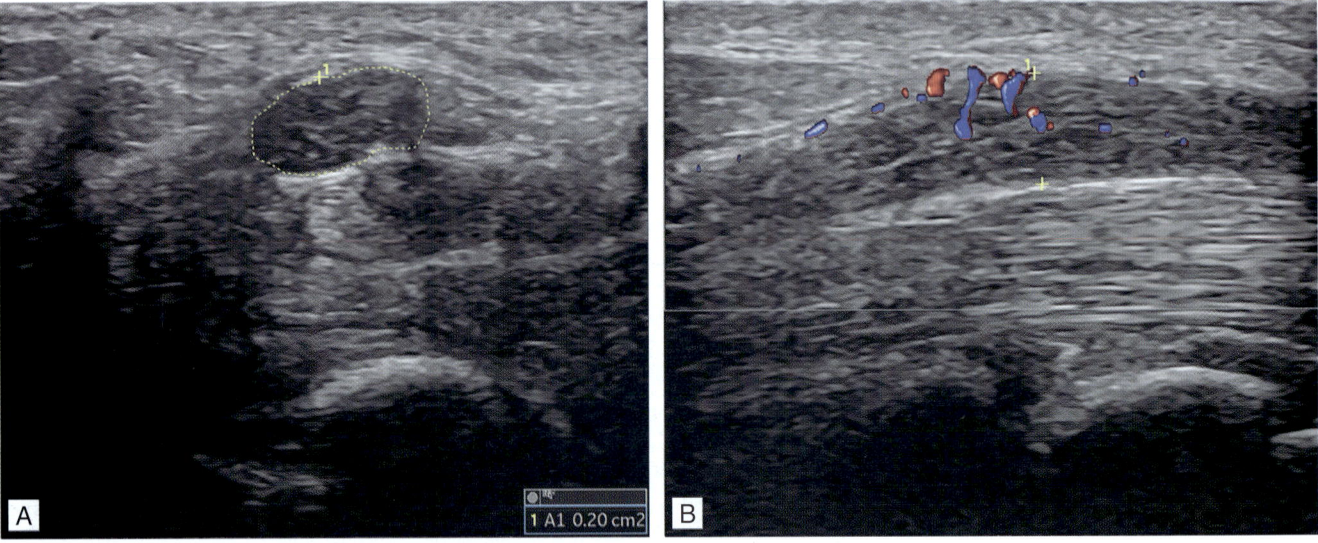

Figure 58.20 Transverse (A) and longitudinal Doppler (B) ultrasound images demonstrate marked thickening of the median nerve, with a maximal cross-sectional area of 20 mm^2 (normal range, 9–11 mm^2), proximal to the flexor retinaculum as well as mild increased vascularity. The patient also had symptoms (volar thumb, index finger, and middle finger paraesthesia) that were compatible with carpal tunnel syndrome.

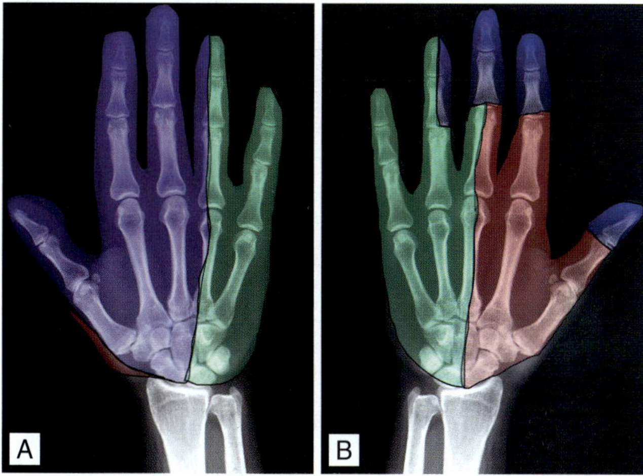

Figure 58.21 Posteroanterior radiograph with a colored overlay demonstrates the median (*blue*), ulnar (*green*), and radial (*red*) nerve sensory distributions to the palmar (A) and dorsal (B) hand.

an accessory artery called the *persistent median artery*, at risk of resection during carpal tunnel release. During carpal tunnel release, the recurrent branch may also be at risk of resection (and litigation, sometimes called the "million-dollar nerve"), particularly with a radial surgical approach or when it has a transligamentous course. The median nerve supplies the thenar muscles (abductor pollicis brevis, flexor pollicis brevis, opponens pollicis) and the radial/lateral two lumbrical muscles. The *median nerve* receives sensory information from the palmar skin of the radial three and a half digits (Fig. 58.21) via the *palmar cutaneous branch*, which travels superficial to the flexor retinaculum and joins the median nerve proximal to the carpal tunnel; therefore, it is spared in carpal tunnel syndrome.

Ulnar Nerve

The *ulnar nerve* (ulnar artery and ulnar veins) traverse the wrist through *Guyon canal* (or the ulnar canal). Guyon canal commences at the proximal border of the *palmar carpal ligament*. It ends distally at the level of the hamate and fibrous arch of hypothenar muscles (*opponens digiti minimi, flexor digiti minimi,* and *abductor digiti minimi*). From proximal to distal, the ulnar border is formed by the flexor carpi ulnaris tendon, pisiform, and abductor digiti minimi. The transverse carpal ligament and hamate form the radial border. The flexor digitorum profundus tendons, transverse carpal ligament, pisohamate ligament, and pisometacarpal ligament form the floor, and the palmar carpal ligament and palmaris brevis muscle form the roof. Because of its close proximity, the ulnar nerve may be damaged when the hamate's hook is fractured.

After Guyon canal, the ulnar nerve bifurcates into *superficial* and *deep branches*. The *superficial branch of the ulnar nerve* supplies the palmaris brevis. Together with the *palmar* and *dorsal cutaneous branches of the ulnar nerve*, which both arise more proximal to the wrist, the ulnar nerve's superficial branch receives the sensory information from the dorsal and palmar skin of the ulnar one and a half digits (see Fig. 58.21). The deep branches of the ulnar nerve supply all the other intrinsic muscles of the hand not supplied by the median nerve or the superficial branch of the ulnar nerve; that is, the hypothenar muscles (opponens digiti minimi, flexor digiti minimi, abductor digiti minimi), the ulnar/median two lumbricals, all the interossei, and adductor pollicis.

Radial Nerve

The *radial nerve* bifurcates in the proximal forearm into *superficial* and *deep branches*. The superficial branch of the radial nerve is dorsal compared to the ulnar and median nerves and lies superficial to the extensor retinaculum, at the level of extensor compartment I, and there is a risk of injury during extensor compartment I surgical release. The superficial branch of the radial nerve then usually bifurcates further into *lateral* and *medial branches*, which receive the sensory information from the dorsal skin of the radial three and a half digits (see Fig. 58.21).

Imaging Modalities and Protocols

Radiographs

Wrist

Radiographs are commonly performed for assessing painful or injured hands or wrists. The wrist *radiograph series* consists of posteroanterior (PA) and lateral projections (with or without oblique projections).

To *assess the wrist's alignment on radiographs* (Table 58.4 and Fig. 58.22), the three normal arcs of the carpal rows should be analyzed to exclude malalignment/dislocation. The three arcs should be parallel to each other and follow the contours of the

TABLE 58.4 Radiography Measurements

Measurement		Normal Range
Radial inclination	The angle the distal radial articular surface makes with a line drawn perpendicular to the diaphysis on the PA view	13–30 degrees
Scapholunate interval	The interval between the scaphoid and lunate (PA view)	<2 mm normal, 2–3 mm borderline, >3 mm abnormal
Volar tilt	The angle the distal radial articular surface makes with a line drawn perpendicular to the diaphysis on the lateral view	4 degrees of dorsal tilt to 11 degrees of volar tilt
Scapholunate angle	The angle between long axes of the scaphoid and lunate on the lateral view	30–60 degrees (DISI = increased, VISI = decreased)
Capitolunate angle	The angle between long axes of the capitate and lunate on the lateral view	<30 degrees (DISI and VISI = increased)

DISI, dorsal intercalated segment instability; *PA*, posteroanterior; *VISI*, volar intercalated segment instability.

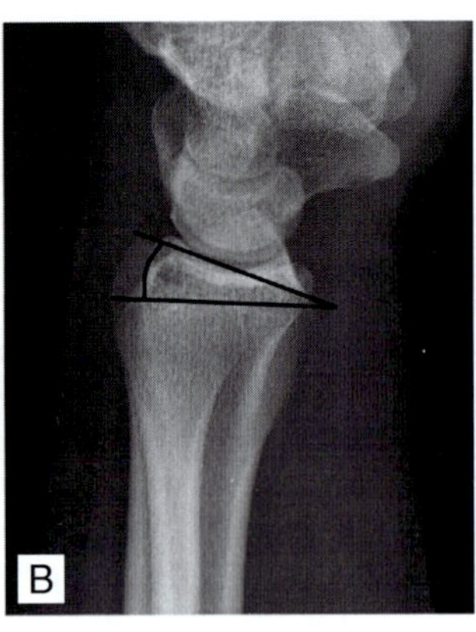

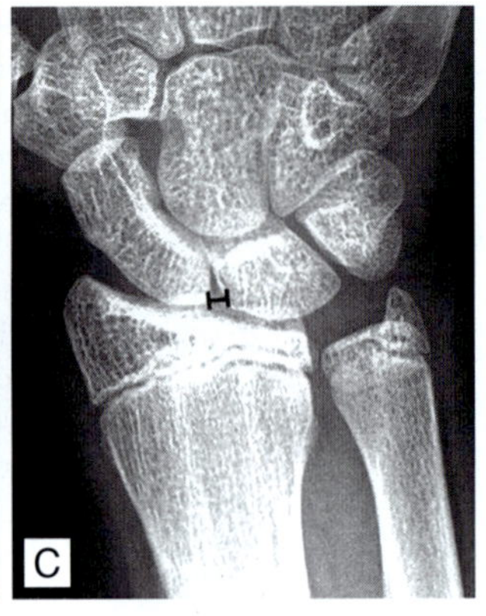

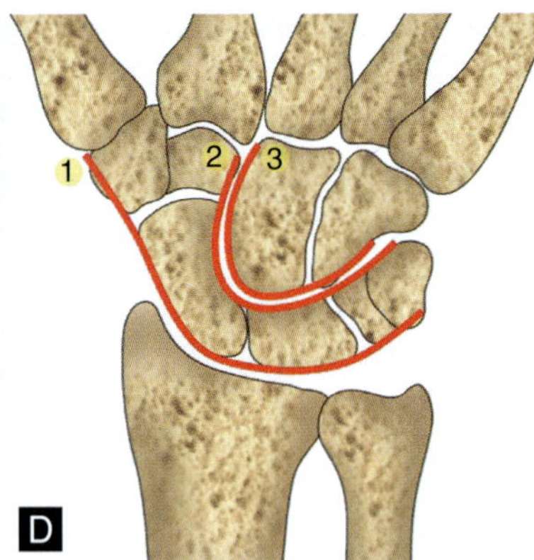

Figure 58.22 Radiographs with a normal (A) radial inclination angle (13–30 degrees), volar tilt angle (4 degrees dorsal tilt to 11 degrees volar tilt) (B), and scapholunate interval (<2 mm normal, 2–3 mm borderline, >3 mm abnormal) (C). (D) Three normal arcs (*1–3*) of the carpal rows.

proximal carpal row proximal articular surface, the proximal carpal row distal articular surface, and the proximal articular surface of the hamate and capitate. Short triquetral bones and a hamate facet on the lunate bone (type II lunate) are normal variants that may disrupt normal arc contours. Ulnar variance should be measured with standard PA views of the wrist, with the arm abducted 90 degrees and the elbow flexed at 90 degrees [5].

To *assess the scaphoid*, oblique projections and an additional PA view with ulnar deviation of the wrist (scaphoid view) are helpful. To profile the ulnar carpal bones, a PA view with radial deviation may be performed. *Carpal tunnel* (or hook of hamate) *views* are obtained in the axial plane of the wrist during wrist extension, augmenting the concavity of the palmar wrist. This view may be used to assess for the hook of hamate, pisiform, and trapezium fractures. In contradistinction, carpal bridge views are performed in the axial plane of the wrist during wrist flexion to assess the dorsal margin of the proximal carpal row.

The semisupination oblique (or pisotriquetral) view is started with true lateral positioning and then supinated 45 degrees from the original position, allowing the pisotriquetral interval to be adequately profiled. When performed by both hands as an anteroposterior projection, it is referred to as catcher (or Norgaard) views (see later). The *clenched fist views* help assess the scapholunate ligament injury, performed as a PA projection with both hands clenched and within the field of view. Other *stress views*, such as wrist flexion and extension, may be performed to assess and augment intercarpal instability.

Hand

The hand, thumb, and finger (or digit) *radiographic series* also consist of PA and lateral projections. To reduce overlapping of the digits when imaging the hand, an additional or alternate lateral fanned view may be performed. For rheumatology patients, both hands are usually included in a single PA projection, and similar catcher (or Norgaard) views are also performed (as earlier), permitting better assessment for erosions. For finger radiographs, it is essential to obtain true lateral projections so that the bifid condyles are properly profiled and the interphalangeal spaces are not obscured because of obliquity.

Magnetic Resonance Imaging and Computed Tomography

When initial radiographs are negative or equivocal, magnetic resonance imaging (MRI) (Table 58.5) and CT are the subsequent imaging modalities of choice. Computed tomography (CT) is usually performed for preoperative planning for complex fractures, suspected nonunion, osteonecrosis, and occult fracture. For most other indications such as posttraumatic pain, tendon or ligament injury, chronic wrist pain, and osteonecrosis and for evaluation of occult fractures, MRI is the modality of choice. Postcontrast MRI, with gadolinium-based contrast, is usually reserved for a workup of tumors or when infection or inflammation is suspected. Unlike other, larger joints throughout the body, magnetic resonance arthrography (MRA) has not been replaced by conventional 3-T MRI when there is suspected ligament, tendon, or TFCC injury. MRA is also beneficial in patients with chronic wrist pain, particularly ulnar-sided-wrist pain. Computed tomography arthrography (CTA) can also be used when there is suspected ligamentous or TFCC injury but is less favorable to MRA (as well as conventional MRI, particularly if performed on 3-T MRI) and is best utilized when MRI or MRA is contraindicated. Four-dimensional CT (4D) CT of the wrist has become available for clinical use to detect distal radioulnar joint and carpal instability. It allows a kinematic assessment of active wrist motion, depicting slight positional bone changes with high temporal and spatial resolution.

TABLE 58.5 Example Wrist or Hand Magnetic Resonance Imaging Protocol

Sequence	Plane
Precontrast: STIR, T1 weighted, PDW FS	Coronal
Precontrast: T1 weighted, T2 weighted FS	Axial
Precontrast: PDW FS	Sagittal
Precontrast: T1 weighted FS[a]	Axial
Postcontrast: T1 weighted FS	Axial
Postcontrast: T1 weighted FS	Sagittal
Postcontrast: T1 weighted FS	Coronal

[a]Additional sequences if contrast is administered.
FS, fat saturated; *PDW*, proton density weighted; *STIR*, short tau inversion recovery.

Ultrasonography

Given the superficial and easily accessible nature of anatomy, dynamic ultrasonography (USG) is preferred when assessing the wrist and hand tendons, ligament and joint anatomy, and pathology. USG is also useful for locating foreign bodies, including those that may be occult on radiography. Ultrasound-guided percutaneous interventions of the hand and wrist are commonly performed. For patients with inflammatory arthritis with equivocal findings on radiography or clinical examination, conventional and Doppler USG is a valuable screening tool looking for active synovitis and marginal erosions. USG is a viable option when patient access to MRI (or CT) is limited because of geographic, mobility, insurance, or financial reasons.

Nuclear Medicine

Technetium-99m methylene diphosphonate (^{9m}Tc MDP) bone scan (triple-phase), ^{9m}Tc m-hexamethyl propylene amine (HMPAO)–labeled white blood cell scans, and indium-111-labeled white blood cell scans are useful tools when osteomyelitis is suspected, particularly when MRI is contraindicated or unavailable or when the presence of metallic prostheses limits assessment. ^{9m}Tc-MDP bone scan (triple phase) may also be beneficial when stress or occult fractures are suspected and for diagnosing complex regional pain syndrome.

Common Clinical Scenarios

Common presenting signs and symptoms include pain and palpable abnormality. Pain can be localized, diffuse, or follow a nerve distribution and may be associated with trauma, localized infection, or inflammation. The palpable abnormality may be asymptomatic, discovered during a clinical examination. For both of these presentations, radiographs are the initial modality. Subsequent investigations, including other imaging modalities, are dependent on the clinical context (see overall approach flow charts).

Wrist Pain

Although fractures are covered in Chapter 83, they warrant mention as a history of recent trauma and can lead to instability or osteonecrosis. Scaphoid fractures are the most common carpal fracture but may also be occult on the initial radiographs (in ~10–40% cases) [6,7]. MRI and bone scan are most sensitive for further assessment (MRI also being more specific). If the scaphoid is fractured and not immobilized, then the risk of *nonunion* (Fig. 58.23) increases. Nonunion or osteonecrosis is more likely to occur for more proximal scaphoid fractures because of a distal to proximal blood supply (via the dorsal carpal artery and, to a lesser degree, the superficial palmar arch).

Carpal osteonecrosis may be posttraumatic or associated with other systemic risk factors, including systemic lupus erythematosus, sickle cell anemia, diabetes, steroid use, alcohol use, and bisphosphonate use. Osteonecrosis most commonly involves the lunate and is also called *Kienböck disease* or lunatomalacia (Fig. 58.24). *Negative ulnar variance* (Fig. 58.25) is associated with osteonecrosis and is present in up to 75% of patients with Kienböck disease [8].

Other common sites of osteonecrosis in the carpal bones include the scaphoid, the capitate, and the hook of hamate. According to Lichtman's modified Stahl classification, osteonecrosis of the lunate can be divided into four stages (Table 58.6) [9]. CT and MRI are more sensitive than radiography [10] with sclerosis (low signal on T1- and T-weighted sequences) first occurring centrally and bone marrow edema (intermediate signal on T1-weighted and high signal on T2-weighted sequences) occurring at the radial margin to differentiate from changes related to *ulnar impaction syndrome*. Nuclear medicine bone scans are not performed as frequently as other modalities for Kienböck disease but may be an adjunct for difficult cases [11].

Early stages may require immobilization, antiinflammatory drugs, leveling procedures (for negative ulnar variance), decompression, or revascularization. Later stages need more extensive surgeries such as proximal row carpectomy and joint fusion.

Injury to the TFCC and lunotriquetral ligament may cause ulnar wrist pain. TFCC injury may be posttraumatic or degenerative; the latter is associated with positive ulnar variance and ulnar impaction syndrome (see later). Both may present with ulnar wrist pain and best evaluated with MRI or MRA after radiographs are negative for fracture. TFCC may be classified according to the Palmer classification [12] (Table 58.7). Treatment varies from conservative (immobilization and antiinflammatory drugs) to arthroscopy intervention (debridement or repair) to various ulnar shortening procedures.

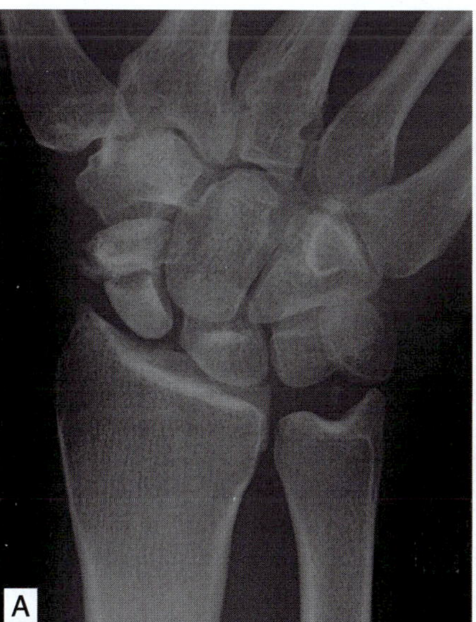

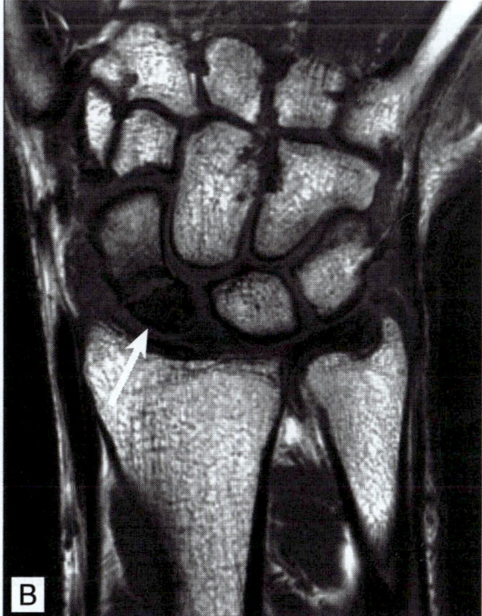

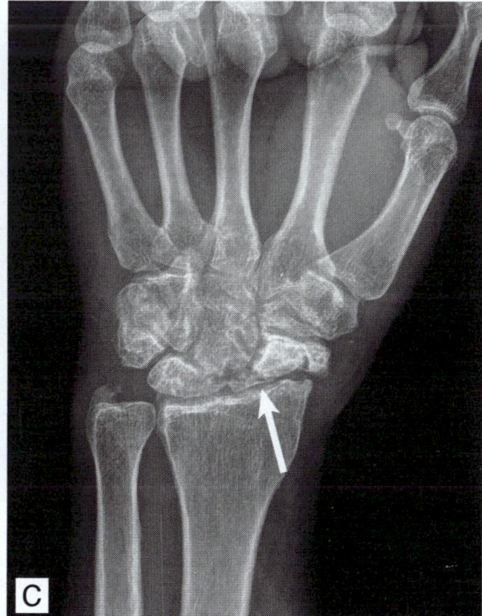

Figure 58.23 Posteroanterior (PA) radiograph (A) of the hand demonstrates nonunion of a scaphoid waist fracture that if left untreated may result in subsequent scaphoid nonunion and proximal bone osteonecrosis, as demonstrated on the coronal T1-weighted MRI (B) (*arrow*) or advanced collapse as demonstrated on the PA radiograph (C) (*arrow*) from two different patients.

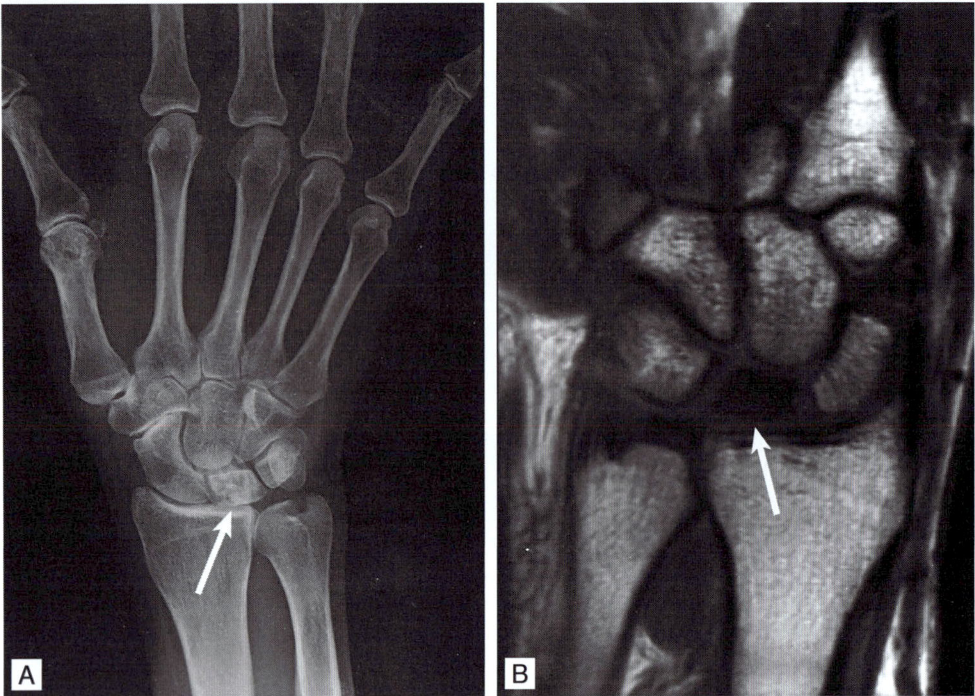

Figure 58.24 (A) Posteroanterior radiograph of the hand demonstrates diffuse sclerosis of the lunate (*arrow*) with mild loss of height or flattening but no fragmentation consistent with Kienböck disease. (B) Coronal T1-weighted MRI in a different patient with Kienböck disease demonstrates diffuse (central and peripheral) T1 low signal throughout the lunate bone (*arrow*) corresponding to sclerosis associated with osteonecrosis.

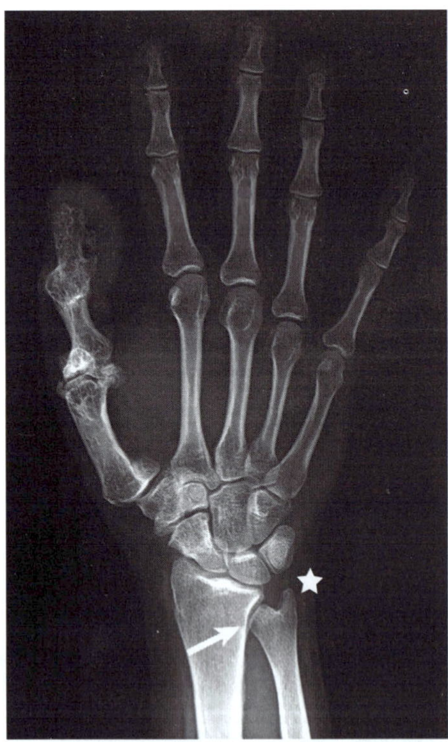

Figure 58.25 Posteroanterior radiograph of the hand demonstrates ulnar impingement syndrome with negative ulnar variance or shortening of the ulnar (*star*) resulting in sclerosis and remodelling of the ulnar margin of the radius at the site of impingement just proximal to the sigmoid notch (*arrow*). These are findings of thumb macrodactyly secondary to macrodystrophia lipomatosa.

TABLE 58.6 Lichtman's Modified Stahl Classification of Lunate Osteonecrosis

Stage	Radiograph Description	Magnetic Resonance Imaging Description
I	Normal radiograph	Edema
II	Increased density of the lunate with possible decrease of lunate height at the radial margin	Partial necrosis but preserved morphology
III	1. Lunate collapse without scaphoid rotation 2. Lunate collapse with scaphoid rotation[a]	Lunate collapse (partial or complete necrosis)
IV	Secondary degenerative changes surrounding the lunate	Secondary degenerative changes surrounding the lunate (partial or complete necrosis)

[a]Scaphoid rotation or palmar angulation can be inferred when the scapholunate angle is greater than 60 degrees.

Ulnar impaction syndrome (or *ulnocarpal abutment*) is associated with positive ulnar variance in addition to TFCC injury and can be exacerbated during ulnar deviation. In contrast to lunate osteonecrosis, *ulnar impaction syndrome* results in bone marrow changes, first edema, and then sclerosis, at the site of impaction or at the radial side of the triquetrum or ulnar margin of the lunate.

TABLE 58.7 Palmer Classification of Triangular Fibrocartilage Complex Injury

Class 1 (Traumatic)	Description
1A	Central disc perforation
1B	Ulnar avulsion (with or without distal ulnar fracture)
1C	Distal avulsion (ulnotriquetral and ulnolunate ligament)
1D	Radial avulsion (with or without sigmoid notch fracture)
Class 2 (Degenerative)	**Description**
2A	Thinning or fraying without perforation
2B	Thinning or fraying with lunate, triquetral, or ulnar chondromalacia
2C	Disc perforation with or without lunate, triquetral, or ulnar chondromalacia
2D	Lunotriquetral ligament perforation with 2A, 2B, or 2C
2E	Any or all of the above (2A to 2D) with ulnocarpal osteoarthritis

Ulnar impingement syndrome (see Fig. 58.25), not to be confused with ulnar impaction syndrome, is associated with *negative ulnar variance.* The ulna compresses against the distal radius, usually proximal to the sigmoid notch, resulting in localized bony remodeling and marrow changes.

Ulnar styloid impaction syndrome (Fig. 58.26) and *hamatolunate impingement syndrome* are less common causes of ulnar wrist pain. Ulnar styloid impaction syndrome may occur because of an elongated ulnar styloid process (>6 mm) or ulnar styloid nonunion impacting the triquetral bone. Hamatolunate impingement syndrome refers to secondary joint degeneration when there is a normal variant articulation between the lunate and hamate (type II lunate).

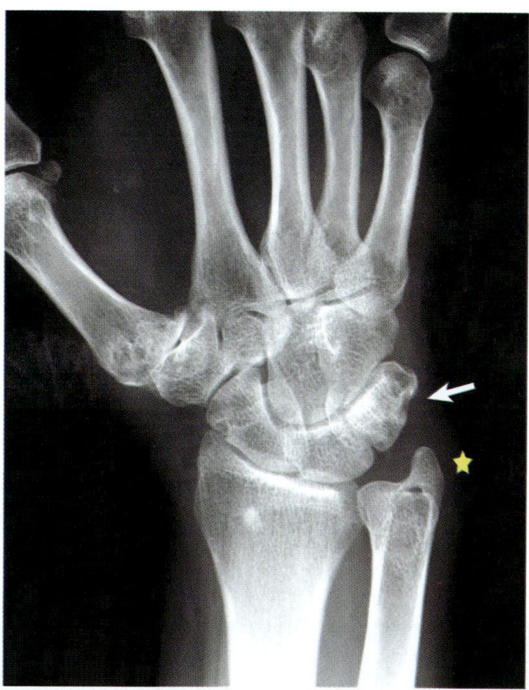

Figure 58.26 Oblique radiograph of the wrist demonstrates an elongated ulnar styloid process (*star*) with well corticated remodelling of the ulnar margin of the triquetrum (*arrow*) consistent with ulnar styloid impaction syndrome. Note severe first carpometacarpal and mild triscaphoid joint osteoarthritis.

The most common form of carpal instability is *scapholunate instability*, occurring because of injury to the *scapholunate ligament* (see Fig. 58.6), *radioscapholunate ligament*, or *ligament of Testut and Keunz.* Scapholunate ligament injury is suspected when the *scapholunate interval* is widened by more than 3 mm (Fig. 58.27) or foreshortening of the scaphoid, causing the *cortical ring sign*

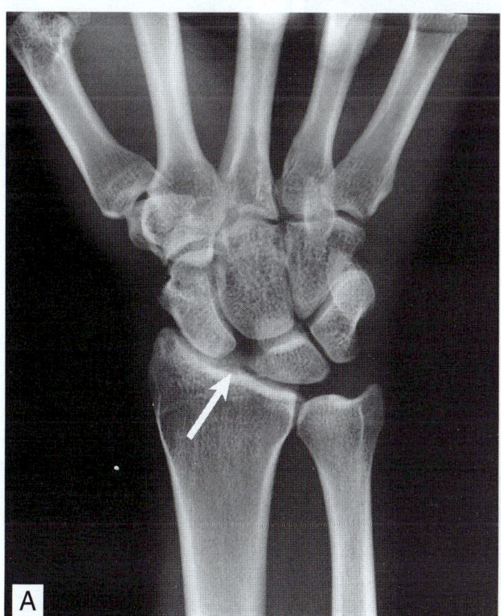

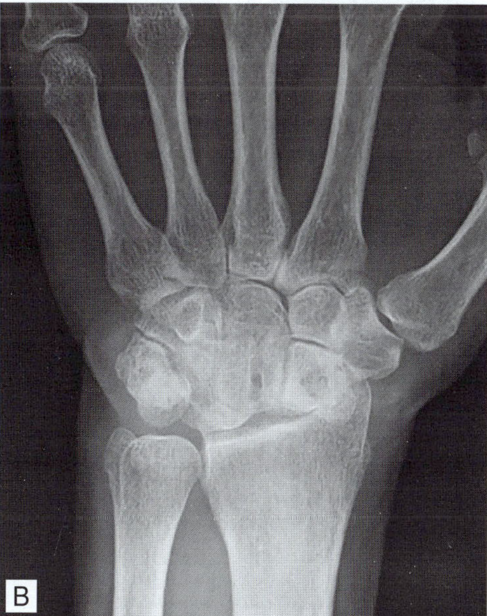

Figure 58.27 Posteroanterior radiograph (A) of the wrist demonstrates widening of the scapholunate interval by greater than 4 mm (*arrow*), consistent with scapholunate ligament tear and if left untreated may result in subsequent scapholunate advanced collapse as demonstrated on the posteroanterior radiograph (B) from a different patient.

(caused by scaphoid rotatory subluxation with an en face scaphoid pole on PA radiographs). MRI and MRA are more sensitive than radiography for scapholunate ligament injury detection. Scapholunate injury may be classified according to the Andersson and Garcia-Elias classification [13,14] (Table 58.8). Treatment again includes conservative management (immobilization and antiinflammatory drugs) and in cases of fracture, immobilization. Other options include ligament repair or reconstruction and fusion.

TABLE 58.8 Andersson and Garcia-Elis Classification of Scapholunate Injury

Type	Description
1	Radial avulsion
2	Ulnar avulsion
3	Mid-substance rupture
4	Partial rupture plus elongation

The alignment on lateral radiograph may be abnormal or become abnormal with increased capitolunate and scapholunate angles (>30–60 degrees, respectively) as a result of posterior displacement of the capitate, lunate dorsal angulation, and scaphoid palmar angulation, also referred to as *dorsal intercalated segment instability* (*DISI*) (Fig. 58.28). DISI alignment may also be associated with prior or remote distal radius or a scaphoid fracture or dorsal intercarpal extrinsic ligament tear.

Volar intercalated segment instability (VISI) (Fig. 58.29) is less common than DISI. It may result from lunotriquetral or dorsal radiocarpal extrinsic ligament injury or be caused by multiligamentous laxity. On lateral radiographs, VISI is demonstrated by increased capitolunate and decreased scapholunate angles (>30 and <30 degrees, respectively) and may also cause lunotriquetral joint widening (although this is less common than scapholunate widening in DISI).

Scapholunate advanced collapse (SLAC) and *scaphoid nonunion advanced collapse (SNAC)* are patterns of posttraumatic osteoarthritis caused by undiagnosed or untreated scapholunate ligament injury or scaphoid fracture nonunion, respectively. SLAC (see

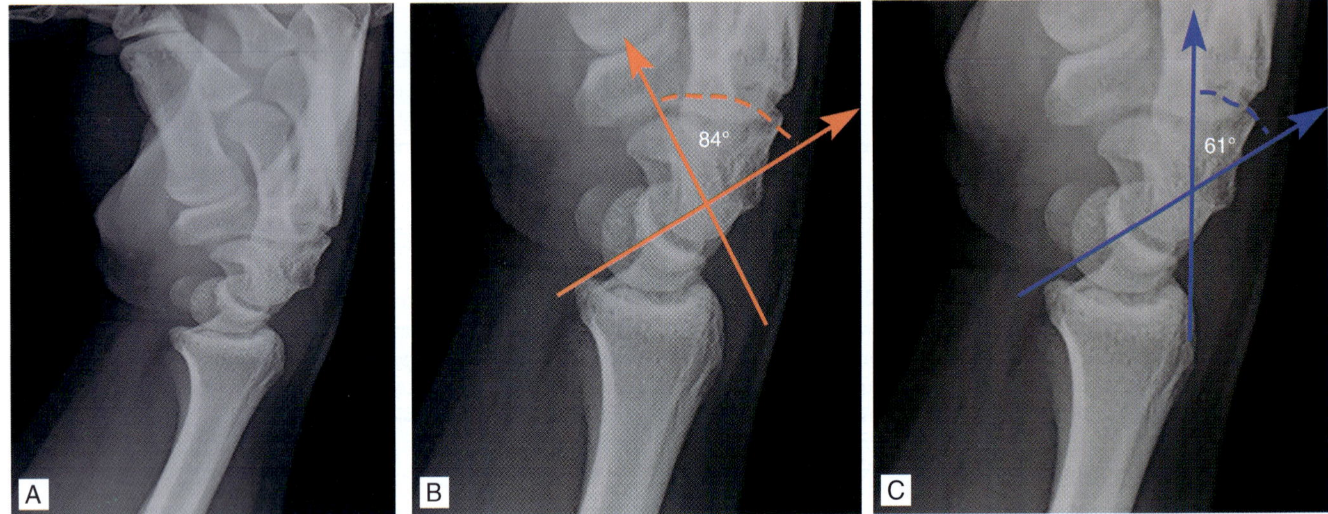

Figure 58.28 Lateral radiograph (A) of the wrist demonstrates dorsal intercalated segment instability caused by a scapholunate ligament tear with dorsal tilt of the lunate resulting in (B) a scapholunate angle of greater than 60 degrees and a capitolunate angle of greater than 30 degrees (C).

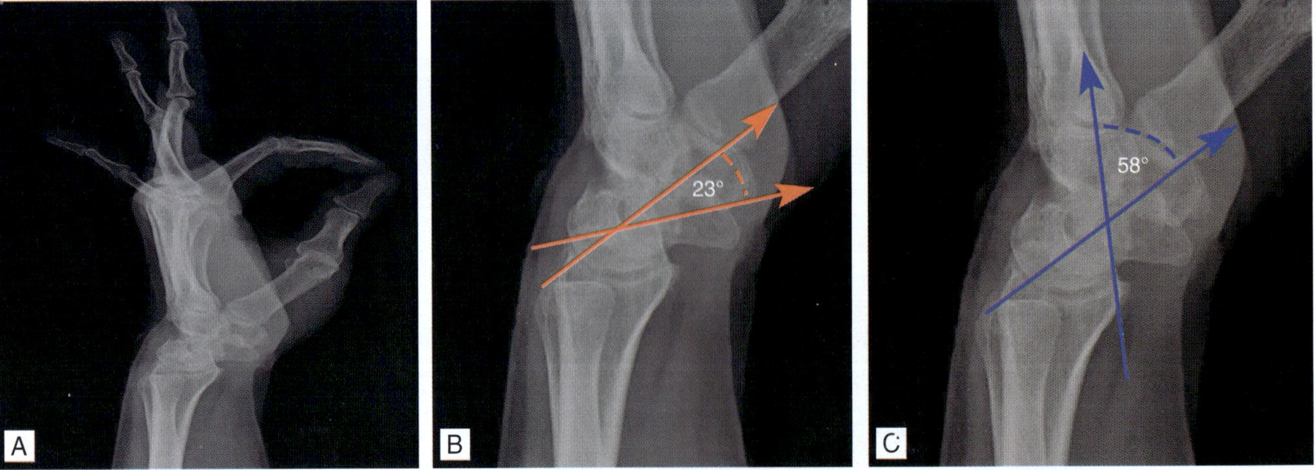

Figure 58.29 Lateral radiograph (A) of the wrist demonstrates volar intercalated segment instability (VISI) that can be caused by laxity or tears of the triquetrocapitate or triquetrohamocapitate ligament (part of the volar arcuate ligament when combined with the scaphocapitate ligament) or the lunotriquetral ligament with volar tilt of the lunate resulting in a scapholunate angle of less than 30 degrees (B) and a capitolunate angle of greater than 30 degrees (C).

Fig. 58.27) begins with scapholunate dissociation after a scapholunate ligament tear followed by proximal migration of capitate in the gap between the scaphoid and lunate. Osteoarthritis is seen initially between the radial styloid and maligned scaphoid and then progresses to the radioscaphoid joint's involvement, capitolunate joint, and then other radiocarpal or intercarpal joints with or without the DRUJ. SNAC (see Fig. 58.23) begins with osteoarthritis between the radial styloid and the distal scaphoid fracture fragment and then between the scaphoid and capitate followed by involvement of the proximal scaphoid and lunocapitate joint. In advanced forms, the capitate begins to migrate proximally toward the distal radius. DISI may occur in combination with either SLAC or SNAC patterns.

Distal radioulnar joint instability may manifest clinically as an inability to supinate or pronate the wrist. On radiographs, it may manifest as a widening of the DRUJ (by >6 mm) with dorsal subluxation or dislocation of the ulna with respect to the sigmoid notch of the distal radius. True lateral radiographs are vital to interpretation as altered angulation may lead to false-negative (or false-positive) interpretation. Even with adequate positioning DRUJ instability can be challenging to diagnose, and CT in supination and pronation may be helpful [15]. Recently, 4D CT has proven to be valuable in this condition. The DRUJ is stabilized by the dorsal more than the palmar radioulnar ligaments and can also be associated with TFCC injuries, making MRI a useful investigation tool.

Carpal Tunnel Syndrome

Extrinsic, direct, or repetitive impaction at specific wrist locations may result in various nerve entrapment or vascular compression syndromes. Pain, sensory change, and later stage weakness are symptoms associated with nerve entrapment syndromes; the distribution varies according to the nerve affected. The most common is *carpal tunnel syndrome* (see Figs. 58.20 and 58.30), with a lifetime incidence of about 10% to 15% [16], occurring most frequently in manual laborers.

The diagnosis of carpal tunnel syndrome is based on the characteristic clinical presentation of numbness and tingling through the median nerve territory that may be provoked with different examination techniques, such as Phalen and Tinel tests. Compression of the nerve is believed to occur as a result of repetition induced synovial inflammation changes to the flexor tendon sheaths that traverse the carpal tunnel. Risk factors for developing carpal tunnel include female gender, diabetes, inflammatory arthritides such as rheumatoid arthritis, aromatase inhibitors, obesity, hypothyroidism, pregnancy, and many more.

Whereas carpal tunnel syndrome results from compression of the median nerve, *Guyon canal syndrome* affects the ulnar nerve (see Fig. 58.30). Thrombosis of the ulnar artery or vein (both follow the ulnar nerve) may present similarly. If the ulnar artery is compressed at the level of the hook of the hamate, directly or repetitively, this may cause *hypothenar hammer syndrome* (Fig. 58.31), presenting with altered temperature sensation and pain or ischemia through the ulnar artery distribution. The ulnar artery may occlude or change caliber, either becoming spindlelike or aneurysmal.

Both USG and MRI are useful during the workup of nerve entrapment syndromes to exclude extrinsic compression by masses and for confirmation by assessing for nerve flattening, enlargement or, in the case of MRI, an altered signal on fluid sensitive sequences. Of the ultrasound diagnostic criteria for carpal tunnel, one of the most sensitive and specific is a wrist-to-forearm ratio of 1.4 or greater [17] (the median nerve is imaged in axial plane at the level of distal wrist crease and 12 cm proximally in the forearm). A more practical way of calculating is an absolute surface area difference of 2 mm^2 when comparing the median nerve area in the carpal tunnel with the level of the pronator quadratus muscle [18].

Hand or Finger Pain

Trauma to the complex hand and finger flexor or extensor mechanisms can result in significant morbidity. Tendon injuries (Fig. 58.32) occur from open to closed injuries, particularly those from lacerations. Both flexor (zones I–V, Tables 58.9 and 58.10) and extensor (zones I–VIII; Table 58.11) tendon injuries are defined by zones, which can be used to determine the tendons likely to be involved, the surgical approach, and the prognosis. The dynamic nature and portability of USG are ideal for assessing tendon injuries throughout the hand and digits.

Tendinosis and *tenosynovitis* (Figs. 58.33 and 58.34) refer to tendon degeneration and synovial membrane inflammation, respectively, and are defined by the tendon involved and location. The two pathologies may occur concurrently or independently and may result from trauma, repetition, or altered biomechanics (including underlying arthritis). If tendinosis is present, the tendon is usually thickened with abnormal echotexture (on ultrasound) or signal (on MRI with increased signal on T1-weighted or T2-weighted sequences). Tenosynovitis is confirmed by the presence of increased fluid within the

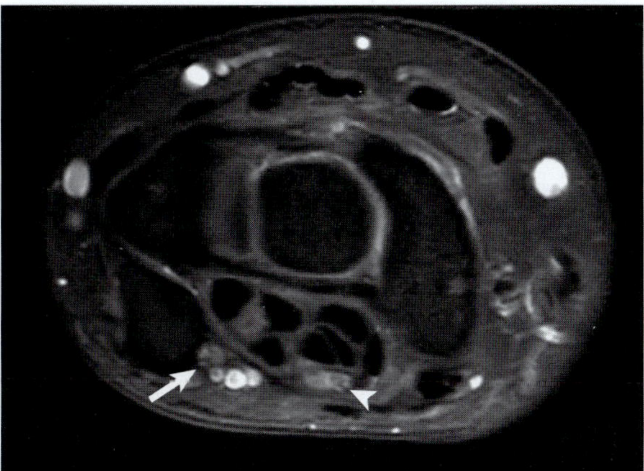

Figure 58.30 Axial T2-weighted fat-saturated MRI of enlarged ulnar (*arrow*) and median (*arrowhead*) nerves with increased T2 signal in Guyon canal and the carpal tunnel, respectively, in a patient with chronic inflammatory demyelinating polyneuropathy

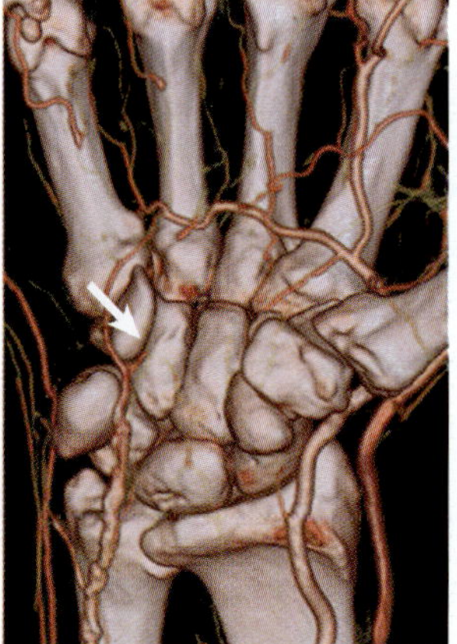

Figure 58.31 Three-dimensional reconstructed computed tomography angiogram of the hand demonstrates occlusion of the super ficial palmar arch artery (*arrow*) associated with hypothenar hammer syndrome.

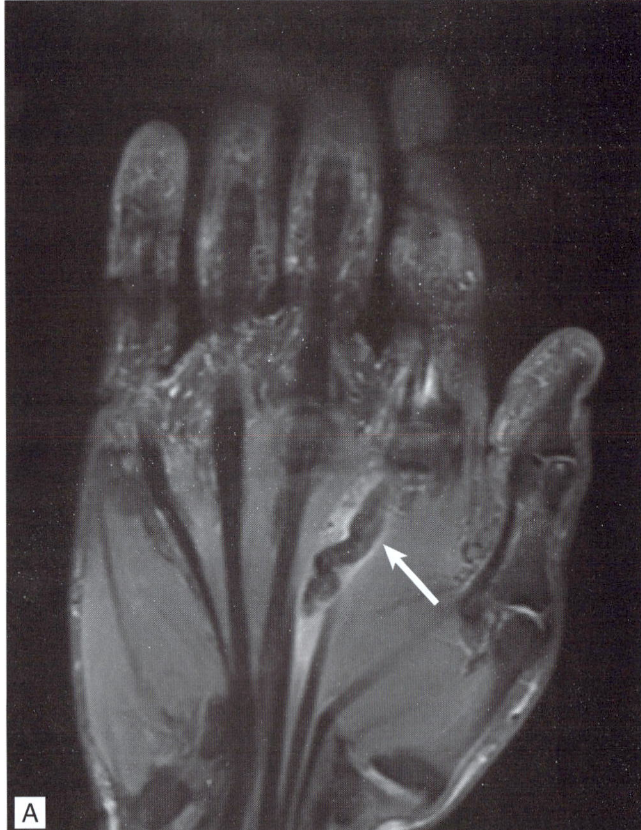

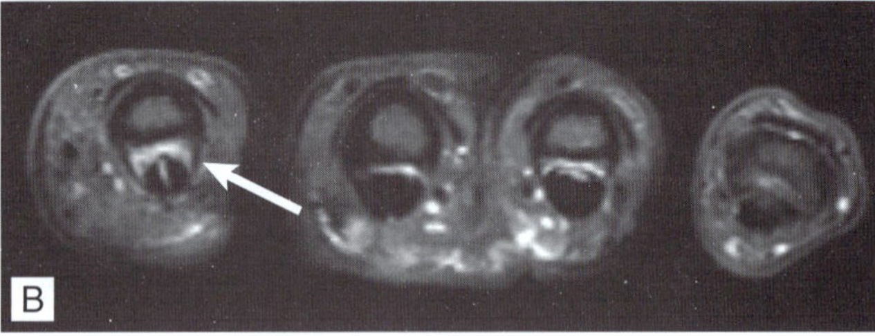

Figure 58.32 (A) Coronal proton density–weighted fat-saturated MRI demonstrates complete tear of the right index finger flexor digitorum profundus tendon (*arrow*) with proximal retraction to the level of the metacarpal head. (B) Axial T2-weighted fat-saturated MRI of the same patient with absence of the retracted flexor digitorum profundus tendon at the level of the intact A2 pulley (*arrow*) with a preserved flexor digitorum superficialis tendon.

TABLE 58.9 Flexor Tendon Injury Zones of the Fingers

Zone	Location	Injury or Tendon Involvement
I	Distal to the FDS insertion (base of the middle phalanx)	Jersey finger
II	Between the A1 pulley and the FDS insertion (the MCP joint to the base of the middle phalanx)	The FDS and FDP may be involved
III	Between the carpal ligament and the A1 pulley (midpalm to the MCP joint)	Associated with neurovascular injury
IV	Carpal tunnel	Carpal tunnel
V	Between the forearm and carpal tunnel	Associated with neurovascular injury

FDP, flexor digitorum profundus; *FDS*, superficialis; *MCP*, metacarpophalangeal.

TABLE 58.10 Flexor Tendon Injury Zones of the Thumb

Zone	Location	Injury or Tendon Involvement
TI	Distal to the FDS insertion (base of the middle phalanx)	Jersey finger
TII	Between the A1 pulley and the FDS insertion (the MCP joint to the base of the middle phalanx)	The FDS and FDP may be involved
TIII	Between the carpal ligament and the A1 pulley (the midpalm to the MCP joint)	Associated with neurovascular injury

FDP, flexor digitorum profundus; *FDS*, superficialis; *MCP*, metacarpophalangeal.

TABLE 58.11 Extensor Tendon Injury Zones

Zone	Location	Injury or Tendon Involvement
I	Distal to the DIP joint of the fingers or the IP joint of the thumb	Terminal extensor tendon (mallet finger)
II	Middle phalanx of the fingers or proximal phalanx of the thumb	Conjoined tendons (and triangular ligament) or EPL of thumb
III	PIP of the fingers or MCP joint of the thumb	Central slip (boutonniere deformity) or EPL and EPB of the thumb
IV	Proximal phalanx of the fingers or metacarpal of the thumb	Extensor digitorum (extensor apparatus, medial band, or lateral band) or EPL and EPB of the thumb
V	MCP joint of the fingers or CMC joint of the thumb	Extensor digitorum and sagittal band or EPL, EPB, and AbdPL of the thumb
VI	1st through 4th metacarpals	Associated with neurovascular injury
VII	Wrist	Tendon or retinaculum
VIII	Distal forearm	Extensor muscle

AbdPL, Abductor pollicis longus; *CMC*, carpometacarpal; *DIP*, distal interphalangeal; *EPB*, extensor pollicis brevis; *EPL*, extensor pollicis longus; *IP*, interphalangeal; *MCP*, metacarpophalangeal; *PIP*, proximal interphalangeal.

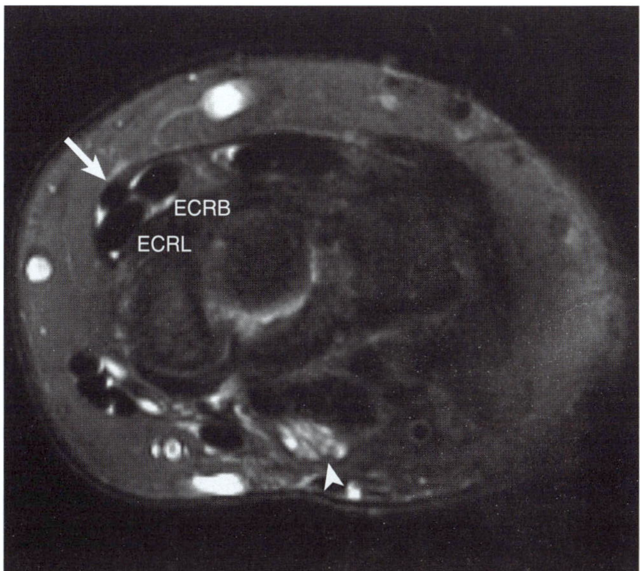

Figure 58.33 Axial T2-weighted fat-saturated MRI demonstrates fluid within the tendon sheaths with mild peritendinous edema dorsally, reflecting tenosynovitis, that is localized to where extensor pollicis longus or extensor compartment 3 (*arrow*) crosses extensor carpi radialis longus (ECRL) and extensor carpi radialis brevis (ECRB) tendons or extensor compartment 2, consistent with distal intersection syndrome. Note the enlarged and mildly edematous median nerve (*arrowhead*) that is associated with carpal tunnel syndrome.

tendon sheath on either modality. Peritendinous edema may also be present on both modalities, and Doppler ultrasound may show increased vascularity within the tendon or peritendinous tissues.

Proximal intersection syndrome occurs at the crossing point of the first and second extensor tendon compartments in the distal forearm. *Distal intersection syndrome* (see Fig. 58.33) occurs where the third crosses the second extensor tendon compartment at the dorsal wrist. *De Quervain tenosynovitis* (see Fig. 58.34) involves the first extensor compartment tendons, usually at the radial styloid, where it is fixated by the extensor retinaculum. This is also *stenosing tenosynovitis* as it is associated with a fibro-osseous tunnel that may also be inflamed or thickened. Another common form of stenosing tenosynovitis is *trigger finger* (or *trigger thumb*) (Fig. 58.35). The digit often locks in flexion (at the MCP or proximal interphalangeal joints), and re-extension is painful or difficult. The A1 pulley, at the level of the metacarpal heads, or the tendons (flexor digitorum profundus or superficialis) becomes thickened, inhibiting the normal gliding function and leading to stenosing tenosynovitis.

The *volar plate* (Fig. 58.36) of the proximal interphalangeal joint may be injured during hyperextension. Findings can mimic synovitis. It may be an isolated injury or associated with a phalangeal palmar base fracture, best demonstrated on lateral radiographs. If the collateral ligaments are only attached to the avulsed fragment, the middle phalanx may subluxate or dislocate dorsally. Two classifications systems, the Eaton and Keifhaber-Stern classifications [19,20], help guide treatment with the stability of the avulsion fracture based on the size or amount of articular surface involved.

The collateral ligaments represent the thickening of the joint capsule mediolaterally. Among other joints, these ligaments also support the first MCP joint. The *ulnar collateral ligament* is more commonly injured than the *radial collateral ligament* because of hyperextension or abduction injuries. Tears of the ulnar collateral ligament, either acute *(skier's thumb)* or chronic *(gamekeeper's thumb)*, may occur with or without an avulsion fracture distally, at the ulnar base of the thumb proximal phalanx, or less commonly at the ulnar margin of the first metacarpal head. *Stener*

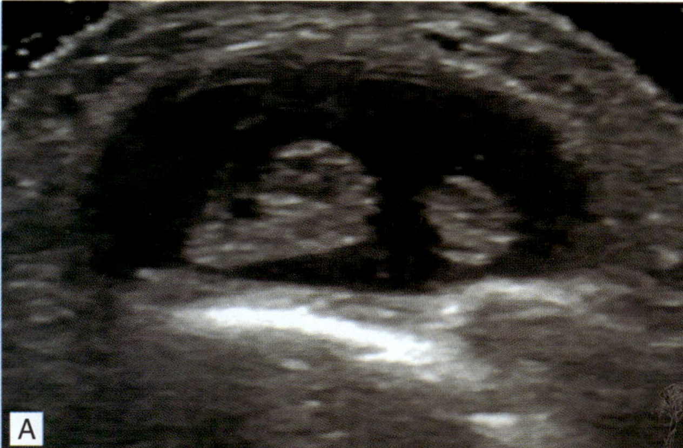

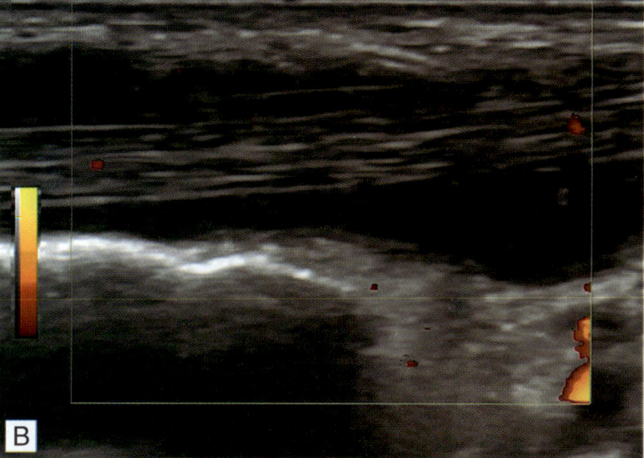

Figure 58.34 Transverse (A) and longitudinal Doppler (B) ultrasound images demonstrate marked fluid distension of extensor compartment 1 with tendon sheath thickening and increased tendon vascularity, consistent with De Quervain tendinitis and tenosynovitis.

lesions (Fig. 58.37) occur when the torn ulnar collateral ligament is displaced superficial or proximal to the *adductor aponeurosis*. Surgical repair is necessary as the torn ligament ends of Stener lesions cannot oppose for healing. MRI and USG with dynamic maneuvers are best for assessing ulnar collateral ligament injury and identifying Stener lesions. Two dynamic USG maneuvers include applying valgus stress to the first MCP joint to exacerbate the defect and thumb interphalangeal joint flexion for differentiating adductor aponeurosis from the ulnar collateral ligament.

Complex regional pain syndrome (specifically type I) (Fig. 58.38), reflex sympathetic dystrophy, and Sudeck atrophy are synonyms for the same clinical entity. There is no confirmatory test, but the diagnosis may be made clinically when there is disproportionate limb pain, with respect to the sentinel event, in addition to vasomotor dysfunction. Imaging findings are often nonspecific and include patchy osteopenia on radiography and heterogeneous bone marrow signal on MRI with soft tissue atrophy (not conforming to a specific nerve territory). On triple-phase bone scans (with blood-flow, blood pool, and delayed phases), complex regional pain syndrome may be positive during each phase with a juxtaarticular distribution on the delayed phase. Again, this is not specific to this entity because triple-phase positive bone scans are associated with osteomyelitis, periprosthetic infection, or loosening and inflammatory arthritides.

Palpable Abnormality

Ganglion cysts (Fig. 58.39) are the most common non-neoplastic "tumor," being cystic and intimately related to joints, tendon

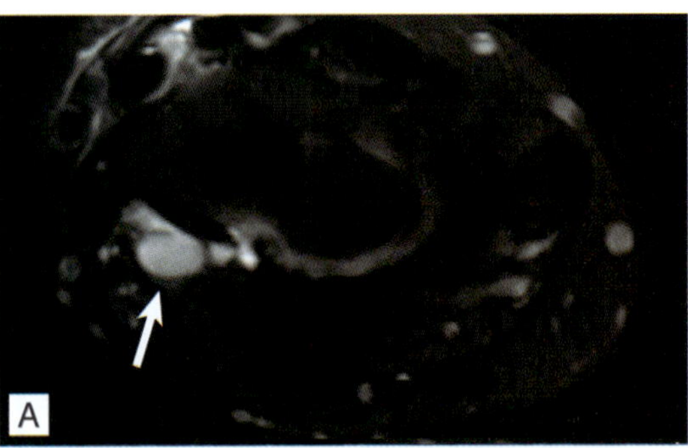

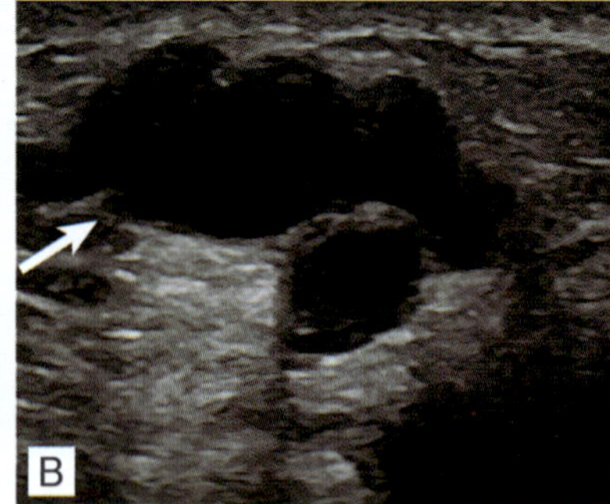

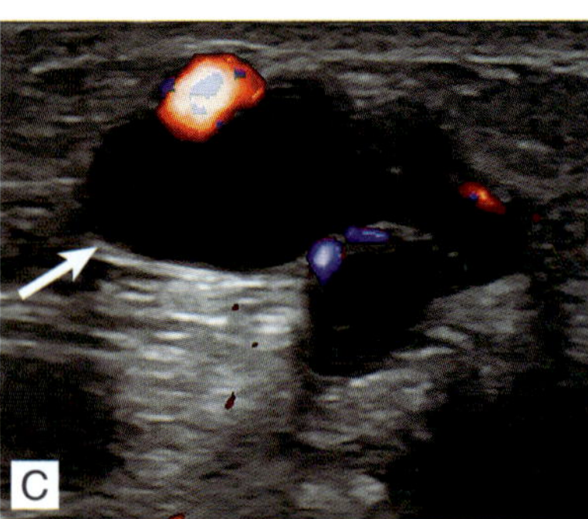

Figure 58.39 Axial (A) T2-weighted fat-saturated MRI demonstrates a T2 high/fluid signal multiseptated structure (*arrow*) arising from the palmar radioscaphoid joint. The corresponding transverse real-time (B) and Doppler (C) ultrasound examination of the same lesion (*arrow*) with no internal echoes, posterior acoustic enhancement, and no internal vascularity, consistent with a radioscaphoid ganglion.

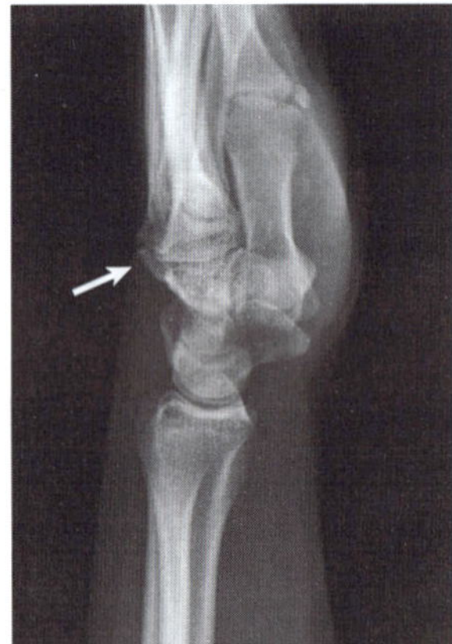

Figure 58.40 Lateral radiograph of the wrist demonstrates a prominent dorsal protuberance (*arrow*) of the third metacarpal base, consistent with carpal bossing.

appear as a bluish nodule on clinical examination. They are less common than other benign tumors such as lipomas, neuromas, nerve sheath tumors, and fibromas; however, they require mentioning here because they most commonly occur in hand, particularly subungual, along the dorsal margin of the distal phalanges. Because of slow growth (like GCTTS), they can cause pressure erosions of the adjacent bone, appreciated on radiographs. The nodule is solid on USG, and on MRI, it is low to intermediate signal on T1-weighted and high on T2-weighted images. The lesion is highly vascular on Doppler USG and hence also avidly enhances with contrast on MRI. They are treated by surgical excision. Endovascular treatment can be technically difficult in achieving complete occlusion, resulting in revascularization.

The most common bone tumors of the hand are *enchondroma* and *osteoid osteoma*, which are discussed in more detail with other bone tumors in Chapter 62. Enchondromas of the hand most commonly involve the proximal phalanges, followed by the metacarpals and middle phalanges. Generally, they lack a radiographically evident chondroid matrix and appear lucent. When multiple enchondromas are present, enchondromatosis such as *Ollier disease* (Fig. 58.43) and *Maffucci syndrome* should be considered; the latter is associated with subcutaneous venous malformation or hemangiomas and a higher incidence of malignant transformation. *Bizarre parosteal osteochondromatous proliferation* (BPOP) (Fig. 58.44), sometimes called Nora lesions, should also be mentioned because they typically occur in the hands (or feet). BPOP is a nonmalignant exophytic osteochondral lesion, similar to osteochondroma except they arise from the cortex without medullary bone continuation, they are not orientated away from the physes, and they may demonstrate osteolysis regions. The

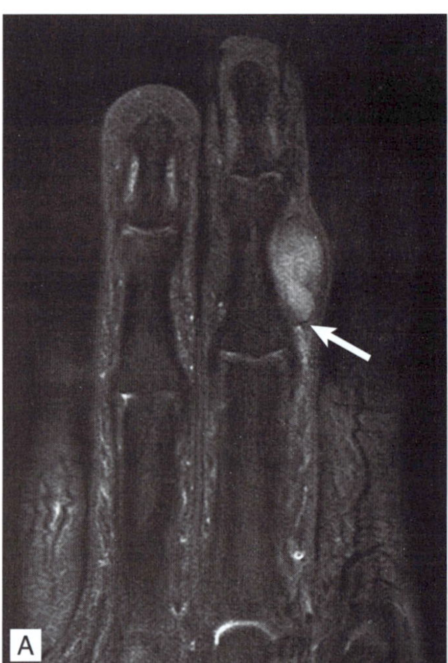

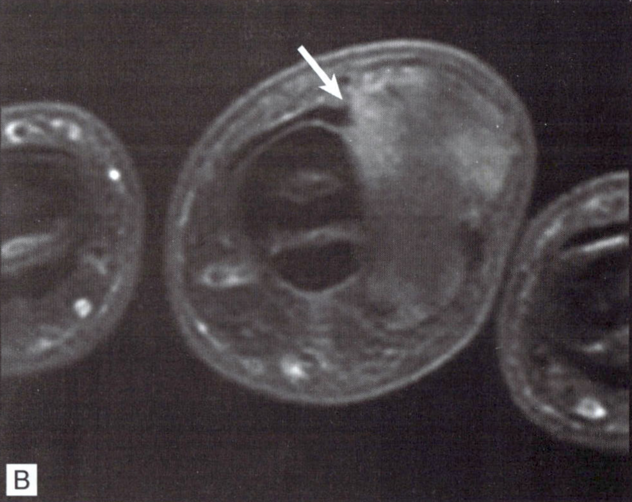

Figure 58.41 Coronal T2-weighted fat-saturated MRI (A) demonstrates homogeneous T2 high signal of a large mass at the ulnar margin of the middle finger middle phalanx with a small focus of susceptibility (*arrow*) and pressure remodeling of the subjacent cortex. Axial postcontrast T1-weighted fat-saturated MRI (B) demonstrates mild diffuse enhancement of the mass that is intimately related to the ulnar margin of the flexor digitorum tendons (*arrow*), a common associated of giant-cell tumors of the tendon sheath.

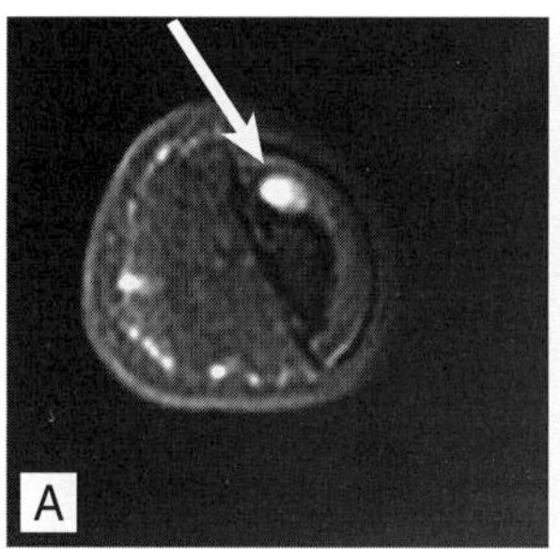

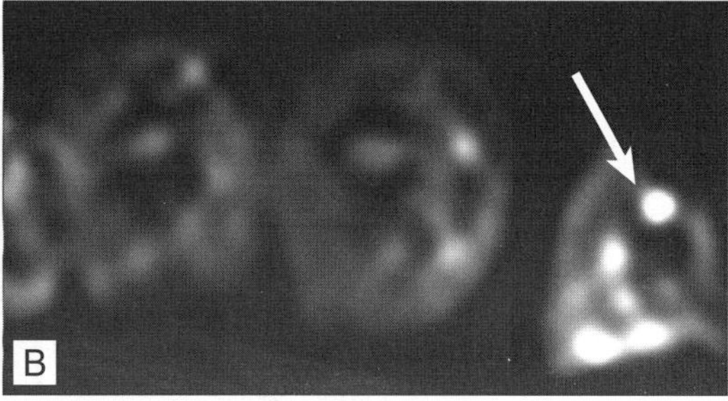

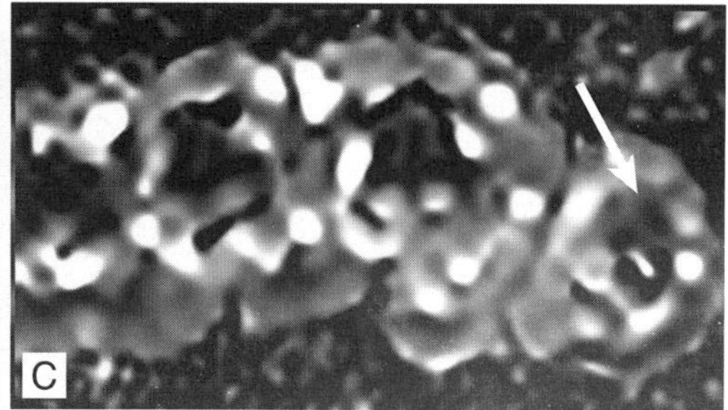

Figure 58.42 Axial postcontrast T1-weighted fat-saturated MRI (A) of the thumb with an avidly enhancing subungual lesion (*arrow*) that demonstrated diffusion restriction, being high signal on (B) diffusion-weighted imaging (at b value of 800 sec/mm^2) (*arrow*) and low signal (C) on apparent diffusion coefficient images (*arrow*). This was resected, and the pathology was consistent with a glomus tumor.

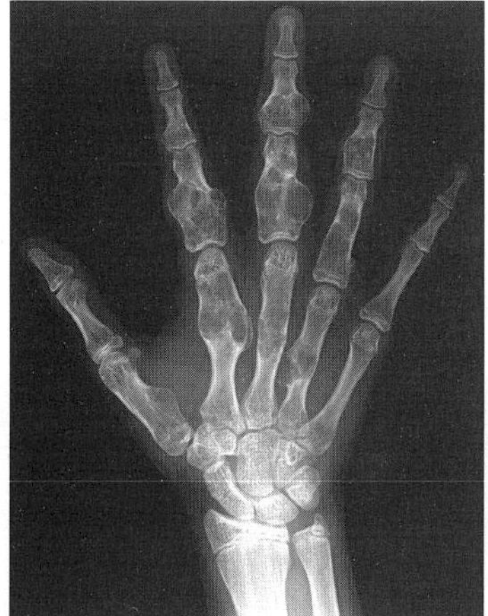

Figure 58.43 Posteroanterior radiograph of the hand with multiple enchondromas in a patient with Ollier disease. Enchondromas of the hand are predominantly lucent, although some of these have faint chondroid matrix or "rings and arcs" calcification, with narrow zones of transition and the larger lesions are also expansile.

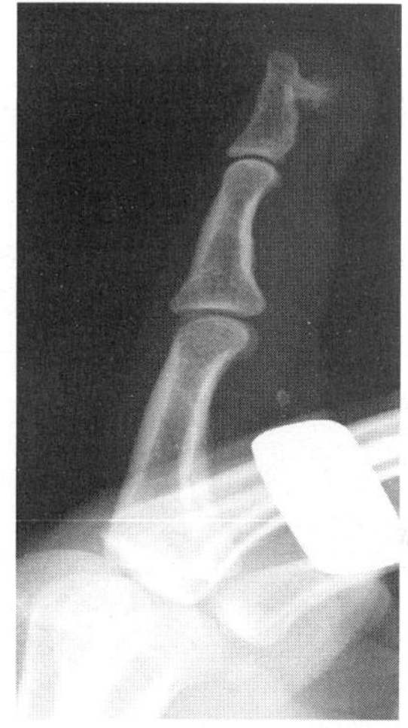

Figure 58.44 Lateral radiograph of the middle finger demonstrates an ossified outgrowth extending from the volar cortex of the distal phalanx with superficial margins that are irregular due to regions of osteolysis, consistent with a bizarre parosteal osteochondromatous proliferation.

hand's malignancies are rare, with cutaneous malignancies being more common than soft tissue or bone malignancies and metastases. Although metastases to the hand are rare, lung cancer is the most common primary malignancy to metastasize to the hand.

Palmar fibromatosis (Dupuytren disease) is a superficial fibromatosis arising from the fascia and aponeurosis. *It is the most common type of fibromatosis.* It is composed of spindle-shaped fibrous cells having a strong tendency for recurrence but never metastasize. It is commonly bilateral with older age group prevalence. It presents as subcutaneous nodules on the palmar surface at the level of the distal crease of the hand. Nodules slowly progress to fibrous cords that attach to and cause traction on the adjacent flexor tendons, resulting in flexion contractures of the digits. *The fourth and fifth rays are commonly affected.* USG shows these nodules to be hypoechoic and located directly superficial to the flexor tendons. Surgery is usually done in mature lesions with less cellularity rather than in hypercellular lesions because of less probability of recurrence in the former. MRI helps in this decision making by staging the lesion. Whereas mature lesions show predominantly low signal intensity on T2-weighted images and low to intermediate signal intensity on T1-weighted images, hypercellular lesions show high or intermediate signal intensity on T2-weighed images.

Infection

Hand infections usually occur after direct inoculation such as known or overlooked trauma. If left untreated, infection may destroy cartilage and impair function, contributing to significant morbidity [23]. Those most prone to hand infections include immunocompromised individuals, people with diabetes, intravenous drug users, and those sustaining bite injuries. The most common microbe is *Staphylococcus aureus*, occurring in up to 60% to 80% [23]. Bites, either from humans or animals, are commonly polymicrobial, and anaerobic infection should also be considered, particularly in those who are immunocompromised.

Hand infections are mostly found either superficially (cellulitis) or in the nail bed (paronychia). MRI and ultrasound may be utilized to exclude abscess formation, with restricted diffusion on MRI considered confirmatory. *Necrotizing fasciitis* (Fig. 58.45) carries a high mortality rate, reported as close to 30% [24] in some studies, even when treatment is instituted. The presence of perifascial gas, related to gas-forming bacteria, particularly anaerobes, is the most specific sign for the diagnosis of necrotizing fasciitis. Still, gas is rarely present and may only be noticed during the disease's advanced stages. CT is more sensitive than radiographs and MRI for the assessment of perifascial gas. The presence of deep or intermuscular fascial thickening and fluid collections on MRI is the most sensitive sign of necrotizing fasciitis and carries a high negative predictive value. Differential includes necrotizing inflammatory fasciitis, cellulitis, and myositis.

Paronychia (Fig. 58.46) involves infection of the soft tissues around the fingernail and may result in abscess formation or extension to the pulp and subsequent felon. *Felon* (Fig. 58.47) is a subcutaneous abscess of the fingertip (or toe tip) pulp and may result in subsequent osteomyelitis of the distal phalanx. Infection may also extend from the subcutaneous soft tissues into the many tendon sheaths, resulting in *septic* or *pyogenic tenosynovitis* (Fig. 58.48) or into the multiple

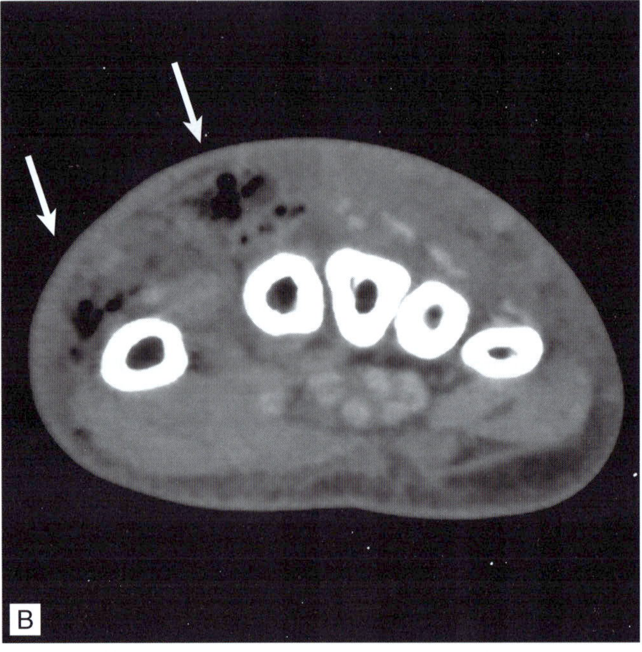

Figure 58.45 Oblique radiograph (A) of the hand with subcutaneous emphysema (*arrow*) surrounding the index finger distal and middle phalanges in a patient with necrotizing fasciitis. Axial postcontrast computed tomography (B) in a different patient with necrotizing fasciitis demonstrates extensive subcutaneous emphysema (*arrows*) and marked subcutaneous edema throughout the dorsum of the hand at the level of the first and second metacarpal diaphyses.

potential spaces of the dorsum and volar hand and wrist. The numerous deep spaces include the *space of Parona* (interposed between pronator quadratus and the flexor digitorum profundus sheaths in the distal forearm), among many others (thenar, midpalmar, hypothenar, dorsal subcutaneous, dorsal subaponeurotic, and interdigital web spaces). Septic arthritis and osteomyelitis may ensue from direct extension from the above locations; direct inoculation, particularly after bite injuries; and less commonly hematogenous spread. MRI (ideally with contrast and diffusion-weighted imaging) is most sensitive for assessing the presence and defining the extent of infections of the hand and wrist and monitoring treatment response. MRI with contrast and

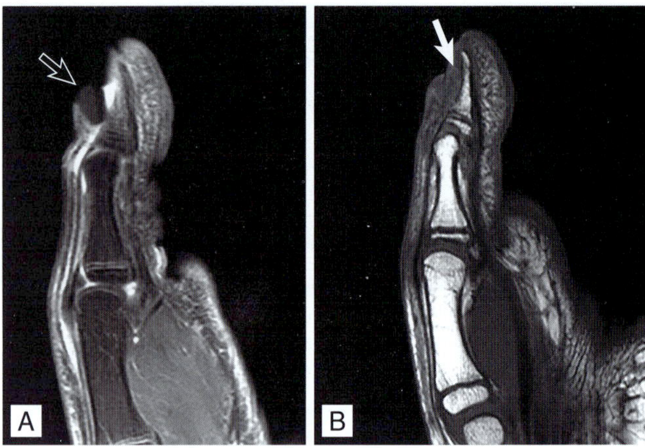

Figure 58.46 Sagittal postcontrast T1-weighted fat-saturated and (A) noncontrast T1-weighted (B) MRI demonstrate subcutaneous soft tissue enhancement adjacent the fingernail of the thumb with a rounded region of non-enhancing tissue or abscess formation (*open arrow*) immediately adjacent the nail bed. These findings are consistent with paronychia, and there is also subungual extension (*closed arrow*) but no marrow fat replacement in *B* to indicate osteomyelitis.

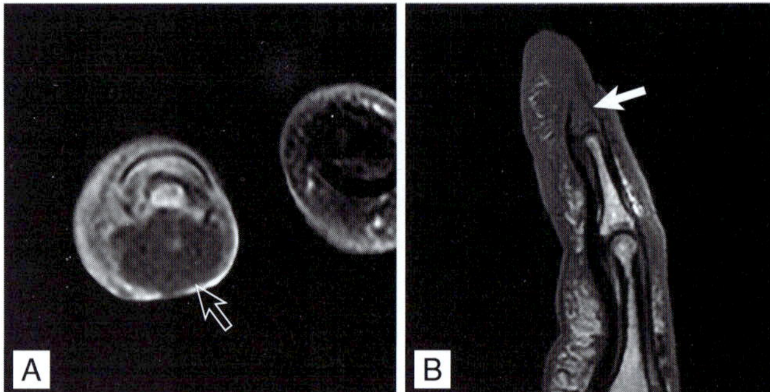

Figure 58.47 Axial postcontrast T1-weighted fat-saturated (A) MRI of the ring finger with nonenhancing tissue or abscess formation involving the pulp, consistent with felon (*open arrow*). The surrounding soft tissues and distal phalanx also demonstrate enhancing edema. The sagittal noncontrast T1-weighted (B) MRI in the same patient demonstrates marrow fat replacement, consistent with secondary osteomyelitis (*closed arrow*).

diffusion-weighted imaging increases reader confidence when diagnosing osteomyelitis, abscess formation, septic arthritis, and physis involvement in children [25].

Inflammation

The small joints of the hand and wrist are often the first to become inflamed, stiff, and painful. The most common arthritis of the hand and wrist are *osteoarthritis* and rheumatoid arthritis (Fig. 58.49), with many other types of arthritis described in more detail in Chapter 52. The hallmarks of osteoarthritis are asymmetric joint space loss, subchondral sclerosis marginal osteophytes, and subchondral cyst formation.

Periarticular soft tissue swelling (often related to underlying *synovitis*), juxtaarticular osteopenia, and later marginal erosions are seen in *rheumatoid arthritis* (see Fig. 58.49) and favor the MCP joints, proximal interphalangeal joints, thumb interphalangeal joint, and between the ulnar styloid and triquetrum. During the later stages of the disease, there may be joint laxity, resulting in subluxation, deformity, secondary osteoarthritic changes, and ankylosis, resulting in significant functional decline and morbidity. *Erosive osteoarthritis* (see Fig. 58.49) should be mentioned as a

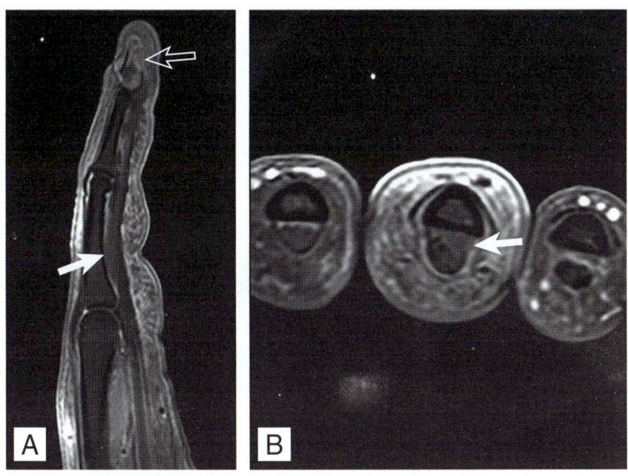

Figure 58.48 Sagittal (A) and axial (B) postcontrast T1-weighted fat-saturated MRI of the middle finger demonstrate destructive enhancing osteomyelitis of the distal phalanx (*open arrow*) with nonenhancing soft tissue or abscess formation extending deep to and within the flexor digitorum tendons (*closed arrows*), consistent with septic tenosynovitis. There is also extensive and enhancing soft tissue edema reflective of cellulitis, in this context.

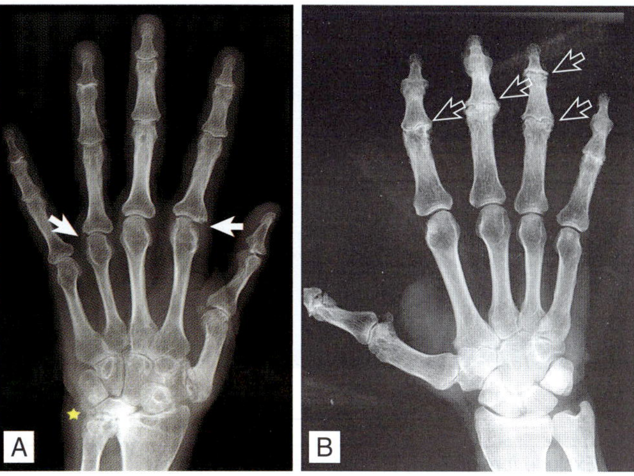

Figure 58.49 Posteroanterior (PA) radiograph (A) of the hand demonstrates periarticular osteopenia with marginal erosions (*closed arrows*) adjacent the second and fourth metacarpophalangeal joints, as well as erosions and remodeling of the ulnar styloid (*yellow star*). There are also features of carpal instability with scapholunate widening and progression towards a scapholunate advanced collapse wrist. These findings are associated with rheumatoid arthritis, which had been previously diagnosed in this patient. PA radiograph (B) of the hand from a different patient demonstrates multiple proximal and distal interphalangeal joint central or paramedian erosions with overhanging marginal osteophytes giving a "gull-wing" appearance (*open arrows*), consistent with erosive osteoarthritis. Note some of the distal interphalangeal joints have fused.

subset of osteoarthritis, and the distribution follows that of conventional osteoarthritis. Similarly, there are joint space loss and subchondral sclerosis, but central or paramedian articular erosions result in typical gull-wing contouring of the articular surfaces.

Conclusion

This chapter has provided an overview of some of the common clinical conditions that may affect the hand and wrist. Please refer to the flow charts provided in Figs. 58.50 to 58.52, adapted from the American College of Radiology appropriateness criteria, when deciding on which imaging modality to use based on the patient's clinical presentation and the clinical context [26].

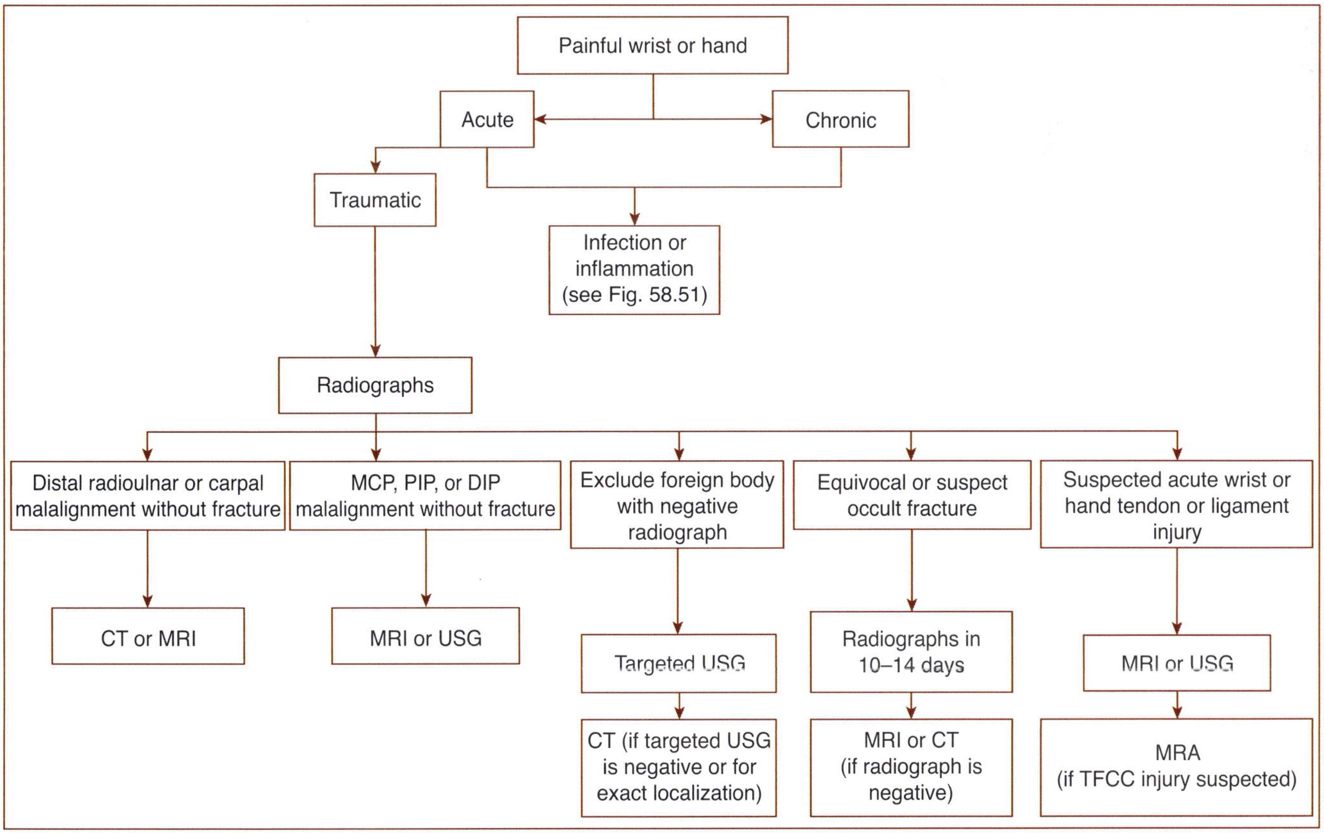

- Painful wrist or hand
  - Acute
    - Traumatic
      - Radiographs
        - Distal radioulnar or carpal malalignment without fracture → CT or MRI
        - MCP, PIP, or DIP malalignment without fracture → MRI or USG
        - Exclude foreign body with negative radiograph → Targeted USG → CT (if targeted USG is negative or for exact localization)
        - Equivocal or suspect occult fracture → Radiographs in 10–14 days → MRI or CT (if radiograph is negative)
        - Suspected acute wrist or hand tendon or ligament injury → MRI or USG → MRA (if TFCC injury suspected)
  - Acute / Chronic
    - Infection or inflammation (see Fig. 58.51)
  - Chronic

Figure 58.50 Painful wrist and hand. *CT,* Computed tomography; *DIP,* distal interphalangeal; *MCP,* metacarpophalangeal; *MRA,* magnetic resonance arthrography; *MRI,* magnetic resonance imaging; *PIP,* proximal interphalangeal; *TFCC,* triangular fibrocartilage complex; *USG,* ultrasonography.

and predispose to arthritis; these will be discussed later. Important parameters to assess imaging include:

- The shape of the femoral head and neck
- The angle of the femoral neck compared with the shaft (normal 120–140 degrees) (Fig. 59.2A)
- Femoral version, which refers to the angle of the femoral neck compared with the acetabulum (a normal angle is 5–20 degrees of anteversion) [10,11] (Fig. 59.2B)

One important anatomic area of the proximal femur is the calcar femorale, also known as the "calcar." This is a region of vertically oriented dense bone that originates from the posteromedial surface of the proximal femoral diaphysis, near the lesser trochanter.

In adults, the epiphysis typically has yellow (fatty) marrow, while there is red (hematopoietic) marrow in the femoral neck and intertrochanteric region. On MRI, yellow marrow follows fat signal, while red marrow is lower on T1-weighted images than fat but higher than muscle, and higher on T2-weighted images than muscle. *Reconversion of red marrow in the adult takes place in a symmetric and predictable pattern, first occurring metaphyses of long bones from proximal to distal and from the metaphysis to the diaphysis, usually sparing the epiphysis* (Fig. 59.3). There can be an area of apparent demarcation in the proximal femoral diaphysis, which is the normal junction of red and yellow marrow, but can mimic a lesion/area of marrow replacement [12].

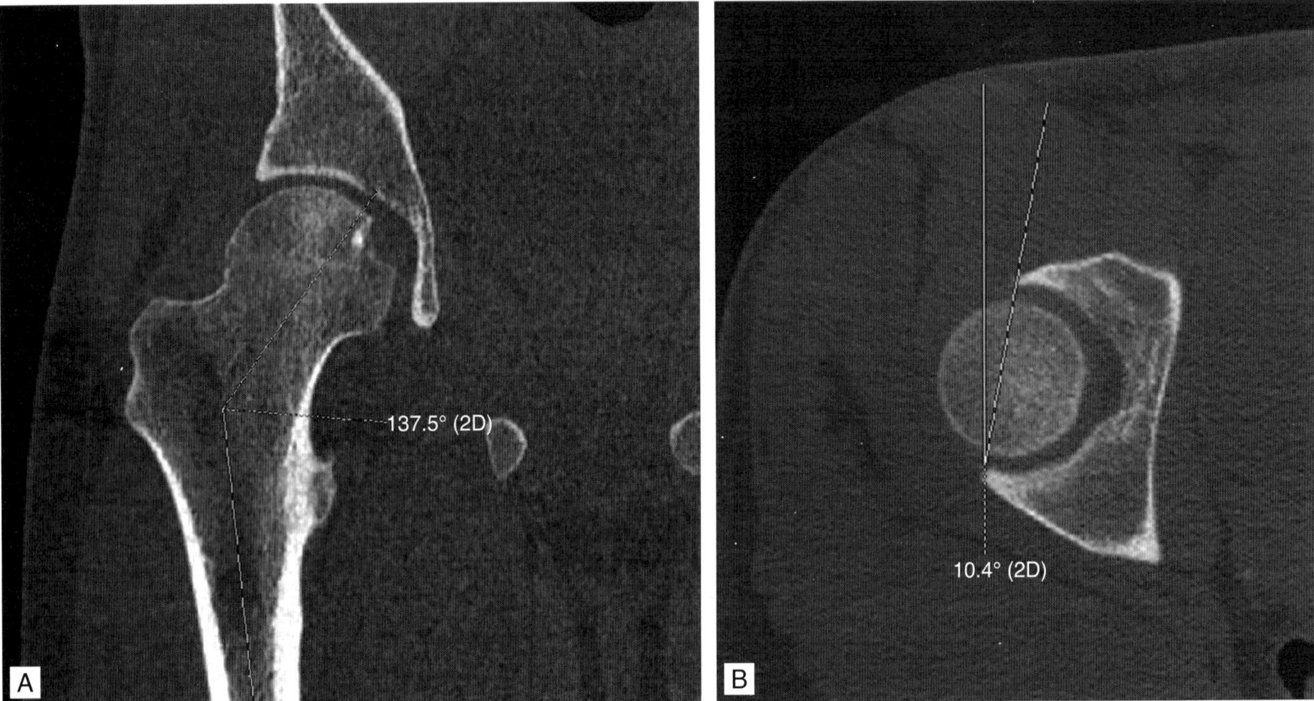

Figure 59.2 CT measurements of hip joint. (A) Coronal CT image shows measurement of the femoral neck–shaft angle (normal is 120–140 degrees). (B) Axial CT image shows measurement of acetabular version; in this case, there are about 10 degrees of anteversion (normal is 5–20 degrees anteversion).

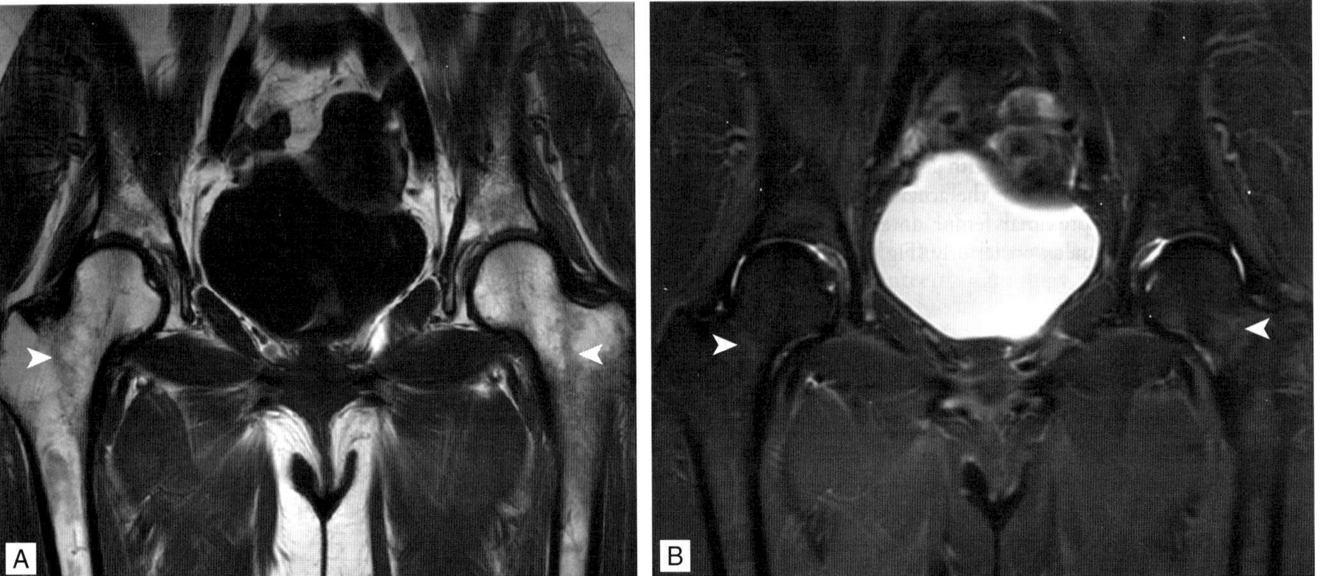

Figure 59.3 Red marrow reconversion in an adult patient. Coronal MR T1-weighted (A) and T2-weighted (B) images show bilaterally symmetric areas of red marrow (*arrowheads*), which are higher in signal than skeletal muscle on T1-weighted and T2-weighted images.

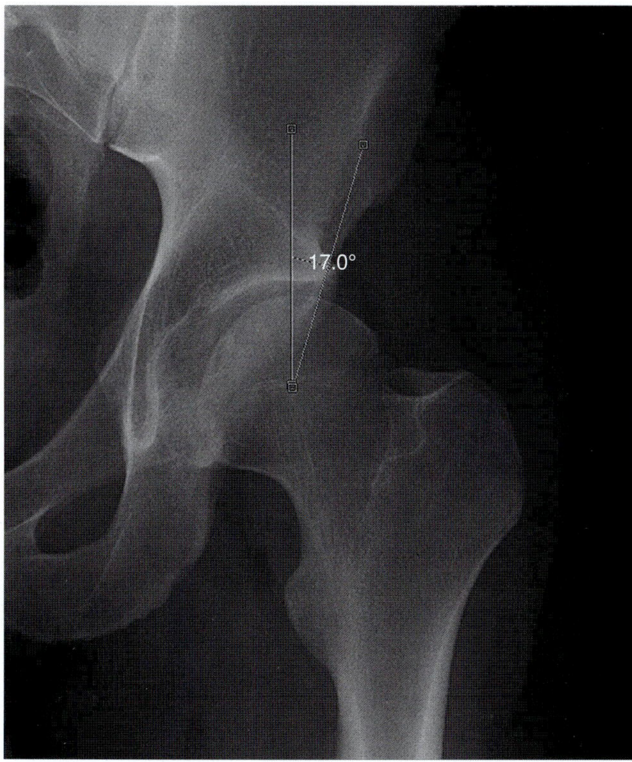

Figure 59.4 Measurement of a center-edge angle, which is calculated by finding the angle between a vertical line through the center of the femoral head and the superolateral acetabulum. This patient has a center-edge angle of less than 20 degrees, which is considered to be within the range of acetabular dysplasia.

The femoral head's main blood supply comes from the medial and lateral circumflex femoral arteries, which are branches of the deep femoral artery. There is also a small contribution from the foveal artery, located adjacent to the ligamentum teres, although this is mostly relevant in the pediatric age group. Femoral neck fractures disrupt the arterial branches extending medially from the circumflex femoral arteries, which puts the femoral head at risk of avascular necrosis, thus necessitating hip arthroplasty. An intertrochanteric fracture does not disrupt blood supply to the femoral head, and therefore can be retained and fracture approximated using surgical screws.

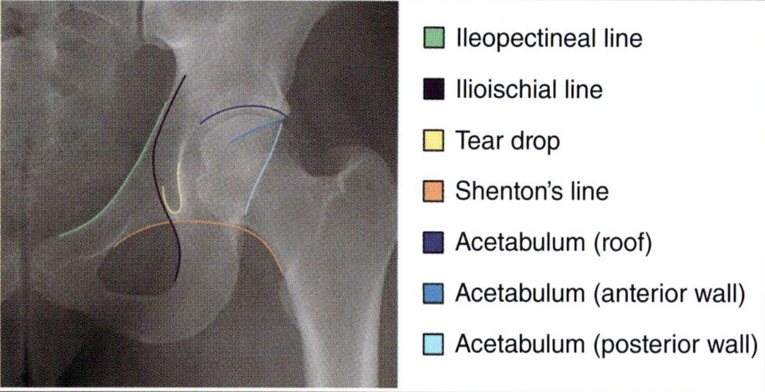

Figure 59.5 Pelvic radiograph with superimposed lines, which should be smooth and uninterrupted when normal. Any irregularity or step-off should prompt investigation for fracture or other pathology.

Acetabulum/Pelvis: The acetabulum is made up of portions of three bones i.e., ilium, ischium, and pubis of the pelvis. Its shape is approximately two-thirds of a sphere, and it usually has mild anteversion and lateral opening. The acetabular socket is open at the inferior aspect, with the transverse ligament spanning the inferior margin and holding the femoral head in place (Fig. 59.1). Just as proximal femoral anatomy variants can cause pathology, abnormal acetabular morphology can also cause chronic issues; these will be discussed in a later section. One standard measurement taken on imaging studies is the center-edge angle, which refers to the angle formed between a vertical line through the center of the femoral head and the most superolateral portion of the acetabulum (Fig. 59.4). A normal angle is above 25 degrees; in dysplasia (acetabular under-coverage) it is less than 20 degrees, and angles over 40 degrees suggest acetabular over coverage [13,14].

On radiographs, multiple lines can be traced on osseous structures on either side of the pelvis, including the main pelvic ring and obturator foramina [15]. These lines should be symmetric bilaterally without step-off or disruption; any deviation from this pattern suggests a fracture or other injury. These lines are illustrated in Fig. 59.5 and are described in Table 59.1.

TABLE 59.1 Pelvic Lines

	Anatomy	Disruption Suggestive of:
Iliopectineal line	Medial border of iliac wing to superior border of pubic bone	Anterior column fracture or pubic bone fracture
Ilioischial line	Lateral border of obturator foramen to medial border of iliac wing	Posterior column fracture
Pelvic teardrop	U-shaped structure along the medial acetabular wall due to an osseous ridge	Increased distance between pelvic teardrop and femoral head is a sign of hip joint effusion (Waldenstrom sign) >11-mm total or >2-mm asymmetry [13]; could also suggest an acetabular fracture
Shenton's line	Inferior border of superior pubic ramus to inferomedial border of femoral neck	Femoral neck fracture or developmental dysplasia of the hip
Acetabular roof	Border of superior acetabulum	Fracture
Anterior acetabular rim	Projects over the posterior rim	If projecting laterally compared with the posterior rim, suggestive of pincer-type deformity ("crossover sign")
Posterior acetabular rim	Posterior portion of acetabular wall	Prominent posterior acetabular rim suggests over-coverage ("posterior wall sign")
Sacral arcuate lines	Inferior surfaces of bone that form the roofs of sacral foramina	Sacral fracture

Cartilage

The femoral head is covered by hyaline cartilage, *except for the fovea, which is a central depression in which the ligamentum teres arises* (Fig. 59.1) [8]. The acetabulum contains horseshoe-shaped hyaline cartilage with a depression in the central roof called the "acetabular fossa." The cartilage in the hip joint can be difficult to evaluate on imaging, as it is a covered curved surface and is relatively thin compared with other large joints like the knee. MR arthrography is typically the imaging study of choice and has a sensitivity of 50–79% and specificity of 77–84% for cartilage defects [16].

Labrum

The labrum is made of *fibrocartilage* and is attached to the osseous rim of the acetabulum. It is thickest superiorly and posteriorly. The labrum blends inferiorly with the transverse ligament along the edges of the acetabular notch (Fig. 59.1). The labrum attaches to the acetabulum near the joint capsule, and *the small gap between the two can be seen on imaging as a perilabral sulcus.* There is controversy over the etiology of a cleft at the interface between the labrum and hyaline cartilage in the anterosuperior quadrant, with some authors considering this to be a normal variant but others report this as a tear [8]. A normal labrum has a triangular configuration in cross section and low signal on T1-weighted images [17] (Fig. 59.6). *Symptomatic tears most commonly involve the anterosuperior labrum.*

Tendons

There are numerous tendon attachments in the pelvis and hips. Table 59.2 gives details regarding these tendons, and Fig. 59.7 shows the tendon attachment sites on a pelvic radiograph. On MRI, tendons should appear as low signal, linear structures. *Any intrasubstance high signal, thickening, or fluid-signal clefts on MRI suggest pathology such as tendinosis or tear* [18]. One potential pitfall on MRI is the "magic angle" artifact. Dense, fibrillary structures, such as tendons, will appear falsely high in signal on

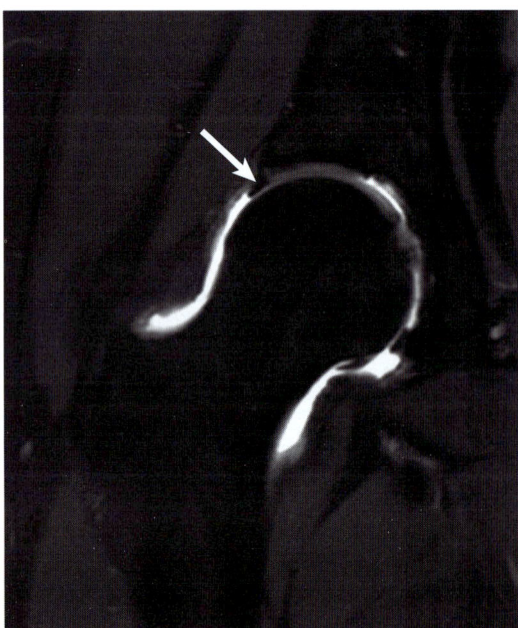

Figure 59.6 Coronal MR arthrogram image shows the normal, low-signal, triangular labrum (*arrow*).

TABLE 59.2 Tendon Attachments in the Pelvis and Hips

	Proximal Attachment	Distal Attachment
Sartorius	Anterior superior iliac spine	Proximal, medial tibia
Quadriceps Tendons		
Rectus femoris	(Heads fuse proximal to muscle belly)	
Direct head	Anterior inferior iliac spine	Patella
Indirect head	Posterior acetabulum	
Vastus lateralis	Greater trochanter, intertrochanteric line, linea aspera	Patella
Vastus intermedius	Anterolateral femoral diaphysis, linea aspera	Patella
Vastus medialis	Intertrochanteric line, linea aspera	Patella
Gluteal Tendons		
Minimus	Lateral ilium	Anterior facet of greater trochanter
Medius	Iliac crest and posterior ilium	Muscular: lateral facet of greater trochanter Tendinous: superoposterior facet of greater trochanter
Maximus	Sacrum, coccyx, and sacrotuberous ligament	Posterosuperior femur and iliotibial tract
Hamstring Tendons		
Semimembranosus	Superolateral facet of ischial tuberosity	Posteromedial femoral condyle
Semitendinosis	Ischial tuberosity (common origin with biceps femoris—conjoint tendon)	Proximal, medial tibia
Biceps femoris	Ischial tuberosity (common origin with semitendinosis—conjoined tendon)	Head of fibula
Adductor Tendons		
Adductor longus	Anterior pubis	Linea aspera
Adductor magnus	Pubofemoral portion: ischiopubic ramus Ischiocondylar portion ("mini hamstring"): tendinous attachment to ischial tuberosity	Pubofemoral portion: lower gluteal line and linea aspera Ischiocondylar portion: adductor tubercle
Adductor brevis	Inferior pubic ramus	Linea aspera
Iliopsoas Tendon		
Iliacus	Iliac fossa/crest, anterior ligaments of SI joint, lumbosacral, and iliosacral ligaments	Lesser trochanter
Psoas	Transverse processes of lumbar vertebrae	Lesser trochanter
Tensor fascia latae	Lateral edge of iliac crest, anterior superior iliac spine, sacrotuberous ligament, sacrum/coccyx	Middle third of the femur
Iliotibial tract	Thickened fascia originates from tensor fascia latae and gluteus maximus muscles	Gerdy's tubercle

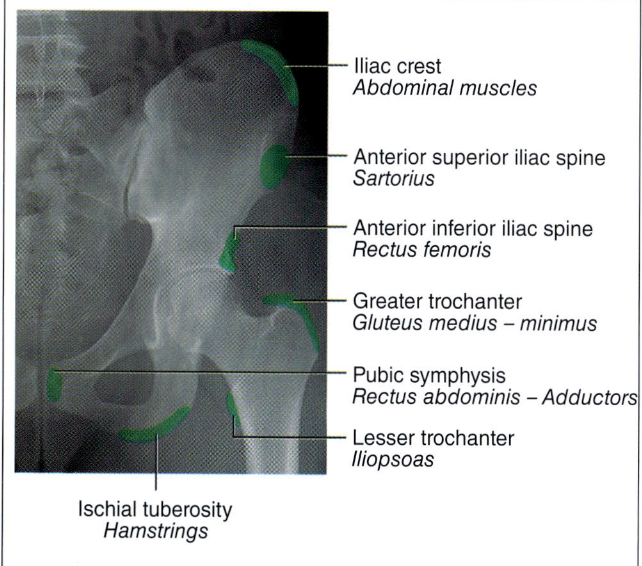

Figure 59.7 Pelvic radiograph with superimposed tendon attachment sites.

specific sequences (proton density, T1-weighted, and gradient echo) when at an angle of 55 degrees to the main magnetic field. Findings should be confirmed or rejected based on cumulative appearances on other sequences, such as T2-weighted sequences. This magic angle artifact on MRI corresponds to the anisotropy artifact on USG. On USG, tendons should have a fibrillar appearance and linear configuration; toggling the USG probe can change the appearance from hypo to hyperechoic, which is an artifact known as anisotropy.

Pubic Symphysis

The pubic symphysis is a nonsynovial joint formed by the confluence of the two pubic bones with an intervening fibrocartilaginous disk (Fig. 59.8). The medial surfaces of the pubic bones are covered by hyaline cartilage, and four ligaments are surrounding the joint (superior, arcuate/inferior, and anterior, posterior). Superiorly, the rectus abdominus and external oblique aponeurosis merge with the superficial layer of the anterior ligament. Inferiorly, the adductor longus and gracilis proximal attachments also merge with the aponeurosis, which attaches to the pubic bone.

Summary of Teaching Points: Functional Anatomy Section

- The hip is a ball-and-socket-type, synovial joint with a capsule extending over a relatively large span, including the femoral head and much of the femoral neck. Capsular thickening (7 mm or more) indicates intra-articular pathology (synovitis, joint effusion, etc.), can have clinical manifestations, including a limited range of motion.
- Normal marrow appearance in the pelvis should be bilateral and symmetric.
- Red marrow reconversion follows a predictable pattern, from first to last: proximal metaphysis, distal metaphysis, diaphysis, epiphysis (usually spared)
- On radiographs, trace symmetric lines on both sides of the pelvis and proximal femurs; if lines are disrupted or asymmetric, consider fracture or another source of pathology
- A normal labrum has a triangular configuration in cross–section and low signal on T1-weighted images. The labrum blends with the transverse ligament inferiorly. Sulci can be formed at the labral–capsular junctions, which can mimic tears. Symptomatic tears most commonly involve the anterosuperior labrum.
- On MRI, tendons should appear as linear, low signal structures; consider "magic angle" artifact on certain MRI sequences when the tendon is at a 55-degree angle.
- At the pubic symphysis, the rectus aponeurosis attaches to bone and blends inferiorly with the adductor aponeurosis.
- Native/anatomic bursas are synovial-lined structures; adventitial bursas develop at sites of friction) and do not have a synovial lining.

Bursas

There are numerous bursas in pelvis and hip region (Fig. 59.9). Anatomic (native) bursas are synovial-lined structures, while adventitial (non-native) bursts do not have a synovial lining and can develop at sites of pressure and friction. *Bursas can be filled with fluid, but the term "bursitis" should not be used unless there is imaging evidence of inflammation* [19]. Some commonly encountered bursas in the pelvis and hips are described in Table 59.3.

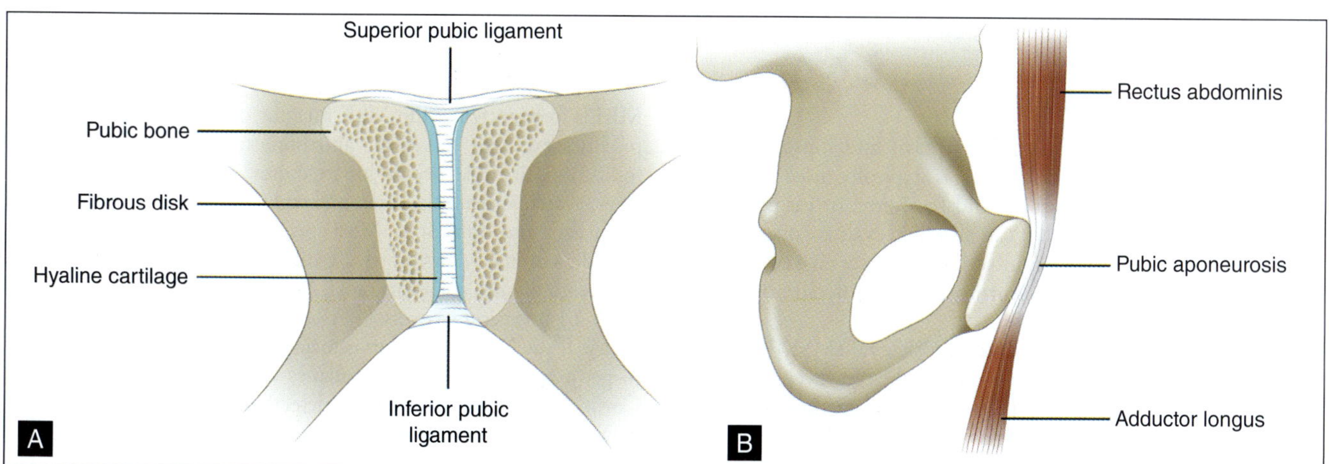

Figure 59.8 Illustration of pubic symphysis anatomy (A) and muscle attachments (B).

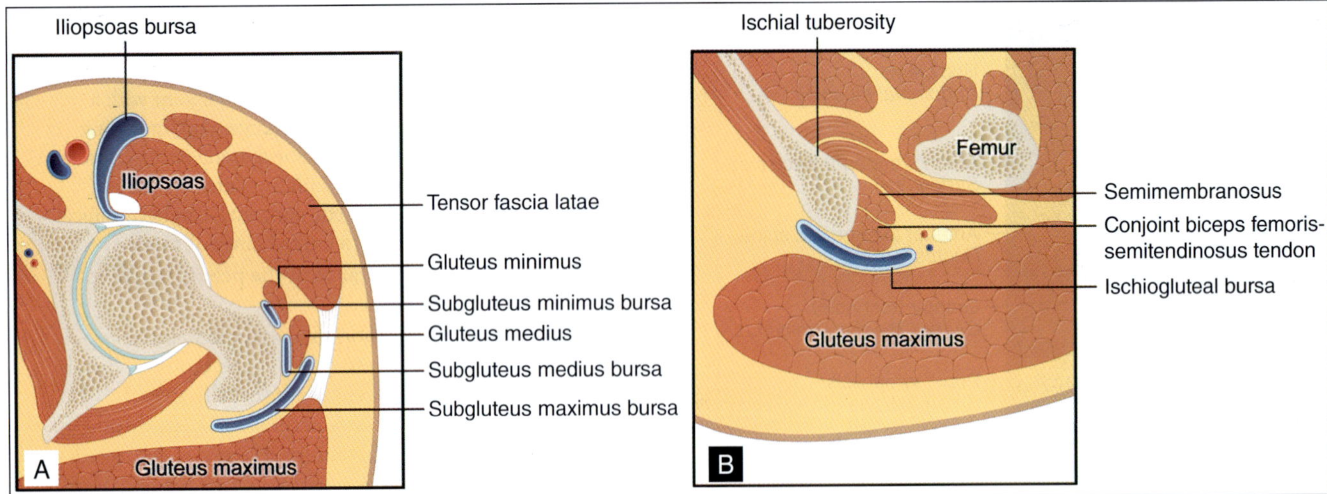

Figure 59.9 Illustration of bursas about the hip (A) and ischial tuberosity (B).

TABLE 59.3 Commonly Encountered Bursas in the Pelvis and Hips

	Associated Tendons	Comments
Iliopsoas	Iliopsoas	Communicates with the joint in 10–15% [20]
Subgluteus minimus	Gluteus minimus	
Subgluteus medius	Gluteus medius	
Subgluteus maximus	Gluteus maximus	Largest in the region; often called "greater trochanteric" bursa
Ischiogluteal	Hamstring tendons	In proximity to sciatic and posterior femoral cutaneous nerves

Imaging Techniques and Protocol

Radiographs

Radiographs remain the first-line study for evaluating most conditions in the pelvis and hip, including acute trauma, chronic conditions, such as arthritis, and the workup of any unknown cause of pain. Table 59.4 lists radiographic views of the hip and describes patient positioning and typical pathology that is best seen on each view [21,22].

Computed Tomography (CT)

CT is a useful tool in evaluating the pelvis and hips, especially when osseous detail is required. It is typically used in acute trauma, to assess fracture healing and hardware, or for preoperative measurements. However, it can also help evaluate osseous and soft-tissue tumors as well as an infection. CT may give even better details than radiographs of the cortex, matrix mineralization, and soft-tissue calcifications [23].

High resolution is crucial in musculoskeletal (MSK) CT, and often the thinnest slices possible are desirable. However, this must be balanced with the need to keep the radiation dose as low as possible. Some considerations are as follows:

- Thin sections can help identify femoral neck and acetabular fractures and help evaluate osseous bridging and fracture healing.
- Three-dimensional reconstructions can be used for preoperative planning and evaluation of fractures.
- Intravenous contrast is typically given for the evaluation of neoplasm and infection; postcontrast images alone are often sufficient in MSK CT to significantly reduce dose in younger patients.
- Metal can cause beam hardening or the loss of lower-energy photons as the beam passes through an object, resulting in streaks and dark bands [24]. Hardware suppression protocols are thus beneficial in the presence of hip arthroplasties and other metallic hardware [24].
- The use of dual-energy CT is limited in the hip due to depth.

Ultrasonography (USG)

Although some structures of the pelvis and hip are relatively deep, USG can be utilized for the evaluation of most of these structures. Typically, a linear 5–12 MHz probe is used in MSK USG. Still, a curvilinear 4–9 MHz probe is often helpful when evaluating the hip, as the lower frequency gives more penetration, although lower resolution. The patient is placed supine to scan the hip and anterior thigh and prone to scan the posterior thigh and hamstring tendons.

Tables 59.5 describes primary indications in which hip USG can be diagnostic and when it can be limited, and Table 59.6 describes common USG interventions.

Magnetic Resonance Imaging (MRI)

MRI is frequently used in MSK imaging of the pelvis and hips and provides excellent soft tissue and bone marrow detail. Common indications include occult hip fractures, stress/insufficiency fractures, avascular necrosis, and labral and tendon pathology, as well as neoplasm and infection. Most pelvis and hip MRI protocols include coronal views of the entire pelvis, typically with both T1-weighted and a fat-saturated, fluid-sensitive sequence, such as short-T1 inversion recovery (STIR). This allows evaluation for symmetry. If the MRI evaluation is focused on a single hip, it is helpful to get a sequence in all three planes (axial, coronal, and sagittal). Coronal sequences are best for detecting hip fractures, but other planes help to confirm the fracture and allow evaluation of other structures. Proton density (PD) sequences, especially with fat-saturation allow excellent evaluation of soft-tissue anatomy, and are

TABLE 59.4 Radiographic Views of the Hip

Radiographic View	Positioning	Helps Evaluate/ Identify
Anteroposterior or AP (standard view)	Internal rotation (toes in)	Femoral neck fracture, arthritis, dysplasia, FAI, effusion
Frog-leg	External rotation, bilateral hips	Shape of femoral head, SCFE, Perthes disease
Horizontal ray/crosstable	Internal rotation, contralateral hip flexed 90 degrees (out of the way)	Injury in trauma patients; head–neck junction and anterior/posterior dislocation
False profile	Patient standing, pelvis rotated at 65 degrees	Shape of acetabulum, anterior coverage of femoral head, impingement, measurement of anterior center-edge angle
Judet	Two projections: ▪ Iliac oblique in which unaffected side is rotated 45 degrees anterior ▪ Obturator oblique in which affected side is rotated 45 degrees anterior	Acetabular fracture; iliac oblique shows anterior acetabulum and ilioischial column, while obturator oblique shows posterior acetabulum and posterior acetabular rim
Inlet–outlet	Supine, beam tilted caudally and cranially	Inlet view: posterior displacement of pelvic ring, pubic symphyseal disruption Outlet view: vertical shift

FAI, femoroacetabular impingement; *SCFE*, slipped capital femoral epiphysis.

TABLE 59.5 Utility of Hip USG

Indications	Limitations
Hip joint effusion	Intra-articular pathology
Fluid collections	Labral tears
Tendons and tendinosis	Posterior hip
Snapping Hip	Osseous evaluation
Bursal distention and bursitis	Patient obesity
Greater trochanteric pain syndrome	Fatty infiltration of muscles
Inguinal and femoral hernias	

TABLE 59.6 Common Hip USG Interventions

Procedure	Clinical Setting
Hip joint aspiration	Suspected infection
Hip joint injection	Hip pain and/or arthritis
Aspiration of fluid collections	Suspected infection
Injection of iliopsoas peritendon	Hip pain
Bursal injection (trochanteric or iliopsoas)	Bursitis/pain
Needling/tenotomy	Tendinosis
Platelet-rich plasma injection	Tendinosis

frequently used. If there is a suspicion of infection or mass, gadolinium contrast can be useful; pre- and postcontrast, fat-saturated, T1-weighted sequences tend to show the contrast better.

Some special sequences can be utilized for problem solving, such as T1 in- and opposed-phase coronal sequences of the entire pelvis, which helps to distinguish red marrow reconversion (loses signal on out-of-phase sequence, appearing dark) from a pathologic process like neoplasm (does not lose signal). MR arthrography of the hip is used in younger individuals to evaluate intra-articular pathology and labral tears. This involves a separate injection of gadolinium contrast into hip joint (under fluoroscopic or USG guidance) just before MRI. The operator should take care to avoid air in the injectate, which appears as low signal areas on the MRI (Table 59.7).

Nuclear Medicine

Although nuclear imaging is less frequently used than other techniques when evaluating the hip, bone scan, typically utilizing technetium-99m-labeled diphosphonate can be helpful in the evaluation of stress and insufficiency fractures, avascular necrosis, osseous metastatic disease, and prosthetic loosening. One finding worth mentioning is that of a "superscan," in which intense, symmetric radiotracer uptake is seen in the bones, with relative paucity of uptake in the soft tissues and kidneys. This condition can be seen in the setting of diffuse osseous metastatic disease and other diffuse processes that affect the bones, such as hyperparathyroidism, renal osteodystrophy, and osteomalacia.

Single photon emission computed tomography (SPECT) can be used for better localization if bladder uptake obscures the

TABLE 59.7 A Sample MRI Reporting Template of Hip

MRI of the hip
Clinical information:
Technique: (description of protocol, sequences, and use of contrast)
Comparison studies:
Findings: Osseous Joints Labrum Tendons Muscles Bursas Other (lymph nodes, neurovascular, incidental findings)
Impression

pathology. A labeled white blood cell (WBC) scan can be useful in evaluating osteomyelitis, especially in patients who cannot undergo MRI because of a pacemaker or other implant.

Summary of Teaching Points: Imaging Techniques and Protocol Section

- Radiographs are the first-line study for most hip and pelvis imaging
- CT is useful to evaluate osseous detail and orthopedic hardware
- US can be especially helpful to evaluate for joint effusion, tendon pathology, fluid collections, and bursitis
- MRI is an excellent tool for soft tissue and bone marrow evaluation
- Nuclear medicine can be helpful for problem solving, including labeled WBC scan for osteomyelitis

Joint Pathology

Central/Hip Joint Region

Patients with pathology in the hip joint and/or central region will often present with groin pain or hip pain. Radiographs are the first-line imaging technique to assess for joint and/or osseous involvement, but cross-sectional imaging, including MRI or potentially an MR arthrogram, may need to be considered.

Hip Joint

Hip joint-based processes, such as arthritis, are well evaluated on imaging, and accurate diagnosis also depends on the clinical scenario. Osteoarthrosis (OA) is due to degeneration and abnormality of hyaline cartilage, and its primary form is usually due to overuse and/or old age. Secondary OA is a similar process but resulting after some insult, such as trauma, hip dislocation, or hip dysplasia. The hallmarks of OA on imaging are:

- Osteophytes
- Joint space narrowing
- Subchondral cysts
- Subchondral sclerosis

Because the hip is a weight-bearing joint, and the cartilage on the weight-bearing surfaces wears out first, there is often asymmetric

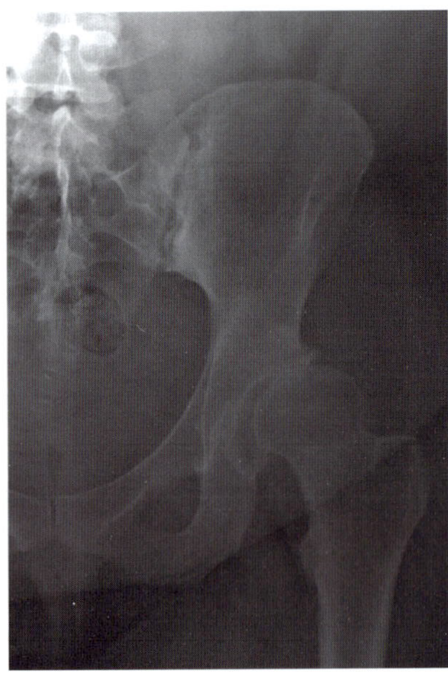

Figure 59.10 Osteoarthrosis. A frontal radiograph of the hip shows complete, asymmetric joint space loss in the superior hip joint with bone-on-bone articulation, sclerosis, and osteophyte formation, consistent with severe osteoarthrosis.

joint space narrowing in the areas of greatest force, usually the superior joint (Fig. 59.10).

Inflammatory arthritis, in contrast, results from inflammation and synovial proliferation in the hip joint, which can lead to erosions and effusion. Marginal erosions occur when inflammatory synovial tissue (pannus) erodes the bone in the "bare area" of the intra-articular bone, where there is no hyaline cartilage. Joint space narrowing is typically concentric or involving the entire joint (Fig. 59.11). In the hip, this can appear as axial femoral head migration and remodeling in the central acetabulum, causing protrusion, or displacement of the

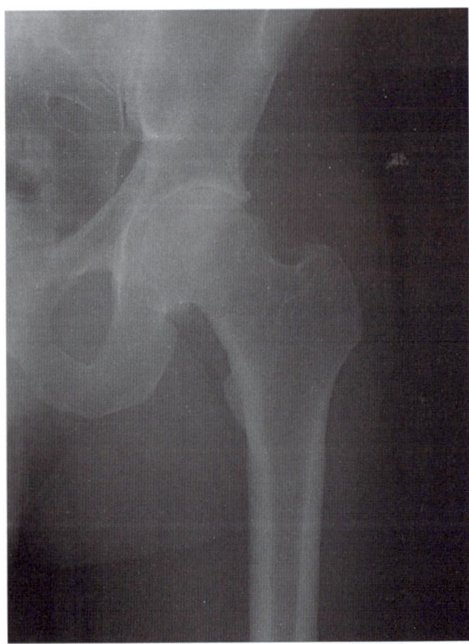

Figure 59.11 Rheumatoid arthritis. An anteroposterior (AP) radiograph of the hip shows severe, concentric joint space narrowing with only mild sclerosis and small osteophytes, atypical for osteoarthrosis. This patient was only 35 years old, but had a history of rheumatoid arthritis.

TABLE 59.8 Imaging Features of Osteoarthrosis Compared to Inflammatory Athritis

	Osteoarthrosis	Inflammatory Arthritis
Radiographic findings	Osteophytes Joint space narrowing Subchondral cysts Sclerosis	Erosions (possibly marginal) Joint space narrowing Periarticular osteopenia
Joint effusion	Sometimes	Yes (often)
Joint space narrowing	Typically worst on weight-bearing surfaces; asymmetric	Entire joint (concentric)
Clinical presentation	Hip pain, often in older/ elderly patients and/or due to previous trauma or overuse	Hip pain and stiffness, worse in the morning, women > men in 20s–40s

femoral head into the pelvis, past the ilioischial line. Coxa profunda, in contrast, refers to the acetabulum being medial to the ilioischial line. A well-centered pelvic radiograph is essential for evaluation.

Rheumatoid arthritis (RA), common inflammatory arthritis, has a different clinical presentation than OA, with:

- Women more affected than men
- Patients typically diagnosed in their 20–40 years of age
- Patients having joint stiffness in the morning with pain and swelling in multiple, symmetric joints
- Positive rheumatoid factor in blood

Seronegative spondyloarthropathies, especially ankylosing spondylitis, may involve the hip, although rheumatoid factor should be negative in these patients.

Table 59.8 lists a comparison of imaging features between OA and RA. It is important to note that some patients with RA will also have secondary OA with osteophytes and more severe joint space narrowing on the weight-bearing surface.

Radiologists should be aware of the recent discussion in the literature of the entity known as rapidly destructive osteoarthritis (RDOA) of hip, which is a progression of degenerative changes over 6–12 months to complete joint destruction [25]. This entity is typically unilateral and most often seen in elderly patients, especially women. Some authors have suggested that RDOA of the hip may be related to steroid injection, with a faster progression to arthroplasty after the procedure [26,27]. Although the literature is not entirely conclusive, the possibility of RDOA should be discussed with patients who underwent hip steroid injection before the procedure and during consent.

Septic Joint

A septic hip is an orthopedic emergency, as an acute infection can irreversibly destroy native hip cartilage within hours. The radiologist can make a difference in clinical management and outcome by helping to identify this entity early in its course. The clinical presentation is crucial when interpreting imaging studies. Patients with an acute septic hip will often present with an acute onset of joint pain, extreme limitation of movement, swelling, redness, and a feeling of heat in the joint. Patients might have a flexion deformity of the hip and be unable to bear weight.

The progression of a septic hip is shown in Fig. 59.12. Although radiographs are the first-line evaluation tool, a negative radiograph does not necessarily exclude a septic joint, and cross-sectional imaging should be considered when there is high clinical suspicion. CT or MRI might show only joint effusion even in the setting of a septic hip (Fig. 59.13). These techniques can also help to rule out other pathologies, such as a hip fracture or soft-tissue process. If there is clinical suspicion of an acute septic hip and a joint effusion is seen, emergent joint aspiration is warranted, and this is frequently done with fluoroscopic or USG guidance. Typically a large-bore needle is used to allow for aspirate that could be viscous, and initially lavage should be avoided to allow for proper cell count. *Lidocaine injection into the joint is contraindicated, as the solution can be antimicrobial.* A positive diagnosis of a septic joint typically prompts a surgical washout procedure, which can prevent additional joint destruction.

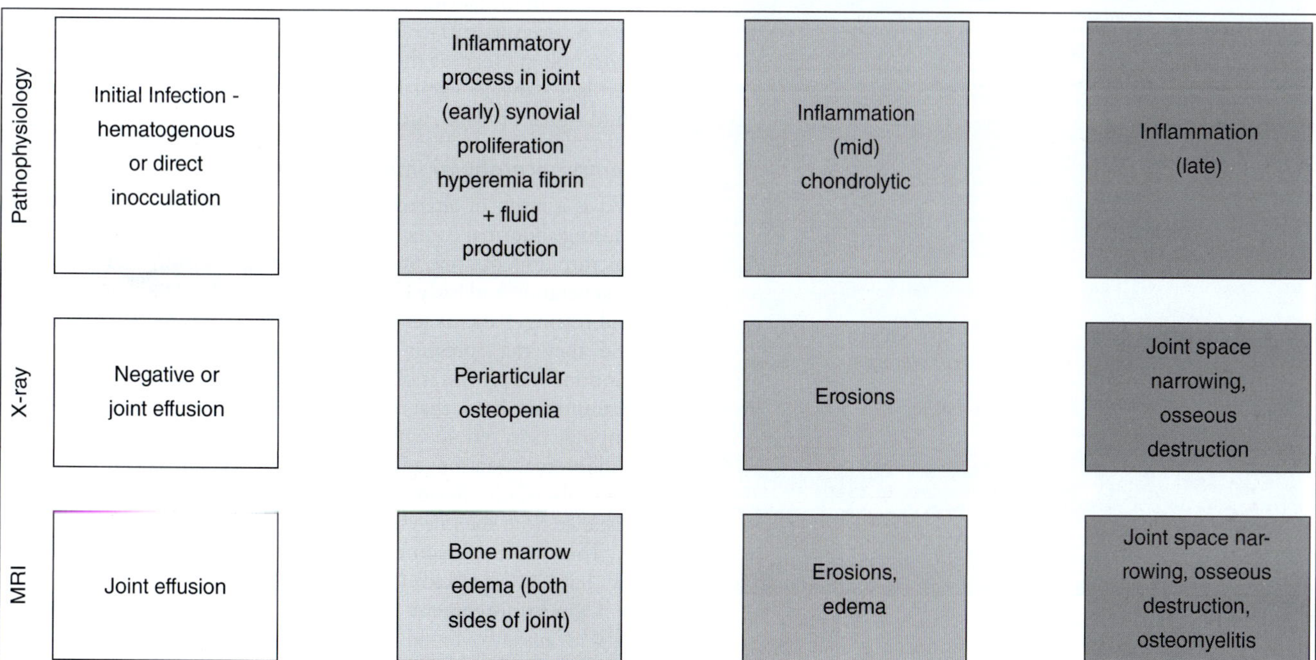

Figure 59.12 Flowchart for pathophysiology of septic hip with imaging correlates.

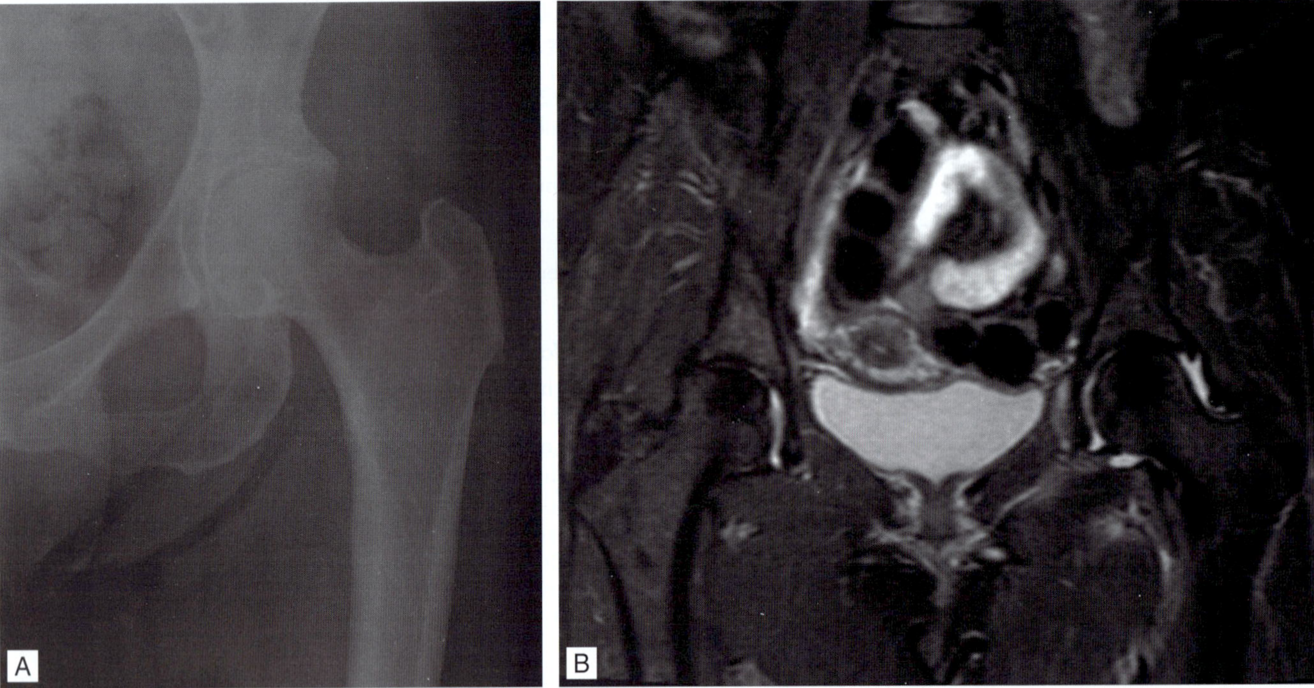

Figure 59.13 Septic hip. Initial radiograph is normal (A). Coronal STIR MR image (B) left hip joint effusion, without marrow signal changes.

Labral Tear

Suspected labral tears are a common indication for hip imaging. Patients tend to be in the younger age group (teens to 30s) and are often active. Presenting symptoms include hip or groin pain with catching and/or locking of the hip. Labral tears can be caused by trauma, overuse, FAI, and hip dysplasia, although labral degeneration is common with increasing age. Especially in patients older than 40, labral tears can an asymptomatic and/or incidental finding, which can add confusion when reviewing the study for a source of pain. It may be prudent to describe the findings with different verbiage than the word "tear" in such situations [28].

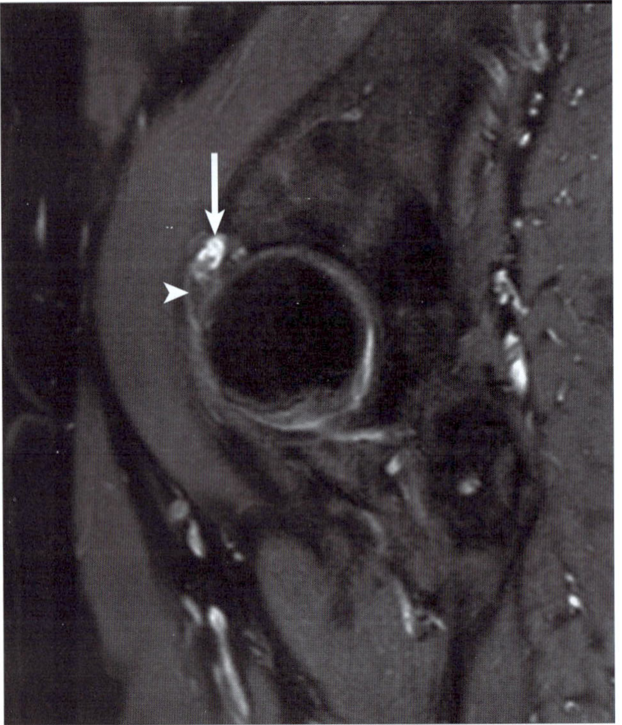

Figure 59.14 Labral tear. Sagittal proton density fat-saturated (PDFS) MR image of the hip shows high signal and abnormal morphology of the anterosuperior labrum (*arrowhead*) with fluid-signal, multiloculated paralabral cyst (*arrow*) emanating from the tear.

MR arthrogram is the study of choice to evaluate for labral tears, on which they will appear as a contrast-filled defect within the normally low-signal labrum (Fig. 59.14) [8]. *Tears are most common in the anterior or anterosuperior region, with some studies showing as many as 86% of tears in this location* [29]. On a non-MR arthrogram, labral tears can appear as linear, increased signal intensity in the labrum or at the chondro-labral junction, but may also be seen as surface irregularity or truncation of the normal morphology. Tears at the chondral junction may suggest adjacent cartilage damage. Paralabral cysts, which appear as multiloculated fluid signal on MRI, are highly suggestive of tears.

Femoroacetabular Impingement

FAI is a result of altered morphology of bone involving the hip, causing abnormal contact of the femur and acetabulum. Repetitive microtrauma of bone on the cartilage and labrum causes cartilage degeneration and early OA of the hip as well as labral degeneration and tearing. Patients tend to be younger (teens to 30s) and active, and they may present with hip pain and restricted range of motion. The process is often bilateral and symmetric [30]. Physical examination tests that might suggest FAI include the anterior impingement test, in which the flexed hip is forced into adduction and internal rotation, and the "FABER" test, in which the patient's leg is placed into flexion, abduction, and external rotation, and the distance from the knee to the examination table is measured [31].

There are two main categories of FAI, although some patients can have both (mixed) (Fig. 59.13A):

- **Cam impingement**
  - Caused by broad osseous protuberance at the anterolateral femoral head–neck junction, causing loss of normal concavity that looks like a pistol grip (Figs. 59.15A1 and 59.15B)

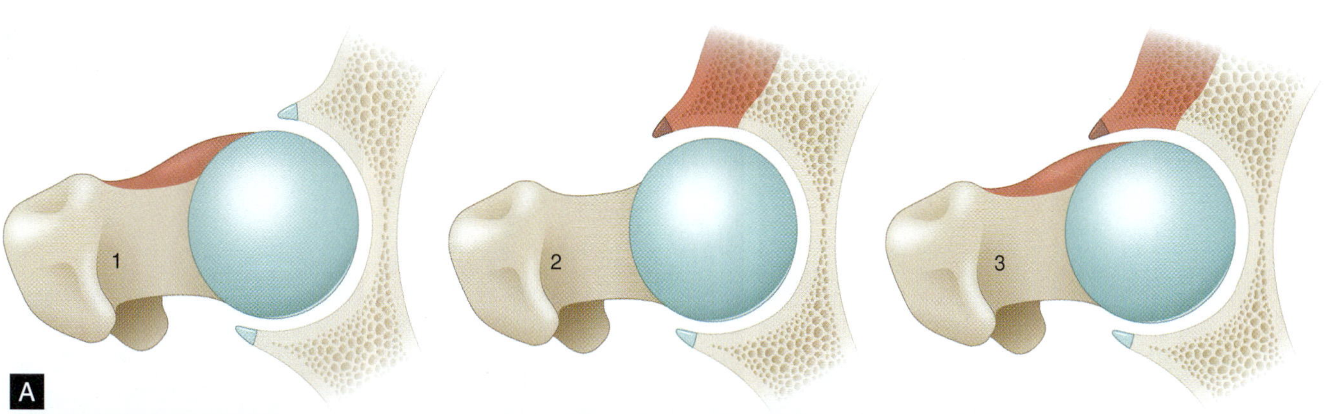

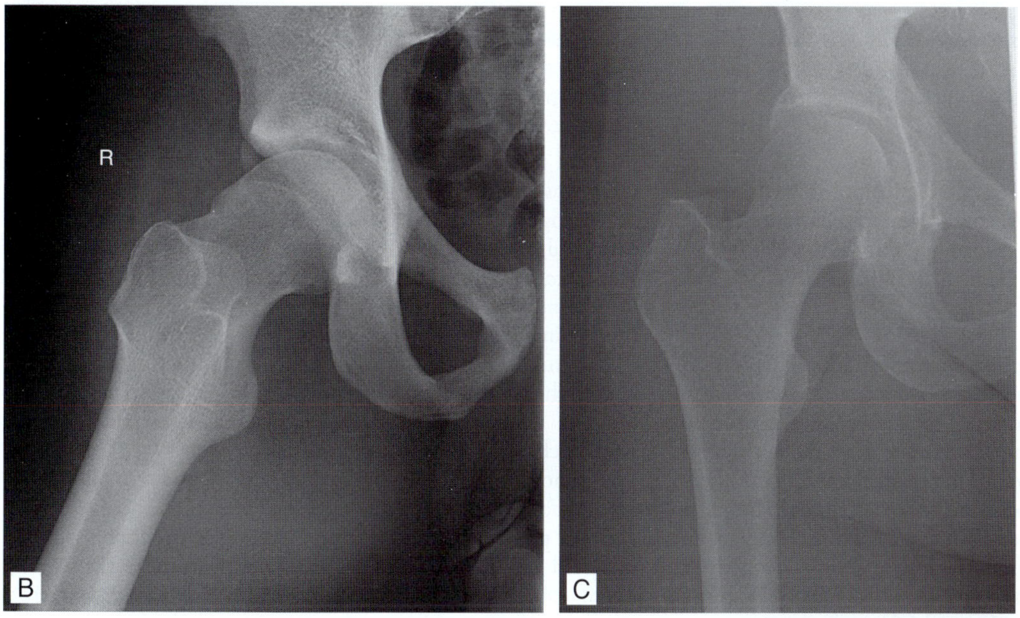

Figure 59.15 Appearance of FAI. (A) Illustration of cam (1), pincer (2), and mixed-type (3) FAI. (B) Cam deformity. Frog-leg radiographic view of the right hip shows osseous protuberance along the femoral head–neck junction. (C) Pincer deformity. Frontal radiograph of the right hip shows over-coverage of the acetabulum, with "crossover sign."

- Protuberant bone repeatedly strikes the labrum and acetabulum during flexion, which can lead to labral tear and eventually osteoarthrosis
- Usually seen in young, active men
- Many patients will develop a small, cystic area at the femoral head–neck junction, called a "synovial herniation pit"
- Decreased femoral head–neck offset

- **Pincer impingement**
  - Overcoverage of the femoral head by the laterally extending superolateral acetabulum, involving the anterosuperior quadrant (Figs. 59.15A2 and 59.15C)
  - Often associated with acetabular retroversion
  - More common in women
  - Underlying labrum and cartilage are pinched during the normal range of motion, resulting in labral tearing and degenerative changes
  - Synovial herniation pits also seen
- **Mixed-type cam/pincer impingement (Fig. 59.15A3)**
  - More common than individual types
  - Slipped capital femoral epiphysis (SCFE) is said to increase susceptibility for future impingement

Radiographic evaluation can help evaluate osseous morphology and allows the radiologist to provide measurements, including the amount of over coverage. The alpha angle issued to assess the presence of a cam deformity, and this is often seen best on CT or MRI (Fig. 59.16). To perform this measurement, two lines are drawn:

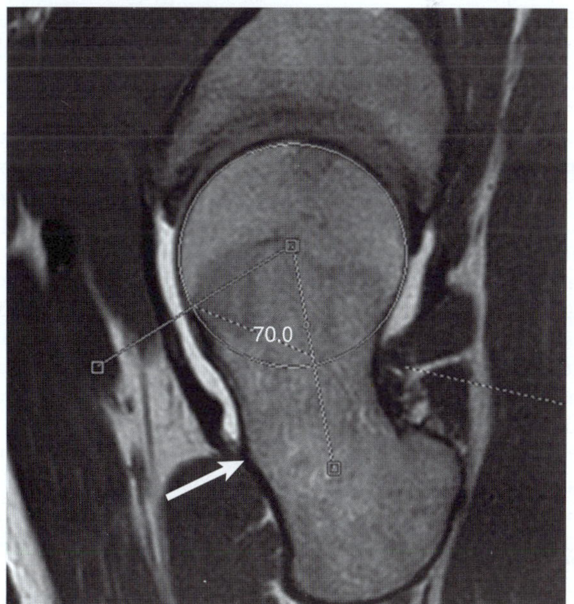

Figure 59.16 Cam deformity with abnormal alpha angle. Sagittal oblique, T1-weighted MR arthrogram image of the hip shows the measurements that reveal an alpha angle of 70 degrees, which is greater than normal (55 degrees), consistent with a cam deformity. The osseous protuberance along the femoral head–neck junction is visible (*arrow*).

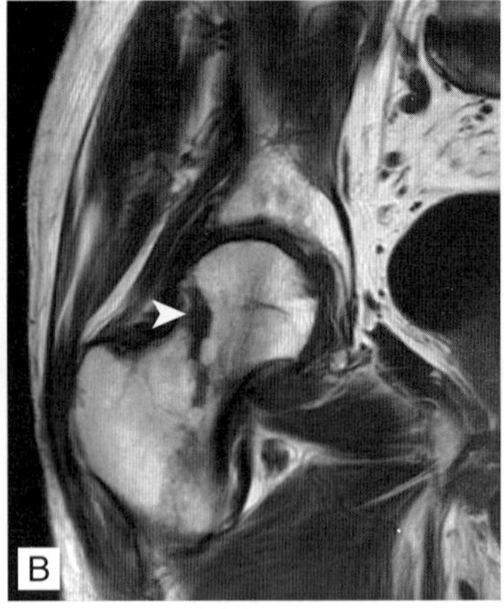

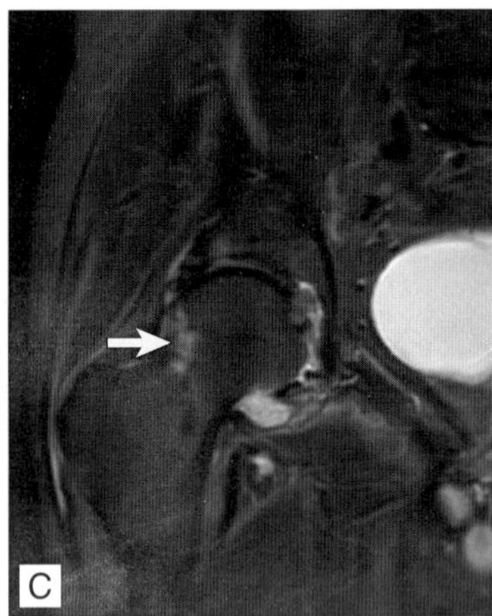

Figure 59.17 Occult hip fracture. (A) Frontal radiograph of the pelvis is normal. MRI shows bone marrow edema (C, *arrow*) and linear, low-signal (B, *arrowhead*) in the right femoral head and neck region, consistent with a nondisplaced fracture.

one along the central axis of the femoral neck on an oblique view and one from the center of femoral head to the point where femoral head sphericity is first lost. An angle greater than 55 degrees is abnormal and confirms a cam deformity; clinical correlation for pain is essential.

Occult Hip Fracture

The osseous structure of the proximal femur includes both cortical and trabecular bone, and both are strongest when exposed to longitudinal force and weaker when exposed to tension and shear forces. Multiple vertically oriented compressive trabeculae radiate superiorly to the weight-bearing portion of the femoral head, while a second group of compressive trabeculae radiates obliquely from the lesser trochanter toward the greater trochanter. Multiple horizontally oriented tensile trabeculae run from the intertrochanteric region to the femoral head. It is these tensile trabeculae that are at increased risk of fracture due to tensile force, which places them at a greater risk of displacement, and thus necessitates surgical fixation [32].

Proper identification of an occult hip fracture is crucial, because a nondisplaced fracture can be stabilized with an intramedullary rod, thus sparing the hip joint, whereas an undiagnosed, nondisplaced fracture can eventually progress to a displaced fracture, which requires a hip arthroplasty. When there is strong clinical suspicion of a hip fracture because the patient is in severe pain, holding the leg in external rotation, and/or unable to bear weight, CT or MRI should be performed if the radiographs are negative. One study showed that 4.4% of patients in the emergency department with clinical suspicion of a hip fracture, but negative radiographs were proved to have an occult fracture on subsequent cross-sectional imaging (Fig. 59.17) [33]. MRI has the best sensitivity for nondisplaced fractures [34], although CT is often adequate, is easy to obtain, and can be used when there is a contraindication to MRI. Nondisplaced fractures are occasionally not detected on CT [35,36], although recent literature has shown that dual-energy CT increases sensitively for nondisplaced hip fractures by showing marrow edema at the occult fracture site [37].

Insufficiency and Stress Fractures

Patients with stress and insufficiency fractures of the hip may present with hip or groin pain that worsens with weight-bearing activity. *Stress fractures occur in patients who experience an abnormal amount of stress on normal bone, such as long-distance runners, while insufficiency fractures occur with normal stress on abnormal (e.g., osteopenic) bone.* The proximal femoral shaft is the most common site, and the fracture line is usually medial, as this is the area of greatest weight bearing.

Radiographs exhibit a progression of bone injury, with focal periosteal reaction relatively early, sclerosis, and eventually a lucent fracture line. Medial femoral neck buttressing, or cortical thickening with an overlying segment of smooth periosteal reaction, is in the differential diagnosis in the early phases of stress-related injury, although a fracture should not be seen; this process is thought due to altered hip mechanics [38]. MRI is the most sensitive technique and allows earlier diagnosis, before radiographic changes are visible (Fig. 59.18).

Bisphosphonate-related insufficiency fractures are a special category of proximal femoral fractures, which have been shown to occur in patients who underwent bisphosphonate therapy due to impaired bone remodeling in small numbers of patients [39]. These tend to be located along the lateral, proximal femoral

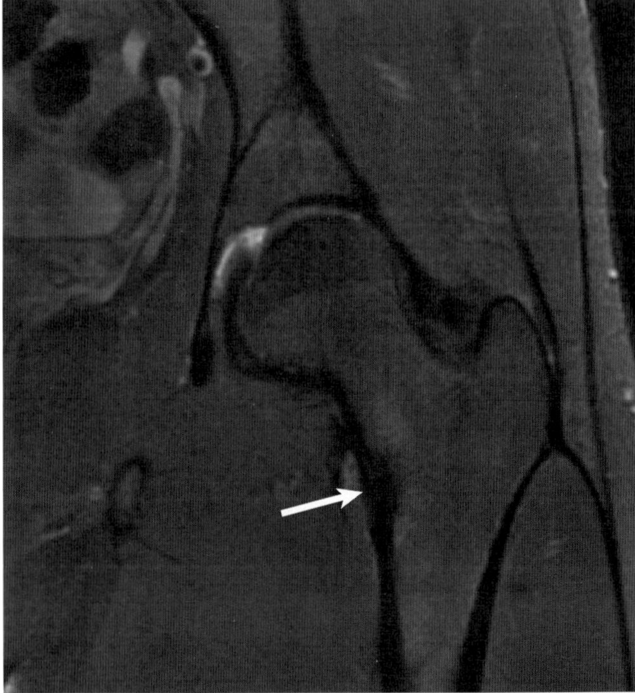

Figure 59.18 Coronal STIR MR image shows bone marrow edema in the medial, proximal left femur with linear, low signal (*arrow*) consistent with a fracture.

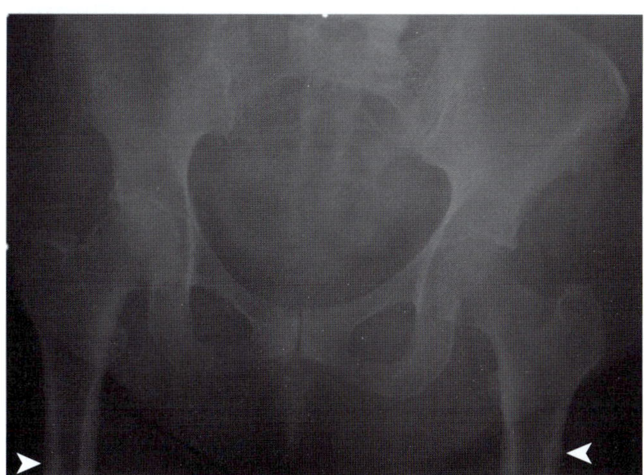

Figure 59.19 Frontal radiograph of the pelvis shows bilateral, focal cortical thickening along with the lateral aspects of the femoral diaphysis in a patient who underwent bisphosphonate therapy. These were later shown to represent insufficiency fractures on MRI.

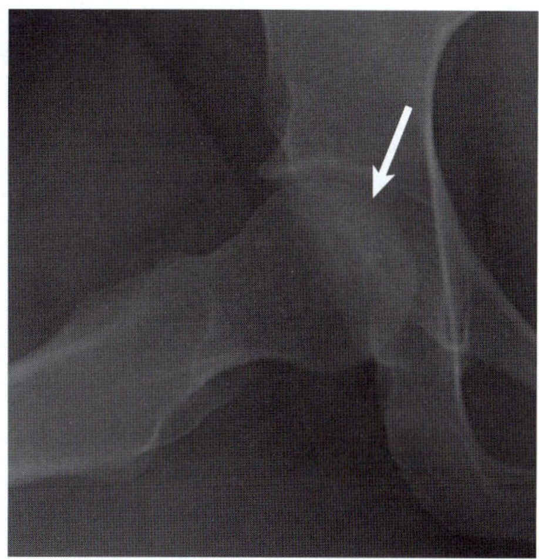

Figure 59.20 Frog-leg radiograph of the pelvis shows a crescentic, subchondral lucency (*arrow*) along with the superior femoral head, also known as the "crescent sign."

diaphysis with cortical thickening and possibly a visible fracture line [40] (Fig. 59.19).

Avascular Necrosis

Patients with avascular necrosis of the hip may present with hip or groin pain. Because the condition results from interruption of the blood supply with resulting necrosis of the marrow, medullary bone, and cortex, certain patients are predisposed, such as those with a history of steroid use, trauma, sickle cell anemia, alcoholism, radiation therapy, chemotherapy, and lupus. *Avascular necrosis is commonly seen in the anterosuperior femoral head, as this is an area of relatively limited blood supply.* Initially, radiographs can appear normal, with a crescentic subchondral lucency (Fig. 59.20) and/or mixed lucency and sclerosis sometimes appearing later in the course. The typical appearance on MRI is that of smooth, linear geographic signal abnormality, typically concave to the articular surface, with central fat and both low- and high-signal lines of demarcation ("double line sign"); there can be marrow edema, and eventual subchondral collapse/fracture is possible. A differential diagnosis could include a subchondral insufficiency fracture, in which the fracture line on MRI tends to be irregular, disconnected to the cortex, and convex to the articular surface, transient osteoporosis of the hip, discussed in the next section, or stress reaction/fracture [41]. Table 59.9 lists the staging of imaging findings on both radiographs and MRI in the Ficat system, the most widely used categorization system; Fig. 59.21 shows the progression of MRI findings. The Mitchell classification system, based on MRI signal characteristics within the center of the lesion, is also used in some instances [42]. Contrast-enhanced MRI can also help with evaluation, with decreased or nonenhancement in the area of avascular necrosis [43].

Depending on the size and location of the lesion, pharmacologic agents can be considered for treatment. Preservation of the femoral head might be attempted in younger patients without head collapse by using core decompression with bone grafts, bone morphogenic proteins, stem cells, or rotational osteotomies. When femoral head collapse is present, arthroplasty is the primary option [44].

Transient Osteoporosis of the Hip

This entity was first described in patients in the third trimester of pregnancy, with onset of hip pain that resolves spontaneously after delivery, but this can also occur in nonpregnant patients. There is controversy as to the pathophysiology, with subchondral stress fracture as well as ischemia that does progress to necrosis offered as possible explanations, among others. Imaging findings include osteopenia of the femoral head on radiographs and CT and edema of the femoral head on MRI, mimicking AVN (Fig. 59.22). *If post contrast sequences are obtained, the area of edema should enhance on postcontrast images in TOH, while in AVN these areas would show decreased or nonenhancement.* TOH also typically spares the subchondral region of the femoral head. These

TABLE 59.9 Ficat and Arlet Staging System for AVN of Hip

Stage	Radiographs/CT	MRI	Clinical Symptoms
0	Normal	Normal	None
1	Normal or minor osteopenia	Bone marrow edema	Pain
2	Sclerosis	Geographic signal abnormality ("double line sign": adjacent low- and high-signal lines)	Pain and stiffness
3	Subchondral lucency ("crescent sign") and flattening	Bone marrow edema, subchondral fracture/fluid	Pain radiating to knee, stiffness, limp
4	Femoral head collapse, evidence of osteoarthrosis	Bone marrow edema, femoral head collapse	Pain, stiffness, limp

(Adapted from Jawad MU, et al., Clin Orthop Relat Res 470 (9) (2012) 2636–2639.)

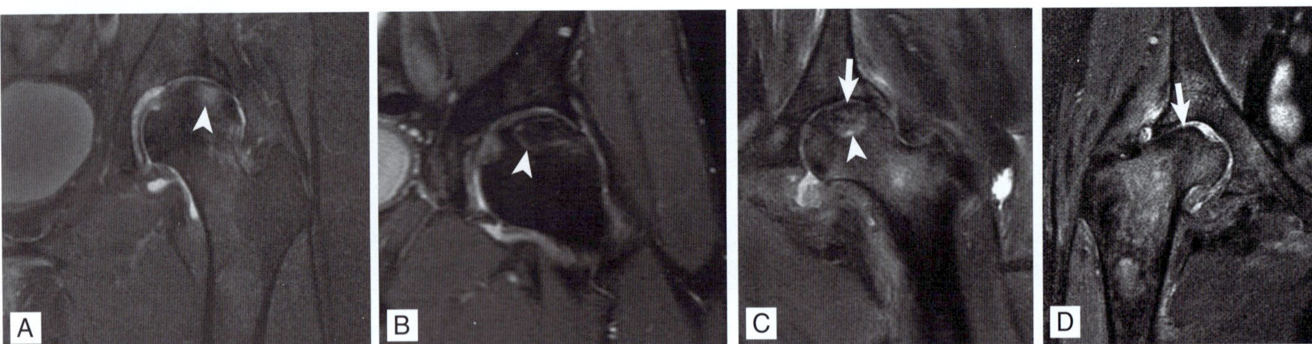

Figure 59.21 Avascular necrosis. (A) Ficat stage 1: bone marrow edema seen in the subchondral region of the femoral head on this coronal PDFS MR image. (B) Ficat stage 2: coronal STIR MR image shows linear, geographic signal abnormality in the bilateral superior femoral heads (*arrows*) with central fat signal, as well as linear high and low signal, representing the "double line sign." (C) Ficat stage 3: coronal PDFS MR image shows subchondral flattening/fracture of the femoral head superior articular surface with underlying marrow edema and fluid. (D) Ficat stage 4: coronal PDFS MR image shows marrow edema, flattening, and remodeling of the superior femoral head, consistent with collapse, with background avascular necrosis that is seen as faint geographic signal abnormality in the superior femoral head.

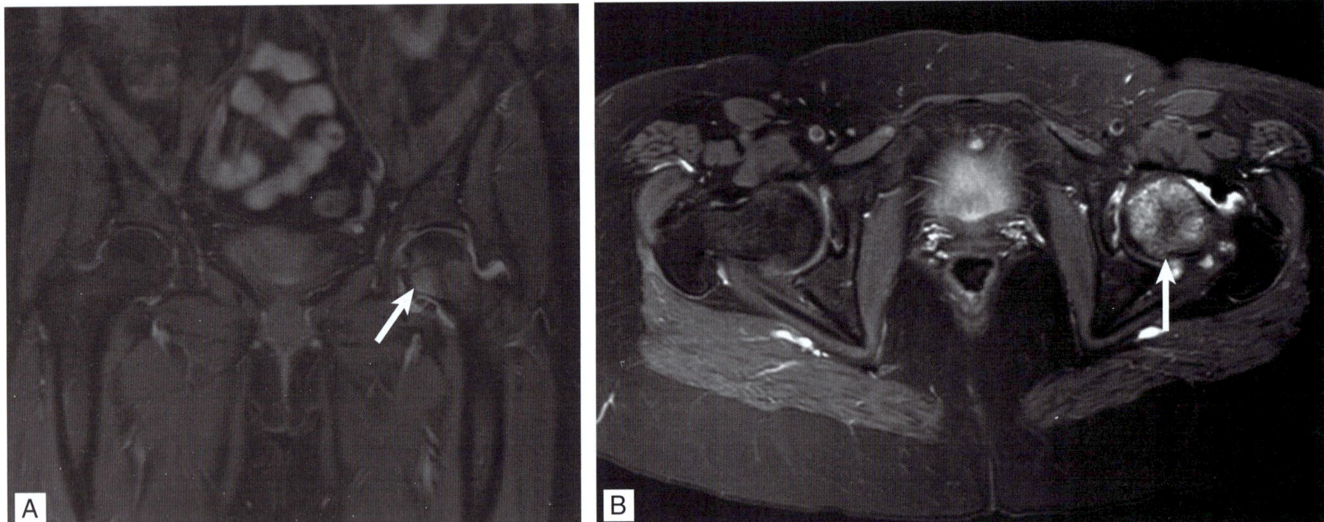

Figure 59.22 Transient osteoporosis of the hip. Coronal STIR (A) and axial T2-fat-saturated (B) MR images of the pelvis show marrow edema in the left femoral head (*arrows*) that resolved spontaneously on follow-up imaging.

findings and the patient's symptoms should eventually resolve spontaneously with conservative management [45,46].

Paget's Disease of Bone

Paget's disease is a non-neoplastic condition that is characterized by abnormal bone remodeling. It can occur anywhere in the body, but the pelvis and proximal femur are common locations. It typically has three stages, as described in Table 59.10. There is often asymmetric involvement of the pelvis with cortical thickening, coarsened trabeculations, sclerosis, and acetabular protrusion. In the proximal femur, there can also be lateral bowing, possibly with the "blade of grass" sign, in which an area of subchondral lucency extends toward the diaphysis in a V-shape (Fig. 59.23) [47]. Although there is cortical thickening and sclerosis, it is essential to note that the bone structure is actually weakened from remodeling, which predisposes to fractures. Metastatic disease should be considered and excluded, especially given the mixed lytic and blastic appearance. There is a low (1%) risk of degeneration to osteosarcoma [48].

TABLE 59.10 Stages of Paget's Disease of Bone

Stage	Pathology
Early	Osteoclasts; active, lytic
Intermediate stage	Osteoblasts and osteoclasts; prominence of osteoblasts
Late stage	Osteosclerotic phase; inactive

Fibrous Dysplasia

Fibrous dysplasia is a non-neoplastic congenital process and is often asymptomatic, but can become symptomatic, such as with a pathologic fracture. As this lesion is classically identified as a "long lesion in a long bone," it is most commonly seen in the pelvis in the proximal femur (Fig. 59.24); *this is the second most common location in the body, after the ribs*. Pathologically, there is replacement of normal bone with fibrous stroma and islands of immature, woven bone [47]. Radiographically, fibrous dysplasia appears as well-defined, bubbly lesion, sometimes with endosteal scalloping and cortical thinning, and there might be central ground-glass matrix and/or sclerosis. In the hip, a large lesion can

Summary of Teaching Points: Central Hip Region

- The hallmarks of OA are: osteophytes, joint space narrowing (asymmetric), subchondral sclerosis, subchondral cysts
- In inflammatory arthritis, joint space narrowing is typically concentric (symmetric)
- A suspected native, septic hip is a true emergency; joint aspiration should be attempted as soon as possible. A negative radiograph does not exclude a septic joint
- Paralabral cysts are highly suggestive of the presence of a labral tear
- In FAI, repetitive microtrauma of bone on the labrum causes labral degeneration and tearing as well as cartilage degeneration and early OA of the hip
- Cam deformity refers to osseous protuberance at the anterosuperior femoral head–neck junction, while pincer deformity refers to acetabular over coverage; some patients have both (mixed-type FAI)
- If there is strong clinical suspicion of a hip fracture, but negative radiographs, MRI, or CT should be obtained
- Proximal femoral stress fractures appear as periosteal thickening, sclerosis, and possibly a linear lucency; these typically occur medially due to weight-bearing stress, with lateral injuries typical of patients with a history of bisphosphonate use
- Avascular necrosis appears as geographic signal abnormality with central fat and both high- and low-signal linear demarcation ("double line sign")
- Transient osteoporosis of the hip will appear as marrow edema, which should spontaneously resolve
- Paget's disease is due to abnormal bone remodeling and appears as cortical thickening and coarse trabeculations; weakened bone structure predisposes to fracture

cause bowing and coxa varus angulation referred to as a "shepherd's crook" deformity.

The differential diagnosis can be broad, as fibrous dysplasia has a variable appearance. Fibro-osseous lesions, such as a nonossifying fibroma, can sometimes have overlapping radiographic features, such as having multiple loculations, a well-defined rim, and peripheral sclerosis. Bone islands are another type of fibro-osseous lesion. However, these are typically distinguishable by their speculated margin and very dense sclerosis, which has been shown to have a mean attenuation over 885 Hounsfield units and a CT [49].

Anterior Hip Region

Tendons

Tendinosis/Tendon Tear/Avulsion Injuries/Calcific Tendinosis: Tendon pathology in the anterior hip can present in several ways, including acute injury (tendon tear or avulsion) or chronic pain (tendinosis or chronic tear). Tendinosis appears as thickening and high signal within the tendon on fluid-sensitive MRI sequences, or similarly as thickening and hypoechogenicity on US. A tendon tear will appear as a fluid-filled gap on MRI or a hypoechoic area on US with the absence of the normal fibrillary pattern. Tears can be partial-thickness, with disruption of only some of the tendon fibers, or full-thickness, in which all tendon fibers are torn. Tears can occur at the attachment site (typically referred to as "avulsions"), in the mid-portion of the tendon, or at the musculotendinous junction.

Avulsion injuries can occur due to forceful muscular contraction. These are common in pediatric patients, in which they are a type of Salter–Harris I injury. These typically occur as a single event and cause acute pain, possibly with loss of function of the involved muscle. Initial radiographs can be normal, although if ossification has occurred, a displaced bone fragment can sometimes be seen. MRI is the most sensitive technique, as the soft-tissue findings of an avulsed tendon stump and marrow and soft-tissue edema are visible as well (Fig. 59.25) [30]. USG can also show the tendon injury with hypoechogenicity in the

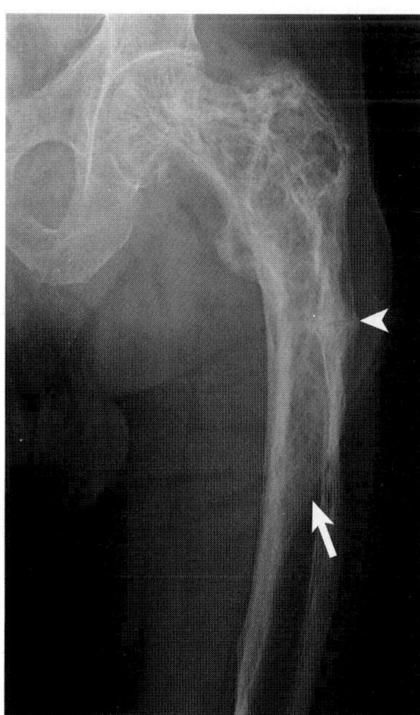

Figure 59.23 Paget's disease of the proximal femur. Frontal radiograph shows cortical thickening, coarse trabeculations, "blade of grass" sign (*arrow*), and an insufficiency fracture of the lateral cortex (*arrowhead*).

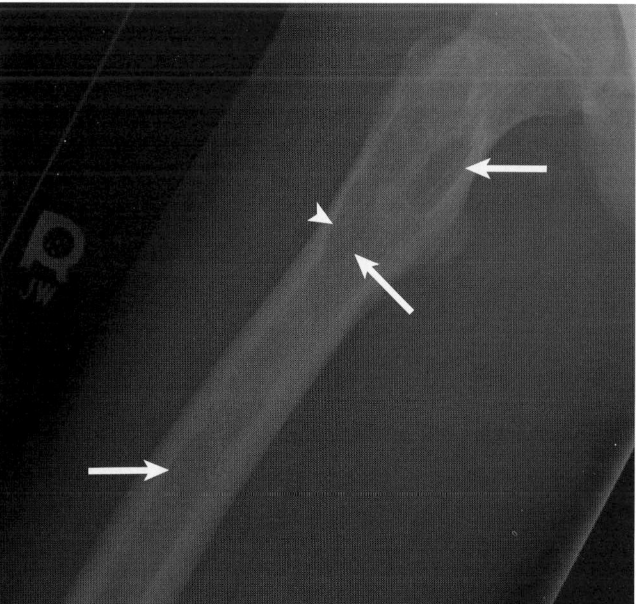

Figure 59.24 Fibrous dysplasia. This patient has multiple lucent, well-defined lesions (*arrows*) in the proximal femur seen on this frog-leg radiograph, some of which show cortical thinning (*arrowhead*).

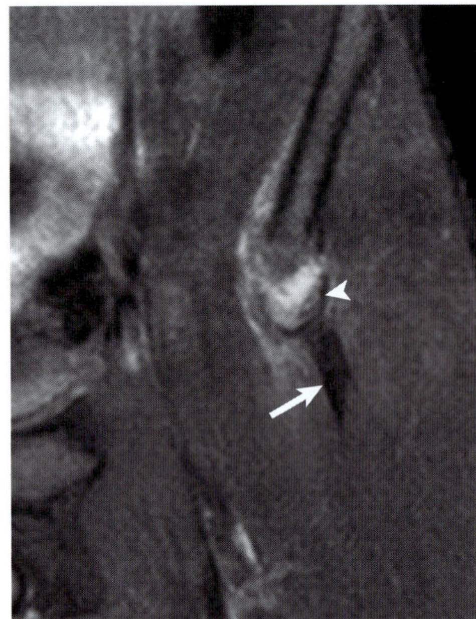

Figure 59.25 Rectus femoris avulsion. This coronal, fat-saturated, proton density MR image shows avulsion of the direct head of the rectus femoris tendon (*arrow*) from the anterior inferior iliac spine. A small osseous fragment (*arrowhead*) remains attached to the proximal tendon stump. There is surrounding soft-tissue edema.

surrounding soft tissues, sometimes with a displaced osseous fragment. Displacement of the fragment by more than 2 cm is often treated surgically [50].

Calcific tendinosis is another common type of tendon pathology in the pelvis and hips and will be discussed later.

Snapping Hip

There are multiple causes of a snapping hip, including extra-articular and intra-articular, with extra-articular being the most common. Extra-articular causes include soft-tissue structures sliding over osseous protuberances, such as the intertendinous iliopsoas tendon snapping or the iliotibial band, the gluteus maximus sliding over the greater trochanter, or the iliofemoral ligament snapping over the femoral head. Intra-articular causes would include such entities as labral tears or intra-articular bodies. USG is a useful evaluation tool given its ability to visualize tendons or ligaments during patient movement, provided that the patient can recreate the snap. MRI is also useful, as it can confirm any intra-articular cause of a snapping hip [51].

Hernia

Patients with lower abdominal/pelvic area hernias can present with groin or hip pain and/or a feeling of pressure or fullness in the hip area, which can prompt an imaging investigation. CT or MRI with and without valsalva can also help to identify hernias. USG is an excellent evaluation tool and allows dynamic imaging, repositioning of patient, and repeated attempts to elicit the hernia. Specific USG findings, such as fluid in the hernia sac, focal pain with transducer pressure, nonreduction of the hernia, or bowel content, suggest a more urgent clinical picture of obstructed hernia that might require immediate surgical intervention. Multiple types of hernias can be assessed, including umbilical hernias, spigelian hernias, indirect inguinal hernias, direct inguinal hernias, and femoral hernias. The locations,

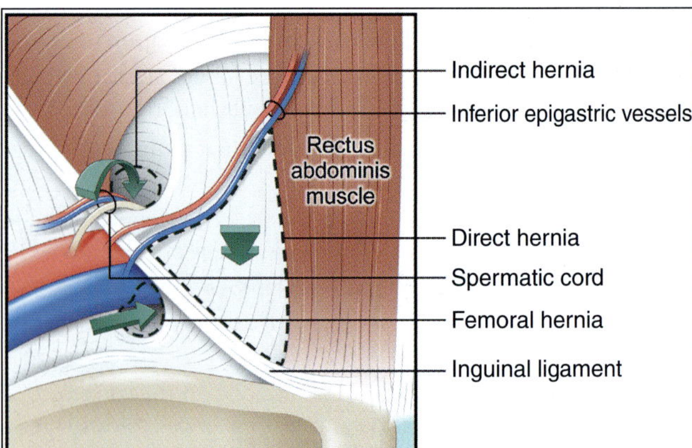

Figure 59.26 Illustration of common hernia locations (in green). This perspective is that of the reader standing within the abdomen, looking in an anterior direction at the abdominal wall.

defined by the where the neck of hernia is present, are better depicted in Fig. 59.26.

Pseudoaneurysm

Vascular pathology can occur anywhere in the body, but one crucial entity in the hip region is a femoral artery pseudoaneurysm. This can happen after catheterization, usually when the puncture is too inferior. The pseudoaneurysm appears as a rounded lesion, contained by a sac with a thin neck/connection to the vessel. Noncontrast CT will show an oval or spherical structure, possibly with high attenuation material adjacent to or within the sac. The contrast-filled sac should be visible on CTA, sometimes with thrombosis, which appears as low attenuation material. On USG, there is typically a to-and-fro pattern on spectral Doppler evaluation. Treatment is often image-guided and can include USG-guided compression, thrombin injection, stent placement, or surgery.

Lymph Nodes

Lymph nodes can be incidentally seen in the pelvic and inguinal region. The main chains are the common, internal, and external iliac, and inguinal. Lymph nodes that measure up to 1.5 cm in shortest dimension in the inguinal area and up to 1 cm in other sites are considered to be in the normal range [52]. Larger nodes, or nodes with abnormal morphology, such as the fatty hilum replacement, should be viewed as suspicious findings, and further imaging and/or biopsy may be warranted.

Summary of Teaching Points: Anterior Hip Region

- Tendinosis appears as a thickening and high signal within the tendon on MRI or as hypoechogenicity on US
- US is an excellent technique to assess for lower abdominal/pelvic region hernias
- On US, pseudoaneurysm will appear as a to-and-fro pattern on spectral Doppler evaluation

Posterior Hip Region

Hamstring Origin Region

Pathology of the hamstring tendons is similar to the discussion above regarding the anterior hip region, but there are a few notable points. Hamstring tendon pathology can present

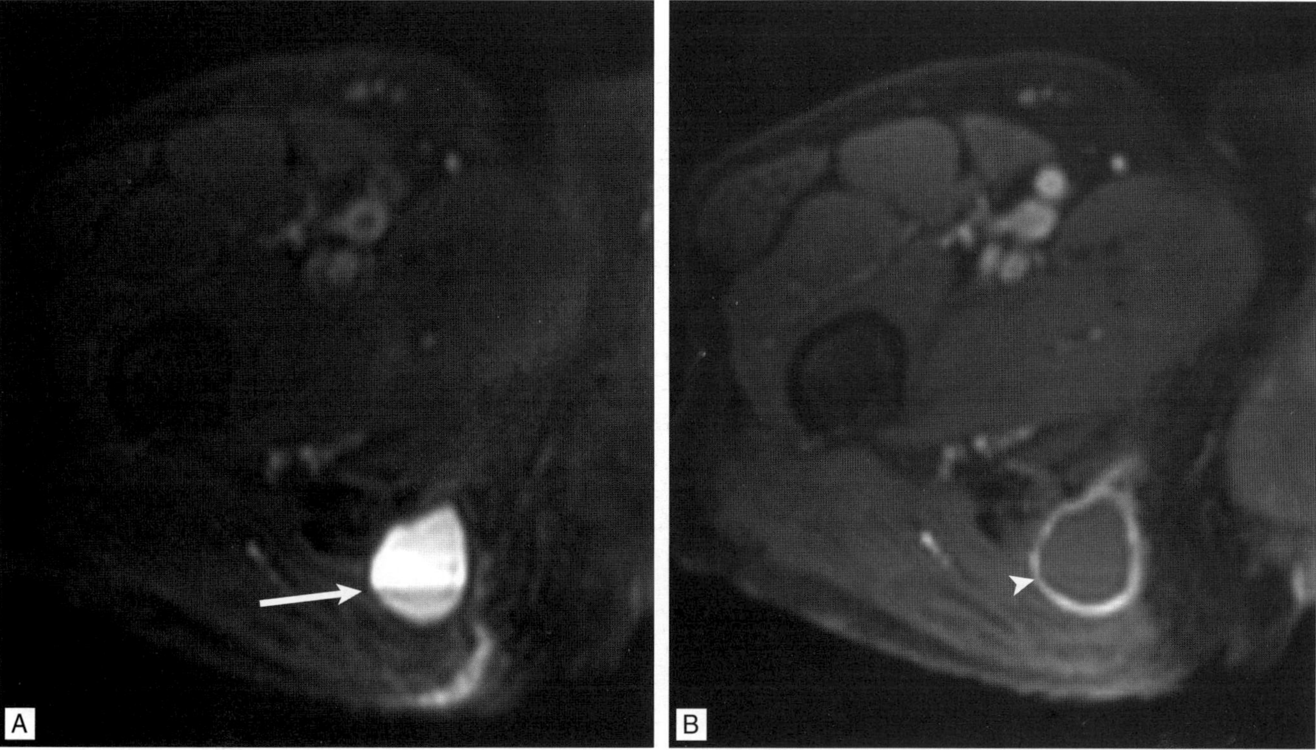

Figure 59.27 Ischiogluteal bursitis. Axial T2 fat-saturated (A) and T1 fat-saturated postcontrast (B) MR images show distention of the ischiogluteal bursa with layering fluid (A, *arrow*) and thin, peripheral postcontrast enhancement (B, *arrowhead*).

clinically as hip or buttock pain, possibly with tenderness over the ischial tuberosity [18]. Injury to the hamstring tendons tends to occur when the hip is flexed and the knee is extended. Ischial bone stress-related injuries can show edema around the proximal hamstring tendon attachments on MRI, so it is important to distinguish this process from a true tendon injury.

The proximal hamstring attachment at the ischial tuberosity consists of the semimembranosus tendon anterolaterally and the conjoint tendon posteromedially. Conjoint tendon is a combination of the biceps femoris and semitendinosis fibers. The proximal semimembranosus tendon is more prone to tendinosis, which can chronically progress to tear, whereas the conjoint tendon is more prone to avulsion following trauma [53]. *Of note, the "mini hamstring," or ischiocondylar portion of the adductor magnus that has a tendinous attachment to the ischial tuberosity, is generally intact after a complete avulsion of the conjoint tendon, and should not be confused as representing an intact conjoint tendon* [54].

The ischial tuberosity/proximal hamstring attachment area also contains the ischiogluteal bursa between the gluteus maximus and ischial tuberosity. Occupations that require prolonged sitting and/or excessive weight loss can predispose patients to ischiogluteal bursitis (Fig. 59.27), which can cause pain in the mid-buttock region. This is often termed "weaver's bottom" because weavers could develop this condition due to many continuous hours of sitting at their job. The differential diagnosis includes a herniated lumbar disk and piriformis syndrome, which refers to a controversial clinical entity that includes a variety of piriformis muscle pathologies resulting in compression of the sciatic nerve and resulting symptoms [55]. Common causes attributed to piriformis syndrome include bulky piriformis (Fig. 59.28) an uncommon anatomic variation with sciatic nerve taking a deviant course through the piriformis muscle. USG or MRI can be useful in distinguishing these entities.

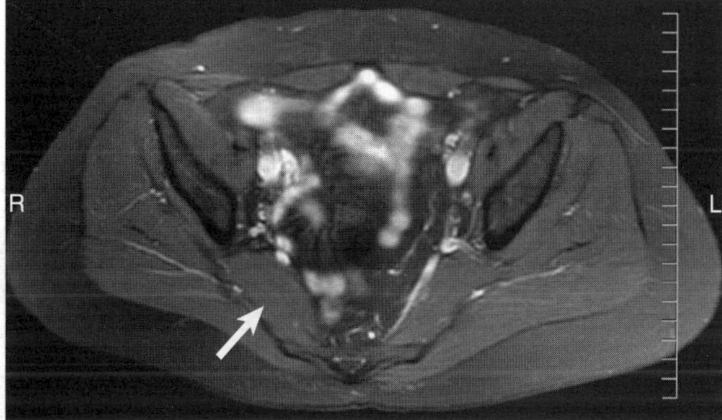

Figure 59.28 Piriformis syndrome. Axial T2 fat-saturated MR image shows thick and edematous right piriformis muscle (*arrow*) compared with left.

Nerves

The sciatic nerve is located in the posterior hip region, exiting the pelvis through the greater sciatic foramen entering the gluteal region. "Sciatica" or sciatic nerve pain is a common clinical problem in which patients have pain, tingling, or numbness in the buttock region, radiating down the posterior leg. This may be caused by compression or inflammation of the sciatic nerve. In some cases, the sciatic nerve will appear enlarged and/or edematous on MRI (Fig. 59.29), or there might be evidence of compression. Other possible abnormalities of the sciatic nerve include transection, which will appear on imaging as a discontinuity with swelling and/or nerve retraction. Because the sciatic nerve is intimately associated with the proximal hamstring attachments, hamstring injuries/tears can cause sciatic nerve damage and resulting symptoms [56]. In the setting of a proximal thigh amputation, sciatic neuromas can develop.

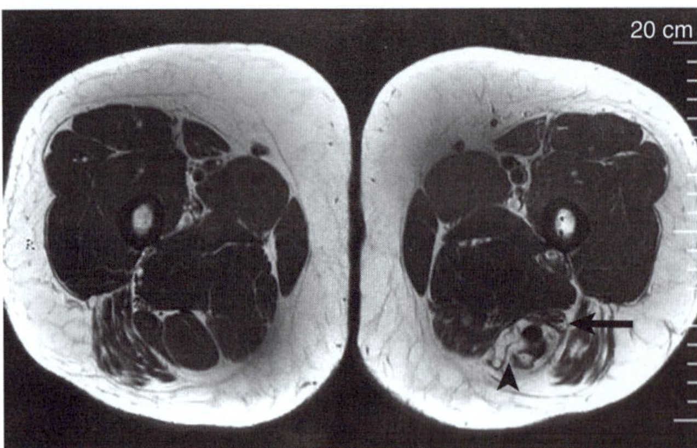

Figure 59.29 Axial T2 MR image shows thickened left sciatic nerve (*arrow*) due to post-traumatic tear of hamstring muscle (*arrowhead*).

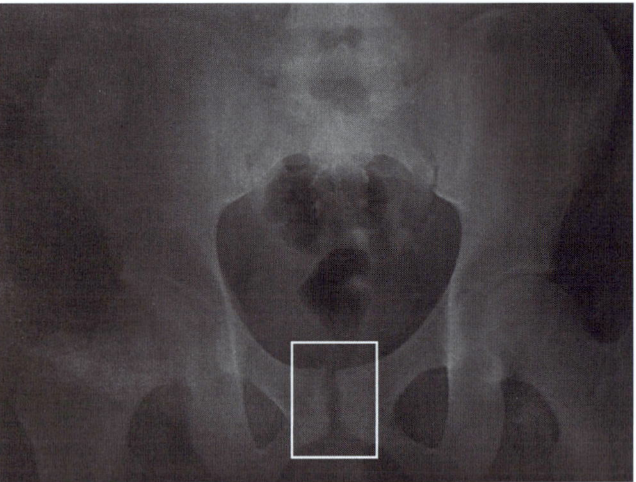

Figure 59.30 Osteitis pubis. Frontal radiograph of the pelvis shows osseous irregularity on both sides of the pubic symphysis.

Summary of Teaching Points: Posterior Hip Region

- Ischiogluteal bursitis can occur due to prolonged sitting
- Posterior hip/buttock pain can be caused by sciatic nerve compression or inflammation; in some cases, there can be enlargement, edema, or compression seen on MRI

Medial Hip Region

Athletic Pubalgia

Athletic pubalgia is the term given to groin pain centered over the symphysis pubis region in athletes, and it can be due to a spectrum of injuries, as described later. The term "sports hernia" is misleading, as there is no true hernia present in this condition. Radiographs are helpful to evaluate the pubic symphysis for fracture and osseous irregularity, but MRI is helpful for the evaluation of soft-tissue injuries and bone marrow edema.

- **Osteitis pubis:** This controversial entity is likely multifactorial and maybe a combination of mechanical and inflammatory processes involving the pubic symphysis and surrounding muscle attachments. Radiographs show osseous irregularity (Fig. 59.30), which can progress to chronic remodeling and osteophyte formation, and there is typically marrow edema on both sides of the symphysis on MRI [57]. Patients can have true instability at symphysis, exacerbated by activity and sometimes made worse by pregnancy. Management is conservative.
- **Rectus abdominis distal attachment injury:** The distal fibers of the rectus abdominis muscle attach to the anteroinferior pubic bone, approximately 1-cm lateral to the symphysis. A tear in the attaching fibers can lead to a fluid-filled gap visible on MRI, best seen on sagittal images (Fig. 59.31); this is also known as the "superior cleft sign," which appears as high signal on fluid-sensitive sequences that runs parallel to the inferior

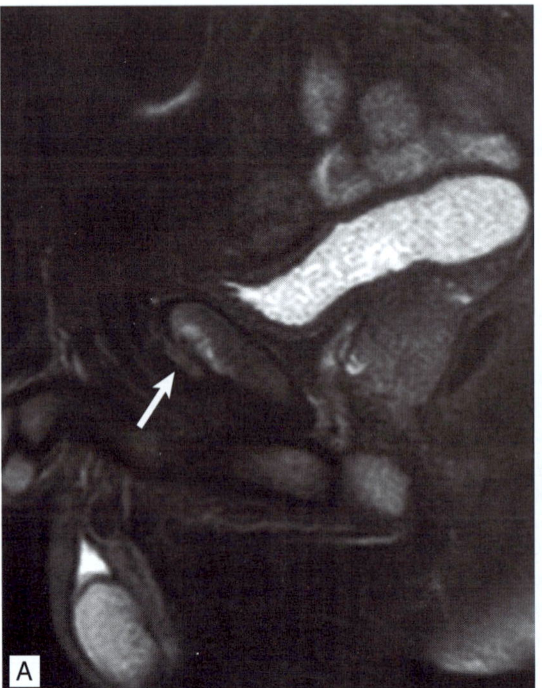

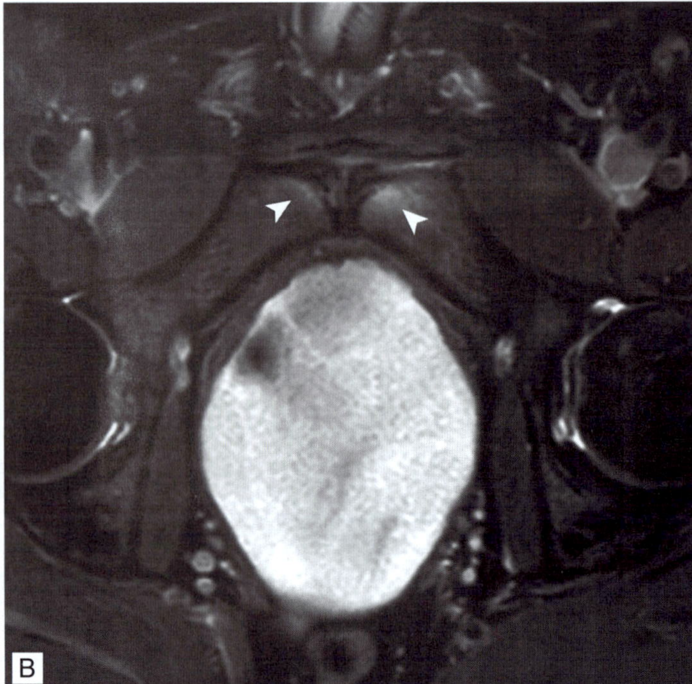

Figure 59.31 Sagittal (A) and axial (B) proton density fat-saturated MR images show separation of the rectus abdominis aponeurosis from the pubic bone with intervening edema (*arrow*). There is an underlying marrow edema (*arrowheads*).

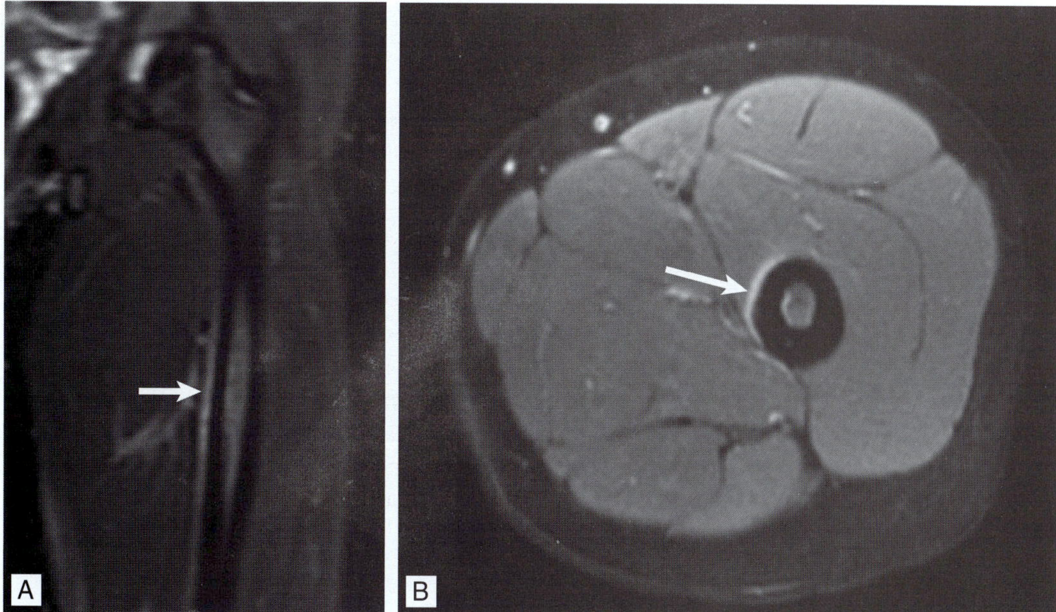

Figure 59.32 Thigh splints. Coronal STIR (A) and axial proton density fat-saturated (B) images of the left thigh show periosteal edema (*arrows*) along the proximal femoral diaphysis with underlying marrow edema.

margin of the superior pubic ramus on coronal MRI [58]. The tear may extend inferiorly to involve the adductor muscle fibers. Bone marrow edema is also sometimes seen, but it tends to be anterior near the muscle attachment, not diffuse like in osteitis pubis.

- **Adductor muscle injury:** This may include chronic, degenerative tendinopathy or acute muscle tears or strains. Patients with adductor longus muscle injury tend not to have bone marrow edema or rectus abdominis insertional disorder. The "secondary cleft sign" refers to microtearing at the short adductor muscle segments and appears as high signal on fluid-sensitive sequences along the inferior margin of the inferior pubic ramus seen on coronal MRI [58]. Muscle and/or tendon injuries typically respond to conservative measures.

Adductor Insertion Avulsion/Thigh Splints

"Thigh splints" refers to a painful condition in which there are repeated avulsive stresses to the adductor muscle attachments of the proximal to the mid femoral diaphysis. Radiographs can be normal, or periosteal reaction can be seen along the femur at the area of muscle attachment. On MRI, there might be soft-tissue edema in the adductor musculature or the adjacent bone (Fig. 59.32). The pain is often relieved with rest, and given that thigh splints might represent an early stage of osseous stress reaction/fracture, athletes with this condition must be cautious about continuing with training [59].

Lateral Hip Region

Greater Trochanteric Pain Syndrome

Patients who experience chronic pain and tenderness along the lateral hip may be given a clinical diagnosis of greater trochanteric pain syndrome, more commonly in women. Although this has often been equated with greater trochanteric bursitis, it is probably more often related to tendinosis and/or tears of the gluteal tendons, possibly in addition to bursitis, with similar imaging findings in regards to tendon pathology as described previously (Fig. 59.33). Other pathologic conditions that might contribute to symptoms at the greater trochanter include thickening of the proximal iliotibial band, which could snap over the greater trochanter.

Summary of Teaching Points: Medial Hip Region

- Athletic pubalgia refers to a spectrum of injuries that result in symphysis pubis pain; the term "sports hernia" is misleading
- A tear in the rectus abdominis aponeurosis can be seen as a fluid-filled cleft on MRI; sagittal images are typically the most revealing
- "Thigh splints" refers to repeated avulsive stress of the adductor muscle attachments at the femoral diaphysis; MRI will typically show periosteal edema

Multiple bursas are surrounding the greater trochanter, and it is important to note that bursal distention with fluid is not equivalent to bursitis. Bursitis indicates an inflammatory or infectious process, with synovial thickening and irregularity plus fluid on MRI and USG, with USG also showing hyperemia. Management of greater trochanteric pain syndrome is typically conservative, targeting the specific reason for pain.

Calcific Tendinosis

Calcific tendinosis is another entity that can affect tendons about the pelvis and hips. This occurs due to the deposition of calcium hydroxyapatite in the tendon fibers. Although it can occur anywhere in the body, the hip tendons that are more likely to be affected include the reflected head of the rectus femoris along superolateral and Gluteus maximus attachment over the posterior proximal femur. Patients can present with acute, severe pain and tenderness around the greater trochanter, which can mimic lumbar radiculopathy, although the pain can also be chronic. On radiographs, there may be calcification in the expected location of a tendon, and these can appear hazy, fluffy, or amorphous in the resorptive (acute) stage of the disease or homogeneous and well defined in the formative/calcific (chronic) stage [60]. Calcifications within the tendon can also be seen on USG or MRI. USG-guided aspiration/lavage (or "barbotage") can be used for treatment, in which a needle is repeatedly inserted into the calcification with an injection of saline or lidocaine solution.

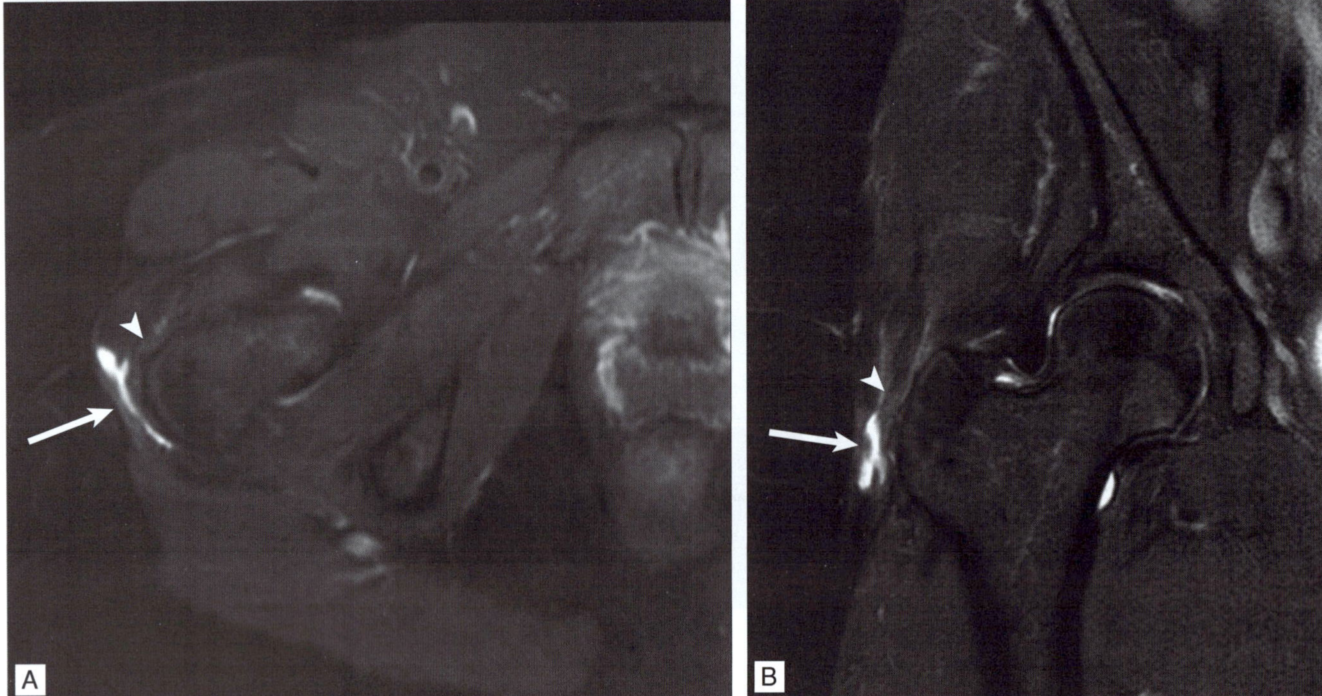

Figure 59.33 Greater trochanteric pain syndrome. Axial (A) and coronal (B) proton density fat-saturated MR images show high signal and thickening of the gluteus minimus tendon (*arrowheads*) and fluid and synovial stranding in the greater trochanteric bursa (*arrows*).

Lateral Femoral Cutaneous Nerve Syndrome

Lateral femoral cutaneous nerve syndrome, or "meralgia paresthetica," is characterized by lateral and anterior thigh-burning, tingling, and numbness, often worsening with standing, walking, hip extension, and lying prone. The course of the nerve is variable. Typically it has a horizontal intrapelvic course along the anterior aspect of the iliacus muscle, courses vertically into the subcutaneous tissues at the level of the inguinal ligament, and branches into the subcutaneous tissues of the upper thigh. When there is clinical suspicion of nerve injury or entrapment, USG can be used for further evaluation. This may show nerve swelling and hypoechogenicity at the entrapment site, most commonly at the inguinal ligament–anterior superior iliac spine junction, which becomes symptomatic with transducer pressure [61].

Sacrum

Insufficiency Fractures

One common type of pathology seen in the sacrum is insufficiency fractures. These often present in an elderly patient with back pain, and an insufficiency fracture might not be clinically suspected. Osteopenia is a significant risk factor, as are before radiation, steroid use, and rheumatoid arthritis. Radiographs can be negative or show vague, roughly linear sclerosis in the location of the fracture. MRI is the best technique for identifying insufficiency fractures, and they appear as linear/band-like low signal intensity on T1-weighted images, with surrounding edema on T2-weighted images (Fig. 59.34) [62]. The fracture lines in the sacrum usually parallel the sacral aspect of the SI joint, although occasionally, there is also a horizontally oriented band (Fig. 59.35) shows common sites in the sacrum, pelvis, and hips). Bone scans can also help identify these fractures, with radiotracer uptake sometimes taking on the "Honda sign," in which uptake at the fracture sites appears similar to the "H" in the brand's logo (Fig. 59.36).

Summary of Teaching Points: Lateral Hip Region

- Greater trochanteric pain syndrome is likely more often related to gluteal tendinopathy, sometimes in addition to trochanteric bursitis
- Bursal distention is not equivalent to bursitis; synovial thickening in addition to fluid and hyperemia on US, are suggestive of bursitis
- US-guided aspiration/lavage ("barbotage") can be used to treat calcific tendinosis, which is most commonly seen involving the gluteal or rectus femoris tendons in the hips

Osteomyelitis

Osteomyelitis can occur in any area of the body, but it often affects the sacrum and pelvis in bedridden patients with pressure ulcers. On imaging, skin ulcers and/or surgical incisions can help guide the radiologist to the underlying osseous involvement. On radiographs, osseous erosion is the key finding to suggest osteomyelitis, and an overlying gas-filled tract leading from the skin surface to the bone is a helpful finding. MRI is typically used both for confirmation and to look for soft-tissue complications, such as abscess, fistula, and cellulitis. Osteomyelitis is confirmed when there is true marrow replacement underlying a known ulcer/soft-tissue infection; this will appear as a signal lower than skeletal muscle on T1-weighted images and higher than muscle on T2-weighted images. Post contrast enhancement of the marrow in this region is helpful, but not necessary, finding to confirm osteomyelitis (Fig. 59.37). Marrow signal changes, such as edema and enhancement, without marrow replacement is suspicious for early osteomyelitis if there is an overlying infection. A tagged WBC scan can be used to confirm osteomyelitis if the patient cannot get an MRI done.

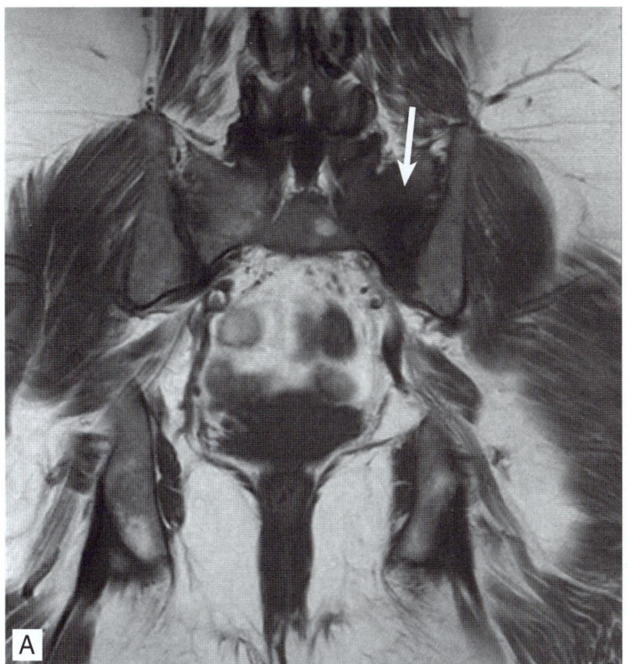

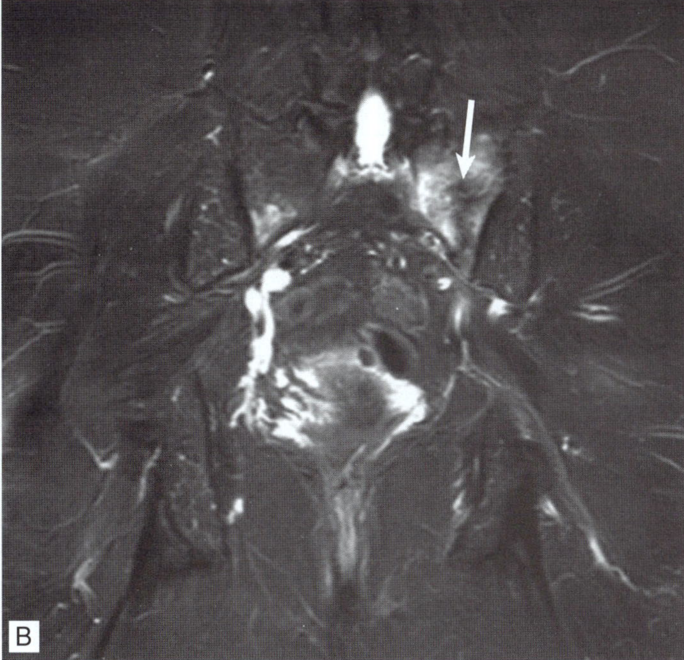

Figure 59.34 Sacral insufficiency fracture. Coronal T1-weighted (A) and STIR (B) MR images of the pelvis show bone marrow edema in the left sacrum (B) with linear, low signal on both sequences (*arrows*).

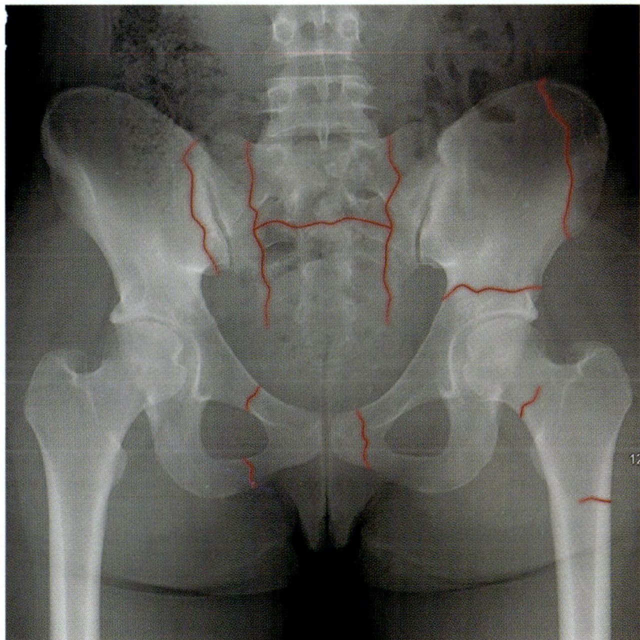

Figure 59.35 Common sites of insufficiency fractures in the pelvis/sacrum and hips. The site in the lateral proximal femoral diaphysis is associated with bisphosphonate use, as described in the text.

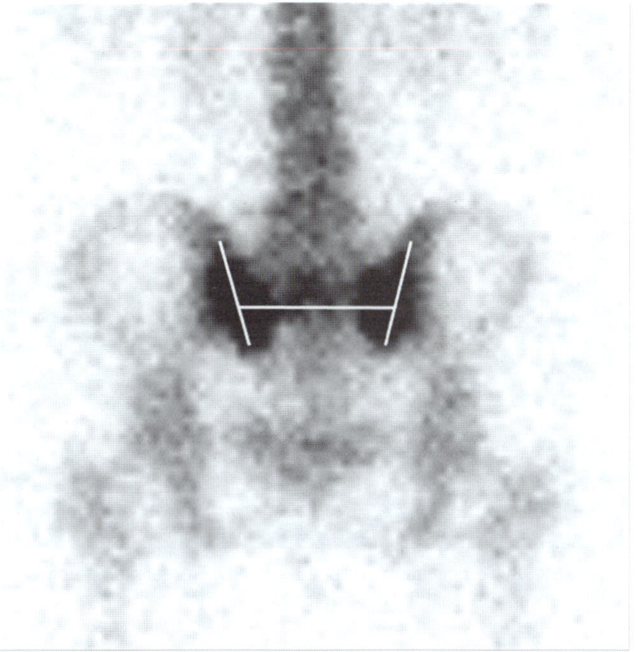

Figure 59.36 "Honda sign" seen on technetium-99m diphosphonate bone scan. Insufficiency fractures in the sacrum, with two vertical lines laterally and a horizontally oriented line in the middle, cause radiotracer uptake (*outlined in white*) that appears similar in configuration to the brand's "H" logo.

Summary of Teaching Points: Sacrum

- Sacral insufficiency fractures can be seen in osteopenic patients; they are often not clinically suspected
- MRI allows excellent evaluation of osteomyelitis and soft-tissue complications
- Marrow signal changes, even without marrow replacement, is suspicious for early osteomyelitis in the setting of overlying soft-tissue changes

Arthroplasties

Hip arthroplasty is a common procedure, and there are many different types of surgical hardware. Radiographs are the first-line study and help detect hardware complications, fractures, and infection (Fig. 59.38). CT without contrast and with metal suppression technique can help evaluate suspected component malposition, particle disease, and other pathology (Fig. 59.39). MRI

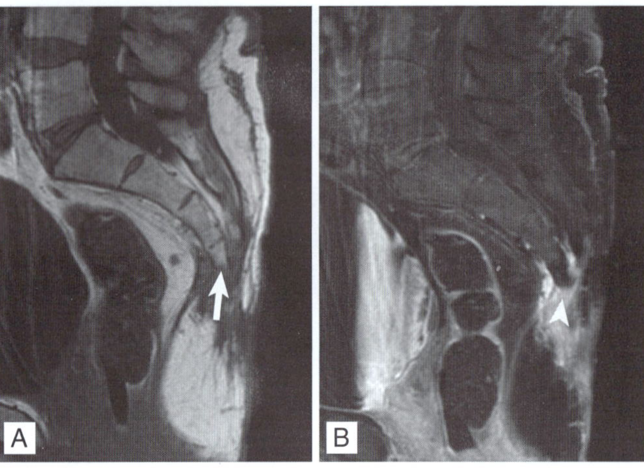

Figure 59.37 Sacral osteomyelitis. Sagittal T1-weighted (A) and T1-weighted fat-saturated postcontrast (B) MR images show marrow replacement at the tip of the residual coccyx (A, *arrow*) consistent with osteomyelitis. There is also postcontrast enhancement in this area (B, *arrowhead*); note that the diagnosis can be made with the A image alone.

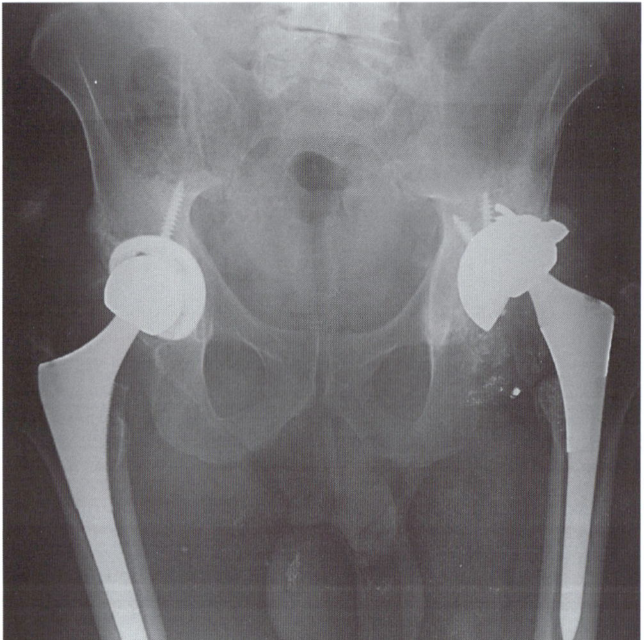

Figure 59.38 Complication of hip arthroplasty. Frontal radiograph of the pelvis shows bilateral total hip arthroplasties. The femoral head component on the left is superiorly located consistent with liner wear, and there are multiple osseous and metallic fragments in the soft tissues.

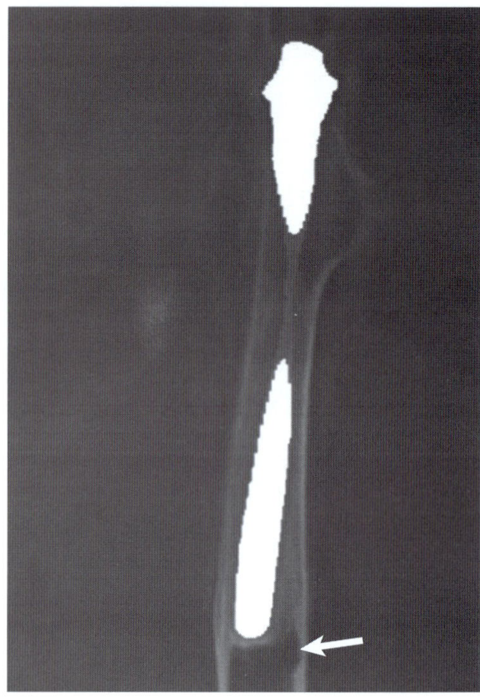

Figure 59.39 Sagittal reconstruction of a noncontrast CT performed with metal suppression protocol, showing a lucent lesion causing cortical thinning (*arrow*) at the tip of the femoral stem component of the hip arthroplasty. Without metal suppression technique, this lesion might have been more difficult, or even impossible, to see.

TABLE 59.11 Common Types of Hip Arthroplasties

	Hemi	Total	Resurfacing
Image			
Femoral head/neck	Replaced	Replaced	Replaced
Acetabulum	Native	Replaced	Replaced (surface only)
Clinical indication	Femoral neck fracture	Osteoarthrosis	Young patients, preserves bone stock

can also be used to detect particle disease, infection, and surrounding abnormalities. To reduce metal susceptibility artifact, MR imaging should utilize intermediate-weighted, fast SE pulse sequences. These sequences provide high-resolution images, fluid sensitivity, and high contrast-to-noise ratio to show periprosthetic tissue and bone. If an infection is suspected, imaging evaluation with radiographs followed by contrast-enhanced CT or MRI should be performed. Aspiration may be needed to confirm infected fluid. In-111 WBC and Tc-99m sulfur colloid scan can also be used to detect infection [63,64].

There are several main types of hip arthroplasties and many different brands and variations. Total hip arthroplasty involves replacing both the acetabulum and femoral head, while with a hemiarthroplasty, only the femoral head and neck are replaced. Total hip arthroplasties typically have a head and an acetabular liner, often made of polyethylene. Some are fixed with screws or cement, while others are cementless with a porous coating for bone ingrowth. Table 59.11 lists the most common types, with example images and primary descriptors [65].

Common Postoperative Complications

- **Periprosthetic fracture**
  - Incidence as high as 18%, during or after surgery
  - The calcar is a frequent site of intra-operative periprosthetic fracture in cementless total hip arthroplasty [66]

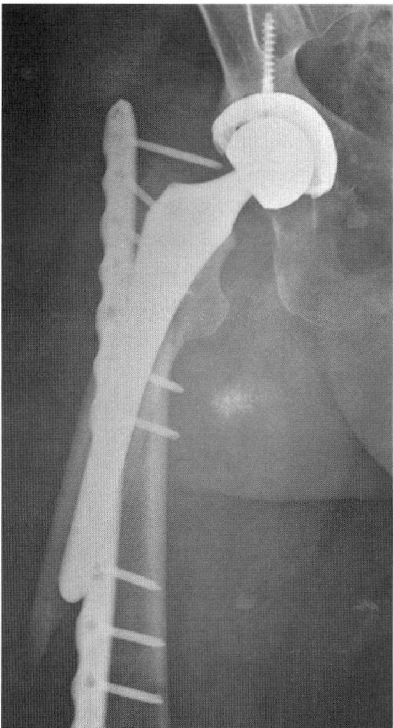

Figure 59.40 Frontal radiograph of the hip shows an oblique, peri-prosthetic fracture through the proximal femoral diaphysis.

- Risk factors: bone resorption, osteolysis, implant loosening, osteoporosis, trauma
- Radiographs are a first-line study (Fig. 59.40)
- On MRI, look for edema in marrow and cortex, fracture line, periosteal thickening
- Potential mimic: edema from reaming, which causes a peri-prosthetic high signal that can persist for months

- **Instability and dislocation**
  - Loosening is seen as lucency on radiographs or CT surrounding the hardware; lucency measuring greater than 2 mm in thickness is usually considered clinically significant
  - A thin fibrous layer, appearing as a lucency of 1–2 mm, often forms at the bone–hardware interface and is considered normal if stable (after 1–2 years) and in some regions of the prosthesis
  - Classification systems help to identify, which areas are involved with lucency/loosening; note that these are targeted for radiographic evaluation
    - Acetabular region: De Lee and Charnley system [63]
      - Zones I, II, and III adjacent to acetabular component (Fig. 59.41A)
      - Zone I (superolateral acetabulum) commonly shows a lucency
      - Zones II (medial) and III (inferomedial) typically should not show lucencies
    - Femoral region: Gruen zones [67]
      - Zones 1–7 surrounding the femoral component (Table 59.12) (Fig. 59.41B)
      - Common to see lucency in zone 1, or occasionally in zone 7
      - Lucency in zones 2–6 should be viewed with suspicion
  - Risk factors: component malposition, implant design, surgical approach, abductor mechanism, extent of soft-tissue dissection at surgery
  - High integrity of posterior joint capsule and musculature can be protective

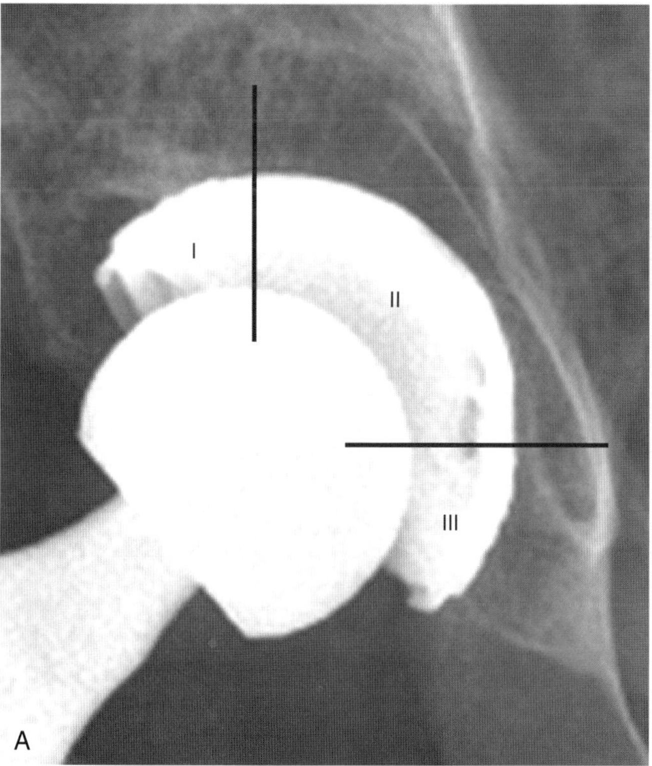

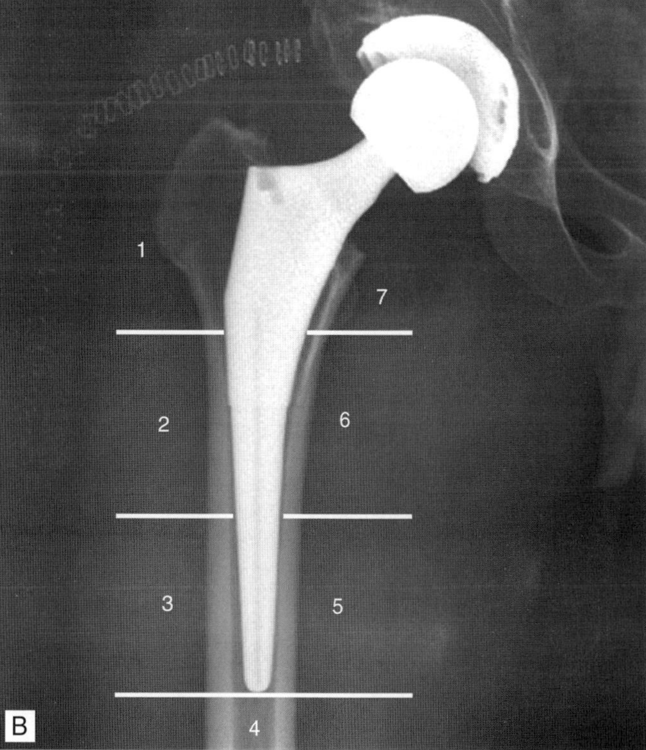

Figure 59.41 Classification systems for the evaluation of loosening on postarthroplasty radiographs. De Lee and Charnley acetabular (A) and Gruen femoral (B) zones help to evaluate and describe areas of lucency on postoperative radiographs.

- **Adverse local tissue reaction**
  - Umbrella term to describe reactions to arthroplasty-related metal products (metallosis) and reactive tissue inflammation (synonymous with pseudotumor)
  - Often resembles type IV hypersensitivity reaction
  - Can cause aggressive soft-tissue destruction
  - Poor correlation between symptoms and metallic ion levels in the blood
  - Prevalence may be as much as 39–66%
- Hematoma formation
- Synovitis
- Infection
- Heterotopic ossification
- Nerve injury

Conclusion/Overall Approach

Imaging of the hip allows the radiologist to evaluate the patient's anatomy and a myriad of pathological conditions. Fig. 59.42 shows an overall approach to the imaging evaluation of hip pain.

TABLE 59.12 Gruen Zones or Radiographic Changes Diagnostic of Loosening of the Femoral Component After Total Hip Arthroplasty

Zone	Area of Proximal Femur
1	Superolateral (involving greater trochanter)
2	Midlateral femur
3	Inferolateral femur
4	Distal tip
5	Inferomedial femur
6	Midmedial femur (includes lesser trochanter)
7	Superomedial (includes calcar)

Summary of Teaching Points: Arthroplasties

- Radiographs are first-line imaging study, but CT with metal suppression can help further to evaluate hardware and the surrounding bone and soft tissues
- Lucency greater than 2 mm in thickness surrounding the hardware is suggestive of clinically significant loosening. De Lee and Charnley (acetabular) and Gruen (femoral) zones help evaluate and describe the perihardware areas of lucency radiographically
- Resurfacing arthroplasty is favored in young patients to preserve bone stock
- Postoperative complications include periprosthetic fracture, instability/dislocation, and adverse local tissue reaction

Summary of Imaging Evaluation of the Hip

Structure/ pathology	*Preferred investigation*	*Secondary option*
Occult fracture	MRI	CT
Tendon pathology (e.g., tendinosis)	MRI or US	
Labral tear	MR arthrography	MRI
Arthritis	Radiograph	MRI or CT
Stress fracture	Radiograph, MRI	Bone scan
FAI	CT, radiographs	
Snapping hip	US	
Bursitis	MRI or US	
Insufficiency fracture	MRI	Bone scan or CT
Hip arthroplasty—no infection	Radiographs	CT, MRI
Hip arthroplasty—infection	Radiographs, aspiration	In-111 WBC and Tc-99m sulfur colloid

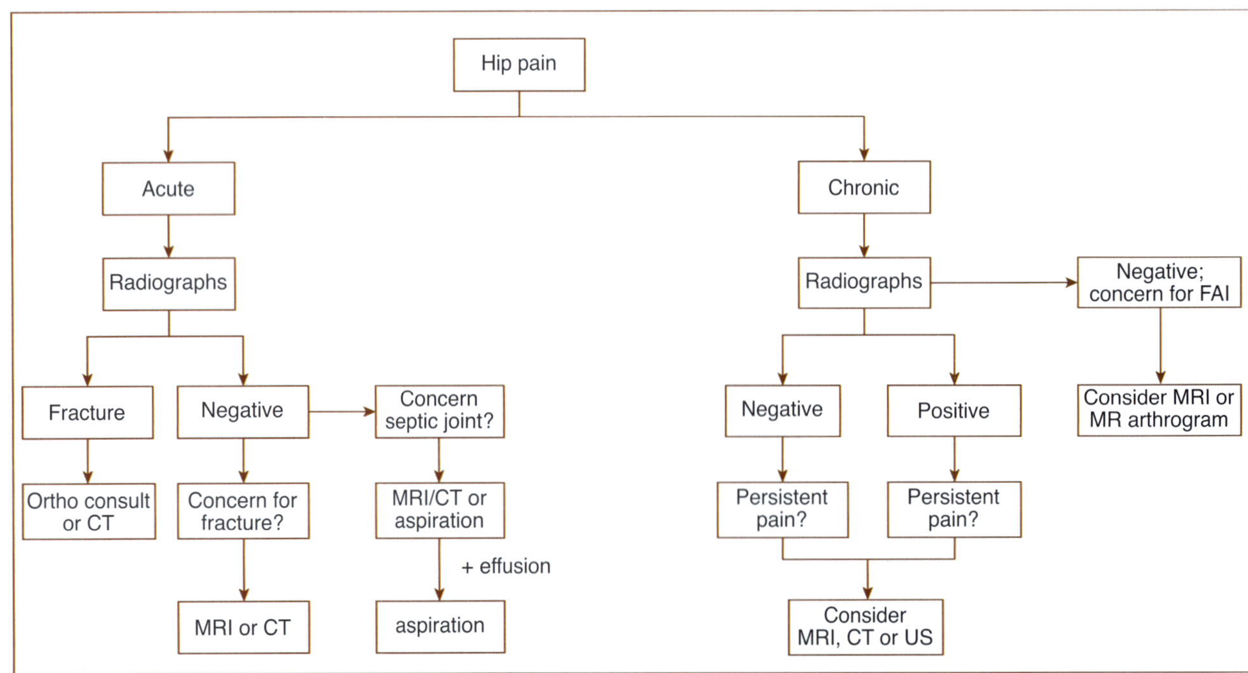

Figure 59.42 Flowchart that shows imaging workup of hip pain.

Suggested Readings

- CA Petersilge, Chronic adult hip pain: MR arthrography of the hip, Radiographics 20 (Suppl_1) (2000) S43–S52 [Internet].
- DR Armfield, JD Towers, DD Robertson, Radiographic and MR imaging of the athletic hip, Clin Sports Med 25 (2) (2006) 211–239.
- H Mulcahy, FS Chew, Current concepts of hip arthroplasty for radiologists: parts 1 and 2, AJR 199 (3) (2012) 559–569 and 570–580.
- TM Hegazi, JA Belair, EJ McCarthy, JB Roedl, WB Morrison, Sports injuries about the hip: what the radiologist should know, Radiographics 36 (6) (2016) 1717–1745.
- S Lim, Y Park, Plain radiography of the hip: a review of radiographic techniques and image features, Hip Pelvis 27 (3) (2015) 125–134.
- M Tannast, KA Siebenrock, SE Anderson, Femoroacetabular impingement: radiographic diagnosis – what the radiologist should know, AJR 188 (6) (2007) 1540–1552.

60

Knee

AMIT KUMAR SAHU

The knee joint is the body's largest synovial joint. Normal knee joint contains less than 5 mL of fluid. Given its significant role in ambulation, it is vulnerable to various mechanical injuries, internal derangements, and osteoarthritis. Knee instability and pain is a common presenting complaint in athletes and nonathletes alike; as well as in young and old. Imaging also has a crucial complementary role to clinical examination in a large number of nontraumatic pathologies associated with the knee joint. The radiograph is the primary imaging technique in most pathology. Ultrasonography (USG) is a readily available technique that is helpful in assessing joint effusion, pathologies of large tendons, and ligaments around the knee, and in guiding intervention. It is gaining a more significant presence in the imaging algorithm. Magnetic resonance imaging (MRI) stands as the gold standard imaging technique for most of the soft tissue and marrow pathologies. CT has an essential role in assessing fractures.

Overview of the Function of the Knee Joint

The knee joint comprises predominantly of the weight-bearing femorotibial articulation and the patellofemoral articulation. The latter creates a frictionless transfer over the knee of the forces generated by contraction of the quadriceps femoris muscle. *In 10% of cases, the knee joint space communicates with the proximal tibiofibular joint* [1]. Movements in the knee joint include flexion, extension, internal, and external rotation. Abduction and adduction movements are limited and can only be achieved in a flexed knee. Any degree of abduction and adduction in an extended knee is considered to be sign of knee laxity. In a large part, the knee joint's stability is maintained by the capsule, intrinsic ligaments and tendons.

Muscles producing movements of the knee are as follows:

- *Flexion*—biceps femoris, semitendinosus, and semimembranosus assisted by the gracilis, sartorius, and popliteus (and with the foot on the ground, the gastrocnemius and plantaris)
- *Extension*—quadriceps femoris, assisted by the tensor fasciae latae
- *Medial rotation of the flexed leg*—popliteus, semimembranosus, and semitendinosus assisted by the sartorius and gracilis
- *Lateral rotation of the flexed leg*—biceps femoris

Anatomy

Osseous and articular anatomy: The three bones forming the knee joint are the femur, tibia, and patella. The knee joint primarily has two components, femorotibial and patellofemoral (Fig. 60.1).

The distal end of the femur has a large, oval medial condyle, and a small circular lateral condyle, separated by the intercondylar region. There are two small bony projections on either side of the distal femur condyles, called the medial and lateral epicondyles. Superior to the medial epicondyle lies the adductor tubercle, which provides the attachment site for the tendinous part of the adductor magnus muscle. The anterior aspect of the distal femur has a saddle-shaped patellar surface called trochlear groove, forming the patellofemoral articulation.

The patella is an oval-shaped sesamoid bone embedded within the tendon of quadriceps femoris. It has no direct role in the weight bearing of the knee joint. The articular surface of the patella is oval and is separated into smaller, more vertical medial, and larger more horizontal lateral facets by a vertical ridge. This vertical ridge fits into the corresponding trochlear groove in the anterior aspect of the femur. Contact between the patellar articular facets and femur varies with different positions of knee. During forced extension of the knee joint, the patella has a tendency to be displaced laterally, given the more horizontal orientation of the lateral facet. The patellar tendon is the inferior

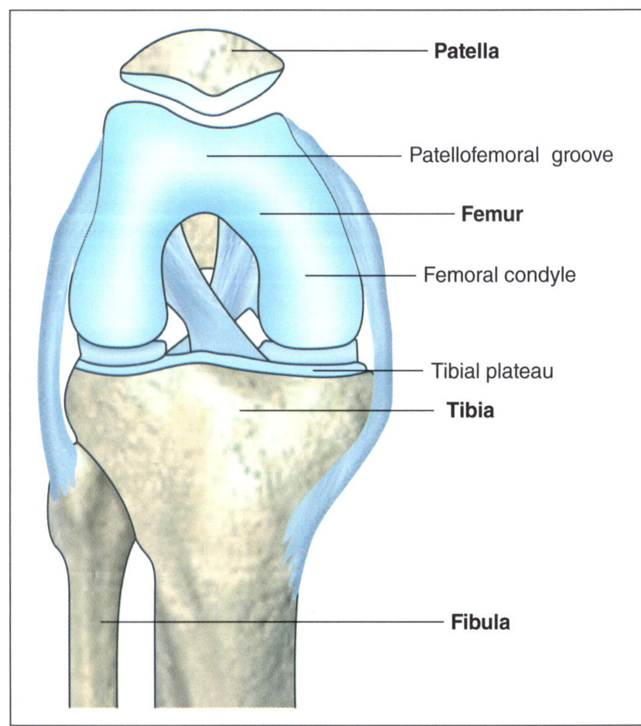

Figure 60.1 Diagrammatic representation of osseous components of the knee joint demonstrating various ligament attachments.

continuation of the quadriceps tendon and attaches to the tibial tuberosity. It is also called patellar ligament, as it extends between two bones.

The proximal tibia has an oval medial tibial condyle with its long axis in the sagittal plane and the circular and the smaller lateral tibial condyle. This topography helps in internal rotation of the femur on the fixed tibia as the knee approaches extension. Between the tibial condyles is the intercondylar area, which, from anterior to posterior, serves as attachments to

- anterior root ligament of the lateral meniscus;
- anterior cruciate ligament (ACL);
- anterior root ligament of the medial meniscus;
- posterior root ligament of the lateral meniscus;
- posterior root ligament of the medial meniscus; and
- posterior cruciate ligament (PCL).

Capsular and Synovial Anatomy

The articular capsule of the knee joint consists of a thick outer fibrous capsule and a thin inner synovial membrane. The knee joint is a common joint space that is subdivided by synovial membranes into several interconnected compartments. Synovial recesses are extensions of the synovial membrane between different anatomical structures that reduce friction during the motion of these structures (Fig. 60.2).

The anatomy of anterior, medial, lateral, and central structures is discussed separately under individual sections later in this chapter.

Imaging Protocols

Radiograph

Radiograph is the primary technique for all knee imaging. Basic radiographic views and their purpose are mentioned in Table 60.1.

TABLE 60.1 Basic Radiographic Views of Knee

Views	Purpose
AP view (weight bearing)	Alignment, femorotibial joint space, fractures, bony erosions, soft-tissue swelling, and calcification
Lateral view	Alignment, patella position, joint effusion, fractures
Axial view or sunrise view (30–45 degrees flexion)	Patella position, patellofemoral joint space, peripheral bony erosions in patella
Intercondylar view	Intercondylar space, tibial plateau fracture

Note: Additional views which can be obtained for patella and patellofemoral joint are Skyline Merchant view (superior-inferior projection of the patella in supine position) and Skyline Laurel view (inferior-superior projection of the patella in semirecumbent position).

USG Protocol

Localized evaluation of a different anatomical aspect of knee is done in both long and short axes (Table 60.2).

CT Protocol (Table 60.3)

- Positioning: Patient supine, knee being imaged is centered in the scanner
- Field of view must include: Entire patella, both femoral condyles, and proximal tibia to just past the fibular head. In the case of a metal prosthesis, scan the entire length of the femoral and tibial components
- Practical indication of the CT scan of the knee is in the evaluation of fractures. In metal prosthesis, projection-based metal artifact reduction (MAR) algorithms are used to better evaluate the hardware and the periprosthetic bone

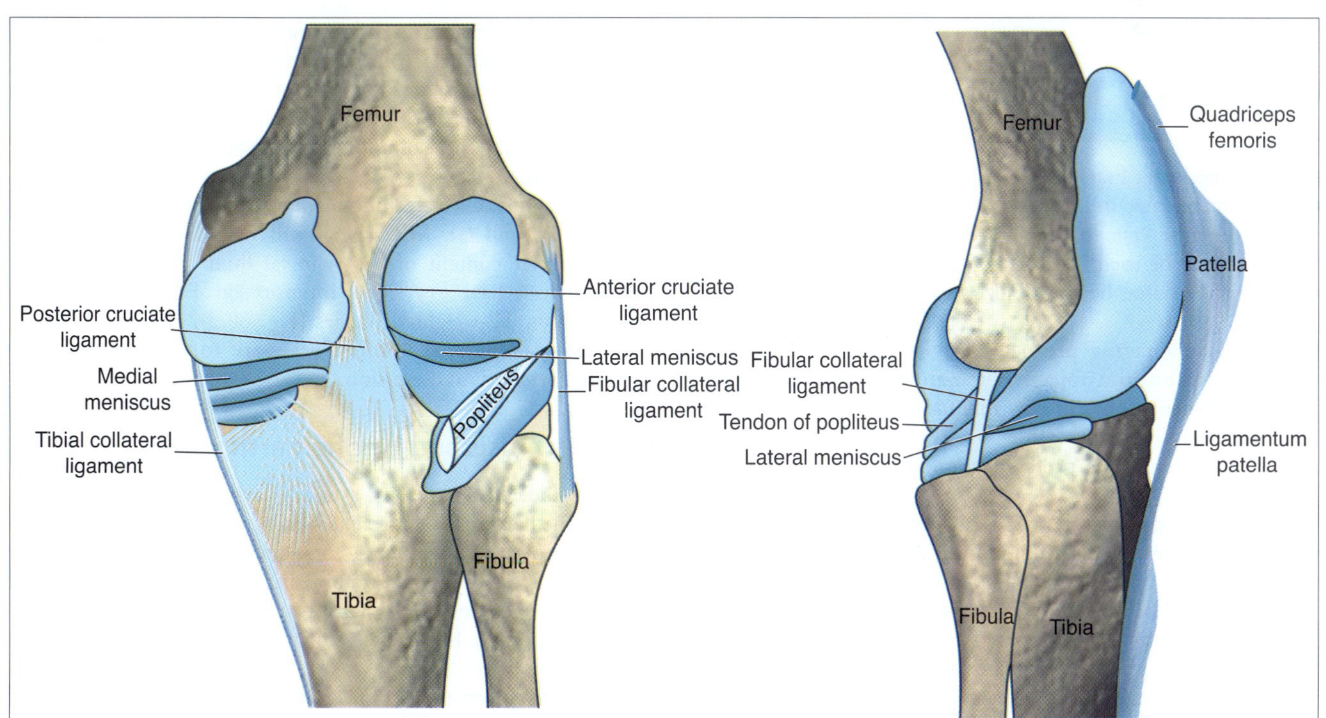

Figure 60.2 Diagrammatic representation of articular capsule attachment and recesses around the knee joint.

TABLE 60.2 Basic Imaging Protocol of USG Knee

Protocol	Structures Evaluated
Anterior knee (patient supine, knee flexed 30 degrees)	Extensor mechanism (quadriceps tendon, patella, and patellar tendon), patellar retinaculum, suprapatellar joint recess, medial and lateral joint recesses, anterior knee bursae, and femoral articular cartilage
Medial knee (patient supine, knee full extension)	Medial collateral ligament, the body and anterior horn of the medial meniscus, and the pes anserine tendons (sartorius, gracilis, and semitendinosus)
Lateral knee (patient supine, knee full extension)	Iliotibial band, lateral collateral ligament, biceps femoris, common peroneal nerve, popliteus, and body and anterior horn of the lateral meniscus
Posterior knee (patient prone, knee full extension)	Baker cyst, the posterior horns of the menisci, posterior cruciate ligament, and the popliteal neurovascular bundle

TABLE 60.3 Basic Imaging Protocol of CT Knee

Plane	Section Thickness	Overlap	Window Width/Level
Source axial	0.625 mm or less	50%	Soft tissue
Reformat axial[a]	2 mm	None	Bone Soft tissue
Reformat coronal[a]	2 mm	None	Bone
Reformat sagittal[a]	2 mm	None	Bone

[a]All reformats should include entire field of view of the source images.

MRI Protocol

Position

- Supine with feet first
- Position the knee in knee coil in 15-degree flexion with cushion below the knee for stability. In unavailability of knee coil, flex coil can be used
- Center the laser beam localizer over the lower border of patella

Although the imaging protocols for knee vary substantially across institutions the objectives remain the same. A representative MR knee protocol may include some combination of the following sequences (this is only a guide as protocols depend on institutional preferences and local practices) (Table 60.4).

MR arthrography of the knee is an invasive procedure that is done by injecting diluted gadolinium contrast into the joint followed by MR imaging. Although not a routine protocol, it is used for the detection of osteochondral lesions and evaluation of postoperative meniscus in current practice.

MR cartigram is used to evaluate the articular cartilage. It uses quantitative cartilage imaging techniques such as T2 mapping sequences to detect changes in the water and collagen content and the three-dimensional ultrastructure of cartilage.

TABLE 60.4 Basic Imaging Protocol of MRI Knee

Sequence	Purpose
PDFS coronal	Synovial pathologies; meniscal tear; collateral ligaments; tendon pathologies; femoral and tibial articular cartilage; and cystic lesions around the knee
PDFS sagittal	Cruciate ligament pathologies; meniscal tear; quadriceps and patellar tendons
PDFS axial	Patellofemoral joint; patellar articular cartilage
T1 coronal	T1 characteristics of any incidental bone or soft-tissue lesion; avulsion fractures; intra-articular bodies
T2 FS coronal (optional)	Meniscal root tear; fat-saturation helps reveal fluid, marrow edema, fat pad edema, bursitis, parameniscal cyst
Gradient (optional)	Calcification and hemorrhage
Pre and Postcontrast T1 FS (optional)	Synovitis, osteomyelitis, tumors

Effusion

Joint Effusion

Physiological fluid is noted in synovial joints, not sufficient to distend the joint cavity. Accumulation of excess fluid within the joint is called synovial effusion and leads to distention of synovial joint recess.

Imaging Features

Radiograph: Properly obtained lateral radiograph of the knee is sensitive for detecting effusion. It is appreciated as distention of the suprapatellar joint recess, leading to separation of the suprapatellar and prefemoral fat pads by more than 5 mm [2] (Fig. 60.3).

USG and MRI are equally sensitive in detecting synovial effusion.

On *USG*, fluid is anechoic, compressible, and displaceable on dynamic evaluation. No intrinsic vascularity is seen. USG is also useful in guiding the aspiration of fluid both for diagnostic as well as therapeutic purposes.

MRI is an excellent technique for assessment, given its sensitivity to fluid and fat. MRI signal will vary depending on fluid, blood, or fat content of the synovial fluid. Both effusion and synovitis can have low signal intensity on T1 and high signal intensity on T2-weighted images (Fig. 60.3). Administration of contrast (gadolinium) is often necessary to tell the difference between synovitis and effusion.

Hemarthrosis and Lipohemarthrosis

The presence of blood in the synovial cavity is termed hemarthrosis. Lipohemarthrosis denotes the presence of marrow fat and blood in the synovial cavity, often a consequence of fracture. This may take 3 hours to appear after trauma. Fat component in the synovial fluid represents seepage of marrow fat (from femur or tibia) into the joint due to fracture, ligament avulsion, or osteochondral abnormality [3].

Other causes of hemarthrosis include:

- Pigmented villonodular synovitis
- Bleeding disorders (hemophilia)

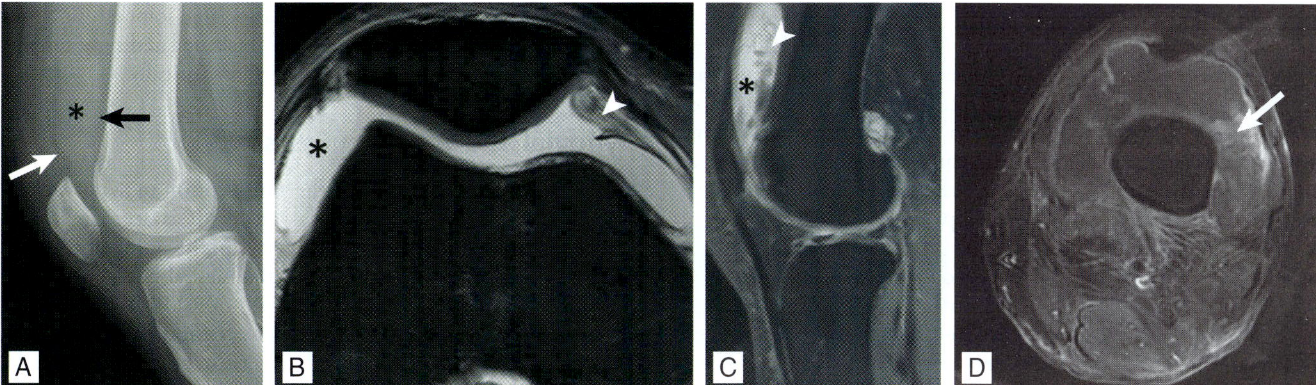

Figure 60.3 Joint effusion versus synovitis. (A and B) Joint effusion: lateral view radiograph shows distension of the suprapatellar space (*asterisk*) separating suprapatellar fat pad (*white arrow*) from prefemoral fat pad (*back arrow*). Axial PDFS MR image showing excess fluid in the knee joint cavity (*asterisk* in B) with smooth synovium (*arrowhead*). (C) Synovitis: sagittal PDFS MR image showing excess fluid in suprapatellar recess (*asterisk*) with thickening of the synovium (*arrowhead*). (D) Axial postcontrast T1FS image of a different patient shows diffuse central enhancement (*white arrow*).

- Intra-articular tumors (synovial hemangioma)
- Neuropathic osteoarthropathy
- Crystal deposition diseases
- Renal osteodystrophy

Imaging Features

Radiograph often cannot differentiate between synovial effusion and hemarthrosis or lipohemarthrosis. However, if a lateral view (erect or supine trans-lateral) is obtained after 5–10 minutes of the patient lying down, fat–fluid levels can be seen in lipohemarthrosis (Fig. 60.4).

USG can differentiate between fat and blood. Fat is seen as echogenic nondependent globules within the synovial fluid and blood appears as floating echoes or as dependent echogenic sediment (Fig. 60.4).

MRI: Three-layer fluid–fluid levels are seen consisting of nondependent marrow fat in the top layer, plasma serum in the middle layer, and dependent blood cells (erythrocytes and leucocytes) in the most dependent portion forming the deepest layer (Fig 60.4). Acute hemorrhagic effusion (<24 hours) may have signal intensity similar to the synovial fluid while subacute hemarthrosis (1–7 days) will demonstrate high signal on both T1- and T2-weighted images. Chronic hemarthrosis (>7 days) will have low signal intensity on both T1- and T2-weighted images due to hemosiderin deposition.

Synovial Pathologies

Synovitis

Synovitis is the inflammation of the synovium, which causes hyperplasia of the synovial lining. It can be focal or diffuse and can lead to the appearance of frond-like projections into the synovial cavity. It is essential to differentiate between joint effusion and synovitis for treatment.

Imaging Features

A radiograph cannot usually differentiate between joint effusion and synovitis.

USG: Areas of synovial hyperplasia can be seen as thick and echogenic synovium with increased color uptake on Doppler study. USG-guided synovial biopsy is performed in the case of nonconclusive imaging features.

MRI holds some advantage in differentiating these two conditions. Synovitis and effusion can coexist. Synovitis is seen as an intermediate signal on T1 as against low signal in joint effusion. T2 signal is higher in synovitis than in joint effusion. Synovitis demonstrates diffuse postcontrast central enhancement (Fig. 60.3), while joint effusion may show peripheral enhancement.

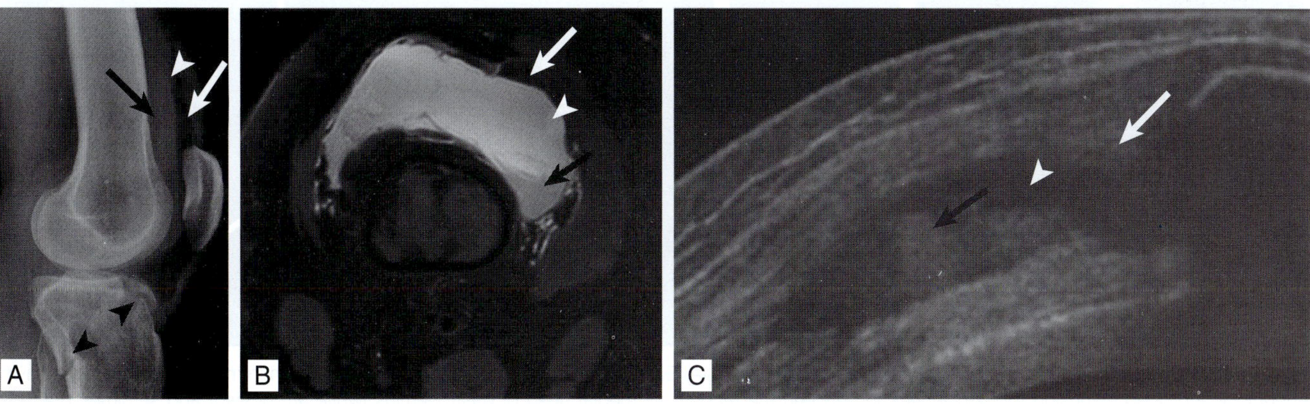

Figure 60.4 Lipohemarthrosis. Radiograph lateral view (A), Axial PDFS MR image (B) and USG (C) in supine position of a traumatic knee showing distension of suprapatellar recess with three-layer appearance of superficial fat (*white arrow*), middle serum (*white arrowhead*), and deep red cells (*black arrow*). There is fracture of tibial plateau (*black arrowheads* in A).

Both menisci are stabilized by the transverse ligament. The meniscocapsular ligaments including the meniscofemoral and meniscotibial ligaments attach the menisci to the posterior femur and posterior tibial plateau. The lateral meniscus is stabilized by the coronary ligament, meniscofemoral ligament, arcuate ligament, and meniscotibial ligament (Fig. 60.11). If any of these supporting ligaments or the meniscus itself degenerates or is torn, the meniscus may become unstable.

Both menisci have anterior horn, body, posterior horn, and roots. Only the periphery of the meniscus remains vascularized in adults (called "red zone"), occupying 15% of the meniscus [10]. Tears that occur within the meniscus' red zone are more likely to heal than those in the avascular, "white zone."

Anatomical Variation in Meniscus

Discoid Meniscus

It is the congenital variable enlargement of the meniscus body, often with thickening of the meniscus. Seen in 3% of knees and is 10–20 times more common in the lateral than in the medial meniscus [11]. Usually asymptomatic but are prone to cystic degeneration and tear. On MRI, the body of discoid meniscus measures 15 mm or more on a midline coronal image and sagittal MR images. The body of meniscus is seen in three or more contiguous slices (Fig. 60.12).

Meniscal Flounce

Wavy appearance of the free inner edge of the meniscus on coronal and sagittal MR images (Fig. 60.12). This is secondary to flexion of the knee where the free edge of the meniscus is redundant. It is more common in the medial meniscus and it may mimic a radial tear in coronal MR images.

Meniscal Ossicle

This is a focus of calcification or ossification seen with a predilection for the posterior horn of medial meniscus (Fig. 60.12). It may be developmental, degenerative, or post-traumatic. On radiographs, the ossicle can be mistaken for an intra-articular body, while at MR imaging, its increased signal intensity can mimic a tear.

Pathologies of Meniscus

A tear is the most common pathology encountered in the meniscus. Developmental, inflammatory, infectious, neoplastic, and metabolic pathologies also affect the meniscus.

Meniscal Tears

Two common categories of pathologies responsible for meniscal tears are traumatic and degenerative. As it is difficult to differentiate between the two, categorization is based on clinical history, age of patient, gross morphology of the meniscus, and secondary imaging findings.

Meniscal tear is defined as linear intrameniscal signal that contacts the superior, inferior or free articular margins of the meniscus or if there is a defect in the normal shape of the meniscus. Once the tear is identified, the description of the tear should be documented to categorize it into specific type. There are different

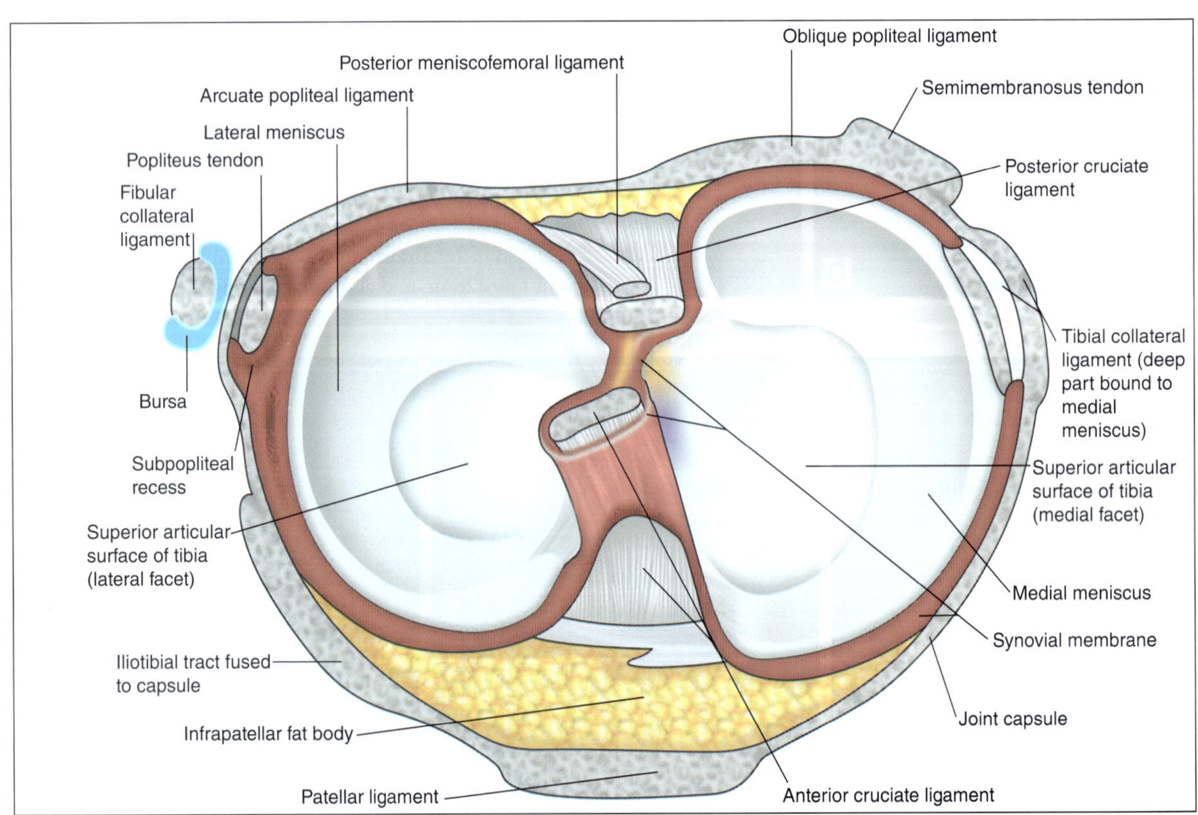

Figure 60.11 Diagrammatic representation of inferior knee through superior view demonstrating normal anatomy of meniscus and various ligaments attached to the menisci.

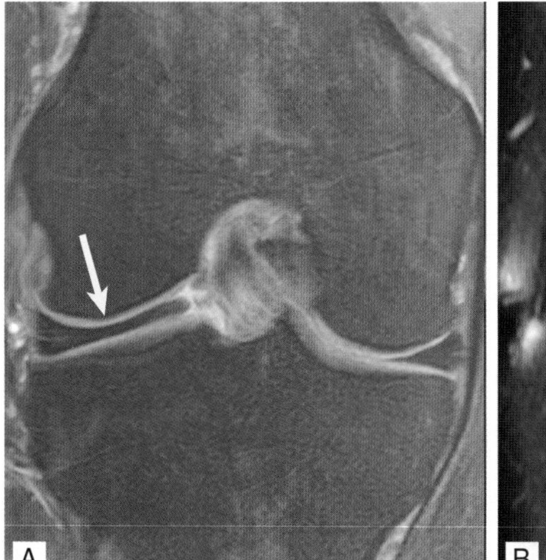

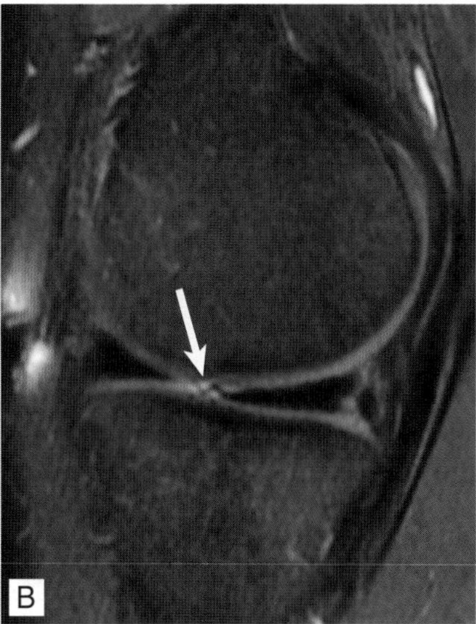

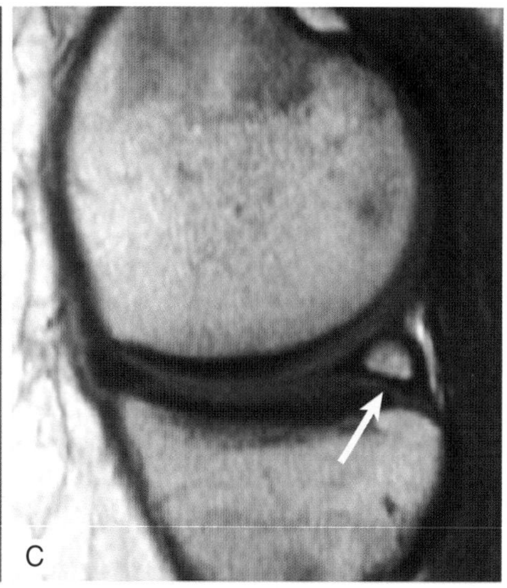

Figure 60.12 (A) Discoid lateral meniscus. There is thickening of the lateral meniscus (*arrow*) as seen in the coronal PDFS MR image of a 28-year male. (B) Meniscal flounce. Wavy appearance of the free inner edge of the medial meniscus (*arrow*) seen in sagittal PDFS MR image. (C) Meniscal ossicle. Focal calcification seen as hyperintense signal in posterior horn of medial meniscus (*arrow*) in sagittal T1 MR image.

terminologies used for meniscal tear classification, without consensus. However, the common classification of meniscal tears is based on the direction of tear [11]:

- Horizontal (parallel or oblique)
- Longitudinal vertical
- Radial

For general consideration: Longitudinal tears and less commonly, horizontal oblique tears are traumatic in nature. Degenerative tears are typically horizontal cleavage lesions that generally occupy the posterior half of the menisci.

Clinical presentation

- Joint pain (at the joint line)
- Giving way on walking
- Clicking on movement
- Joint effusion
- Locking (which may occur immediately after displacement of a meniscal fragment)
- Pseudolocking (secondary to hamstring muscle spasms)

Imaging Features

Radiograph is not useful in the diagnosis of meniscal injuries. However, it may be indicated in elderly patients to obtain a differential diagnosis of osteoarthritis, which often develops in association with meniscal degeneration. AP and lateral radiographs may show joint space narrowing in clinically symptomatic meniscal injury. A radiograph can also exclude unsuspected lesions such as osteochondritis or intra-articular bodies.

CT is less sensitive in diagnosing meniscal tears. However, CT arthrography provides an accurate diagnosis of meniscal and cartilage injuries in patients who cannot undergo MRI.

USG is not a routine test for meniscal imaging. Secondary signs such as extrusion and parameniscal cyst can be detected. Therapeutic USG-guided aspiration is performed in the symptomatic parameniscal cysts.

MRI is the gold standard in diagnosing meniscal tears. It also helps in the evaluation of associated injuries, complications, and the postoperative meniscus. MRI characteristics of pathological meniscus [12] include:

(A) Alteration in signal: Normal meniscus is characterized by low signal intensity on all sequences. Abnormal high signal on T2 and PDFS images is graded as shown in Fig. 60.13.

(B) Alteration in morphology: Normal morphology of a meniscus is triangular with a sharp central tip apparent in both the coronal and sagittal planes (bow-tie configuration). This triangular configuration is distorted in tear.

Indirect signs of meniscal tear:

- Subchondral bone marrow edema beneath a meniscus in the absence of meniscectomy
- Presence of a parameniscal cyst
- Meniscal extrusion (when the meniscus is >3 mm outside the peripheral margin of the tibial plateau)

Nuances in the diagnosis of meniscal tear [12]

- *Two-slice-touch rule*: If intrameniscal signal contacts the meniscus surface on two or more images, there is 90–96% likelihood that a meniscal tear would be identified at arthroscopy. The signal to the surface must be in the same area of the meniscus on the two images, but one image can be in the coronal plane and other in the sagittal plane
- *Meniscal Fraying* is not a typical tear and may involve the free edge of the meniscus. This may appear as ill-defined margin of meniscus with horizontal signal alteration on one or two sequential MR images (sagittal or coronal)

Mimics of meniscal tears

Normal anatomical variations:

- Anterior transverse meniscal ligament of the knee
- Oblique meniscomeniscal ligaments of the knee
- Lateral inferior genicular artery
- Popliteus tendon
- Meniscofemoral ligaments
- Bursa of the medial collateral ligament (MCL)
- Tibial attachment site of the ACL
- Meniscal root ligaments

Physiological appearance:

- Meniscal flounce

Horizontal Tear

It runs parallel or oblique to the tibial plateau, contacts the articular surface(s) or the central free edge, and extends toward the

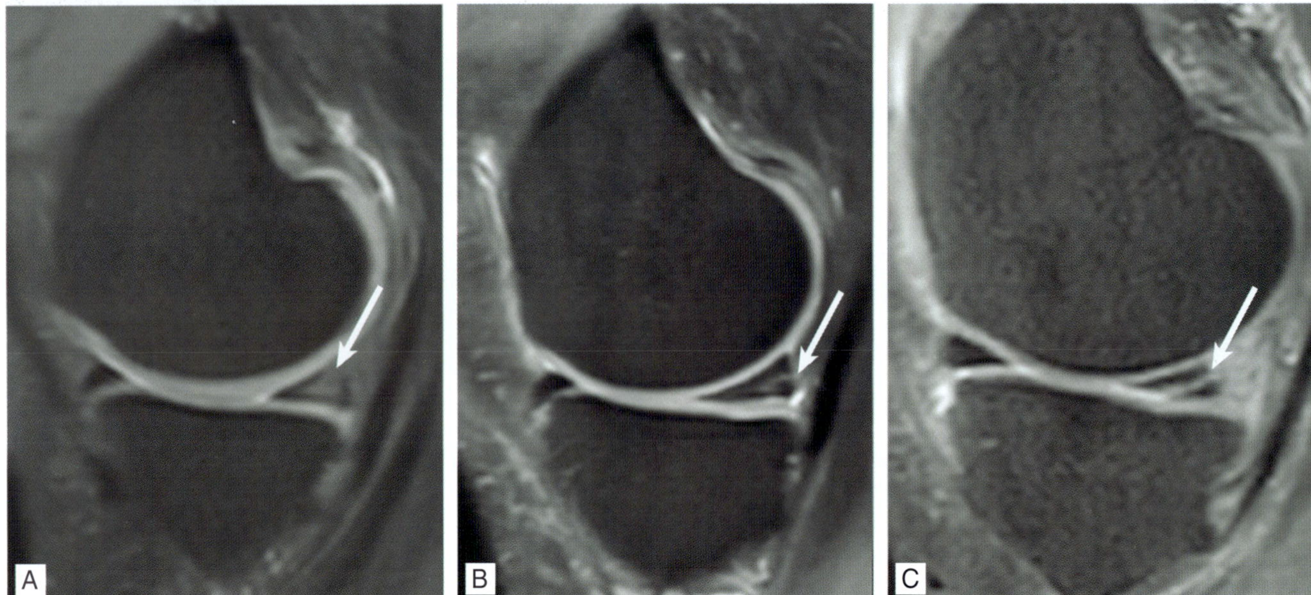

Figure 60.13 MRI grading of meniscus signal represented by *arrows* in sagittal PDFS images. (A) *Grade 1*—nonarticular focal or globular intrasubstance increased signal intensity. This signal correlates with early meniscal degeneration. Myxoid or hyaline degeneration are both used to describe these signal alteration. (B) *Grade 2*—horizontal, linear intrasubstance increased signal intensity usually extending from the capsular periphery of the meniscus without involving an articular meniscal surface. (C) *Grade 3*—area of increased signal intensity communicating or extending to at least one articular surface. Grade 3 signal is considered to be meniscal tear and a meniscus may contain multiple areas of grade 3 signal intensity.

periphery, dividing the meniscus into superior and inferior halves (Fig. 60.14). It usually occurs in patients older than 40 years in the setting of underlying degenerative joint disease. However, horizontal oblique tears can be post-traumatic. Typical MRI appearance is a horizontally oriented line of high signal intensity that contacts the meniscal surface or free edge. Parameniscal cyst (Fig. 60.15) formation is associated with complete horizontal tears that extend to the periphery, presumably secondary to direct communication with the joint fluid.

Longitudinal Vertical Tear

It runs perpendicular to the tibial plateau and parallel to the long axis of the meniscus and divides the meniscus into central and peripheral halves (Fig. 60.14). Unlike horizontal or radial tears, pure longitudinal tears do not involve the free edge of the meniscus. Often occur in younger patients after knee trauma and usually involve the peripheral third of the meniscus and posterior horns. Typical MRI appearance is a vertically oriented line of high signal intensity that contacts one or both articular surfaces. They usually involve the peripheral red zone and occur in posterior horn. There is a close association between peripheral longitudinal tear of either or both menisci and ACL tear.

Longitudinal vertical tear of the peripheral capsular attachment of the posterior horn of the medial meniscus at the meniscocapsular junction is termed as *Ramp lesion.* This lesion most frequently occurs in the setting of a pivot shift mechanism of injury. It is possibly due to disruption of the meniscotibial ligaments, or as a result of a tear of the peripheral attachment of the posterior horn of the medial meniscus.

Radial Tear

It runs perpendicular to both the tibial plateau and the long axis of the meniscus and extends from the free edge toward the periphery (Fig. 60.14). In contrast to horizontal and longitudinal tears, radial tears disrupt the meniscal hoop strength, resulting in a dramatic loss of function and possible meniscal extrusion. These commonly involve the posterior horn of the medial meniscus or the junction of the anterior horn and body of the lateral meniscus. Surgical repair is usually not considered because they are located within the avascular "white zone."

MRI signs of radial tear:

- *Truncated meniscus* represents a truncation of the free edge, with preservation of its peripheral portion, often due to a partial-thickness tear
- *Ghost meniscus* has no in-plane residual normal meniscus, often as a result of a full-thickness tear
- *Marching cleft*: tear that appears to progress away from the free edge on contiguous MR images and is seen in the junction of the horn and body (obliquely oriented to both coronal and sagittal planes)

On coronal MR images, if the cleft is within the body, it results from a longitudinal tear. If the cleft is within the horn, it is the result of a radial tear. The opposite combination holds true on sagittal MR images.

Root Tear

It is typically a radial-type tear and has received increased recognition in recent years, partially because of its previous underdiagnoses at both MR imaging and arthroscopy. On coronal MRI, if the root is not seen over its respective tibial plateau on at least one image, tear is suspected (Fig. 60.16). On sagittal MRI, if the posterior root of the medial meniscus is not detected just medial to the PCL, a root tear should be suspected. Complete root tears have a high association with meniscal extrusion, mainly when the tear occurs in the medial meniscus. When an ACL tear is present, there is an increased incidence of lateral root tears.

Complex Tear

It includes radial, horizontal, and longitudinal components (any two or all three). Often the meniscus appears fragmented, with the tear extending in more than one plane (Fig. 60.16).

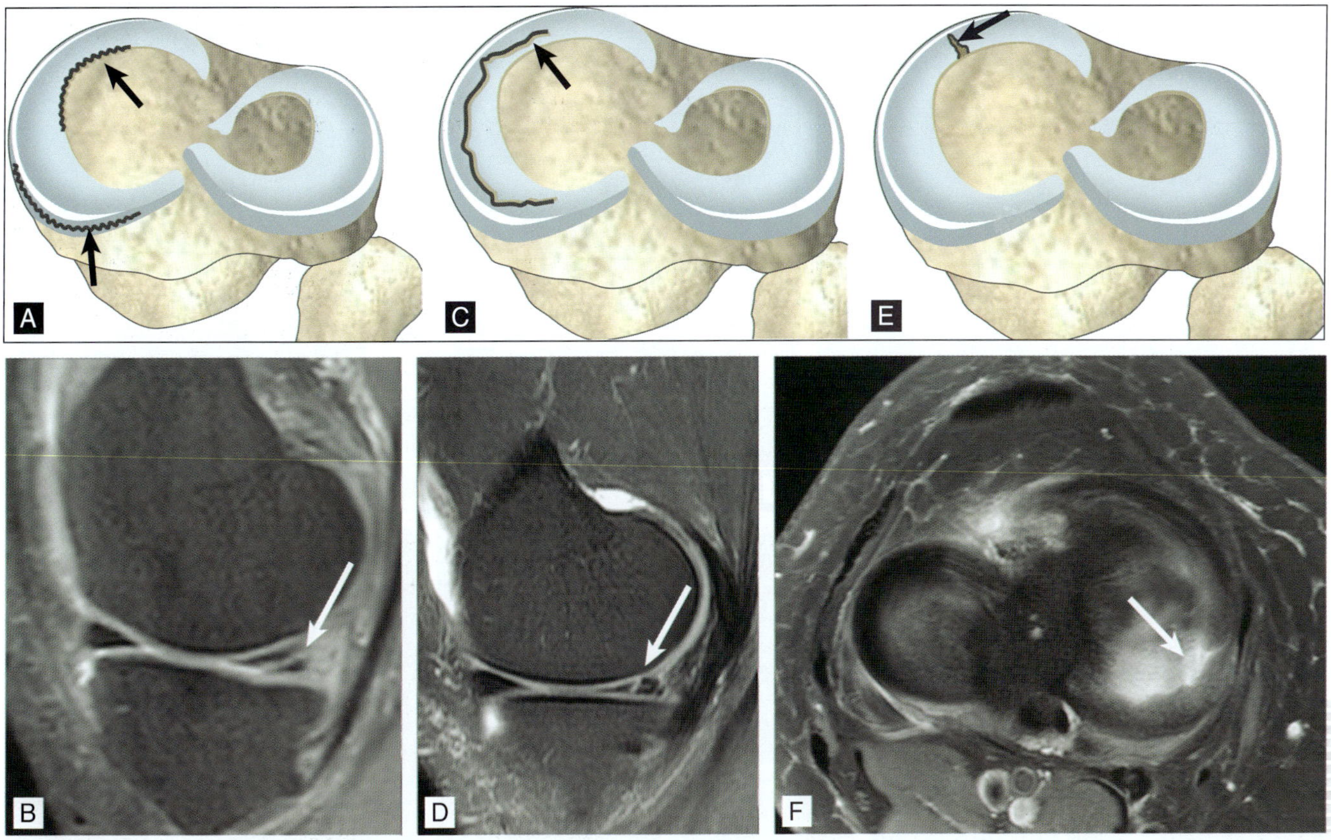

Figure 60.14 Types of meniscal tear based on direction of tear as indicated by arrows. Diagrammatic representation (first row), sagittal (B, D) and axial (F) PDFS MR images (second row) showing tear in posterior horn of medial meniscus in three different patients. (A and B) Horizontal oblique tear, (C and D) longitudinal vertical tear, and (E and F) radial tear.

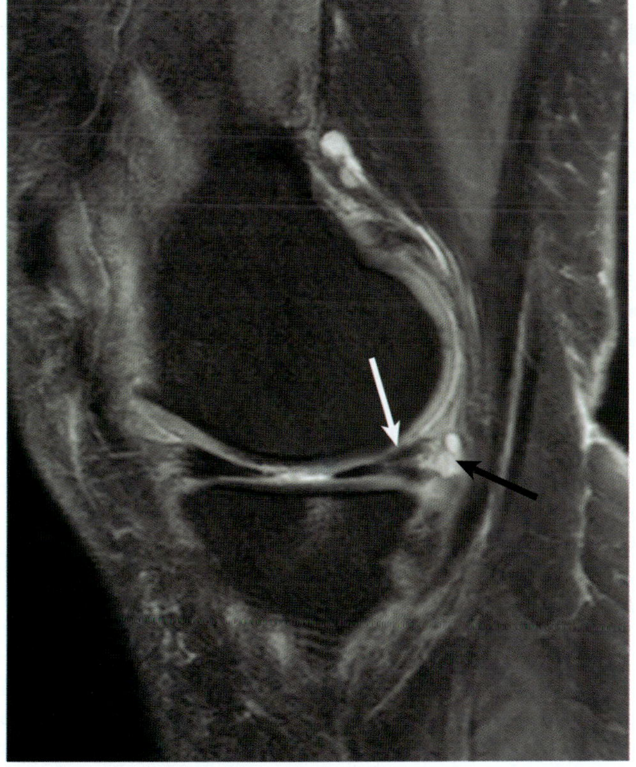

Figure 60.15 Sagittal PDFS MRI image shows horizontal tear of posterior horn of medial meniscus (*white arrow*) with parameniscal cyst formation (*black arrow*).

Displaced Tear

Displaced tears are categorized into: free fragments, displaced flap tears, and bucket-handle tears.

Small free fragments and flaps can be missed at arthroscopy, and retention of a meniscal flap often results in persistent pain and potential knee locking. Flap tears occur more frequently in the medial meniscus. In two-thirds of cases, fragments are displaced posteriorly, near or posterior to the PCL; in the remaining cases, fragments course into either the intercondylar notch or superior recess (Fig. 60.16).

Bucket-Handle Tear

It is a longitudinal tear with central migration of the inner "handle" fragment. This tear pattern occurs more frequently in the medial meniscus.

> *MRI signs of bucket-handle tear* (Fig. 60.16):
> - Absent normal bow-tie configuration
> - Torn fragment within the intercondylar notch
> - Double PCL appearance (PCL and centrally migrated meniscus fragment are seen parallel to each other on sagittal image)
> - Double anterior horn or flipped meniscus
> - Disproportionally small posterior horn

A bucket-handle tear of the lateral meniscus can rarely manifest with a double ACL sign, where the fragment is located just posterior to the ACL.

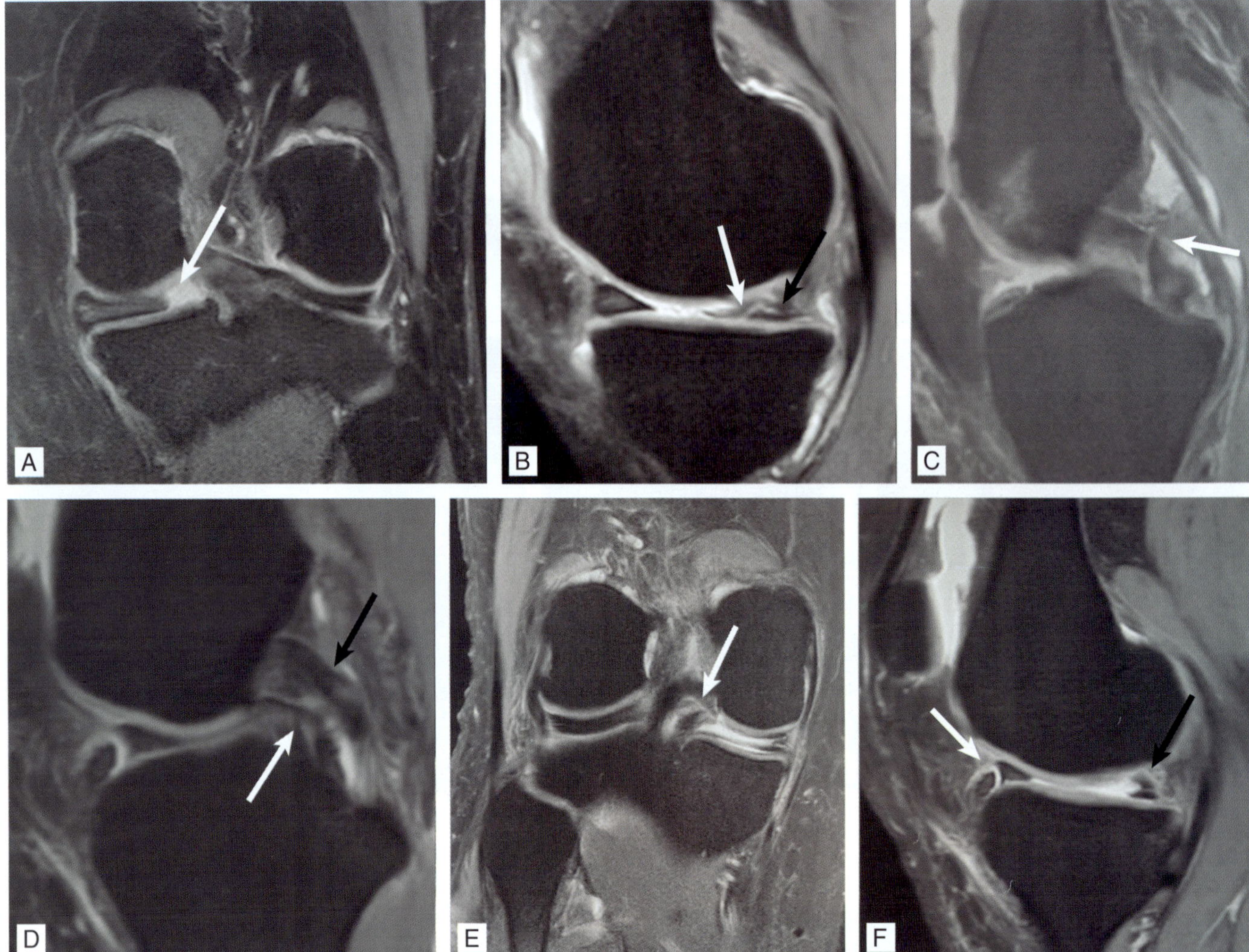

Figure 60.16 PDFS MR images demonstrating different types of meniscal tear. (A) *Root tear*: there is tear at the posterior root attachment of medial meniscus (*white arrow*) as seen in coronal image. (B) *Complex tear*: sagittal image showing tears in horizontal (*black arrow*) as well as in vertical orientation (*white arrow*). (C) *Displaced tear:* tear of the posterior horn of medial meniscus with posterior displacement of the torn fragment (*white arrow*) as seen in sagittal image. (D–F) *Bucket-handle tear* of the medial meniscus leading to PCL (*black arrow* in D) and centrally migrated meniscus fragment (*white arrow* in D) seen parallel to each other (double PCL appearance) on sagittal image. Coronal image shows torn fragment displaced in intercondylar notch (*white arrow* in E). Sagittal image shows double anterior horn (*white arrow* in F) and small posterior horn (*black arrow* in F) resulting in absent of normal bow-tie configuration.

Mimics of the above signs:

- Absent bow-tie configuration: small meniscus; pediatric patient; radial tear of the body; macerated meniscus; or previous partial meniscectomy
- Double PCL sign: prominent ligament of Humphry; menisco-meniscal ligament; or intercondylar osseous bodies

Treatment: Principles of treatment focus on meniscal conservation, selective intervention, only intervening if there are symptoms of locking, displaced fragment, or potential for displacement. Surgical options include open meniscal repair, meniscectomy, and meniscal transplantation.

Postoperative Appearance and Complications of the Meniscus

The postoperative evaluation of partial meniscectomies and primary repair offers unique challenges in diagnosing a retear or persistent tear or normal healing response to the meniscal fibrocartilage. Attenuated but intact meniscus without any cleft rules out re-tear or persistent tear. Intrinsic signal abnormality can persist for few weeks as a normal healing response.

Signs of re-tear include [13]:

- Displaced meniscal fragment(s)
- Increased signal intensity on PDFS or T2-weighted images at a new location or site relative to the repair (Fig. 60.17)

Cruciate Ligaments

The anterior and posterior cruciate ligaments are intracapsular extra synovial structures being enveloped by a synovial fold. Generally, PCL is longer and stronger than ACL.

Anterior Cruciate Ligament

Anatomy

ACL is proximally attached to a fossa on the posterior aspect of the medial surface of the lateral femoral condyle and distally to the tibial intercondylar eminence. Its tibial attachment is stronger than femoral attachment. It has two groups of fascicles:

- the anteromedial bundle is longest in flexion and resists anterior displacement of the tibia in flexion

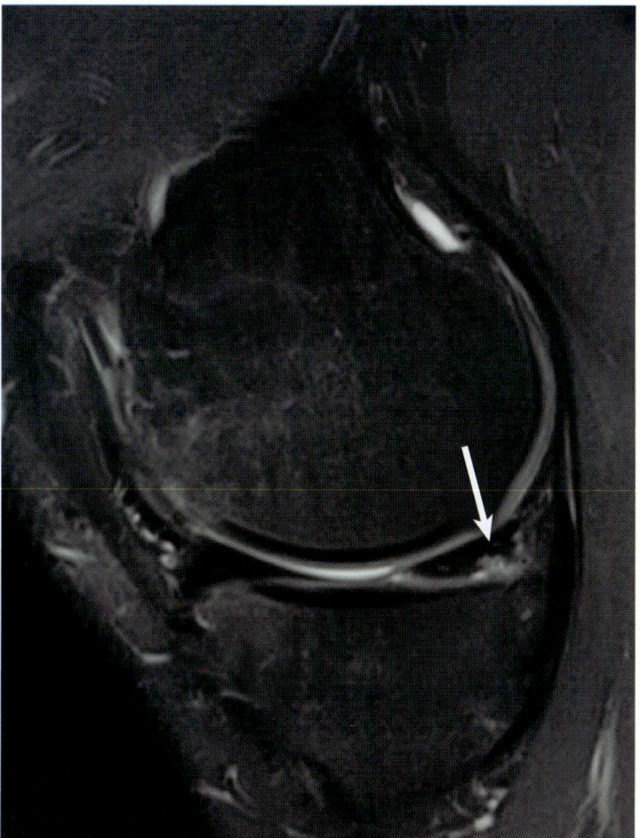

Figure 60.17 Re-tear in repaired meniscus in a 25-year male seen as high signal intensity in the posterior horn of medial meniscus reaching inferior articular margin (*arrow*) in sagittal PDFS MR image.

- posterolateral bundle is longest in extension and resists hyperextension.

It is the primary restraint to anterior displacement of tibia; secondary restraint to internal tibial rotation in full extension and minor restraint to varus-valgus angulation in full extension.

Mechanism of Injury

Classic mechanism of injury is pivot-shift injury where there is indirect trauma related to deceleration, hyperextension, or twisting forces, which is frequently seen in skiers and American football players. Other mechanisms involve dashboard injury (applied force to anterior proximal tibia with knee in flexion); hyperextension injury (direct force applied to the anterior tibia with a planted foot); clip injury (contact injury secondary to pure valgus stress to a partially flexed knee).

Clinical Presentation

- Pain which varies with the severity of injury
- Swelling is usually due to hemarthrosis and 41–75% of knee hemarthrosis is attributed to ACL injury [14]. However, this cause of swelling takes 6–24 hours to develop and in the case of rapidly developing hemarthrosis, osteochondral fracture should be considered as the primary differential diagnosis
- Sensation of "pop" is usually the most common clinical presentation in ACL tear than in any other ligament tear of the knee
- True locking is due to displacement of the distal segment of the torn ligament into the intercondylar region
- Pseudolocking is related to hematoma in posterior joint capsule, collateral ligament rigidity, and extrinsic muscle spasm
- Two important tests for ACL integrity are the *Lachman test* and the *pivot shift test*

Imaging Features

Radiograph and CT

- Anterior tibial translation: when the tangential line drawn along the posterior margin of femoral condyle does not intersect with the posterior aspect of tibia
- Avulsion fracture of the tibial site of attachment is common in children and adolescents rather than in older age (Fig. 60.18). Avulsion fracture at the femoral attachment site is rare
- Segond fracture: discussed later
- Subtle posterior fractures of the lateral or medial tibial plateau due to avulsion at the attachment site of posterior portion of joint capsule and attachment site of semimembranosus which is seen in lateral radiographs

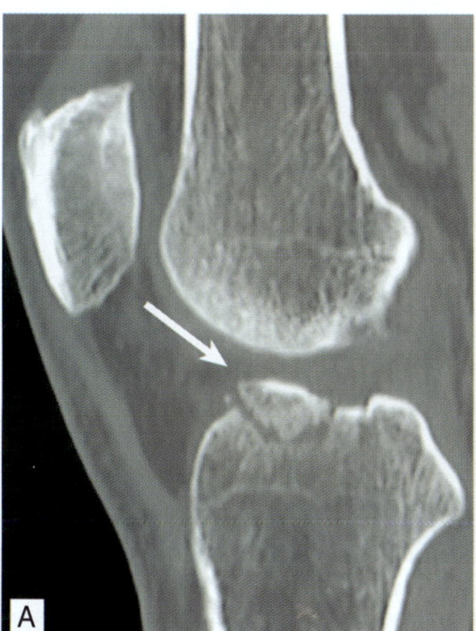

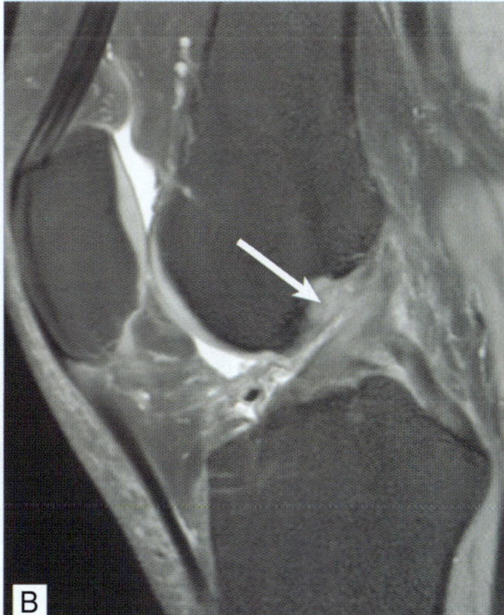

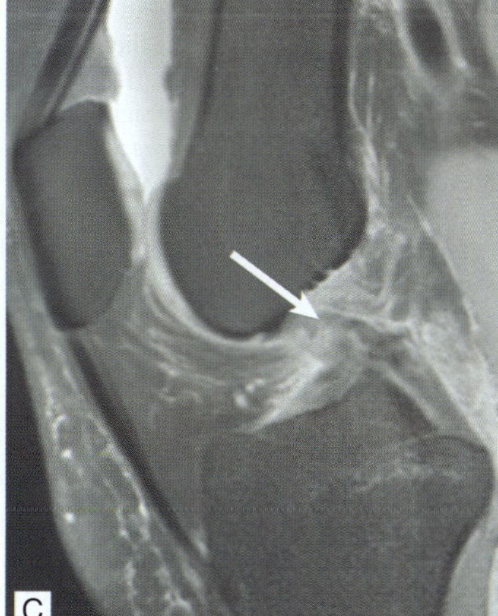

Figure 60.18 Anterior cruciate ligament (ACL) injury. (A) ACL avulsion fracture. Sagittal CT image shows avulsed bone fragment (*arrow*) from the tibial attachment site of ACL. Sagittal PDFS MR image shows (B) high signal in ACL with tear in anteromedial bundle (*arrow*), suggesting partial thickness tear while in (C) there is nonvisualization of ACL due to full-thickness tear (*arrow*).

- Osteochondral fracture of the lateral femoral condyle (lateral notch sign) is considered to be 100% specific for complete tear of ACL when the depth of the notch is more than 2 mm. However, it is less sensitive as it is only seen in 5% of ACL tear [15]

MRI: ACL is best seen in sagittal images as low signal band of fibers in all sequences which usually has high signal than the PCL. The posterolateral fascicle bundle has relatively higher signal than the anteromedial fascicle bundle.

MRI diagnosing of ACL injury is documented by the following:

(a) Abnormalities within the ACL: there are two types of alterations in the ligament itself that indicate injury—*alteration in morphology or orientation* and *alteration in signal intensity* (Fig. 60.18).

Full-thickness tear is evident by complete disruption of fibers and wavy appearance on sagittal images. Complete absence of ACL in coronal images through the intercondylar notch (empty notch sign) is an important indicator of complete tear. Partial tear is sometimes difficult to diagnose and one should be dependent on secondary signs. Anteromedial bundle is commonly involved. Focal or long segment edema within the ligament and in surrounding fat planes seen as high signal intensity in PDFS and T2-weighted images. In chronic tears edema is usually absent, but fluid in the joint cavity may mimic edema within the ligament.

False-positive diagnoses may occur because of the following:

- mucinous or myxoid change in the ligament,
- partial volume averaging of the ACL with the lateral femoral condyle or with periligamentous fat, and
- suboptimal selection of the sagittal imaging plane.

False-negative diagnoses may result from the following:

- formation of scar tissue and adherence to the PCL, and
- partial tears in which residual intact fibers lead to the appearance of a normal ACL.

(b) Alteration in appearance of other soft-tissue structures is attributed to the anterior displacement of the tibia in relation to femur and includes the following:

- Uncovered lateral meniscus sign—tangential line drawn along the posterior cortical margin of lateral tibial plateau in sagittal MR images intersects any part of the posterior horn of lateral meniscus. This sign is negative if the line does not intersect the meniscus or lie posterior to it
- Positive posterior cruciate sign—line drawn along inferior portion of PCL when extended superiorly on sagittal MR images goes parallel to the femur and does not intersect it. Normally this line is seen to intersect the medullary cavity of femur
- Lateral collateral ligament (LCL) seen in entirety in single coronal image is a valuable sign for ACL tear

(c) Abnormalities from bone impaction and avulsion forces can be categorized as follows:

- Chondral, subchondral, and osteochondral lesions-sites being mid-portion of the lateral femoral condyle and posterior aspect of lateral tibial plateau. The involvement of the posterior aspect of the medial femoral condyle and posterior aspect of medial tibial plateau, can be attributed to countercoup injury
- Avulsion fractures—Segond fracture, avulsion at tibial attachment, and avulsion of the tibial insertion of the semimembranosus tendon

(d) Miscellaneous abnormalities include:

- Hoffa's fat pad injury—linear high signal intensity in the middle of the infrapatellar fat pad body in sagittal MR images
- Fluid in the extra synovial triangular space between the cruciate ligaments is seen in the tear of any or both of the cruciate ligaments

Treatment: Conservative management involves functional bracing and modification in lifestyle. In cases of associated injuries to the meniscus and collateral ligament, surgical management is usually

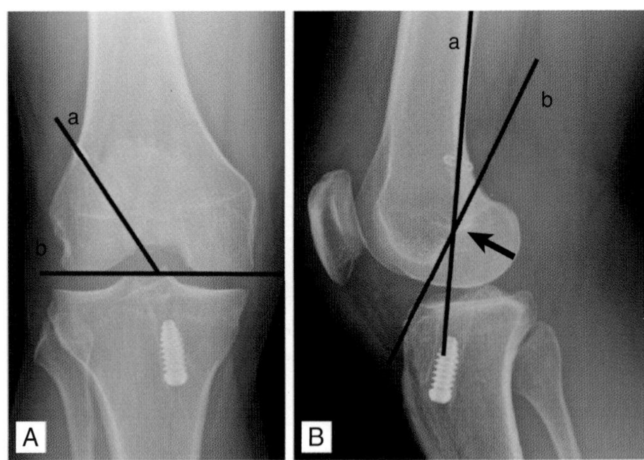

Figure 60.19 Femoral tunnel positioning must be assessed in both the sagittal and coronal planes. (A) In AP radiograph the femoral tunnel (line a) should open superiorly above the lines joining femoral condyles (line b) at the 10–11-o'clock position in the right knee (A) and at the 1–2-o'clock position in the left knee (not shown). (B) In lateral radiograph a line along the posterior cortex of the femur and another line along the roof of the intercondylar notch (Blumensaat line) is drawn. The inferior portion of the tunnel should be located at the intersection of these two lines (*arrow*).

opted. Autogenous, allograft, and synthetic tissues are used. Patellar tendon (bone-tendon-bone [BTB]), quadrupled hamstring tendon, and double-bundle reconstruction using hamstring are the commonly used autografts.

Imaging Appearance of Anterior Cruciate Ligament Reconstruction [16]

In ACL reconstruction, the graft is placed in the newly drilled femoral and tibial tunnels. Correct positioning of these tunnels (Figs. 60.19 and 60.20), mimicking the direction of native ACL is essential for maintaining the isometry and stability of the graft.

MRI Appearance of Anterior Cruciate Ligament Graft

High signal intensity is seen in the early postoperative period (<4 months) on PDFS and T2 images. Intermediate signal is seen

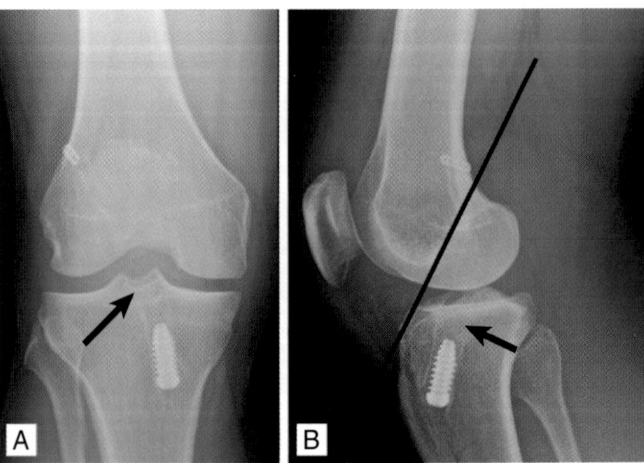

Figure 60.20 Tibial tunnel should be oriented parallel to the projected slope of the intercondylar roof (the Blumensaat line). (A) In AP radiograph the tibial tunnel should open at the intercondylar eminence (*arrow*). (B) In lateral radiograph the opening of the proximal tibial tunnel (*arrow*) should be posterior to the intersection of the Blumensaat line and the tibia (*black line*).

from approximately 4 to 8 months, decreasing with time and usually completely low signal by 12 months. This normal intermediate or high signal is always oriented along the fibers of a graft and is distinguishable from a tear that is perpendicular to the graft (Fig. 60.21).

Complications of ACL reconstruction are mentioned in Table 60.7.

Cystic Mucinous Disease

Encountered in middle-aged and elderly but can also be seen in young and adolescents, suggesting that the term mucinous change is appropriate over degeneration. It is more common in ACL than in PCL. Etiopathogenesis is uncertain and this entity is incidentally diagnosed in MRI knee indicated for some other cause. Typical MR imaging findings include increased girth of ACL with internal longitudinal regions of increased PDFS signal intensity (celery stalk appearance) (Fig. 60.22A). It resembles those of a partial tear of the ligament. However, violation of collagen fibers, as may be seen with partial tears, is not characteristic of this entity, although the determination of whether the altered regions violate or separate collagen fibers is often not possible at the time of MR imaging.

Posterior Cruciate Ligament

Anatomy

PCL is proximally attached to the lateral surface of the medial femoral condyle and distally to the posterior intercondylar area of the tibia. Meniscofemoral ligaments of Humphry and Wrisberg

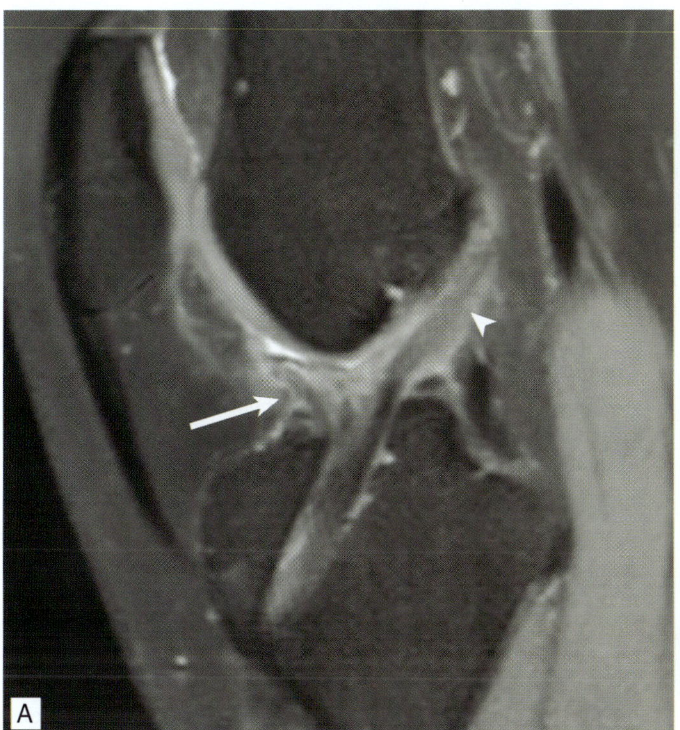

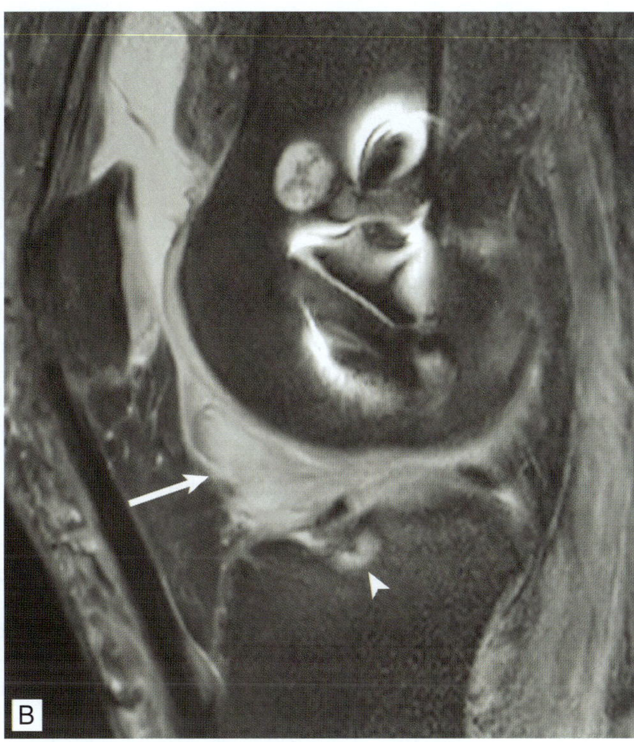

Figure 60.21 Complications of anterior cruciate ligament (ACL) reconstruction. (A) Graft tear. Sagittal PDFS MR image shows high signal in ACL (*arrowhead*) with attenuation of fibers and anterior displacement (*arrow*) of torn anterior fibers (partial thickness tear), 14 months after reconstruction. (B) Focal arthrofibrosis (cyclops lesion). Sagittal PDFS MR image shows a high signal nodular lesion (*arrow*) anterior to the distal end of graft (*arrowhead*), 8 months after reconstruction.

TABLE 60.7 Complications of Anterior Cruciate Ligament Reconstruction [17,18]

Graft impingement	MRI Shows persistent high signal changes more than a year
Graft tear (Fig. 60.21)	Altered graft thickness and graft discontinuity
Arthrofibrosis (Fig. 60.21)	Focal form (cyclops lesion): nodular lesion anterior to the distal end of graft Diffuse form: ill-defined spiculated area of intermediate low signal on all sequences within the Hoffa fat pad or a mass like area of decreased signal anterior and posterior to the graft
Cystic degeneration	Ganglion cyst formation
Intra-articular bodies	Secondary to an associated chondral injury that occurred during the initial trauma
Septic arthritis	Rare complication
Fractures	Due to failure of fixation hardware
Donor site abnormalities	Patellofemoral pain, rupture of the remaining portion of the tendon, and patellar fractures

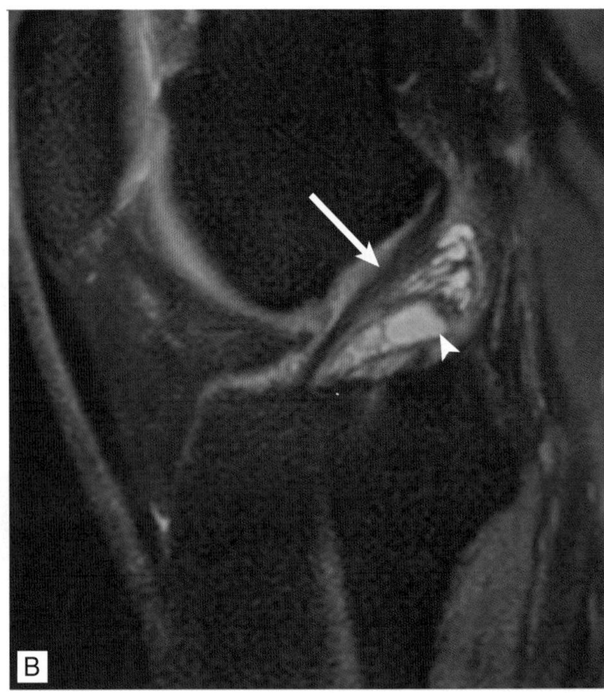

Figure 60.22 Sagittal PDFS MR images. (A) Cystic mucinous disease of ACL. Diffuse thickening and high signal intensity within the ACL (*arrow*) with intact fibers. Cystic change is also seen in the posterior fibers (*arrowhead*). (B) Ganglion cyst. Lobulated cystic area seen within the posterior fibers of ACL (*arrowhead*) with intact fibers (*arrow*). *ACL*, anterior cruciate ligament.

are intimate with the femoral attachment site of the PCL. Fascicles of PCL are also divided into two bundles, the anterolateral and posteromedial. The PCL is primary restraint to posterior displacement of tibia; secondary restraint to external tibial rotation and minor restraint to varus-valgus angulation.

Mechanism of Injury

Force applied to the anterior aspect of the proximal portion of the tibia with the knee flexed. Other mechanisms include extreme hyperextension or hyperflexion of the knee or from rotational or valgus forces applied to the knee. It can occur as an isolated phenomenon or in association with other capsular, ligamentous, or meniscal injuries.

Clinical presentation: Pain and swelling. Two fundamental tests used to evaluate the integrity of the PCL are 90-degree quadriceps active test and posteromedial pivot shift test.

Imaging Features

Radiograph: Avulsion fracture can be seen at tibial attachment (Fig. 60.23). Posterior translation of tibia is evident on axial radiograph of the knee in supine position. Joint effusion may be present.

MRI

PCL normally appears as a band of low signal intensity in all sequences and best seen in sagittal images. Meniscofemoral ligament consisting of anterior (ligament of Humphry) and posterior (ligament of Wrisberg) branches, are seen as ovoid regions of low signal intensity on the surfaces of the PCL (Fig. 60.24). Magic angle effect often leads to a region of intermediate signal in the ligament in short TE sequences. In elderly persons, mucoid or eosinophilic degeneration in the PCL may also lead to regions of intermediate signal intensity. Full-thickness or partial thickness tear of PCL can be seen as disruption of all or

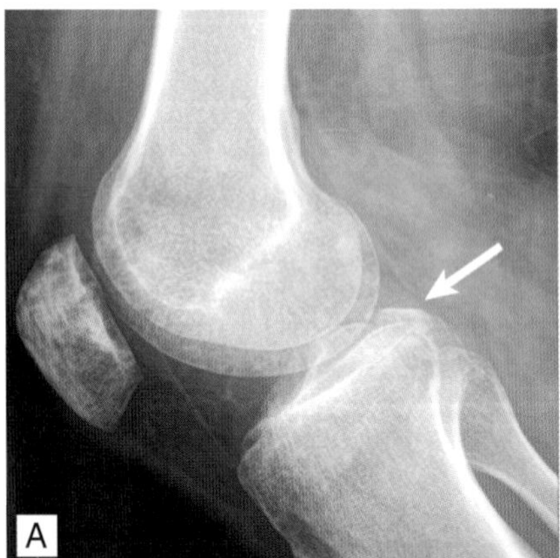

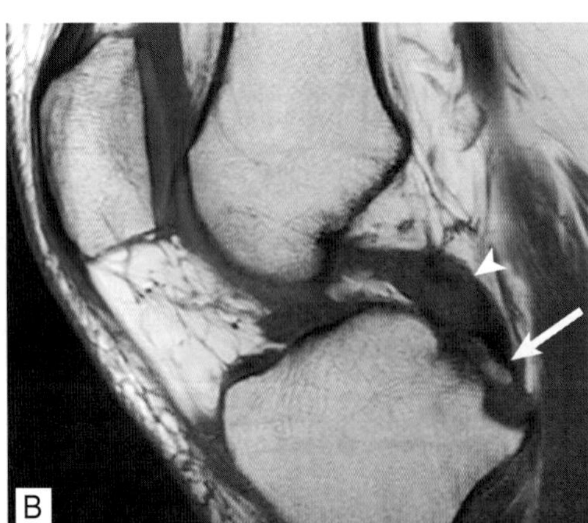

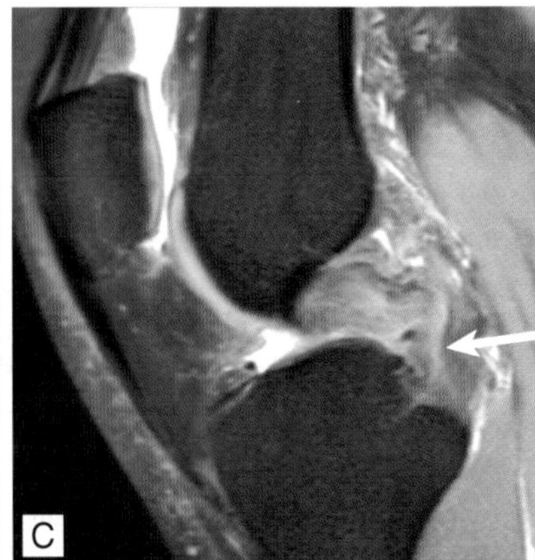

Figure 60.23 Posterior cruciate ligament (PCL) injury. Radiograph lateral view (A) and sagittal T1 MR image (B) show avulsed bone fragment (*arrows*) at tibial attachment of PCL with diffuse thickening of the ligament (*arrowhead*). (C) Sagittal PDFS MR image shows full-thickness tear of the PCL at tibial attachment (*arrow*) with diffuse high signal within the ligament.

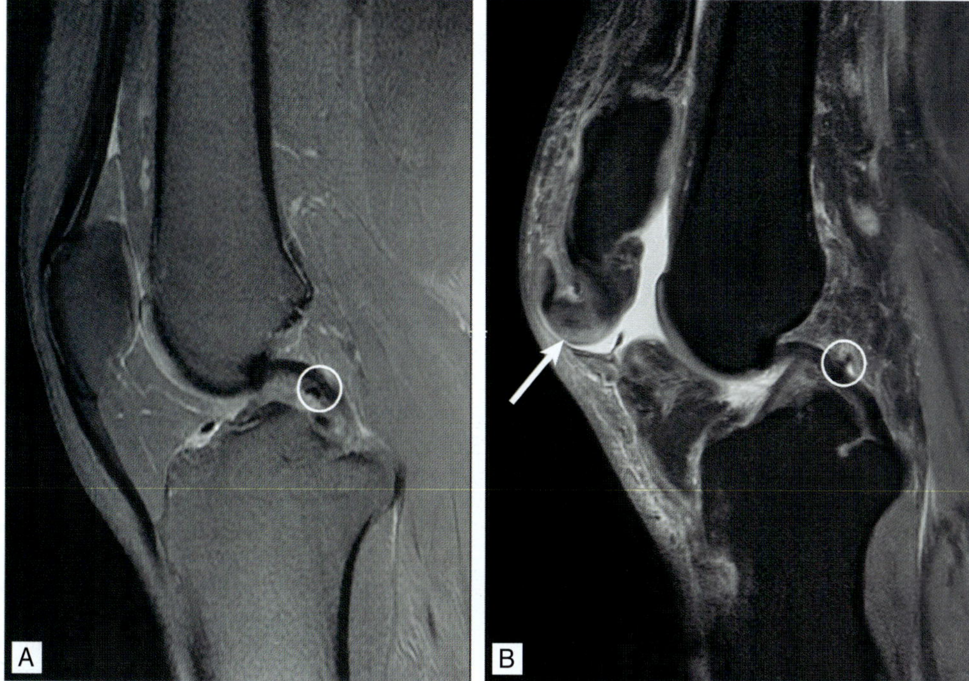

Figure 60.24 PDFS sagittal MRI image of two different patients showing meniscofemoral ligaments consisting of (A) anterior (ligament of Humphry) and (B) posterior (ligament of Wrisberg) branches, are seen as ovoid regions of low signal intensity (circles) on the surfaces of the PCL. Note is made of an additional finding of complete patellar ligament tear (*arrow*) in image B.

some of the fibers as change in morphology and or signal intensity of the ligament (Fig. 60.23). Secondary findings include bone bruises and osteochondral lesions; avulsion fractures and soft-tissue avulsions of PCL. Associated tears of the meniscofemoral ligaments, menisci, and other supporting structures may be seen.

Treatment: Acute tears isolated to the PCL are usually treated conservatively, whereas those involving multiple ligaments and avulsion injuries often require surgical reconstruction.

Postoperative appearance: The revascularization phenomenon of PCL graft is similar to that in ACL graft, which may account for increased intraligamentous signal during the first postoperative year.

Ganglion Cysts

Pericruciate ganglion cysts are encountered in some cases of pain, clicking, and restriction of joint motion. It is more frequently associated with PCL than ACL (Fig. 60.22B). It may be related to the mucinous change in the cruciate ligaments. Intraosseous cystic lesion at the site of tibial attachment of cruciate ligaments can be associated finding. MR imaging characteristics include fluid collection of variable size applied to the surface of the ligament or located a short distance from it. Major differential diagnoses include central extension of a meniscal cyst arising from the posterior horn of the medial meniscus and distension of a posterior recess of the medial femorotibial compartment related to a joint effusion.

Developmental Anomalies

Developmental anomalies are rare and include aplasia, hypoplasia, alteration in shape, and anomalies at ligament attachment sites. They can also be associated with other anomalies like short femur, malformed tibia, fibular hemimelia, absent menisci, congenital thrombocytopenia and absent radius, Ehlers–Danlos, and Larsen's syndromes.

Anterior Knee

Anatomy

Structures forming the anterior knee include (Fig. 60.25):

- Superiorly—Quadriceps muscles (from anterior to posterior includes rectus femoris, vastus lateralis, vastus medialis, and vastus intermedius), which merge few centimeters above patellar attachment to form quadriceps tendon
- Inferiorly—Patellar tendon (strongest anterior knee structure)
- Medially—medial retinaculum (discussed in section on medial knee) and vastus medialis muscle
- Laterally, lateral retinaculum; vastus lateralis muscle; and iliotibial tract.

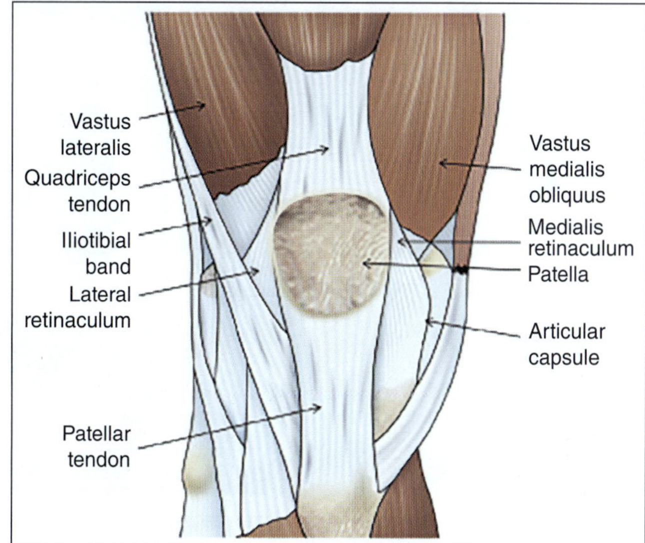

Figure 60.25 Diagrammatic representation of the structures of the anterior knee.

Pathologies of Anterior Knee

Abnormalities of the anterior knee are mostly contributed to the constant complex movements occurring in patellofemoral joint. Clinical manifestation of most of these abnormalities is anterior knee pain (patellofemoral pain syndrome).

Patellar Tendinosis

It is usually a result of a sudden or repetitive extension of the knee that is commonly seen in athletes and is also called as *Jumper's knee*. Histologically, patellar tendinosis is associated with fiber failure, mucoid degeneration, and fibrinoid necrosis rather than inflammation and thus the term "tendinitis" is inappropriate. The proximal portion of the tendon is usually involved rather than the distal portion.

Imaging Features

Radiography: lateral view provides indirect signs of localized soft-tissue swelling, thickening of the patellar tendon, and obscuration of infrapatellar fat.

USG shows a thickened and hypoechoic tendon, predominantly its proximal part.

CT shows an enlarged and thickened tendon at its proximal patellar attachment with decreased attenuation.

MRI is the most useful technique for diagnosis where the entire tendon can be assessed in a sagittal plane. Constellation of MRI findings includes thickening of the proximal tendon (>7 mm in sagittal diameter) with high signal (but not fluid strength) on PDFS and T2 images within the tendon (Fig. 60.26), adjacent proximal infrapatellar fat, and inferior pole of the patella [19]. As patellar tendon does not have a tendon sheath but only a paratenon composed of loose areolar tissue, the earliest changes (<2 weeks) are seen only as paratenon edema with normal-appearing fibers. In subacute to chronic tendinosis (>6 weeks) there is thickening of tendon fibers with low to equivocal signal on T1 images and high signal on PDFS and T2 images.

The patellar tendon can also appear thickened after arthroscopy.

Treatment: Conservative management (patient education, modifications in physical activity, exercises that lead to increased muscle strength) is the rule.

Patellar and Quadriceps Tendon Tear

This is usually due to chronic tendinosis, direct trauma, or underlying systemic cause such as rheumatoid arthritis, gout, renal failure, diabetes, and systemic lupus erythematosus. Quadriceps tendon tear is more common than patellar tendon tear. Most common site for the tear is adjoining the patella. Full-thickness quadriceps tendon tear (Fig. 60.26) leads to an inferior position of the patella (patella Baja). In contrast, full-thickness patellar tendon tear leads to a superior position of the patella (patella alta). Partial tears are not associated with abnormal position of the patella.

Imaging Features

Radiograph in partial tears has a similar appearance as tendinosis. Full-thickness tear may show the abnormal position of the patella. Avulsion fracture can also be appreciated.

USG: Partial-thickness will show hypoechoic areas within the tendon, while in full-thickness tear, there will be full-thickness disruption of the fiber continuity.

MRI: Partial tear will have increased PDFS signal in the tendon with fluid strength. Edema will be seen in the fat pad and at the attachment site of patella. Full-thickness tear will have complete disruption with residual tendon retracted and wavy in appearance (Fig. 60.26). Bony fragments, with or without marrow edema, can be identified in an avulsion injury with gradient images being more sensitive to small avulsed bony fragments.

Treatment: Partial tears may be managed conservatively based on the extent of instability on clinical examination. Complete tears are intervened by direct tendon repair, reconstruction with the semitendinosus tendon, or bony reattachment. Rupture, chronic pain, and dysfunction are complications of repair.

Patellar Malalignment and Instability

The major stabilizers of the patella are the quadriceps and patellar tendons and the medial and lateral patellao-femoral ligaments. Abnormality in these components leads to abnormal patellar position. *Patellar malalignment* is the term used when there is rotational or translational deviation relative to the long axis. It can be attributed to extensor mechanism abnormality, arthritis, infection, bursitis, plica, and stress fractures.

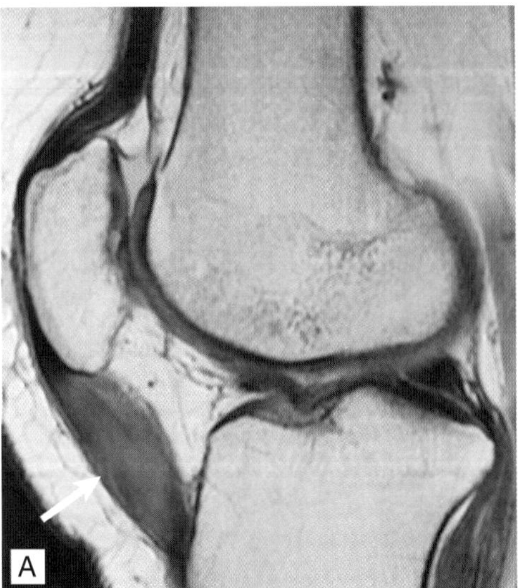

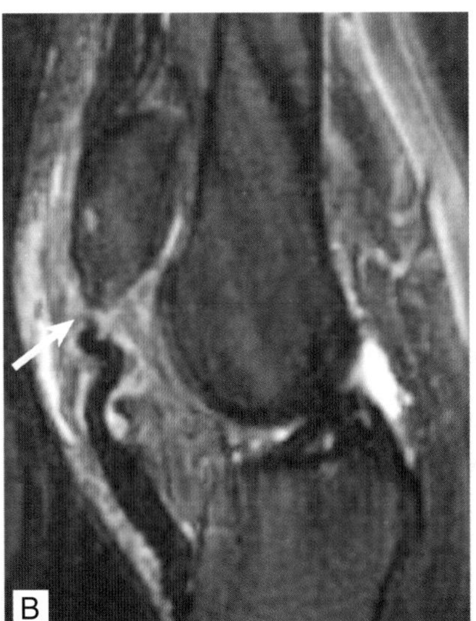

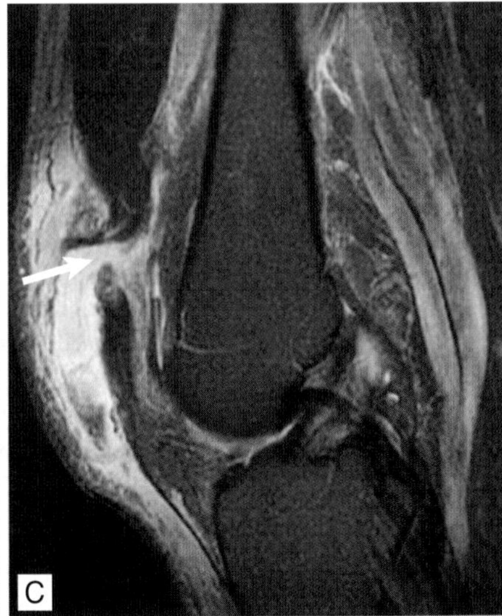

Figure 60.26 (A) Patellar tendinosis. T2 sagittal image of a young patient showing diffuse thickening of the patellar tendon (*arrow*) with intermediate signal intensity. (B) Patellar tendon tear. Sagittal STIR MR image of a young patient with history of recent trauma showing full thickness tear of the patellar tendon (*arrow*) at its attachment to inferior pole of patella. The tendon is retracted and appears wavy. (C) Quadriceps tendon tear. Sagittal PDFS MR image shows full thickness tear of quadriceps tendon (*arrow*) at its patellar attachment.

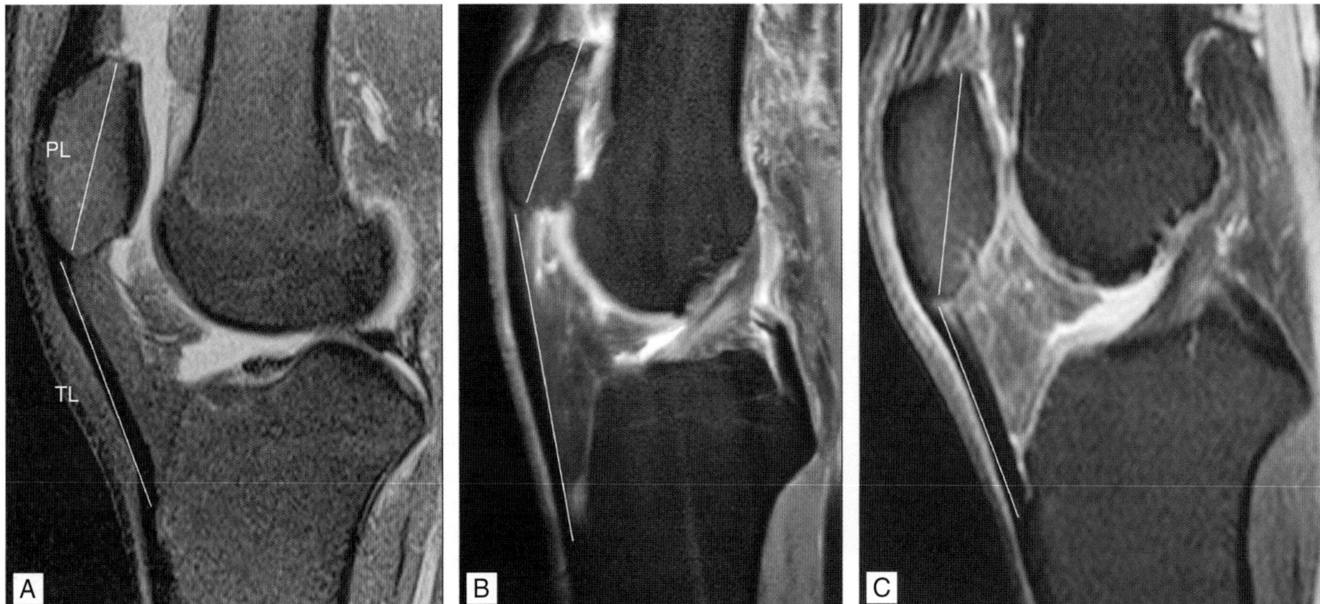

Figure 60.27 (A) Normal vertical position of patella: Insall–Salvati ratio [patellar tendon length (*TL*) to patellar length (*PL*)] is normal (1:1). (B) Patella alta: ratio is greater than 1.32. (C) Patella baja: ratio is less than 0.74.

Patellar instability is a specific condition where there is subluxation or dislocation of the patella. This has a mechanical basis and can be caused by injury, congenital abnormality in patellar position and shape of the trochlea (trochlear dysplasia), ligament laxity, adjoining muscle abnormality, or malalignment of the whole lower limb. Patellar instability can be classified based on pattern of dislocation (superior, inferior, medial, lateral), acute or chronic; and single or recurrent episodes.

Patella Alta and Patella Baja

Vertical position of the patella has clinical significance in assessing the stability of the anterior knee. High-riding patella (patella alta) is considered when the inferior pole of patella is above the femoral trochlear groove while low-riding patella (patella baja or patella infera) is considered when the whole of patella is below the femoral trochlear groove.

Patella alta is attributed to recurrent patellar dislocation, chondromalacia patellae, Sinding–Larsen disease, full-thickness patellar tendon tear, and large joint effusion. Patella baja is identified in achondroplasia, neuromuscular disorders, full thickness quadriceps tendon tear, and surgical transfer of tibial tuberosity.

Imaging Features

Insall-Salvatiratio is ratio of the length of the patellar tendon to the maximum length of patella. Value of 1:1 is considered to be normal. Ratios defined for patella alta and baja are 1.52 and 0.79, respectively, in females and 1.32 and 0.74 in males (Fig. 60.27) [20].

Patellar Shape

Patellar shape is not constant. Three different patellar types have been described by Wiberg (types I, II, and III) based on the asymmetry between the medial and lateral patellar facets (Fig. 60.28). Increasing number type indicates a larger degree of asymmetry and type III is thought to be associated with trochlear dysplasia (described later).

Acute Patellar Dislocation and Subluxation

Complete displacement of patella from the trochlear groove is termed dislocation while partial displacement from the trochlear groove is termed subluxation, with both the terms used interchangeably on clinical examination. Lateral patellar dislocation is a more common entity than medial dislocation.

Lateral Patellar Dislocation

Flexed knee in internal rotation on planted foot and valgus component is the usual mechanism of injury. The process of dislocation and relocation causes injury to the medial retinaculum, medial patellofemoral ligament (MPFL) along with osseous and cartilaginous injuries.

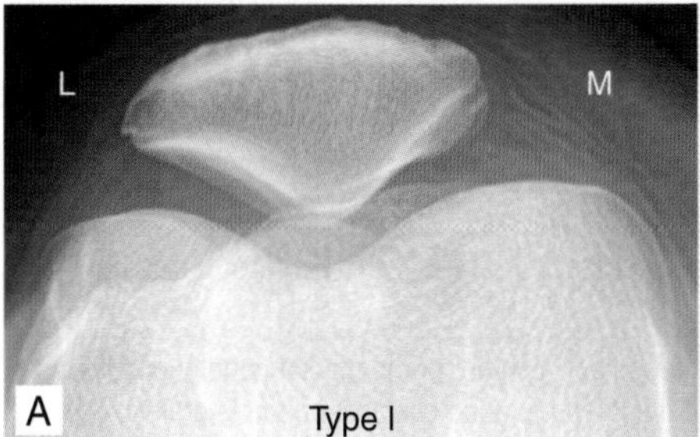

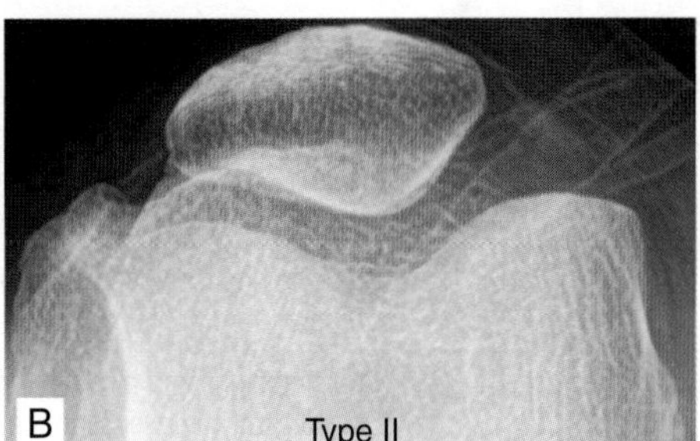

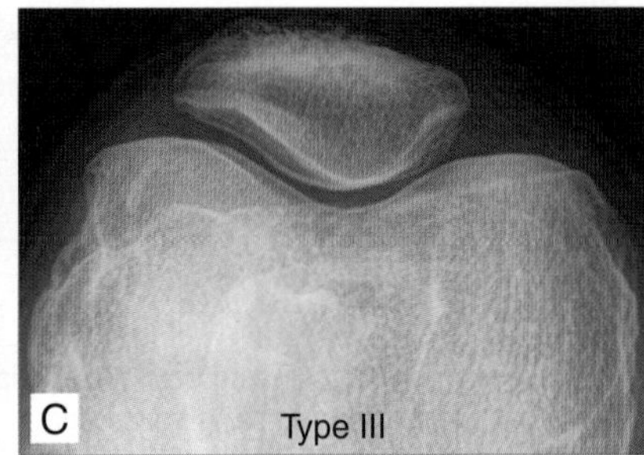

Figure 60.28 Wiberg classification of patellar shape. (A) Type I: medial (M) and lateral (L) patellar facet length are equal. (B) Type II: slightly smaller size of medial facet. (C) Type III: Significantly smaller size of medial patellar facet.

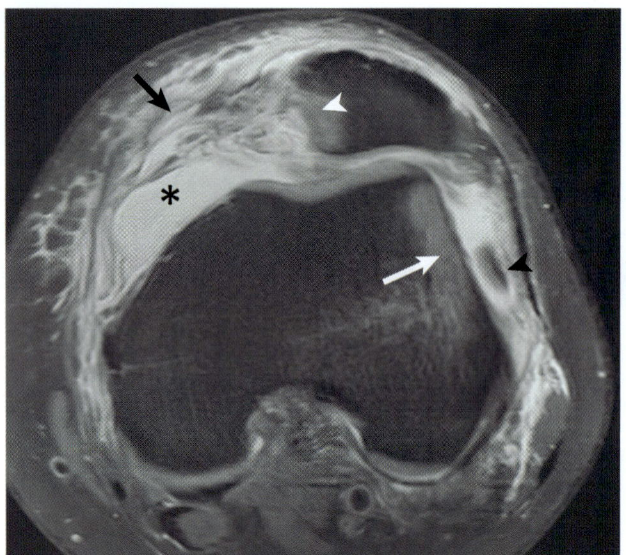

Figure 60.29 Acute lateral patellar dislocation: Axial PDFS MR image showing lateral subluxation of patella. There is cortical breach and marrow edema in medial pole of patella (*white arrowhead*), marrow edema in lateral condyle of femur (*white arrow*); full thickness tear of the MPFL (*black arrow*) and joint effusion (*asterisk*). A fractured bone fragment is also seen in lateral joint space (*black arrowhead*).

Imaging Findings

Radiograph: Axial view demonstrates laterally placed patella in relation to trochlear groove. Occasionally avulsion fracture from the lateral surface of the patella, intra-articular bodies, and joint effusion are seen.
USG: Full thickness or partial thickness tear of the MPFL can be seen. An avulsed bone fragment may be present at the site of injury. Joint effusion can be appreciated when present.
MRI helps to detect the abnormalities and determine mechanism of injury, as the clinical examination is confusing in this scenario (Fig. 60.29) [21].
Bone and cartilage injury: Marrow edema is seen in the anterior aspect of lateral femoral condyle and in medial patellar facet. Fractures or avulsed bone and chondral intra-articular bodies are present. Osteochondral injury can be present in the lateral aspect of femoral trochlea, the dome of the patella and medial patellar facet.
Medial patello-femoral ligament (MPFL) Injury: Partial or full-thickness tear of the MPFL can be seen at its anterior third (patellar attachment), middle third (mid substance), or posterior third (femoral attachment). Partial-thickness tear leads to attenuation of the ligament with high signal on PDFS images. Full-thickness tear demonstrates complete disruption of the ligament with wavy and retracted fibers surrounded by soft-tissue edema and fluid.
Other findings: Joint effusion is reported in 55–95% [21]. Injury to the distal fibers of vastus medialis (where it confluences with MPFL) can be seen as intramuscular edema and surrounding fluid intensity. MPFL tear, when associated with O'Donoghue triad (injury to ACL, medial meniscus, and medial collateral ligament), is termed as O'Donoghue tetrad.
Treatment: Nonsurgical management includes bracing, physical therapy, and strengthening of medial muscles for a first-time dislocation with the absence of complete MPFL tear. However, cases of recurrent dislocations, severe trochlear dysplasia, and presence of complete MPFL tear are usually managed surgically.

Recurrent Lateral Patellar Dislocation

These patients are usually young, and anatomic factors are usually associated with such recurrent episodes. It has been found that more than 85% of patients with a history of a true patellar dislocation had evidence of trochlear dysplasia [22]. The findings pertaining to injury are the same as in acute dislocation but are of more severity.

Trochlear Dysplasia

It is defined as pathologic alteration in the shape of the femoral trochlea, which may be shallower than usual or even flat or convex, thus predisposing the patella to lateral subluxation or even dislocation.

Imaging Findings

Radiograph: Based on different findings, trochlear dysplasia has been classified into four morphological types [23,24]. Radiographic findings of each type are detailed in Table 60.8 and demonstrated in Fig. 60.30.
CT and MRI: These modalities have higher sensitivity in diagnosing trochlear dysplasia than a radiograph. MRI features of trochlear dysplasia include reduction in the trochlear depth, lateral trochlear inclination, and facet asymmetry [25]. These are evaluated on the most cranial axial image showing cartilage, approximately 3 cm above the joint line.

- *Facet asymmetry* is determined by calculating the asymmetry in the length of the medial to the lateral femoral facets and expressed in percentage (Fig. 60.31A). Asymmetry of <40% suggests trochlear dysplasia
- *Lateral trochlear inclination* is the angle between a line tangential to the subchondral bone of the posterior aspect of the femoral condyles and a line along the lateral trochlear facet subchondral bone (Fig. 60.31B). An inclination angle of <11° indicates trochlear dysplasia
- *Trochlear depth* is calculated by measuring the mean of the maximum anteroposterior (AP) distance of the medial and

TABLE 60.8 Classification of Trochlear Dysplasia and Their Radiographic Findings

Type A (shallow trochlear groove)	"Crossing sign" in the lateral view (line which represents the deepest part of the trochlear groove crosses the anterior border of the two condyles), a shallow trochlea, and a sulcus angle >145 degree on the 30 degree flexion axial view
Type B (flat or convex trochlea)	"Crossing sign" and supratrochlear spur (angular projection of the most proximal portion of the trochlea) on lateral view
Type C (asymmetric trochlear facets, with the lateral facet being too high and the medial facet being hypoplastic)	"Crossing sign" and a "double contour sign" (contour of the medial femoral condyle is significantly smaller than that of the lateral femoral condyle) on the lateral view
Type D (asymmetry of trochlear facets plus vertical join and cliff pattern)	"Crossing sign," supratrochlear spur, and "double contour sign"

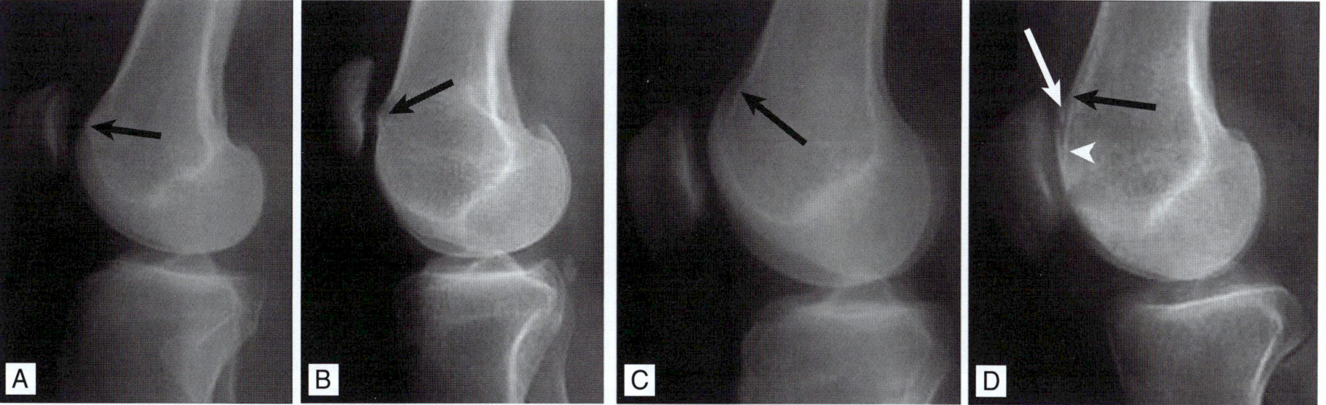

Figure 60.30 Classification of trochlear dysplasia. (A) Type A dysplasia. The "crossing sign" (*black arrow*) is evident. (B) Type B dysplasia. Evidence of crossing sign and supratrochlear spur (*black arrow*). (C) Type C dysplasia. Evidence of crossing sign and double contour (*black arrow*). (D) Type D dysplasia. Concomitant presence of crossing sign (*white arrowhead*), supratrochlear spur (*white arrow*), and double contour (*black arrow*).

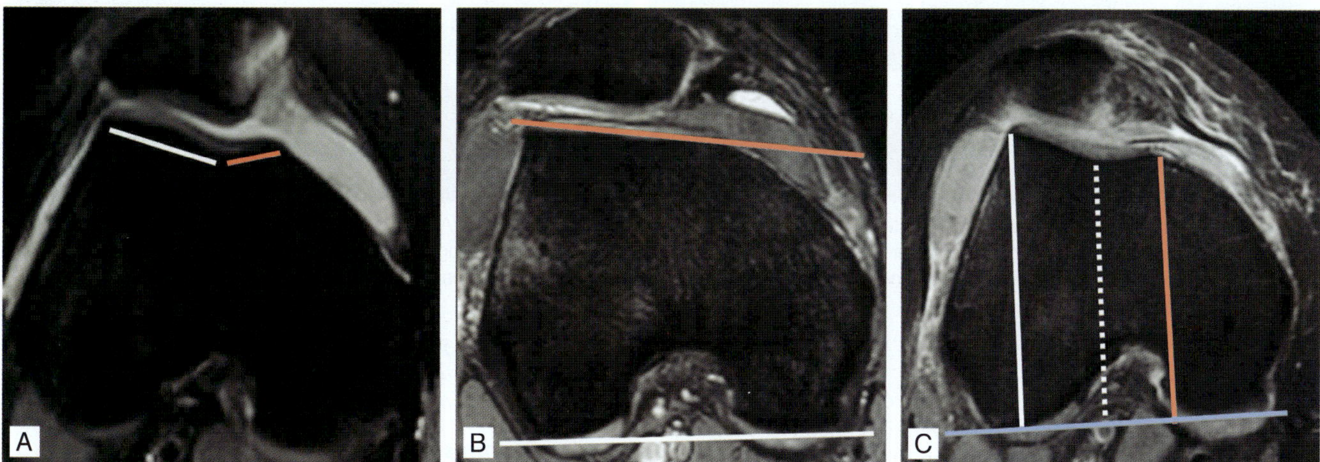

Figure 60.31 Trochlear dysplasia assessed on axial PDFS MR images. (A) *Trochlear facet asymmetry*: ratio of the length of medial facet (*red*) to lateral facet (*white*). Image shows a dysplastic trochlea with ratio <40%. (B) *Lateral trochlear inclination*: angle between line drawn along the subchondral bone of the lateral trochlear facet (*red*) and line along the posterior aspect of the femoral condyles (*white*). This inclination angle is <11°. (C) *Trochlear depth*: line drawn parallel to the posterior aspect of the femoral condyles serves as reference line (*blue*). The lines drawn perpendicular to the reference line indicate the largest anteroposterior diameters of the lateral (*white*) and medial (*red*) trochlear facets and the deepest point of the sulcus (dotted). Trochlear depth is calculated as follows: ((*white* + *red*)/2) – (*dotted*). Image shows a dysplastic trochlea with marked flattening, indicated by a trochlear depth of 1.7 mm.

lateral femoral condyles minus the distance between the deepest point of the trochlear groove and the line paralleling the posterior femoral condyles surfaces (Fig. 60.31C). Less than 3-mm trochlear depth indicates trochlear dysplasia (sensitivity of 100%, specificity of 96%) [25]

- Ventral trochlear prominence: Protrusion of the cartilaginous trochlear floor >8 mm anterior to a line drawn along the most distal 10 cm of the anterior cortex of the femoral diaphysis on mid-sagittal image

Treatment: Surgical treatment is indicated for a symptomatic patient with recurrent patellar instability, which has failed nonoperative management. Several techniques of trochleoplasty have been described to correct trochlear anatomy.

Medial Patellar Dislocation

It is also called Patella Adentro and is diagnosed when the median patellar ridge is displaced medially from the trochlear groove. It is seen in overcompensated surgical release of the lateral retinaculum, tight medial retinaculum, insufficient lateral retinaculum, and quadriceps imbalance. Symptomatic dislocations need redo surgery for correction.

Chronic Habitual Patellar Dislocation

It is commonly seen in children and is described as episodes of lateral patellar dislocation each time the knee is flexed or as permanent lateral dislocation [65]. It is caused by shortening of the quadriceps tendon due to contracture, which may be congenital or due to repeated intramuscular injections or trauma. Treatment of the primary etiology is opted.

Chondromalacia Patellae

The term is applied to the abnormality of articular cartilage of the patella leading to patellofemoral pain. Common causes are trauma, chronic stress, malalignment, prolonged immobilization, and postsurgical reconstruction of ACL. The disorder begins as cartilage softening and progresses through stages of fissuring, fibrillation, and full-thickness loss leading to exposure of subchondral bone.

Imaging Features

For all practical purposes, radiograph, CT, and USG are insensitive for this entity's diagnosis while MRI is the technique used to detect the cartilage changes.

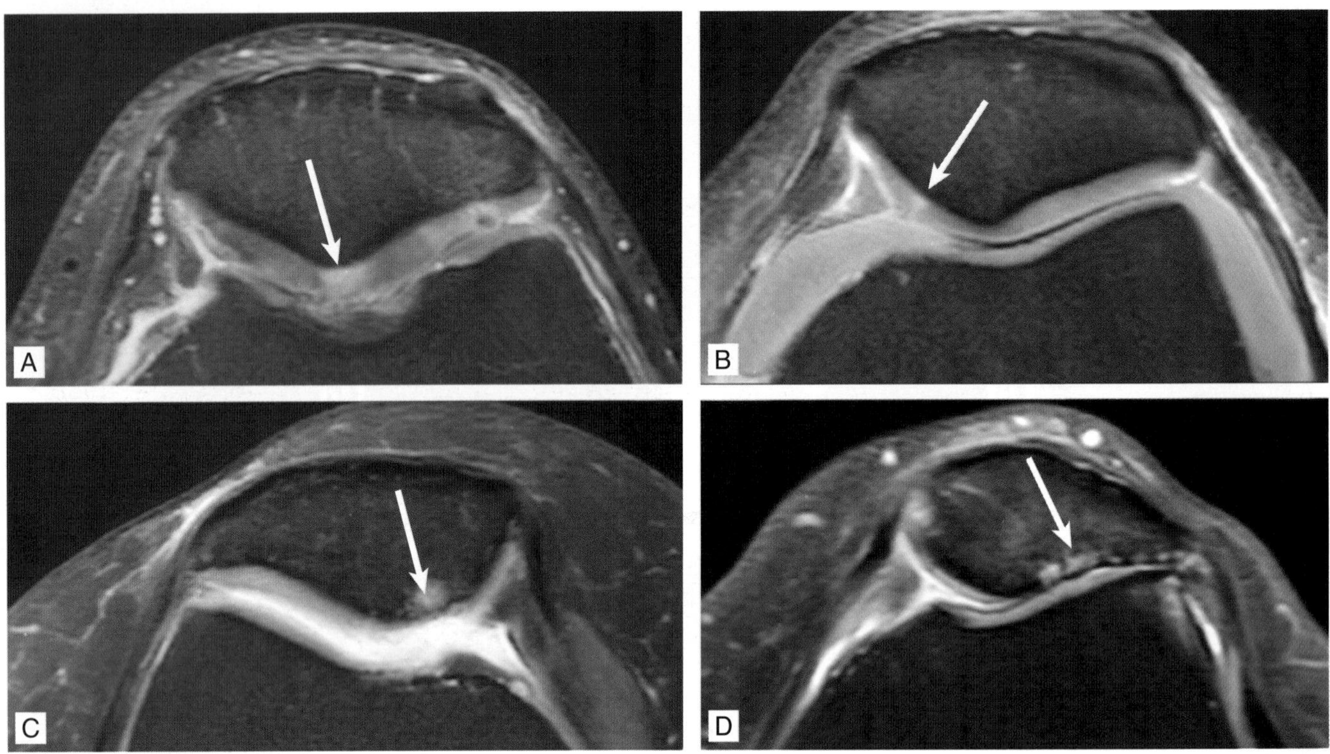

Figure 60.32 MRI grading of chondromalacia patellae represented by *arrows* in axial PDFS images. (A) *Grade 1*—focal areas of high signal in the articular cartilage with normal contour. (B) *Grade 2*—blister-like swelling or fraying of articular cartilage extending to surface. (C) *Grade 3*—partial thickness cartilage loss with focal ulceration. (D) *Grade 4*—full thickness cartilage loss with underlying reactive bone changes.

MRI grading on PDFS images is based on modified outerbridge classification [26] (Fig. 60.32).

Treatment: Operative treatment is usually chosen when there is failure of conservative management. Surgical methods include elevation or transfer of the tibial tuberosity or patellar tendon; lateral retinacular release; excision of chondral surface; and patellectomy, as a last resort.

Osgood–Schlatter Disease

The term is used for traction apophysitis of the tibial attachment of patellar tendon. It usually occurs in adolescents, between the ages of 11 and 15 years. The condition can be bilateral in up to 50% of cases [27]. A relation of this disease with patella alta has been suggested.

Imaging Features

Radiograph: Soft-tissue prominence in the infrapatellar fat, indistinctness of the posterior margin of the lower aspect of the patellar tendon, and irregular ossification of the developing tibial tuberosity (Fig. 60.33).

USG and *MRI* show a thickened distal portion of the patellar tendon, fluid in the deep infrapatellar bursa, soft-tissue edema,

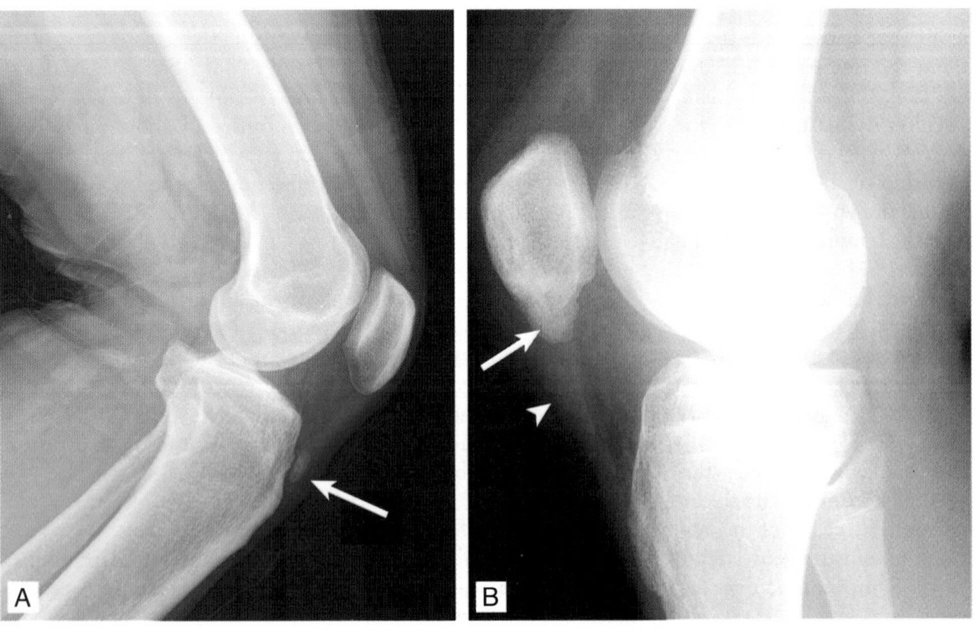

Figure 60.33 (A) Osgood–Schlatter disease: lateral radiograph of the left knee showing ossification (*arrow*) at the tibial attachment of patellar tendon (B) Sinding–Larsen–Johansson disease: lateral radiograph of right knee showing inferior beaking of patella (*arrow*) with thickening of the proximal patellar tendon (*arrowhead*).

TABLE 60.9 Anatomic Components of the Medial Knee

Anterior portion	■ Medial retinaculum and MPFL. MPFL attaches to femur immediately below adductor tubercle and to patella at its upper medial two-thirds. ■ Pes anserinus tendons (sartorius, gracilis, and semitendinosus) attach to the anteromedial aspect of proximal tibia
Middle portion	■ Superficial medial collateral ligament. Femoral attachment is adjoining medial epicondyle; tibial attachment has two sites, semimembranosus tendon attachment site and deep to pes anserinus tendon attachment ■ Deep medial collateral ligament consists of meniscofemoral and meniscotibial (coronary) ligaments. Posteriorly it blends with POL (posterior oblique ligament) ■ Superficial medial collateral ligament acts as primary restraint to valgus force while deep medial collateral ligament acts as secondary restraint to valgus force as well as to the internal rotation of tibia
Posterior portion (posteromedial corner of the knee: PMC)	■ Consists of POL, oblique popliteal ligament, semimembranosus tendon, and posterior horn of medial meniscus ■ PMC is considered to be an important stabilizer for anteromedial rotational instability of the knee

and fragmentation of the tuberosity. There may be associated edema in the tuberosity.

Treatment: Conservative treatment is usually successful, although resection of the ossicles or a portion of the tibial tuberosity is occasionally necessary.

Sinding–Larsen–Johansson Disease

It is indicated by bone fragment inferior to the lower pole of patella either due to calcification of an injured patellar tendon or due to avulsion injury of the lower pole of the patella. It occurs in adolescents between the ages of 10 and 15 years.

Imaging Features

Radiograph shows bone fragmentation inferior to lower pole of patella (Fig. 60.33). USG and MR imaging can used as a supplement to radiography to substantiate the diagnosis.

Treatment: It is generally self-limiting condition and responsive to conservative treatment.

Medial Knee and Posteromedial Corner of Knee

Anatomy

Medial structures act as primary restraint to limit the valgus angulation and internal rotation at knee and secondary restraints to anterior displacement of tibia. There is a practically accepted anterior to posterior approach to the medial structures of the knee [28] (Table 60.9 and Fig. 60.34). The posterior portion is more specifically called as the posteromedial corner (PMC) of the knee.

Injuries to Medial Knee

Injuries to the MCL and PMC are common in contact and noncontact sports. In contact sports such as football, soccer, rugby, and martial arts, there is direct impact onto the lateral knee with a valgus force resulting in isolated injuries to the superficial and deep MCL. Valgus injuries with higher impact can cause posterior oblique ligament (POL) injury as well as concomitant cruciate ligament injuries. In sports in which a cutting action is common, there is external rotation of the tibia in addition to a valgus force, resulting in injury to the PMC in addition to tears of the superficial and deep MCL. Combined tears of the superficial and deep MCL, as well as the PMC, produce anteromedial rotatory instability.

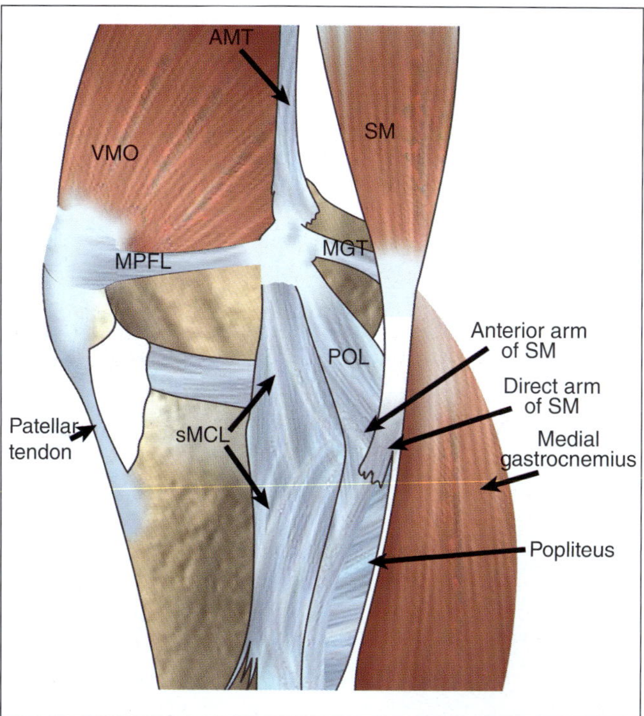

Figure 60.34 Diagrammatic representation of medial knee structures. *AMT*, adductor magnus tendon; *MGT*, medial gastrocnemius tendon; *MPFL*, medial patellofemoral ligament; *SM*, semimembranosus; *sMCL*, superficial MCL; *VMO*, vastus medialis obliquus muscle.

Clinical Presentation

Pain and swelling. Local edema and tenderness along medial aspect is good indicator. In valgus stress test, the extent of opening of the medial side of the knee in comparison to the contralateral normal knee indicates the severity of injury.

Imaging Features

Radiograph and CT: Soft-tissue swelling is seen along medial aspect of the knee with or without effusion. Small avulsion fractures may be present rarely. Associated avulsion fracture of ACL may be present. There can be a calcified focus in soft-tissue adjoining medial femoral condyle, representing calcification or ossification in the torn MCL (Pellagrini–Steida lesion) (Fig. 60.35).

USG can easily demonstrate joint effusion or hemarthrosis. The superficial and deep components of medial collateral ligament are normally seen as hypoechoic bands separated by thin bursa. Tear is seen as discontinuity in the fibers.

MRI: MCL is best visualized in coronal plane as a low signal intensity band like structure. Fluid signal between the superficial and deep components of the ligament and between the deep component and medial meniscus can be normal or represent bursitis and should not be misinterpreted as tear. The posterior

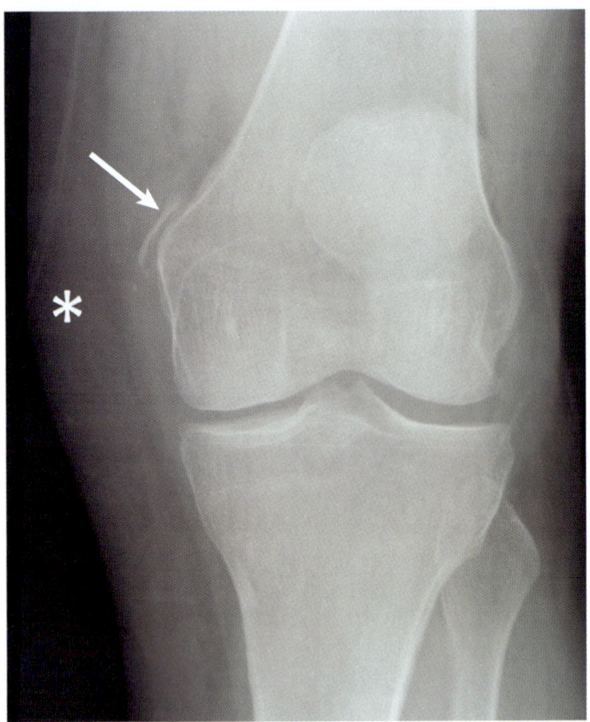

Figure 60.35 Pellegrini–Stieda. Calcification in soft-tissue (*arrow*) adjoining medial femoral condyle with soft-tissue swelling (*asterisk*).

oblique ligament can be assessed on coronal oblique plane at 25-degree angulation. The grading of MCL injury is demonstrated in Fig. 60.36.

Other findings include avulsion from femoral or tibial attachment causing marrow edema; bony contusions in lateral femoral condyle and lateral tibial plateau; and injuries of medial meniscus and ACL. Post-traumatic ossification in the MCL complex (Pellegrini–Stieda lesion) develops in few months to years and the expected location is above the joint line. Injury to posterior oblique ligament (a cause of instability) is diagnosed on MRI as tear of the ligament; edema and hemorrhage superficial to the course of ligament; edema in the meniscosynovial junction of the posterior horn of medial meniscus; edema or tear of the semimembranosus tendon and oblique popliteal ligament and edema in the fascia of the pes anserinus.

Treatment: Isolated MCL tear usually heals by conservative management. Avulsion tears at femoral or tibial attachment can be surgically sutured to the bone. In the case of associated injury to the medial meniscus and ACL, surgical management depends on the degree of instability of the knee.

Lateral Knee and Posterolateral Corner of Knee

Anatomy

Lateral knee structures are major restraints to the varus injury to knee. There is a practically accepted three-layer approach to lateral knee (Table 60.10 and Fig. 60.37).

For all practical purposes, the three most critical structures of the posterolateral corner of the knee are the lateral collateral ligament (LCL), popliteus tendon, and popliteofibular ligament (PFL) (Fig. 60.37).

- LCL is an extracapsular structure and extends from the lateral epicondyle of the femur to the proximal lateral surface of the fibular head. Deepest part of LCL continues as coronary ligament posterior to the lateral meniscus and terminates as arcuate ligament
- Popliteus muscle originates from posterior surface of proximal tibia and its tendon attaches to the lateral femoral condyle (distal and posterior to the attachment of LCL). In its course, it attaches to the posterior horn of lateral meniscus, arcuate ligament, and proximal fibula
- PFL is an inverted Y-shaped structure with its anterior division attaching to posterior part and posterior division to the anterior

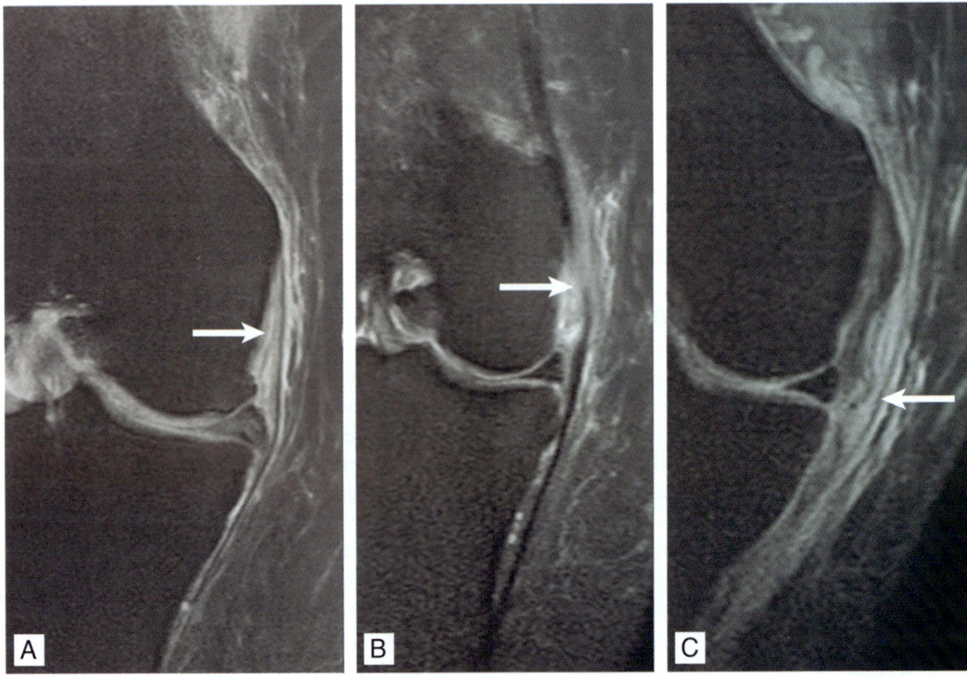

Figure 60.36 MRI grading of medial collateral ligament (MCL) injury represented by *arrows* in coronal PDFS images. (A) Grade I injury shows periligamentous edema and fluid. The ligament is intact throughout its length. (B) Grade II injury shows attenuation of the ligament due to partial thickness tear. (C) Grade III injury shows full thickness disruption of the ligament with retraction of fibers from tibial attachment.

TABLE 60.10 Anatomic Components of Lateral Knee

Superficial layer	■ Iliotibial band and its anterior expansion. It is attached in part to Gerdy's tubercle and some fibers are continuous with vastus lateralis to form lateral patellar retinaculum ■ Superficial portion of the biceps femoris tendon with its posterior expansion which attaches distally to the head and styloid process of fibula
Intermediate layer	Lateral patellar retinaculum; patellofemoral and patellomeniscal ligaments
Deep layer (posterolateral corner of the knee: PLC)	Lateral capsule; lateral collateral ligament; lateral meniscotibial ligament (coronary ligament); arcuate ligament; popliteus muscle-tendon unit; popliteofibular ligament; and when present fabellofibular ligament

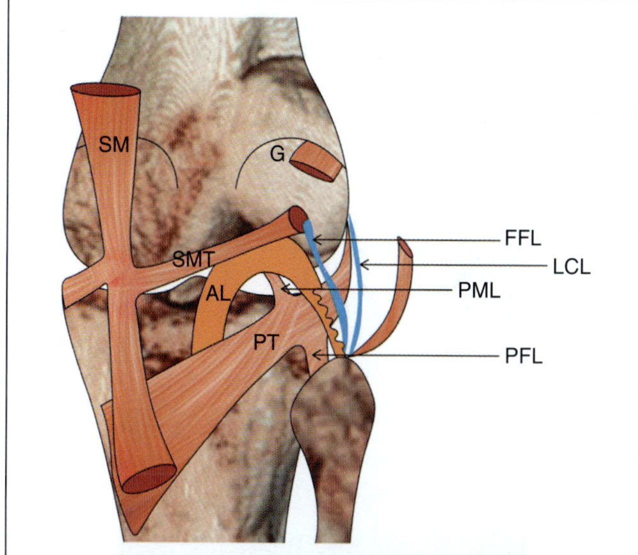

Figure 60.37 Diagrammatic representation of lateral knee structures. *AL*, arcuate ligament; *FFL*, fabellofibular ligament; *G*, gastrocnemius muscle; *LCL*, lateral collateral ligament; *PFL*, popliteal fibular ligament; *PML*, popliteal meniscal ligament; *PT*, popliteus muscle and tendon; *SM*, semimembranosus tendon; *SMT*, recurrent fascicle of the semimembranosus tendon.

part of styloid process of fibula. It resists posterior translation, varus angulation, and external rotation at the knee

There has been a recent proposal on a distinct ligament in the anterolateral aspect of the knee, called as anterolateral ligament (ALL). It is proximally attached to the prominence of the lateral femoral epicondyle, slightly anterior to the origin of the LCL and distally to the anterolateral aspect of the proximal tibia (between Gerdy's tubercle and the tip of the fibular head), with firm attachments to the lateral meniscus. This ligament along with ACL is responsible for rotational stability of the knee, resisting internal tibial rotation and anterior tibial translation. Injury to ALL is related to pivot-shift injuries with ACL tear, and can result in lateral meniscus tear and Segond fracture (described later).

Injuries to Lateral Knee

Mechanism of injury is by varus and external rotational stress to the knee. Isolated injury to single lateral structure is rare and is usually associated with injury to ACL, PCL, and lateral meniscus.

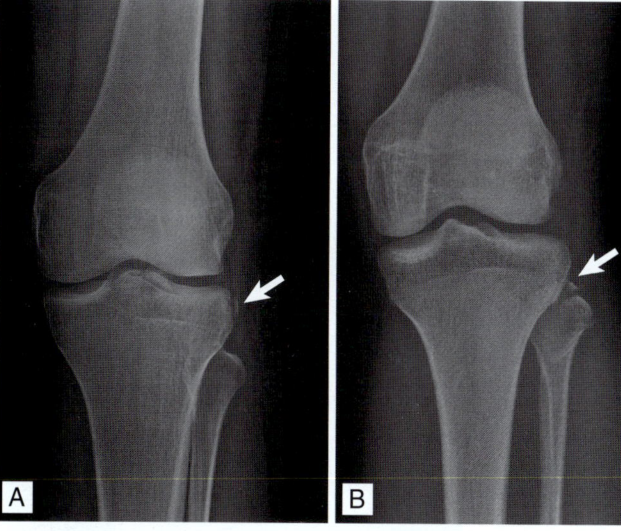

Figure 60.38 AP radiographs of (A) Segond fracture. Fracture of lateral margin of tibia (*arrow*), below the level of joint (B) Arcuate fracture. Avulsion fracture of the fibula tip (*arrow*).

Clinical presentation: buckling of the knee during full extension and difficulty in ascending and descending stairs.

Imaging Features [29,30]

Radiograph: Role of radiography in injury to lateral supporting structures is in identifying the fractures:

- Segond fracture—lateral margin of tibia, below or at the level of joint due to avulsion of the tibial attachment of lateral capsular ligament. Usually indicates association of ACL disruption (Fig. 60.38)
- Arcuate fracture—avulsion fracture of the fibula and the term is reserved only when associated with arcuate ligament injury (Fig. 60.38)
- Gerdy's tubercle avulsion fracture
- Anteromedial tibial margin fracture

USG identifies LCL tear as discontinuity in the fibers and can occasionally detect avulsion fractures.

MRI is the cornerstone in identifying lateral structure injuries (Fig. 60.39). The grading system of injury is the same as followed in medial knee structure injury (discussed previously). *LCL* and *biceps femoris tendons* join to form conjoint tendon and their injuries are usually combined. They are normally seen as dark bands on all sequences and are best visualized in coronal and axial planes. Signs of injury include:

- periligamentous edema resulting from a sprain,
- partial or full-thickness tears,
- soft-tissue avulsions from the femoral and fibular attachment sites,
- osseous avulsion from the fibular head, and
- thickening of the ligament in chronic injuries.

Popliteus myotendinous complex is best seen on axial and coronal images as low- and intermediate-signal-intensity structures, respectively. Myotendinous junction is commonly involved in its injury and rarely there can be avulsion fracture from femoral attachment. Partial tears of the musculotendinous junction appear as amorphous high signal intensity on PDFS images within the tendon and muscle.

PFL is stout tendinous band having similar cross-sectional area as popliteus tendon [30]. It is best assessed in coronal and sagittal

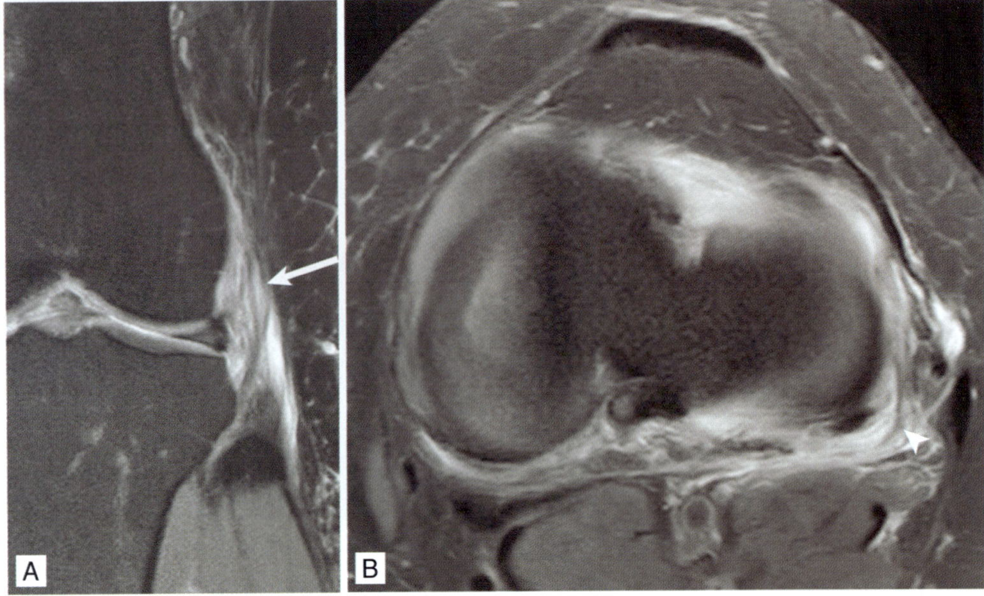

Figure 60.39 Lateral collateral ligament injury. MRI PDFS coronal (A) and axial (B) images show Grade II injury at the femoral attachment of lateral collateral ligament (*arrow*) with injury to the posterolateral corner (*arrowhead*).

planes, deep to the inferior lateral genicular vessels. *Fabellofibular ligament* is best seen on coronal or sagittal images posterior to the arcuate ligament and inferior lateral genicular vessels. On axial images, it is seen immediately anterior to the lateral head of the gastrocnemius tendon. *Arcuate ligament* is seen as a thin low-signal-intensity structure coalescing with the posterolateral capsule and located deep to the inferior lateral genicular artery, overlying the popliteus tendon in general, on axial and sagittal images. Injury to these structures can be seen as partial or full-thickness tear or as avulsion injuries.

Treatment: Patients with grade I and grade II LCL injuries have good prognosis on conservative management and do not develop posttraumatic osteoarthritis even in late follow-up. Patients with either isolated or combined grade III injuries are advocated for surgical treatment in view of gradual development of degenerative arthritis.

Tennis Leg

This is a well-known entity in athletes who complain of acute onset leg pain. There is tearing of the medial head of gastrocnemius, commonly at its myotendinous junction (Fig. 60.40). USG and MRI can demonstrate the tear with adjoining fluid and hematoma formation. It is usually managed conservatively and surgical decision is taken if the patient develops instability or persistent pain.

Osteoarthritis of Knee

Being a large weight-bearing joint with complex anatomy and multidirectional mobility, the knee joint is one of the common joint involved in continuous wear and tear, leading to its degeneration. It leads to various pathological findings including degeneration of menisci, degeneration of cruciate ligaments, osteochondral lesions, and synovial effusion. Detailed discussion is done in the chapter on arthritis (Chapter 52).

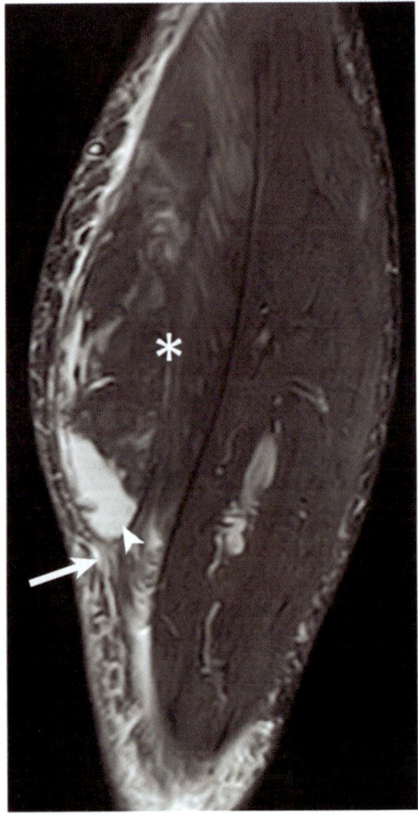

Figure 60.40 Tennis leg. Coronal PDFS MR image of left leg shows tear and retraction (*arrow*) of medial head of gastronemius (*asterisk*) at myotendinous junction. Fluid is also seen at the torn end (*arrowhead*).

Knee Arthroplasty

Surgical replacement of the knee by prosthesis (implants) also called as knee arthroplasty (knee replacement) is definitive treatment for end-stage osteoarthritis. Various types of knee arthroplasty include unicompartmental, bicompartmental, and tricompartmental (total knee replacement) arthroplasty.

Two main groups of implants are [31]:

- *Constrained implants*—or hinged implants are used in severely damaged knees where femur and tibia are bound together by hinge mechanism implant, allowing flexion and extension movement of the knee
- *Nonconstrained implants*—or sliding implants allow normal physiological knee movements and depend on the patient's collateral ligaments for stability

They are further classified as follows:

- *Unicompartmental implants:* only one bony compartment is replaced, either tibiofemoral or patella-femoral compartment. The ACL of the patient must be intact
- *Bicompartmental implants:* the medial and lateral tibio-femoral bony components are replaced while the native patella is retained
- *Tricompartmental implants:* used in total knee arthroplasty where all tibial, femoral, and patellar bony components are replaced by:
  - Metal femoral component
  - Metal tibial base plate
  - Polyethylene insert to tibial base plate
  - Polyethylene patella shield

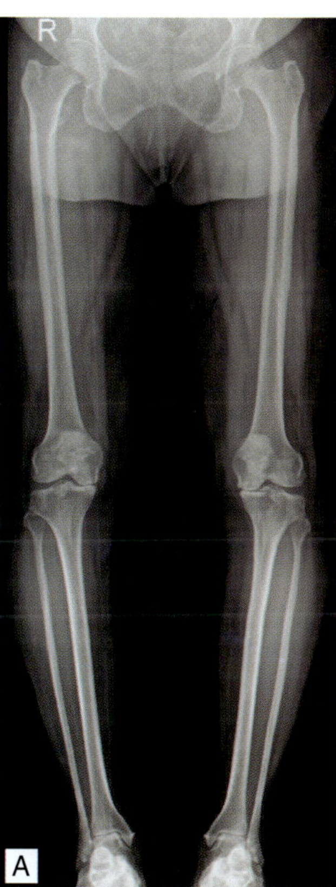

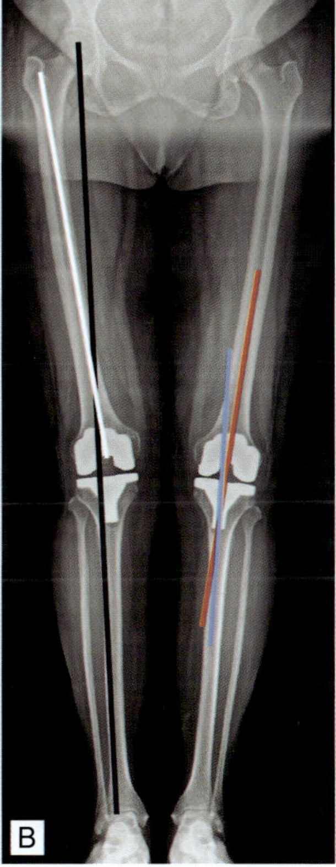

Figure 60.41 Weight-bearing three joint (hip, knee, and ankle) AP radiograph images of preoperative (A) and postbilateral total knee arthroplasty (B) in a patient with knee osteoarthritis. (B) Line drawn from center of femoral head to center of talar body is mechanical axis (*MA*) (*black solid line*), and it should intersect center or just medially to center of prosthetic knee. The femoral and tibial components should be perpendicular to this line. Anatomic axis of femur (*AA*) is line along femoral shaft that passes through center of distal femur (*white line*). On femur, angle between MA and AA is between 4° and 7°. Femorotibial angle is angle intersecting femoral anatomic axis (*red line*) with tibial anatomic axis (*blue line*). Femoral component should be placed 7° ± 3° valgus, and tibial component should be 90° ± 3° relative to AA of tibia on AP radiograph, allowing overall 4–7° valgus angulation.

Preoperative imaging

Weight-bearing three joint (hip, knee, and ankle joints) AP radiograph (Fig. 60.41) and lateral radiographs of both knees are obtained for planning of surgery and determining the size of implants. The following are assessed [31,32]:

- Mechanical axis of lower limb—center of femoral head to center of talar body
- Mechanical axis of femur—center of femoral head to intercondylar fossa
- Anatomical axis of femur—along the femoral shaft
- Tibial axis—along the tibial shaft (anatomical and mechanical axis are identical)
- Angle between the anatomical axis of femur and tibia (valgus angle)

Postoperative imaging

Depending upon local institutional practices, regular interval follow-up is preferred in first year, followed by yearly follow-up. The radiographs to be obtained are weight-bearing three joint AP view (Fig. 60.41), lateral view, and axial view (30–45 degrees flexion) of the knee.

Commonly used criteria to assess successful arthroplasty on radiograph are demonstrated in Fig. 60.41 [31,32]. Rotational malalignment of femoral and tibial components are best assessed by CT imaging. MRI may indicate some postoperative complications and modified pulse sequences called metal artefact reduction (MAR) sequences are performed to reduce metallic artifacts. Specific techniques include section encoding for metal artifact correction, multiacquisition variable-resonance image combination, and orthopedic metal artifact reduction (O-MAR).

Complications of knee arthroplasty include bone resorption or loosening, polyethylene wear and osteolysis, instability, periprosthetic fracture, infection, arthrofibrosis, patellar clunk syndrome, recurrent hemarthrosis, and extensor mechanism injury [31,32].

Summary

Tables 60.11 and 60.12 summarize the mechanical forces causing injury to knee; stabilizing structures; mechanism of injury with associated soft tissue and bony injury.

The flow chart demonstrates the clinical approach to knee swelling.

TABLE 60.11 Summary of Mechanical Forces Causing Injury to the Knee and Structures Stabilizing These Forces

Mechanical Forces	Primary Stabilizers	Secondary Stabilizers
Anterior translation	ACL	MCL, LCL
Posterior translation	PCL	None
Varus	LCL	ACL, PCL
Valgus	MCL	ACL, PCL
Internal rotation	LCL	Anterior cruciate ligament, joint capsule
External rotation	MCL	PCL, joint capsule
Hyperextension	PCL	Anterior cruciate ligament, posterior joint capsule

ACL: anterior cruciate ligament; *LCL*: lateral collateral ligament; *MCL*: medial collateral ligament; *PCL*: posterior cruciate ligament.

TABLE 60.12 Summary of Mechanism of Injury With Associated Soft-Tissue and Bony Injury

Mechanism of Injury	Soft-Tissue Injury	Bony Injury
Pure hyperextension	Posterior cruciate ligament, posterior capsule, anterior cruciate ligament	Bruise: Anterior central tibia, anterior femoral condyles
Hyperextension with varus	Posterolateral corner, anterior cruciate ligament, popliteal tendon, posterior capsule	Bruise: Anteromedial tibia, femoral condyle Avulsion: posterolateral corner, proximal fibula
Hyperextension with valgus	Medial collateral ligament, posteromedial corner, posterior capsule, posterior cruciate ligament	Bruise: Anterolateral tibia, femoral condyle Avulsion: posteromedial tibia
Pure valgus	Medial collateral ligament, anterior cruciate ligament, posterior cruciate ligament	Bruise: Lateral tibia, lateral femoral condyle
Pure varus	Iliotibial band, lateral collateral ligament	Bruise: Medial tibia, femoral condyle
Flexion valgus external rotation (most common)	Medial collateral ligament, anterior cruciate ligament	Bruise: Lateral femoral condyle, posterolateral tibia Avulsion: Posteromedial tibia, femoral condyle
Flexion varus, internal rotation	Anterior cruciate ligament, posterolateral corner	Bruise: Lateral femoral condyle, posterolateral tibia Avulsion: Posterolateral tibia (Segond), fibular head
Flexion with posterior tibia translation	Isolated posterior cruciate ligament, posterior dislocation with severe force	None
Patellar dislocation (flexion and internal rotation of femur on fixed tibia)	Medial patellar retinaculum, medial collateral ligament, anterior cruciate ligament	Bruise: Medial patella, lateral condyle

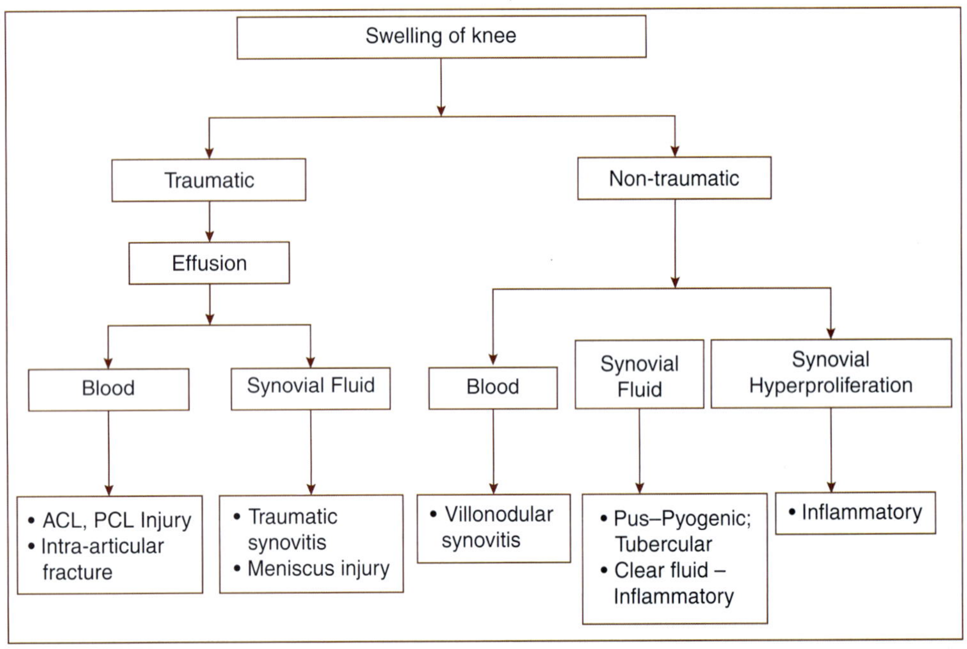

Flowchart: Clinical Approach to Knee Swelling. (Courtesy: Dr. Mantu Jain, Associate Professor, Orthopedics, AIIMS Bhubaneshwar.)

Suggested Readings

- G Tetyana, M Yulia, C Micah, WC Brett, Osteochondral lesions of the knee: differentiating the most common entities at MRI, Radiographics 38 (5) (2018) 1478–1495.
- JC Nguyen, AA De Smet, BK Graf, HG Rosas, MR imaging–based diagnosis and classification of meniscal tears, Radiographics 34 (2014) 981–999.
- CW Pfirrmann, M Zanetti, J Romero, J Hodler, Femoral trochlear dysplasia: MR findings, Radiology 216 (3) (2000) 858–864.
- AS Tadros, TB Nguyen, BR Curtis, BK Huang, DL Resnick, Medial supporting structures of the knee with emphasis on the medial collateral ligament, MRI Web Clinic 2018.
- HG Rosas, Unraveling the posterolateral corner of the knee, Radiographics 36 (6) (2016) 1776–1791.
- AM Naraghi, LM White, Imaging of athletic injuries of knee ligaments and menisci: sports imaging series, Radiology 281 (1) (2016) 23–40.

61

Ankle and Foot

JULIA CRIM

Introduction

Ankle and foot pain are common. This chapter will cover the diagnosis of pain due to nonosseous injury, overuse, abnormal alignment, instability, tarsal coalition, and nerve abnormalities. Imaging evaluation of the foot and ankle requires analysis of a daunting number of small anatomic structures. Moreover, injury to one area often causes the patient to develop an abnormal gait, which may lead to abnormalities in other regions of the foot and ankle. Considering the biomechanical forces acting on the foot will aid in the evaluation of imaging studies. Weight-bearing radiographs should always be the first imaging study performed. Weight bearing shows abnormal alignment, which is often not evident on magnetic resonance imaging (MRI), computed tomography (CT), and ultrasonography (USG). In addition, x-ray (XR) shows abnormal calcifications, which are sometimes difficult to discern on MR because they are low-signal intensity on all sequences, blending with ligaments, tendons, and cortical bone. USG allows excellent visualization of the soft tissues in this region. It is the ideal method to evaluate tendon abnormalities because of the ability to detect tendon instability by performing dynamic maneuvers. A precise and detailed knowledge of normal anatomy is needed to accurately image the small soft tissue structures of the foot on USG. USG and MR are equal in their ability to evaluate ligaments, except for the deep deltoid ligament, which is not well seen on USG. MRI provides excellent static imaging of tendons, and has an advantage over USG in its ability to evaluate bone and cartilage abnormalities.

Imaging Techniques and Protocol

X-Rays

First study obtained in all patients (Figs. 61.1 and 61.2).

- Foot: Anteroposterior (AP) oblique, and lateral views
- Ankle: AP, mortise (20° internal rotation), and lateral views
- Obtain weight-bearing radiographs so that alignment can be assessed
- Stress radiographs may be obtained using manual stress or gravity

CT

- Investigation of choice for the evaluation of complex traumas, tarsal coalition, and some bone tumors
- Inferior to USG and MRI for tendon abnormalities
- Thin sections, reformatted in sagittal and coronal planes
- Dynamic maneuvers useful to assess ligament integrity and tendon subluxation

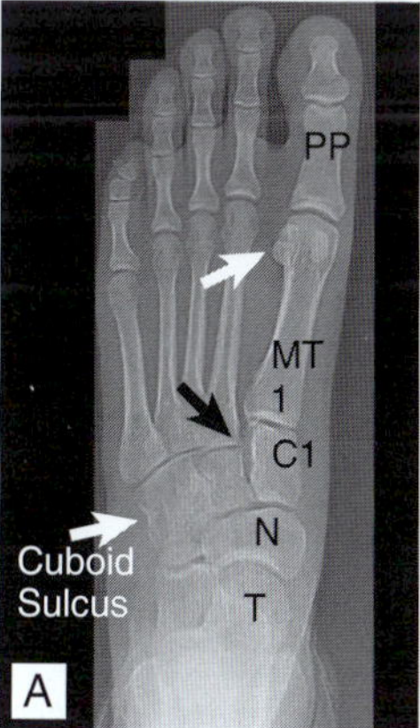

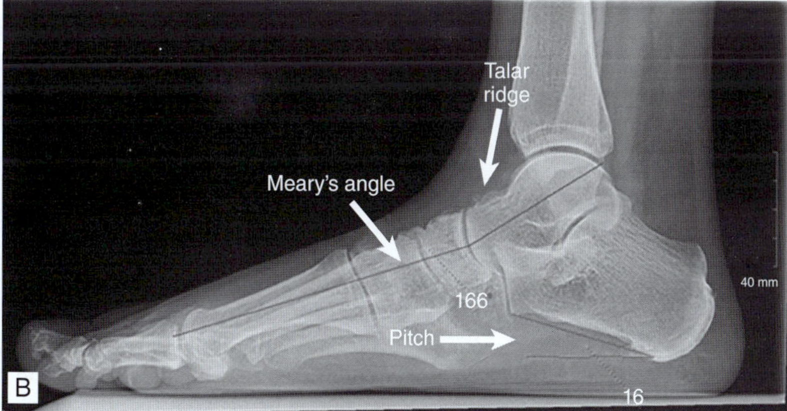

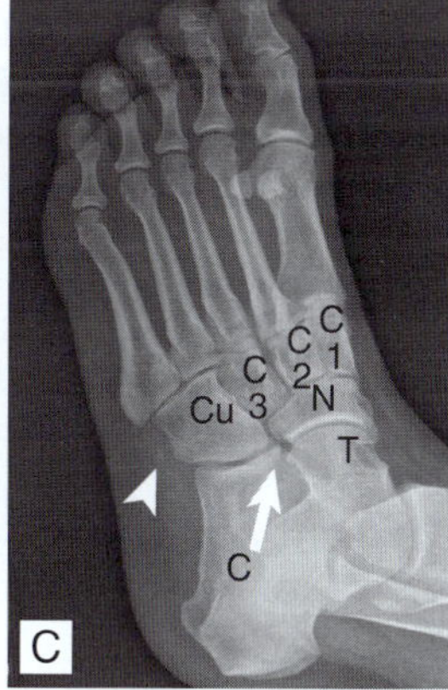

Figure 61.1 Radiographic anatomy of the foot. (A) AP XR shows the axis of the talus is aligned with the axis of the first metatarsal. The angle between the first and second metatarsal (MT) is <10°, and the angle between the first MT and first proximal phalanx (PP) is <15°. Cuboid sulcus is the location where the peroneus longus curves under the foot toward its insertion. Note the medial borders of the second cuneiform and second MT (*black arrow*) are exactly aligned; any lateral shift of the second MT indicates disruption of the Lisfranc ligament. The lateral sesamoid of the great toe is bipartite (*white arrow*) in this patient, a normal variant. (B) Lateral XR shows mild pes planus. The axis of the talus extends below the axis of the first MT (Meary's angle). The inferior border of the calcaneus (calcaneal pitch) is less than 20°, where normal is between 20° and 25°. The talar ridge (*white arrow*) is a normal variant at the insertion of the ankle joint capsule. (C) Oblique XR provides an additional view of the bony relations of the hindfoot and midfoot. Note that the anterior process of the calcaneus (*white arrow*) tapers to a sharp point, and is slightly separated from the lateral margin of the navicular. The styloid process of the fifth MT extends lateral to the lateral margin of the cuboid. There is a small os peroneum (*arrowhead*) in this patient, an ossicle in the peroneus longus tendon. *C,* calcaneus; *C1,* first (also called medial) cuneiform); *C2,* second (middle) cuneiform; *C3,* lateral cuneiform; *Cu,* cuboid; *N,* navicular; *T,* talus.

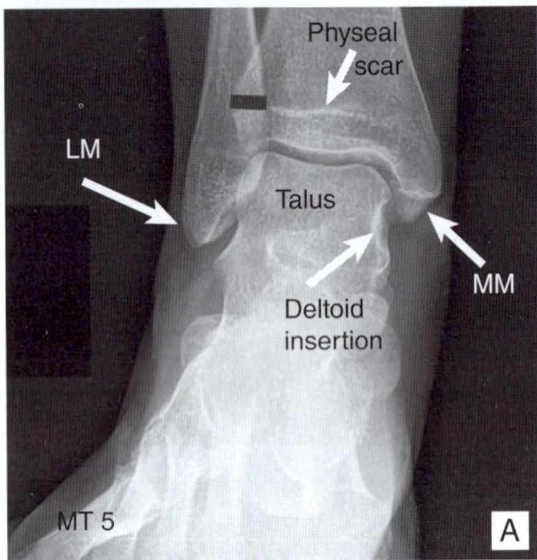

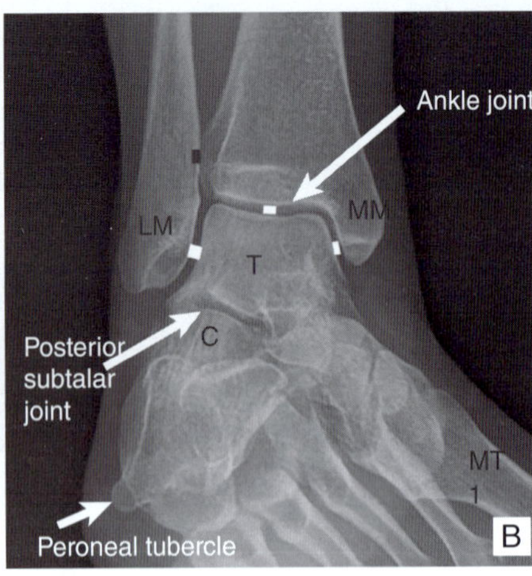

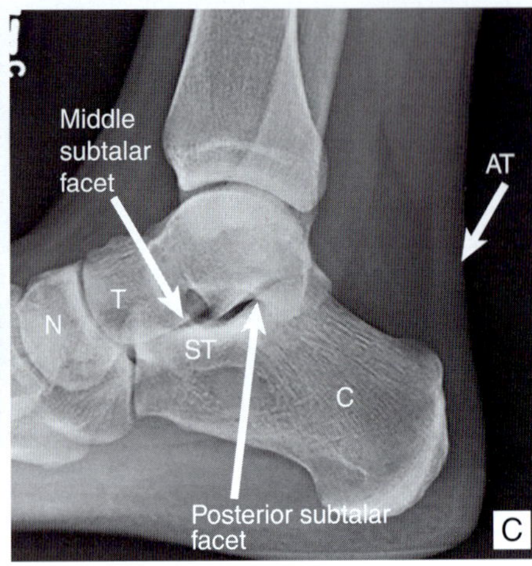

Figure 61.2 Radiographic anatomy of the ankle. (A) AP XR shows the fibula and tibia overlap by 1 cm (gray line). The lateral malleolus extends further caudally than the medial. Note that "talar dome" is a misnomer, because the articular surface of the talus is concave centrally when viewed in the frontal projection, and "talar trochlea" is a better term for this portion of the talus. The dense physeal scar marks the closed physis and is a normal finding. (B) Mortise XR shows that the joint spaces medially, laterally, and superiorly (white lines) are equal, and <4 mm in width. There is 1 mm overlap of tibia and fibula (gray line). (C) Lateral XR shows optimal patient positioning. This view is easily poorly positioned, which can lead to misdiagnosis. In a well-positioned lateral view, the fibula is aligned along the posterior portion of the talus, and the two sides of the talar trochlea are superimposed. The surfaces of the tibial plafond (distal articular surface of tibia) and talar trochlea are congruent. The posterior and middle subtalar joints are well seen. The Achilles tendon contour is sharply demarcated next to the lucent pre-Achilles fat (Kager's fat). *AT*, Achilles tendon; *C*, calcaneus; *LM*, lateral malleolus; *MM*, medial malleolus; *MT*, metatarsal; *N*, navicular; *ST*, sustentaculum tali; *T*, talus.

MRI

- Performed for the evaluation of tendons, ligaments, joints, infection, and masses (Fig. 61.3)
- Dedicated surface coil, centered on the region of concern
- FOV 12–16 cm (avoid too small a FOV because abnormalities often involve multiple structures)
- Contrast used in cases of infection, masses
- MRI imaging planes and recommended sequences are provided in Table 61.1

Ultrasonography

- Preferred for the evaluation of tendons and ligaments, masses, nerves, joint effusions [1] (Fig. 61.4). USG is best employed for a focused examination of a specific clinical question
- Linear array 8–18 MHz (or similar high frequency) transducer most useful
- Obtain long- and short-axis views of structures of concern
- Unique advantage—Use active and passive dynamic maneuvers to show abnormal motion

Normal Anatomy

Joints

Ankle Joint

Also called the mortise or talocrural joint, ankle joint is an articulation between tibia, fibula, and talus. It is a hinge joint allowing only dorsiflexion and plantar flexion. The body of the talus is held within the mortise formed by the tibia and fibula. The mortise is stabilized by the deltoid ligament medially and the syndesmotic and lateral collateral ligaments laterally (Figs. 61.2–61.4A).

Subtalar Joint

Inversion, eversion, and glide occur at the posterior subtalar joint, an articulation between talus and calcaneum. The subtalar joint has three facets: posterior, middle, and anterior (Figs. 61.3 and 61.5).

- The posterior subtalar joint forms a separate joint cavity, and sometimes communicates with the ankle joint
- The middle and anterior subtalar facets form a common joint cavity with the talonavicular joint

Chopart Joint

The talonavicular and calcaneocuboid joint act together in pronation and supination and are often referred to as the Chopart joint.

- On nonweight-bearing examinations, the cuboid moves slightly inferiorly relative to the calcaneus, which can lead to an erroneous diagnosis of subluxation. Alignment should be assessed on weight-bearing XR only

Lisfranc Joint

The tarsometatarsal (TMT) joints, often collectively referred to as the Lisfranc joint, provide only slight motion.

Forefoot joints

The metatarsophalangeal (MTP) and interphalangeal joints are hinge joints allowing dorsiflexion and plantar flexion.

- Bursae lie between the metatarsal heads, and when enlarged, are sometimes mistaken for Morton neuroma

Bones

There are *three subdivisions of the bones of the foot from posterior to anterior*: hindfoot (talus and calcaneus); midfoot (navicular, cuboid, and cuneiforms); and forefoot (metatarsals and phalanges).

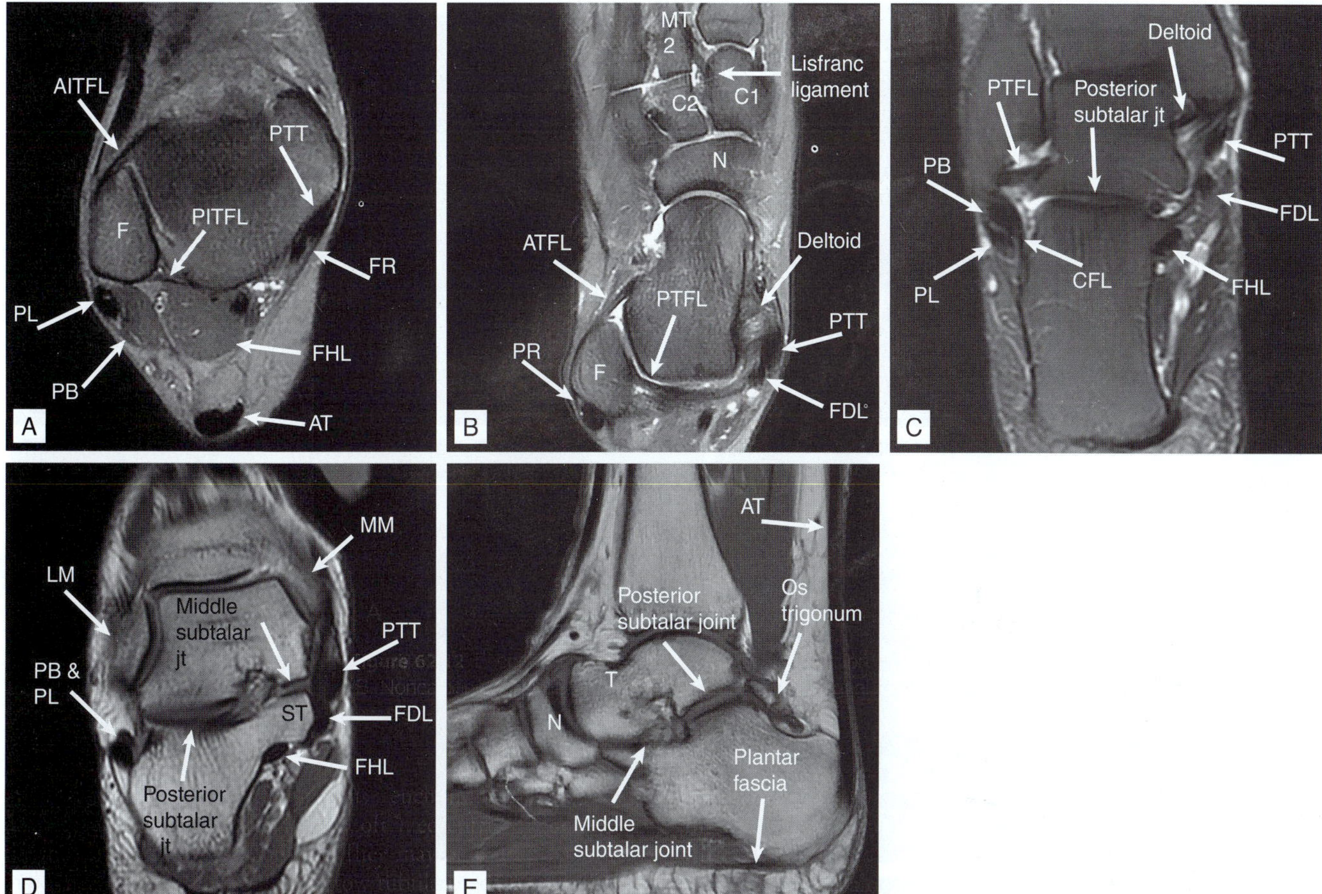

Figure 61.3 MR anatomy of the ankle and foot. (A) Axial proton density with fat suppression (PDFSW) MR is obtained parallel to the long axis of the talus. At the level of the tibial plafond we see two components of the syndesmotic ligaments, the AITFL and PITFL. The interosseous ligament lies between them at a more cephalad level. The PTT is held tightly behind the medial malleolus by the flexor retinaculum. (B) Axial PDFSW MR with the same orientation shows normal appearance of multiple ligaments. The Lisfranc ligament has dorsal, interosseous, and plantar bands. The interosseous band is shown here and is the most important functionally. (C) Coronal PDFSW MR shows the CFL and deep deltoid ligaments. The CFL is part of the floor of the peroneal tendon sheath. Depending on the obliquity of the imaging plane, the entire CFL may not be seen on a single image. The large posterior subtalar facet is well seen. (D) Coronal T1W MR anterior to 4C shows the posterior subtalar facet is smaller at this level, and the middle facet has come into view. The sustentaculum tali, a medial projection from the calcaneus, forms a horizontally oriented support for the middle facet. (E) Sagittal T1W MRI through the mid ankle shows the normal appearance of the Achilles tendon and plantar fascia, attaching to the posterior process of the calcaneus. This patient has an os trigonum, a normal variant. *AITFL,* anterior inferior tibiofibular ligament; *AT,* Achilles tendon; *ATFL,* anterior talofibular ligament; *C1,* first (also called medial) cuneiform); *C2,* second (middle) cuneiform; *CFL,* calcaneofibular ligament; *F,* fibula; *FDL,* flexor digitorum longus tendon; *FHL,* flexor hallucis longus tendon; *FR,* flexor retinaculum; *LM,* lateral malleolus; *MM,* medial malleolus; *MT,* metatarsal; *N,* navicular; *PB,* peroneus brevis; *PL,* palmaris longus; *PITFL,* posterior inferior tibiofibular ligament; *PR,* peroneal retinaculum; *PTT,* posterior tibial tendon; *PTFL,* posterior talofibular ligament; *ST,* sustentaculum tali; *STIR,* short tau inversion recovery; *T,* talus.

TABLE 61.1 MRI Imaging Planes and Recommended Sequences

Imaging Plane	Orientation	Sequences	Shows These Structures and Pathologies Well
Sagittal	Along long axis of talus in hindfoot, second MT in forefoot	T1, STIR	Ankle and subtalar joints, tarsal coalition, some stress fractures (except navicular), plantar fascia, osteomyelitis, neoplasms
Coronal	Perpendicular to talus in hindfoot, second MT in forefoot	T1, PDFS	Ankle and subtalar joints, tarsal coalition, stress fractures, extrinsic tendons, intrinsic muscles, plantar fascia, tarsal tunnel, osteomyelitis, neoplasms, Morton neuroma
Axial	Along long axis of talus in hindfoot, second MT in forefoot	T1, T2FS	Joints of midfoot and forefoot, stress fractures, extrinsic tendons, intrinsic muscles, tarsal tunnel, Lisfranc ligament, osteomyelitis, neoplasm, Morton neuroma

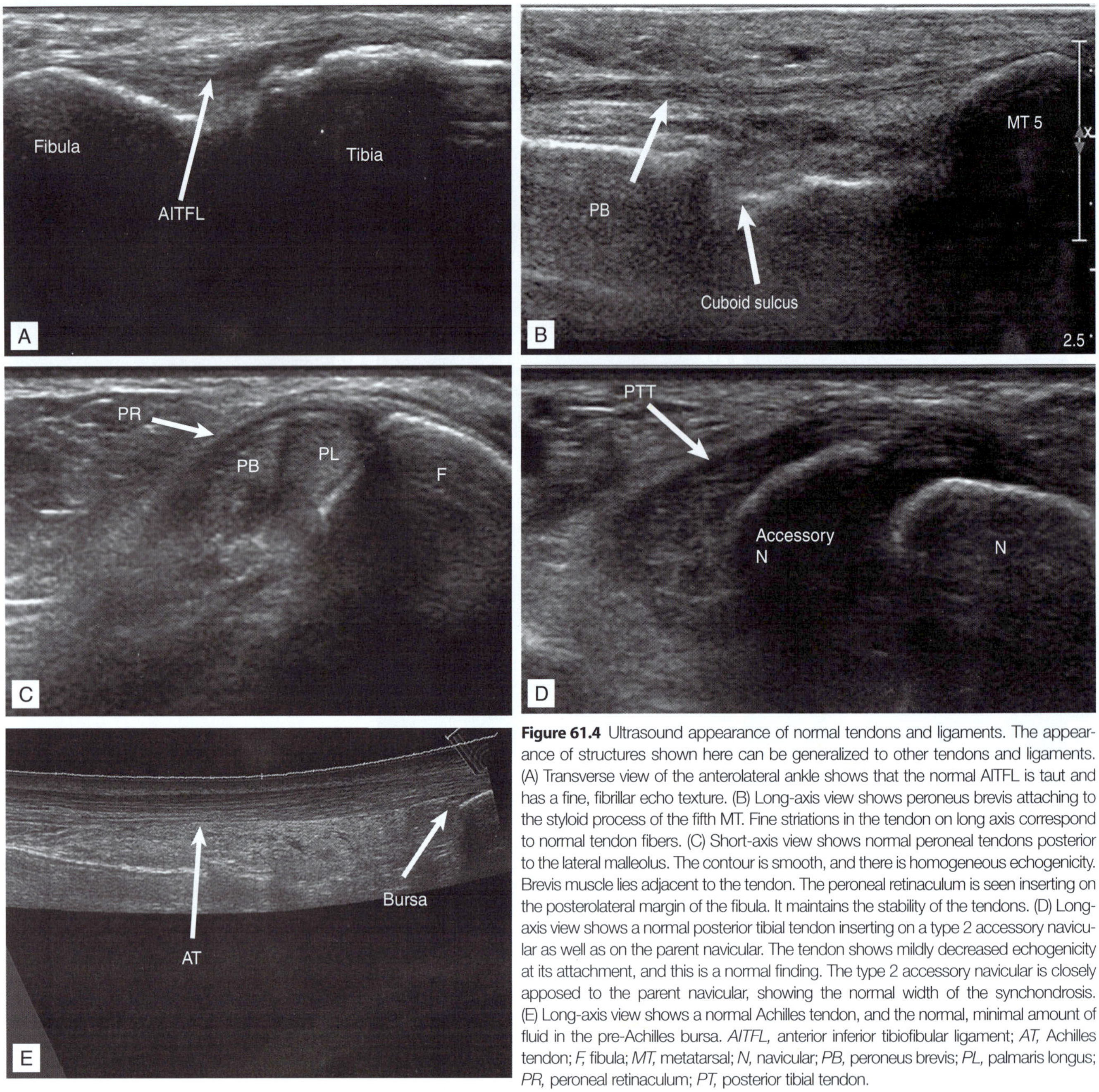

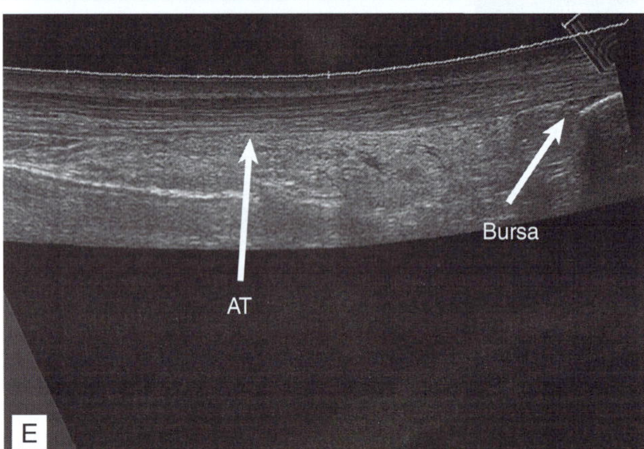

Figure 61.4 Ultrasound appearance of normal tendons and ligaments. The appearance of structures shown here can be generalized to other tendons and ligaments. (A) Transverse view of the anterolateral ankle shows that the normal AITFL is taut and has a fine, fibrillar echo texture. (B) Long-axis view shows peroneus brevis attaching to the styloid process of the fifth MT. Fine striations in the tendon on long axis correspond to normal tendon fibers. (C) Short-axis view shows normal peroneal tendons posterior to the lateral malleolus. The contour is smooth, and there is homogeneous echogenicity. Brevis muscle lies adjacent to the tendon. The peroneal retinaculum is seen inserting on the posterolateral margin of the fibula. It maintains the stability of the tendons. (D) Long-axis view shows a normal posterior tibial tendon inserting on a type 2 accessory navicular as well as on the parent navicular. The tendon shows mildly decreased echogenicity at its attachment, and this is a normal finding. The type 2 accessory navicular is closely apposed to the parent navicular, showing the normal width of the synchondrosis. (E) Long-axis view shows a normal Achilles tendon, and the normal, minimal amount of fluid in the pre-Achilles bursa. *AITFL,* anterior inferior tibiofibular ligament; *AT,* Achilles tendon; *F,* fibula; *MT,* metatarsal; *N,* navicular; *PB,* peroneus brevis; *PL,* palmaris longus; *PR,* peroneal retinaculum; *PT,* posterior tibial tendon.

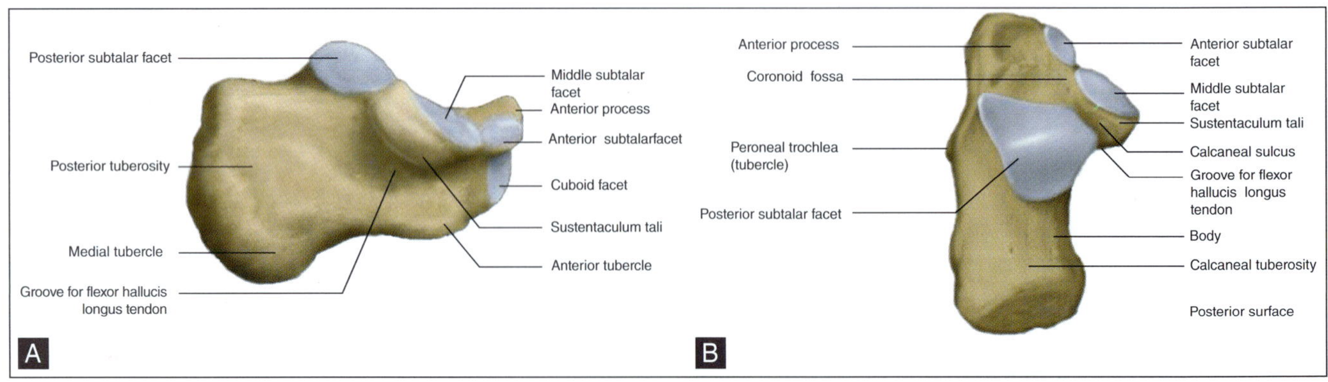

Figure 61.5 The anatomy of the subtalar joint is complex, and the relation between the three facets is perhaps best understood through these drawings, which show the calcaneal joint surfaces. (A) Medial view of the calcaneus (from Imaging Anatomy: Musculoskeletal, 2nd Edition, p. 258). (B) Superior view of the calcaneus (from Imaging Anatomy: Musculoskeletal, 2nd Edition, p. 257).

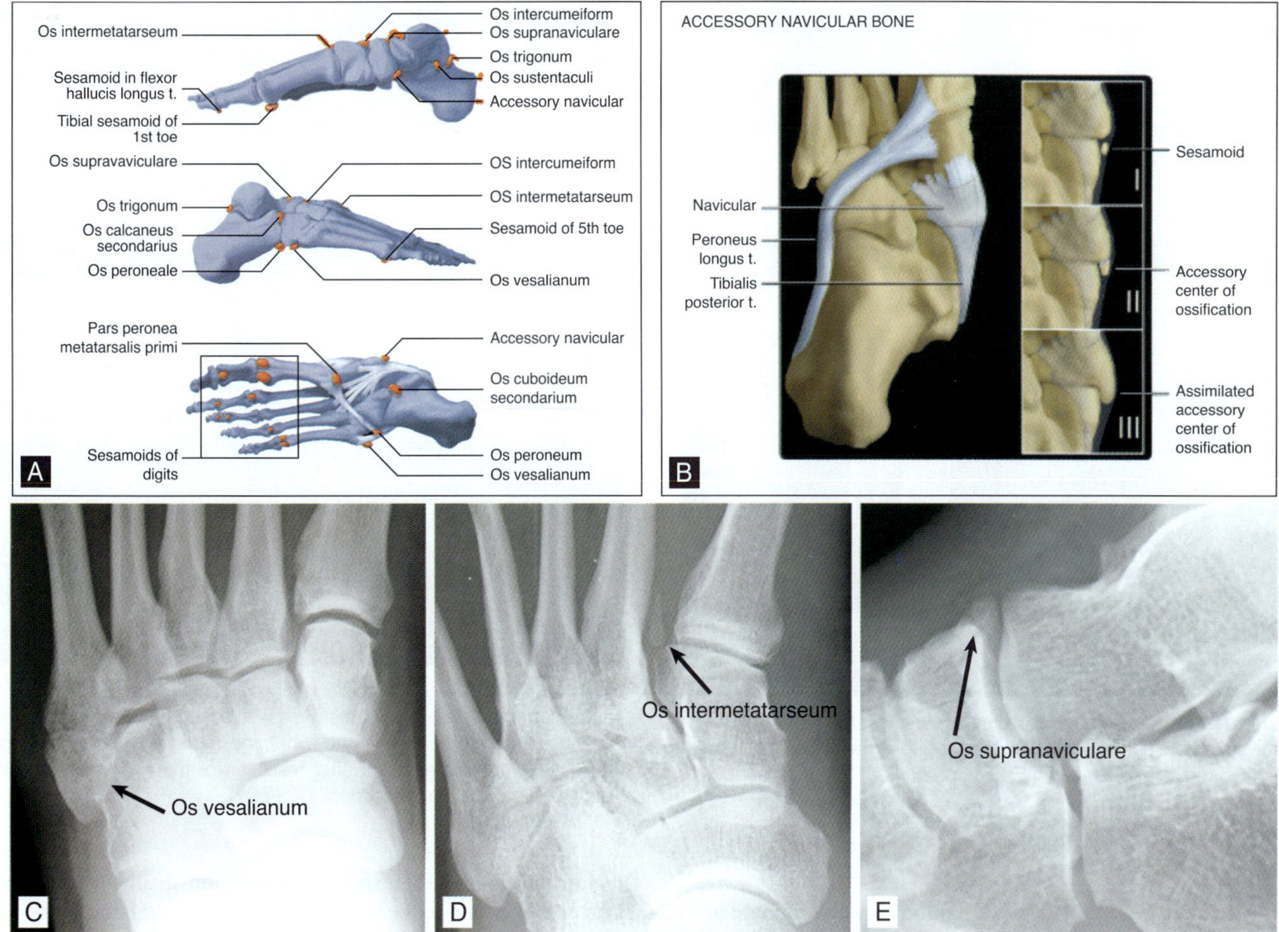

Figure 61.6 (A) Accessory centers of ossification and sesamoids (from "foot & ankle normal variants and imaging pitfalls"; Elsevier Anatomy, p. 1101). Accessory centers of ossification are often mistaken for fractures. Examples shown here exemplify the characteristics which distinguish them from fractures. First, they are corticated and have smooth, usually obtuse margins. Second, they usually enlarge the bone contour, while a chip fracture is subtracted from the normal bone contour. (B) Types of accessory navicular (from "foot & ankle normal variants and imaging pitfalls"; Elsevier Anatomy, p. 1110). (C) Os vesalianum is often mistaken for avulsion of the styloid process of the fifth MT by the peroneus brevis tendon. However, it is larger and more bulbous in contour than the normal styloid process. It is well corticated, and has obtuse margins. (D) Os intermetatarseum is often mistaken for an avulsion fracture of the Lisfranc ligament attachment to the second MT base. However, note that the contour and alignment of the second MT base are normal in the presence of this accessory ossicle. The ossicle has a teardrop shape. (E) Os supranaviculare is often mistaken for chip fracture of the dorsal navicular. Note that the ossicle enlarges the bone contour, rather than being subtracted from the normal contour as occurs with chip fractures.

Here are *three columns of the foot, from medial to lateral.* The medial column is the most mobile column and is formed by the talus, navicular, first cuneiform, and first toe. The middle column is the mid and lateral cuneiforms and second to third MT. The lateral column is formed by the calcaneus, cuboid, and fourth to fifth MT.

Variant Ossifications

Sesamoids (ossicles in a tendon) and accessory centers of ossification associated with a bone are common in the foot (Fig. 61.6).

- Sesamoids may be bipartite or multipartite
- *A multipartite sesamoid has a smooth, round, corticated contour. A fractured sesamoid has irregular margins, and if acute, the margins will not be corticated*

There are three different types of accessory navicular: type 1 is a sesamoid in the posterior tibial tendon (PTT), type 2 is an accessory center of ossification united through a synchondrosis with the parent navicular, and type 3 is assimilated into the parent navicular, creating a prominent medial contour (cornuate navicular).

- *Type 2 accessory navicular is associated with PTT dysfunction*
- The posterior process of the talus may form a separate ossification center, called the os trigonum. It can be associated with posterior ankle impingement
- The first MTP joint has two sesamoid bones at its plantar surface. The medial sesamoid arises in the abductor hallucis and the medial head of the flexor hallucis brevis. The lateral sesamoid arises in the adductor hallucis and the lateral head of the flexor hallucis brevis. The sesamoids are embedded in the plantar plate and attach to the base of the first proximal phalanx. The flexor hallucis longus runs between the sesamoids
- A bipartite MTP sesamoid is usually larger than a unipartite one, and this finding helps to distinguish it from a fractured sesamoid
- Sesamoids are variably present in the lesser toes
- The peroneal tubercle is a variably present projection from the lateral margin of the calcaneal body. When present, it lies between the peroneus brevis and longus tendons

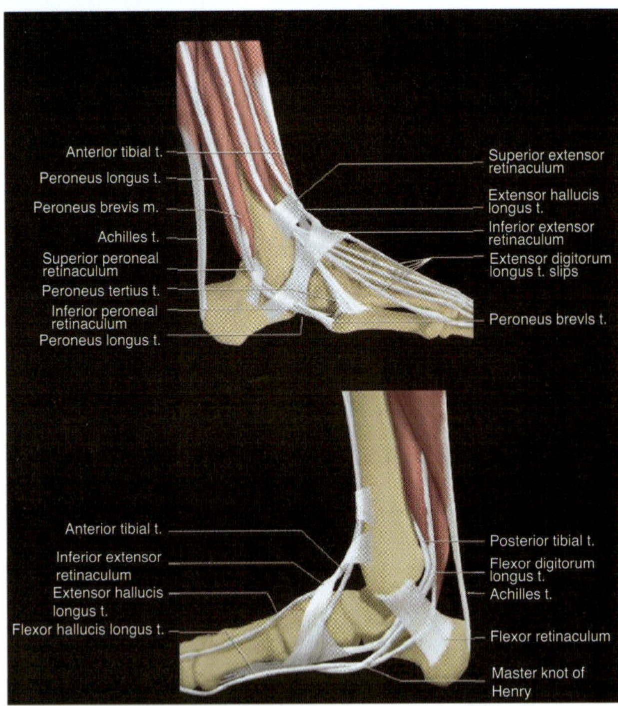

Figure 61.7 Drawing showing course of extrinsic tendons. (A) View of lateral side of the ankle. (B) View of medial side of the ankle (from Imaging Anatomy: Musculoskeletal, 2nd Edition, p. 263).

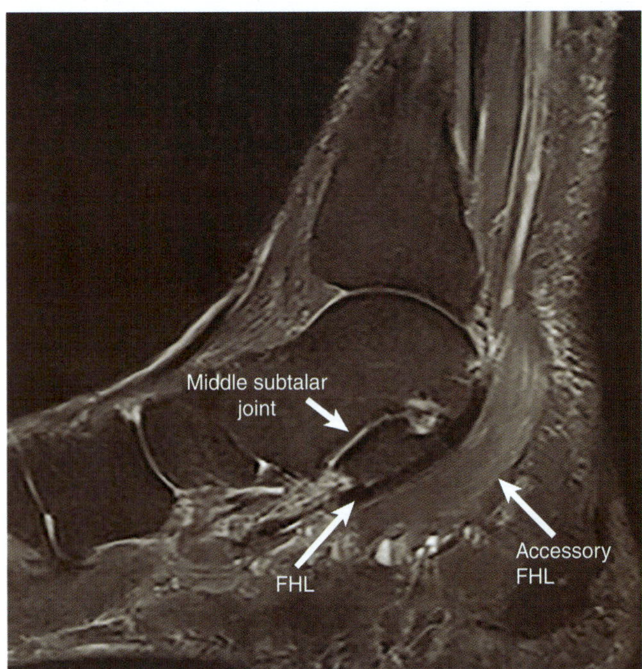

Figure 61.8 Accessory flexor hallucis longus muscle on sagittal STIR MRI. The fusiform muscle belly creates a mass effect in the tarsal tunnel. This patient presented with tarsal tunnel syndrome, and difficulty plantar flexing the foot. Symptoms resolved after resection of the accessory muscle. *FHL,* flexor hallucis longus tendon.

Extrinsic Tendons

There are three groups of extrinsic tendons which originate in the calf and insert on foot: flexors, extensors, and peroneal tendons. They are shown in Fig. 61.7.

The **flexor tendons** originate in the posterior compartment of the calf. They are further divided into superficial (Achilles and plantaris) and deep.

- The Achilles tendon, the conjoint tendon of the gastrocnemius and soleus muscles, is subcutaneous in the posterior ankle. It inserts on the posterior process of the calcaneus. The small pre-Achilles bursa, also known as retrocalcaneal bursa, separates the tendon from the superior portion of the posterior calcaneal process. The plantaris tendon is variably present. It inserts medial to the Achilles on the posterior process of the calcaneus, and when present, can be located alongside medial Achilles tendon
- The deep flexor tendons are from medial to lateral at the level of the posterior malleolus: the posterior tibial, flexor digitorum longus, and flexor hallucis longus. They are stabilized behind the medial malleolus by the overlying flexor retinaculum
  - The flexor hallucis longus tendon sheath communicates with the ankle joint, and for that reason a small amount of fluid is often seen in the tendon sheath. This should not be mistaken for tenosynovitis
- Accessory flexor muscles may be present and are inconsistently named for the closest tendon, or often merely called designated as an accessory flexor (Fig. 61.8). *Accessory muscles may increase pressure in the flexor compartment, and can lead to exertional compartment syndrome or to tarsal tunnel syndrome*

The **extensor tendons** are from medial to lateral the anterior tibial, the extensor hallucis longus, and the extensor digitorum longus. The peroneus tertius is often present lateral to the extensor digitorum longus. The extensor retinaculum maintains the position of the tendons close to the ankle. An extensor bursa is present and can become inflamed.

There are two **peroneal tendons**, the longus and the brevis, which originate in the lateral compartment of the calf. The peroneus brevis inserts on the styloid process of the fifth MT. The peroneus longus extends plantar to the cuboid sulcus of the cuboid, and inserts on the plantar aspect of the first and second MT bases. They share a common tendon sheath.

- An accessory peroneus brevis muscle may be present and may predispose to posterolateral impingement

Intrinsic Muscles

These are divided into four plantar layers and two layers of extensor muscles. Extrinsic tendons lie adjacent to the intrinsic muscles in each layer. They extend from the calcaneus to the MTP joints. The peroneus longus courses across all layers. The plantar fascia is a superficial aponeurosis with three separate bands (central, lateral, and medial) overlying each of the muscles of the superficial layer. It extends from medial calcaneal tuberosity along the inferior calcaneus toward the MTP joints and the toes.

- First plantar layer: abductor hallucis, flexor digitorum brevis, abductor digiti minimi, peroneus brevis
- Second plantar layer: quadratus plantae, flexor digitorum, lumbricals, flexor hallucis longus
- Third plantar layer: flexor hallucis brevis, adductor hallucis, flexor digiti minimi, tibialis posterior
- Fourth plantar layer: plantar and dorsal interossei
- Superficial dorsal layer: anterior tibial, extensor hallucis longus, extensor digitorum longus, peroneus tertius
- Deep layer (hindfoot and midfoot only): extensor hallucis brevis, extensor digitorum brevis

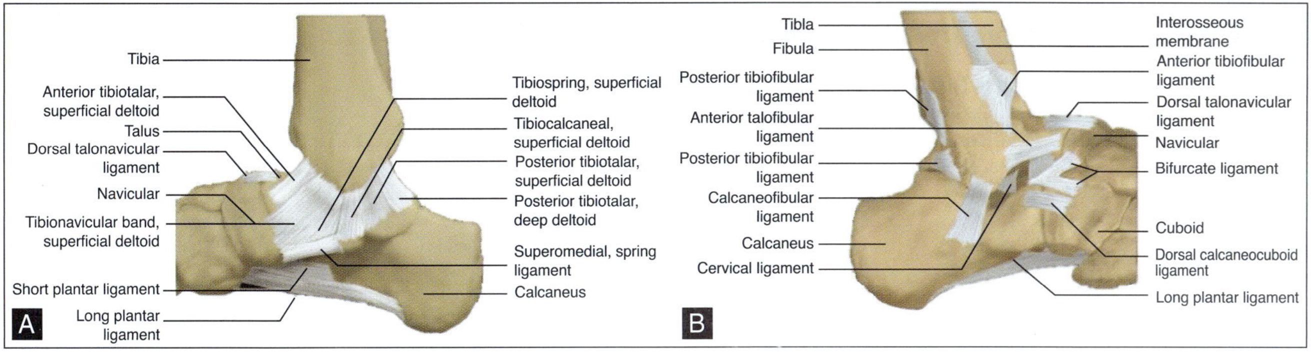

Figure 61.9 Drawing shows the ligaments of the hindfoot from the medial (A) and lateral (B) view (from Imaging Anatomy: Musculoskeletal, 2nd Edition, p. 261 (A), 260 (B)).

Ankle Ligaments

There are three sets of ligaments stabilizing the ankle (Figs. 61.3 and 61.9).

- The **lateral collateral ligament** has three components, the anterior talofibular, the calcaneofibular, and the posterior talofibular. It stabilizes the ankle against abnormal inversion and internal rotation
- The **syndesmotic ligament** also has three components, the anterior and posterior inferior tibiofibular and the interosseous. It maintains close apposition of the tibia and fibula, and protects the ankle against eversion and internal and external rotation
- *It is important to remember that although the lateral collateral and syndesmotic ligaments lie in close proximity to each other, their functions are quite different. The lateral collateral ligament stabilizes against inversion, and the tibiofibular ligament stabilizes against eversion*
- The **deltoid ligament** is divided into deep and superficial components
    - The **deep deltoid ligament** extends from the deep surface of the anterior colliculus of the medial malleolus to a concavity at the medial surface of the talar body. It normally has a striated appearance, similar to the anterior cruciate ligament of the knee. It prevents lateral displacement of the talus
    - The **superficial deltoid ligament** fans out widely from the superficial surface of the medial malleolus to the medial hindfoot. It provides rotational stability to the ankle. It has multiple bands, named for their attachments, to the talus, navicular, and calcaneus. The most important component is the tibiocalcaneal ligament

Hindfoot Ligaments

- The inter**osseous and cervical ligaments** between the talus and calcaneus help maintain subtalar stability (Figs. 61.3 and 61.9)
- The **bifurcate ligament** extends from the anterior process of the calcaneus to the navicular and cuboid and provides inversion stability
- **Intertarsal ligaments** are also present and are named for their attachments
- **Spring Ligament** or plantar calcaneonavicular ligament connects the calcaneus and navicular and supports talus

Tarsometatarsal Ligaments

- The TMT or Lisfranc joint is essentially straight from medial to lateral, except for the variable recession of the second MT base. Its stability is heavily dependent on ligaments
- The second to fifth MT bases are joined by interosseous ligaments, but there is no ligament between the first and second MT bases
- The **Lisfranc ligament** stabilizes the second TMT joint. It extends from the first cuneiform to the base of the second metatarsal (Fig. 61.3B)
- The Lisfranc ligament is critical to maintaining the alignment of the TMT joints and the longitudinal arch of the foot

Metatarsophalangeal Ligaments

The plantar plate is a thickening of the joint capsule important for preventing dorsal subluxation. Each MTP joint also has medial and lateral collateral ligaments.

Abnormal Alignment

Infants are born with flat feet. The longitudinal and transverse arches are important for normal function and develop when the child begins to walk. Abnormal foot and ankle alignment can lead to chronic foot pain and premature osteoarthritis. Corrective shoes and shoe inserts are the first lines of treatment for foot deformities. Severe, symptomatic deformities can be treated with a variety of osteotomies or with fusion. Radiograph views and measurements of alignment abnormalities are provided in Table 61.2.

Pes planus refers to a flat longitudinal arch of the foot (Fig. 61.1B), *and pes cavus to an abnormally high longitudinal arch* (Fig. 61.10A). Planus is often associated with hindfoot valgus, where the heel is tilted away from the midline of the body in the vertical plane, while cavus is often associated with hindfoot varus (Fig. 61.11).

Rocker bottom deformity of the foot refers to the reversal of the normal upward arch and can develop in adults due to neuropathic arthropathy (Fig. 61.12).

Toe deformities are much more common in women than in men and are related to the choice of shoes.

The terms valgus and varus are used to evaluate toe alignment, but unlike the usage of the terms in other joints, the deformity is in the horizontal plane (Fig. 61.10B).

Metatarsus primus varus is present when the angle between the first and second MT is >9°.

Hallux valgus is an increased angle between the first MT and first proximal phalanx. Hallux valgus is classified as mild (16–25°), moderate (26–34°), or severe (>35°). *Bunion* refers to a medial bony prominence of first metatarsal head. In severe cases, the first and second toes may show crossover, which should be noted in reports.

Bunionette refers to a lateral bony prominence of fifth MT head, often associated with >5° difference in the axis between fifth MT and proximal phalanx.

TABLE 61.2 Evaluation of Abnormal Alignment on Weight-Bearing XR

Alignment Abnormality	View of Foot Where Measured	Measurement #1	Measurement #2
Pes planus	Lateral	Meary angle <–4°	Calcaneal pitch <20°
Pes cavus	Lateral	Meary angle >4°	Calcaneal pitch >25°
Hindfoot valgus	AP	Talus axis extends medial to first MT	Talocalcaneal angle >40°
Hindfoot varus	AP	Talus axis extends lateral to second MT	Talocalcaneal angle <25°
Metatarsus primus varus	AP	Intermetatarsal angle: angle between first and second MT >9°	
Hallux valgus	AP	Hallux angle: angle between first MT and first PP > 15°	

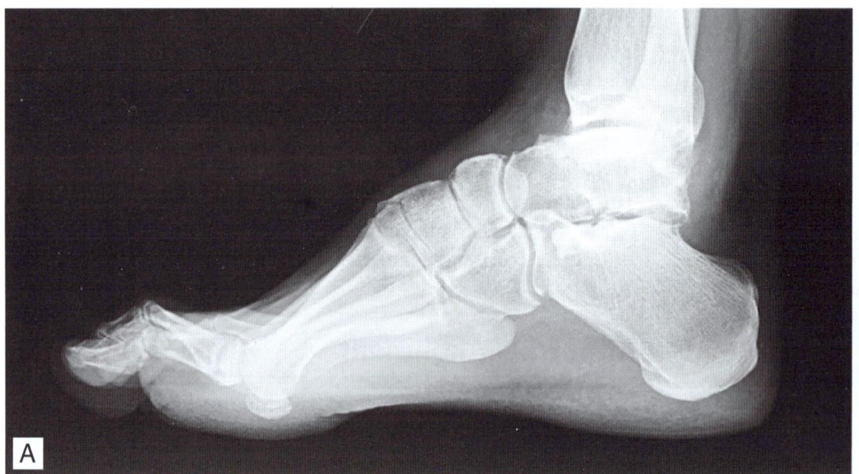

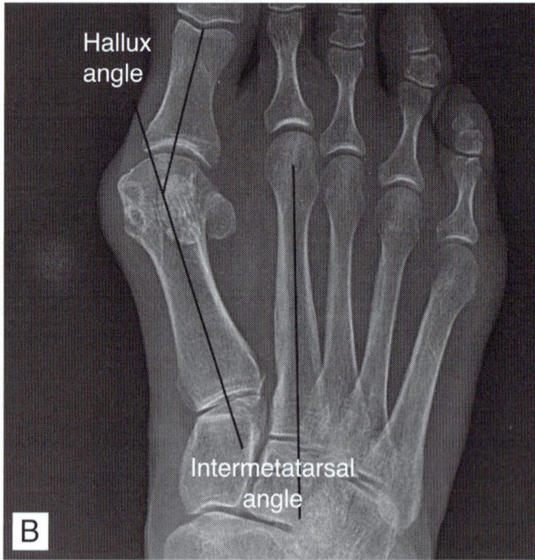

Figure 61.10 Abnormal alignment on radiographs. (A) Lateral XR of a patient with Charcot–Marie–Tooth neuropathy shows severe pes cavus, with elevated calcaneal pitch and the axis of the talus superior to the first MT axis (Meary's angle). There are flexion deformities of the toe. (B) AP weight-bearing XR shows intermetatarsal angle >9° (metatarsus primus varus) and hallux angle >15° (hallux valgus). There is a prominent bony bunion. Cysts are seen in the medial MT head and are a common finding related to pressure of shoes on the bunion. Bunionette of the fifth toe is also present.

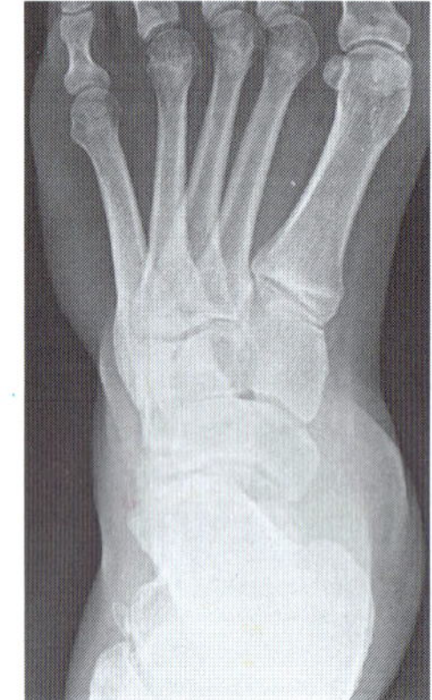

Figure 61.11 Hindfoot varus. AP radiograph in a patient with Charcot–Marie–Tooth disease shows that the axis of the talus is deviated laterally, nearly parallel to the calcaneus, indicating hindfoot varus. The normal talar axis should extend either along the axis of the first metatarsal, or between the first and second metatarsals. Varus of the forefoot is also present, and is evident as increased overlap of the bases of the toes.

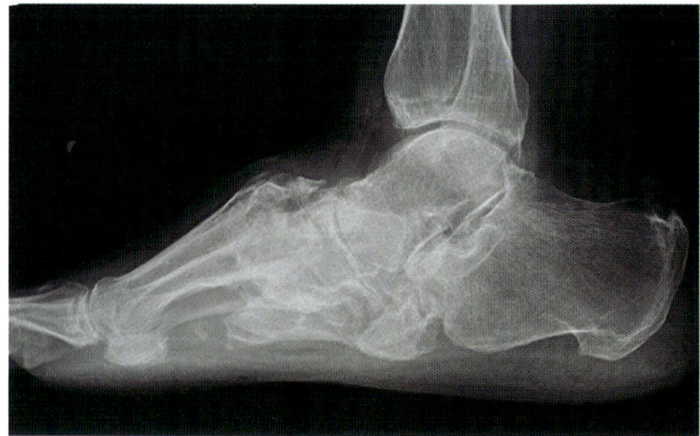

Figure 61.12 Rocker bottom deformity due to neuropathic arthropathy. Lateral radiograph shows the normal convex superior longitudinal arch of the foot has become reversed, and is convex inferiorly. Ulcers often develop at the site of the cuboid, which is now at the plantar margin of the foot.

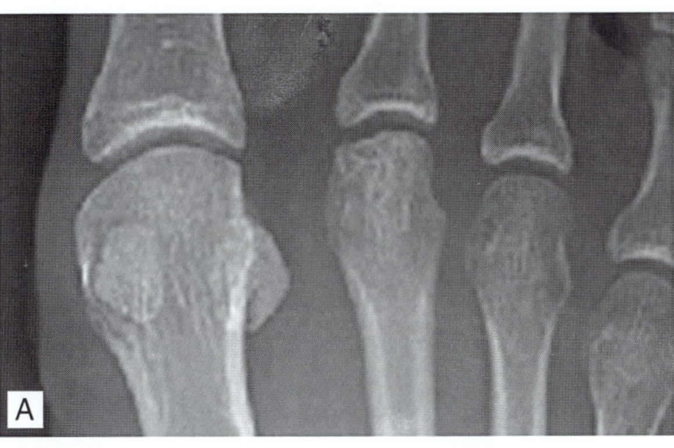

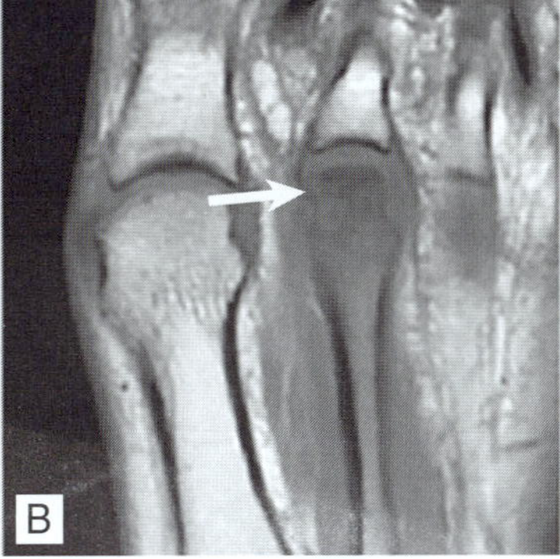

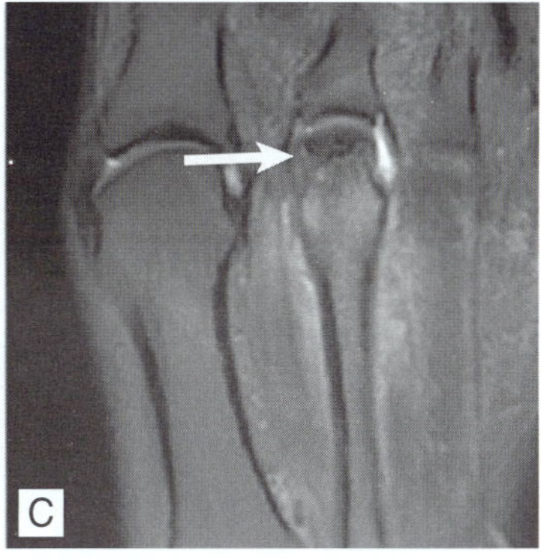

Figure 61.13 Freiberg infraction. (A) AP radiograph shows mottled sclerosis of the second metatarsal head, indicative of Freiberg infraction. In this case, a fracture is visible through the area of abnormality, and there is slight cortical depression. (B) Axial 1WI shows low-signal intensity edema in the second metatarsal head and neck. The fracture line (*arrow*) is visible as a jagged line of lower signal within the edematous region. (C) Axial T2WIFS shows the fracture line (*arrow*). The bone marrow distal to the fracture is low-signal intensity, due to sclerotic reaction. The bone marrow proximal to the fracture shows high-signal intensity edema. Note edema is also present in the soft tissues around the metatarsal.

Flexion deformities of the lesser toes are divided into claw and hammer toes. Both types show dorsiflexion (extension) at the MTP joint, usually due to the laxity of the MTP plantar plate. *Claw toes* are flexed at the PIP and DIP joints. *Hammer toes* are flexed at the PIP joint but extended at the DIP joint.

Causes of pes planus: normal variant, tarsal coalition, PTT, and spring ligament insufficiency, neuromuscular disorder (most commonly cerebral palsy), neuropathic arthropathy.

Causes of pes cavus: normal variant, neuromuscular disorder (most commonly cerebral palsy or Charcot–Marie–Tooth disease).

Causes of hallux valgus: genetic predisposition, tight shoes, unstable first TMT joint, pes planus, the medial inclination of first cuneiform, inflammatory arthritis, cerebral palsy.

Causes of flexion deformities of the toes: tight shoes, neuromuscular disorders, inflammatory arthritis, gout, or connective tissue disorders. They are often associated with pes cavus.

Morton foot configuration is significant shortening of first MT than the second; different criteria are used for diagnosis. A short first MT transfers weight-bearing stress to the second and third digits.

- This can result in *transfer metatarsalgia* (painful second and third digits) metatarsal stress fracture, Freiberg infraction (Fig. 61.13), and instability of second and third MTP joints

Tarsal Coalition

A tarsal coalition is an abnormal bony, cartilaginous, or fibrous bridge between two or more tarsal bones [2], *and is found in about 1–3% of the population.* The coalition restricts motion and causes pain. About 50% of cases show flatfoot deformity. Traditionally, these were believe to present in the second decade of life, but the presentation is often later. A common presentation is repeated ankle sprains. The two most common coalitions are talocalcaneal and calcaneonavicular.

Talocalcaneal Coalition

Talocalcaneal coalition is detectable on lateral radiographs of the ankle utilizing several, variably present signs (Fig. 61.14A). The **talar beak** is a superior flaring of the articular surface of

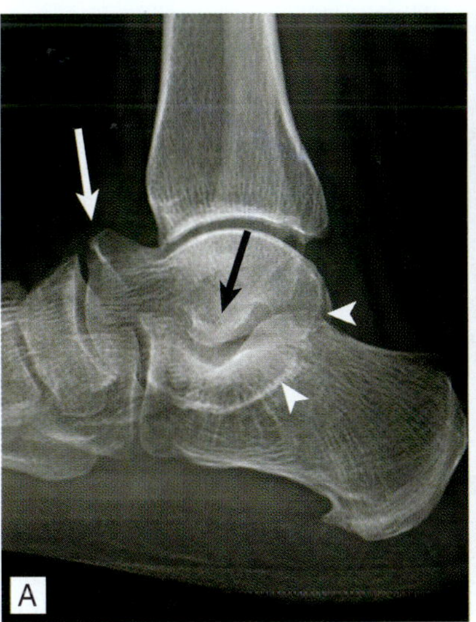

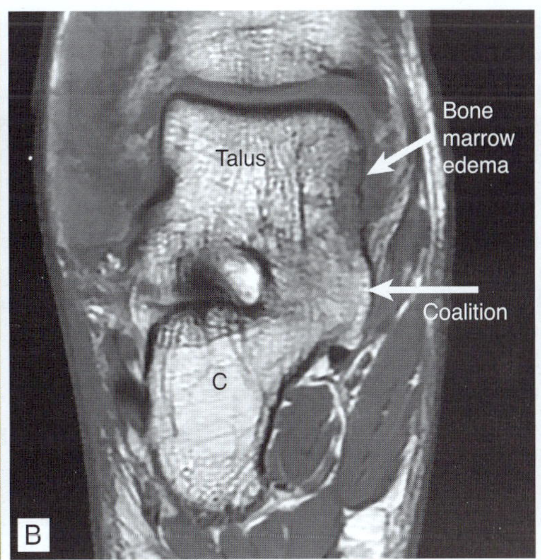

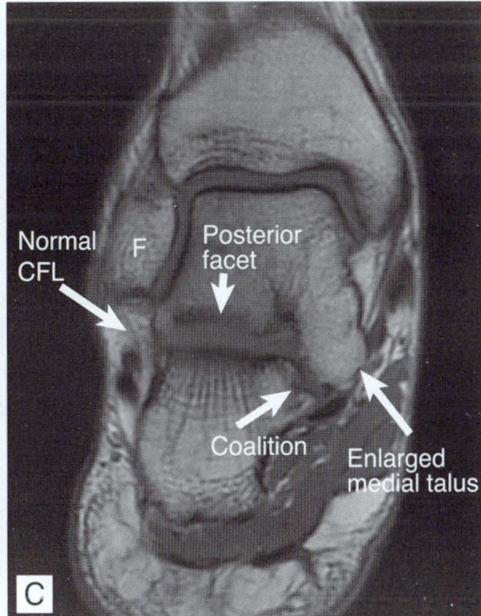

Figure 61.14 Talocalcaneal coalition. (A) Lateral XR shows the classic signs of subtalar coalition. The C-sign (*arrowheads*) is a continuous contour from the medial margin of the talar body along the sustentaculum tali. This sign can also be seen in the absence of coalition, if the patient has a pronated foot. The white arrow marks the talar beak, and the blunting of the lateral process is shown by the black arrow. (B) Coronal T1W MRI shows bony continuity between the medial talus and the sustentaculum tali. The bone marrow edema reflects altered hindfoot stresses because of the coalition. The patient had multiple ankle ligament tears. (C) Coronal T1W MRI shows malformed medial talus and sustentaculum tali. An oblique, fibrous, or cartilaginous bridge is seen. It is strikingly different from the normal, smooth, horizontal contour of the middle facet (compare Fig. 61.3D).

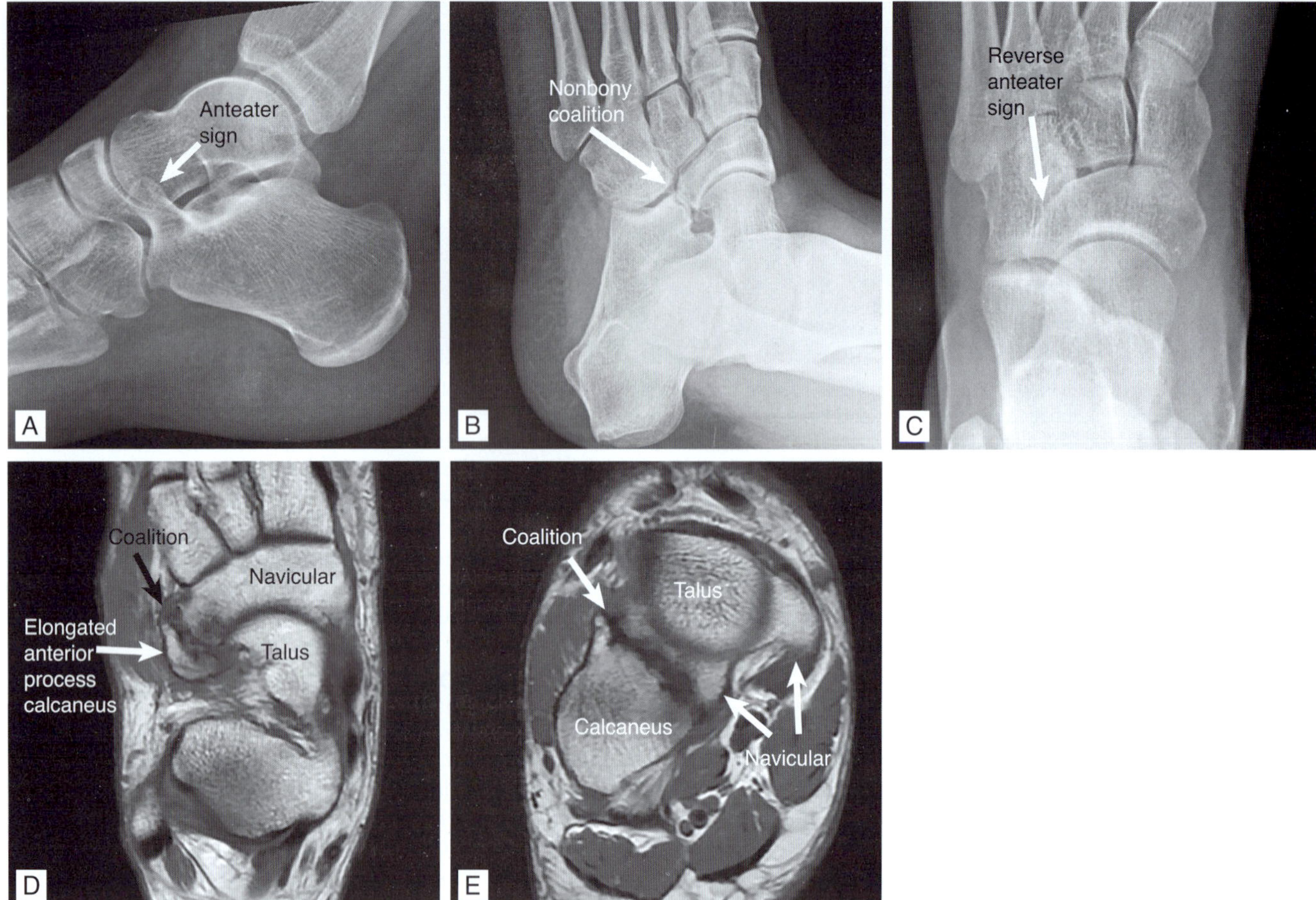

Figure 61.15 Calcaneonavicular coalition. (A) Lateral XR show the broadened, blunt tip of the anterior process of the calcaneus, referred to as the anteater sign. (B) Oblique XR shows the abnormal articulation between the broadened anterior process of the calcaneus, and the elongated lateral margin of the navicular, called the reverse anteater sign. Compare with normal anterior process as shown in Fig. 61.1C. (C) AP XR shows the lateral navicular elongation, and the irregularly contoured coalition, which partly overlies the calcaneocuboid joint. (D) Axial T1 MR shows the elongated, broad anterior process of the calcaneus abutting the lateral margin of the navicular. The nonbony coalition has a characteristic, irregular contour which looks quite different from a normal, smooth articular surface. (E) Coronal T1 MR shows the navicular abutting the enlarged anterior process of the calcaneus. The navicular and calcaneus normally lie in close proximity without contacting each other.

the talar head, which develops because of restricted subtalar motion. It must be distinguished from the normal talar ridge (Fig. 61.1B). The **C-sign** is a curved, continuous contour of the medial posterior talus and the enlarged sustentaculum tali, which has an inferior convex contour. It can also be seen in a pronated foot, without a coalition [3]. **Blunting of the lateral process of the talus** compared with its normal sharp "V" shape inferiorly is an underutilized but useful sign as well. A bony coalition is easily spotted on coronal MRI or CT, which shows bony continuity between an enlarged medial talus and the sustentaculum tali (Fig. 61.14B). A nonbony coalition is more common than a bony one, and is evident on MRI or CT as an overgrown medial articulating facet of the talus, which forms an oblique and irregular bridge to a malformed sustentaculum tali (Fig. 61.14C).

Calcaneonavicular Coalition

Calcaneonavicular coalition can be seen on all three routine views of the foot. Normally, the calcaneus does not articulate with the navicular. The space between the anterior process of the calcaneus and the navicular varies, but a small space is normally present.

The most characteristic finding is the **anteater sign**, where the anterior process of the calcaneus is elongated and has a blunt tip analogous to an anteater's snout (Fig. 61.15A, B). Older patients with flatfoot deformity may develop bony remodeling of the anterior process due to impingement against the navicular, which may mimic coalition.

The **reverse anteater sign** (Fig. 61.15C) refers to the elongation of the lateral margin of the navicular, seen on the AP radiograph. *Calcaneonavicular coalitions are often less conspicuous on advanced imaging* (Fig. 61.15D) than on radiographs.

Ligament Abnormalities

Lateral Collateral Ligament

Lateral collateral ligament sprain is a very common injury due to ankle inversion. Most cases heal with conservative management, although some patients develop chronic instability.

The components of the lateral collateral ligament typically tear in a defined order: anterior talofibular ligament (ATFL) is torn first, then calcaneofibular ligament, then posterior talofibular ligament. Isolated ATFL tear is common, and often asymptomatic.

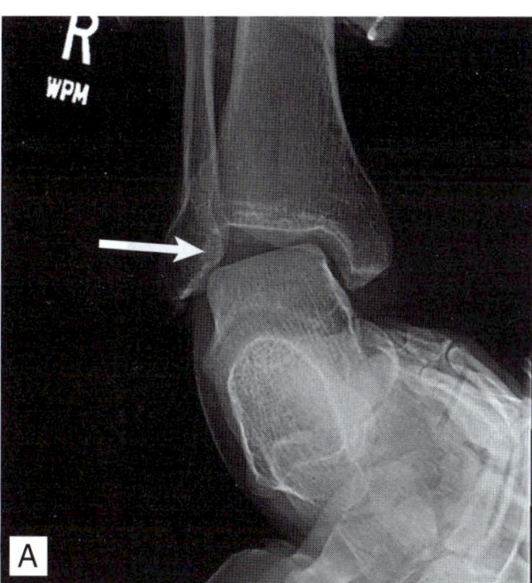

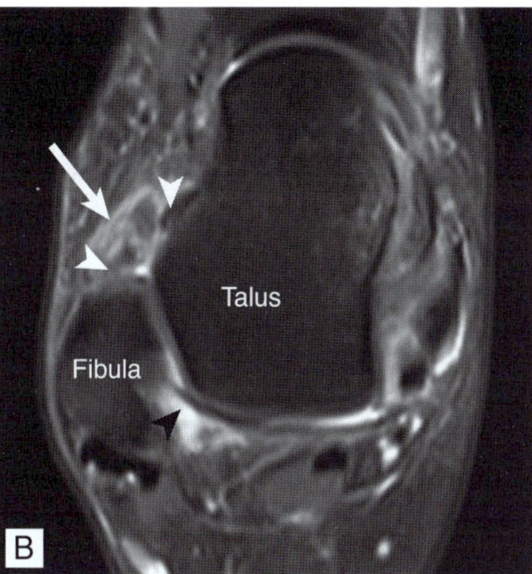

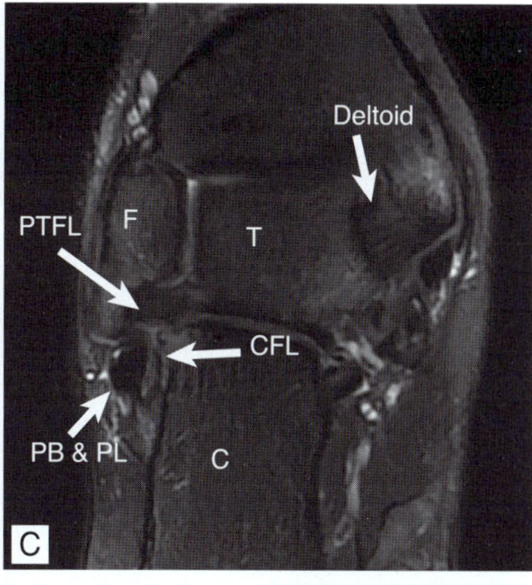

Figure 61.16 Lateral collateral ligament injury. (A) AP XR with inversion stress manually applied shows tibiotalar tilt. The operator's hands are not gloved, but a glove should be used to reduce radiation exposure. The weight-bearing portion of the joint is widened laterally (*arrow*), indicating insufficiency of the CFL. (B) Axial PDFSW MR aligned with axis of talus shows amorphous high-signal intensity in the expected course of the ATFL (*arrow*). White arrowheads point to the stumps of the torn ligament. PTFL (*black arrowhead*) is rarely torn, and is intact in this case. (C) Coronal T2FSW MR shows the CFL is wavy and discontinuous, displaced medially from its normal attachment to the tip of the fibula. The peroneal tendons are displaced slightly medially, a useful secondary sign of CFL tear. PTFL is intact. Note normal deep deltoid is taut and well defined, and has a striated appearance due to multiple ligamentous bands. Multifocal bone bruises are present. *C,* calcaneus; *CFL,* calcaneofibular ligament; *PB,* peroneus brevis; *PL,* palmaris longus; *PTFL,* posterior talofibular ligament; *T,* talus.

XR shows lateral soft-tissue swelling centered at the tip of the lateral malleolus, and often a joint effusion. A tiny avulsion fragment of the tip of the fibula by the calcaneofibular ligament is still generally considered an ankle sprain. Stress radiographs may show tibiotalar tilt (superior joint space widened from medial to lateral, Fig. 61.16A), and an anterior drawer sign (talus subluxates anteriorly when anterior stress is applied).

MRI (Fig. 61.16B, C) shows ligament discontinuity either at attachment or midsubstance [4], and often shows medial and superior displacement of the peroneal tendons beneath the tip of the fibula.

Deltoid Ligament

Deltoid ligament sprain [5] usually occurs due to eversion injury, in which case it may be associated with syndesmosis injury, posterior malleolar fractures, or Maisonneuve fracture of the proximal fibula. Injuries are usually treated conservatively. XR may be normal or may show widening of the medial clear space of the ankle more than 6 mm. This can be better shown on the stress view (Fig. 61.17A). The deep deltoid ligament is sparsely accessible to USG, but is well seen on coronal MRI images (Fig. 61.17B). Superficial deltoid injury is usually an avulsion from the medial malleolus and can be evaluated on both USG and MRI (Fig. 61.17C). An alternative injury mechanism leading to tearing of the superficial deltoid ligament is inversion + twist injury, in which case the deep deltoid ligament is often intact, but the lateral collateral ligament is injured [6].

Syndesmotic Ligament

Syndesmotic ligament sprain (high ankle sprain) occurs due to eversion injury, often in association with a deltoid ligament injury. Depending on the severity, it may be treated conservatively or with fixation screw or fiber tape fixation between the tibia and fibula to restore the normal width of the syndesmosis. XR shows soft-tissue swelling centered at the level of the syndesmosis (i.e., superior to the soft-tissue swelling visible on ankle sprains), and may show syndesmosis widening (Fig. 61.17A). Discontinuity of the ligaments is visible on MRI or USG (Figs. 61.17C–E).

Lisfranc Ligament

Lisfranc ligament tear (midfoot sprain) occurs due to severe plantar flexion of the TMT joints, occurring when the forefoot folds under the hindfoot, either in sports or due to injury going downstairs or stepping off a curb. *Although disruption of the Lisfranc ligament is a seemingly small injury, it destabilizes the TMT joint and needs to be fixed surgically* [7].

Weight-bearing XR in cases of Lisfranc ligament tear usually shows slight lateral displacement of the second metatarsal relative to the middle cuneiform (Fig. 61.18A). A small bony avulsion fragment may be present. MRI shows discontinuity of the ligament on axial and coronal images (Fig. 61.18B).

Stress Fractures

Stress fractures are common in the calcaneus, navicular, and metatarsals, and may not be visible on XR for 1–2 weeks after onset of pain. At that time, a sclerotic or lucent line is usually discernible, and there may be a cortical break and periosteal callus formation (Fig. 61.19A). Most are readily diagnosed clinically when patients present with sharp, focal pain after increased activity. It is good management to treat these patients presumptively with a flat bottom, stiff shoe/boot, and to repeat radiographs to confirm the diagnosis, rather than performing an expensive MRI. An exception is the navicular stress fracture, which occurs in runners, and presents with vague midfoot soreness; XR is negative until late in the clinical course, and MRI or CT is useful for the diagnosis (Fig. 61.19B). *If left untreated, navicular stress fractures can progress to complete fracture and to osteonecrosis of the navicular (Mueller Weiss syndrome)* [8].

Abnormal Tendons

Tendinosis (also called tendinopathy) is collagen degeneration of a tendon due to overuse and aging. Tenosynovitis is seen as abnormal fluid within a tendon sheath, due to inflammation or overuse.

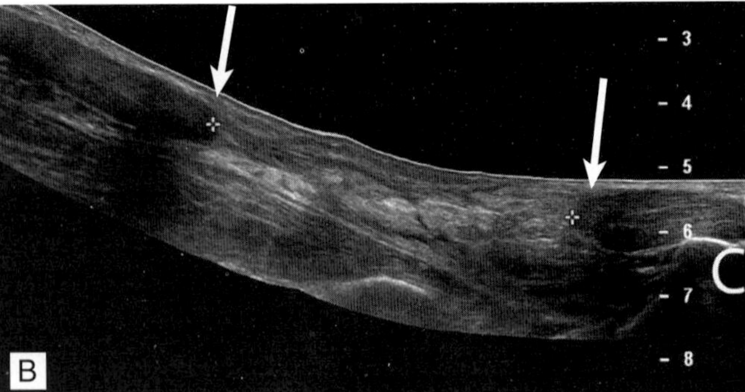

Figure 61.20 Abnormal Achilles tendon on USG. (A) Achilles tendinosis. Long-axis panoramic USG shows severe tendon thickening. The tendon is considered abnormally thickened when the AP diameter is >8 mm. There is a focal area suggestive of low-grade partial tear (*arrow*) at the anterior margin of the tendon. A small rim of fluid around the tendon is indicative of peritendinosis. (B) Achilles tendon tear. Long-axis panoramic USG shows a 6-cm defect in the tendon. Arrows point to the torn tendon ends. Amorphous material between the tendon ends represents blood and injured tissue.

Imaging of Tendons

Imaging can be performed well on both USG and MRI [9–13]. *Ultrasound has the advantage of dynamic imaging to evaluate tendon stability with provocation maneuvers.*

Ultrasound: Normal tendons should have a uniform, fine, fibrillar appearance. Anisotropy may mimic tendon abnormality and can be corrected for by varying transducer angle. Tendinosis results in a thickened, heterogeneous tendon containing hypoechoic regions.

MRI: Normal tendons are low-signal intensity on all sequences. Magic angle phenomenon, where tendons curve around 45–55° relative to the main magnetic field, may mildly increase tendon signal and mimic abnormality; correlate between different planes to confirm. Tendinosis results in increased signal within the tendon in fluid sensitive sequences. An early, interstitial partial tear is evident as longitudinal stripes of fluid within the tendon. A more advanced partial tear will show focal tendon thinning, and a full-thickness tear will show tendon discontinuity.

Key Points for Tendon Imaging on MRI and USG

- Follow each tendon from above ankle to its insertion (supramalleolar, malleolar, and inframalleolar portions)
- Be aware of artifacts due to magic angle on MR, and to anisotropy on USG
- Fluid around tendon suggests tenosynovitis, except around flexor hallucis longus where a small amount of fluid is normally seen due to the connection of the tendon sheath to the ankle
- A slight decrease in echogenicity at tendon insertions is normal
- Mild splitting of tendon substance may enlarge tendon, while more severe partial tears show focal tendon thinning
- When tear is complete, measure length of the gap between torn tendon ends
- Fluid or amorphous tissue fills the gap in complete tears and is compressible on USG
- Stress maneuvers are useful to elicit instability of the posterior tibial or peroneal tendons when retinacular tears are present

Achilles Tendon

Achilles tendon is the conjoined tendon of the gastrocnemius and soleus muscles and acts as a strong plantar flexor of the foot. It attaches to the posterior process of the calcaneus. It lacks a tendon sheath and is surrounded by a loose paratenon, which may become inflamed (paratenonitis, peritendonitis).

Middle-aged patients frequently develop a degenerative Achilles tendinopathy (Fig. 61.20A), *which may progress to a tear when they engage in unaccustomed vigorous physical activity* (Fig. 61.20B). Patients with a torn Achilles present with inability to plantarflex the foot, except in cases when the patient maintains a functional plantaris tendon. Degenerative tears usually occur in the midsubstance of the tendon. In contrast, young athletes may develop a tear within the substance of the gastrocnemius or soleus muscle or at the musculotendinous junction (commonly medial). Tear may be treated conservatively with casting, with the foot in plantar flexion. Surgical repair is usually performed, sometimes augmented with transfer of the flexor hallucis longus tendon to the Achilles. Insertional tendinosis, at the insertion of the tendon onto the calcaneus, is painful but generally does not progress to tear. It is treated with debridement and excision of Haglund deformity. Acute tears may occur in young athletes, and generally involve the junction of the Achilles and soleus, or maybe interstitial tears of the soleus muscle.

Unique imaging findings of Achilles tendon injury: Enlargement of the superior margin of the calcaneus posterior process is known as a Haglund deformity (Fig. 61.21), and is associated with insertional tendinosis. Congenital and stress response has been attributed as a cause of this deformity. Symptomatic patients usually show marrow edema within the deformity on MRI. Pre-Achilles bursitis is seen on USG or MRI as a focal fluid collection between the calcaneus and Achilles. An adventitious bursa, the retro-Achilles bursa, may develop in patients with tendon impingement. Together, it is termed as Haglund syndrome.

Posterior Tibial Tendon

PTT acts to invert and plantarflex the foot, maintain the medial arch and provide dynamic foot stability. It is held behind the medial malleolus by the flexor retinaculum. It attaches primarily to the median eminence of the navicular, with small slips to multiple bones of the midfoot.

PTT dysfunction is most commonly seen in obese, middle-aged women with a pre-existing flatfoot deformity [14]. PTT is also very commonly involved in rheumatoid arthritis. Dysfunction

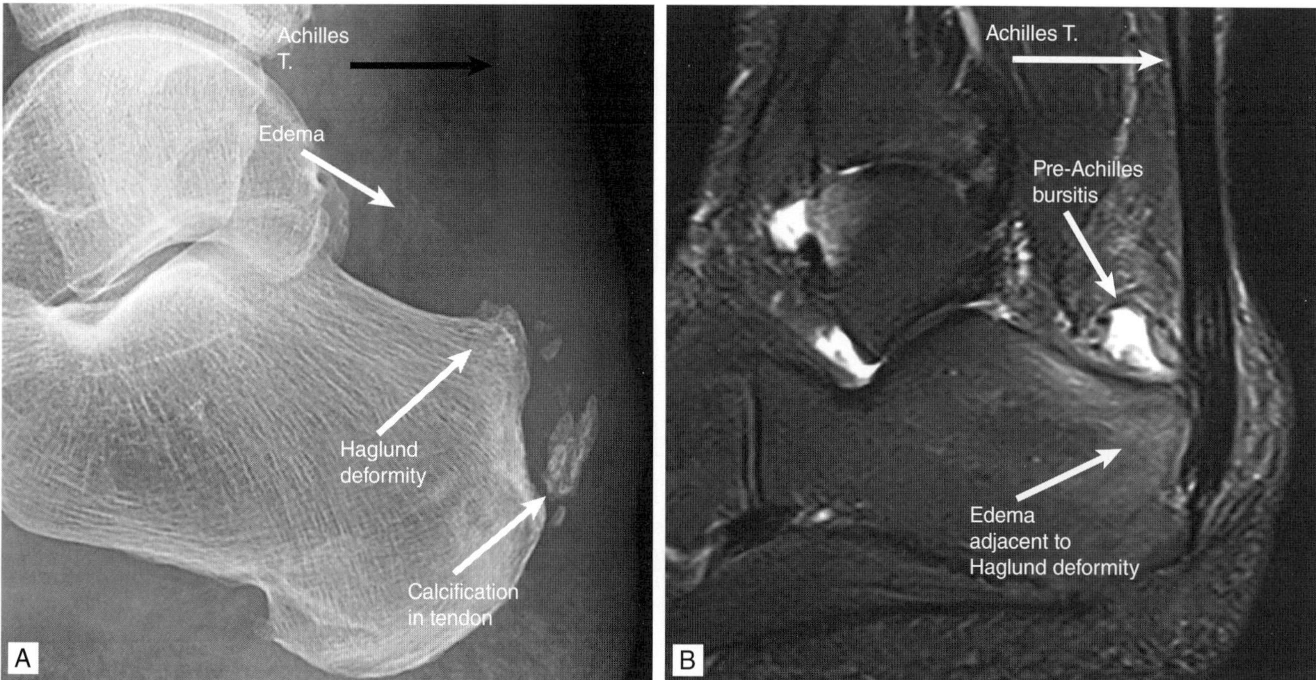

Figure 61.21 Haglund deformity. (A) Lateral XR. The Haglund deformity refers to bony overgrowth of the superior margin of the posterior process of the calcaneus, and is a response to chronic stress. Achilles tendon is sharply outlined against the pre-Achilles fat. It becomes progressively thickened as it extends caudally toward its insertion. It contains calcifications and ossifications consistent with insertional tendonitis. Edema is seen as increased density in the pre-Achilles fat. (B) Sagittal STIR MR. There is bone marrow edema secondary to impingement by the Haglund deformity. The pre-Achilles bursa is distended. Thickening and streaks of high signal within the Achilles tendon indicate insertional tendinitis and early interstitial tearing.

progresses from tenosynovitis and tendinopathy to partial tear (Fig. 61.22) to complete tear. Elongation and insufficiency of the spring ligament also develops. *Tears of the PTT lead to adult-acquired flatfoot, hindfoot valgus deformity, and dorsolateral peritalar subluxation* (Fig. 61.23). Mild dysfunction may be treated with orthotics, walking boot, or brace. Partial or complete tears may be treated with surgical repair, corrective osteotomies to realign the hindfoot, and tendon transfers.

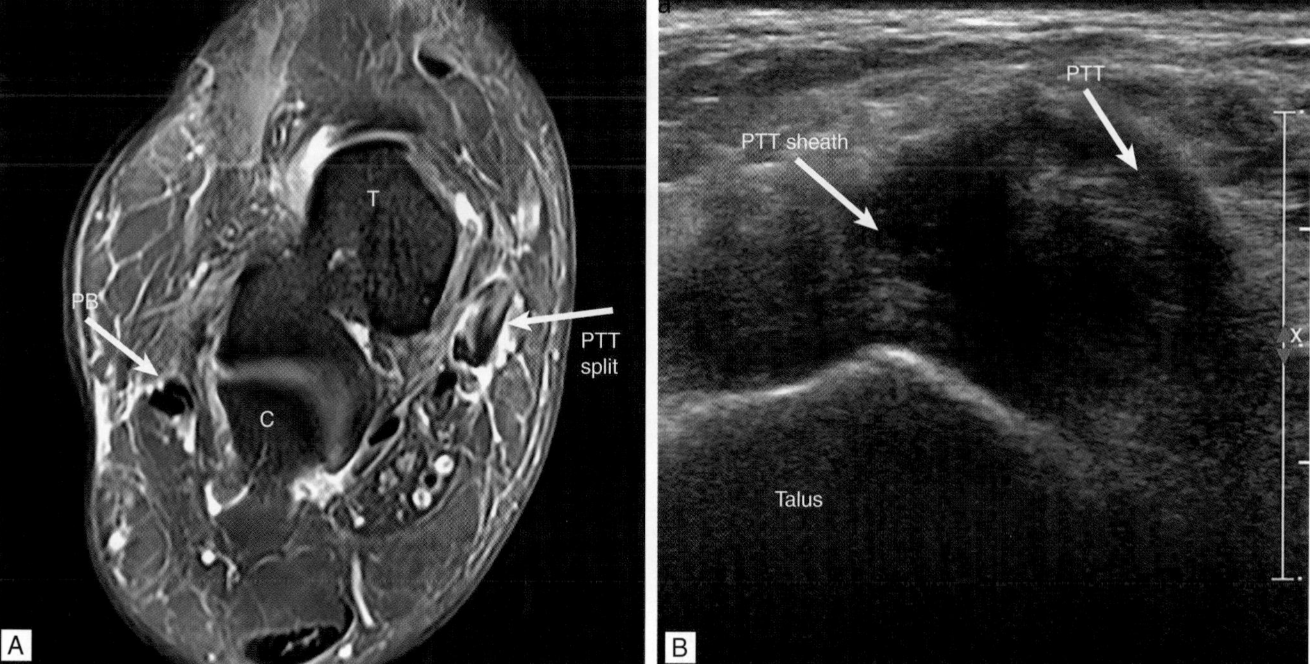

Figure 61.22 High-grade partial tear of posterior tibial tendon. (A) Axial PDFS MRI shows severe thinning of the PTT (*arrow*) and fluid in the tendon sheath surrounding the tendon. The peroneus brevis tendon PB (*arrow*) also shows mild splitting, which is often asymptomatic. (B) Short-axis USG at the level of the talar neck shows an irregularly shaped PTT within a tendon sheath which is distended with anechoic fluid. *C,* calcaneus; *PB,* peroneus brevis; *PTT,* posterior tibial tendon; *T,* talus.

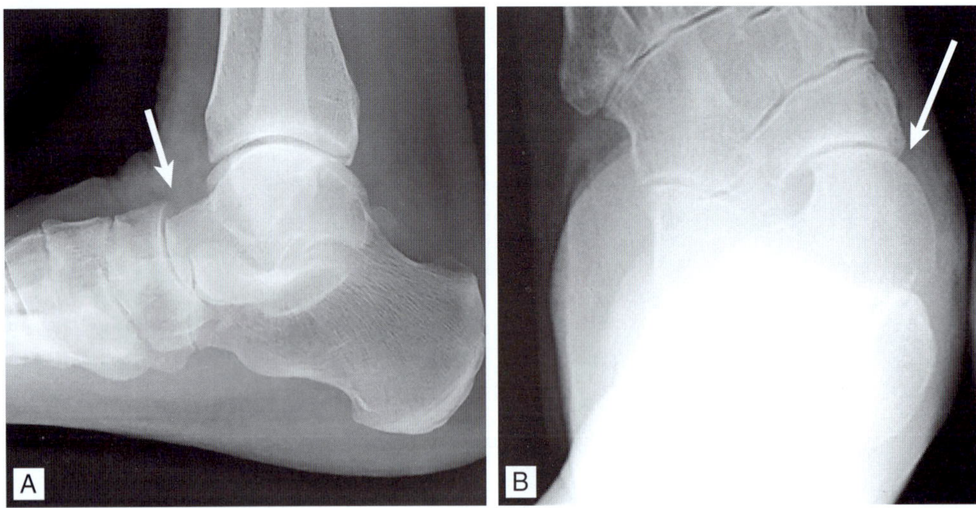

Figure 61.23 XR findings of advanced PTT dysfunction. Although the talus is the bone which is displaced, by convention malalignment is designated by the distal part affected. Therefore, this deformity is known as dorsolateral peritalar subluxation. (A) Lateral XR shows the head of the talus is positioned inferior to the dorsal margin of the navicular, due to loss of support by the PTT and the spring ligament. (B) AP XR shows the head of the talus is rotated, and subluxated medially (*arrow*).

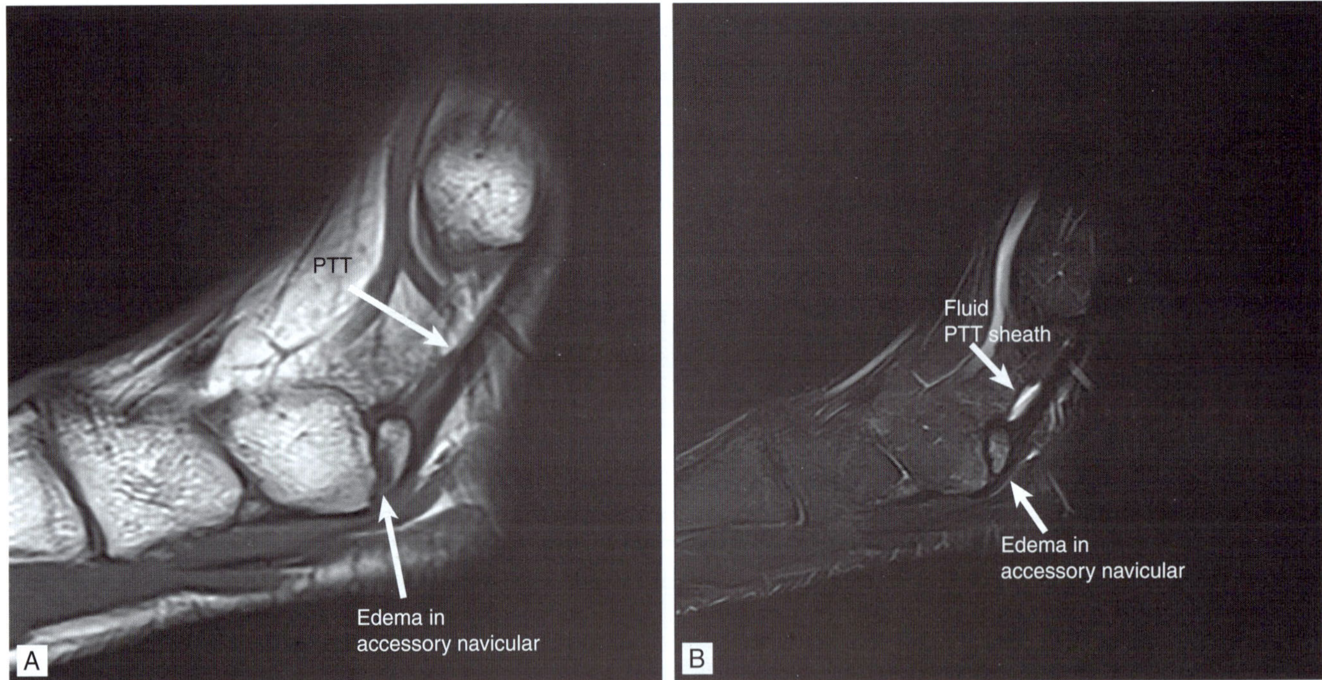

Figure 61.24 Painful accessory navicular. Sagittal T1W (A) and STIR (B) MR show edema in the type II accessory navicular, and fluid in the PTT sheath. Patient was treated with excision of the ossicle and reattachment of the tendon. *PTT,* posterior tibial tendon.

Unique imaging findings of PTT injury: *The type 2 accessory navicular predisposes the PTT to injury.* If the patient has a type 2 accessory navicular, PTT injury may disrupt the synchondrosis between the navicular and the ossicle, leading to edema in the ossicle or proximal displacement (Fig. 61.24). Radiographs of advanced PTT dysfunction show lateral and dorsal subluxation of the navicular relative to the head of the talus (Fig. 61.23). Rarely, the traumatic tear of the flexor retinaculum may destabilize the tendon as it passes behind the medial malleolus. Dynamic USG with inversion maneuver will show anteromedial subluxation of the tendon.

Peroneal Tendons

Peroneal tendons act to evert and plantarflex the foot and assist in maintaining ankle stability. They are held behind the lateral malleolus by the peroneal retinaculum. A sesamoid bone, the os peroneum, is often present in the peroneus longus tendon distal

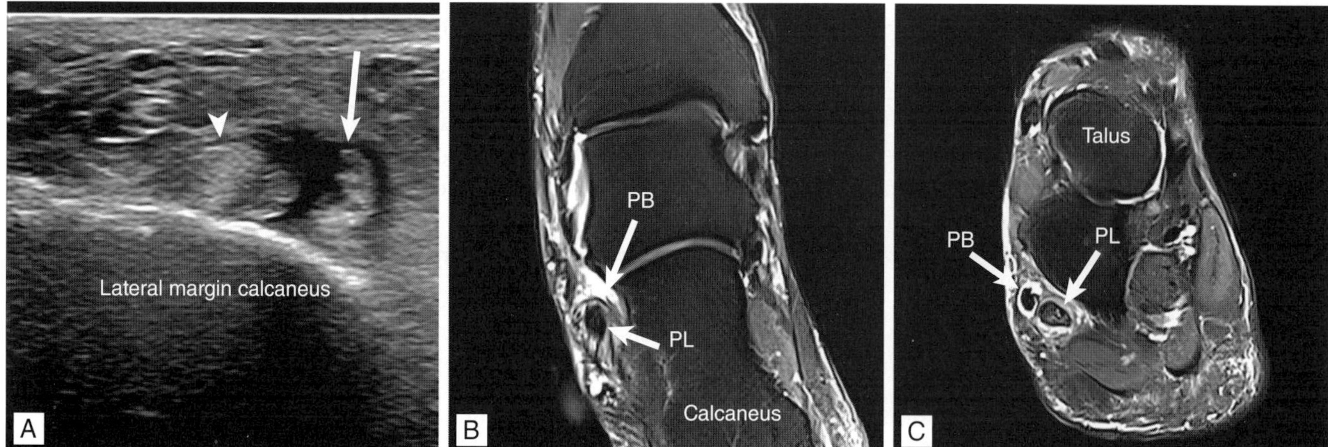

Figure 61.25 Splitting of the peroneal tendons. (A) Short-axis USG along lateral margin of calcaneus shows the PB (*arrow*) has an irregular contour due to longitudinal splitting. The PL (*arrowhead*) shows mildly irregular contour. Fluid surrounds the tendons within their shared tendon sheath. (B) Coronal T2FS MR at the level of the posterior subtalar joint in a different patient shows that the PB is severely split, and forms a V-shape which cups the peroneus longus tendon. Fluid and amorphous material are seen in the tendon sheaths. (C) Coronal T2FS MR (same patient as Fig. 61.22B) at the level of the anterior subtalar joint shows that splitting involves the PL as well as the PB. The PB is less severely affected at this level. *PB,* peroneus brevis; *PL,* palmaris longus.

to the calcaneal–cuboid joint line. It may be bipartite or multipartite, and can sometimes develop a painful sesamoiditis. *Peroneal tendon tears often develop in patients with chronic ankle instability or injury to the peroneal retinaculum.* Longitudinal splits (Fig. 61.25) may be repaired ("tubularized") to regain a rounded contour. More severe injuries are often treated with tenodesis of the torn tendon to its companion peroneal tendon. Peroneal tendon abnormalities can also be seen in inflammatory arthropathy.

Unique imaging findings of peroneal tendon injury: Severe splits of the PB tendon often cause it to form a V-shape, with tendon fibers lying on either side of the PL tendon inferior to it (Fig. 61.25B). *Peroneal retinaculum injury may result in anterolateral dislocation of the peroneal tendons.* Instability may not be visible on MRI and is best seen on dynamic ultrasound when the foot is everted (Fig. 61.26). *An os peroneum displaced proximal to the calcaneocuboid joint indicates tear of the peroneus longus* (Fig. 61.27). Peroneus brevis tendon normally becomes thin and ribbonlike near its insertion, and this should not be mistaken for partial tear.

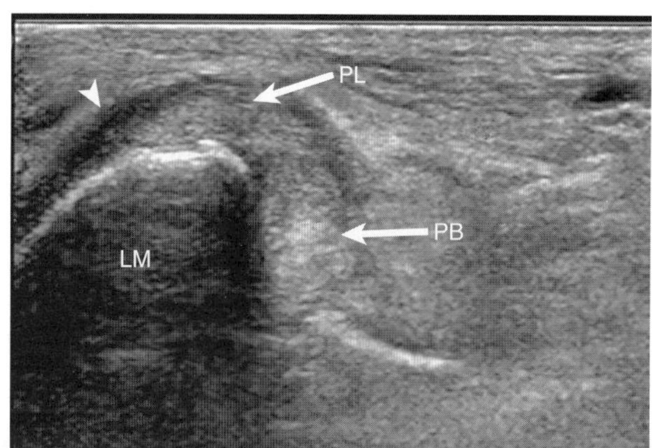

Figure 61.26 Lateral subluxation of the peroneus longus on short-axis USG. The retinaculum (*arrowhead*) has been previously injured, and has reattached along the lateral margin of the lateral malleolus. This allows dynamic subluxation of the tendon around the corner of the fibula into the lateral subcutaneous region, when the foot is everted. *LM,* lateral malleolus; *PB,* peroneus brevis; *PL,* palmaris longus.

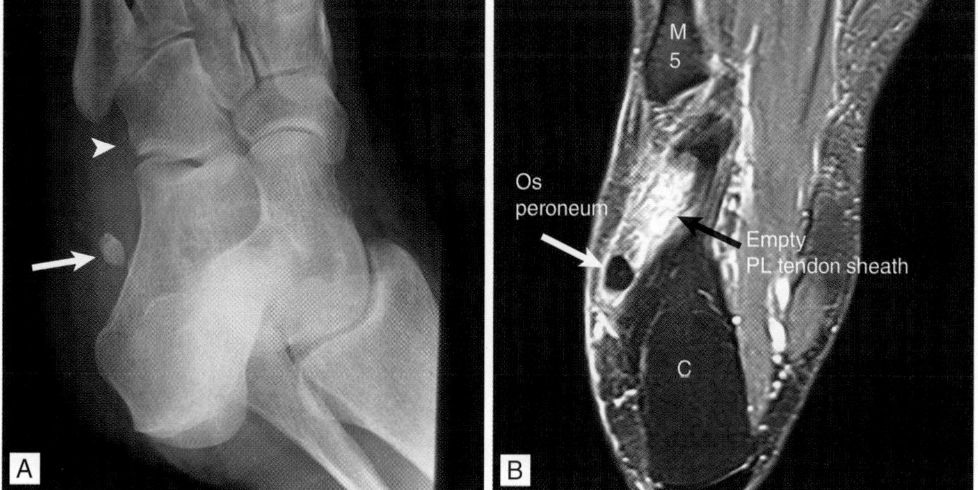

Figure 61.27 Complete tear of the peroneus longus tendon. (A) Oblique XR shows os peroneum (*arrow*) along the lateral margin of the calcaneus. Arrowhead points to its normal location, at the level of the calcaneocuboid joint or slightly distal to it. Proximal displacement is a reliable XR sign of complete tear. (B) Axial MR T2FS shows the displaced ossicle (*white arrow*) and the empty PL tendon sheath distal to it (*black arrow*). *PL,* peroneus longus.

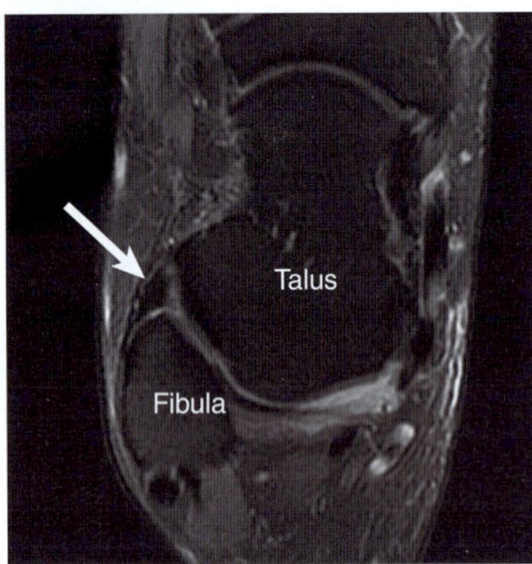

Figure 61.28 Anterolateral impingement. Axial PDFS MR shows meniscoid lesion (*arrow*) representing scarring of chronically torn anterior talofibular ligament. This can cause pain and limit motion when the patient dorsiflexes and everts the foot.

Ankle Impingement Syndromes

Limitation of ankle motion may occur in a variety of locations around the joint, and from a variety of causes [15]. In addition to the causes listed below, also consider decreased motion due to tarsal coalition, synovitis, or intra-articular bodies. Imaging can never diagnose impingement, which is a clinical diagnosis. Imaging can only suggest that findings are present, which may result in impingement.

Anterior Impingement

Anterior impingement refers to limited ankle dorsiflexion, usually due to anterior osteophytes of the tibiotalar joint.

Anterolateral Impingement

Anterolateral impingement refers to lateral pain and limited ankle dorsiflexion + eversion. It is caused by scarring in the anterolateral joint recess after chronic tear of the ATFL or the AITFL. Axial MRI shows a "meniscoid" lesion, a triangular scar, in the anterolateral joint recess (Fig. 61.28).

Anteromedial Impingement

Anteromedial impingement refers to anteromedial ankle pain and limited motion with ankle dorsiflexion + inversion. It is caused by osteophytes or by chronic tear and scarring of the superficial deltoid ligament. Axial MRI or USG show rounded scar at the anterior margin of medial malleolus, at the level of the joint.

Posterior Impingement

Posterior impingement refers to posterior ankle pain and limited plantar flexion (Fig. 61.29). It is seen primarily in athletes who repeatedly maximally plantarflex the foot, for example, dancers and basketball players. It may be due to posterior ligament scarring and synovitis, or to a large os trigonum (os trigonum syndrome). The FHL tendon suffers impingement at the level of the posterior process of the talus. MRI signs of os trigonum syndrome include bone marrow edema in the os trigonum, and focal fluid in the FHL sheath adjacent to the ossicle.

Other Hindfoot Abnormalities

Osteochondral Lesion of the Talus

Osteochondral lesion (OCL) of the talus (Figs. 61.30 and 61.31) is a general term referring to a spectrum of acute and chronic

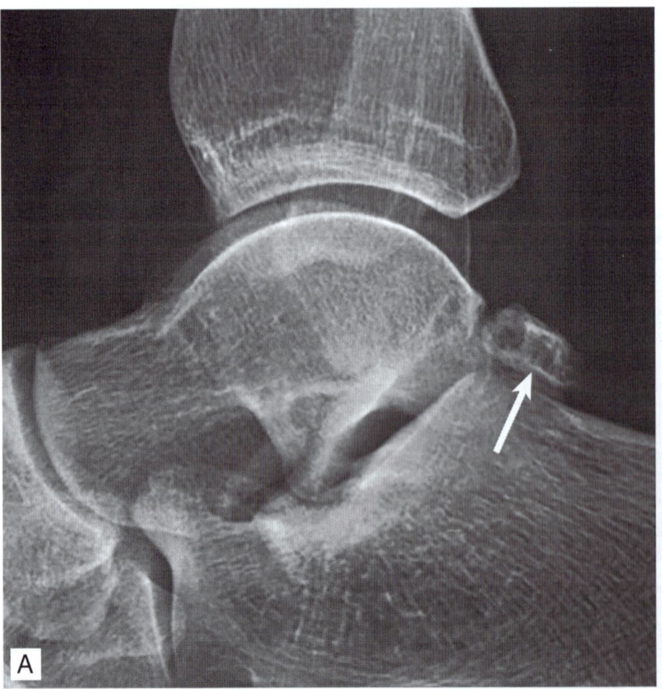

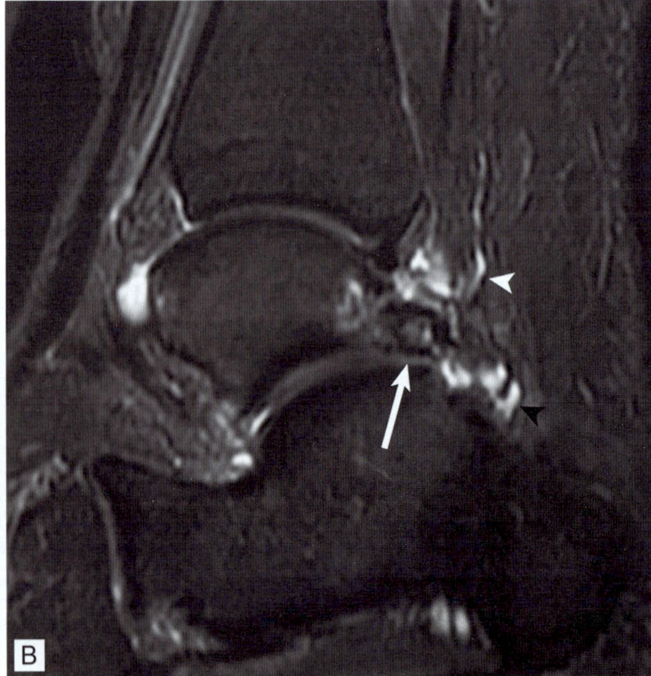

Figure 61.29 Os trigonum syndrome. (A) Lateral XR shows os trigonum (*arrow*). Cysts within the ossicle suggest abnormal motion. (B) Sagittal STIR MR shows high signal bone marrow edema in the os trigonum (*arrow*) and subjacent talar body. There is focal fluid in the FHL tendon sheath (*white arrowhead*) and the posterior subtalar recess (*black arrowhead*). Although it is normal to see a small amount of fluid in the FHL tendon sheath, a focal collection extending superiorly from the level of the os trigonum is suggestive of impingement.

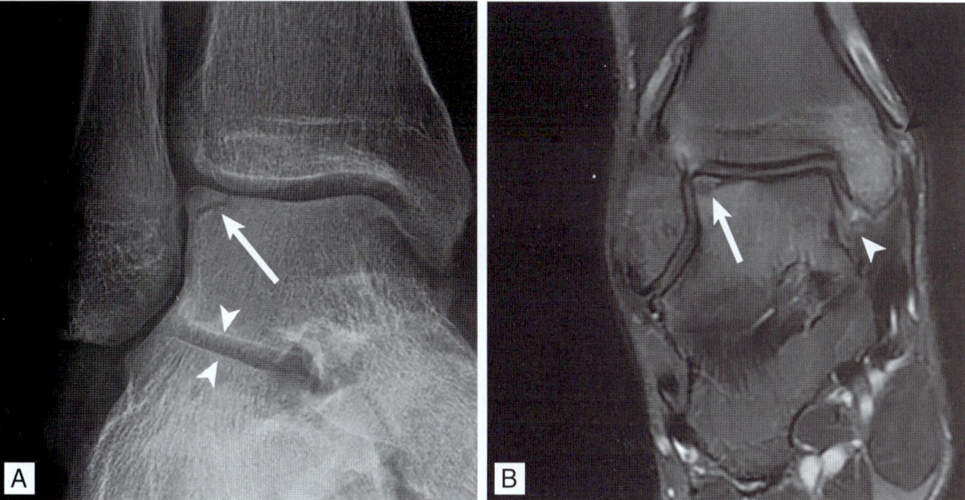

Figure 61.30 Stable OCL talus. (A) Mortise XR shows fracture line (*arrow*) across lateral margin of talar dome, which may be due to acute or chronic injury. Arrowheads point to normal subtalar joint. (B) Coronal T2FS MR shows that the fracture (*arrow*) is stable, because there is no fluid-filled cleft around it. Patient also has injuries of the deep (*white arrowhead*) and superficial (*black arrowhead*) deltoid ligament. Although OCL is associated most strongly with LCL injury, other ligament injuries commonly occur as well. Note also the multiple areas of bone bruising.

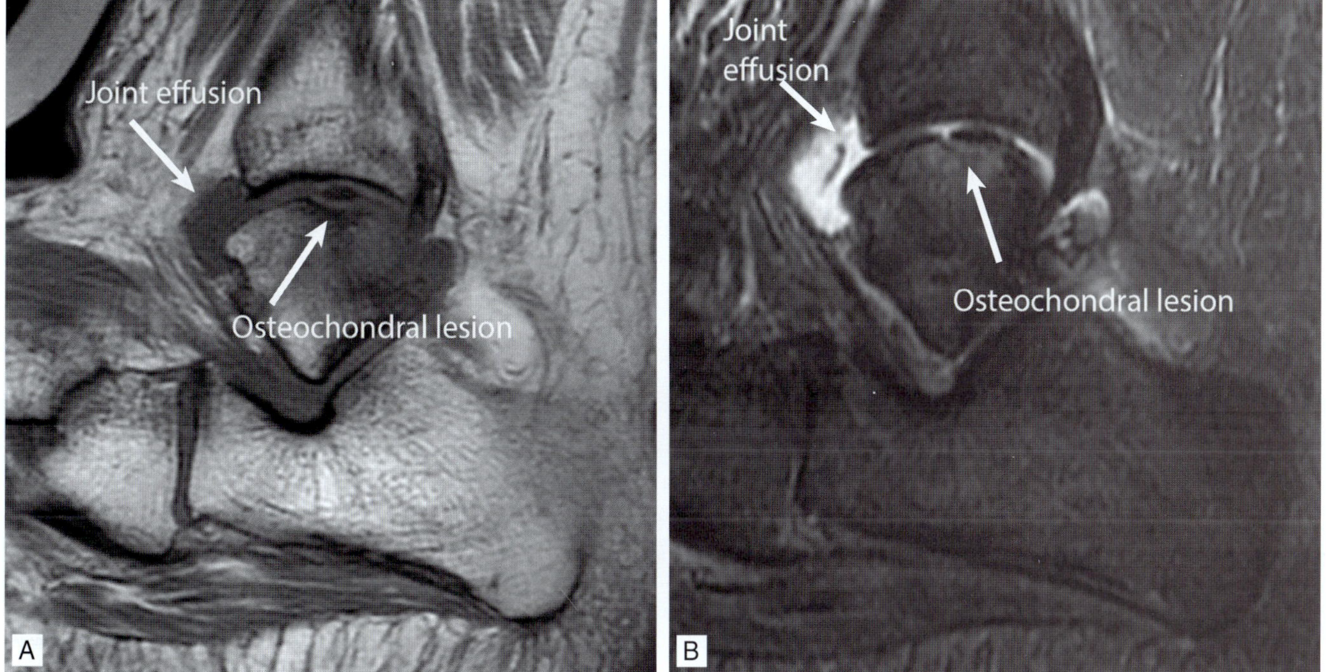

Figure 61.31 Unstable OCL talus. (A) Sagittal T1W MRI shows a bowl-shaped transchondral fracture line (*arrow*). Low signal in the central fragment suggests a chronic lesion which has undergone osteonecrosis. A joint effusion is present. (B) Sagittal STIR shows the central fragment is surrounded by fluid, indicating the fragment is unstable, and vulnerable to displacement.

injury to articular cartilage together with the underlying subchondral bone. On imaging, OCL can be characterized as stable lesions (Fig. 61.30), where a bone bruise or fracture line is present but is not complete, and unstable lesions (Fig. 61.31), where the osteochondral fragment is separated from the underlying bone. The unstable fragment may displace and present as a loose body in the ankle joint. *Chronic OCL may develop central cystic degeneration, and this is a sign that the lesion is unlikely to heal.*

The most common site for OCL in the foot is the medial or lateral talar dome. It may also occur in the tibia. Both injuries occur with ankle sprains. OCL is rare in other locations.

Heel pain *may occur due to abnormalities of the Achilles tendon, tarsal tunnel syndrome, stress fracture, plantar fasciitis, tarsal sinus syndrome, or heel pad syndrome* [16].

Plantar Fasciitis (or Plantar Fasciosus)

It is a commonly seen painful condition of the plantar fascia, due to chronic stress. The central band, overlying the flexor digitorum brevis, is most commonly affected, and the abnormality is centered at the origin of the fascia close to calcaneal tuberosity. Plantar fasciitis is seen most commonly in obese patients and runners,

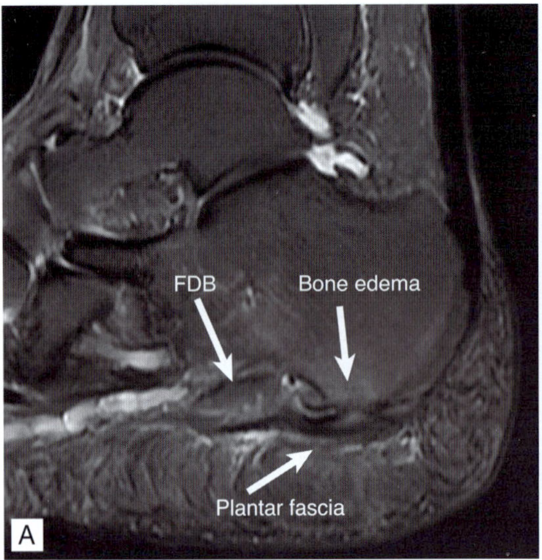

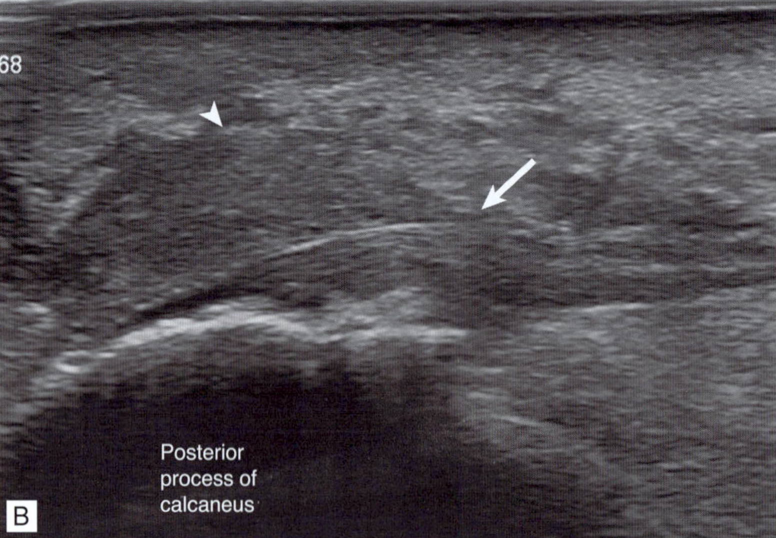

Figure 61.32 Plantar fasciitis. (A) Sagittal STIR shows thickening of the plantar fascia at the calcaneal origin. Edema is present not only in the fascia, but also the subjacent fat, flexor digitorum brevis muscle, and calcaneus. (B) Long-axis USG shows thickening of the plantar fascia at its origin from the posterior process of the calcaneus. A small bone spur is visible, and there are small calcifications in the fascial origin. Note edema in the fat pad (*arrowhead*) adjacent to the plantar fascia origin. *FDB,* flexor digitorum brevis.

but it can also be associated with seronegative spondyloarthropathy. It is treated with stretching exercises or corticosteroid injection.

The XR finding of a heel spur does not have a strong association with plantar fasciitis. MR in cases of plantar fasciitis shows thickened plantar fascia and increased T1 and T2 signal of the fascia as well as the underlying muscle, adjacent bone marrow edema (Fig. 61.32A). Ultrasound shows thickened origin (>4 mm)of the plantar fascia, decreased echogenicity in the affected region, and edema in the superficial soft tissues (Fig. 61.32B). Plantar fasciitis may cause impingement of Baxter's nerve (the inferior calcaneal nerve which is the first branch of the lateral plantar nerve), which leads to isolated atrophy of the abductor digiti minimi muscle.

Plantar Fascia Tear

Plantar fascia tear is rare. It may be caused by steroid injection or athletic activity (Fig. 61.33).

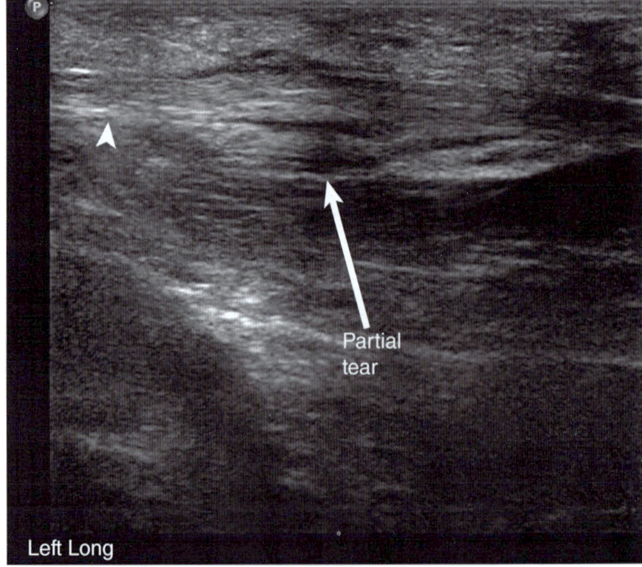

Figure 61.33 Partial tear of plantar fascia on USG in a patient complaining of a painful nodule. Long-axis view in area of patient's pain shows focal thickening of fascia in the center of the image, fiber discontinuity, and low echogenicity fluid between the torn fibers. Compare with the normal appearance of the fascia on the left side of the image (*arrowhead*).

Tarsal Sinus Syndrome (Sinus Tarsi Syndrome)

Sinus tarsi is a cylindrical cavity located between the talus and calcaneus on the lateral aspect of the foot, distal and slightly anterior to the lateral malleolus. The syndrome is a poorly defined entity where patients have pain in the lateral hindfoot, which can be attributed to inflammation or scar in the tarsal sinus. There is often a subjective feeling of instability. The cervical ligament in the sinus tarsi is sometimes injured (Fig. 61.34). Synovitis emanating from the posterior subtalar joint may also contribute to pain. It is commonly associated with lateral ankle ligament sprain.

Chronic Instability

Chronic instability occurs when ligament tears fail to heal. *Bone marrow edema patterns are useful to suggest abnormal motion, usually at the tibiotalar joint, but sometimes at the subtalar joint* (Fig. 61.35). The presence of bone marrow edema should prompt a careful evaluation of ligamentous integrity.

Heel Pad Syndrome

Heel pad syndrome is atrophy of the fat of the plantar heel pad, generally due to obesity and diabetes. MR shows replacement of normal fat with fibrous tissue (low T1, intermediate to high T2 signal).

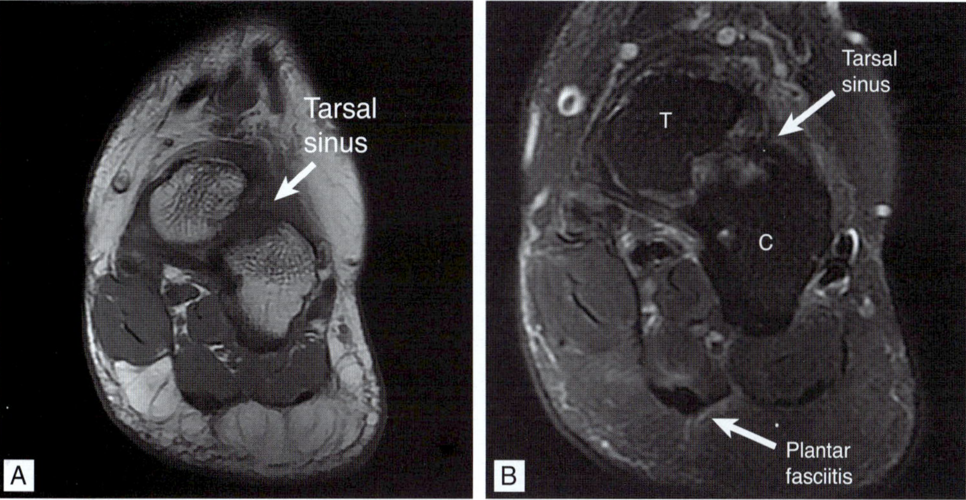

Figure 61.34 Tarsal sinus syndrome. (A) Coronal T1 MR shows that the normal high-signal intensity fat in the tarsal sinus has been replaced with low-signal intensity material. (B) Coronal T2 MR at the same level shows heterogeneous material filling the tarsal sinus. The patient also has plantar fasciitis. *C,* calcaneus; *T,* talus.

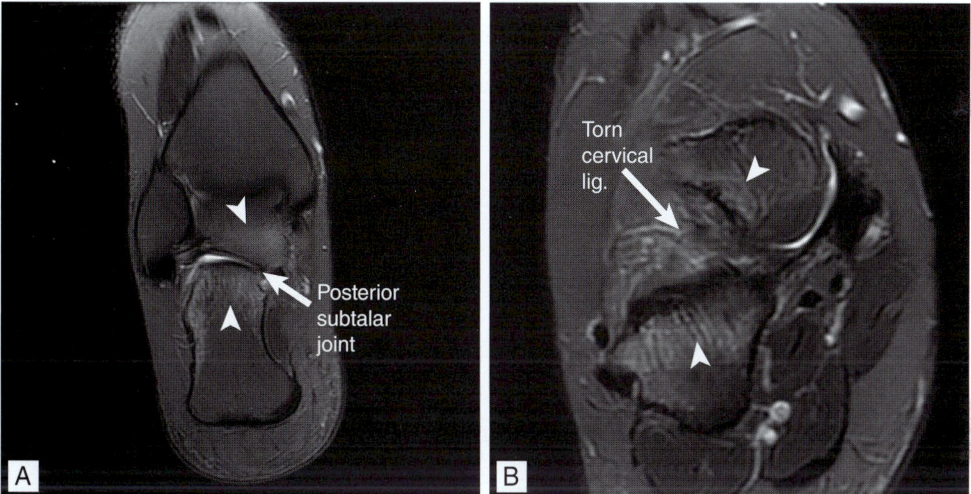

Figure 61.35 Subtalar instability. An 18-year-old male athlete with feeling of "giving way." Ankle ligaments were intact. (A) Coronal T2FS image shows bone marrow edema (*arrowheads*) on both sides of the posterior subtalar joint, suggesting abnormal motion. (B) Coronal T2FS image anterior to previous image, through tarsal sinus, shows absent cervical ligament, and shows bone marrow edema centered at the ligament attachments.

Abnormalities of the Forefoot

Plantar Fibromatosis

Plantar fibromatosis is a nodular thickening of the plantar fascia, which usually occurs in the forefoot. It causes a palpable lump and is painful when the patient bears weight. The nodules may be single or multiple. Treatment starts with cushioning pads around the lesion to decrease pressure. Corticosteroid injection and surgical removal are sometimes used. USG and MRI show focal, fusiform nodules in the plantar fascia (Fig. 61.36).

Sesamoiditis

Sesamoiditis refers to pain resulting from chronic stress on one or both of the sesamoids lying plantar to the first metatarsal head. The condition may progress to stress fracture. Treatment centers on offloading stress to the sesamoids. MRI shows bone marrow edema in the affected sesamoid.

Lesser Metatarsalgia

Lesser metatarsalgia refers to pain in the MT other than the first. It most commonly affects the second and third MT. *Lesser metatarsalgia is usually due to increased stress.* The increased stress may occur because the first MT is either short or affected by hallux valgus, and in these cases the pain in the lesser metatarsals is often called transfer metatarsalgia. Pointed toe, high-heeled shoes also contribute to lesser metatarsalgia. Imaging may show stress fractures, Morton neuroma, Freiberg infraction, or dorsal subluxation of the MTP joint.

Freiberg Infraction

Freiberg infraction is an osteochondral injury (some authors believe it represents osteonecrosis) of the MT head, usually the second or third (Fig. 61.37).

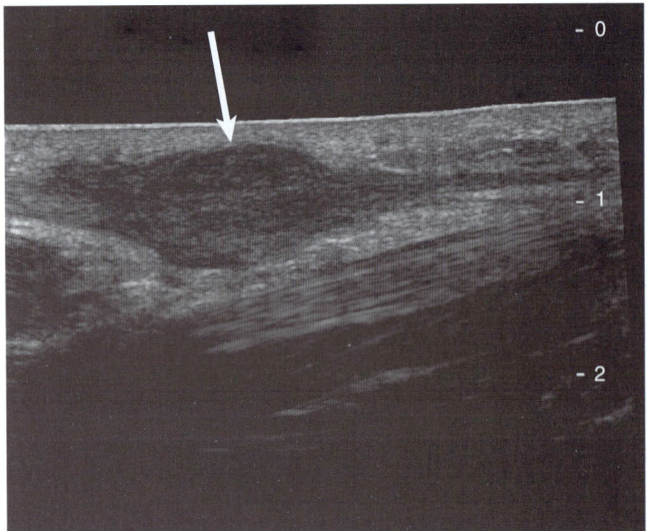

Figure 61.36 Plantar fibroma. Long-axis USG shows a fibroma (*arrow*) arising from the plantar fascia. It has a fusiform shape. Its margins taper into the normal adjacent fascia. It is usually isoechoic to the fascia.

Nerve Abnormalities

Patients with symptoms related to nerve abnormalities present with altered sensation and/or muscle weakness. A Tinel's sign (tingling in the distribution of the abnormal nerve when the nerve is tapped) is typical. Nerve abnormalities may occur due to peripheral neuropathy, nerve injury, or entrapment.

Imaging of Nerves

Neuritis is evident on USG or MRI as nerve enlargement and edema of the nerve fascicles (Fig. 61.38) [17]. MRI shows changes in muscles innervated by a nerve. The first MR sign is a high T2 signal, "denervation edema," in the affected muscles. Diffuse muscle fatty atrophy occurs later in the course.

- *Denervation edema can be distinguished from increased T2 signal related to infection and muscle trauma because, unlike in those entities, the normal architecture of the muscle is preserved (Fig. 61.38C, D).*

Tarsal Tunnel Syndrome

Tarsal tunnel syndrome is entrapment of the tibial nerve or its branches and is the most common location for nerve impingement in the foot. The tarsal tunnel lies deep to the flexor retinaculum in the hindfoot, and contains the tibial nerve and its branches, as well as vessels, flexor tendons, and quadratus plantae muscle. Compression of nerve may occur due to neoplasm, venous varicosities, synovial cysts, tenosynovitis, accessory muscles, tarsal coalition, osteophytes, post-traumatic deformity, or scar (Fig. 61.38).

Baxter Neuropathy

Baxter neuropathy refers to isolated neuropathy of the nerve to the abductor digiti minimi, which is innervated by the first branch of the tibial nerve in the tarsal tunnel. It is often due to plantar fasciitis, with the nerve getting compressed between plantar fascia and underlying calcaneum. MRI shows isolated edema and fatty atrophy of the abductor digiti minimi.

Peripheral Neuropathy

Peripheral neuropathy is common in diabetic patients, also seen in Charcot–Marie–Tooth syndrome. It is often described as a "stocking-glove" pattern and involves the small peripheral nerves. Patients experience burning pain and decreased sensation and proprioception. The intrinsic muscles of the foot show diffuse atrophy (Fig. 61.39).

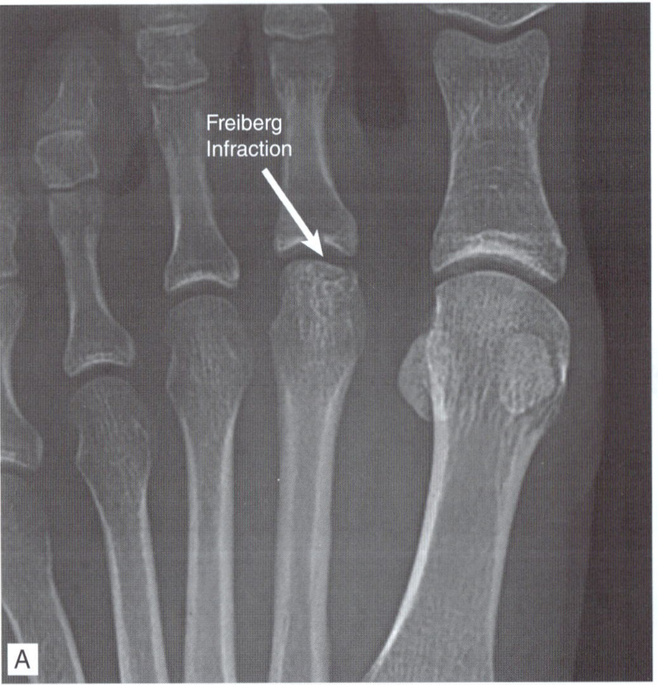

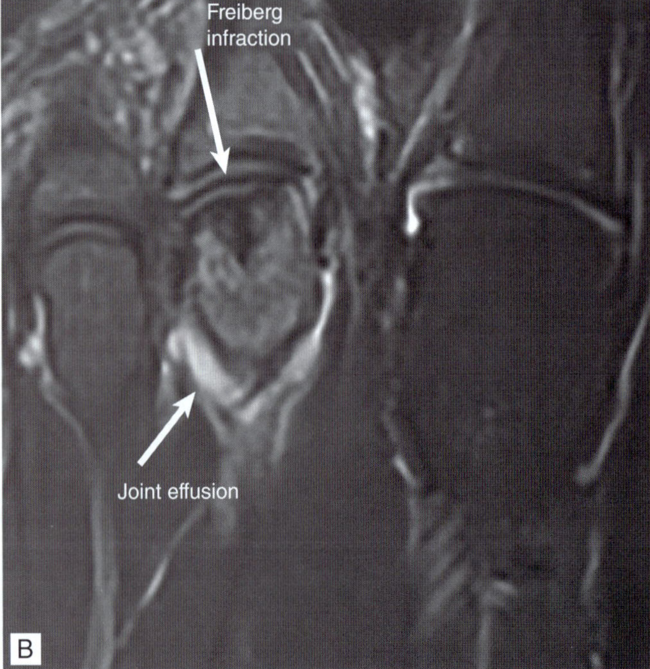

Figure 61.37 Freiberg infraction. (A) AP XR shows concave contour of the MT head articular surface, and mottled subchondral sclerosis, surrounded in more advanced cases such as this one by a bowl-shaped sclerotic rim. Note that the lateral sesamoid of the first MT is bipartite, a normal variant. (B) Axial T2FS MRI in same patient shows the collapsed, sclerotic, low signal intensity area of Freiberg infraction, with surrounding high signal representing reactive edema and/or reparative tissue.

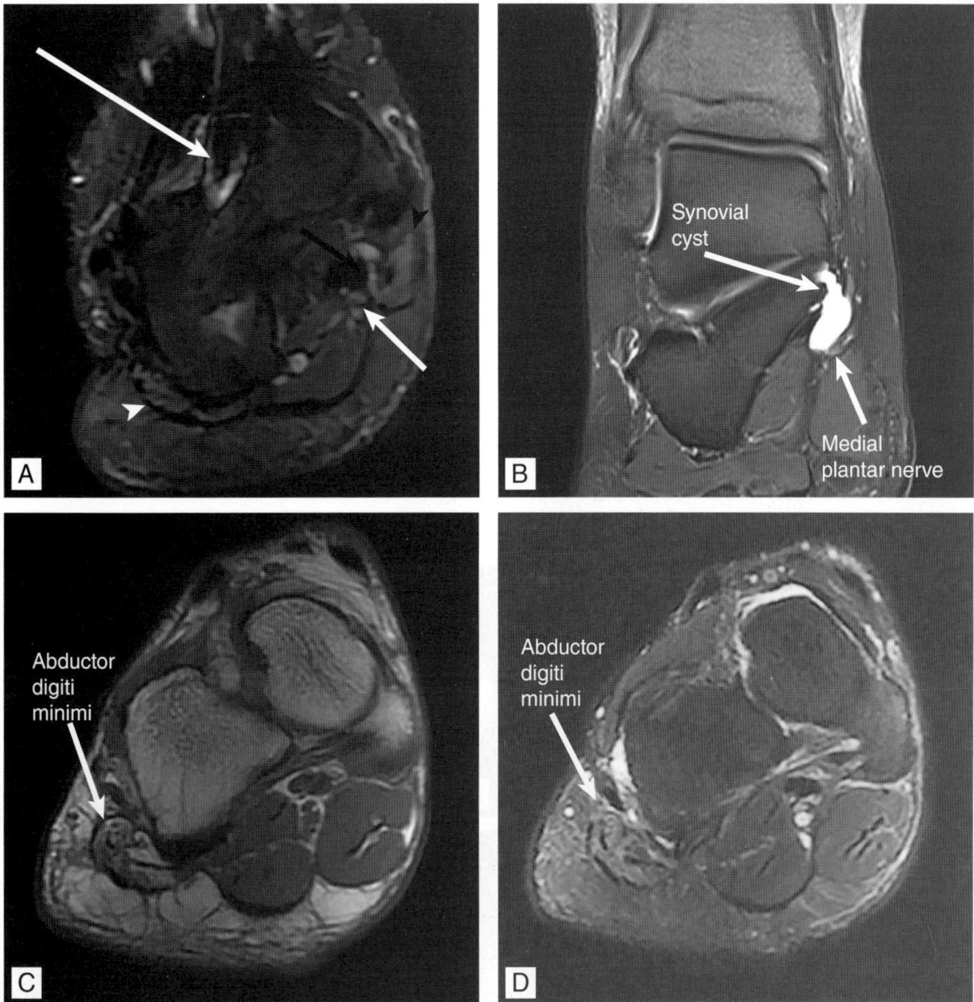

Figure 61.38 Tarsal tunnel syndrome. (A) Coronal STIR MR shows the enlarged medial (*black arrow*) and lateral (*short white arrow*) branches of the tibial nerve. Denervation edema is visible in the abductor hallucis (*black arrowhead*) and abductor digiti minimi (*white arrowhead*) muscles. Note degradation of image by artifact from fixation hardware (*long white arrow*). Becoming proficient at MR interpretation requires learning to "read around" artifacts such as this, in addition to altering technique to reduce artifact. (B) Coronal PDFSW MR in another patient shows a synovial cyst arising from the subtalar joint, and deviating the medial plantar nerve. The patient had pain and a positive Tinel sign, but no changes are seen in the plantar muscles. (C) Cor T1W MRI shows fatty atrophy which is limited to the abductor digiti minimi muscle. This is due to impingement of the Baxter nerve, the first nerve branch of the lateral plantar nerve. (D) Coronal T2FSW MRI shows diffusely increased signal in the abductor digiti minimi. This pattern is characteristic of denervation edema.

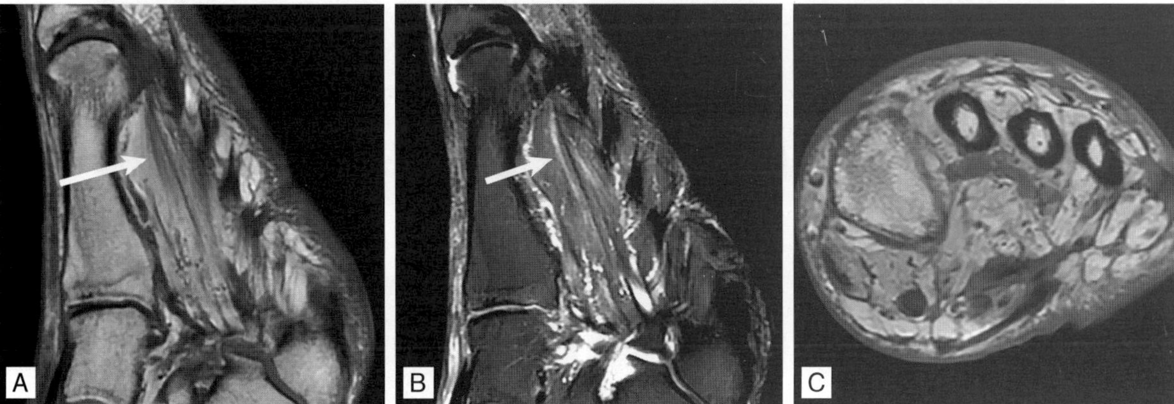

Figure 61.39 Advanced denervation changes in the forefoot due to peripheral neuropathy. (A) Axial T1 shows nearly complete fatty replacement of the oblique head of the adductor hallucis muscle (*arrow*). The few fibers of remaining muscle are intermediate-signal intensity. (B) Axial PDFS shows that the remaining muscle fibers (*arrow*) are high-signal intensity, reflecting denervation edema. Denervation edema occurs rapidly after muscle denervation, while fatty atrophy is a chronic finding. Note that the residual muscle fibers have a straight course, and do not show the focal disruption that will be present in muscle injury. (C) Coronal T1 shows the fatty atrophy involves all of the intrinsic muscles of the forefoot. The distribution of muscle involvement is a helpful clue to etiology.

Morton Neuroma

Morton neuroma is a traumatic neuroma due to chronic compression of the interdigital nerves at the level of the metatarsal (Fig. 61.40A, B) along the plantar aspect. It is most common in women, due to compression from pointed-toe and high-heel shoes. Common differential is an intermetatarsal bursa (Fig. 61.40C) which is a fluid distension in the web space.

Arthroplasty, Arthrodesis, and Alignment Correction Surgeries

Arthroplasty is not commonly employed in the foot and ankle to treat arthritis; arthrodesis remains more desirable. There are a large number of arthroplasty designs that have been developed for the ankle, however (Fig. 61.41), as in other joints, the concern of the radiologist is to monitor for particle disease, subsidence, loosening, and infection. *Particle disease refers to a granulomatous reaction due to release of small polyethylene, cement, or metal particles from the prosthesis* and manifests as more than 2-mm periprosthetic lucency.

Arthrodesis can relieve pain but can increase stress on adjacent joints. Radiographs and CT are utilized to evaluate for bony bridging across a joint and hardware failure (Fig. 61.42), and for accelerated osteoarthritis in adjacent joints.

Hindfoot valgus or varus can be corrected by osteotomies of the calcaneus and often the medial cuneiform. Hallux valgus correction varies according to the site of abnormality. The bony prominence (bunion) is resected at the same time that the deformity of the first digit is corrected. If the patient has an oblique or hypermobile first TMT joint, the fusion of the TMT joint may be performed. The orientation of the first MT and first PP can be corrected with a variety of osteotomies (Fig. 61.43).

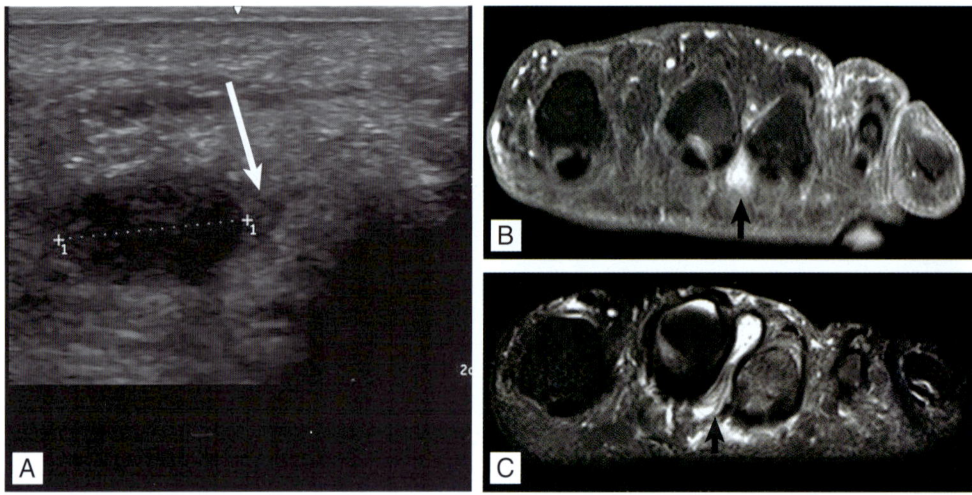

Figure 61.40 Morton neuroma. (A) Long-axis USG shows a hypoechoic, 1-cm fusiform mass (between the calipers) which tapers (*arrow*) into the interdigital nerve. The neuroma lies between the MT heads, and visualization especially of smaller neuromas is improved using a small hockey-stick transducer, imaging from the plantar side of the foot, and applying pressure to the dorsum of the foot with the other hand to push the MT heads apart. (B) Axial postcontrast T1 fat-saturated MR image shows an enhancing nodular lesion in second web space (*arrow*). (C) Intermetatarsal bursa. Axial STIR MR image shows a fluid signal lesion in second web space (*arrow*).

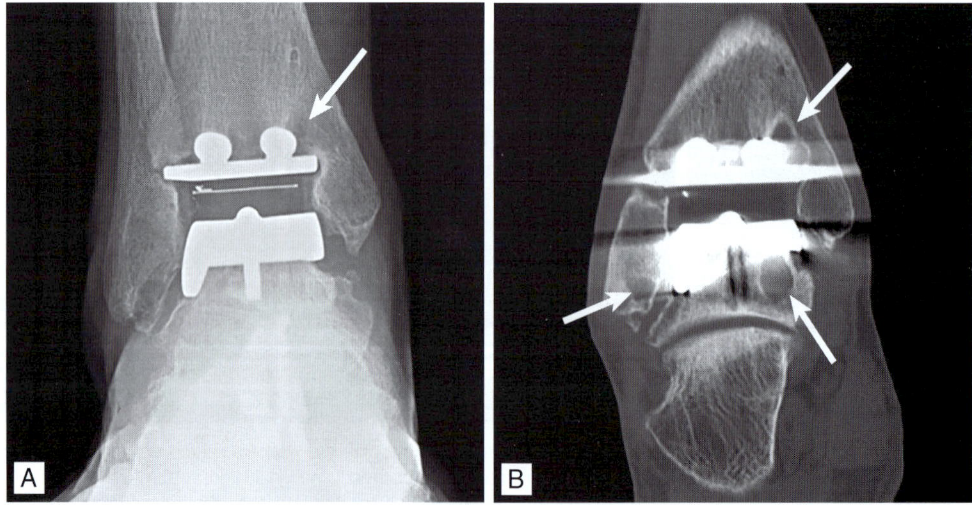

Figure 61.41 Ankle arthroplasty. (A) AP XR shows arthroplasty which appears well positioned. A lucency above the tibial component (*arrow*) is suspicious for particle disease. (B) Coronal CT performed at the same time shows the extent of the particle disease (*arrows*) is much greater than evident on radiographs.

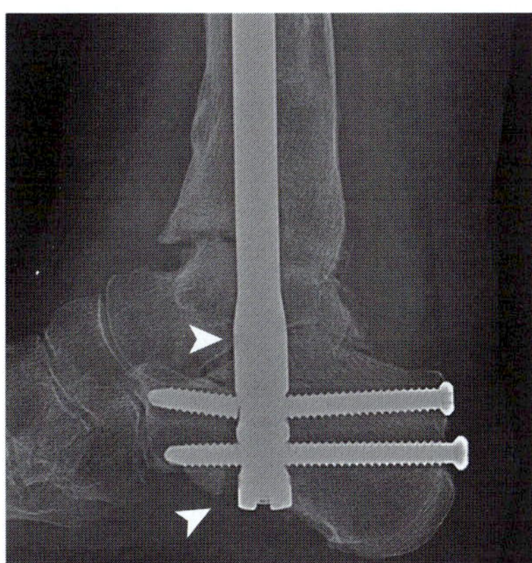

Figure 61.42 Failed ankle and subtalar arthrodesis. Lateral radiograph shows a retrograde nail has been placed from the plantar surface of the calcaneus, across the subtalar and tibiotalar joints. Both joints show no bridging bone. One of the interlocking screws is fractured, and there are lucent haloes (*arrowheads*) around the nail and the more inferior screw. These signs indicate motion across the sites of attempted arthrodesis.

Foreign Bodies

The foot is vulnerable to puncture by foreign bodies, and it can be difficult to localize on physical exam. In some cases, they are visible on XR or MRI. However, foreign bodies may be obscured on MRI due to the high-signal intensity of the surrounding inflammatory reaction. Glass can be commonly identified on radiographs. The technique of choice to image foreign bodies is USG (Fig. 61.44). Thin slivers can be detected when the USG transducer is aligned along their long axis. In our clinic, the skin is marked at the site of the foreign body seen on ultrasound. The patient then goes to the clinic for removal, and removal is guided by the mark.

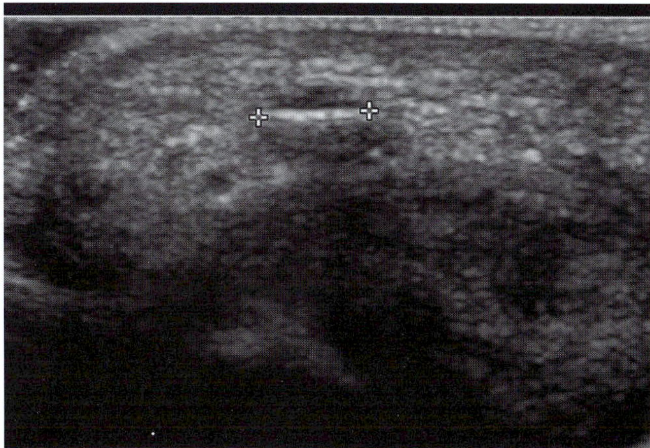

Figure 61.44 Foreign body (thorn) on USG. The thorn is outlined by calipers. It shows moderate shadowing deep to it.

Practical Approach to Imaging the Foot and Ankle

Always start with weight-bearing radiographs. These will give the best evaluation of alignment, and will additionally provide a good screening for bone trauma, bone tumors, infection, and arthritis, important causes of pain which are not covered in this chapter. Ultrasound is an excellent tool, but to utilize it effectively, the operator needs to have a high level of understanding of normal anatomy to visualize the small, obliquely oriented structures of the foot. Another advantage of ultrasound is the ability to perform dynamic maneuvers. MRI is best for evaluating bony abnormalities and for obtaining a global picture of the entire region.

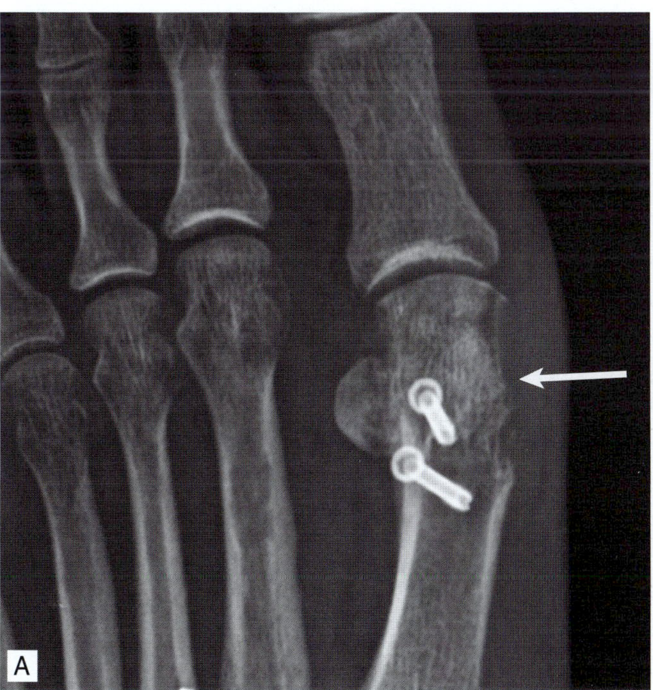

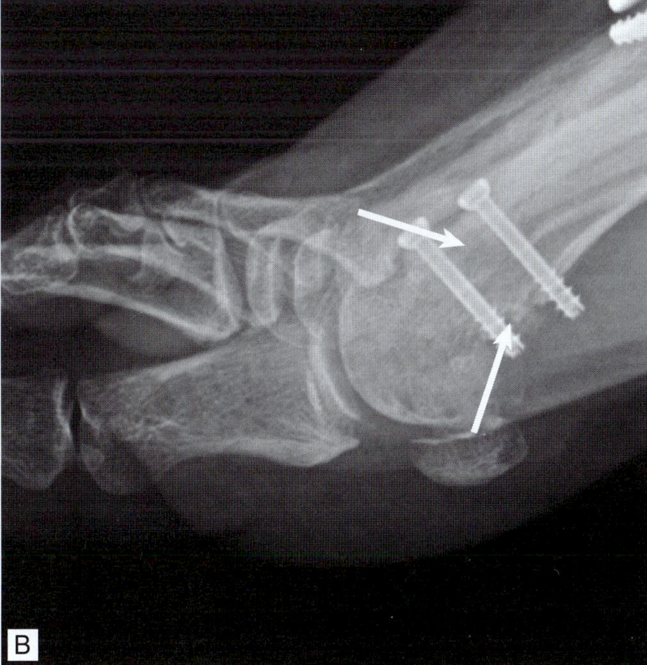

Figure 61.43 Hallux valgus surgery. (A) AP XR shows a straight contour of the medial first MT head (*arrow*), indicating the bony bunion has been resected. Fixation screws are in place across a chevron (V-shaped) osteotomy, which is poorly seen on this view. (B) Lateral XR shows a chevron osteotomy (*arrows*). The distal MT can be moved medially across the chevron.

The MRI template given here can be used as a guide to reviewing MRIs in a systematic fashion. Evaluating every study using the same search pattern, in the same order, reduces errors. It is also important to remember that one problem in the foot and ankle can lead to other problems. For example, hallux valgus can lead to Freiberg infraction.

MR Template

Technique: Describe area of coverage, contrast if given.

Comparison: Always compare with previous radiographs, and advanced imaging.

Lateral collateral ligament: Describe injuries to components separately.

Syndesmotic and deltoid ligaments: Describe injuries to components separately.

Intertarsal and TMT ligaments: Always specify Lisfranc ligament intact or injured. Can group other ligaments together as being normal, without naming specific ligaments, unless injured.

Achilles tendon: Describe as normal, tendinopathy, peritendinosis, or tear. Give AP diameter of tendon if abnormal. Describe bursitis, Haglund deformity, and pre-Achilles fat if abnormal.

Deep flexor tendons: Describe as normal, or describe tenosynovitis, tendinopathy, partial or complete tear. Describe any injury to flexor retinaculum here. Describe accessory navicular if present.

Peroneal tendons: Describe as normal, or describe tenosynovitis, tendinopathy, partial or complete tear. Describe any injury to peroneal retinaculum here. Describe os peroneum if present.

Extensor tendons Describe as normal, or describe tenosynovitis, tendinopathy, partial or complete tear. Describe extensor bursitis if present.

Intrinsic muscle and plantar fascia: Describe as normal, or describe injury or denervation edema.

Joints: Describe as no evidence of articular abnormality, or precisely and briefly describe osteophytes, erosions or joint effusions. Describe any evidence of impingement on a joint.

Bones: Describe fracture, bone marrow edema, stress fracture, or marrow replacement process.

Neurovascular structures: Describe as normal, or describe vascular abnormalities or evidence of nerve injury/impingement.

Impression: This should be a short, succinct, numerical list, in order of importance of findings.

Suggested Readings

- J Crim, Imaging of tarsal coalition, Radiol Clin North Am 46 (2008) 1017–1026, vi.
- T Alves, Q Dong, J Jacobson, C Yablon, G Gandikota, Normal and injured ankle ligaments on ultrasonography with magnetic resonance imaging correlation, J Ultrasound Med 38 (2019) 513–528.
- A Donovan, ZS Rosenberg, JT Bencardino, ZR Velez, DB Blonder, GA Ciavarra, et al., Plantar tendons of the foot: MR imaging and US, Radiographics 33 (7) (2013) 2065–2085.
- SB Soliman, PJ Spicer, MT van Holsbeeck, Sonographic and radiographic findings of posterior tibial tendon dysfunction: a practical step forward, Skeletal Radiol 48 (2019) 11–27.
- DV Flores, C Mejia Gomez, M Fernandez Hernando, MA Davis, MN Pathria, Adult acquired flatfoot deformity: anatomy, biomechanics, staging, and imaging findings, Radiographics 39 (2019) 1437–1460.

62

Bone Tumors

JAMES KHO, RAJESH BOTCHU, STEVEN JAMES

Introduction

Imaging plays a central role in the diagnosis and management of suspected bone tumors. For many suspected bone tumors, a definitive diagnosis or narrow differential diagnosis is possible from the imaging appearances alone. It is imperative that a radiological diagnosis is made as far as possible to avoid unwarranted biopsies of lesions with pathognomic radiological appearances, such as bone cysts. In other bone lesions, correlation with histopathological examination of the lesion may be required to establish the diagnosis. However, even in these cases, imaging should be regarded as complementary to histopathological opinion, particularly if this is based on biopsy material rather than the sectioning of a resection specimen. Inadequate investigations have occasionally been responsible for erroneous diagnoses of benign lesions as malignant, resulting in unnecessary surgical procedures, including iatrogenic disasters, such as amputation. Beyond establishing the diagnosis, imaging is important for surgical planning, oncological staging, and image-guided treatment such as radiofrequency ablation and follow-up.

It is recognized that bone tumors can present as a considerable diagnostic challenge. Although benign and innocuous lesions such as fibrous cortical defects are common, and may occur in up to 30% of normal children, primary malignant tumors of bone are *relatively rare* and are responsible for only 1% of all deaths from neoplasia. Consequently, most radiologists will see comparatively few cases. Furthermore, there are a large number of recognized types of primary bone tumors, with varying radiological appearances.

With these challenges in mind, this chapter begins with a discussion of a general diagnostic approach to bone lesions, irrespective of etiology. Following this, the clinical and imaging characteristics of individual primary bone tumors (i.e., bone lesions of neoplastic or uncertain etiology) will be discussed, followed by metastatic bone disease. However, it is important to recognize that neoplastic bone lesions, whether benign or malignant, only represent a subset of bone lesions. Bone lesions may also arise from a myriad of non-neoplastic pathophysiological processes, including trauma, hematological diseases, autoimmune disorders, and metabolic disorders.

General Diagnostic Approach to Bone Tumors

Radiographic Features

The radiograph is *vital* in establishing the diagnosis or differential diagnosis of a bone lesion and is supplemented where necessary by further imaging including magnetic resonance imaging (MRI), computed tomography (CT), and nuclear medicine studies. Many of the characteristic imaging features of bone lesions were initially described on conventional radiographs given the long history of this technique. Radiographs are most frequently the initial technique used and it is therefore important to be able to assess bone lesions on radiographs to decide if further imaging is indicated. Finally, many of the principles of assessing a lesion on radiographs such as nature of periosteal reaction and lesion margins are applicable across imaging techniques.

A *systematic approach* should be adopted in the radiographic assessment of any bone lesion. The key features that need to be assessed are the age of the patient, the location of the lesion, and the lesion appearances (Table 62.1).

Age of the Patient

The patient's age should always be taken into account when formulating the differential diagnosis of any bone lesion because the *prevalence of different bone lesions changes considerably with age*. For example, a lytic lesion confined to the epiphysis is likely to reflect infection or chondroblastoma in a child before growth plate fusion, whereas if this is encountered in an adult over 50 years, alternate diagnosis such as a geode needs to be considered. As a general rule, with increasing age, bone metastasis, and myeloma become more likely causes of bone lesions than primary bone tumors. Nonetheless, on very rare occasions, lesions may be found outside the typical age groups. Some tumors such as osteosarcomas classically have a dual peak in incidence—the primary idiopathic form occurring in younger patients, and the secondary form occurring in older patients in association with Paget's or

TABLE 62.1 Systematic Assessment of Bone Lesions

Features to Be Assessed on Any Bone Lesion
Age of patient
Location of lesion ■ Which bone is affected? ■ Where is the lesion within the bone?
Lesion appearances ■ Is lesion lytic or sclerotic? ■ Is there matrix calcification? ■ Are there any aggressive features? ○ Margins within the bone ○ Cortex ○ Periosteum ○ Soft-tissue

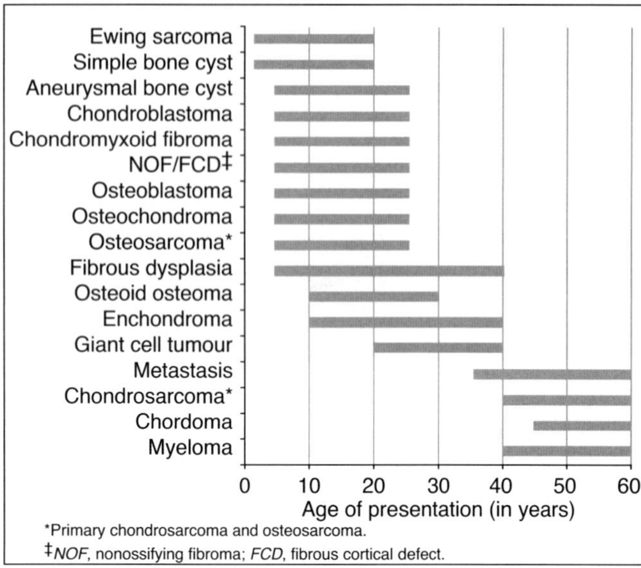

Figure 62.1 Incidence of bone tumors by age.

previous irradiation. In clinical practice, the patient's age should be readily available clinical information, but in the absence of this, the approximate patient's age may be discerned from the state of physeal closure and the presence or absence of degenerative joint disease. The following diagram summarizes the tumors by age (Fig. 62.1).

Lesion Location

The prevalence of bone lesions varies between *different bones* and between *specific locations within bones.* Primary bone lesions often show a predilection for certain types of bones (e.g., osteoid osteomas usually occur in long bones, not flat bones). Some lesions almost always occur in a specific bone (e.g., osteofibrous dysplasia [OFD] and adamantinoma in the tibia). The importance of considering the location in formulating a differential is exemplified by the example of central cartilage tumors—intramedullary cartilage-forming lesions with no aggressive imaging features in the phalanges, proximal humeri, and distal femur are most likely to be enchondromas, but lesions with similar imaging appearances in the axial skeleton should be considered suspicious for low-grade chondrosarcomas. The specific bone favored by each lesion will be discussed under the relevant subsection for that lesion later in this chapter.

The location of the lesion *within a bone* should be noted in relation to the physis (diaphysis, metaphysis, epiphysis, apophysis), and in relation to the cortex and medulla (surface or periosteal lesion, intracortical, intramedullary). Intramedullary lesions may also be described as either central or eccentric. For example, nonossifying fibroma and fibrous cortical defects are cortically based lesions, located at the metadiaphysis of a long bone. The following diagrams summarize the distribution of bone lesions by their location (Figs. 62.2 and 62.3).

Epiphyseal lesions also occur in *epiphyseal equivalents* which include apophyses (e.g., greater trochanter of the femur) and certain bones such as the patella, talus and calcaneum. For example, the most common primary bone tumors of the patella are chondroblastoma and giant cell tumor (GCT).

In addition to the location of the lesion, the radiograph should also be reviewed for any further bone lesions. Most primary bone tumors are *confined to a single bone* at the time of presentation in

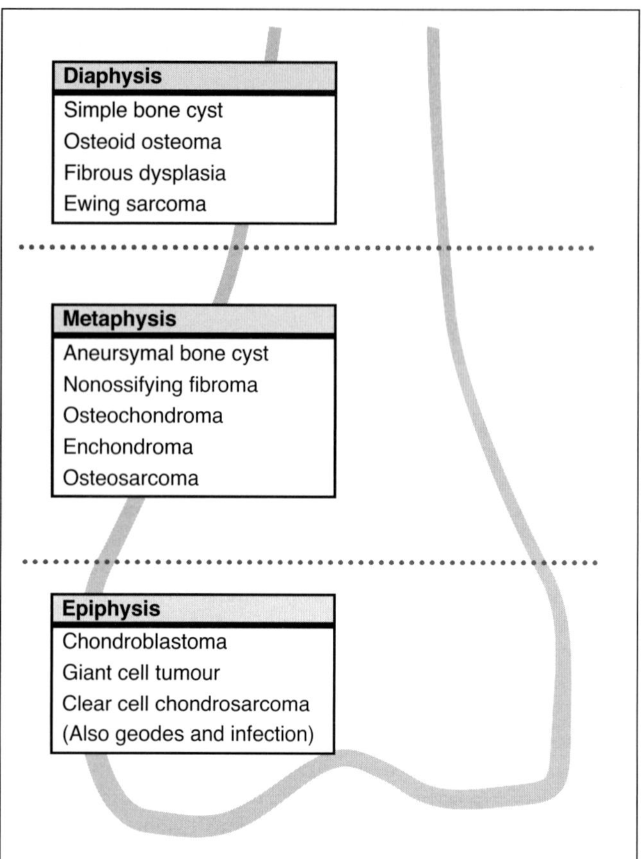

Figure 62.2 Distribution of bone tumors by location relative to the physis.

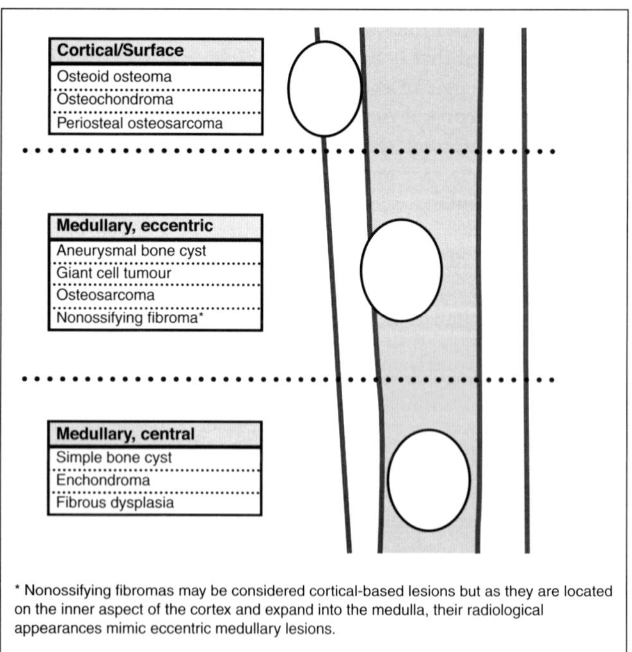

Figure 62.3 Distribution of bone tumors by location relative to the cortex and medulla.

the absence of an underlying syndromic predisposition such as the multiple osteochondromas of hereditary multiple exostosis (HME) and multiple cartilage tumors in Ollier disease/Maffucci syndrome. Direct tumoral spread across a joint is rare but is well described at the sacroiliac joints with benign lesions such as GCT of the bone, as well as malignant tumors such as osteosarcoma. Imaging should include the *entirety of the bone* containing the lesion (i.e., from the joint proximal to the lesion, until the joint distal to the lesion), to evaluate for skip metastasis or multifocal lesions within a bone. *Skip metastases* refer to metastatic lesions either within the same bone of the primary lesion or across a single joint in an adjacent bone, in the absence of widespread systemic metastatic disease. Skip metastases can occur in all high-grade sarcomas arising from the bone, but are most typically associated with osteosarcoma, chondrosarcoma, and Ewing sarcoma.

Lesion Appearances

A comprehensive description of the radiographic appearances of a suspected bone tumor, in combination with the age and location of the lesion as described earlier, will often allow the radiologist to narrow the differential down to one or a few possibilities. The radiographic appearances can be subdivided and each category should be assessed for and described in every lesion.

Is the Lesion Lytic or Sclerotic?

This is, essentially, whether the lesion results in increased or decreased density relative to normal bone. Some lesions will be of mixed lytic and sclerotic components. Sclerotic components in a bone lesion are not a sign of benignity, as a gamut of lesions of varying aggressiveness, ranging from benign bone islands to malignant high-grade osteosarcoma may be sclerotic in nature. Likewise, the differential for lytic lesions includes completely benign entities such as simple bone cyst, and highly malignant entities such as Ewing sarcoma.

Is There Matrix Calcification or Mineralization?

The matrix refers to the internal substance of a lesion. On radiographs, the terminology matrix is usually applied to the *pattern of calcification or mineralization*, from which the nature of a lesion may be inferred. Two primary patterns of mineralization are recognized—*chondroid* and *osteoid* (Fig. 62.4). A chondroid matrix refers to ring, arc, or popcorn pattern of calcification and implies a cartilage-forming lesion. An osteoid matrix refers to denser mineralization in a rounded or amorphous pattern, and implies a bone-forming lesion. If the lesion extends into the surrounding soft-tissue, matrix calcification may be visualized better in the extraosseous component than in the intraosseous component. The terminology *"ground-glass matrix"* is sometimes used to refer to the relatively homogenous hazy density characteristically seen in fibrous dysplasia.

Are There Any Aggressive Features?

It is generally preferable to describe lesions based on the presence or absence of aggressive features rather than having malignant or benign features. Infection and histologically benign lesions such as GCT can have aggressive features on imaging. Conversely, small intramedullary bone metastases may not show any aggressive appearances. With regard to the aggressive features, the lesion should be reviewed in terms of its margins within the bone, followed by any changes in surrounding tissue starting from the closest to most distant (namely the bone cortex, periosteum, and soft-tissue). In practice, the presence of *any single aggressive feature* in a lesion generally warrants concern, requiring further clinical and radiological workup, although it should be emphasized that not all lesions demonstrating aggressive features will be malignant.

Margins Within the Bone (Zone of Transition)

The margins of a bone lesion are often described based on the width of the *zone of transition*, that is the region between normal bone and the lesion (Fig. 62.5). An abrupt change at the margin of the lesion to normal bone is a narrow zone of transition. Some lesions have a thin surrounding rim of sclerosis which by definition is a narrow zone of transition. If the margin with normal bone is ill-defined, with a gradual change from lesional tissue to normal bone, this is a wide zone of transition. Occasionally, lesions will have a permeative pattern, where the lesion and normal bone appear interspersed with no boundary between normal and abnormal bone. A wide zone of transition and a permeative pattern are both considered aggressive features in a focal bone lesion, although a permeative pattern may also be seen in metabolic diseases such as osteoporosis.

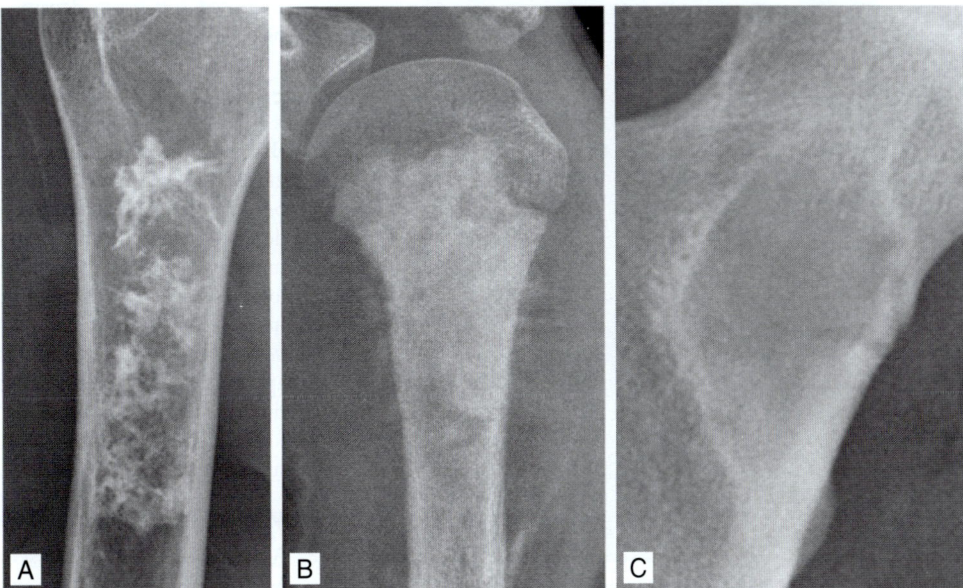

Figure 62.4 Matrix. (A) Ring and arc calcification of chondroid matrix, (B) dense mineralization of osteoid matrix, and (C) homogenous hazy density of ground-glass matrix.

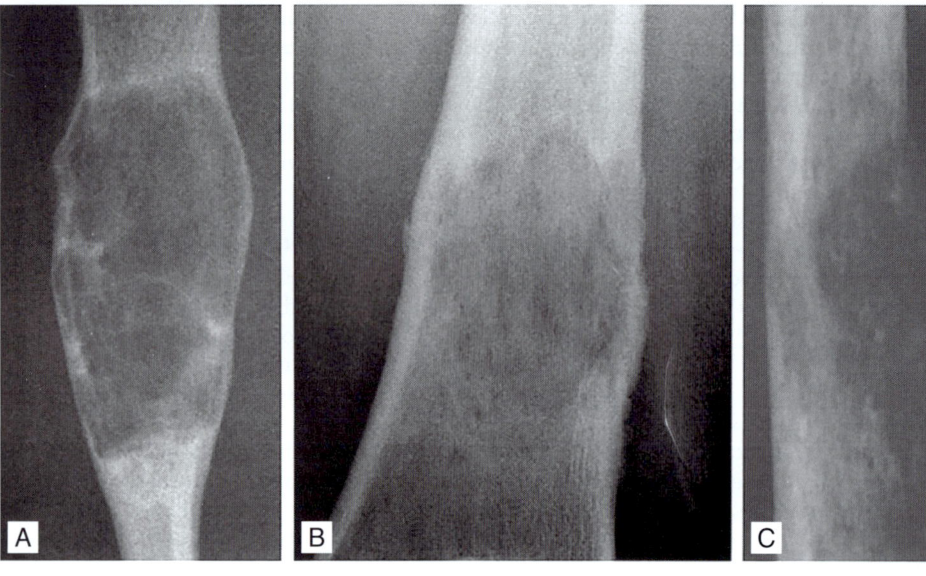

Figure 62.5 Zone of transition. Narrow (A), wide (B), and permeative pattern (C).

Cortex

The cortex should be examined to determine if it is intact, or whether there is endosteal scalloping or cortical destruction (Fig. 62.6). *Cortical destruction* is an aggressive feature. *Endosteal scalloping* generally implies a slow-growing bone lesion but in the setting of a central cartilage tumor, endosteal scalloping raises the possibility of a low-grade chondrosarcoma.

The cortex should also be reviewed for other changes that do not imply aggressiveness or otherwise but may help narrow the differential diagnosis. Expansile lesions result in *bowing* (outward convexity) of the cortex, often associated with *cortical thinning*. Cortical thickening suggests exuberant periosteal bone formation, and is associated with osteoid osteomas, infection, and stress fractures. A focal step or linear lucency in the cortex overlying the lesion should raise concern for a *pathological fracture*. Pathological fractures occur in both benign and malignant lesions and are not an indicator of lesion aggressiveness. Lesions arising from the surface of the bone or in the adjacent soft-tissue can cause smooth scalloping or remodeling of the cortex of the bone that is sometimes referred to as saucerization.

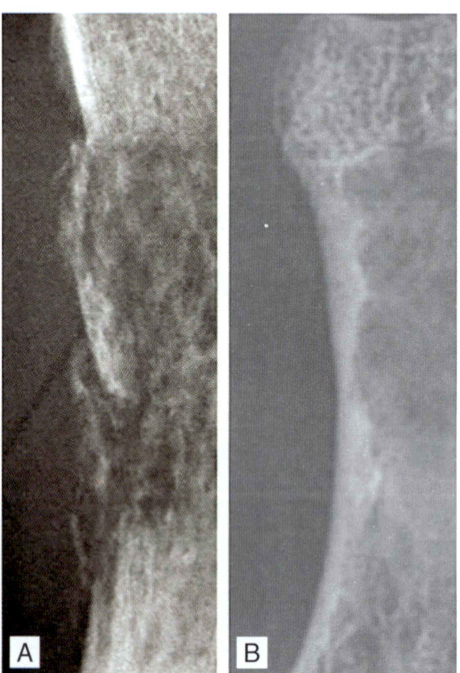

Figure 62.6 Cortical destruction (A) and endosteal scalloping (B).

Periosteum

The periosteum is a layer of thick connective tissue that covers the surface of all bones, except in its intra-articular portion. Periosteal reaction that is *lamellated*, *spiculated*, or *interrupted* are considered to be aggressive features, as is the *Codman's triangle* (Fig. 62.7). Continuous, smooth, or wavy periosteal reactions are not considered to be indicative of an aggressive pathology, and are sometimes referred to as "benign" periosteal reactions. A pathological fracture is a possible cause of a periosteal reaction in proximity to a bone lesion but periosteal reactions resulting from fracture callus formation should never display aggressive morphology on radiographs.

Soft-Tissue

Increased soft-tissue density around a bone lesion implies extraosseous extension into the soft-tissue which is an aggressive feature.

Further Imaging and Biopsy

Based on the age of the patient, the lesion location and its radiographic appearances, a diagnosis or differential diagnosis should be formulated. At this stage, further imaging may be warranted depending on the differential diagnosis. Indications for further imaging include further characterization of the lesion, for oncological staging, treatment planning, and follow-up. Imaging investigations for lesion characterization should be *performed before any biopsy* of a lesion as such procedures may alter imaging appearances. The role of biopsies will also be briefly discussed in this section as image-guided biopsies are increasingly being performed by radiologists under imaging guidance rather than by surgeons in the operating theatre.

Magnetic Resonance Imaging

Although radiograph is essential for the diagnosis of bone tumor, MRI defines better, the extent of involvement in terms of marrow

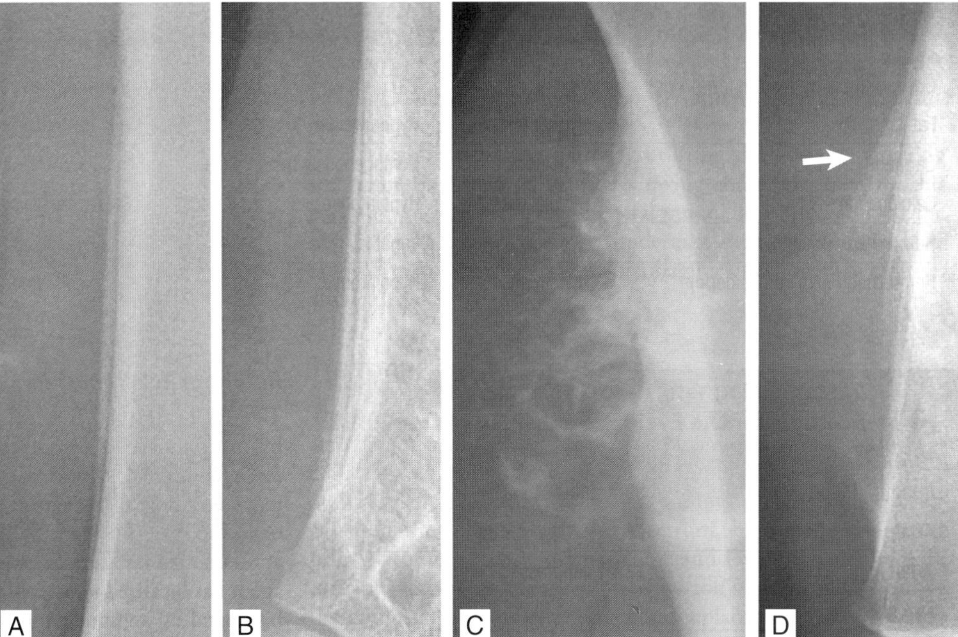

Figure 62.7 Periosteal reaction. (A) Smooth, thin, (B) lamellated, (C) spiculated, and (D) interrupted with Codman's triangle (*arrow*).

and soft-tissues. Therefore, tumor measurements, radiation, and resection planning are more accurately undertaken based on MRI (usually with contrast). MRI provides high spatial resolution images with excellent tissue discrimination in multiple planes. In terms of lesion characterization, the following imaging features are particularly well visualized on MRI, and are helpful in discriminating between different lesions.

- Precise anatomical location and extent of the lesion
- Extent of perilesional edema—both bone marrow edema and soft-tissue edema
- Extent of extraosseous extension into surrounding soft-tissue, and assessment of neurovascular and joint involvement
- Signal characteristics of lesion to identify specific tissue components

The precise delineation of lesion from perilesional edema can be challenging, particularly on fluid-sensitive sequences, and therefore T1-weighted images are often most helpful for this (Fig. 62.8). Neurovascular involvement should be considered when there is loss of the normal fat plane separating these structures lesion, particularly when there is encasement. Signal characteristics help distinguish between solid and cystic lesions, and allow for the identification of specific components that may be present within a lesion, namely fat, cartilage, hemorrhage, and calcification (Table 62.2). However, in the absence of these specific tissue types within a lesion, bone lesions on MRI can *show considerable overlap in signal characteristics*.

Imaging protocols vary between institutions, but a combination of *T1 imaging and fluid-sensitive sequences* (e.g., T2, PDFS, STIR) in different planes are required at the minimum. An example of an imaging protocol at the authors' institution is provided in Table 62.3.

Gadolinium-enhanced MRI sequences can provide additional information, in particular, to distinguish between solid components within a lesion that generally enhance and necrotic/cystic components within a lesion that do not enhance. Dynamic contrast enhancement may also help in discriminating higher grade from lower-grade lesions, based on the principle that higher-grade lesions enhance more rapidly than lower-grade lesions. There is, however, debate as to whether routine use of contrast-enhanced sequences is necessary.

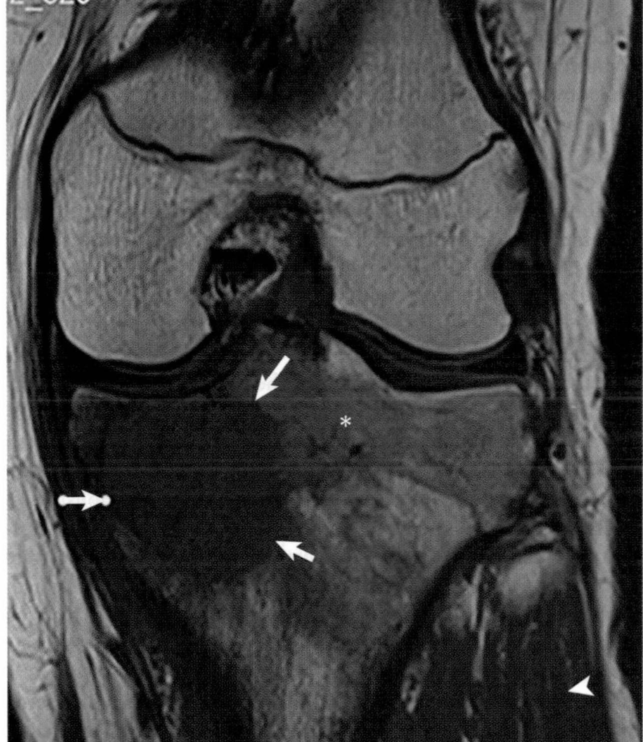

Figure 62.8 Lesion delineation on T1-weighted MRI image. Replacement of normal high signal fat in bone marrow by low-signal tumoral tissue (*white arrows*). Perilesional edema (*asterisk*) typically remains hyperintense relative to the skeletal muscle (*arrowhead*) on T1 as fat remains present.

Whole-body MR imaging is sometimes used for oncological staging of bone tumors, particularly childhood bone tumors such as Ewing sarcoma. Whole-body MRI briefly involves acquisition of wide-field of view images over large body regions using limited

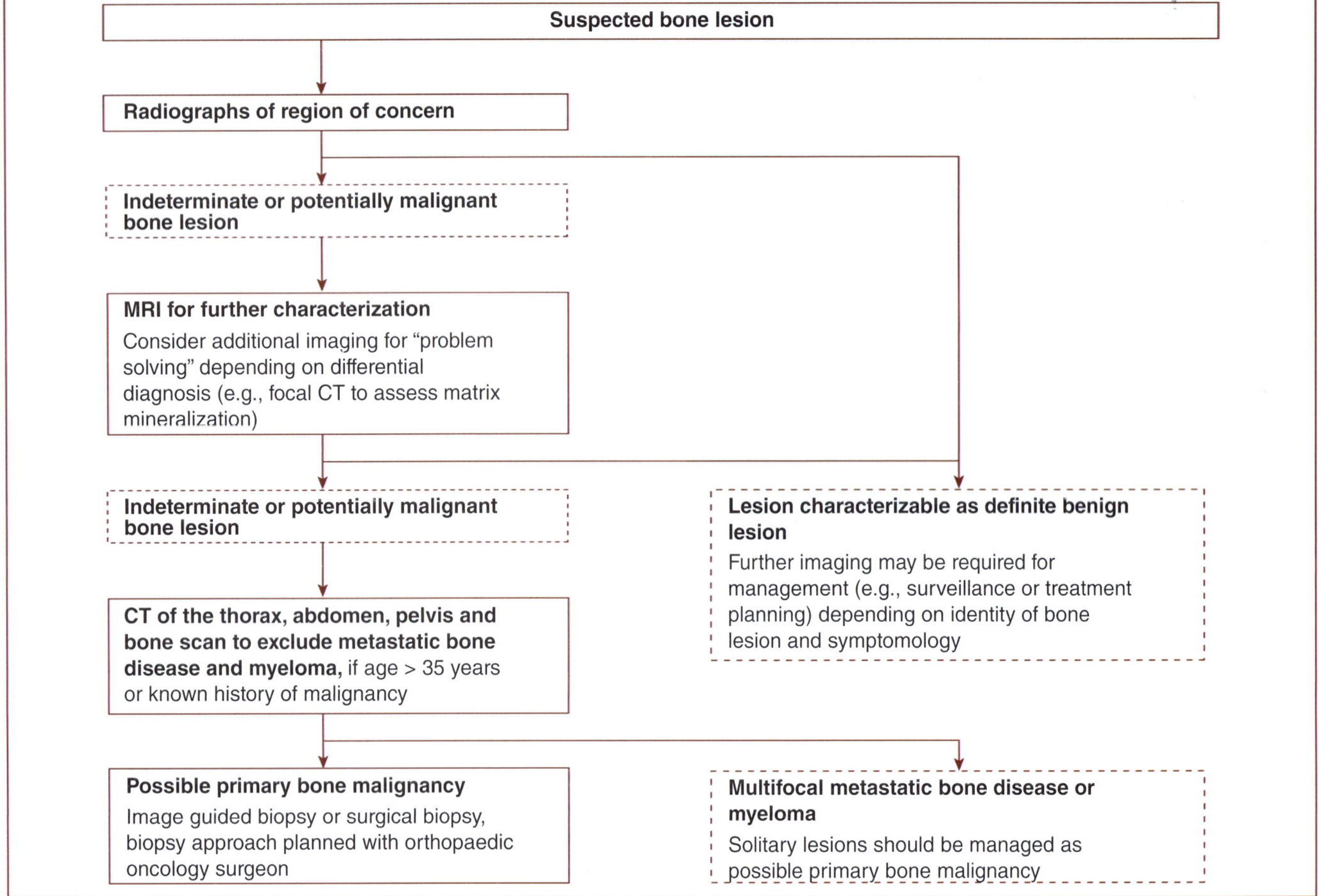

Figure 62.10 Diagnostic imaging pathway for a suspected bone lesion.

TABLE 62.4 Classification of Primary Bone Lesions

	Benign[a]	Malignant
Cartilage-forming	Chondroma (enchondroma/ periosteal chondroma) Chondroblastoma Chondromyxoid fibroma Osteochondroma	Chondrosarcoma
Bone-forming	Bone island (enostosis) Osteoma Osteoid osteoma Osteoblastoma	Osteosarcoma
Fibrous	Nonossifying fibroma/fibrous cortical defect Fibrous dysplasia Osteofibrous dysplasia Desmoplastic fibroma	Fibrosarcoma
Cystic	Simple bone cyst Aneurysmal bone cyst	–
Ewing sarcoma	–	Ewing sarcoma
Others	Hemangioma Intraosseous lipoma Giant cell tumor	Chordoma Adamantinoma

[a] Includes locally aggressive lesions with nonexistent or very low metastatic potential.

A brief description of the clinical features of individual primary bone tumors, followed by their imaging features and differential diagnosis are presented in the following section. It is advised that equal emphasis should be placed on reviewing the images as the text, to get a "feel" for the appearances of each lesion.

Cartilage-Forming Tumors

Chondromas

Chondromas are benign cartilaginous tumors, consisting histologically of well-differentiated cartilage with low mitotic activity. Chondromas are commonly subclassified according to their location; *enchondromas* when they occur within a bone, and *periosteal chondromas* when they arise from the surface of a bone. Chondromas can also arise within the soft-tissues, as soft-tissue chondromas.

Enchondromas

Enchondromas present clinically either as an incidental imaging finding or occasionally as a pathological fracture. Classically, these lesions are thought of as being most common in the hands and feet, based on conventional radiographs. With increasing MRI utilization, it is now apparent that up to 2–3% of all knee MRIs demonstrate incidental enchondromas, many of which may be occult on radiographs [3,4]. Treatment is *conservative*, except in rare circumstances where the risk of fracture is considered to be high.

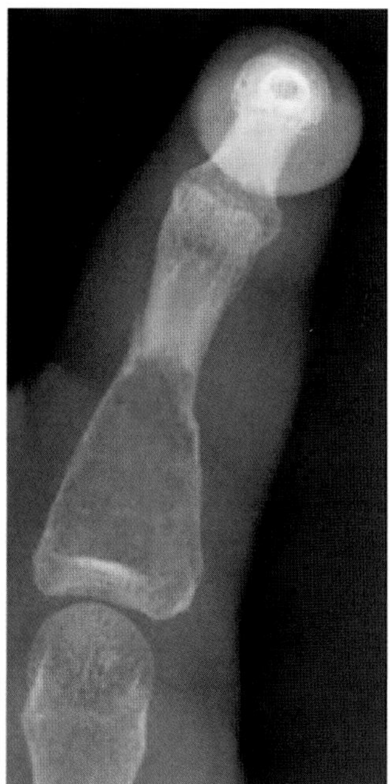

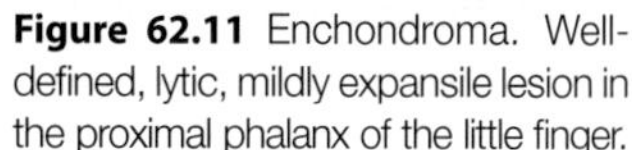

Figure 62.11 Enchondroma. Well-defined, lytic, mildly expansile lesion in the proximal phalanx of the little finger.

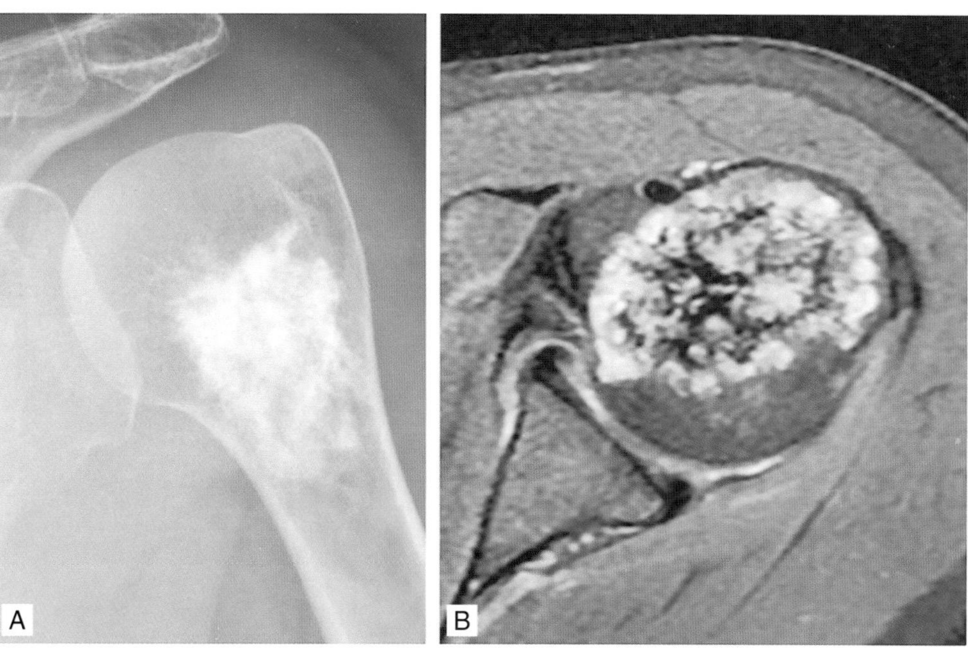

Figure 62.12 Enchondroma. (A) Ring and arc calcification in proximal humeral enchondroma on radiograph. (B) Noncalcified cartilage within enchondroma is high signal on fluid-sensitive images, while calcified cartilage is low signal.

Imaging Features: On radiographs, enchondromas are well-defined metadiaphyseal lytic lesions, often eccentrically located in the medullary cavity (Fig. 62.11). They may be mildly expansile, particularly when located in a narrow tubular bone, for example, fibula or phalanges, with associated endosteal scalloping and cortical thinning. A chondroid (ring and arc) pattern of matrix mineralization is almost invariably present, except in the small bones of the hands and feet, where they may be purely lytic. As a benign lesion, an enchondroma should exhibit *no aggressive features* radiologically. Any aggressive feature such as cortical destruction, extraosseous extension, or periosteal reaction (in the absence of a fracture) is in keeping with a chondrosarcoma.

On MRI, enchondromas demonstrate low T1 and high T2 signals in keeping with well-differentiated cartilage (Fig. 62.12). The lesion is usually uniform in signal, aside from small foci of low signal on all sequences representing chondroid calcification. No perilesional edema should be present. Peripheral enhancement occurs after administration of contrast. Enchondromas may show uptake on the bone scan but uptake is more often demonstrated with chondrosarcomas.

Sometimes, intramedullary cartilaginous tumors do not demonstrate gross aggressive imaging features but exhibit more clinically aggressive behavior. These lesions represent atypical cartilaginous tumors or low-grade chondrosarcomas, rather than enchondromas. Low-grade chondrosarcomas rarely metastasize to the lungs and the bones, with an 83–89% 10-year survival rate [5].

In practice, distinguishing between enchondroma and low-grade central chondrosarcoma can sometimes be difficult, as both these lesions *may demonstrate similar features radiologically and histologically* [6]. There are however several imaging features that can be helpful. It is critical to appreciate that enchondromas are common in tubular bones, but uncommon in flat bones, such that an "enchondroma" of a flat bone should be regarded as a probable low-grade chondrosarcoma. Conversely, it is very unusual for central cartilaginous tumors in the hands and feet to demonstrate aggressive behavior, and the diagnosis of enchondroma in these sites can often be made on radiographs alone. Second, any interval change in size or radiological appearances on serial imaging should raise concern for chondrosarcoma. Third, larger lesions, particularly greater than 5 cm, are more likely to represent chondrosarcomas. Lastly, deep (>2/3 cortical thickness) or circumferential endosteal scalloping favors chondrosarcoma over enchondroma (Fig. 62.13).

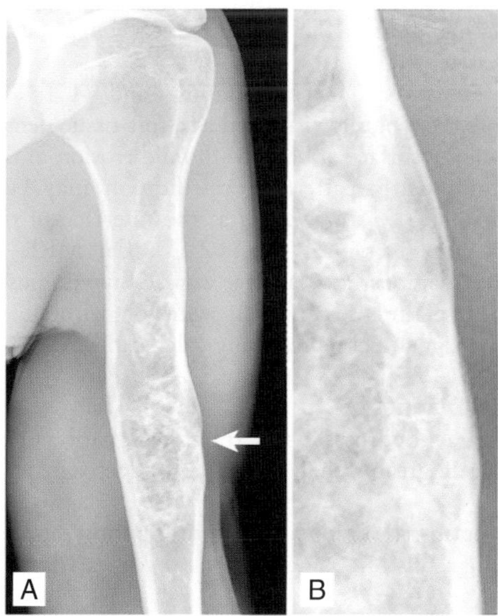

Figure 62.13 Low-grade chondrosarcoma in the humerus demonstrating marked craniocaudal extension within the proximal-to-mid diaphysis and deep endosteal scalloping along the lateral cortex (*arrow*, A), which is magnified in the image (B).

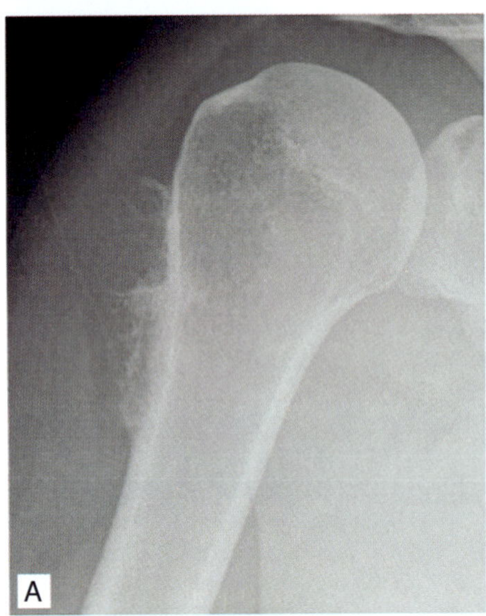

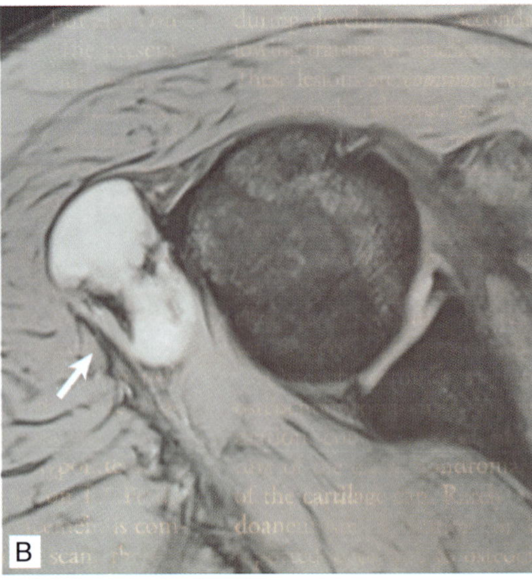

Figure 62.14 Periosteal chondroma, proximal humerus. (A) Periosteal reaction and mild cortical erosion at the interface of the lesion with the bone cortex. (B) Axial MRI T2 image demonstrates the lesion comprises largely of hyperintense signal of well-differentiated cartilage (*arrow*), with small internal hypointense regions representing calcification. Note absence of medullary involvement.

Differential Diagnosis

- Low-grade central chondrosarcoma (consider if large >5 cm, deep endosteal scalloping, interval change, or uncommon location).
- High-grade central chondrosarcoma (aggressive features present).
- On radiographs alone, if purely lytic in small tubular bones, consider GCT (if subarticular) or aneurysmal bone cyst (ABC). MRI differentiates.
- Occasionally serpiginous calcification of bone infarcts may be confused for ring and arc calcification of enchondroma.

Periosteal Chondroma

Periosteal chondromas, also known as juxtacortical or surface chondromas, are much less common than enchondromas. These benign lesions are *histologically similar to enchondromas* and have predilection to the same bones as enchondromas. Given their more superficial location, periosteal chondromas tend to present clinically as hard lumps. They occur frequently in association with Ollier disease.

Imaging Features: On radiographs and CT, periosteal chondromas are typically visualized as a soft-tissue density lesion arising from the surface of bone, with mild erosion of the cortex. A chondroid matrix pattern of calcification may be present. *Reactive periosteal bone formation* at the interface of this lesion with the cortex is typical (Fig. 62.14). On MRI, periosteal chondromas demonstrate cartilage signal (hypointense on T1, uniformly hyperintense on T2), with or without markedly hypointense signal foci representing calcification.

Differential Diagnosis

- Periosteal chondrosarcomas (rare malignant counterpart), consider if greater than 3 cm or if deep cortical surface erosion.
- Other periosteal lesions may mimic periosteal chondroma on radiographs but these do not exhibit cartilage signal on MRI.

Syndromic Forms

- *Ollier disease (Enchondromatosis)* is a sporadic (nonhereditary) syndrome characterized by multiple enchondromas, although periosteal chondromas may also be present (Fig. 62.15). Enchondroma distribution is usually similar to nonsyndromic solitary enchondromas, with additional involvement of other sites such as the pelvis. The severity of the presentation varies between patients but may be large with associated deformity and limb growth abnormality. An increased risk of chondrosarcomatous change has been reported, with an estimated lifetime risk of chondrosarcoma of 25–40% [7,8]. Chondrosarcoma should be considered if *interval change occurs in a lesion after skeletal maturity.* Lesions of Ollier disease are more hypercellular than nonsyndromic enchondromas, and can mimic chondrosarcoma histologically.
- *Maffucci syndrome* is the association of multiple enchondromas with multiple soft-tissue hemangiomas. On radiographs, the soft-tissue hemangiomas are characteristically recognized by the presence of soft-tissue masses containing phleboliths (Fig. 62.16). An increased lifetime risk of chondrosarcoma of 15–50% has been reported [7–9].

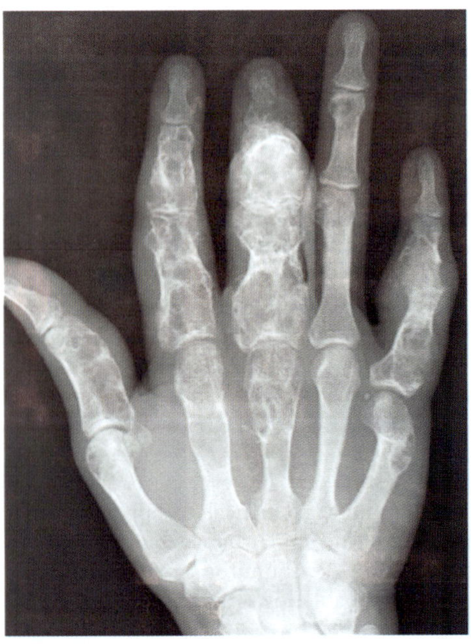

Figure 62.15 Ollier disease. Multiple enchondromas with associated deformity are present. A periosteal chondroma is also present on the third metacarpal.

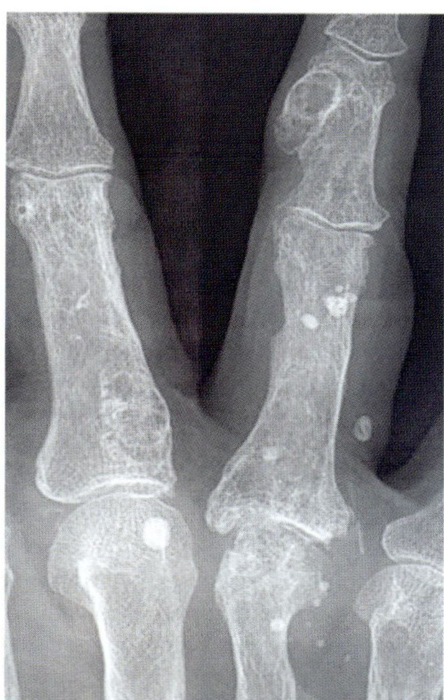

Figure 62.16 Maffucci syndrome. In addition to multiple enchondromas, note the ovoid calcific densities within the soft-tissues which are phleboliths within soft-tissue hemangiomas.

Chondroblastoma

This chondroid tumor arises in the epiphysis of the tubular bones, or epiphyseal equivalent (e.g., apophysis or patella). Chondroblastoma usually occurs in children or young adults before growth plate fusion [10], in contrast to GCTs which occur after growth plate fusion. Presentation is of pain around the joint which may be of long duration and there may be limitation of joint movement. Treatment is by image-guided ablation for small lesions or curettage for larger ones.

Imaging Features: On radiographs, a chondroblastoma is typically a rounded or oval lytic lesion with a thin sclerotic rim in the epiphysis or other epiphyseal equivalent. Larger lesions may *extend into the metaphysis* (Fig. 62.17). Approximately half of lesions will have a demonstrable chondroid matrix pattern of calcification [10]. No aggressive features are present, but a benign periosteal reaction and joint effusion in the adjacent joint may be demonstrated [11].

On MRI, chondroblastomas demonstrate variable signal characteristics. In addition to its epiphyseal location, a distinguishing imaging feature is the *presence of a local surrounding inflammatory response*. Surrounding marrow edema is common, as is soft-tissue edema (Fig. 62.17). Fluid–fluid levels may be present in some chondroblastomas reflecting secondary ABC formation. On bone scans, there is marked increased uptake on blood-pool phase.

Differential Diagnosis: Other epiphyseal lesions in patients of a young age are the main differentials:

- GCT does not typically demonstrate such florid edema and is uncommon before growth plate fusion. No sclerotic rim or matrix mineralization is present with GCT.
- Osteomyelitis is usually readily distinguished from chondroblastoma on MRI due to the presence of a peripheral rim of mildly increased T1 signal (penumbra sign) around the intraosseous abscess, the presence of a sequestrum, sinus, or soft-tissue collection.

Chondromyxoid Fibroma

Chondromyxoid fibroma (CMF) is a very rare benign chondroid tumor, comprising <1% of bone tumors [11,12].

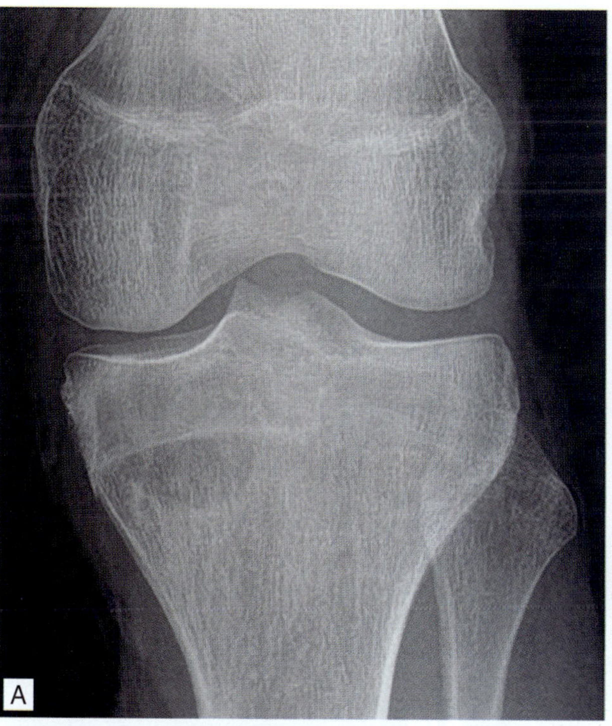

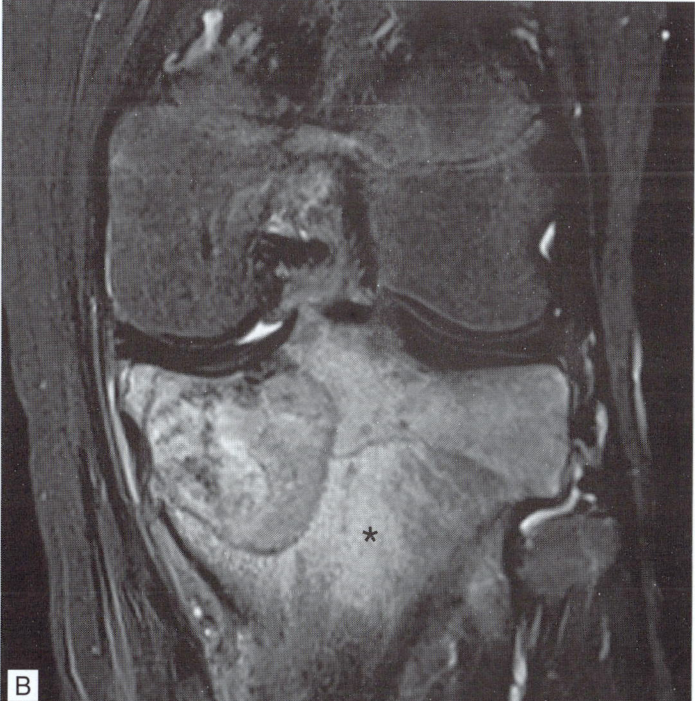

Figure 62.17 Chondroblastoma in the proximal tibia. Although chondroblastomas arise in the epiphysis, extension into the metaphysis is not uncommon, as depicted in (A). Florid surrounding marrow edema (*asterisk*) typical of chondroblastomas is demonstrated on the coronal MRI STIR image in (B).

Histologically, CMF is predominantly chondroid, but also contains myxomatous and fibrous tissue components. The presenting complaints are of localized pain with or without swelling. The peak age incidence is between 20 and 30 years [2,11,12]. The lesion occurs *around the knee joint in two-thirds of cases*, with a particular affinity for the proximal end of the tibia. Other sites include the pelvis, small tubular bones of the hands, and feet and facial bones.

Imaging Features: CMF occurs in the metaphysis, but may extend into the epiphysis. Typical radiographic appearances are of an eccentric, well- defined lytic lesion, with or without a sclerotic margin (Fig. 62.18). No aggressive features are present but the overlying cortex may be markedly thin secondary to the expansile nature of CMF. Chondroid matrix is not usually evident on radiographs, but internal trabeculations may be present.

MRI signal is a fairly nonspecific; CMF is hypointense to isointense on T1 and hypointense to hyperintense on T2. Perilesional edema is usually minimal or absent. Enhancement is common, although the pattern is variable. On bone scan, there is increased uptake peripherally with reduced uptake centrally.

Differential Diagnosis: Other lytic lesions in the metaphyseal–epiphyseal region need to be considered.

- Nonossifying fibroma (NOF) can be indistinguishable radiologically but often asymptomatic.
- Chondroblastoma is centered on the epiphysis rather than metaphysis and typically demonstrates prominent marrow edema, unlike CMF.
- GCT is subarticular and may demonstrate some aggressive features.
- ABC may be similar on radiographs but has characteristic fluid–fluid levels on MRI that are not a feature of CMF.

Osteochondroma

Osteochondromas are osseous outgrowths (exostosis) from the surface of bone, which are capped with cartilage. Osteochondromas may represent developmental lesions rather than neoplastic lesions, arising from the separation of a portion of the growth plate cartilage during development. Secondary osteochondromas can occur following trauma or irradiation to the growth plate during childhood. These lesions are *commonly solitary*, except in the setting of HME.

Osteochondromas grow slowly during childhood and adolescence with endochondral ossification, the central spongiosa merging with that of the medullary cavity of the bone from which it is derived. *Growth should cease with skeletal maturity*. Osteochondromas arise mainly in tubular bones near the metaphyses. They are particularly common around the knee and the proximal end of the humerus. Less commonly, flat bones also may be affected, particularly the pelvis and scapula. Osteochondromas can be very large, particularly when arising from the flat bones.

Osteochondromas are usually *asymptomatic*. Pain from an osteochondroma may arise from overlying adventitial bursa formation, compression of adjacent neurovascular structures, fracture of the osteochondroma, or rarely malignant transformation of the cartilage cap. Rarely, vascular complications such as pseudoaneurysm formation or deep vein thrombosis have been reported secondary to osteochondromas. Imaging is necessary to exclude these complications in a symptomatic osteochondroma.

Transformation of the cartilaginous cap to peripheral chondrosarcoma is a *rare* (1% of solitary osteochondromas) but well-recognized phenomenon [13]. Therefore, enlargement or increasing pain in any lesion, particularly after skeletal maturity warrants at least imaging if not surgical removal.

Imaging Features: On radiographs, an osteochondroma is typically recognized as an exostosis that is directed away from the joint (Fig. 62.19). To confidently diagnose an osteochondroma, the medullary cavity within the exostosis should be clearly seen as continuous with the *medullary cavity* of the bone that it is arising from. Visualization of the cartilage cap is variable on radiographs, particularly in children when the radiolucent cartilage cap may be similar in radiodensity to the surrounding soft-tissue. In adults, the cartilage cap usually shows chondroid calcification, but may also completely ossify such that no residual cartilage is present. Osteochondromas may be either sessile or pedunculated.

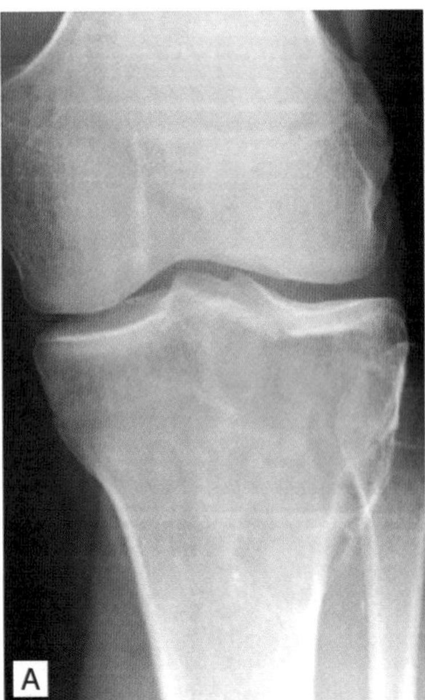

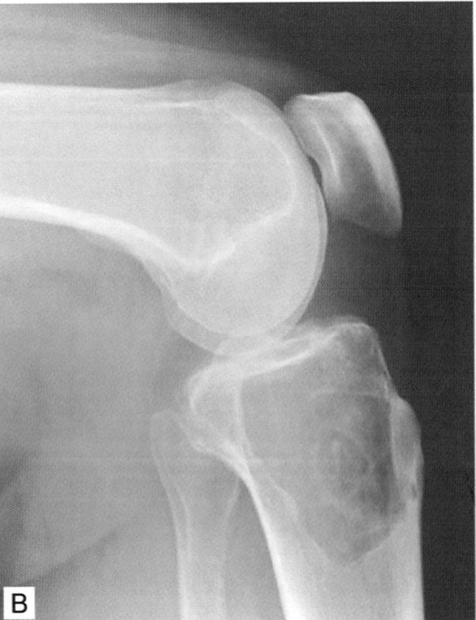

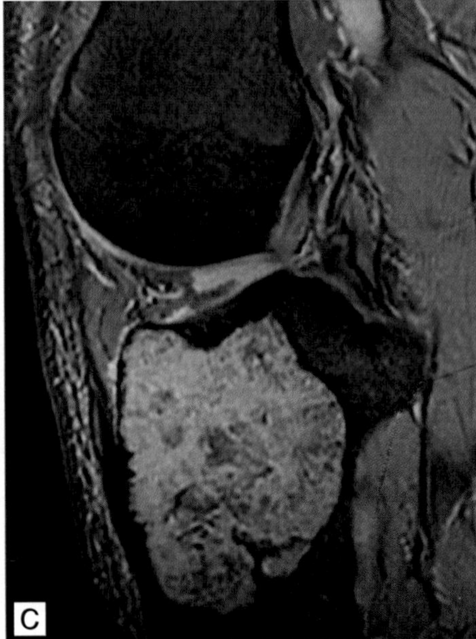

Figure 62.18 Chondromyxoid fibroma. (A) and (B) Frontal and lateral radiographs of knee demonstrating a mildly expansile, eccentric lesion involving the metaphysis and epiphysis. (C) The lesion is heterogeneously hyperintense on fluid-sensitive MRI sequence.

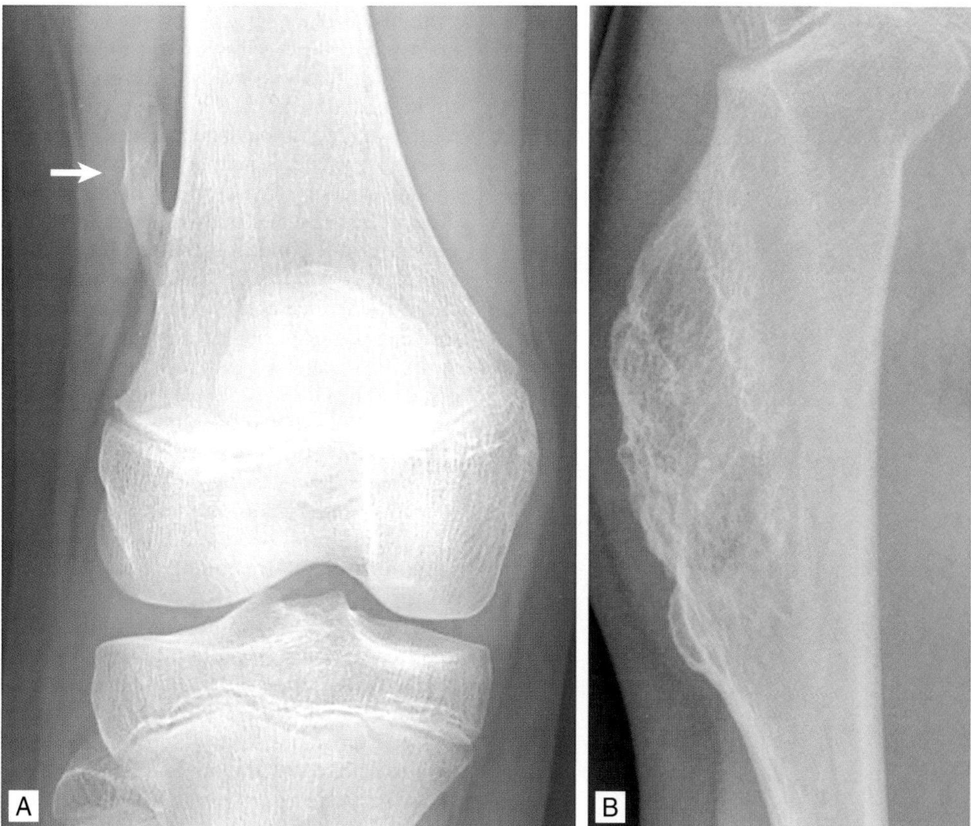

Figure 62.19 Osteochondromas. (A) Pedunculated osteochondroma (*arrow*) directed away from the knee joint. (B) Sessile osteochondroma on the humeral shaft.

MRI optimally demonstrates the cartilage cap, although the cap may also be visualized on CT. The cartilage cap is hypointense on T1 and uniformly hyperintense on T2, as typical of well-differentiated cartilage. The *thickness* of this cartilage cap should be measured, as a thickness of greater than 1.5 cm should raise concern for sarcomatous change [13,14]. The superior soft-tissue contrast on MRI is also particularly helpful to assess for complications such as overlying bursa formation and neurovascular compression (Fig. 62.20).

Aside from a thick cartilage cap, the development of lytic regions within an osteochondroma, or any other *interval change after skeletal maturity*, are suspicious for development of peripheral chondrosarcoma.

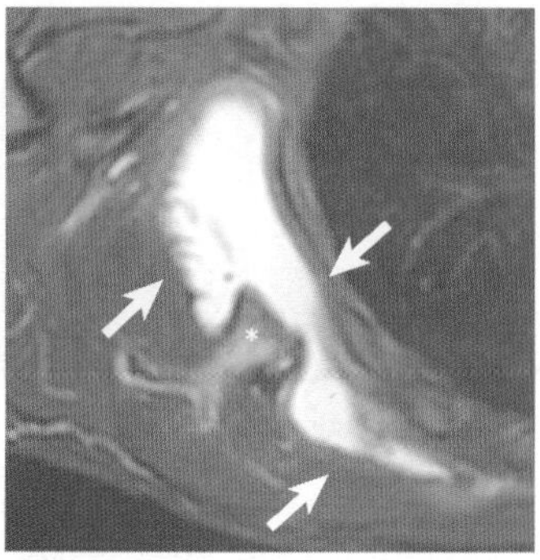

Figure 62.20 Osteochondroma. Bursitis, depicted as distension of the scapulothoracic bursa, (*arrows*) secondary to irritation from a scapular osteochondroma (*asterisk*).

Differential Diagnosis

- Other surface lesions of the bone including benign parosteal osteochondromatous proliferation, parosteal osteosarcoma, and periostitis ossifications may mimic osteochondroma.
- Other surface lesions lack true medullary continuity, although some may have cortical continuity.

Syndromic Forms

- *HME*, also previously known as diaphyseal aclasis, is a relatively common hereditary skeletal dysplasia characterized by the presence of *multiple osteochondromas* (Fig. 62.21). The osteochondromas of HME are more frequently sessile rather than pedunculated and are most common around the knee,

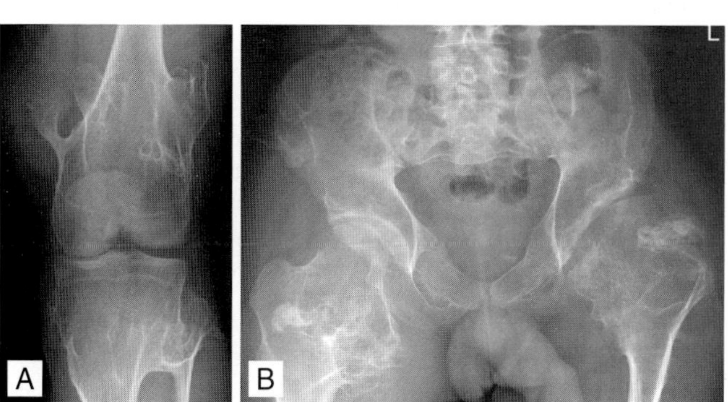

Figure 62.21 Hereditary multiple exostoses. Multiple sessile and pedunculated osteochondromas around the knee (A), hips, and pelvis (B).

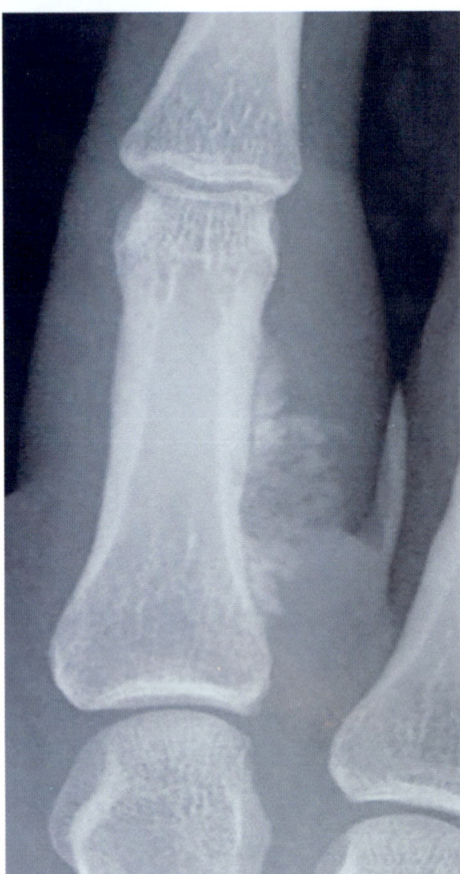

Figure 62.22 Bizarre parosteal osteochondromatous proliferation. Ossified surface lesion on the proximal phalanx.

but may affect nearly any bone with the only notable exception being the calvarium [15]. Aside from multiple osteochondromas, short stature, and limb deformity are typical, and most patients will be diagnosed in the first decade of life. The prevalence of malignant transformation in HME is higher than the solitary form and is estimated at 3–5% [13].

Bizarre Parosteal Osteochondromatous Proliferation and Turret Exostosis: Bizarre parosteal osteochondromatous proliferation (BPOP), also known as the Nora lesion, is characterized by heterotopic ossification along from the periosteal surface of the bone. This benign lesion is of uncertain etiology, but maybe reactive or post-traumatic in nature [16]. It is most commonly described in the phalanges of the hand (Fig. 62.22). The typical radiographic appearances are of a well-circumscribed focus of ossification arising from the periosteal or cortical aspect of the phalanges. Biopsy may be necessary to differentiate BPOP from other surface lesions when the location or radiological appearances are atypical [17]. The term turret exostosis is used to describe a dome-shaped osteochondromatous lesion, typically of the dorsal aspect of the phalanx or metacarpal of the hand. Turret exostoses are thought to arise from previous subperiosteal hemorrhage, and may be represent a spectrum of reactive periosteal ossification, along with BPOP [18]. *Neither BPOP nor turret exostoses demonstrate medullary continuity*, unlike osteochondromas.

Chondrosarcoma

Chondrosarcomas are a *heterogeneous* group of tumors that exhibit a spectrum of malignant behaviors, which is best predicted by their histologically grade. Low-grade (grade 1) chondrosarcoma has a very low propensity to metastasize and a 5-year survival of 82–99%, but can be locally aggressive [19]. High-grade (grade 3) chondrosarcoma behaves in an aggressive pattern with metastases to the lungs. Various subtypes of chondrosarcoma have been described, including primary central chondrosarcoma, secondary chondrosarcoma, juxtacortical chondrosarcoma, clear cell chondrosarcoma, and mesenchymal chondrosarcoma.

Conventional Chondrosarcoma (Primary Central Chondrosarcoma): Conventional chondrosarcoma represents 90% of all chondrosarcomas and is the most common malignant cartilage-forming tumor of bone. Conventional chondrosarcoma occurs mainly between the ages of 30 and 70 years and is relatively rare distal to the elbow and knee joints [11]. The pelvis and ribs are the most common sites, followed closely by the proximal end of the femur. Because of this distribution, virtually all *central chondroid lesions arising in flat bones including the pelvis* should be regarded as *potential chondrosarcomas*. The diagnosis may be delayed because of slow growth or relatively mild symptomatology. The tumor, therefore, may be very large when it is first recognized.

Imaging Features: The imaging features of conventional chondrosarcoma vary according to histological grade. Low-grade lesions demonstrate *overlapping imaging features with enchondromas*, and have been discussed with enchondromas.

On radiographs, conventional chondrosarcomas are typically lesions centered on the medulla, with aggressive features such as soft-tissue extension or cortical destruction (Figs. 62.23 and 62.24). There is usually a chondroid matrix, although in some lesions chondroid calcification may only be apparent on CT. Some high-grade lesions may demonstrate a permeative pattern or absence of calcification.

On MRI, intralesional *cartilage signal* (hypointense on T1, hyperintense on T2) is usually present, although the lesion may contain areas of noncartilaginous components such as hemorrhage. Low signal areas corresponding to matrix calcification are also commonly seen. Enhancement is typical, although unlike benign cartilage tumors, may be diffuse or nodal in pattern.

The majority of chondrosarcomas demonstrate marked increased uptake on bone scintigraphy.

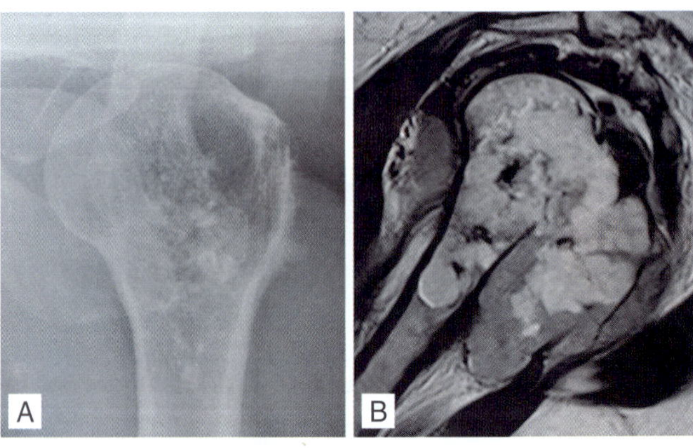

Figure 62.23 Conventional chondrosarcoma. (A) Shoulder radiograph demonstrating intramedullary chondroid matrix calcification in the proximal humerus, with spiculated periosteal reaction anterolaterally. (B) Sagittal oblique MRI T2 image demonstrating extraosseous extension into the soft-tissue of the chondrosarcoma. The extraosseous component is poorly visualized on radiographs due to minimal calcification.

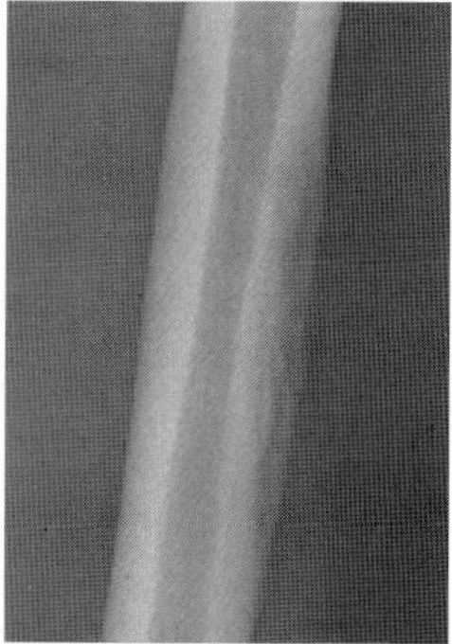

Figure 62.64 Femoral shaft cortical metastasis from bronchogenic carcinoma.

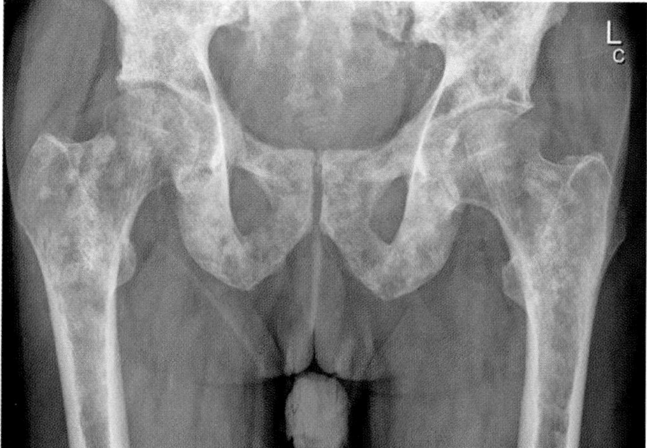

Figure 62.65 Diffuse sclerotic metastasis of prostate carcinoma.

Breast

Not only is this the most common primary tumor in women, but its metastases show a particularly affinity for bone, the skeleton being the most common site of metastatic breast cancer. The lesions are usually osteolytic and commonly multiple. Diffuse infiltration, however, may cause an apparently coarse trabecular pattern without an obvious area of bone destruction. The condition should be suspected in the presence of vertebral compression fractures in older women. Differentiation of these from osteoporotic collapse may be difficult, although, in the latter, evidence of focal areas of bone destruction on CT and MRI is usually lacking. Multiple lytic lesions may also resemble diffuse myeloma, but in that condition, the margins of the lucencies are sharply defined with endosteal scalloping and the serum alkaline phosphatase is usually normal.

About 10–20% of metastases from carcinoma of the breast produce osteoblastic lesions and in another 10% the lesions are mixed [46]. Sclerosis may occur in lytic lesions following successful hormone or radiation therapy.

Difficulty may be experienced in differentiating between intense disuse osteoporosis following radiotherapy and metastatic disease. This problem arises particularly around the shoulder where the bones have been included in the radiation field. The lesions of intense disuse osteoporosis tend to be sharply defined and ellipsoid in the long axis of the bone. Similarly, multiple rib fractures secondary to radiation therapy should not be mistaken for metastases. Often such fractures occur at the edge of the radiation field and consequently tend to be in a line, a distribution observed also in acute trauma and osteomalacia.

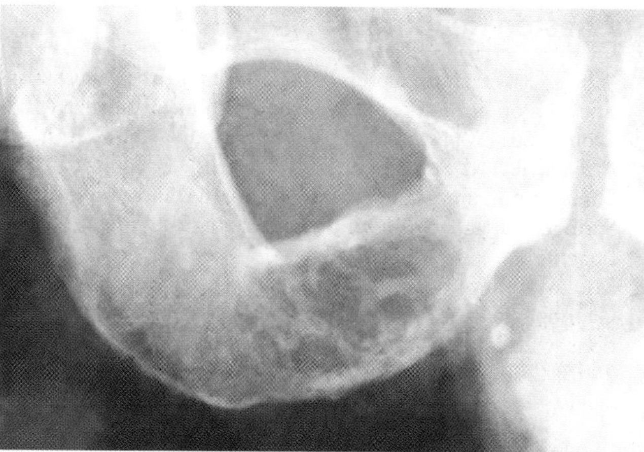

Figure 62.66 Example of solitary metastasis in pubic bone from renal cell carcinoma. The lesion is expansile and have crenellated margins, with trabeculation in the lesion.

Prostate

This is the commonest secondary bone tumor in men and, in contrast to breast deposits; almost all these metastases are sclerotic. They appear as round or oval areas of increased density, particularly in the pelvis and spine, growing slowly and merging so that widespread and diffuse increase in bone density may ensue. Periosteal new bone formation and/or apparent expansion of bone may occur, so that the differentiation from Paget's disease may be difficult. The deposits may be shown to regress with hormone therapy. In some patients, metastases from the prostate may be osteolytic.

Lung

This tumor is the third most common cancer to spread to bone, with such bone lesions occurring eventually in about a third of patients. These metastases are almost always lytic and may develop in unusual locations, occurring in the small bones of the hand or eccentrically in the cortex of a long bone.

Kidney

The skeleton is the second most common site of renal cell carcinoma metastasis after the lung. Renal cell carcinoma metastases have a predilection for the pelvis and lumbar spine. These lesions are typically expansile with a crenelated margin and usually have a typical radiological appearance (Fig. 62.66). They are often purely lytic in nature and thus may be occult on the delayed phase images of bone scintigrams. On MRI, the rich vascularization of renal cell carcinoma metastases may be manifested as flow voids, scattered, or tubular foci of low signal on all sequences. Transcatheter embolization of a renal cell cancer metastasis should be considered before surgical treatments in view of this rich vascularity.

Alimentary Tract

Bone metastasis from colorectal carcinoma is uncommon, and usually lytic or mixed in radiographic appearances. Gastric carcinoma and carcinoid metastasis are typically sclerotic.

Thyroid Carcinoma

Bone metastasis in thyroid carcinoma is typically lytic, expansile, and hypervascular in a similar manner to renal cell carcinoma.

Suggested Readings

- WHO Classification of Tumours Editorial Board. WHO Classification of Tumours of Soft Tissue and Bone, fifth ed., IARC, Lyon 2020. (WHO classification of tumours; vol. 3).
- AM Davies, M Sundaram, SJ James, Eds., Imaging of Bone Tumors and Tumor-like Lesions: Techniques and Applications, Springer-Verlag, Berlin and Heidelberg 2009. (Diagnostic Imaging).
- MD Murphey, JJ Choi, MJ Kransdorf, DJ Flemming, FH Gannon, Imaging of osteochondroma: variants and complications with radiologic-pathologic correlation, Radiographics. 20 (5) (2000) 1407–1434.
- H Douis, A Saifuddin, The imaging of cartilaginous bone tumours. II. Chondrosarcoma, Skeletal Radiol 42 (5) (2013) 611–626.
- JW Chai, SH Hong, J-Y Choi, YH Koh, JW Lee, J-A Choi, et al., Radiologic diagnosis of osteoid osteoma: from simple to challenging findings, Radiographics 30 (3) (2010) 737–749.
- G Yarmish, MJ Klein, J Landa, RA Lefkowitz, S Hwang, Imaging characteristics of primary osteosarcoma: nonconventional subtypes, Radiographics 30 (6) (2010) 1653–1672.
- R Erlemann, Imaging and differential diagnosis of primary bone tumors and tumor-like lesions of the spine, Eur J Radiol. 58 (1) (2006) 48–67.
- GJ O'Sullivan, FL Carty, CG Cronin, Imaging of bone metastasis: an update, World J Radiol 7 (8) (2015) 202–211.

63

Bone Tumor Mimics

RAMANAN RAJAKULASINGAM, STEVEN JAMES, RAJESH BOTCHU

Introduction

Focal bony lesions are encountered very frequently by all radiologists. Although some may be true lesions, many are normal variants, developmental, congenital, metabolic, infection, and trauma related. A classical location and imaging appearances usually allow the vast majority to be dismissed as a "pseudolesion," mimicking a bone tumor. If misdiagnosed, it may lead to unnecessary imaging follow-up and even invasive investigations such as biopsy, resulting in increased patient anxiety. We outline the most common pseudolesions, stating how they can be differentiated from more concerning pathology. The majority can be diagnosed purely on radiographs, stressing the importance it plays in being the first-line investigation and often only technique needed for diagnosis.

Normal Variants

Ward's Triangle of the Femur

- *Ward's triangle is a space within the center of the femoral neck formed by the intersection of principal compressive, secondary compressive, and tensile trabecular bundles* (Fig. 63.1) [1]. The quantity of trabeculation changes with patient age and follows that of underlying osteoporosis. Singh et al. have proposed a grading system to reflect the changes ranging from grade 6 (normal) to grade 1 (severe osteoporosis) [2]. Grade 4 is considered between borderline osteoporotic and normal skeleton.
- In the lower grades, there is a lack of trabecular structure and so the ward's triangle lucency is less well seen. In the higher grades, it is more well defined giving the appearance of an underlying lytic lesion. Radiologists should be aware that alternating areas of more and less trabeculae can give rise to a pseudolesion in this area.

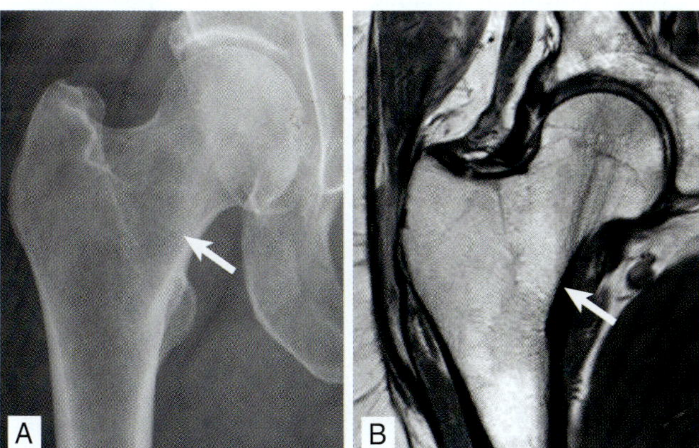

Figure 63.1 X-ray of the right hip joint shows an apparent lucency (*arrow*) at the femoral neck (A). This is formed by the intersection of compressive, secondary compressive, and tensile trabecular bundles in the femur and is termed "ward's triangle." Corresponding MRI shows normal marrow signal (*arrow* in B).

Humeral Pseudocyst

- *The superolateral portion of the proximal humeral head can appear lucent* suggesting an underlying lesion, such as giant cell tumor or chondroblastoma. This is a normal pseudolucency which can appear pathological, with some cases depicting ill-defined borders. It should be noted that the inferomedial margin of the lucency is centered over the fusion line between the greater tuberosity, humeral head, and humeral shaft (Fig. 63.2) [3].
- As with Ward's triangle of the femur, the lucency may be less apparent in osteoporotic patients due to the lack of surrounding trabeculae. In some cases, subsequent MR images will show prominent fatty marrow signal at this location (Fig. 63.2C) [4].

Calcaneal Pseudocyst

- *The outlining trabecular pattern in the anterior calcaneus can give rise to a pseudolucency* (Fig. 63.3). However, many pathologies such as simple bone cysts and intraosseous lipomas also occur in this location which have their own defining features. Intraosseous lipomas are perhaps the most common lesion in this area and are identified by their sclerotic margin and areas of punctuate central calcification in chronic cases (Cockade sign).

Prominent Radial Tuberosity

- *The radial tuberosity is a normal anatomical structure where the biceps tendon inserts distally*. However, it can appear as a poorly defined lucent area, especially on a lateral projection radiograph (Fig. 63.4) [5]. Variations in appearances are due to a broad or thin insertion of the distal biceps tendon.
- The abnormality typically disappears or becomes less apparent on anterior posterior (AP) radiographs therefore reviewing all the projections is crucial in avoiding a misdiagnosis.

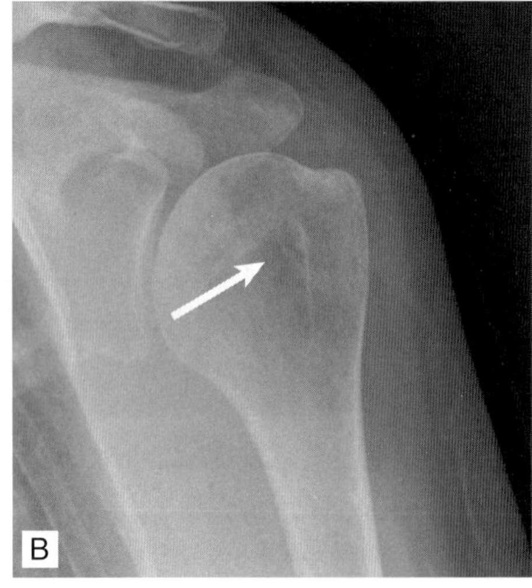

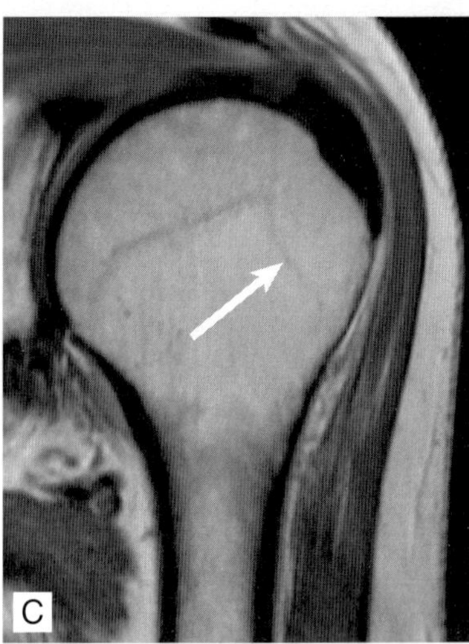

Figure 63.2 An apparent lucent lesion is seen to occupy the superolateral portion of the humeral head involving the greater tuberosity (A). The location is classical for a pseudocyst. Although most have a well-defined demarcation to the surrounding bone, some can appear ill defined (B). MRI (C) may show decreased traversing trabeculae and prominent marrow fat content.

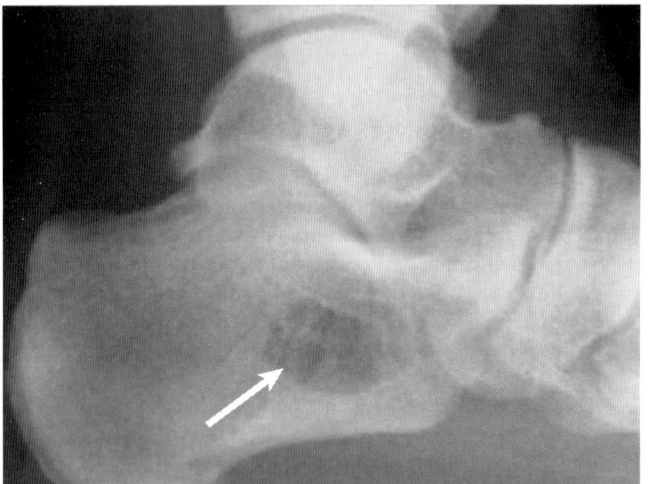

Figure 63.3 This figure shows an apparent lucency at the anterior calcaneum with normal traversing trabeculae. Please note, however, that actual bone lesions can develop in this region including intraosseous lipoma and cysts. The central dystrophic calcification is typical and, if present, helps to distinguish this lesion from a bone cyst or pseudolesion.

Prominent Deltoid Tuberosity

- *The deltoid tuberosity is an elongated v-shaped area on the anterolateral portion of the mid humeral shaft which corresponds to the deltoid muscle attachment* (Fig. 63.5). In roughly 10% of cases, it can appear very prominent giving the appearances of a pseudolesion. This area if prominent commonly shows uptake on bone scintigraphy and is termed the "delta sign [6]." It is believe to be due to increased affinity of the tracer for cortical thickening at the tuberosity [6].

Focal Nodular Marrow Hyperplasia

- Diffuse red marrow hyperplasia is a relatively common finding on magnetic resonance imaging (MRI) and has been attributed to patients with underlying chronic anemia, malignancy and various other medical conditions [7]. Focal nodular marrow hyperplasia (FNMH) displays a limited but similar imaging appearance reflecting proliferation of focal red marrow. Although entirely benign, it has the appearances of a pseudotumor potentially resulting in misdiagnosis, especially in the setting of a patient with known primary malignancy.

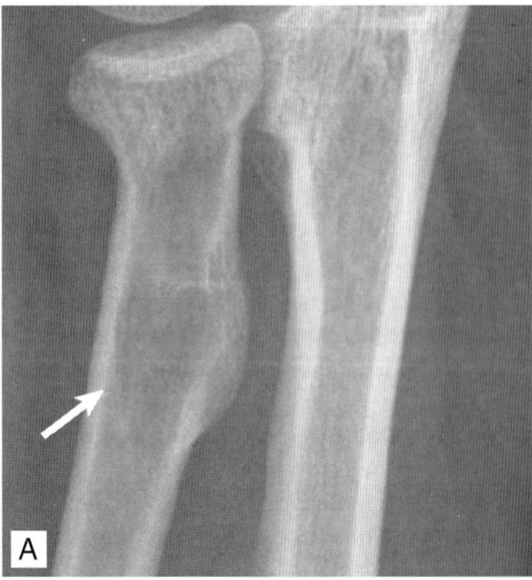

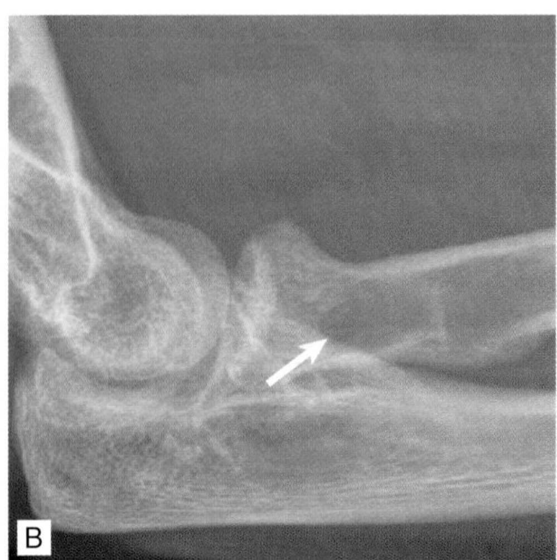

Figure 63.4 This figure shows an apparent lucency at the radial tuberosity. Note how the pseudolesion appears slightly less defined on the AP projection (A) compared to the lateral projection (B) where it is viewed enface. This landmark relates to the insertion of the distal biceps tendon.

Figure 63.5 X-ray shows bony irregularity and lucency at the deltoid muscle insertion on the proximal humerus. Smooth, well-defined borders and characteristic location are pathognomonic for a pseudolesion here. Differing appearances in the amount of cortical thickening may be due to irregularity and thickness at the level of the deltoid insertion. Some have suggested the lucency may even represent a focal herniation pit.

- It is commonly seen in the vertebra, but also in the femur and pelvic bones [7].
- *Iso- to hyperintense T1 signal of the lesion compared with skeletal muscle is crucial in first identifying the absence of marrow infiltration* (Fig. 63.6) [7]. *Second, chemical shift imaging (CSI) can be used to highlight microscopic fat content, showing signal drop off more than 20% between in and out of phase MRI sequences* (Figs. 63.6 and 63.7) [8]. In cases when there is less than 20% drop off; computed tomography (CT) is useful to look for areas of obvious or subtle sclerosis to possibly account for this (Fig. 63.6) [8].

Congenital and Developmental Abnormalities

Synovial Herniation Pit of the Femur

- A well-defined round- or oval-shaped lucency at the junction of the proximal femoral head and neck is called a synovial herniation pit (Fig. 63.8). It is believe to represent herniation of synovium into cortical defects at the head–neck junction due to subtle erosions of the hip joint capsule into the femoral neck [5]. Radiologically, they are typically less than 1 cm in size and lucent with a sclerotic margin. *Importantly, no central nidus is seen differentiating it from an osteoid osteoma.*
- Although once considered asymptomatic and a normal anatomical variant, there has been an association with femoroacetabular impingement. *They are now considered a radiological indicator of possible femoroacetabular impingement* [9]. On MRI the lesion is seen to show uniform low T1 signal, and tends to have anterior cortical extension [10]. *The anterosuperior lateral quadrant of the femoral neck, ovoid shape, and 1-cm size are quite classical imaging appearances for a synovial herniation pit.*

Dorsal Defect of the Patella

- *Dorsal defect of the patella represents a focal subchondral defect in the superolateral portion of the patella.* It appears as a rounded 1–2-cm lucency in the upper outer quadrant, a similar location to where a bipartite patella is seen (Fig. 63.9) [11]. *The location is important in distinguishing this from a focal area of*

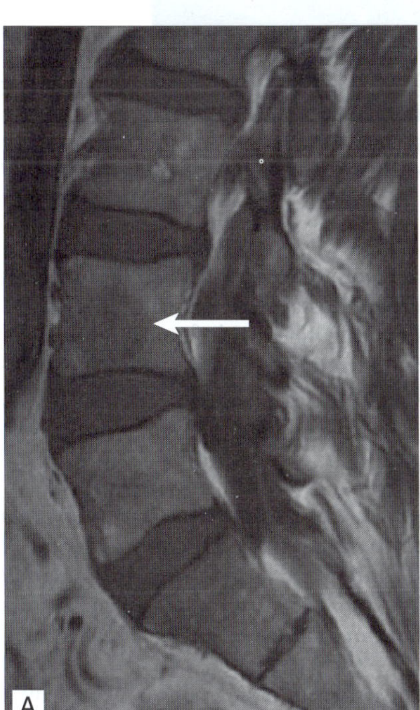

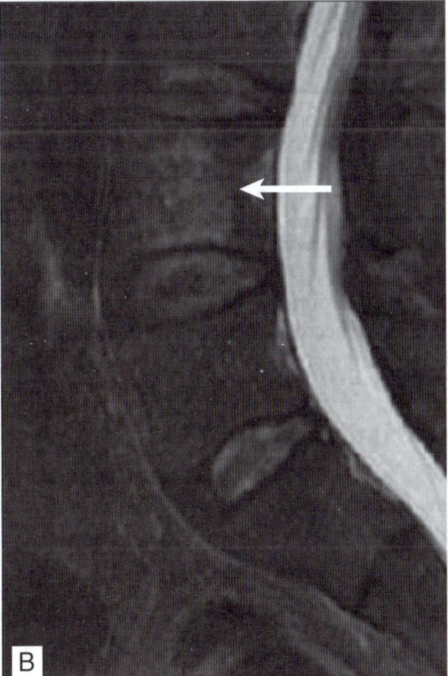

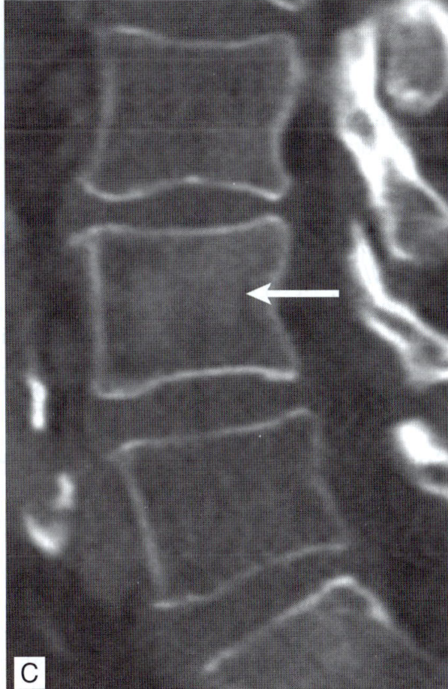

Figure 63.6 Sagittal T1W image (A) shows a poorly defined lesion with reduced signal but slightly hyperintense to skeletal muscle in the L4 vertebral body. It demonstrates mildly increased short tau inversion recovery (STIR) signal (B). A similar lesion in a different patient at L4 (C) shows mild medullary sclerosis consistent with FNMH which may account for CSI drop <20% on out of phase MRI sequences.

TABLE 63.3 Differential Diagnosis of Radiation Osteitis

Differential Diagnosis	Differentiating Imaging Features
Paget disease	Focal bony expansion
Radiation-induced sarcoma	Possible soft-tissue mass, aggressive changes appear years after therapy
Recurrent malignancy	Bone destruction and/or soft-tissue mass

- The differential diagnosis of radiation osteitis includes radiation-induced sarcoma, recurrent malignancy, and Paget disease. Table 63.3 outlines some useful differentiating features. Clearly, a history of radiation therapy and stability of imaging appearances over time would also support radiation osteitis.

Hemophilic Pseudotumor

- In hemophilia patients, minimal trauma can cause bleeding into muscles, joints, and bony cavities. This can result in pseudotumors which initially occur as areas of post-traumatic or spontaneous hemorrhage [50]. Repetitive bleeding into the hematoma can lead to rapid expansion of the mass.
- On radiographs, pseudotumors appear as areas of soft-tissue density (Fig. 63.33), with possible internal calcific foci and ground glass appearance. Repetitive bleeding over time may cause erosion of the adjacent bone or denervation of adjacent muscle [51]. Pathological fracture with uncontrolled bleeding is the most severe consequence.
- The pseudotumors are usually in the muscle themselves adjacent to bone with the bones being secondarily involved.

Sarcoidosis

- The musculoskeletal manifestations of sarcoidosis are rather nonspecific and ill-defined unlike its thoracic counterpart. However, small bone imaging features especially in the hands are well documented.
- Changes typically affect the second and third phalanges and include dactylitis if acute [52]. The classic lace like, honeycomb pattern of osteolysis is said to be pathognomonic (Fig. 63.34) [52]. On MRI, lesions display low T1w, high T2w signal making sure to look for extra cortical involvement which is usually under visualized on radiographs [52].

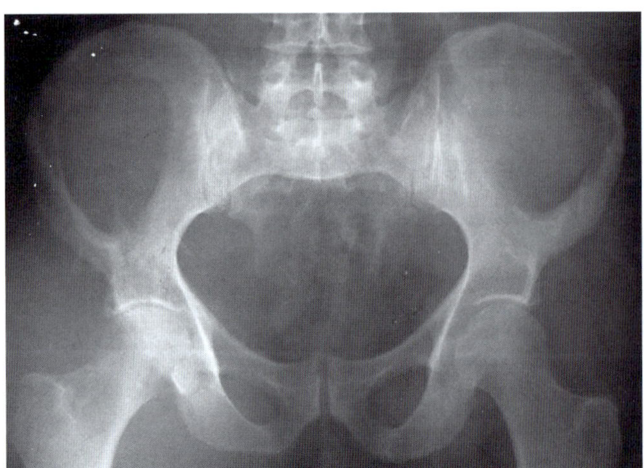

Figure 63.33 Radiograph showing lobulated lucencies with traversing septations projected over the iliac wings bilaterally consistent with intramuscular hemophilic pseudotumors.

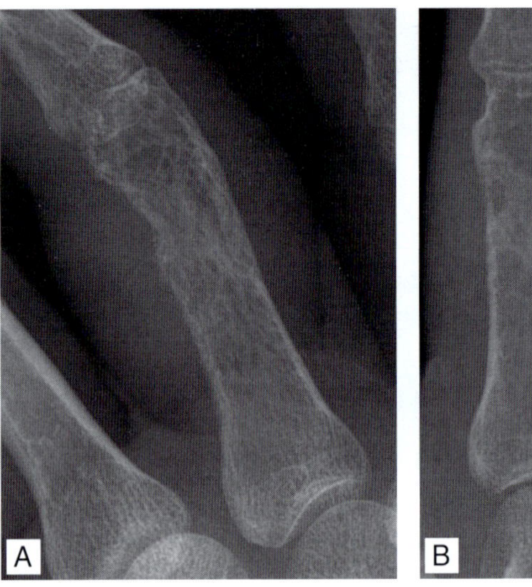

Figure 63.34 Oblique (A) and anteroposterior (B) radiographs of the third metacarpal showing a lytic lace like trabeculation pattern. No erosions or areas of cortical destruction are seen, consistent with sarcoidosis.

- Nail thickening may also be seen. Large bone sarcoidosis is usually seen as focal areas of lysis without cortical involvement in the long bones [53,54]. MRI shows round and irregular areas of confluent marrow infiltration of intermediate T1w and T2w signal [53,54].
- Soft-tissue nodules are far commoner than bone changes.
- Periarticular calcification due to hypercalcemia occurs in 20–45% of cases of sarcoid.
- Arthritis is a common manifestation, occurring in up to 37% of patients, most commonly in females. In the acute form, joint destruction does not occur but, in chronic disease, a destructive arthropathy of large joints does rarely occur due to local granulomas.

Intraosseous Muscle Transfer

- Local muscle flap transfers/transposition are commonly used to provide soft-tissue cover for bony defects in reconstructive surgery. In the pelvis, common muscle flaps are harvested from the sartorius or rectus abdominus muscles. Another common surgery is termed posterior lateral iliopsoas transplantation [55]. Here, the iliopsoas muscle is transferred to the posterolateral proximal femur. This is often bilateral and so surgical augmentation from posterior lateral iliopsoas transplantation can result in seeing bilateral lucent lesions projected over the iliac bones on radiographs.
- A rare lower limb procedure is gastrocnemius muscle transfer [56]. Here, the gastrocnemius muscle is used to cover defects around the knee including the proximal tibia where surgery can result in large osseous defects (Fig. 63.35).
- The flap often shows similar signal characteristics and striations to surrounding muscles, and radiologists should look for a vascularized pedicle. Over time, there may well be progressive peripheral ossification, internal muscular fatty atrophy with some T1- and T2-weighted signal changes especially in cases were radiation has been used [57].

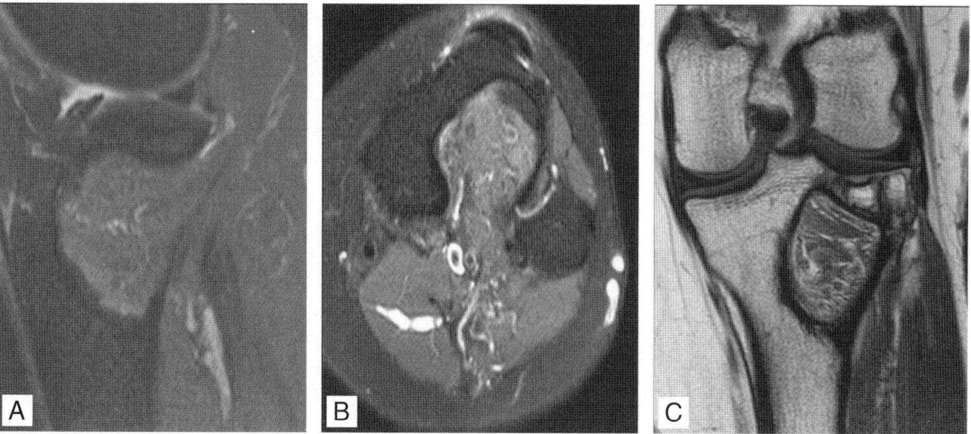

Figure 63.35 Sagittal PD FS (A) and axial STIR (B) images of the proximal tibia showing a pedicled lateral gastrocnemius intraosseous muscle transfer. (C) demonstrates internal muscular striations with a sclerotic rim.

Langerhans Cell Histiocytosis

- LCH has been previously described as *mimicking any bony lesion, in particular Ewing sarcoma*. Radiological manifestations in the spine and skull vault are well documented consisting of vertebra plana (Fig. 63.36) and a lucent lesion with a beveled edge, respectively (Fig. 63.37) [58].
- LCH in the pelvis, extremities, and long bones presents as an expansile lytic lesion with a moderately aggressive bone destruction pattern (Lodwick Type 1b or 2) [59], an intact but expanded cortex and either absent or laminated periosteal response (Fig. 63.38) [13].
- The lesion itself tends to be small, with *florid surrounding marrow edema, typically many times the size of the lesion* not typical of Ewings sarcoma [33]. A soft-tissue component if present is usually eccentric and not circumferential.
- MRI signs include a hypointense rim, so-called "budding" and "bulging" sign (Fig. 63.38). Rare features include subacute hemorrhage, fluid–fluid levels, the penumbra sign and even more rare is matrix calcification similar to that of a chondral lesion [33,60].

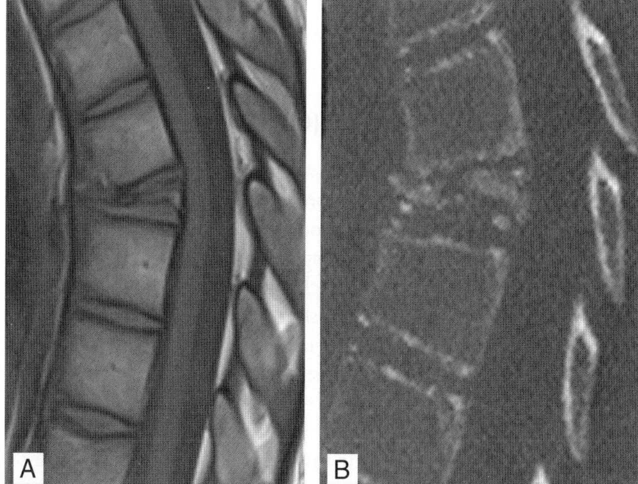

Figure 63.36 Sagittal T1 MRI (A) shows complete collapse of the T7 vertebral body, with fragmentation and resulting sclerosis better visualized on CT (B). Imaging appearances are consistent with vertebra plana.

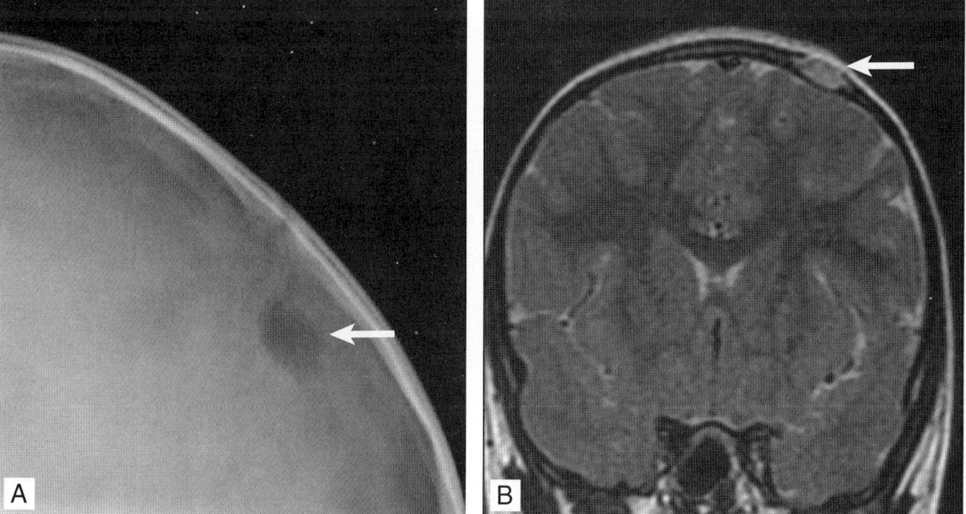

Figure 63.37 Skull radiograph shows an irregular focus of lucency (*arrow*) (A) within the left frontal bone with minimal surrounding sclerosis. MRI confirms that the abnormality is arising from the skull vault itself, with mild indentation of the underlying frontoparietal brain parenchyma (B). The appearances are classical for LCH.

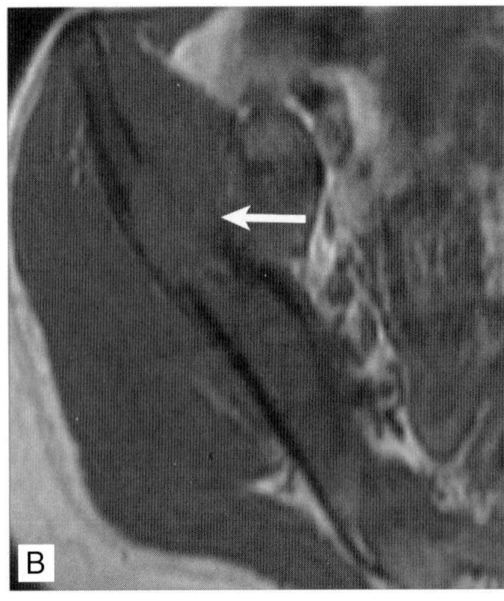

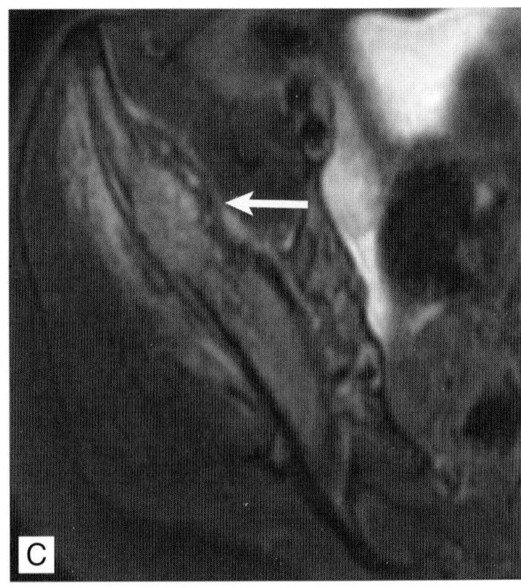

Figure 63.38 AP radiograph (A) demonstrates a slightly ill-defined lobular lytic lesion (*arrow*) in the iliac wing and acetabulum. Axial T1 (B) MRI shows a slightly hyperintense T1 lesion with a relatively sharp margin to surrounding bone. (B) and axial T2FS (C) show bulging of the medial and lateral bony margins of the ilium with focal medial cortical break through or "budding," (*arrow* in B). Note the extensive soft-tissue and bone marrow edema with associated periosteal reaction. CT biopsy confirmed Langerhans cell histiocytosis as the underlying diagnosis.

Vanishing Bone Disease (Gorham Stout Disease)

This relatively rare syndrome is a variant of angiomatosis of bone in which vascular proliferation predominates. Its origin is unknown. It is recognized usually in childhood, but more than one-third of patients is over the age of 35. Progressive weakness and limitation of movement of the affected area characterize the onset. Pain is not an early feature, although obviously occurring with a pathological fracture. After a period of months or years the limb becomes useless or flail. The course is unpredictable, either stabilizing or progressing fatally with the development of chylothorax.

Radiologically an ill-defined area of radiolucency may be observed in a single bone, but this destructive process progresses slowly to involve adjacent bones without respect for intervening joints (Fig. 63.39). Symptoms, however, may be so insidious that extensive absorption of many adjacent bony structures may be revealed at the initial examination. Arteriography and lymphography have shown no connection of these lesions to either the vascular or lymphatic circulations.

The radiological appearance is consequently that of a diffuse increase in translucency with progressive absorption of the affected structures. In the course of the process, deformity is likely to develop and may be crippling. Although local recurrence is a major hazard, slow progression is the rule.

Similar massive osteolysis may occur with tumorous masses of lymphatic origin (*lymphangiomatosis*). Histological differentiation of the cavernous spaces that are found may be difficult and the radiological features are virtually identical.

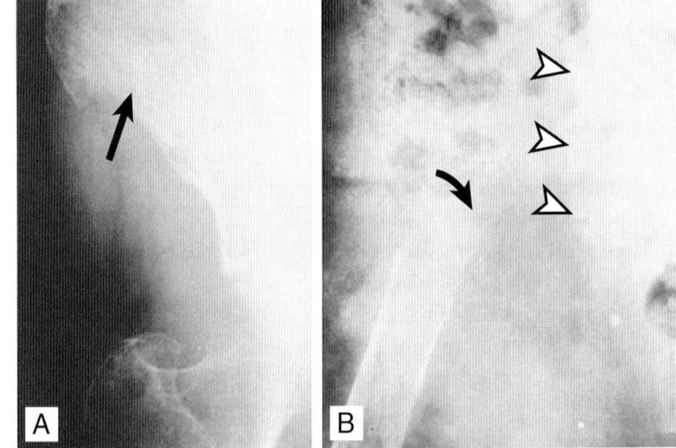

Figure 63.39 Radiograph of hip (A) shows lucency over the right iliac bone (*arrow*). Follow-up radiograph (B) shows progressive bony resorption in iliac bone (*arrowheads*). A corresponding pathological femoral fracture is also seen (*curved black arrow*). Findings are consistent with Gorham Stout disease.

Implantation Dermoid Cyst

These rare lesions usually follow a penetrating wound associated with a crush fracture, when it is assumed that epithelial cells are carried into the underlying bony structure. Typically, they arise in distal phalanges of adolescents or young adults, the left middle finger being the single commonest site. The lesion grows slowly over many years.

Radiologically a well-defined translucency results, with slight expansion and sharply defined margins around which a minimal sclerotic reaction may be visible (Fig. 63.40). Subungual fibromas

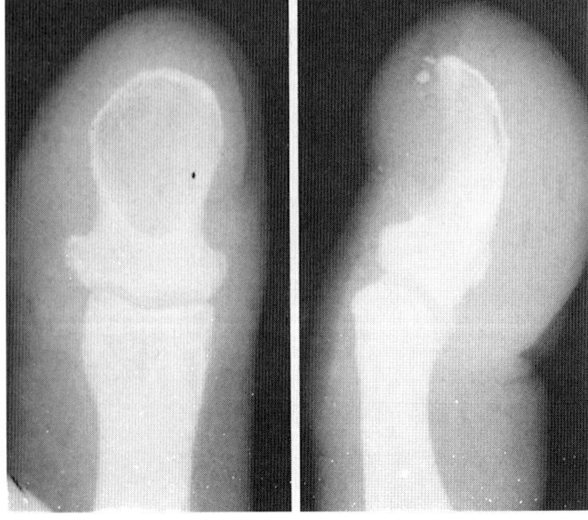

Figure 63.40 There is an expansile lytic lesion in the distal phalanx with a thin intact cortical rim, in keeping with an epidermoid cyst.

represent the only serious differential diagnostic possibility. A glomus tumor is almost invariably extraosseous.

Overall Approach

We have highlighted a number of pseudolesions commonly encountered. In most, the location and radiographic appearances are enough to confirm them as pseudolesions. However, if there is clinical concern then dedicated cross-sectional imaging, usually MRI should be obtained to allow for further characterization. Some of these are considered "do not touch," lesions and so the radiologist should be vigilant of these mimics to avoid unnecessary scanning and invasive procedures.

Suggested Readings

- V De Wilde, M De Maeseneer, L Lenchik, et al., Normal osseous variants presenting as cystic or lucent areas on radiography and CT imaging: a pictorial overview, EJOR 51 (1) (2004) 77–84.
- JN Mhuircheartaigh, YC Lin, JS Wu, Bone tumor mimickers: A pictorial essay, Indian J Radiol Imaging 24 (3) (2014) 225–236.

64

Soft Tissue Tumors

JENN SHIUNN WONG, RADHESH LALAM

Introduction

Soft tissue lesions are commonly encountered in the practice of radiologists, whereupon imaging findings together with a host of clinical features come together to allow characterization of these lesions. Soft tissue tumor is a heterogenous group of tumors derived from mesenchymal tissues, arising from either the multipotent mesenchymal stem cells, or from one of its many differentiated cell types (osteoblasts, chondrocytes, adipocytes, myocytes, cardiomyocytes, and neuronal cells). Soft tissue sarcoma is rare, while benign mesenchymal soft tissue tumors are more common (benign to malignant ratio of 18:1) [1]. Soft tissue sarcoma represents approximately 1% of all cancers in adults, incidence of which increases with increasing age. In the pediatric population however, while incidence is much lower, soft tissue sarcoma makes up a larger proportion (around 20%) of all pediatric cancers.

Imaging Techniques

Every imaging technique has a role in the assessment of soft tissue tumors, and there is no single perfect imaging technique for assessing every single lesion. Imaging features are often nonspecific, and histological correlation may be required for definitive diagnosis.

Ultrasonography (USG) is the preferred first-line technique in assessing a soft tissue lump. Following this, if required, magnetic resonance imaging (MRI) is usually the next preferred technique. Between these two techniques, majority of lesions can be managed appropriately before deciding if a lesion is benign or malignant (and will therefore need intervention), or indeterminate (which often need a biopsy or follow-up imaging). Radiography, computerized tomography (CT), and nuclear medicine can provide useful information and may clinch the diagnosis in certain situations, and these will be discussed in subsequent section.

Ultrasonography

USG is undoubtedly the best first-line imaging technique to investigate a new superficial soft tissue lump. It is relatively affordable, widely available, radiation free, and does not carry any contraindications. One of the greatest benefits lies in the opportunity for a face-to-face interaction between the radiologist and the patient. This brings about numerous advantages including ability to extract a targeted clinical history, carry out clinical examination, and perform dynamic imaging of the lump (such as compressibility and determining relationship with adjacent structures). All of these will provide invaluable clues leading to the final diagnosis.

USG can also differentiate between a cystic-appearing mass (such as a myxoid tumor) from a true cystic lesion. While a cyst appears anechoic, a myxoid lesion will appear heterogeneously hypoechoic, and these areas may demonstrate internal Doppler flow.

It is useful to have a clear strategy before embarking on an USG scan:

1. The main value lies in the ability of USG to provide a specific diagnosis to a wide range of benign conditions. The primary objective of the USG examination is to identify these conditions thereby decisively concluding the patient's workup and avoiding any further unnecessary investigations or interventions. Examples of such conditions are listed in Table 64.1
2. If imaging features are equivocal or suspicious during the initial USG scan, further imaging or referral will be required

When performing an examination of a lump on USG, several features should be assessed for (Table 64.2). There are a few notable features worth expanding on, which may either be of diagnostic value or may change subsequent management:

- *Location:* Location of certain lesions can be specific enough for USG to make a confident diagnosis. These include palmar and plantar aponeurosis (Dupuytren's nodule and plantar fibroma respectively); subscapular location (elastofibroma); intermetatarsal location (Morton's neuroma)
- *Relationship to a nerve or tendon sheath:* Oval lesion arising from a nerve points to peripheral nerve sheath tumor (PNST). Giant cell tumor (GCT) of tendon sheath has an intimate

TABLE 64.1 List of Presenting Benign Lumps That Can Be Accurately Diagnosed Based on USG Features Alone

Normal variants	Asymmetry in rib contours, accessory muscles, asymmetrical muscle hypertrophy
Nontumoral lumps	Ganglion, tenosynovitis, bursa, foreign bodies, degenerative and hypertrophic asymmetric sternoclavicular joint, muscle hernias, rheumatoid nodules, gouty tophus, muscle tears, neuroma's including traumatic or Morton's neuroma, epidermoid cyst, hematoma, Morel–Lavallée lesion, cysticercosis
Benign tumors	Lipoma, Dupuytren's nodule and plantar fibroma, peripheral nerve sheath tumor, vascular malformation

TABLE 64.2 List of USG Characteristics That Should Be Assessed for During Examination of a Soft Tissue Lump

Features	Assessment
Location	Superficial (dermal, epidermal, subcutaneous, fascial), or deep (subfascial, intermuscular, intramuscular), subungual
Appearance and morphology	Size (all three dimensions), shape, well or poorly defined margin, echopattern, solid/cystic, acoustic transmission, calcification
Compressibility	Compressible or noncompressible
Relationship to adjacent structures	Neurovascular bundle, tendon (including dynamic imaging), bone
Vascularity	Presence and degree of vascularity, peripheral or intralesional
Invasion	Invading between different planes of tissue
Others	Compare with contralateral side if applicable, multiplicity

relationship with the tendon sheath and does not move during tendon flexion or extension (Fig. 64.1)

- *Clinical assessment:* Superficial nodules in a patient with clinical features of rheumatoid arthritis may represent rheumatoid nodules. Similarly, gouty tophi have a yellow–white appearance (Fig. 64.2). Tinel's sign points to PNST. A soft tissue lump close to a caesarean scar may suggest an endometrioma
- *Calcification:* Presence of calcification in a lesion brings with it a wide range of differentials, both benign and malignant (including benign ossifying fasciitis, synovial chondromatosis, myositis ossificans, hemangioma, lipoma variant, gout, tumoral calcinosis, foreign bodies, chondrosarcoma, synovial sarcoma) (Fig. 64.3). One should consider performing at least a radiograph in the first instance for further characterization. The pattern of calcification/ossification can sometimes be useful (centripetally progressing ossification in myositis ossificans, ring-shaped calcifications (phleboliths) in hemangiomas and vascular malformations)
- *Underlying bone:* A soft tissue lesion may cause underlying bone erosion, for example, foreign body granuloma, gout. Soft tissue lump may arise from underlying bone. If there is suspicion of underlying bone involvement, further imaging may be warranted, starting with a radiograph (Fig. 64.4)
- *Compressibility:* Cystic-appearing spaces on USG, if compressible, may suggest a venous vascular malformation (Fig. 64.5). Lymphatic vascular malformation on the other hand is not compressible [2]. Other apparently compressible lesions include lipoma and Morel–Lavallée lesions
- *Twinkling artifact on Doppler USG:* Twinkling artifact in a well-defined soft tissue lump is highly specific for epidermoid cyst (Fig. 64.6). It can also be seen in trichilemmal cyst

USG findings are often able to differentiate a malignant soft tissue tumor from a benign lesion. If features have not been characteristic enough to provide a specific benign diagnosis, one should now determine the likelihood of the lesion being malignant. Features raising concern for malignancy are:

- Rapid growth clinically
- Presence of pain
- Size >5 cm
- Deep location (situated deep to the deep fascia)
- Significant intralesional vascularity (especially if chaotic and disorganized pattern) [3]
- Ill-defined margins (Fig. 64.7)
- Fascial plane invasion
- Known history of primary malignant tumor
- Recurring lump at site of surgery, regardless of previous histology

Presence of one or more of the above features should prompt further imaging, usually with an MRI. Needless to say, none of

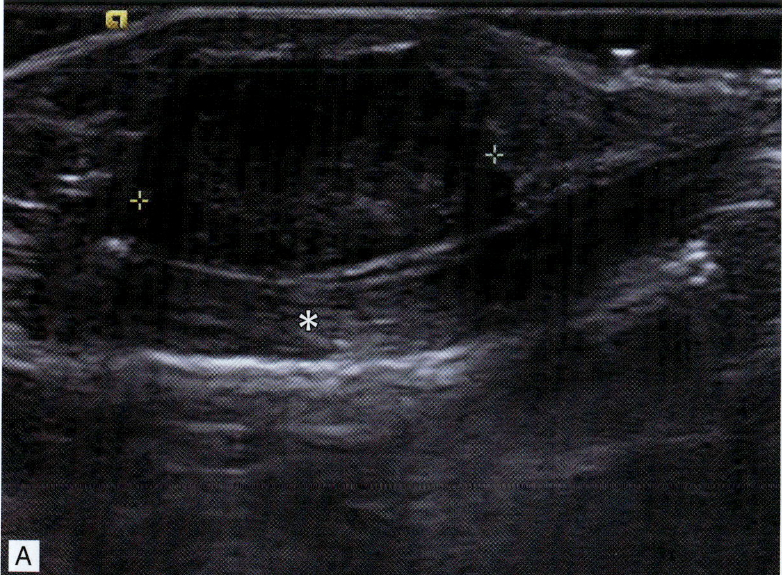

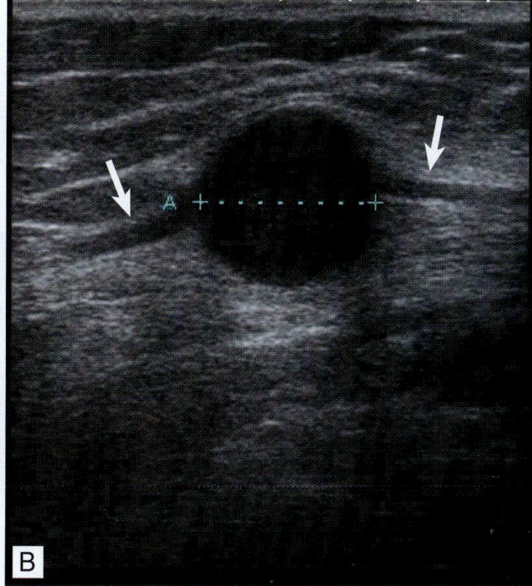

Figure 64.1 Close relationship of soft tissue lesions provides clue to the underlying etiology. (A) USG image shows a solid lobulated lesion intimately related to the underlying flexor tendon sheath. GCT of tendon sheath is the top differential (and was indeed histologically proven). As the lesion is attached onto the tendon sheath, rather than the tendon (*asterisk*), the lesion should remain static during flexion/extension of the finger. (B) PNST typically has a round or oval morphology, and a nerve can often be traced to enter and exit (*arrows*) the lesion on USG.

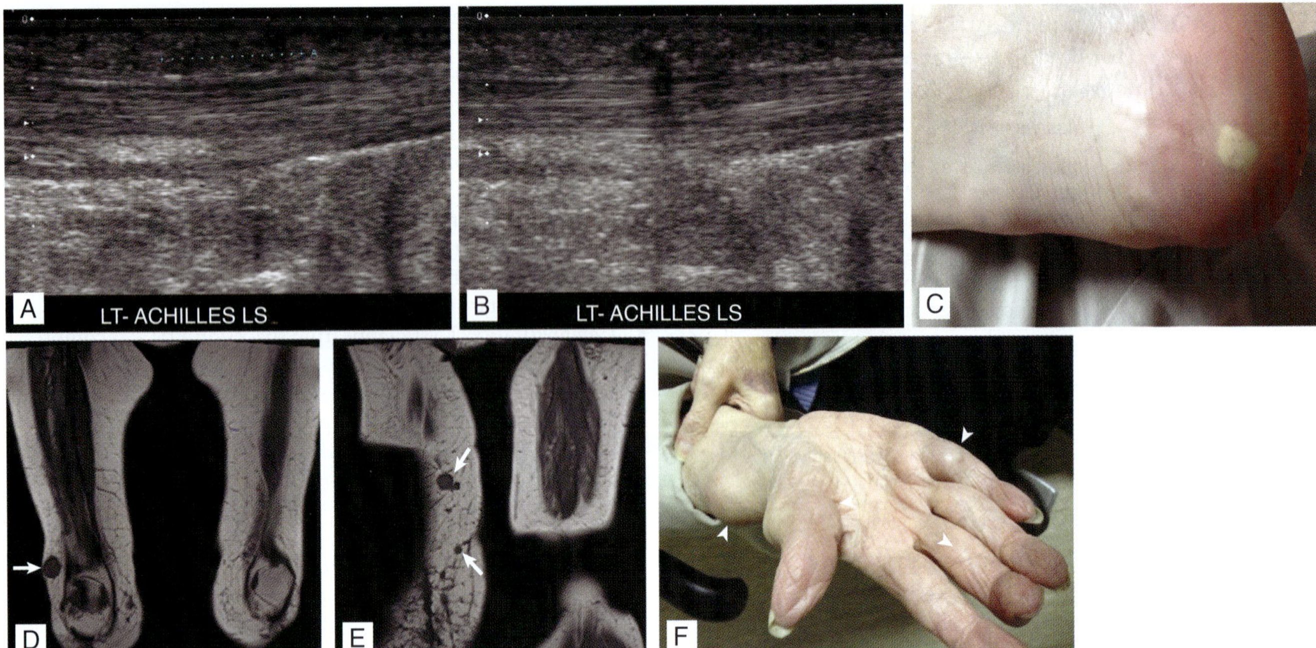

Figure 64.2 Correlate lumps with clinical inspection and medical history. (A) and (B) USG images demonstrating nonspecific superficial calcification in the subcutaneous tissue over the heel. (C) On inspection, the lump has the typical yellow–white appearance, allowing confident diagnosis of a gouty tophus. In a another patient, (D) and (E) are T1w coronal images of the thighs, demonstrating multiple superficial nodules (*arrows*). Appearances were nonspecific, so the patient was recalled for USG examination. (F) When the patient attended her appointment, on clinical inspection, it was evident the patient suffers from rheumatoid arthritis and that these are multiple rheumatoid nodules, also seen in her hands (*arrowheads*).

these features are perfect. For example, many benign lesions will have ill-defined margins (including hemangioma, scar tissue, and inflammatory mass). Furthermore, benign vascular malformation and hemangioma will demonstrate intralesional Doppler flow. A lesion showing invasion through the deep fascia should also raise concern; however invasive nature can also be seen in benign lesions (including fibromatosis, vascular malformation).

Elastography

Elastography is an emerging technique centered around estimating tissue stiffness, providing another layer of assessment over that of B-mode and Doppler imaging. There are a few elastography techniques available, with the main two being strain elastography and shear wave elastography. Elastography has clinical applications across different subspecialties including imaging of liver fibrosis, distinguishing malignancies in breast, thyroid, and prostate. Within musculoskeletal imaging, it is being investigated for a wide range of areas such as imaging of tendons, fascia, ligaments, carpal tunnels, and musculoskeletal soft tissue tumors.

There is currently no uniform consensus in the use of elastography in the assessment of soft tissue lesions with mixed results in both strain and shear wave elastography [3,4]. Some authors reported that the addition of shear wave elastography has not improved diagnosis accuracy over what can already be achieved with B-mode and Doppler USG [3,4] (Fig. 64.8).

Part of the difficulty with elastography in musculoskeletal soft tissue lesions lies in the fact that sarcoma is a vastly heterogenous group of tumors, with a wide-ranging tissue lineage such as adipose, fibrous, cartilage, muscles, nervous, and vascular tissues. Therefore, to dictate a cutoff value of elasticity whereby a lesion is considered malignant is arbitrary and cannot

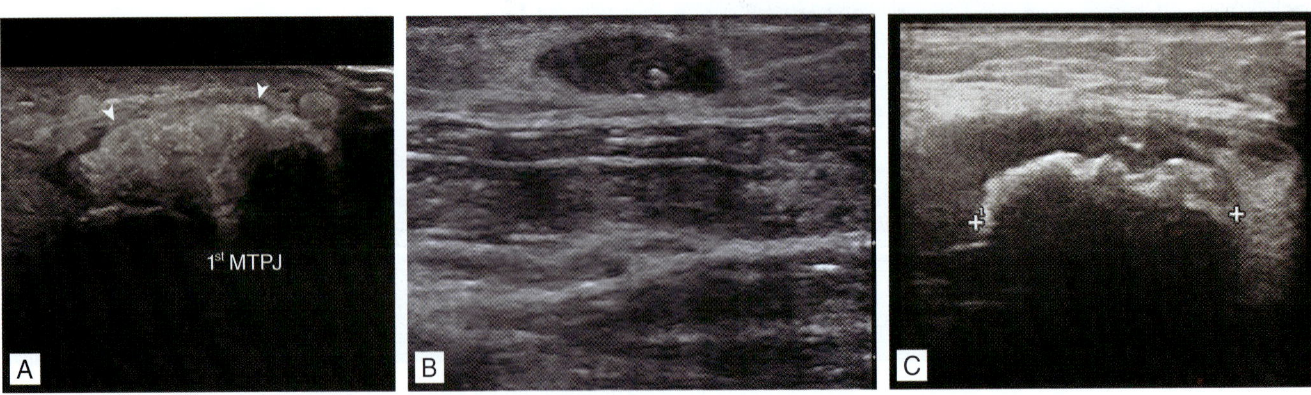

Figure 64.3 Calcification on USG. (A) Amorphous calcification (*arrowheads*) adjacent to the first metatarsophalangeal joint (MTPJ), proven histologically, to be crystal deposition. (B) Focus of phlebolith in a soft tissue mass which is slightly compressible and has internal vascularity (not shown), in keeping with a hemangioma. (C) Layer of ossification seen in this soft tissue mass (chondrosarcoma).

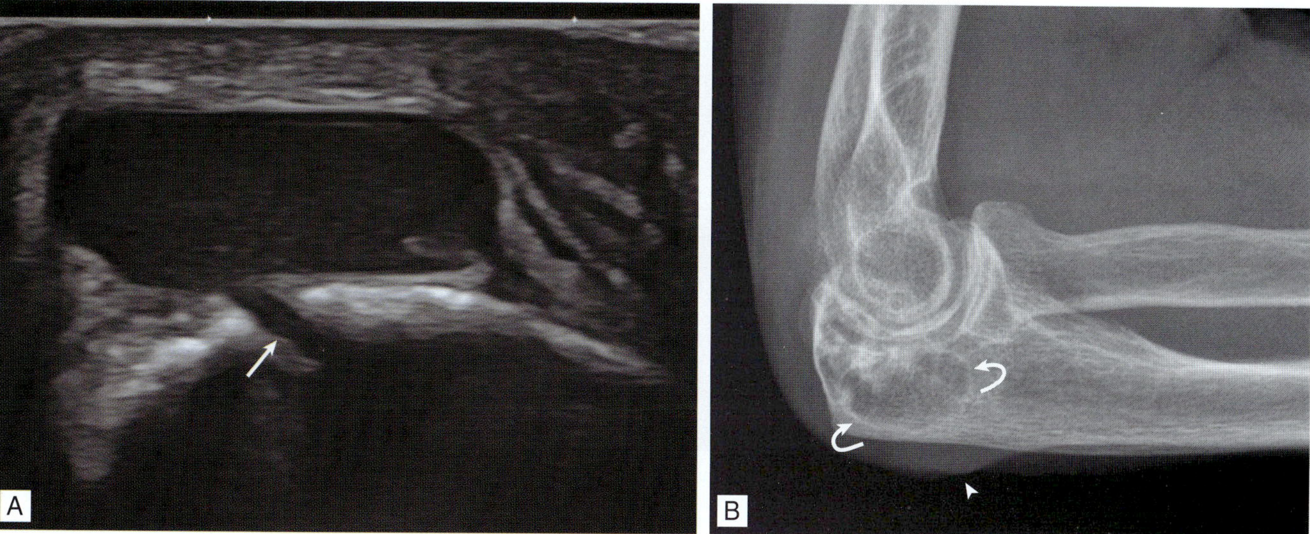

Figure 64.4 A 64-year-old female presenting with a lump on the dorsal aspect of the elbow. (A) USG revealed a well-defined hypoechoic, almost anechoic lump. Careful interrogation revealed the lump to have a neck (*arrow*) arising through the cortex of the underlying ulna. (B) This prompted a radiograph which also demonstrated the soft tissue lump (*arrowhead*), revealing a large geode (*curved arrows*) in the olecranon on background of osteoarthritis. Appearance is that of a geode with extraosseous extension.

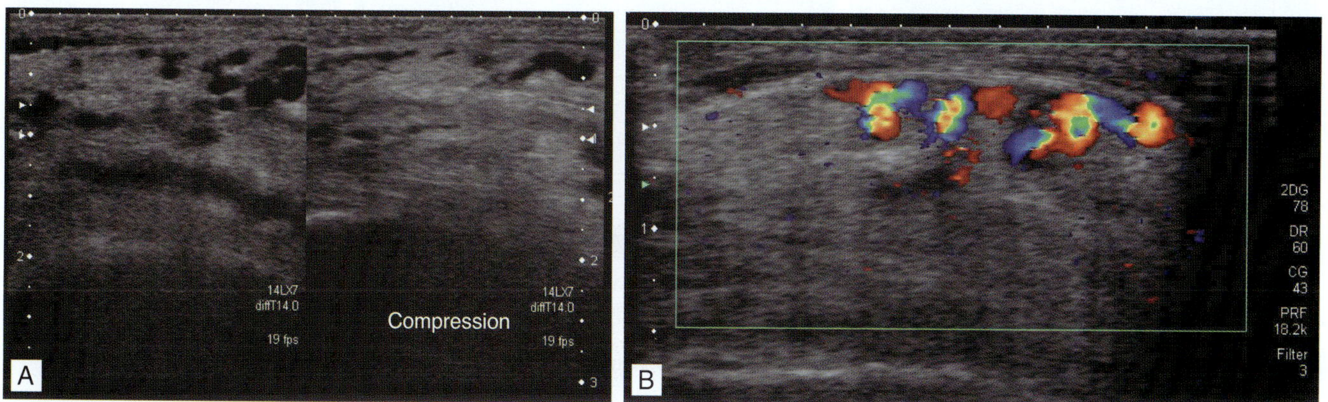

Figure 64.5 (A) USG image of a vascular malformation demonstrated as anechoic cystic spaces which are compressible. (B) Presence of serpiginous Doppler flow in both directions reflect the tortuosity of the vessels.

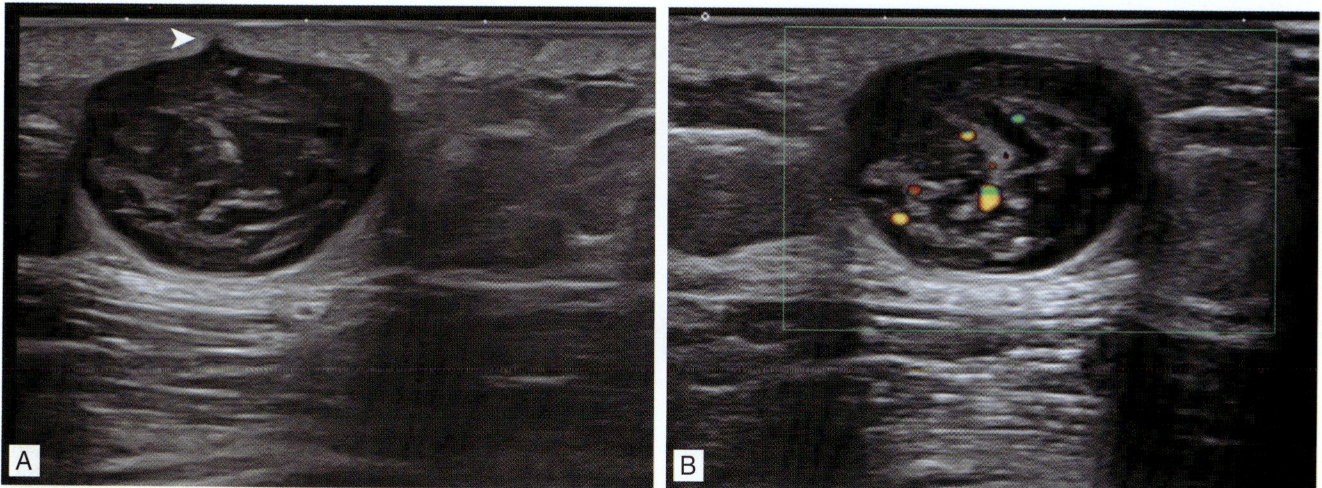

Figure 64.6 Epidermoid cyst. Characteristic appearance of an epidermoid cyst, of an ovoid morphology and heterogenous echotexture. Posterior acoustic shadowing reflects its cystic nature. More specifically, presence of punctum (*arrowhead* in A), (B) and twinkling artifact (alternating colors on Doppler signal) allows confident diagnosis of an epidermoid cyst. There is often a preceding history of a "spot" or an insect bite.

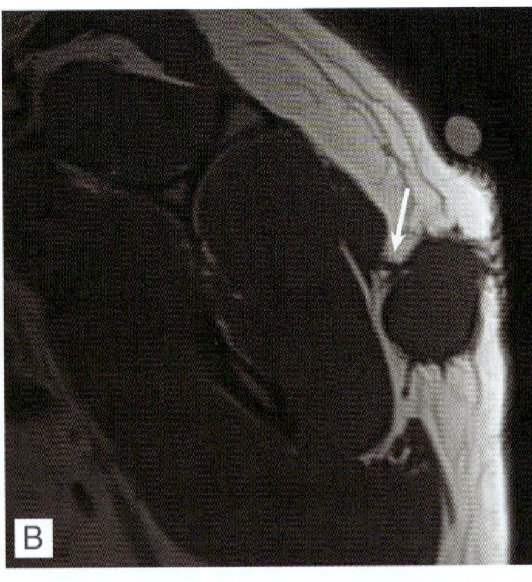

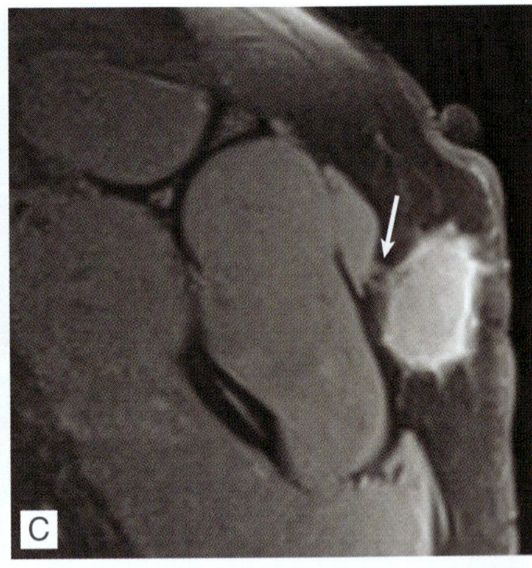

Figure 64.7 Deep fascial involvement can be seen on (A) USG as a small extension to the deep fascia, also seen on (B) T1w sagittal and (C) PD FS sagittal images (*arrows*). This is a desmoid-type fibromatosis, with an irregular spiculated margin seen on all techniques. This lesion is categorized as locally aggressive without metastatic potential.

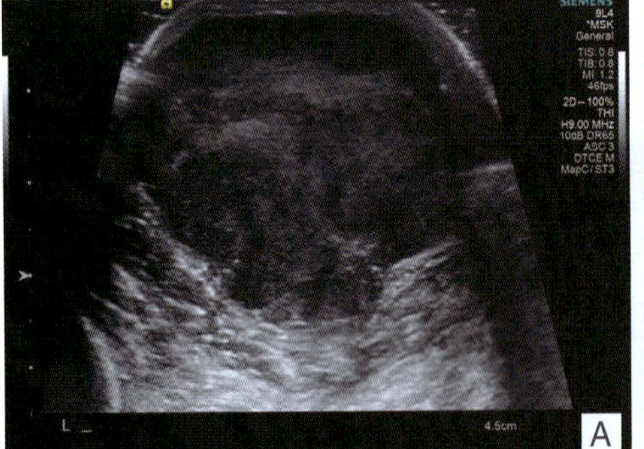

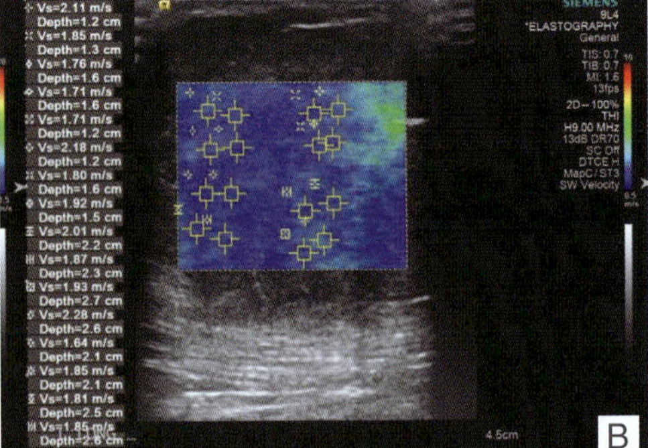

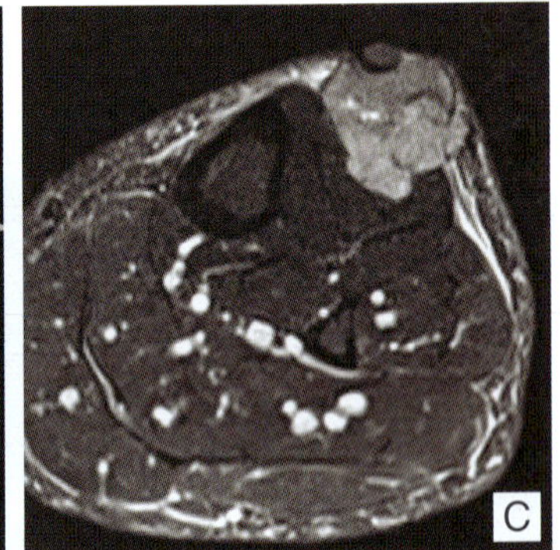

Figure 64.8 Undifferentiated pleomorphic sarcoma in the leg of an 80-year-old patient. (A) USG image demonstrates a heterogenous and irregular lesion in the leg. (B) Shear wave velocity USG image showing a lesion of medium stiffness, seen with a blue color representation and with multiple regions of interests (providing quantitative shear wave velocity measurements). The lesion is also seen on (C) STIR axial images. There is substantial overlap of shear wave velocities, limiting the use of elastography in differentiating malignant from benign lesions.

be uniformly applied to all tumor types. This is in contradistinction to lesions in other organs such as breast and thyroid where neoplasms generally fall in a more homogenous spectrum. Furthermore, focal areas of hemorrhage, necrosis, cystic degeneration, calcification, or fibrosis can also influence the stiffness of the lesion. Finally, in some tumors, a diagnosis of malignancy is not even possible with histological analysis alone, and is only made after cytogenetic or molecular analysis. In summary, elastography has an exciting future within musculoskeletal soft tumor imaging, and further research focusing on specific sarcoma subtypes will no doubt reveal this to be a promising technique.

Magnetic Resonance Imaging

MRI is a great imaging technique for assessing a soft tissue lesion, not least because MRI has exceptional soft tissue contrast and the ability to assess the true local extent of the tumor. In addition, MRI is not operator dependent. There is also a huge array of MRI techniques available, including the use of different pulse sequences to achieve not only anatomical imaging, but also functional and metabolic imaging. The addition of contrast enhancement (static or dynamic) also adds another layer of interpretation.

Soft tissue tumor MRI involves a few standard principles:

1. Skin markers

   When imaging a palpable superficial lump, skin markers MUST be applied on the patient in the vicinity of the lump. This is especially relevant if the lump is small and may not be immediately evident on the scan (Fig. 64.9), or if there is more than one lump incidentally which may distract the reporter from the main lump.

2. Imaging both limbs (or full width of the torso)

   It may sometimes be useful to not just image the lump on the ipsilateral limb, but to include the contralateral limb (or full width of the torso) for comparison. This may be relevant in cases where the lump is due to asymmetry in muscle bulk.

3. Standard imaging sequences

   Example of a standard soft tissue tumor imaging protocol includes axial T1w, axial T2w (or PDFS, T2w FS or STIR), coronal/sagittal T1w, and coronal/sagittal PDFS (or STIR). Axial plane is the mainstay of interpretation, allowing accurate assessment of tumor margin, and relationship with nearby structures (such as fascia and neurovascular bundle). Longitudinal plane, either sagittal or coronal plane depending on the location of the tumor, gives an overview of the extent of the lesion and its anatomical landmark.

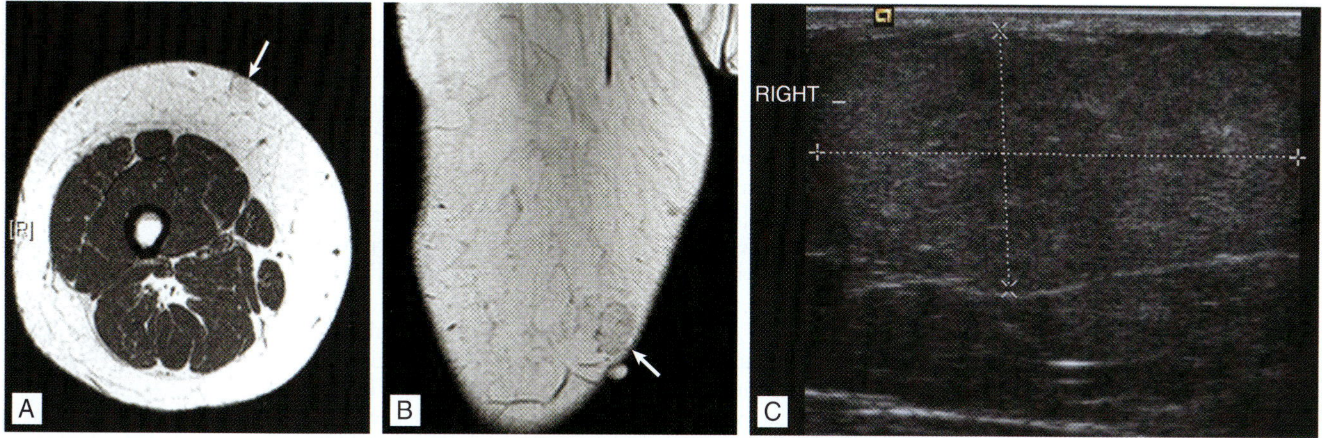

Figure 64.9 Using skin marker to mark the location of the lesion. (A) T1w axial and (B) T1w coronal images showing a subcutaneous lipoma (*arrows*) in the right thigh which is not immediately evident without a skin marker. (C) On the other hand, the lipoma is readily visible on USG.

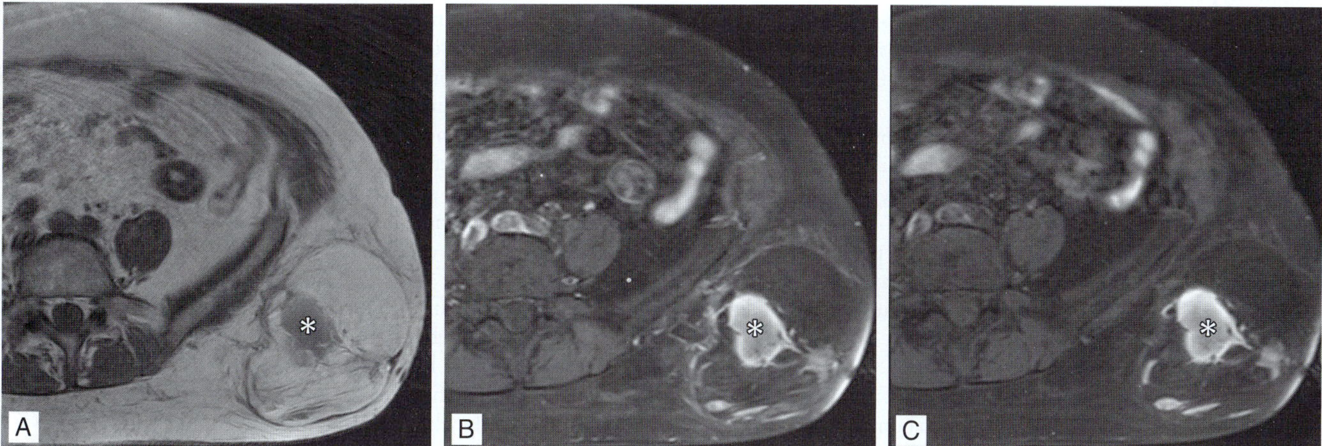

Figure 64.10 Comparing contrast enhancement on equivalent precontrast sequences (either FS or non-FS T1w sequences). (A) T1w, (B) T1w FS precontrast, (C) T1w FS postcontrast axial images demonstrating a lipomatous lesion with a large nonfatty central nodule (*asterisk*). (C) Interpreting contrast enhancement should always be accompanied with a similarly fat-saturated precontrast sequence, as in image (B), which in this case did not show any enhancement. In the absence of (B) T1w FS precontrast image, comparing images (A) and (C) can easily lead to false interpretation of enhancement being present.

4. Intravenous contrast agent

The use of intravenous contrast agent is recommended when performing MRI for tumor workup [5], but may not necessarily be part of the routine protocol for every institution. Assessment for contrast enhancement should only be performed on equivalent sequences; in other words, a fat suppressed T1w postcontrast image should be compared with a precontrast fat suppressed T1w image (and not with a nonfat suppressed precontrast T1w image). This is because fat suppression triggers rescaling of values across the grayscale, and some nonfatty areas may now appear brighter. This apparent increase in signal intensity may be falsely interpreted as enhancement when it is actually secondary to rescaling effect (Fig. 64.10). Interpretation of postcontrast enhancement can also be performed using subtraction postprocessing, where precontrast image is digitally subtracted from a postcontrast image. This technique can increase conspicuity of contrast enhancement.

Differentiating Malignant From Benign Lesions

MRI can differentiate between malignant and benign lesions with high sensitivity and specificity, reported at 93% and 82%, respectively [6], although this was documented by a group of researches with abundant experience in musculoskeletal soft tissue imaging, achieved by analyzing the tumors in a nonquantitative manner. Unfortunately, there is no single quantitative MRI feature, if utilized in isolation, that could reliably distinguish between benign and malignant soft tissue tumor [7]. Nevertheless, certain MRI features or parameters should raise concern for a malignant lesion [8,9]. Notice how some of these features overlap those described in the "*USG*" section above:

- Mean diameter >3.3 cm (which provides better sensitivity); or >6.6 cm (better specificity)
- Irregular margins
- Fascial invasion
- Presence of tumor necrosis
- Perilesional edema
- Bone involvement
- Neurovascular involvement

Contrast-enhanced MRI can be helpful in distinguishing between benign and malignant lesions, but similarly, it is not a perfect parameter. Enhancement, either moderate or intense, can be seen in both benign and malignant lesions. Dynamic contrast enhancement has also been studied. Generally, malignant lesions tend to demonstrate rapid contrast uptake compared to benign lesions [9]. Van der

Woude et al. reported a sensitivity of 91%, specificity 72% based on start of early enhancement ≤6 seconds [10].

Histological Characterization of Tumor

The success of histological characterization of a soft tissue tumor based on MRI appearances is generally poor [6,7]. Gielen et al. reported success rate at predicting the histology on MRI in 50%, which decreases to 38% if benign lesions were excluded [6]. Nevertheless, it is worthwhile to consider some of the listed features below which can be useful to help arrive at a sensible differential diagnosis:

1. Masses with very high T1w signal

There are five types of material (listed below) that can produce very high T1w signal, almost similar to subcutaneous fat. In the presence of high T1w signal, one should correlate with a fat suppressed sequence—fat-containing lesions will demonstrate decreased signal intensity, whereas other materials (proteinaceous, methemoglobin, melanin, and gadolinium) will remain hyperintense.

- *Fat.* Fat-containing lesions include lipoma, lipoma variants, liposarcoma, lipoblastoma, lipomatosis of nerve, hibernoma, hemangioma, marrow-containing lesions such as mature myositis ossificans
- *Proteinaceous material.* Ganglion or abscess can sometimes contain enough protein content to exhibit high T1w signal
- *Methemoglobin* in subacute hematoma, or even hemorrhage secondary to underlying tumor
- *Melanin.* High T1w signal reflecting presence of melanin can be seen in melanotic melanoma (Fig. 64.11), clear cell sarcoma (in around half of the cases), melanotic schwannoma
- Gadolinium contrast material

2. Masses with very low T2w signal

Lesions with lower T2w signal similar to bony cortex can generally be considered to contain one or more of these components:

- *Fibrosis,* such as plantar fibroma, GCT of tendon sheath, desmoid, fibroma, fibrosarcoma
- *Calcification,* such as gouty tophi, chondroid mineralization, phleboliths (venous malformation)
- *Hemosiderin,* such as GCT of tendon sheath, pigmented villonodular synovitis (PVNS), hematoma. It is worth keeping in mind that not all of these lesions have sufficient hemosiderin at the time of scanning to produce a low T2w signal. Hemosiderin will also produce a blooming artifact on T2*-weighted gradient-echo images (Fig. 64.12)
- *Flow-voids,* seen in high flow lesions such as arterial malformation and hemangioma

3. Masses with very high T2w signal

Majority of soft tissue lesions demonstrates high T2w signal in a heterogenous fashion which does not particularly lead to a specific characterization. However, a very high T2w signal (similar to water) can help with characterization of lesions. Some lesions have homogenous bright T2w signal, and can represent true cystic lesions (such as ganglion and bursa), or cyst-appearing lesion which are actually solid lesions (such as myxoid tumors, PNST, vascular tumors, glomus tumors, synovial sarcoma) (Table 64.3). True cystic lesions can demonstrate enhancement in the periphery of the lesion (but not internally). Myxoid lesions on the other hand will have internal enhancement. Focal areas of high T2w signal in otherwise solid tumors are suggestive of necrosis, the presence of which may indicate a high-grade malignant tumor.

4. Diagnosis based on location and relationship with particular structures

- As discussed in the "*USG*" section above, there are several tumors whereby a diagnosis can be made based on their characteristic location. They include Dupuytren's nodule and plantar fibroma in palmar and plantar aponeurosis respectively; elastofibroma in a subscapular location; PNST arising from a nerve.

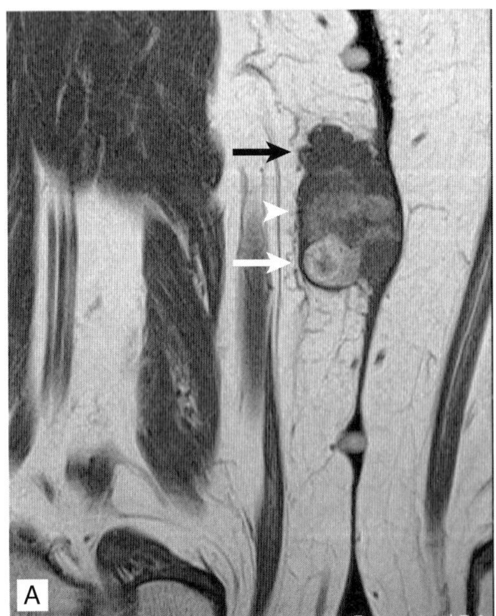

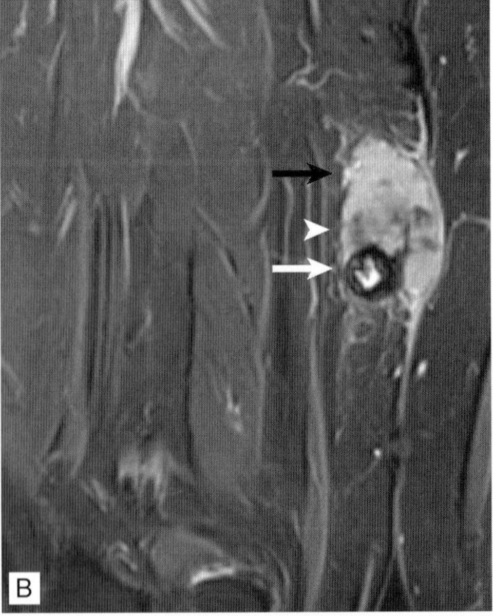

Figure 64.11 Example of a melanoma with high T1w signal in the right thigh, seen in (A) T1w and (B) STIR coronal images. This lesion has a varying degree of melanin distribution. In the caudal aspect of the lesion (*white arrow*), there is a round focus of high T1w signal, corresponding with a rim of very low STIR signal (reflecting signal drop out due to paramagnetic property of melanin). At the middle level (*arrowhead*), there remains some patchy areas of increased T1w, corresponding with patchy varying high and low STIR signal, reflecting presence of patchy distribution of melanin, but not as dense as the former. Finally, at the cranial third (*black arrow*), there is low T1w area, corresponding to increased STIR, reflecting an amelanotic portion of this lesion.

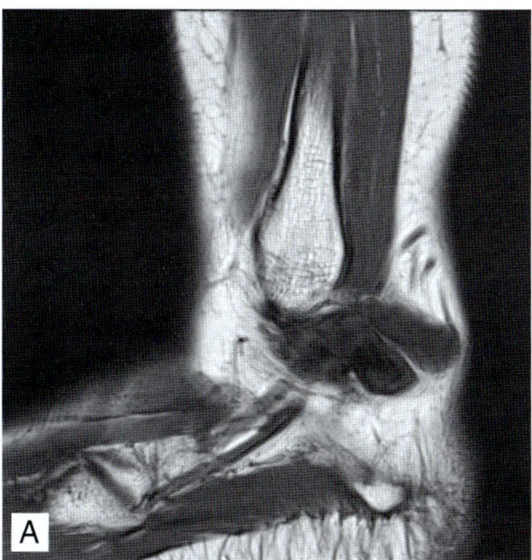

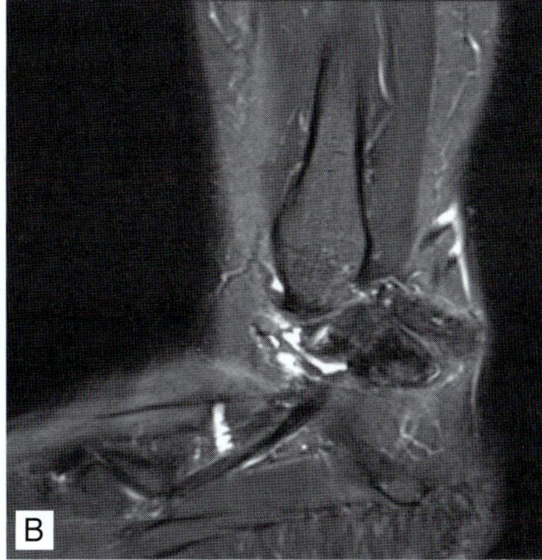

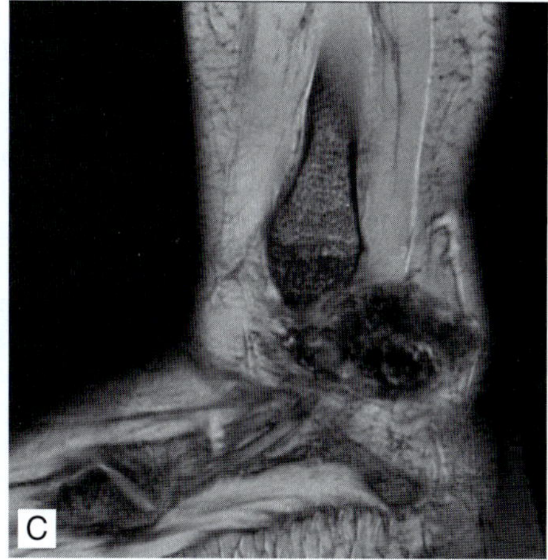

Figure 64.12 Blooming artifact. (A) T1w and (B) STIR sagittal images demonstrating a synovial-based mass in the ankle joint posterolateral recess. (C) Note the blooming artifact on the T2*w sagittal sequence, reflecting presence of superparamagnetic hemosiderin, lending confidence to the diagnosis of PVNS.

Local Staging

There are two main staging systems for soft tissue sarcoma: TNM system (by the American Joint Committee on Cancer Staging), and Enneking system (by Musculoskeletal Tumour Society), the former of which is more widely utilized. There are a few differences between the two systems. For example, Enneking system takes into account the site of tumor (intracompartmental or extracompartmental), and disregards presence of nodal involvement (in contradistinction to TNM system).

Regardless of which staging system is used by the institution, the reporting radiologist should consistently report on the following:

- Size of tumor (in three dimensions)
- Location (superficial/deep to the deep fascia, retroperitoneal, mediastinum; intra- or extracompartmental)
- Extracompartmental invasion
- Bone or joint involvement
- Neurovascular bundle involvement
- Lymph node involvement

DWI/ADC

Diffusion-weighted imaging (DWI) is a functional imaging technique that measures the Brownian motion of water molecules. During acquisition of a DWI image, different amount of diffusion weighting (expressed as *b* values) can be applied. The higher the *b* value, the more sensitive the image is to molecular motion. DWI should be performed with at least two or three different *b* values ($b = 50$, $b = 400$, $b = 900$ s/mm^2, for example). The signal intensity of every voxel will decrease in an exponential manner with increasing *b* values; and the rate of this decrease can be

TABLE 64.3 Masses With Cystic-Appearing Hyperintense T2W Signal and Their Differentiating Features

Category	Types of Lesions	Differentiating Imaging Features
True cystic lesions (benign)	Ganglion, bursa	Both ganglion and bursa will occur in typical locations. For example, typical location for a ganglion is in the hands and wrists.
	Epidermoid cyst	This has twinkling artifact on USG.
	Abscess, hematoma, postsurgical seroma	Differentiation is possible based on accompanying history. High T1w areas can be seen in abscess and hematoma (due to proteinaceous or blood products respectively).
Myxoid tumors (benign and malignant)	Intramuscular myxoma	The solid nature of this lesion is reflected by the presence of contrast enhancement. Lesions can have internal T2w hypointense septal and nodular areas. USG will demonstrate a hypoechoic solid lesion, rather than a truly anechoic cystic lesion.
	Myxoid liposarcoma	Fat can be seen in the lesion on T1w images, but not always.
	Extraskeletal myxoid chondrosarcoma	Matrix mineralization can be seen on MRI and even USG, but better appreciated on radiograph or CT.
	Myxofibrosarcoma	Curvilinear extension or "tails" along fascial planes.
Others (benign and malignant)	Vascular lesions	Lymphatic malformation can be truly cystic or multiseptated. Flow voids in high-flow malformation. Phleboliths in venous malformation and hemangioma. Hemangioma can have interspersed fat in the lesion seen on T1w images.
	Peripheral nerve sheath tumor	Round or ovoid lesions arising along the nerves. Target sign.
	Synovial sarcoma	This lesion typically occurs near a joint (but not intra-articular), most commonly near the knee.

calculated, voxel by voxel, using logarithmic regression analysis to produce an apparent diffusion coefficient (ADC) value. The ADC values are displayed as an image (also known as ADC map), which can then be analyzed in a quantitative manner.

There are a few applications for DWI/ADC, all of which bring a new layer of information that can be used to augment routine MRI sequences. These DWI/ADC can be used to:

1. Differentiate malignant from benign lesions

This operates on the premise that malignant lesions are more cellular than benign lesions, thereby causing significant restriction to the diffusion mobility of water. Malignant tumors have been shown to have significantly lower ADC values than benign lesions. For example in one study, a threshold ADC value of 1.34×10^{-3} mm^2/s has been proposed to differentiate between malignant and benign lesions with 94% sensitivity and 88% specificity [11]. Nevertheless, others have found significant overlap in the ADC values in malignant and benign lesions [12].

2. Differentiate cystic from solid masses

Using a minimum ADC value of 1.8×10^{-3} mm^2/s or mean value of 2.5×10^{-3} mm^2/s yielded 100% specificity in determining a cyst from a solid tumor. This can be useful in differentiating a myxoid tumor (which has cyst-like appearances) from true cysts [13], providing an alternative from using MRI contrast enhancement or USG (Fig. 64.13).

3. Monitor disease response following chemotherapy or radiotherapy

DWI/ADC can be used to monitor response to chemotherapy or radiotherapy [14]. This operates on the premise that malignant lesions following chemotherapy or radiotherapy will have lower tumor cell density, thereby allowing greater water molecule motion, reflected in an increase in ADC values. An increase in ADC value can also be seen in necrotic area post-therapy [12]. Interestingly, Moustafa et al. have reported that they found an inverted trend in fibromatosis lesions, where lesions with favorable response would show lower ADC values than those with progressive disease. The authors suggested that fibromatosis with favorable response will lead to progressive collagenization, which typically have low ADC values [14].

4. Differentiate true recurrence/residual tumor from postsurgical scar tissue

Detection of tumor recurrence on static contrast-enhanced MRI has a reported sensitivity 87.5–100%, but with a poor specificity of 52–55.6% owing to their similar appearance of mass-like enhancement. However, with the addition of DWI/ADC, specificity is increased to 97–100% [15,16]. Further, larger studies will be required to substantiate the value of functional imaging in tumor follow-up. Of note, the value of DWI/ADC does not extend to myxoid sarcomatous tumor recurrence which may show elevated ADC similar to that seen in postoperative changes, thereby providing false reassurance [15].

Role of Contrast-Enhanced MRI

Gadolinium contrast-enhanced MRI can be part of the routine sequences in a tumor workup protocol, but this is not universal across every institution. Some institutions choose to omit this from their routine protocol because:

a. they use USG for initial workup of all soft tissue tumors which can assess the vascularity and cystic nature of tumors;
b. majority of lesions can be adequately characterized on routine sequences, for example, lipoma, PNST, vascular malformation, to name a few.

Patients can of course be recalled if it later transpires that there are unexpected findings or uncertainties requiring a contrast-enhanced study. This approach vastly reduces the number of patients receiving gadolinium injections and their associated risks.

In general, there are a few instances where contrast-enhanced MRI is useful, or indeed strongly advised:

1. Postneoadjuvant chemotherapy or radiotherapy

While contrast-enhanced MRI is not routinely performed during initial tumor work up, contrast-enhanced sequences must be performed after neoadjuvant chemotherapy or radiotherapy. Following neoadjuvant therapy, as many as 31% of lesions can increase in size, the majority of which correlates with histopathological changes such as intralesional necrosis,

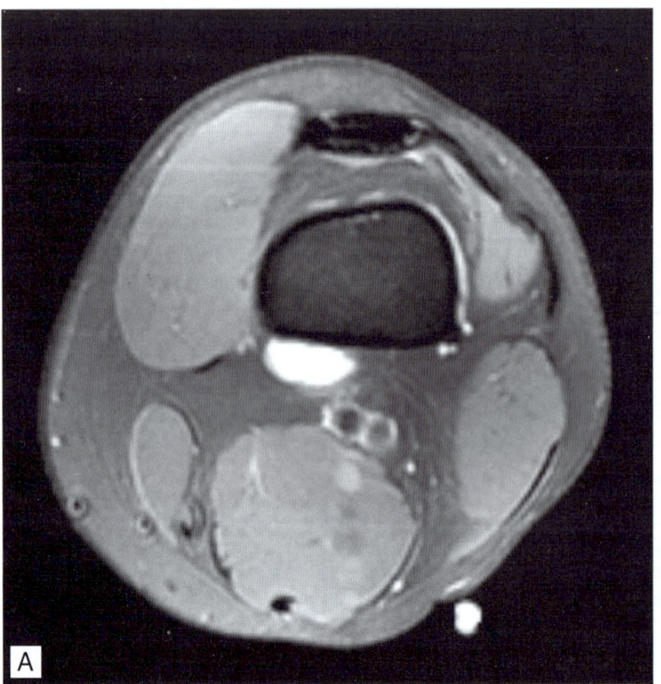

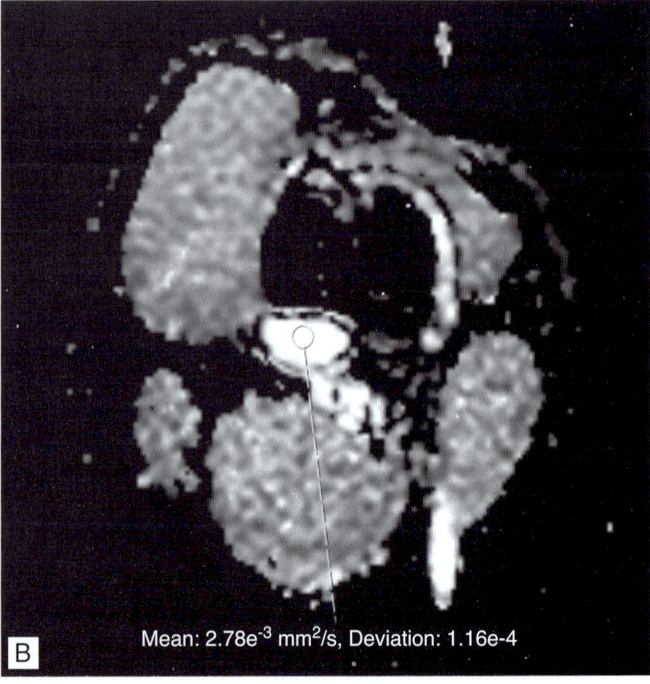

Figure 64.13 Use of ADC in determining cystic nature of a soft tissue mass. (A) PD FS axial image of the distal femur demonstrated a high signal lesion. (B) Mean ADC value of this lesion is 2.8×10^{-3} mm^2/s, above the quoted minimum threshold ADC value, reflecting its cystic nature.

cystic change, or hemorrhage [17]. Contrast-enhanced MRI sequences will be able to accurately distinguish viable tumor from nonviable areas. Nevertheless, the true challenge lies in distinguishing viable tumor from post therapy granulation tissue, due to similar T1w and T2w characteristics and their enhancing nature. For this purpose, dynamic-enhanced contrast MRI may be more useful, being able to differentiate early contrast uptake in viable tumor, from slower contrast uptake in granulation tissue [18].

2. Postoperative follow-up

MRI is the preferred technique if follow-up imaging for locoregional recurrence is required postoperatively. The challenge is differentiating postoperative inflammation and scarring from true tumor recurrence. Tumor recurrence may have a more nodular or mass-like postcontrast enhancement, although scar tissue may have the same appearance on static postcontrast-enhanced study. Dynamic postcontrast study can resolve this as tumor recurrence will show rapid arterial enhancement (Fig. 64.14).

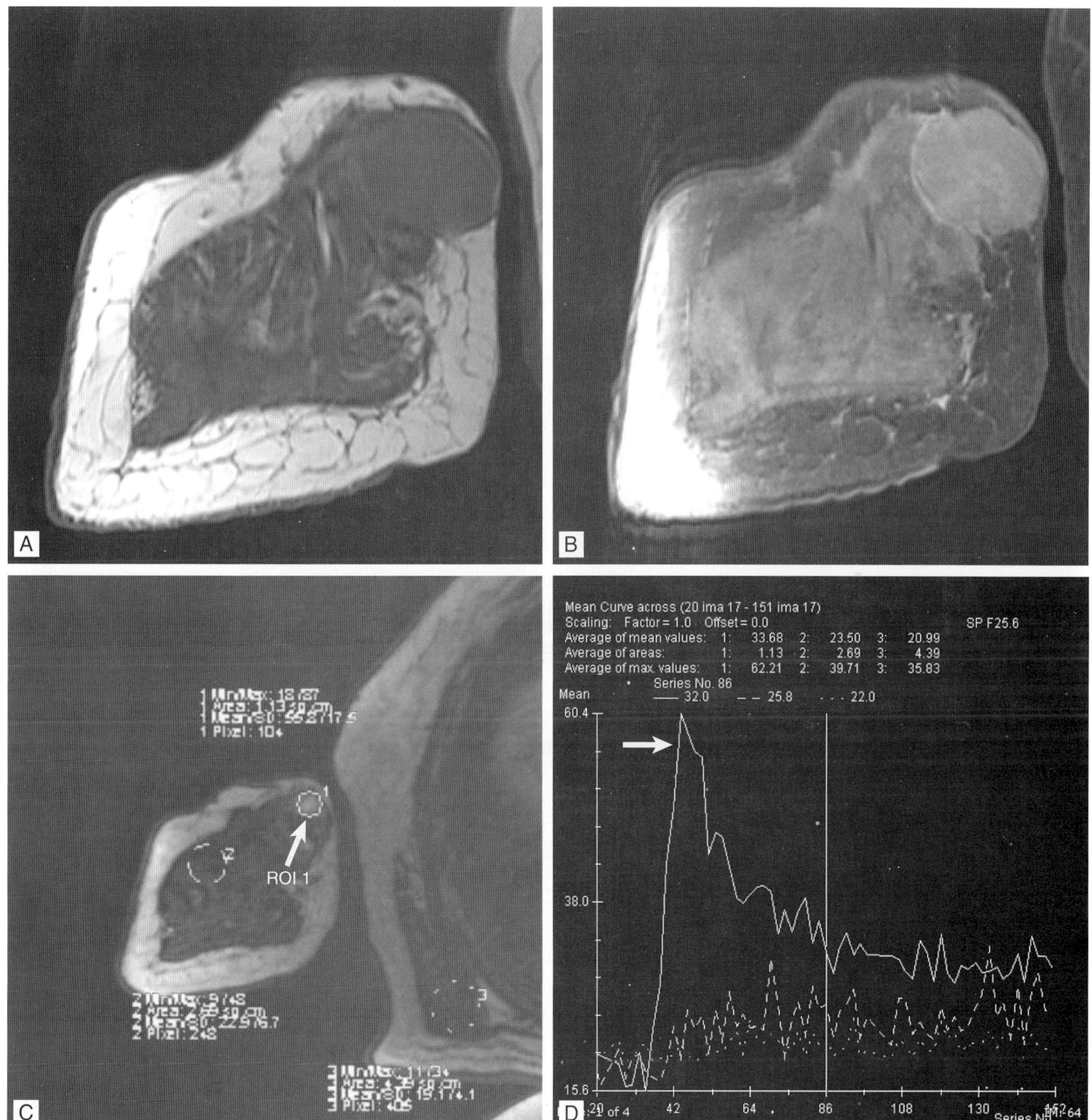

Figure 64.14 Recurrence of myxofibrosarcoma. (A) T1w and (B) PD FS axial images demonstrating a new mass a few months after surgical resection. (C) ROI 1 (*arrow*) placed over the lesion demonstrates early contrast uptake and washout on the (D) time intensity curve (*solid line*), in keeping with a recurrence. ROI 2 and 3 (*dashed and dotted lines*, respectively) are placed in normal muscles and are used as controls, demonstrating general slow uptake.

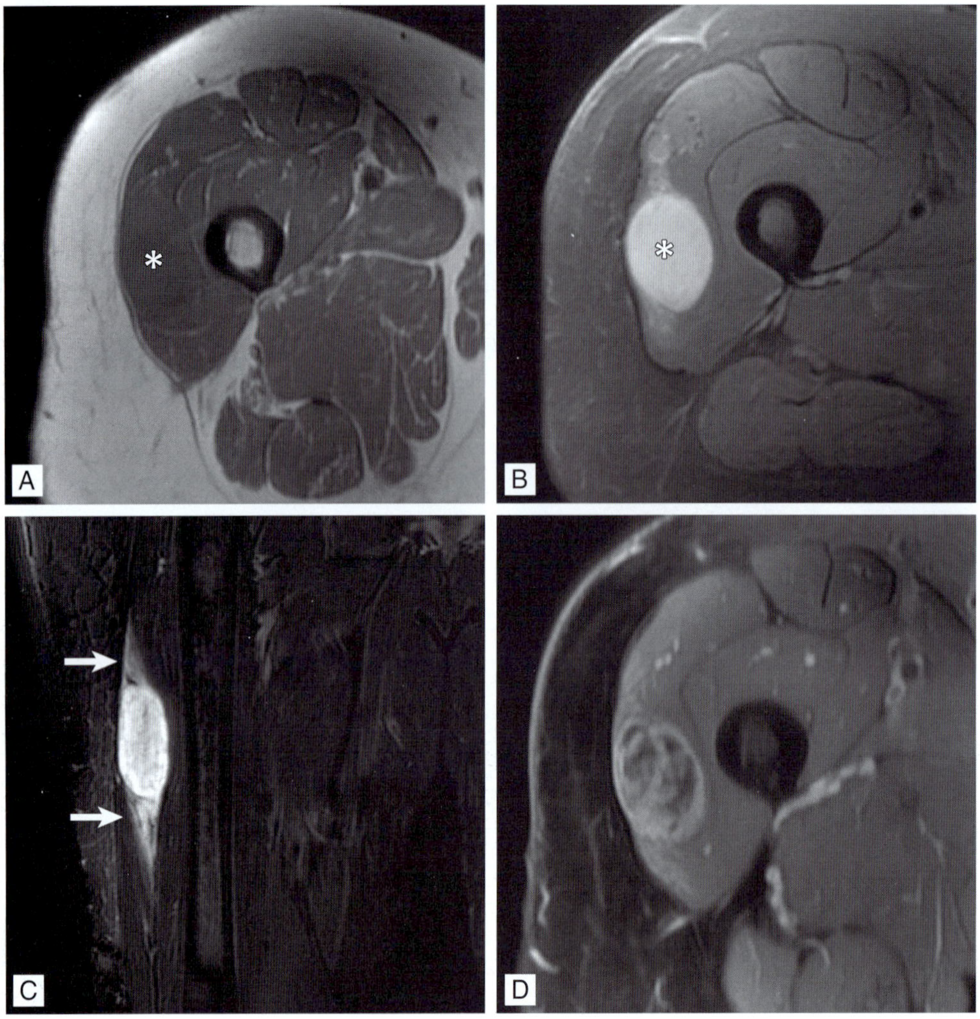

Figure 64.15 Intramuscular myxoma mimicking a cyst. (A) T1w, (B) PD FS axial images demonstrating an ovoid, well-defined lesion with low T1w and high PD FS signal, mimicking a cyst (*asterisks*). (C) STIR coronal image demonstrates internal complexity, reflecting that this is not a simple cyst. Perilesional edema is typically seen at the poles of an intramuscular myxoma (*arrows*). (D) T1w FS postcontrast image demonstrates typical enhancement in a peripheral and septal pattern, confirming the solid nature of this mass.

Contrast enhancement with subtraction imaging can also improve detection of tumor recurrence.

3. Distinguishing cystic from solid (but cystic appearing) lesion

Some solid tumors may have high T2w signal, mimicking a cyst. When faced with such lesions, solid tumors will have features such as thick-wall or internal complexity (inhomogeneity, thick septation, or nodularity), whereupon postcontrast MRI should be performed to assess for lesional enhancement to confirm its solid nature (Fig. 64.15). While USG can perform this assessment for superficial tumors, MRI with contrast is preferable for deeper lesions to assess cystic versus solid areas.

Another circumstance to consider contrast enhancement is in the presence of a hemorrhage—a tumor may hemorrhage and lead to a large hematoma which may be incorrectly dismissed as a simple hematoma. Contrast enhancement is sometimes necessary to unveil the tumor nodule.

4. Selecting an appropriate site for biopsy

Contrast-enhanced MRI can identify solid and well-vascularized areas in the lesion, which should be targeted during biopsy. Nonviable, nonenhancing, necrotic areas should be avoided (Fig. 64.16).

Radiograph

Radiograph has poor contrast resolution when it comes to assessing a soft tissue lesion. Vast majority of soft tissue lesions are isodense to muscles, therefore generally not appreciable on radiograph—unless when the lesion is large, which by extension makes it more likely to be a malignant tumor. About 64% of soft tissue lesions visible on radiographs are malignant [19]. Fat-containing lesions on the other hand are hypodense relative to adjacent muscles.

Radiograph is often unfairly dismissed as unimportant in the assessment of soft tissue lesions. However, despite its shortcomings, there are instances where it can be useful, specifically by assessing for lesional calcification and underlying bone involvement.

Presence of calcification in a soft tissue lesion can provide invaluable information in narrowing the differential diagnoses of the lesion, and even clinching the diagnosis in some instances. There are a few patterns of calcification (Fig. 64.17):

- Ossification

The term ossification refers to bone formation and is reserved for when bony trabeculae are visible. Ossification can be seen in myositis ossificans where the mineralization is focused on the

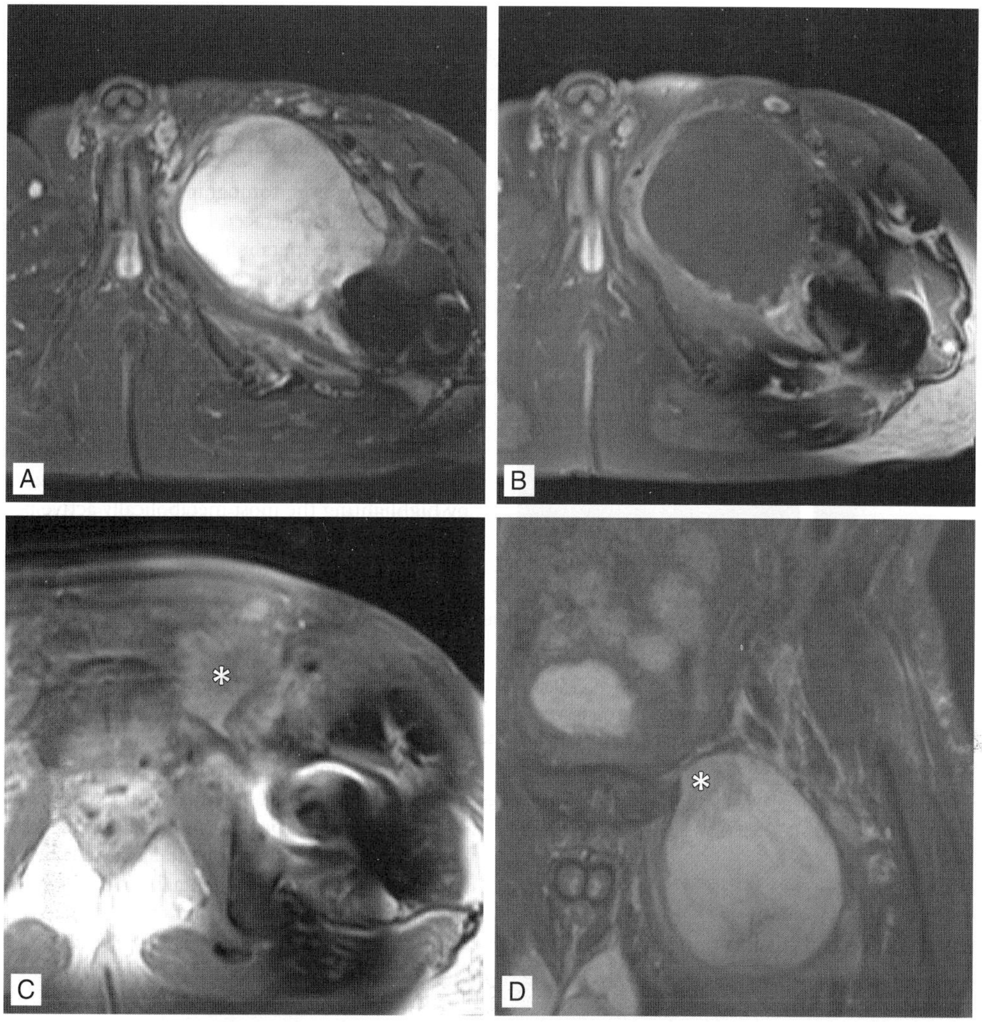

Figure 64.16 Prebiopsy planning. Large mass in the left proximal thigh, with (A) high STIR signal mass and (B) peripheral enhancement on this T1w FS image, in keeping with a necrotic mass. Presence of necrosis is suggestive of a high-grade lesion, as in this grade 3 rhabdomyosarcoma. Biopsy of the necrotic component should be avoided due to low diagnostic yield. (C) On the cranial aspect of the lesion, this T1w FS image shows an area of viable, enhancing tissue (*asterisk*), correlating with (D) intermediate signal on this coronal STIR image. This is the area that should be targeted for biopsy.

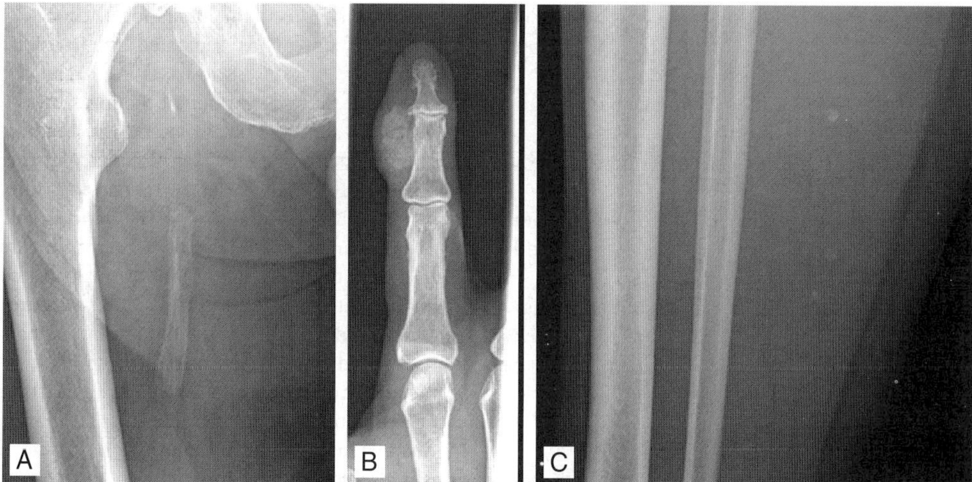

Figure 64.17 Different types of calcification on radiographs. (A) Ossification with internal marrow and trabecular formation, seen in this long-standing myositis ossificans. (B) Chondroid calcification in a soft tissue chondroma of the finger demonstrating an amorphous appearance. (C) Several rounded phleboliths with lucent center in a vascular malformation in the calf.

tumor (depending on the staging system used) and is an independent adverse prognostic factor [21]. On the other hand, oncological outcome for de novo extracompartmental space sarcoma is inconsistent; poor outcome has been reported, but several studies have shown a comparable outcome with intracompartmental lesions when managed with adjuvant therapy and surgical excision after adjusting for lesion size, presence of metastasis and histologic grade [26].

Examples of true extracompartment spaces are the axilla, antecubital fossa, popliteal space, subsartorial canal, and femoral triangle. In general, extracompartmental space lesions are not restrained by the tight muscle fascia, allowing the lesions to extend with little resistance. Extracompartmental space lesions are surgically challenging due to their close proximity to vessels and nerves, limiting the ability to obtain a wide surgical margin.

WHO Classification

The 2020 World Health Organization (WHO) Classification of Tumours of Soft Tissue and Bone lists more than 100 histological subtypes of soft tissue tumors. This long list is intimidating, but it is less daunting to appreciate that in practice, the majority of tumors, either benign (70%) or malignant (80%), are made up of only a handful of tumors (Table 64.5) [29,30]. The list of tumors in Table 64.5 is based on referral to a specialist tumor center. In a more generalist practice, lesions such as ganglia, lipoma, post-traumatic lesions, skin gland lesions, and normal variants form an even higher proportion of the soft tissue lumps assessed.

The 2020 WHO Classification of Tumours of Soft Tissue and Bone is the fifth and latest edition, published in the first half of year 2020. Every edition brings with it updated classifications and diagnostic criteria, detailing new knowledge ranging from genetic markers to immunohistochemistry advances. For example, one of the changes in this latest edition is the introduction of a new entity called atypical spindle cell/pleomorphic lipomatous tumor, an adipocytic tumor with a nonaggressive clinical course. One noteworthy change introduced in the previous fourth edition released in 2013, was the removal of the term malignant fibrous histiocytoma (MFH). MFH had previously been thought to be a distinct tumor category, but with evolving knowledge in immunohistochemical and molecular genetics, a lot of previously diagnosed MFH can actually be reclassified into a specific tumor category [31]. In addition, tumors that do not exhibit any identifiable line of differentiation were classed under a newly introduced category of "undifferentiated/unclassified sarcomas" in the 2013 edition.

TABLE 64.5 Most Frequent Benign and Malignant Soft Tissue Tumors Constituting the Majority of Tumors Encountered in Practice

Benign Tumors	Malignant Tumors
Lipoma (16%)	Malignant fibrous histiocytoma (24%) (see following paragraph)
Fibrous histiocytoma (13%)	Liposarcoma (14%)
Nodular fasciitis (11%)	Leiomyosarcoma (8%)
Hemangioma (8%)	Malignant schwannoma (6%)
Fibromatosis (7%)	Dermatofibrosarcoma protuberans (6%)
Neurofibroma (5%)	Synovial sarcoma (5%)
Schwannoma (5%)	Adult fibrosarcoma (5%)
Giant cell tumor of tendon sheath (4%)	Extraskeletal chondrosarcoma (2%)
Myxoma (3%)	Not further specified (12%)

The following section will discuss lesions from different categories of soft tissue tumors. It is not intended to be an all-inclusive write-up but aims to provide an overview of these lesions, where diagnosis of some can be suggested based on imaging features.

Adipocytic Tumors

Benign Adipocytic Tumors

Lipoma

Lipoma is the commonest benign soft tissue tumor, making up just under half of all the benign soft tissue tumors [1]. Histologically, they are lobules of mature adipocytes. They are most frequently located superficially in the subcutaneous plane, with around 5% located deep to the deep fascia, either intra- or intermuscularly. Lipoma is generally painless. They can increase in size during their initial growth period but should only demonstrate minimal increment after that. Patients who have lost weight may also report their lipoma becoming larger, which is made more prominent due to reduced surrounding fat.

USG is a useful technique to diagnose a superficial lipoma with diagnostic accuracy of 96% [32]. On USG, a benign lipoma is (Fig. 64.24)

- typically ovoid or spindle in shape;
- homogenous;
- variable echogenicity, ranging from hypoechoic, to isoechoic, or hyperechoic compared to either adjacent subcutaneous tissue or skeletal muscle [32];
- can have minimal internal blood flow seen on Doppler USG.

MRI features are:

- Homogenous high T1w signal, and completely suppresses on fat-suppressed sequences
- Thin septa can be seen, and should be <2 mm
- MRI contrast agent, if administered may produce minor strand-like enhancement in these septa and is acceptable
- Superficial lipoma is classically described to have a well-defined margin, with or without a surrounding pseudocapsule. This pseudocapsule may or may not be evident on imaging. When this capsule is absent, it can often be difficult to identify a lipoma (hence the need for skin markers for all soft tissue tumor MRI scans)
- Intramuscular lipomas can also have a well-defined margin, but more commonly shows interdigitation with the muscle, producing a striated appearance

Radiograph has little role in the evaluation of a lipoma although a large lipomatous lesion can be visualized as an ovoid lesion of similar density to subcutaneous fat, and lower to that of adjacent muscles.

Benign Lipoma Variants

Conventional lipoma is the most common form of lipomatous tumor seen in practice. There are however several variants of lipoma, all benign in nature, and are named according to the histological elements found admixed with the mature adipocytes. They include (but not limited to) angiolipoma, spindle cell

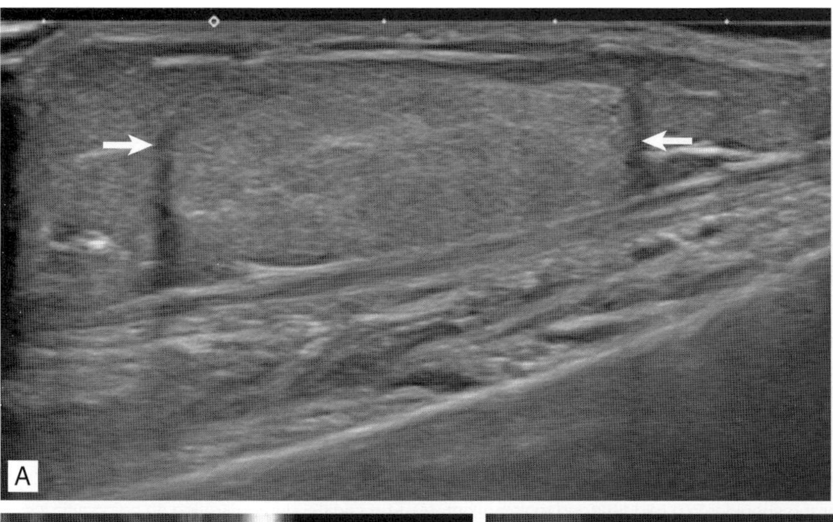

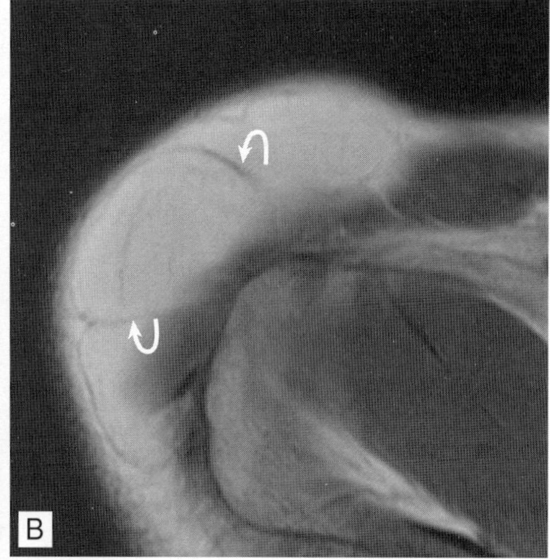

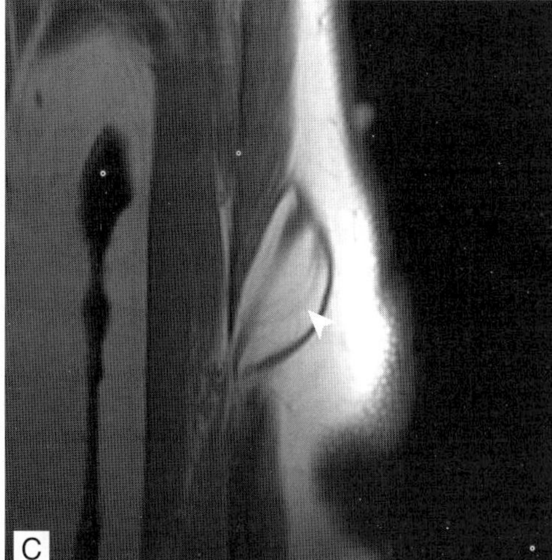

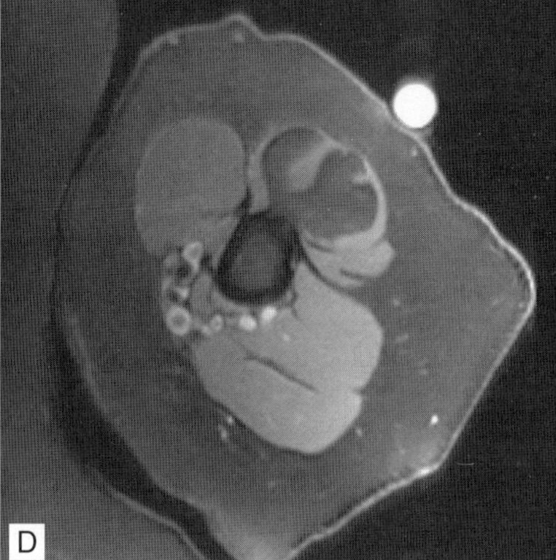

Figure 64.24 Benign lipomas (in different patients). (A) On USG, lipomas typically have an ovoid or spindle shape (*arrows*) with homogenous echotexture. This lesion has a isoechoic echogenicity to adjacent subcutaneous tissue, but they can be variable. (B) Lipomas can have thin septations, as shown in this axial T1w of the right shoulder (*curved arrows*). (C) Intramuscular lipomas can demonstrate interdigitation with muscles (*arrowhead*), as seen on this coronal T1w image of the left forearm (deltoid muscle). (D) They should have complete fat suppression as seen on this PD FS axial image.

lipoma, chondroid lipoma, and myolipoma. We will limit our discussion to the former three.

Angiolipoma: Angiolipoma consists of mature adipocytes and vessels. The proportion of vessels is variable and can even make up the majority of the lesion. These vessels are thin-walled and of the size of capillaries which often contain fibrin microthrombi [33]. Like a simple lipoma, they are always benign, do not recur after surgical excision, and have no malignant potential. Angiolipoma is unique among lipoma variants in that it can be tender on palpation. Recognizing this is useful, as it provides an explanation, or even reassurance to the patient.

Angiolipoma is commonly found in the forearm, with a predilection for male patients. On imaging, they are (Fig. 64.25)

- hyperechoic (rather than isoechoic) to adjacent subcutaneous fat;
- ovoid (rather than spindle-shaped);
- lateral tumor capsule being less well-visualized;
- smaller (mean length around 2 cm, rather than more than 4 cm);
- presence of vascularity.

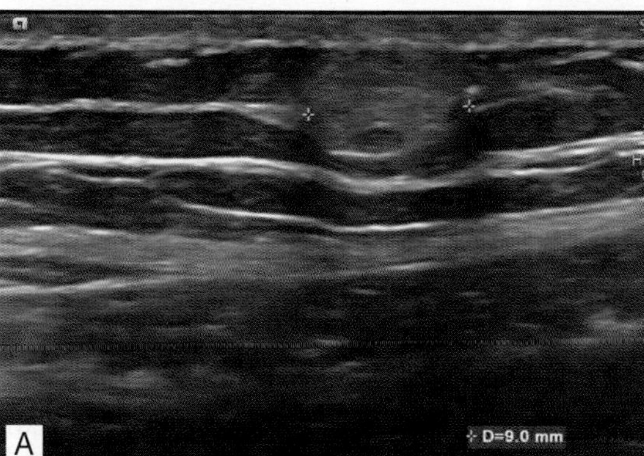

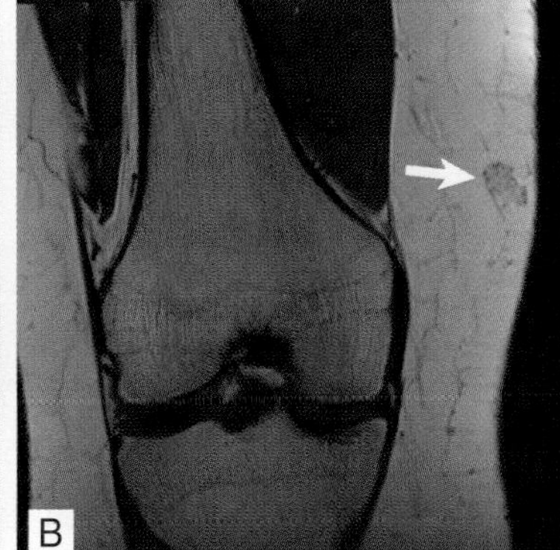

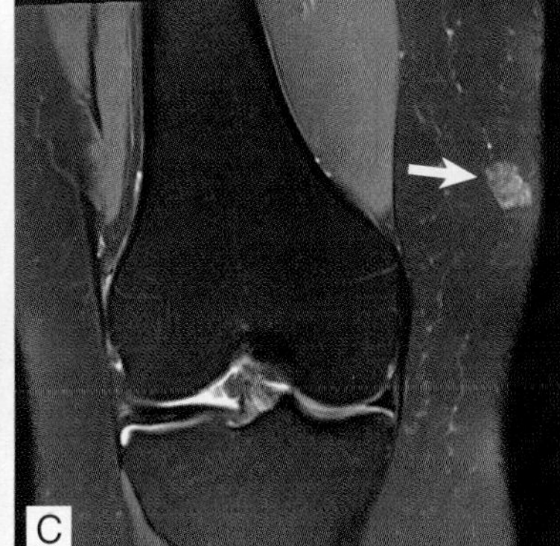

Figure 64.25 Angiolipoma (images are from different patients). (A) Angiolipoma typically appears hyperechoic to adjacent subcutaneous fat and has an ovoid configuration. (B) and (C) are T1w and PD FS coronal images, respectively. On MRI, angiolipoma can appear as a nodule with fat, interspersed with low T1w signal and increased fluid-like signal which corresponds to the vascular proliferation in the lesion (*arrows*).

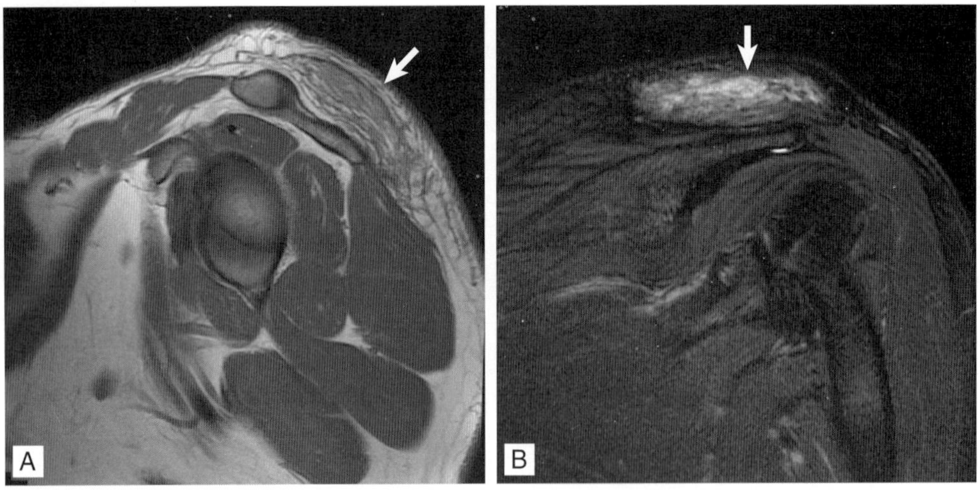

Figure 64.26 Spindle cell lipoma in a typical location over the shoulder in a middle-aged male patient. (A) T1w sagittal demonstrating an adipocytic lesion (*arrow*) with multiple thick septae. On image (B) T2w FS, there is little to no signal suppression in the lesion, suggesting dominating nonadipose material in the lesion. Imaging appearances warrants a biopsy, and was shown to be a spindle cell lipoma, containing dense collagenous tissue in a myxoid stroma.

Spindle Cell Lipoma: Spindle cell lipomas are most commonly found in the shoulder and posterior neck region, mostly in men (>90%) in their middle-age (mean >55 years) [34]. They consist of mature adipocytes and bland spindled cells, on background of collagen fibers or myxoid matrix [33]. The proportion of these bland spindled cells is variable, ranging from a few spindle cells to a lesion with predominant spindle cell and little fat cells. This will affect the amount of fat visible on MRI, with some lesions demonstrating little to no T1w signal. In addition, MRI appearance of a spindle cell lipoma varies greatly (Fig. 64.26), and unfortunately overlaps with that of a liposarcoma:

- The septa in the lesion can be thin or thick, and there may be nonadipose areas in the lesion
- Both the septa and nonadipose area can demonstrate enhancement

While presence of the above imaging features should always prompt a biopsy, one should however consider this benign variant of lipoma when faced with a well-defined fatty mass, even though complex appearing, in the subcutaneous plane at the posterior neck, in a middle-aged male patient.

Chondroid Lipoma: Chondroid lipoma consists of adipocytes on a background of myxoid/chondroid matrix. On MRI, the lesion is well-defined and lobulated, with variable and nonspecific signal properties. Visualization of T1w signal will depend on the proportion of the adipocytic component. T2w signal can be prominent owing to the myxoid/chondroid components in the lesion (Fig. 64.27). Calcification can be present on radiographs and CT. Similar to spindle cell lipoma, a specific diagnosis cannot be made with confidence based on imaging alone, and biopsy should be considered.

Lipomatosis of Nerve: Lipomatosis of nerve is also known as neural fibroma, or fibrolipomatous hamartoma (or variations thereof such as lipofibromatous hamartoma, or lipofibrohamartoma) of a nerve. It is a benign neoplastic process, characterized by proliferation of adipose or fibrous tissue within the epineurium of a nerve. The median nerve is by far the most involved nerve (upward of 80%), and has also been reported

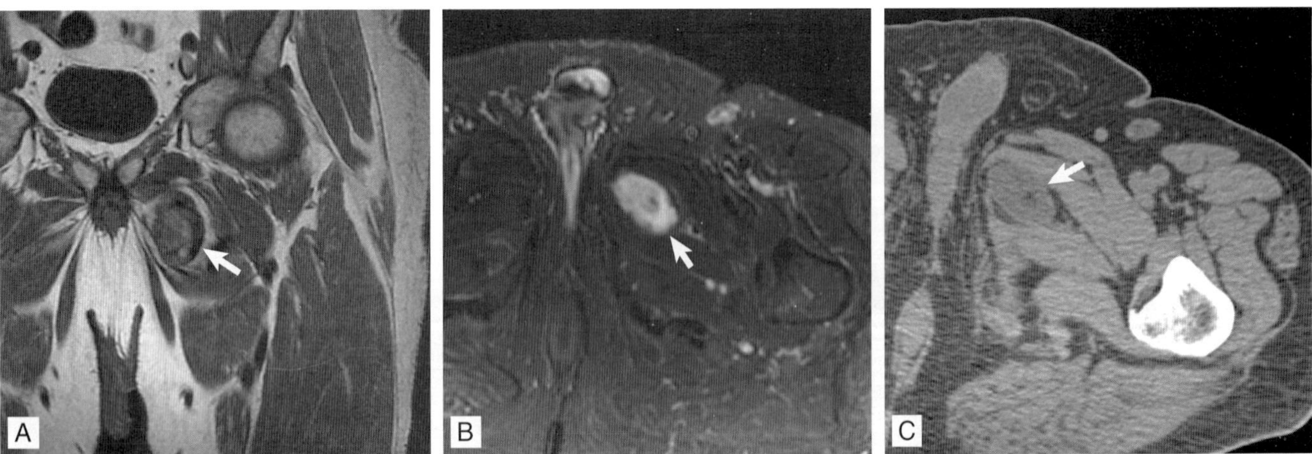

Figure 64.27 Chondroid lipoma. This is a rare benign lipoma variant, seen as a lesion (*arrows*) with little area of fat on this (A) T1w coronal. (B) Note the predominant high signal intensity on this STIR axial image, reflecting the background myxochondroid matrix. Small punctate areas of fat can be seen as low signal focus, also seen on (C) CT image. There is no mineralization seen in this lesion.

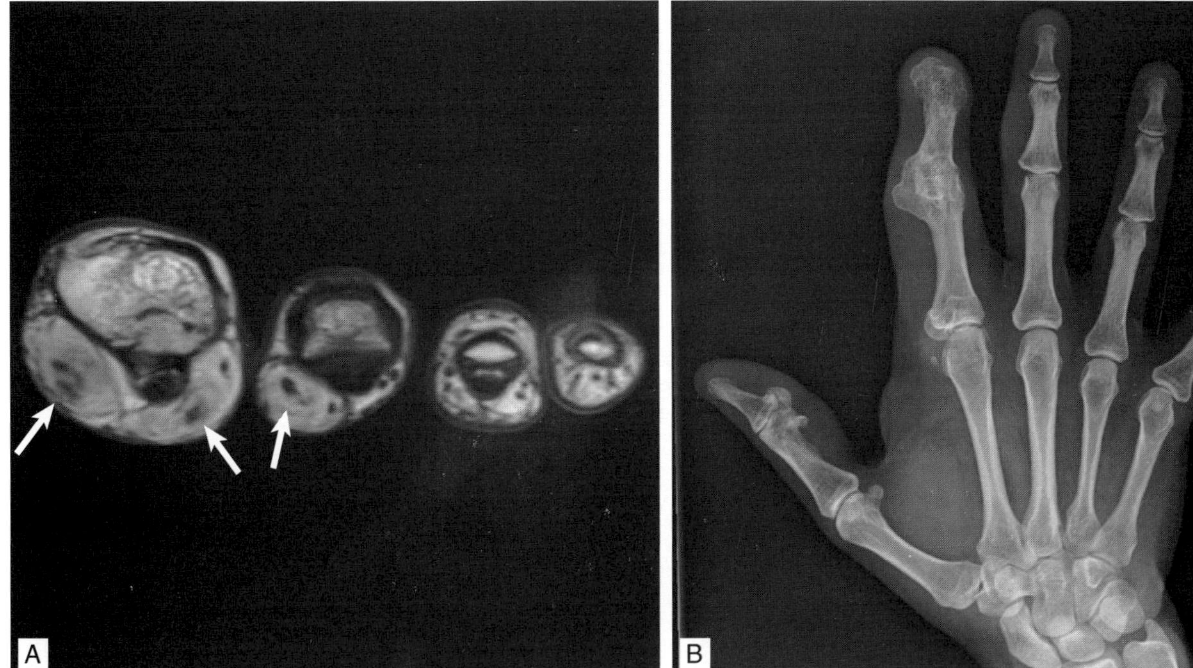

Figure 64.28 Lipomatosis of the median nerve. (A) T1w axial image (at the level of the PIPJ) demonstrating thickened digital branches of the median nerve (*arrows*) in the index and middle finger (radial side only), enveloped by hypertrophied adipose tissue. As on the MRI, macrodactyly can also be seen on the radiograph (B), affecting mainly the index finger, and a little of the middle finger (radial side) and thumb. Association with exostosis formation is recognized (seen in the thumb IPJ; and index finger MCPJ, IPJs).

to involve the ulnar nerve, radial nerve, brachial plexus, cranial nerve, and sciatic nerve.

There are several characteristic features in lipomatosis of nerve (Fig. 64.28):

- Macrodactyly can occur in 32% of cases (leading to another synonym of macrodystrophia lipomatosa) [35], where there is hypertrophy of the skin, subcutaneous tissue, and bones of the affected nerve territory
- MRI appearance is pathognomonic whereby one can see the hypointense (T1w and T2w) and thickened nerve fascicles, interspersed within hypertrophied fibroadipose tissue, producing a characteristic cable-like appearance
- USG can also be used to visualize the thickened nerve fascicle

Management of this condition is mainly conservative, with surgical intervention focused on decompressing the compromised nerve to relieve pain and paraesthesia, for example, by carpal tunnel decompression in the context of the median nerve involvement.

Hibernoma: Hibernoma is rare, accounting for only 1.6% of all benign lipomatous tumors [33]. It is composed of mature adipose tissue with variable proportions of brown fat cells. The thigh is the commonest site for hibernoma (though with a wide range of reported frequency in the literature (29–83%), followed by the shoulder) [36,37].

Imaging features of hibernoma (Fig. 64.29):

- On CT, a hibernoma can be visualized as a fat-containing lesion, though is typically of higher attenuation than the subcutaneous fat

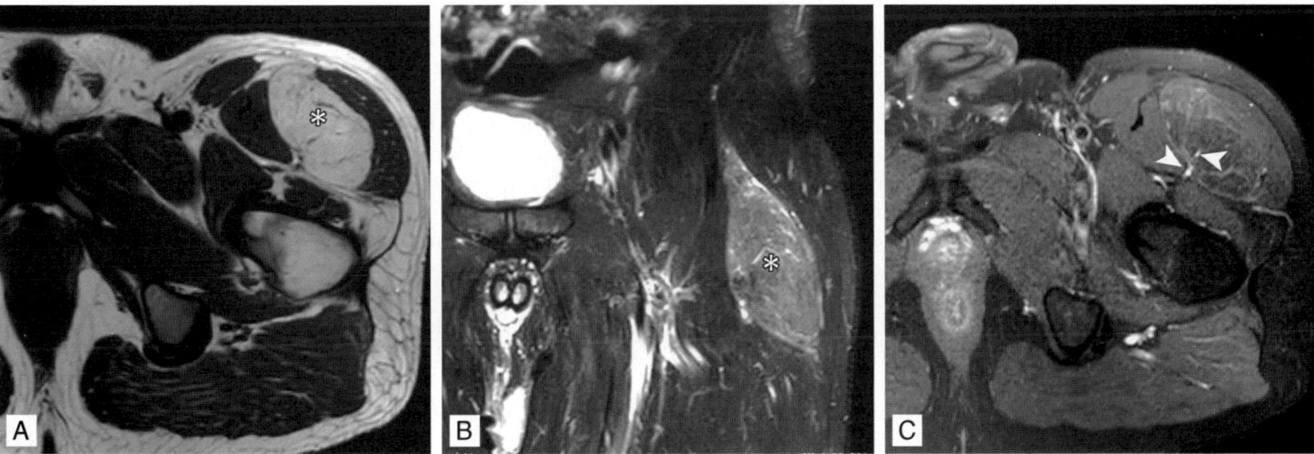

Figure 64.29 Hibernoma. Commonly found in the thigh, hibernoma (*asterisks*) has characteristics (A) high T1w signal (but just slightly lower than subcutaneous fat), (B) and signal suppression (though not as suppressed as subcutaneous fat) as seen on this T2w SPAIR coronal image. (C) T1w FS post-contrast demonstrates heterogenous enhancement, with a feeding/draining vessel visible (*arrowheads*).

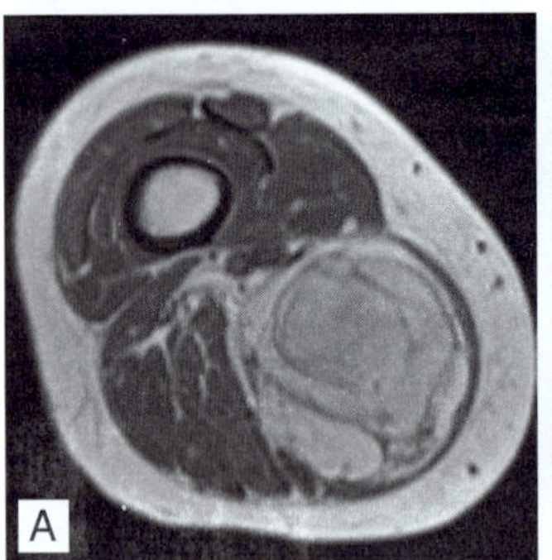

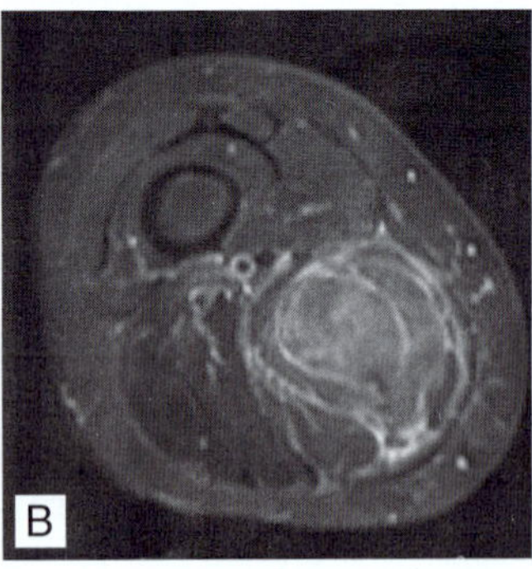

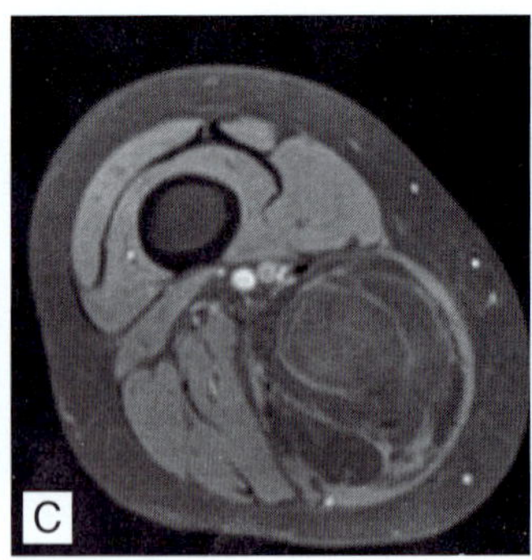

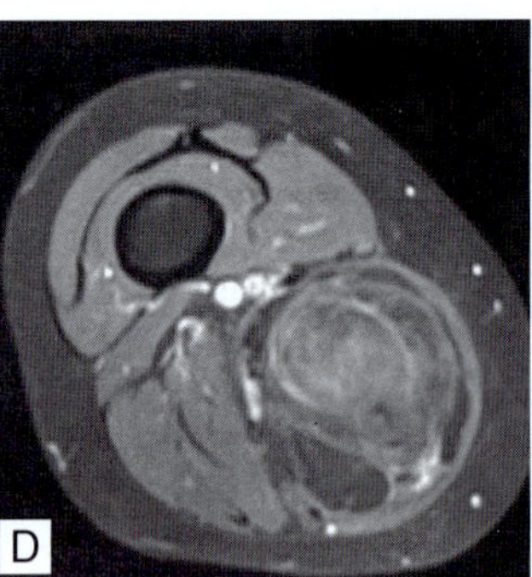

Figure 64.30 Atypical lipomatous tumor/well-differentiated lipoma-like liposarcoma. (A) T1w image demonstrates a large lipomatous tumor with thick septae, which are hyperintense on the (B) STIR sequence. T1w FS (C) precontrast and (D) postcontrast images demonstrate enhancement about the lesion and the septae. There is also background inhomogeneity which also enhances.

- On T1w MRI, it is of high signal, but slightly lower than that of subcutaneous fat, with partial suppression on fat-suppressed sequences. Hibernoma typically appear homogenous on imaging, though a small proportion can be heterogenous
- Contrast enhancement is present on both CT and MRI, and can be heterogenous, reflecting its hypervascularity. Indeed prominent serpentine vessels can sometimes be seen in the lesion, and may demonstrate flow-void on MRI [37]. Some investigators advocate using MR angiography to visualize the feeding and draining vessels to aid surgical planning [38]
- On PET/CT, hibernomas demonstrate intense uptake, much higher than that reported in lipoma and liposarcoma. This reflects the vascularity and large number of mitochondria, which interestingly lends itself to a feeling of warmth during clinical examination over a hibernoma, in contradistinction to the cool feeling over a lipoma

Malignant Adipocytic Tumors (Liposarcoma)

Liposarcoma is the second most common soft tissue sarcoma, comprising of 14% of all malignant soft tissue tumors, trailing behind MFH (24%) (this entity does not exist anymore, now renamed to undifferentiated pleomorphic sarcoma) [30]. WHO recognizes four subtypes of malignant lipomatous neoplasm. They are:

1. atypical lipomatous tumor (ALT), also known as well-differentiated lipoma-like liposarcoma (WDLLL);
2. dedifferentiated liposarcoma (DDL);
3. myxoid liposarcoma;
4. pleomorphic liposarcoma [33].

Atypical Lipoma/Well-Differentiated Lipoma-Like Liposarcoma

ALT/WDLLL is the most common form of liposarcoma. Like lipoma, they are composed of mature adipocytes, but they are distinct in that there is significant variation in cell sizes and presence of hyperchromatic nuclei. They occur most commonly in the thigh (intramuscular) and in the retroperitoneum, and rarely superficially in the subcutaneous plane [33]. They have no metastatic potential if they remain as ALT/WDLLL.

It is important to distinguish an ALT/WDLLL from a simple lipoma for two reasons. First, ALT/WDLLL has the potential to dedifferentiate and therefore metastasize (lungs being the most common target). Second, and more relevant to a "central-body" ALT/WDLLL (retroperitoneum, mediastinum, spermatic cord), is the extreme difficulty to obtain a clear surgical margin in these locations. This translates to a high recurrence rate (86–92%) and can occasionally cause morbidity. This is in contradistinction to extremity lesions where the risk of recurrence is much lower (9–43%) [39,40]. While ALT/WDLLL are synonyms, it is for this reason that in practice, the term WDLLL should be reserved for "central-body" lesions, and ALT for extremity lesions.

On CT and MRI examinations, an ALT/WDLLL can have attenuation and signal intensities similar to that of subcutaneous fat, and differentiating an ALT/WDLLL from a lipoma may not always be straightforward. MRI is the preferred technique to assess an ALT/WDLLL, whereby presence of features listed here may increase the likelihood of the lesion being a ALT/WDLLL, rather than a lipoma (Fig. 64.30):

- Thick and nodular septa (>2 mm), hyperintense septa or nodules on STIR or fat-suppressed T2w sequences
- Avidly enhancing septa (rather than weakly enhancing)
- Nonadipose areas in the lesion
- Large tumor size >10 cm

These imaging feature are not perfectly specific to ALT/WDLLL and can sometimes overlap with benign lipoma variants. However, this overlap should not impact our immediate management, that is, any lesions with suspicious imaging features should lead to the lesion being regarded as such, and biopsied at the very least.

It is worth discussing briefly the use of immunohistochemical and molecular testing, specifically the role of MDM2 in the diagnosis of ALT/WDLLL. Just as there is limitation in the ability of imaging in differentiating lipoma from ALT/WDLLL, histologically the degree of cytologic atypia can be equivocal and fall short in clinching the diagnosis of an ALT/WDLLL; this is one of the circumstances when MDM2 is useful. MDM2 amplification is a characteristic feature of ALT/WDL and DDL (also present in some nonadipocytic sarcomas), and is not present in a benign lipoma or lipoma variant. MDM2 protein overexpression can be detected with immunohistochemistry, though a more superior test is utilizing fluorescence in situ hybridization to demonstrate amplification of the MDM2 gene (100% sensitivity and 100% specificity) [41], though at higher cost, slower turnaround time, and not available to every center. Fluorescence in situ hybridization testing is also recommended for recurrent lipoma, large deep lipomas >15 cm without features of atypia, to rule out possibility of ALT/WDLLL [42].

Dedifferentiated Liposarcoma

DDL describes a lesion which was originally an ALT/WDLLL, which has undergone nonlipogenic sarcomatous dedifferentiation. A previously resected ALT/WDLLL can also transform into a DDL at the time of recurrence. The risk of dedifferentiation is thought to be higher in lesions located in a "central body location" (retroperitoneum, mediastinum, spermatic cord) (22%), compared to extremity lesions (7%) [40]. However, it is thought more likely that this risk of dedifferentiation is "time-dependent" rather than "site-dependent," due to the higher risk of persistent disease in the retroperitoneum.

Most DDL is located in the retroperitoneum (70%), followed by 21% in the extremities and trunk, and the rest in scrotum/spermatic cord (9%) [43]. DDL can also occur in the subcutaneous tissue, although rare. Risk of metastasis from DDL is widely variable in the literature, ranging from 2% to 17% [43,44]. Local recurrence and disease-related mortality are reported at 41% and 28%, respectively, with lesions in the retroperitoneum carrying the worst survival [43].

On imaging, DDL (Fig. 64.31):

- Often have features of an ALT/WDL, with focal variably sized areas of dedifferentiation. Occasionally, the original lipomatous areas may not be visible on imaging
- The dedifferentiated area will appear as a nodular, nonlipomatous component on both MRI and CT
- On MRI, the dedifferentiated area will reflect the signal characteristics specific to the dedifferentiated tissue, but generally is low/intermediate on T1w, and intermediate-high on T2w
- On CT, this component can have a variable CT attenuation and is nonspecific
- This dedifferentiated component will enhance on either CT or MRI
- Mineralization can sometimes be appreciated on CT or on radiographs

Myxoid Liposarcoma

Myxoid liposarcoma is the second most common form of liposarcoma, accounting for around 25% of all liposarcoma, trailing behind the most common well-differentiated type (48%) [30]. It typically represents as a painless mass, affecting patients of mean age 42 years. It can also occur in younger patients; indeed, while rare in the pediatric population, it is the most common subtype of liposarcoma in patients <22 years of age [45]. Majority of lesions (>75%) are located in the lower extremity, with the thigh being the most common location [30].

Myxoid liposarcoma has a prominent myxoid matrix with a delicate vascular network, admixed with variable amount of lipoblasts, and round or oval nonlipogenic cells. The amount of fat is variable and can range from <5% to 90% of the tumor volume. On MRI, myxoid liposarcoma has (Figs. 64.32 and 64.33)

- well-defined multilobulated appearance with septations;
- prominent myxoid appearance appearing as low T1w, high T2w areas;
- little to no visible fat. When visible, they appear as lacy, linear, or amorphous high T1w areas;
- heterogenous postcontrast enhancement.

Histological grading of myxoid liposarcoma depends on the amount of round cells in the lesion—low (pure myxoid liposarcoma with no round cells), intermediate (up to 5% of round cells), and high grade (>5% of round cells). Tateishi and colleagues reported that presence of significant contrast enhancement, and with globular and nodular pattern, are predictive of an intermediate or high-grade tumor, probably a reflection of the amount round cells in the lesion. This will in turn influence prognosis

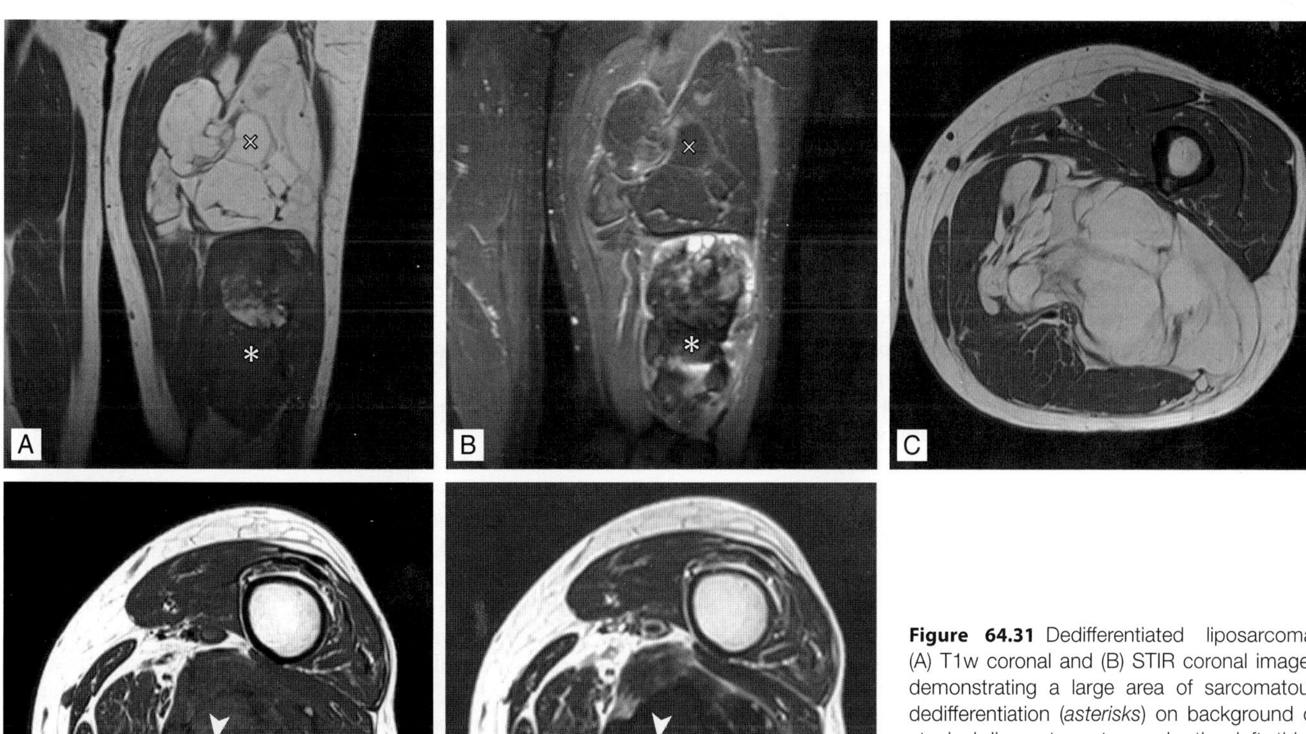

Figure 64.31 Dedifferentiated liposarcoma. (A) T1w coronal and (B) STIR coronal images demonstrating a large area of sarcomatous dedifferentiation (*asterisks*) on background of atypical lipomatous tumor in the left thigh (cross). (C) T1w axial demonstrating the ALT/WDLLL component with thick nodular septae. More caudally, (D) T1w and (E) T2w axial through the dedifferentiated component with low signal, which on histology is composed of "fibrotic" tissue with few vacuolated adipocytes (*arrowheads*).

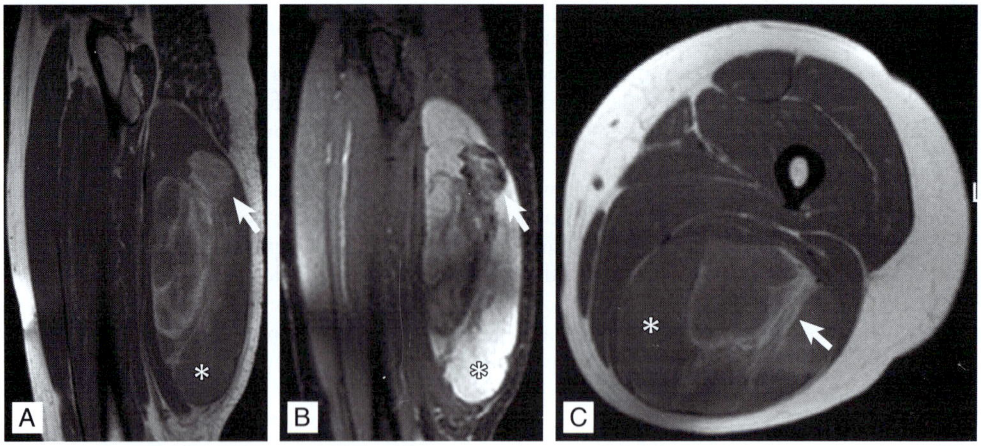

Figure 64.32 Myxoid liposarcoma. (A) T1w sagittal, (B) STIR sagittal, (C) T1w axial images of the left thigh. In this example, the diagnosis of myxoid liposarcoma can be arrived radiologically given the presence of prominent myxoid matrix (*asterisks*), fat (*arrows*), and a well-defined, multilobulated and septated appearance.

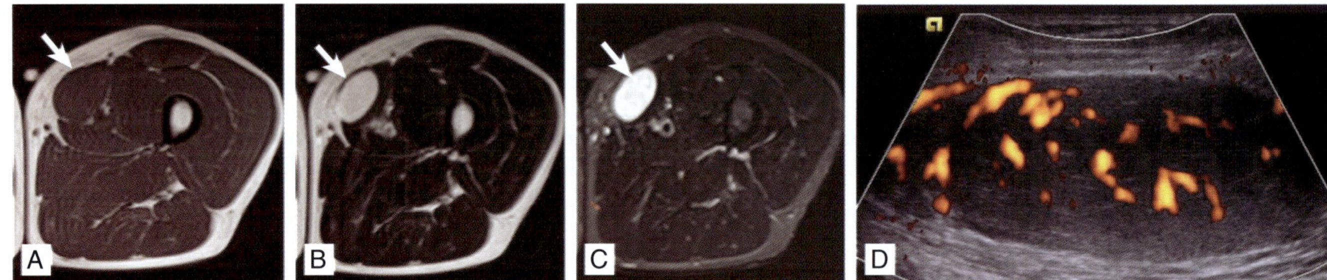

Figure 64.33 Myxoid liposarcoma can masquerade as a myxoma or cyst. Myxoid liposarcoma (*arrows*) can have so little fat that it is not seen on imaging. (A) T1w axial image showing a homogenous low signal lesion with no presence of fat. Furthermore, its prominent myxoid matrix leads to a homogenous high (B) T2w and (C) STIR signal, and can be misinterpreted as a simple cyst. (D) However, with USG, one can easily demonstrate the intralesional vascularity, confirming its solid nature and quickly discount a simple cyst.

adversely. Low-grade tumors on the other hand are likely to have thin septa or has a tumor capsule.

Myxoid liposarcoma metastases are more likely to be extrapulmonary, in contradistinction to most other sarcomas and other forms of liposarcoma which tend to metastasize to the lungs first. For example, in a series, 81% of first metastatic site from myxoid liposarcoma are extrapulmonary, involving a variety of areas including limb muscles, subcutaneous tissue, retroperitoneal, and chest wall [46]. For this reason, staging for this type of sarcoma often involves whole-body imaging in the form of MRI, CT, or PET/CT. At the senior author's institution, we perform whole-body MRI for routine staging of myxoid liposarcoma (Fig. 64.34).

Myxoid liposarcoma, given their substantial myxoid stroma, can mimic a cyst or other myxoid tumor on imaging, such as intramuscular myxoma or myxoid chondrosarcoma and myxofibrosarcoma.

Pleomorphic Liposarcoma

Pleomorphic liposarcoma is the rarest of all liposarcoma, accounting for 6% of all cases, affecting patients with mean age of 60 years [30]. The lower extremity is the most common location (38–47% of cases). Other sites include the upper limb (14–18%), retroperitoneum (7–15%), and trunk (8–14%) [30,47]. Around a quarter of cases can occur superficially (in the subcutaneous tissue or skin) [47].

On MRI, imaging features may be similar to that of other high-grade sarcomas (heterogenous high T2w signal, with postcontrast enhancement). Furthermore, there may only be a little amount of fat visible, in line with histological findings of variable amount of lipoblasts even between areas within the same tumor [33]. This highlights the importance of intralesional targeting during biopsy, to also sample the lipogenic component to enable histological diagnosis of pleomorphic liposarcoma, which otherwise may be interpreted as undifferentiated pleomorphic sarcoma.

Fibroblastic/Myofibroblastic Tumors

Nodular Fasciitis

Nodular fasciitis is a benign proliferation of fibroblasts and myofibroblasts. It usually presents as a rapidly growing mass or nodule in a span of few weeks, and together with high cellularity and mitotic activity, leads to common misdiagnosis as sarcoma [48]. The nodules can be a little painful, and measure around 2 cm in size. It is more commonly found in adults (20–50 years), and most frequently located in the forearm (27%), thigh (17%), upper arm (12%), followed by trunk, and head and neck [49,50].

Nodular fasciitis, as the name suggests, involves the fascia (either superficial or deep fascia). Lesions can be sited in the subcutaneous plane (most common), intramuscular plane, or along the fascia. Intramuscular lesions are usually slightly larger (around 2.5 cm in size).

On MRI, nodular fasciitis appears (Fig. 64.35):

- Variable MR signal depending on the amount of myxoid and fibrous stroma, and also the cellularity of the lesion. Myxoid stroma will produce iso T1w, high T2w signal; fibrous stroma

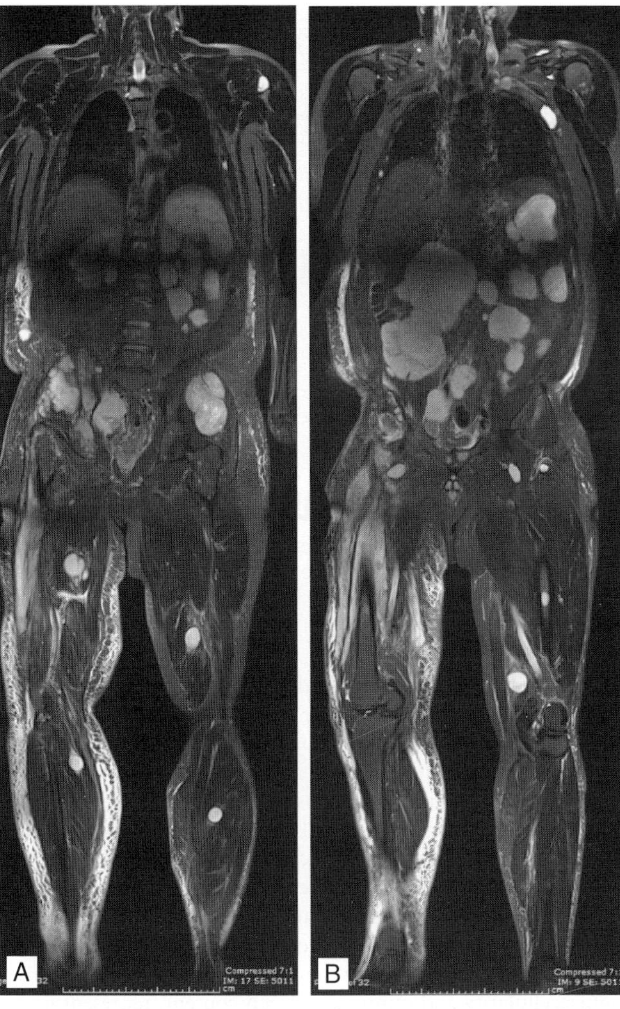

Figure 64.34 Myxoid liposarcoma and their tendency for extrapulmonary metastases. (A and B) STIR coronal of whole-body MRI of a patient with myxoid liposarcoma diagnosed 2 years earlier. Despite the diffuse skeletal and soft tissue metastases, there is no pulmonary metastasis demonstrated on the concurrent CT thorax (not shown).

low T1w and T2w signal; cellular lesion has slightly increased T1w, high T2w signal
- Round or oval in shape
- Fascial tail
- Variable contrast enhancement. Enhancement patterns documented include homogenous (myxoid lesions), heterogenous (cellular lesions), and periperal (fibrous lesions)

Differential diagnoses for nodular fasciitis include extra-abdominal desmoid lesion, fibrous histiocytoma, PNST, and sarcoma (myxofibrosarcoma or fibrosarcoma). Nodular fasciitis has a few rare variants, one of which is ossifying fasciitis where metaplastic ossification can be seen, bringing in other differentials such as extraosseous osteosarcoma and myositis ossificans.

Elastofibroma

Elastofibroma is a benign proliferation of fibrocollagenous tissue with prominent elastic fibers, characteristically located deep to the inferomedial border of the scapula and superficial to the posterior chest wall. It has a reported prevalence as high as 18% in an autopsy study (although a separate CT study revealed a prevalence of only 2%) [51,52]. It is a disease affecting patients almost exclusively over the age of 55 years old, with higher prevalence in female. Elastofibroma can be bilateral in about half of the cases [51]. Up to half of the patients will experience enough symptoms (pain, stiffness, "clunking" sensation) to require surgical excision.

On imaging (Fig. 64.36):
- The lesion lies deep to the scapula and muscles, and superficial to the ribs
- It can have a convex posterolateral margin [52]
- On MRI, the lesion is demonstrated as a nonencapsulated heterogenous soft tissue mass, with low T1w and T2w signal (reflecting its fibrous content), and interlaced with areas of fat
- Enhancement can be subtle on MRI
- On CT, the lesion has attenuation similar to that of muscles, again interlaced with areas of fat
- USG will demonstrate interspersed linearities within the lesion, similar to that of the overlying muscles. Dynamic USG is useful by asking the patient to perform movements that will elicit the symptoms, typically by abducting the shoulder (while

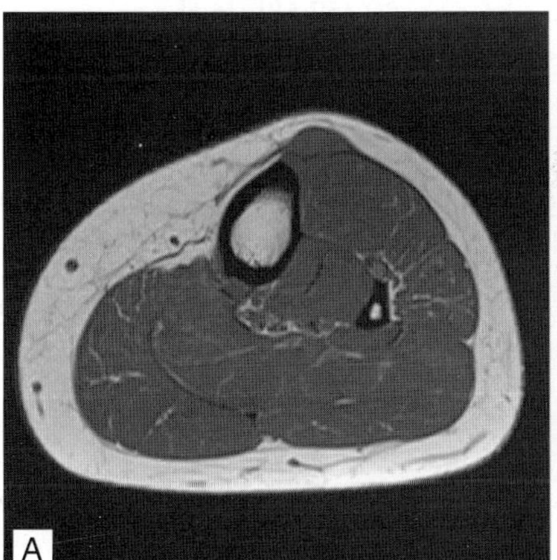

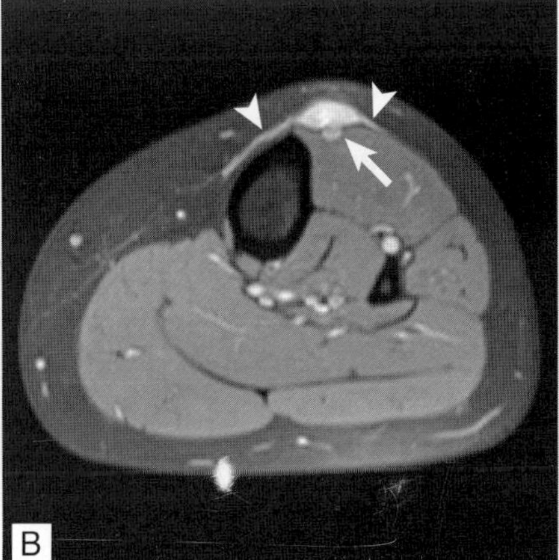

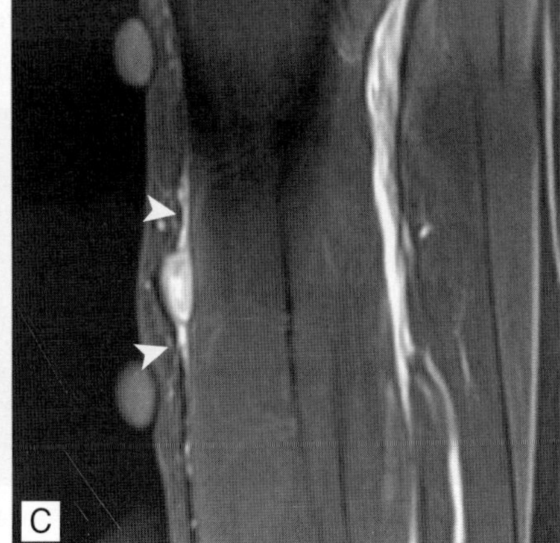

Figure 64.35 Nodular fasciitis in the leg of a 39-year-old patient. (A) T1w axial, (B) PD FS axial, (C) STIR sagittal images demonstrating a lesion based on the deep fascia, with a nodule penetrating through this fascia into the tibialis anterior muscle (*arrow*). Note the fascial tails (*arrowheads*) extending from the nodule.

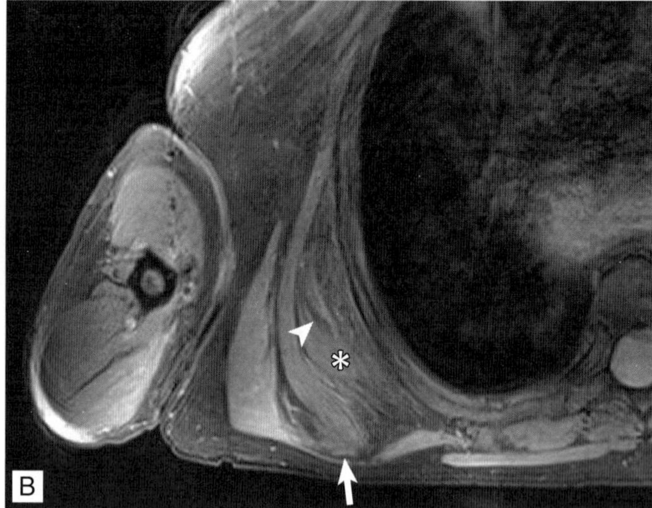

Figure 64.36 Elastofibroma. (A) T1w and (B) PD FS axial images demonstrating a nonencapsulated mass (*asterisks*) lying in between serratus anterior and the ribs, on the inferomedial border of the scapula (*arrow*). The fibrocollagenous content of elastofibroma has a relatively isointense signal to muscles. Interlaced areas of internal fat (*arrowheads*) can also be seen as slivers of signal suppression on image (B).

the patient is lying prone), to protrude the mass beyond the inferior border of the scapula

Superficial Fibromatoses

Both palmar and plantar fibromatoses are superficial fibromatoses, characterized by infiltrative fibroblastic proliferation of the palmar and plantar aponeurosis, respectively. These are classified as intermediate malignancy by WHO, being locally aggressive though without metastatic potential [33].

Palmar Fibromatosis

Palmar fibromatoses (Dupuytren's contracture) represent the most common form of superficial fibromatoses. There is a predilection or male patients, with increasing prevalence with increasing age, ranging from 2% under 40 years old, to 20% in over 60 years old in a study [53]. It can also occur bilaterally. Palmar fibromatosis initially manifests as a palpable firm nodule, most commonly on the ulnar side on the fourth digit (36%), followed by the third (29%) and fifth digits (20%) [54], and mostly occurring at the level of the distal metacarpal. With time, there may be bands or cordlike indurations developing between the nodules and adjacent fingers, leading to the characteristic flexion contracture.

Diagnosis of palmar fibromatosis can be made on USG. It has:

- a hypoechoic nodular or cord appearance;
- majority of palmar fibromatosis lies at the level of the distal metacarpal, directly superficial to the flexor tendons;
- intralesional vascularity or calcification can be seen rarely.

On MRI (Fig. 64.37), the nodules or cords are mostly low signal on T1w and T2w images, shown to represent the hypocellular and dense collagen nature of the lesion [55]. However, some lesions can be of intermediate T1w and T2w signals, reflecting their higher cellularity and minimal collagen content, representing the earlier proliferative stage of the disease [48,55].

Treatment-wise, there is limited evidence in conservative measurements in preventing progression to contracture. Intralesional corticosteroid injection, for example, has been reported to soften and decrease the size of the nodules (although 50% risk of recurrence), but has not been shown to improve or prevent a contracture [56]. Radiation therapy is another form of noninvasive option which can improve pain related to the nodules (also for plantar fibromatosis) [57,58]. In the presence of contracture, percutaneous needle fasciotomy to rupture the

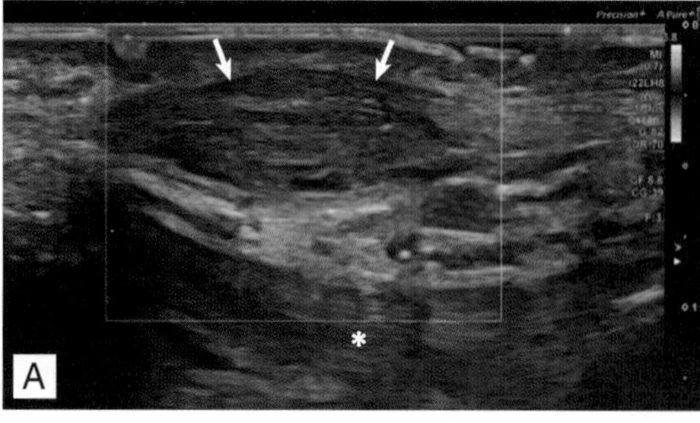

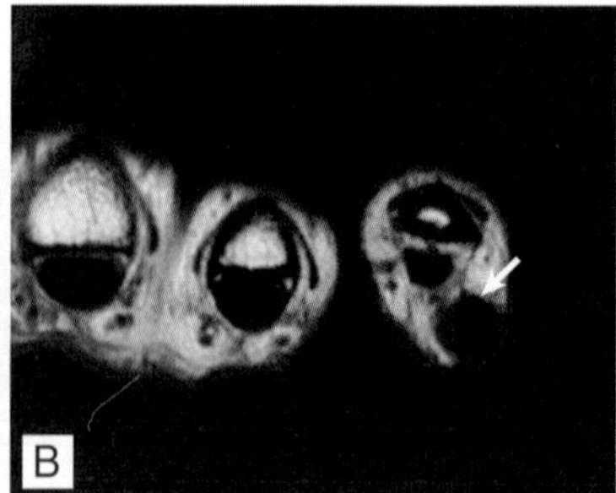

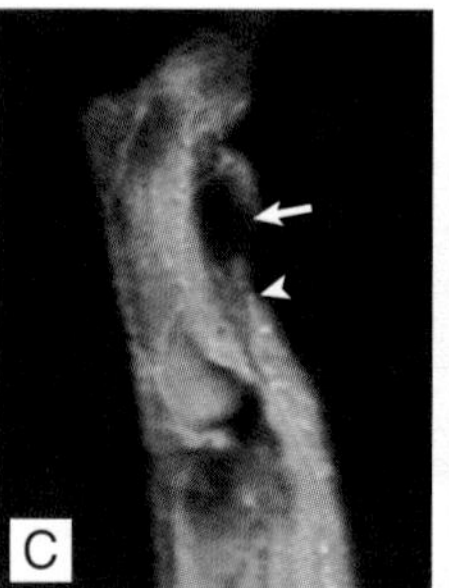

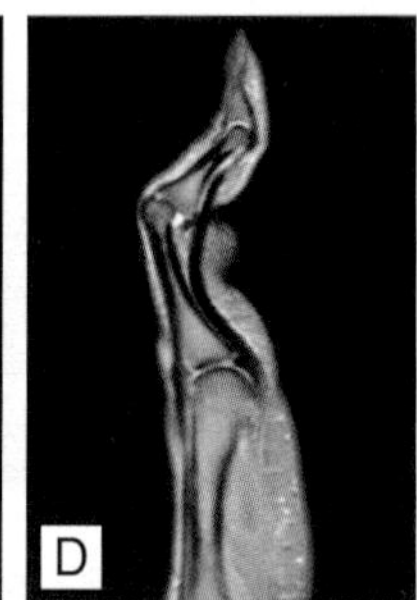

Figure 64.37 Dupuytren's nodule. A 56-year-old female presented with a painless, slow-growing, solitary lump in her little finger, at the level of the proximal phalanx neck. (A) USG demonstrated a superficial solid fusiform mass (*arrows*), a distance away from the underlying flexor tendon (*asterisk*). No intralesional vascularity. (B) T1w axial, (C) PD SPIR MRI demonstrate the lump (*arrows*) to have a low signal intensity, which can be seen to be related to a thickened palmar aponeurosis (*arrowhead*). (D) PDW SPIR sagittal image demonstrates the resultant contracture of the finger. The patient reported another lump in her contralateral palm a few months later (not shown).

cord is a minimally invasive option, with recurrence of around 50% [59]. Surgical fasciectomy is the mainstay treatment and can range from regional fasciectomy to more extensive dermofasciectomy requiring skin grafting; there is a wide range in the risk of recurrence reported in literature. Another form of treatment is enzymatic fasciotomy with collagenase injection, which is proving to be a promising nonsurgical alternative, shown to improve contracture and improve hand function, and may have a role as first-line intervention for contracture [60].

Plantar Fibromatosis

Plantar fibromatosis (Ledderhose disease) usually arises in the central or medial cord of the plantar arch. There is a higher incidence in younger population, with up to 44% of cases seen before 30 years old [61]. Patients can complain of pain which can be exacerbated by walking or standing, or just of a palpable lump without actual symptoms [62]. In contradistinction to its palmar counterpart, contracture is not a typical feature in plantar fibromatosis, and can be seen rarely in the hallux.

On USG, plantar fibromatosis:

- Appear as a fusiform nodule of hypo- or mixed echogenicity
- Located on either the medial or central bands of the fascia at the mid- or forefoot [62,63]
- A fifth of the lesions can have moderate or marked vascularity, with the remaining majority demonstrating little to no vascularity [63]
- Larger lesions can demonstrate the comb-sign where there is alternating bands of hypo- and isoechoic bands in the lesion (relative to plantar fascia) [63]

On MRI, the lesion appears (Fig. 64.38):

- As a well-defined nodule located along the plantar fascia
- Similar to palmar fibromatosis, the signal characteristics depends on the amount of collagen and cellularity, varying between low and intermediate on T1w and T2w images

Symptoms of plantar fibromatosis generally improve over time. Therefore, it is best managed conservatively with physiotherapy and orthotics. Other noninvasive management for painful nodules includes intralesional corticosteroid injection and radiation therapy. Surgical intervention can be offered for severe intractable cases, with a variable risk of recurrence depending on the extent of the surgery; local excision is associated with 100% recurrence rate, compared with 25% in total plantar fasciectomy [64].

Deep Fibromatoses

Deep fibromatoses are also known as desmoid tumors. These are rare, accounting for around 0.4% of all benign soft tissue tumors [1]. Similar to superficial fibromatoses, these are also of intermediate malignancy being locally aggressive with no potential for metastasis. Deep fibromatoses demonstrate a more aggressive behavior compared to superficial fibromatoses with infiltrative growth pattern and high risk of recurrence. Lesions can also be multicentral and metachronous [65]. Deep fibromatoses are composed of spindle-shaped myofibroblastic cells embedded in a collagenous matrix. There can also be a variable degree of myxoid matrix [48].

Deep fibromatoses can be divided into three subtypes based on their location:

1. *Extra-abdominal fibromatosis.* This is commonly found in the lower limbs (particularly the foot, followed by hip and thigh, and the lower leg), shoulder, chest wall, and back (Fig. 64.39). Metachronous lesions can be seen in around 10% of cases, and tend to arise in the same limb in a more proximal location [65,66]
2. *Abdominal fibromatosis.* This has a tendency to affect women of child-bearing age, and can arise or demonstrate rapid growth during pregnancy or in the postpartum period. Lesions can arise from the aponeuroses or muscles of the anterior abdominal wall, particularly the rectus abdominis and internal oblique muscles or fascia (Fig. 64.40)
3. *Intra-abdominal fibromatosis.* Lesions typically arise from the mesentery of the small bowels or from the retroperitoneum. As a whole, majority of desmoid lesions are incidental, but there is an association with familial adenomatous polyposis (Gardner syndrome), where around 10% of patients can develop desmoid lesions, the majority of which are intra-abdominal desmoids [67]

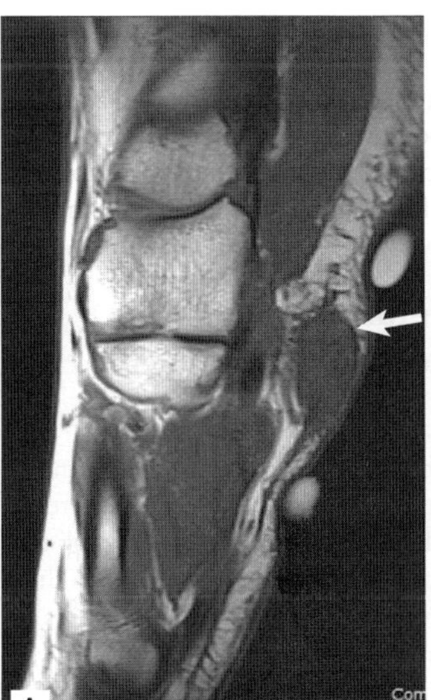

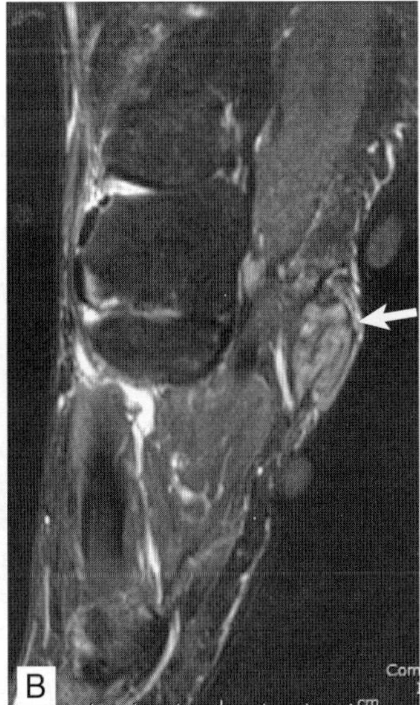

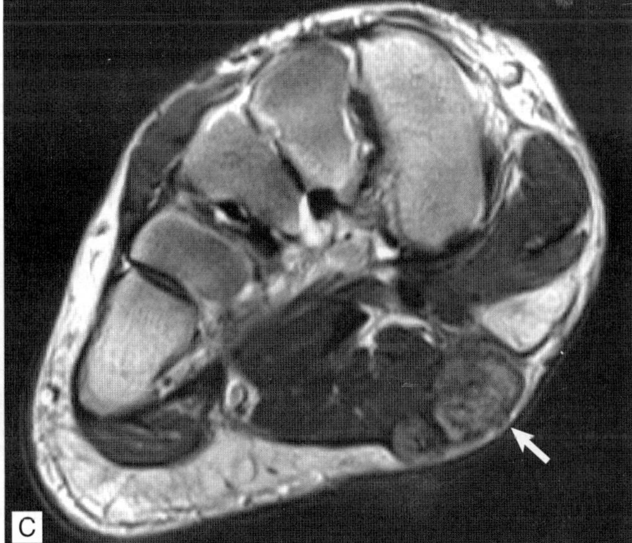

Figure 64.38 Plantar fibromatosis. (A) T1w sagittal, (B) STIR sagittal, (C) T2w short axial images showing a fusiform mass (*arrows*) arising from the central band of the plantar fascia. It has a low T1w signal and intermediate/high signal on STIR and T2w images. This patient also has bilateral plantar fibromas (not shown).

MRI findings are generally nonspecific. They can appear:

- Low/isointense on T1w, moderate to high on T2w
- Band-like or septated areas of low T2w in the lesion [73]
- Marked peripheral contrast enhancement, some with spoked-wheel appearance [8,73]

Myxofibrosarcoma

Myxofibrosarcoma (previously known as myxoid MFH) is a malignant fibroblastic tumor with a variable myxoid stroma. Myxofibrosarcoma most commonly affects older patients with median age 61 years, and found most often in the lower extremities [74].

MRI findings:

- Homogenous T1w, high T2w, reflecting the prominent myxoid stroma in the lesion
- Curvilinear extension or "tails" along fascial planes. This finding illustrates the infiltrative nature of its growth. When applied in the assessment of myxoid-predominant lesions, this sign has a reported sensitivity of 64–77%, and a specificity 79–90% in diagnosing myxofibrosarcoma [74]. These "tumor tails" should be recognized and conveyed to the surgeons to ensure complete surgical resection (Fig. 64.42)
- Postcontrast enhancement

Fibrohistiocytic Tumors

Giant Cell Tumor of Tendon Sheath

GCT of tendon sheath is a group of tumors arising from the synoviocytes which line the surface of synovial membrane (which in turn lines joints, tendon sheaths, and bursae). There are two main types of GCTs of tendon sheath:

1) Localized type, also known as tenosynovial GCT (TS-GCT)
2) Diffuse type, also known as PVNS

Typically, localized type TS-GCT is an extra-articular lesion closely related to the tendon sheath, whereas diffuse type PVNS is an intra-articular lesion. Less commonly however, localized type can also present as an intra-articular location, and diffuse type PVNS in an extra-articular location (either as an extra-articular extension from an intra-articular lesion, or as a purely extra-articular lesion).

Localized Type Tenosynovial Giant Cell Tumor

This commonly affects patients between 20 and 50 years old (mean 32 years), with a predilection for female patients (70%). Large majority of lesion is located in the hand, affecting most commonly the thumb (20–37%) and index finger (19–23%) [75,76]. Less commonly affected areas include ankle and

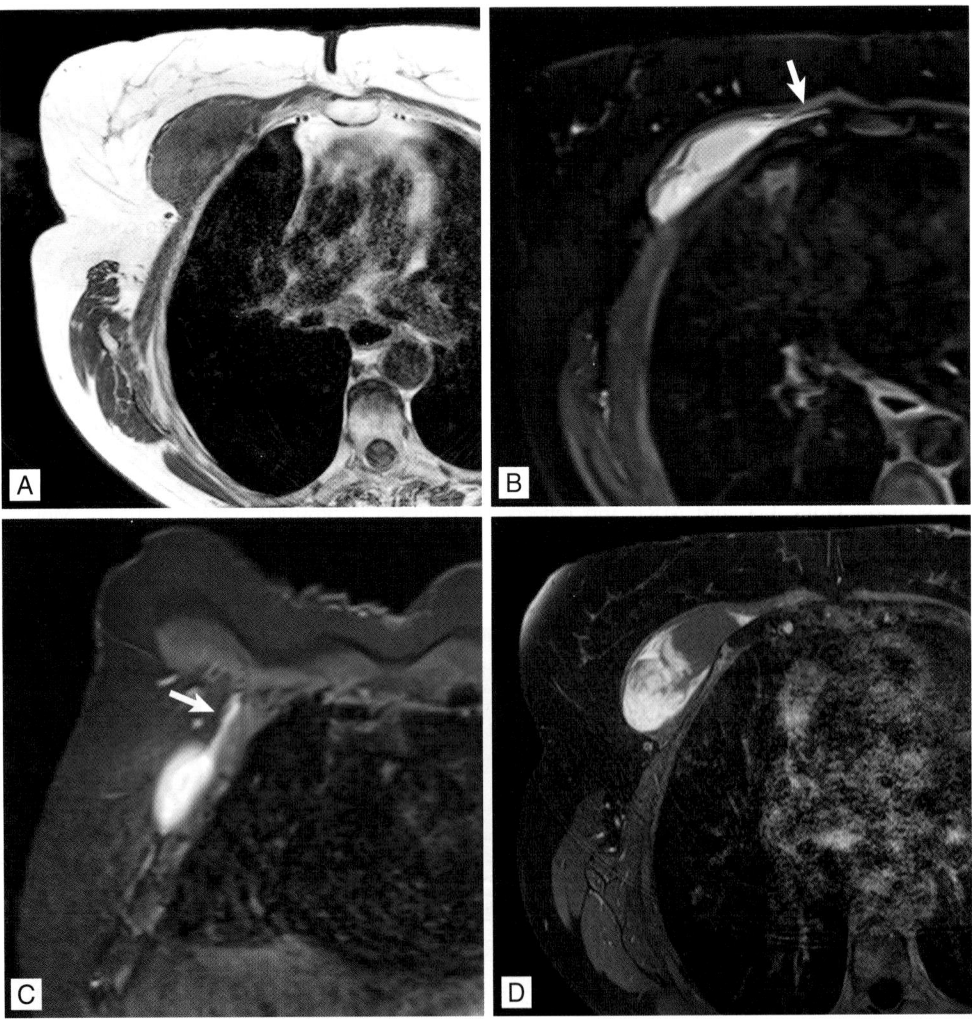

Figure 64.42 Myxofibrosarcoma in a 71-year-old patient. (A) T1w axial, (B) PD FS axial, (C) T1w STIR coronal image demonstrating a well-defined mass with tumoral tails (*arrows*) seen on the medial and cranial portion of the mass. (D) T1w FS axial image demonstrating postcontrast enhancement. It has a fairly homogenous fluid-like signal on images (A) and (B), reflecting its myxoid stroma.

foot [77]. While typically extra-articular, localized GCT can also present as an intra-articular lesion (Fig. 64.43), typically in the knee joint, and should not be confused as a diffuse type GCT.

Localized type GCT usually presents as a painless, slow-growing nodule in the hand, usually on the volar surface, measuring 1–2 cm in size [75]. Pressure erosion of the underlying bone can occasionally be seen.

On USG, tenosynovial GCT appears:

- Well-defined, solid, hypoechoic, and homogenous
- Posterior acoustic shadowing can sometimes be present
- Vascularity is present on Doppler USG
- Closely related to tendon, but does not move with tendon excursion, given that the tumor is arising from tendon sheath, rather than from the tendon

On MRI, tenosynovial GCT appears (Fig. 64.44):

- Isointense on T1w relative to muscle. It can be variable (hypo-, iso-, or hyperintense on T2w imaging
- Blooming artifact on gradient-echo sequences due to the presence of hemosiderin
- Close relation to tendon, either partially or completely enveloping the tendon
- Postcontrast enhancement can be heterogenous, or less commonly homogenous [77]

Diffuse Type Giant Cell Tumor (Pigmented Villonodular Synovitis)

PVNS is a rare proliferative disorder of the synovium. This is a benign but locally aggressive neoplastic process. It usually affects young adults, between age 20 and 50 years, with equal gender predilection. The knee joint is by far the most commonly affected site, followed by the hip, and less commonly other joints including ankle, shoulder, and elbow joints. Patients typically present with joint swelling and symptoms of stiffness and popping sensation, with occasionally locking and instability.

Joint effusion can be readily appreciated on radiographs and can occasionally appear dense reflective of hemorrhagic effusion. On MRI, there is (Fig. 64.45):

- large joint effusion;
- variable degree of diffuse synovial thickening, which will have low T1w and T2w signal intensity;
- abnormal synovium will also demonstrate blooming artifact on gradient-echo images due to presence of hemosiderin;
- diffuse postcontrast enhancement of the abnormal synovium;
- there may be underlying bony erosion.

The bony erosion can also be seen on radiograph or CT, which will often have well-defined sclerotic margins. The extent of erosion is also dependent on the capacity of the joint—the smaller the joint, the more likely the presence of erosions. Diffuse PVNS in the hip joint, for example, has erosion documented in 93% of cases, compared to only 26% in the knee joint (which has a large suprapatellar bursa) [78]. Prevalence of erosions is also relatively high in other joints (75% in shoulder, 63% in elbow, and 56% in ankle joints) [78].

Malignant Tenosynovial Giant Cell Tumor

Malignant tenosynovial GCT is extremely rare, and can occur primarily (as an area of sarcoma coexisting with benign TS-GCT), or secondarily (as a sarcomatous recurrence following treatment of a benign TS-GCT). Literature on malignant TS-GCT is sparse, although unpredictable rapid progression or extensive marrow infiltration should raise concern (Fig. 64.46). Pulmonary metastasis has also been reported.

Vascular Tumor and Malformation

The terms "hemangioma" and "vascular malformation" are often incorrectly used interchangeably when they are in fact two distinct entities. Hemangioma is a true neoplasm originating from

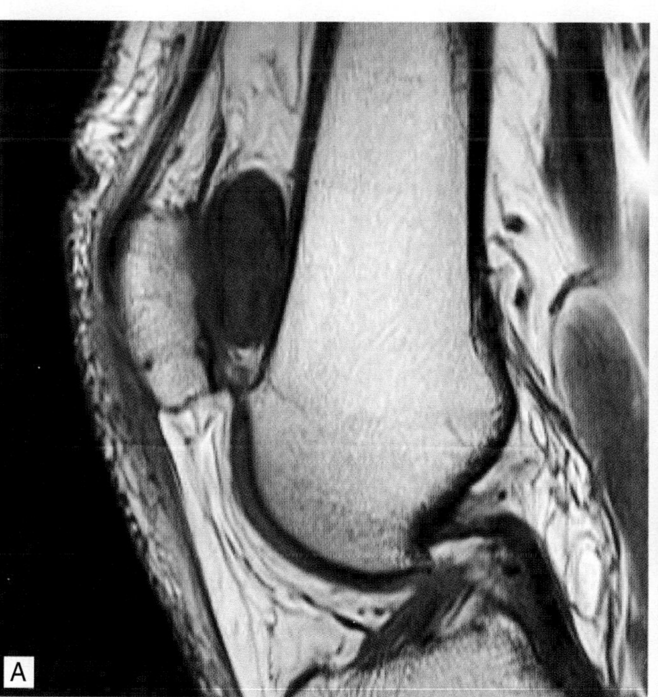

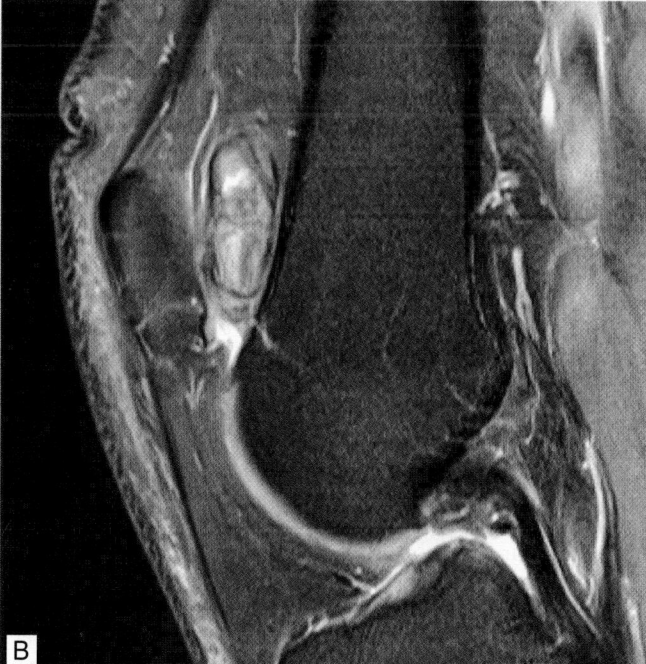

Figure 64.43 Localized type intra-articular tenosynovial GCT. (A) T1w and (B) PD FS sagittal images demonstrate a well-defined mass in the retropatellar region. Note the low signal internal foci and particularly the rim, reflecting hemosiderin.

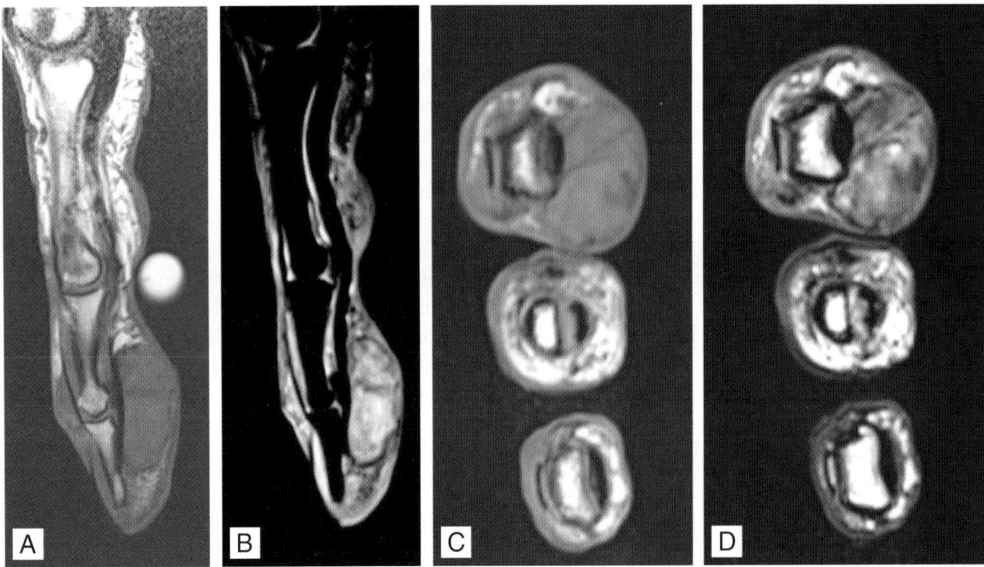

Figure 64.44 Tenosynovial GCT. (A) and (C) T1w sagittal and axial images demonstrating an iso/hypointense lesions partially enveloping the flexor tendon of the middle finger. (B) STIR sagittal image low signal in the lesion and particularly in the rim, representing hemosiderin. (D) The rim and patchy foci of intralesional low signals can be better appreciated on this T2*w axial image.

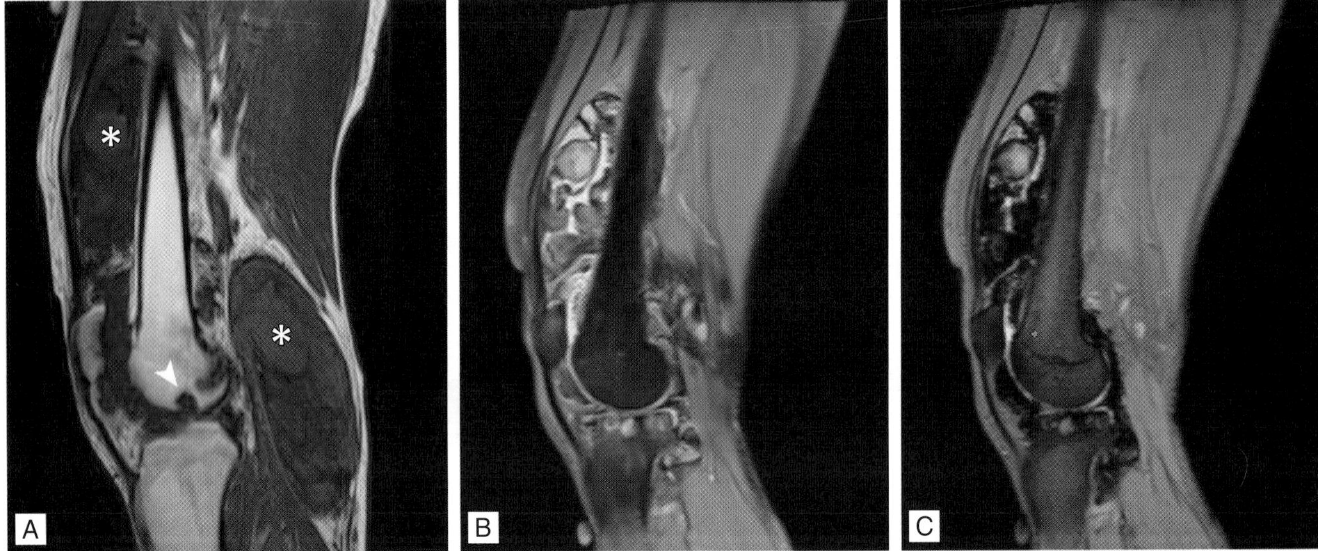

Figure 64.45 Diffuse PVNS in the knee. (A) T1w sagittal, and (B) PD FS sagittal images demonstrating a large knee joint effusion with diffuse synovial thickening in the suprapatellar and semimembranosus bursa (*asterisks*). Erosions can also be seen in the distal femur (*arrowhead*). (C) The lobules of synovial thickening demonstrate low signal rims in keeping with hemosiderin deposition, seen with blooming artifact on the (C) T2*w gradient-echo image.

endothelial cells and represent the benign spectrum of vascular tumors. Vascular malformation on the other hand is a developmental defect occurring in utero with little to no proliferative activity.

Hemangioma

Hemangioma is the most common soft tissue tumor in infancy and childhood. Hemangioma can be divided into several subtypes, the main two being infantile and congenital hemangioma. Infantile hemangioma develop in early postnatal period is red in color, and grow to become elevated and protruding, producing a "strawberry" appearance. Congenital hemangioma, on the other hand, will be fully formed at birth. Broadly speaking, both infantile and congenital hemangiomas can involute (although certain forms can be static, or demonstrate an initial period of rapid growth), whereas vascular malformations tend to grow proportionately with the patient (although can enlarge rapidly in the presence of thrombosis, infection, or trauma) [2].

Hemangiomas are typically located in the head and neck, followed by the trunk and extremities [79]. Imaging of hemangioma is rarely needed as they are diagnosed clinically based on their clinical features, unless when they occur in dangerous areas such as the orbit or airway where crucial anatomical delineation is required. Imaging features are laid out in Table 64.6.

Another noteworthy form of hemangioma is intramuscular hemangioma (Fig. 64.47). This form of hemangioma typically occurs in the lower limbs particularly the thigh [48], and may produce pain. The typical diagnostic cutaneous features are absent in intramuscular hemangioma, and therefore imaging is required for assessment.

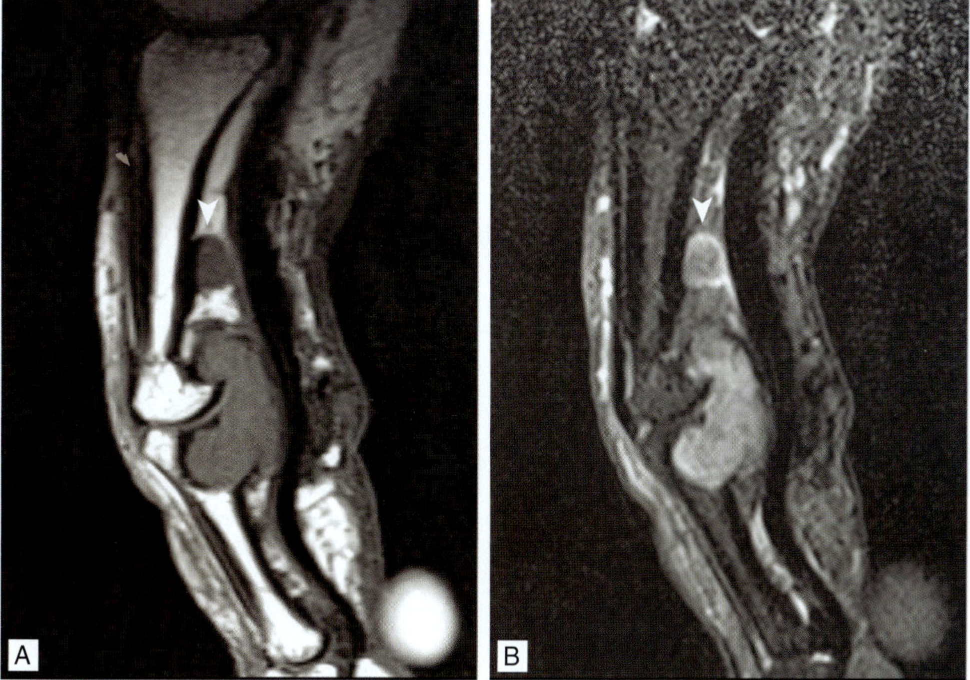

Figure 64.46 Recurrence of GCT of tendon sheath, possibly low-grade malignant. (A) T1w and (B) STIR sagittal images demonstrating a mass with close relationship with the flexor tendon sheath, eroding into the base of the proximal phalanx. There is an additional tumor nodule more proximally (*arrowheads*). Recurrence and aggressive radiological features should raise concern for malignant GCT of tendon sheath. Histologically in this patient, although this lesion did not meet the frank criteria for malignancy, there was high mitotic rate and a degree of nuclear atypia.

On MRI intramuscular hemangioma appears:

- Isointense to muscle on T1w MRI, and heterogenous high signal on T2w
- Fat can be present either within the lesion, or around the lesion
- The lesion will demonstrate homogenous contrast enhancement

On USG, intramuscular hemangioma appears:

- Isoechoic (occasionally hypoechoic) to the adjacent muscle
- Presence of fat can be appreciated as area of hyperechogenicity
- Doppler USG can demonstrate a high-flow lesion with an arterial waveform

Vascular Malformation

Vascular malformation is broadly divided into fast-flow (arterio-venous) and slow-flow lesions (venous, capillary, and

TABLE 64.6 MRI and USG Findings of Hemangioma and Vascular Malformations

	Hemangioma	AV Malformation	Venous Malformation	Lymphatic Malformation
USG	Variable echogenicity mass. Vessels may be too small to be seen on gray scale USG. However, abundance of vessels can be easily appreciated on color Doppler, also demonstrating high flow [81].	Heterogenous lesion. Abundant vessels with high flow. However, unlike hemangioma, vessels in AVM are larger with pulsatile draining veins. Presence of high systolic flow and high diastolic flow, with low resistive index <0.5, reflecting arteriovenous shunting [81].	Variable appearance. Can have anechoic vascular spaces which are compressible, or appear as a heterogenous lesion. Phleboliths, if present, can be identified. Doppler USG will demonstrate either low flow, or lack of flow (due to thrombosis).	Multilocular cystic mass. Look out for fluid–fluid level. Lymphatic malformation can also be in the form of multiple microcysts, in which case the mass will be hyperechogenic rather than cystic appearing.
MRI	Soft tissue mass with intermediate T1w and increased T2w signal. Flow-void can be present.	No well-defined mass lesions. Enlarged feeding arteries and draining veins, with early venous filling on time-resolved contrast-enhanced MRI angiography. Flow-void present. Punctuate areas of high T1w signal cause by hemorrhage and thrombosis.	Normal sized feeding arteries and draining veins, without early venous filling (on time-resolved contrast-enhanced MRI angiography). No flow-voids. Phlebolith is characteristics of venous malformation. Care should be taken so as not to mistake this as flow-voids. Thrombosis can also mimic flow-voids. Variable signal on T1w and T2w because of hemorrhage and thrombosis. High T2w and STIR signal. Fluid–fluid level can be present [2].	Multilocular, septated, cystic lesion. Variable T1w signal due to varying amount of protein. High T2w and STIR signal. Fluid–fluid level can be present. Rim and septa enhancement, sparing the central cystic area.

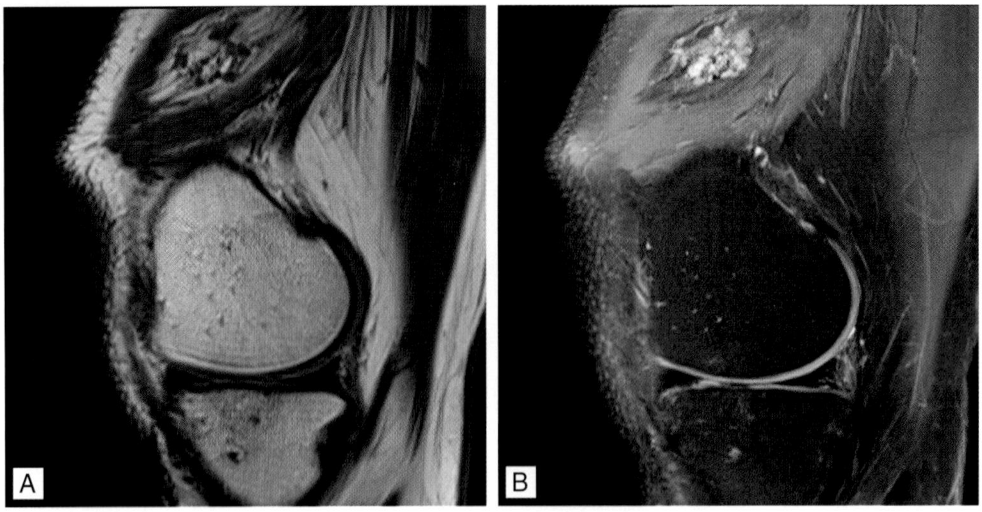

Figure 64.47 Intramuscular hemangioma. Lesion interspersed between the individual muscle fibers of vastus medialis. Note the presence of fat on (A) T1w sagittal image, which suppresses on (B) PD FS sagittal image. Tiny low foci signal on both images is compatible with flow-voids which can be seen in hemangioma.

lymphatics), the latter being more common accounting for 90% of all lesions. A combination of the different vessel types can also occur. Superficial venous malformations have typical clinical appearance of a blue-tinted, puffy, mass (due to dilated vessels), which is compressible and nonpulsatile. They may expand with Valsalva maneuver and easily flattened with pressure. Arteriovenous malformation (AVM) on the other hand, when superficial, can exhibit palpable thrill and pulsatility with increased skin temperature.

Determining a fast-flow lesion from a slow-flow lesion is pivotal in guiding management strategy. As a general rule, a slow-flow malformation is managed with sclerotherapy, whereas a fast-flow lesion will require some form flow control either with tourniquet application or embolization before sclerotherapy, lest the sclerotherapy agent is rapidly washed out of the lesion.

Imaging features of high-flow malformations:

- *Flow-voids on MRI.* Flow-voids on spin echo sequences reflect high-flow nature of the lesion (Fig. 64.48), and is absent in slow-flow lesions. Flow-void can be seen in AVM or hemangioma. However, one must be careful not to mistake a phlebolith for flow-void (Fig. 64.49). Radiograph is invaluable to circumvent this pitfall. In addition, gradient-echo MRI can resolve this; phleboliths are low signal on all pulse sequences, while flow-void is low signal on spin echo but high signal on gradient-echo imaging
- *Early venous filling.* This feature is seen in AVM, which consists of variable proportion of intercommunicating large arteries and veins. There is shunting of the capillary bed, which leads to early enhancement of draining veins, not seen in slow-flow lesions. This feature can be demonstrated on dynamic time-resolved contrast-enhanced MRI angiography, depicting the feeding and draining vessels in detail
- *High systolic flow and low resistive index on spectral USG.* This is seen in AVM and can be variably present in hemangioma too. It can be difficult to ascertain the orientation of the vessel accurately, so the exact peak velocity is difficult to be determined. A mean peak arterial velocity of 32 cm/s has been

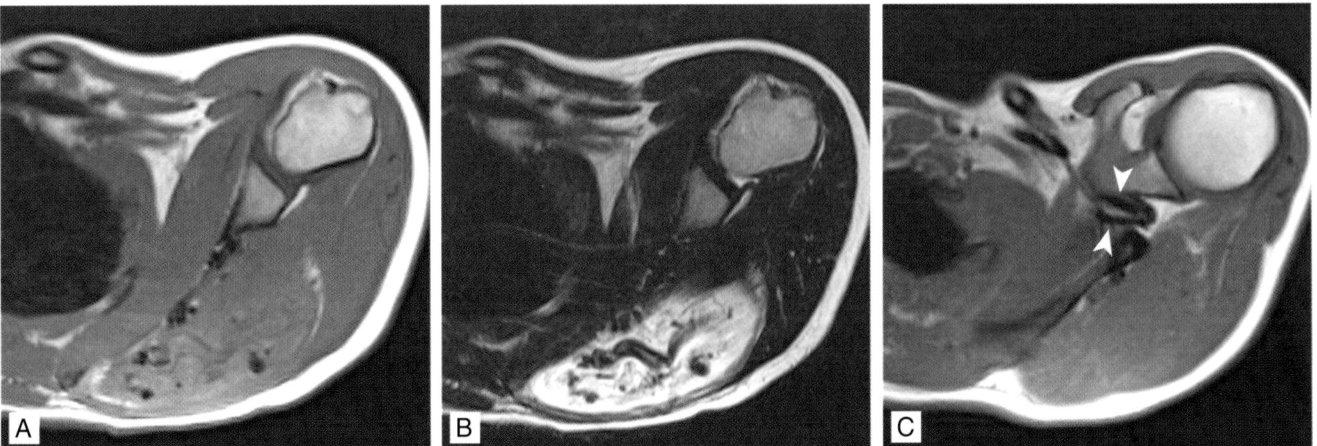

Figure 64.48 AV malformation. (A) T1w and (B) T2w demonstrating a large intramuscular mass in the infraspinatus muscle. Serpentine and tubular flow-voids are reflective of high-flow nature of the vessels on these spin echo sequences. (C) A few slices cranially, the feeding suprascapular vessels can be seen (*arrowheads*) on this T1w axial image.

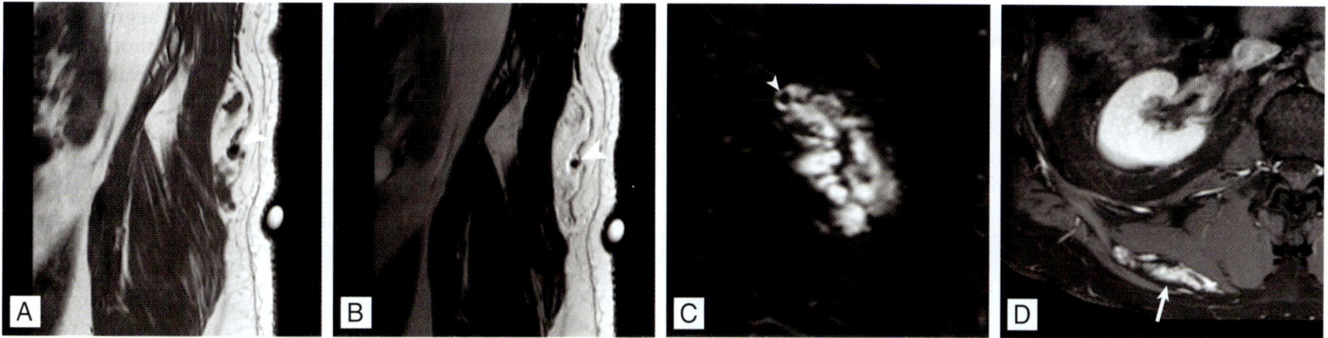

Figure 64.49 Slow-flow venous malformation. (A) T1w sagittal image demonstrates an oval mass adjacent to the right paraspinal muscles where there is serpinginous tubular structures, surrounded by fat, less well seen on (B) T2w sagittal image due to isointensity of its fluid content with adjacent fat. (C) The vascular spaces are also appreciated on this STIR coronal image. (D) Enhancement of these vascular spaces is demonstrated on this T1w FS postcontrast axial image (*arrow*). (C) Of note is presence of signal-void foci (*arrowhead*) which can be mistaken as flow-voids, and are shown to be phleboliths on concurrent CT (not shown).

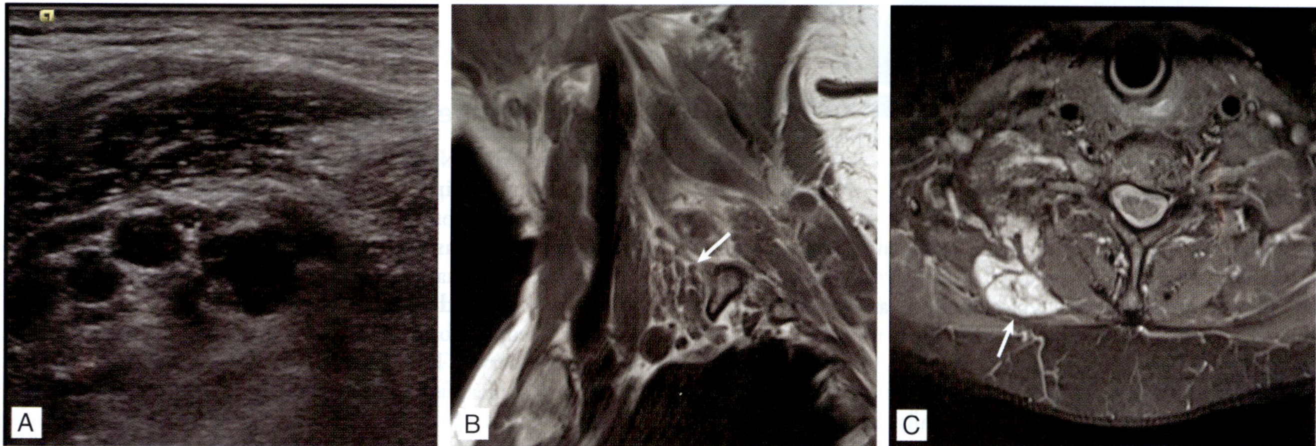

Figure 64.50 Lymphatic malformation. (A) USG and (B) T1w sagittal images demonstrating lobulated cystic space with no Doppler flow (not shown), closely related to the brachial plexus and extending along the intermuscular plane of posterior neck muscles. It is noncompressible. (C) STIR axial images demonstrating the cystic and septated mass (*arrows*).

reported in AVMs [80]. Resistive index threshold of <0.5 has also been reported [81]

- *Earlier contrast enhancement on dynamic MRI.* A high-flow vascular malformation has been shown to demonstrate a significantly earlier maximal enhancement time (5.8 seconds), compared to a slow-flow lesion (88.4 seconds) [82]

Other imaging features in vascular malformations include:

- *Presence of phlebolith.* Phleboliths are characteristic for venous malformation. The slow-flow nature of venous malformation predisposes to formation of thrombi, calcification, and phleboliths, the latter two of which can be appreciated the easiest on radiograph or CT, and also seen on MRI and USG
- *Lobulated or multiloculated cystic mass in lymphatic malformations.* This is better seen on MRI or USG (Fig. 64.50). Lymphatic malformations will also demonstrate rim and septal enhancement, leaving the central cystic component unenhanced
- *Fluid–fluid level.* Lymphatic malformations can have variable amount of protein or hemorrhage, leading to presence of fluid–fluid level, best appreciated on MRI. Venous malformation may also demonstrate this appearance owing to pooling of blood due to its slow-flow nature (Fig. 64.51)

Chondro-osseous Tumor

Soft Tissue Chondroma

Soft tissue chondroma, also known as extraskeletal chondroma, is a benign neoplastic lesion composed of chondrocytes surrounded in a hyaline cartilaginous matrix. About 72% of the lesions are located in the upper limb, 24% in the lower limb. In fact, almost 50% of all soft tissue chondromas are located in the fingers [83]. The lesion arises in the soft tissue (e.g., in the subcutaneous tissue, or attached to the tendon or tendon sheath), and is not attached to the periosteum. Nevertheless, an intimate relationship with the adjacent bone may potentially cause pressure erosion or bone remodeling.

On imaging, the soft tissue chondroma is (Fig. 64.52):

- Typically less than 3 cm
- Has well-defined and lobulated margins
- Mineralization is present in 83% of all lesions in a small series [84], with a morphology typical of that seen in a chondroid lesion, which is ring-like, curvilinear, punctate, or granular. This can be appreciated on CT, radiograph, and even MRI
- On MRI, the nonmineralized area of the lesion has an intermediate to low T1w, and intermediate to hyperintense T2w

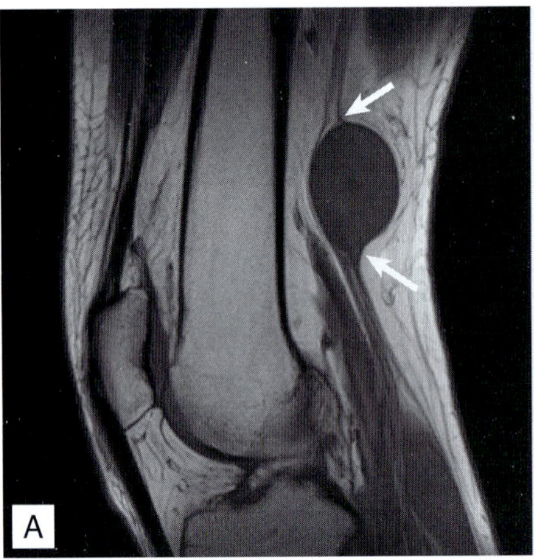

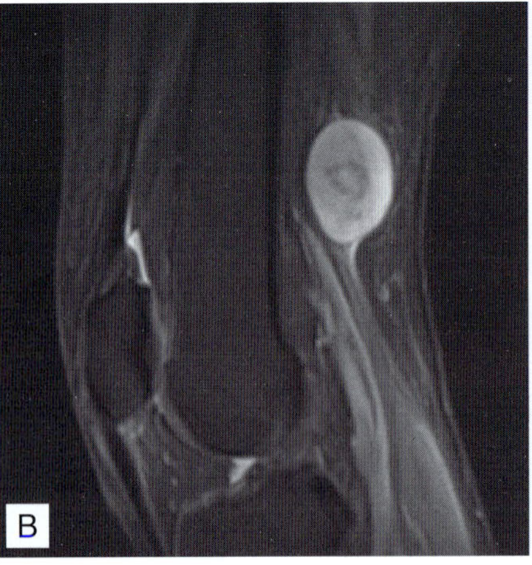

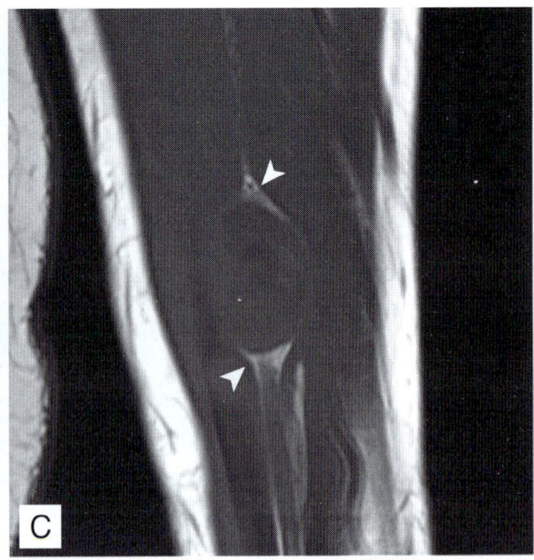

Figure 64.55 Features of a PNST (from different patients). (A) T1w sagittal image demonstrating an eccentric location of this PNST in relation to the sciatic nerve (*arrow*), in keeping with histologically proven schwannoma. (B) STIR sagittal image demonstrating the typical "target sign" of this schwannoma. (C) T1w coronal image demonstrating "split fat" sign (*arrowheads*) in a PNST of the forearm.

There are a few imaging features that will help radiologist suggest a diagnosis of nerve sheath tumor (Fig. 64.55). These features do not necessarily equate to a benign lesion; in fact, differentiating between malignant and benignity is challenging, and will be discussed subsequently.

1. *Anatomical relation to a nerve.* The lesion can be seen to arise from a peripheral nerve. This can be established with either USG or MRI and CT, although may not be possible in a small peripheral branch of the nerve. In addition, differentiating a neurofibroma from a schwannoma is sometimes possible given the way the tumor grows—a schwannoma will arise eccentrically in relation to the nerve, whereas a neurofibroma is located centrally
2. *Ovoid or fusiform shape of the lesion.* Neurofibroma and schwannoma are characteristically fusiform or ovoid in shape
3. *Split-fat sign.* This sign occurs when the nerve courses either inter- or intramuscularly, whereby the presence of fat around the neurovascular bundle is preserved as the growing PNST displaces the adjacent muscle fibers
4. *Target sign.* This sign describes central area of T2w hypointensity with peripheral hyperintensity in the lesion. This reflects the presence of fibrocollagenous content centrally, and myxoid changes peripherally. Contrast enhancement will also be more prominent in the center of the lesion. Presence of target sign is considered to be a benign feature, being less frequently exhibited by malignant PNST [92]
5. *Fascicular sign.* This sign describes the appearance of multiple small ring-like structures with peripheral higher signal intensity, representing the fascicular bundles of the nerve
6. *Associated muscle atrophy.* Muscle atrophy of the surrounding or distally innervated area can be present though subtle. This is best appreciated on T1w (as fatty streaks) and even better if comparison with contralateral unaffected side is available

Malignant PNST

Malignant PNSTs can arise de novo, from malignant degeneration in a pre-existing benign PNST, or secondary to radiation therapy. The risk of MPNST is increased in patient with NF1, with a lifetime risk of around 10% (compared with the general population of 0.01%) [93]. Indeed, around 50% of MPNSTs in a series were found in patients with NF1 [94]. Presentation of MPNSTs is much earlier in patients with NF1 at median of 26 years, compared to 62 years in sporadic MPNST [95]. Symptoms of MPNST include severe rest pain or neurological deficit. Rapid increase in the size of a pre-existing benign PNST should also raise concern for MPNST.

Differentiation of MPNST from a benign PNST is not always straightforward. Several features should raise the suspicion of a MPNST, including (Fig. 64.56):

- large lesion size (>5 cm) [96];
- perilesional edema [96];
- intratumoral cystic change or central necrosis [92,96];
- marked heterogeneity [92];
- infiltrative margin, thereby rendering the split-fat sign less common in MPNST than in BPNST (35% vs 77%) [97];
- prominent enhancement [92];
- lack of target sign (target sign being generally regarded as a sign of benignity, and is rarely seen in MPNST) [98].

DWI/ADC mapping can be of value as well, with MPNSTs demonstrating lower ADC values than benign PNSTs. Using a threshold value of $ADC_{min} \leq 1 \times 10^{-3}$ mm^2/s, a 100% sensitivity and 94% specificity can be achieved in diagnosing MPNSTs. MPNST will also show a higher FDG-PET uptake than benign PNST, with SUV_{max} >3.2 achieving 100% sensitivity and 83% specificity [99].

Muscle Tumors

Muscle tumors are divided into smooth muscle and skeletal muscle tumors. Within these two groups, they can be divided into benign (leiomyoma for smooth muscle, rhabdomyoma for skeletal muscle) and malignant tumors (leiomyosarcoma and rhabdomyosarcoma, respectively).

Leiomyoma

Benign smooth muscle tumors can be categorized into cutaneous leiomyomas, angioleiomyomas, leiomyomas of deep soft tissue, and leiomyomatosis peritonealis disseminata.

Cutaneous leiomyoma is the most common group of benign smooth muscle tumors (Fig. 64.57), and is largely managed outside the remit of radiology, although multiple cutaneous leiomyomas can be part of an autosomal dominant hereditary leiomyomatosis

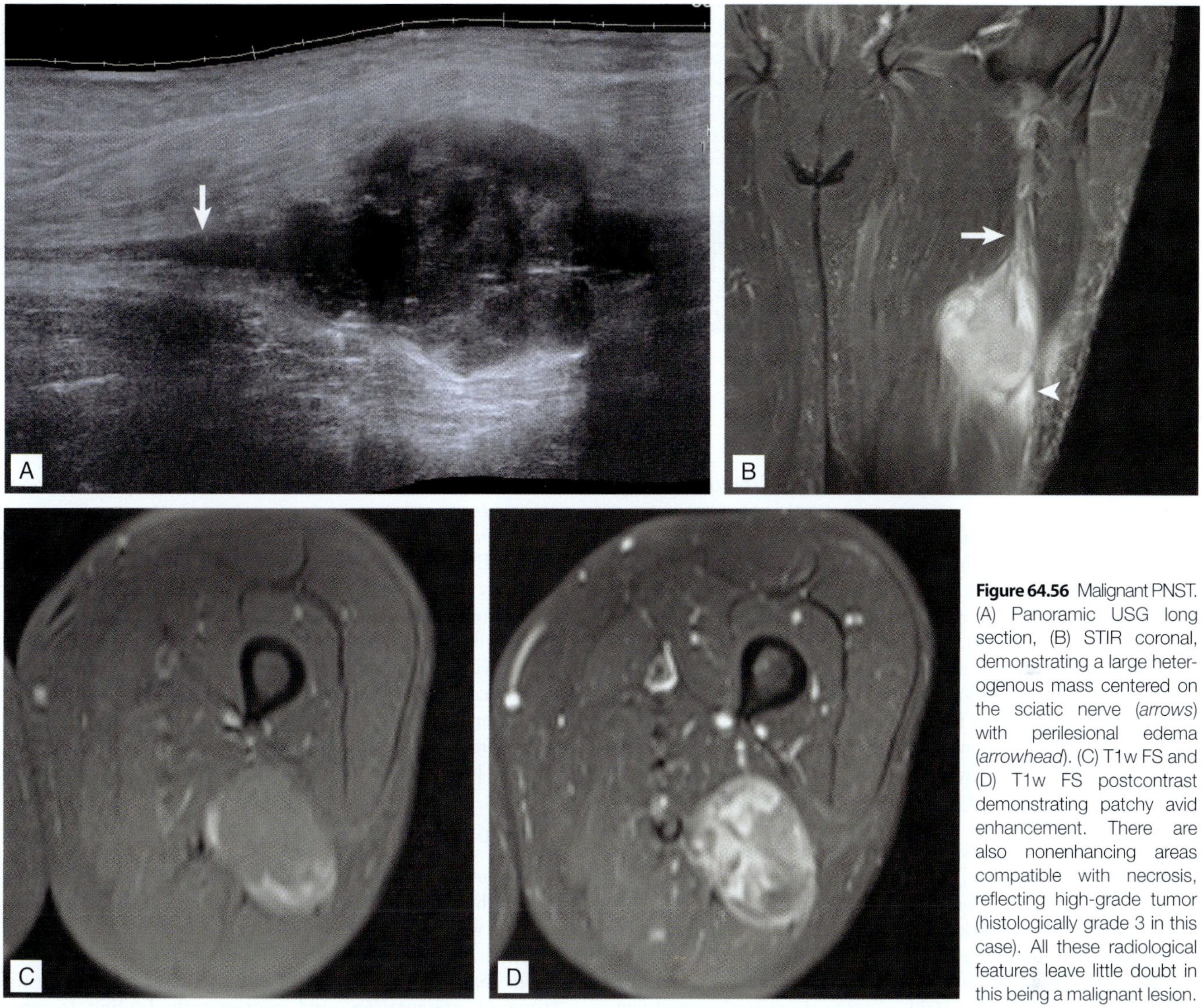

Figure 64.56 Malignant PNST. (A) Panoramic USG long section, (B) STIR coronal, demonstrating a large heterogenous mass centered on the sciatic nerve (*arrows*) with perilesional edema (*arrowhead*). (C) T1w FS and (D) T1w FS postcontrast demonstrating patchy avid enhancement. There are also nonenhancing areas compatible with necrosis, reflecting high-grade tumor (histologically grade 3 in this case). All these radiological features leave little doubt in this being a malignant lesion.

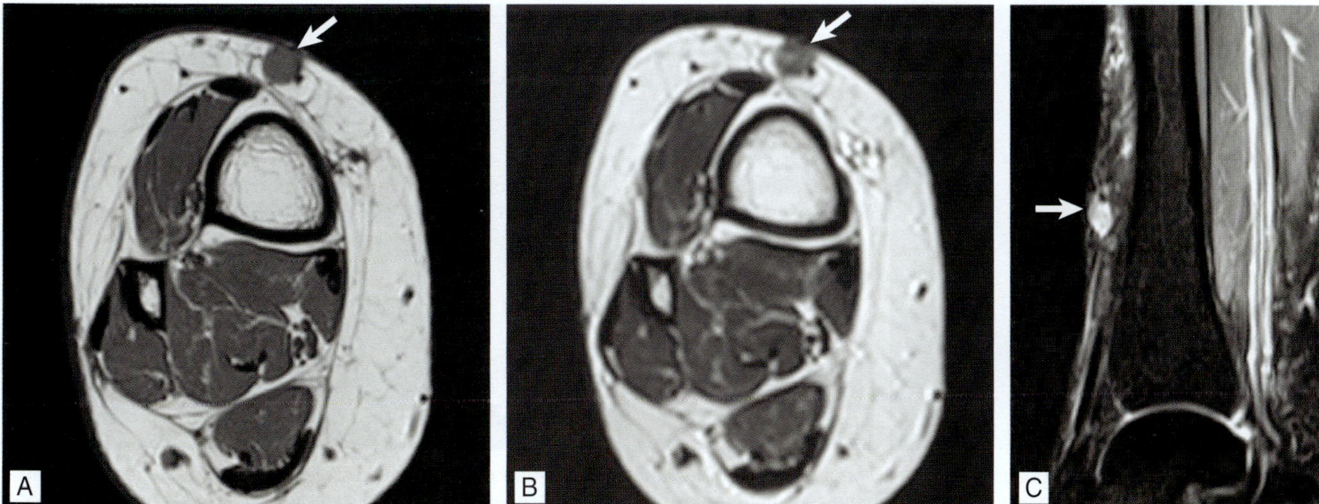

Figure 64.57 Superficial leiomyoma. (A) T1w, (B) T2w, and (C) STIR sagittal images showing a nodule (*arrows*) in the subcutaneous tissue just deep to the dermis with nonspecific features.

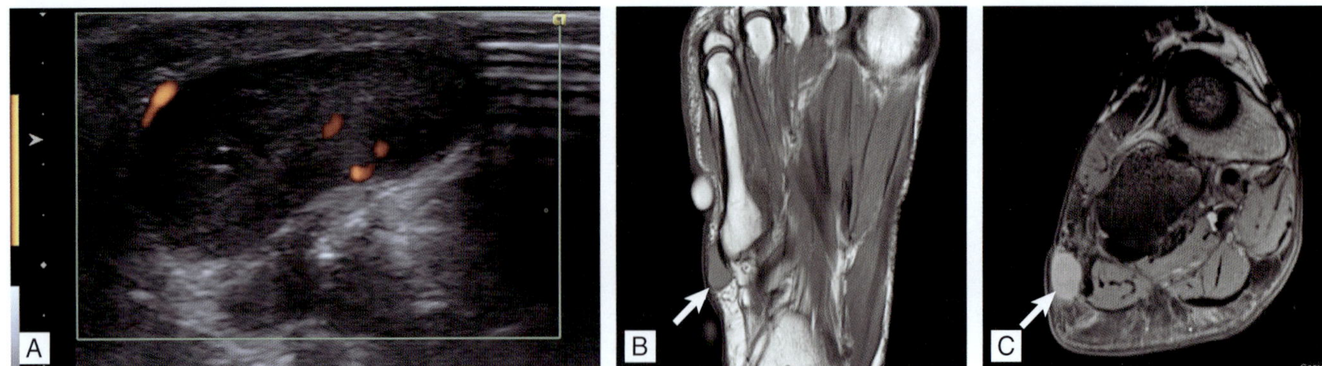

Figure 64.58 Angioleiomyoma in the foot. (A) USG demonstrates a superficial, ovoid, solid lesion with a homogenous echotexture. The lesion has pulsatile arterial vascularity, with an entering and exiting vessel seen at the time of scanning. (B) T1w long axial demonstrates a slightly hyperintense nodule compared to muscles, and (C) a hyperintense signal on this PD FS short axis image.

and renal cell cancer where imaging surveillance of the kidneys may be required.

Angioleiomyoma is most commonly found in the limbs—67% in the lower, 22% in the upper extremity [100]. Pain is a common feature. Angioleiomyomas are mostly <2 cm in size, well-circumscribed, oval, or round in shape, and is found in the subcutaneous plane [100,101] (Fig. 64.58). If sited close to a bone, its slow-growing nature may produce pressure erosion [101]. On USG, angioleiomyoma is hypoechoic with a homogenous echotexture and has linear vascularity within. On MRI, it is iso- or slightly hyperintense on T1w, and hyperintense on T2w relative to muscle, and has homogenous contrast enhancement [101]. *One should look out for a close relationship with a vessel which can give clue to its etiology.*

Leiomyoma of deep tissue is a rare entity, accounting for only 0.18% of cases in a series [102]. Leiomyoma of deep tissue can be divided into two groups based on their locations:

- *Retroperitoneum or abdominal/pelvic cavity*, occurring mostly in women, with mean age of 45 years. There is marked histological resemblance to uterine leiomyomas. These lesions can demonstrate hyaline, myxoid, or cystic degeneration, and few may show areas of calcification. On imaging, leiomyoma is isointense to muscles on T1w and T2w imaging, and demonstrates contrast enhancement
- *Peripheral deep soft tissue* (where there is equal gender distribution). The lesion can be heavily calcified, which can be radiologically mistaken for myositis ossificans, calcific myositis, chondrosarcoma (Fig. 64.59). On MRI, the nonmineralized areas will demonstrate isointense T1w and hyperintense T2w areas, with prominent contrast enhancement

Leiomyomatosis peritonealis disseminata is a rare benign proliferation of smooth muscle nodules in the peritoneum. CT and MRI may reveal multiple tumor nodules of varying sizes from 1 cm to 11 cm [103], and can mimic a diffuse metastatic process.

Leiomyosarcoma

Leiomyosarcoma accounts for around 10% of all soft tissue sarcoma, with a median age of 65 years [104]. There are broadly three sites where leiomyosarcoma can arise from:

- *Retroperitoneum and pelvis.* Leiomyosarcoma in these locations may be left undetected until it is large >10 cm by the time of presentation, and consequently leading to poor prognosis.

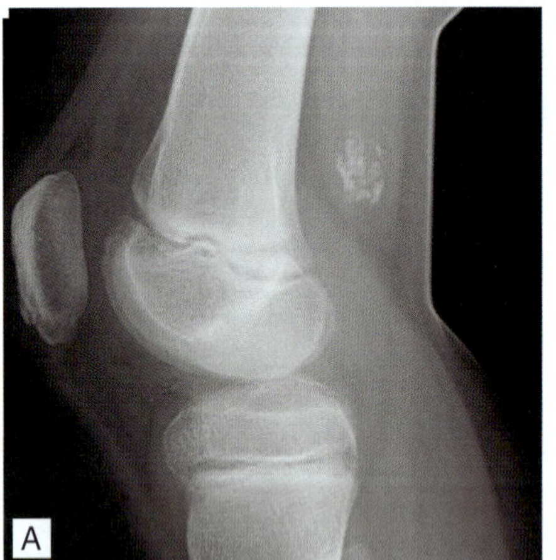

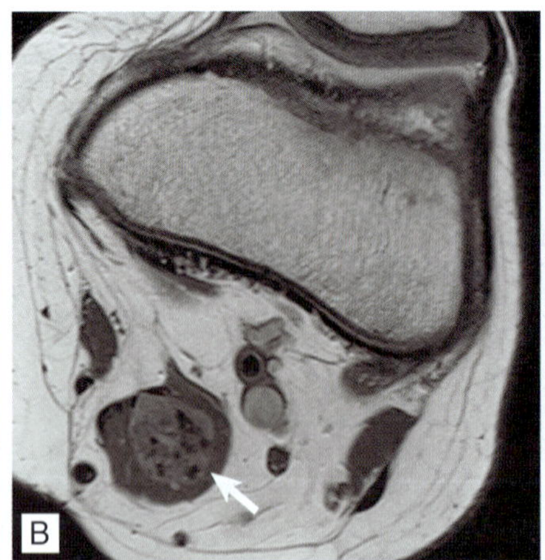

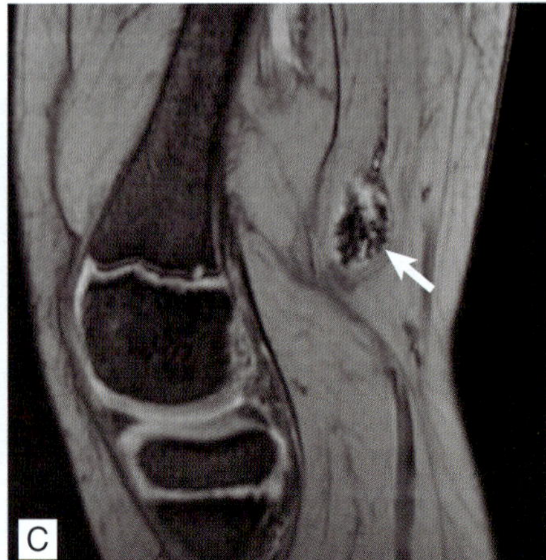

Figure 64.59 Leiomyoma of deep tissue in a 10-year-old patient. (A) Lateral radiograph demonstrates a calcified lesion posterior to the distal femur. (B) T1w axial demonstrating a lesion within the semimembranosus muscle, with heavy intralesional calcification, also seen as dense signal void on the (C) T2*w sagittal image (*arrows*). Heavy calcification can raise differentials including soft tissue chondroid lesion or myositis ossificans.

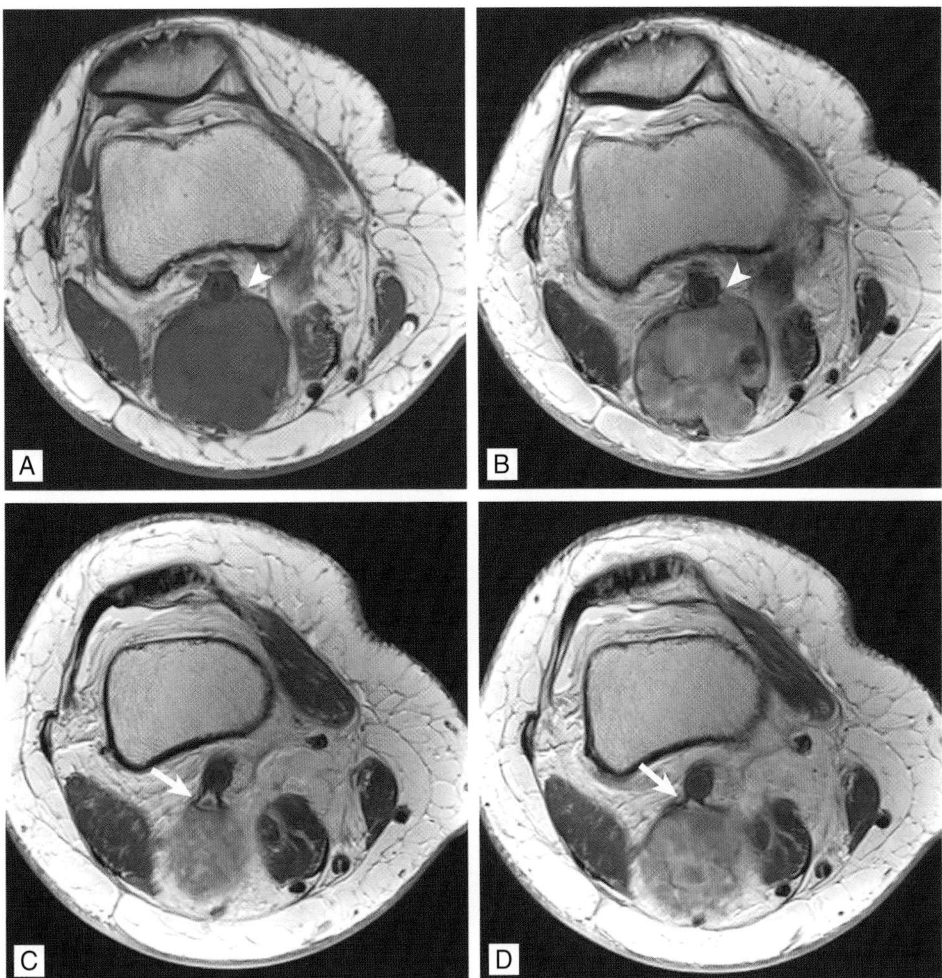

Figure 64.60 Leiomyosarcoma. (A) T1w and (B) T2w axial images demonstrating a large heterogenous mass in the popliteal fossa. (C) and (D) are consecutive T2w axial images at the cranial end of this lesion, demonstrating its origin from the femoral vein (*arrows*). There is broad contact of the lesion with the femoral artery (*arrowheads* in A and B).

- *Large blood vessels* (arising from the muscular wall), most commonly the inferior vena cava (IVC) (40%). Another 40% arise from other medium–large sized veins (Fig. 64.60). Arteries are less commonly affected, with pulmonary artery around 10% of all cases [105]
- *Nonretroperitoneal soft tissue*, mainly in lower extremity. This can arise either in the subcutaneous tissue or the muscle [33]

Imaging of retroperitoneal and nonperitoneal soft tissue is generally nonspecific. On MRI, leiomyosarcoma demonstrates iso- to hyperintense T1w signal to muscle, high T2w signal, and marked gadolinium enhancement. Similarly, CT appearances are nonspecific, and can demonstrate areas of necrosis. Calcification is not seen. Retroperitoneal lesions are mostly large >10 cm, and can have areas of hemorrhage, fibrosis, myxoid, or necrotic changes [48]. These changes can be appreciated on CT and MRI. Nonperitoneal soft tissue on the other hand is smaller (median 6 cm) [104].

Leiomyosarcomas of vascular origin most commonly arise from the IVC, and can have a predominantly extraluminal (76%) or intraluminal (20%) growth with variable degree of luminal obstruction. IVC leiomyosarcoma can be divided into three groups depending on which segment of the IVC is involved: segment 1 (infrarenal), segment 2 (inter- and suprarenal), segment 3 (suprahepatic veins and including intracardiac extension). Segments 1 (36.7%) and 2 (43.1%) are more commonly involved than segment 3 [106]. Symptoms would depend on the segment of the IVC involved. For example, segment 3 (suprahepatic veins) involvement would cause hepatic dysfunction including Budd–Chiari syndrome, jaundice, and ascites. Imaging would show a lesion arising from the vessel, which may be expanded in the presence of tumor thrombus. *Differentiation from a bland thrombus should be made.* Vascular leiomyosarcoma will demonstrate heterogenous contrast enhancement, and the vessel expanded several times the original diameter; bland thrombus on the other hand should not enhance, and vessel expansion should not be more than twice the diameter [8].

Rhabdomyoma

Rhabdomyoma is broadly divided into *cardiac* and *extracardiac* rhabdomyomas. Within extracardiac rhabdomyomas, there are three subgroups: adult type, fetal type, and genital type. Adult and fetal rhabdomyomas most commonly affect the head and neck region.

Adult rhabdomyoma occurs in patients with median age of 60 years, with a 3:1 male to female ratio. The sites most commonly affected are the pharynx, oral cavity, and larynx leading to symptoms such as dysphagia, hoarseness of voice, and airway obstruction. On imaging, appearance of rhabdomyoma is nonspecific, with slight hyperintensity on T1w, and slight to clear hyperintensity on T2w relative to muscle, and exhibits homogenous contrast enhancement [8,107]. It tends to displace adjacent structures rather than invade them while preserving fat planes [107]. They can occasionally present as multifocal masses.

Fetal and genital rhabdomyomas are very rare. Fetal rhabdomyoma occurs in young patients (median age of 4.5 years), also most commonly located in the head and neck region. The most common site is the preauricular, followed by the postauricular regions. Genital rhabdomyoma occurs mostly in woman of mean age 50 years, and affects most commonly the vagina. It has also been reported in male patients [33].

Rhabdomyosarcoma

Rhabdomyosarcoma is the most common form of soft tissue sarcoma in the pediatric population (<14 years), accounting for around 50% of all cases [108]. In contrast, it is much rarer in adults, accounting for <5% of all soft tissue sarcomas [48]. The most commonly affected sites are head and neck, followed by the genitourinary tract [48]. There are four main recognized subtypes of rhabdomyosarcoma [33,48]:

1. *Embryonal.* This is the most common subtype, accounting for nearly half of all rhabdomyosarcomas. Head and neck is the most commonly affected site. Around 40% of cases occur by age 4 years, and 70% by 9 years old
2. *Alveolar.* This is the second most common subtype, accounting for 20–30% of all rhabdomyosarcomas. This subtype is most commonly found in the peripheral intramuscular location. In contrast to embryonal subtype which preferentially affects <9 years, alveolar subtype has a more uniform incidence across the first two decades
3. *Pleomorphic.* Rare subtype, accounting for 15% of rhabdomyosarcomas, in patients of median age 64 years, and most commonly located in the thigh
4. *Sclerosing/spindle cell.* Rare subtype, accounting for <10% of rhabdomyosarcomas, in patients of median age 76 years. This subtype has a strong male predilection, and can be found in paratesticular region, head and neck, and in the limbs

Rhabdomyosarcoma has nonspecific appearances on imaging (Fig. 64.61). They have either lobulated or ill-defined margins, and demonstrate mostly isointense (or slightly hyperintense) T1w signal, and moderate to very hyperintense T2w signal relative to muscles. Contrast enhancement is seen on MRI and CT. *Regional lymph node involvement is frequent, especially in alveolar subtype* [109]. An imaging study of adult rhabdomyosarcoma has documented some subtle differences between the forms of rhabdomyosarcoma [110]:

- Embryonal has a more homogenous MRI signal compared to the more heterogenous appearance of alveolar and pleomorphic rhabdomyosarcoma.
- Pleomorphic rhabdomyosarcoma tends to have a very high T2w/STIR images.

Tumor of Uncertain Differentiation

Intramuscular Myxoma

Intramuscular myxoma is a rare benign tumor (annual incidence 0.11 cases per 100,000 people) [111], consisting of sparse, bland spindle-shaped cells in an abundant myxoid matrix. It affects patients with median age of 54 years, most commonly involving the thigh or buttock, and there can be a female predominance (2:1 ratio) [111]. *Intramuscular myxoma is mostly a solitary finding, but can coexist with fibrous dysplasia, that is, Mazabraud syndrome* (Fig. 64.62). In this syndrome, the number of intramuscular myxomas can be single or multiple (50:50 ratio), with the vast majority of lesions found next to the fibrous dysplasia.

On MRI, intramuscular myxoma (Fig. 64.63):

- Can either be well-defined or partially ill-defined in its borders
- Ovoid or less commonly lobulated in shape [112]
- Has fluid-like signal, with homogenous low T1w and high T2w signal. Some lesions can have a nodular septal pattern [112]
- Perilesional rim of fat best seen at the poles of the lesion
- Peripheral edema, also best seen at the poles of the lesion
- Postcontrast enhancement can be either heterogeneously diffuse, or demonstrate a septal/peripheral nodular enhancement pattern

Owing to its abundant myxoid matrix, intramuscular myxoma can be misdiagnosed as a simple cyst on MRI. *However, a ganglion is expected to arise from a typical location such as the wrist joint and is located in the extramuscular plane (as opposed to intramuscular location of myxoma).* USG is also invaluable to differentiate a cyst from a cyst-like lesion. Other imaging

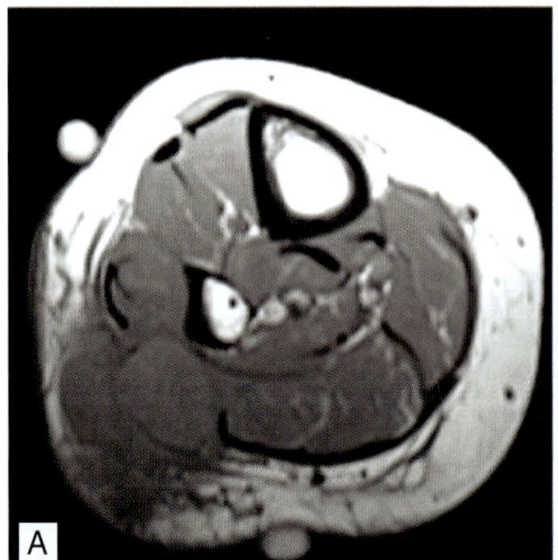

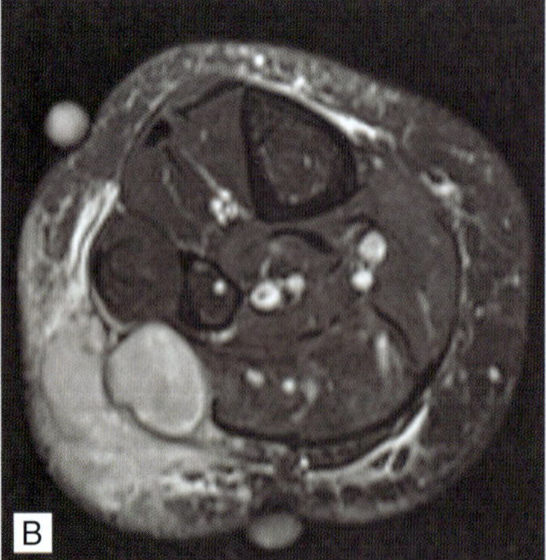

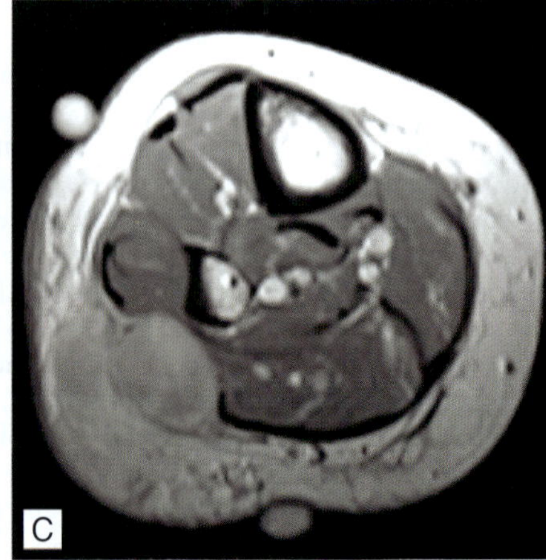

Figure 64.61 Pleomorphic rhabdomyosarcoma in a 61-year-old female patient. (A) T1w and (B) T2w FS image demonstrating a large ill-defined mass in the lateral calf, occupying the subcutaneous tissue and breaching the deep fascia. (C) T1w shows avid contrast enhancement. In this case, there are no specific imaging appearance to allow radiological diagnosis of rhabdomyosarcoma.

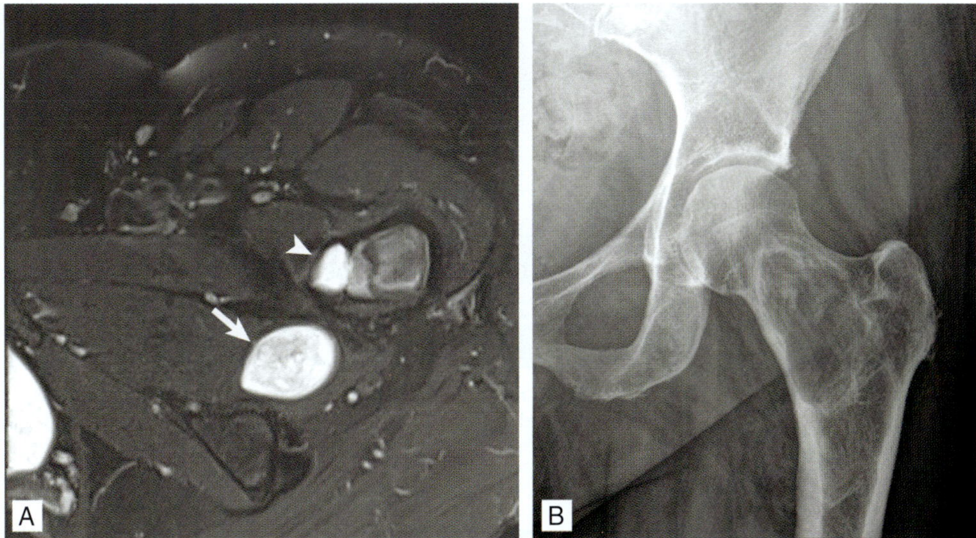

Figure 64.62 Mazabraud syndrome. (A) PD FS transverse oblique image demonstrating an intramuscular myxoma (*arrow*). Note the partially imaged fibrous dysplasia of the left femur (*arrowhead*), also seen on the radiograph (B).

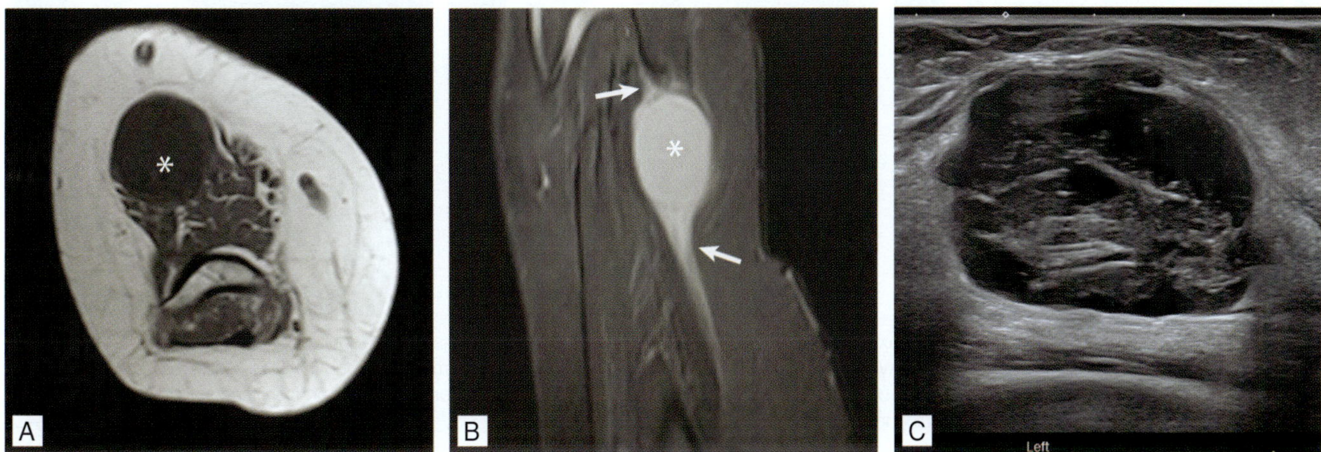

Figure 64.63 Intramuscular myxoma in the volar aspect of arm. This lesion can easily be misdiagnosed as a simple cyst on MRI given its homogenous texture on (A) T1w axial and (B) T1w STIR coronal images (*asterisks*). (C) USG is invaluable to show that this is in fact a solid lesion. (B) Note the typical edema on the poles of the myxoma (*arrows*).

differentials for intramuscular myxoma include PNST and other myxoid lesions such as myxoid liposarcoma. To help differentiate from myxoid liposarcoma, presence of perilesional fatty rim or peripheral edema strongly favors a diagnosis of intramuscular myxoma rather than myxoid liposarcoma [112].

Extraskeletal Chondrosarcoma

Extraskeletal chondrosarcoma is a rare tumor, making up only 2% of all soft tissue sarcomas [113]. Despite its name, WHO has grouped this tumor under tumors of uncertain differentiation because there is no definite cartilaginous differentiation. Lesions are frequently found in the lower limbs (85%), with the thigh making up a third, and the knee 18% of all cases [114]. There are three subtypes of extraskeletal chondrosarcoma, namely, myxoid, mesenchymal, and well-differentiated chondrosarcoma, in order of decreasing frequency. Mesenchymal form is the most aggressive, with a 10-year survival of 42.8% [115], while myxoid has a survival higher rate of 70% [116]. Well-differentiated extraskeletal chondrosarcoma is very rare, and prognosis is considered good.

On MRI, extraskeletal chondrosarcoma appears well-demarcated mass with lobular architecture and internal septations, with low T1w and high T2w signals. It has a large size, with a mean of 8.9 cm [117]. Extracompartmental invasion, cortical destruction, and vascular encasement can be seen [117]. Enhancement is typically seen in the periphery of the lesion and in the septae. Differentiation between the subtypes of extraskeletal chondrosarcoma is generally not feasible. However, matrix mineralization (best seen on radiograph or CT) is reported to be a frequent feature in the mesenchymal subtype [115] (Fig. 64.64), and rare in the myxoid subtype [117]. In addition, hemorrhage is often seen in the myxoid form [114], demonstrated as high T1w on fat-suppressed images or with fluid–fluid level (Fig. 64.65). Well-differentiated subtype has been reported to show dense and homogenous mineralization [113].

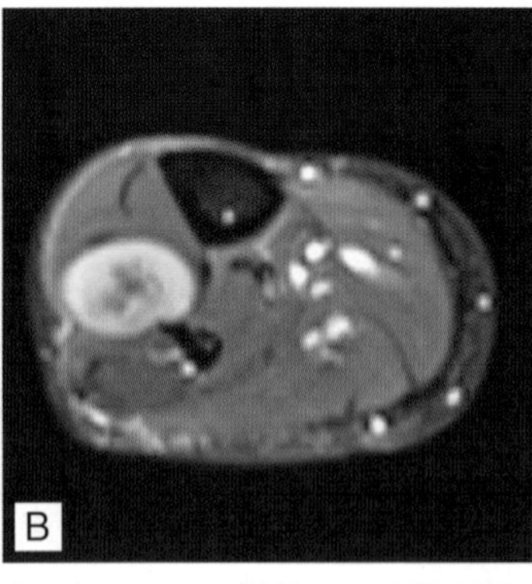

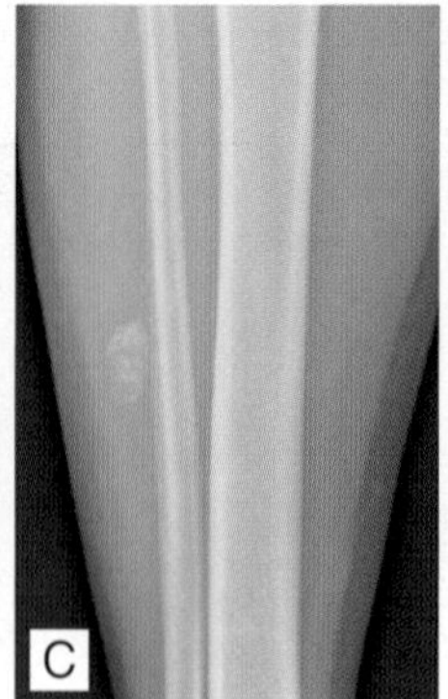

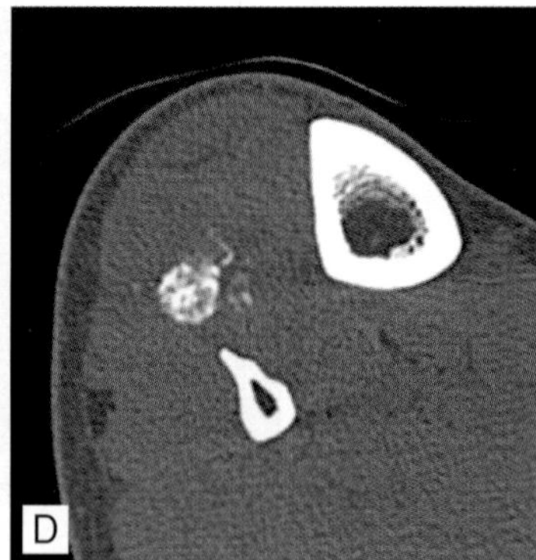

Figure 64.64 Mesenchymal extraskeletal chondrosarcoma. (A) T1w and (B) STIR axial images demonstrating a well-defined mass with central very low signal representing areas of mineralization, better appreciated on (C) radiograph and (D) CT. Matrix mineralization can frequently be seen in the mesenchymal subtype of extraskeletal chondrosarcoma.

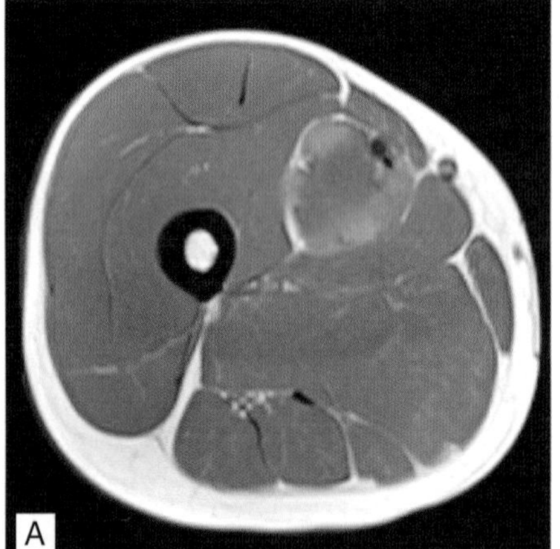

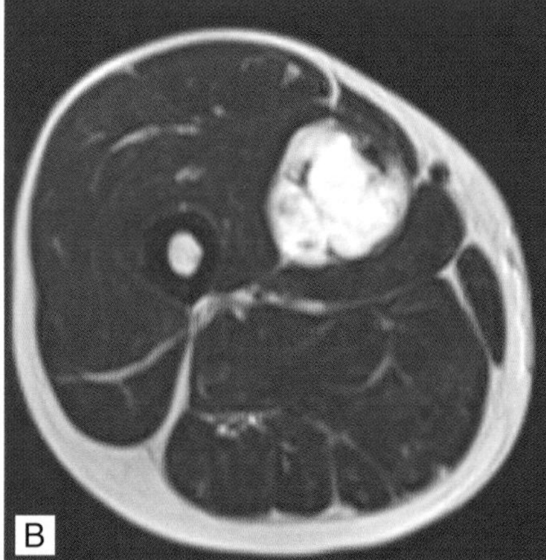

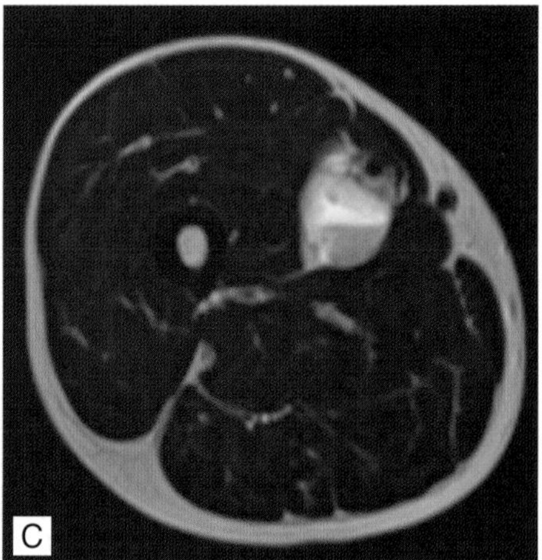

Figure 64.65 Myxoid chondrosarcoma. (A) T1w axial and (B) T2w axial images demonstrating a mass in the adductor canal, with a lobular architecture and internal septations. The fluid-like signals of low T1w and high T2w images are in keeping with a myxoid tumor. (C) Fluid–fluid level can also be seen on this T2w axial image, representing internal hemorrhage, a common feature in myxoid chondrosarcoma. There is no calcification in this lesion on radiograph (not shown). Mineralization is a rare finding in myxoid chondrosarcoma.

Synovial Sarcoma

The term synovial sarcoma is really a misnomer—not only is synovial sarcoma unrelated to synovial differentiation, but it rarely arises from within the joint (around 5%) [118]. Synovial sarcoma is typically found in the vicinity of a joint (most commonly the knee). Majority of lesions are found in the lower limb (71%) and the upper limbs (24%), and also less commonly the head and neck, and trunk region. The thigh and knee are the most commonly affected sites (42%), followed by foot, hand, and leg [118]. Patients typically present with a slow-growing lump which can be painful.

Imaging features of synovial sarcoma (Fig. 64.66):

- Majority of lesions (>85%) are large, measuring >5 cm [119,120]
- Relatively well-defined with multilobulation to its margins
- It can have multilocular appearance with fluid–fluid levels reflecting hemorrhage, seen in 18–25% of lesions [119,121]. This can produce a "bowl of grape" appearance
- *Triple signal sign on MRI.* This sign is seen on T2w images, and denotes the presence of hyper-, iso-, and hypointense areas in the lesion relative to fat [119]. This signal heterogeneity reflects the different elements contained within the lesion—hemorrhage, necrosis, or myxoid change (hyperintense); solid cellular component (isointense); calcified, fibrous, or collagenous area (hypointense). This sign can be seen in 35–50% of cases [119,120,122], and is associated with poorer prognosis [122]
- Calcification is present in synovial sarcoma in around 30% of cases [118], and is commonly seen peripherally about the soft tissue lesion, seen either on radiograph or CT. Various descriptions to the appearance of the calcification have been described, including discrete, nodular, crumbly, and amorphous [8]. Some lesions can have extensive calcification or ossification, which has been associated with better prognosis [122]. Presence of soft tissue calcification is certainly not unique to synovial sarcoma, but its presence should raise the differential of synovial sarcoma, particularly if the lesion is sited in the thigh and near the knee joint
- Adjacent bone involvement can be seen in variable frequency (14–63%), producing either pressure erosion, or invasion/destruction
- Diffuse contrast enhancement presents in the solid components, and peripheral enhancement in the cystic components

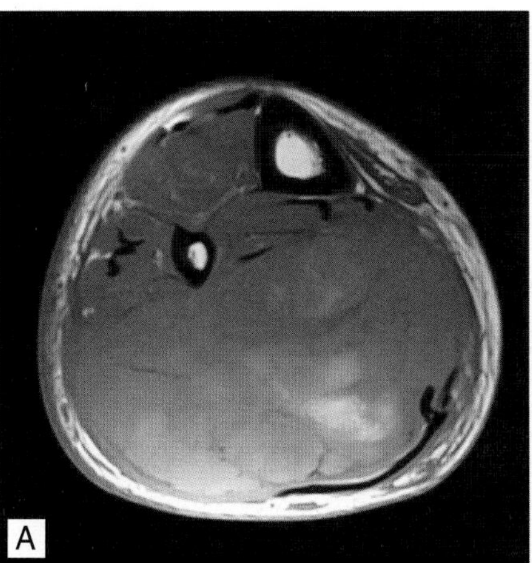

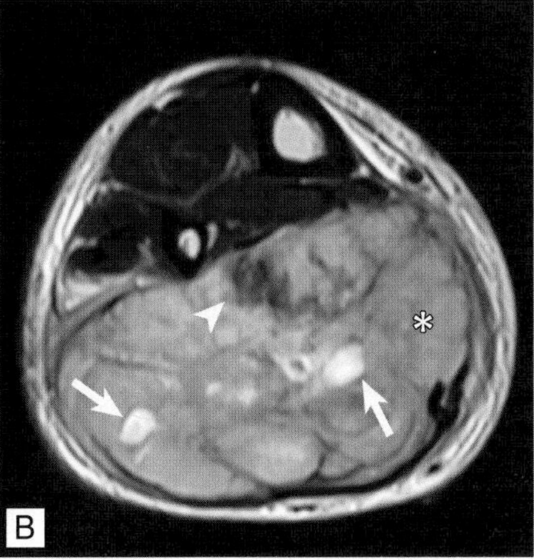

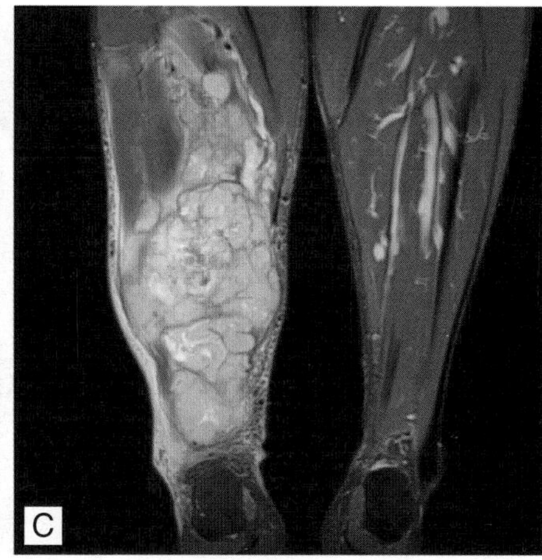

Figure 64.66 Synovial sarcoma in the right calf. (A) T1w axial, (B) T2w axial, and (C) STIR coronal images demonstrating a large multilocular lesion in the calf, producing a "bowl in grape" appearance. (B) Triple signal sign can be seen on this T2w image, with hyperintense areas (*arrows*, reflecting hemorrhage, necrosis, or myxoid change), intermediate signal (*asterisk*, reflecting solid cellular area), and hypointense area (*arrowhead*, reflecting calcified, fibrous, or collagenous area).

Synovial sarcoma can be mistaken for a benign lesion on imaging when it is small and with homogenous internal signal on MRI. Presence of calcification and close relationship to a bone or joint may mimic other lesions including myositis ossificans, extraskeletal, or parosteal osteosarcoma, and soft tissue chondroma.

Tumor Mimics

Hematoma

Hematoma has a variable imaging appearance and can change with time (Fig. 64.67). On USG, acute hematomas can have a complex cystic appearance due to the presence of uncoagulated blood, fibrin strands, clot formations with other granulation, and inflammatory infiltrates. Hematoma can also organize, being surrounded by a fibrous capsule, and appears as a solid heterogenous mass. Either of these appearances can easily lead to misinterpretation as a soft tissue sarcoma on USG. Misinterpretation can also occur on MRI with hematoma appearing as a well-defined heterogenous mass.

A particular form of post-traumatic collection is the Morel–Lavallée lesion, which is secondary to a degloving injury, separating the subcutaneous tissue from the underlying fascia, creating a space where blood, lymph, and debris can accumulate. Morel–Lavallée lesion was originally described for hematoma found adjacent to the greater trochanter of the femur and upper thigh, but this phenomenon can be found adjacent to any bony protuberances including scapula, knee, flank, and lumbar region.

Unfortunately, soft tissue sarcoma can also initially present as a hematoma. Intratumoral hemorrhage may occur, usually in high-grade sarcoma, masking the underlying soft tissue tumor, and be misinterpreted as a simple hematoma (Fig. 64.68).

It is therefore important to have a low threshold of suspicion in unprovoked hematoma (unless patient is on anticoagulant); and if the hematoma increases or persists in size. In these instances, MRI with contrast can be useful to demonstrate any enhancing tumoral nodules. A nontumoral hematoma will only have peripheral enhancement without internal enhancement. If there is any doubt, biopsy should be considered.

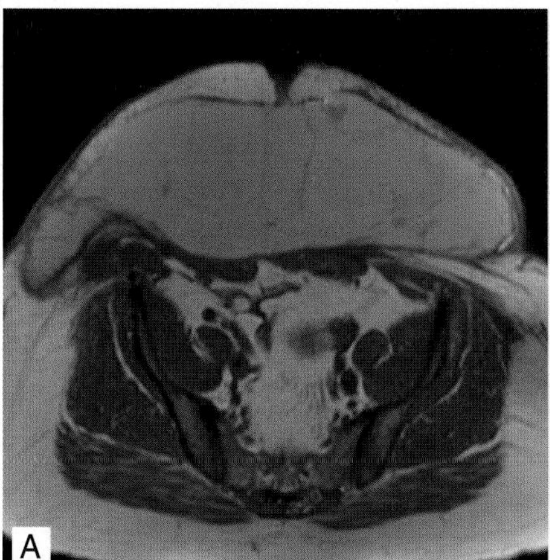

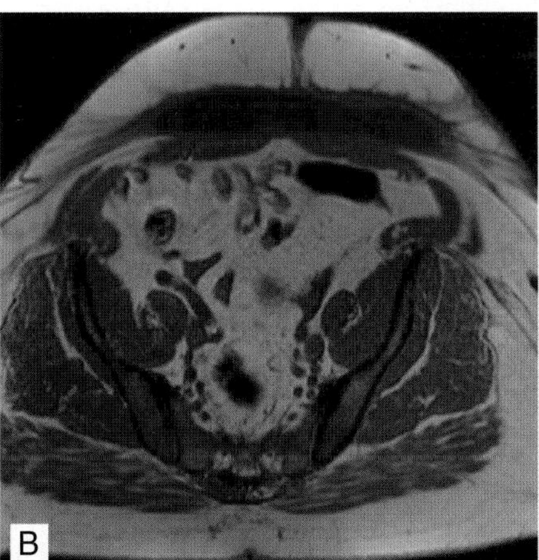

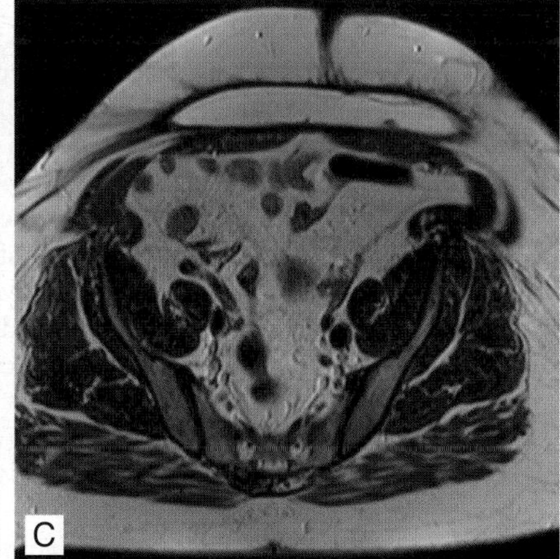

Figure 64.67 Seatbelt injury. (A) T1w FLASH axial image, performed less than 2 weeks after initial injury demonstrating a large Morel–Lavallée lesion with high T1w content reflecting presence of methemoglobin in this subacute hematoma. (B) T1w FLASH and (C) T2w axial images performed a few years later, showing a smaller but persistent Morel–Lavallée lesion. (C) Note the peripheral low T2w signal reflecting a combination of fibrous and hemosiderin-laden capsule.

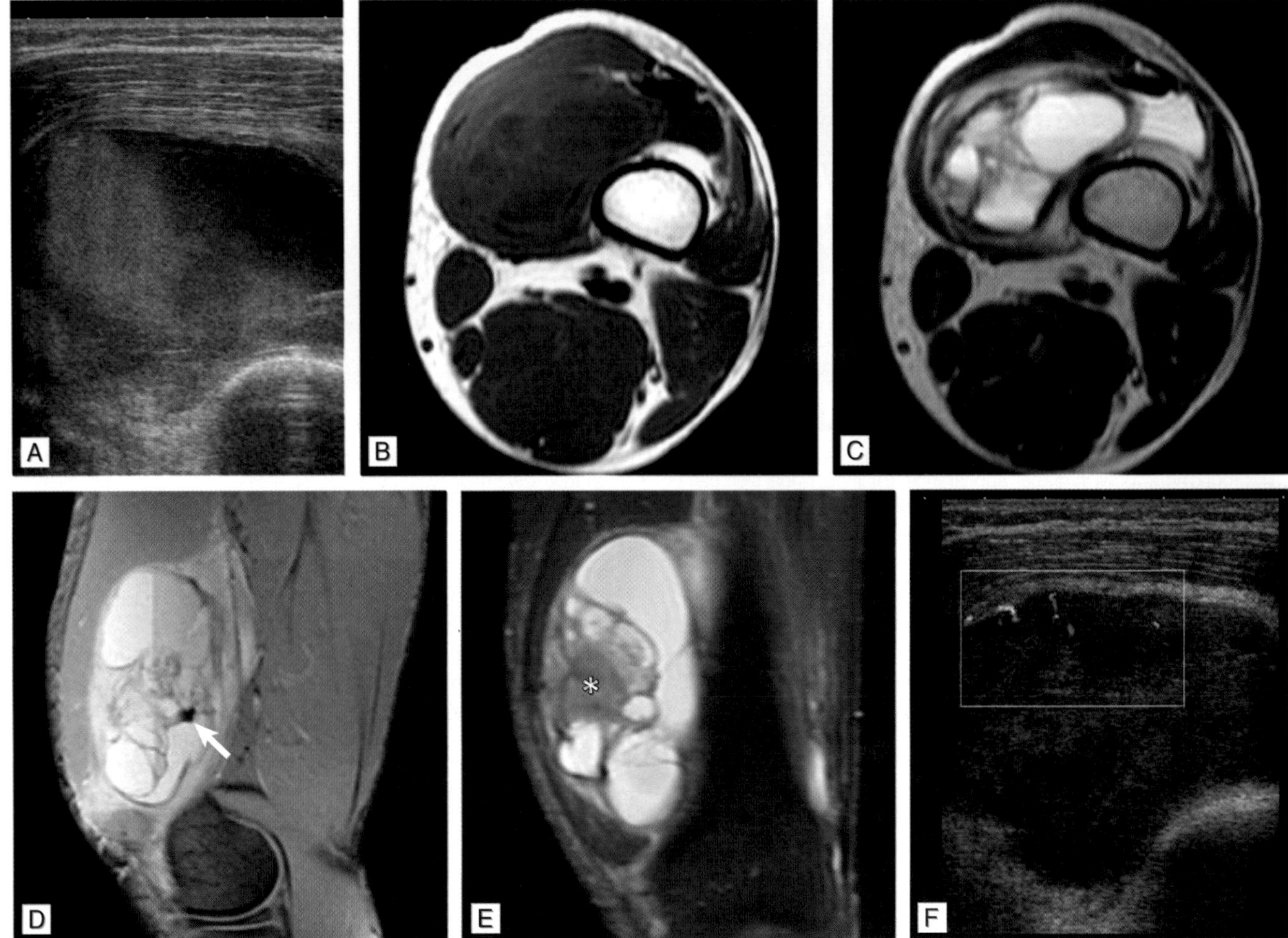

Figure 64.68 Sarcoma masquerading as hematoma. A 44-year-old footballer presenting to his local hospital with a swelling in the thigh, and was misdiagnosed with a simple hematoma following USG (A) and MRI (B)–(E). (A) USG demonstrated a large cystic mass with echogenic material, in keeping with hemorrhage. (B) T1w axial, (C) T2w axial, and (D) sagittal T2* GRE demonstrating a large mass with dominant fluid component demonstrating fluid–fluid level, in keeping with hemorrhage. A solid component had not been appreciated, which can be seen on (E) STIR coronal image (*asterisk*). Administration of contrast material may have facilitated detection of this solid component. (F) Subsequent USG also detected a solid mass lesion with vascularity. This was histologically proven to be synovial sarcoma. Indeed, the "triple sign" of synovial sarcoma can be seen in this lesion on the fluid-sensitive sequences (C), (D), and (E)—hyperintense hemorrhage, isointense solid component (*asterisk*), hypointense focus (*arrow*, representing either calcified, fibrous, or collagenous area).

Tumoral Calcinosis

Tumoral calcinosis is characterized by deposition of calcium hydroxyapatite most commonly affecting young adults, found in a periarticular location, particularly in the hip and buttock (where they make up more than half of all cases). Shoulder and elbows are also commonly affected areas. Lesions can be solitary or multiple (and symmetrical). There are three forms of tumoral calcinosis: sporadic (idiopathic), familial, and secondary (to conditions such as chronic renal failure with hyperparathyroidism, systemic sclerosis, and sarcoidosis). There is a predilection for black patients.

The amount of cellularity and calcification varies depending on the stage of the disease process, where cystic cavities are gradually filled with calcified material surrounded by inflammatory cells [123].

On CT or radiographs (Fig. 64.69):

- The calcifications typically have an amorphous appearance
- The calcifications can appear as cystic calcified globules, where CT or upright radiograph can demonstrate layering, reflecting sedimentation of the calcium deposits
- Commonly found in extensor surfaces

On MRI:

- Areas of calcification will be demonstrated as low T1w nodular areas and T2w signals
- Lesions can have high T2w cystic spaces

Patients with tumoral calcinosis can present with a soft tissue mass where it can be mistaken for a soft tissue sarcoma with calcifications, such as synovial sarcoma and extraskeletal chondrosarcoma.

Accessory Muscles

Accessory muscles are usually asymptomatic, but can occasionally cause pain with palpable swelling, which can lead to suspicion of a local soft tissue tumor. Examples of accessory muscles are listed in Table 64.7. In particular, accessory soleus muscles in the past decades have led to unnecessary open surgery (Fig. 64.70). However, with increasing ubiquity of MRI and USG, these are becoming less of an issue. MRI and USG will demonstrate isointense signal on all pulse sequences and similar echotexture to adjacent muscles, respectively.

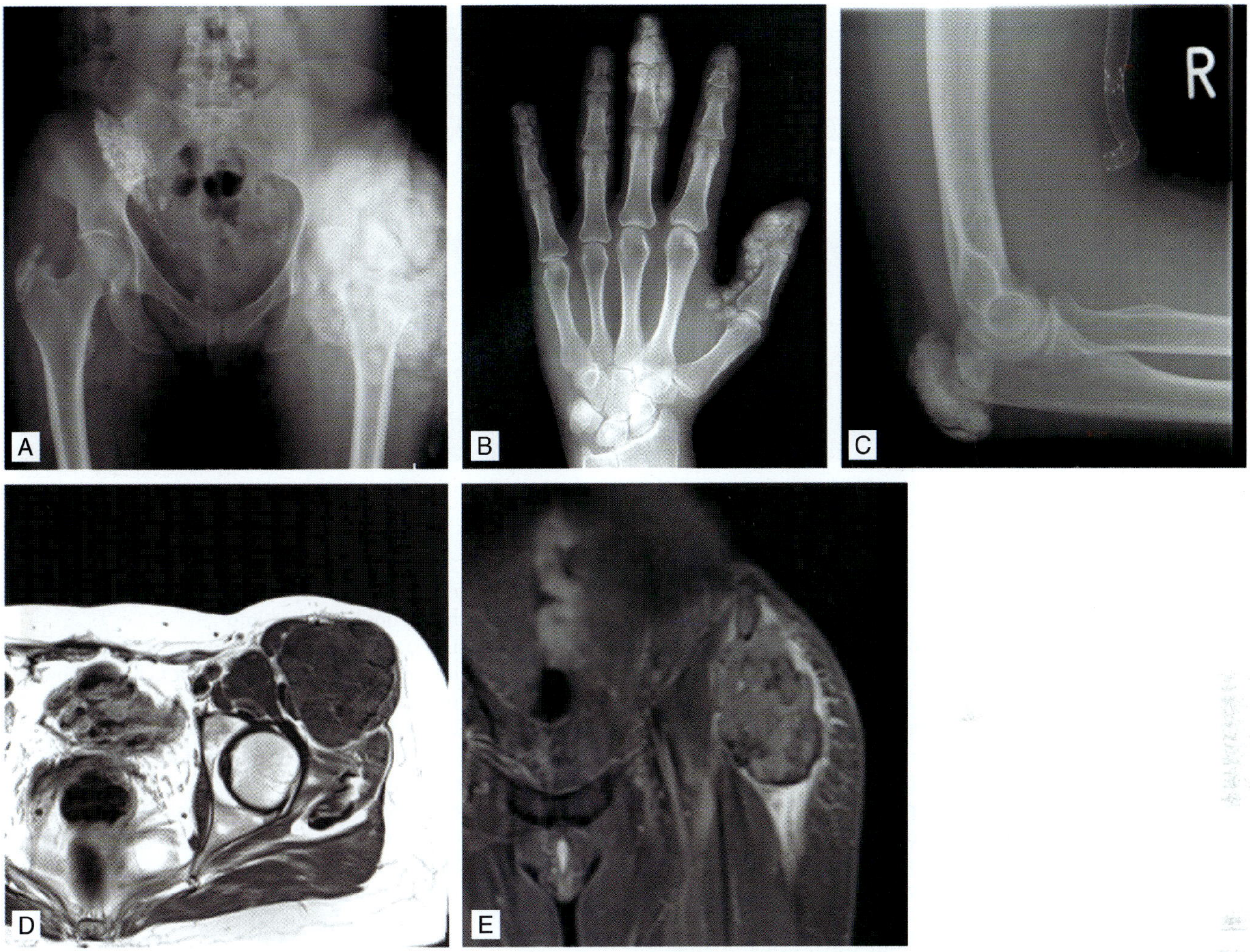

Figure 64.69 Tumoral calcinosis in a patient with chronic renal failure. (A) Pelvis, (B) hand, (C) elbow radiographs demonstrating globular calcification seen about both hips, several fingers, and olecranon bursa. Note the stent in the arteriovenous fistula. (D) Axial T2w and (E) STIR coronal image demonstrating nodular low signal areas.

TABLE 64.7 Example of Accessory Muscles [124]

Elbow	Knee
Accessory brachialis	Accessory slip of medial and lateral gastrocnemius
Anconeus epitrochlearis	Accessory popliteus
Accessory head of flexor pollicis longus	
Hand and Wrist	**Ankle**
Accessory flexor digitorum superficialis indicis	Accessory peroneal muscles
Accessory abductor digiti minimi	Flexor digitorum accessorius longus
Accessory extensor carpi radialis brevis	Accessory soleus

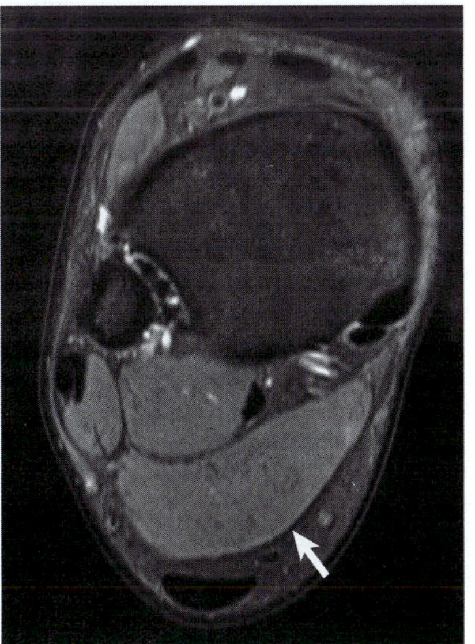

Figure 64.70 Accessory soleus muscle. PD FS image demonstrates a accessory soleus muscle (*arrow*) which is usually asymptomatic. If the muscle is large, as in this case, patient can present with a soft tissue mass in the posteromedial aspect of the ankle.

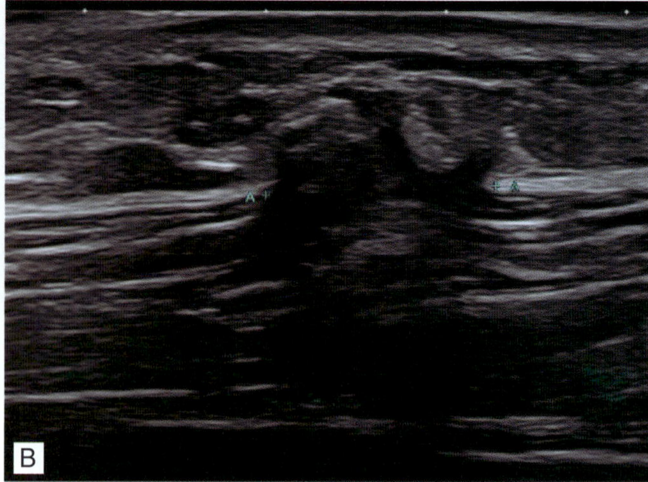

Figure 64.71 Muscle hernia. USG (A) axial and (B) longitudinal images of the leg, demonstrating a defect in the fascia (measured), allowing the underlying muscle (tibialis anterior in this case) to herniate through.

Muscle Hernia

Muscle hernia is a focal protrusion of the muscle through a focal defect in the overlying fascia. The hernia presents as a lump, and can occasionally be painful, mimicking a soft tissue tumor. Lower and upper limbs are the most frequently reported site. There is frequently a preceding history of trauma, either direct or indirectly. In the lower limb, herniation of tibialis anterior in the anterior compartment is frequently reported (Fig. 64.71). Lateral compartment of the leg while less commonly involved can occur at the point where the superficial peroneal nerve pierces the deep fascia. Peroneus brevis muscle herniation here may compress on the nerve leading to neuropathy.

Muscle hernia is best diagnosed with USG, demonstrating a protruding muscle through a visible defect of the fascia. *It is important to utilize light probe pressure, and if required, a gel-standoff, to prevent inadvertent effacement or reduction of the hernia.* Active contraction of the muscle may also accentuate the hernia during USG. MRI can delineate the fascial defect. Muscle hernia can also be visualized, although may not necessarily be present at the time of scanning. The affected muscle may also show focal edema.

Myositis Ossificans

Myositis ossificans is characterized by a non-neoplastic ossifying process in the soft tissue. While it is considered to be a post-traumatic reaction, a specific trauma may not always be evident (Fig. 64.72). There is a male predominance, with the thigh being the most commonly affected location, and also frequently found in the arm [125].

In the early stages (0–4 weeks), the lesion can be easily confused with an extraskeletal osteosarcoma:

- Imaging with MRI can show a markedly heterogenous soft tissue mass with high T2w signal and significant surrounding edema
- Contrast-enhanced MRI frequently shows rim enhancement, although diffuse enhancement has also been reported [126], adding to the confusion
- This confusion can occur on histology as well due to presence of immature and high levels of cellularity. It is for this reason that close correlation with a traumatic history be sought, and that biopsy should not be rushed into

In the intermediate stage (4 weeks to 6 months after onset):

- Follow-up with imaging with radiograph or CT will show the reassuring progression of calcification at its periphery
- Detecting this rim of calcification while possible is difficult on MRI, and is seen as rim of low T1w and T2w signal

In the mature stage (>6 months):

- There will be progression of the peripheral calcification into mature well-corticated bone, best seen on radiograph and CT, and also on MRI
- Adjacent soft tissue edema should also gradually resolve on MRI

Biopsy

The definitive diagnosis of a soft tissue lesion is made on histology. However, this does not mean that every soft tissue lesion require a biopsy. Benign lesions (such as lipoma, benign fibrous tumors, hemangioma) with typical clinical and imaging features can be diagnosed confidently and managed appropriately without a biopsy. However, if a specific benign diagnosis cannot be made either clinically or on imaging, then biopsy should be considered.

At this juncture, one should strongly consider prompt referral to a sarcoma center where there is a full complement of a multidisciplinary team (including but not limited to radiologist, pathologist, sarcoma surgeon, and oncologist) for further management. *A biopsy should not be performed in the absence of pathological support.* Sarcoma, being a rare and diverse group of tumors, can be difficult to accurately diagnose by nonspecialized pathologists. Discrepancy in the accuracy of the histology report can be as high as 42% when reported by a nonspecialist pathologist [127]. The discrepancies were centered around tumor type and grade, and can influence whether neoadjuvant chemotherapy or radiotherapy is utilized. It is not a surprise then that patient outcome is also better when treated at sarcoma center, with lower recurrence rate (19% at sarcoma center, compared to as high as 40% at district general hospital) and better survival advantage [128,129].

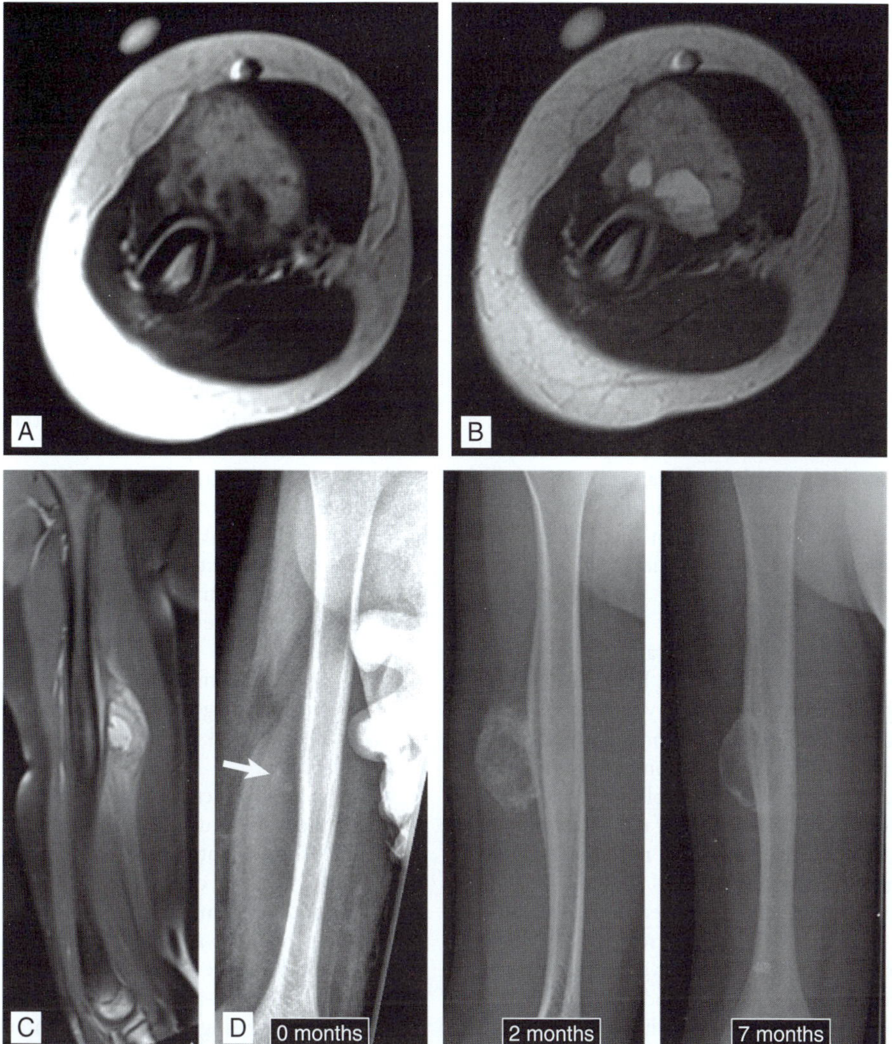

Figure 64.72 Myositis ossificans and periosteal hematoma in a 12-year-old girl. (A) T1w axial, (B) T2w axial, and (C) PD FS sagittal of the humerus demonstrating an aggressive-appearing mass with fluid–fluid level and underlying periosteal reaction. Presence of significant accidental trauma leading to a bruise in prior weeks had not been specifically appreciated, leading to referral to sarcoma center with a working diagnosis of osteosarcoma. (D) First radiograph performed 2 months prior had demonstrated a hint of mineralization (*arrow*). Serial radiographs demonstrated progressive peripheral ossification and maturation. There is also periosteal thickening in keeping with ossified periosteal hematoma. This case illustrates the role of radiograph because MRI findings of myositis ossificans can be unnecessarily alarming. Close correlation of imaging findings with history is also essential.

Soft Tissue Biopsy Techniques

Percutaneous Approach

Core needle biopsy is the preferred method in obtaining tissue from a suspected soft tissue sarcoma, capable of providing adequate tissue for histological analysis and also for ancillary tests (such as immunohistochemistry, molecular cytogenetics, and molecular diagnosis). Compared to surgical incisional biopsy, core needle biopsy is less traumatic to the patient, does not require general anesthesia, quicker patient recovery, and less costly.

Core needle biopsy is most commonly performed under USG guidance. Compared to other imaging-guidance, USG is quick, easily available and radiation free. Its "free-plane" imaging allows flexibility on the needle approach (but within limitation of surgical field as discussed in section "*Compartmental anatomy*"). Neurovascular structures can be identified, and care taken to avoid them. Color Doppler can also be applied to identify areas with neovascularity which may be of higher yield. Linear high-frequency probes are suitable for extremity and superficial lesions. The "hockey stick" probe, with its small footprint may be particularly useful for lesions in the finger where there is limited skin contact. For deeper lesions, curvilinear abdominal probe can sometimes be of use, although case can be argued that CT-guided biopsy may be a better option.

A study has shown no difference in diagnostic yield in between needle gauges (from 14G to 18G), as long as three or four cores are obtained [130]. *We advise the routine use of 14G or 16G, and obtaining a minimum of three cores if the patient allows.*

Imaging guidance under CT is another option and is reserved for lesions deep in abdomen when visualization with USG can be difficult. MRI-guided biopsy can also be performed (though not widely available, requiring new set of equipment to say the least), in the rare instances where lesions cannot be seen on other techniques. Example cases include when viable tumor after chemotherapy or radiotherapy is suspected, suspected lesion near surgical hardware, in pregnant or pediatric population when CT radiation exposure should be minimized.

Blind percutaneous biopsy is another option, reserved for superficial and easily palpable tumors, which should also be homogenous on imaging, that is, there is no particular area that needs to be specifically targeted for histological assessment.

Another percutaneous biopsy technique is fine-needle aspiration. While FNA is generally accepted as a method in diagnosing tumor recurrence or metastasis (especially when there is previous material available for comparison), its role in primary preoperative diagnosis is controversial and heavily debated. FNA provides only cytology without information on architecture of the tumor. It may be difficult to subtype certain sarcomas on FNA alone. Grading a tumor can also be challenging for certain tumors, especially low-grade sarcomas, which may be falsely classified as a benign lesion. As such, FNA is not commonly accepted as the sole source of pathology on which oncological management is based upon [5]. Nevertheless, it should be noted that when led by experienced cytopathologists and with utilization of ancillary techniques, a high diagnostic accuracy can be achieved [131].

Surgical Approach

Core needle biopsy has largely replaced surgical incisional biopsy, which was historically the mainstay approach. Incisional biopsy is associated with higher complications such as wound breakdown, bleeding, and hematoma. These complications can have detrimental oncological consequences: complication with wound healing will prevent neoadjuvant radiotherapy; bleeding and hematoma formation may lead to contamination of the adjacent tissues leading to high risk of recurrence, and may necessitate a wider definitive resection, or even amputation.

Excisional biopsy is not routinely performed in the workup of suspected soft tissue sarcoma. It is usually reserved for highly selected, superficial, small ≤3 cm lesions, after judicious consideration has been given regarding the location and orientation of the biopsy incision. However, in the event of an unplanned excisional biopsy, for an unexpected malignancy, a second, more extensive surgery will be required which will need to include the whole of the previous excisional biopsy bed. This is not only potentially more debilitating for the patient, but is also associated with worse prognosis.

Prebiopsy Planning

All available imaging should be reviewed before performing the biopsy. It goes without saying that all desired imaging should be obtained before embarking on a biopsy, lest confusing the imaging appearances. Prebiopsy considerations are:

1. Intralesional targeting to sample the most diagnostic or representative portion of the lesion. For example, in a DDL, the intended target should include both the dedifferentiated component and nondedifferentiated area. In addition, necrotic area should be avoided due to low diagnostic yield (Fig. 64.73).
2. Choosing the correct needle approach is essential. This is to allow the biopsy tract to be resected en bloc during the definitive surgery, even though the risk of tract contamination is low with core needle biopsy. There are a few considerations for the biopsy access point or route:
   - Ideally the needle entry point be sited along the expected definitive surgery incision. In the extremities, the biopsy tract should be longitudinally oriented, as is the standard surgical incision during definitive surgery, making it easier for the tract to be incorporated in the resection
   - In cases of proximal extremity lesions, care should be taken to avoid placing the biopsy entry site on the trunk. This is to prevent trunk contamination should limb amputation be considered
   - In contradistinction to extremity lesions, surgical incision on the trunk is usually transversely oriented, and the biopsy tract should match this as well
   - Stay within the compartment of the tumor without traversing another compartment. This applies not only in extremity lesions, but also in retroperitoneal lesions where effort should be made to biopsy a retroperitoneal lesion without traversing intra-abdominal space
   - Avoid traversing, injuring or contaminating the neurovascular bundle. Sarcoma can potentially spread between compartments along the neurovascular bundle, thereby precluding limb-sparing surgery. Epithelioid sarcoma is an example with tendency to spread along nerves (and along fascial planes and tendons) [132]

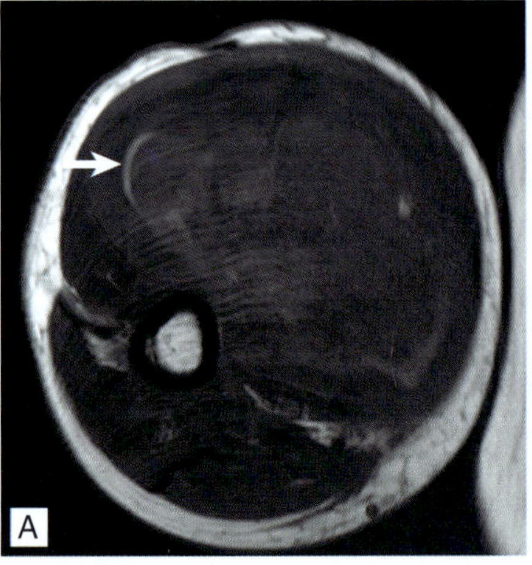

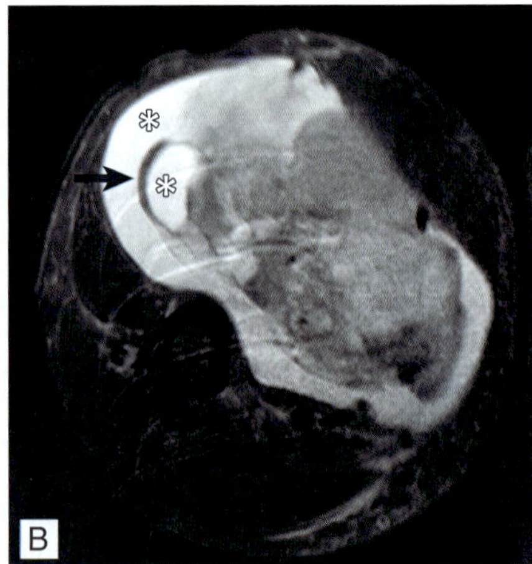

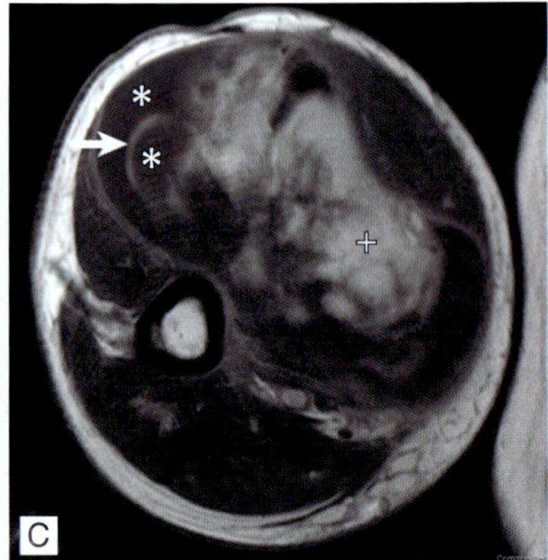

Figure 64.73 Pleomorphic liposarcoma in a 78-year-old male patient. (A) T1w axial image demonstrates a large lesion in the anterior compartment of the forearm. There is a thin rim of fat present (*arrow*), supported by fat suppression on (B) STIR axial image (*arrow*). There is surrounding area of necrosis (*asterisks*), supported by a homogenous nonenhancing area (C) seen on T1w axial postcontrast image, and should not be biopsied due to low yield. Care should be taken to plan the biopsy route, incorporating both the small layer of fat (*arrow*) and the viable enhancing component (*cross*).

Staging

Staging should be performed in accordance to the American Joint Committee on Cancer Staging Manual. Local staging has been discussed in earlier section. For metastatic disease, *all patients with soft tissue sarcoma should be imaged with CT thorax—the lungs are the most common site for metastatic spread* (seen in 56–72% of all patients with metastases [133–135]). This is much higher than the next most common location for metastasis, which is the bones, seen in around 17% of all patients with metastases [133,134]. In addition, further imaging is warranted depending on the likely sites of metastasis, and this is laid out in Table 64.8 and in the remainder of this section.

Regional Lymph Node

Regional lymph node involvement is rare in soft tissue sarcoma (2–5% as a whole) [136,137]. *However, there are a few histological types where higher incidence of regional lymph node spread is recognized, namely, rhabdomyosarcoma (around 20%) (Fig. 64.74), epithelioid sarcoma (17–53%), clear cell sarcoma (around 50%), angiosarcoma (14%)* [136–138].

TABLE 64.8 Recommended Staging Imaging for Different Histological Types

Recommended Imaging	Histological Types
CT or MRI for regional lymph nodes	Rhabdomyosarcoma, epithelioid sarcoma, clear cell sarcoma, angiosarcoma
CT thorax (unenhanced)	All soft tissue sarcomas
CT abdomen/pelvis	Myxoid liposarcoma, leiomyosarcoma, epithelioid sarcoma, alveolar soft part sarcoma
Brain CT or MRI	Alveolar soft part sarcoma
MRI spine or whole-body MRI	Myxoid liposarcoma

CT Abdomen/Pelvis

Abdominal metastases are less common, present on average in 3% of patients with metastatic disease [134]. However, higher incidence of abdominal metastasis can be seen in certain histological types, *particularly myxoid liposarcoma where abdominal involvement (Fig. 64.75) is seen in up to 50% of all patients with metastases* [139,140]. Other histological types with frequent abdominal metastases are leiomyosarcoma, epithelioid sarcoma, and alveolar soft part sarcoma [141–143]. The liver, mesentery, retroperitoneal are the most commonly affected sites [134,142].

MRI Spine

Bony metastases from myxoid liposarcoma are often occult on CT and can only be seen on MRI [144]. They can also be occult on bone scan and PET (even when primary lesion is PET-positive). *Therefore, to assess for extrapulmonary metastasis from myxoid liposarcoma, the patient should at least have an MRI of their whole spine. Whole-body MRI should also be considered if presence of other occult lesions would change oncological management* [144].

Brain Imaging

Brain metastasis from soft tissue sarcoma is rare, occurring in 1% of all cases [145]. However, alveolar soft part sarcoma (which is a rare tumor) demonstrates a higher incidence of brain metastasis (20–30% of cases) [145–147]. The increased incidence could be explained by the slow-growing nature and longer disease duration of alveolar soft part sarcoma [147]. Other histological types where cases of brain metastases have been reported include leiomyosarcoma, liposarcoma, rhabdomyosarcoma; the occurrences of intracranial metastases from these histological types are likely due to their higher prevalence [145].

There is no uniform consensus on the imaging of the brain in the context of soft tissue sarcoma. Brain metastasis mostly occurs when there is already metastatic disease elsewhere [145–147]. *However, given the high incidence of intracranial metastases, brain imaging should be part of the initial staging scan for alveolar soft part sarcoma.*

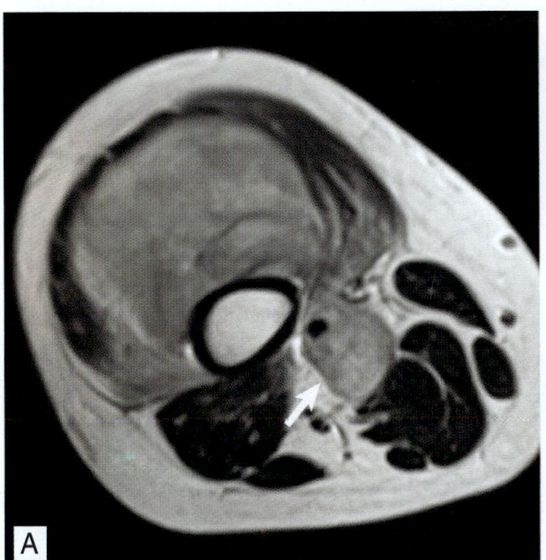

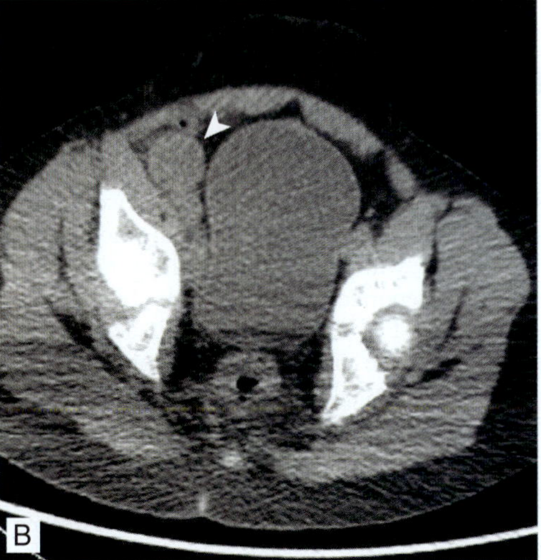

Figure 64.74 Regional lymph node involvement in a 10-year-old patient with embryonal rhabdomyosarcoma. (A) T2w axial image demonstrating a large soft tissue mass in the distal right thigh with popliteal (*arrow*) and (B) external iliac lymph nodes involvements seen on CT (*arrowhead*).

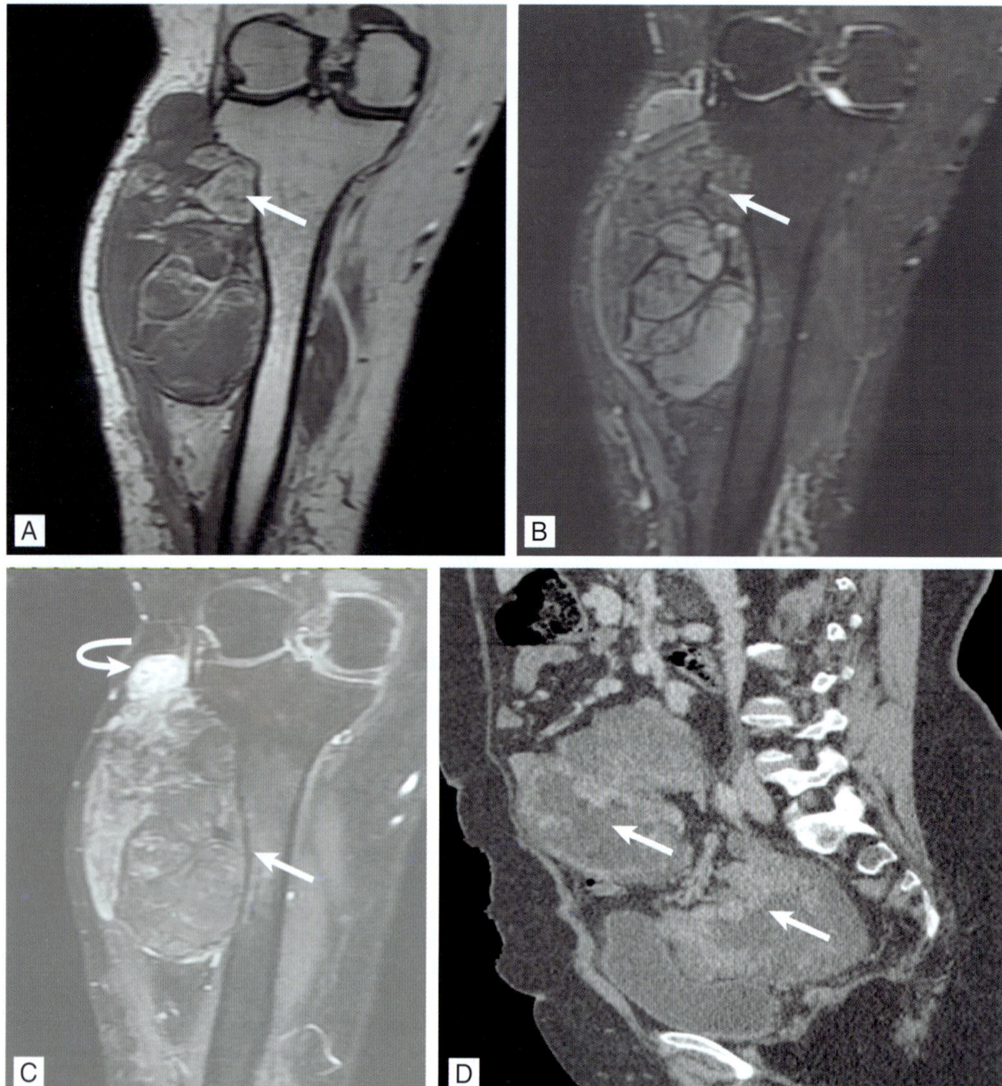

Figure 64.75 Myxoid liposarcoma. Coronal MRI T1w (A), STIR (B), and postcontrast (C) images show a large heterogeneous fat-containing soft tissue mass lesion in lateral aspect of proximal leg (*arrows* in A and B) and demonstrates postcontrast soft tissue nodular enhancement (*curved arrow* in C). Large mass is causing scalloping of the adjacent lateral cortex of proximal tibia and mild unusual enhancement of the marrow is also seen (*arrow* in C). Sagittal CT image of the same patient shows multiple intra-abdominal metastases (*arrows* in D).

Positron Emission Tomography

There are a few studies focusing on the pediatric population regarding the use of PET in soft tissue sarcoma staging [148,149]. In a study of pediatric rhabdomyosarcoma, Federico et al. reported higher sensitivity of PET/CT in detecting nodal and marrow disease compared with conventional imaging [149]. Similar findings were also reported by Volker et al. [148]. There may therefore be a role for PET in certain soft tissue sarcoma known to have a predilection to metastasize to lymph nodes (as listed in earlier section) or bones (alveolar soft part, DDL, angiosarcoma, rhabdomyosarcoma) [150]. Unfortunately, the high sensitivity of PET compared to conventional imaging is not a universally replicated [151]. Furthermore, PET has been shown to upstage only a small minority of adult soft tissue sarcoma (<5%) [152]. Overall, more studies are required to determine the prognostic value afforded by the addition of PET in the staging of soft tissue sarcoma.

Postoperative Imaging

Assessment for local recurrence of soft tissue sarcoma is performed with imaging in tandem with clinical examination. American College of Radiology (ACR) recommends for high-risk patients (size >5 cm), imaging (MRI being the preferred technique) every 3 months for first 2 years, every 4 months for next 2 years, every 6 months for the fifth year, and then annually thereafter. In low-risk patients, imaging may not be required in the limbs where clinical examination may be sufficient; however in less accessible areas such as trunk or retroperitoneum, imaging may be required at every 3–4 months for 2 years, 4–6 months for next 2 years, and annually thereafter for up to 10 years [153]. For systemic surveillance, National Comprehensive Care Network recommends for Stage I patients, chest imaging (CT preferred over radiograph) every 6–12 months. For Stage II to IV patients, chest imaging and other known sites of metastatic disease be performed every 2–6 months for 2–3 years, then every 6 months for the next 2 years, and then annually thereafter [154]. The likelihood of developing a recurrence is low after 10 years, and follow-up can be tailored individually.

Postoperative seroma is a fairly common finding, and easily identified on USG as an anechoic, avascular structure and compressible on probe pressure. Tumor recurrence on the other hand is solid. On MRI, tumor recurrence generally has similar signal to the original tumor, serving as a reminder to always refer and compare to the original preoperative images. The challenge with postoperative MRI is the difficulty in differentiating true tumor recurrence from postoperative inflammatory change and scarring. Comparison with postoperative baseline imaging is invaluable, as well as utilization of MRI techniques including static or dynamic contrast-enhanced MRI and DWI/ADC (as discussed earlier in the chapter).

Summary

We have discussed a wide range of soft tissue tumors and tumor mimics, focusing on their imaging appearances and how imaging features from different techniques complement each other to allow either a specific benign diagnosis, or a well-grounded list of differential diagnoses when lesions appear indeterminate or malignant. Specific histological diagnosis is often not possible on imaging features alone, and biopsy is almost always required preoperatively to guide and tailor management. We have also discussed few important considerations around imaging-guided biopsy including compartmental anatomy, but more importantly highlighting the need for prompt referral to a sarcoma tertiary center when sarcoma is suspected.

Suggested Readings

- MW Anderson, HT Temple, RG Dussault, PA Kaplan, Compartmental anatomy: relevance to staging and biopsy of musculoskeletal tumors, AJR Am J Roentgenol 173 (6) (1999) 1663–1671.
- JS Wu, MG Hochman, Soft-tissue tumors and tumorlike lesions: a systematic imaging approach, Radiology 253 (2) (2009) 297–316.
- MJ Kransdorf, MD Murphey, Imaging of soft-tissue musculoskeletal masses: fundamental concepts, Radiographics 36 (6) (2016) 1931–1948.
- A Chhabra, T Soldatos, Soft-tissue lesions: when can we exclude sarcoma? AJR Am J Roentgenol 199 (6) (2012) 1345–1357.

65 Oral Cavity and Pharynx

ANAGHA RAJEEV JOSHI, DIVA SIDDHARTH SHAH, RAJENDRA SOLANKI

Section 1: Oral Cavity

Introduction

The oral cavity is the anterior most part of aerodigestive tract, located anterior to oropharynx and inferior to the sino-nasal region. Though a wide spectrum of abnormalities are seen in this region, squamous cell carcinoma (SCC) is the most frequent disease of the oral cavity. While the oral cavity is fairly accessible to clinical examination, imaging plays an important role to evaluate deeper extent of the lesions and also to provide space based differentials.

Anatomy

The oral cavity is bounded superiorly by the hard palate and the maxillary alveolar ridge, laterally by the cheek, posteriorly by the soft palate and anterior tonsillar pillars, inferiorly by the mylohyoid muscle and alveolar mandibular ridge and anteriorly by lips.

Anatomically, oral cavity is subdivided into lateral part or the "oral vestibule" and the "oral cavity proper." The vestibule is a slit like space between cheeks and gums, lined by gingival and buccal mucosa. Oral cavity proper includes the space within the alveolar margins of mandible and maxilla, and contains the oral tongue (Fig. 65.1) [1–3].

The mucosal area of the oral cavity is broadly divided into the following anatomic subsites:

1. Gingivobuccal mucosa
2. Retromolar trigone
3. Floor of the mouth
4. Oral tongue
5. Hard Palate

In terms of spaces, the sublingual space is located within the oral cavity and forms an essential component of the floor of the mouth. The submandibular space (SMS) is located inferolateral to the mylohyoid muscle and hence is actually not a part of the oral cavity. However due to the close anatomical relationship with the oral cavity and frequent extension of the disease processes from the floor of mouth (FOM) into the SMS, it will be briefly described here.

Gingivobuccal mucosa: Oral vestibule is lined by buccal mucosa laterally, the gingival mucosa medially, and superiorly and inferiorly by reflections of buccal mucosa on mandible and maxilla known as upper and lower gingivobuccal sulci. SCCs arising from this mucosa spread into adjacent buccomassteric and masticator space.

Retromolar trigone (RMT): RMT is a triangular-shaped mucosal fold that is located behind the last molar tooth. It extends from the level of maxillary last molar to the mandibular last molar. RMT considered as a "cross road" from where cancer can spread into adjacent suprahyoid neck spaces [1]. It is best seen in oblique sagittal CT reformations [5] (Fig. 65.2).

Floor of mouth: FOM is a U-shaped region of the oral cavity, formed by the mylohyoid muscle on either side and fibrous median raphe in the midline. Pair of anterior bellies of digastric muscle and pair of geniohyoid muscles below the mylohyoid sling are additional supporting structures for the FOM. The mylohyoid muscle sling is best demonstrated in coronal plane on cross-sectional imaging. The sublingual space is located superomedial to the mylohyoid sling and the SMS is located inferolateral to it (Fig. 65.3). The root of tongue (ROT) is the deep midline aspect of the oral tongue above the mylohyoid sling and below the

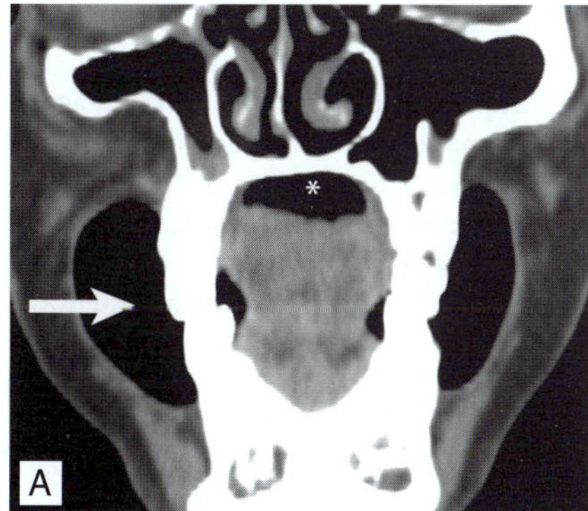

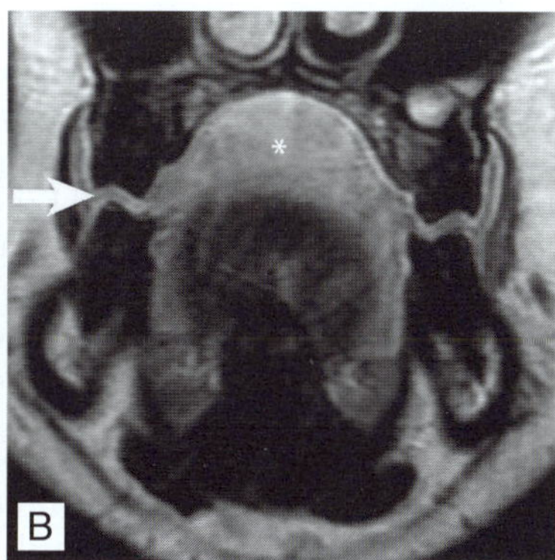

Figure 65.1 Oral cavity anatomy. Coronal puffed cheek CT image (A) and T2W MRI (B) with water distension maneuver shows oral cavity proper (*asterisk*) and oral vestibule (*arrow*).

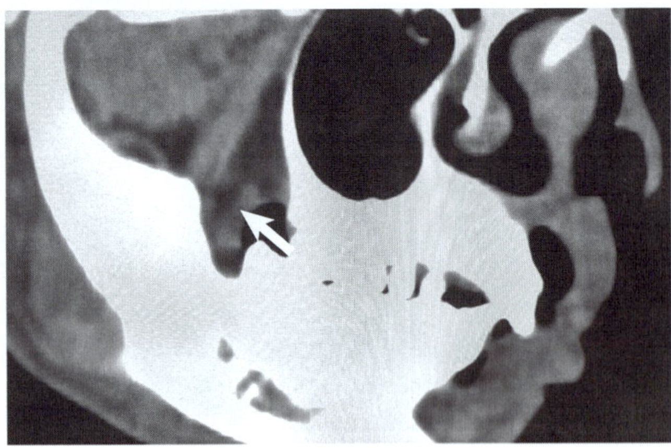

Figure 65.2 Retromolar trigone. Oblique sagittal reformatted CT image shows a triangular mucosal fold behind the upper and lower molar teeth (*arrow*).

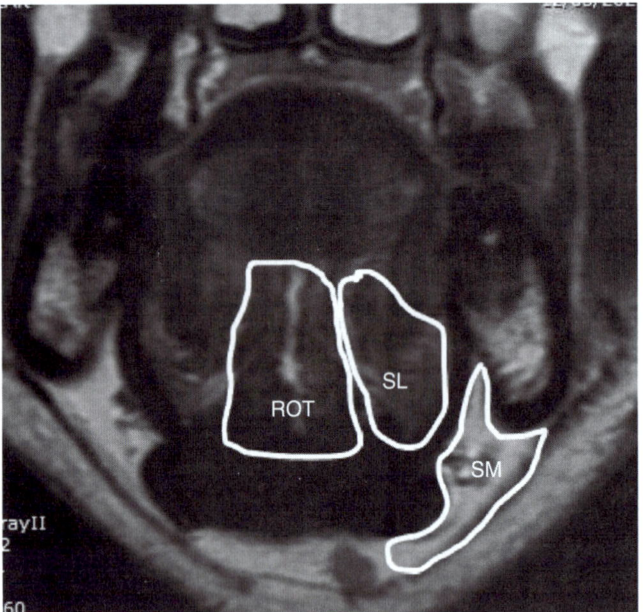

Figure 65.3 Oral cavity anatomy. Coronal T2W image shows root of tongue (ROT), adjacent sublingual (SL), and submandibular space (SM).

extrinsic muscles of the tongue, anteriorly bounded by mandibular symphysis. It consists of paired genioglossus muscles and the fibrofatty lingual septum. ROT is relatively resistant to neoplastic and infective processes due to lack of significant lymphatics and abundance of skeletal muscle [3–5].

Oral tongue: This refers to the anterior two-third portion of the tongue that is anterior to the circumvallate papillae. It is a major content of oral cavity proper. On imaging, in midsagittal cross-sectional plane, the oral tongue lies anterior to a line running through the posterior margin of hard palate; the portion of the tongue posterior to this line is referred to as oropharyngeal tongue and will be discussed later (Fig. 65.4). Superior, inferior, and transverse longitudinal muscles are intrinsic muscles of the tongue and are supplied by hypoglossal nerve. These muscles are very well demonstrated on magnetic resonance imaging (MRI) in coronal and sagittal planes as low signal intensity bundles surrounded by high signal intensity fibrofatty tissue. Extrinsic muscles of tongue include pair of genioglossus, hyoglossus, palatoglossus, and styloglossus muscles. These muscles allow attachment of tongue to mandible, hyoid bone inferiorly, and styloid process of skull base superiorly (Fig. 65.5).

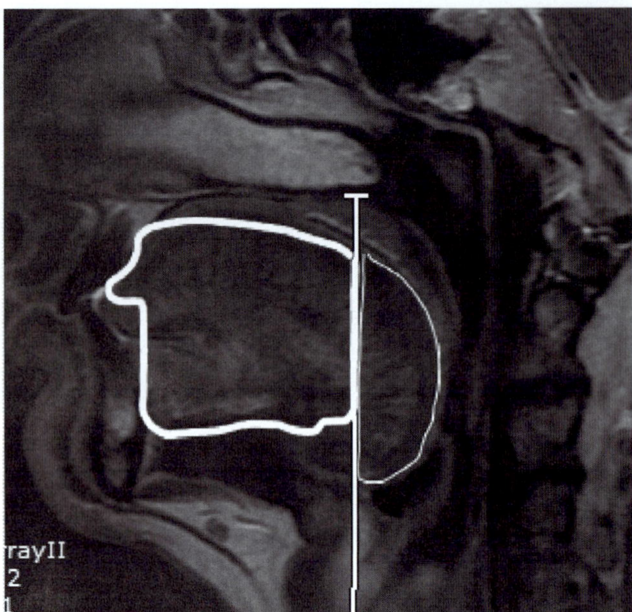

Figure 65.4 Oral and oropharyngeal tongue. Sagittal T2W MRI shows oral tongue (*thick white outline*) and base of tongue (*thin white outline*) by a perpendicular line that passes from posterior margin of hard palate (hard palate–soft palate junction).

Hard palate: Hard palate is bound anteriorly by the upper alveolar ridge and is continuous posteriorly with the soft palate which is a part of the oropharynx. There is abundance of minor salivary gland present in palatal submucosa and hence most of the minor salivary gland tumors of oral cavity are arise from the hard palate.

Imaging Techniques

Majority of oral cavity lesions are clinically evident. Imaging plays a crucial role in differential diagnosis of various benign diseases, assess the deeper extent of oral cavity lesions and staging of malignant lesions.

Multidetector computed tomography (MDCT) and MRI are the most commonly used imaging techniques for evaluation of various oral cavity lesions. Ultrasonography (USG) with high frequency transducers is also valuable in lesions of FOM and SMS. MDCT scans allow faster acquisition time, multiplanar reformations, and excellent depiction of anatomy and bone. MDCT is generally preferred for gingivobuccal and RMT cancers. MRI offers superior contrast and spatial resolution when compared with computed tomography (CT) and is preferred especially for small mucosal lesions, lesions of the tongue and FOM and assessment of perineural spread in hard palate cancers. MRI is also superior in evaluation of extent of marrow disease in SCC.

Positron emission tomography (PET-CT) is the imaging technique of choice in staging and restaging of oral cancers and National Comprehensive Cancer Network (NCCN) (Version 1.2020) recommends routine use of PET-CT in stage III and IV oral cancers. However, the use of PET-CT varies from institution to institution.

Pearls and pitfalls:

- "Puffed cheek" and water distension technique at MDCT is preferred in patients with severe submucosal fibrosis or evaluation of small buccal mucosa and RMT lesion (Fig. 65.6A and B)
- "Open mouth" maneuver adds value for small palatal lesions or upper alveolar lesions (Fig. 65.7). Tongue protrusion helps in delineating small lesions along ventrolateral aspect of oral tongue
- Pitfalls in evaluation of oral cavity lesions on cross-sectional imaging include dental amalgam, beam hardening, and motion artifacts that may obscure the entire lesion

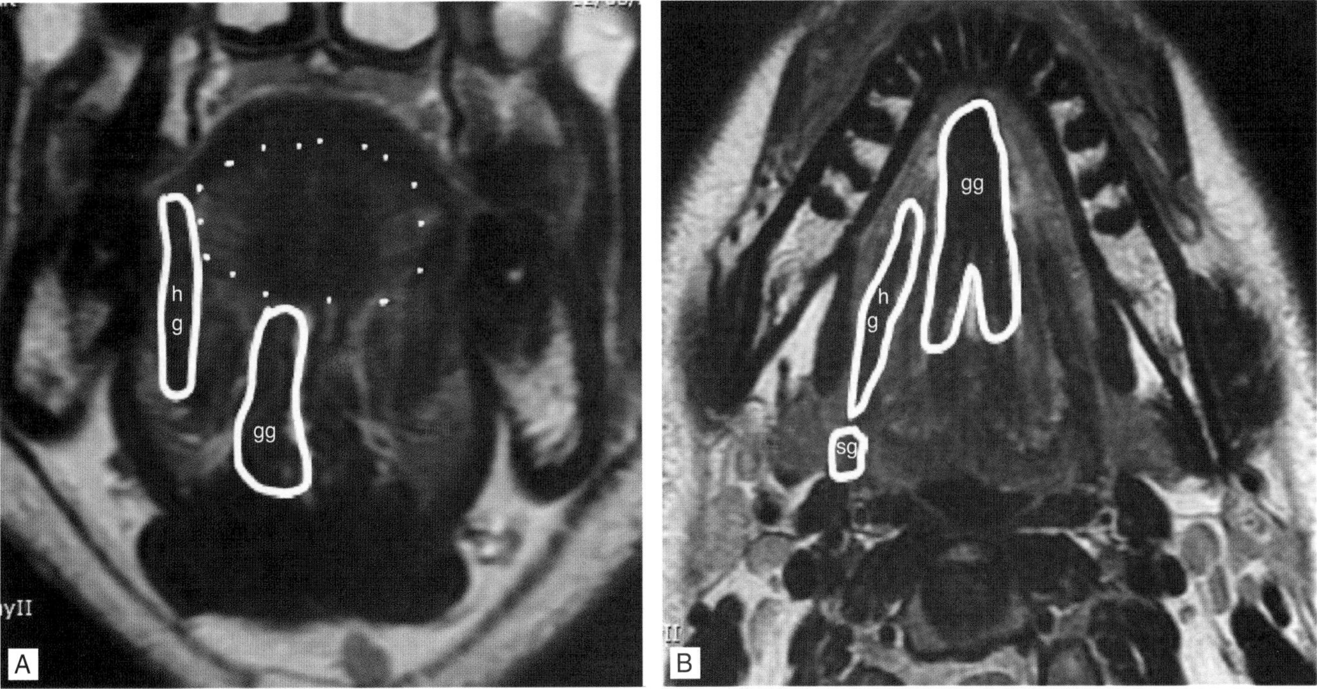

Figure 65.5 Oral tongue anatomy. Coronal (A) and axial T2W (B) MRI shows intrinsic (*dotted line*) and paired extrinsic muscles of tongue—genioglossus (gg), hyoglossus (hg), and styloglossus muscles (sg).

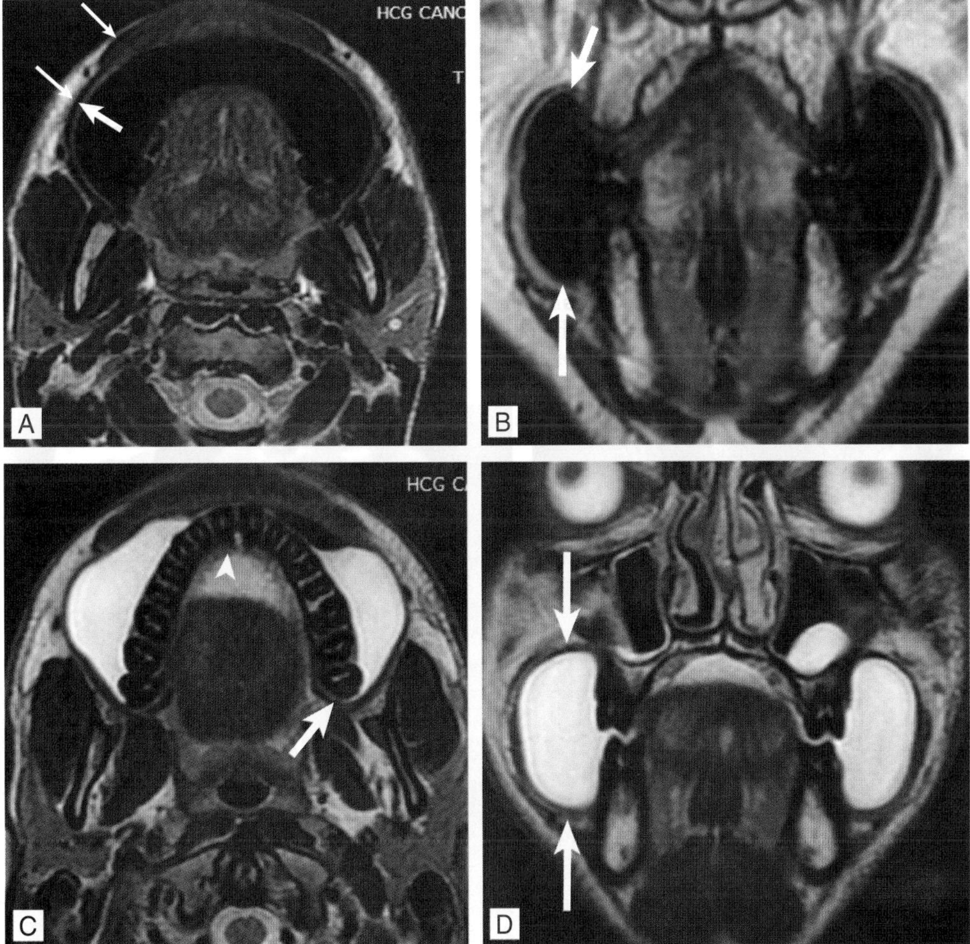

Figure 65.6 Gingivobuccal mucosa and sulci anatomy. (A) Axial T2W MRI with puffed cheek maneuver showing mucosa–submucosa (*thick arrow*) and buccinator orbicularis oris muscles (*small arrows*). Coronal T2W MRI (B) with puffed cheek maneuver showing well-distended upper and lower gingivobuccal sulci (*arrow*). (C) Axial T2W MRI with water distension maneuver showing RMT (*arrow*) and alveolar mucosa (*arrowhead*), coronal T2W. (D) MRI with water distension maneuver showing well-distended upper and lower gingivobuccal sulci (*arrow*).

Metastases: These are extremely rare tumors of oral cavity and arise from primary malignancies of the lung, breast, kidney, thyroid melanoma, and kidneys [31,33]. Imaging findings are nonspecific and often associated with findings of metastatic deposits elsewhere in the body.

Postoperative Oral Cavity

Imaging of the postoperative oral cavity is crucial and radiologist must have knowledge of various imaging appearances of post-treatment oral cavity including anatomic distortion, appearance of flap reconstructions as well as postsurgical fibrosis from recurrent disease. Goals of postoperative imaging include:

1. Evaluation of postoperative bed
2. Evaluation of post-treatment short-term and long-term complications
3. Evaluation of disease recurrence at operative bed side and at flap mucosal junction

Imaging pearls of postoperative bed evaluation on cross-sectional imaging [34].

- Any asymmetry or thickening at operative site or nodular/irregular contour of operated area raises the suspicion of recurrent malignant disease and should always be correlated with clinical examination findings
- Enhancing soft tissue lesion at operative bed or involving the flap mucosal junction is almost definitive of recurrent malignant lesion (Fig. 65.21)
- DW-MRI and delayed contrast-enhanced MDCT/MRI (taken after 10 minutes of contrast injection) helps at times to differentiate benign changes from recurrent disease spread (Fig. 65.22)
- FDG PET-CT is valuable tool to evaluate recurrence and restaging for oral cavity cancers, metastatic neck node of unknown primary; however dental streak artifacts hinder the evaluation of oral cavity. Combining PET and MRI gives unique metabolic information and excellent soft tissue contrast as well as morphologic data [35,36] (Fig. 65.23)

Section 2: Pharynx

Pharynx is a long musculomembranous tube which extends from base of the skull cranially to the lower border of cricoid cartilage. It is subdivided into three parts, nasopharynx, oropharynx, and hypopharynx.

Anatomy

Nasopharynx: It is the superior most part of pharynx which is situated below the skull base, posterior to the nasal cavity, anterior to clivus and bound by parapharyngeal space laterally and carotid space posterolaterally on either side and extends inferiorly up to the level of the line passing through the hard and soft palates. The lateral wall of nasopharynx shows two fossae and one mucosal projection on either side. The eustachian tube (ET) opening is located along the upper part of its lateral wall through which nasopharynx communicates with middle ear. Torus tubarius, a mucosal projection formed by cartilaginous portion of ET is located posterior to ET opening and the fossa of Rosenmuller is situated posterior to the torus tubarius (Fig. 65.24). The fossa of Rosenmuller and surrounding area is a frequent site for origin of nasopharyngeal carcinoma (NPC).

Oropharynx: Oropharynx is located behind the oral cavity, and comprises the palatine tonsils with anterior and posterior pillars which are made up of palatoglossus and palatopharyngeus muscles, respectively, base of tongue and lingual tonsil, soft palate, posterior oropharyngeal wall related to second and third cervical vertebral bodies and vallecula formed by median glossoepiglottic fold and laterally by lateral glossoepiglottic fold [1] (Figs. 65.25 and 65.26). Oropharyngeal subsites usually contain lymphoid tissue in variable degree. This is the reason for lymphoma being a common diagnostic differential of oropharyngeal SCC (OPSCC).

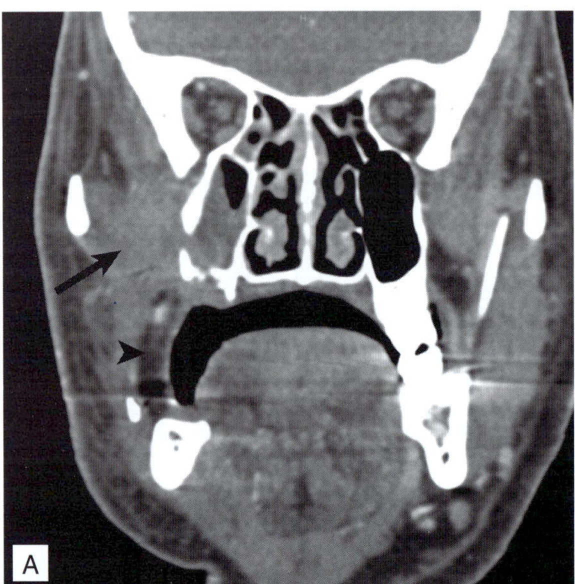

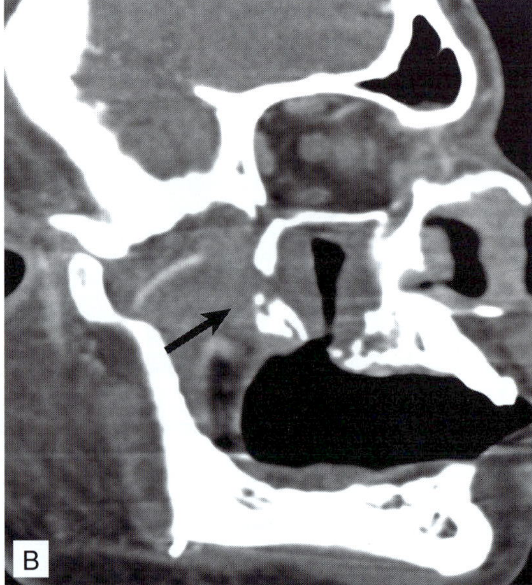

Figure 65.21 Operated case of right buccal mucosa with flap reconstruction. Reformatted coronal (A) and sagittal (B) postcontrast CT images showing enhancing soft tissue (*arrows*) in superior aspect of flap (*arrowhead*) with intrasinus extension in residual right maxilla.

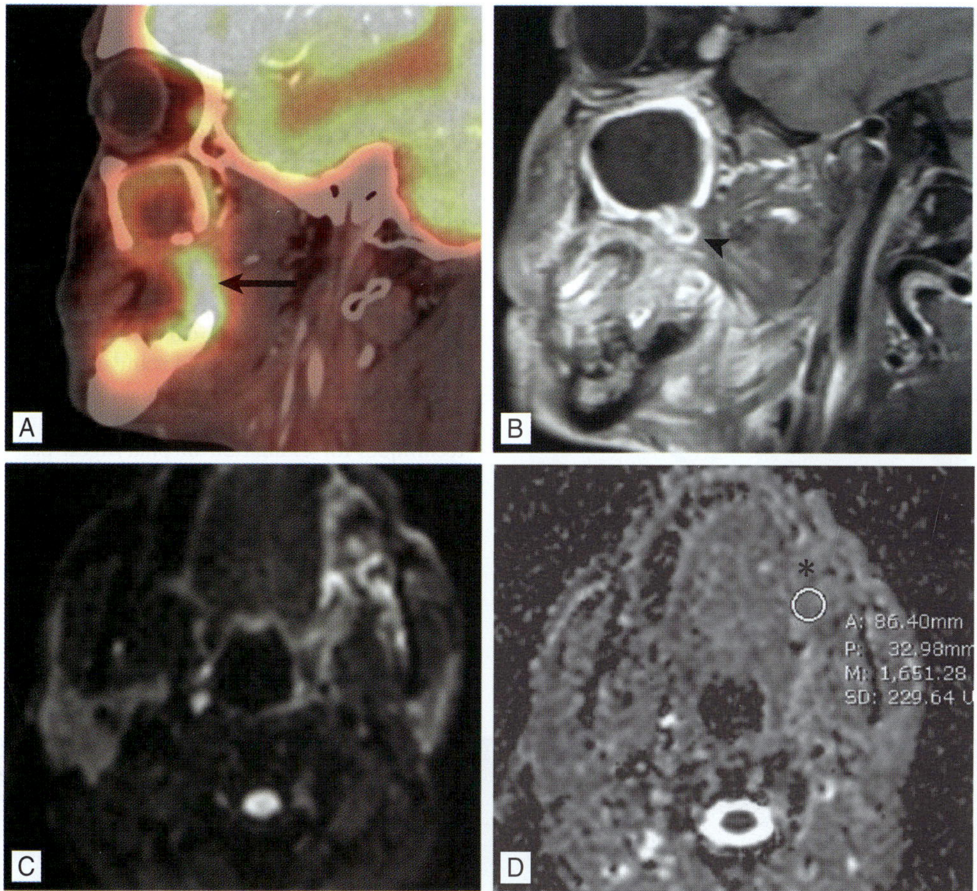

Figure 65.22 Operated case of carcinoma of left buccal mucosa, presented with pus discharge from oral cavity. (A) Sagittal PET-CT image shows hypermetabolic area at flap site (*arrow*). Postcontrast sagittal T1 fat suppressed image (B) shows inflamed flap with peripherally enhancing oroantral fistula (*arrowhead*) and DWI (C) with ADC (D) images show no restriction with high ADC value (*asterisk*).

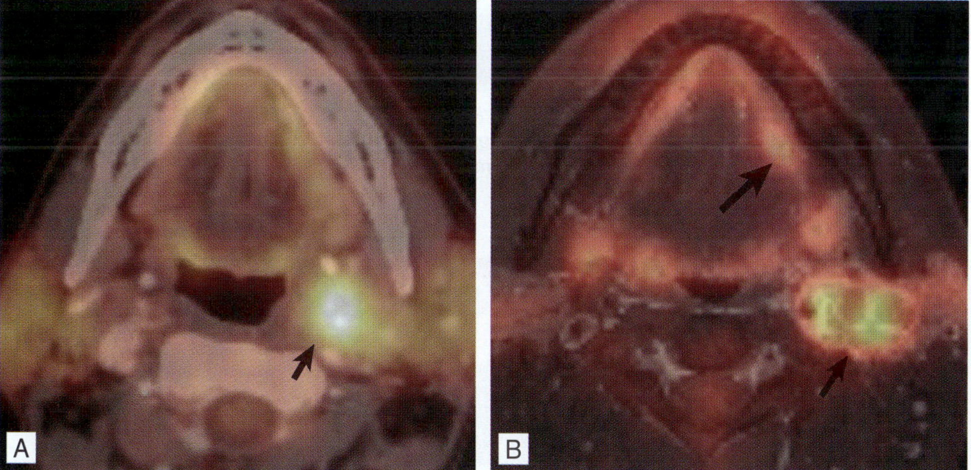

Figure 65.23 Floor of mouth cancer. Axial PET-CT image (A) shows metabolically active metastatic left level II (*arrow*), axial PET-MRI fusion (B) shows metabolically active metastatic left level II node (*arrow*) and small lesion in left side of floor mouth (*large arrow*). Biopsy showed moderately differentiated SCC from ulcer in floor of mouth.

Hypopharynx: Hypopharynx is located below oropharynx and extends caudally till the inferior margin of cricoid cartilage (Figs. 65.27, 65.28, and 65.29). It continues below as cervical esophagus. Hypopharynx is made up of three components namely pyriform fossa, postcricoid region, and posterior hypopharyngeal wall.

Visceral fascia is located behind the constrictor muscle of pharynx, posterior to which is retropharyngeal fat plane. Fat plane in retropharyngeal region is an important landmark while evaluating prevertebral fixation in cases of malignancy [37,38].

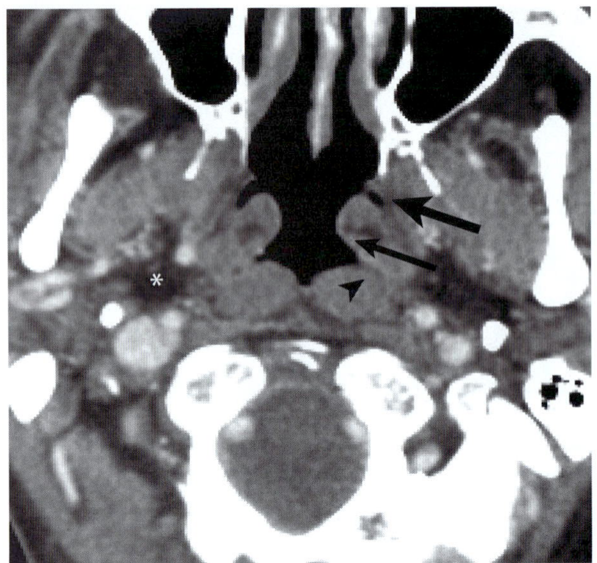

Figure 65.24 Normal anatomy of the nasopharynx. Axial CT section shows (1) Eustachian tube opening (*thick black arrow*), (2) torus tubarius (*thin black arrow*), (3) fossa of Rosenmuller (*arrowhead*), (4) and parapharyngeal space (*asterisk*).

Imaging Techniques

In the era of CT scan and MRI, plain radiographs and barium procedures are almost obsolete for imaging of these malignancies, except for screening [39-42].

USG can be used to detect metastatic lymphadenopathy and for performing a few ultrasound-guided interventional procedures. MDCT and MRI are well-established imaging techniques for evaluation of pharyngeal pathologies. Mucosal abnormality of pharynx can be demonstrated on clinical evaluation or by endoscopy. The primary goal of imaging is to define the submucosal spread and locoregional extent into adjacent spaces. PET-CT is very useful and a gold standard for staging in conditions like lymphoma as well as residual, recurrent, and postoperative cases of pharyngeal malignancies. Commonly used imaging techniques for evaluation of pharyngeal pathology are given in Table 65.3.

Nasopharynx

Various pathologies that affect the nasopharynx are given in Table 65.4.

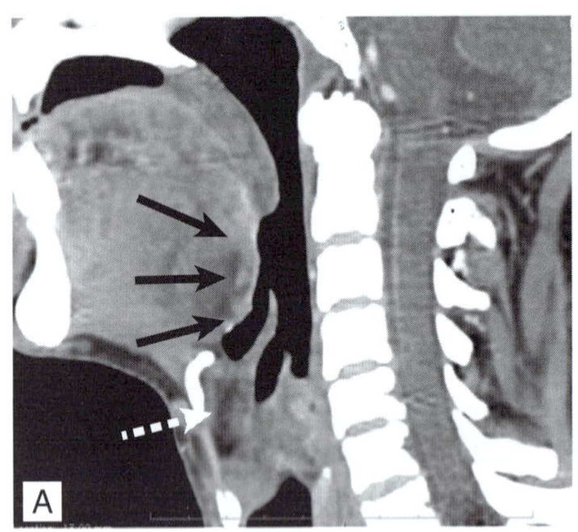

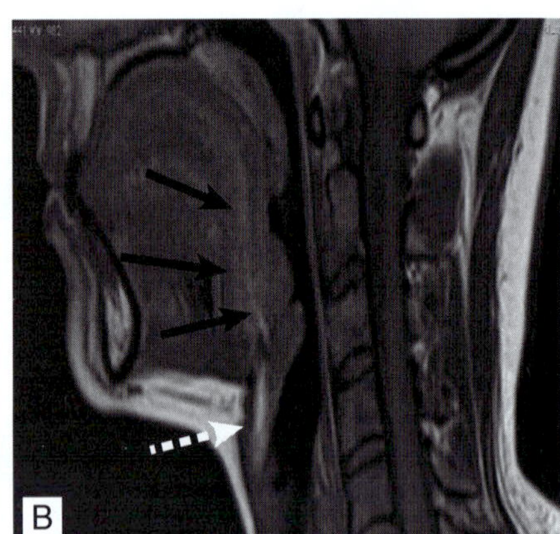

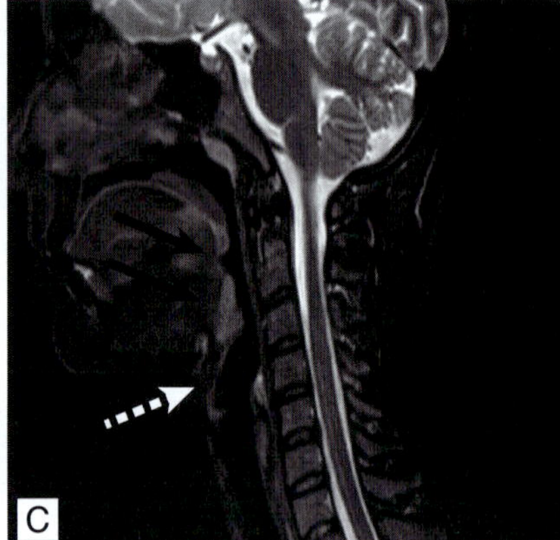

Figure 65.25 Normal anatomy of oropharynx. (A) Base of tongue (*solid black arrows*). Postcontrast CT image showing differential enhancement than rest of the tongue due to presence of lymphoid tissue. It is located just above preepiglottic fat (*dotted white arrow*). On T1 W image (B) and on T2 fat saturated image (C), differential signal in base of tongue is seen due to presence of lymphoid tissue. Junction of soft and hard palate demarcates anterior boundary of oropharynx superiorly.

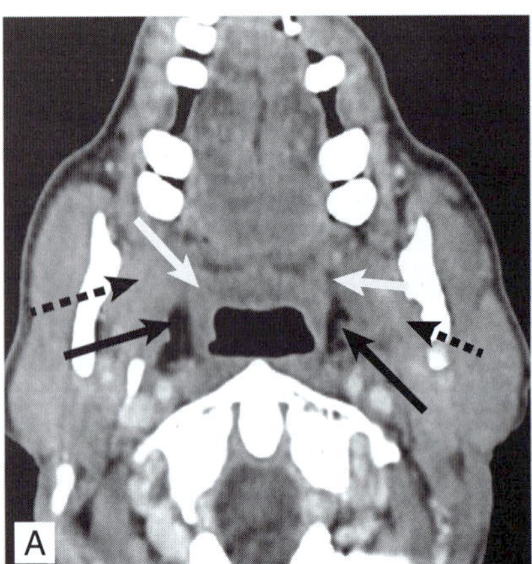

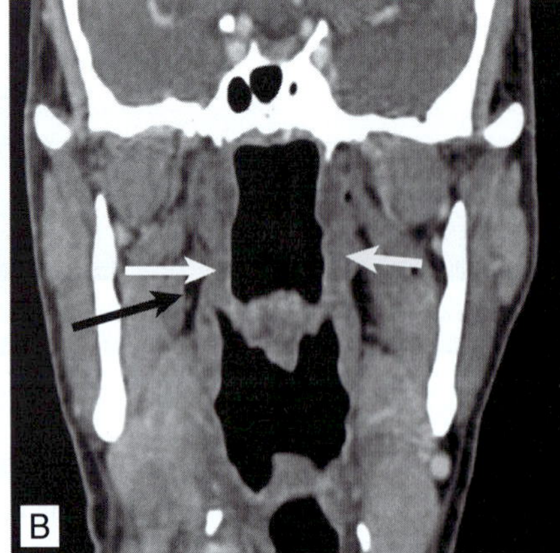

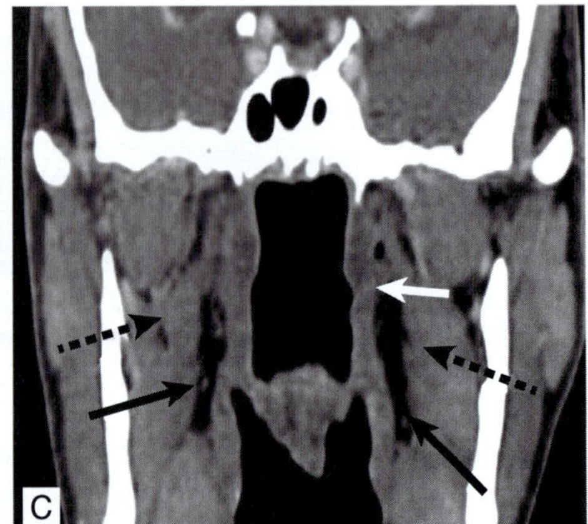

Figure 65.26 Normal anatomy of oropharynx. Axial (A) and coronal (B and C) anatomy shows bilateral palatine tonsils (*solid white arrows*) on medial aspect of parapharyngeal fat (*solid black arrows*). Medial pterygoid muscles (*dotted black arrows*) are located just lateral to parapharyngeal fat. Anterolaterally, retromolar trigone comes in relation with palatine tonsils.

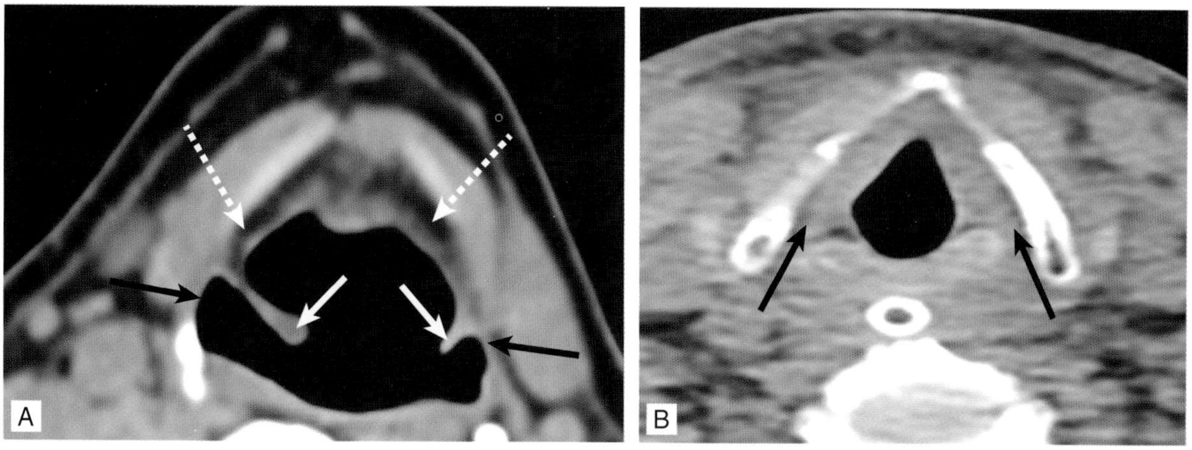

Figure 65.27 Pyriform fossa anatomy. Pyriform fossa is indicated by *solid black arrows*. Anteriorly, it comes in relation with paraglottic fat (*dotted white arrows*). Medially, it is related to aryepiglottic fold (*solid white arrows*). Laterally, it comes in relation with thyrohyoid membrane superiorly. In inferior part, pyriform fossa tapers as pyriform apex. Pyriform apex is located at the level of true vocal cord and cricoarytenoid joint. In image B, normal pyriform apex is seen on either side (*solid black arrows*).

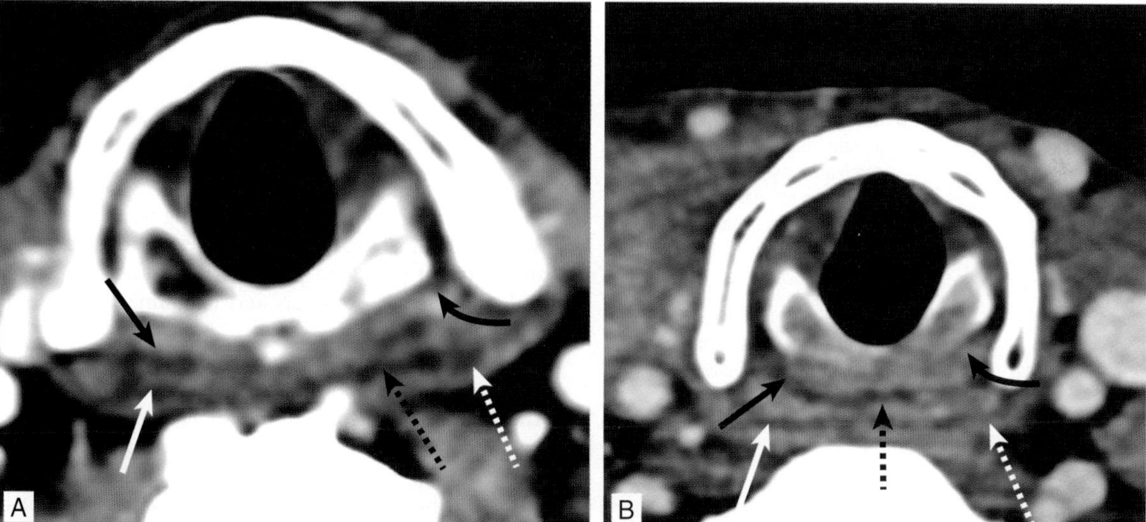

Figure 65.28 Postcricoid region layered arrangement. Comparison of two different patients in axial CT scan images. Just behind the cricoid cartilage, first layer is posterior cricoarytenoid muscle (*curved black arrows*). Second layer is anterior submucosal fat plane (*solid black arrows*). Third layer is hypopharyngeal mucosa/opposed lumen (*dotted black arrows*). Fourth layer is second submucosal fat plane (*solid white arrows*). Inferior constrictor muscle of pharynx (*dotted white arrows*) is located behind second submucosal fat plane and anterior to longus capitis muscle.

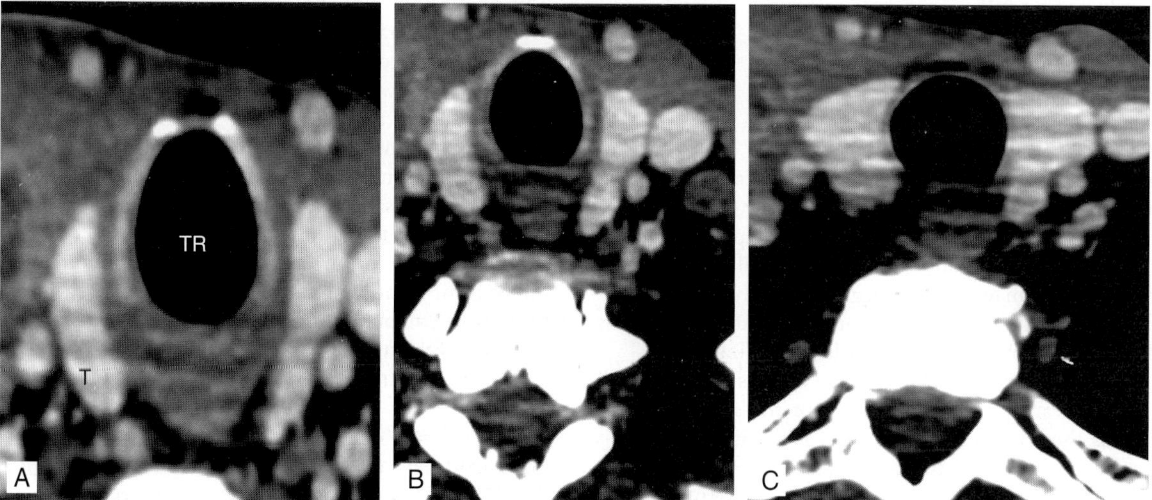

Figure 65.29 Postcricoid region. (A) Sections at the level of thyroid gland (T) and trachea-esophageal groove. (B) As we go toward esophagus from hypopharynx, hypopharynx starts to change shape from flat to round and (C) becomes completely round in shape at level of esophagus. *TR*, trachea.

TABLE 65.3 Commonly Used Imaging Techniques for Evaluation of Pharyngeal Pathology

Subsites	Technique
Nasopharynx	MRI is preferred over CT PET CT
Oropharynx	MRI is preferred over CT Contrast CT combined with MR imaging has highest degree of sensitivity [1]
Hypopharynx	CT is preferred over MRI

TABLE 65.4 Nasopharynx—Common Diseases

Non-neoplastic	Neoplastic
Congenital/developmental ■ Tornwaldt's cyst ■ Encephalocoele, meningocoele	Benign ■ Juvenile nasopharyngeal angiofibroma (JNA) ■ Pleomorphic adenoma/benign mixed tumor
Infective/inflammatory ■ Adenoid hypertrophy ■ Retropharyngeal abscess ■ Mucous retention cyst ■ Pharyngitis	Malignant ■ Nasopharyngeal carcinoma (keratinizing squamous cell carcinoma, nonkeratinizing squamous cell carcinoma) ■ Nasopharyngeal lymphoma ■ Nasopharyngeal rhabdomyosarcoma ■ Metastasis
Others ■ Antro-choanal polyp ■ Trauma	Direct extension of malignant sino nasal tumors or skull base tumor, e.g., chordoma, Extramedullary plasmacytoma

Common pathologies involving nasopharynx in the pediatric age group are adenoid hyperplasia and juvenile nasopharyngeal angiofibroma (JNA), while in adult it is NPC. An adult presenting with metastatic neck node(s) with carcinoma from unknown primary as initial presentation or nonresolving serous otitis media must be evaluated for NPC.

Neoplastic Lesions

Juvenile Nasopharyngeal Angiofibroma

It is commonest benign, but locally aggressive vascular tumor that may extend into the nasopharynx and exclusively occurs in adolescent males. Nasal obstruction and recurrent epistaxis are the commonest clinical presentations. Cross-sectional imaging (CT and/or MRI) are the main stay of imaging not only for confirmation of diagnosis of JNA but for its locoregional extension. This is followed by preoperative angiography with embolization.

JNA originates from a vascular nidus in the posterolateral wall of nasal cavity near the superior margin of the sphenopalatine foramen, thus the term "nasopharyngeal" is a misnomer as it is only secondarily involved by this tumor [43,44].

The role of imaging is to determine exact site, extent and very importantly to know feeding arteries of this tumor before surgery, since surgery is the mainstay of treatment. Contrast-enhanced

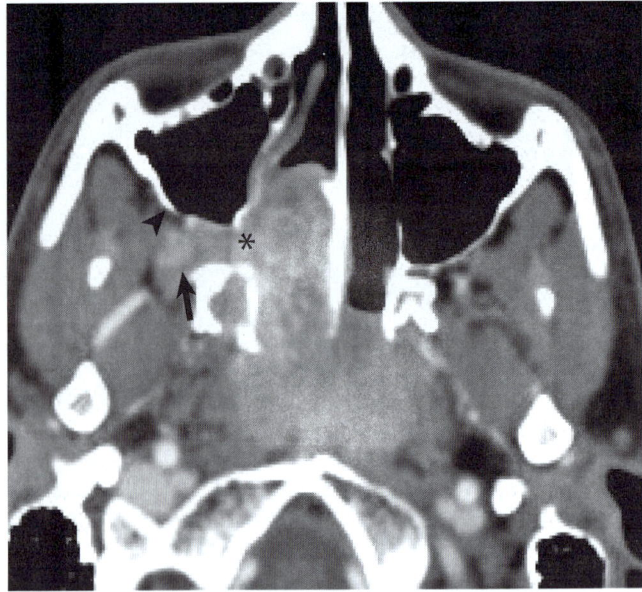

Figure 65.30 Juvenile nasopharyngeal angiofibroma (JNA). Postcontrast axial CT scan shows classical signs of JNA. Widening of right sphenopalatine foramen (*asterisk*) with extension of tumor into pterygopalatine fossa and pterygomaxillary fissure (*large arrow*) and anterior bowing of posterolateral wall of right maxillary sinus (*arrowhead*).

MDCT is the primary baseline imaging technique for mapping of tumor as well as to see intracranial extension, skull base erosion, and status of pterygoid plates. MRI should be reserved in cases with intracranial extension and engulfment of internal carotid artery [43–45].

On cross-sectional imaging JNA has a classical appearance of soft tissue density polypoidal mass showing avid enhancement. The lesion is centered at the sphenopalatine foramen. It can extend anteriorly into nasal cavity and nasopharynx, laterally into infratemporal fossa, masticator space through pterygopalatine fossa, and pterygomaxillary fissure. It causes anterior bowing of posterior wall of maxillary sinus known as "Holman–Miller sign" (Antral sign) [43,44] (Fig. 65.30). In 2017, Janakiram et al. have analyzed imaging findings of 242 patients of JNA and suggested that all primary cases of JNA show marked widening of pterygoid wedge which is a junction of medial and lateral pterygoid plates. This sign is known as "Ram–Haran" sign (Fig. 65.31), and in follow up postoperative imaging shows two parallel lines of pterygoid plates due to drilling of cancellous bone in pterygoid wedge. This sign is known as "chopstick sign" [45]. At the time of imaging, most of the tumors are fairly large in size. They show signals that are isointense to muscle on T1 images and are heterogeneously hyperintense on T2 images. Presence of prominent flow voids leads to "salt and pepper" appearance at MRI. Moderate enhancement is seen on the contrast study.

The purpose of preoperative angiography in this vascular tumor is for identifying the feeding vessels of the tumor, followed by elective embolization of feeders, which helps to reduce intraoperative bleeding (Fig. 65.32) [46].

Arterial feeders in JNA are given in Table 65.5.

Nasopharyngeal Carcinoma

NPC is a silent head and neck malignant tumor with approximately 60–85% presenting as metastatic neck nodes. Other presenting symptoms include headache, nasal obstruction, epistaxis, and cranial nerve palsy. The tumor occurs in adults, with male to

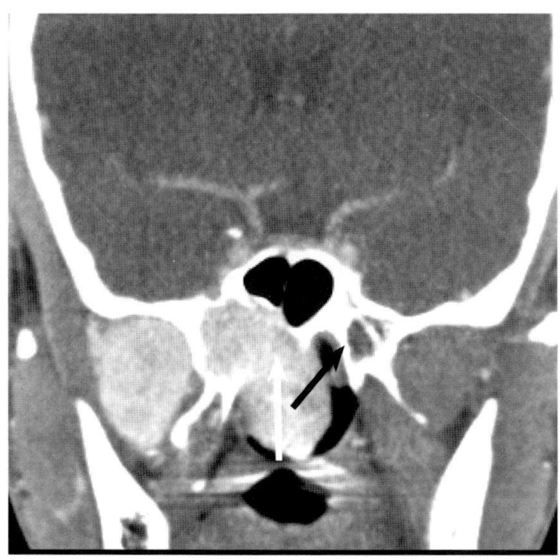

Figure 65.31 Juvenile nasopharyngeal angiofibroma (JNA). Coronal CT reformatted image shows an intensely enhancing JNA (stage II) with marked widening of right pterygoid wedge—"Ram–Haran sign" (*white arrow*) and normal pterygoid wedge on left side *(black arrow)*.

female ratio being 3:1 and shows bimodal peak between second and sixth decades. It rarely affects children below 6 years of age. The diagnosis of NPC is usually done by endoscopy and biopsy. NPC starts in fossa of Rosenmuller and spreads submucosally. The primary goal of imaging is to know the entire extent of spread, especially in patients with ambiguous endoscopy findings, where tumor resembles hypertrophied lymphoid tissue or if the lesion is entirely submucosal.

On CT, very early NPC may not be appreciated or can be seen fossa of Rosenmuller obliteration while in advanced NPC, the tumor is seen as a soft tissue density homogenously or heterogeneously enhancing lesion. On MRI it is seen as low signal intensity lesion on T1-weighted images and intermediate to hyperintense signal mass on T2-weighted images with hypoenhancement than the normal mucosa on contrast T1-weighted images. Patterns of spread of NPC are shown in Table 65.6.

Post-Treatment NPC Evaluation: NPC is a radiosensitive malignancy and radiation therapy is the mainstay of treatment for early disease and chemoradiation is preferred in locally advanced cases. Post-treatment MRI in NPC reveals diffusely thickened enhancing mucosa and submucosa of nasopharynx due to radiation induce edema and mucositis [49] (Fig. 65.34). Contrast-enhanced

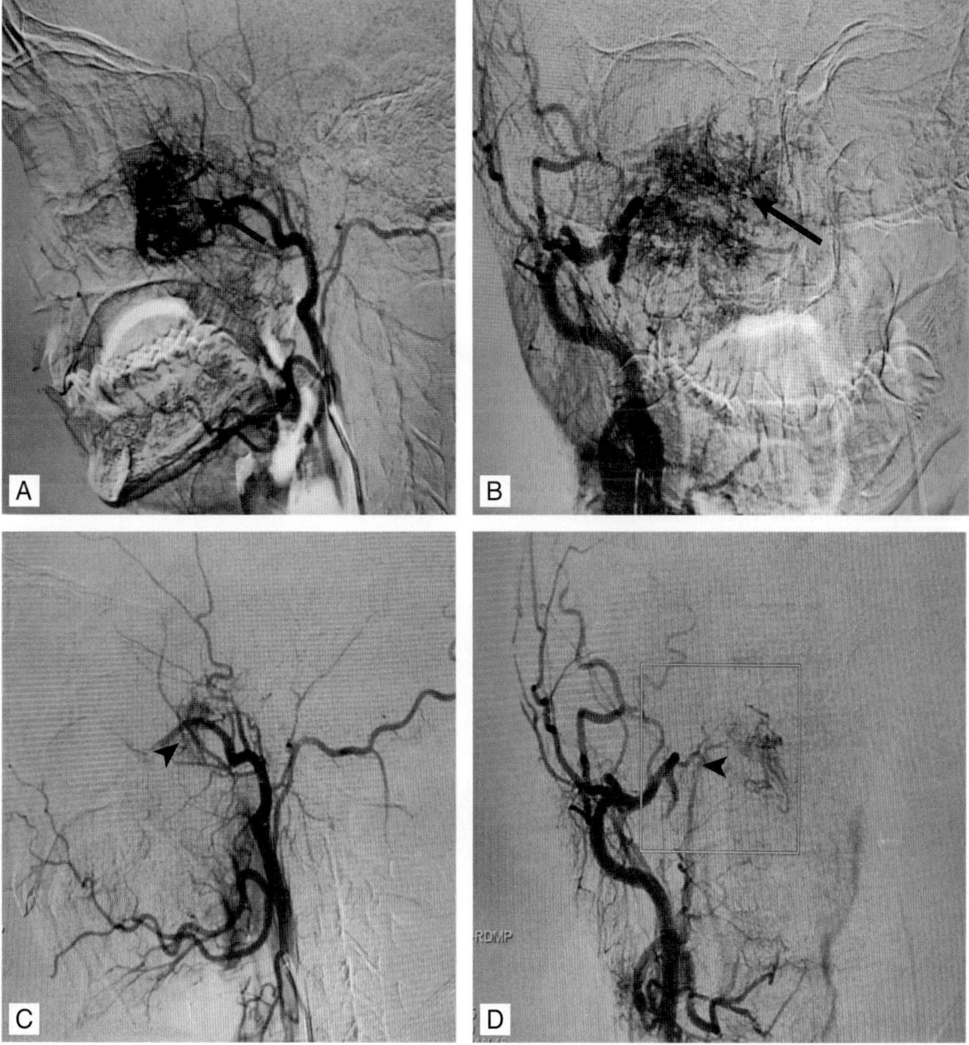

Figure 65.32 Juvenile nasopharyngeal angiofibroma (JNA). Sagittal (A) and coronal (B) digital subtraction angiography images show blush of contrast in JNA (*arrows*), postembolization, sagittal (C) and coronal (D) digital subtraction angiography images show no blush of contrast at tumor site (*arrowheads*).

TABLE 65.5 Arterial Feeders in JNA

ECA—external carotid artery (major)	ICA—internal carotid artery (minor)
Internal maxillary artery ▪ Sphenopalatine branches ▪ Descending palatine branches	Ophthalmic artery
Ascending pharyngeal artery	Sphenoidal branches

MRI is superior in evaluating post-treatment changes and recurrent nasopharyngeal tumors. PET-CT or PET-MRI is superior imaging techniques in equivocal follow-up cases of NPC, where MRI findings are not clearly diagnostic [50,51] (Fig. 65.35). Apart from information about distant metastasis, PET-CT is also valuable when MRI shows equivocal neck nodes. Recurrent or residual disease shows uptake of radionuclide tracer on PET imaging while on MRI, it appears as intermediate to high T2 signal intensity with inhomogeneous postcontrast enhancement. Combining PET and MRI significantly improves diagnostic accuracy in evaluation of recurrent disease with an advantage of combined metabolic and morphologic information.

Lymphoma of Nasopharynx

This is the second most common malignancy of nasopharynx. On imaging, it appears as a diffuse homogenous symmetrical enlargement of walls of nasopharynx with bulky masses and florid lymphadenopathy [52]. PET-CT is valuable in staging and restaging of lymphoma. Lymphoma is usually differentiated from NPC on the basis of midline location with symmetrical involvement and uncommon bony invasion. On MRI, lymphoma shows low ADC values due to high cellularity.

Non-Neoplastic Lesions

Adenoid Hyperplasia

It is the commonest benign lesions of children and one of the common causes of upper airway obstruction. Lateral radiograph in an extended neck is sufficient to demonstrate adenoid hyperplasia, seen as a radio-opacity in the roof of nasopharynx. No

TABLE 65.6 Patterns of Spread of NPC

Extension	Involvement
Anterior	Posterior aspect of nasal cavity. It can cause widening and/or erosion of sphenopalatine foramen with further spread of tumor into pterygopalatine fossa and pterygomaxillary maxillary fissure. NPC with limited spread to nasal cavity is considered as T1 stage. Inferior extension of the tumor into oropharynx rarely occurs.
Lateral	Extension through levatorpalatini muscle and pharyngobasilar fascia into the parapharyngeal space (PPS) [47]. Invasion of this space can lead to high incidence of distant metastasis and from this space the lesion can encase or invade internal carotid artery and further anterolateral spread occurs into the masticator space and infratemporal fossa. PPS extension is considered as T2 stage.
Superior	Invasion of the skull base and skull base foramina (foramen lacerum, ovale, and vidian canal) is best appreciated on coronal and axial postcontrast T1W fat saturated images. Erosion of clivus, body of sphenoid, and pterygoid bones is fairly common and better seen on MDCT. Paranasal sinus involvement occurs as direct extension, with sphenoid sinus involvement being the commonest. MRI can differentiate intrasinus extension from retained secretions [47]. Skull base and paranasal sinus extension of NPC is considered as stage T3 disease. Intracranial dural extension or infiltration, meningeal involvement or extension into the cavernous sinus are considered as T4 disease (Fig. 65.33)
Posterior	NPC infiltrates the prevertebral muscle posteriorly via infiltration of longus coli muscle. Hematogenous spread occurs frequently after infiltration of prevertebral space by the lesion as space is rich in the venous plexus [48]. Extensively rich submucosal capillary lymphatic plexus of nasopharynx explains high incidence of cervical nodal metastasis. Nodal metastases occur commonly to retropharyngeal nodes followed by jugulodigastric nodes from level II to V.

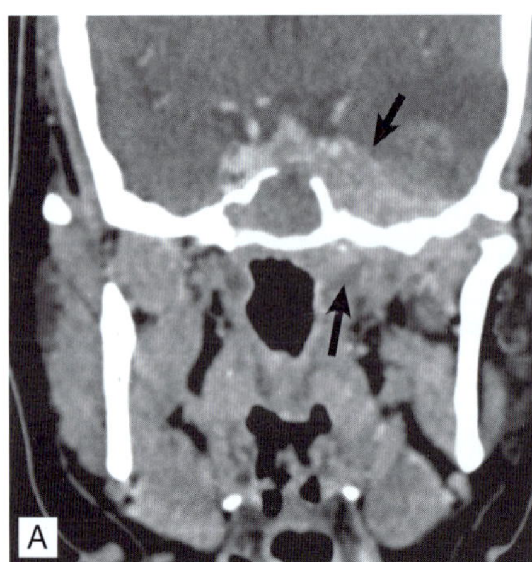

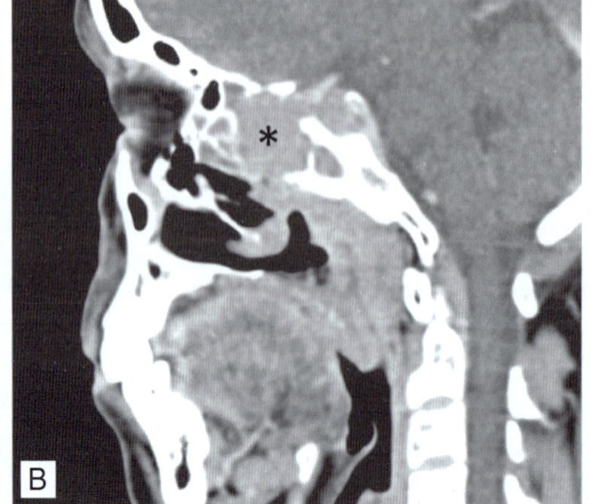

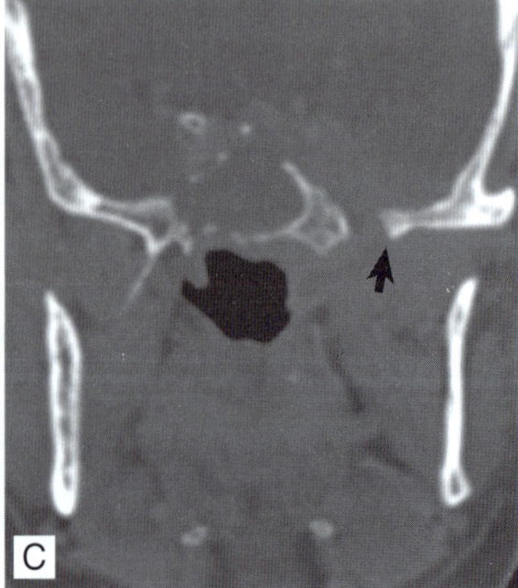

Figure 65.33 Nasopharyngeal carcinoma. Coronal (A) and sagittal (B) postcontrast reformatted CT images show stage IV nasopharyngeal carcinoma with intrasinus (*asterisk*) and intracranial (*long arrows*) extension on left side and bone reformatted image (C) shows erosion of foramen ovale (*short arrow*).

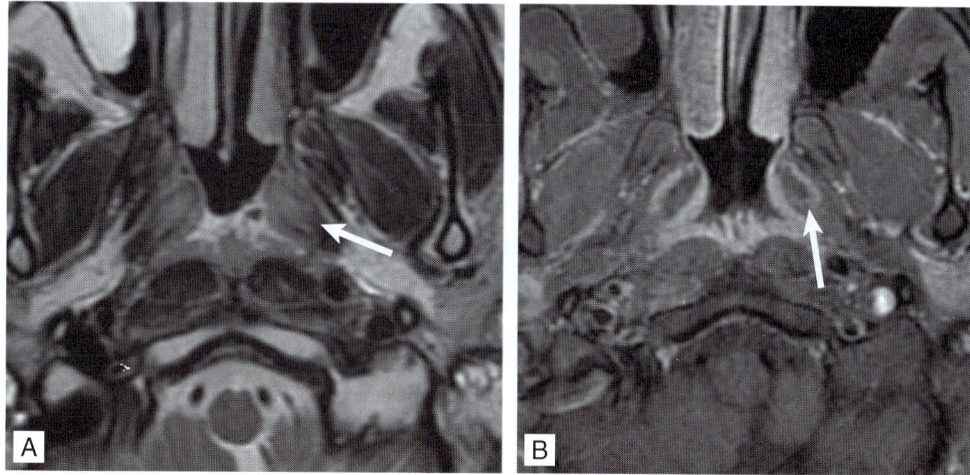

Figure 65.34 Nasopharyngeal cancer post-treatment. Axial T2W (A) and postcontrast T1W (B) images show diffusely enhancing edematous symmetrical thickened nasopharyngeal wall (*arrows*) following chemoradiation for nasopharyngeal cancer.

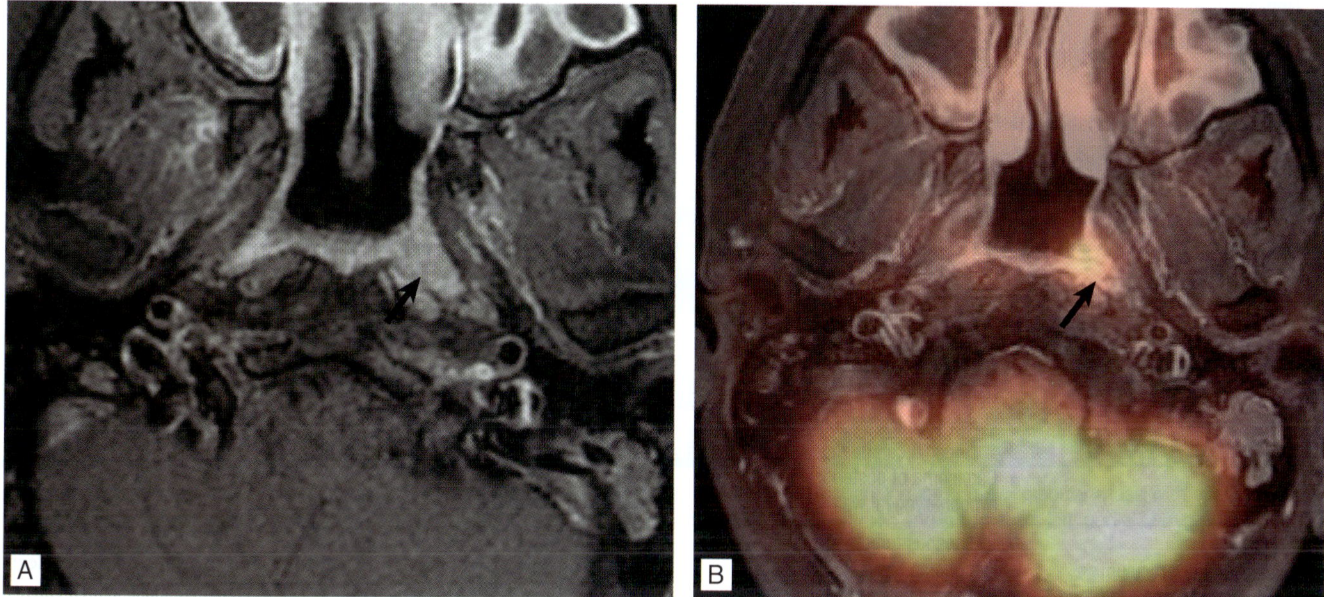

Figure 65.35 Recurrent nasopharyngeal cancer. Follow-up MRI postcontrast T1W fat saturated (A) image shows mild asymmetric thickening of posterolateral wall of nasopharynx (*arrow*). PET MRI fusion image (B) shows focal metabolic activity in the thickened left posterolateral wall (*arrow*). Biopsy was suggestive of recurrent squamous cell carcinoma.

other imaging is generally required. It is often seen as incidental finding in CT and MRI scans of the brain in children performed for various other reasons.

Nasopharyngeal Cysts

Cystic lesions like mucous retention cyst and Thornwaldt's cysts are incidentally seen on head and neck imaging. Mucous retention cyst is seen in posterolateral wall of nasopharynx, while Thornwaldt's cyst is a developmental cyst seen in midline due to failure of closure of nasopharyngeal bursa [53].

Encephalocoele/Meningocoele

These are uncommon pathologies involving the nasopharynx [54]. Encephalocoele/meningocoeles are more commonly seen in nasal, frontoethmoidal regions, or occipital region, and are usually associated with a defect in the skull base. CT is good to identity the bony defect and MRI for the contents and its intracranial connection.

Antrochoanal Polyp

These are sinonasal polyps which originate from the maxillary sinus and extend from the maxillary ostium, nasal cavity, and posterior choana into the nasopharynx. CT shows a hypodense well-defined mass with associated widening of the maxillary ostium (Fig. 65.36). Contrast-enhanced computed tomography (CECT) may show peripheral enhancement. MRI reveals a T1 hypointense and T2 homogenously hyperintense mass which shows peripheral enhancement.

Oropharynx and Hypopharynx

Various pathologies that affect the *oropharynx* and *hypopharynx* are given in Table 65.7.

TABLE 66.5 T-Staging of Subglottic Cancers

Tx	Primary tumor cannot be assessed
Tis	Carcinoma in situ
T1	Tumor limited to subglottis
T2	Tumor extends to vocal cord(s) with normal or impaired mobility
T3	Tumor limited to larynx with vocal cord fixation or invasion of paraglottic space or inner cortex of the thyroid cartilage
T4a	Moderately advanced local disease: invades through the outer cortex thyroid cartilage, invades cricoid cartilage or invades tissues beyond the larynx (e.g., trachea, soft tissues of neck including deep extrinsic muscle of tongue, strap muscles, thyroid, or esophagus)
T4b	Very advanced local disease: invades prevertebral space, encases carotid artery or invades mediastinal structure

Laryngeal SCC in each laryngeal compartment exhibits some characteristic spread patterns that have been detailed in the following paragraphs [24–27].

Supraglottic SCC: Supraglottic cancers constitute about 30% of all laryngeal cancers. These patients often present in advanced stage because hoarseness due to vocal cord involvement occurs late. Neck lumps due to nodal metastases (level II and III nodes) are frequent as the supraglottis enjoys a rich lymphatic network.

Supraglottic SCC have three main subsites and are categorized as anterior compartment (epiglottis) or the posterolateral compartment (aryepiglottic fold and false cords) cancers.

Epiglottic cancers are anterior midline cancers that are likely to invade into the PES through the tiny perforations in the epiglottis. While the SCCs arising from the mobile portion of the epiglottis may spread from the PES further into the base of tongue and laterally into the aryepiglottic fold and PGS, those arising from the caudal portion often invade the low PES and via the anterior commissure, reach the glottis or subglottis (Figs. 66.4 and 66.5). The primary sign of PES invasion at imaging is replacement of the normal fat by abnormal enhancing soft tissue and is very well delineated at CT and MR imaging (Figs. 66.5B, G, 66.7A, C). Aryepiglottic fold (AE fold) cancers present as exophytic or infiltrative posterolateral masses. They expand the AE fold and spread into the PGS (Figs. 66.4C, 66.5C, 66.6, 66.7A, 66.8A). They may spread further anteriorly into the PES or posteriorly to invade the piriform sinus (Fig. 66.7A). False cord cancers are lateral masses with a strong predilection for submucosal spread into the PGS (Fig. 66.5D, 66.7B, 66.8B, 66.9). More extensive tumor may destroy the thyroid cartilage and spread into the extralaryngeal soft tissues or transglottically into the glottis and subglottis (Fig. 66.5, 66.8, 66.9). Tumor spread to the PGS on CT or MRI is seen as replacement of the normal paraglottic fat by the enhancing tumor (Figs. 66.5C, D, H, 66.6, 66.7A, B, 66.8A, B, C, 66.9).

Glottic SCC: About 65% of laryngeal cancers arise in the glottis and patients present early with hoarseness due to early involvement of true cords. Metastatic nodal disease is rare due to sparse lymphatic drainage. The anterior third of the cords is more commonly involved with spread of disease to anterior commissure identified on cross-sectional imaging as soft tissue thickening of more than 1 mm. From the anterior commissure, the tumor may spread further into the contralateral cord and the thyroid cartilage or posteriorly into the posterior commissure, the arytenoids, cricoarytenoid joint, and the cricoid. Involvement of cricoarytenoid joint or interarytenoid space suggests vocal cord fixation. The tumor may spread superiorly to access the PES and the PGS, or inferiorly reach the subglottis along the cricothyroid membrane. Extralaryngeal spread may occur through the cricothyroid membrane (Figs. 66.8C, 66.10, 66.11).

Subglottic SCC: Primary subglottic cancers are rare, accounting for only 5% of all laryngeal cancers, clinically silent, present late in the course of the disease and have a poor prognosis. Nodal metastases are common and affect the pre and paratracheal nodes. Subglottic cancer is usually a caudal spread of the glottis cancer. Subglottic cancer is diagnosed if any tissue thickening more than 1 mm is noted between the airway and the cricoid ring (Figs. 66.5F, 66.8D, 66.10B). Due to their late presentation, invasion of the thyroid cartilage, cricoid cartilage, trachea, the cervical esophagus with extralaryngeal spread are common findings at imaging. Spread may occur through the cricothyroid membrane.

Laryngeal Cancer—Structuring a Clinically Relevant Report

The treatment options for patients with laryngeal cancers include primary radiation, surgery, chemotherapy, and combinations of these depending on the cancer staging. While mapping the deep extent of the tumor on the neck scans, accurate assessment of a few key areas and patterns of disease spread is fundamental to generate a report that impacts the staging and hence the prognosis and management options of a patient with laryngeal cancer [24–27].

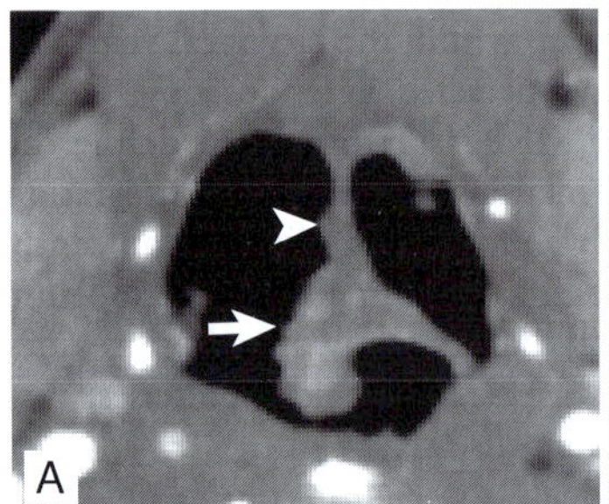

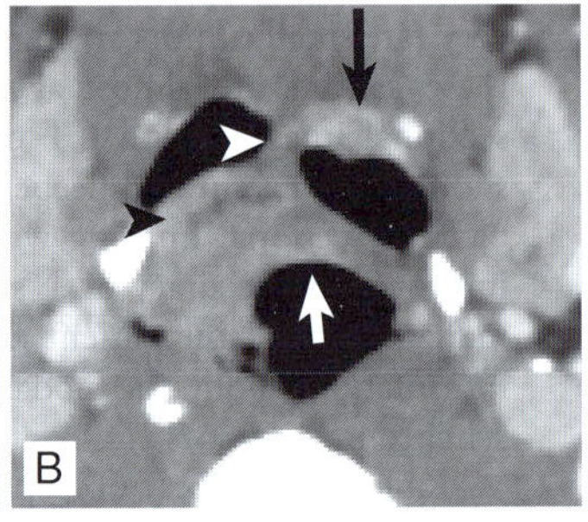

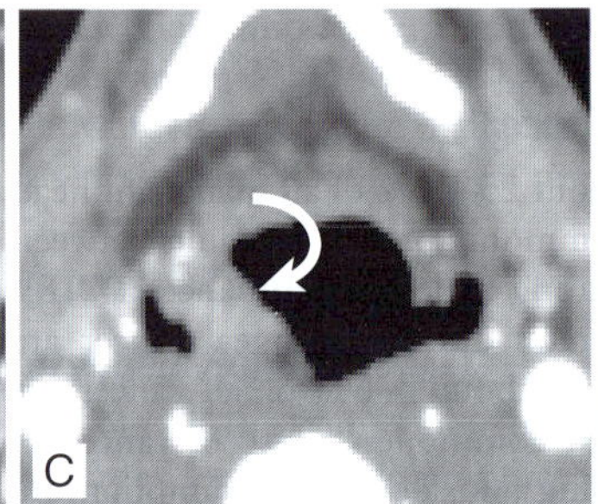

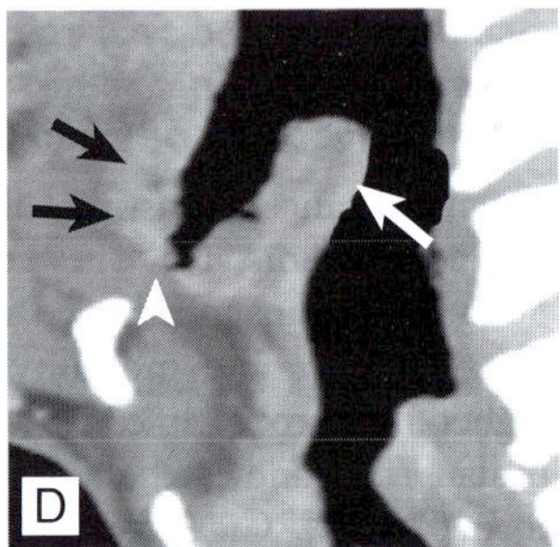

Figure 66.4 Supraglottic cancer—epiglottis and aryepiglottic fold. (A) Axial CECT image shows the abnormal thickened enhancing free edge of the epiglottis (*straight white arrow*) and the thickened median glossoepiglottic fold (*white arrowhead*). (B) The thickened enhancing free edge of epiglottis (*straight white arrow*) is seen with enhancing mass invading the right vallecula (*black arrowhead*), the median glossoepiglottic fold (*white arrowhead*) and the base of tongue (*straight black arrow*). (C) The tumor extends into the right aryepiglottic fold that is thickened and enhancing (*curved white arrow*). (D) Midline sagittal section shows the epiglottic tumor (*straight white arrow*) with enhancement along the glossoepiglottic fold (*white arrowhead*) extending into the base of tongue (*straight black arrows*).

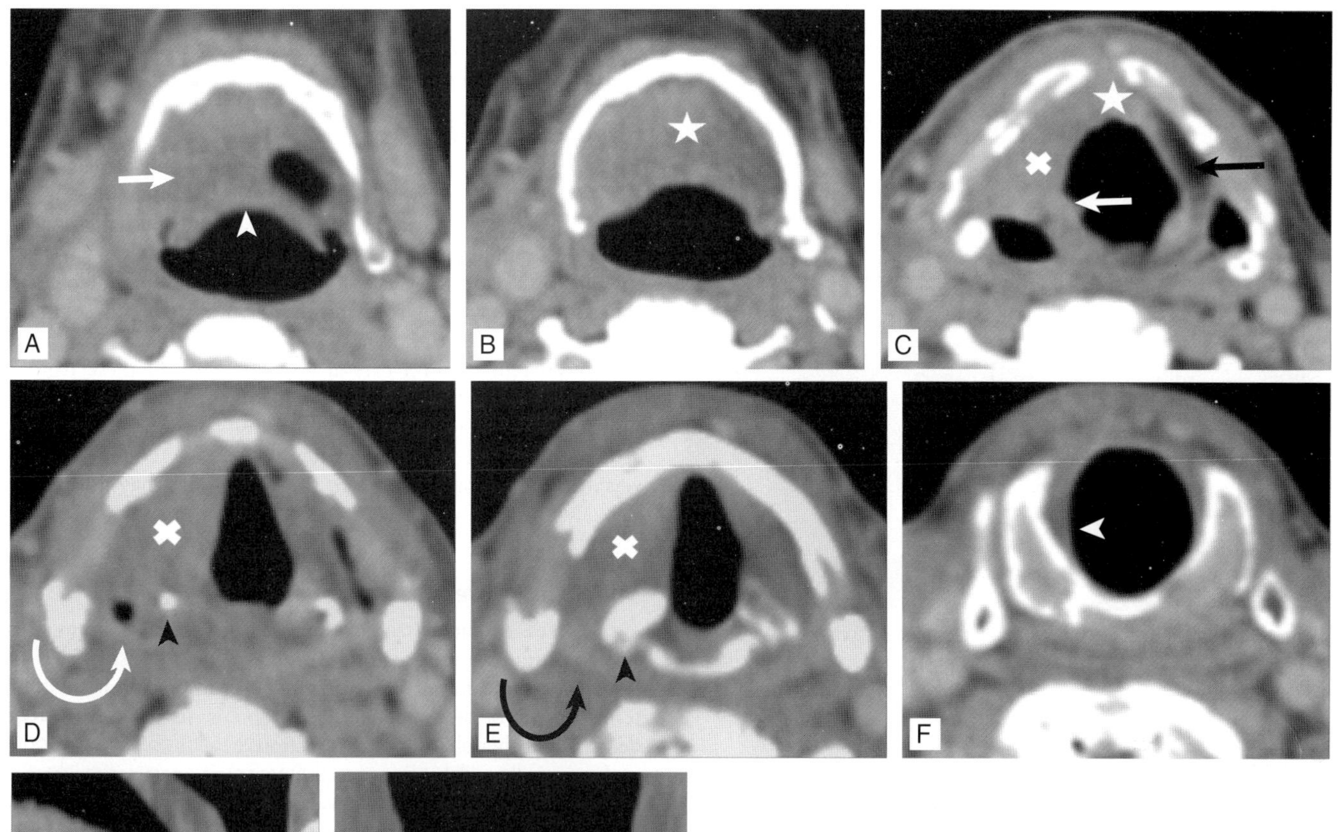

Figure 66.5 Transglottic cancer. (A) Axial CECT image shows abnormal thickening of the epiglottis (*white arrowhead*) with the soft tissue mass filling the right vallecula (*straight white arrow*). (B) The soft tissue mass is seen in fairly central location within the pre-epiglottic fat (*white star*). (C) Caudal image shows the soft tissue extending into the pre-epiglottic fat (*white star*), the right paralaryngeal fat (*white cross*) and the right ary-epiglottic fold (*block white arrow*). Note the normal left paralaryngeal fat (*straight black arrow*). (D) Extension of the mass into the paraglottic fat deep to the right false cord is seen (*white cross*). The right piriform sinus is narrowed (*curved white arrow*). The tip of right arytenoid cartilage shows mild sclerosis (*black arrowhead*). (E) Mass extends into the right true cord (*white cross*). Note the sclerosis of right arytenoid cartilage (*black arrowhead*) and widened right thyroarytenoid space (*curved black arrow*). (F) There is subglottic spread of the mass to the right lateral wall of subglottis (*white arrowhead*). (G) Sagittal image very nicely shows the mass in the pre-epiglottic fat (*white star*) with thickened free edge of the epiglottis (*white arrowhead*). (H) Coronal image depicts the transglottic tumor with mass in the right paraglottic space (*white cross*).

Submucosal Spread of Tumor Into PES and PGS

While disease spread into the PGS is fairly common in supraglottic and glottic cancers, involvement of the PES is commoner in supraglottic cancers. Tumor in these spaces upstages the disease to T3 has increased incidence of nodal metastases and high risk of recurrence following radiation. Bulky tumor in these spaces precludes radiotherapy, local laser resections, and partial laryngectomy procedures. This form of disease spread cannot be assessed clinically or at endoscopy, but is very well seen at imaging. Hence, it is imperative to assess this tumor spread accurately on the scan.

Cartilage Invasion

Cartilage disease in laryngeal cancer cannot be assessed at endoscopy and is associated with a higher risk of tumor recurrence, poor response to radiation, and increased risk of later complications. Depending on the extent of the erosion, the tumor is upstaged to T3 or T4 disease and thus impacts the therapeutic options. Cricoid cartilage invasion always requires a total laryngectomy. Both CT and MRI can depict cartilage disease very well. MRI has a high sensitivity, lower specificity, and a very high negative predictive value for detection of cartilage disease as compared to CT, the overall accuracy of CT and MRI is nearly the same for cartilage invasion [22]. Box 66.3 summarizes the CT and MRI features of cartilage invasion in laryngeal cancer [28].

Very recently, the use of dual energy CT using iodine overlay images has been found to have higher specificity and acceptable sensitivity when compared with MRI for assessment of neoplastic cartilage invasion [29]. USG is also reported to be comparable in sensitivity and specificity to CT or MRI in the detection of cartilage invasion [5].

Figure 66.6 Supraglottic cancer—aryepiglottic fold. Tumor is seen in the right aryepiglottic fold (*white star*) extending into the right paralaryngeal fat (*white arrowhead*).

Transglottic Spread of Cancer

Laryngeal SCC encroaching on both, the glottis and supraglottis, with or without subglottic component and when the site of origin is unclear, is termed as transglottic tumor. This tumor spread is frequently submucosal through the PGS and hence may be missed at endoscopy. It is readily identified on coronal and axial images (Figs. 66.5, 66.8). This type of disease spread is again, a negative indicator for primary radiotherapy, contraindicates partial laryngectomy procedures and is frequently accompanied by nodal disease.

Spread Across the Commissure

This disease is best assessed at axial images obtained during quiet breathing. Thickening of more than 1 mm is suggestive of disease (Fig. 66.11). Diagnosis of this spread impacts the options of voice conserving surgeries available for the patient. Spread of a glottis cancer across the anterior commissure to involve more than a third of the contralateral cord precludes a vertical hemilaryngectomy and disease in the posterior commissure may obviate a supracricoid laryngectomy.

Extralaryngeal Spread

Extralaryngeal spread implies deep spread beyond the laryngeal boundaries into the soft tissues of the neck and represents T4 disease that contraindicates primary radiation or partial laryngectomy and requires extensive surgery.

This form of spread can occur through the thyroarytenoid gap posteriorly, the cricothyroid and thyrohyoid membranes anterolaterally and across the thyroid and cricoid cartilages and hence it is important to do a careful assessment of all these regions while interpreting the neck scans [30] (Figs. 66.8, 66.9, 66.10). Furthermore, if the extralaryngeal disease surrounds the carotid artery subtending an angle greater than 270°, it must be conveyed to the operating surgeon, since the artery may not be salvaged at surgery [31].

Nodal Metastases

While assessing the T-stage of the disease in the neck scans, it is very important to look for cervical nodal metastases since it is an important indicator of prognosis and has implications on long term survival of these patients. This topic is discussed in further detail in another chapter in this section.

Lungs followed by liver are the common metastatic sites for laryngeal cancer and these are usually seen in advanced cases.

Box 66.4 summarizes the key assessment areas while interpreting neck scans in patients with laryngeal cancer.

Submucosal Tumors

Although the vast majority of laryngeal tumors are mucosal, a bunch of nonsquamous cell tumors arising from the nonepithelial elements of the larynx may present as submucosal laryngeal masses—Table 66.2. These do not present with obvious mucosal abnormalities at endoscopy and are seen as a submucosal bulge under an intact mucosa necessitating cross-sectional imaging to characterize them and guide an appropriate site for biopsy. When such a mass is referred for imaging, a good approach is to begin by first assessing the possibility of a cartilaginous or a vasculogenic neoplasm because these tumors have fairly characteristic imaging

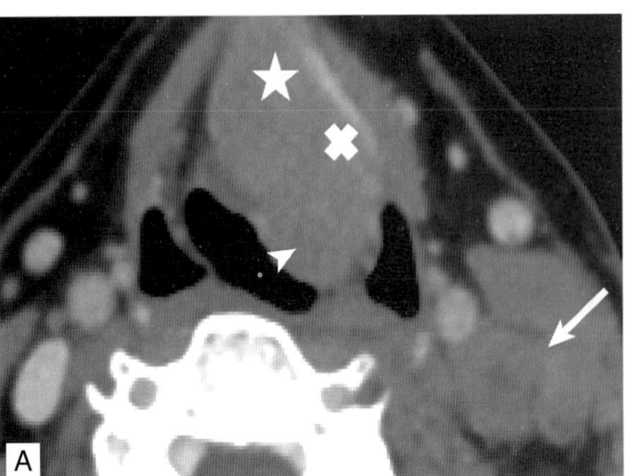

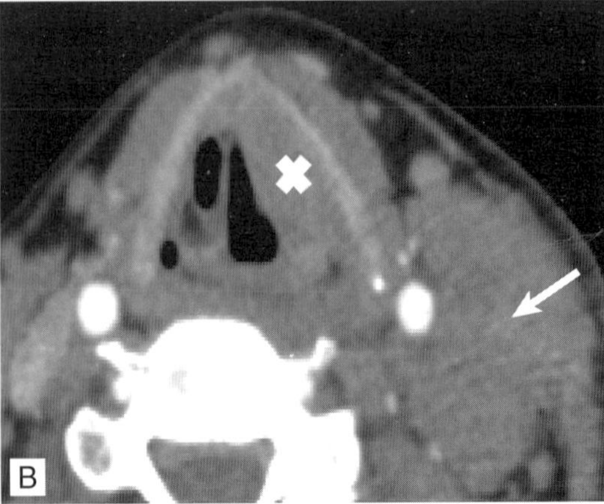

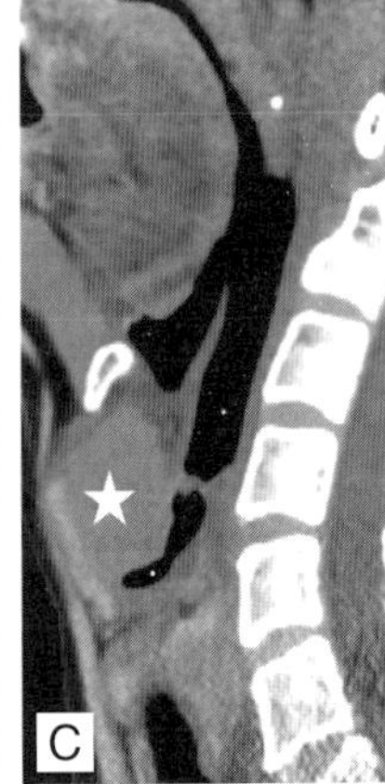

Figure 66.7 Supraglottic cancer—aryepiglottic fold and false cord. (A) Large lobulated enhancing mass is seen in the left aryepiglottic fold (*white arrowhead*) extending into the epiglottis and filling the pre-epiglottic fat (*white star*). Tumor is also seen in the left paraglottic space (*white arrowhead*). Note the enlarged level II nodes (*white arrow*). (B) Tumor extends into the false cord and is seen in the paraglottic fat and the laryngeal ventricle (*white cross*). Note the enlarged level II nodes (*white arrow*). (C) Sagittal CT section shows a large tumor in the pre-epiglottic fat (*white star*).

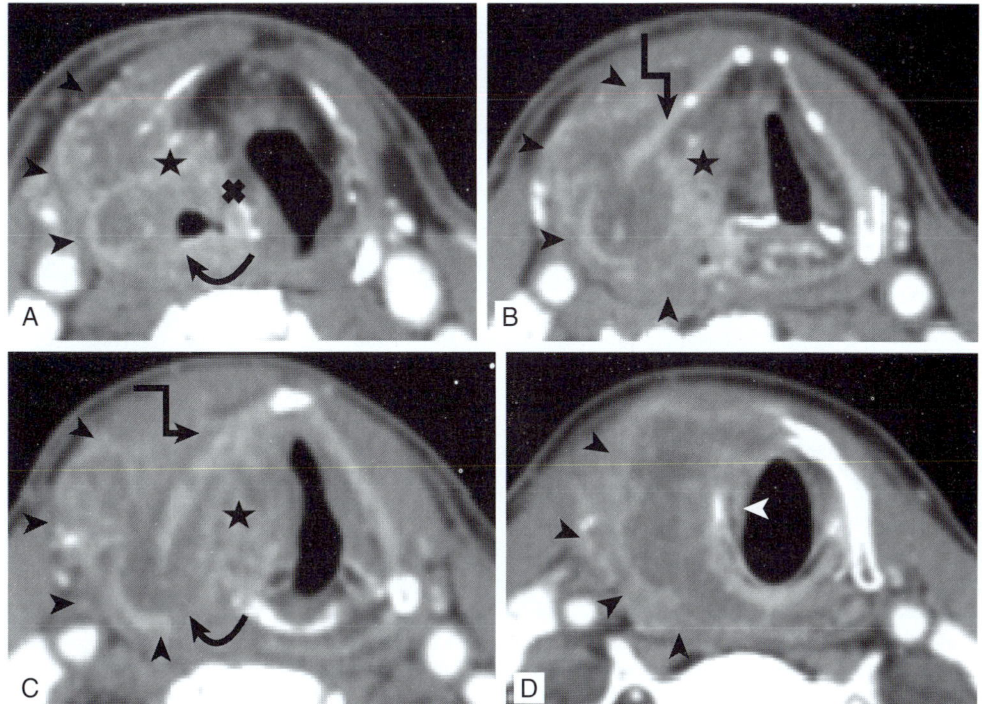

Figure 66.8 Transglottic cancer with extralaryngeal spread. (A) Heterogeneously enhancing tumor in right aryepiglottic fold (*black cross*) extending into the right paralaryngeal fat (*black star*) and further posterolaterally to encase the walls of the right piriform sinus (*curved black arrow*). Note the erosion of the right thyroid lamina and extralaryngeal tumor spread into the overlying strap muscles (*black arrowheads*). (B) Large heterogenously enhancing tumor is seen in the right paralaryngeal fat (*black star*) with erosion of the right lamina of thyroid cartilage (*black elbow arrow*) and extralaryngeal extension of the mass into the strap muscles of the neck (*black arrowheads*). (C) The tumor involves the right true cord (*black star*) with erosion of the right lamina of thyroid cartilage (*black elbow arrow*) and extralaryngeal extension of the mass into the strap muscles of the neck (*black arrowheads*) across the cartilage and the widened thyroarytenoid gap (*curved black arrow*). (D) *White arrowhead* shows subglottic tumor in right lateral wall of subglottis. Complete erosion of the right lamina of thyroid cartilage is seen with deep subglottic extension into the soft tissues of the neck (*black arrowheads*).

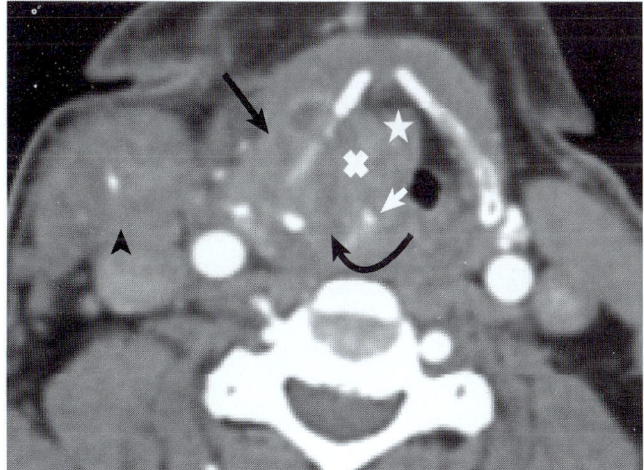

Figure 66.9 Supraglottic cancer—false cord. Bulky tumor is seen in the right false cord and the paraglottic fat (*white cross*) with erosion of the right lamina of the thyroid cartilage and extralaryngeal extension into the overlying strap muscles (*straight black arrow*). Enhancing soft tissue extends into the pre-epiglottic fat (*white asterisk*). Sclerosis of the right arytenoid is seen (*small white arrow*). The right thyroarytenoid gap is widened (*curved black arrow*). Note level II adenopathy with extranodal disease spreading into right sternocleidomastoid muscle (*black arrowhead*).

features that allow a precise diagnosis to be made [31,32]. The other soft tissue submucosal tumors do not display any specific imaging characteristics.

Chondroid tumors of the larynx show a striking male predilection and are commonly seen in older men between 50 and 70 years of age. About 70% arise in the cricoid cartilage, the next common site being the thyroid cartilage. They are seen as hypodense masses at CT, with stippled or coarse calcifications which are the diagnostic feature of these tumors. The cartilage may be expanded suggesting that the lesion is arising from within the cartilage rather than eroding the cartilage from outside (Fig. 66.13). CT scores over plain radiography and MRI in detection of even very subtle intratumoral calcifications and is easily the preferred investigation [33,34].

On MRI, the tumor is intensely hyperintense on T2W images due to high water content and low cellularity of hyaline cartilage. Small foci of T1 and T2 hypointensity may be seen that represent stippled calcifications. While chondrosarcomas are commoner

BOX 66.3 Cartilage Disease in Laryngeal Cancer [28]

CT	MRI
■ Cartilage sclerosis Highly sensitive but lacks specificity as it may be due to reactive bone formation adjacent to tumor Specificity is highest for thyroid cartilage (Figs. 66.5D, E, 66.10)	Unenhanced and enhanced T1W images Tumor invasion is seen as abnormal soft tissue intensity within the bright signal of medullary fat of ossified cartilages, that enhances on the contrast study similar to the adjacent tumor (Fig. 66.12)
■ Cartilage erosion, lysis and extralaryngeal spread High specificity but lower sensitivity as they are seen later in the course of the disease (Figs. 66.8, 66.9, 66.11)	T2W images Tumor invasion is seen as hyperintense signal within the cartilage, paralleling the signal of the tumor. If the hyperintensity is more than the tumor, it is likely to suggest peritumoral edema

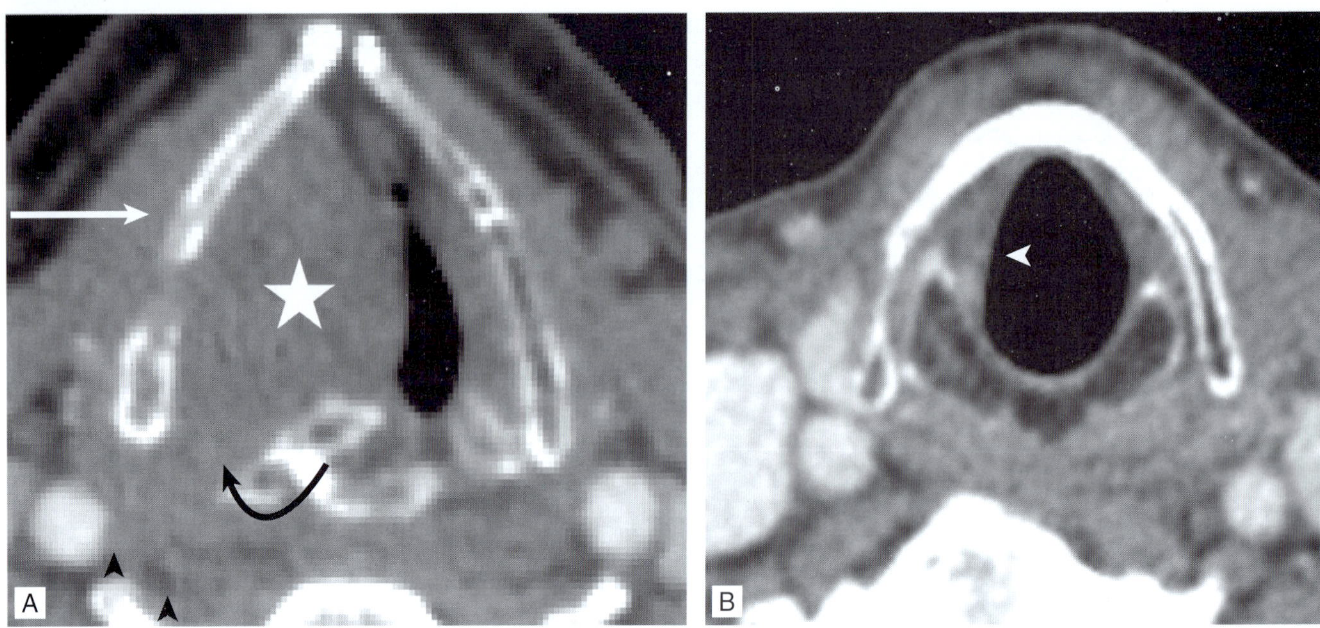

Figure 66.10 Glottic cancer with subglottic extension. (A) Axial CECT image shows a large enhancing tumor in the right true cord (*white star*) with widening of the thyroarytenoid gap (*curved black arrow*) and extralaryngeal spread of tumor abutting the right carotid artery (*black arrow heads*). Mild sclerosis of the right lamina of thyroid cartilage is seen (*white arrow*). (B) Caudal extension of the mass is seen in the right lateral wall of the subglottis (*white arrowhead*).

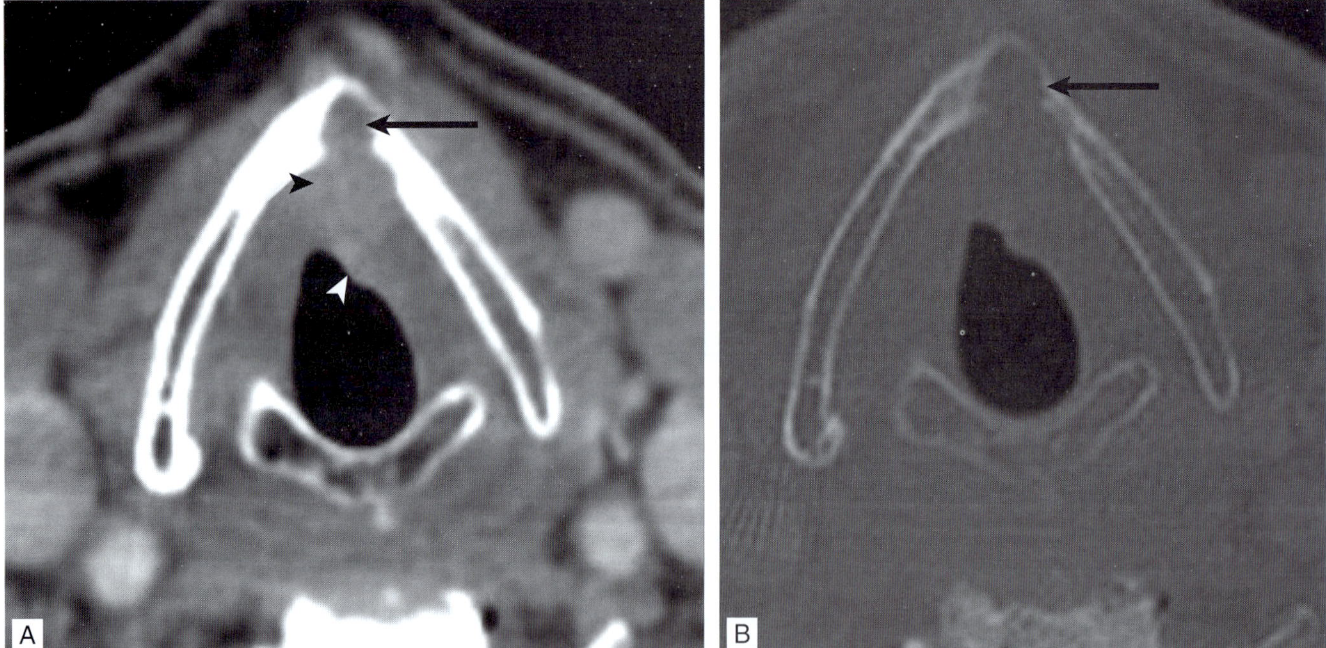

Figure 66.11 Glottic cancer. CECT scan of the larynx in a patient with clinically staged T1 glottis cancer. (A) Axial CECT image shows an enhancing mass in the anterior third of left true cord (*white arrowhead*) reaching the anterior commissure (*black arrowhead*). Note the cartilage erosion (*black arrow*). (B) CT image in bone algorithm confirms erosion of the inner cortex of the thyroid cartilage (*black arrow*) upstaging the tumor to T3.

than chondromas, it may be difficult to differentiate between them at imaging. Laryngeal chondrosarcomas are low grade tumors and rarely metastasize.

Laryngeal hemangiomas are seen as characteristic intensely enhancing submucosal masses due to the rapid filling of vessels within [35] (Fig. 66.14). Any narrowing of the airway is clearly depicted at imaging. Infantile and adult types are described. Infantile hemangioma is commoner in girls and generally presents before 6 months of age with some form of respiratory distress. It is commonly located in the subglottic region. Adult hemangiomas are commoner in males. An association between the subglottic hemangioma and a cutaneous hemangioma elsewhere in the body particularly in the head and neck in the "beard" distribution and cardiovascular anomalies like coarctation and right-sided aortic arch has been described [36].

Non-Tumorous Lesions

A few important nontumorous diseases where imaging plays an important role will be discussed here. Laryngeal trauma has been discussed under the section of "Trauma and emergency radiology."

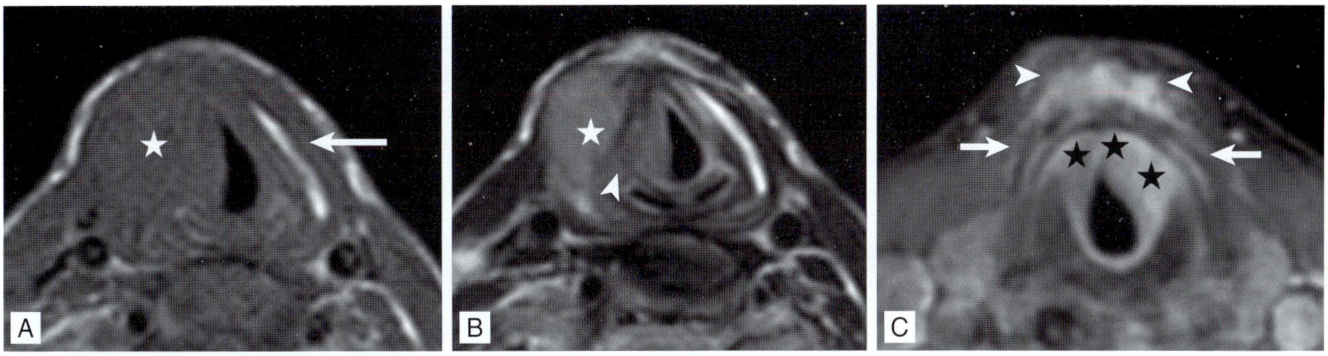

Figure 66.12 Cartilage invasion and extralaryngeal spread—MRI. (A) Axial T1W image shows a large right false cord tumor with extralaryngeal spread (*white star*). The right lamina of cartilage is not seen separate from the soft tissue. Note the appearance of normal ossified left lamina of thyroid cartilage (*straight white arrow*). (B) Axial T2W image shows the hyperintense signal of the mass. Note the erosion of the right lamina of thyroid cartilage with irregular cortical margins and near similar intramedullary signal as the soft tissue mass (*white arrowhead*). (C) Contrast T1 axial image with fat suppression in another patient shows enhancing tumor in the subglottis (*black stars*). Note the enhancement in the cartilage (*white arrows*) along with the extralaryngeal soft tissue enhancement (*white arrowheads*), the intensity being similar to the tumoral enhancement.

BOX 66.4 Imaging Checklist While Reporting Scans for Laryngeal Cancers

- Submucosal disease in PES and PGS
- Cartilage invasion
- Transglottic spread
- Commissure spread
- Extralaryngeal spread
- Nodal metastases
- Submucosal tumors

Laryngocele

Laryngocele is an abnormal dilatation of the saccule of the laryngeal ventricle that extends upward within the false vocal cord and is in communication with the laryngeal lumen. Laryngoceles are commonly unilateral and seen in adults. They may be spontaneous or a sequelae to increased intralaryngeal pressures as in glass blowers and wind instrument players. Another important cause is a mechanical obstruction at the outlet of the saccule due to a tumor or chronic inflammation [37,38].

CT shows the laryngocele as an air or fluid density blind-ending tubular lesion extending cranially into the paraglottic fat. When this is confined to the PGS medial to the thyrohyoid membrane, it is called as internal laryngocele. When the laryngocele herniates upward across the thyrohyoid membrane above the superior border of the thyroid cartilage into the soft tissues of the neck, it is called as a combined laryngocele (Fig. 66.15). Hence, combined laryngocele has an internal component medial to the thyrohyoid membrane and an external component that is lateral to the thyrohyoid membrane. Fluid-filled laryngocele is also called a laryngomucocele and when it gets infected a pyolaryngocele forms. CT is useful not only for the diagnosis but to map the entire extent, differentiate the internal and mixed varieties and delineate any enhancing tumor or obstruction at the saccular outlet. Pyolaryngoceles additionally show mucosal thickening, rim enhancement, and inflammatory changes in paralaryngeal soft tissues. Air-filled laryngoceles show a signal void on T1W and T2W images with blooming on susceptibility imaging. Fluid-filled laryngoceles are hypointense on T1W

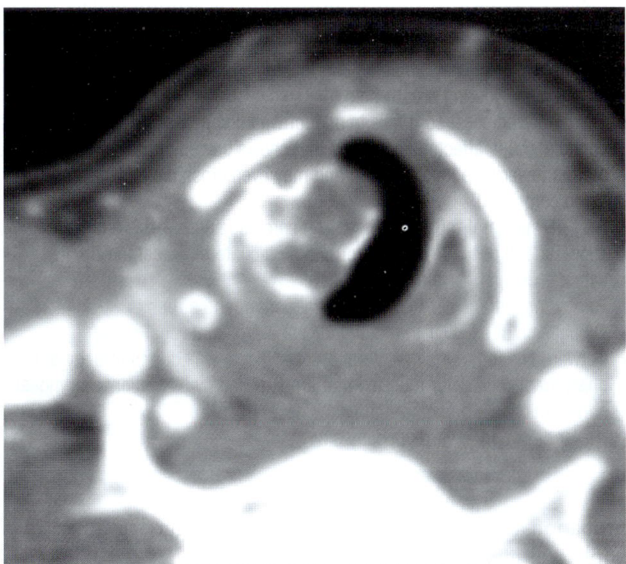

Figure 66.13 Chondroid tumor. Axial CECT image shows a calcified expansile tumor arising from the right lateral wall of the cricoid ring. (Courtesy: Suresh Mukherji.)

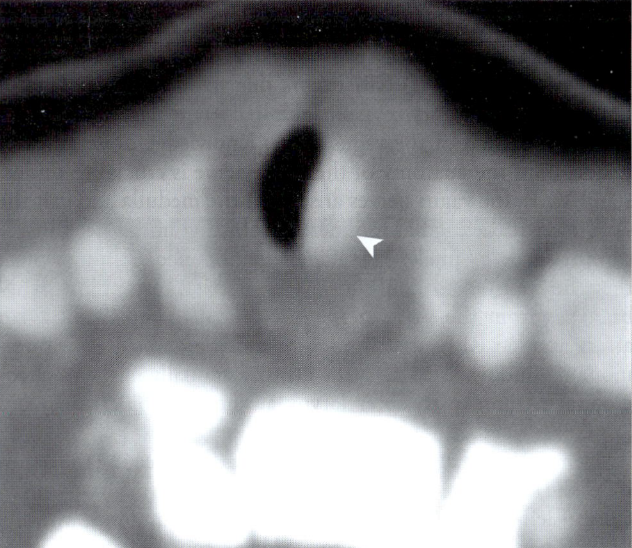

Figure 66.14 Subglottic hemangioma. Axial CECT image in a neonate who presented with stridor shows an intensely enhancing lesion in the subglottis on the left side, bulging slightly into the lumen (*white arrowhead*).

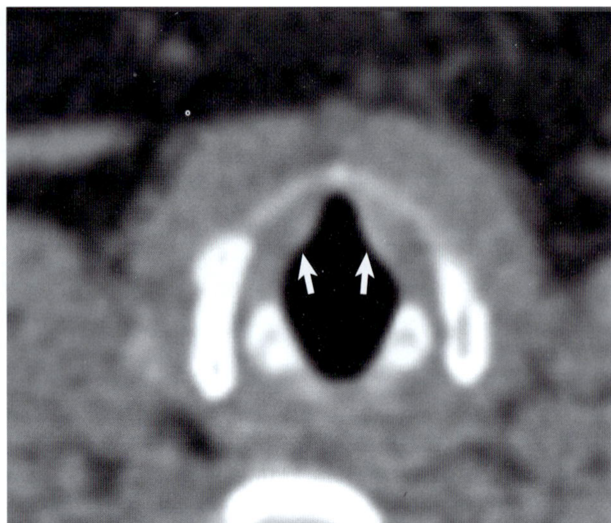

Figure 66.18 Vocal nodules. Axial NECT image shows small symmetric bulges (*white arrows*) along the undersurface of the anterior thirds of the true cords on either side.

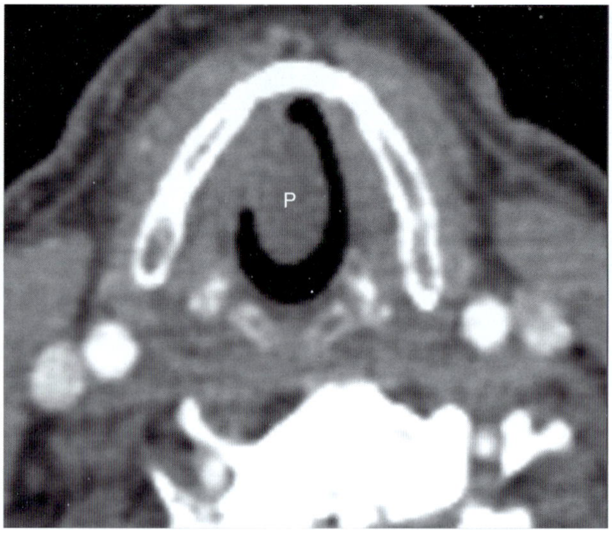

Figure 66.19 Vocal cord polyp. Axial CECT image through the glottis shows a well-defined hypodense polypoid lesion (P) arising from the anterior aspect of the medial margin of the right vocal cord, protruding into the laryngeal lumen.

Post-Treatment Evaluation

Interpretation of post-treatment neck scans can be challenging because of the postsurgical anatomical distortion and radiation induced changes in the soft tissues of the neck. Knowledge of these expected alterations and an optimal imaging interval following treatment can help the radiologist to avoid misinterpretation of normal post-treatment changes as recurrent or persistent disease.

Postirradiation changes are seen within all the soft tissues that are included within the radiation port and have been enlisted in Box 66.6. If the patient has been operated upon, it is always good to know the type of resection and any reconstruction performed and assess the appearance of structures that are visualized or not visualized. Scans following a total laryngectomy will show the absence of all laryngeal structures leaving behind a remnant of the thyroid gland, midline position of the neopharynx, and esophagus in place of the larynx just below the subcutaneous fat and a characteristic "rounded" appearance of the esophagus that mimics the larynx, due to lack of compression by the cartilaginous supporting structures and the thyroid gland [46] (Fig. 66.20).

The best time to obtain a post-treatment scan has been recommended approximately 3–4 months following the completion of the treatment [47–49]. While complete resolution of the primary mass strongly suggests a positive result, a persistent unchanged mass indicates treatment failure and a partial resolution of a mass on the post-treatment CT study is an indeterminate finding and requires further imaging [47,48] (Fig. 66.21). Stability of the mass on follow-up imaging over a 2-year period is suggestive of fibrosis and scarring [47,48].

Recurrent disease following radiation is seen as a nodular thickening or soft tissue at the primary site. Postsurgical recurrence manifests as focal areas of nodularity or soft tissue in the surgical bed, commonly at the cut margins of the surgery where the tumor was previously located (Fig. 66.22). Progressive sclerosis of laryngeal cartilages on post-treatment scans is likely to suggest local tumor recurrence whereas resolution of pretreatment cartilage sclerosis favors disease control [47,48]. While CT and diffusion-weighted imaging at MRI are used for assessment of post-treatment patients, FDG PET/CT imaging is a highly sensitive technique with superior diagnostic accuracy compared with CT and MRI in detection of recurrent head and neck cancer [50–53].

BOX 66.6 Normal Postradiation Changes in the Neck at Imaging [45,47,48]

A. Early reactions (within 90 days)
- Thickening of the skin and platysma muscle
- Reticulation of the subcutaneous fat
- Enhancement of the pharyngeal mucosa, thickening of the posterior pharyngeal wall, retropharyngeal space edema
- Increased enhancement and size of the major salivary glands
- Thickening of the laryngeal structures with increased density and stippling of the fat in the pre-epiglottic and paralaryngeal spaces.

B. Late reactions (after 90 days)
- Atrophy of the salivary glands
- Thickening of the skin and platysma
- Thickening of the pharyngeal muscles

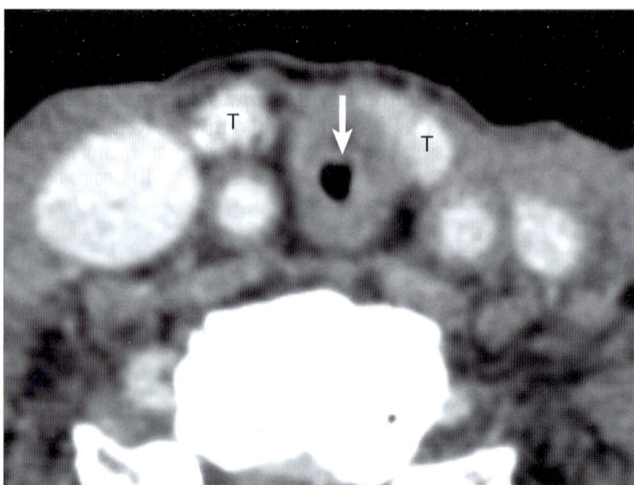

Figure 66.20 Postlaryngectomy CT. Axial CECT image shows the normal appearance at CT following a total laryngectomy. The neopharynx is seen in the midline with a rounded appearance (*white arrow*). The isthmus of thyroid gland is not seen. Only small remnants of the thyroid gland (T) are seen. (Courtesy: Saugata Sen.)

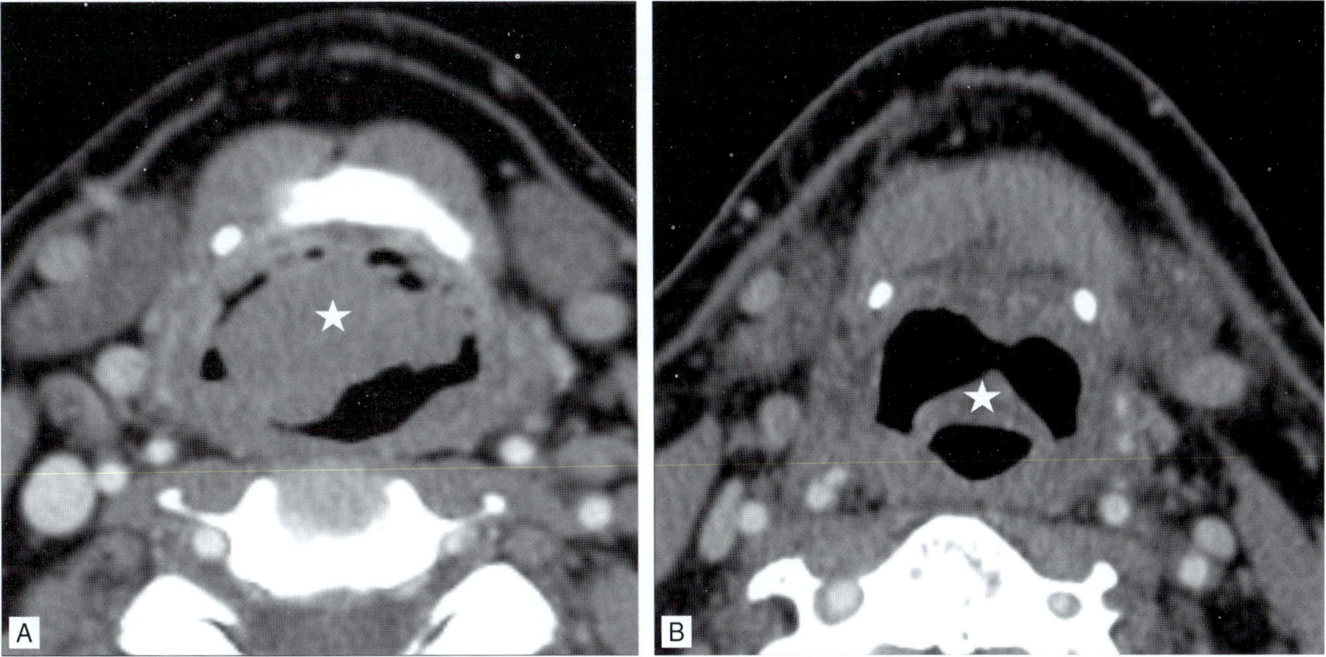

Figure 66.21 Postradiation response. (A) Axial CECT image shows a midline lobulated epiglottic tumor (*white star*). (B) Axial CECT image obtained after radiation shows a smooth slightly thickened epiglottis indicating a successful control of primary tumor (*white star*). (Courtesy: Suresh Mukherji.)

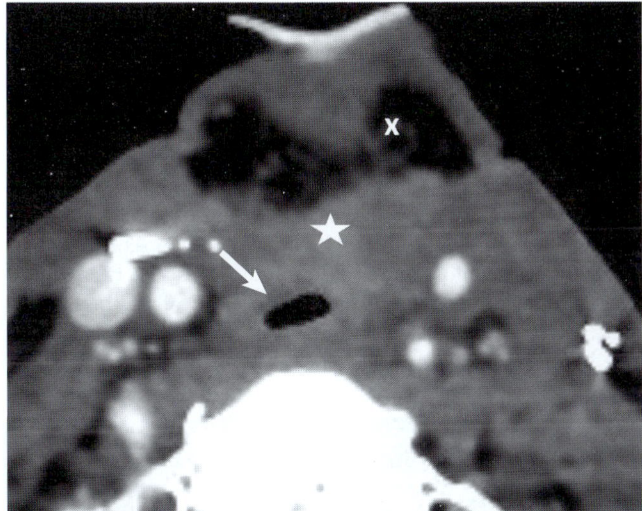

Figure 66.22 Postlaryngectomy CT—recurrence. Post total laryngectomy axial CECT shows a recurrence in the operative bed (*white star*) flattening the rounded neopharnx (*white arrow*). A myocutaneous flap is seen (*white cross*). (Courtesy: Suresh Mukherji.)

Summary

Cross-sectional imaging plays an indispensable complementary role to clinical endoscopy in imaging of laryngeal diseases. Determination of the precise extent of cancer spread within the larynx (T staging) is the single-most critical factor guiding the management in patients with localized laryngeal cancer. A clear understanding of the standard imaging techniques and protocols for imaging the larynx, and familiarity with the key anatomical features and characteristic patterns of tumor spread within the different regions of the larynx, are fundamental to the interpretation of CT and MRI scans of these patients.

Suggested Readings

- V Joshi, V Wadhwa, S Mukherji, Imaging in laryngeal cancers, Indian J Radiol Imaging 22 (3) (2012) 209–226.
- S Connor, Laryngeal cancer: how does the radiologist help? Cancer Imaging 7 (1) (2007) 93–103.
- CM Paquette, DC Manos, BJ Psooy, Unilateral vocal cord paralysis: a review of CT findings, mediastinal causes, and the course of the recurrent laryngeal nerves, Radiographics 32 (3) (2012) 721–740.
- SK Mukherji, WJ Weadock, Imaging of the post-treatment larynx, Eur J Radiol 44 (2002) 108–119.
- V Saito, RN Nadgir, M Nakahira, M Takahashi, A Uchino, F Kimura, et al., Posttreatment CT and MR imaging in head and neck cancer: what the radiologist needs to know, Radiographics 32 (2012) 1261–1282.

67

Neck Nodes

SAUGATA SEN, ANISHA GEHANI, ARGHA CHATTERJEE, PRIYA GHOSH

Introduction

Neck nodes are ubiquitous and there are reports of over 300 nodes in the neck out of the 800 odd, which are present in the body [1]. Hence, 40% of the nodes of the human body are located in 20% of the volume of the body [2]. This very high concentration of nodes in the neck is related to exposure of the aerodigestive tract to environmental infective agents and carcinogens [2]. Nodes can be pathologically involved for a variety of reasons, such as infection, malignancy, or even as a reaction to acute systemic inflammation.

Due to the very high prevalence of pathological involvement of neck nodes, a thorough knowledge is essential for diagnosis, description, and intervention. A radiologist is expected to recognize and report a pathological node from various criteria described in the literature. Localization and staging are mandatory for planning therapy and prognostication. Image-guided sampling is also within the domain of the radiologist.

This chapter will discuss the techniques of imaging and their optimal use, the criteria of a pathological node, localization and staging of malignant nodes, and certain important clinical scenarios. Metastatic neck nodes are key to disease prognosis and treatment in malignancies of the head and neck region. This topic has been studied and published extensively. We will deal with metastatic neck nodes in detail in this chapter.

Imaging Techniques and Appropriateness

Even though cervical lymph nodes can easily be palpated, imaging is essential in assessing the extent of disease due to the following reasons:

1. Many regions in the neck are not palpable, for example, retropharyngeal nodes (RPNs) (Fig. 67.1A and B).
2. Postsurgery and radiotherapy, neck can be difficult to palpate (Fig. 67.2).
3. Clinical palpation is inadequate for pretreatment assessment and may result in suboptimal management.
4. Oftentimes, imaging guidance is required to sample a lymph node (Fig. 67.3).
5. Imaging helps exclude other neck disorders, for example, a branchial cleft cyst.

Ultrasonography

The initial and sometimes only technique required to assess the neck nodes is ultrasonography (USG). This technique is comparatively less expensive and easily available. Linear transducers of 7–12 MHz are used for the studies. USG has very high sensitivity and specificity to diagnose abnormal cervical nodes [3]. Even in the setting of postsurgical or postradiation neck, USG has high sensitivity and specificity for detection of abnormal nodes [3]. It is very

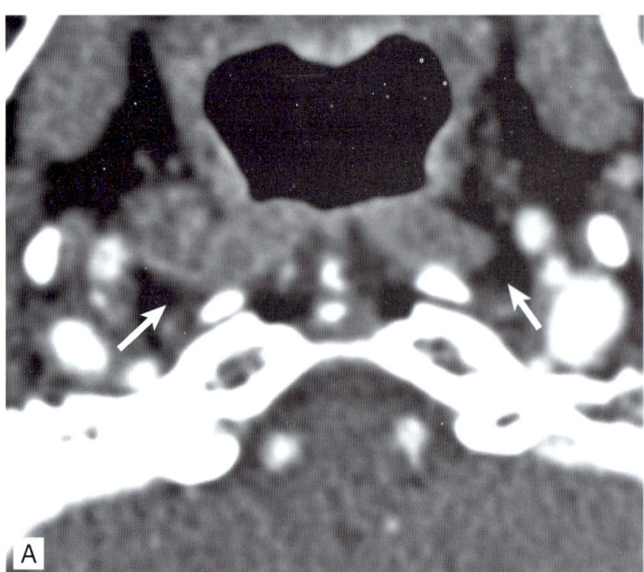

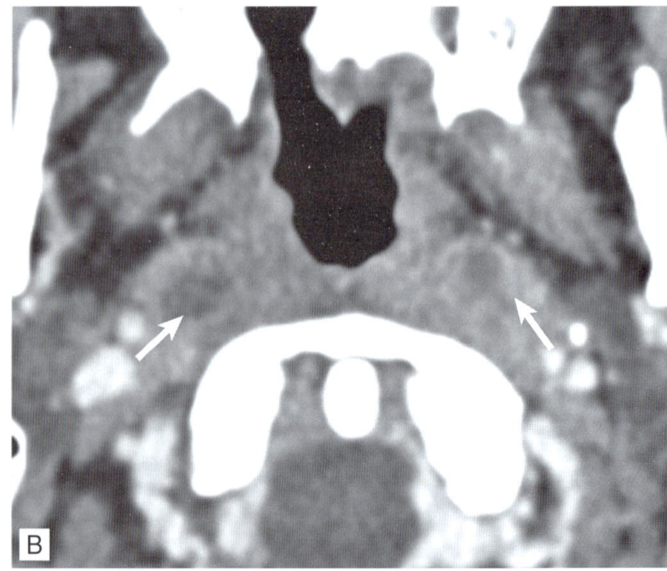

Figure 67.1 (A) Axial CECT image shows bilateral retropharyngeal spaces (*white arrows*). (B) Axial CECT image shows necrotic bilateral retropharyngeal nodes (*white arrows*) medial to the internal carotid arteries.

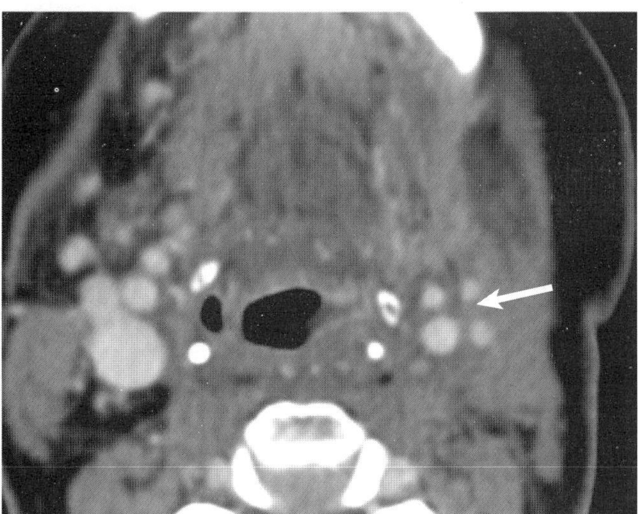

Figure 67.2 Post modified radical left neck dissection. Axial CECT image shows soft tissue cuffing around the left carotid sheath (*white arrow*) which can cause small nodes to be impalpable in the region.

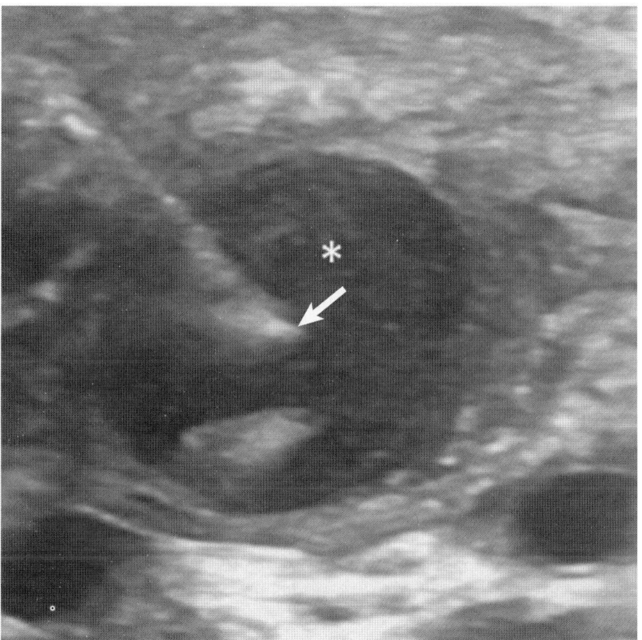

Figure 67.3 USG-guided FNAC from a pathological cervical node. Note the advancing needle tip (*white arrow*) within the thickened cortex of the node (*asterisk*).

useful for nodal sampling and can also be used as a problem-solving tool when computed tomography (CT) or magnetic resonance imaging (MRI) provide equivocal information.

US elastography is a relatively new technique that also has the ability to characterize nodes, on the premise, that malignant (carcinomatous) nodes are stiffer [4–6]. Contrast-enhanced USG is another new technique with limited use for assessment of neck nodes [7]. The drawback of USG is its inability to examine deep areas such as the retropharyngeal region.

Computed Tomography

Contrast-enhanced CT (CECT) has been the most widely used technique for evaluating cervical lymph nodes for a

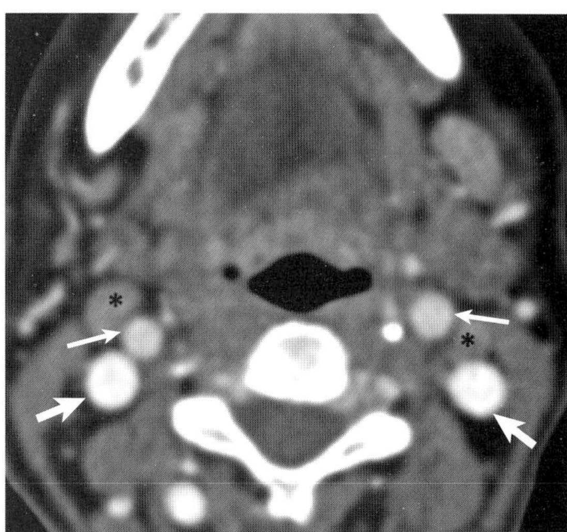

Figure 67.4 Axial CECT image shows bilateral cervical level II nodes (*asterisks*) distinctly visualized from carotid arteries (*thin white arrows*) and internal jugular veins (*thick white arrows*).

malignant etiology and can evaluate any region in the neck unlike palpation or USG. Since malignant etiologies of the head and neck region are some of the commonest causes of cervical lymphadenopathy, both the primary site and the regional nodes can be staged in a single exam. The contrast delivery (90–120 mL in adults) is crucial and must follow one of the following protocols (Fig. 67.4).

a. Image with a 60-second delay after beginning contrast injection with a flow rate of 2–3 mL/s [8].
b. Initial bolus of 60 mL at 2–3 mL/s. A delay of 30 seconds followed by another 30 mL of contrast at 2–3 mL/s. Image after another 10–12 seconds delay. A saline chase can be used, but is not mandatory [8].

On CT, cervical nodes should be differentiated from the vascular structures. The above protocols are optimum with the fast scanners that are in use in modern times. As per American College of Radiology guidelines, caution should be exercised before administration of contrast to an individual with estimated glomerular filtration rate of less than 60 mL/s.

There have been many controversies about radiation exposure in CT scans. In the head and neck region, concerns were raised about exposure to the lens and the thyroid gland. It has, however, conclusively been proven that even after multiple scans, the risks are significantly low, especially in the era of multidetector CT [9].

Magnetic Resonance Imaging

The lack of ionizing radiation and better soft tissue resolution are advantages of MRI in cross-sectional imaging. Higher expenses and motion artifact (swallowing and respiration related) as well as long scan durations are some of the limitations.

Thyroid cancers (papillary) and human papilloma virus (HPV) positive oropharyngeal cancers develop cystic lymph nodes that appear as hyperintense on T2WI. T1 hyperintensities are seen in thyroid cancers due to the presence of hemorrhagic or proteinaceous products. Contrast-enhanced MRI (CEMRI) is also a competent technique in detecting subtle extranodal extension (ENE) [10].

(18F) Fluorodeoxyglucose Positron Emission Tomography-Computed Tomography

(18F) Fluorodeoxyglucose positron emission tomography-computed tomography (FDG PET-CT) is a more recent addition to imaging and has a major role in malignancies. The technique has the ability to detect and stage disease, detect recurrence, and assess response. It has a higher specificity and sensitivity than CT or MRI for pathological neck nodes [11].

However, reactive nodes may also show FDG avidity [12]. For nodes less than 1 cm in size, the sensitivity of FDG PET-CT is much lower than the larger nodes [13] (Fig. 67.5A and B).

Choice of Appropriate Imaging Technique

The choice of imaging technique depends on the presentation, clinical features, and probable treatment of the primary pathology. Infective or inflammatory nodes may only be imaged if there is no response to initial therapy to document extent of disease and for sampling. This may be achieved by USG. If a malignant etiology is suspected, USG is used to sample the node, but staging would require cross-sectional imaging.

The following scenarios are envisaged in the setting of malignant disease.

a. *Nasopharyngeal carcinoma (NPC)*: MRI is usually the first imaging method used. CT sections may be made available to assess skull base invasion by NPC. If size of node is more than 6 cm or nodes are observed below the level of the lower border of the cricoid cartilage, the disease is at high risk of distant metastasis. In such conditions, either PET-CT or CT scan of Thorax, Abdomen and Pelvis is recommended [14–16].
b. *Thyroid cancer*: Initial imaging technique is USG, which is also used for sampling. Before surgery, CT scan of neck is commonly performed as a roadmap. If thyroid cancers show nodal disease in the retropharyngeal region, the disease is at high risk of distant metastasis and CECT scan of thorax, abdomen, and pelvis is recommended. Imaging to search for distant metastasis is also warranted in cases of locally invasive disease, bulky or extensive nodal disease, symptoms of distant metastasis and anaplastic thyroid cancers [17].
c. *Head and neck squamous cell carcinoma (HNSCC)*: CECT scan is preferred for most subsites. CEMRI is recommended for the tongue and also for laryngeal cancers to exclude the involvement of thyroid cartilage. However, practice differs between institutions and both techniques are used as per local expertise and preference.
d. *Lymphoma*: FDG PET-CT scan is the imaging technique of choice. In lymphoma, excision biopsy is the standard practice. If excision biopsy is not possible, USG-guided neck node biopsy may be recommended.
e. *Recurrence*: For HNSCC, NPC, and thyroid cancers, CT and MRI can both be used. FDG PET-CT may be used for HNSCC. For lymphoma, FDG PET-CT is always the first choice.

Imaging Technique

Any cross-sectional imaging of the head and neck region should cover the region between skull base and the carina to image level VII nodes and retrosternal thyroid. CT sections should be between 0.6 and 1.25 mm. On MRI, 3 mm sections are recommended. A small field of view is standard practice for optimal resolution. T1, T2, and contrast images are obtained on MRI on all three axes along with a fat saturated sequence in at least one axis [8].

Anatomical Location of Nodes

The first detailed description of the human lymphatic system was published by Prof. H. Rouviere in 1938 in Paris, France (Anatomie des Lymphatiques de l'Homme) [1]. His description included a craniocaudal and transverse set of chains for a superficial system. The transverse chains consisted of occipital, mastoid, parotid, facial, RPN, submaxillary, and sublingual nodes. Two craniocaudal chains described were the anterior and lateral cervical chains. The deep system consisted of the internal jugular chain, the spinal accessory chain, and a transverse cervical chain. The final pathway of drainage of the lymph from the cervical region is the IJV chain.

Anatomic location of nodes is principally important from the surgical standpoint. The Memorial Sloan Kettering surgical group proposed a simplified labeling of neck nodes as a set of seven levels [18] (Fig. 67.6). This was modified over time by imaging groups [19]. This system has been accepted by the American Joint Committee for Cancer (AJCC) system [17] as well, and is commonly used for staging of malignant neck nodes. Table 67.1 enumerates the levels of neck nodes as described by Som et al. [19] (Fig. 67.7A–C).

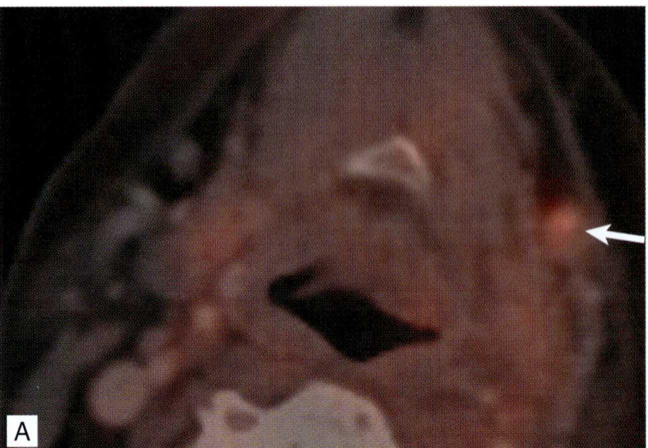

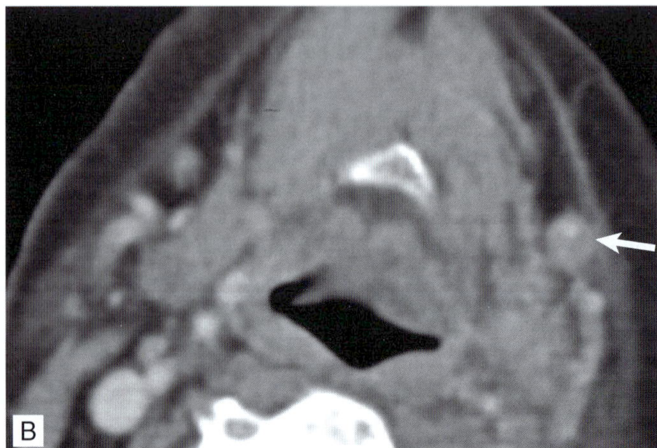

Figure 67.5 A 58-year-old woman with carcinoma right lateral border of tongue. (A) Axial PET CT and (B) corresponding axial CECT images show a rounded left cervical level IB node (*arrow*) showing FDG avidity. FNAC suggested reactive changes without any malignant cells.

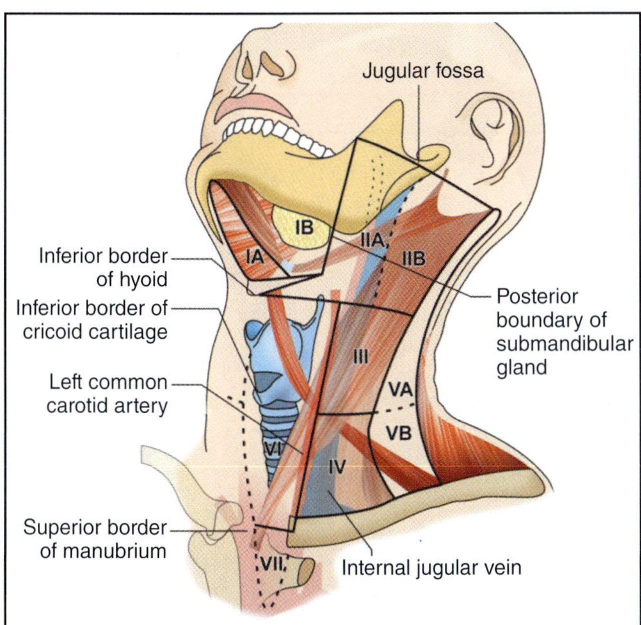

Figure 67.6 Cervical neck node levels.

Several regions that were surgically not amenable and not included in the above-mentioned system are still termed according to the anatomic location. They are as follows:
1. RPN
2. Facial
3. Pre- and postauricular and parotid
4. Occipital

Lymphatic Drainage of the Head and Neck Region

Table 67.2 is adapted from the 8th edition of AJCC and shows the lymphatic drainage pathways of the head and neck region [17].

Differentials of a Neck Mass and How to Ascertain That the Lesion is a Node

When a patient presents with a neck mass, it must be determined if the lesion is indeed a lymph node. In the pediatric population, branchial cleft cysts and various venolymphatic malformations are among the differentials. In adults, infective and inflammatory masses may mimic lymph nodes. An enlarged submandibular gland is commonly mistaken for a lymph node. USG is a great technique to solve the problem and sample the lesion (Fig. 67.8A and B).

Suboptimal cross-sectional imaging can lead to vascular structures and muscles to be incorrectly diagnosed as nodes. The imaging techniques and administration of contrast must be standardized to mitigate the errors (Fig. 67.4).

Imaging Features of a Normal and an Abnormal Node

The normal node has a reniform shape with an eccentrically placed hilum containing fat. The other parts of a node are the cortex placed at the periphery and medulla placed centrally. There is a covering by capsule, which is pierced by lymphatic and blood

TABLE 67.1 Levels of Neck Nodes

Level	Location Description
Level I	These nodes lie above the hyoid bone, below the mylohyoid muscle and anterior to the back of the submandibular gland (previously classified as the submental and submandibular nodes).
Level IA	These nodes lie between the medial margins of the anterior bellies of the digastric muscles above the hyoid bone and below the mylohyoid muscles (previously known as submental nodes).
Level IB	On each side of the neck, these nodes lie lateral to the level IA nodes and anterior to the back of each submandibular gland.
Level II	These nodes extend from the skull base to the level of the bottom of the body of the hyoid bone. They are posterior to the back of the submandibular gland and anterior to the back of the sternocleidomastoid muscle.
Level IIA	These nodes are level II nodes that lie either anterior, lateral, medial, or posterior to the internal jugular vein. If posterior to the vein, the nodes are inseparable from the vein (previously classified as upper internal jugular nodes).
Level IIB	These are level II nodes that lie posterior to the internal jugular vein with a fat plane separating the nodes and the vein (previously classified as upper spinal accessory nodes).
Level III	These nodes extend from the level of the bottom of the body of the hyoid bone to the level of the bottom of the cricoid arch. They lie anterior to the back of the sternocleidomastoid muscle (previously known as the mid-jugular nodes).
Level IV	These nodes extend from the level of the bottom of the cricoid arch to the level of the clavicle. They lie anterior to a line connecting the back of the sternocleidomastoid muscle and the posterior-lateral margin of the anterior scalene muscle. They are also lateral to the carotid arteries (previously known as the low jugular nodes).
Level V	These nodes lie posterior to the back of the sternocleidomastoid muscle from the skull base to the level of the bottom of the cricoid arch. From the level of the bottom of the cricoid arch to the level of the clavicle as seen on each axial scan, they lie posterior to a line connecting the back of the sternocleidomastoid muscle and the posterior-lateral margin of the anterior scalene muscle. They also lie anterior to the anterior edge of the trapezius muscle.
Level VA	Upper level V nodes extend from the skull base to the level of the bottom of the cricoid arch. They are posterior to the back of the sternocleidomastoid muscle.
Level VB	Lower level V nodes extend from the level of the bottom of the cricoid arch to the level of the clavicle as seen on each axial scan. They are posterior to a line connecting the back of the sternocleidomastoid muscle and the posterior-lateral margin of the anterior scalene muscle.
Level VI	These nodes lie between the carotid arteries from the level of the bottom of the body of the hyoid bone to the level of the top of the manubrium (previously known as the visceral nodes).
Level VII	These nodes lie between the carotid arteries below the level of the top of the manubrium and above the level of the innominate vein (previously known as the superior mediastinal nodes).

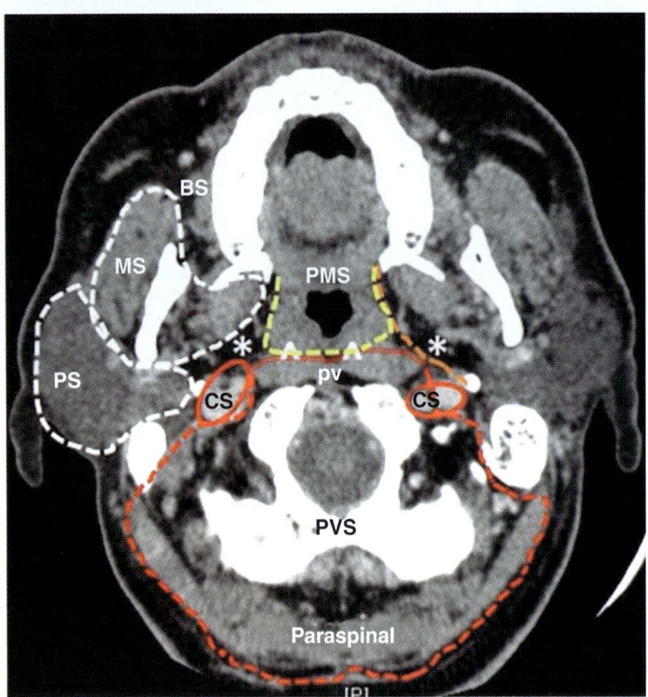

Figure 68.1 Axial CT image of the suprahyoid neck at the level of palate shows layers of deep cervical fascia as dashed lines. Investing layer (*white*), middle layer (*yellow*), and deep layer (*red*). The fascial layers enclose spaces, *BS*, buccal space; *CS*, carotid space; *MS*, masticator space; *PMS*, pharyngeal mucosal space; *PS*, parotid space; *PVS*, perivertebral space which has an anterior prevertebral compartment (pv) and posterior paraspinal compartment. The *asterisk* on each side shows the parapharyngeal space (PPS). The tensor vascular styloid fascia is a slip of middle layer (orange) passing from medial pterygoid plate to styloid process, which separates PPS from CS. The *caret symbol* shows the potential retropharyngeal space between the middle layer and prevertebral fascia. The CS sheath is composed of all three layers, but predominantly the deep layer.

pharyngeal mucosal space, which is discussed as nasopharynx, and oropharynx in a separate chapter. Two other spaces, *sublingual space* (SLS) and *submandibular space* (SMS), are part of the oral cavity but will be discussed in this chapter.

Infrahyoid Neck Spaces: Overview

The cervical fascial layers cleave the infrahyoid neck into five tightly packed spaces (Fig. 68.3). The central space is the *visceral space* surrounded by the middle layer of deep cervical fascia and contains not only the hypopharynx (which is a continuation of the suprahyoid pharyngeal mucosal space), but also the larynx, thyroid, parathyroid glands, trachea, and esophagus. These contents will be discussed elsewhere. The other spaces continuing from the suprahyoid neck are the *CS*, the *RPS*, the *PVS*, and the *PCS*. The *PCS* is a triangular fat-filled space between the carotid vessels anteriorly, sternocleidomastoid muscle laterally, and paraspinal muscles posteromedially. Table 68.1 shows the various spaces of the suprahyoid and infrahyoid neck.

Approach to Diagnosis of a Suprahyoid Neck Space Mass [1,2]

The head and neck region usually has exquisite symmetry. The absence of symmetry should alert the radiologist to the region of asymmetry, which is often the location of the lesion. After identification of the lesion, the next step is to localize its epicenter to a neck space if possible. In the suprahyoid neck, the fat-filled PPS has a crucial location being surrounded by other spaces. Displacement of the PPS is a useful clue to the epicenter of the mass. For example, a MS mass will displace the PPS posteromedially while a CS mass will displace it anteriorly. A PS mass will displace it anteromedially while a pharyngeal mucosal space mass will displace it laterally. Deciding the epicenter between the two midline

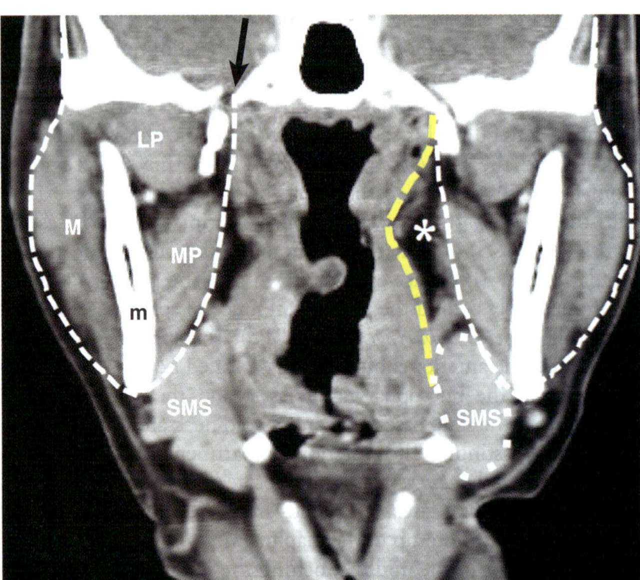

Figure 68.2 Coronal CT reformation shows the investing fascia splitting at the lower border of the mandible to medial and lateral slips (*dashed white lines*) to enclose the masticator space containing the ramus of mandible (m) and the muscles: masseter (M), medial pterygoid (MP), and lateral pterygoid (LP) with the foramen ovale in the roof (*arrow*). The parapharyngeal space (*asterisk*) is seen between the middle layer of the deep cervical fascia (*yellow dashed line*) and the medial slip of the investing layer; and communicates with the submandibular space (SMS) inferiorly that contains the submandibular gland (*outlined*).

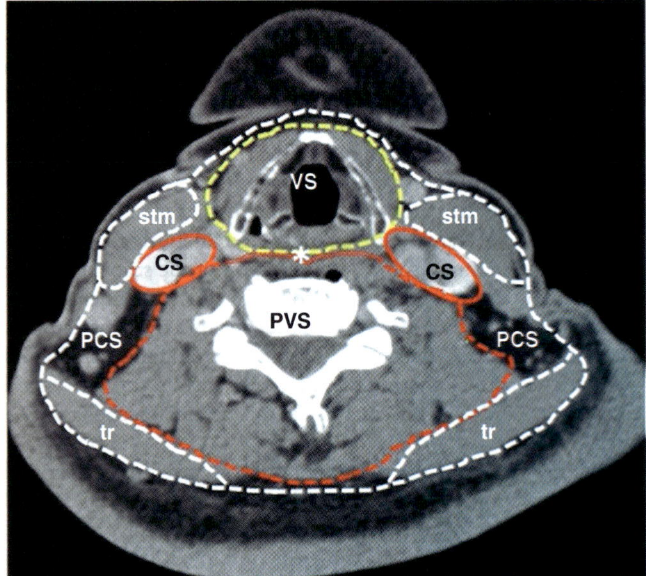

Figure 68.3 Axial CT image of the infrahyoid neck at the level of supraglottic larynx shows layers of deep cervical fascia as dashed lines. Investing layer (*white*); middle layer (yellow), and deep layer (red). The fascial layers enclose spaces. *CS*, carotid space; *PCS*, posterior cervical space; *PVS*, perivertebral space; *VS*, visceral space; the *asterisk* shows the potential retropharyngeal space between the middle layer and deep layer/prevertebral fascia. The investing layer encloses the sternomastoid (stm) and trapezius (tr). The CS sheath is composed of all three layers, but predominantly the deep layer.

TABLE 68.1 Spaces of the Neck[a]

	Suprahyoid Neck	Infrahyoid Neck
Median spaces	Pharyngeal mucosal space/visceral space	Visceral space
	Retropharyngeal space	Retropharyngeal space
	Perivertebral space	Perivertebral space
Lateral spaces	Masticator space	
	Parotid space	
	Buccal space	
	Parapharyngeal Space	
	Carotid space	Carotid space
	Posterior cervical space	Posterior cervical space

[a]Sublingual space and Submandibular space are parts of the oral cavity.

spaces, PVS and RPS, requires examination of the location of the prevertebral muscles. RPS masses displace the prevertebral muscles posteriorly while PVS masses displace them anteriorly. The origin of a mass from the SLS or SMS is decided by studying its relationship with the mylohyoid muscle (in the floor of the mouth). SLS masses are located superomedial to the mylohyoid muscle while SMS masses are seen inferior and lateral to it.

Once the epicenter is located, the differential diagnosis can be formed based on the knowledge of the various contents of that space and the list of lesions characteristic to that location. The differential diagnosis can be further narrowed, using a combination of the patient's age, clinical history, and specific imaging features of the lesion. For example, an intensely enhancing nasopharyngeal mass in an adolescent male is typically a juvenile nasopharyngeal angiofibroma. An aggressive destructive pediatric soft tissue tumor in the MS is often a rhabdomyosarcoma. Hence, thorough knowledge of the boundaries and contents of the spaces, lesions specific to them and their imaging features together with the clinical history help devise a systematic approach to a neck mass.

TABLE 68.2 Lesions of the Masticator Space

Developmental	*Vascular anomalies* a. Hemangioma* (pediatric) b. Vascular malformations ■ High flow (AVMs and AVFs) ■ Low flow* (venous/lymphatic/mixed malformation)
Inflammatory	a. Masticator space abscess from odontogenic focus*/spread from adjacent spaces b. Mandibular osteomyelitis
Benign tumor	*Nerve origin* a. Schwannoma* b. Neurofibroma *Bony origin* a. Odontogenic origin* Dentigerous cysts, odontogenic keratocyst, ameloblastoma b. Nonodontogenic Simple bone cysts, aneurysmal bone cysts *Fibro-osseous lesions* Fibrous dysplasia, ossifying fibroma *Soft tissue lesions* Lipoma, rhabdomyoma, leiomyoma
Malignant tumor	*Intrinsic* a. Neurogenic origin—malignant peripheral nerve sheath tumor b. Bony origin—osteosarcoma, chondrosarcoma, Ewing's sarcoma, and metastases c. Soft tissue—rhabdomyosarcoma* (in children), malignant fibrous histiocytoma, fibrosarcoma, synovial sarcoma d. Non-Hodgkin's lymphoma *Extrinsic* a. Tumor spread from adjacent spaces*—oral cavity, pharynx, parotid space, skull base b. Perineural tumor spread along V3 to the foramen ovale (via inferior alveolar nerve or auriculotemporal nerve)
Miscellaneous/ pseudolesions	a. Benign masseteric hypertrophy* b. Accessory parotid gland* c. V3 denervation atrophy (acute and subacute phase)

*Represents the more common lesions.
AVF, arteriovenous fistula; *AVM*, arteriovenous malformation.

Masticator Space

Boundaries

MS has its floor at the lower border of the mandible and its roof at the skull base (Fig. 68.2). The foramina ovale and spinosum are located in the roof of the MS. Medially, it is limited by the medial layer of investing fascia (also called medial pterygoid fascia). The lateral layer of investing fascia, which closely abuts the superficial part of the masseter and reaches up to the zygomatic arch, forms the lateral boundary of the MS. This layer continues further cranially over the temporalis muscle. Hence, laterally the MS extends further above the zygomatic arch, as a recess, called the suprazygomatic MS or the temporal fossa (by the surgeons). Anteriorly, the MS has an incomplete boundary with the BS. Posteriorly, it is bounded by the PS [1,2].

Contents

The contents of the MS are:

- Ramus and body of the mandible
- Muscles of mastication
- Mandibular nerve and branches
- Inferior alveolar nerve
- Inferior alveolar artery and vein

The ramus and body of the mandible form the central strut in the MS. The muscles of mastication are the medial pterygoid muscle, lateral pterygoid muscle, temporalis, and masseter. The mandibular nerve or V3 nerve (third division of the trigeminal nerve) gives branches to the masticator muscles. The mandibular nerve trunk is located in the central part of MS in between the medial and lateral pterygoid muscles. The inferior alveolar nerve, the largest division of the mandibular nerve, is a sensory nerve that accompanies the inferior alveolar artery and vein. These structures enter the mandibular foramen to run within the inferior alveolar canal in the mandibular shaft [1,2].

Lesions of the MS

The lesions of the MS can be classified as developmental, inflammatory, tumors, and miscellaneous (Table 68.2) [3].

Imaging Methods for MS Lesions

CT and MRI are the commonly used methods for imaging MS lesions, except in case of vascular malformations where USG is the first-line diagnostic imaging. CT is superior for detecting cortical erosion and characterizing tumor matrix and mineralization. CT is the investigation of choice in suspected MS infection as it demonstrates mandibular osteomyelitis and MS abscess along with the cause of infection (odontogenic focus/parotid calculi). However, MRI is the preferred investigation in neoplasia as it depicts muscle and soft tissue invasion better due to superior soft tissue resolution. MRI is also superior for demonstrating mandibular marrow invasion and perineural tumor spread [1–4].

Imaging Features of Common MS Lesions

Infections

Infections are more common than tumors and are usually due to odontogenic causes, such as dental caries, gingivitis, or tooth extraction. Less commonly, the infection can also extend from an infected parotid gland or a tonsillar focus. Well-defined fluid collections with enhancing walls may be seen in the MS representing abscesses that may extend into adjacent spaces [3]. Masseteric abscess may not always be seen as a collection, instead, the muscle may appear enlarged, show heterogeneous enhancement, and the adjacent mandible may show sclerosis [5]. Suppurative osteomyelitis of the mandible is seen as an osteolytic pattern in the mandible with a lamellated periosteal reaction.

Developmental Lesions

The developmental lesions seen in the MS are vascular anomalies (Table 68.2). USG is the first-line imaging method for these and can differentiate between hemangioma and vascular malformations by depicting the parenchymal component in the former. Color Doppler USG (CDUSG) can also demonstrate the high-velocity flow in arteriovenous malformations and the low-velocity flow in venous and lymphatic malformations (LMs) [4].

The commonest benign pediatric tumor of the MS is a hemangioma. Two types exist, infantile hemangioma (a true neoplasm) and congenital hemangioma. USG with CDUSG is used for superficial lesions and shows a highly vascular soft tissue mass. Cross-sectional imaging is useful for studying large or deeply located masses. On MR imaging, hemangioma is seen as a soft tissue mass, which in the proliferating phase is seen as a lobulated, well-circumscribed, homogeneous mass that is intermediate in signal on T1-weighted images. Homogeneous hyperintense signal on T2-weighted images is noted with homogeneous postcontrast enhancement. Heterogeneity is seen in the involutional phase [4].

Venous malformations (VMs) appear as compressible lesions with poorly defined margins on USG without arterial waveform on CDUS. Calcified phleboliths, best seen, as high attenuation foci on CT, are diagnostic of VMs (Fig. 68.4). Remodeling of adjacent bone may be typically seen in VMs, that is unusual in hemangiomas. On MRI, hypo to isointense homogeneous signal on T1-weighted images is usual except when thrombosis or hemorrhage is seen. T2-weighted images show high signal intensity when the vascular channels are large and intermediate signal when these are smaller. Heterogeneous delayed enhancement is seen on the postcontrast study (Fig. 68.5). Flow voids are not seen [4].

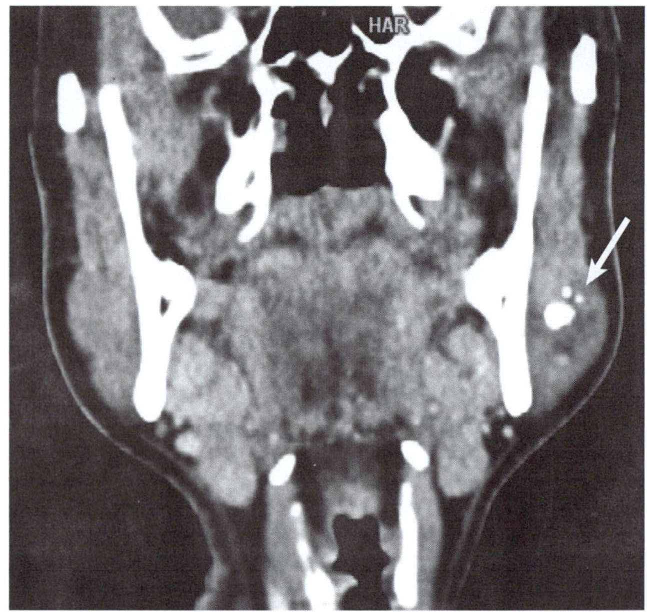

Figure 68.4 Venous malformation (VM), coronal CT reformation in a clinically soft compressible swelling of the left jaw shows mild heterogeneous enhancement in the masseter with phleboliths (*arrow*), which are pathognomonic of VM.

LMs can be microcystic, macrocystic, or mixed types. Macrocystic lesions appear as septated cystic structures on both MRI and USG with fluid–fluid levels when there is hemorrhage within. A T1-weighted postcontrast fat-saturated sequence shows that the cysts do not enhance while the internal septae do and is useful to differentiate from a VM which shows delayed heterogeneous enhancement. Microcystic LMs have tiny cysts within and appear hyperechoic on USG. The tiny cysts show crowding of the walls, which are T2 hypointense and show postcontrast enhancement and this may make the lesion appear enhancing and solid on MRI [4]. Mixed malformations show a combination of all the above components.

Arteriovenous malformations show a tangle of vessels without any parenchymal component and large flow voids on both T1- and T2-weighted images. They do not show high signal on T2-weighted sequences. Large feeding arteries and draining veins without intervening capillary components are characteristic, with intense early venous enhancement. The posterior body and ramus of the mandible may also be involved resulting in bony expansion and erosion of margins [4].

Benign and Malignant Tumors

The common benign tumor of the MS is a schwannoma of the mandibular nerve or its branches. It is seen as a fusiform well-defined soft tissue intensity mass appearing hypointense on T1-weighted and hyperintense on T2-weighted images. Cystic degeneration is common in large tumors, which appear heterogeneous. Postcontrast enhancement can be homogenous or heterogeneous. Extension intracranially produces a dumbbell-shaped tumor with a waist at the foramen ovale (Fig. 68.6) [2].

Neurofibromas (NFs) may be solitary or multiple (when associated with neurofibromatosis type 1). NFs show high T2 signal intensity and may exhibit either strong or heterogeneous postgadolinium enhancement (Fig. 68.7). Solitary NFs may show the typical target sign with central low signal intensity on T2-weighted images and peripheral hyperintense rim [6]. Plexiform NFs can involve multiple adjacent spaces.

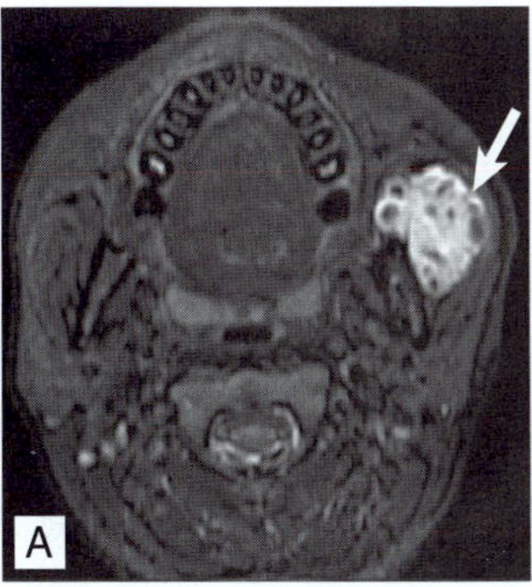

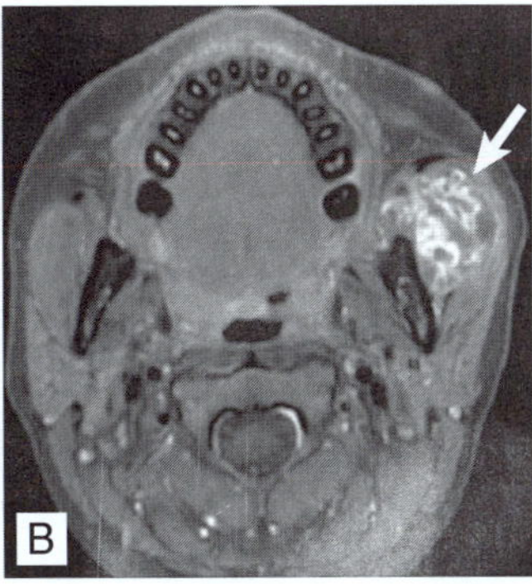

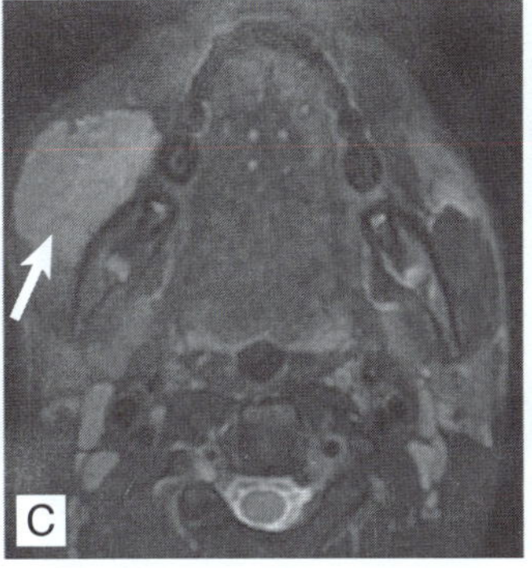

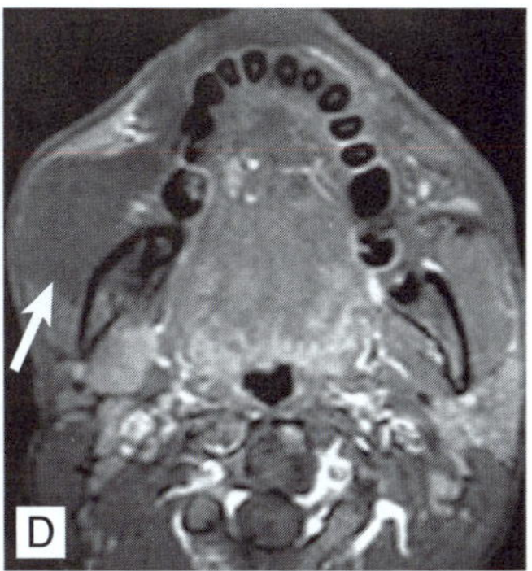

Figure 68.5 (A and B) MRI in venous malformation. (A) Fat-suppressed T2W axial image shows high signal intensity lesion (*arrow*) in the masticator space within the substance of the masseter muscle. (B) Fat-suppressed postcontrast T1W axial image shows delayed heterogeneous enhancement in the lesion (*arrow*), not usually seen in the cysts of lymphatic malformation. (C and D) MRI in lymphatic malformation (macrocystic). (C) Fat-suppressed T2W axial image shows a cystic lesion (*arrow*) in the masticator space within the substance of the masseter muscle. (D) Fat-suppressed postcontrast T1W axial image shows no enhancement of the cystic spaces which is typical of a lymphatic malformation.

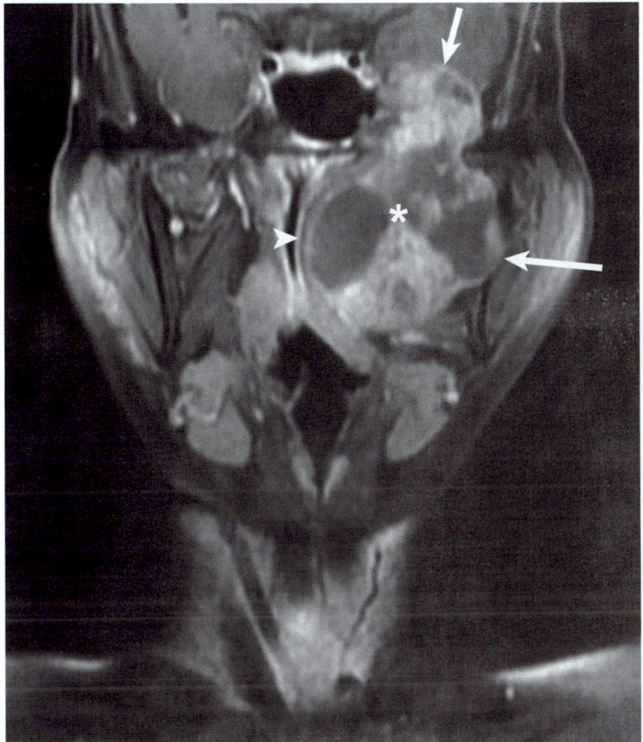

Figure 68.6 Schwannoma with cystic degeneration. Coronal fat-suppressed postcontrast T1W MRI shows a dumbbell-shaped solid-cystic mass (*asterisk*) in the masticator space (MS) closely apposed to the mandibular ramus (*long arrow*) extending through the foramen ovale intracranially (*short arrow*). Parapharyngeal fat that is compressed medially (*arrowhead*) confirms epicenter in the MS.

Malignant peripheral nerve sheath tumor that arise de novo from schwannomas or NFs may have similar imaging appearance, but greater heterogeneity, foraminal erosion, and rapid increase in size may suggest malignant peripheral nerve sheath tumor [1,2].

Rhabdomyosarcoma is the most common malignant tumor of MS in children. It appears as an infiltrating soft tissue mass with bony destruction or erosion. Non-Hodgkin lymphoma (NHL) occurs as a part of systemic NHL and has no specific imaging features; the mass is fairly homogenous with well-defined margins, is more likely to mould than infiltrate bone, destruction being rare. Soft tissue sarcomas of the MS have no specific imaging features [1,2]. Odontogenic and nonodontogenic bone lesions are beyond the scope of this chapter.

Tumor extension into the MS from the adjacent oral cavity, particularly from buccal and retromolar trigone cancers, is common and this causes upstaging of the primary disease. Other tumors that can spread into MS are nasopharyngeal carcinoma, tonsillar carcinomas, and parotid malignancies. This may be seen as direct tumor extension or as perineural spread (PNS) that is seen along the nerves, either in continuity with the primary in the adjacent space or as skip lesions. Malignant parotid tumors can spread along the auriculotemporal nerve and oral cavity tumors along the inferior alveolar nerve to reach the V3 nerve extending up to the foramen ovale and beyond (Fig. 68.8). Contrast-enhanced MR imaging best demonstrates the direct signs of PNS as nerve enlargement, excessive enhancement of the nerve, and loss of fat adjacent to the foraminae. Fullness and enhancement of Meckel's cave and cavernous sinus may be seen. CT demonstrates more advanced cases, showing foraminal erosion and soft tissue density obliterating the fat adjacent to foraminae.

Miscellaneous Lesions (Pseudolesions)

Indirect signs of PNS are denervation atrophy of the masticator muscles. These show increased enhancement, T2 hyperintensity, and enlargement in the acute–subacute phase that should not be misinterpreted as a tumor.

Benign masseteric hypertrophy may be unilateral or bilateral. The etiology remains unclear although bruxism, jaw malocclusion, and temporomandibular joint disorders have been implicated. Homogeneous enlargement of the entire muscle is seen on imaging without any focal mass-like lesion. There may be associated hypertrophy of the pterygoid and temporalis muscles too (Fig. 68.9).

An accessory parotid gland is seen just superficial to the masseter muscle and is usually unilateral. It is morphologically identical with the main parotid gland and should not be mistaken for a mass lesion. The characteristic density/intensity similar to the adjacent parotid gland is an important clue to correct diagnosis [1,2].

Teaching Points

- MS lesion is either located anterior/anterolateral to the PPS and when large displaces the PPS posteriorly/posteromedially
- Optimal imaging of an MS lesion extends from above the skull base (level of the pons) to below the

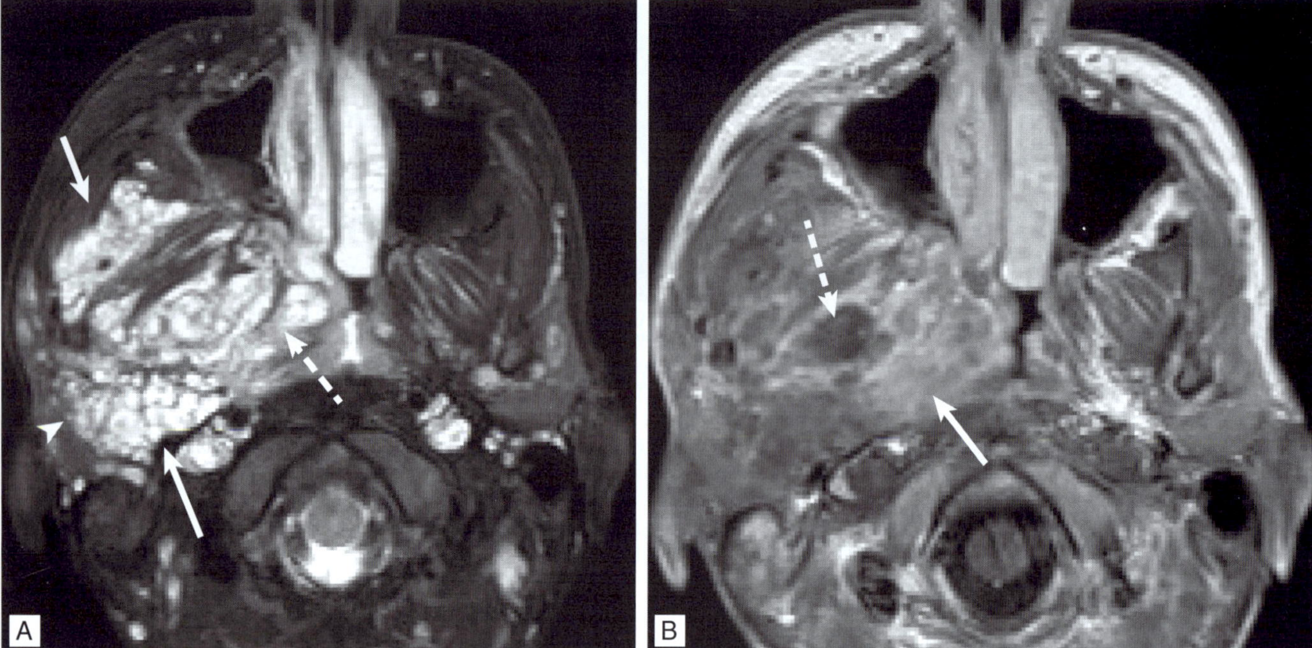

Figure 68.7 Neurofibroma in the masticator space. (A) Axial T2W MRI shows a hyperintense mass with epicenter in the masticator space (*solid arrows*), also extending laterally into the parotid gland (*arrowhead*) and medially into the parapharyngeal space (*dashed arrow*). (B) Contrast-enhanced axial T1W MRI shows heterogeneous enhancement in the lesion (*solid arrow*) with a focus of cystic degeneration (*dashed arrow*). (Courtesy: Suresh K. Mukherji.)

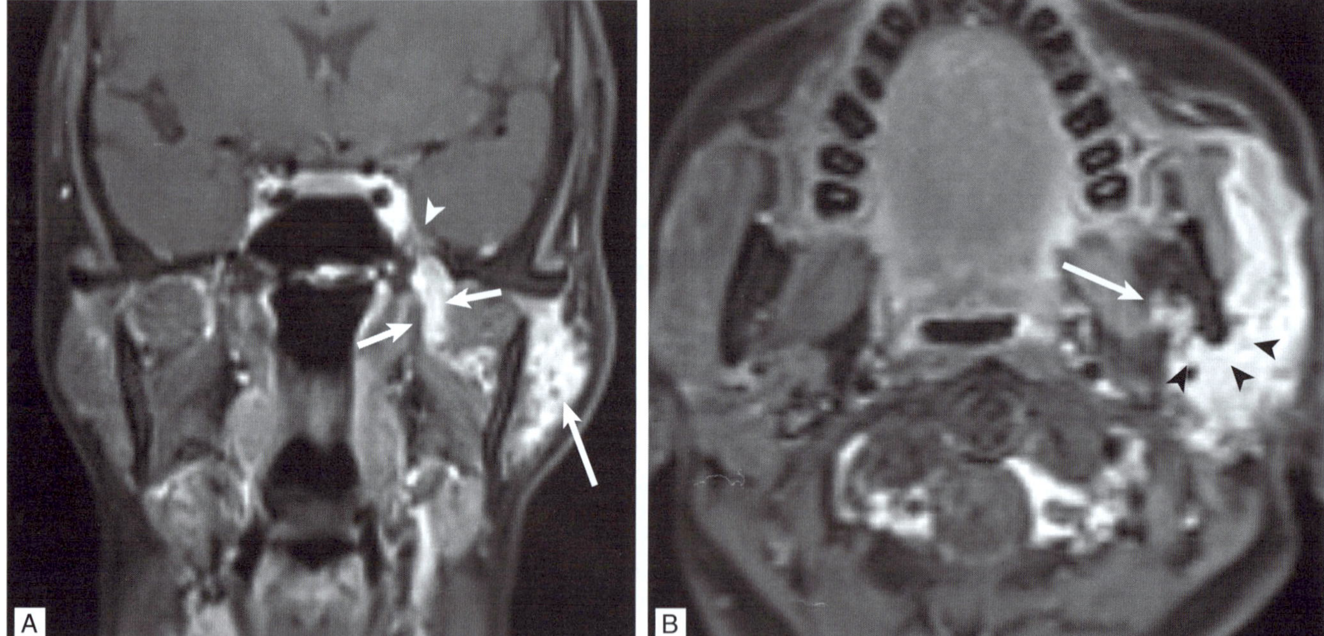

Figure 68.8 Adenoid cystic carcinoma with perineural spread (PNS). Fat-suppressed postcontrast T1W MRI. (A) Coronal image shows enhancing parotid mass (*long arrow*) and PNS along V3 (*short arrows*) reaching foramen ovale (*arrowhead*). (B) Axial section. *Arrowheads* show the PNS along auriculotemporal nerve course (behind mandibular ramus) to reach V3 at mandibular foramen (*white arrow*).

mandible and in case of suspected malignancy up to the root of the neck

- MRI is the preferred method of imaging for suspected malignancy and CT is the preferred method of imaging for suspected infection of the MS

Buccal Space

Boundaries

The BS is located anterior to the MS and separated from it by an incomplete fascial boundary. It lies lateral to the buccinator muscle (and oral cavity) and medial to the zygomaticus major (Fig. 68.10).

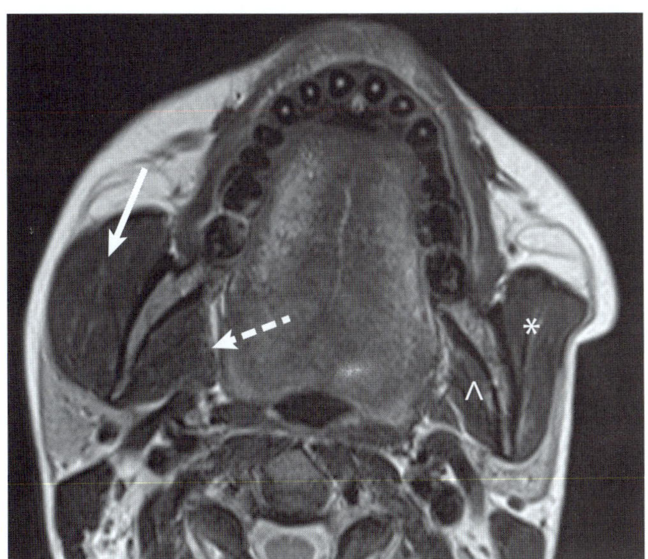

Figure 68.9 Benign hypertrophy of right masseter (*solid arrow*) and medial pterygoid (*dashed arrow*) seen on axial T2W MRI. Note the normal left-sided masseter (*asterisk*) and medial pterygoid (*caret symbol*).

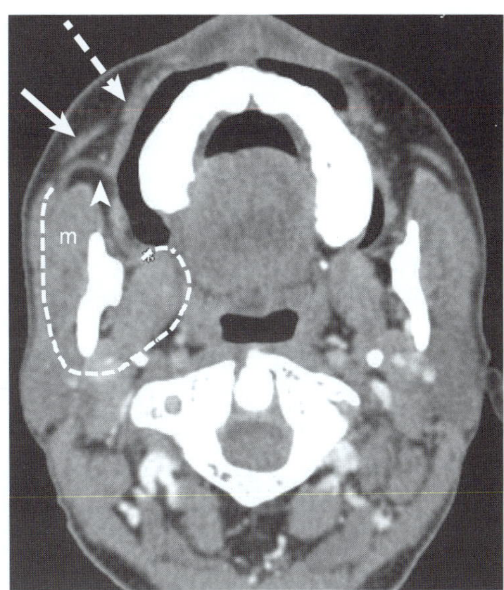

Figure 68.10 Buccal space (BS) anatomy. Axial CT image shows BS bounded by zygomaticus major muscle (*solid arrow*), buccinator muscle (*dashed arrow*), and masseter (m) in the masticator space (*outlined*). The terminal end of the parotid duct (*arrowhead*) divides the buccal fat pad into anterior and posterior parts.

Lateral to the zygomaticus major muscle lies the subcutaneous fat under the skin of the cheek and this is not a part of the BS. Superiorly, the BS fat merges with the retroantral fat (part of infratemporal fossa) while inferiorly the BS merges with the SMS [1,7].

Contents

The contents of the BS are:

- Adipose tissue
- Parotid duct
- Minor salivary gland rests
- Accessory parotid lobules
- Facial and mandibular nerve branches
- Facial artery and vein
- Buccal artery
- Lymphatic channels
- Lymph nodes

The central adipose tissue is called the buccal fat pad. The terminal end of the parotid duct traverses the buccal fat pad transversely to pierce the buccinator opposite the upper second molar. This divides the buccal fat pad into two equal anterior and posterior compartments (Fig. 68.10). The buccal fat pad has other extensions. A lateral extension is seen along the parotid duct, a medial and superior extension is seen between the posterior wall of maxillary sinus and ramus of the mandible and an anterior extension is seen anterior to the maxillary sinus. The minor salivary gland rests, the nerves and lymphatic channels are not seen on imaging [7]. Lesions of the BS are listed in Table 68.3.

TABLE 68.3 Lesions of the Buccal Space

Developmental	*Vascular anomalies* a. Hemangiomas b. Vascular malformations* ■ High flow (AVMs and AVFs) ■ Low flow* (venous/lymphatic/mixed malformation)
Inflammatory/ infection	*Cellulitis/abscess* due to* a. Dental infections/salivary calculi b. Spread of infection from complicated sinusitis c. Spread of infection from masticator space
Benign tumor	*Minor salivary gland tumor* a. Pleomorphic adenoma* *Nerve origin* a. Schwannoma b. Neurofibroma* *Soft tissue lesions* a. Lipoma b. Rhabdomyoma
Malignant tumor	*Intrinsic* a. Adenoid cystic carcinoma b. Non-Hodgkin lymphoma c. Rhabdomyosarcoma (children) *Extrinsic* a. Tumor spread from adjacent spaces*—oral cavity, masticator space b. Nodal metastases from SCC*

*Represents the common lesions.
AVF, arteriovenous fistula; *AVM*, arteriovenous malformation.

Imaging Features of BS Lesions

Infections

BS infections are either from adjacent infected dental foci/ parotid calculi or extension of infection from adjacent MS. Invasive fungal sinusitis of the maxillary antrum is another focus of infection and all the above cause buccal fat infiltration. Cellulitis is manifested as stranding of the buccal and overlying subcutaneous fat with thickening of skin and enlargement of adjacent muscles while abscess appears characteristically as a fluid collection with enhancing walls.

Vascular Anomalies

Vascular malformations encountered in the BS could be VMs (more frequent) or LMs (Fig. 68.11).

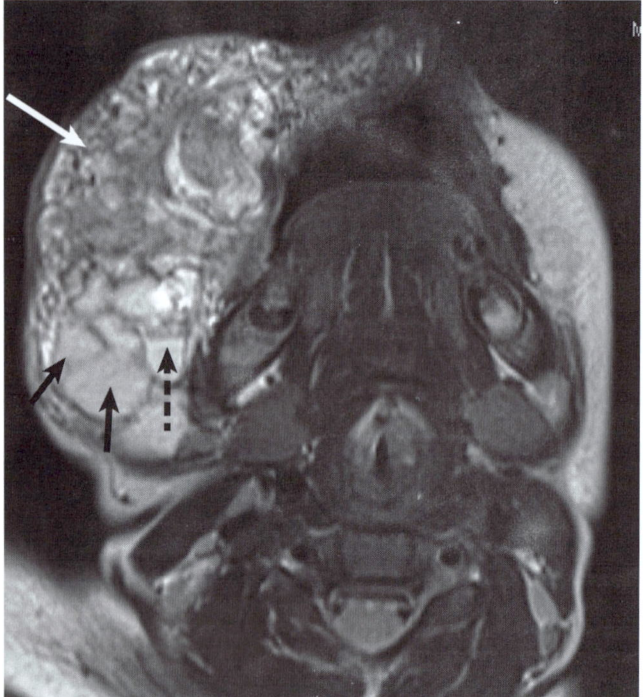

Figure 68.11 Lymphatic malformation (macrocystic and microcystic components) in the right buccal space. Axial T2W MRI. Cystic components (*black arrows*) with fluid–fluid level (*dashed arrow*) indicate the macrocystic component. The anteriorly located intermediate signal intensity areas (*white arrow*) represent crowded walls of tiny cysts in the microcystic component.

Benign and Malignant Tumors

Minor salivary gland rests (not seen on imaging) could give rise to the benign pleomorphic adenoma or the malignant adenoid cystic carcinoma (ACC) or mucoepidermoid carcinoma (MEC). MRI is the preferred method for characterizing neoplasms of the BS. The pleomorphic adenomas typically have low signal on T1-weighted images and high signal on T2-weighted images and are often homogeneous when small. Ill-defined infiltrative margins and areas of low signal intensity are seen in malignant salivary neoplasms [7]. Lipomas show the typical fat density or intensity.

Malignancies of the oral cavity vestibule (gingival-buccal mucosa and retromolar trigone) when advanced, invade the BS after invading the buccinator. Further spread can reach the skin laterally or MS posteriorly (Fig. 68.12) upstaging the "T" category of the oral cancer.

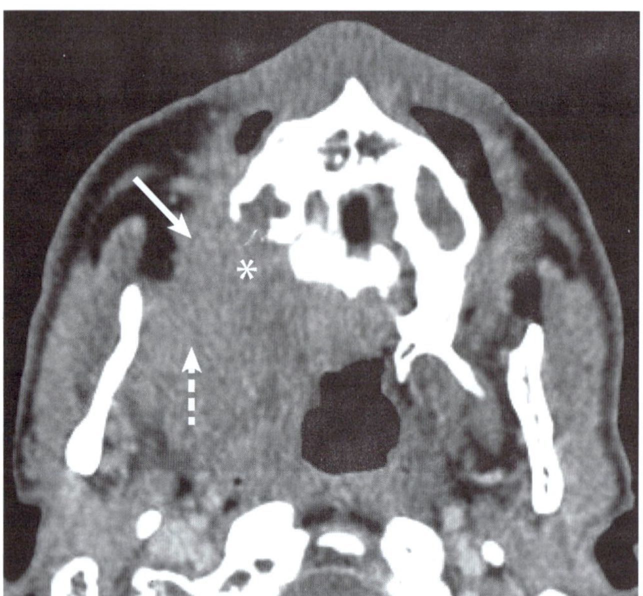

Figure 68.12 Oral cancer extension. Axial CT section at the level of upper alveolus shows tumor extension into the buccal space (*solid arrow*) and masticator space (*dashed arrow*) from an advanced right upper alveolar oral cancer that destroys the bony alveolus (*asterisk*) and pterygoid plates.

Teaching Points

- BS is anterior to the MS and separated by an incomplete fascia
- BS is located lateral to the buccinator and oral cavity
- BS can be a conduit for the spread of squamous carcinoma from the oral cavity to MS, which upstages disease (to T4b category)

Parapharyngeal Space

Boundaries

The PPS is an inverted pyramidal-shaped space with its base superiorly at the skull base (undersurface of temporal bone) and its apex inferiorly at the junction of the greater cornu of hyoid bone and the posterior belly of digastric muscle. On coronal imaging, it is seen located between the MS (lined by the medial slip of investing fascia) and the naso-oropharynx lined by the buccopharyngeal fascia; and communicates inferiorly with the SMS of the oral cavity (Fig. 68.2).

On the axial imaging section, the pterygoid muscles and mandibular ramus (in the MS) are located anterolateral to it while posteriorly the tensor–vascular styloid fascia, a slip of the middle layer of cervical fascia (not seen on imaging), separates the PPS from the CS (Fig. 68.1). The posterolateral border of the PPS abuts the PS in the region of the deep lobe of the parotid [1,2,8].

Contents

The contents of the PPS are:

- Fat
- Minor salivary gland rests
- Internal maxillary artery
- Ascending pharyngeal artery
- Pteryoid/pharyngeal venous plexus

The pterygoid venous plexus is a cluster of venules that are counterparts of branches of the maxillary artery. It is located in the PPS along the medial margin of the lateral pterygoid muscle and eventually forms the retromandibular vein [2].

Lesions of the PPS

The lesions of the PPS can be classified as developmental, pseudomasses, inflammatory lesions, and tumors (Table 68.4) [1,2].

Imaging Features of Common PPS Lesions

Infections

Infections of the PPS are always due to spread from adjacent spaces and hence abscesses seen are multicompartmental (Fig. 68.13).

Developmental Lesions

An atypical second branchial cleft cyst (BCC) is seen in the PPS. This entity encountered in the pediatric age group or young adults is seen as

TABLE 68.4 Lesions of the Parapharyngeal Space

Developmental	Atypical second branchial cleft cyst*
Pseudomass	Asymmetric pterygoid venous plexus*
Inflammatory	Abscess spreading from adjacent deep spaces* a. masticator space (dental focus) b. parotid space (calculous disease) and c. pharyngeal mucosal space (tonsillar focus)
Benign tumor	*Minor salivary gland tumor* Pleomorphic adenoma* *Fat* Lipoma
Malignant tumor	*Intrinsic* a. Adenoid cystic carcinoma b. Mucoepidermoid carcinoma *Extrinsic* a. Tumor spread from adjacent spaces*—parotid space, masticator space, and pharyngeal mucosal space

*Represents the more common lesions.

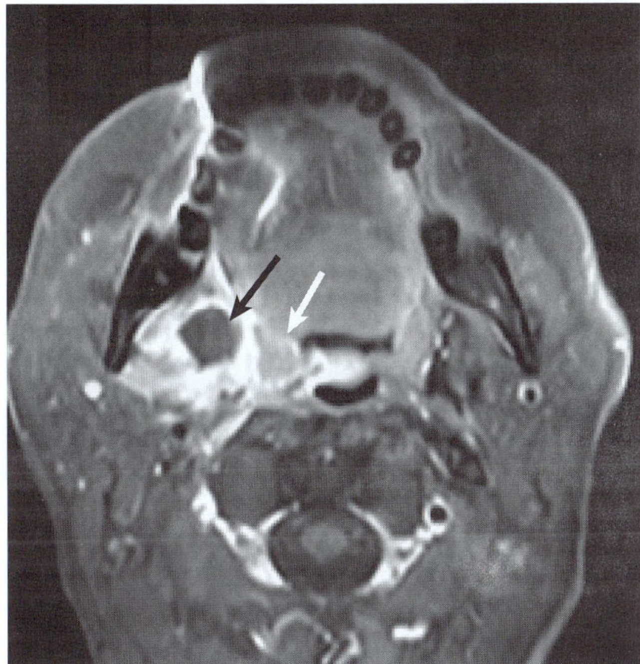

Figure 68.13 Tonsillar and peritonsillar abscess reaching the parapharyngeal space (PPS) and masticator space. Contrast-enhanced axial MRI shows the PPS abscess as a fluid-containing cavity (*black arrow*) with surrounding enhancement reaching up to the mandible. The right tonsil is enlarged and shows a nonenhancing central focus (*white arrow*) suggestive of a tonsillar abscess.

an ovoid cystic mass of water density/intensity, within the PPS, reaching the skull base superiorly. Inferiorly, it abuts the pharyngeal wall.

Pseudomass

When the pterygoid venous plexus is asymmetrically enlarged on one side, it appears as an enhancing cluster of vessels and should not be mistaken for a vascular tumor (Fig. 68.14).

Benign and Malignant Tumors

As a general rule, the larger the salivary gland, the lower the incidence of malignancy with the highest incidence observed in the

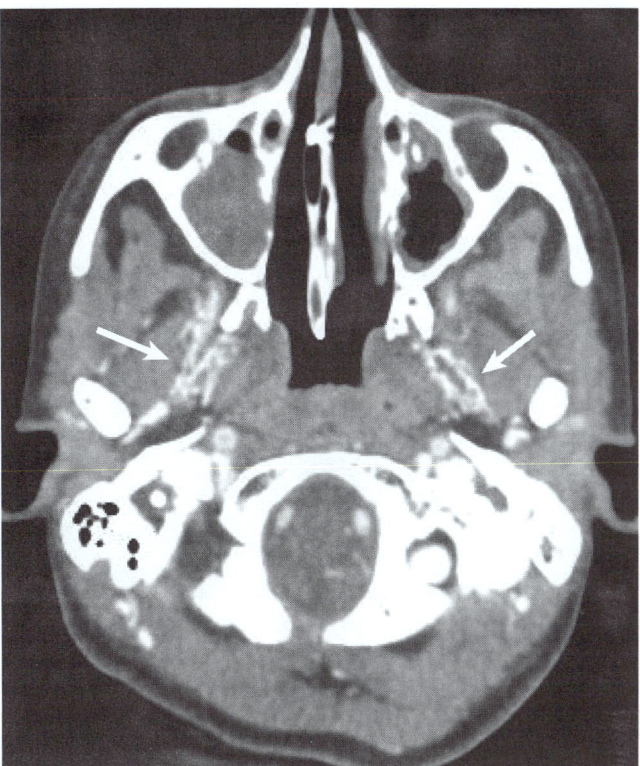

Figure 68.14 Axial CT section at the level of nasopharynx shows prominent pterygoid venous plexus (*arrows*) in parapharyngeal spaces (normal content). An asymmetrically enlarged plexus should not be misinterpreted as a tumor.

minor salivary gland rests. However, when it comes to the PPS salivary rests, benign tumors are much more common than malignant tumors [8]. Pleomorphic adenoma of the PPS is seen as round or oval soft tissue density mass on CT with very high signal on T2-weighted images. The mass is sharply circumscribed, centered in the PPS, and shows a well-defined fat plane all around the periphery if arising de novo from the PPS rests (Fig. 68.15A). On the other hand, a pleomorphic adenoma arising from the adjacent deep lobe of the parotid and extending secondarily into the PPS shows a fat plane only along the medial margin of the mass and would be inseparable from the deep parotid lobe (Fig. 68.15B). This difference is important to recognize and convey, as the surgical approach for a parotid mass is trans-parotid, while a de novo PPS mass can be approached from an oral or submandibular approach. A large de novo PPS mass may push the parotid deep lobe laterally, however is very unlikely to reach the superficial parotid lobe (which is very likely with a deep lobe tumor). Also, multifocal masses are more likely to be parotid in origin while PPS masses are unifocal [1,2].

Adenoid cystic or mucoepidermoid cancers of the PPS can show infiltrative margins. PNS to foramen ovale if visible is diagnostic of a malignant tumor (Fig. 68.16) [8].

Malignant lesions of the nasopharynx and tonsil (squamous carcinomas, lymphomas, and minor salivary gland malignancies) can also invade the PPS fat and displace it laterally. Sarcomas of the MS may extend into the PPS displacing the fat posteriorly and medially.

Teaching Points

- PPS mass has a strategic location on each side of the suprahyoid neck. Its displacement helps decide the epicenter of a lateral suprahyoid neck lesion

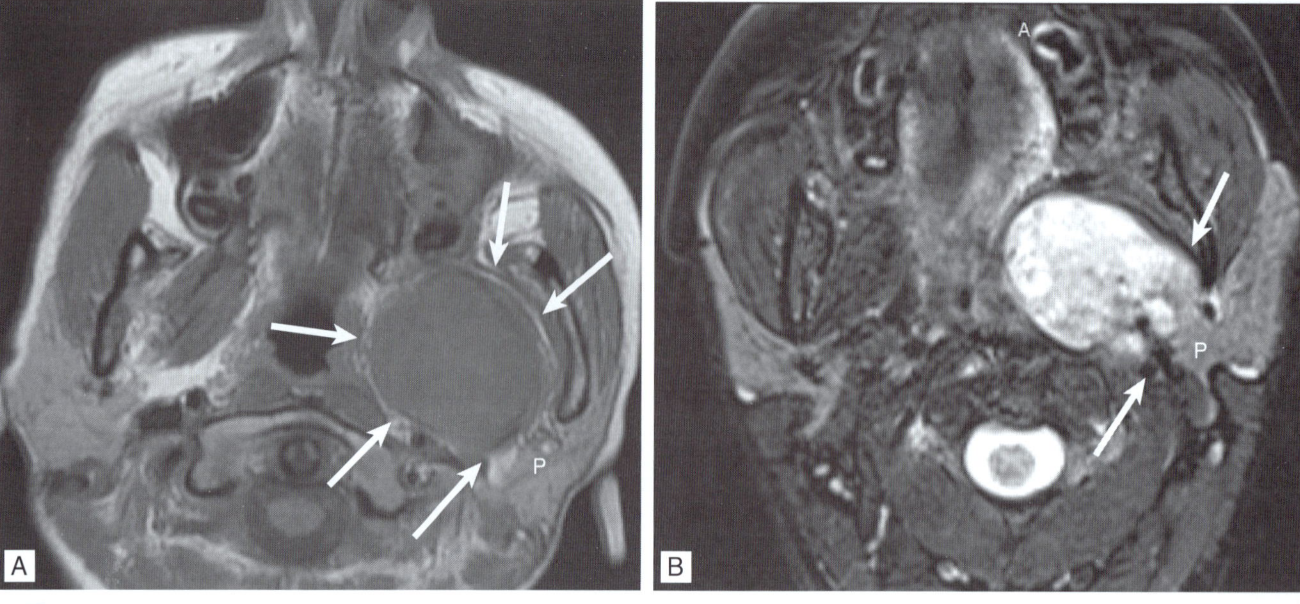

Figure 68.15 De novo parapharyngeal space (PPS) mass versus parotid mass. (A) Noncontrast axial T1W MRI shows a de novo left PPS mass with fat plane all around the mass (*arrows*), also separating it from the deep lobe parotid (P). (B) Axial T2W fat-suppressed image shows a hyperintense tumor (pleomorphic adenoma) inseparable from the deep lobe of the left parotid gland (P) extending into left PPS with widening of the stylomandibular tunnel (*arrows*).

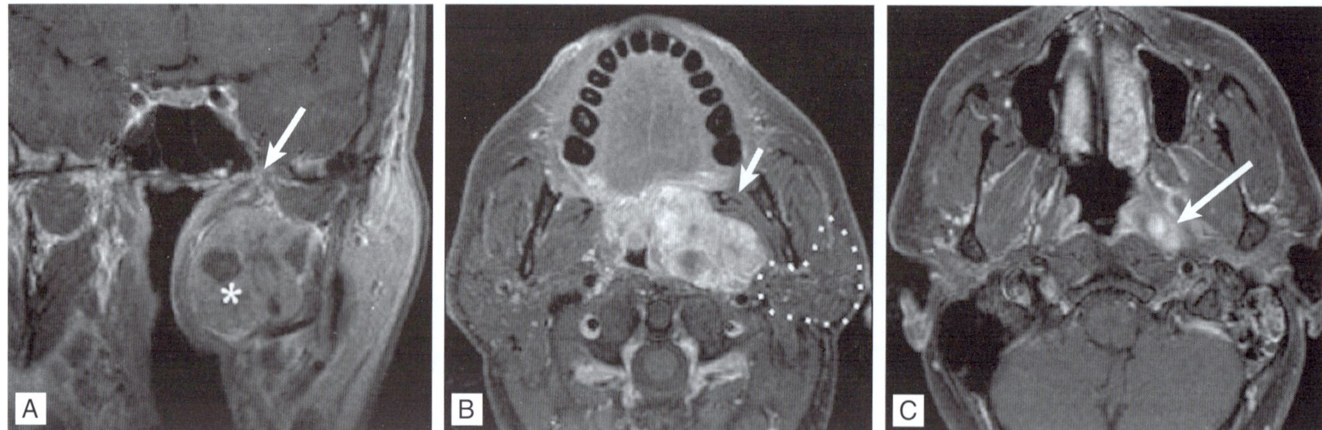

Figure 68.16 Mucoepidermoid carcinoma of parapharyngeal space (PPS). A. Coronal T2W MRI and B & C. Axial contrast enhanced T1W MRI, show a well-defined heterogeneously enhancing mass in the left PPS in A (*asterisk*) and B. Subtle perineural spread (PNS) to the foramen ovale (*arrow* in A) is confirmed in C (*arrow*). The mass is separate from the parotid (*outlined* in B), displaces medial pterygoid muscle anterolaterally (*arrow* in B) establishing the epicenter in the PPS. Salivary neoplasms of the PPS are rarely malignant, but the presence of PNS is a pointer to malignancy.

- It is important to differentiate between a salivary tumor arising de novo from the PPS salivary rests and a deep lobe parotid tumor as this can change the surgical approach
- MRI is the preferred method of imaging for suspected malignancy and CT is the preferred method of imaging for suspected infection of the PPS

Parotid Space

Boundaries

The PS extends superiorly from the external auditory canal and mastoid tip to the angle of the mandible inferiorly. The superficial layer of the deep cervical fascia encloses the PS; and the MS lies directly anterior to it (Fig. 68.1). PPS lies anteromedial to the PS while the CS which is posteromedial to it is separated by the posterior belly of the digastric muscle [1,2].

Contents

The contents of the PS are:

- Parotid gland
- Facial nerve
- External carotid artery branches
- Retromandibular vein
- Lymph nodes

The PS contains the parotid gland, the largest salivary gland in the body. The facial nerve passes through this gland entering through its posterior border and arbitrarily divides the parotid gland into the superficial and deep lobes. The facial nerve divides into five terminal branches within the gland that innervate the muscles of facial expression; however, the parotid does not receive innervation from the VII

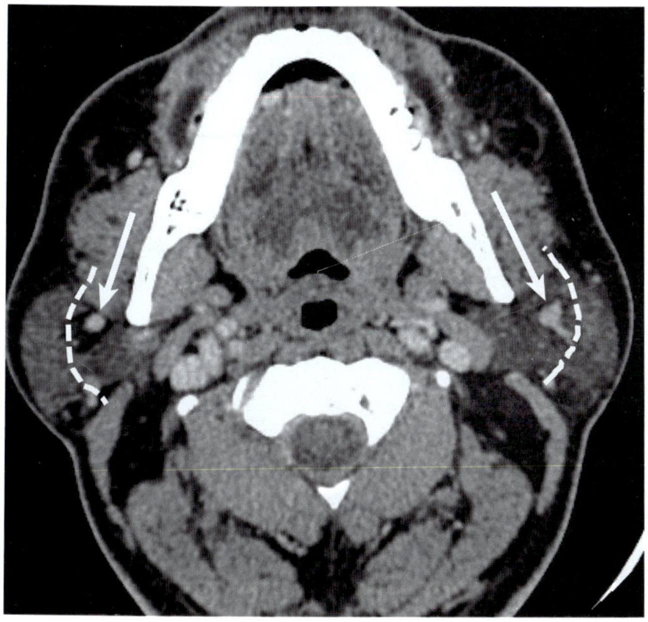

Figure 68.17 Parotid space anatomy. Axial CT shows fatty replacement in the parotid gland. Arrows show the retromandibular veins (RMV) and approximate location of the facial nerve (*curved dashed lines*) lateral to the RMV. The facial nerve divides the gland into a deep lobe (medial) and superficial lobe (lateral).

nerve. The facial nerve is not identified on standard imaging. Hence, the retromandibular vein that passes through the parotid and lies just medial to the facial nerve is used as an imaging landmark to demarcate the superficial from the deep lobe. This information is important as a benign tumor localized only to the superficial lobe requires superficial parotidectomy alone. A line passing along the lateral margin of the retromandibular vein extending up to the posterior belly of digastric approximates the plane of the facial nerve (Fig. 68.17) [9]. The external carotid artery also passes through the parotid gland, and divides into its terminal branches, the superficial temporal and internal maxillary artery. The retromandibular vein is seen lateral to the external carotid artery (Fig. 68.17).

The parotid gland also contains about 20 intraparotid lymph nodes, which receive drainage from the adjacent scalp, cheek, and external auditory canal. This is the only salivary gland to contain lymph nodes within, owing to late encapsulation of the gland embryologically. Lesions of the PS are shown in Table 68.5.

TABLE 68.5 Lesions of the Parotid space

Developmental	*Epithelial cyst* a. First branchial cleft cyst *Vascular anomalies* a. Hemangiomas* (in infants) b. Vascular malformations* ▪ High flow (AVMs and AVFs) ▪ Low flow (venous/lymphatic/mixed malformation)
Infections and inflammatory	a. Parotitis—acute and chronic b. Benign lymphoepithelial lesions in HIV c. Sjogren's syndrome d. Reactive adenopathy e. Sarcoidosis
Benign tumor	a. Benign mixed tumor* b. Warthin tumor* c. Oncocytoma d. Myoepithelioma e. Monomorphic adenoma f. Basal cell adenoma g. Schwannoma/neurofibroma (seventh nerve) h. Lipoma
Malignant tumor	a. Mucoepidermoid carcinoma* b. Adenoid cystic carcinoma* c. Acinic cell carcinoma d. Adenocarcinoma e. Squamous cell carcinoma f. Lymphoma g. Metastases
Pseudolesion	Asymmetric fatty replacement of parotid gland*

*Represents the more common lesions.
AVF, arteriovenous fistula; *AVM*, arteriovenous malformation.

Imaging Methods for PS Lesions

CT, MRI, and USG have nearly completely replaced plain films and sialograms for imaging PS lesions. CT is the technique of choice for inflammatory lesions of the PS. CT is superior for detecting calcifications and calculi within the parotid gland and its ductal system. For evaluation of salivary gland masses, contrast-enhanced MRI is the preferred technique, although CT may also be used. MRI is superior in depicting the perineural and intracranial spread of disease. Diffusion-weighted imaging with apparent diffusion coefficient (ADC) value calculation helps differentiation between benign and malignant tumors. Dynamic contrast enhanced MR imaging is another promising tool to aid differentiation of benign and malignant tumours using time intensity curve pattern of enhancement and washout.

USG can well delineate the pathology of the superficial parotid gland but cannot demonstrate lesions of the deep lobe of the parotid gland. However, USG is a useful technique to evaluate superficial parotid lesions in pregnant women and children. USG is also useful to guide fine needle aspiration cytology/biopsy.

Imaging Features of Common PS Lesions

Developmental Lesions

The imaging features of vascular anomalies have already been discussed in earlier sections. Hemangiomas are the most common salivary gland masses in infants. First BCC is seen within the parotid and around the parotid/external auditory canal region. It appears as a cystic lesion when uncomplicated. When the cyst is infected, enhancing wall thickening and fluid levels may be seen and a sinus tract may be seen up to the external auditory canal [9].

Inflammatory Lesions/Infections

Parotitis or inflammation of the parotid gland may be acute or chronic in nature. Acute parotitis can result from infection or obstruction of the parotid duct due to a calculus. Obstructive causes are not as common in the inflammation of the parotid gland as in the submandibular gland. This is because the submandibular gland has more viscous and alkaline secretions and an uphill course of its duct that predisposes to calculi formation, unlike the parotid gland. Infectious causes include bacteria (*Staphylococcus aureus*), and viruses (*Paramyxovirus*), and uncommonly, *mycobacteria* and *fungi* [10].

Bacterial parotitis predominates in neonates and adults greater than 50 years of age. Bacterial parotitis is usually unilateral, often

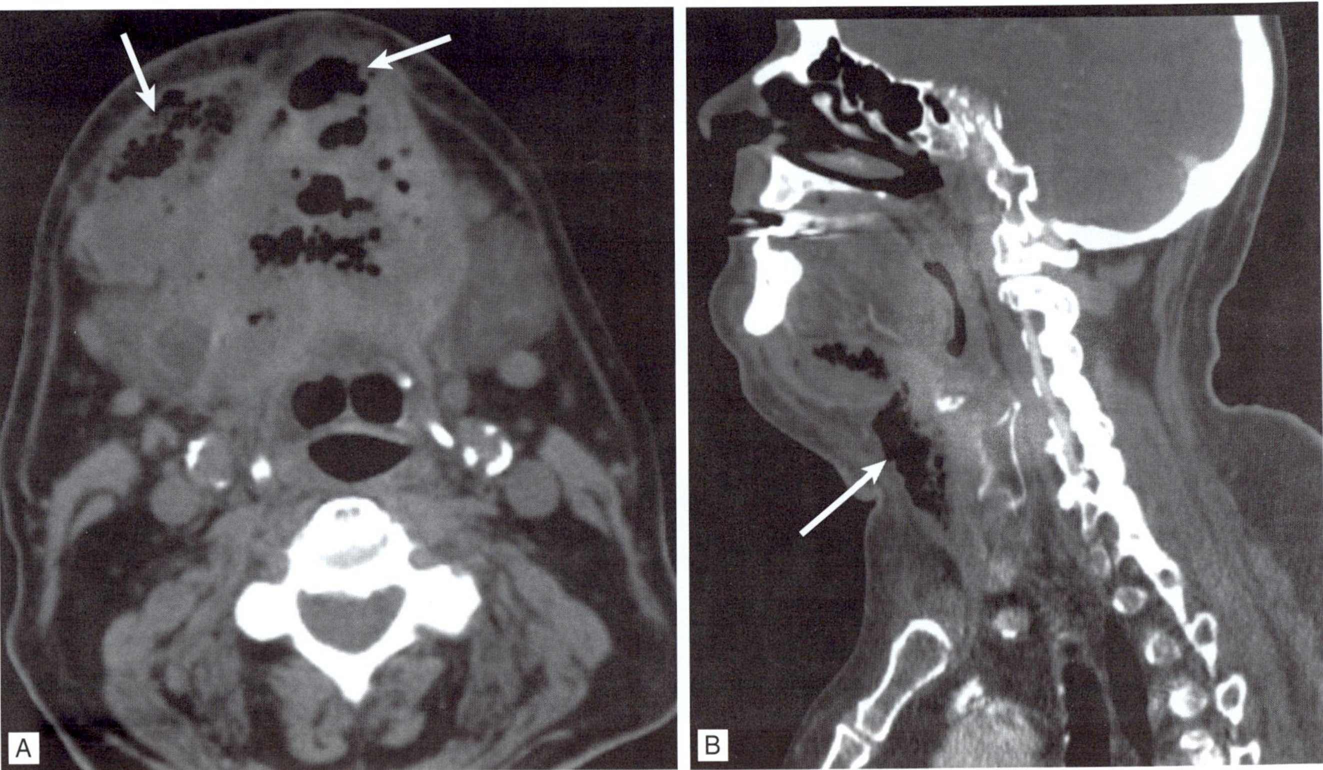

Figure 68.36 Ludwig's angina with necrotizing fasciitis. (A) Axial Contrast enhanced CT shows swelling in the submandibular space with gas formation (*arrows*). (B) Sagittal CT reformation shows extension into the infrahyoid neck (*arrow*). (Courtesy: Suresh K. Mukherji.)

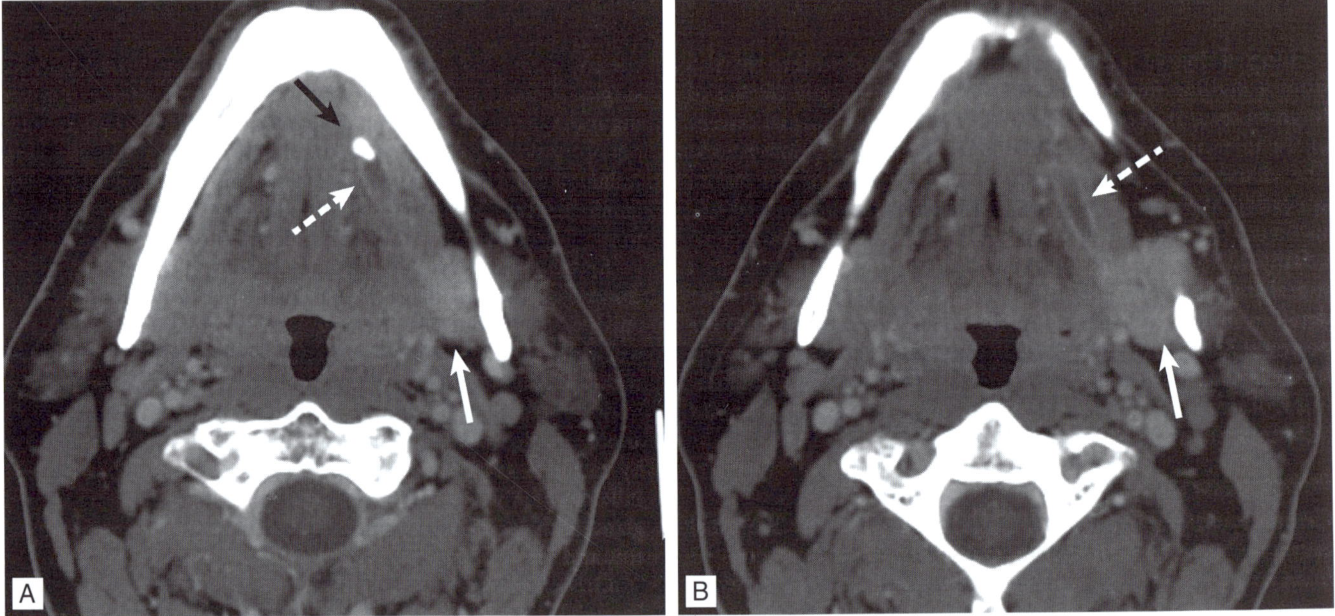

Figure 68.37 Contrast-enhanced axial CT showing sialolith with obstructive sialadenitis. A shows a radiodense calculus in the left Wharton's duct (*black arrow*) with proximal ductal dilatation (*dashed arrows* in A and B). Note the left submandibular gland (*solid white arrows* in A and B) shows increased enhancement and appears enlarged as compared to the right gland. It also shows indistinct medial margins in A; all the above features suggest resultant sialadenitis. (Courtesy: Suresh K. Mukherji.)

submandibular glands that appear homogeneous in signal intensity with low to intermediate T2 signal and homogeneous enhancement. USG examination in Kuttner tumor shows enlarged submandibular glands with a poorly demarcated mass showing increased vascularity (Fig. 68.38). End-stage chronic adult sialadenitis and postradio-iodine therapy sialadenitis show small shrunken glands with low to intermediate T2 signal intensity (due to fibrosis) and ductal ectasia [38].

A common lesion in the SLS is a simple ranula, which is a postinflammatory retention cyst of the sublingual gland and is lined by epithelium. It appears as a unilocular cystic lesion in the SLS and cannot be differentiated from an epidermoid cyst or a

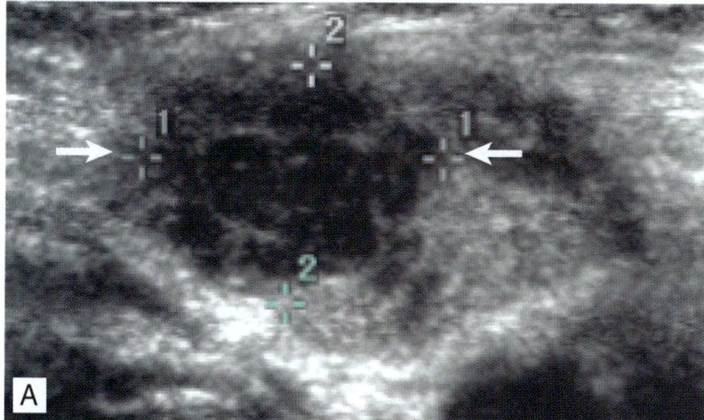

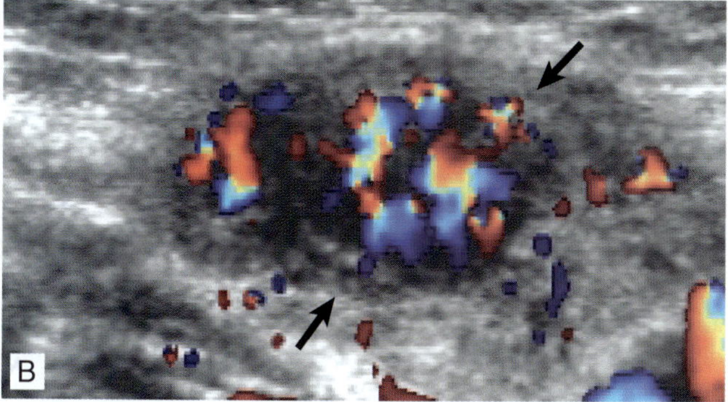

Figure 68.38 Ultrasound (USG) features of Kuttner tumor. (A) Grayscale USG shows poorly marginated hypoechoic mass in the submandibular gland (*arrows*). (B) Color Doppler USG shows increased vascularity seen as increased color signal (*arrows*). (Courtesy: Suresh K. Mukherji.)

unilocular LM (Fig. 68.39A). Infected simple ranulas can appear like abscesses. A simple ranula can rupture if it becomes large and extend posteriorly and inferiorly into the SMS (and even further into the PPS) and is then called a diving or plunging ranula (Fig. 68.39B–D). Once the ranula ruptures, the bulk of it is seen in the SMS (Fig. 68.39B) with a collapsed sublingual portion showing the origin from the SLS and this is called the "tail sign" of the diving ranula (Fig. 68.39C). Diving ranula is not epithelial lined and is a pseudocyst [2].

Tumors

Squamous cell carcinoma is the commonest lesion of the SLS [1] and is an extension from the mucosal component in the dorsum/lateral border of the oral tongue or the mucosa of the base tongue. Contrast-enhanced MRI best shows the complete extent of the tumor. The tumors appear infiltrating with invasion of the neurovascular bundle and spread across the midline (Fig. 68.40). Minor salivary gland tumors of the sublingual gland such as ACC or MEC are rare lesions [2]. Infrequently neurogenic tumors (schwannomas) may be seen arising from the lingual or hypoglossal nerve [1]. They appear well defined with smooth margins, hypovascular, and may show cystic degeneration. Benign pleomorphic adenomas of the sublingual gland are extremely rare with a reported incidence ratio of 1 sublingual tumor to 100 parotid tumors [39].

Tumors of the SMS can be benign or malignant. The benign tumors include lipoma and pleomorphic adenoma (BMT) of the submandibular gland. Pleomorphic adenomas are infrequent with only 8% involving the submandibular gland, while 84% are seen in the parotid [40]. Small tumors are homogeneous with marked enhancement, while larger pleomorphic adenomas appear as well-defined heterogeneous masses involving the submandibular gland and may show delayed enhancement, areas of cystic degeneration and foci of calcification [40].

Malignant tumors of the submandibular gland are rare, the commonest being an ACC [2]. SMS is more likely to be involved by oral tongue squamous cell carcinoma by direct invasion across the mylohyoid muscle. The commonest malignancy of the SMS though is metastatic adenopathy from squamous cell carcinoma of the oral cavity [1]. On imaging, a metastatic node appears enlarged and rounded (rather than ovoid) with increased enhancement on CT (Fig. 68.40) and internal heterogeneity on MRI and the hilum may not be seen. Necrosis when present is the most reliable criterion of metastasis. Presence of ill-defined or indistinct margins suggests extracapsular spread. The other common malignant lesion of the SMS is nodal lymphoma in which multiple enlarged homogenous nodes with well-defined margins are seen not only at level IA and level IB but also at other levels (II–V) bilaterally.

Pseudomass

Occasionally, cranial nerve palsies may cause ipsilateral denervation atrophy that can result in the contralateral side being mistaken for a tumor. Injury to the hypoglossal nerve can cause ipsilateral volume loss of the tongue with fat replacement in the tongue muscles. On imaging, the contralateral normal tongue can be mistaken for a tumor in the SLS. When the mandibular

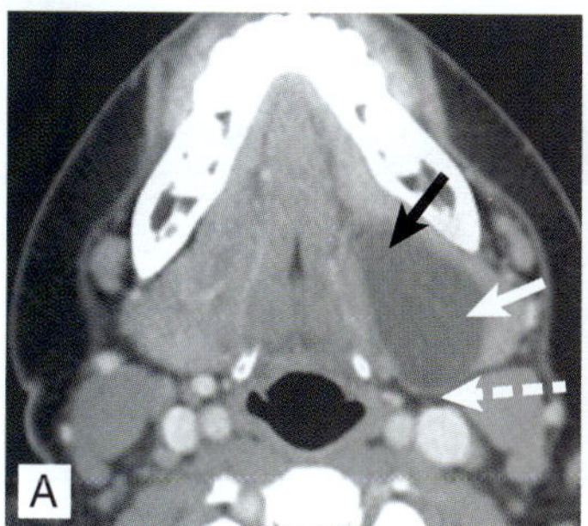

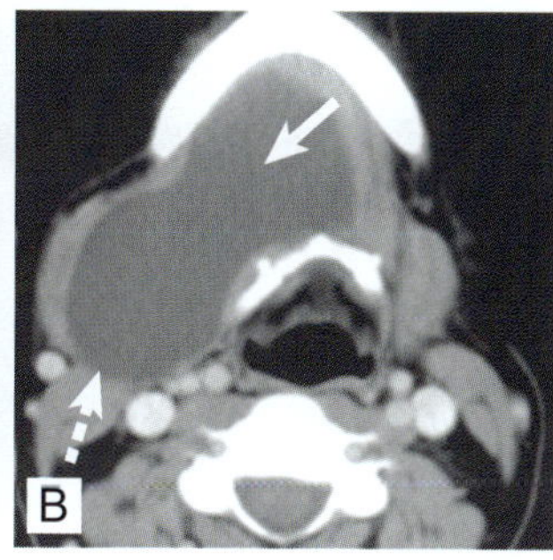

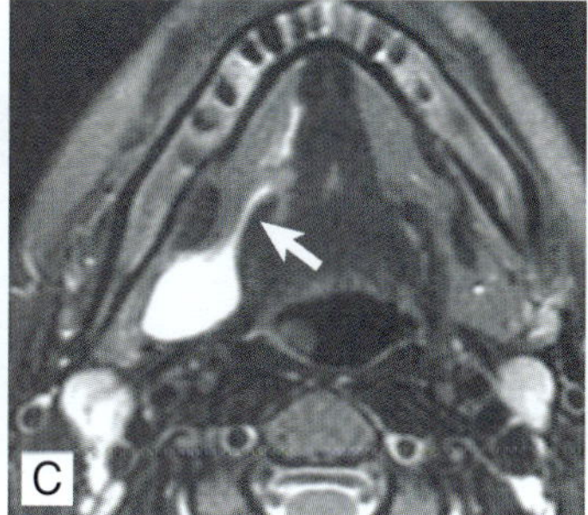

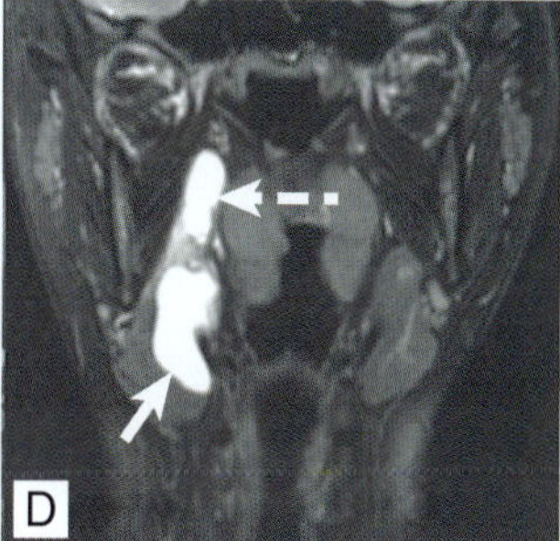

Figure 68.39 Ranula of the sublingual space (SLS) and its extensions into the submandibular space (SMS) and parapharyngeal space (PPS). (A) Contrast enhanced axial CT shows a well-defined unilocular cyst with thin walls (ranula) beginning in the SLS (*black arrow*) with extension into the SMS (*white arrow*) but not reaching the lower limit of PPS (*dashed arrow*). B Diving ranula. The bulk of the cystic lesion is in the SMS (*solid arrow*) and also extends into the adjacent lower PPS (*dashed arrow*). (C) Axial T2W MRI. Arrow shows the collapsed sublingual portion of the diving ranula, demonstrating its origin from the SLS and this is called the "tail sign" of the diving ranula. (D) Coronal T2W MRI shows extension of the diving ranula from the SMS (*solid arrow*) into the PPS (*dashed arrow*). (Courtesy: Suresh K. Mukherji.)

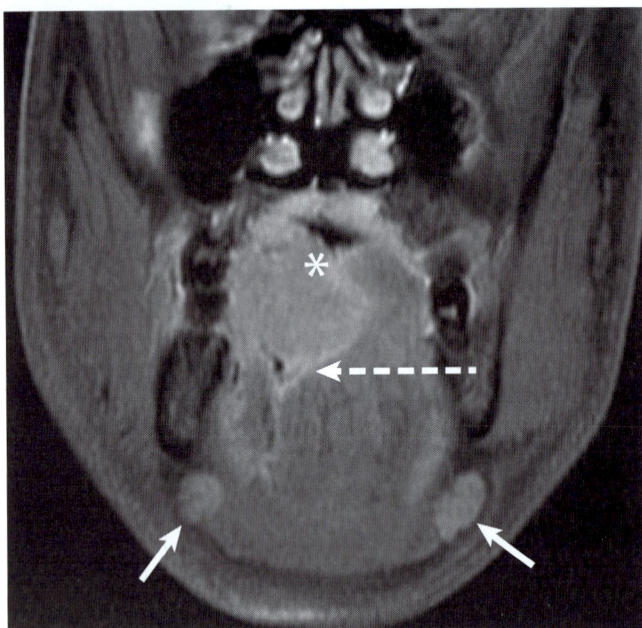

Figure 68.40 Contrast-enhanced coronal MRI shows squamous cell carcinoma (SCC) of the mucosa of the oral tongue with epicenter on the right but crossing midline and showing ulceration in the dorsum (*asterisk*). The SCC is seen reaching inferiorly into the sublingual space and encasing the lingual artery flow void (*dashed arrow*). Solid arrows show bilateral level IB nodes in the submandibular space. The nodes are enlarged, rounded, enhancing, without visible hila and the inferior margin of the left IB node is slightly lobulated. Nodal features suggest metastatic nodes. SCC of the tongue that crosses midline can give rise to contralateral nodal metastases.

division of the trigeminal nerve is injured/invaded by the tumor, the mylohyoid muscle and anterior belly of the digastric supplied by the mylohyoid branch undergo atrophy and fatty infiltration. The contralateral normal nonatrophied muscles should not be mistaken for a tumor [2].

Teaching Points

- A lesion is primary to the SLS if it is seen superomedial to the mylohyoid muscle, while a lesion is primary to the SMS if it is located inferolateral to the muscle
- SLS and SMS communicate with each other along the free posterior edge of the mylohyoid muscle and hence, lesions can extend from the SLS to the SMS. A diving ranula typically extends from the SLS to the SMS
- Primary involvement of the sublingual and submandibular glands by benign and malignant tumors is not very common; secondary invasion by squamous cell carcinoma of the oral cavity is the commonest tumor of the SLS
- A second BCC is the commonest SMS lesion in children while metastatic adenopathy from squamous carcinoma of the oral cavity is the commonest SMS lesion in adults

Conclusion

The neck spaces represent elegant natural barriers while protecting vital structures. For the radiologist too, it is useful to divide the complex region of the neck into various spaces to devise a systematic approach to a neck lesion. Knowledge of the anatomic boundaries and contents of each space helps generate a list of differential diagnoses unique to each space. The characteristic imaging findings and clinical information can help further refine the diagnosis.

Suggested Readings

- SK Mukherji, M Castillo, A simplified approach to the spaces of the suprahyoid neck, Radiol Clin North Am 36 (5) (1998) 761–780.
- AH Baer, HA Parmar, MA DiPietro, SJ Kasten, SK Mukherji, Hemangiomas and vascular malformations of the head and neck: a simplified approach, Neuroimaging Clin 21 (3) (2011) 641–658.
- A Abdullah, FFR Rivas, A Srinivasan, Imaging of the salivary glands, Semin Roentgenol 48 (1) (2013) 65–74.
- S Arya, V Rao, S Juvekar, AK Dcruz, Carotid body tumors: objective criteria to predict the Shamblin group on MR imaging, Am J Neuroradiol 29 (7) (2008) 1349–1354.
- VFH Chong, YF Fan, Radiology of the retropharyngeal space: pictorial review, Clin Radiol 55 (10) (2000) 740.

69 Thyroid and Parathyroids

SNEHA DESHPANDE, ANUJ JAIN, SUPREETA ARYA

THYROID

Introduction

Thyroid lesions are very common, which include focal lesions to generalized parenchymal involvement. Focal lesions range from benign "touch-me-not" lesions to aggressive malignancies with locoregional and distant spread. Accurate characterization of thyroid lesions aids in institution of timely and appropriate treatment. Also, thyroid hormonal imbalance is a major cause of morbidity, ranging from subclinical disease to florid thyroid dysfunction.

Embryology

Thyroid gland consists of two types of cells: thyroxin (T4) and triiodothyronine (T3) producing *follicular cells* and calcitonin producing *parafollicular cells ("C" cells)*. Thyroid follicular cells originate from the median thyroid anlage, which arises during the third week of embryonic development as an endodermal thickening between the first and second pharyngeal arches [1]. This thickening then forms the thyroid bud, a small pit which elongates into a bilobed diverticulum. *It courses anteriorly to the primordial hyoid bone, loops inferiorly and posteriorly to the hyoid (due to rotation and fusion of hyoid anlage) and descends caudally, reaching its anatomical position in the anterior midline infrahyoid neck by the end of seventh week* [1]. A small channel, the thyroglossal duct, temporarily persists as a connection between the pharynx and the caudally migrating thyroid primordium which later involutes. The inferior portion of the thyroglossal duct may differentiate into the pyramidal lobe. The lateral thyroid anlagen, known as the ultimobranchial bodies, arise laterally along the fourth pharyngeal pouch and give rise to parafollicular cells. The lateral anlagen merge with median anlage after descent into the infrahyoid neck [1,2].

Anatomy

Thyroid is an anterior midline neck structure composed of two lobes connected by the isthmus, which crosses the trachea anteriorly at the level of second and third tracheal rings. Thyroid gland and the posteriorly located trachea and esophagus are bound by the pretracheal fascia (part of middle layer of cervical fascia) and located within the visceral space of the neck. Thyroid is bound anteriorly by the sternothyroid and sternohyoid (strap) muscles, superior belly of omohyoid and anterior border of sternocleidomastoid and posterolaterally by the common carotid arteries and internal jugular veins, on either side. Thyroid gland size varies with age, gender, pregnancy, and disease states. Average dimensions of a thyroid lobe are 4–6 cm in height and 1–2 cm in width and thickness [1]. The isthmus varies from 1 to 2 cm in height [1].

Superior thyroid artery which is a branch of external carotid artery and the inferior thyroid artery which is a branch of the thyrocervical trunk provide a rich blood supply to the thyroid gland. In few individuals, there is an additional artery known as the thyroid ima artery which has variable origin, commonly from the aortic arch or brachiocephalic trunk. Venous drainage of thyroid is via the superior, middle, and inferior thyroid veins.

Imaging Methods

Ultrasonography (USG)

USG is a noninvasive, nonionizing widely available tool with high sensitivity and spatial resolution for thyroid evaluation. Also, superficial location of the thyroid gland makes it easily accessible to USG. Hence, USG is the first radiological investigation of choice in all suspected thyroid lesions [3]. All patients are scanned in supine position with hyperextended neck, using a high-frequency linear-array transducer and both, grayscale and color Doppler imaging (CDI) techniques are used. On USG, normal thyroid appears homogenous with a medium to high-level echogenicity with an echogenic thin capsule.

According to the American Thyroid Association (ATA) 2015 guidelines, USG with survey of the cervical lymph nodes should be performed in all patients with known or suspected thyroid nodules (strong recommendation, high-quality evidence), to confirm the presence, to localize, to accurately measure and characterize the lesion/s; thus assess the risk of malignancy and guide fine-needle aspiration (FNA) from suspicious thyroid nodules [3]. USG also helps to differentiate thyroid nodules from other cervical masses. In thyroid malignancies, preoperative USG is required to assess the status of the contralateral lobe and detect suspicious cervical lymphadenopathy while postoperative USG is indicated to detect residual or recurrent disease in the thyroid bed or the lymph nodes. USG is used to screen high-risk patients for thyroid malignancy with history of multiple endocrine neoplasia (MEN) type II, familial thyroid cancer, and neck irradiation in childhood. USG helps in assessing gland size, parenchymal echotexture, and vascularity in diffuse thyroid diseases. USG is also the initial technique of choice for evaluation of congenital neck masses, suspected to be of thyroid origin. USG is the technique of choice to evaluate thyroid incidentalomas (TI) seen on other imaging techniques.

Computed tomography (CT) and magnetic resonance imaging (MRI)

Normal thyroid appears hyperdense to adjacent muscles on CT, due to high intrinsic iodine content. On contrast-enhanced CT, it shows homogenous avid enhancement. On MRI, thyroid appears isointense to mildly hyperintense on T1-weighted images (T1WI), mildly hyperintense on T2-weighted images (T2WI), and shows homogenous avid enhancement on gadolinium-enhanced MR.

According to the ATA 2015 guidelines, use of cross-sectional imaging studies (CT, MRI) with intravenous contrast is recommended as an adjunct to USG in (a) assessment of the extent of advanced thyroid malignancies including invasive primary tumor, (b) clinically suspected multiple or bulky cervical lymph nodes to look for involvement of atypical lymph node stations and extra-nodal spread, and (c) clinically suspected distant metastases (Fig. 69.1) [3]. The initial nodal metastases from thyroid malignancy are to the central compartment nodes, level VI and VII (which include pretracheal, paratracheal, prelaryngeal/Delphian nodes, or upper mediastinal nodes). It can also metastasize to lateral compartment lymph nodes (level I–V). A peculiar metastatic spread may also occur to the retropharyngeal nodes (Fig. 69.2). Cross-sectional imaging has limited role in diffuse thyroid diseases, except in more extensive forms like Riedel's thyroiditis (RT) or acute suppurative thyroiditis. Congenital thyroid abnormalities like ectopic thyroid or thyroglossal duct cysts (TDCs), are often evaluated with CT or MRI to confirm the diagnosis, assess the extent, and associated complications.

Scintigraphy

Radionuclide scan/scintigraphy produces a visual display of functional thyroid tissue by selective uptake of injected radionuclides, thus providing both, anatomical and functional information. *It has an essential role in evaluating clinically suspected thyroid nodule with low serum thyrotropin (TSH) levels (seen in hyperfunctioning or "hot" nodule)* [3]. Other common clinical indications include evaluation of thyrotoxicosis to differentiate diffuse thyroid disease and toxic nodule/s and congenital thyroid disorders. Due to easy availability, low cost, less radiation exposure, and good imaging characteristics, Tc99m pertechnetate is the most commonly used radiopharmaceutical. Tc99m pertechnetate is trapped by thyroid

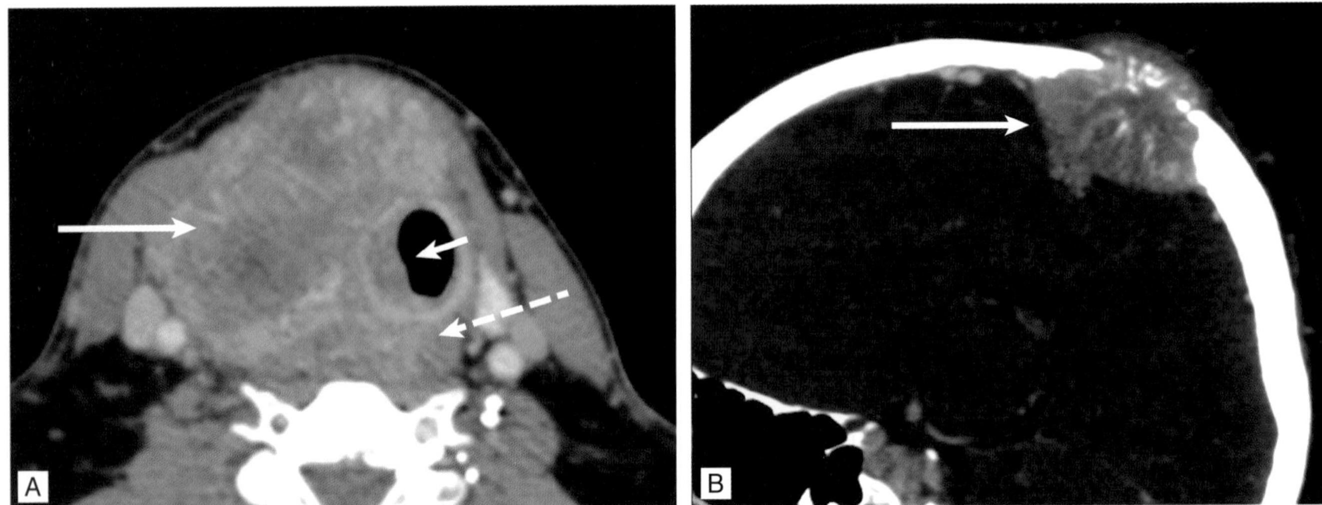

Figure 69.1 Invasive thyroid carcinoma. (A) Axial postcontrast CT image showing heterogeneously enhancing mass in the right thyroid lobe and isthmus (*long solid arrow*) with extrathyroidal extension, tracheal invasion (*short solid arrow*), and esophageal infiltration (*dashed arrow*). (B) Sagittal postcontrast CT brain showing an osseous calvarial lesion with associated soft tissue (*long solid arrow*) suggestive of osseous metastases.

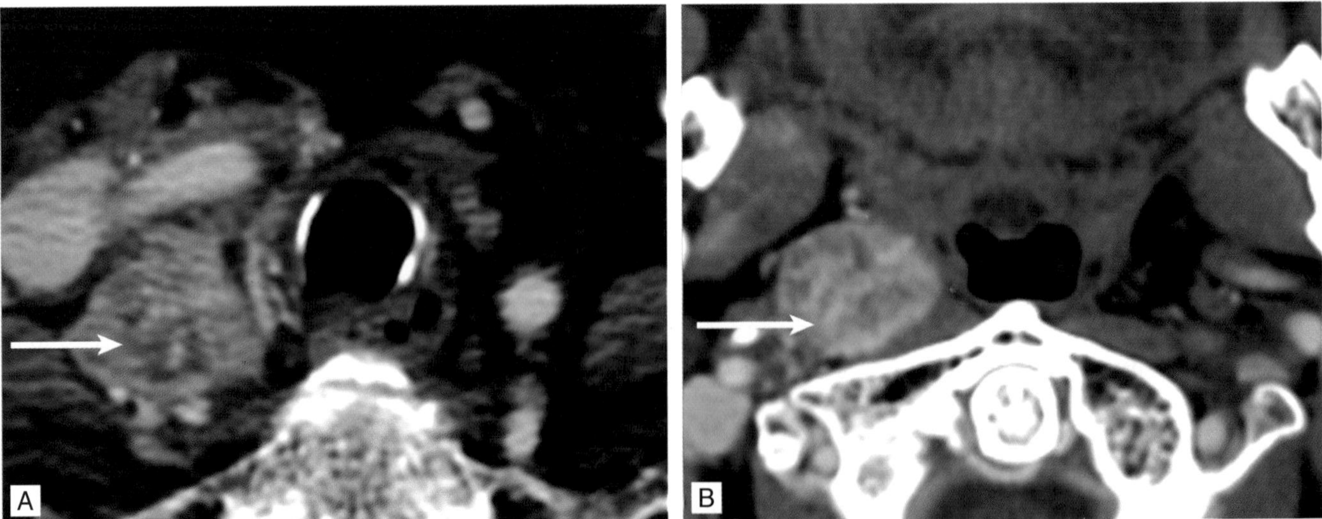

Figure 69.2 Papillary thyroid carcinoma with retropharyngeal nodal metastasis. (A) Axial postcontrast CT image showing a heterogeneously enhancing lesion in the lower pole of the right thyroid lobe (*arrow*). (B) Axial postcontrast CT image showing a heterogeneously enhancing enlarged right retropharyngeal node (*arrow*).

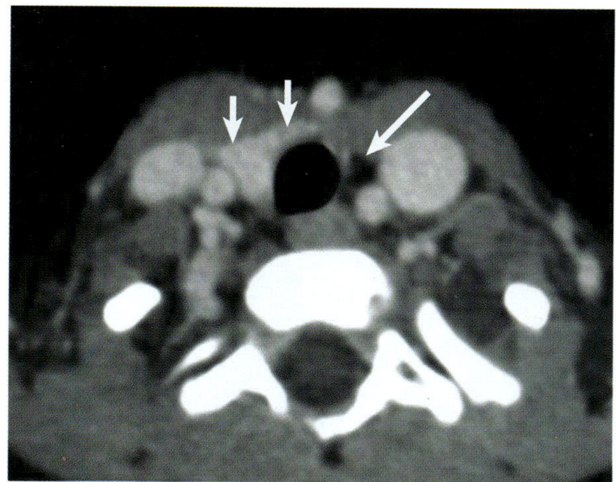

Figure 69.3 Axial postcontrast CT image showing left thyroid lobe agenesis (*long arrow*) with normal right thyroid lobe and isthmus (*short arrows*).

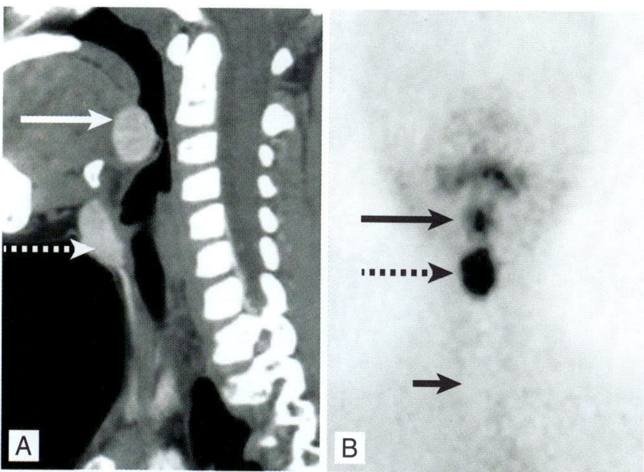

Figure 69.4 Ectopic thyroid (dual ectopia). (A) Sagittal reformation CT image showing homogenously enhancing well-defined ectopic thyroid tissue at the base of the tongue (*solid white arrow*) and adjacent to hyoid bone in infrahyoid location (*dashed white arrow*). (B) Radionuclide thyroid scan shows functioning thyroid tissue in these corresponding regions (*black long solid arrow* and *dashed black arrow*, respectively) with no functioning thyroid tissue in thyroid bed (*short black solid arrow*).

gland in an identical manner as iodide, but is not organified or incorporated into thyroid hormone. Thyroid image is acquired after 20–30 minutes of intravenous injection of 3–5 mCi of Tc99m pertechnetate, which shows uptake in the thyroid gland along with some normal uptake in salivary glands and oral cavity. The other radiopharmaceuticals for thyroid scintigraphy are I^{131} and I^{123}. Due to high radiation dose, clinical use of I^{131} is largely limited to the postoperative therapeutic and whole-body diagnostic scanning of differentiated thyroid carcinoma (DTC). I^{123}, if available, can be used in place of Tc99m pertechnetate and I^{131}.

Positron Emission Tomography/Computed Tomography (PET/CT)

Use of 18F-fluoro-2-deoxyglucose (18F-FDG)-PET/CT and other PET tracers in the evaluation of thyroid disorders is limited. ATA guidelines state that use of 18F-FDG-PET/CT for routine evaluation of nodules suspicious for malignancy on USG or for staging of diagnosed DTC is not recommended [3]. It is however recommended for staging of anaplastic carcinomas [4]. An incidentally detected focal uptake in the thyroid, seen on a PET scan is suspicious for malignancy [3]. Diffuse PET uptake in a thyroid is usually inflammatory, especially if USG too is corroborative.

Pathology

Thyroid Dysgenesis

Congenital developmental defects of the thyroid gland like aplasia (absent gland), hypoplasia (small gland), hemiagenesis (absent lobe; Fig. 69.3), and ectopia (abnormal location) are collectively called thyroid dysgenesis.

Ectopic Thyroid Tissue

Stalled migration at any stage of the migratory path of the thyroid during embryological development or erroneous migratory course can lead to variant locations of thyroid tissue [5]. *Thyroid ectopia is commonly seen at: (1) the base of the tongue, being the most common site; (2) adjacent to the hyoid bone; (3) the midline infrahyoid portion of the neck* [2]. Ectopic thyroid tissue has rarely been reported in locations such as the lateral part of the neck, pharynx, esophagus, trachea, mediastinum, heart, lungs, breast, adrenal glands, bowel, and ovaries [2,5].

Ectopic thyroid tissue appears identical to the native thyroid gland on all imaging techniques, except the characteristic shape. *It may show parenchymal nodules and can develop any of the abnormalities akin to thyroid gland, including malignancy.* Orthotopic thyroid tissue is absent in 70–80% of the cases [2,5]. USG demonstrates absent orthotopic thyroid tissue and may indicate presence of ectopic thyroid. Ectopic thyroid is often evaluated with CT or MRI to confirm diagnosis and evaluate complications. Radionuclide scans are usually confirmatory to demonstrate ectopic thyroid tissue and absence of functioning orthotopic thyroid tissue (Fig. 69.4).

Thyroglossal Duct Cyst (TDC)

TDC is the most common congenital neck mass, which results from remnants of the thyroglossal duct, anywhere along its course and may be associated with ectopic thyroid tissue [2,6]. It manifests usually in childhood as gradually increasing painless neck swelling which moves with deglutition and tongue protrusion. It may present in infrahyoid, suprahyoid or juxtahyoid and rarely intralingual locations [6]. Suprahyoid TDCs are usually midline, while infrahyoid TDCs may be paramedian in location, usually deeply embedded within or splaying the strap muscles.

Preoperative imaging is performed to identify the anatomic extent of the cyst, identify ectopic thyroid tissue, and evaluate for potential malignancy within the cyst. USG reveals a well-circumscribed anechoic cyst with posterior enhancement, with some internal debris due to proteinaceous contents and may sometimes show a pseudo-solid echogenic pattern. At CT, TDCs are seen as thin-walled well-circumscribed lesions with fluid attenuation or may sometimes show higher attenuation (Fig. 69.5). At MR imaging, they appear hypointense to isointense on T1WI and hyperintense on T2WI. Infected TDCs may show thick enhancing wall and internal septations on CT and MRI. Fistula may develop in cases of external cyst rupture, recurrence after resection, or may rarely be congenital. Malignancy in TDCs is rare; most common type being papillary carcinoma. Imaging features which warrant evaluation for malignancy are enhancing wall nodularity and calcification (Fig. 69.5).

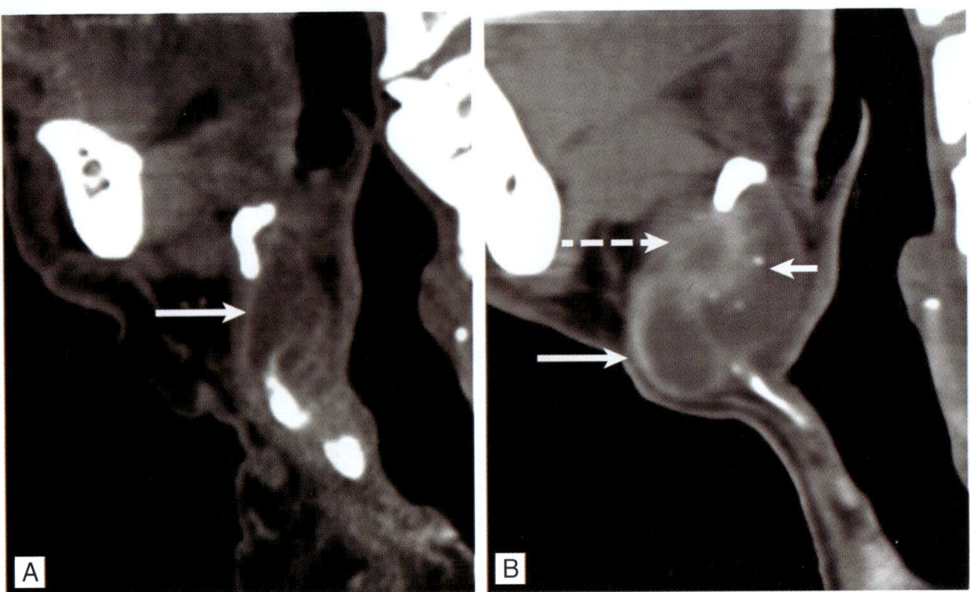

Figure 69.5 (A) Sagittal reformation CT image showing a well-defined thin-walled fluid density cystic lesion (*arrow*) in the juxtahyoid location reaching the posterior aspect of the hyoid bone suggesting a thyroglossal duct cyst (TDC). (B) Sagittal reformation CT image showing a juxtahyoid TDC (*long solid arrow*) with enhancing solid mural nodule (*dashed arrow*) and multiple foci of calcifications (*short solid arrow*). A case of papillary carcinoma in TDC.

Pearls

- Ectopic thyroid and TDC are common differentials of anterior neck masses presenting in children and young adults
- Typical location along the line of decent of thyroid primordium and characteristic imaging features clinch the diagnosis

Focal Thyroid Lesions/Thyroid Nodules

A thyroid nodule is defined by the ATA as "*a discrete lesion within the thyroid gland that is radiologically distinct from the surrounding thyroid parenchyma*" [3]. Thyroid nodules can be completely asymptomatic, may present with hormonal imbalance, compressive symptoms due to mass effect, or may harbor malignancy.

During the initial evaluation of a patient with a clinically suspected thyroid nodule, serum TSH is measured [3]. If the serum TSH is subnormal (hyperthyroidism), the ATA guidelines recommend a radionuclide thyroid scan to assess whether the nodule is hyperfunctioning ("hot"), isofunctioning ("warm"), or nonfunctioning ("cold") [3]. Hyperfunctioning nodules rarely harbor malignancy, and hence, no cytologic evaluation is recommended. In all patients with nodularity detected on thyroid scintigraphy, USG should be performed to confirm the presence of nodules corresponding to the hyperfunctioning areas on the scan and to evaluate other "warm" and "cold" nodules. In patients where the serum TSH is normal or elevated, a radionuclide scan should not be performed. Instead, USG of the thyroid and neck nodes is recommended in all such patients, as elevated serum TSH level is associated with increased risk of malignancy in a thyroid nodule, as well as a more advanced stage of thyroid cancer [3].

Thyroid nodules can be benign or malignant, with the incidence of benign nodules being significantly higher than malignancies. Various benign pathologies affect thyroid gland, like benign follicular nodules, follicular adenomas, or focal thyroiditis [7]. The malignant pathologies affecting thyroid are papillary thyroid carcinomas (PTCs) and follicular thyroid carcinomas (FTCs), which together are called differentiated thyroid malignancies (DTCs), medullary and anaplastic carcinomas, lymphomas, and metastases [7]. However, due to the high incidence of thyroid nodules, low incidence of thyroid malignancy, patient anxiety, and economic point of view, it is not feasible to biopsy every thyroid nodule. Hence, recommendations have been put forth by numerous committees for risk stratification and management decision making. One of them is the Thyroid Imaging Reporting and Data System (TI-RADS), which has several versions, the most widely used being that put forth by American College of Radiology (ACR).

ACR TI-RADS

ACR TI-RADS is based on the evaluation of USG features of thyroid nodules in five lexicon categories—composition, echogenicity, margin, shape, and echogenic foci (Table 69.1) [8]. Features in the first category (composition) are assigned 0–2 points while that in the other four categories are assigned 0–3 points, with more suspicious features awarded more points. When evaluating a thyroid nodule, one feature is selected from each of the first four categories, and all the features that are applicable to the nodule are selected from the fifth category (echogenic foci). The total score, which is a sum of points assigned to all five categories, determines the ACR-TIRADS risk level (TR level) of the nodule, and the nodule is categorized as benign (TR1), not suspicious (TR2), mildly suspicious (TR3), moderately suspicious (TR4), or highly suspicious for malignancy (TR5). TR level in conjunction with the maximum nodule diameter dictates the management recommendations, like FNA, follow-up USG, or no further action [8]. ACR TI-RADS recommends reporting up to four thyroid nodules with the highest TR level [8,9]. Associated suspicious cervical lymphadenopathy or distant metastases suspected to be of thyroid origin are important factors guiding the decision to sample a thyroid nodule, irrespective of the size. The USG evaluation of each of these ACR-TIRADS lexicon categories is discussed below.

Composition: *According to ACR-TIRADS, the composition of a thyroid nodule is classified as cystic or almost completely cystic*

TABLE 69.1 **USG Evaluation of a Thyroid Nodule According to ACR-TIRADS**

ACR TIRADS				
Composition (Choose Any 1)	**Echogenicity (Choose Any 1)**	**Margins (Choose Any 1)**	**Shape (Choose Any 1)**	**Echogenic Foci (Choose All Features That Apply)**
Cystic or almost completely cystic: 0 points Spongiform: 0 points Mixed solid-cystic: 1 point Solid or almost completely solid: 2 points	Anechoic: 0 points Iso or hyperechoic: 1 point Hypoechoic: 2 points Very hypoechoic: 3 points	Smooth: 0 points Ill-defined: 0 points Lobulated/irregular: 2 points Extrathyroidal extension: 3 points	Wider-than-tall: 0 points Taller-than-wide: 3 points	None or large comet-tail artifacts: 0 points Macrocalcifications: 1 point Peripheral (rim) calcifications: 2 points Punctate echogenic foci: 3 points
Sum of Points Assigned to All Five Categories				
0 points	2 points	3 points	4–6 points	7 points or more
TR1 Benign	TR2 Not suspicious	TR3 Mildly suspicious	TR4 Moderately suspicious	TR5 Highly suspicious
No FNA required	No FNA required	FNA if ≥2.5 cm Follow if ≥1.5 cm	FNA if ≥1.5 cm Follow if ≥1 cm	FNA if ≥1 cm Follow if ≥0.5 cm

Adapted from ACR-TIRADS White Paper 2017 [8].

(0 points), spongiform (0 points), mixed solid-cystic (1 point), and solid or almost completely solid (2 points) [8]. Purely cystic or almost completely cystic lesions are highly likely to be benign [3]. As per the ACR TIRADS lexicon, a "spongiform" appearance of a thyroid nodule, defined as the aggregation of multiple microcystic components in more than 50% of the volume of the nodule, is strongly correlated with benignancy (Fig. 69.6) [3,8,9]. Majority (82–91%) of thyroid cancers are solid or almost completely solid [3]. Solid nodule that contains minimal cystic component, which occupies no more than approximately 5% of the overall volume, should be classified as "almost completely solid" and is given similar points as a solid nodule [9]. Also, nodules with dense shadowing calcifications that preclude assessment of their composition are assumed to be solid [8,9]. If nodule contains both solid and cystic components, it is classified as a mixed solid-cystic nodule and the appearance of the solid component with the nodule's maximum dimension, determines management (Fig. 69.6) [3,9]. The features of a solid-cystic thyroid nodule, which are suspicious for malignancy, are an eccentric hypoechoic solid component forming an acute angle with the cyst wall, microcalcifications, irregular margins, and extrathyroidal spread [3,9]. Lobulated margins and increased vascularity in the solid component are suspicious features, though less robust [3].

Echogenicity: *According to ACR-TIRADS, echogenicity of a nodule is classified as anechoic (0 points), iso or hyperechoic (1 point), hypoechoic (2 points), or very hypoechoic (3 points)* [8]. Anechoic nodules represent cystic or almost completely cystic nodules. Isoechoic or hyperechoic solid nodules (Fig. 69.7) prompt low suspicion for malignancy since only approximately 15–20% of thyroid cancers

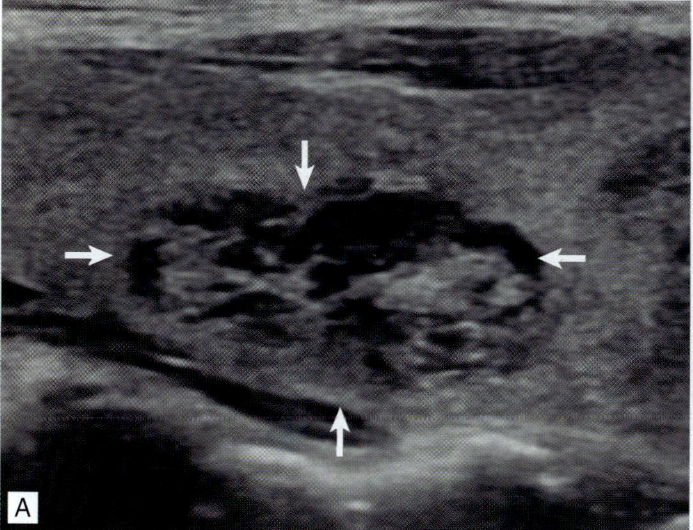

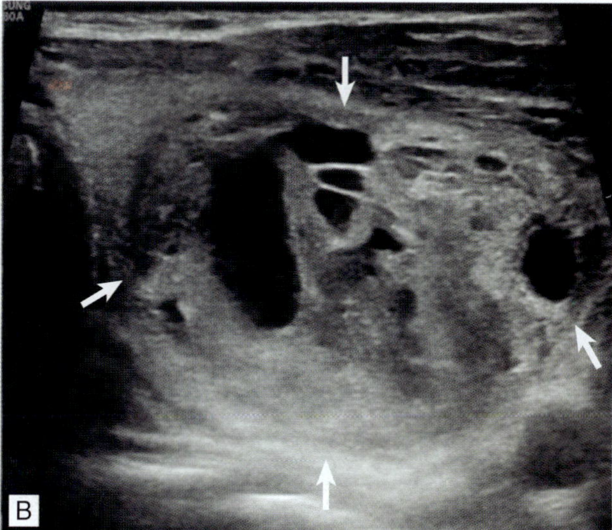

Figure 69.6 USG image showing: (A) A well-defined nodule (*arrows*) with smooth margins and aggregation of multiple microcysts in the entire nodule which suggests a "Spongiform nodule." (B) A well-defined mixed solid-cystic nodule (*arrows*) in the left thyroid lobe with isoechoic solid component, shows smooth margins, wider-than-tall shape and no echogenic foci. The nodule was assigned a total of 2 points (TR2).

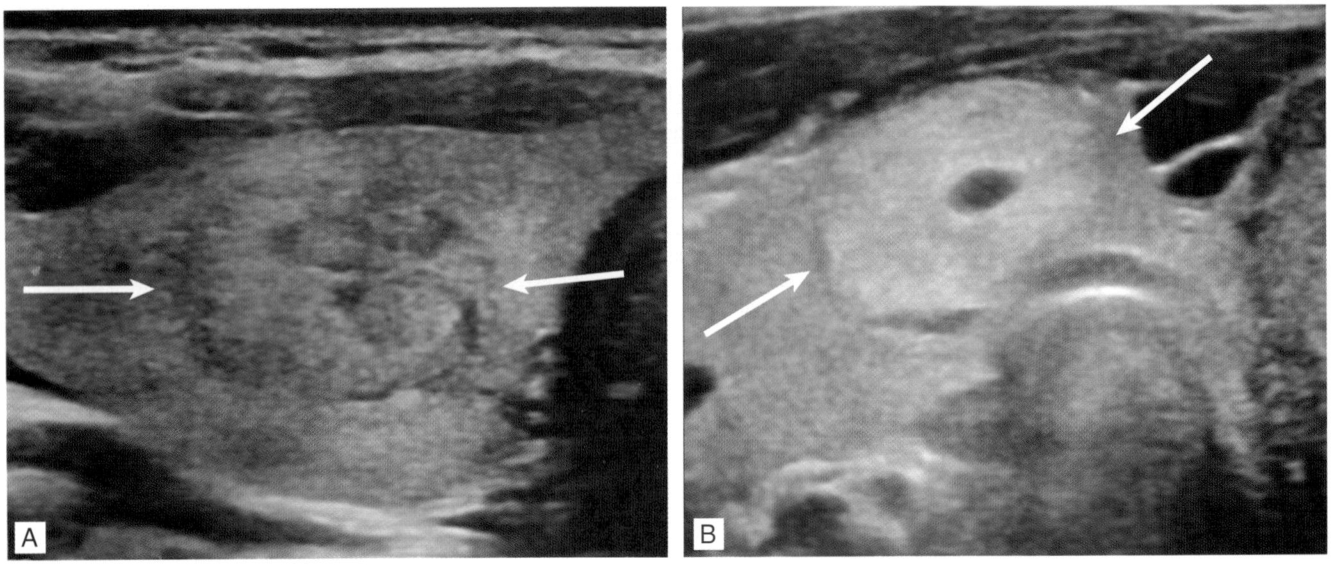

Figure 69.7 USG image showing almost completely solid nodules (<5% cystic component) (*arrows*) (A) isoechoic nodule (B) hyperechoic nodule, both showing smooth margins, wider-than-tall shape and no echogenic foci. The nodules were assigned a total of 3 points each (TR3).

are iso- or hyperechoic, and are generally the FTCs or follicular variant of PTCs [3]. Nodules that are less reflective than the adjacent thyroid parenchyma are classified as hypoechoic, while those that are less reflective than the strap muscles are classified as very hypoechoic (Fig. 69.8) [8,9]. Mixed echogenicity nodules are assessed based on the predominant echogenicity, and described as predominantly hypoechoic, isoechoic, or hyperechoic [8]. If dense calcification precludes the assessment of a nodule's echogenicity, it is assumed to be at least isoechoic or hyperechoic and is assigned 1 point [9].

Margins: *Margin of a nodule constitutes its interface with intra- or extrathyroidal tissue, and according to ACR-TIRADS, it is classified as smooth (0 points), ill-defined (0 points), lobulated/irregular (2 points), or extrathyroidal extension (3 points)* [8]. Smooth margin is characterized by a well-defined regular sharp curvilinear border (Figs. 69.6 and 69.7). It is generally observed in benign thyroid nodules; however, some malignancies may also show smooth margins. The nodule margin is characterized as ill-defined if more than 50% of its margin is not clearly depicted on imaging or demarcated from the adjacent parenchyma; and is not considered a discriminatory feature [9,10]. Lobulated or irregular margins, defined as infiltrative, microlobulated, angulated, or spiculated interface, which suggests infiltration of the nodule's solid component into the adjacent normal thyroid parenchyma; are highly suspicious of malignancy (Fig. 69.8). Extrathyroidal extension is characterized by invasion of adjacent structures and is unequivocally suggestive of malignancy.

Shape: Shape of a nodule refers to the relationship of the nodule's anteroposterior dimension and transverse dimension on an axial image. *According to ACR-TIRADS, it is classified as wider-than-tall (0 points) or taller-than-wide (3 points)* [8]. The "taller-than-wide" appearance of a malignant thyroid nodule implies that the nodule has violated tissue planes (Fig. 69.9). Nodules that are perfectly round are reported as either wider-than-tall or not taller-than-wide [9].

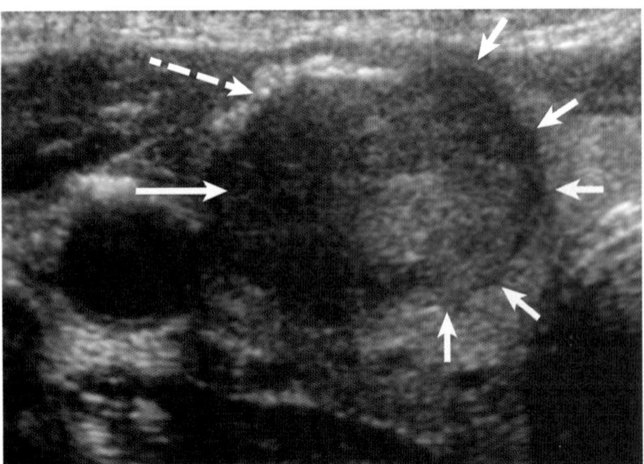

Figure 69.8 A solid very hypoechoic nodule (*long solid arrow*) in the right thyroid lobe with lobulated margins (*short solid arrows*), wider-than-tall shape and with peripheral calcification (*dashed arrow*) causing posterior shadowing. The nodule was assigned a total of 9 points (TR5). Histopathology was suggestive of follicular carcinoma.

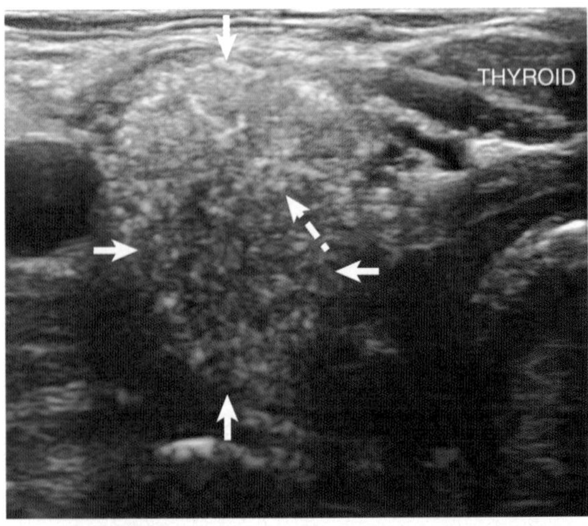

Figure 69.9 Papillary thyroid carcinoma. USG image showing a solid hypoechoic nodule (*solid arrows*) in the right thyroid lobe with taller-than-wide shape and multiple punctate echogenic foci (microcalcifications), one of which is shown by the *dashed arrow*.

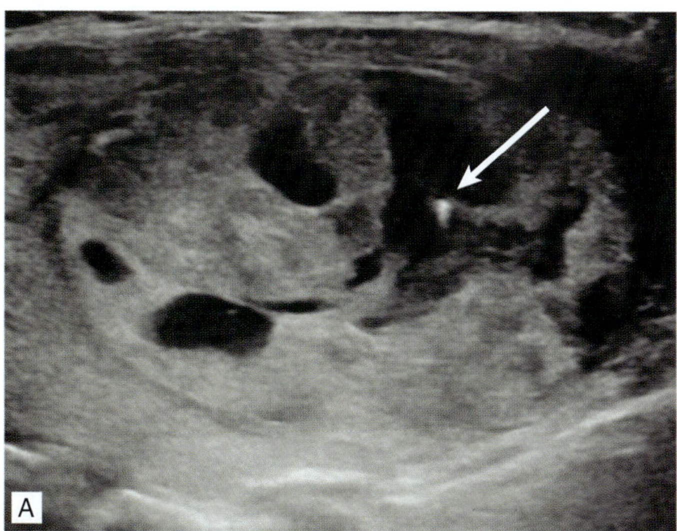

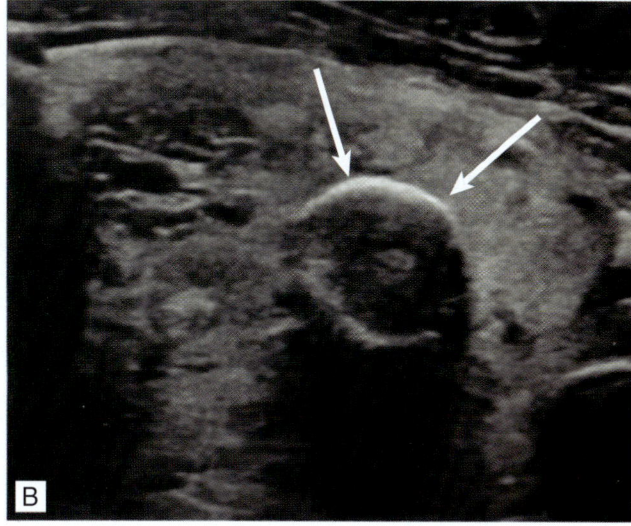

Figure 69.10 USG image showing: (A) Mixed solid-cystic nodule with "large comet-tail artifact" (*arrow*). (B) A nodule with rim calcification (*arrows*) leading to posterior shadowing which precludes evaluation of the nodule.

Echogenic Foci: *According to ACR-TIRADS, thyroid calcifications are classified as none or large comet-tail artifacts (0 points), macrocalcifications (1 point), peripheral (rim) calcifications (2 points), or punctate echogenic foci (PEFs) (3 points)* [8]. ACR-TIRADS classifies comet-tail artifacts as small and large comet-tail artifacts; with "large comet-tail artifacts" defined as "echogenic foci with V-shaped echoes more than 1 mm deep to them" (Fig. 69.10) [8]. These are usually associated with colloid and seen in benign nodules [10]. Macrocalcifications appear as large irregularly shaped echogenic foci with posterior shadowing (Fig. 69.11). These are areas of dystrophic calcifications which are postulated to be secondary to tissue necrosis [10]. They are commonly seen in benign diseases like multinodular goiter (MNG); however, when noted in solitary thyroid nodules, they may be associated with a high rate of malignancy. Peripheral (rim) calcifications deter detailed evaluation of a thyroid nodule due to dense posterior shadowing (Fig. 69.10). This type of calcification may be seen in malignancy or benign MNG. Focal interruption of peripheral calcification with extrusion of soft tissue through it is considered a highly sensitive sign of malignancy [8]. PEFs, often termed as microcalcifications, are discrete and nonshadowing, and may represent psammoma bodies, which are 10–100 μm round laminar crystalline calcific deposits [9,10]. They are highly suspicious of malignancy, mainly PTCs (Figs. 69.9 and 69.12). This category (PEF) also includes the "small comet-tail artifacts" mentioned earlier. PEF may rarely be seen in spongiform nodules, which represent back walls of minute cysts and are not suspicious [8].

Measurement of Nodule Size

ACR TI-RADS recommends measuring a nodule in three axes: Maximum dimension in axial image, longest dimension perpendicular to the previous measurement on same image, and the maximum craniocaudal dimension on a sagittal image [8,9].

Growth

ACR TI-RADS and ATA guidelines define clinically significant growth as a 20% increase in at least two nodule dimensions with a minimal increase of 2 mm, or greater than 50% increase in volume [8,9]. Nodules that do not grow significantly over a

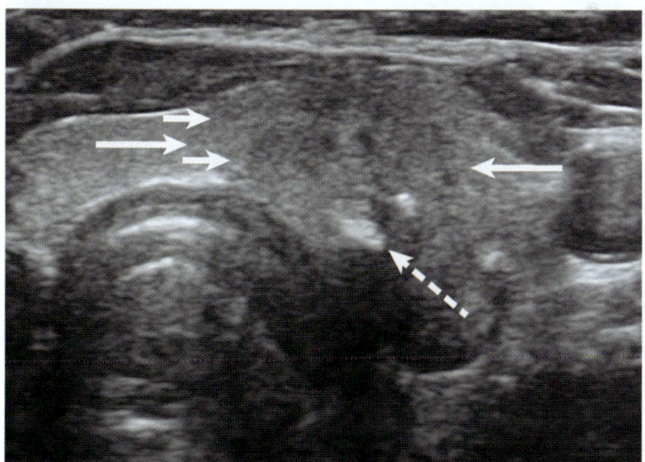

Figure 69.11 Medullary thyroid carcinoma. USG image showing a solid hypoechoic nodule (*long arrows*) in the left thyroid lobe with irregular margins (*short arrows*) and macrocalcifications (*dashed arrow*).

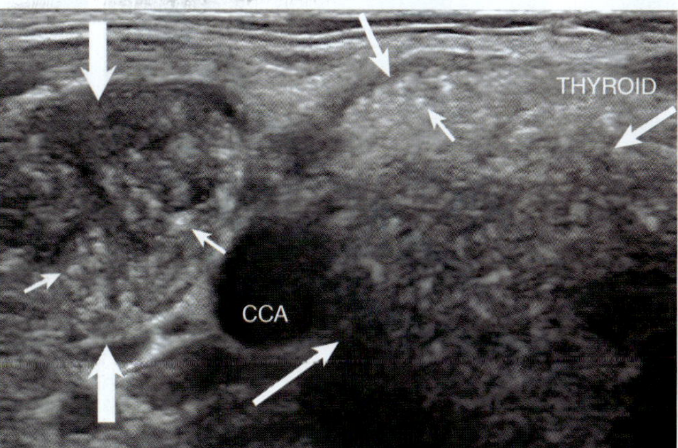

Figure 69.12 Papillary thyroid carcinoma. USG image showing a solid hypoechoic nodule (*long thin arrows*) in the right thyroid lobe associated with an enlarged right level IV lymph node (*block arrows*), both showing punctate echogenic foci/microcalcifications (*short arrows*).

period of 5 years may be considered benign [8]. Rapid growth is suspicious of malignancy; however, it does not reliably distinguish between benign and malignant nodules.

There are other features not included in ACR-TI-RADS. These are discussed below.

Perinodular Halo

The "halo" around a thyroid nodule represents the nodule capsule or pseudocapsule formed by compressed thyroid parenchyma and chronic inflammatory infiltrates. A completely uniform perinodular halo is frequently associated with benign nodules; however, it is not highly specific and may be found in neoplasms [8].

Nodular Vascularity

CDI detects intranodular or perinodular vascularity, with marked intranodular flow being the most common pattern of vascularity in malignancy [10]. Perinodular flow, which is defined as the presence of vascularity around at least 25% of the circumference of a nodule, is more likely to be seen in a benign thyroid nodule [10]. However, these findings have low specificity due to significant overlap [10]. Complete absence of vascularity is a more reliable sign of benignancy.

USG Elastography

USG elastography (USGE) is a noninvasive technique, which measures "tissue stiffness"; usually performed as an extension of conventional USG evaluation in focal thyroid nodules. Two types of USGE techniques are used, "strain elastography" and "shear wave elastography." Malignant thyroid tissue is usually firmer than a benign nodule or normal thyroid parenchyma. USGE is a promising cancer-risk stratification tool; however, its performance is highly variable and operator dependent. Also, USGE can only be effectively applied to solid nodules. Obesity, MNGs with overlapping or coalescent nodules and posteriorly or inferiorly located nodules pose difficulty in optimal evaluation. *Thus, ATA does not presently recommend its universal use or widespread adoption, neither is it incorporated in ACR-TIRADS assessment* [3,8]. USE may be performed when available and in patients in whom accurate assessment is feasible; however, its results should not modify the recommendations for traditional USG.

Pearls

- Morphological features and size of a focal thyroid nodule together dictate management decision
- Solid composition, hypoechoic or very hypoechoic echogenicity, irregular margins, taller-than-wide shape, presence of PEFs, peripheral calcifications or macrocalcifications are considered as suspicious features

Thyroid Malignancies

Papillary Thyroid Carcinoma (PTC)

PTC is the most common thyroid malignancy [7], and is associated with history of neck irradiation, family history of thyroid cancer, or familial thyroid cancer syndromes like familial adenomatous polyposis, Carney complex, Werner syndrome, and PTEN-hamartoma tumor syndrome [3]. *On USG, it characteristically presents as solid hypoechoic or markedly hypoechoic, taller-than-wide nodule with lobulated or irregular margins, and shows PEFs within (Figs. 69.9 and 69.12).* Multifocal PTCs have been reported in 18–87% of the cases in the literature [11]. PTCs have many documented variants. Follicular variant of PTCs, which is the most common type following the classic PTC, more often presents as iso to hyperechoic solid nodules with smooth margins and no calcifications [3]. PTC may also present as diffuse sclerosing variant which is characterized by diffuse involvement of one or both lobes of thyroid, without formation of a mass and commonly with scattered PEFs. PTCs commonly metastasize to cervical lymph nodes (Fig. 69.13) with distant metastases being uncommon in classic PTCs.

Follicular Thyroid Carcinoma (FTC)

FTC is the second most common thyroid malignancy [7]. Differentiation between FTC and follicular adenoma is suboptimal on imaging, and hence are reported as follicular neoplasms (Fig. 69.8). FTC exhibits differences in sonographic features compared to PTC; with

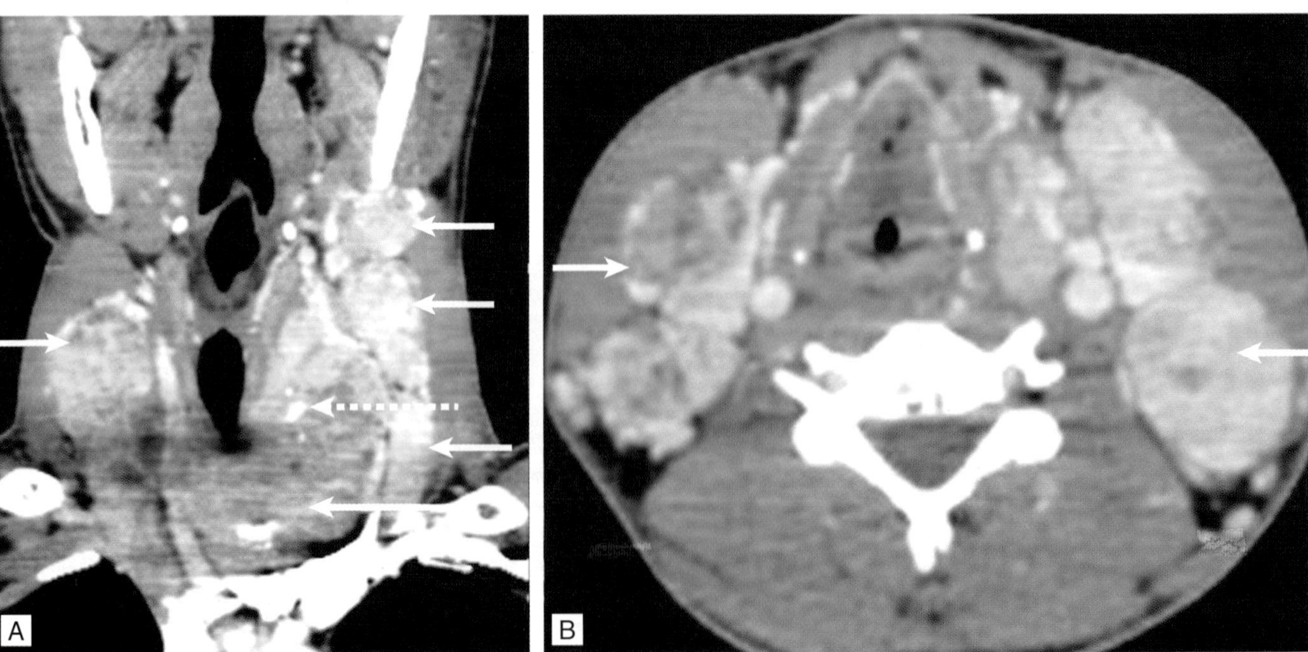

Figure 69.13 Papillary thyroid carcinoma. (A) Coronal postcontrast CT image showing heterogeneously enhancing mass in the left thyroid lobe and isthmus (*long solid arrow*) with macrocalcifications (*dotted arrow*). (B) Axial postcontrast CT image showing multiple enlarged hyperenhancing nodes at bilateral levels II, III, and IV (*short solid arrows* in A and B) suggestive of nodal metastases.

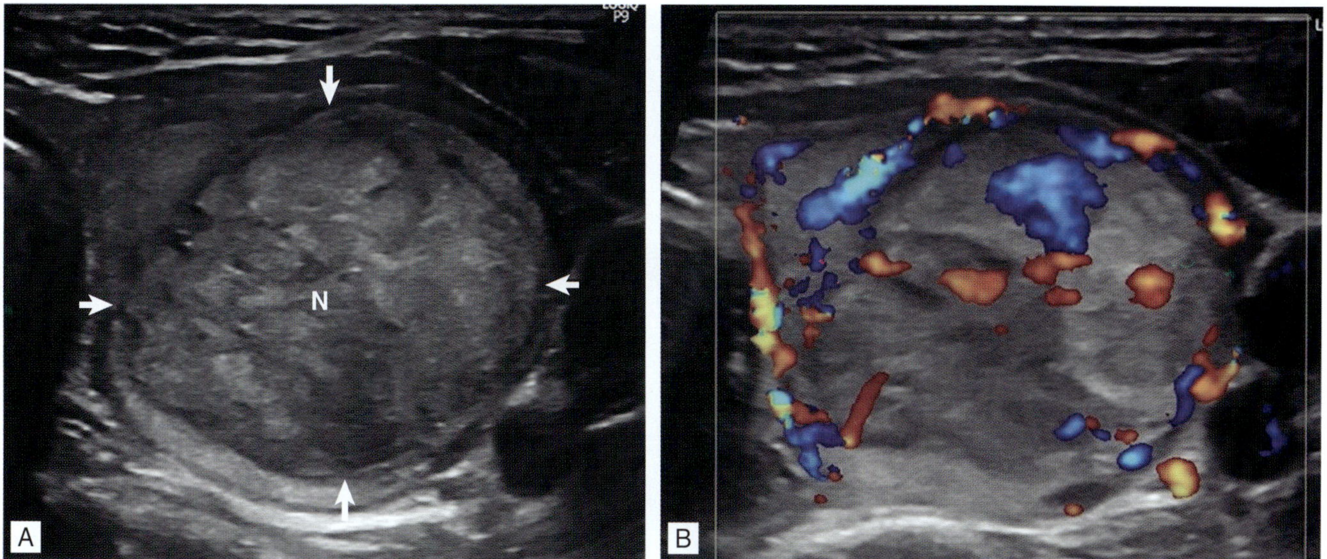

Figure 69.14 Follicular thyroid carcinoma. (A) USG image showing a solid predominantly hypoechoic nodule (N) with isoechoic areas in the left thyroid lobe with smooth margins (*arrows*), wider-than-tall shape and no echogenic foci. (B) Color Doppler imaging shows intranodular and peripheral vascularity.

FTC more likely to present as iso- to hyperechoic, round nodule with smooth margins and less likely to show calcifications (Fig. 69.14) [3]. FTC more commonly shows hematogenous spread with distant metastases and nodal metastases are less frequent. Hürthle cell carcinoma, a variant of FTC, has greater propensity for nodal metastases.

Medullary Thyroid Carcinoma (MTC)

MTC is a malignant neuroendocrine neoplasm arising from parafollicular cells (C cells) that secrete calcitonin. Majority of the cases are sporadic; however, MTC can be hereditary and are found in MEN type 2A or 2B syndromes or as part of familial MTC. MTCs more commonly present as hypoechoic or markedly hypoechoic, ovoid to round solid nodules which may show dense and irregular macrocalcifications as well as PEFs (Fig. 69.11) [12]. They may show extrathyroidal extension; nodal and distant metastases are common.

Anaplastic (Undifferentiated) Carcinoma (ATC)

ATC is a highly malignant neoplasm, which commonly presents with rapidly enlarging neck mass and symptoms of mass effect or local invasion. On USG, ATC usually appears as a large, hypoechoic, heterogeneous, solid mas with vascularity which may show calcifications and features of extrathyroidal spread and local invasion. CT reveals a large necrotic heterogeneously enhancing mass involving the entire gland with ill-defined margins, extrathyroidal spread, and local invasion (Fig. 69.15). Nodal and distant metastases are common.

Lymphoma

It is a rare primary thyroid malignancy, typically encountered in elderly women with long-standing goiter or Hashimoto thyroiditis (HT). The disease commonly manifests as a solid hypoechoic or markedly hypoechoic mass at USG. CT shows lymphoma as a homogeneously enhancing solid mass without calcification or necrosis (Fig. 69.16).

Metastatic Tumor

Metastases to thyroid are extremely rare, and commonly originate from primary tumors of lung, breast, or renal cell carcinoma [7,10]. Head and neck squamous cell carcinomas can also rarely metastasize to the thyroid gland.

Post-Treatment Imaging of DTCs

Following completion surgery for thyroid malignancy, disease-free status is indicated by no evidence of tumor on clinical examination

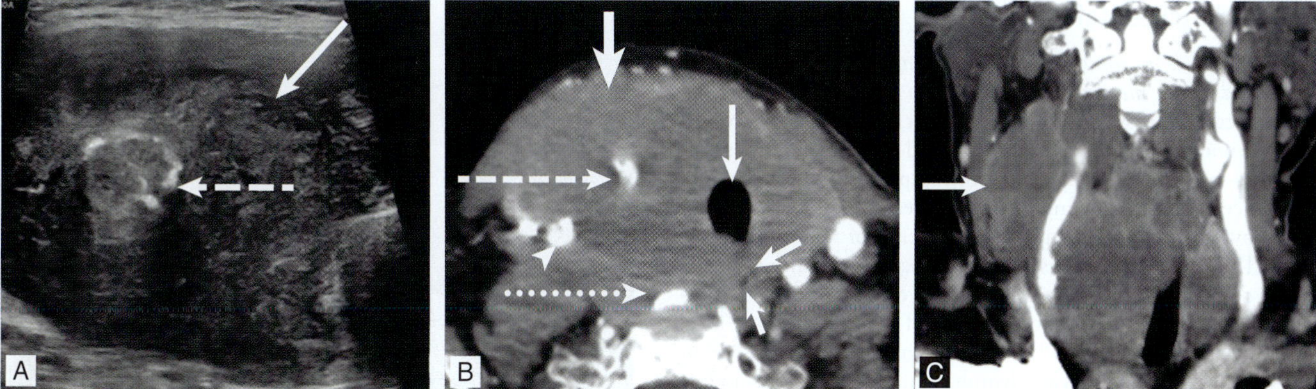

Figure 69.15 Anaplastic carcinoma. (A) USG showing a very hypoechoic large mass (*solid arrow*) with heterogenous echotexture, irregular margins, and macrocalcifications (*dashed arrow*). (B) CT reveals a large heterogeneously enhancing mass (*block arrow*) with necrosis, involving the entire thyroid with foci of calcifications (*dashed arrow*). It shows tracheal encasement and luminal narrowing (*long solid arrow*), esophageal infiltration (*short arrows*), encasement of the right carotid artery (*arrow head*). The mass is contacting the vertebral body which is suggestive of prevertebral space invasion (*dotted arrow*). (C) Coronal reformation CT image showing a large necrotic nodal mass at right level II and III (*arrow*).

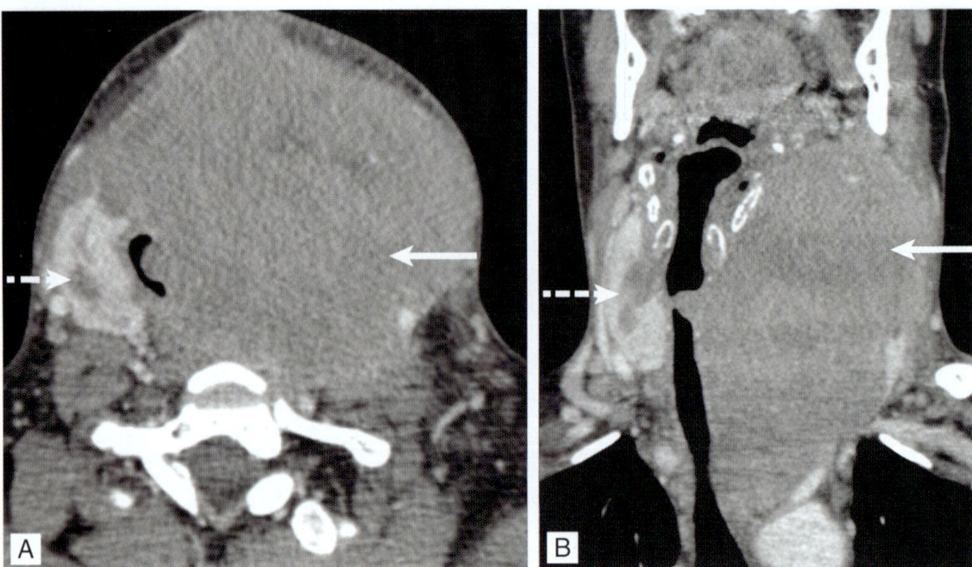

Figure 69.16 Thyroid lymphoma. (A) Axial (B) coronal reformation CT images showing a large homogenously enhancing mass (*solid arrow*) involving the left thyroid lobe and isthmus. Similar smaller focal lesions are also noted in the right thyroid lobe (*dashed arrow*). (Courtesy: Suresh K. Mukherji, MD, MBA, FACR.)

and imaging with a low serum thyroglobulin (Tg). The standard imaging approach used in the post total thyroidectomy evaluation of DTC is a combination of USG neck and whole-body radio-iodine scanning; which have complementary roles. Scintigraphy shows thyroid bed disease, while USG is highly sensitive in detecting lymph node metastases in both central and lateral compartments. USG may not always distinguish between thyroid bed recurrences and benign nodules. *On USG, the normal postoperative thyroid bed between the trachea and carotid arteries shows no intervening tissue or appears uniformly echogenic due to fibrofatty connective tissue. Any hypoechoic nodule in this region is suspicious of recurrence, with the rate of malignancy being higher if the nodule shows microcalcifications, irregular margins, or a shape not parallel to the surrounding tissue planes* [13]. Mimics of recurrence in the thyroid bed include remnant thyroid tissue, postoperative changes including suture granulomas or reactive lymph nodes. 18F FDG PET/CT scanning is indicated in a small subset of postoperative DTC cases with high serum Tg levels (>10 ng/mL) and negative whole-body radio-iodine scanning [3].

Thyroid Incidentalomas (TI)

TI is defined as an unsuspected, asymptomatic thyroid lesion that is discovered on an investigation unrelated to the thyroid gland [14]. TIs detected on USG are managed similar to a clinically apparent thyroid nodule, according to the standard recommendations. TIs on cross-sectional imaging are a growing problem due to its high incidence and lack of definitive imaging feature to identify malignant thyroid nodules, except in the presence of frank local invasion. The ACR (2015) has proposed recommendations, which states that an incidentally detected thyroid nodule is recommended for further evaluation by thyroid USG, if it shows focal thyroid uptake on FDG-PET, shows signs of local invasion or associated suspicious cervical lymphadenopathy, thyroid nodule ≥1 cm (in axial plane) in patients <35 years or thyroid nodule ≥1.5 cm in patients ≥35 years [15]. The ATA (2015) recommends thyroid USG for all patients in whom another imaging study suggests the presence of a thyroid nodule >1 cm [3].

Diffuse Thyroid Diseases

Multinodular Goiter (MNG)

MNG results due to recurrent episodes of hyperplasia and involution leading to irregular enlargement of the thyroid gland, caused by variations in response of follicular cells to external stimuli such as trophic hormones. *USG reveals focal or diffuse irregular enlargement of the thyroid with a heterogeneous appearance due to conglomeration of multiple nodules with variable composition and echogenicity, without or with minimal intervening normal parenchyma* (Fig. 69.17). The nodules may show presence of calcification, cystic changes, and hemorrhage. Calcifications (present in 15–25%) may be peripheral or macrocalcifications; few nodules showing "large comet-tail artifacts," which are suggestive of colloid nodules [16]. The nodules show variable vascularity on Doppler imaging; however, most commonly show peripheral vascularity. Role of USG in MNG is to detect suspicious nodules, cervical lymphadenopathy, to

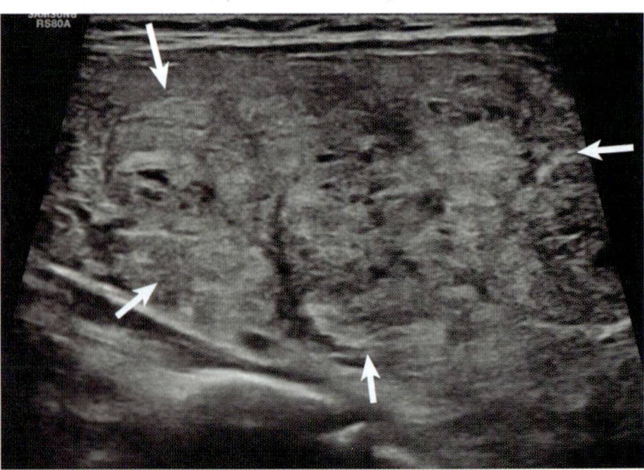

Figure 69.17 Multinodular goiter. USG reveals diffuse enlargement of the thyroid with a heterogeneous appearance due to conglomeration of multiple spongiform and iso to hyperechoic solid nodules (*arrows*) without intervening normal parenchyma.

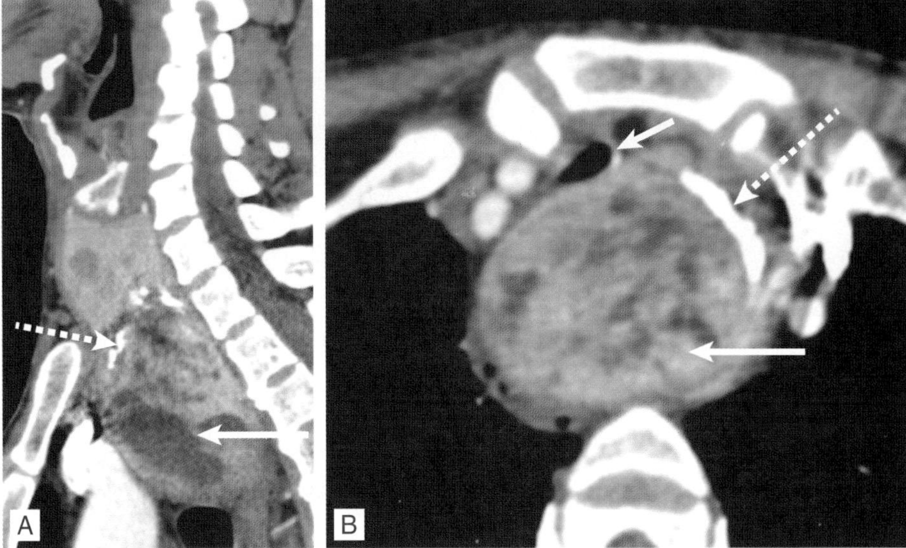

Figure 69.18 (A) Sagittal and (B) axial postcontrast CT images showing multinodular goiter with a large hypodense heterogeneously enhancing nodule (*long arrow*) arising from the inferior pole of the left thyroid lobe which shows rim calcification (*dotted arrow*). It shows retrosternal extension with significant tracheal compression (*short solid arrow*).

guide FNA and assess the extent of enlargement in cases presenting with mass effect. Each nodule in MNG is evaluated individually, based on its internal features and managed accordingly. Papillary carcinoma is the most common cancer in MNG [16]. CT and MRI, though not routinely used, aid in assessment of large goiters with suspected substernal extension, and/or those with mass effect leading to obstructive or pressure symptoms (Fig. 69.18).

Hashimoto's Thyroiditis (HT) (Chronic Lymphocytic Thyroiditis)

HT is a chronic, autoimmune-mediated lymphocytic inflammatory disease leading to hypothyroidism, frequently affecting older women [16]. *In early stages, USG reveals diffusely enlarged hypoechoic gland with heterogenous, coarse echotexture, and fine linear echogenic fibrotic bands. Multiple hypoechoic solid micronodules or pseudonodules with ill-defined margins may be seen ranging from 1 to 7 mm in size representing focal lymphocytic infiltration surrounded by echogenic rim of fibrosis (Fig. 69.19).* This appearance is highly specific for HT with a positive predictive value of 95% [17]. CDI shows mild- to markedly increased gland vascularity. The hypoechoic pseudonodules do not show increased vascularity, while isoechoic normal thyroid parenchyma, especially along areas of fibrosis shows increased vascular flow. In late stages, USG shows heterogenous atrophic gland due to intense fibrosis with reduced or absent vascularity. It may also present with diffuse gland enlargement with or without formation of nodules. Nodular form of HT is also described, which has variable USG appearance; however, studies have reported solid hyperechoic nodules with regular or ill-defined margins to be common [18,19]. USG aids in detecting focal lesions in HT and differentiating them from PTC and primary thyroid lymphoma, which are possible complications of HT (Fig. 69.19).

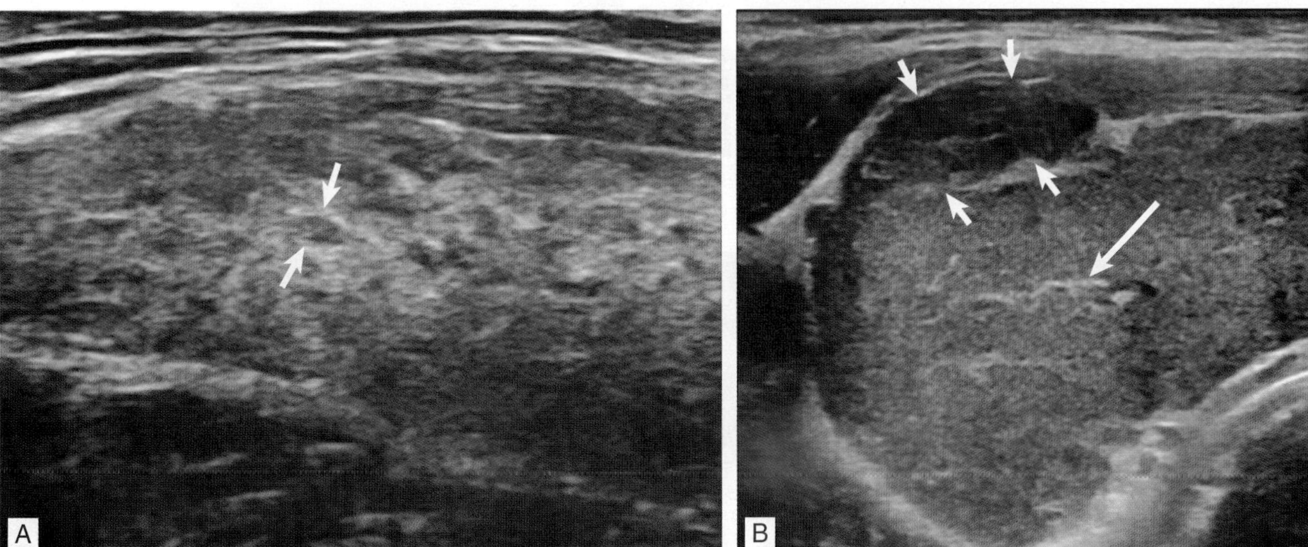

Figure 69.19 Hashimoto's thyroiditis. (A) USG reveals hypoechoic gland with heterogenous echotexture and multiple hypoechoic solid micronodules with ill-defined margins surrounded by echogenic rim of fibrosis (*arrows*). (B) USG reveals enlarged thyroid gland with heterogenous echotexture and fine linear echogenic strands (*long arrow*). A solid very hypoechoic nodule, wider-than-tall showing lobulated margins and no echogenic foci, is noted in the right thyroid lobe (*short arrows*). Hashimoto's thyroiditis with papillary carcinoma.

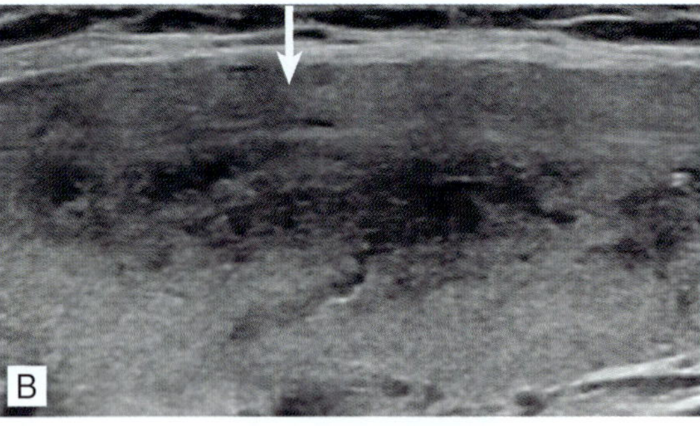
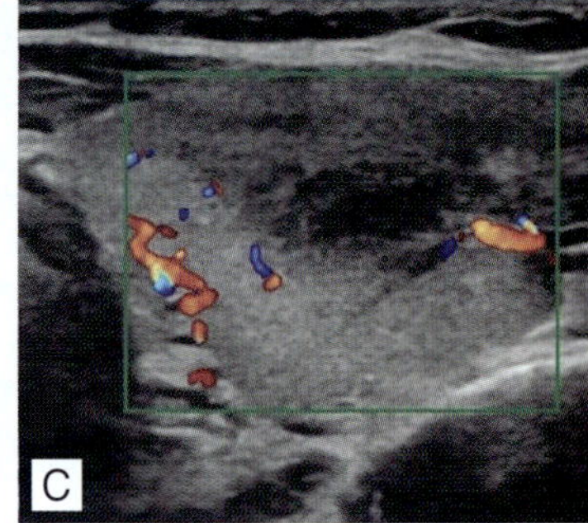

Figure 69.20 Subacute thyroiditis. (A) Transverse (B) longitudinal USG image reveals ill-defined hypoechoic heterogeneous predominantly subcapsular confluent areas showing centripetal reduction in echogenicity (*arrows*). (C) Color Doppler image shows no significant internal vascularity.

Subacute Thyroiditis (De Quervain's Thyroiditis)

Subacute thyroiditis is a self-limiting disease presumed to be triggered by viral infection [16]. It presents as painful goiter with the anterior neck pain radiating to the ears and jaw; and may be accompanied by systemic symptoms like fever, fatigue, and weight loss. USG reveals diffuse tender thyroid enlargement, with initial unilateral involvement followed by symmetric or asymmetric involvement of contralateral lobe. Ill-defined hypoechoic heterogeneous predominantly subcapsular confluent areas showing centripetal reduction in echogenicity are noted, with no discrete mass formation, characteristically defined as "lava flow." CDI shows no significant internal vascularity (Fig. 69.20) [16,20]. Follow-up USG reveals resolution of radiological changes on recovery or gland atrophy. Scintigraphy commonly shows diffusely reduced tracer uptake in thyroid gland.

Graves' Disease

Graves' disease is an autoimmune disease characterized by stimulatory autoantibodies to the TSH receptors (long-acting thyroid-stimulating antibodies) and is the most common cause of hyperthyroidism. It is clinically characterized by diffuse goiter, ophthalmopathy with exophthalmos, and pretibial myxoedema (dermopathy). *USG reveals diffuse nontender, symmetrical thyroid enlargement with hypoechoic, heterogeneous, and coarse parenchymal echotexture. Hypoechoic micronodular appearance may be noted. CDI shows markedly increased parenchymal vascularity (turbulent flow with arteriovenous shunting), which is called "thyroid inferno"* (Fig. 69.21) [16,21]. Scintigraphy shows diffusely enlarged both lobes of thyroid gland with significantly increased tracer uptake and suppressed background and salivary gland activity (Fig. 69.21).

Acute Suppurative Thyroiditis

Acute suppurative thyroiditis and thyroid abscesses are rare since thyroid has rich blood supply and lymphatic drainage, a high iodine level which has bactericidal effects and a complete fibrous capsule that contributes to the high resistance of thyroid to infection. Acute suppurative thyroiditis is more commonly seen in immunosuppressed individuals, due to local or hematogenous spread of infection or in children with third or fourth branchial

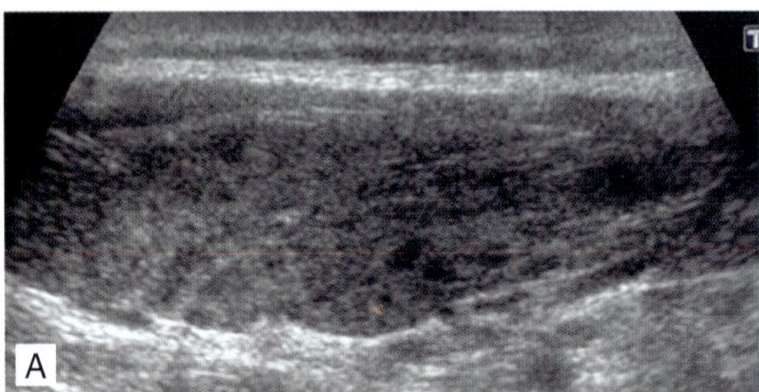
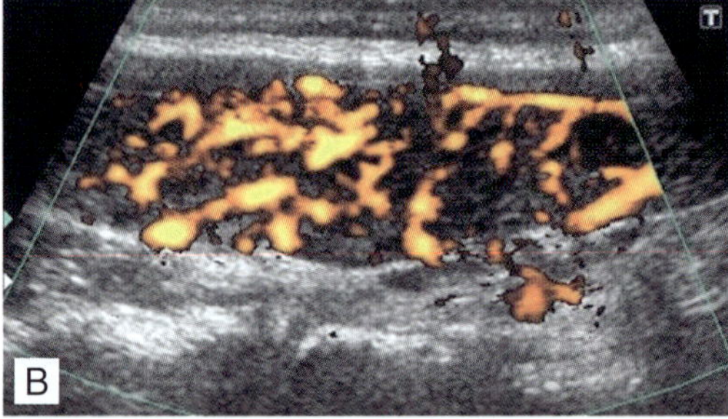
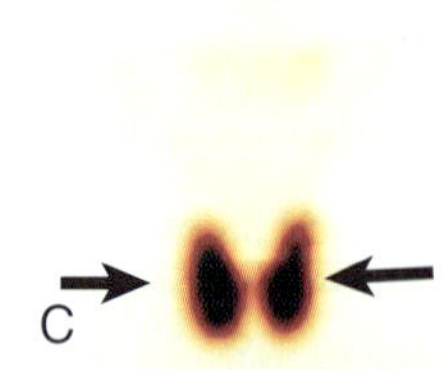

Figure 69.21 Graves' disease. (A) USG reveals hypoechoic thyroid gland with heterogenous echotexture. (B) Power Doppler image showing marked vascularity within the gland. (C) Radionuclide thyroid scan showing intense uptake in thyroid (*black arrows*) with suppressed uptake in salivary glands.

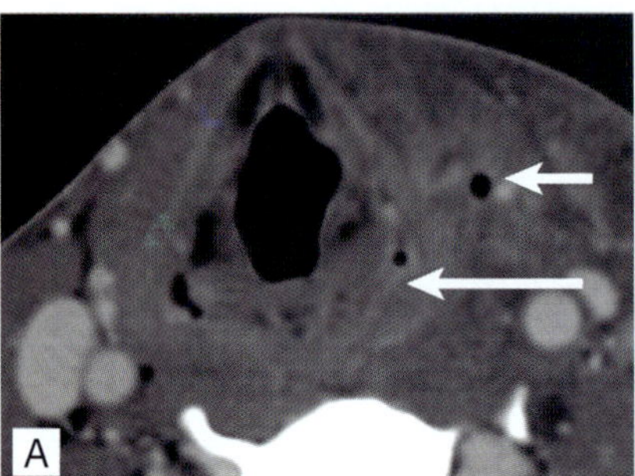
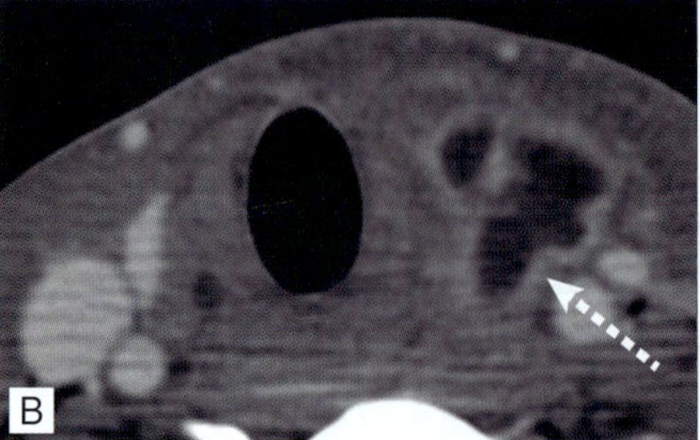
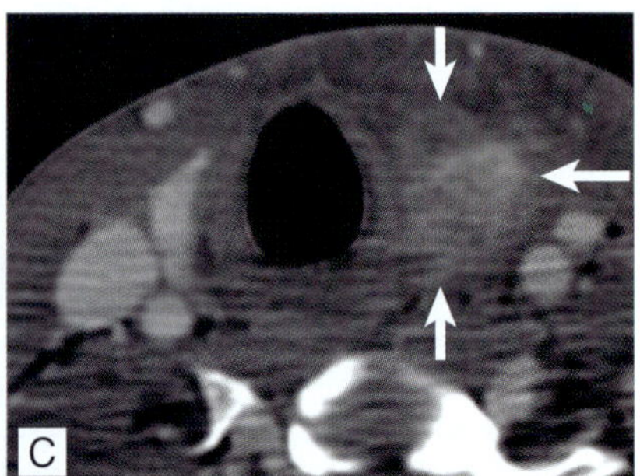

Figure 69.22 Acute suppurative thyroiditis secondary to pyriform sinus fistula. Axial postcontrast CT images showing: (A) Soft tissue swelling and enhancement involving the left pyriform sinus (*long solid arrow*) and adjacent soft tissues with an air focus (*short solid arrow*). (B) Peripherally enhancing abscess noted in the perithyroidal region (*dotted arrow*). (C) The left thyroid lobe appears enlarged, shows heterogeneous enhancement with few hypoattenuating areas and poorly defined margins (*short solid arrows*). (Courtesy: Suresh K. Mukherji, MD, MBA, FACR.)

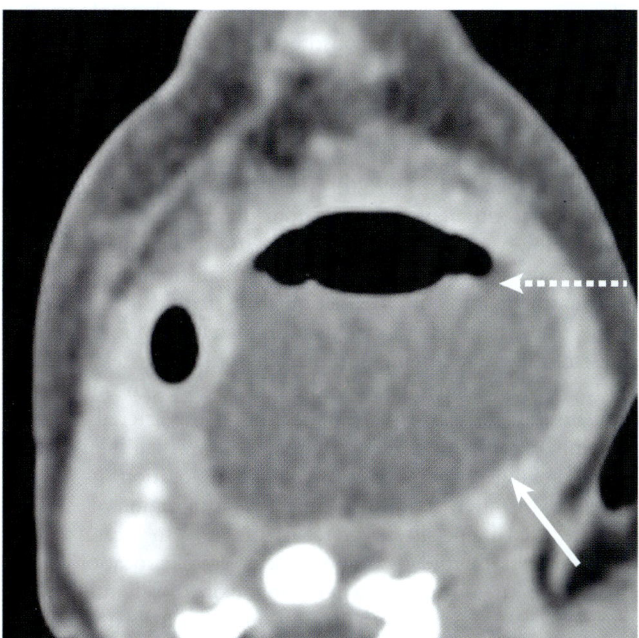

Figure 69.23 Acute suppurative thyroiditis. Axial postcontrast CT images showing a peripherally enhancing abscess involving the left thyroid lobe and perithyroidal region (*arrow*) which shows air fluid level (*dotted arrow*). (Courtesy: Suresh K. Mukherji, MD, MBA, FACR.)

fistula (pyriform sinus fistula), where infection tends to be recurrent (Fig. 69.22) [16,22]. *USG reveals diffuse goiter with heterogenous parenchymal echotexture. Focal poorly defined hypoechoic lesions or localized heterogenous fluid collections with internal echoes and septations may be seen suggesting abscess formation, with or without air foci within; air foci leading to posterior shadowing. CDI shows normal or increased gland vascularity, and no significant internal vascularity within the parenchymal abscesses. Inflammatory changes may be noted in the strap muscles and periglandular area* [16]. CT, preferred over MRI, is done to delineate and assess extent of inflammatory lesions, depict thyroid gland involvement, look for sinus or fistulous tracts, and detect air foci (Fig. 69.23).

Riedel's Thyroiditis (RT)

RT, also known as invasive fibrosing thyroiditis, is characterized by densely fibrotic inflammatory process involving thyroid and the surrounding structures. RT has been proven with immunohistochemical staining to be part of the IgG4-related disease spectrum and may be associated with mediastinal and retroperitoneal fibrosis, orbital pseudotumor, or sclerosing cholangitis [23]. RT presents as stony hard nontender goiter, with or without symptoms of adjacent organ involvement. *USG reveals hypoechoic, homogenous, or heterogeneous hypovascular mass which may show extrathyroidal extension characterized by encasement of vessels or involvement of trachea and esophagus* [24]. CT or MRI is done to assess vascular and adjacent organ involvement. CT reveals an enlarged heterogeneous thyroid gland with lower to normal density. MR signal and postcontrast enhancement on CT and MR may change with the activity of inflammation. Presence of mature fibrosis leads to hypointense signal on both T1 and T2WI and decreased postcontrast enhancement while immature fibrosis with inflammation in the early stages leads to variable heterogenous signal intensity on T2WI and variable postcontrast enhancement depending on its vascularity [24]. Differentials of RT include invasive thyroid carcinoma, lymphoma or fibrotic variant of HT.

Pearls

- Clinical, biochemical, immunological, and radiological evaluation together contribute to the final diagnosis of diffuse thyroid diseases

PARATHYROID

Anatomy, Embryology, and Physiology

In 85% individuals, there are four parathyroid glands, two superior and two inferior, oval in shape, measuring approximately 3–6 mm in length, 2–4 mm in width, and 1–3 mm in thickness [1]. Supernumerary fifth gland can occur in 2.5–13% of the population with few studies reporting higher incidence [1,25]. Normal parathyroid glands are not seen on imaging, and are visualized if pathological. Superior parathyroid glands arise from fourth branchial pouch, migrate caudally along with thyroid gland, and are located along the posterior aspect of the upper pole or mid portion of the thyroid lobes. Inferior parathyroid glands arise from the third branchial pouch, have a common origin and migrate with the thymus gland, and most commonly found inferior to the posterior aspect of the lower poles of thyroid lobes [1]. The common locations of ectopic parathyroid glands are mediastinal, retropharyngeal, retroesophageal, or trachea-esophageal grove [1,26].

Chief cells of the parathyroid gland produce parathyroid hormone (PTH), which is largely responsible for maintenance of calcium homeostasis. PTH leads to increase in serum calcium level by enhancement of renal tubular calcium reabsorption, inhibition of renal tubular phosphate reabsorption, and stimulation of osteoclastic bone resorption. PTH stimulates the renal hydroxylation of 25-hydroxy–vitamin D, which further increases calcium absorption from intestines.

Pathology

Hyperparathyroidism

Hyperparathyroidism (HPT) is subdivided on the basis of etiopathogenesis into primary, secondary, and tertiary HPT. *Primary HPT represents autonomous overproduction of PTH, resulting from parathyroid adenomas (PTAs; approximately 80% of cases), primary parathyroid hyperplasia (PH; less than 20% of cases), or parathyroid carcinoma (PaTC; approximately 1%)* [1]. Secondary HPT is caused by any condition associated with chronic low levels of serum calcium, most commonly from chronic renal insufficiency. Vitamin D deficiency and dietary calcium deficiency can also lead to secondary HPT. When one or more hyperplastic glands in a case of secondary HPT become autonomously functioning, it is called as tertiary HPT.

Definitive treatment for primary HPT is surgery. Traditional bilateral cervical dissection or four-gland exploration requires no preoperative imaging. However, preoperative imaging for accurate localization of pathological parathyroid gland and establishment of solitary or multigland involvement is vital for minimally invasive/focused parathyroidectomy. Other subgroup which requires imaging evaluation is patients with persistent/recurrent HPT. In general, USG and Tc^{99m}-sestamibi scanning are more commonly used as primary techniques. 4D CT, MRI, and PET/CT are used in more difficult, recurrent cases or when results of primary imaging techniques are not helpful.

Parathyroid Adenoma (PTA)

PTAs are benign parathyroid tumors; commonly involving a single gland; however multigland involvement has been described. Various "anatomical" and "functional" imaging techniques are used in conjunction to detect and localize PTAs.

Ultrasonography: USG accurately evaluates PTAs in eutopic glands and also assesses multigland involvement/multiple areas of uptake on radionuclide scanning, concomitant thyroid disease, and cervical lymphadenopathy. USG may also aid in cases of persistent or recurrent HPT postsurgery and in MEN syndromes. *On USG, PTA appears as round to oval or rarely multilobulated, homogenously hypoechoic solid mass with well-defined margins. Some PTAs may show heterogeneous echotexture and cystic areas within. An echogenic line is seen separating thyroid and parathyroid tissue* (Fig. 69.24). On CDI, these lesions are highly vascular and show a prominent "polar feeding vessel" that arises from the branches of the inferior thyroidal artery. This vessel tends to branch along the periphery of the lesion before penetrating the lesion, covering 90–270° arc and gives the characteristic appearance of a "*vascular arc*"; which is a specific sign of PTA (Fig. 69.24) [27]. The adjacent thyroid parenchyma may also show asymmetrically increased vascularity.

Imaging differentials of PTA on USG are enlarged cervical lymph nodes and thyroid nodules. Cervical lymph nodes show hilar vascularity and are more lateral in the neck. Thyroid nodules are usually of mixed echogenicity, including calcification and cystic component, are within the echogenic thyroid capsule and show variable peripheral or intranodular vascularity.

Dual Phase Tc^{99m}-Sestamibi Scan: Tc^{99m}-sestamibi is a cationic complex which localizes into cellular mitochondria. Since PTAs have larger number of mitochondria, Tc^{99m}-sestamibi is taken up more avidly in adenomatous tissue than the thyroid or normal parathyroid gland and is followed by slower release. Dual phase Tc^{99m}-sestamibi scan involves acquisition of early and delayed planar images of neck and thorax after an intravenous injection of Tc^{99m}-sestamibi. Abnormal parathyroid gland shows increased focal uptake in early images and retained tracer in delayed phase, while thyroid or normal parathyroid gland show physiological uptake of tracer in early phase and faster washout. SPECT or SPECT/CT images can be performed for better localization (Fig. 69.25).

4D-Computed Tomography: 4D-computed tomography (4D-CT) is a technique used for preoperative localization of PTAs in eutopic or ectopic locations. Multiplanar CT (axial acquisition with coronal and sagittal reformations) forms the first three "dimensions" of 4D-CT and provides the anatomical information. Change in enhancement from non–contrast-enhanced, arterial, and venous phase imaging constitutes the fourth "dimension" of 4D-CT and provides the perfusion information [28]. *Characteristic imaging appearance of PTAs on 4D-CT is low attenuation on the non–contrast-enhanced images, peak enhancement on the arterial phase (greater than thyroid gland) and contrast washout seen on venous phase images* (Fig. 69.26). These characteristic imaging features help to differentiate PTAs from thyroid nodules or lymph nodes. However, other enhancement patterns that may be noted in PTAs are—not higher in attenuation than thyroid in the arterial phase but lower in attenuation than thyroid in the delayed phase; or neither higher in attenuation than thyroid in the arterial phase nor lower in attenuation than thyroid in the delayed phase [29]. CT may also demonstrate the "polar vessel sign" in the form of a prominent vascular channel seen on the arterial phase of imaging, terminating in a parathyroid lesion, which is larger than contralateral neck vessels in a corresponding location.

MRI: MRI is rarely used for preoperative localization of PTAs. It may be used in persistent or recurrent HPT to locate residual abnormal parathyroid tissue, in neck or ectopic locations. Parathyroid appears isointense to hypointense on T1WI and hyperintense on T2WI. Attempts have been made to evaluate 4D-MRI to localize PTAs, where they show similar enhancement characteristics as that on 4D-CT [30].

PET-CT: Few PET tracers like F^{18} choline and C^{11} methionine have been employed for preoperative planning of parathyroid surgery, however these are considered second-line techniques. F^{18} choline appears to be a promising tracer due to excellent detection rates and better availability as compared to C^{11} methionine.

Parathyroid Carcinoma (PaTC)

PaTC is an extremely rare malignant tumor and presents with palpable neck mass with severe HPT. *On USG, PaTC tends to be larger than PTAs with an average size of 3 cm or more [31]. It appears as a round to oval hypoechoic mass, with heterogeneous echotexture, irregular shape, lobulated or noncircumscribed margins, thick capsule, internal vascularity, and may show intralesional calcifications and cystic changes* [31]. It commonly shows features of local invasion and may be associated with metastatic cervical lymphadenopathy [31]. CT and MRI may be used to assess for local invasion, metastatic disease, and postsurgical recurrence.

Parathyroid Hyperplasia (PH)

PH involves symmetric or asymmetric enlargement of two or more glands, most commonly seen secondary to chronic renal

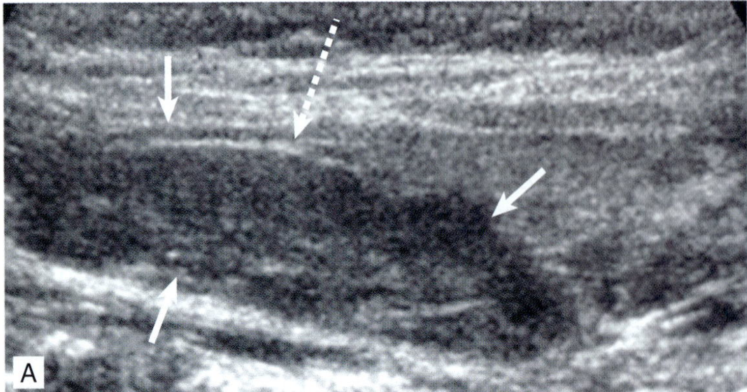

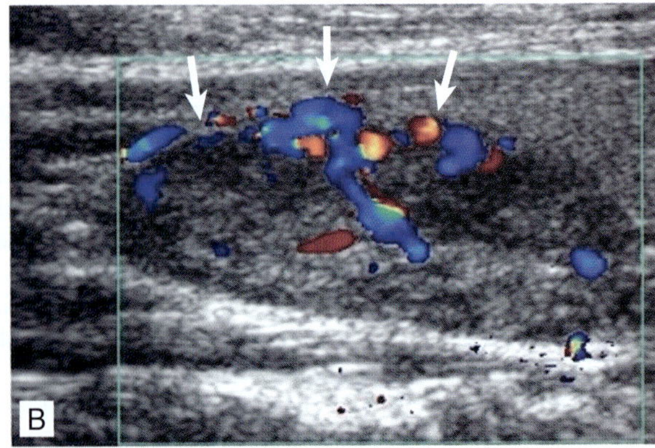

Figure 69.24 Parathyroid adenoma. (A) USG reveals an oval hypoechoic solid mass posterior to the thyroid lobe, with lobulated margins (*solid arrows*). An echogenic line is seen separating thyroid and parathyroid tissue (*dashed arrow*). (B) Color Doppler image shows a peripheral "vascular arc" (*arrows*).

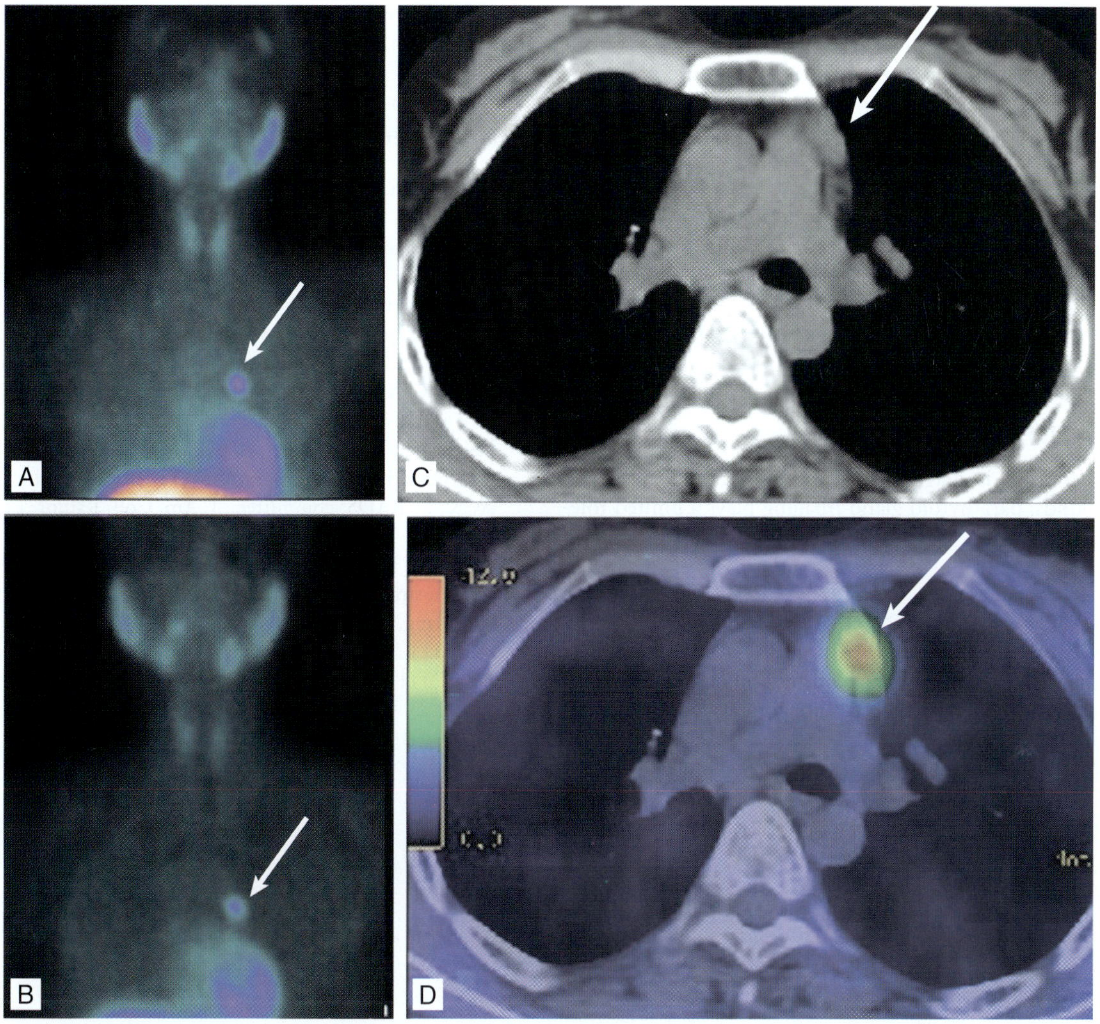

Figure 69.25 Parathyroid adenoma. (A) Early and (B) delayed planar images of Tc^{99m}-sestamibi scan show focal tracer uptake in mediastinum in the early phase (*arrow*) with retained tracer uptake in delayed phase (*arrow*). Corresponding (C) CT and (D) SPECT/CT axial sections show a well-defined soft tissue density lesion (*arrow*) with increased tracer uptake in anterior mediastinum (*arrow*) suggestive of ectopic parathyroid adenoma.

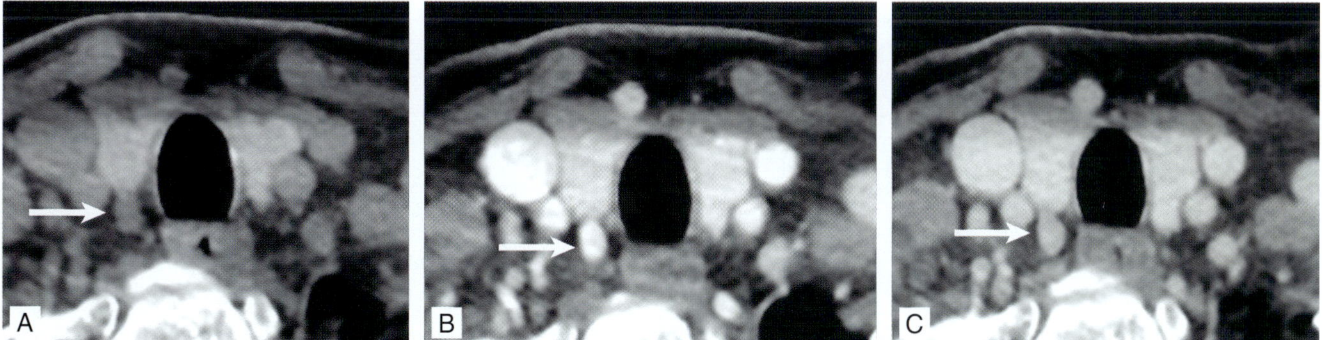

Figure 69.26 Parathyroid adenoma. (A) Noncontrast CT shows the thyroid gland which appears hyperdense on NCCT. A well-defined hypodense lesion is noted posterior to the right thyroid lobe (*arrow*). The lesion (*arrow*) is (B) hyperattenuating to thyroid on arterial and (C) hypoattenuating to thyroid on venous phase.

insufficiency. *Differentiation of PTA and hyperplasia on USG is difficult due to similar morphological features, however each gland tends to be smaller in PH than adenoma.* 4D-CT shows similar features as that of PTAs and may be used for preoperative evaluation.

Parathyroid Cyst (PC)

PCs are rare lesions which may be found in the neck or mediastinum; majority arising from the inferior parathyroid glands. They are classified as functioning or nonfunctioning PCs; nonfunctioning PCs being more common. On USG, PCs appear as anechoic round to oval well-circumscribed lesions at the sites of parathyroid glands and may show an echogenic capsule. CT and MRI show a well-circumscribed cystic lesion and are useful in mediastinal lesions.

Pearls

- Hyperparathyroidism is a more common clinical entity than hypoparathyroidism, with PTA being the commonest cause
- USG and Tc^{99m}-sestamibi scanning are the commonly used primary imaging techniques to evaluate PTAs

Hypoparathyroidism

Hypoparathyroidism is diagnosed mainly on clinical and biochemical grounds; parathyroid gland imaging plays a limited role in its evaluation.

Conclusion

Thyroid and parathyroid diseases are common in clinical practice. A detailed clinical history, methodical imaging evaluation with a thorough knowledge of the recommendations, is pivotal in accurate diagnosis and management.

Suggested Readings

- BR Haugen, EK Alexander, KC Bible, et al., 2015 American Thyroid Association management guidelines for adult patients with thyroid nodules and differentiated thyroid cancer: the American Thyroid Association guidelines task force on thyroid nodules and differentiated thyroid cancer, Thyroid 26 (1) (2016) 1–133.
- AC Nachiappan, ZA Metwalli, BS Hailey, RA Patel, ML Ostrowski, DM Wynne, The thyroid: review of imaging features and biopsy techniques with radiologic-pathologic correlation, Radiographics 34 (2) (2014) 276–293.
- FN Tessler, WD Middleton, EG Grant, et al., ACR thyroid imaging, reporting and data system (TI-RADS): white paper of the ACR TI-RADS committee, J Am Coll Radiol 14 (5) (2017) 587–595.
- HY Yuen, KT Wong, AT Ahuja, Sonography of diffuse thyroid disease, Australas J Ultrasound Med 19 (1) (2016) 13–29.
- JK Hoang, W Sung, M Bahl, CD Phillips, How to perform parathyroid 4D CT: tips and traps for technique and interpretation, Radiology 270 (1) (2014) 15–24.

70 Paranasal Sinuses

PRIYA GHOSH, ADITI CHANDRA, SAUGATA SEN

Introduction

The sinonasal space consists of the nose, the nasal cavity, and the paranasal sinuses, namely, the paired maxillary, ethmoid, frontal, and sphenoid sinuses. The sinonasal spaces share a common embryological development pathway. The entire sinonasal region consists of mucous lined closely connected air-filled spaces that show commonality of pathology, as well as easy regional spread of disease processes. Being exposed to the external environment, they are vulnerable to a variety of traumatic, infectious, inflammatory, and neoplastic diseases.

Imaging Techniques

Radiography

The indication and the need for plain x-rays in diagnosis and further management have declined over the last decade as cross-sectional imaging with multiplanar reconstructions create a near-perfect anatomical simulation for the treating physician. There is still a limited role for plain films of the paranasal sinuses in acute infection. This is limited to a single occipitomental view (Fig. 70.1), which is considered adequate for the basic assessment of the maxillary antra, the frontal sinuses, and the sphenoid sinus but is poor at excluding pathology of the ethmoid air cells or providing minute bony detail.

Computed Tomography (CT) Scan

CT is the initial and most common technique for imaging the sinonasal space. Modern CT scanners are fast, readily available, and have very little radiation exposure. Excellent detail is available regarding the anatomy, anatomical variants, and pathology. Both soft tissue and bony detail can be observed in respective windows.

Technique

Modern multidetector scanners can reconstruct images in any plane from the raw data with no loss of detail. Hence, only axial sections are acquired followed by multiplanar reconstructions in coronal and sagittal planes. The lesser scan time and radiation dose results in better patient compliance. The scan plane being parallel to the hard palate helps obviate dental artifacts to a large extent as well. This was not possible when direct coronal images were acquired with older single detector scanners. Images are usually reconstructed at 2.5–3 mm and 0.625–1 mm intervals. Reconstructions in both bone and soft tissue algorithms are required.

For diseases such as congenital abnormalities, infections, inflammations, and granulomatous pathologies, the scan extends from the hard palate to the skull base. The decision to administer intravenous contrast should depend on the disease entity and should be performed for the evaluation of neoplasms and aggressive infectious and inflammatory disorders.

Magnetic Resonance Imaging (MRI)

In the sinonasal region, MRI is reserved for neoplasms and any other sinonasal pathology that involves the orbits or brain. The assessment of the brain, meninges, and orbits, as well as perineural spread is superior with contrast-enhanced MRI. MRI is superior to CT due to better soft tissue resolution and multiparametric imaging, but is expensive and has longer acquisition times. CT is superior to MRI for evaluating bony architecture, calcification, and periosteal reaction.

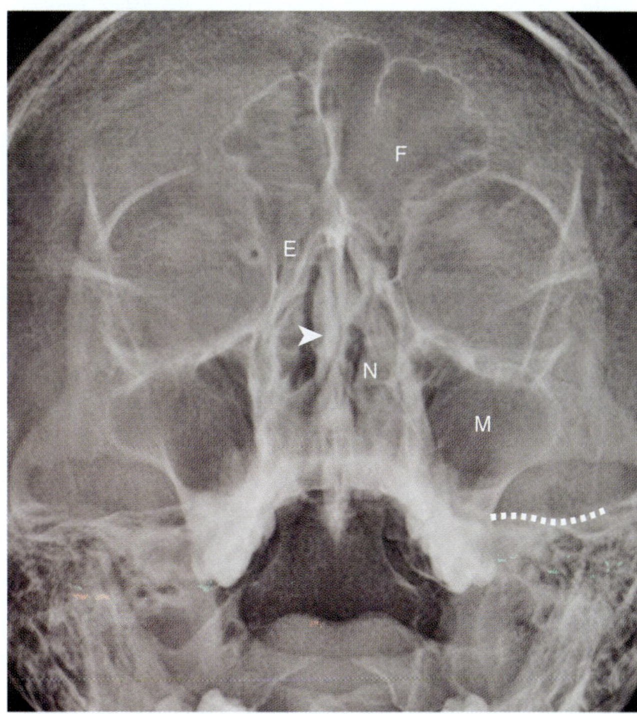

Figure 70.1 X-ray occipitomental view showing normal aerated paranasal sinuses in a 54-year-old woman. *F*, left frontal sinus; *M*, left maxillary sinus; *E*, right ethmoid sinuses; *N*, left nasal cavity; *white arrowhead*, nasal septum. Correct positioning is indicated by projection of the petrous ridge (*dotted line*) inferior to the maxillary sinus (M).

Standard head coil is used for MR imaging of the sinonasal region using a 1.5T or 3T magnet. High-resolution T1-weighted and T2-weighted FSE sequences performed in the axial, coronal, and sagittal planes are the mainstay of sinonasal imaging. T2-weighted fat-saturated or STIR sequences are used as an adjunct to increase tumor conspicuity. Slice thickness of 3 mm is maintained, with interslice gap of 0–0.3 mm. Axial images are obtained parallel to the hard palate and the other sections perpendicular to the axial plane. Diffusion-weighted imaging is also routinely performed with images acquired at three *b* values, usually *b*50, *b*500, and *b*1000 that also generate apparent diffusion coefficient (ADC) maps. Most malignant tumors show diffusion restriction due to high cellularity. T1-weighted fat-saturated pre- and post-IV-gadolinium images are obtained, which help identify tumor extension, perineural, intraorbital, and intracranial spread, meningeal involvement. MRI is also helpful for assessing intracranial complications of infectious or inflammatory diseases, such as intracranial abscesses or orbital cellulitis.

Nuclear Medicine

18F-fluorodeoxyglucose (FDG) positron emission tomography/computed tomography (PET/CT) is not indicated for routine sinonasal imaging. In oncology, FDG-PET is not useful for evaluating the primary site, but it is useful for assessing distant disease ("M stage"). FDG-PET is commonly used to assess recurrent or residual neoplastic disease following treatment, and also in monitoring response [1] (Fig. 70.2). A key disadvantage of FDG PET CT in the sinonasal region is its high false-positive rate, as inflammatory changes following therapy may also show FDG avidity [2].

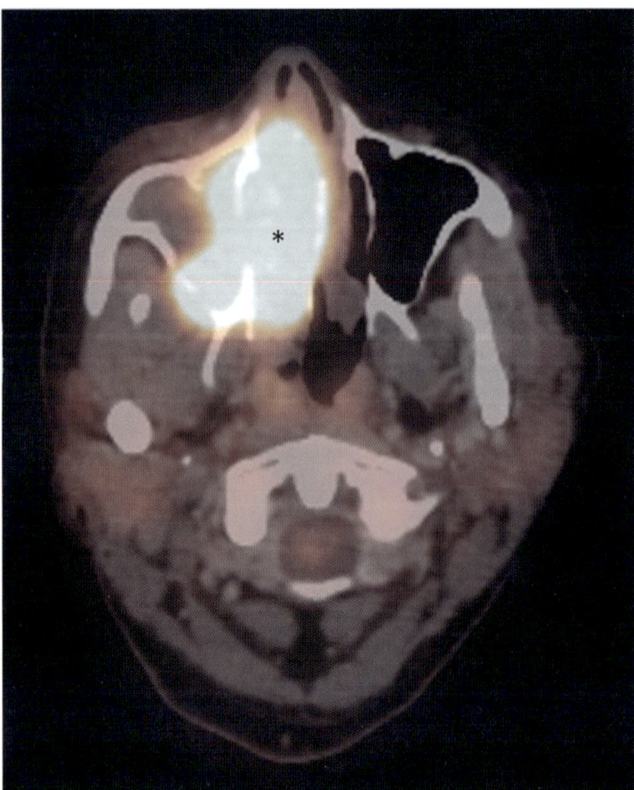

Figure 70.2 Axial PET-CT image in a 40-year-old woman with sinonasal PNET (peripheral neuroectodermal tumor) shows mass in the right nasal cavity invading right maxillary sinus with high metabolic activity signified by increased FDG uptake (*asterisk*).

American College of Radiology (ACR) appropriateness criteria for imaging in sinonasal diseases [3] are shown in Table 70.1.

Sinonasal Anatomy, Anatomical Variants, and Physiology

The nasal cavity and paranasal sinuses have a common developmental pathway (Fig. 70.3). The nasal cavity and olfactory system begin to develop as early as fourth to fifth gestational week and are completely developed at birth. The turbinates and paranasal sinuses have a common origin from the cartilaginous nasal capsule [4]. The paranasal sinuses begin to develop around sixth gestational week as outpouchings from the lateral nasal wall. The paranasal sinuses are rudimentary at birth and their development continues through childhood. There are usually only 3–4 ethmoid sinuses at birth and progressively increase in number and size [5]. The maxillary, frontal, and sphenoid sinuses are small sacs at birth and progressively enlarge reaching an adult configuration by 12–14 years [6].

Nasal Cavity and Septum

The nasal cavity communicates with the exteriors through the anterior nares. Posteriorly, the nasal cavity communicates with the nasopharynx through the paired posterior choanae. The nasal cavity is divided into two halves by the nasal septum, having a posterior bony part formed by vomer and perpendicular plate of ethmoid, and an anterior cartilaginous part formed by the septal cartilage [7]. The lateral wall of the nasal cavity is formed by medial walls of the maxillary and ethmoid sinuses. The lateral nasal wall has three C-shaped or scroll-shaped structures attached to it, named superior, middle, and inferior turbinates, which curl inferolaterally and divide the nasal cavity into superior, middle, and inferior meatuses (Box 70.1).

The paired nasal cavities may be asymmetric due to deviation of the nasal septum. *Nasal septal deviation* is very common and is seen in up to 80% of healthy adults, commonly at the inferior part near the junction of bony and cartilaginous parts [8] (Fig. 70.4). Deviation may be simple or S-shaped, involving the cartilaginous septum, bony septum or both. A deviated nasal septum may compress the middle turbinate and uncinate process to narrow the infundibulum and obstruct the drainage of the maxillary, frontal, and anterior ethmoid sinuses. Septal deviation may need to be corrected to improve drainage and get better access during endoscopic surgery. *Septal spurs* are projections arising from the nasal septum that may form adhesions or impinge upon the turbinates (Figs. 70.4 and 70.5). These are common and resection may be necessary to improve endoscopic surgical access to the sinuses. One anatomical variant that may be confused with septal deviation or spur is the nasal septal swell body, which is a thickened area of nasal septum consisting of cartilage and bone anterior to middle turbinate near the internal nasal valve [9]. The nasal septum may occasionally be *pneumatized*, narrowing the sphenoethmoid recess and access to sphenoid ostium (Fig. 70.4). The pneumatized part of septum may arise from anterior aspect through crista galli or from posterior aspect through sphenoid sinus. Rarely, nasal septum may be aplastic, or its posterior part may be absent.

The roof of the nasal cavity is formed by the cribriform plate. Superior to the cribriform plate is the olfactory fossa containing the paired olfactory bulbs. The olfactory fossa is formed by crista galli medially, medial lamella of cribriform plate inferiorly, and

TABLE 70.1 **ACR Appropriateness Criteria for Imaging in Sinonasal Diseases**

Clinical Presentation	Usually Appropriate Investigation	May be Appropriate Investigation	Summary
Acute (<4 weeks) uncomplicated rhinosinusitis	None	■ CT PNS without IV contrast ■ CT Cone beam PNS without IV contrast	No imaging required
Possible surgical candidate. Recurrent acute rhinosinusitis, chronic rhinosinusitis, sinonasal polyposis, or noninvasive fungal sinusitis.	■ CT PNS without IV contrast ■ CT cone beam PNS without IV contrast	■ CT PNS with IV contrast ■ MRI maxillofacial without IV contrast ■ MRI maxillofacial without and with IV contrast	Noncontrast CT PNS is the usual imaging required
Acute rhinosinusitis. Suspected orbital or intracranial complication	■ MRI maxillofacial without and with IV contrast ■ MRI head without and with IV contrast (complementary to above) ■ CT PNS with IV contrast (next best alternative in case of contraindications to MRI) ■ CT PNS without IV contrast		Both CT and MRI may be necessary to better define the soft-tissue structures, orbital contents, and brain to guide appropriate treatment
Sinonasal obstruction. Suspected mass	■ MRI maxillofacial without and with IV contrast ■ CT PNS without IV contrast (complementary to above) ■ CT PNS with IV contrast (if MRI cannot be done)	■ MRI maxillofacial without IV contrast ■ CTA head with IV contrast ■ CTA neck with IV contrast ■ MRA head with IV contrast ■ MRA head without IV contrast ■ MRA Neck with IV contrast ■ Arteriography craniofacial ■ FDG-PET/CT skull base to mid thigh	Complete evaluation of the extent of disease usually requires both CT and MRI sinus evaluation without contrast and, in certain cases, with contrast Angiography studies may be needed for preoperative planning, preoperative embolization or treatment of epistaxis
Suspected invasive fungal sinusitis	■ MRI maxillofacial without and with IV contrast ■ CT PNS without IV contrast (complementary to above) ■ CT PNS with IV contrast (if MRI cannot be done)	■ MRI maxillofacial without IV contrast ■ MRA head without IV contrast ■ CTA head with IV contrast ■ MRA head with IV contrast	Both CT and MRI of the sinuses, including evaluation of the adjacent brain and orbits, may be needed to fully define the extent of disease and orbital or intracranial extension

ACR, American College of Radiology; *CT*, computed tomography; *CTA*, computed tomography angiography; *IV*, intravenous contrast; *MRA*, magnetic resonance angiography; *MRI*, magnetic resonance imaging; *PNS*, paranasal sinus.

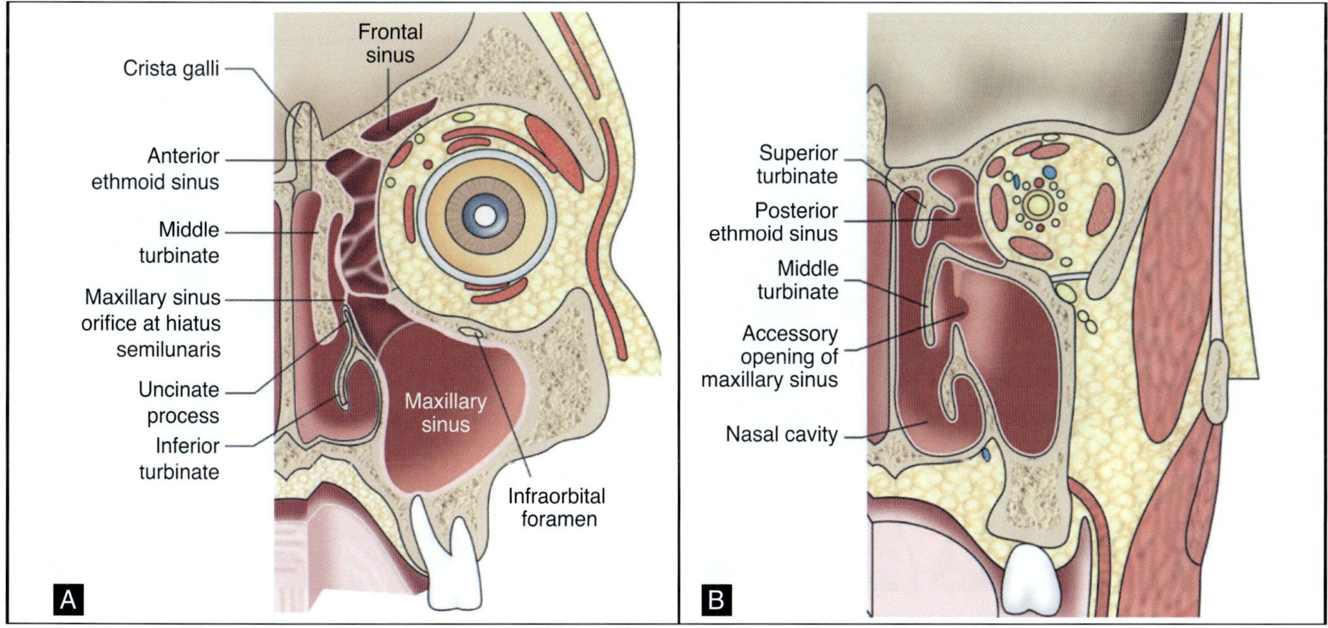

Figure 70.3 Diagram showing anatomy of the nasal cavity and paranasal sinuses. (A) Anterior section. (B) Posterior section.

BOX 70.1 Openings in the Meatuses

Superior Meatus

Openings of posterior ethmoid air cells, the sphenoethmoid recess drains the sphenoid sinus and posterior ethmoid air cells posterosuperior to the superior meatus

Middle Meatus

Drains the frontal sinus via FSDP*, maxillary sinus via maxillary ostium, and the anterior ethmoidal air cells

Inferior Meatus

Opening of the nasolacrimal duct

**FSDP*, frontal sinus drainage pathway.

lateral lamella of cribriform plate laterally. The cribriform plate, together with the roof of ethmoid sinuses (fovea ethmoidalis) form a vulnerable segment of the anterior skull base related to the sinonasal space. *The lateral lamella of the cribriform plate is the thinnest bone of the anterior skull base.* This may be dehiscent, increasing the risk of complications during endoscopic surgery. Keros classified olfactory fossae into Types 1 (1–3 mm), 2 (4–7 mm), and 3 (8–16 mm) based on the vertical height of the lateral lamella [10]. Type 3 is predisposed to intraoperative injury. Asymmetry of the level of olfactory fossa also predisposes to intraoperative injury on the "deeper" side. Another risk classification by Gera et al. measures the angle between the lateral lamella of cribriform plate and the horizontal line along medial lamella. This classification divides the nasal cavities into low, medium, and high risk of intracranial penetration [11].

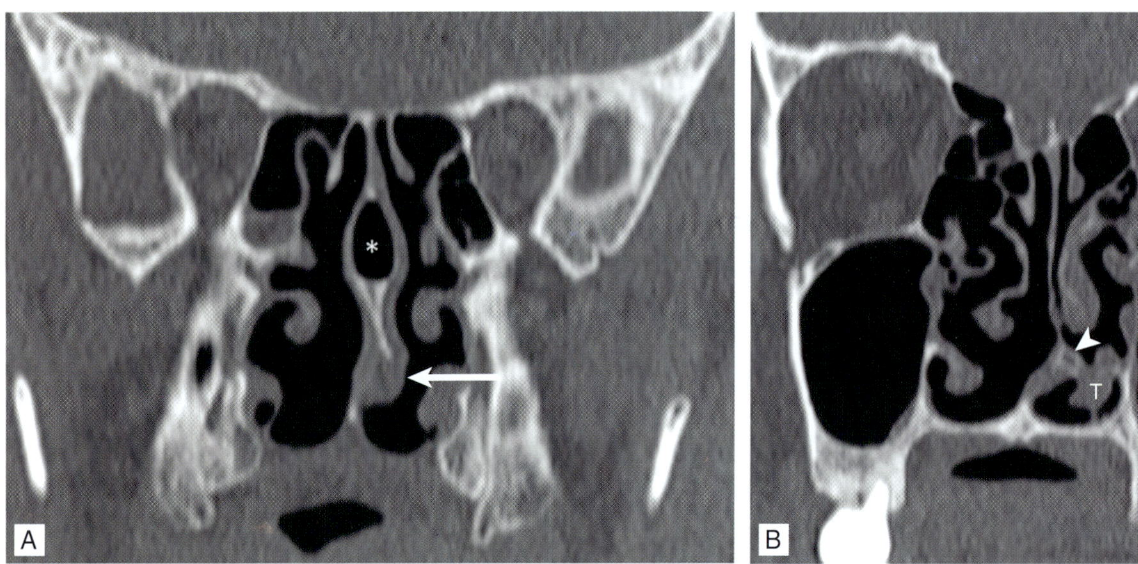

Figure 70.4 Coronal CT scan showing septal deviation (*white arrow* in A) with septal pneumatization (*asterisk*) and spur (*white arrowhead* in B) indenting inferior turbinate (T) in a 62-year-old man.

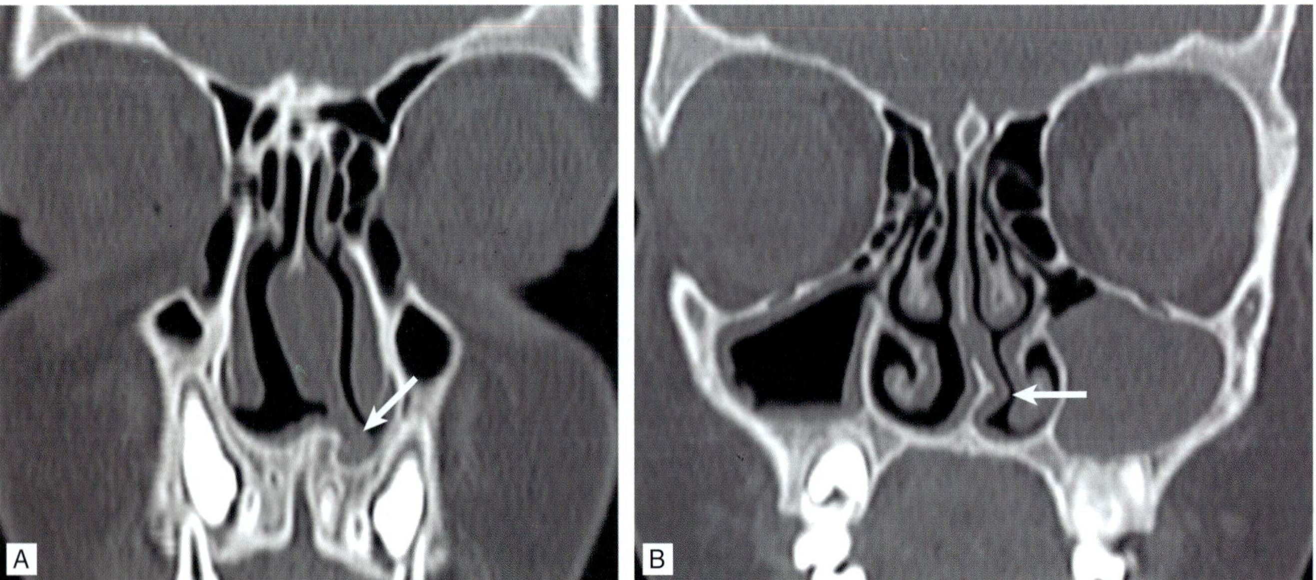

Figure 70.5 Coronal CT of a 14-year-old showing vomeroseptal deviation (*white arrow* in A) and septal spur (*white block arrow* in B).

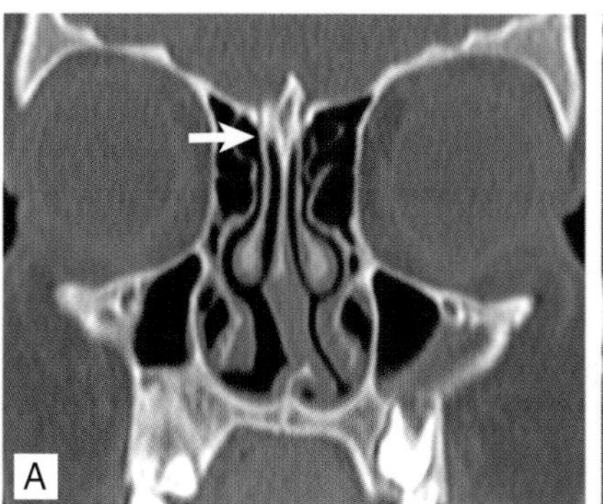

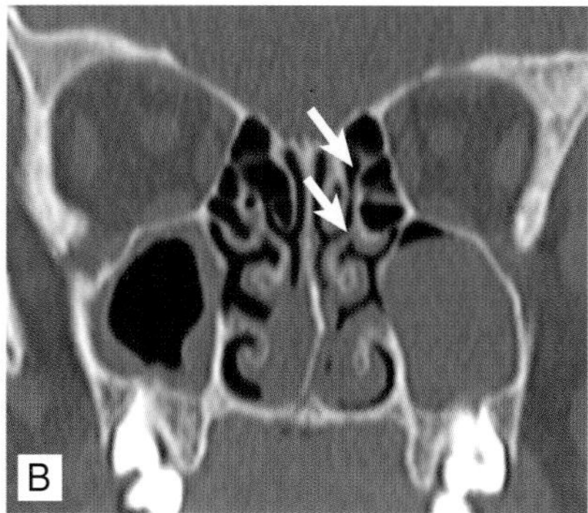

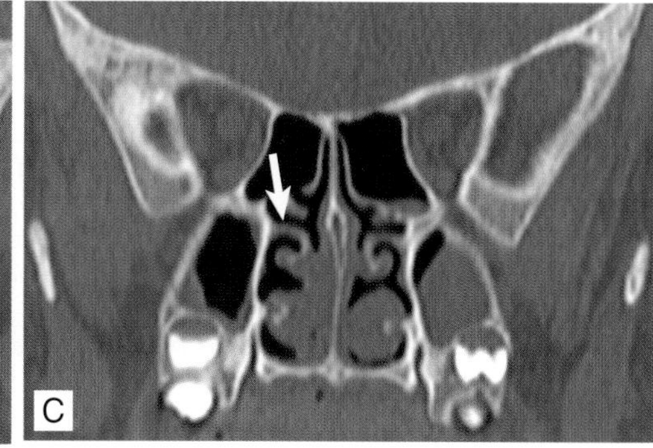

Figure 70.6 Attachments of middle turbinate in coronal CT scan (bone window). (A) Anterior vertical attachment (*white arrow*) to the anterior skull base at the lateral end of the cribriform plate. (B) Middle oblique attachment, that is, basal lamella (*white arrow*), which penetrates through the ethmoid labyrinth and is attached obliquely to the lamina papyracea. (C) Posterior horizontal attachment (*white arrow*) to the medial wall of maxillary sinus.

The middle turbinate deserves special description due to its surgical importance and anatomical variants. Its attachment to the nasal cavity walls is in three orientations (Fig. 70.6) [12]. Anterior attachment to the lateral end of the cribriform plate is vertical and there is risk of injury to the floor of anterior cranial fossa during surgical resection. The middle oblique attachment to the lamina papyracea is known as basal lamella, and if this is manipulated during surgery, the thin lamina papyracea may be damaged leading to orbital penetration. The basal lamella may be pneumatized. The posterior attachment of the middle turbinate to the medial wall of maxillary sinus is in the coronal plane. *Concha bullosa* (Fig. 70.7) is pneumatization of the middle turbinate and is present in 13–53% patients [13]. It is not seen during endoscopy as the turbinates are covered by mucosa. Concha bullosa may be asymptomatic, may become infected, cause septal deviation, or narrow the openings of sinuses in the middle meatus causing chronic sinusitis. According to the location of pneumatization, concha bullosa is classified into bulbous (inferior end), lamellar (vertical lamellar part above the level of ostiomeatal complex, also known as interlamellar cell of Grunwald), and extensive types [14]. The middle turbinate may have *paradoxical curvature* (Fig. 70.8), with lateral convexity, present in 5–26% of the population [15]. This may cause obstruction of the ostiomeatal complex (OMC) and restrict surgical access. Other variants are *turbinate sinus, accessory, secondary, and furcated middle turbinate.*

Ostiomeatal Complex or Unit

The ostiomeatal complex or unit (OMC/OMU) (Fig. 70.9) is the functional unit or region where the frontal, anterior ethmoid, and maxillary sinuses drain. This includes the middle meatus, uncinate process, hiatus semilunaris, ethmoid bulla, the infundibulum, maxillary ostium, anterior ethmoid sinus ostia, and the frontal recess. Disease at the OMC is the major cause of recurrent acute or chronic sinusitis. The uncinate process is a thin crescent-shaped plate of bone covered with mucosa situated lateral to the middle turbinate, attached to the lateral wall of nasal cavity at inferior and anterior aspects. The superior attachment of the uncinate process is variable. It may be attached to the lamina papyracea, anterior skull base, middle turbinate, or have multiple attachments to these structures. This bone has a free upper border posteriorly, known as the hiatus semilunaris, and a channel lateral to it, known as the infundibulum. The infundibulum connects the maxillary and anterior ethmoid sinus ostia to the hiatus semilunaris. The bulla ethmoidalis is a single prominent ethmoid air cell projecting inferomedially at the upper border of hiatus semilunaris.

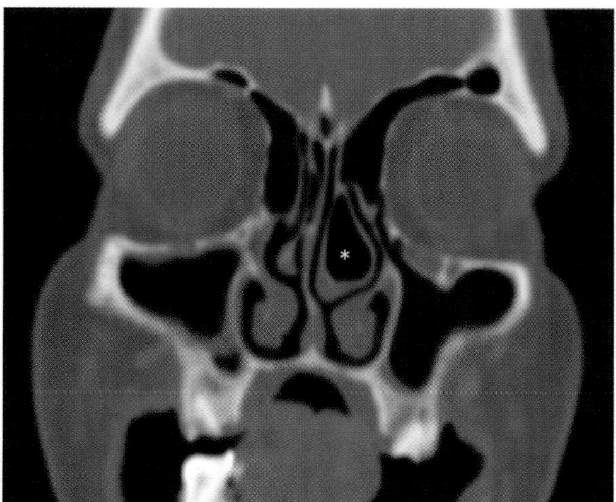

Figure 70.7 Coronal CT scan image showing pneumatization of left middle turbinate, known as concha bullosa (*asterisk*).

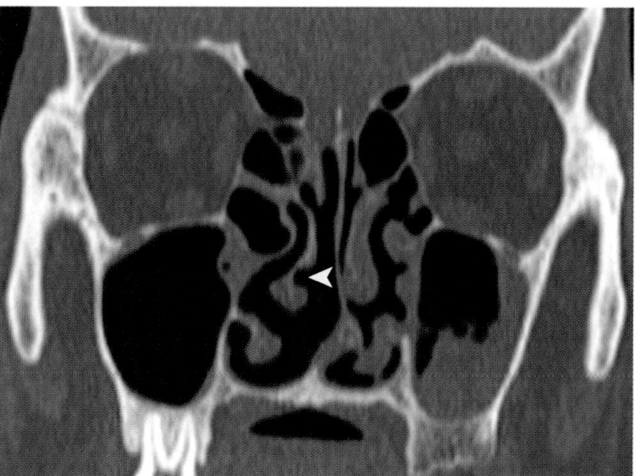

Figure 70.8 Coronal CT scan showing paradoxical curvature of right middle turbinate.

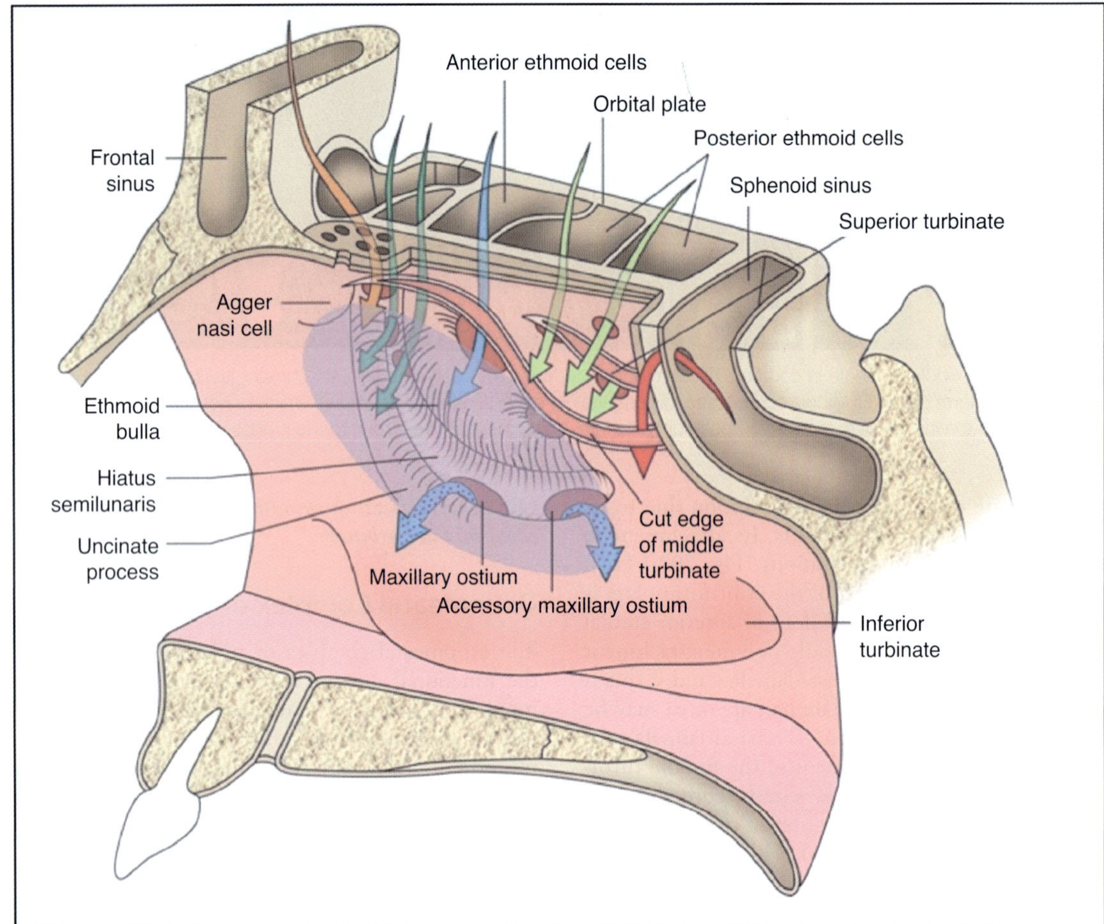

Figure 70.9 Drainage pathways of the paranasal sinuses shown with *arrows*. Area shaded in violet, ostiomeatal complex/unit. *Orange arrow*, frontal sinus drainage pathway; *dark green arrows*, drainage of anterior ethmoid air cells; *blue arrow*, drainage of bulla ethmoidalis; *light green arrows*, drainage of posterior ethmoid air cells; *red arrow*, drainage of sphenoid sinus; *dotted blue arrows*, drainage of maxillary sinus.

Variations of the uncinate process, such as *pneumatization* (*uncinate bulla*) or *eversion*, result in narrowed infundibulum, hampering sinus ventilation. *Atelectatic uncinate process* is closely apposed to inferior and medial orbital wall and may lead to orbital penetration during endoscopic surgery.

Maxillary Sinus

The maxillary sinuses are the largest paranasal sinuses and occupy the body of the maxilla. The maxillary sinus is a pyramidal sinus, with the base at the lateral wall of nasal cavity and three recesses, the alveolar recess inferiorly, the zygomatic recess superolaterally, and the infraorbital recess superiorly. The superior wall of the maxillary sinus forms the orbital floor, inferior wall forms the alveolar process of maxilla and the posterior wall forms the anterior border of pterygopalatine fossa (PPF). The maxillary sinuses drain via the ostium into the posterior aspect of the infundibulum, and eventually into hiatus semilunaris of the middle meatus [16].

The maxillary sinuses may be *hypoplastic*, but *aplasia* is rare. A hypoplastic maxillary sinus increases the risk of orbital injury during endoscopic surgery. *Hyperpneumatized maxillary sinus* results in a deficient bony floor, and roots of teeth project into the maxillary sinus, separated only by mucosa. This increases the chance of maxillary sinusitis from dental source, and chance of oroantral fistula after tooth extraction. The infraorbital nerve runs through the roof of maxillary sinus, opening anteriorly into premaxillary fat just below the inferior margin of orbit. If the bony wall of the infraorbital nerve canal is dehiscent, the nerve becomes exposed to sinus pathologies and surgery. Other variations of maxillary sinus include *septation* and *duplication*, which may hamper drainage and cause recurrent sinusitis.

Frontal Sinus

The frontal sinuses are paired structures, located between the outer and inner cortex of the frontal bone, superior to the orbits and nasal cavities. The configuration and pneumatization of frontal sinuses vary considerably in the population. These may be *hypoplastic*, *aplastic*, *septated*, *hyperpneumatized*, *asymmetric*, or *overlapping*. The frontal sinus may be absent bilaterally in 3–5% patients and the incidence of unilateral aplasia ranges from 1% to 7%, with geographical and racial variation [17]. Posterior wall of the frontal sinus forms the anterior boundary of anterior cranial fossa, and small *dehiscences* in this wall may cause meningeal involvement during sinus irrigation. Lateral aspects of frontal sinuses cannot be accessed endoscopically, and imaging provides important information regarding inflammatory diseases in these hidden areas.

The frontal sinuses drain through the frontoethmoidal recess or frontal sinus drainage pathway (FSDP), into the anterior frontal recess of the middle meatus. Frontal beak is a focal thickening at the frontonasal process of maxilla. This is well visualized in parasagittal images and marks the level of frontal sinus ostium. Frontal sinus

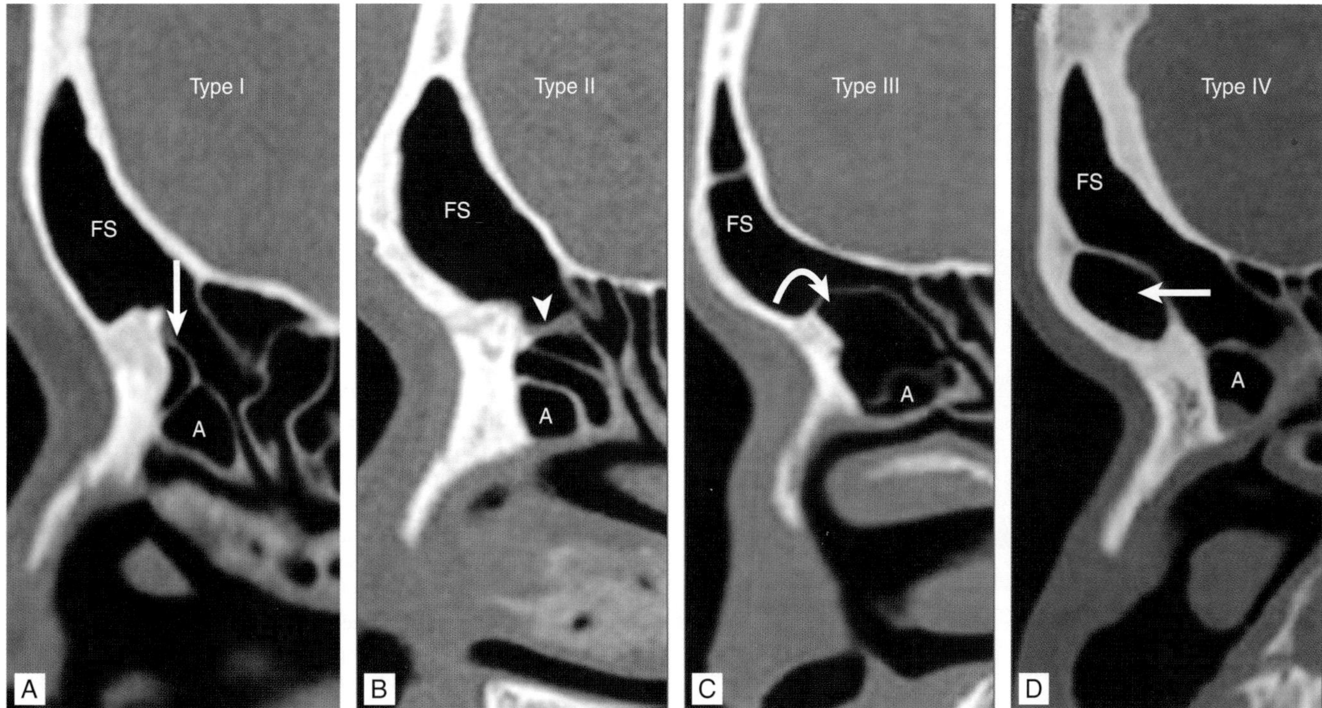

Figure 70.10 Sagittal CT scan showing types of frontal cells. *FS*, frontal sinus; *A*, agger nasi cell. According to Kuhn's classification, Type I: single frontal cell above an agger nasi cell (*vertical white arrow*); Type II: a tier of cells in the frontal recess above the agger nasi cell (*white arrowhead*); Type III: large cell pneumatizing from the frontal recess into the frontal sinus (*curved white arrow*); Type IV: a totally isolated cell within the frontal sinus (*horizontal white arrow*). (Courtesy: Dr. Varsha Joshi.)

extends above the frontal beak, and FSDP lies inferior to it. The thickness of the frontal beak determines the size of the ostium, and drilling is required to widen the ostium during endoscopic surgery. Also, the superior attachment of the uncinate process determines variations of FSDP. *Agger nasi* is the anteriormost ethmoid air cell, lies within the FSDP and is present in 90–98.5% patients [18,19]. Certain other anterior ethmoidal cells may be closely related to the FSDP, and these are called *frontal cells or frontoethmoidal cells*. They are present in 20–41% patients [19,20] and have been classified by Kuhn et al. into four types (Fig. 70.10) [21].

- Type I frontal cell signifies a single cell in the frontal recess above the agger nasi
- Type II signifies multiple cells in this region
- Type III is a single large frontal cell from the frontal recess into the frontal sinus
- Type IV frontal cell is an isolated cell within the frontal sinus

Type III and IV cells require surgery of the frontal ostium. Other variants, such as *frontal bullar cell* and *interfrontal sinus septal cell*, may be present.

Ethmoid Sinus

The ethmoid air cells are usually 3–18 in number [22] and classically grouped into anterior, middle, and posterior according to their drainage. The anterior ethmoid air cells drain into the anterior aspects of hiatus semilunaris in the middle meatus; the middle ethmoid air cells drain on or above the ethmoid bulla; and the posterior ethmoids drain into the superior meatus via multiple ostia and sometimes into sphenoid sinus. Surgically, the ethmoid sinuses are grouped into anterior and posterior ethmoid sinuses, divided by the middle oblique attachment of the middle turbinate to lamina papyracea, known as the basal lamella [7]. Laterally, the ethmoid sinuses are closely related to the medial wall of orbit and separated only by a thin layer of bone named lamina papyracea. Small *dehiscences in lamina papyracea* are common, but larger defects along the posterior aspect of the bone increase the risk of orbital injury during endoscopic surgery. Normally, the lamina papyracea lies in the same sagittal plane as the maxillary sinus ostium. Medialization of lamina papyracea predisposes the orbit to surgical penetration during functional endoscopic sinus surgery (FESS). The fovea ethmoidalis and the ascending lateral lamella of the cribriform plate form the roof of the ethmoid sinus and separate the ethmoid air cells from cranial cavity. This is contiguous with the horizontal medial lamella of the cribriform plate.

The largest anterior ethmoid air cell is the bulla ethmoidalis, which is a specialized air cell lying in relation to the uncinate process and lamina papyracea, and a part of the OMC as described above. If the *bulla is small*, there is risk of orbital injury during endoscopic surgery. The anterior ethmoid air cell extending along the roof of orbit is called *supraorbital cell*. These may be confused with the frontal sinus but lie posterior to it, separated by an intact posterior wall of the frontal sinus. A large supraorbital cell can cause posterior displacement of the canal for anterior ethmoidal artery, described below. The anterior ethmoid cells extending along the floor of orbit lateral to the lamina papyracea are called *Haller cells* (Fig. 70.11). These may narrow the maxillary ostium and manipulation of Haller cells carries the risk of orbital injury.

As described above, the posterior ethmoid air cells are located posterior to the basal lamella. If the height of the posterior ethmoid cells are reduced in reference to the roof of maxillary sinus, it may lead to intracranial penetration during endoscopic surgery. *Onodi cells* (Fig. 70.12), also known as sphenoethmoidal cells, signify those posterior ethmoid cells located superior and lateral to the sphenoid sinus and best seen on coronal CT. Prevalence of Onodi cells has been variably reported to be 7–42% [23]. The points for identification of Onodi cells are cruciform septa within

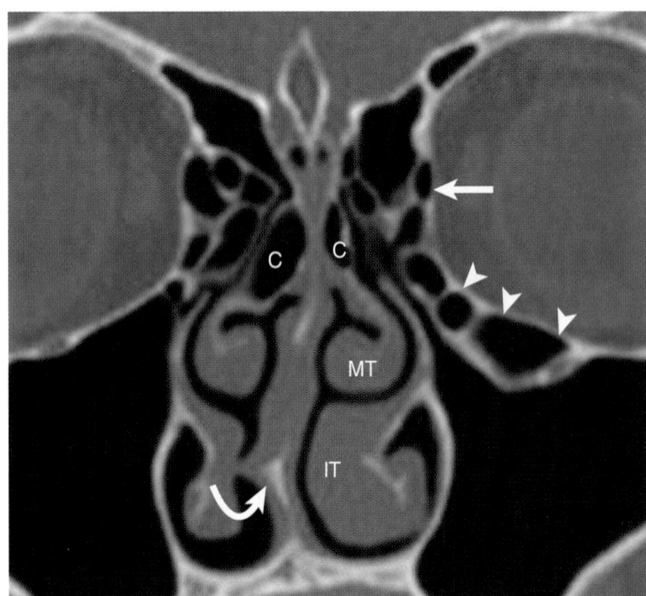

Figure 70.11 Haller cells. Coronal CT scan showing Haller cells (*white arrowheads*), which are anterior ethmoid cells extending along the floor of orbit lateral to the lamina papyracea (*white arrow*). *C*, interlamellar cells of Grunwald; *MT*, middle turbinate with paradoxical curvature; *IT*, inferior turbinate; *curved white arrow*, septal spur. (Courtesy: Dr. Varsha Joshi.)

sphenoid sinus at the level of choana, or an oblique/horizontal septum within sphenoid sinus in coronal CT. Onodi cells are critical as the internal carotid artery and optic nerve are in close proximity and at risk of injury during endoscopic surgery. Pneumatization of anterior clinoid process may occur from the posterior ethmoid air cells, and surgical manipulation may lead to optic nerve injury due to their close proximity.

Lamellar Anatomy

There are five bony lamellae, normally best seen on parasagittal reformats, which extend from lateral wall of nasal cavity to skull base and orbit (Fig. 70.13). From anterior to posterior, these are the uncinate process, anterior margin of bulla ethmoidalis, basal lamella, lamella of superior turbinate, and lamella of supreme turbinate/anterior wall of sphenoid sinus. These lamellae are intact in benign pathologies and are destroyed or distorted in aggressive pathologies.

Sphenoid Sinus

The sphenoid sinuses are paired midline structures with a septum usually dividing it into two unequal halves. The sphenoid sinus ostium and posterior ethmoid air cells drain into the sphenoethmoid recess which is posterosuperior to the superior meatus. The sphenoid sinus is within the sphenoid bone and contributes to the central skull base. The roof of the sphenoid sinus is closely related to the sella turcica, cavernous sinus, and internal carotid artery. Anterior relations of the sphenoid sinus are the nasal cavity, nasopharynx, and posterior ethmoid air cells. Laterally, the posterior part of the orbit and the optic nerve come in close relations to the sphenoid sinus [24].

Sphenoid sinus pneumatization can be variable and has been classified according to the extent of pneumatization in relation to the floor of sella. The most common type is the sellar type (76.9–79.9%) in which pneumatization extends beneath the sella. The less common varieties are the presellar type (18.7–20.6%) where pneumatization extends superiorly to the anterior margin of sella, and the conchal type (1.3–2.3%), where only the anterior part of sphenoid body is pneumatized [25]. *Attachment of the intrasinus septum* to the walls of optic nerve canal or internal carotid artery canal needs to be identified to prevent intraoperative injury to the structures. If the sphenoid sinus is *excessively pneumatized*, the vidian canal and foramen rotundum may lie within the sinus, connected to the wall with bony stalks. In addition, the walls of the bony canals may be dehiscent, increasing the chance of injury during sphenoid sinus exploration. The relations of the optic nerve with the posterior ethmoid sinuses and sphenoid sinus also vary and have been classified by DeLano et al. as Types I–IV. The optic nerve variation which indents the sphenoid sinus (Type II) or passes through it (Type III) are vulnerable during endoscopic surgery [26].

Vascular Supply

Arterial Supply

The sinonasal cavity receives arterial supply from both internal and external carotid circulation (Fig. 70.14):

i. *Sphenopalatine artery*: This is the most important supply and is a branch of internal maxillary artery from external carotid circulation. It exits from the pterygopalatine fossa (PPF) medially through sphenopalatine foramen, and enters the nasal cavity behind the middle turbinate.

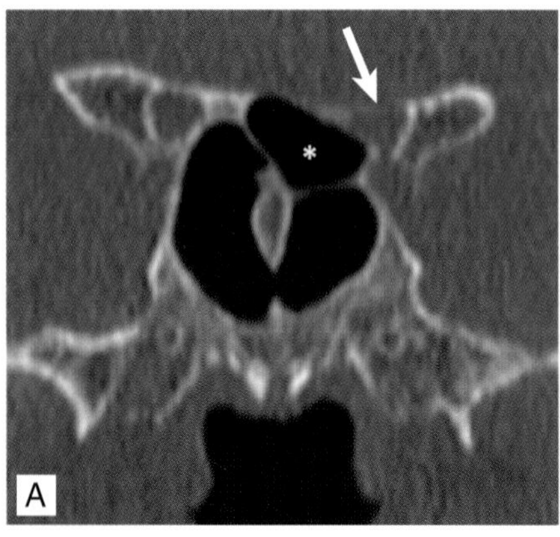

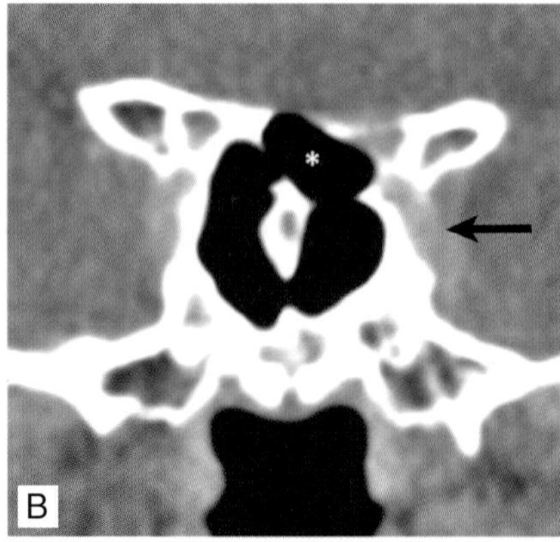

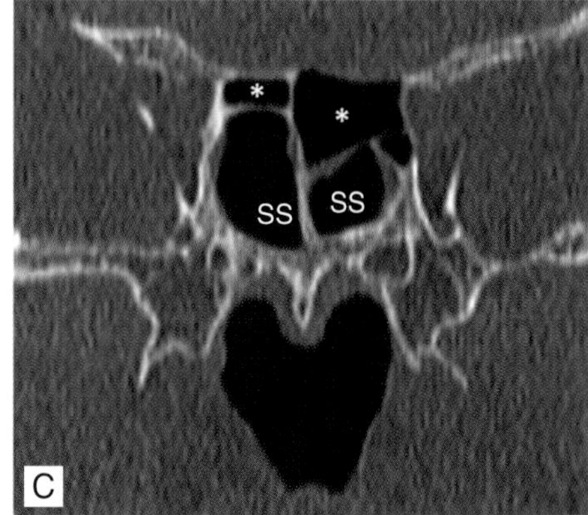

Figure 70.12 Onodi cells. Coronal CT scan images show Onodi cells (*asterisk*), which are posterior ethmoid cells located superior and lateral to the sphenoid sinus (SS). Close relation with internal carotid artery (*black arrow* in B) and optic nerve (*white arrow* in A) is demonstrated. Cruciform septa within sphenoid sinus at the level of choana, as seen in C, is an important point for identification of Onodi cells.

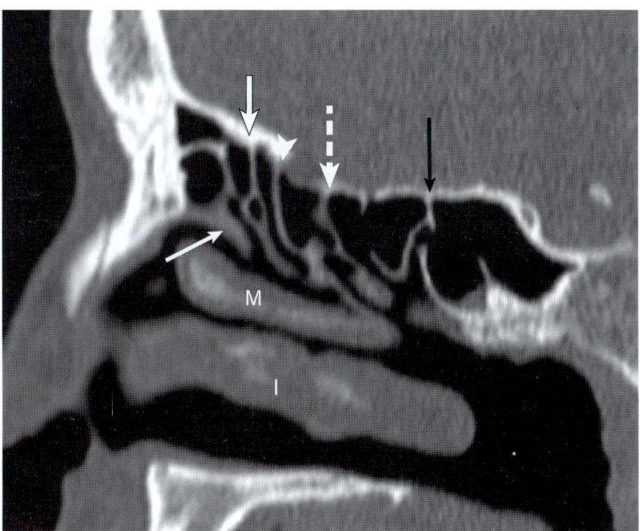

Figure 70.13 Normal lamellar anatomy in parasagittal plane CT scan image. From anterior to posterior: uncinate process (*thin white arrow*), anterior margin of bulla ethmoidalis (*block white arrow*), basal lamella (*white arrowhead*), lamella of superior turbinate (*dashed white arrow*), lamella of supreme turbinate/anterior wall of sphenoid sinus (*thin black arrow*). *M*, middle turbinate; *I*, inferior turbinate.

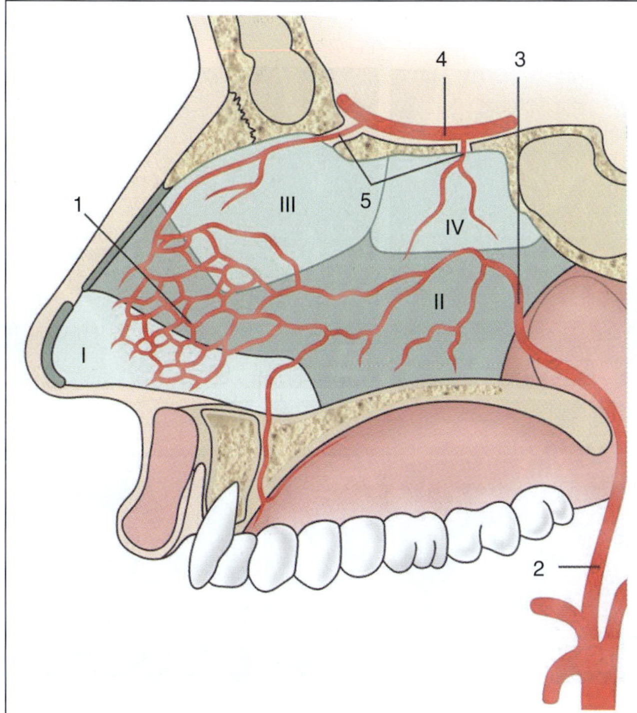

Figure 70.14 Arterial supply of the nasal cavity and sinuses. 1, Kiesselbach's area. 2, internal maxillary artery. 3, sphenopalatine artery. 4, ophthalmic artery. 5, anterior and posterior ethmoid arteries. Areas supplied by arteries: I, facial artery; II, sphenopalatine artery; III and IV, anterior and posterior ethmoidal arteries.

ii. *Anterior and posterior ethmoidal arteries*: These originate from the ophthalmic artery, which is a branch of internal carotid artery. They enter the nasal cavity at the level of cribriform plate via the anterior and posterior ethmoidal canals and anastomose with the nasal branches of sphenopalatine artery. Anterior ethmoidal artery arises from the orbit and usually passes through a bony canal across the upper third of lamina papyracea at the level of anterior ethmoidal sinuses. This bony canal is seen as a beaking or bony projection from the medial orbital wall behind the bulla ethmoidalis in coronal CT images. If this bony canal wall is dehiscent, the artery lies within the ethmoid air cells and is predisposed to injury during endoscopic surgery, leading to rapid development of intraorbital hematoma and loss of vision. The posterior ethmoid artery passes through another bony canal in close relations to the posterior ethmoidal sinuses and optic nerve canal.

iii. *Septal branch of superior labial artery*: Branch of facial artery.

iv. *Greater palatine artery*: Branch of internal maxillary artery.

Little's area is an area at the anteroinferior extent of nasal septum, which contains rich anastomosis of multiple branches of the facial, sphenopalatine, and greater palatine arteries (*Kiesselbach's plexus*). This is the most common site of epistaxis [27].

Venous Drainage

Veins from the sinonasal cavity drain into anterior facial vein and eventually into internal jugular vein. The anterior facial vein has communications with ophthalmic veins, which drain into the cavernous sinus, and also with the pterygoid venous plexus via deep facial vein. This is the pathway through which rapid spread of sinonasal infection may occur intracranially [28].

The CT anatomy of the sinonasal space has been demonstrated in Figs. 70.15–70.17.

Physiology

The sinonasal space is lined by two types of mucosa. The superior most part of the nasal cavity is lined by olfactory mucosa, which is nonciliated in nature. Pseudostratified columnar ciliated epithelium lines the rest of the nasal cavity [29]. The normal sinonasal secretions (1–2 L of serous secretions daily) are cleared by the cilia [30]. The cilia direct the sections toward the natural ostia of the sinuses. Each sinus has its own opening as a drainage pathway and hence its own characteristic pattern of mucociliary clearance. Adequate normal secretions, normal ciliary action, and patent ostia are necessary for normal physiological function, and alteration in any of the above will result in pathology.

Nasal cycle is the phenomenon of alternating air-flow through only one of the nasal cavities during inspiration, the other remaining quiescent. This cycle alternates approximately every 30 minutes to a few hours [31]. The turbinates and mucosa of the inactive side are congested and engorged and can be identified on imaging (Fig. 70.18). Only a thin sliver of air space is preserved between the turbinates and the nasal wall on the quiescent side. This air channel may be lost in case of hypertrophied turbinates.

Diseases Affecting Sinonasal Space

Classification Chart

Classification chart is presented in Table 70.2.

Infectious, Inflammatory, and Granulomatous Diseases

Sinusitis

Sinusitis is the most common disease affecting the sinonasal space. The preferred term by otorhinolaryngologists is "rhinosinusitis" and it signifies inflammation of the nasal cavity and the

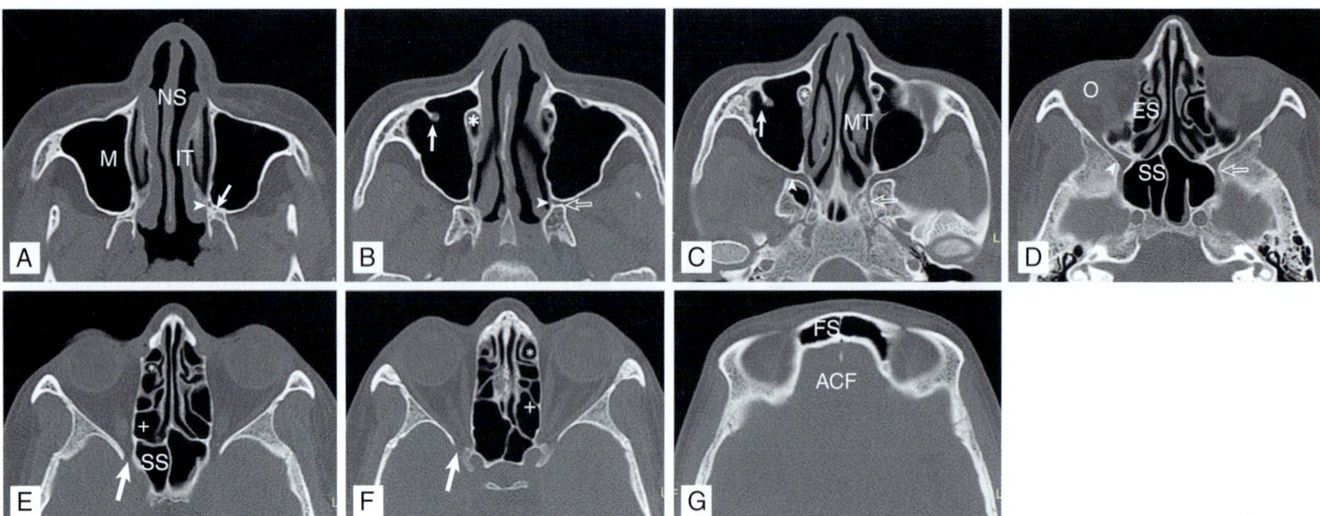

Figure 70.15 Serial axial CT scan images of the sinonasal space showing normal anatomical structures: inferior to superior. (A) *M*, maxillary sinus; *NS*, nasal septum; *IT*, inferior turbinate; *arrowhead*, greater palatine canal; *arrow*, lesser palatine canal. (B) *Arrow*, infraorbital canal; *asterisk*, nasolacrimal duct (NLD); *arrowhead*, sphenopalatine foramen; *outline arrow*, pterygomaxillary fissure; linear space between *arrowhead* and *outline arrow*, pterygopalatine fossa (PPF). (C) *Arrow*, infraorbital canal; *asterisk*, NLD; *MT*, middle turbinate; *arrowhead*, PPF; *outline arrow*, vidian canal. (D) *O*, Orbit; *ES*, ethmoid sinus; *SS*, sphenoid sinus; *arrowhead*, PPF; *outline arrow*, foramen rotundum. (E) *asterisk*, anterior ethmoid sinuses; +, posterior ethmoid sinuses; *SS*, sphenoid sinus; *arrow*, optic canal. (F) *asterisk*, anterior ethmoid sinuses; +, posterior ethmoid sinuses; *arrow*, superior orbital fissure. (G) *FS*, frontal sinus; *ACF*, anterior cranial fossa.

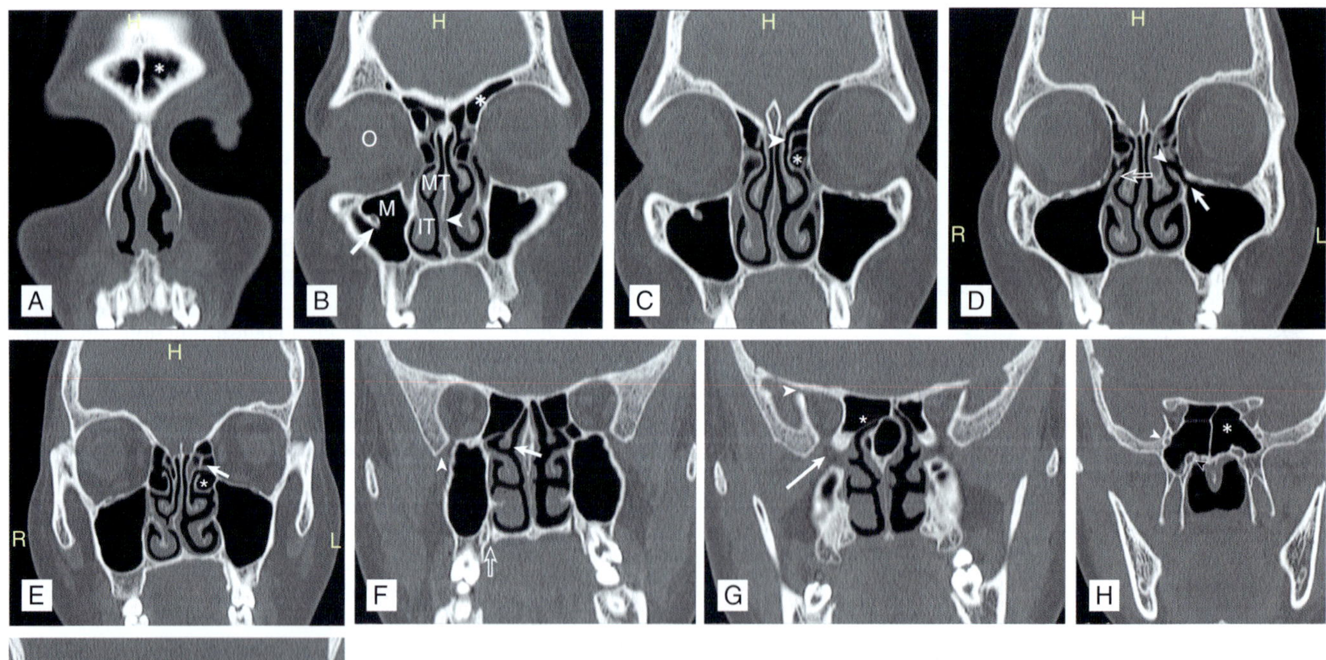

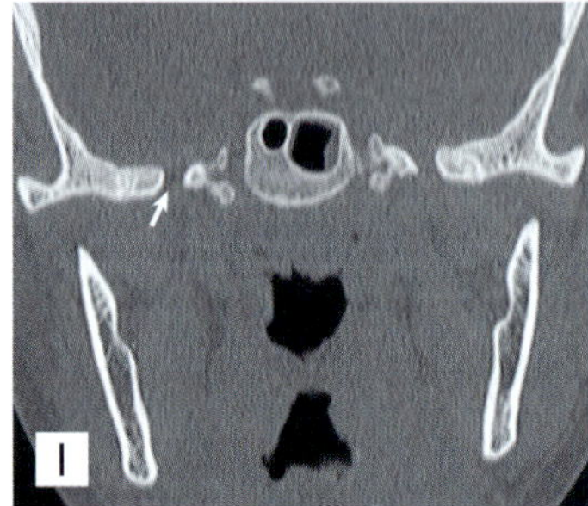

Figure 70.16 Serial coronal CT scan images of the sinonasal space showing normal anatomical structures: anterior to posterior. (A) *asterisk*, frontal sinus. (B) *asterisk*, frontal sinus; *O*, orbit; *M*, maxillary sinus; *MT*, middle turbinate; *IT*, inferior turbinate; *arrowhead*, nasal septum; *arrow*, infraorbital canal. (C) *Arrowhead*, frontal sinus drainage pathway; *asterisk*, anterior ethmoid sinus. (D) *Outline arrow*, uncinate process; *arrowhead*, hiatus semilunaris; *arrow*, maxillary sinus ostium; narrow channel between *arrowhead* and *arrow*, infundibulum. (E) *Arrow*, basal lamella; *asterisk*, bulla ethmoidalis. Serial coronal CT scan images of the sinonasal space showing normal anatomical structures: anterior to posterior. (F) *Arrow*, superior turbinate; *arrowhead*, inferior orbital fissure; *outline arrow*, greater palatine foramen. (G) *Arrowhead*, superior orbital fissure; *asterisk*, sphenoid sinus; *arrow*, pterygopalatine fossa. (H) *White arrowhead*, foramen rotundum; *black arrowhead*, vidian canal; *asterisk*, sphenoid sinus. (I) *Arrow*, foramen ovale.

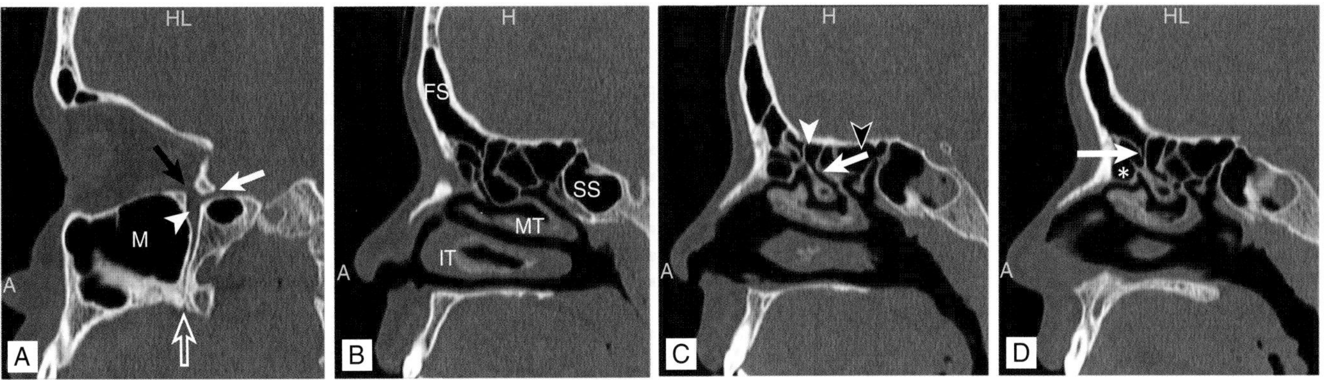

Figure 70.17 Sagittal and parasagittal CT scan images of the sinonasal space showing normal anatomical structures (lateral to medial). (A) *M*, maxillary sinus; *arrowhead*, pterygopalatine fossa; *black arrow*, inferior orbital fissure; *white arrow*, foramen rotundum; *outline arrow*, greater palatine foramen. (B) *FS*, frontal sinus; *SS*, sphenoid sinus; *MT*, middle turbinate; *IT*, inferior turbinate. (C) *Arrow*, basal lamella; *white arrowhead*, anterior ethmoid sinuses; *black arrowhead*, posterior ethmoid sinuses. (D) *Arrow*, frontal sinus drainage pathway; *asterisk*, agger nasi cell.

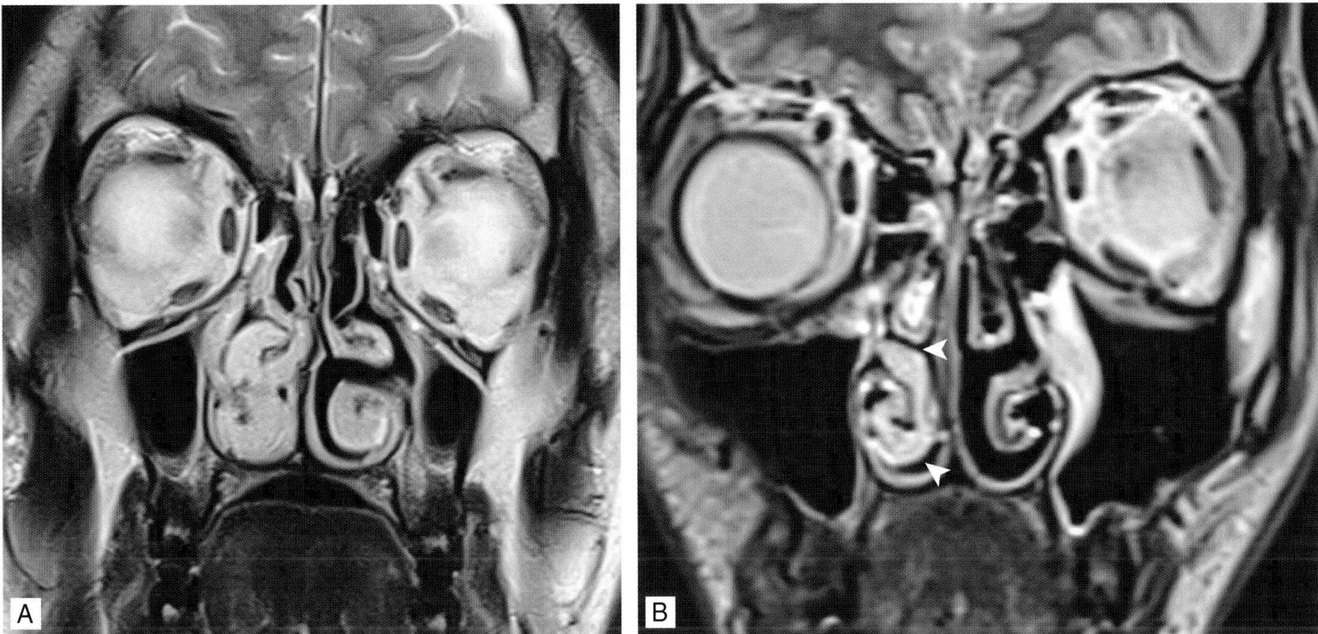

Figure 70.18 (A) Coronal T2-weighted MR images in different patients showing right middle and inferior turbinate hypertrophy (A) and nasal cycle with enlarged right middle and inferior turbinate (B). Note the maintained narrow air channels (*white arrowheads*) surrounding the turbinates in B, which are lost in A.

contiguous paranasal sinuses, which almost always accompany each other [32]. Sinusitis is classified according to the duration of symptoms. In the acute form of the disease, duration of symptoms is less than 4 weeks, while in chronic form the duration is more than 12 weeks [33]. Traditionally, sinusitis lasting for 4–12 weeks was called subacute sinusitis, but more recent guidelines suggest individualizing this group of patients into acute or chronic varieties [32]. The term recurrent acute sinusitis is used if there are four or more acute episodes in a year, with intermittent periods of resolution. Acute episodes may be superimposed on chronic sinusitis.

Sinusitis may also be classified according to etiology, such as viral, bacterial, fungal, allergic, and vasomotor. In this chapter, further discussion will be under the heads of acute sinusitis, chronic sinusitis, and special varieties such as fungal, allergic, and vasomotor sinusitis.

Acute Sinusitis: The duration of symptoms in acute sinusitis is typically less than 4 weeks. Patients present with nasal discharge, obstruction, sneezing, loss of smell, pain, or sense of pressure over sinuses. Acute sinusitis is also a common cause of headache. Majority of patients recover without treatment within 2 weeks. The usual causative agents are "common cold" viruses, such as rhinovirus, parainfluenza or influenza viruses, adenoviruses, respiratory syncytial virus, coronaviruses, enteroviruses, and metapneumovirus [34]. Bacteria may contribute to acute sinusitis, either as a primary agent, or secondary to viral rhinosinusitis. Acute bacterial sinusitis is commonly caused by *Streptococcus pneumoniae* and *Haemophilus influenzae* in immunocompetent hosts, and staphylococci or *Pseudomonas* in immunosuppressed hosts [35,36].

Imaging: *"Sinusitis" is a clinical diagnosis based on signs and symptoms, not a radiological diagnosis.* Indications of imaging in

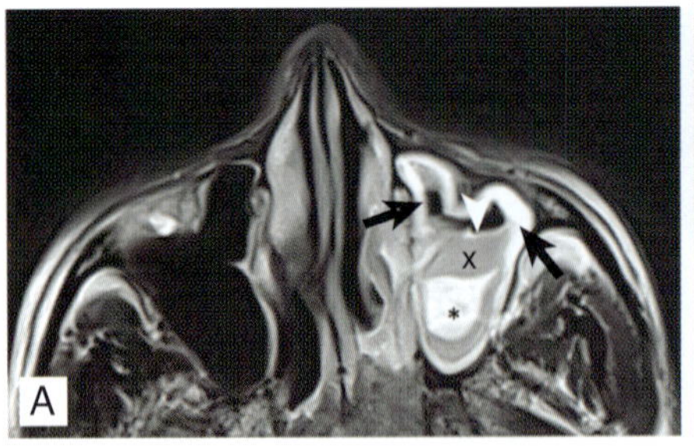

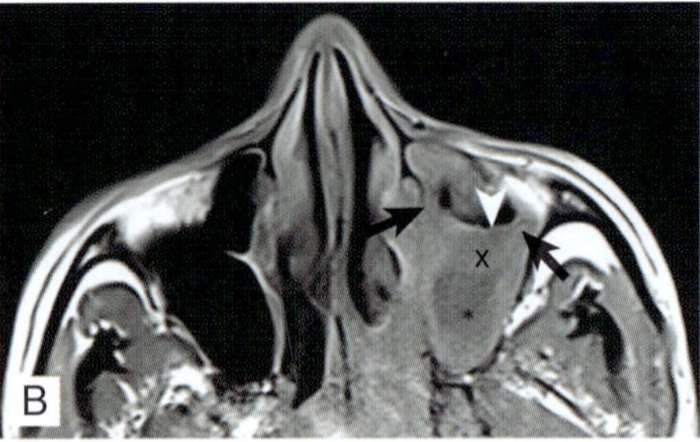

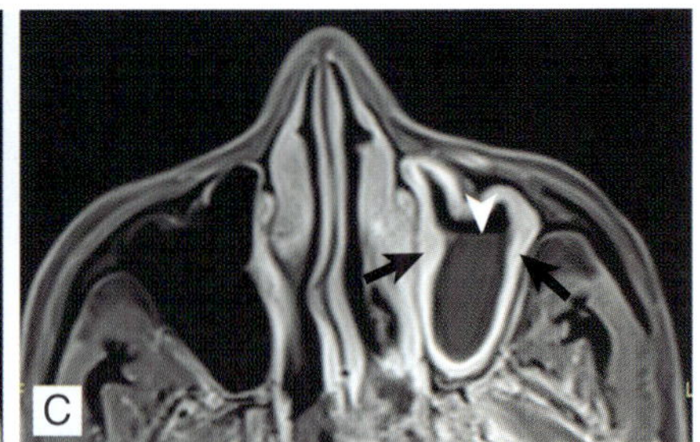

Figure 70.22 Acute sinusitis in a 54-year-old man. (A) Axial T2-weighted, (B) axial T1-weighted, (C) axial postcontrast fat-saturated T1-weighted MR images showing air–fluid level (*white arrowheads*), mucosal thickening (*black arrows*) seen as smooth sinus lining hyperintense in T2, isointense to muscles in T1 and enhancing in postcontrast images. Differing intensities of fluid are seen in left maxillary sinus signifying different protein content-dependent fluid (*asterisk*) is hyperintense in T2, hypointense in T1, and supernatant fluid (x) is hypointense in T2, isointense to mucosa in T1-weighted images. Fluid is not enhancing in postcontrast images.

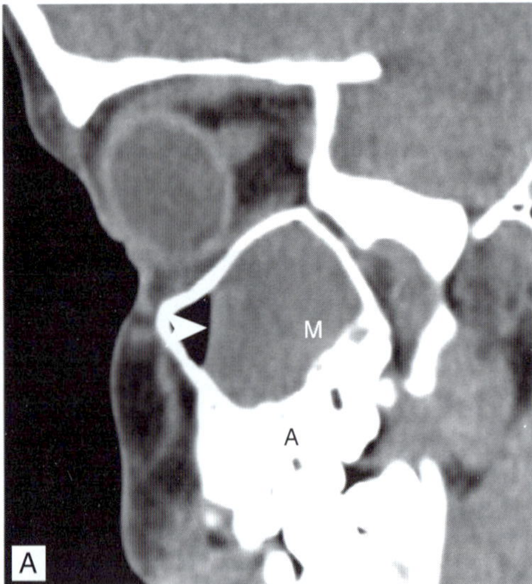

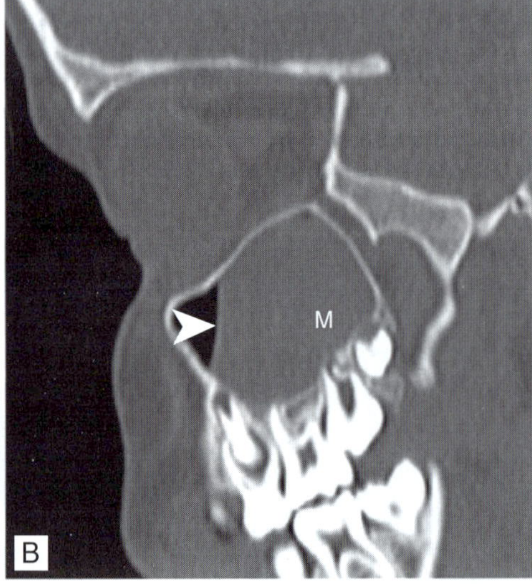

Figure 70.23 Noncontrast CT: (A) soft tissue window and (B) bone window, showing air–fluid level (*white arrowhead*) in left maxillary sinus (M). Note that the patient is supine during the scan and these are sagittal reformations, thus explaining the appearance.

BOX 70.2 Differential Diagnosis of Air–Fluid Levels in Paranasal Sinuses

i. Acute bacterial sinusitis: air–fluid levels are seen in 25–50% of such cases [39]
ii. Trauma, barotrauma
iii. Hemorrhage in patients with bleeding disorders
iv. Intubated patients, patients with nasogastric tube—in sphenoid sinus
v. Lavage of maxillary sinus—rare cause nowadays
vi. In children, may not be pathological—because of tears, normal retained secretions, normal redundant mucosa

BOX 70.3 Differential Diagnosis of Unilateral Paranasal Sinus Opacification

i. Acute bacterial sinusitis
ii. Chronic sinusitis
iii. Sinonasal polyposis
iv. Benign and malignant neoplasms
v. Mucocele
vi. Dentigerous cyst
vii. Ameloblastoma
viii. Silent sinus syndrome

Contrast-enhanced CT and MRI show meningeal enhancement, rim enhancing extradural, subdural, or cerebral lesions with edema. Cavernous sinus thrombosis is seen as heterogeneous filling defects within the sinus and may be accompanied by thrombosis of superior ophthalmic vein and dural venous sinuses [38].

iii. Osteomyelitis: Bony walls of the sinuses or adjacent bones may be involved by the infectious process, causing osteomyelitis, but this is rare in the present era of antibiotics. Imaging may show periosteal reaction, osteolysis, and sequestrum formation.

Chronic Sinusitis: Repeated attacks of acute sinusitis may result in chronic sinusitis. The main factors contributing to chronic sinusitis are inadequate drainage through natural ostia, impaired ciliary function, and thickened secretions.

Chronic sinusitis results in more "permanent" changes. The mucosa may show areas of hypertrophy, polypoidal thickening, atrophy, and fibrosis [40]. These mucosal changes result in impaired ciliary function which further predisposes the patient to repeated infection.

Collections within the sinuses vary in their appearance according to chronicity. Chronic sinusitis may be associated with polyp formation and reactive periostitis of the involved sinus wall, which appear as sclerosis (Fig. 70.25).

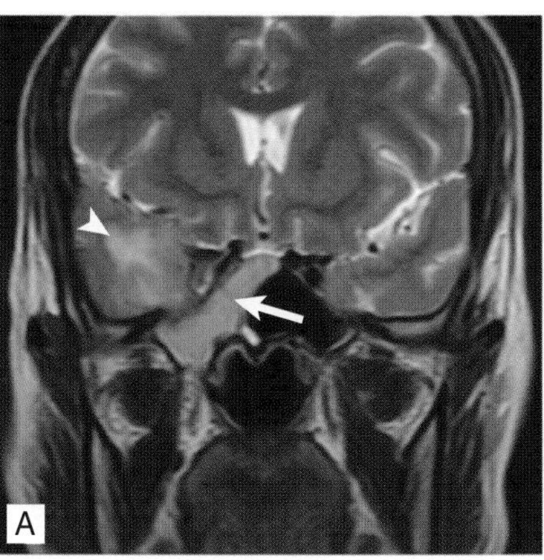

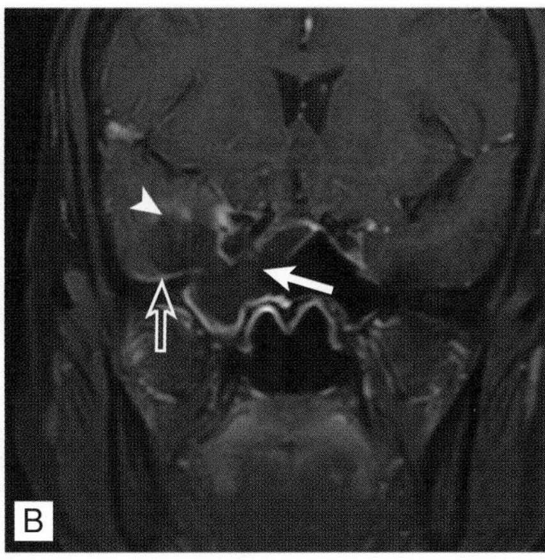

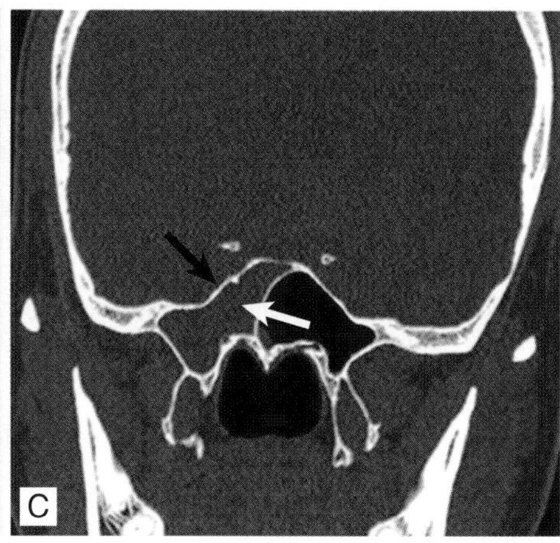

Figure 70.24 Intracranial spread of acute sinusitis in a 32-year-old man presenting with headache. (A) Coronal T2-weighted MR image shows collection within the right sphenoid sinus (*white arrow*) and hyperintensity within adjacent cerebral parenchyma at right temporal lobe (*arrowhead*). (B) Coronal post-contrast fat-saturated T1-weighted image shows mucosal enhancement in right sphenoid sinus (*white arrow*), adjacent meningeal enhancement (*outline arrow*), and nonenhancing Hypointense lesion in the temporal lobe (*arrowhead*), suggesting developing cerebral abscess. (C) CT scan (*bone window*) shows opacified right sphenoid sinus (*white arrow*) and intact bony wall (*black arrow*). (Courtesy: Dr. Manisha Agrawal. Jai Prakash Hospital and Research Centre, Rourkela.)

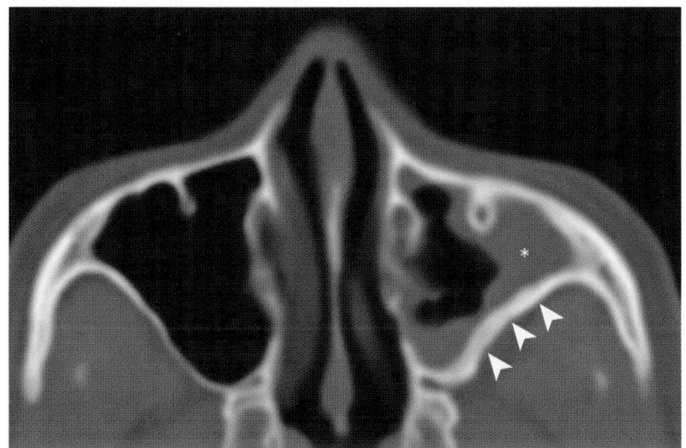

Figure 70.25 A 61-year-old man with history of chronic sinusitis. Noncontrast axial CT scan (bone window) shows mucosal thickening (*asterisk*), sclerosis of left maxillary sinus walls (*white arrowheads*) with inward bowing of lateral wall.

Imaging Appearance of Secretions in Sinusitis: The appearance of sinus secretions in inflammatory diseases depends on the chronicity and protein content. Initially, the contents are fluid or mucoid, appearing as hypodense on CT (0–25 HU). As chronicity develops, water content decreases and protein content increases, resulting in progressively thick secretions. The density in CT scan increases to 20–45 HU. On MRI, secretions in acute diseases are hypointense on T1-weighted images and hyperintense on T2-weighted images. Secretions with protein content between 5% and 30% appear hyperintense on T1-weighted images. With further increase in protein concentration, both T1 and T2 signal intensity falls and eventually may appear as signal void similar to air in sinuses. This may cause MRI to underestimate the disease extent in chronic sinusitis, and CT is helpful to visualize the actual extent of disease in such cases [41–43].

Patterns of Sinonasal Inflammatory Disease: Sinonasal inflammatory disease has been classified into five patterns for better identification and prognostication [44,45].

- Pattern 1 or "infundibular pattern" has obstruction at the level of inferior infundibulum and maxillary ostium, with involvement of the ipsilateral maxillary sinus
- Pattern 2 or "ostiomeatal unit pattern" has obstruction at the middle meatus, with involvement of one or more components of ipsilateral maxillary, frontal, and anterior ethmoid sinuses

These two varieties are common and are considered simple surgical patterns.

- Pattern 3: Obstruction at the level of sphenoethmoid recess, with involvement of sphenoid sinus and posterior ethmoid sinuses is described as the "sphenoethmoid recess pattern"
- Pattern 4: Polyposis involving nasal cavity and paranasal sinuses is defined as "sinonasal polyposis pattern"
- Pattern 5 is the "sporadic pattern" with random involvement of sinuses not attributable to known pathways and includes mucoceles and retention cysts

Patterns 3, 4, and 5 are usually felt to represent complex surgical patterns.

Fungal Sinusitis: There are various types of fungal sinusitis with some forms being very aggressive, leading to a fulminant course especially in immunocompromised patients. Fungal sinusitis may be classified in several ways (Box 70.4).

The most common classification of fungal sinusitis is according to the degree of tissue invasion and clinical course [47,48]:

1. *Noninvasive fungal sinusitis—mycetoma/fungal ball*: This is a conglomeration of fungal hyphae in a sinus cavity without invasion into surrounding tissues (Fig. 70.26). Risk factors are previous surgery or radiotherapy, impaired mucociliary clearance, ostial blockage. Maxillary sinus is involved in the majority of cases (84%) [47]. Immunocompetent middle-aged to elderly females are most commonly affected, and patients present with sensation of pressure in the sinuses.

   Imaging: Single sinus cavity is affected, unlike most other fungal sinusitis. Focal intrasinus high attenuation material is noted within the sinus on CT and is often associated sinus wall thickening and "periosteitis." On MRI, the fungal elements appear hypointense on both T1- and T2-weighted images due to absence

BOX 70.4 Classification of Fungal Sinusitis

Classification according to causative fungus:

1. Fungal hyphal disease—caused by mucor (violent clinical course) or *Aspergillus* (varied presentation from mycetoma to invasive disease)
2. Fungal yeast disease—caused by *Candida* (in the immunocompromised and postantibiotic setting), histoplasma (AIDS defining feature), *Cryptococcus* (in AIDS patients), *Coccidioides* (rare, extremely infectious, lethal)

Classification according to duration of symptoms [46]:

1. Acute—symptoms <30 days
2. Subacute—symptoms 30–90 days
3. Chronic—symptoms >90 days

Classification according to degree of invasion into tissue and clinical course:

1. Noninvasive fungal sinusitis—mycetoma/fungal ball
2. Noninvasive—allergic fungal sinusitis
3. Acute invasive fungal sinusitis
4. Chronic invasive fungal sinusitis
5. Granulomatous invasive fungal sinusitis

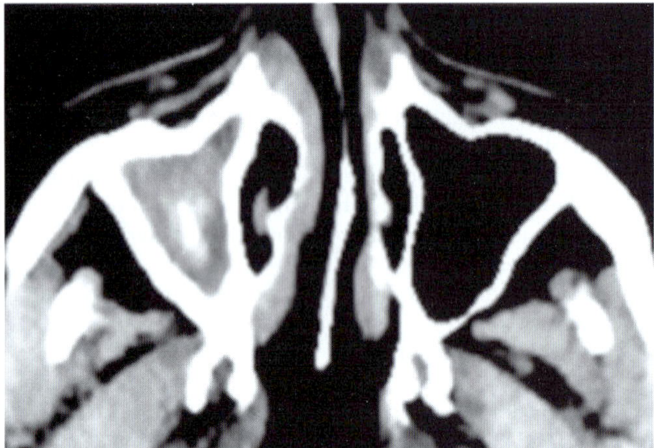

Figure 70.26 Fungal ball. Axial noncontrast CT scan shows single sinus involvement in the form of opacified right maxillary sinus with central high-density material suggesting fungal contents, surrounding secretions and mucosal thickening. Right maxillary bony wall shows sclerosis and thickening signifying chronic sinusitis. (Courtesy: Dr. Varsha Joshi.)

of water and presence of calcification and other paramagnetic substances, such as manganese, magnesium, and iron [49]. The fungal ball does not enhance, but surrounding thickened mucosa is hyperintense on T2-weighted images and enhances.

2. *Noninvasive—allergic fungal sinusitis*: Allergic fungal sinusitis is the most common form of fungal sinusitis and it represents IgE-mediated chronic inflammatory response of the sinus mucosa to fungal elements rather than true infection [49] (Fig. 70.27). Patients are young, immunocompetent, atopic, asthmatic, and this entity is more common in warm humid climate zones. Patients present with signs and symptoms of polyposis, such as facial dysmorphism, hypertelorism, and anosmia. Sinus contents are gray, green, brown inspissated thick mucus. Serum IgE is elevated.

   Imaging: Bilateral multiple sinuses are involved in an asymmetric fashion. The maxillary and ethmoid sinuses are most commonly involved. Noncontrast CT shows hyperdense areas surrounded by hypodense inflamed mucosa. The MRI signals vary according to the content and composition of mucin and can be both hypointense or hyperintense on T2-weighted images.

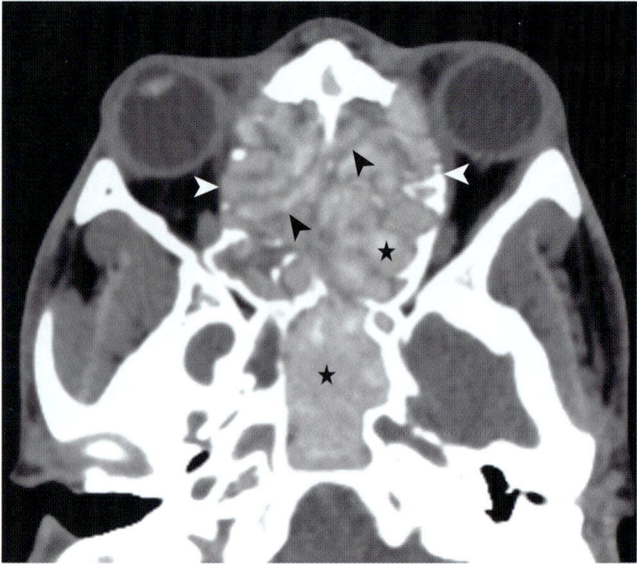

Figure 70.27 Allergic fungal sinusitis. Axial noncontrast CT scan shows opacification of ethmoid and sphenoid sinuses containing hyperdense material (*black stars*), suggesting inspissated secretions and fungal material. Intervening linear hypodense mucosa (*black arrowheads*) is seen in the ethmoid sinuses, and bony expansion is present (*white arrowheads*). (Courtesy: Dr. Varsha Joshi.)

   Enhancement is variable. Although this is a form of noninvasive sinusitis, it is usually associated with bony expansion and remodeling of the sinus walls. This form of sinusitis is usually treated with topical steroids and surgical exploration.

3. *Acute invasive fungal sinusitis*: This is the most aggressive and rapidly progressive form of fungal sinusitis, with a high mortality rate of 50–80% [49] (Fig. 70.28). Immunosuppressed and severely diabetic patients are predisposed to acute invasive fungal sinusitis. Disease onset is less than 4 weeks, and patients are acutely ill. Clinical features are similar to acute bacterial sinusitis, with fever, headache, facial pain, rhinorrhea, and nasal mucosal ulceration. In the COVID-19 pandemic, patients treated with systemic steroids have shown a predisposition to acute invasive sinusitis caused by mucor, leading to a grave prognosis [50] (Fig. 70.29).

   Imaging: Nasal cavity and multiple sinuses are affected, with associated bone destruction and extension of inflammation to the surrounding soft tissue, such as orbits, subcutaneous fat, and masticator space. Intracranial extension may be seen. CT is superior for assessment of the bony walls, and MRI is preferred for evaluating orbital and intracranial involvement. A characteristic feature of early disease is lack of enhancement of the mucosal lining of nasal cavity and turbinates (black-turbinate sign) due to the angioinvasive nature of the disease [51]. Treatment is debridement and antifungal therapy.

4. *Chronic invasive fungal sinusitis*: This is an indolent disease, with duration of symptoms more than 4–12 weeks. Patients are immunocompetent or mildly immunosuppressed, and present with sinus pain, discharge, and low-grade fever.

   Imaging: Imaging shows soft tissue thickening and collections within the sinuses, usually hyperdense in noncontrast CT scan, hypointense in T1- and T2-weighted images. Imaging features may mimic malignancy, with destruction of bone and extrasinus extension, involvement of orbital apex and cranial nerves. Bony sclerosis may be present due to chronicity [49]. Irregular calcification may also be seen in some cases [52].

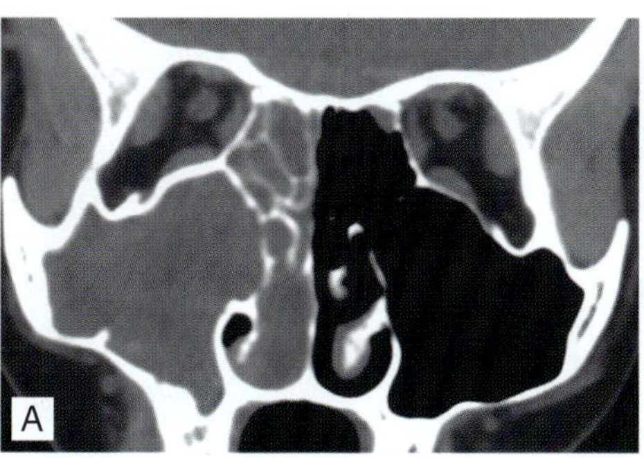

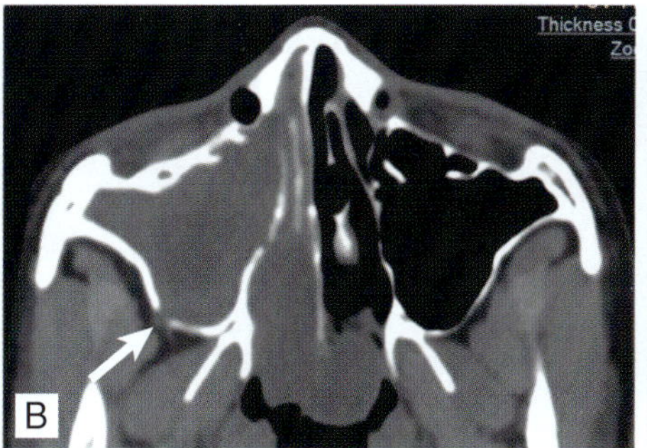

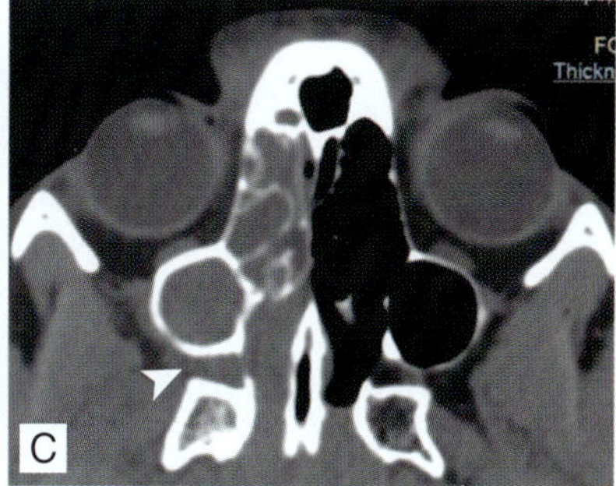

Figure 70.28 Acute invasive fungal sinusitis in a 14-year-old girl with leukemia on chemotherapy. Noncontrast coronal (A) and axial (B, C) CT scan shows opacification of right maxillary and ethmoid sinuses, right nasal cavity. Invasive nature of the disease is demonstrated by erosion of right lateral maxillary wall with soft tissue in the retromaxillary fat (*white arrow* in B) and in right pterygopalatine fossa (*white arrowhead* in C). (Courtesy: Dr. Varsha Joshi.)

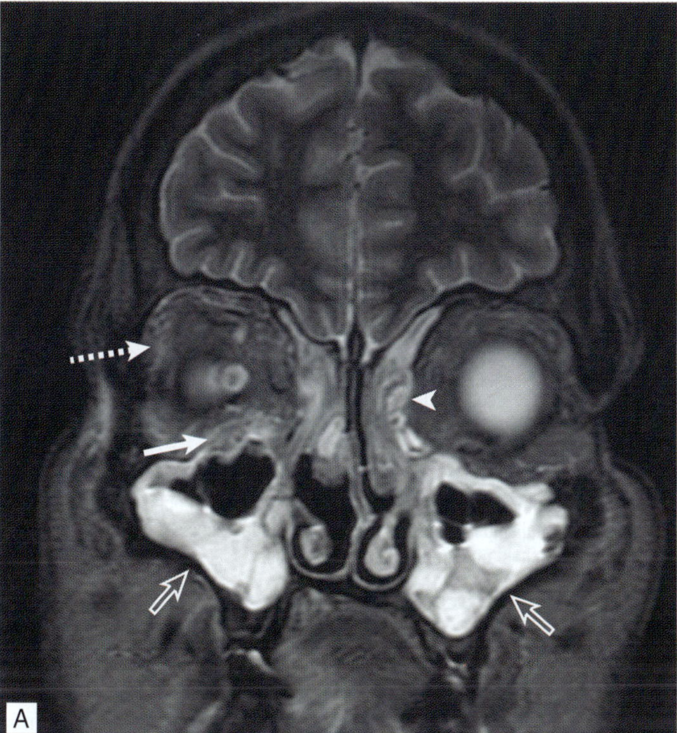

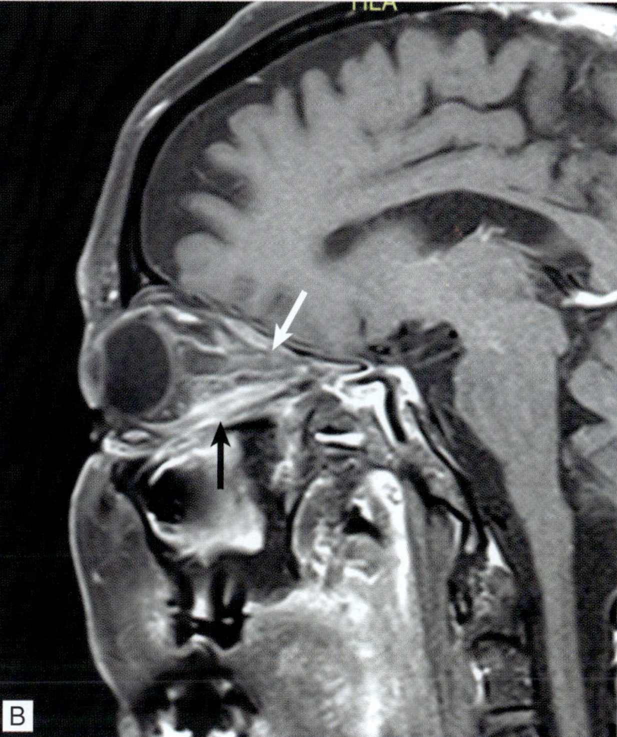

Figure 70.29 Acute invasive fungal sinusitis—mucormycosis in a post-COVID-19 patient. (A) Coronal T2-weighted fat-saturated coronal MR image shows mucosal thickening and collections involving bilateral maxillary (*outline arrows*) and ethmoid sinuses (*white arrowhead*). Right-sided intraorbital fat shows stranding (*dashed arrow*) and inferior rectus shows hyperintensity (*white arrow*). (B) Sagittal fat-saturated postcontrast T1-weighted image shows enhancement of right inferior rectus (*black arrow*), intraorbital fat and optic nerve sheath complex (*white arrow*), indicating the invasive nature of the disease and orbital spread of inflammation. (Courtesy: Dr. Anandamoyee Dhar Bankata. Max Superspeciality Hospital, New Delhi.)

5. *Granulomatous invasive fungal sinusitis*: Seen in immunocompetent patients, this disease is characterized by submucosal noncaseating granulomatous inflammation induced by sparse fungal elements (*Aspergillus*) [48]. Clinically, patients present with features of chronic sinusitis. Disease course is more indolent than chronic invasive fungal sinusitis.

   Imaging: Imaging features are similar to chronic invasive form and may mimic malignancy. Usually one or two sinuses are involved, bony destruction and extrasinus extensions are characteristic (Box 70.5 enumerates the reporting checklist for rhinosinusitis).

Allergic Sinusitis: Usually presenting with symmetric polypoid mucosal thickening, multiple paranasal sinuses are commonly involved in this condition. Children presenting with allergic sinusitis and polyps should be evaluated for cystic fibrosis [53].

BOX 70.5 Checklist for Reporting Rhinosinusitis

- Enumerate the sinuses involved, with laterality
- Assess degree of mucosal involvement in each sinus
- Some features may indicate acute disease, such as air–fluid level, and some features may indicate chronic disease, such as sclerosis, but do not provide final report as "acute" or "chronic" as overlapping features are present
- Mention nasal cavity findings separately. Thickening of unilateral turbinates may be attributable to nasal cycle/deviated nasal septum, and as long as some air can be demonstrated around the turbinates and septum, patient does not present with obstruction
- Small bilateral crenated inferior turbinates usually indicate the use of nasal decongestant
- Other structures to be routinely mentioned: skull base, orbits, visualized intracranial structures, visualized soft tissue under skull base

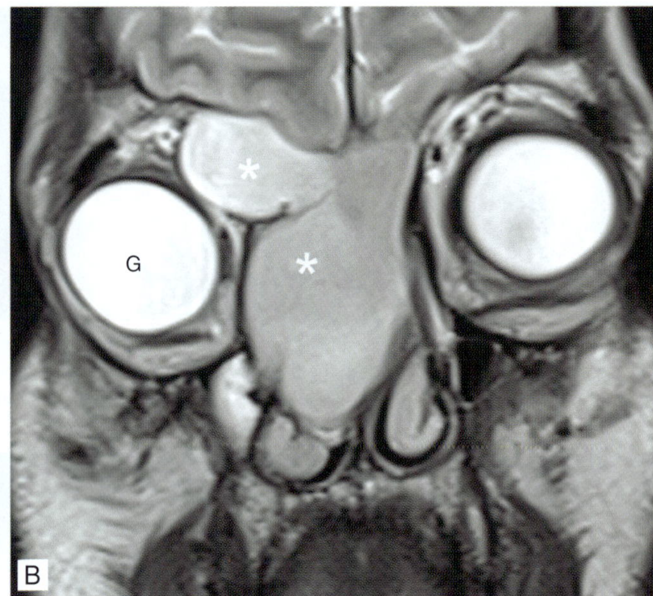

Figure 70.30 (A) Mucocele involving right frontal and anterior ethmoid sinus in a 36-year-old man presenting with right eye proptosis. (A) Coronal CT scan shows soft tissue filling the entire right frontal and anterior ethmoid sinuses (*asterisk*), expansion of the walls and bone remodeling (*black arrowheads*). At some places, the bony wall appears deficient. (B) Corresponding coronal T2-weighted MR image shows hyperintense contents within the mucocele. The mucocele bulges into right orbit and right globe (G) is displaced downward and outward.

Vasomotor Sinusitis: This is a clinical diagnosis, often one of exclusion. Nasal congestion, watery discharge, and polyps may occur in the absence of allergy, obstruction, or infection. Thickening of turbinates, serous secretions, and mild mucosal thickening of the sinuses are the common morphological changes, but there are no characteristic imaging findings.

Mucocele

A commonly encountered entity that expands the sinuses is mucocele (Fig. 70.30). Mucoceles usually present in adults of third and fourth decades and are slightly more common in males [54]. Mucoceles involve the frontal, ethmoid, maxillary, and sphenoid sinuses in decreasing frequency. Frontoethmoid varieties constitute 70–90% mucoceles, maxillary sinus approximately 10%, but sphenoid sinus involvement is rare [55]. Mucoceles result from obstruction of the ostium of a sinus or a septated compartment, resulting in retention of mucosal secretions, expansion of the entire sinus with bone remodeling. They are lined by the mucosal lining of the sinus. Clinically, mucoceles present because of their mass effect on the surrounding structures. Large frontal and maxillary sinus mucoceles may displace the globe. Anterior ethmoid mucoceles may result in a bulge at inner canthus, proptosis, and epiphora in case of lacrimal sac compression. Sphenoid sinus mucoceles are rare but can have serious complications if not treated early, and imaging plays a key role. Involvement of optic nerve, cavernous sinus, and oculomotor nerve may occur due to proximity, and patients may present with headache, blurring of vision and diplopia. Pain is a feature of an infected mucocele or a mucopyocele.

Imaging: CT scan is usually sufficient for the diagnosis of mucoceles. It shows an expanded, airless sinus with outward bowing of walls. Very large mucoceles have deossification of walls, and these parts of the bony wall may not be visualized in imaging, giving the impression of bone erosion. MRI may be needed for assessment of the contents and complications. The appearance of mucocele depends on the protein content. Faint enhancement may be seen at the periphery if contrast is administered (Box 70.6).

BOX 70.6 Checklist for Reporting Mucocele

- Type of secretion, as higher protein content/thicker secretions are difficult to drain for the surgeon.
- Integrity of wall: walls of frontal and sphenoid sinus are commonly deossified but intact, rendering them invisible in CT or MRI.
- Direction of displacement of globe, relationship with optic nerve.
- For frontal sinus mucocele: whether an orbital recess of the sinus is present, which is a common site of recurrence.

Mucus retention cysts result as a blockage of the duct of a seromucinous gland within the sinus. As a result, these cysts fill a part of the sinus, the rest of the sinus remaining aerated. Expansion of the sinus and bony remodeling is unusual. Majority of retention cysts occur in maxillary sinuses and are asymptomatic incidental findings.

Important differential diagnoses of mucoceles are cysts of dental or odontogenic origin, such as radicular (periapical) cysts and dentigerous (follicular) cysts. Odontogenic cysts may expand to involve a large part of the maxillary sinus and contain mucoid secretions. The presence of the "double bony wall" sign may help distinguish a large odontogenic cyst from a mucocele (Fig. 70.31).

Chronic obstruction of sinus ostium can also result in inward bowing of the sinus wall, commonly maxillary sinus, resulting in enophthalmos [56]. This entity is called the "silent sinus syndrome."

Sinonasal Polyps

Sinonasal polyps are the most common expansile masses of the nasal cavity. Polyps are pedunculated soft tissue masses arising from edematous hyperplastic upper respiratory mucosa.

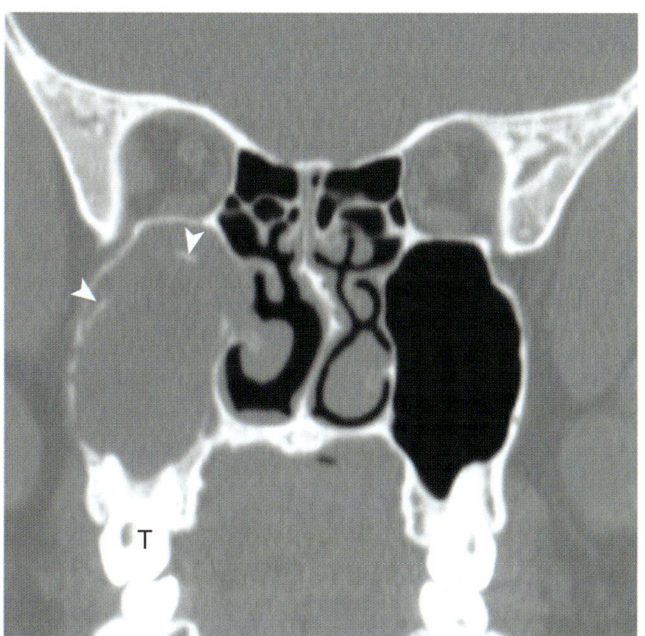

Figure 70.31 Odontogenic cyst. Coronal CT scan showing expansile soft tissue mass within the right maxillary sinus in relation to the roots of a tooth (T), signifying a radicular cyst—a type of odontogenic cyst. Dental origin is demonstrated by the thinned bony wall (*white arrowheads*) seen separately from maxillary sinus walls (*double bony wall*).

Polyps differ from serous retention cysts in the layer of fluid accumulation, which occurs in the deeper layers of lamina propria of the nasal cavity or sinus mucosa. These are associated with allergy, asthma, infections, vasomotor rhinitis, diabetes, cystic fibrosis, aspirin intolerance, and nickel exposure. These are usually small, with little vascularity, but if neglected, may lead to expansion, mass effect on orbits, bony remodeling and erosion, and even intracranial extension. Antrochoanal polyps arise from and fill the maxillary sinus, enlarge the ostium, prolapse into nasal cavity through sinus ostium and may even extend into nasopharynx and oropharynx.

Imaging: Polyps most commonly arise in the maxillary sinus [57]. These appear as homogeneous soft tissue masses within sinuses and/or nasal cavity with convex margins (Fig. 70.32), may be single or multiple (as in polyposis). Associated features are widening of the infundibulum, thinning of sinus walls and the nasal and ethmoid septa, bulging of the lamina papyracea, leading to displacement of the eyeballs, and hypertelorism. MRI features are similar to inflammatory disease in T1- and T2-weighted images.

Antrochoanal polyps may cause deossification or destruction of medial maxillary sinus walls, but the rest of the walls are unaffected (Fig. 70.33).

Granulomatous Diseases

Granulomatous inflammation of the sinonasal cavity may either be an isolated local disease or a part of systemic disorders. Infectious, inflammatory, autoimmune, substance abuse, and even traumatic and neoplastic diseases may cause granulomatous rhinosinusitis. These conditions may be indolent or severely destructive.

Actinomyces, tuberculosis, syphilis, rhinoscleroma, blastomycosis, paracoccidioidomycosis, leprosy, rhinosporidiosis, and leishmaniasis may cause granulomatous inflammation of the sinonasal cavity. Actinomyces infection of sinonasal cavity is a part of cervicofacial disease [58]. The process is destructive, mimicking malignancy. Soft tissue abscesses, multiple draining fistulas,

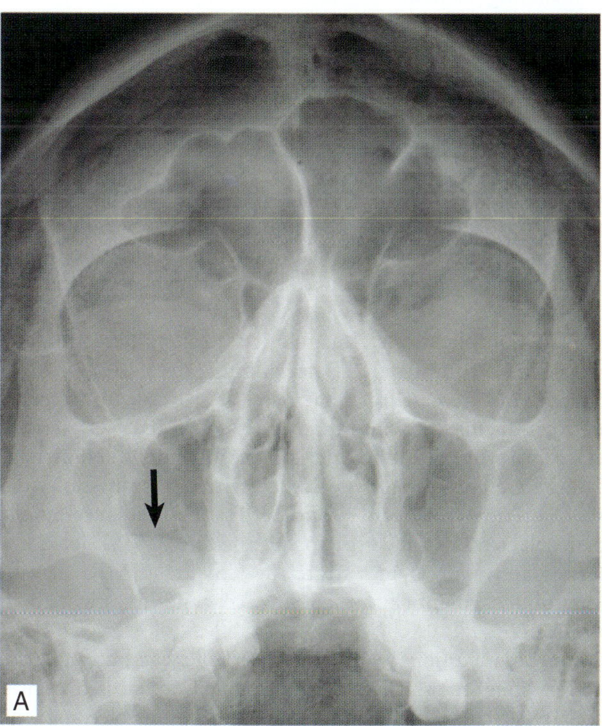

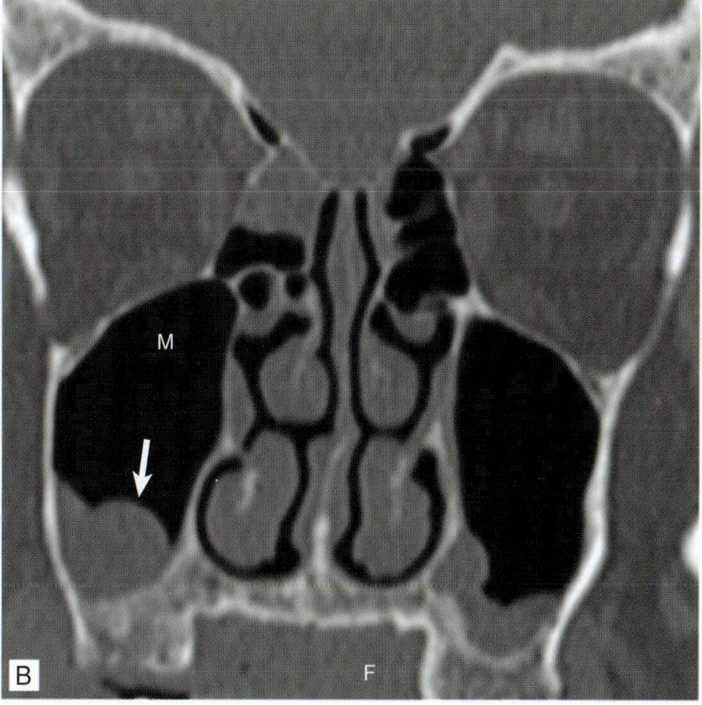

Figure 70.32 A 71-year-old man with right maxillary sinus polyp. (A) X-ray OM view showing opacity at lower aspect of right maxillary sinus with convex upper margin (*black arrow*). (B) Coronal noncontrast CT (*bone window*) shows homogeneous soft tissue mass within right maxillary sinus (M) with convex superior margin (*white arrow*).

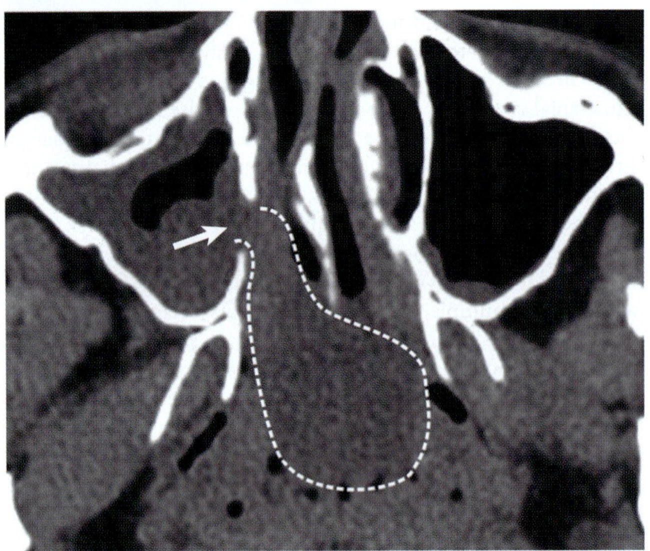

Figure 70.33 Antrochoanal polyp—axial CT scan. Outline of the polyp is marked with *dashed white line* and maxillary sinus ostium is marked with *white arrow*. (Courtesy: Dr. Varsha Joshi.)

and "sulfur granules" are characteristic morphological features. *Mycobacterium tuberculosis* and *M. bovis* rarely affect the sinuses, and may simulate granulomatosis with polyangiitis in both clinical features and histology. Atypical mycobacterial infections may involve the sinuses in end stage human immunodeficiency virus (HIV) patients.

Granulomatosis with polyangiitis, previously known as Wegener's granulomatosis, is a necrotizing granulomatous vasculitis affecting the sinonasal space, upper and lower respiratory tracts as well as the kidneys [59]. Elevated cytoplasmic antineutrophil cytoplasmic antibodies (cANCA) levels are observed. Sarcoidosis in the head and neck region may involve the sinonasal cavity and rest of the upper respiratory tract mucosa, neck nodes, orbits, and parotids. Beryllium exposure and cocaine abuse can also cause granulomatous disease of the sinonasal cavity.

Imaging: The granulomatous disorders most commonly involve the nasal cavity followed by paranasal sinuses. Focal or diffuse thickening of nasal septum are early observations that may progress to erosion and perforation. Nonspecific inflammatory sinus mucosal thickening is seen and maxillary and ethmoid sinuses are most commonly involved. Bony changes may range from chronic periostitis to destruction. On MRI, soft tissue within the sinonasal cavity is intermediate to hyperintense on T2W sequences, hypointense on T1W, and enhances with contrast. The findings are nonspecific and may mimic a malignancy.

Surgical Considerations for Infectious and Inflammatory Diseases: FESS and Imaging

FESS is a term coined by Kennedy et al. [60] and popularized by Stammberger [61]. The principal indication of FESS is refractory chronic sinusitis not responding to medical treatment. Other indications are recurrent acute sinusitis, nasal polyposis, antrochoanal polyps (arising from the maxillary antrum), sinus mucoceles, cerebrospinal leak closure, orbital decompression, choanal atresia repair, optic nerve decompression, control of epistaxis, and dacryocystorhinostomy [62]. FESS addresses the major factor contributing to chronic sinusitis, which is inadequate drainage (Box 70.7).

BOX 70.7 Overview of Steps of FESS [39]

- Endoscopic septoplasty, if needed, to relieve obstruction and facilitate access
- Uncinectomy: Removal of the uncinate process to gain access to bulla, maxillary ostium, and anterior ethmoids
- Maxillary antrostomy: Maxillary sinus ostium and infundibular widening, ostium is widened posteriorly and inferiorly
- Anterior ethmoidectomy: Removal of ethmoid bulla, removal of septa within the anterior ethmoid sinus complex
- Frontal sinusectomy: Frontal recess mucosa and obstructing cell removal
- Further exploration of sphenoid sinus may be done if required
- The surgery is customized, according to the need of the individual patient depending on the preoperative imaging findings
- The surgery may be unilateral or bilateral, minimal or extensive, involving single or multiple sites

Imaging: *Preoperative CT scan provides excellent visualization of the extent of disease and bony involvement.* Information about the anatomical variants helps the surgeon avoid potentially disastrous complications. The timing of CT should be after acute infection has subsided.

A pre-FESS CT scan needs to be reported using a structured format to mention all points and to make it easy for surgeons to review the report. The format of the report should follow the order of surgical steps and contain all the anatomical regions of the sinonasal space and related structures. The report should begin with the status and degree of involvement of each sinus and their drainage pathways, and move on to the description of sinus disease including content, mucosa, and bony walls. Anatomical variants and sequelae of previous surgery should be described in the report. In addition, complications of sinusitis and involvement of surrounding important structures, such as the brain and orbits, should be detailed. The radiologist should also look for a possible cause of sinusitis, such as an obstructing tumor. The relevant structures of the sinonasal space and their common anatomical variations have been discussed in the anatomy section. The most critical areas are the floor of anterior cranial fossa (cribriform plate), lamina papyracea, sphenoid sinus, Onodi cells, and anterior ethmoidal artery, and should be highlighted [63–65] (Box 70.8).

Post-FESS Complications: Imaging has a role in detection and evaluation of complications developing after FESS. Major complications are cerebrospinal fluid (CSF) leak, optic nerve injury, extraocular muscle injury, damage to the nasolacrimal duct, cribriform plate fracture, and perioperative hemorrhage and these are best initially evaluated with CT scan. Bony defect of anterior cranial fossa and soft tissue/fluid level at the site of defect raises the suspicion of the site of CSF leak. CT cisternography may demonstrate the CSF tract. MRI may be further done to demonstrate meningocele and investigate ocular injuries.

Minor complications which may occur following FESS are periorbital swelling or orbital emphysema, small orbital hematomas, temporary olfactory dysfunction, minor self-limiting bleeding (epistaxis), and tooth pain. Most of these resolve without intervention and imaging may not be required.

BOX 70.8 Pre-FESS Imaging Checklist: What the Surgeon Wants to Know

- Previous FESS/surgical changes
- Status of the sinuses:
  - Hypoplasia/excessive pneumatization
  - Involvement of each sinus
  - Description of sinus disease
- Complications of sinusitis
- Nasal cavity and septum
  - Turbinates
  - Septal deviation
  - Septal spur
  - Pneumatization
- Middle turbinate:
  - Concha bullosa/interlamellar cell of Grunwald
  - Pneumatized basal lamella
  - Paradoxical curvature, turbinate sinus
- Anterior skull base:
  - Cribriform plate
  - Asymmetry of olfactory fossa
  - Fovea ethmoidalis
- Ostiomeatal complex/unit and maxillary sinus:
  - Status of OMC
  - Ostium and accessory ostia
  - Infraorbital nerve canal
  - Superior attachment of uncinate process
  - Pneumatization/atelectasis of uncinate process
  - Status and pneumatization of maxillary sinus
  - Septate/duplicated maxillary sinus
- Frontal sinus drainage pathway and frontal sinus:
  - Status and pneumatization of frontal sinus
  - Frontal sinus wall dehiscences
  - Frontal beak and ostium
  - Frontal cells (types)
- Anterior ethmoidal sinuses and lamellar anatomy:
  - Bulla ethmoidalis
  - Supraorbital cells
  - Haller cells
  - Lamellar anatomy distortion
- Posterior ethmoidal sinuses
  - Height
  - Onodi cells
  - Pneumatization of anterior clinoid process
- Lamina papyracea and anterior ethmoidal artery
  - Defects/gaps
  - Vertical plane in relation to maxillary ostium
  - Dehiscence of bony canal of anterior ethmoidal artery
- Sphenoid sinus and optic nerve:
  - Sphenoid sinus pneumatization pattern
  - Intrasinus septum
  - Optic nerve canal, variations
  - Carotid canal, vidian canal, foramen rotundum
- Brain, orbit, upper neck

Sinonasal Neoplasms: Tumors and Tumor-Like Conditions

Epidemiology

Sinonasal neoplasms are rare and comprise approximately 5% of all head and neck cancers. The low incidence (1 per 100,000) [66] and commonality of clinical features with infective/inflammatory diseases result in low clinical suspicion, delayed diagnosis, and advanced stage of presentation. The majority (60%) involve the maxillary sinus, 20–30% occur in the nasal cavity, 10–15% in ethmoid sinuses, and 1% in frontal and sphenoid sinuses [67]. The global incidence varies, with certain parts of the world experiencing higher incidence, such as Japan, parts of China, and India. Most sinonasal cancers are more common in males with the male:female ratio varying from approximately 2:1 in squamous cell carcinoma (SCC) to 6:1 in intestinal type adenocarcinoma (ITAC) [68].

Clinical Presentation

Clinical presentation is similar to infective and inflammatory disease of the sinonasal space, namely, nasal stuffiness, congestion, obstruction, and epistaxis. Some lesions in the maxillary sinus may involve the alveolar margins causing loosening of tooth or pain. Headaches, visual disturbances, anosmia, and facial swelling are suggestive of advanced disease.

Classification

Discussion on the World Health Organization (WHO) classification of head and neck tumors, 2017, is beyond the scope of this chapter [69]. Broad subgroups are malignant epithelial, benign epithelial, soft tissue, hematolymphoid, germ cell, bone and cartilage, neuroectodermal and secondary tumors. The most common entities will be discussed here.

Imaging Features to Suspect Sinonasal Neoplasm (Fig. 70.34)

Clinical features of neoplastic and inflammatory disease overlap considerably. On imaging, certain observations increase the

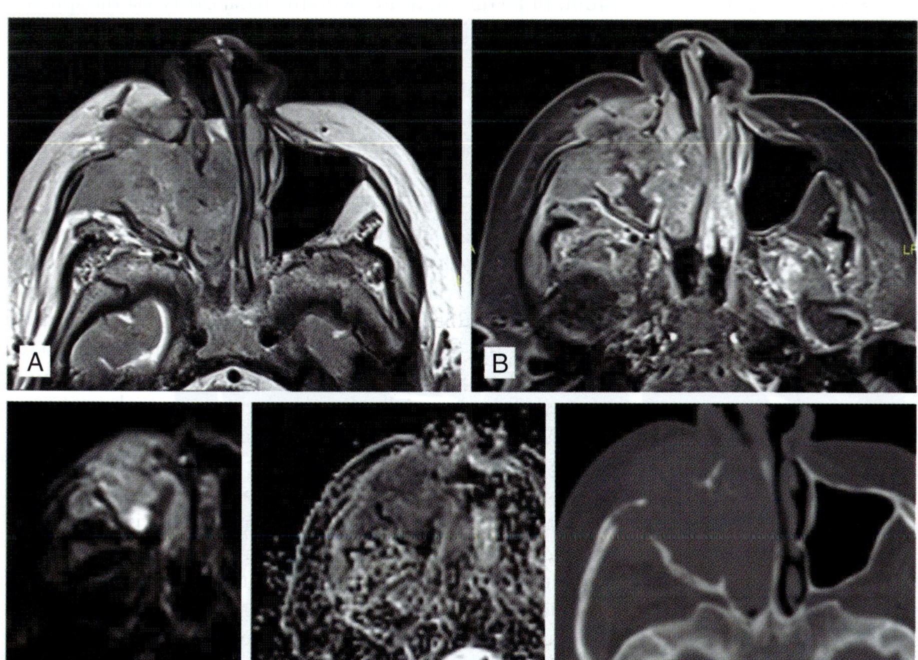

Figure 70.34 Features of sinonasal malignancies. (A) Axial T2-weighted MR image showing right maxillary mass (single site of origin), intermediate signal intensity. (B) Axial fat-saturated postcontrast T1-weighted MR image shows heterogeneous enhancement with necrotic areas. (C and D) High *b* value DWI and corresponding ADC image show restricted diffusion (hyperintense in C, hypointense in D). (E) Axial CT scan shows bone destruction.

suggests true dural involvement. Cerebral parenchymal involvement is suspected when there is parenchymal edema adjoining the tumor.

Involvement of Pterygopalatine Fossa and Related Neural Foramina: Contiguous tumoral involvement of PPF and its communicating pathways, namely, pterygomaxillary fissure, sphenopalatine foramen, foramen rotundum, vidian canal, and the greater and lesser palatine foramina are harbingers of poor prognosis. Careful inspection of these structures helps stage the disease and plan surgical approach as well as radiotherapy fields. On CT, replacement of fat density in these regions by enhancing or necrotic tumor tissue in contiguity with primary disease is the hallmark of involvement. Foraminal widening is also a very useful sign to detect disease encroachment. On MRI, replacement of fat is observed with tumor signals (Fig. 70.39). Enhancement is usually seen, but is variable and dependent on the amount of necrosis of the primary tumor.

Perineural Spread: The involvement of nerve sheath by a pathological process is known as perineural spread and is most commonly seen in malignancies. The phenomenon is different from perineural invasion, which is involvement of a nerve by a tumor and is a pathological diagnosis. Perineural spread may be contiguous (antegrade or retrograde) or may present as skip lesions. Perineural spread from sinonasal cavity may involve the branches of trigeminal nerve (CN V), more commonly maxillary (V2) and mandibular (V3) divisions.

The tumors commonly having higher propensity for perineural spread are adenoid cystic carcinoma (ACC), melanoma, lymphoma, and rhabdomyosarcoma [73]. SCCs have a low propensity for perineural spread, but as they are the commonest cancers in the sinonasal cavity, they are responsible for the majority of cases of perineural spread.

Perineural spread on imaging appears as thickening of the nerve on MRI with enhancement. The enhancement should not be confused with the normal enhancement seen along the perineural vascular plexus, in which case the nerve is not thickened. On CT, apart from a thickened and enhancing nerve, there is evidence of foraminal widening and loss of normal fat density at the skull base. In case of ambiguity, comparison with the contralateral side helps clinch the diagnosis.

The most helpful MRI sequence to detect perineural spread is volumetric contrast-enhanced fat-saturated T1-weighted images, obtained with high resolution, small field of view. Thin section axial and coronal T1- and T2-weighted images with and without fat suppression are also helpful [72]. Specialized MRI sequences, such as CISS help in visualization of intracranial courses of the nerves.

The key principle of imaging perineural spread is to image the entire course of the nerves. Perineural spread may have "skip lesions," and asymmetric enhancing soft tissue within *Meckel's cave* or cavernous sinus [74] on the ipsilateral side of the tumors may be the only indication of perineural spread. An additional evidence of perineural spread of tumor is denervation changes in the muscles supplied by the nerve. Early denervation changes are characterized by muscle edema and increased enhancement. Chronic denervation changes result in atrophy of the muscles. These changes are most commonly seen in the muscles of mastication in patients with V3 involvement.

Nasolacrimal Duct Involvement: Any malignant lesion in the inferior meatus of the nasal cavity can extend along the nasolacrimal duct to the preseptal compartment of the orbit. In such cases, the nasolacrimal duct is expanded and contains enhancing tumor which is best appreciated on contrast-enhanced T1W sequences.

Skin Involvement: Involvement of the subcutaneous fat in maxillary sinus carcinoma upstages the tumor to T3. Skin involvement further upstages the tumor to T4. This is usually evident clinically, and imaging may help to differentiate tumor extension to the skin from overlying edema.

Nodal Involvement: Staging of neck nodes is best performed by cross-sectional imaging. Of particular importance is detection of adenopathy in nonpalpable locations, such as retropharyngeal nodes. Signs of nodal involvement are size more than 1 cm, necrosis, and extranodal extension.

Common Benign Sinonasal Neoplasms

Schneiderian Papilloma: The mucosal lining of sinonasal cavity is termed as Schneiderian mucosa and is composed of stratified ciliated columnar epithelium. This mucosa is predisposed towards hyperplastic change, and may give rise to papillomas. These are uncommon and comprise approximately 0.5–4% of nasal neoplasms, typically present in males between fourth and seventh decade [75].

Three varieties are seen:

1. Exophytic papilloma (fungiform, squamous variety): The most common variety, comprising almost half of the cases, arises from nasal septum unilaterally, and is not associated with malignant transformation.
2. Inverted papilloma (endophytic variety): This is the second most common form and arises from the lateral wall of nasal cavity with extension into sinuses. Malignant transformation is seen in 5–15% cases [76], most commonly to squamous cell carcinoma (SCC).
3. Oncocytic papilloma (cylindrical variety): Rarest (3–5%) of all papillomas [77], this entity arises from the lateral nasal wall and has some malignant potential.

Imaging: On CT, papillomas present as unilateral masses with thinning or bowing of the sinus wall. Inverted papillomas may show foci of hyperostosis and osteitis at the site of origin which need to be resected to prevent recurrence. The classical feature in MRI is the cerebriform pattern best appreciated on T2W and postcontrast T1W sequences (Fig. 70.43). Features suggesting malignant transformation are bone destruction, necrotic area with loss of cerebriform pattern, and extrasinonasal extension.

Neurogenic Tumors

Schwannoma. These are benign tumors composed of Schwann cells and supporting neural elements and are more common in females of 30–60 years age.

Imaging: Schwannomas are ovoid, encapsulated, slow growing tumors causing bone remodeling (Fig. 70.44). Bone destruction is rare, and should raise the suspicion of malignant transformation. Enhancement is variable, depending on cellularity. MRI shows intermediate signal on T1-weighted images, intermediate signals on T2-weighted images if cellular, or hyperintense signals if cystic and stromal. Schwannomas may mimic juvenile nasopharyngeal angiofibroma by bowing of maxillary sinus wall but tend not to involve the pterygomaxillary fissure.

Neurofibroma. These are benign tumors composed of fibroblasts and neural elements. They may be single or multiple and may occur sporadically or in patients with genetic predisposition, such as neurofibromatosis.

Imaging: Imaging features are similar to schwannomas. One feature of neurofibromas is the extent of low density nonenhancing

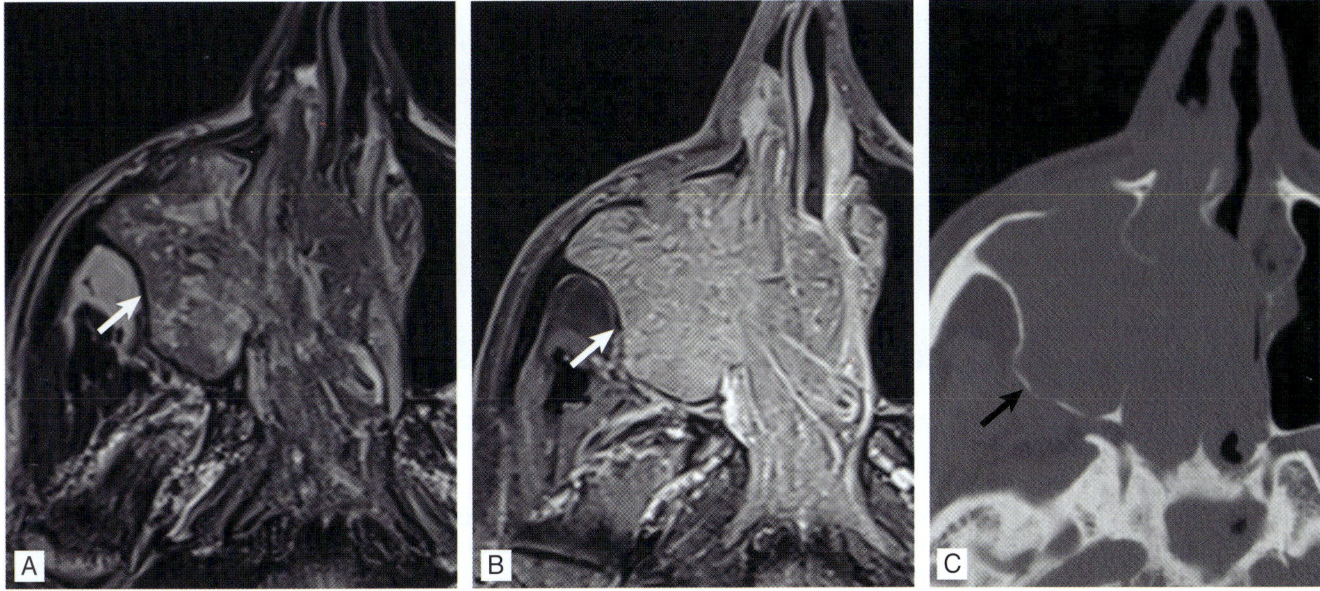

Figure 70.43 Inverted papilloma. Mass in the right maxillary sinus and nasal cavity (*white arrow*) showing fine linear pattern of alternating hypointense and hyperintense lines in axial T2-weighted MR image (A) and in corresponding postcontrast fat-saturated T1-weighted MR image (B). Bone remodeling of the maxillary sinus walls (*black arrow*) is seen in axial CT scan (C).

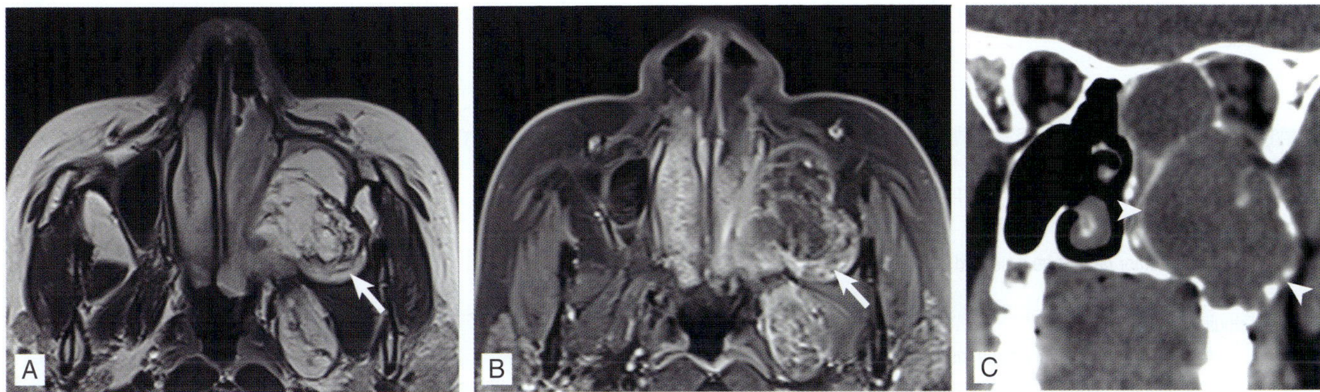

Figure 70.44 Schwannoma in a 44-year-old lady. (A) Axial T2-weighted MR image and (B) axial postcontrast fat-saturated T1-weighted MR image shows an encapsulated mass (*white arrows*) in the left maxillary sinus with hyperintense signals in A, heterogeneous enhancement in B. (C) Coronal CT scan image shows bone remodeling (*white arrowheads*).

areas in CT scan are more than schwannomas. Plexiform variety of neurofibromas are seen as large lesions, hyperintense on T2W images, infiltrating from superficial to deep, and have the appearance of "bag-of-worms."

Osteoma, Fibrous Dysplasia, Ossifying Fibroma, Ameloblastoma, Jaw Cysts. Please refer to the maxillofacial imaging section.

Juvenile nasopharyngeal angiofibroma: Please refer to the pediatric section (Chapter 81).

Common Malignant Sinonasal Neoplasms

Squamous Cell Carcinoma: SCCs are the most common cancers of sinonasal cavity and comprise nearly 65–70% of all sinonasal malignancies [78].

They are more common in males in the sixth to seventh decade. Risk factors include long-term exposure to nickel, chromium, mustard gas, isopropyl alcohol, coexistent inverted papillomas, prior radiation exposure and immunosuppression. The clinical findings of early lesions are nonspecific and overlap with infective and inflammatory lesions. Typical features include nasal stuffiness and obstruction, epistaxis, facial deformity, and visual changes. Clinical presentation is often late and patients present with advanced disease with involvement of the adjacent nasal cavities, sinuses, and orbits. SCC most commonly involves the maxillary sinuses (25–58%), nasal cavities (25–35%), ethmoid sinuses (10%), frontal and sphenoid sinuses (<1%) [79,80].

Imaging: On CT, these tumors usually present as soft tissue mass with bone destruction and extension to adjacent structures (Fig. 70.45). Rarely bone sclerosis might occur, but this is usually in the setting of a pre-existing inverted papilloma. The role of imaging is in the diagnosis and staging, excluding the various

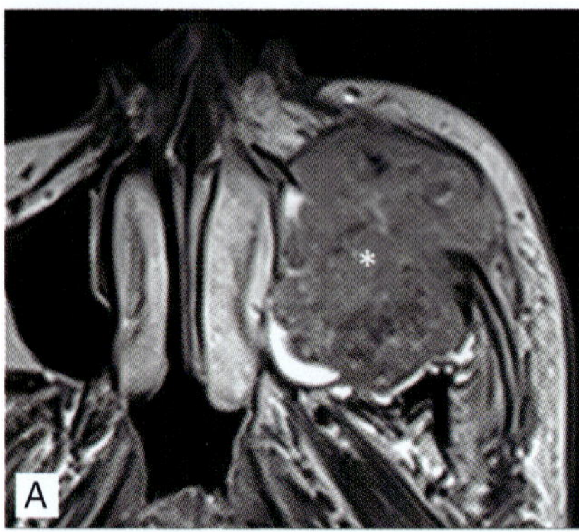

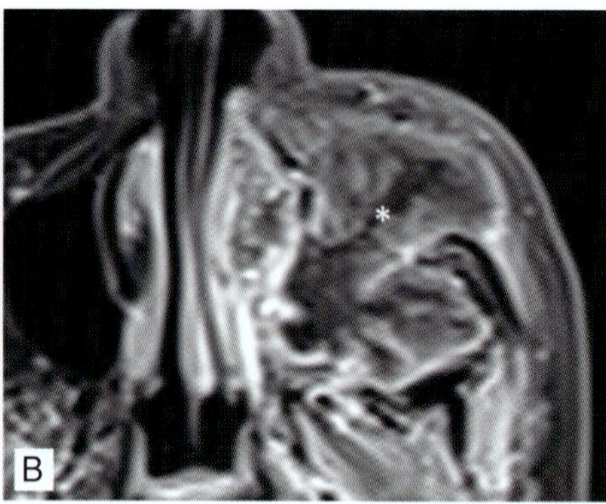

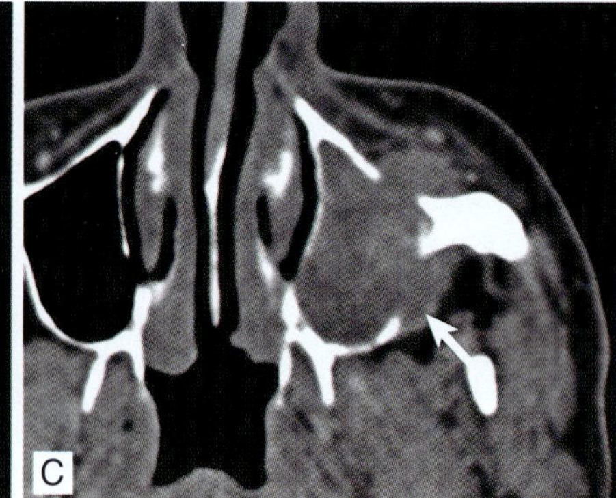

Figure 70.45 Squamous cell carcinoma in a 53-year-old man. (A) Axial T2-weighted MR image shows a destructive mass (*asterisk*) with intermediate signals. Heterogeneous enhancement with necrosis is seen in postcontrast T1-weighted MR image (B) and bone destruction (*arrow*) is seen in corresponding CT scan image (C).

subtle routes of extension such as perineural spread, and treatment planning. On MRI, SCCs are intermediate to mildly hypointense in T2-weighted images and may enhance. Small tumors enhance heterogeneously. Advanced tumors show large areas of necrosis.

Staging. The American Joint Committee on Cancer (AJCC) staging classification is summarized below and is separate for maxillary sinus and nasal cavity/ethmoid sinus (Box 70.10) [81]. Cancers at sphenoid and frontal sinuses are rare, hence no separate staging system exists for these sites. Nodal staging is detailed in Box 70.11.

Adenocarcinoma: Adenocarcinomas constitute 10% of sinonasal malignancies [79]. Adenocarcinomas are of two varieties: intestinal type (ITAC) and nonintestinal type (non-ITAC). ITAC may be related to occupational exposure to wood dust or sporadic, and are more common in males of 55–60 years age. Sporadic ITAC tend to occur more commonly in maxillary sinus and have a poorer prognosis. On the other hand, occupational exposure-related ITAC are more common in nasal cavity or ethmoid sinuses, present at an earlier stage, and have a better prognosis. Sinonasal non-ITAC are usually low grade.

BOX 70.10 American Joint Committee on Cancer

TNM staging system for the nasal cavity and paranasal sinuses (8th ed., 2017).

Primary tumor (T)

Tx	Primary tumor cannot be assessed
Tis	Carcinoma in situ
Maxillary sinus	
T1	Tumor limited to maxillary sinus mucosa with no erosion or destruction of bone
T2	Tumor causing bone erosion or destruction including extension into the hard palate and/or middle meatus, except extension to posterior wall of maxillary sinus and pterygoid plates
T3	Tumor invades any of the following: bone of the posterior wall of maxillary sinus, subcutaneous tissues, floor or medial wall of orbit, pterygoid fossa, ethmoid sinuses
T4	Moderately advanced or very advanced local disease
T4a	Moderately advanced local disease Tumor invades anterior orbital contents, skin of cheek, pterygoid plates, infratemporal fossa, cribriform plate, sphenoid or frontal sinuses
T4b	Very advanced local disease Tumor invades any of the following: orbital apex, dura, brain, middle cranial fossa, cranial nerves other than maxillary division of trigeminal nerve (V2), nasopharynx, or clivus
Nasal cavity and ethmoid sinus	
T1	Tumor restricted to any one subsite, with or without bony invasion
T2	Tumor invading two subsites in a single region or extending to involve an adjacent region within the nasoethmoidal complex, with or without bony invasion
T3	Tumor extends to invade the medial wall or floor of the orbit, maxillary sinus, palate, or cribriform plate
T4	Moderately advanced or very advanced local disease
T4a	Moderately advanced local disease Tumor invades any of the following: anterior orbital contents, skin of nose or cheek, minimal extension to anterior cranial fossa, pterygoid plates, sphenoid or frontal sinuses
T4b	Very advanced local disease Tumor invades any of the following: orbital apex, dura, brain, middle cranial fossa, cranial nerves other than V2, nasopharynx, or clivus

Note: For staging, the nasoethmoidal complex has been divided into two sites by American Joint Committee on Cancer, that is, nasal cavity and ethmoid sinuses. The ethmoids are further divided into two subsites, left and right, separated by nasal septum. The nasal cavity is divided into four subsites, the septum, floor, lateral wall, and the edge of nares to mucocutaneous junction. The maxillary sinus is divided into two subsites, left and right [81].

BOX 70.11 American Joint Committee on Cancer

TNM staging system for the nasal cavity and paranasal sinuses (8th ed., 2017).

Regional lymph nodes (N): clinical N (cN)

Nx	Regional lymph nodes cannot be assessed
N0	No regional lymph node metastasis
N1	Metastasis in a single ipsilateral lymph node, 3 cm or smaller in greatest dimension and extranodal extension (ENE)(−)
N2	
N2a	Metastasis in a single ipsilateral node larger than 3 cm but not larger than 6 cm in greatest dimension and ENE(−)
N2b	Metastases in multiple ipsilateral nodes, none larger than 6 cm in greatest dimension and ENE(−)
N2c	Metastases in bilateral or contralateral lymph nodes, none larger than 6 cm in greatest dimension and ENE(−)
N3	
N3a	Metastasis in a lymph node larger than 6 cm in greatest dimension and ENE(−)
N3b	Metastasis in any node(s) with clinically overt ENE (ENE_c)

Imaging: CT features of adenocarcinoma resemble those of other aggressive tumors such as SCC (Fig. 70.46). Calcification may rarely be seen, reflecting its mucin content [82]. Tumors with high mucin content are hyperintense on T2WI with gradual enhancement in postcontrast MRI. Tumors with low mucin content show intermediate to low T2 signals.

Sinonasal Undifferentiated Carcinoma: Sinonasal undifferentiated carcinomas, as the name suggests, are poorly differentiated carcinoma of the sinonasal cavity. These are rare, constituting 3–5% of sinonasal cancers [82]. These are more common in males and in the sixth decade, usual sites being ethmoid sinus and upper nasal cavity. The CT and MRI characteristics are indistinguishable from SCCs and usually present at an advanced stage and similar spread patterns as SCC.

Adenoid Cystic Carcinoma: Salivary gland carcinomas have been classified by WHO as a separate entity, and ACCs are the most common variety (35%) [83]. ACCs are typically known for their propensity to have perineural spread, either contiguous or as skip lesions, and may recur long after treatment, along the course of the involved nerve or at the surgical margins. Other salivary gland-like carcinomas include acinic cell carcinoma, mucoepidermoid carcinoma, carcinoma ex pleomorphic adenoma, epithelial–

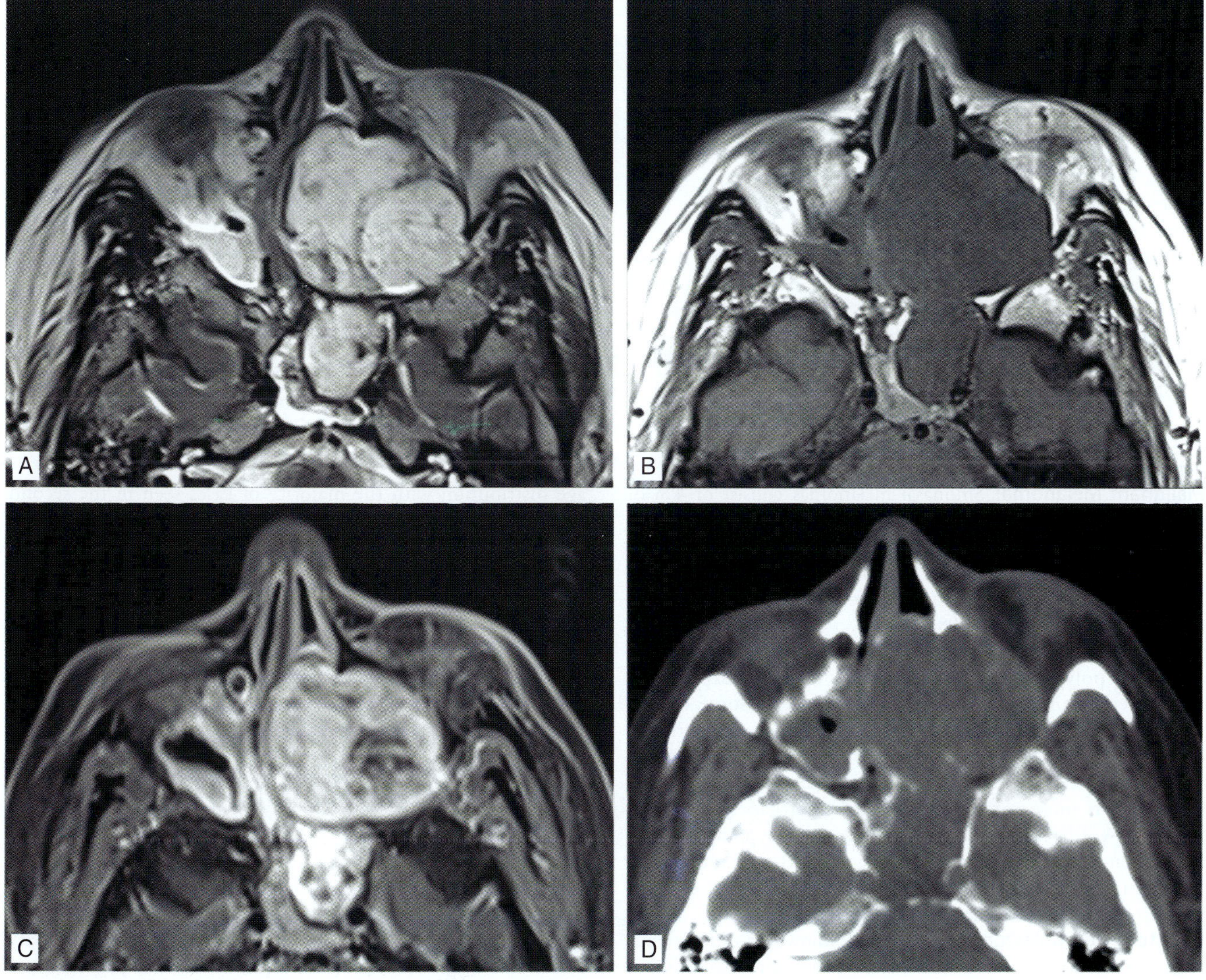

Figure 70.46 Adenocarcinoma of left ethmoid and maxillary sinuses in a 62-year-old lady with nasal bleeding. Axial T2-weighted MR image (A) shows predominantly hyperintense mass, which is hypointense in T1-weighted image (B), heterogeneously enhancing in postcontrast T1-weighted image (C). Bone remodeling with erosion is seen in axial CT scan image (D).

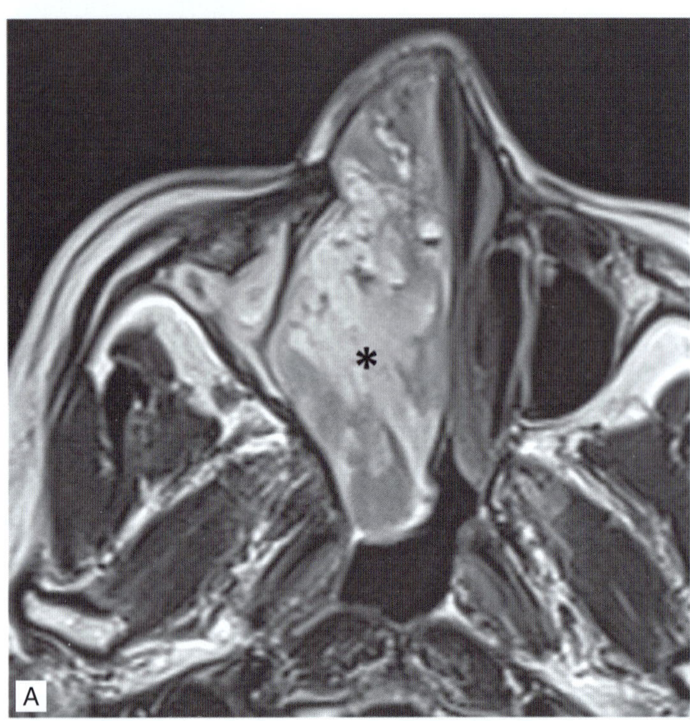

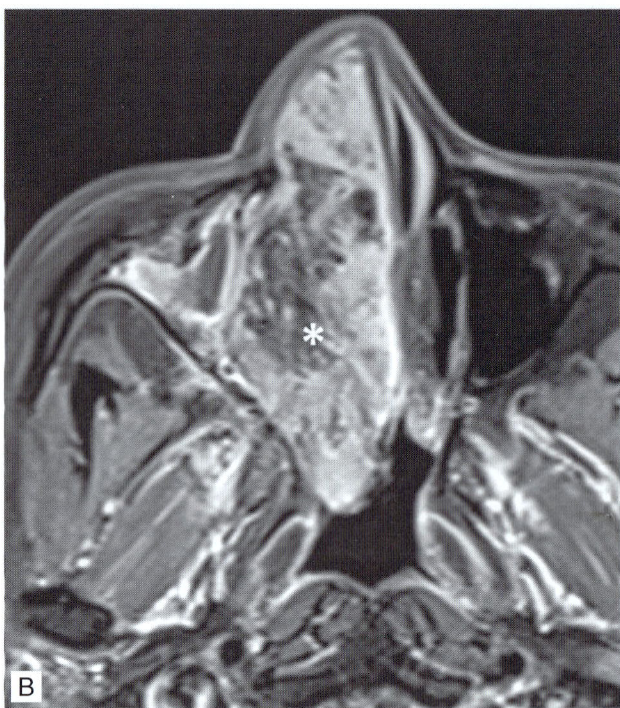

Figure 70.47 Adenoid cystic carcinoma in a 50-year-old lady with nasal bleeding. (A) Axial T2-weighted MR image shows a heterogeneous right nasal cavity mass (*asterisk*) with expansion. (B) Heterogeneous enhancement within the mass (*asterisk*) is seen in postcontrast fat-saturated T1-weighted MR image.

myoepithelial carcinoma, clear cell carcinoma N.O.S. The most common site is palate followed by the maxillary sinus.

Imaging: Low-grade ACCs are polypoid soft tissue masses on CT and may mimic a simple polyp (Fig. 70.47). High-grade ACCs present as large heterogeneous destructive masses [1]. Low-grade ACCs show hyperintense signals on T2WI. The moderate and poorly differentiated ones show progressive hypointensities on T2WI.

ACCs have widespread local invasion. Perineural spread is best detected on MRI, with the maxillary segment of the trigeminal nerve being most commonly affected in sinonasal ACCs.

Malignant Melanoma: Sinonasal melanomas consist of 4% of sinonasal malignancies and are a subset of extracutaneous mucosal melanomas arising from melanocytes of neural crest origin [84]. Patients may present with nasal stuffiness, facial deformities, and lymphadenopathy. These tumors are associated with poor prognosis, 5-year survival being <30% [85,86].

Imaging: The morphology of sinonasal melanoma may vary from polypoid to mass-like lesions that may expand the sinus cavities and destroy bony walls. On CT, some lesions show increased attenuation due to melanin or hemorrhagic contents.

Characteristic MRI finding is the presence of T1 hyperintensity which is more commonly due to hemorrhage rather than melanin. A T1-septate pattern of alternating hypointense and hyperintense lines in T1-weighted images has been described in melanomas, similar to T2 and T1 postcontrast "cerebriform pattern" in inverted papillomas [87] (Box 70.12).

BOX 70.12 Differential Diagnosis of T1-Hyperintense Lesions in Sinonasal Cavity

1. Melanotic melanomas
2. Hemorrhagic primary neoplasms: JNA, hemangioma, olfactory neuroblastoma
3. Hemorrhagic metastases from: renal cancer, thyroid cancer
4. High protein content secretions

Olfactory Neuroblastoma: Historically known as esthesioneuroblastoma, these tumors arise from the neuroepithelial lining of the olfactory mucosa which lines the cribriform plate, upper third of nasal septum, and superior turbinate. There is bimodal age distribution with the majority of cases seen in the second and sixth decades. The Kadish staging is often used to help assess extension and predict outcome [88].

Imaging: In CT, esthesioneuroblastoma are homogeneous enhancing soft tissue masses which contain focal areas of calcification (Fig. 70.48). These tumors often erode bone and extend into the anterior cranial fossa, adjacent paranasal sinuses, and orbits. CT plays an important role in determining the integrity of cribriform plate, fovea ethmoidalis, and lamina papyracea. Cervical nodal (20–25%) and distant metastases (10–40%) may occur. On MRI, these tumors are hyperintense on T2W images and enhance on contrast administration. The characteristic imaging findings are a "figure-8" appearance with "waist" occurring at the cribriform plate, and peritumoral cysts. The cysts are often seen at the tumor brain interface [89].

Lymphomas: Lymphomas involving the sinonasal space are part of extranodal presentation of lymphomas, primarily non-Hodgkin's lymphomas (NHLs). They represent 2–5% of total primary extranodal lymphomas [90]. Sinonasal NHLs are classified into B cell lymphomas, more common in western countries, and NK-T cell lymphomas, more common in Asian countries

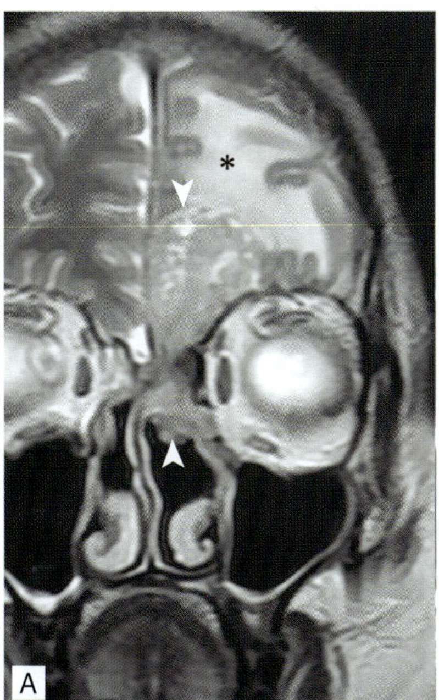

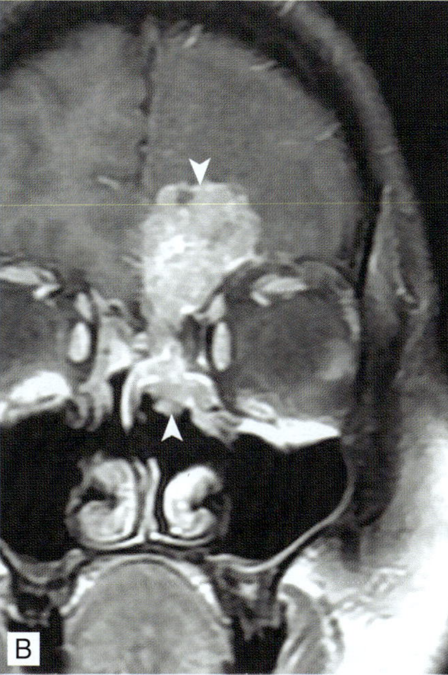

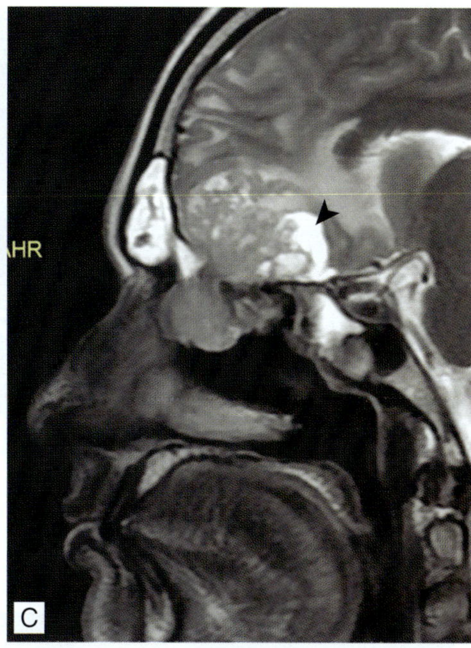

Figure 70.48 A 44-year-old man with olfactory neuroblastoma. The patient presented with headache, facial puffiness, seizure for 2 months. (A) Coronal T2-weighted MR image shows soft tissue mass (*white arrowheads*) at roof of left nasal cavity–cribriform fossa region and left anterior ethmoid air cells with invasion into anterior cranial fossa and frontal lobe involvement, signified by brain edema (*asterisk*). (B) Coronal postcontrast fat-saturated T1-weighted image shows avid enhancement of the mass (*white arrowheads*). (C) Sagittal T2-weighted MR image shows peritumoral cysts (*black arrowhead*) at tumor–brain interface.

TABLE 70.3 Comparison of Features of Sinonasal DLBCL and NK-T Cell Lymphomas

	DLBCL	NK-T Cell Lymphomas
Epidemiology	More common in Europe and North America	More common in Asian, Central, and South American countries Strong association with Epstein–Barr virus [92]
Site [93–95]	Maxillary sinus more commonly involved	Nasal cavity location is more common
Clinical course	Less aggressive, better prognosis	More aggressive, poorer prognosis
Imaging features	Homogeneously enhancing mass	Areas of necrosis may be seen Sheet-like appearance may be seen
Association with systemic lymphoma	Uncommon	Common

DLBCL, diffuse large B cell lymphoma; *NK-T*; natural killer/T-cell.

(Table 70.3). NHL most commonly involves the maxillary sinus while Burkitt's lymphoma may involve maxilla, mandible, and other facial bones.

Imaging: Lymphomas are destructive enhancing soft tissue mass often associated with bony remodeling or erosion (Figs. 70.49 and 70.50). Lymphomas typically have intermediate T1W signals and are mildly hyperintense on T2W images. Lymphomas have been shown to have lower ADC values compared to SCC [91].

Leukemia: Granulocytic or myeloid sarcomas, previously known as chloromas, are soft tissue deposits of myeloid precursor cells associated with acute myeloid leukemia, and 12% of these are seen in the head and neck region [96]. In the head and neck region, myeloid sarcomas may involve bones of the skull base, orbits, and paranasal sinuses. Imaging features are nonspecific, but most common appearance is a soft tissue mass, isointense to muscle in T1-weighted images, mildly hyperintense in T2-weighted images, with strong homogeneous contrast enhancement, slightly infiltrative margins [97].

It is important to note that imaging of the sinonasal space in hematologic malignancies is most commonly performed to rule out infection. Fungal infections are common in hematologic malignancies and also as a complication of immunosuppressive treatment.

Plasma Cell Neoplasms: Sinonasal cavity may be involved by *extramedullary plasmacytomas* as a part of initial presentation of multiple myeloma or as a part of disseminated disease. Bony lesions may be seen as single (*solitary plasmacytoma*) or multiple punched out lytic lesions (*multiple myeloma*). More than 80% of extramedullary plasmacytomas are seen in the upper

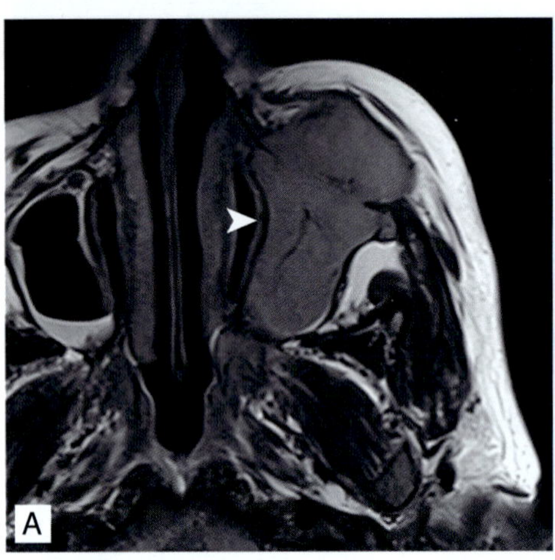

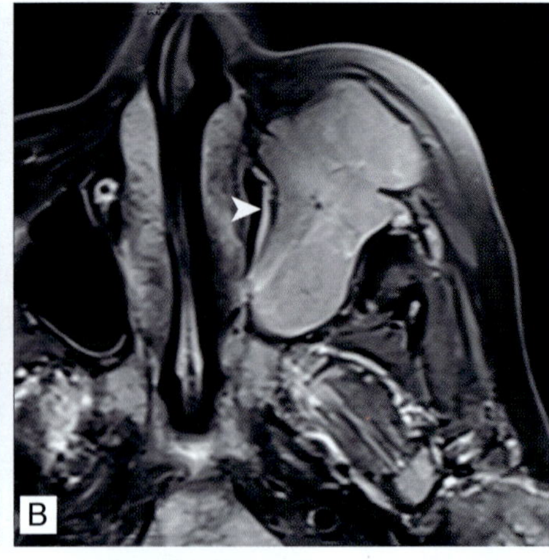

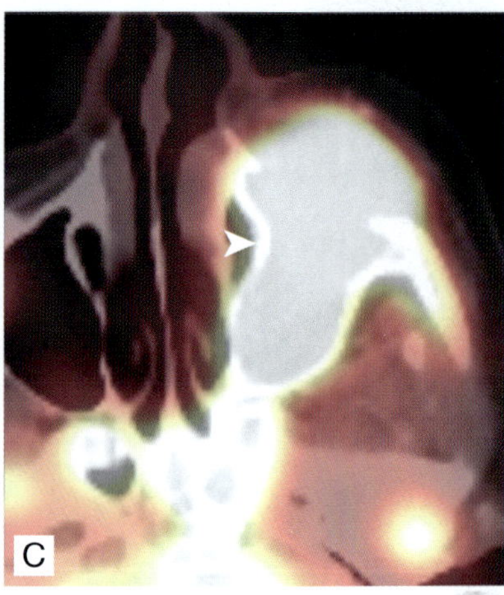

Figure 70.49 A 36-year-old lady with B-cell lymphoma. (A) Axial T2-weighted MR image shows an expansile soft tissue mass (*arrowhead*) in left maxillary sinus with homogeneous intermediate signals showing bone remodeling as well as destruction. (B) Homogeneous enhancement (*arrowhead*) is seen in postcontrast fat-saturated T1-weighted MR image. (C) Corresponding axial PET-CT image shows high metabolic activity in the mass (*arrowhead*).

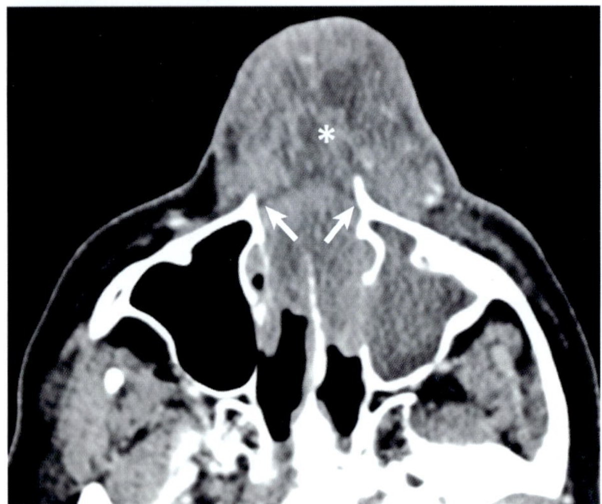

Figure 70.50 NK-T cell lymphoma in a 32-year-old lady. Axial CT scan image shows large nasal cavity mass (*asterisk*) with heterogeneous enhancement and bone remodeling (*white arrows*).

aerodigestive tract of which 80% involve the sinonasal cavity [98]. Nasal cavity involvement is more common than paranasal sinuses. If solitary plasmacytoma is encountered in the sinonasal cavity, systemic dissemination may be investigated with PET-CT or whole body MRI, and biochemical studies.

Imaging: CT scan shows polypoidal enhancing masses with bone remodeling, and MRI shows intermediate signal intensity lesions in all sequences with variable enhancement.

Soft Tissue Sarcomas: This is a heterogeneous group of malignant neoplasms arising from fibrous, vascular, myogenic, cartilaginous, and osseous tissues. Relatively common entities include rhabdomyosarcomas, chondrosarcomas, osteosarcomas, and Ewing's sarcomas/PNET. Their features are summarized in Table 70.4.

Secondary Tumors: Metastases to the sinonasal cavity are uncommon. Usually a single sinus is involved and imaging features may mimic a primary. Primary malignancies metastasizing to the sinonasal cavity are renal cell cancer (50%), breast, colon, prostate, thyroid, female genital tract cancers [99]. Renal cell cancer metastases are often hypervascular and patients may present with epistaxis.

TABLE 70.4 Features of Different Types of Soft Tissue Sarcomas Involving the Sinonasal Space

	Rhabdomyosarcoma (RMS) (Fig. 70.51)	Chondrosarcoma (CS)	Osteosarcoma (OS)	Ewing's Sarcoma (ES)/ PNET
Age	Wide age range, more common in children	Fifth decade, later than OS	Peak is 1–2 decades later than skeletal OS	5–30 years
Epidemiology [39]	Sinonasal RMS are a rare location of head and neck RMS (8% of head and neck RMS) May be secondarily involved from orbital RMS	5% of CS arise in head and neck Site: Maxilla > nasal cavity, ethmoid, sphenoid > mandible/ nasal tip. Associations: Irradiation, Maffucci's syndrome, Ollier's disease	7% of OS arise in head and neck Site: Maxilla > mandible involvement Associations: Paget's disease, retinoblastoma, irradiation Poorer prognosis of radiation induced OS	1–4% of ES arise in head and neck Site: Mandible > maxilla > calvarium > cervical spine. Rare within sinonasal cavities Associations: Irradiation following retinoblastoma
Imaging	Nonspecific features: usually homogeneous, enhancing, associated with bone remodeling/destruction	Marginal bone erosion seen, characteristic chondroid calcification is diagnostic if present High T2 signals, intense enhancement	Sunburst periosteal reaction, bone destruction seen, dense sclerotic bone may be present T1 and T2 signals vary depending on bone content Enhancement is less than CS	Destructive soft tissue mass, rarely expansile mass Onion-peel periosteal reaction

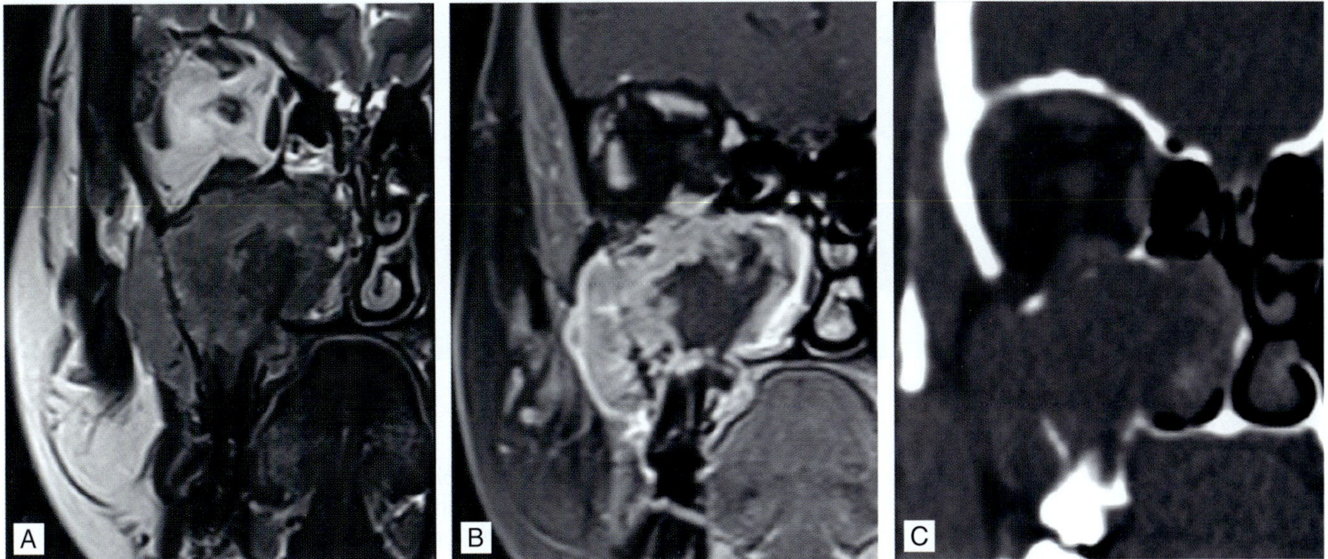

Figure 70.51 Rhabdomyosarcoma in a 15-year-old boy. Coronal T2-weighted (A) and postcontrast fat-saturated T1-weighted (B) MR images show a heterogeneous signal intensity enhancing mass with necrotic areas in right maxillary sinus. Extensive associated bone destruction is seen in coronal CT scan (C). (Permission from: S Sen, A Chandra, S Mukhopadhyay, P Ghosh, Sinonasal tumors, Neuroimaging, Clin N Am 25 (2015) 595–618.)

Suggested Readings

- S Vaid, N Vaid, S Rawat, AT Ahuja, An imaging checklist for pre-FESS CT: framing a surgically relevant report, Clin Radiol 66 (5) (2011) 459–470.
- WT O'Brien Sr, S Hamelin, EK Weitzel, The preoperative sinus CT: avoiding a "CLOSE" call with surgical complications, Radiology 281 (2016) 10–21.
- VM Joshi, R Sansi, Imaging in sinonasal inflammatory disease, Neuroimaging Clin N Am 25 (2015) 549–568.
- S Sen, A Chandra, S Mukhopadhyay, P Ghosh, Imaging approach to sinonasal neoplasms, Neuroimaging Clin N Am 25 (2015) 577–593.
- S Sen, A Chandra, S Mukhopadhyay, P Ghosh, CT and MRI in imaging sinonasal neoplasms, Neuroimaging Clin N Am 25 (2015) 595–618.

71 Orbit

ALLAN MIDYET, DEEPAK BHATT, SURESH K. MUKHERJI

71.1 Technique

While the orbit's observable share of skull volume sometimes seems small, their central role in visual function clearly causes them to commandeer a critical function. Modern orbital imaging has come to rely on a current a triad of tried and true techniques of ultrasonography (USG), computed tomography (CT), and magnetic resonance imaging (MRI). Imaging techniques tried in yesteryear have largely been replaced, although they are sometimes resurrected in special circumstances, including catheter angiography, fluoroscopy, plain film radiography, nuclear medicine, orbital venography, and dacryocystography. Within CT & MRI there are powerful specialized subtechniques, including CT angiography (CTA) and MR angiography (MRA). With the choice of multiple techniques, it is more important than ever that orbital imaging is directed by individuals who can correlate clinical history and physical examination to perform and interpret these often elaborate examinations.

CT is frequently the first technique performed in trauma cases, often because these patients have trauma to more than just the orbit, and CT is their initial study. CT excels in cases needing exquisite bony detail. In complex orbital cases, CT and MRI are commonly complimentary.

MRI: Probably the procedure of choice for evaluation of visual impairment or suspected cranial nerve abnormality allowing assessment of entire cranial nerves and visual pathways. While T1 Gd images with fat saturation are sometimes superb, most neuroradiologists have found that fat is the imager's friend and that T1 images without contrast are essential in evaluating marrow signal in skull base and orbital foramina. Continued progress in protocols and coil design show significant strides shifting some avoid artifacts while others exploit them. Every effort should be made to eliminate eye makeups which contain ferromagnetic particles. As always, all absolute contraindications to MRI should be observed including but not limited to noncompliant intracranial devices. Imaging sequences should be tailored to the individual imaging situation but in general include T1, T2, and T1 Gd. Postcontrast fat saturation frequently improves conspicuity of subtle lesions. MRA and/or MRV sometimes show abnormality involving the arteries and veins. 2D and 3D time of flight and phase contrast techniques should be tailored to the suspected abnormality.

USG is discussed in detail elsewhere in this text.

Various lesser used techniques for the orbit include plain films, dacryocystography, angiography, PET CT, and PET MRI and are discussed further in this chapter and elsewhere in this text.

Anatomy

Bony orbits: Resemble conical cones, with ice cream at its base and a small posterior apex. The four sides form a *floor*, a *roof* with *lateral and medial walls* which are loosely lined with periorbital periosteum contiguous with intracranial dura.

- The orbital *roof* is formed anteriorly by the frontal bone and posteriorly by the sphenoid's lesser wing
- The lateral wall forms from the zygoma anteriorly and the sphenoid's greater wing posteriorly
- The orbital floor and medial walls exhibit complex embryologic origins evolving from several segments of sphenoid, maxilla, zygoma, palatine, ethmoid, lacrimal bones. These are thinner and predisposed to fracture, particularly the paper-thin *lamina papyracea* of the medial wall

Principal posterior openings include the optic canal, as well as superior and inferior orbital fissures (IOFs). Cylindrical optic canals connect the middle cranial fossa to the orbit and convey the ophthalmic artery and optic nerve with supplementary sympathetic fibers. Located lateral and caudal to the optic canal, the superior orbital fissure (SOF) comprises a craggy orbital apex cleft connecting the orbit to the middle cranial fossa conveying essential structures, including CN III, IV, V_1, VI. The IOF enters the orbit caudal the SOF opening onto the posterolateral orbital floor. The IOF transmits the infraorbital and zygomatic nerves, the infraorbital artery (and vein), orbital ganglionic branches of the pterygopalatine ganglion, a branch of the inferior ophthalmic vein and various venous emissaries to the pterygoid plexus. The supraorbital and infraorbital foramina are important structures superiorly and inferiorly. Important medial foramina include the anterior and posterior ethmoidal foramina which convey the anterior and posterior ethmoidal nerves, arteries, and veins. Embryologically, the bony orbits manifest a montage of no less than seven different bones including the frontal, ethmoid, sphenoid, maxilla, zygoma, lacrimal, and last but not least, the palatine bones [1].

Optic pathway: The posteriorly pointing orbital apex conveys the ophthalmic (artery and veins) and cranial nerves (II, III, IV, V_1, and V_2, VI) through three optic openings including the optic canal and outlets through the superior and IOFs which form a V with a medially pointing apex. Before forming the base of the anterior clinoid process, the optic strut separates the optic canal from the SOF. CN II is surrounded by meninges continuous with visceral dura forming the optic nerve sheath containing varying quantities of CSF within the perioptic subarachnoid space. Retinal axions pierce the choroid and sclera to connect with the optic nerve. The ophthalmic artery courses into the optic canal inferior to the optic nerve then crosses over its midsegment coursing anteriorly and medially supplying terminal twigs to the globe, nerve sheath, eyelid, muscles, and lacrimal gland. Small vessels pierce the sclera to supply the posterior choroid. The superior ophthalmic vein (SOV) connects the facial venous plexus to the orbit joining the inferior ophthalmic vein at the orbital apex to the SOF into the cavernous sinus [2].

Extraocular muscles (EOMs) comprise the group of muscles which move they eye and include the inferior, superior, lateral, and medial recti, the superior and inferior obliques, and the levator palpebrae. Fascia forms a familiar anatomic "muscle cone" around the four rectus muscles, with the two extraconal oblique muscles in the superomedial and inferomedial orbit. The fascial muscle cone extends posteriorly to form a dense fibrous band (the annulus of Zinn) which surrounds the optic nerve, ophthalmic artery, CN III, V_1, VI, and related structures. It attaches anterior to the globe's equator at Tenon's capsule [1].

Orbital septum formed by palpebral fascia is a membranous sheet which anchors at Tenon's capsule extending peripherally to the orbital rim's periosteum forming three spaces. The preseptal space is contiguous with the face. The intraconal and extraconal spaces are postseptal. It is extremely important for imagers to identify pathologic processes which violate the orbital septum.

Innervation: CN IV (Trochlear) supplies the superior oblique muscle. CN VI (Abducens) supplies the lateral rectus muscle. All other EOMs are innervated by CN III (Oculomotor), including the levator palpebrae. The globe is formed from a fibrous tunic outer sclera, an in inner neural retina, and a middle layer of uveal/vascular tunic. The interleaved layer of choroid, ciliary body, and iris is collectively called the uvea. The ciliary body assists the lens to focus transmitted light from the cornea onto the retina. The anterior and posterior chambers contain aqueous humor. The lens separates the smaller anterior and posterior chambers from the larger vitreous chamber posteriorly which is conspicuously imaged with its collection of vitreous humor. Like in a camera's lens, the iris regulates light reaching the retina [3].

Lacrimal glands: The paired elliptical lacrimal glands lodge in the lacrimal fossa's superolateral postseptal extraconal space supplying lubrication to the anterior globe. Tears traverse the globe anteromedially storing surplus in the lacrimal sacs via upper and lower puncta. The preseptal lacrimal sacs drain through nasolacrimal ducts into the inferior meatus caudal to the inferior turbinates [4].

Trauma

It has long been acknowledged that the orbit seems to be a "sitting duck" inviting an assortment of trauma. While a plethora of protective equipment has been devised, alas, unfortunate patients are often not wearing protective gear when the offending occasion occurred. The orbit appears plagued with blunt and penetrating injury with equal incidence. *CT* shows soft tissue and bony injury, air, and some foreign bodies. While CT excels when foreign bodies have high or low Hounsfield units, it sometimes struggles when foreign bodies are isodense to surrounding structures as is sometimes seen with wood, most glass, and some plastics. *MRI* can be complementary to CT in many cases but is clearly contraindicated in cases with metallic foreign bodies [5].

There are two commonly held theories for blow-out fractures. The "hydraulic theory" contends that pressure on orbital contents raises to the point that contents "blow-out" through the weakest point. The "buckling theory" purports that direct force proceeds through the orbit to cause the fracture. Whichever theory is correct, "blow-out fractures" are common and are frequently found medially (Fig. 71.1) and inferiorly (Fig. 71.2), although they occasionally involve the orbital roof. As originally described by Smith and Regan in 1957, blow-out fractures occur with intact orbital rims [5]. It is the radiologist's responsibility to define the anatomy and identify which patients have significant extrusion and/or entrapment of orbital structures. Orbital "trapdoor" fractures are reported more frequently found in children ostensibly related to better bone elasticity. Whatever the cause, prompt identification of these fractures is important as urgent surgical repair reduces morbidity (and malpractice suits) [6]. There is a significant spectrum of post-traumatic global injury which ranges from minor to severe. Laceration, rupture, global deformity, and decreased ocular volume are conspicuous while anterior chamber leaks and lens dislocations are sometimes subtle and initially overlooked (Figs. 71.3 and 71.4).

Ruptured globe is usually well depicted by imaging and modern diagnostic and surgical techniques have increased the chances of visual salvage (Fig. 71.5). However, phthisis bulbi is the unfortunate end-result of various vicious orbital oddities showing a small, shrunken, misshapen globe which is insensitive to light revealing redundant, thickened, dense scleral calcifications. The characteristic imaging appearance is shown in Fig. 71.6.

Ocular prostheses present a gamut of finding for imagers ranging in conspicuity from blatantly obvious to virtually invisible depending on the material and the technique. In general, many are hyperdense on CT demonstrating a signal void on MRI and some show artifacts on one or more techniques.

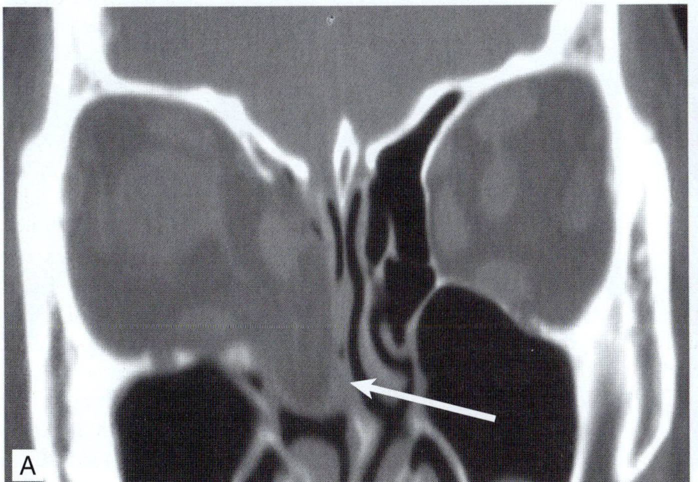

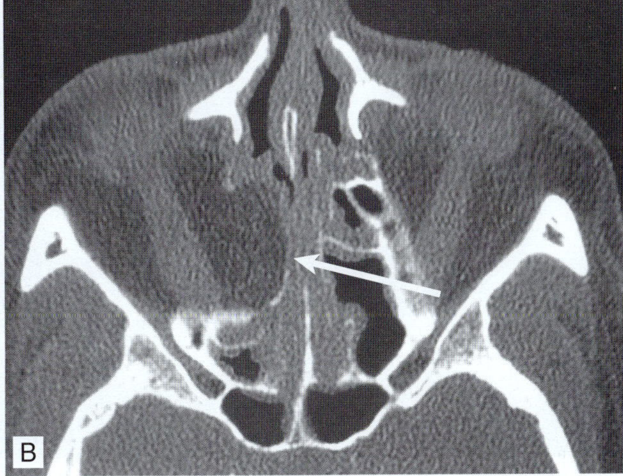

Figure 71.1 Medial blow-out fracture. Coronal (A) and axial (B) noncontrast CT shows dehiscent medial wall with orbital contents herniating inferiorly and medially (*arrows* in A & B resepectively).

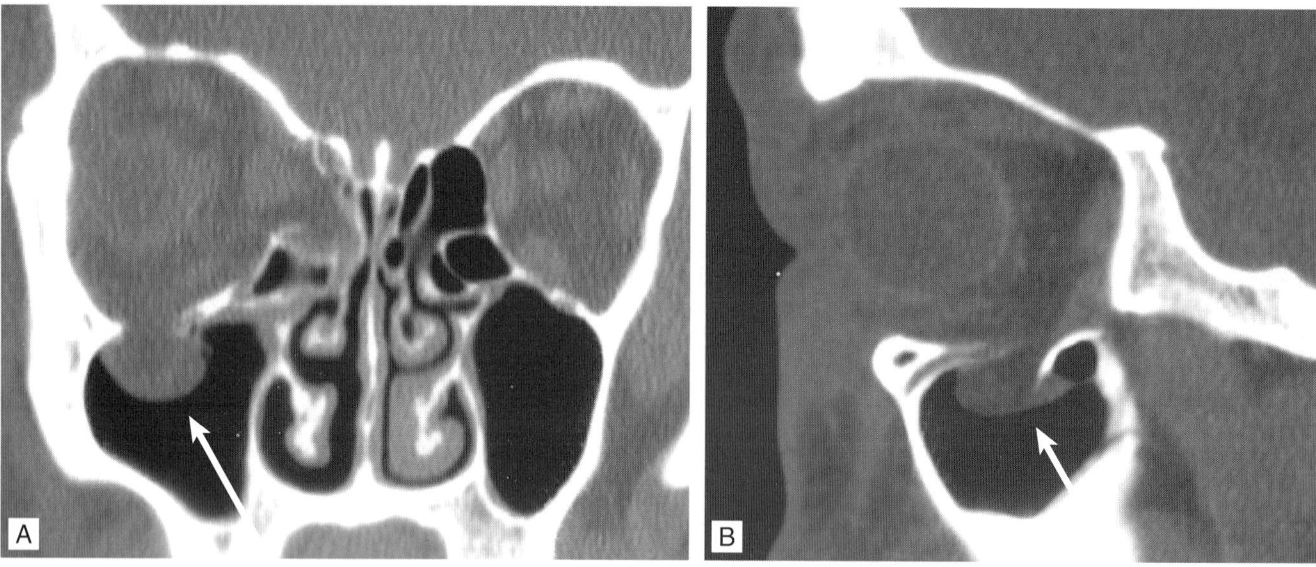

Figure 71.2 Inferior blow-out fracture. Coronal (A) and sagittal (B) Noncontrast CT shows comminuted depressed left orbital floor fracture (*arrows* in A & B).

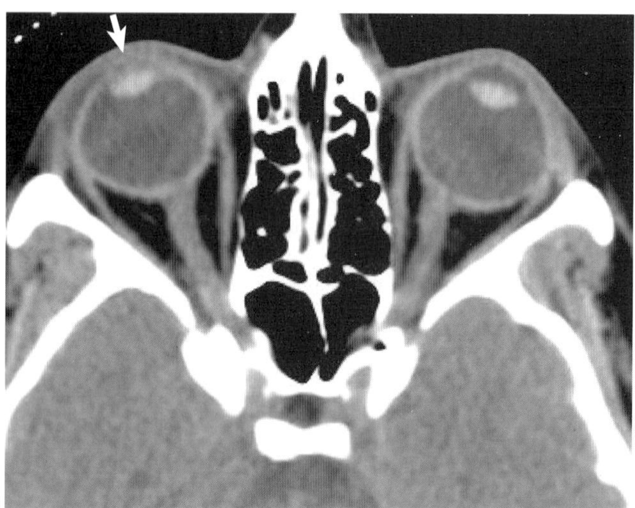

Figure 71.3 Anterior chamber perforation. Axial NECT shows narrowing of the space between right lens and cornea secondary to loss of fluid from anterior chamber perforation (*arrow*).

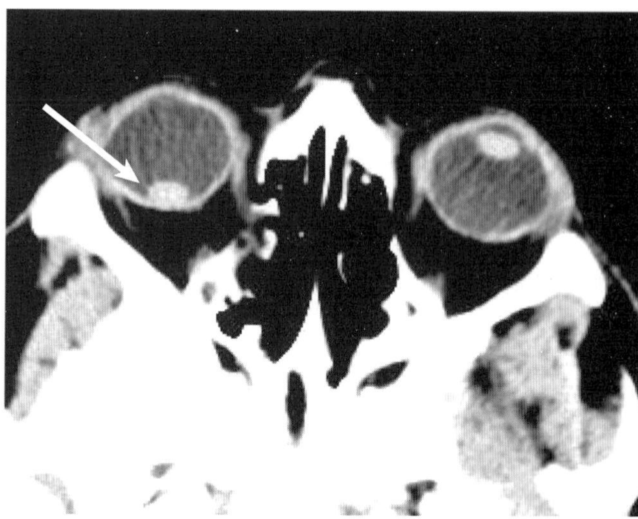

Figure 71.4 Ocular lens displacement. Axial NECT shows clear posterior displacement of calcified right lens (*arrow*).

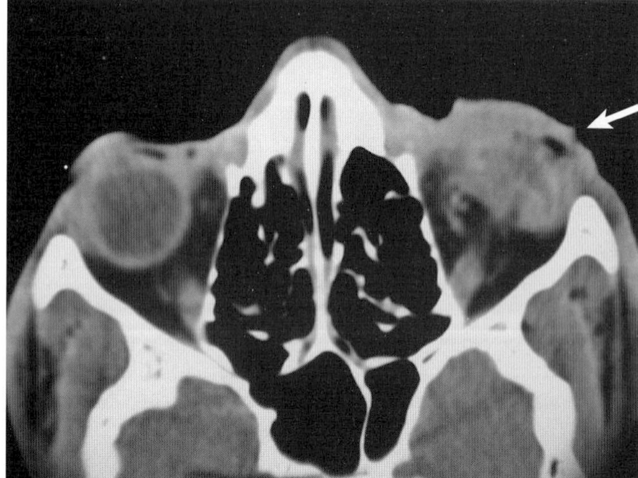

Figure 71.5 Ruptured globe. Axial NECT demonstrates traumatic rupture of the left globe (*arrow*).

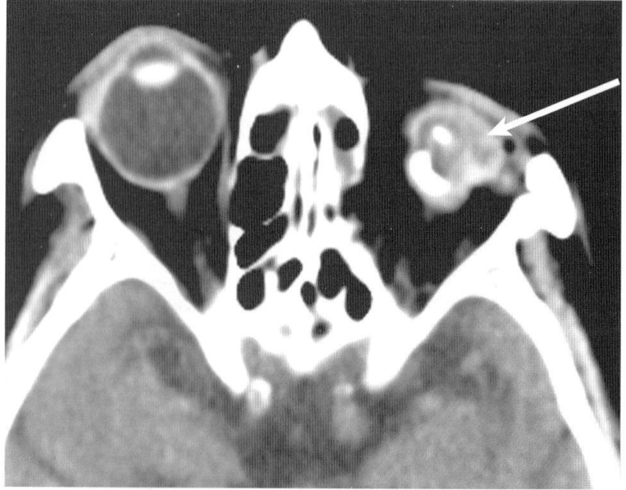

Figure 71.6 Phthisis bulbi. Axial NECT 1A shows a small shrunken, left globe with thickened sclera, large coarse dystrophic calcifications, increased vitreous attenuation, and enophthalmos from phthisis bulbi (*arrow*).

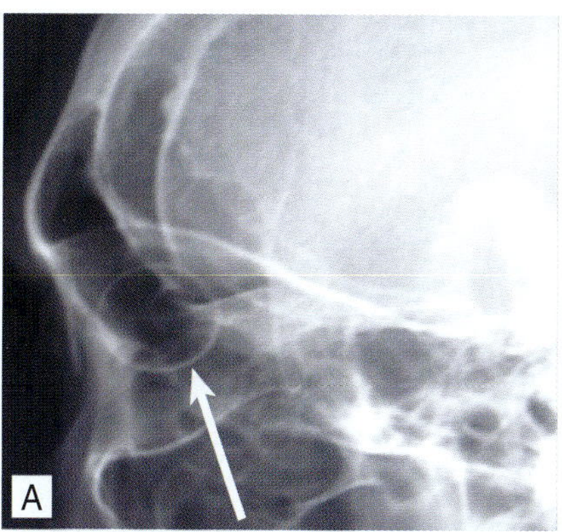

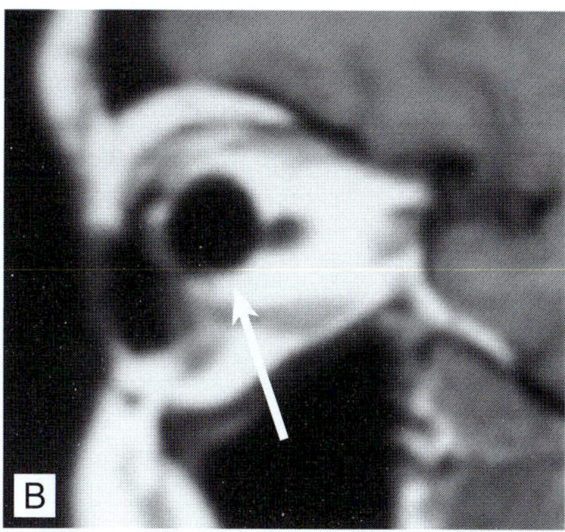

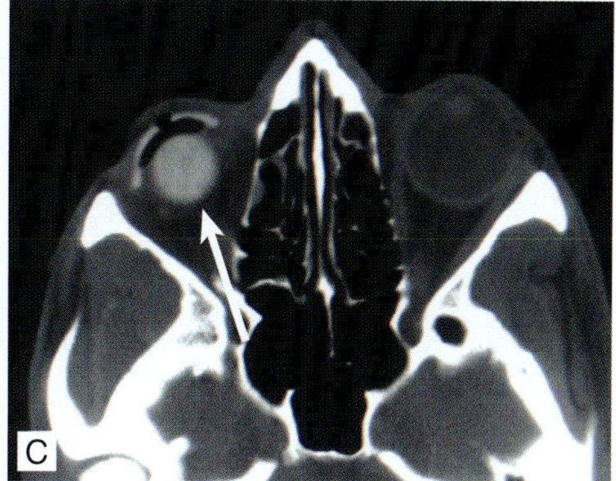

Figure 71.7 Ocular prosthesis. (A) Lateral radiograph reveals an opaque, spherical aluminum oxide right orbital prosthesis (*arrow*). Sagittal T1 (B) an ocular implant surrounded by orbital fat (*arrow*). Noncontrast CT (C) obtained in a different patient shows a high attenuation ocular implant (*arrow*).

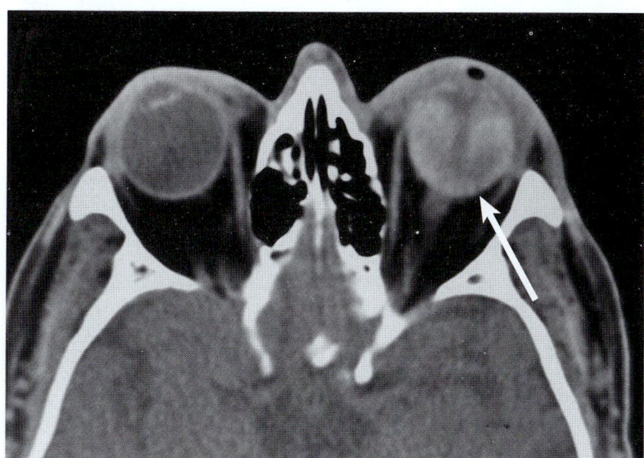

Figure 71.8 Retinal detachment. Axial NECT conveys classic "tulip" appearance of retinal detachment containing both high attenuation blood and low attenuation vitreous humor beneath detached retinal stopping at the ora serrata and not extending to limbus (*arrow*). Prior cataract removal of the right globe with lens replacement.

While glass and plastic spheres have been mainstays, newer low attenuation integrated hydroxyapatite implants made of denatured coral have allowed direct attachment to the EOMs with fibrovascular ingrowth. Evaluation of this implant's assimilation is sometimes assessed on T1 Gd or nuclear medicine uptake (Fig. 71.7).

Retinal detachments occur when the globes inner retinal layer peals away from the middle choroidal layer permitting fluid accumulation in the previously present potential space. This is a true medical emergency which progresses to permanent vision loss and blindness if not repaired in 24–72 hours. The retina is tethered posteriorly to the optic nerve's insertion and anteriorly to the ora serrata at the retinal/scleral junction. This results in retinal detachments demonstrating a "tulip-shaped" intraocular mass on USG, CT, and MRI (Fig. 71.8) [7].

Neoplasms

Cavernous venous malformations of the orbit (AKA orbital cavernous hemangiomas) comprise the most common orbital vascular lesion in adults. Newer nomenclature by International Society for Study of Vascular Anomalies classifies them as "slow flow venous malformations." These are benign, slow growing, encapsulated, vascular abnormalities usually presenting with progressive, painless proptosis. These are associated with Sturge–Weber syndrome and may result in spontaneous hemorrhage and retinal detachment. Venous malformations are typically unilateral, well circumscribed, enhancing, intraconal masses in adults. CT shows an intraconal mass that may have delayed enhancement. MRI shows T1 isointense, T2 hyperintense, avidly enhancing lesions that may have "blooming" effect on gradient echo or susceptibility-weighted imaging [8] (Fig. 71.9).

Optic nerve gliomas (ONGs) are usually grade I juvenile pilocytic astrocytomas and most commonly present in children and young adults. In adults, they often appear as aggressive malignant optic gliomas arising from foci near the optic chiasm and have a poor prognosis. Contrast-enhanced MRI is the preferred technique for evaluating the optic nerves and chiasm. Since 90% of ONGs arise outside the orbit, the field of view must include the entire visual pathway. The characteristic findings are diffuse enlargement of this optic nerves which avidly enhances. The retrobulbar optic nerve is most commonly involved, but the lesion can extend posteriorly to the chiasm in more advanced cases. Bilateral ONGs are pathognomonic for neurofibromatosis type 1 [9] (Fig. 71.10).

Optic nerve meningiomas are rare, benign tumors arising from arachnoid cap cells in the meninges covering the optic nerve. CT shows a high attenuation mass surrounding the optic nerve causing calcification in 20–50% of cases. Optic nerve meningioma is usually idiopathic, however, 10% of patients with ONM may have neurofibromatosis type 2. The "tram track" or "sandwich" sign is the characteristic finding best appreciated on fat-suppressed contrast-enhanced T1W images. While "tram track" perineural enhancement is classic, it is not pathognomonic and this findings can be mimicked by pathologies that cause diffuse leptomeningeal enhancement, such as lymphoma, sarcoid, and leptomeningeal metastases [10] (Fig. 71.11).

Orbital schwannomas usually present in middle-aged adults as well defined, encapsulated, slowly growing benign tumors arising from peripheral nerve Schwann cells and comprise 1% to orbital tumors. Orbital schwannomas do not arise from the optic nerves since the optic nerve is not a "real" cranial nerve and is not surrounded by schwann cells. Rather, orbital schwannomas are thought to arise from distal branches of cranial nerves which innervate the extraocular muscles and felt to most likely arise from intraorbital branches of cranial nerve III [11] (Fig. 71.12).

Orbital lymphoma is a frequent orbital tumors in adults and account for 50% of all orbital malignancies. These malignancies usually arise in older patients presenting with progressive ptosis, exophthalmos, diplopia, and restricted extraocular movement. Imaging shows restricted diffusion. ADC may represent a noninvasive surrogate biomarker to measure treatment response [12] (Fig. 71.13).

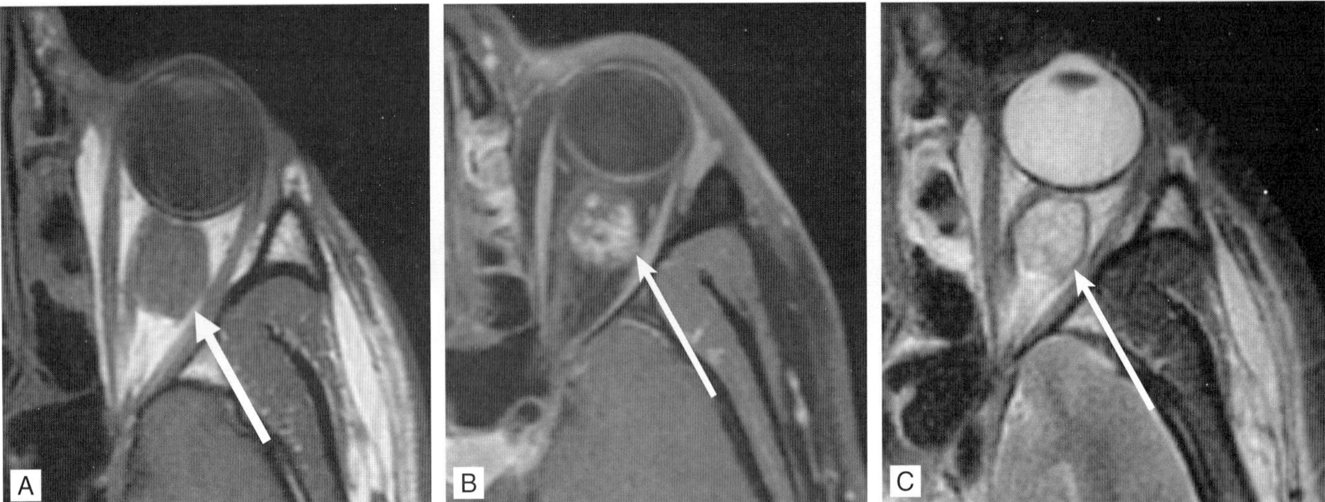

Figure 71.9 Cavernous venous malformation (*arrows*). (A) Axial T1 confirms well-circumscribed intraconal mass isointense to muscle. (B) Axial T1 Gd parades pattern of "mulberry" enhancement. (C) Axial T2 confirms characteristic sharp, low signal pseudocapsule.

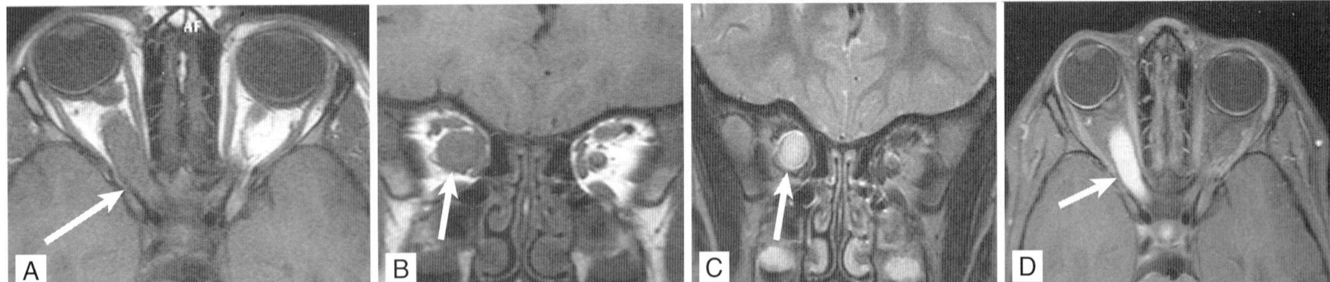

Figure 71.10 Optic nerve glioma (*arrows*). (A) Axial T1 shows fusiform enlargement of right ON from the globe through the orbital apex. (B) Coronal T1 exhibits enlargement of right ON with mass effect on adjacent structures. (C) Coronal T2 shows increased signal within the mass. (D) Axial T1 Gd exhibits avid, homogeneous enhancement of ON through the orbital apex.

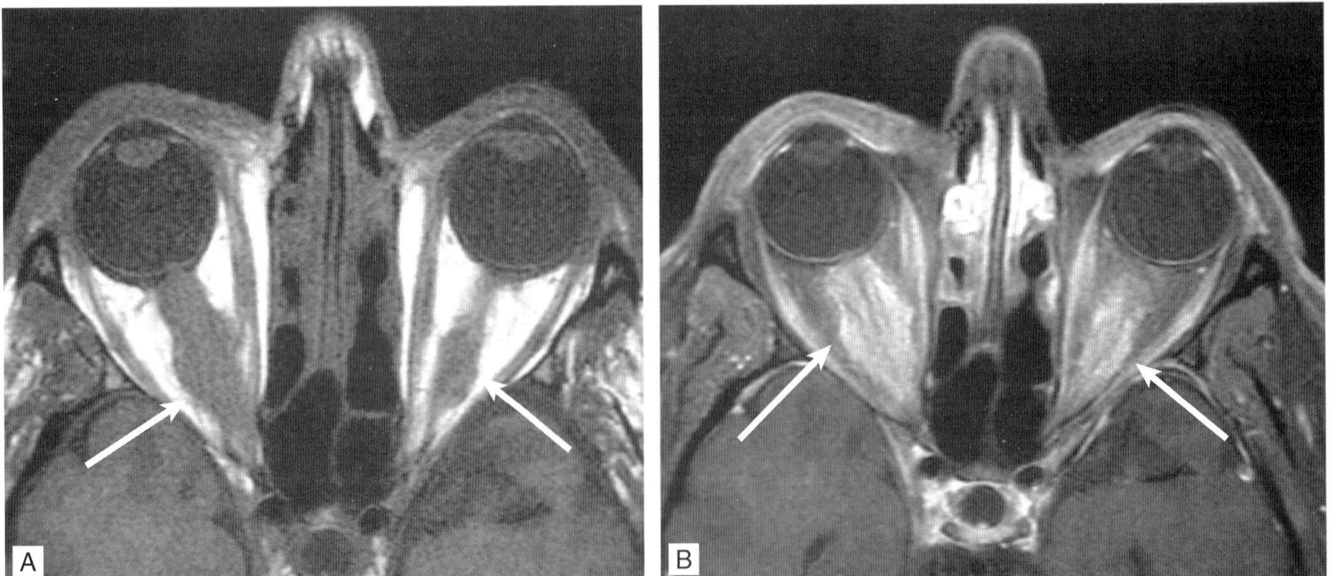

Figure 71.11 Optic nerve meningioma. (A and B) Axial T1 images exhibit tubular enlargement of ON's from globe through the orbital apices (*arrows*).

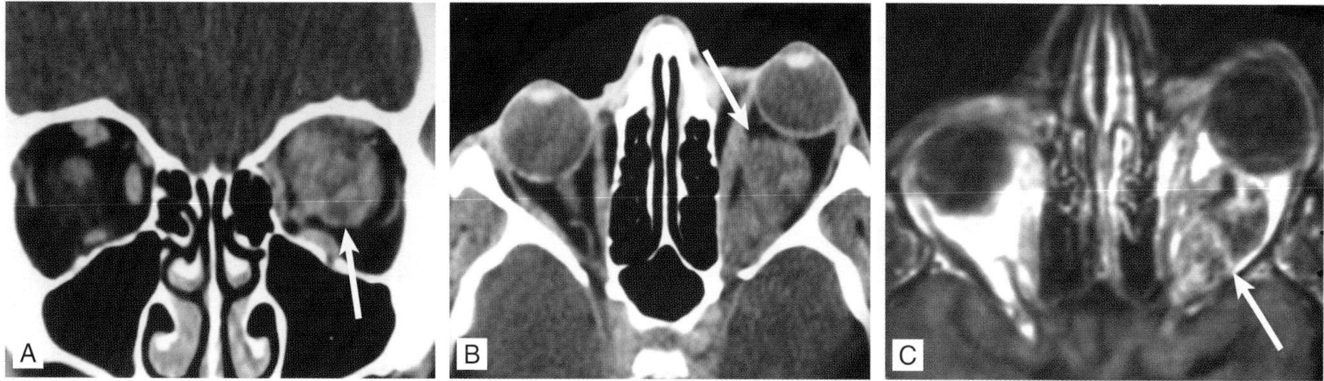

Figure 71.12 Orbital schwannoma. (*Arrows*) (A) Coronal NECT shows large heterogeneous left intraconal mass. (B) Axial CECT exhibits large mildly enhancing heterogeneous oval intraconal mass extending from posterior globe to orbital apex. (C) Axial T1 Gd exhibits large isointense mass with areas of avid "ring" enhancement extending from the posterior globe to the orbital apex producing exophthalmos.

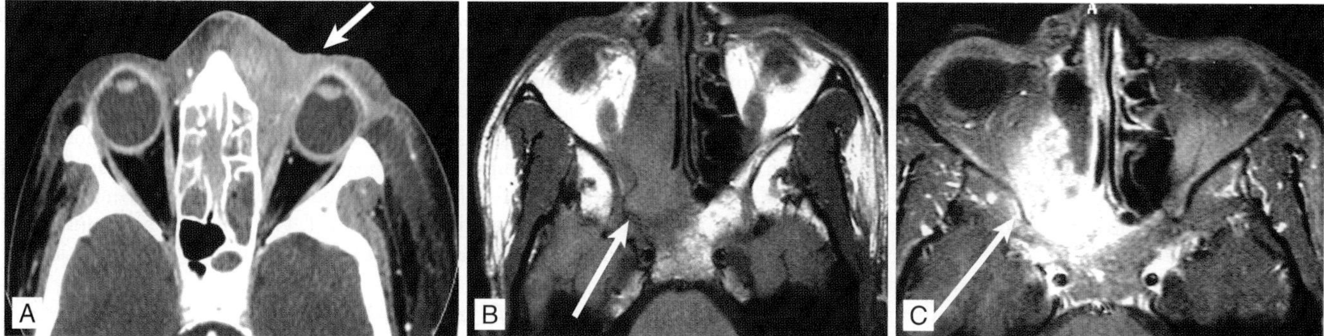

Figure 71.13 Orbital lymphoma. (A) Axial CECT shows ill-defined infiltrative enhancing mass invading the medial left orbit, deforming and deviating left globe and medial rectus muscle with pre- and postseptal involvement (*arrow*). Axial T1 (B) and (C) T1 Gd performed in a different patient demonstrate an avidly enhancing aggressive mass invading the right orbit and ethmoid sinus extending posteriorly through the orbital apex (*arrows*).

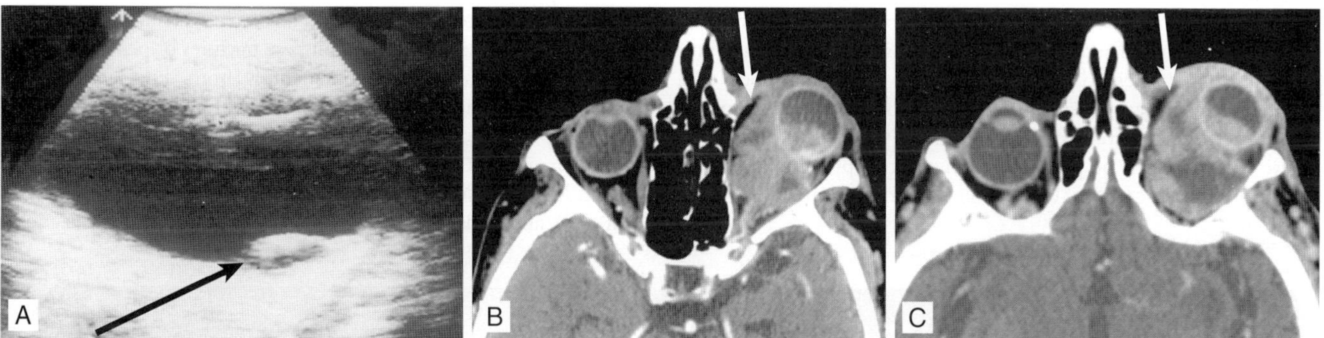

Figure 71.14 Ocular melanoma (*arrows*). (A) Real-timeUSGsector scan shows small, focal, raised melanoma protruding into posterior vitreous chamber. Axial contrast-enhanced CT (B and C) shows a large heterogeneously enhancing soft tissue mass filling a significant portion of the vitreous chamber, and extending into the retrobulbar region exhibiting exophthalmos.

Ocular melanoma (OM) is the most common adult intraocular malignancy. OM can be detected on both CT and MR as either focal or en plaque lesion abutting the retina. OMs are sometimes seen as an incidental findings on CT and are usually high attenuation masses that enhance with contrast. While there are variations between melanotic and amelanotic tumors, OM typically shows bright T1, dark T2, and moderate enhancement on T1 Gd. MRI is the technique of choice for complete evaluation, particularly when the lesion is large. Amelanotic tumors resemble other soft tissue masses like metastases. MRI is excellent in sorting out effusions which are sometimes slightly bright on T1 [13] (Fig. 71.14).

Retinoblastoma (RB) is the most common intraocular tumor in children. The most common clinical finding is loss of the red reflex resulting in leukocoria. Most cases are autosomal recessive with a mutation in RB1 on chromosome 13. One-third of patients present with bilateral lesions with autosomal dominant inheritance. Sporadic (<1%) cases of trilateral RBs reveal a concurrent PNET in the pineal or suprasellar region. RBs are highly malignant with hematogenous, intraocular, and trans-scleral spread. When tumor is confined, radiation and enucleation can be curative, but extensions into orbital vascular or subarachnoid spaces portend a particularly poor prognosis with a 5-year disease-free survival of >90% with only intraocular disease but <10% with extraocular involvement. CT characteristically shows a calcified posterior intraocular mass in 90% of cases with characteristic punctate or sparsely speckled calcifications. Therefore,

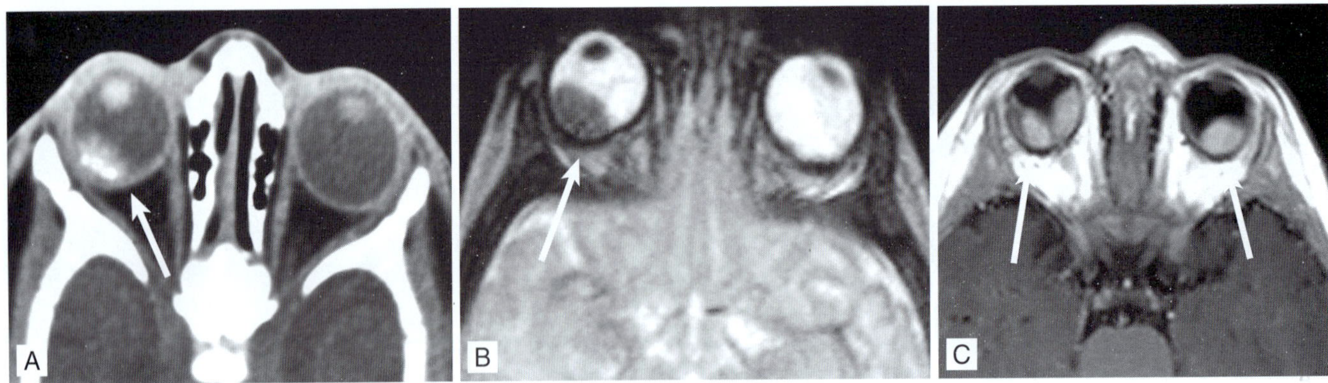

Figure 71.15 Retinoblastoma. (A) Axial NECT demonstrates a calcified intraocular mass (*arrow*). (B) Axial T2 connotes conspicuous low signal "filling defect" within high signal intraocular fluid (*arrow*). (C) Axial contrast-enhanced T1W images in a different patient show bilateral enhancing retinoblastomas (*arrows*).

any intraocular calcifications in an infant or young child should suggest RB until proven otherwise. CT is preferred to MR due to the ability to detect calcification. However, the superior contrast resolution is essential to identify tumor spread and involvement of adjacent structure. Currently, CT and MRI are considered complimentary. RB is typically intermediate signal on T1 and avidly enhances with contrast. DWI shows restricted diffusion at high *b* values with low ADC contrasting to high intensity vitreous [14] (Fig. 71.15).

Optic disk drusen is the most common cause of ocular calcifications in adults. Considered degenerative in origin, optic disk drusens are tiny yellow (or white) globules of hyaline-like material deposited on or below the surface of the optic disk which progressively calcify causing visual field defects. While one is a "druse," they commonly present in pairs (of drusen) varying from 1 mm to 4 mm.

There are various other system hematologic processes that can involve the orbit. These include metastases, leukemia, and lymphoma. All of these disorders can either present as focal soft tissue masses or leptomeningeal disease. Focal leukemic deposits are sometimes referred to as chloromas (Fig. 71.16). However, these disorders can be purely leptomeningeal process and result in disuse enhancement of the optic nerve sheath [15] (Fig. 71.17).

Rhabdomyosarcoma is the most common pediatric orbital malignancy with the majority of children presenting by 6 years of age. Approximately half of orbital cases arise in the orbit while the remainder are metastatic. The most common presentation is an enlarging mass with progressive exophthalmos. The tumors often have bone erosion and may extend into the adjacent paranasal sinus. One of the classic findings is rhabdomyosarcoma involving an EOM and are isodense to muscle on CT. On MR, they are isointense to muscle on T1W sequences and avidly enhance [16] (Fig. 71.18).

Vascular Abnormalities

Carotid-cavernous fistulas (CCFs) are commonly classified as direct or indirect fistulas between the arterial supply and venous drainage. A fistula that communicates directly between the ICA and cavernous sinus form is a "direct" fistula while an "indirect" CCFs is when ICA or ECA *branches* communicate with the cavernous sinus. CCFs are felt to arise from trauma, such as skull base fractures or penetrating injuries. They may also arise spontaneously from dural arteriovenous malformations, aneurysm rupture, or fibromuscular hyperplasia. Patients present acutely with unilateral pulsatile exophthalmos, scleral injection, and chemosis. Venous distention is apparent on USG, CT, CTA, MRI, and MRA, while muscle enlargement is best appreciated on CT and MRI. CTA is currently considered the diagnostic

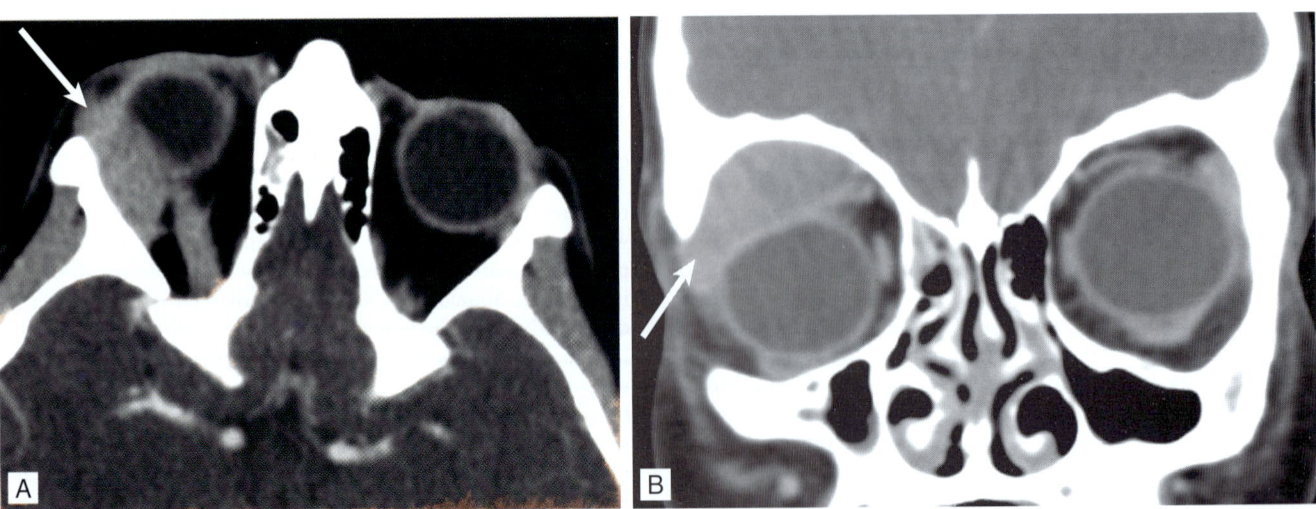

Figure 71.16 Orbital leukemia (*arrows*). (A) Axial CECT shows relatively dense homogeneous oval soft tissue mass in upper outer quadrant of the right orbit. (B) Coronal CECT in the same patient shows the mass to inferiorly displace the globe.

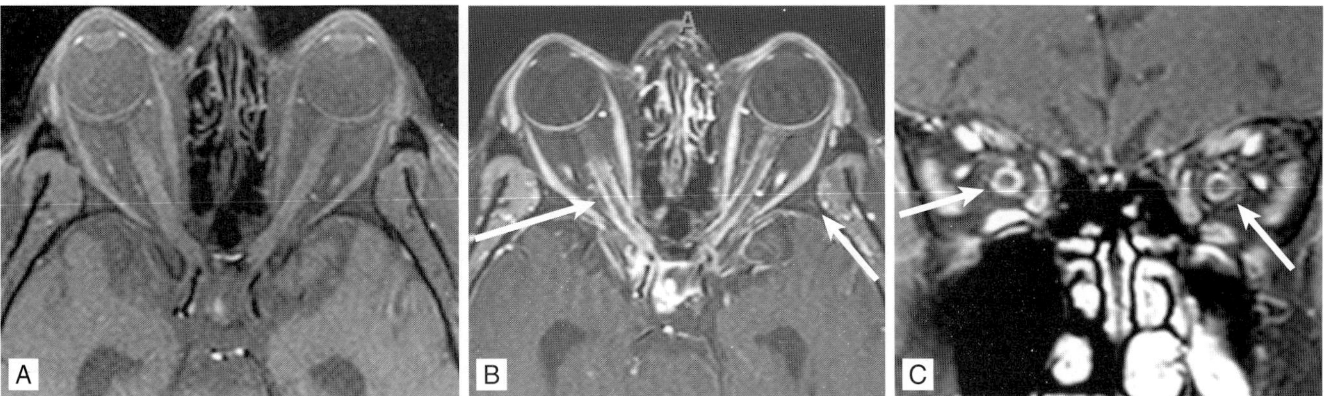

Figure 71.17 Optic nerve metastasis. (A) Axial T1 FatSat shows proptosis with prominent ON complexes bilaterally with sheaths showing slightly higher signal than adjacent ON's. (B) Axial T1 Gd FatSat shows proptosis with avid abnormal enhancement of both ON sheaths extending smoothly from globes to optic chiasm (*arrows*). (C) Coronal postcontrast T1W images exhibit abnormal enhancement of ON sheaths and some central ON portions (*arrows*).

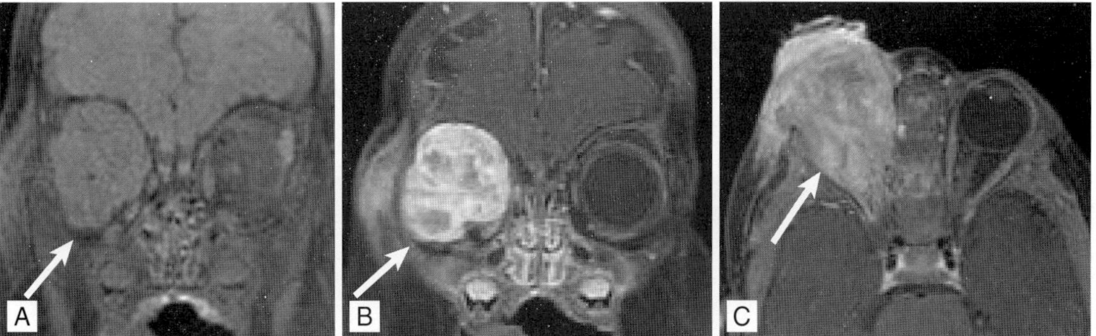

Figure 71.18 Rhabdomyosarcoma (*arrows*). (A) Coronal T1 fat-suppressed images show a large mass involving the right orbit. Postcontrast T1W images (B and C) show the heterogeneous enhancement within this very aggressive tumor with extension into the adjacent periorbital soft tissues.

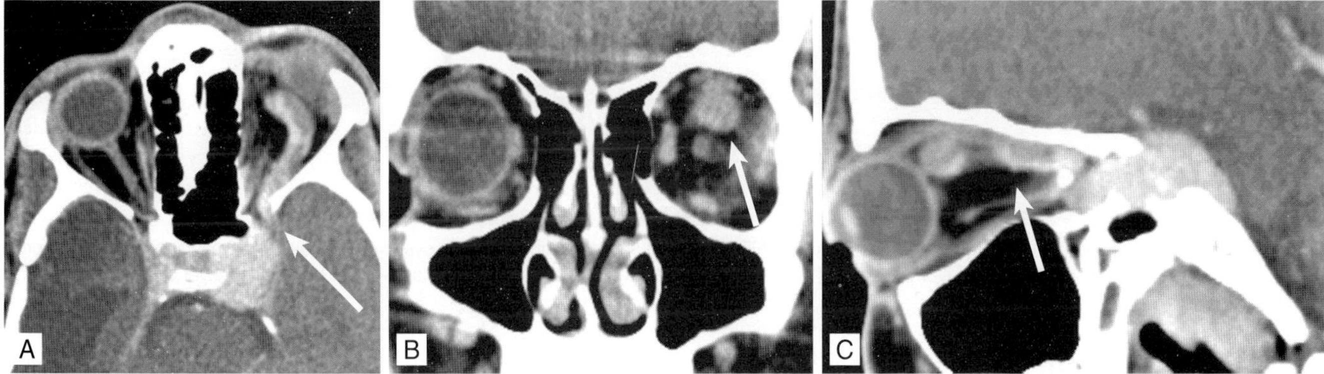

Figure 71.19 Carotid-cavernous fistula. (A) Axial contrast-enhanced CT angiography demonstrates dilated and tortuous L SOV and asymmetrically enlarged cavernous sinus (*arrow*). (B) Coronal CECT shows enhancing dilated SOV (*arrow*). (C) Sagittal CECT shows enhancing SOV displacing the superior rectus muscle cranially with exophthalmos (*arrow*).

procedure of choice for detecting early cavernous sinus and jugular vein enhancement [17,18] (Fig. 71.19).

Orbital venous varix is an uncommon vascular malformation composed of enlarged single or multiple venous channels that communicate with the systemic venous system. While mild prominence and asymmetry of the SOVs are normal variants, patients presenting with exophthalmos or acute intraorbital hemorrhage who are found to have a mass causing painful proptosis aggravated by a dependent head position, coughing, sneezing, or Valsalva maneuver. Contrast-enhanced CT or MR shows a focally dilated SOV (Fig. 71.20). These findings can be confirmed with time-resolved magnetic resonance or conventional angiography [19].

Venolymphatic malformations may arise in the retrobulbar region and have a tendency to undergo rapid expansion due to spontaneous hemorrhage resulting in sudden exophthalmos. The classic presentation is a young patient with upper respiratory infection presenting with proptosis and decreased eye movements. The spontaneous hemorrhage may also result in vision loss from optic nerve compression. The hemorrhage is felt to be due to intrinsic vascularity and many of these lesions are thought to be low-flow venolymphatic malformations as opposed to pure lymphatic malformations. These lesions are typically cystic and have a "fluid–fluid" level(s) after spontaneous hemorrhage [19] (Fig. 71.21).

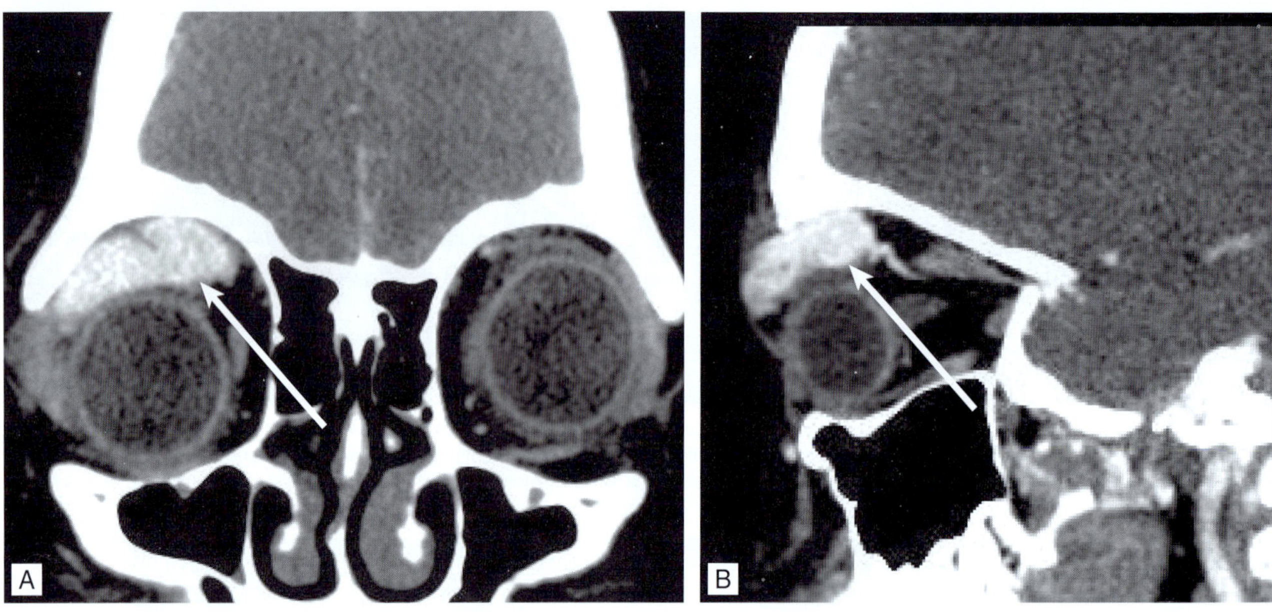

Figure 71.20 Orbital venous varix (*arrows*). Coronal (A) and sagittal (B) contrast-enhanced CT shows an enhancing focally dilated superior ophthalmic vein indicative of an orbital varix. (Courtesy of Varsha Joshi, MD.)

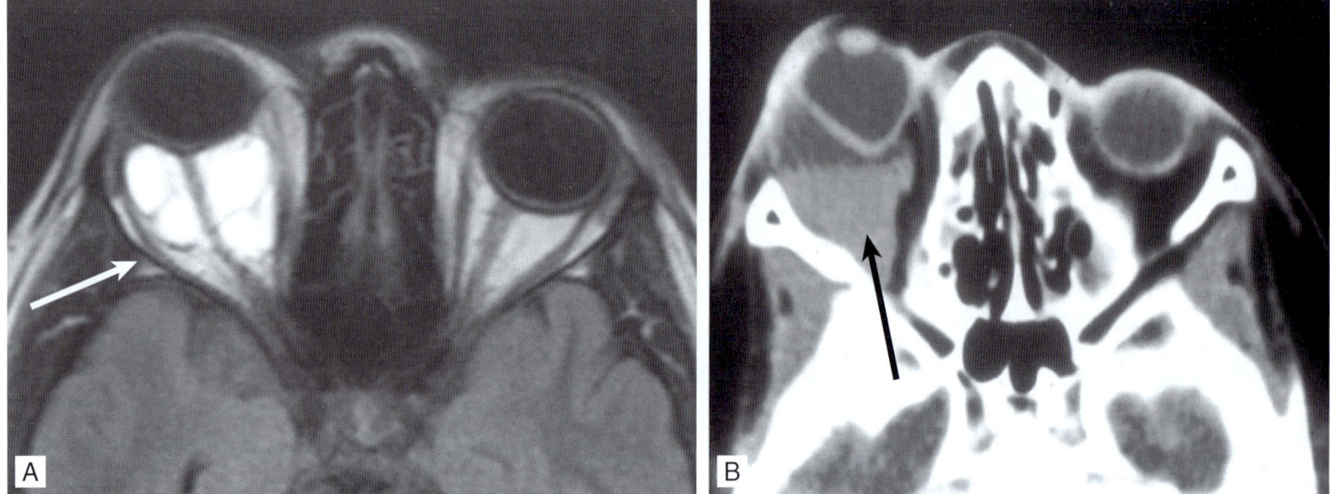

Figure 71.21 Venolymphatic malformation (*arrows*). (A) Axial FLAIR sequence shows a multiseptated cystic retrobulbar mass causing right ocular proptosis. (B) Axial CT of a venolymphatic malformation with spontaneous hemorrhage shows a cystic mass with a blood–fluid level causing a "tension" globe and proptosis.

Infection and Inflammatory Processes

Infection is the most common orbital pathology in children secondary to spread from an adjoining paranasal or skin infection or sequela of prior trauma. While most are bacterial, always remember that diabetic and immunocompromised patients are prone to debilitating fungal infections. Preseptal cellulitis is usually due to a skin infection or a "bug bite." The Chandler classification is often used to describe the spectrum of orbital infection that arise from the adjacent paranasal sinuses and potential complications [20]. Preseptal cellulitis is defined by the inflammation being anterior to the orbital septum, whereas postseptal cellulitis extends posterior to the orbital septum [21]. The attachment of the orbital septum is the posterior lacrimal crest which forms the medial border of the lacrimal sac [3].

Subperiosteal and intraorbital abscesses are later stages of untreated periorbital infections. Subperiosteal abscess usually arise from direct extension from an untreated paranasal sinus infection. Contrast-enhanced CT is the preferred technique. The typical finding is a lenticular fluid collection that abuts the orbital wall of the sinus. Bone algorithms should routinely be performed to evaluate for bone erosion [22] (Fig. 71.22).

Orbital abscess are rare complications of untreated sinus or orbital infections and typically present with fever, proptosis, and chemosis. MR with contrast preferred for evaluating patients for possible orbital abscess [23] (Fig. 71.23). Any patients with orbital infections and reduced ocular motions should be specifically evaluated for cavernous sinus thrombosis. Either CT venogram or MR venogram can be performed. We prefer CT venogram since the exam is quicker and can be easier to differentiate the normally enhancing veins from nonenhancing veins dues to thrombosis (Fig. 71.24).

Graves ophthalmopathy is considered an autoimmune inflammatory disorder with leukocytic infiltration causing erythema,

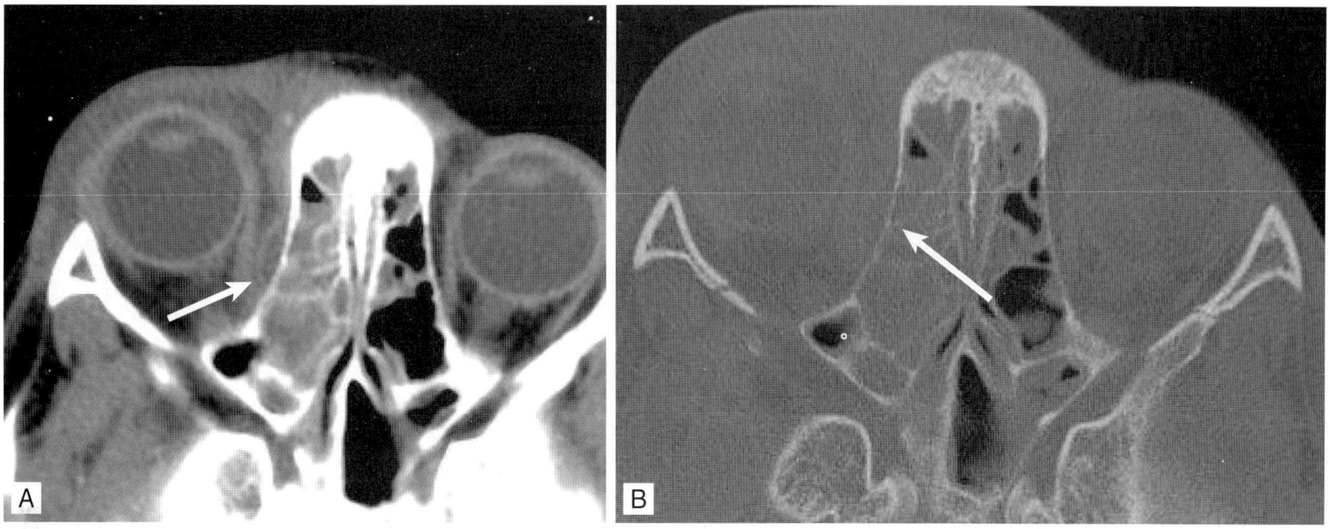

Figure 71.22 Subperiosteal abscess. (A) Contrast-enhanced CT shows a subperiosteal abscess arising from right ethmoid sinus (*arrow*). Bone algorithm (B) shows no evidence of erosion of the lamina papyracea (*arrow*).

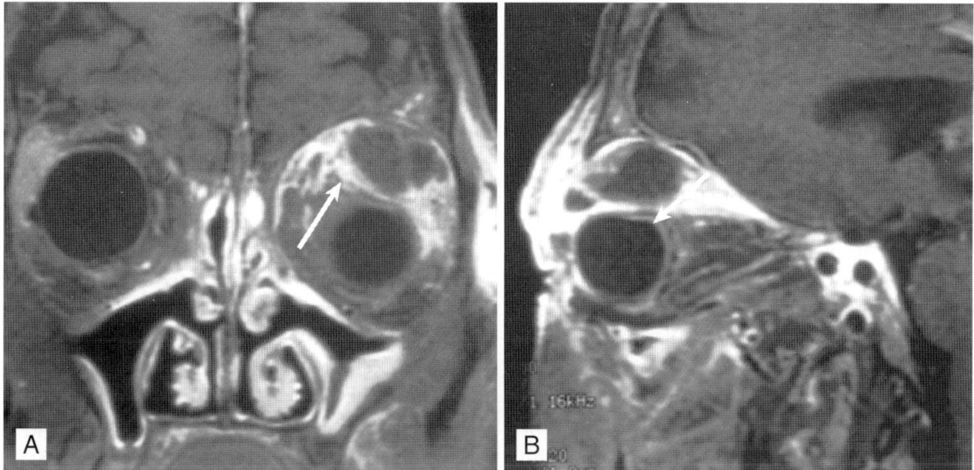

Figure 71.23 Orbital abscess. Fat-suppressed contrast-enhanced T1W image illustrates an abscess in the superior aspect of the orbit (*arrow* in A) with surrounding enhancing phlegmon inferiorly displacing the globe (*arrow* in B).

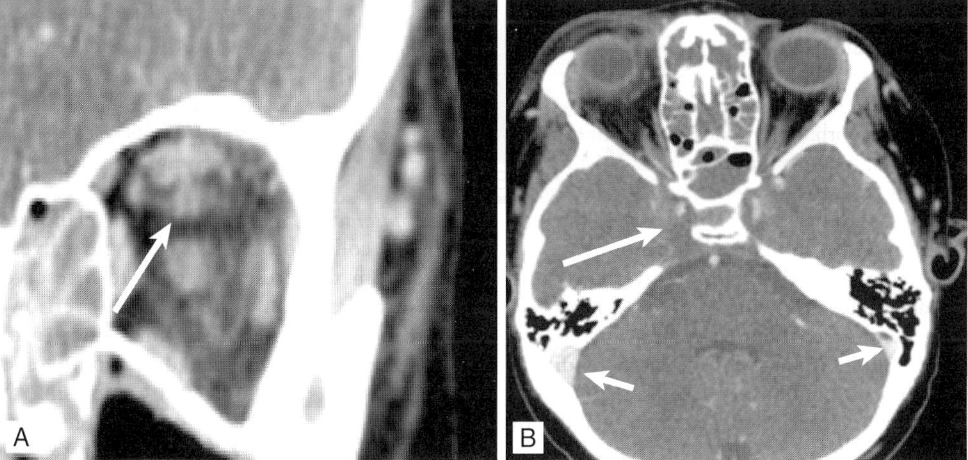

Figure 71.24 Cavernous sinus thrombosis. (A) Coronal contrast-enhanced CT shows no opacification of the superior ophthalmic vein (*arrow*) in a patient with a left sixth nerve palsy. CT venogram in the same patient shows enhancement of the transvers sinus (*short arrows*) and no enhancement in the cavernous sinuses (*long arrow*) indicative of cavernous sinus thrombosis.

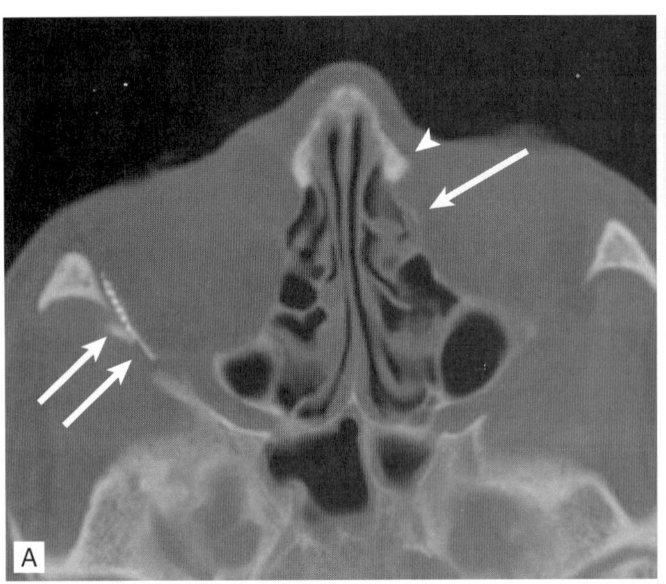

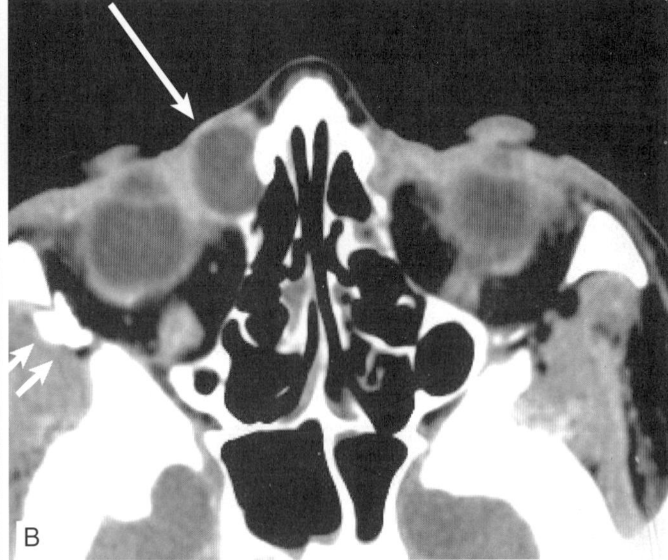

Figure 71.28 Dacryocystocele. (A) Axial bone algorithms obtained through the orbit show the borders of the lacrimal sac. The *arrowhead* identifies the anterior lacrimal crest and the *large arrow* shows the posterior lacrimal crest. (B) Axial soft tissue algorithms in the same patient show a dacryocele involving the lacrimal sac (*arrow*). This was probably post-traumatic since the patient has undergone surgical repair of the right lateral orbital wall fracture (*small arrows* in A & B).

of the orbit. While the fascial planes surrounding the lacrimal fossa provide a relatively resistant barrier to spread, serious pathologic entities may arise and spread from this location.

The lacrimal glands contain true lymphoid tissue and may reveal lymphoid hyperplasia (pseudolymphoma) or primary lymphoma, usually NHL. These present with soft masses conforming to the globe and orbital wall rarely resulting in bony destruction or marked proptosis and pose problematic differentials for both imagers and pathologists. Lacrimal glands predictably portray pathologic changes similar to other minor salivary glands and half are epithelial in origin. The other half have inflammatory or lymphoid origins. Keep in mind that minor salivary glands have a higher incidence of malignancy than major salivary gland tumors [30].

Pleomorphic adenomas (benign mixed-cell tumors) are classically well-defined homogeneous soft tissue masses. They are slow glowing lesions and do not usually have substantial mass effect on the adjacent globe often resulting in a diagnostic delay of 1–2 years before individuals seek medical attention. Calcifications are infrequently found. Enhancement is mild and variable on CT and MRI. Preferred treatment is complete excision and recurrences are uncommon. Malignant transformation rarely occurs when individuals are untreated for extended periods [30].

Dermoid and epidermoid tumors are benign, well-defined, encapsulated neoplasms, which occasionally occur in the lacrimal fossa causing proptosis. Epidermoids are fluid-filled cystic lesions while dermoids contain fat [1] (Fig. 71.29).

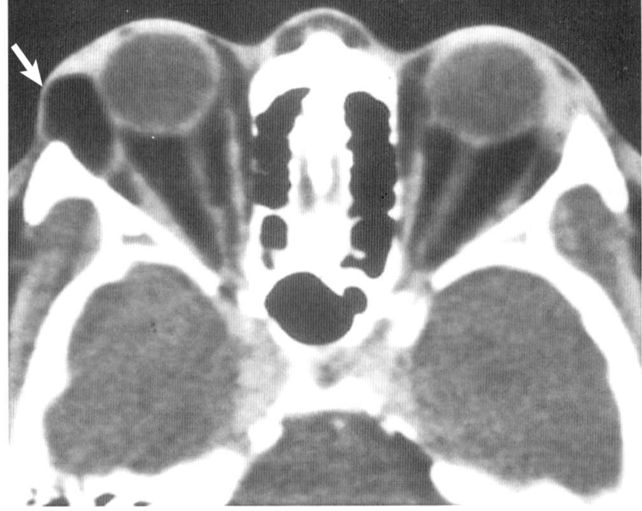

Figure 71.29 Lacrimal gland dermoid. Axial NECT shows well-circumscribed ovoid right lacrimal gland mass filled with fat attenuation material in this typical noninfected dermoid (*arrow*). The mass exhibits exophthalmos and medial globe displacement.

Adenoid cystic carcinoma is the *most common lacrimal gland malignancy* and favors middle-aged women. Involvement of an adjacent lateral rectus muscle or globe can cause pain or limited motion. CT sometimes shows erosion of the adjacent lateral orbital wall. A poorly defined inhomogeneous soft tissue mass is shown on both CT and MRI, frequently exhibiting exuberant focal enhancement. Imagers must look carefully for characteristic perineural tumor spread which portends a particularly poor prognosis [31] (Fig. 71.30). Rarely, squamous cell carcinoma can also arise from the lacrimal gland. Both the clinical and imaging findings are nonspecific with patients typically presenting an orbital mass epiphora and recurrent dacryocystitis. The imaging findings are similar to those previously described for adenoid cystic carcinoma [31].

Various autoimmune and inflammatory processes can involve the lacrimal gland. The majority of these are systemic disorders that result in bilateral involvement and include sarcoidosis and Sjögren's disease (Fig. 71.31). Patients are most commonly between age 40- and 60-years and present with bilateral symptoms of dry eyes or painless proptosis for less than 1 year [1].

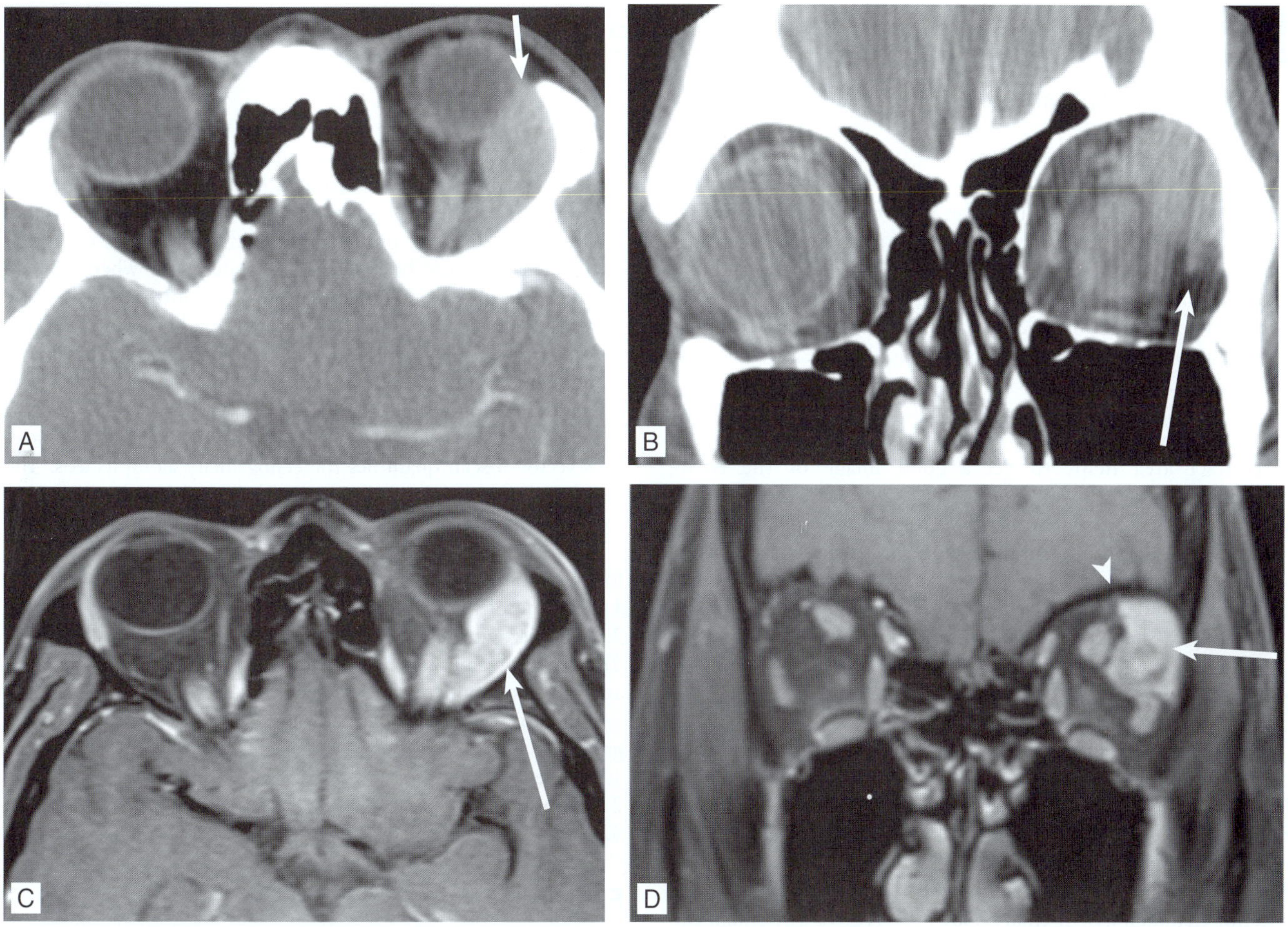

Figure 71.30 Lacrimal gland ACC (*arrows*). (A) Axial (A) and coronal (B) contrast-enhanced CT shows homogeneously enhancing soft tissue mass involving the left lacrimal gland abutting the adjacent globe. Axial (C) and coronal (D) fat-suppressed contrast-enhanced T1W images show the mass (*arrow*) to be avidly enhancing without evidence of retrograde perineural spread along the expected locations of the ophthalmic division of the trigeminal nerve (*arrowhead*).

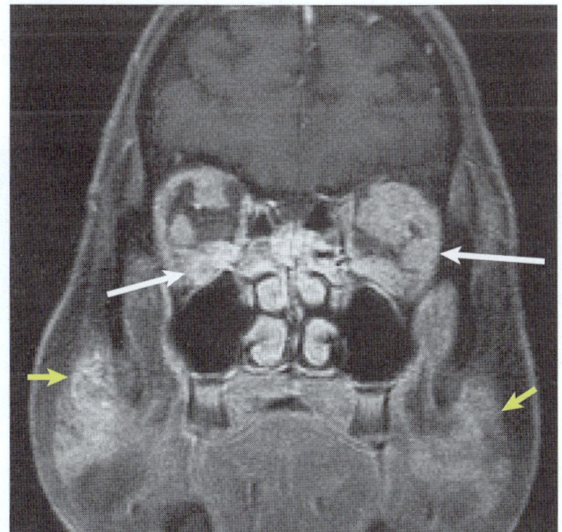

Figure 71.31 Sarcoidosis. Contrast-enhanced coronal T1-weighted images with fat suppression show diffuse enhancement of multiple extraocular muscles (*white arrows*). There is also diffuse irregularity and enhancement of the parotid glands bilaterally (*yellow arrows*).

71.2 Ultrasonography of the Orbit

Deepak Bhatt, Kalpana Bhatt, Vaidehi Bhatt

Introduction

Ultrasonography (USG) of the orbit is an important noninvasive diagnostic tool that helps in the examination of the ocular tissues, especially in the presence of diseases that make a routine eye examination difficult due to the presence of opaque media [32]. A dedicated ophthalmic USG machine is a must for complete evaluation of the eye and the orbit. It should have the following characteristics [33,34]:

1. A 10 or 20 MHz B-mode probe with a very narrow contact area (<1 cm). Since the eye has a curved surface, a small contact area helps to get a good image of the entire eyeball
2. It should have a synchronized vector A-scan, which helps to study the amplitude of the echoes in any quadrant of the image
3. There should also be a facility for amplification of the A-mode in a log, S-shaped, and a stepwise pattern

Normal Ultrasonography Anatomy of the Eye

The eye is divided into the anterior segment, comprising of the cornea, anterior chamber, iris, ciliary body, and the crystalline lens, and the posterior segment containing the vitreous cavity, retina, choroid, and sclera [33]. A 10 or 20 MHz probe is not ideal to comment on the anterior segment structures as it does not have the resolution to differentiate pathologies of the cornea, anterior chamber, iris, or ciliary body [35]. A gross assessment can be made of the position of the lens, but it is not the ideal investigation of choice. The ideal investigation of choice for anterior segment is ultrasound biomicroscopy (with a 35 or 50 MHz probe) [35].

The natural anechoic vitreous acts as an ideal medium for USG evaluation (Fig. 71.32). All pathologies within the vitreous are echogenic and hence there is an excellent interface between them and the vitreous cavity [34].

On a normal USG image, the three ocular coats (retina, choroid, and sclera) cannot be separated from each other [33,34,36]. The thickness of these coats is roughly around 500–700 μm; therefore a 10 or 20 MHz probe cannot differentiate between them [34]. These coats can be identified separately only when they are thickened secondary to inflammation or hemorrhage. The optic nerve is seen as an echo-lucent shadow extending from the optic disk posteriorly. It is advisable not to include the lens shadow in the B-mode image to prevent artifacts in the vitreous cavity. The B-mode image should ideally be studied with a vector A-scan. In Fig. 71.32, vector A-scan is seen overlapping the B-scan image. This vector A-scan quantifies the echogenicity along its axis. The vector A-scan reflectivity of vitreous cavity is low (almost flat) as there are no interfaces noted in the normal vitreous cavity.

Any lesion detected in the vitreous cavity is studied under the following headings:

1. Relation of the lesion with the optic nerve
2. Mobility with respect to the movement of the eyeball

Tips: Do not comment on pathologies of the anterior chamber and the ciliary body on the B-scan

On basis of USG, ocular pathologies can be divided into three groups:

1. Echoes
2. Membranes
3. Tumors

Echoes

Vitreous Floaters

Vitreous floaters or vitreous syneresis are produced due to liquefaction of vitreous gel [37,38]. This liquefaction could be secondary to degeneration of the vitreous [38]. Vitreous floaters should not be considered pathological unless they produce visual disturbances. They are commonly seen in old age or high myopia [38] (Fig. 71.33).

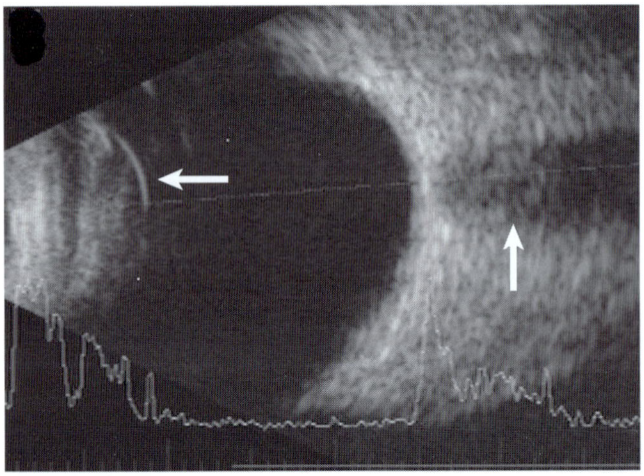

Figure 71.32 The real-time normal B-mode image of the eye shows the posterior capsule of the lens anteriorly (*left arrow*) followed by a clear anechoic vitreous. The optic nerve is seen as an echo-lucent linear shadow (*up arrow*).

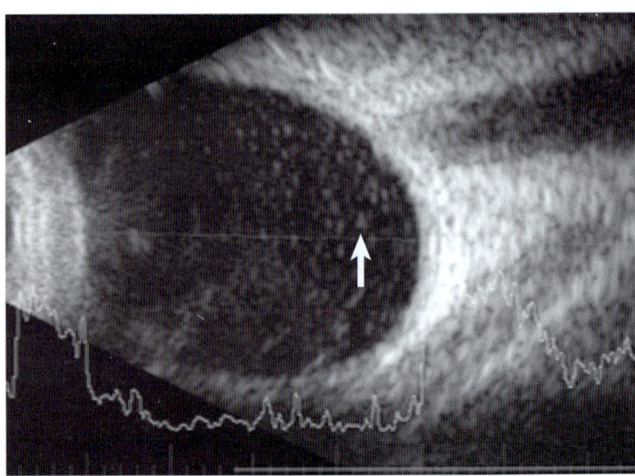

Figure 71.33 The real-time B-mode image of the eye showing few scattered low-intensity vitreous echoes (*white arrow*) which are uniformly distributed in the vitreous cavity. On A-scan, the reflectivity of the vitreous floaters is low.

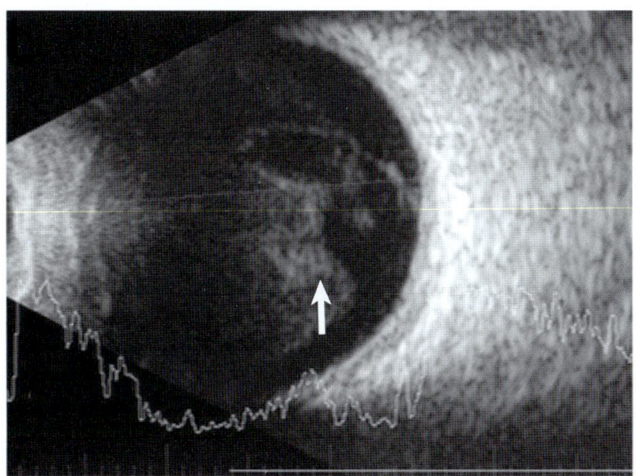

Figure 71.34 The real-time B-mode image of the eye showing fresh vitreous hemorrhage as vitreous echoes in the form of a small dot or short lines (*white arrow*).

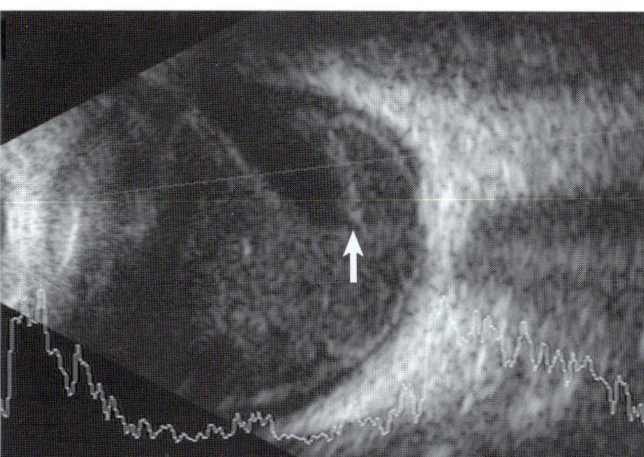

Figure 71.35 The real-time B-mode image of the eye showing resolving vitreous hemorrhage as homogenous hypo- to isoechoic vitreous echoes clumped together with distinct after movements (*white arrow*). On A-scan, resolving vitreous hemorrhage produces low to moderate reflectivity (40–60%).

Vitreous Hemorrhage

Vitreous hemorrhage is the commonest condition encountered in routine B-scan ultrasonography (USG) [33,37]. It can occur due to multiple disorders such as retinal vascular diseases (diabetic retinopathy, retinal vein occlusion, and retinal macroaneurysm), trauma, posterior vitreous detachment (PVD), retinal tears, age-related macular degeneration, etc. [39].

The diagnostic criteria of vitreous hemorrhage depend on the stage of evolution of the hemorrhage namely fresh, resolving, and organized.

Fresh Vitreous Hemorrhage

Normally within the first 12 hours, the RBCs are uniformly spread in the vitreous fluid. Hence, they do not cause any interface with the vitreous fluid. This lack of interface is the cause of nonvisualization of hemorrhage in the first 12 hours on USG. As soon as the RBCs conglomerate, vitreous hemorrhage is seen as low-intensity mobile echoes within the vitreous cavity on a B-scan [33,39] (Fig. 71.34).

It may be difficult to differentiate fresh vitreous hemorrhage from vitreous floaters. On dynamic B-scan, fresh vitreous hemorrhagic echoes show distinct after movements. On real-time USG when vitreous echoes continue to move even after the movement of the eyeball stops it is called after movements. On A-scan, the reflectivity of fresh vitreous hemorrhage is less than 25%.

Resolving Vitreous Hemorrhage

After 24–48 hours the RBCs within the hemorrhage, conglomerate to form a homogenous mass-like lesion within the vitreous cavity (Fig. 71.35).

Organized Vitreous Hemorrhage

Long-standing vitreous hemorrhage resolves with deposition of fibrin within it. Fibrin produces multiple vitreous membranes and bands (Fig. 71.36).

These bands have no movements due to the presence of fibrin within them. The sites of attachment of the vitreous membranes to the retina should be noted and carefully evaluated, as these are potential sites for tractional retinal detachment.

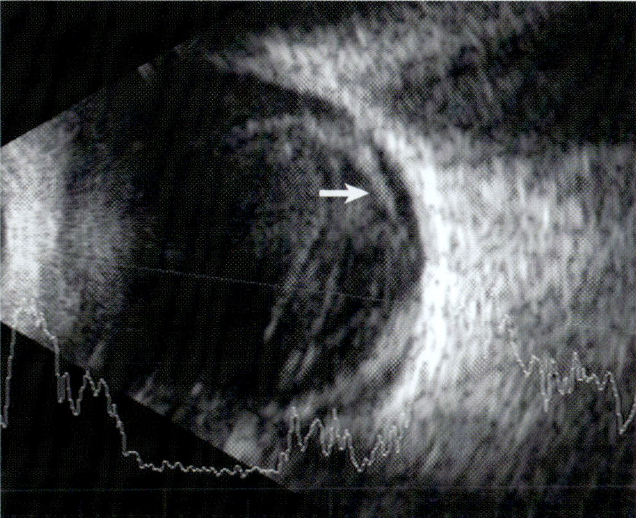

Figure 71.36 The real-time B-mode image of the eye showing organized vitreous hemorrhage as multiple dense vitreous membranes and bands (*white arrow*). On A-scan, the reflectivity of the membrane is high (70–80%) due to fibrin content within the vitreous membranes.

Subhyaloid Hemorrhage

Subhyaloid hemorrhage occurs in a potential space created between the PVD and retina. As subhyaloid hemorrhage occurs in a potential space, it remains in a fluid state till it is absorbed.

Due to the peripheral layering, the subhyaloid hemorrhage has a classical "BOAT-SHAPED" appearance on USG (Fig. 71.37).

Cysticercosis

Cysticercosis is an infestation caused by the larval stage of taenia solium. The commonest area to be affected within the eye is the subretinal space. However intravitreal and retro-ocular spaces can also be involved [40].

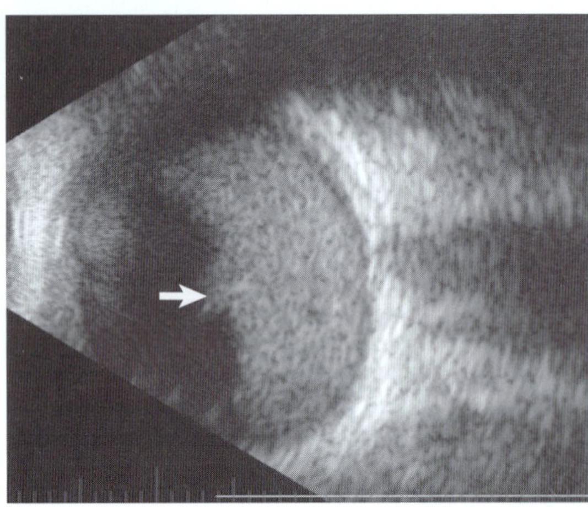

Figure 71.37 On real-time B-mode image of the eye, the subhyaloid hemorrhage is seen as low-intensity homogenous echoes with peripheral layering (*white arrow*). On A-scan subhyaloid hemorrhage has low reflectivity of around 20–30%.

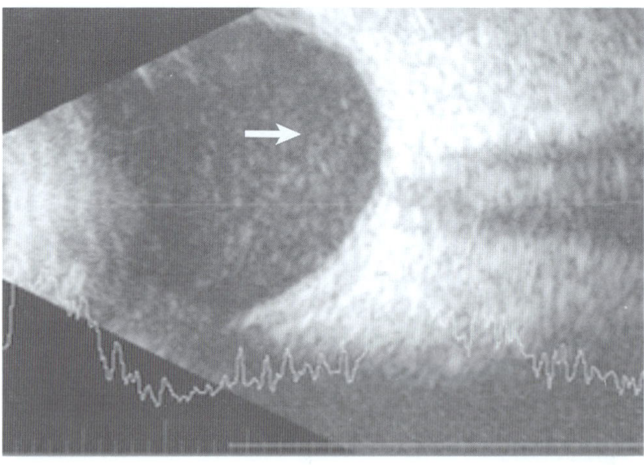

Figure 71.39 On real-time B-mode image of the eye, vitritis is seen as small discrete dot-like lesions with free after movements within the vitreous cavity (*white arrow*). The A-scan reflectivity is generally less than 20%.

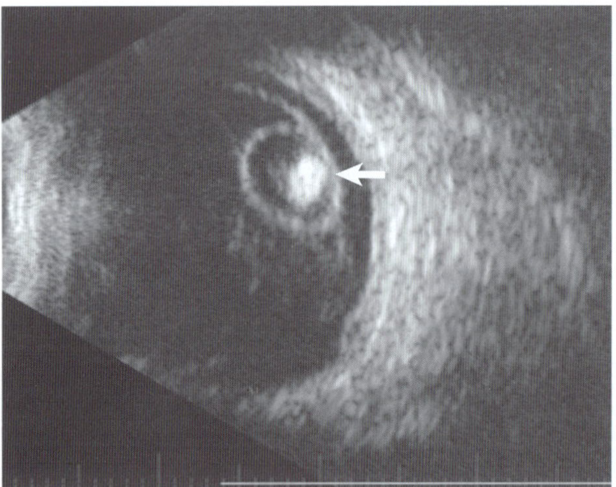

Figure 71.38 On real-time B-mode image of the eye, the cysticercosis is seen as a thin-walled cystic mass lesion within the vitreous cavity or in the subretinal space (*white arrow*).

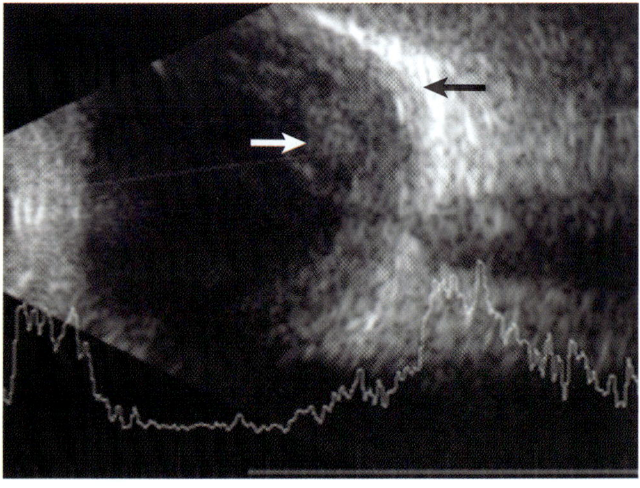

Figure 71.40 The real-time B-mode image of the eye showing progression of vitritis to endophthalmitis (*white arrow*: vitritis; *black arrow*: thickening of the choroid).

During dynamic B-scan, the cyst wall may show some undulating movements. A dense echogenic lesion is seen within the cyst (often eccentrically located) representing the scolex (Fig. 71.38).

Endophthalmitis

Endophthalmitis is an inflammation of the tissue or fluid inside the eyeball, which is usually due to an infection [41]. Vitritis is an initial phase of endophthalmitis. On B-scan vitritis is seen as small discrete dot-like lesions with free after movements within the vitreous cavity (Fig. 71.39).

It may not be possible to differentiate between vitreous hemorrhage and vitritis only on their USG appearance. The echoes within the vitreous need to be correlated with the clinical state.

Endophthalmitis on B-scan is seen as vitritis with thickening of the ocular coats (mainly chorioretinal layer; Fig. 71.40). Endophthalmitis may progress to panophthalmitis. Infection may extend to the Tenon's space, leading to widening of the Tenon's space and the optic nerve. Tenon's space is a potential space between the sclera and orbital fat. Panophthalmitis on B-scan is seen as vitritis with chorioretinal thickening and fluid in the Tenon's space (Fig. 71.41).

Tips: On USG, the appearance of vitreous echoes cannot differentiate between degenerative, hemorrhagic, or inflammatory echoes. Vitreous echoes need to be correlated with the clinical findings.

Membranes

Posterior Vitreous Detachment

Any derangement in the vitreous cavity leads to the detachment of the posterior vitreous from the retina [37,38] (Fig. 71.42).

Retinal Detachment

Retinal detachment can be rhegmatogenous (primary; Fig. 71.43) or nonrhegmatogenous (secondary to other pathologies, e.g., choroidal melanoma).

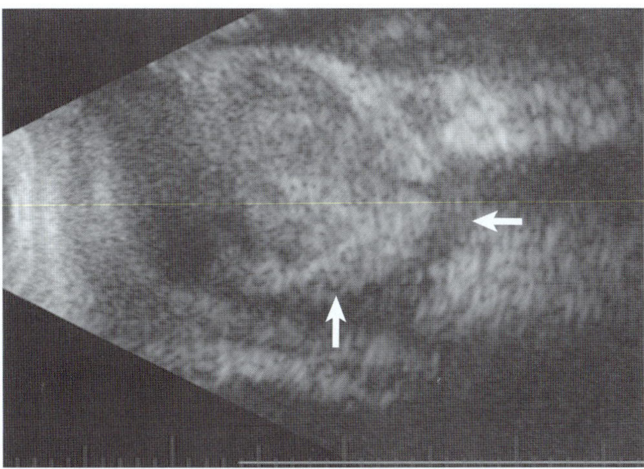

Figure 71.41 On real-time B-mode image of the eye, panophthalmitis is seen as vitritis (*up arrow*) with chorioretinal thickening and fluid in the Tenon's space (*left arrow*).

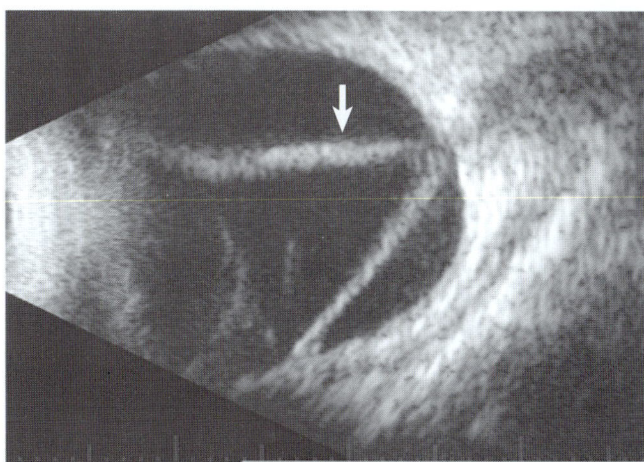

Figure 71.43 On real-time B-mode image of the eye, retinal detachment is seen as a highly reflective, V-shaped membrane attached to the optic disk (*white arrow*). This membrane classically has restricted mobility.

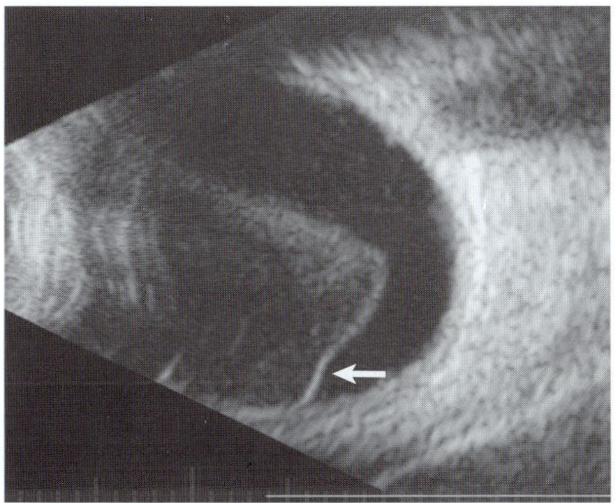

Figure 71.42 On real-time B-mode image of the eye, PVD is seen as a thin irregular membrane with distinct after movements (*white arrow*). The presence of after movements is a hallmark of PVD.

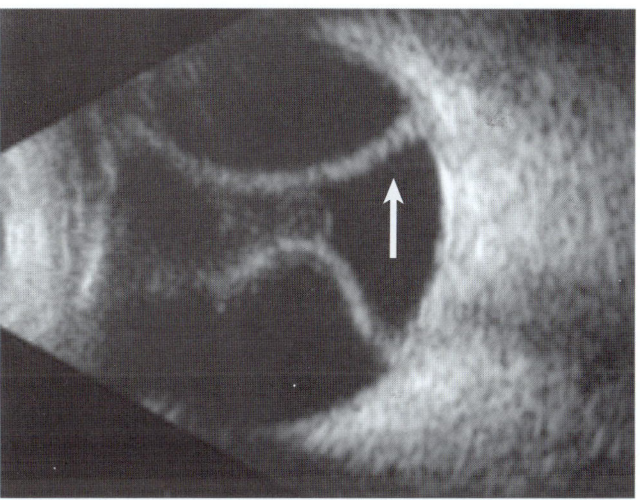

Figure 71.44 On real-time B-mode image of the eye, serous choroidal detachment is seen as a thick dome-shaped membrane, not attached to the optic disk (*white arrow*).

It is very important to differentiate retinal detachment from a thick PVD attached to the optic disk.

The differential diagnosis of membranes attached to the optic disk:

Retinal Detachment	Posterior Vitreous Detachment
Thick uniform fixed membrane	Thin undulating membrane
No after movements	Free after movements

Choroidal Detachment

A choroidal detachment occurs due to the collection of fluid in the potential suprachoroidal space, which is located between the choroid and the sclera [33,41]. Choroidal detachments are of three types, namely, serous, exudative, and hemorrhagic. Of these, a serous choroidal detachment is the commonest type (Fig. 71.44).

Hemorrhagic choroidal detachment may occur secondary to trauma or postoperatively. In acute hemorrhagic choroidal detachment the choroidal membrane may not be seen separately from the hemorrhage (Fig. 71.45).

The role of USG in cases of hemorrhagic choroidal detachment is to access whether the hemorrhage is in a solid or fluid state, as it will determine the treatment procedure (Fig. 71.46).

Tips: USG evaluation of membranes in the vitreous cavity is never complete without kinetic USG evaluation. It is important to determine the presence or absence of after movements before differentiating membranes.

Tumors

Intraocular tumors are divided into two major groups.

A. Retinoblastoma and conditions simulating retinoblastoma, seen in the young age group
B. Choroidal melanoma and conditions simulating melanoma, seen in older age group

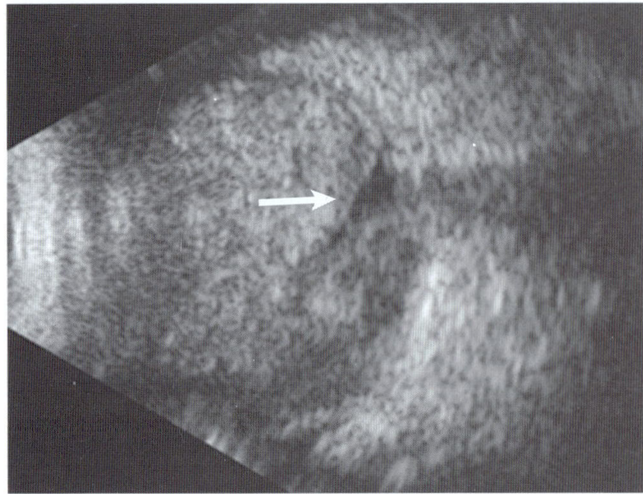

Figure 71.45 On real-time B-mode image of the eye, the acute phase of hemorrhagic choroidal detachment is seen as a choroidal mass lesion (*white arrow*). Please note that the choroidal membrane cannot be separated from hemorrhage at this stage.

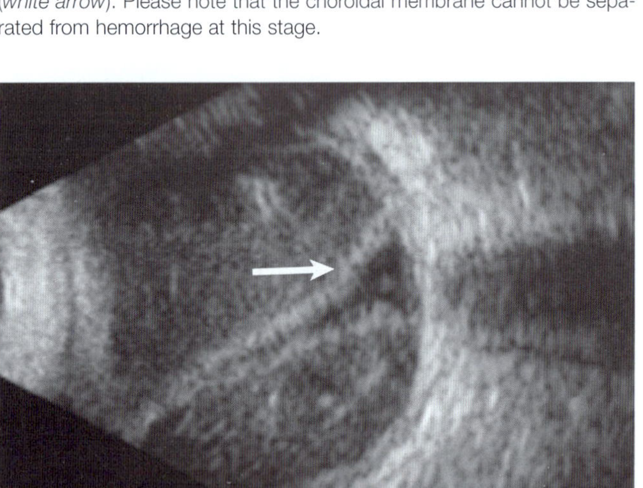

Figure 71.46 On follow-up real-time B-mode image of the eye of the same patient as in Fig. 71.45 with hemorrhagic choroidal detachment, there is gradual change in the hemorrhage noted from solid to fluid state. The choroidal membrane is now distinctly visualized (*white arrow*).

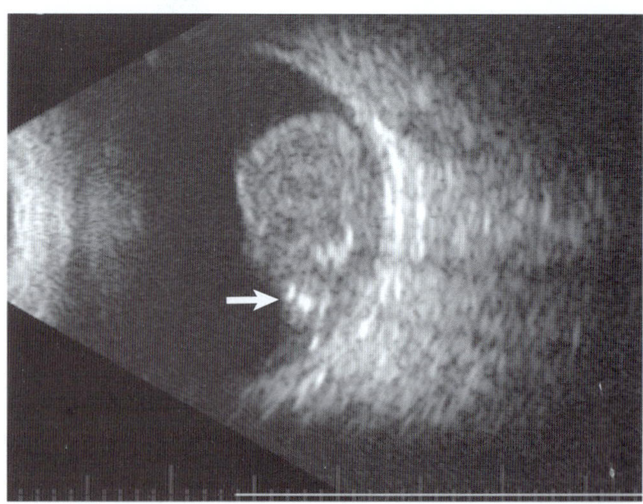

Figure 71.47 On real-time B-mode image of the eye, retinoblastoma is seen as an irregular echogenic mass lesion in the posterior segment with a broad base. Calcification is seen in 50% of retinoblastomas (*white arrow*).

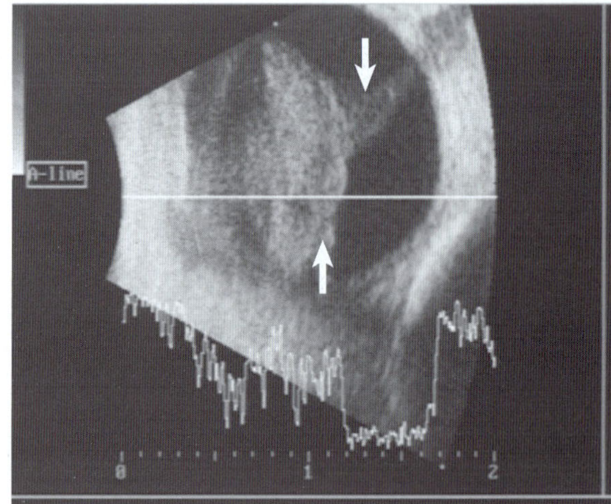

Figure 71.48 On real-time B-mode image of the eye, stage 4 and stage 5 of retinopathy of prematurity is seen either as a V-shaped retinal detachment (*down arrow*) with a dense fibrotic membrane in the retrolental space (*up arrow*). There may be associated hemorrhage in the subretinal space. On A-scan, there is high reflectivity noted due to fibrosis.

Retinoblastoma and Its Differential Diagnosis

Retinoblastoma is a tumor usually seen in the first decade of life [33].

Calcification whenever present in a tumor is typically diagnostic of retinoblastoma, but the absence of calcification does not rule out retinoblastoma (Fig. 71.47).

On A-scan, there is typically a high irregular reflectivity, which is diagnostic of retinoblastoma.

Extension into the optic nerve or retro-orbital space is accurately evaluated on a CT scan rather than USG.

Retinoblastoma is the most important cause of leukocoria (white pupil) in children.

The differential diagnosis of leukocoria include [42]

1. Retinopathy of prematurity
2. Persistent hyperplastic primary vitreous
3. Coat's disease
4. Cysticercosis
5. Endophthalmitis

Retinopathy of Prematurity

This condition is seen in premature children and/or after oxygen therapy in the neonatal age group (Fig. 71.48). It is always a bilateral condition, although it can be asymmetrical [42].

Persistent Hyperplastic Primary Vitreous

Persistent hyperplastic primary vitreous is a developmental disorder of the eye, where the embryonic hyaloid artery fails to completely regress. It is a unilateral condition where a fibrotic band is seen extending from the posterior capsule of the lens to the optic disk [42] (Fig. 71.49). Due to the fibrotic band, the axial length of the eye is reduced. There may be associated retinal detachment. It is sometimes possible to detect the presence of blood flow in this band due to the presence of a persistent hyaloid artery.

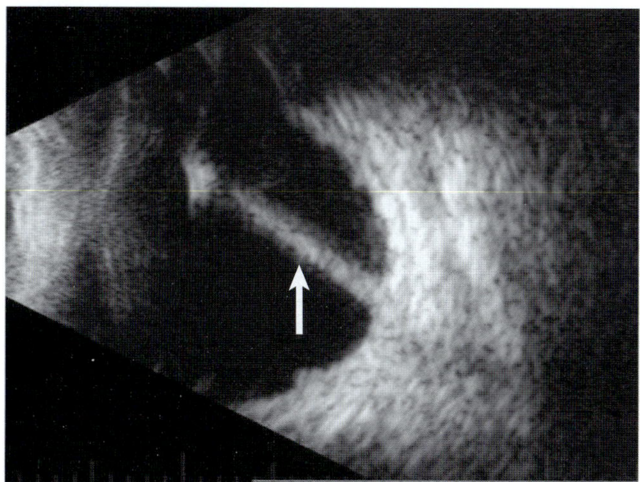

Figure 71.49 On real-time B-mode image of the eye, persistent hyperplastic primary vitreous (PHPV) is seen as a band extending from the posterior capsule of the lens to the optic disk showing high reflectivity (*white arrow*).

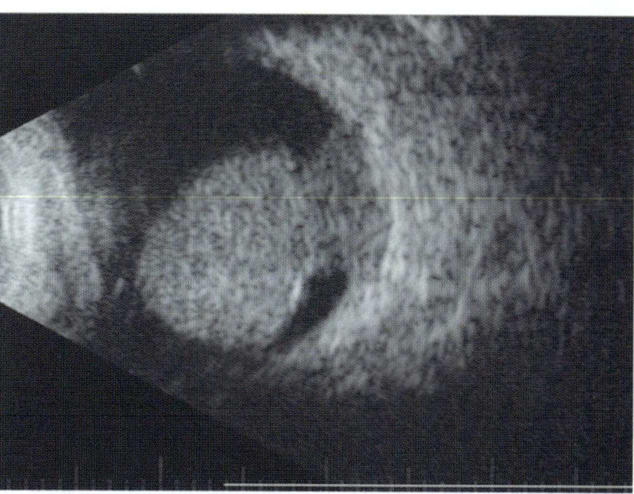

Figure 71.51 On real-time B-mode image of the eye, the collar button shape is pathognomonic of melanoma.

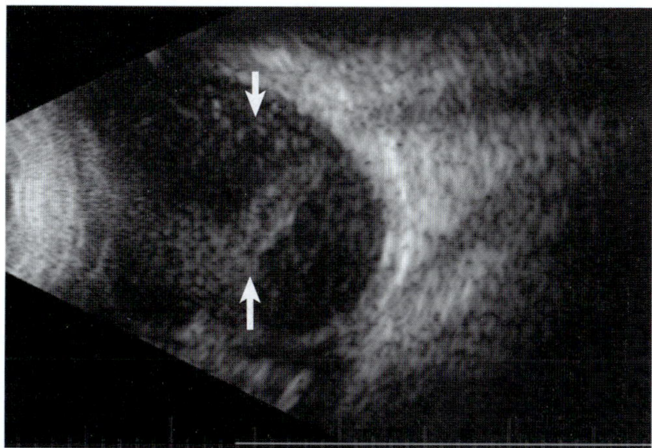

Figure 71.50 On real-time B-mode image of the eye, Coat's disease is seen as an open or closed funnel retinal detachment (*up arrow*) with dense subretinal exudates (*down arrow*).

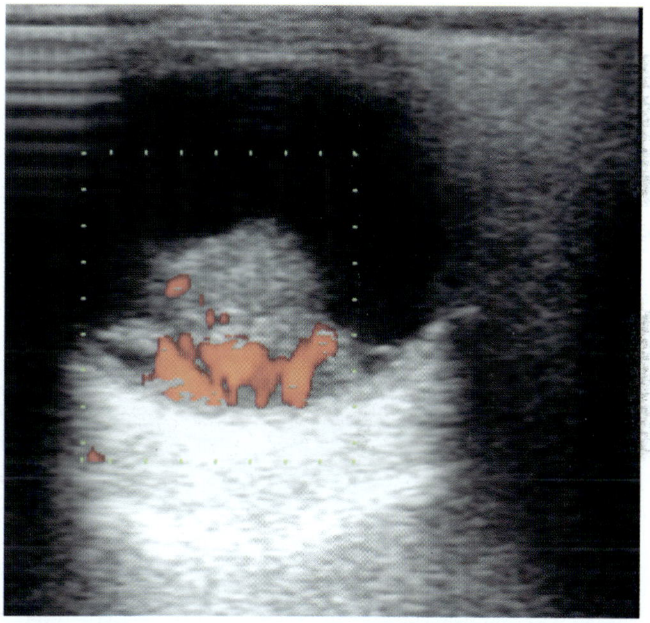

Figure 71.52 A melanoma demonstrating high vascularity.

Coat's Disease

Coats disease is a telangiectatic neovascular disease of the retina. This is a unilateral condition presenting with an exudative retinal detachment (Fig. 71.50). There are cholesterol crystals noted in the subretinal fluid. It is commonly seen in young males.

Tips: It is important to rule out the presence of retinoblastoma in cases of leukocoria. Try changing gains to rule out calcification. In the absence of calcification use A-scan to study the echogenicity of the mass lesion.

Choroidal Tumors

Choroidal Melanoma

Choroidal melanoma is the most common tumor of the eye in the middle-age group [41]. Melanomas on B-scan are seen as a dome-shaped or collar button-shaped tumor with the base over the choroid (Fig. 71.51). The collar button shape is due to the break in the Bruch's membrane. Bruch's membrane is a thick layer of the choroid, which resists choroidal contents from entering retinal layer.

Melanomas are highly vascular tumors (Fig. 71.52). On B-scan, the vascularity is seen as a fast-flickering motion within the tumor. This motion is more marked at the base of the tumor (Fig. 71.53).

Choroidal Metastases

The commonest primary which metastasizes to the choroid is an oat cell tumor of the lung in males and breast in females [41] (Fig. 71.54). On B-scan, choroidal metastasis shows heterogenous echotexture and irregular anterior surface. On A-scan, the reflectivity of choroidal metastasis is high and irregular, these features help to differentiate between choroidal metastasis and melanoma.

Choroidal Hemangioma

Choroidal hemangiomas may occur as a solitary lesion or as a part of Sturge–Weber syndrome [41].

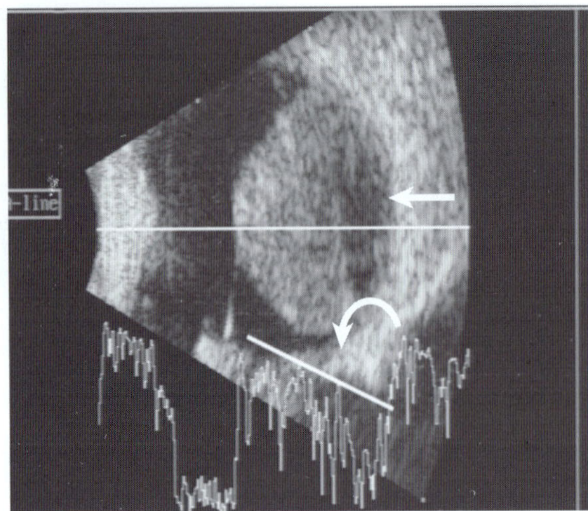

Figure 71.53 On real-time B-mode image of the eye, melanomas usually demonstrate choroidal excavation at the base of the tumor (*left arrow*). On A-scan, it shows is a high anterior surface spike followed by low internal reflectivity with a typical cascading effect (*curved arrow*).

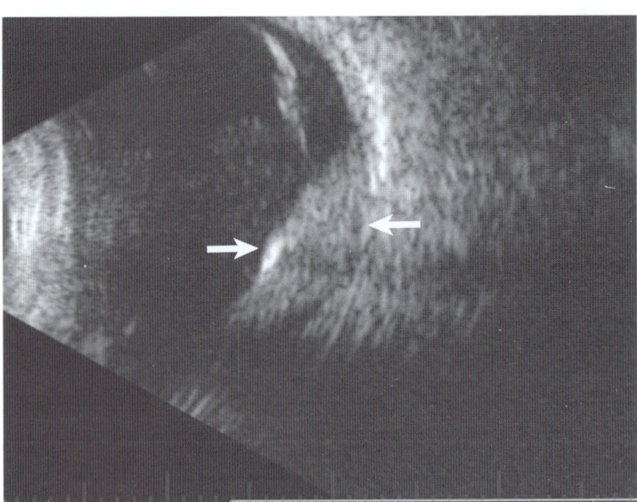

Figure 71.55 The real-time B-mode image of an eye shows a choroidal hemangioma (*left arrow*) with a calcific area (phlebolith) in choroidal hemangioma (*right arrow*).

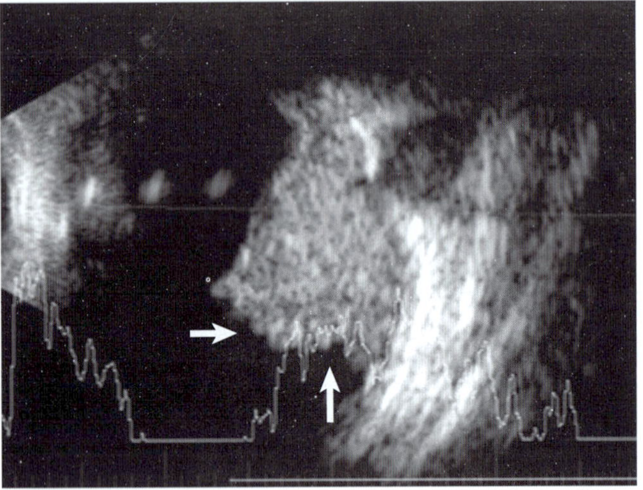

Figure 71.54 On real-time B-mode image of the eye, choroidal metastasis is seen as an irregular lobulated mass lesion arising from the choroid with heterogenous echotexture (*horizontal arrow*). On A-scan, there is a high irregular reflectivity noted because of multiple interfaces (*vertical arrow*).

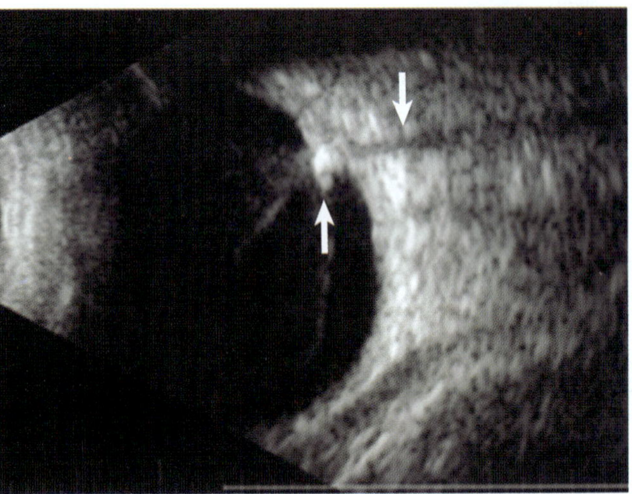

Figure 71.56 The real-time B-mode image of an eye illustrating a foreign body (*up arrow*), which is seen as a localized echogenic lesion with posterior shadowing (*down arrow*).

On B-scan, a choroidal hemangioma may have various shapes, but they all have a broad base over the choroid.

The echotexture of choroidal hemangioma is heterogeneous due to the multiple interfaces within the tumor. A small calcific area is occasionally noted over the surface of choroidal hemangioma, known as a phlebolith (Fig. 71.55). It may or may not produce shadowing depending on the density of calcium within the phlebolith. The presence of phlebolith is diagnostic of hemangioma, but the absence does not rule out a hemangioma.

Tips: The A-scan evaluation is extremely important in the differential diagnosis of choroidal tumors.

Trauma

USG evaluation in ocular trauma is very challenging due to following reasons [43].

a. The patient may have extreme pain and hence he does may not cooperate for a thorough USG evaluation.
b. There is a possibility of rupture of the globe when excessive pressure is applied while performing USG and this may lead to disastrous consequences.
c. The presence of vitreous hemorrhage and retinal detachment may mask the classical appearance of an intraocular foreign body.

Intraocular Foreign Body

USG has a role in ruling out the presence or absence of a foreign body [44] (Fig. 71.56).

Shadowing is the hallmark of a foreign body but in the presence of vitreous hemorrhage or choroidal hemorrhage foreign body may not show classical shadowing. In such cases reducing gains help in highlighting the foreign body (Fig. 71.57).

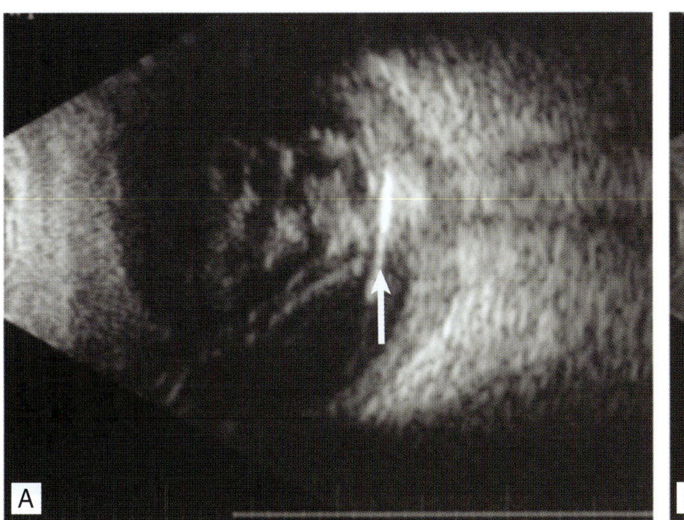

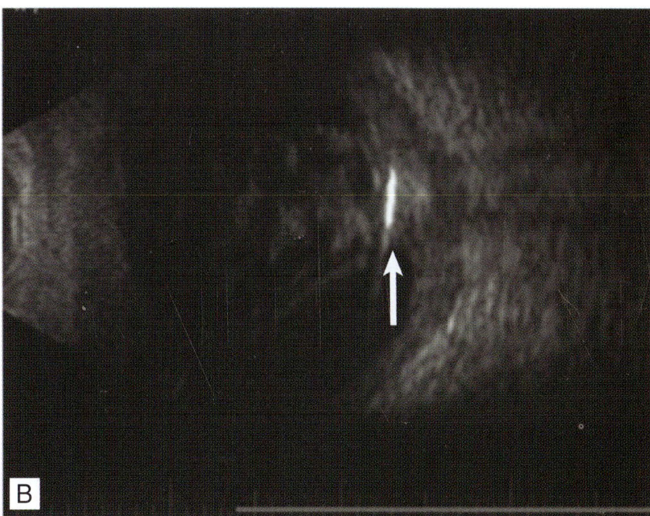

Figure 71.57 The real-time B-mode image of an eye (A) with high gain and (B) with low gain. Note that a foreign body is illustrated better (*white arrow*) after reducing the gain setting.

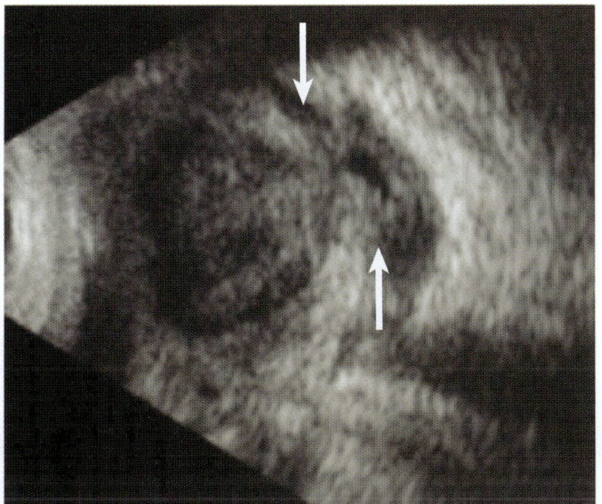

Figure 71.58 The real-time B-mode image of an eye illustrating the two cardinal signs of scleral rupture, that is, vitreous incarceration (*down arrow*) and hemorrhage in Tenon's space (*up arrow*).

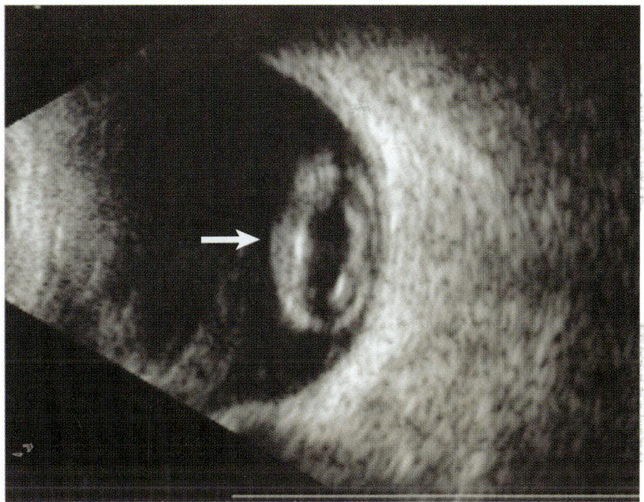

Figure 71.59 The real-time B-mode image of an eye illustrating a dislocated lens, which is seen as an oval echogenic lesion in the vitreous (*white arrow*).

Scleral Tear

Detecting scleral tear in open globe injuries is a big challenge on USG. The exact location and extent of the tear may be difficult to ascertain on USG. The main reason for this is the distortion of the ocular anatomy in the presence of trauma. This problem is further compounded with the presence of vitreous, retinal, and choroidal hemorrhage. The two most important signs which help us detect scleral rupture are vitreous incarceration and hemorrhage in the Tenon's space. The presence of these signs guides to the site of scleral tear (Fig. 71.58).

Tips: In cases of trauma take a complete history to ascertain the exact nature of trauma and intraocular foreign body. Take a plain radiograph of the orbit before doing an USG.

Dislocated Lens and Intraocular Lens

The dislocated lens may be fixed or mobile. It may be difficult to identity dislocated lenses in the presence of dense vitreous hemorrhage (Fig. 71.59). If there are dense echoes within the dislocated lens it may mimic cysticercosis.

Tips: Please look for normal lens shadow anteriorly before looking for a lens in the vitreous cavity.

Ultrasonography of the Extraocular Region

The extraocular region is generally evaluated with a CT scan or MR. However, USG has a definite role in the preliminary evaluation of the extraocular region. USG helps to rule out the presence of a retro-orbital lesion in patients with proptosis (Fig. 71.60).

The orbital cavity is divided into three parts by the muscular coats, namely intraconal, conal, and extraconal spaces.

Intraconal Ultrasonography

The most important structure in the intraconal space is the optic nerve.

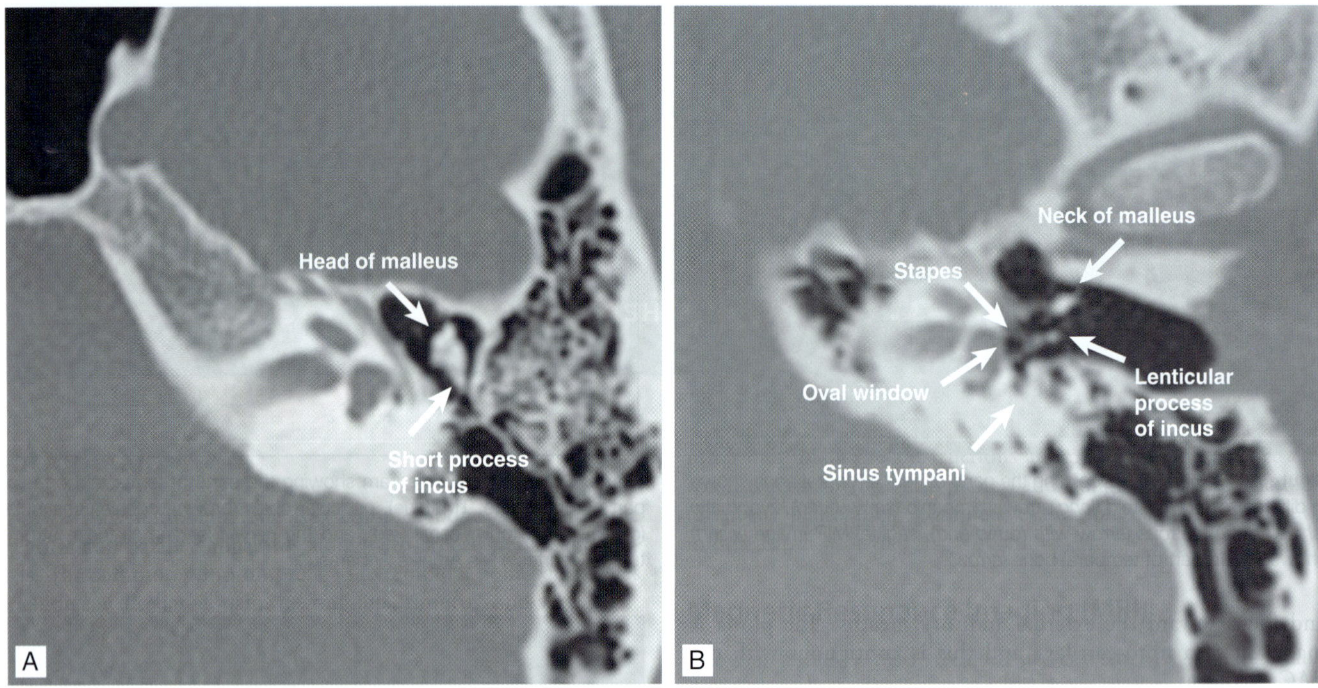

Figure 72.4 (A and B) Axial HRCT of right temporal bone showing the ossicular chain and middle ear anatomy.

The lateral epitympanic recess is located at the epitympanum lateral to the ossicular chain, best seen in the coronal plane. The inferior aspect of the lateral epitympanic recess is called the Prussak's space. This is located just medial to the scutum, and regarded as the classic location of pars flaccida Cholesteatoma. The coronal plane also shows the "roof" of middle ear and mastoid—called the tegmen tympani and tegmen antri respectively. This bony roof can be of variable thickness and sometimes dehiscent.

Ossicular chain:

The ossicular chain is important conducting mechanism that carries the sounds in the form of vibrations from the TM to the oval window membrane. Malleus, incus, and stapes are the three ossicles (Fig. 72.4).

The malleus has the following components—head, neck, manubrium (also known as handle). The manubrium is attached to the TM and the tip of the manubrium is also called umbo located at central part of the TM.

Superiorly, there are two tiny processes seen arising from the just below the neck of malleus providing attachment of the ligaments suspending the malleus in position.

The incus is an anvil-shaped structure. The head of the malleus articulates with the body of incus (malleo-incudal joint). The body of incus extends posteriorly as a short process and reaches the fossa incudis, almost the same level as the anterior aspect of the Aditus ad antrum.

Inferiorly, the long process of incus extends toward the stapes and ends in a small nodular thickening called the lenticular process or lenticular nodule. The lenticular process articulates with stapes forming an incudostapedial joint.

The stapes comprises a head, neck, anterior and posterior crura, and foot plate. The foot plate is seen as a single structure with oval window membrane. The anterior and posterior crura are obliquely oriented and can be asymmetrical.

Multiplanar reconstructions of CT volume data in axial, coronal, sagittal, and oblique planes are important steps in assessing the ossicular chain (Fig. 72.5).

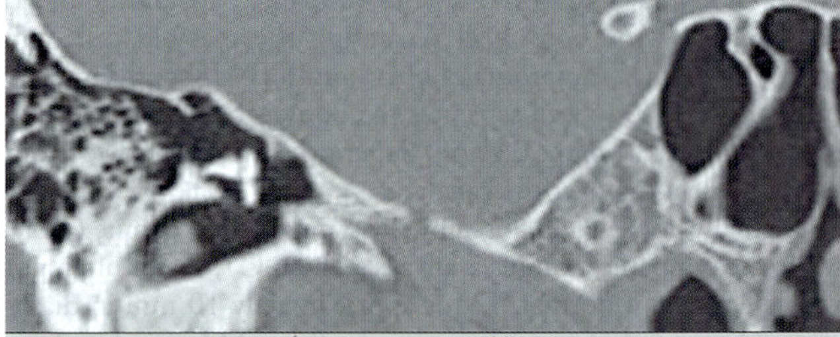

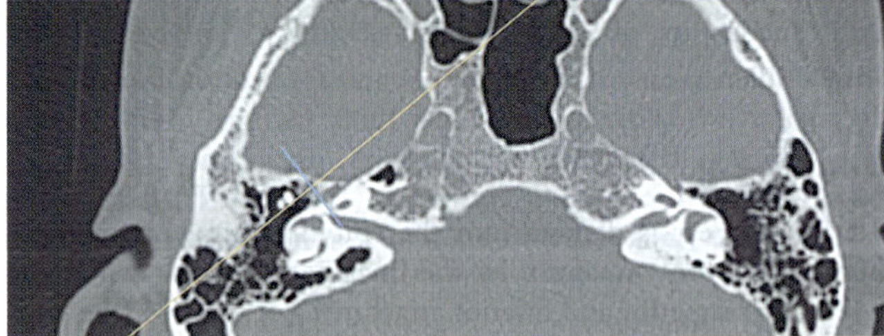

Figure 72.5 Axial HRCT with yellow line (*bottom*) depicting the oblique coronal plane (*top*) showing the malleo-incudal articulation in its true sagittal plane for the *right side*.

Inner Ear

Inner ear is made of bony labyrinth that houses membranous labyrinth; bony labyrinth is the bony cavity structure, such as cochlea, vestibule, and semicircular canals; it contains perilymph that surrounds the membranous labyrinth that contains endolymph.

The cochlea is located anteriorly and slightly inferiorly, and the semicircular canals are located more posteriorly and superiorly in relation to the horizontal plane with vestibule in between.

The cochlea has about $2^{1/2}$ to $2^{3/4}$ turns (Fig. 72.6A–D). The central bony pillar of cochlea is called the modiolus; spiral lamina is the outward bony projections from the modiolus that gives attachments to membranes; the membranes divide the cochlea

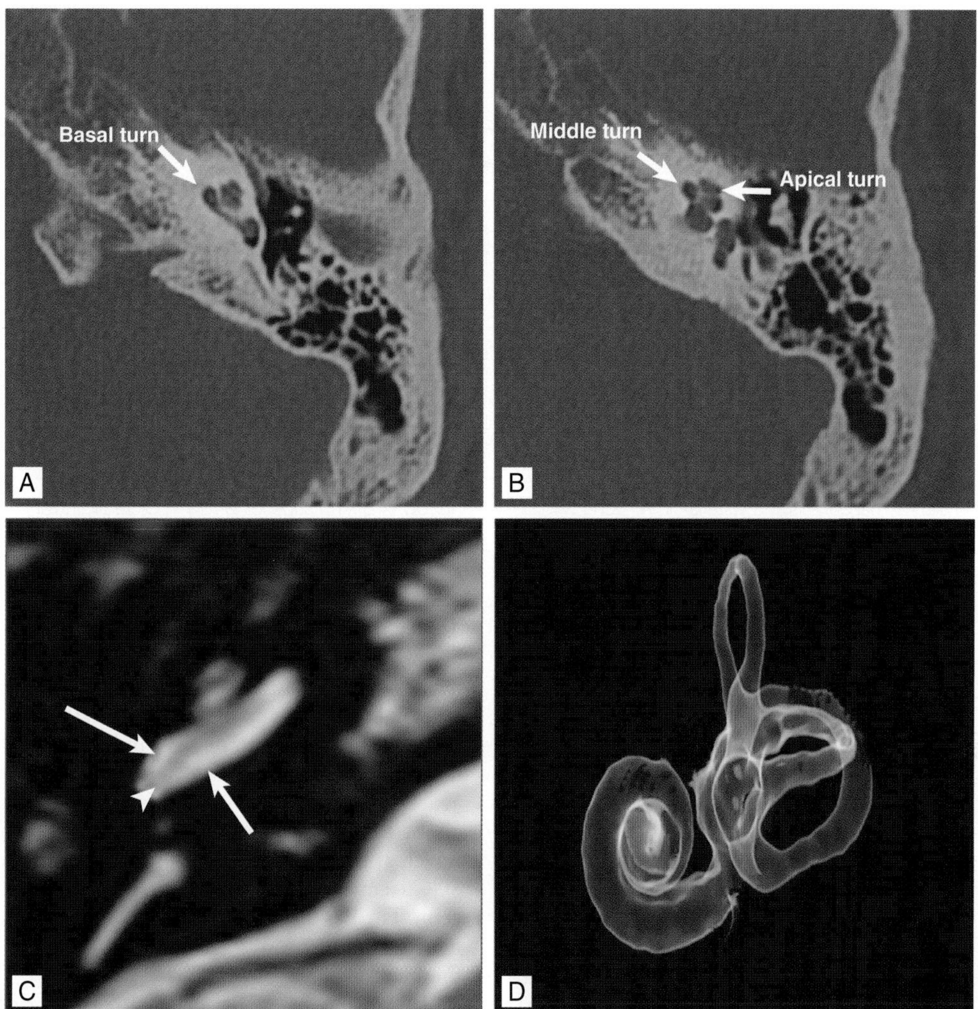

Figure 72.6 Axial HRCT temporal bone showing the turns of cochlea (A, B); high-resolution T2W MRI image (C) showing the scala tympani (*short arrow*), scala vestibuli (*long arrow*), and basilar membrane (*arrowhead*); 3-D MinIp images (D) of the inner showing the cochlea, vestibule, and semicircular canal.

into three fluid-filled spaces; the scala vestibuli and scala tympani (containing perilymph) and scala media in between (also called the cochlear duct, containing endolymph). The scala tympani is located at the inferior aspect, relative to apex and the scala vestibuli is located at the superior aspect, both communicate at the apex (at helicotrema).

Reissner's membrane separate scala vestibuli and scala media, and basilar membrane separates the scala tympani from scala media; the basilar membrane holds the organ of corti—the cells of hearing are connected to the cochlear nerve and the tectorial membrane.

The movement of stapes transmitted the waves through the perilymph, which depends on the frequency distorting the basilar membrane and Reissner's membrane, transmitting the wave to scala media; thus, moving the haircells at organ corti and tectorial membrane, resulting in depolarization and formation of nerve impulse.

The vestibule contains utricle (superiorly located) and saccule (inferiorly located)—both contains endolymph. The saccule connects with the cochlear duct and the utricle, the larger structure connects to all the semicircular canal structures.

The semicircular canals are named anterior, lateral, and superior and contains endolymph that circulates through this structures and plays role in position sense related to linear acceleration (Fig. 72.7).

The endolymph from utricle and saccule drains through endolymphatic duct. This is located at the posterior part of petrous temporal bone and courses posteriorly and inferiorly. The bony part that houses endolymphatic duct is called the vestibular aqueduct. The duct ends in a broader structure that houses the endolymphatic sac.

The cochlea is best seen in axial, coronal CT planes, and 3-D reconstructions. The ossicles are best assessed on axial, coronal, and sagittal planes. Vestibular aqueduct is seen best in sagittal oblique plane. Superior semicircular canal is seen best on sagittal oblique plane; lateral semicircular canal seen best on corona and off-axial planes.

Internal Auditory Canal, Jugular Fossa, Carotid Canal

Internal auditory canal is an obliquely oriented structure and measures approximately 8–9 mm in length. It tapers toward the apex that is located at the lateral aspect. Important structures, including seventh and eighth nerve cranial nerves, are seen traversing through this canal.

There is a small bony projection called falciform crest (crista falciformis) located at the fundus of internal auditory canal (IAC) and divides canal into superior and inferior parts. Bill's bar is a

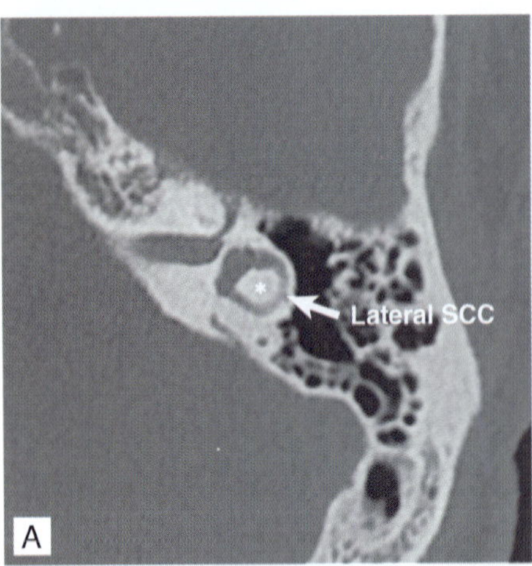

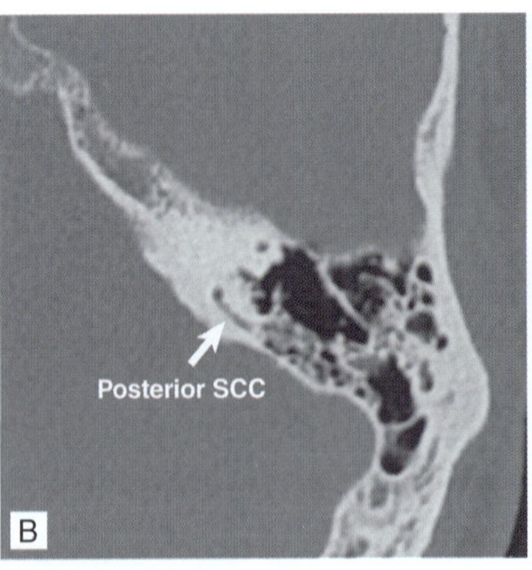

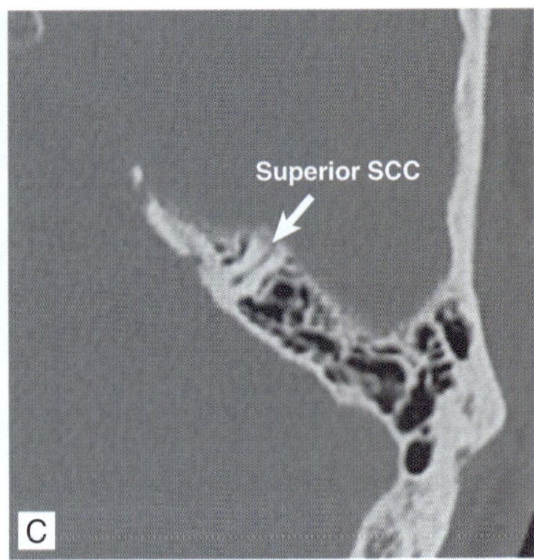

Figure 72.7 (A–C) Axial HRCT: Vestibule and semicircular canals—left temporal bone HRCT images show the complete ring of vestibule, lateral semicircular canal (*arrow* in A), and the normal bone island (*asterisk* in A) along with posterior (*arrow* in B) and superior (*arrow* in C) semicircular canals.

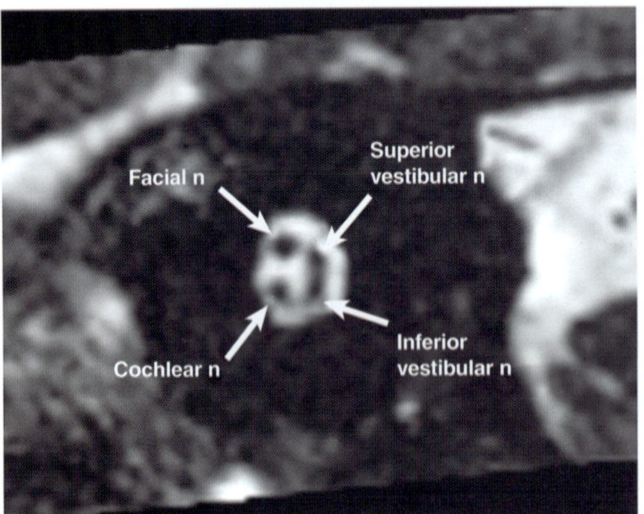

Figure 72.8 High-resolution T2W in oblique sagittal plane showing divisions of the eighth nerve (n – nerve) in respective compartments at lateral aspect internal auditory canal.

vertical bony crest that divides the superior compartment into anterior and posterior.

The cochlear nerve is located at anteroinferior compartment and enters through the lamina cribrosa into the modiolus. The facial nerve is located at anterosuperior compartments. The superior and inferior vestibular nerves are noted, respectively, at the posterosuperior and posteroinferior aspects and are seen extending towards the vestibule (Fig. 72.8).

The jugular fossa and carotid canal are two impartment structures situated at the inferior aspect of the middle and inner ear region. The carotid canal is partly outlined by the eustachian tube margin and partly by the petrous temporal bone and is seen reaching the apex of the petrous before it curves into the cavernous sinus.

The jugular fossa collects blood from the sigmoid sinus and is focally dilated at its origin called the jugular bulb. There is a bony process called carotico-jugular spine or septum separates the carotid canal from jugular bulb. Cranial nerves IX, X, and XI are located within the pars nervosa part of the jugular fossa and descend along the internal jugular vein (IJV) and internal carotid artery (ICA) at the skull base into the carotid space of the neck. Within the carotid canal, there is ICA and sympathetic chain—which is not seen in routine scans.

Facial Nerve Canal

The facial nerve follows a unique course through the temporal bone; after exiting from the cerebello pointine (CP) angle, the nerve is located anterior to the vestibuloochclear nerve at the CP angle cistern and IAC; the facial nerve is located at the anterosuperior portion of IAC and enters the bone to form the labyrinthine segment. The nerve acutely turns posteriorly by acute angle of about 70 degrees at the level of geniculate ganglion, to run as a tympanic segment. The tympanic segment travels at the superior aspect of middle ear, inferior to the lateral SCC (semicircular canal), close to stapes to reach the posterior genu. Further 90-degree turn inferiorly at this level leads to the mastoid segment of facial nerve, reaching the stylomastoid foramen.

The greater superficial petrosal nerve starts at geniculate ganglion and runs medially. The chorda tympani arises from the mastoid segment and runs superiorly around the TM to exit anteriorly at petrotympanic fissure.

Normal Variants

External Ear

EAC can be slightly narrow, usually due to hypoplasia; however, atresia is a pathological condition. Foramen of Huschke [1] (persistent foramen tympanicum) is due to nonossification of the anteroinferior bony canal, this may sometimes communicate with the TM joint (3–25%). Patency of the foramen of Huschke is usually asymptomatic, but can present with ear pain, discharge during mastication, and soft tissue protrusion into EAC due to bulging of the TMJ. There is an area of narrowing located 6 mm proximal to the TM within the bony; this area is called isthmus; sometimes foreign body located medial to this isthmus can be difficult to remove by routine examination, and specialized surgical approaches may be needed.

Middle Ear

Ossicular variations do not cause major clinical issue, except when there is moderate-to-severe hypoplasia. Asymptomatic variations include curved appearance of the long process of the incus. Stapes can have asymmetric and uneven crura which sometimes even dehiscence or the absence of bone crura.

The oval window membrane usually of 2.5 sq. mm sized and sometimes there can be stenosis leading to oval window hypoplasia. Mastoid pneumatization can be variable from minimal pneumatization up to hyperpneumatization involving petrous apex and also extending into the squamous temporal bone.

Inner Ear/Petrous Apex

Internal ear variations are often pathological; however, many times the lateral semicircular canal can be hypoplastic without major symptoms. The vestibular aqueductis is usually less than the size of the semicircular canal or less than 1.5 mm as measured in the mid part. The cochlea apical turn can be slightly hypoplastic with asymmetric partition but can be asymptomatic.

The petrous apex can show, asymmetric pneumatization with variable asymmetric marrow fat; retained fluid at one petrous apex with pneumatization on the other side, can be mistaken for pathology.

External Ear Pathologies

Clinical Factors

The external ear is the most accessible subsite, with most conditions are diagnosed clinically and treated without imaging. Common clinical presentations include ear discharge, pain, swelling, and not infrequently retained foreign body. A most common indication for imaging includes a high index of suspicion for necrotizing otitis externa to assess its presence, extent, and evaluate associated complications. Other indications include soft tissue mass of obliterating visualization of the TM, hard bony swellings, and EAC atresia [2].

Soft tissue attenuation lesions are common. Cerumen/wax appears as soft tissue attenuation in the external ear, and often an unwary radiologist may confuse this for pathology. The presence of air pockets between the lesion and the external auditory walls is a diagnostic clue to the possibility of ceruminous deposits. Differential diagnosis and density based approach of external ear disease is listed under Table 72.1.

External Otitis and Necrotizing Otitis Externa (NOE)

External otitis is a common condition due to infection involving the external ear and presents with pain and ear discharge. The imaging is to assess for the presence of complications and associated disease.

In susceptible individuals, especially diabetics and immunosuppressed patients, the infection is usually due to pseudomonas.

TABLE 72.1 Differential Diagnosis of External Auditory Canal Lesions

Soft tissue density lesions—cerumen/wax, KO, external otitis, external auditory canal cholesteatoma
Bone density lesions—atresia, exostosis, osteoma
Soft tissue lesion with bone erosion or destruction—necrotizing otitis externa, cholesteatoma, carcinoma

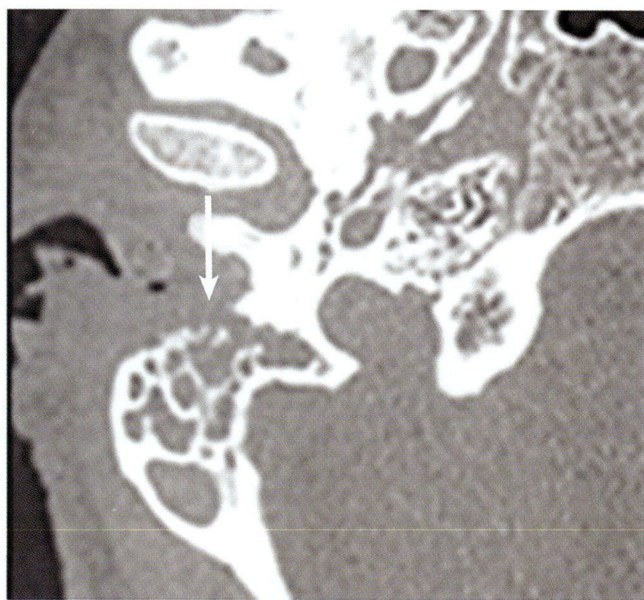

Figure 72.9 Necrotizing otitis externa (NOE): Axial HRCT, *right side*, showing external ear soft tissue eroding the posterior wall (*arrow*); in addition associated mastoid fluid attenuation changes; this can also erode into EAC and thus cause external otitis with changes similar to NOE.

It may involve the EAC's bony margins resulting in erosion, periostitis, new bone formation, and bony necrosis. In severe cases, the disease process can extend into the adjacent structures, including perimastoid soft tissue, around the auricle, parapharyngeal space, and TMJ with rare skull base involvement. This appearance of extensive soft tissue changes with bone erosion, centered in the EAC in immune-suppressed patients, suggests necrotizing otitis externa.

- High resolution computed tomography (HRCT) of the temporal bone is the investigation of choice. CT depicts bony erosion of EAC margins (Fig. 72.9) with enhancing inflammatory soft tissue, extending into the infratemporal region, masticator space, around the TMJ and skull base/nasopharynx regions with occasional small rim enhancing areas suggesting necrotic areas and abscess (Fig. 72.10).
- MR imaging with contrast-enhanced studies better depicts the soft tissue changes and small infected fluid collections.
- In complex cases, radionuclide bone scans or labeled WBC scans may help, especially in follow-up studies to diagnose persistent active or recurrent disease.

Keratosis Obturans (KO)

KO is a rare EAC lesion that mimics otitis externa or EAC cholesteatoma. This is due to accumulation of keratin in the EAC, especially the bony canal resulting in widening and remodeling with thickening of the TM. The patients present with a clinical history of severe ear pain and conductive hearing loss; this is common in young patients, and bilateral in up to 50% of cases. It is known to be associated with other skin diseases, bronchiectasis, and sinusitis. The pathology is felt to be related skin debris causing keratin accumulation and subsequent obstruction resulting in the term keratosis obturans (Fig. 72.11).

EAC soft tissue with widening of bony canal but no bony erosions suggest KO and this helps to separate this entity from EAC cholesteatoma or carcinoma.

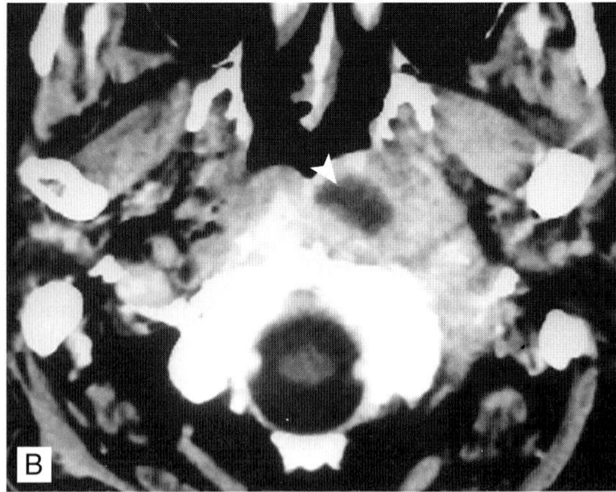

Figure 72.10 (A and B) Necrotizing otitis externa leading to skull base osteomyelitis: Axial HRCT, *left side*, showing erosion of external ear walls (*long arrow*), with soft tissue along the skull base eroding the clival cortex (*short arrows*); CT with contrast show abscess (*arrowhead*) skull base level with extensive surrounding inflammatory changes.

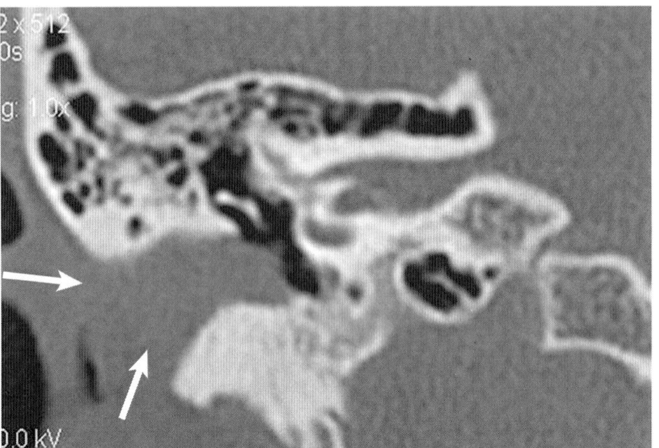

Figure 72.11 Keratosis obturans. Coronal HRCT, *right side*. Soft tissue filling (*arrow*) the external ear bony canal with mild expansion but no erosion or destruction.

EAC Cholesteatoma

EAC cholesteatoma is a chronic disease and usually presents with otorrhoea and dull aching pain. It appears as a whitish pearly mass on clinical examination and is characterized by the presence of keratinized stratified squamous epithelium on pathology.

Imaging is primarily to assess the extent of disease, the presence of bone erosion, and extension into the middle ear. HRCT demonstrates soft tissue mass coursing erosion of bony walls of the EAC. Similar imaging findings are also seen in necrotizing otitis externa and malignancy and need histology and microbiological examinations for optimal diagnosis.

Exostosis (Surfer's Ear/Coldwater Ear)

Exostosis is an osseous overgrowth from the medial aspect of the EAC resulting in the formation of sessile bony masses. Prolonged exposure to cold wind and water in swimmers and surfers, and long-standing chronic exposure to irritants may lead to exostosis.

CT demonstrates bony overgrowth having the same density as adjacent bone in the medial aspect of the EAC. It is usually bilateral (Fig. 72.12) but can be asymmetric with no invasive features and erosion. Imaging evaluation should include size, location, the status of the middle, and the EAC medial to the exostosis.

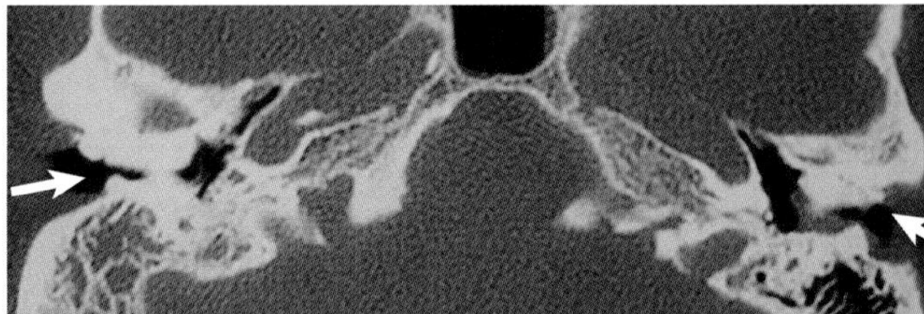

Figure 72.12 Surfer's ear. Axial HRCT. Bilateral EAC bony wall asymmetric thickening (*arrows*) and narrowing of the lumen. Density similar to the surrounding cortical bone.

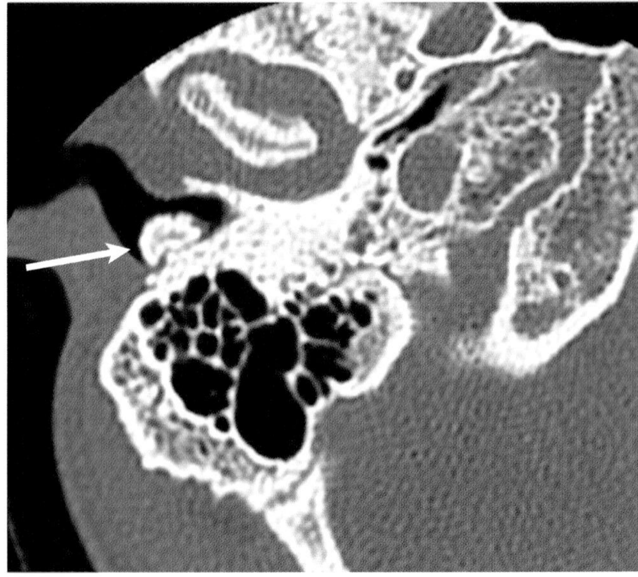

Figure 72.13 Osteoma. Axial HRCT. Nodular bony projection from posterior wall of EAC, *right side* (*arrow*).

Osteoma

Osteoma is a solitary, unilateral, pedunculated osseous growth from the outer bony canal, usually at the bony cartilaginous junction. These are generally asymptomatic, incidentally detected, and infrequently cause pain, conductive hearing loss, and secondary infection.

On CT, they appear as unilateral pedunculated osseous lesions with mature bone, located in the outer bony canal and lack invasive features (Fig. 72.13).

EAC Carcinoma

Squamous cell carcinoma (SCCA) is the most common histological subtype, followed by basal cell carcinoma, adenoid cystic carcinoma, adenoid carcinoma, and melanoma.

Both CT and MR imaging with contrast are needed to assess the extent of disease and the presence of skull base erosion. CT findings are nonspecific and demonstrate a soft tissue mass with heterogeneous enhancement. SCCA can spread along the periosteum, can also extend anteriorly into the parotid gland through the fissures of Santorini at the osteocartilaginous junction, to the TMJ through the foramen of Huschke and posteriorly eroding into the mastoid. The imaging report should also specifically comment on the presence of middle ear involvement, mastoid air cells, extension into the inner ear, and the presence of intracranial extension.

The presence of adjacent invasion and cervical lymphadenopathy favors EAC carcinoma over NOE, and histopathology is conclusive.

Trauma

EAC trauma is often associated with facial bone fractures causing posterior displacement of the mandibular condyle, leading to tympanic bone fractures, TMJ dislocation, and condylar fractures. CT delineates the fracture of the tympanic bone with or without displacement and rarely air pockets in the TMJ. It is necessary to highlight the presence of fractures of the tympanic bone due to increased risk of acquired EAC atresia due to delayed diagnosis and management.

EAC Atresia

The first branchial arch cartilage anlage forms the head and body of malleus, short process of incus, tensor tympani; the second branchial arch cartilage anlage forms manubrium of malleus, body and long process of incus, stapes (except footplate) and stapedius. EAC atresia occurs in 1 in 10,000 to 20,000 live births and can be bilateral in up to 30% of cases; this anomaly can either be unilateral or bilateral and partial.

HRCT is the investigation of choice and helps assess the entire temporal bone (Figs. 72.14 and 72.15).

The CT findings include dysplastic or malformed pinna (microtia—best seen on 3-D images), stenosis or atresia, bony bar or bony plate separating the skin and the stenotic area from the middle ear cavity, narrow middle ear cavity, decreased

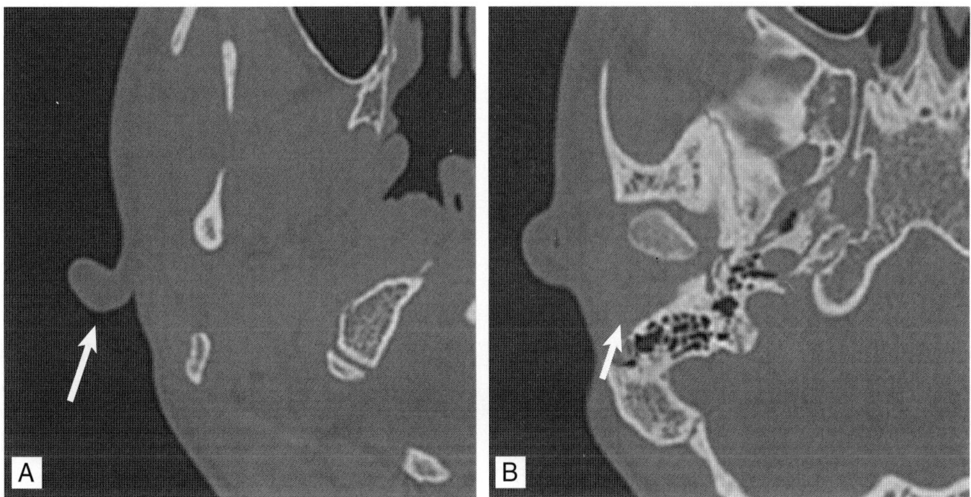

Figure 72.14 (A and B) Developmental malformation of external ear and middle ear. Axial HRCT. Right temporal bone. Hypoplastic and malformed pinna—microtia (*long arrow*); absent EAC with soft tissue filling the expected location (*short arrow*).

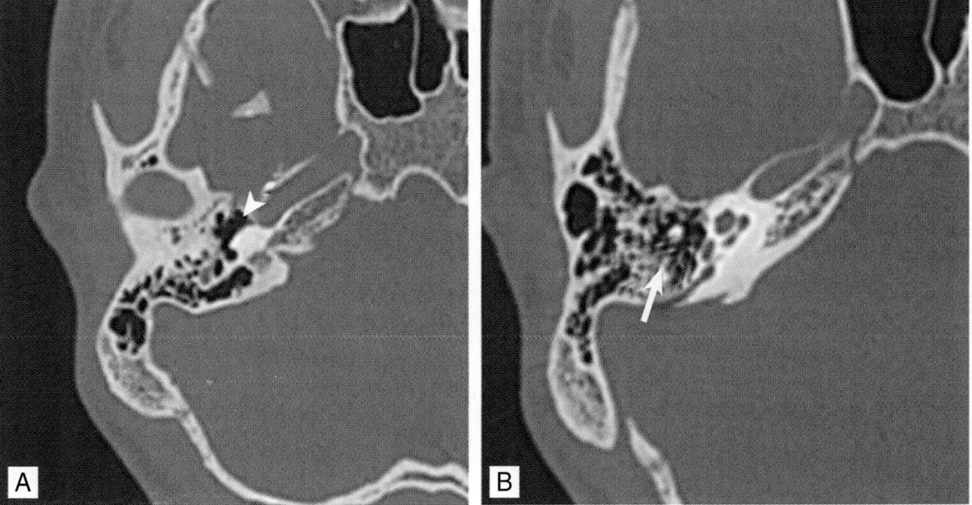

Figure 72.15 (A and B) Developmental malformation of external ear and middle ear (axial HRCT—same patient as Fig. 72.14): small middle ear cavity (*arrowhead*). Note the malformed and fused ossicles (*short arrow*).

or absent mastoid pneumatization, more anterior course of mastoid segment of facial nerve and malformed ossicles.

The extent of ossicular involvement is variable, ranging from near-normal ossicles to partial or complete ossicular dysplasia with the asymmetric fusion of the ossicles and with the adjacent bone.

The ossicular findings predominantly involve malleus and incus as they share the same embryologic origin. Rarely, the ossicles show abnormal rotation or complete aplasia. The inner ear is usually normal as it develops from the otic capsule.

Other important associated findings include congenital cholesteatoma and a superimposed infectious or inflammatory process.

EAC malformations are associated with anomalous course of the facial nerve. Thus, the imaging report should specifically comment on the course of tympanic and descending segments low facial nerve. This affect the surgical approach if the patient is being considered for meatoplasty.

Pearls and Pitfalls in EAC Imaging

External ear disease is often diagnosed clinically and treated without imaging, Soft tissue mass in the external ear with bone erosion and inflammatory changes in an immunosuppressed individual should raise concern for necrotizing otitis externa. Soft tissue mass in the external ear when associated with cervical lymphadenopathy raises the possibility of malignancy, although recurrent infections may be associated with reactive lymphadenopathy, EAC soft tissue mass with the widening of the bony canal is a clue to KO. In microtia evaluation, the extent of auricular dysplasia is proportional to middle ear anomalies.

Middle Ear and Mastoid Pathologies

The middle ear disease may clinically manifest with ear discharge, hearing loss, pain, tinnitus, and vertigo. HRCT of the temporal bone is the technique of choice for evaluating the extent of involvement of the middle ear and adjacent structures. MR imaging is a problem-solving tool, primarily the non-echo planar diffusion weighted imaging (non-EPI DWI) technique and post-contrast imaging, are reserved for specific indications [3].

Systematic evaluation of HRCT in temporal bone includes assessing the middle ear in both axial and coronal planes. In addition, coronal and sagittal oblique planes are essential for evaluating specific structures, particularly the tegmen tympani and arcuate eminence. A differential diagnosis of soft tissue attenuating lesions within the middle ear and its differentiation based on approach is useful (see Table 72.2).

Acute Otitis/Middle Ear Effusions (Serous Otitis/Glue Ear)

Otitis media and otomastoiditis are among the most common childhood infections, closely associated with repeated respiratory infections and eustachian tube dysfunction. Acute otitis typically presents with ear pain as the primary symptom; other clinical manifestations include ear discharge through the TM defect, headache, hearing loss, and fever. Clinical examination reveals bulging TM with fluid or pus on otoscopy [4].

Isolated middle ear effusions are often seen as incidental findings on CT and MR imaging, especially in children. They should not be misdiagnosed as otitis media (infection/inflammation) unless symptomatic, as effusions lack clinical evidence of inflammation in 80–90% of cases.

However, in elderly individuals with recurrent middle ear and unilateral mastoid opacification should alert the radiologist to assess the nasopharynx for possible mass lesion obstructing the eustachian tube.

Acute otitis is typically seen in children less than 5 years of age and usually due to eustachian tube dysfunction from enlarged adenoids and is often caused by Streptococcus and Haemophilus.

The role of imaging is limited in acute otitis as it is primarily a clinical diagnosis. CT of the temporal bone demonstrates soft tissue or fluid attenuation in the middle ear with or without extension into the mastoid air cells and lacks ossicular erosion. Acute otitis is generally treated with a tympanostomy tube and shows an adequate response to antibiotic therapy.

In adhesive otitis, the retracted TM is partly or entirely adherent to the medial wall of the middle ear. Although TM perforation is a clinical diagnosis, CT may demonstrate a defect in the TM.

TABLE 72.2 Soft Tissue Density Lesions of the Middle Ear Based on Location

Epitympanum—cholesteatoma, otitis
Mesotympanum—cholesteatoma, otitis, facial nerve schwannoma, glomus tympanicum
Hypotympanum—fluid, inflammatory tissue, dehiscent jugular bulb, aberrant course of the internal carotid artery

Acute Mastoiditis

Acute mastoiditis presents with pain, ear discharge, retroauricular swelling, and associated inflammatory changes in a patient with recent otitis. It is often a complication of otitis media and resolves with antibiotic therapy. Inadequate or delayed antibiotic therapy may result in complications.

Imaging is mainly performed to exclude intratemporal complications, including coalescent mastoiditis, subperiosteal abscess, petrous apicitis, facial nerve palsy, and rarely intracranial complications, including dural venous sinus thrombosis, meningitis, empyema, and cerebral abscess.

Coalescent mastoiditis is due to the breakdown of intervening septae within the mastoid air cells that leads to the formation of small or large cavity (Fig. 72.16). It may also be associated with erosion of the sigmoid plate or the lateral mastoid cortex, resulting in a subperiosteal abscess. CT shows erosion of external mastoid wall with a purulent collection extending laterally into the postauricular region, extending to the external ear, zygomatic bone, inferiorly to involve the sternomastoid or trapezius muscles (Bezold's abscess).

Petrous apicitis is a rare complication of otomastoiditis which occurs due to the extension of mastoid disease into the pneumatized petrous apex. It can present with a classic triad of abducens nerve palsy, deep facial pain, and ipsilateral ear discharge (Gradenigo syndrome). The deep facial pain is due to inflammation of meningeal layers, related to Gasserian ganglion (trigeminal nerve), located adjacent to the petrous apex.

Intracranial complications associated with mastoid inflammation include extradural abscess or subdural empyema formation around the sigmoid sinus, venous sinus thrombosis (Fig. 72.17), cerebritis, and cerebral abscess.

Rare involvement of the ICA may result in hemiplegia or Horner's syndrome. MR imaging may demonstrate arterial spasm or enhancement along the arterial walls suggesting arteritis.

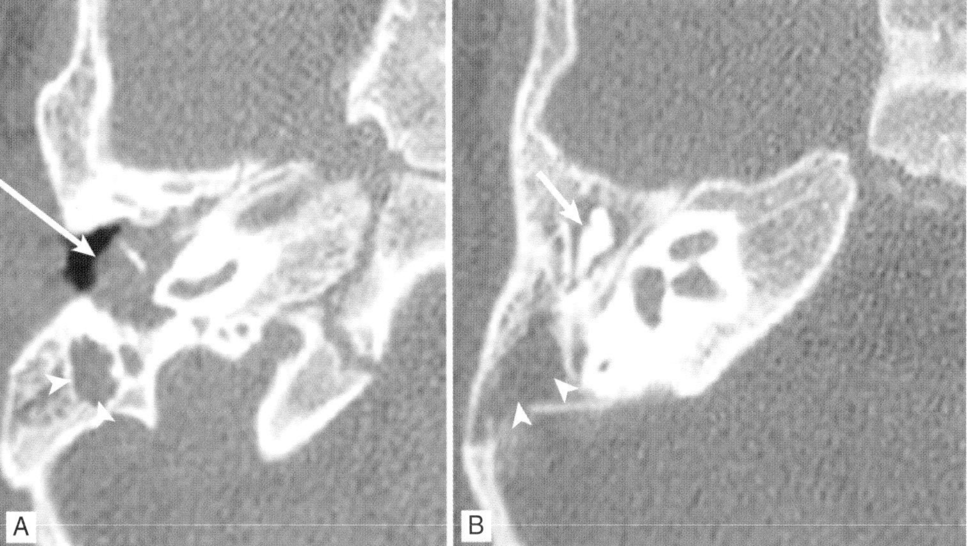

Figure 72.16 (A and B) Otitis and mastoiditis. Axial HRCT, *right side*. Soft tissue filling the middle ear with bulging of tympanic membrane (*long arrow*). Ossicular chain is intact (*short arrow*). Mastoid cells show coalescence, loss of septation, and cavity filled with soft tissue (*arrowheads*).

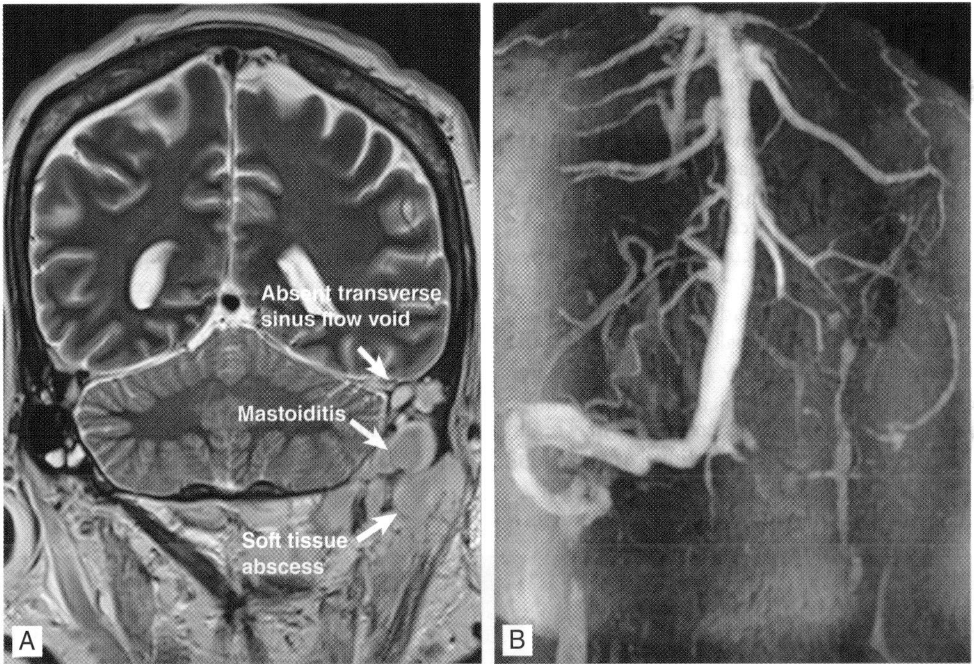

Figure 72.17 (A and B) Coronal T2W MRI and corresponding MR venogram (MRV). Abnormal high signal at left middle ear and mastoid region with thrombosis of left sigmoid sinus superiorly and soft tissue abscess at inferior aspect. MRV shows no flow signal at left sigmoid and transverse sinuses—consistent with venous sinus thrombosis.

Chronic Otitis and Mastoiditis

Chronic suppurative otitis media refers to symptoms of more than 6–12 weeks with ear discharge through a TM perforation. It is commonly associated with mastoiditis and is encountered in both children and adults. Chronic otitis presents with ear discharge, hearing loss, and feeling of pressure sensation within the ear along with occasional vertigo and tinnitus.

HRCT of the temporal bone is the imaging technique of choice to assess the appearances and complications associated with chronic otomastoiditis. These include

- fluid/soft tissue attenuation in the middle ear;
- thickening/ defect or retraction of the TM;
- soft tissue/air-fluid levels within the middle ear;
- extension of inflammatory changes in the attic, antrum, and mastoid air cells;
- deossification of ossicular density, commonly involving the long and lenticular process of incus;
- bone erosions are rare, seen in less than 10%—tegmen, sinus plate, and bony labyrinth can be affected with intracranial extension of disease.

Chronic otitis is often associated with mastoiditis and may lead to sclerosis.

Long-standing inflammation may be complicated by granulation tissue and cholesteatoma formation. Cholesteatoma is often associated with scutum erosion, bony or

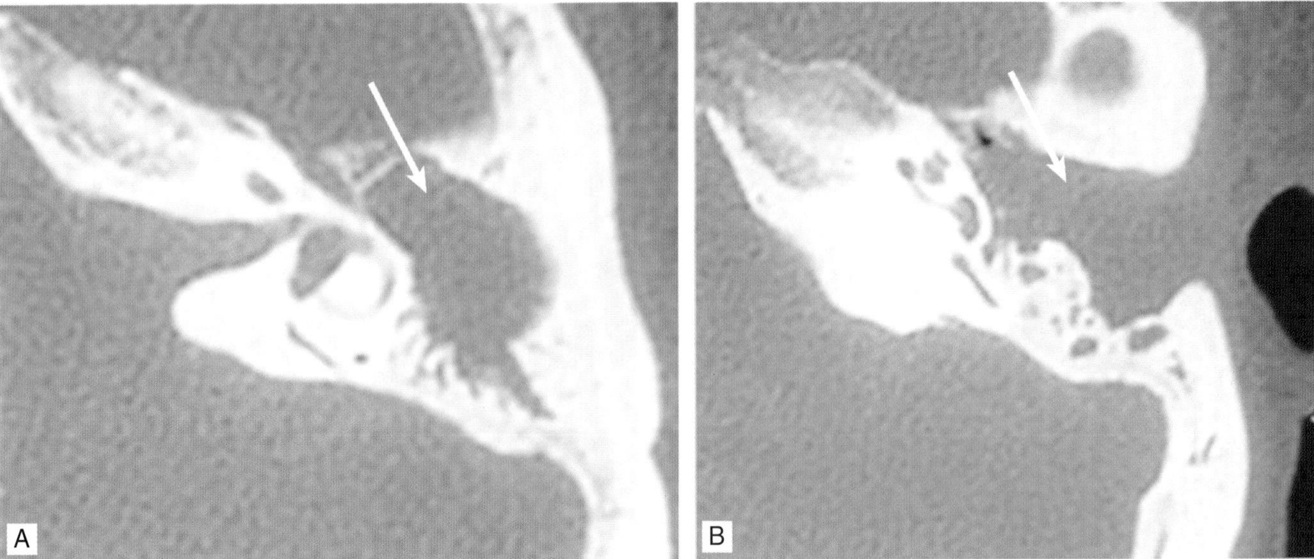

Figure 72.22 (A and B) Cholesterol granuloma. Axial HRCT, *left side*. Soft tissue filling the mastoid post surgical cavity (*arrow*). Infection, granulation, cholesteatoma can mimic this appearance (see Fig. 72.23).

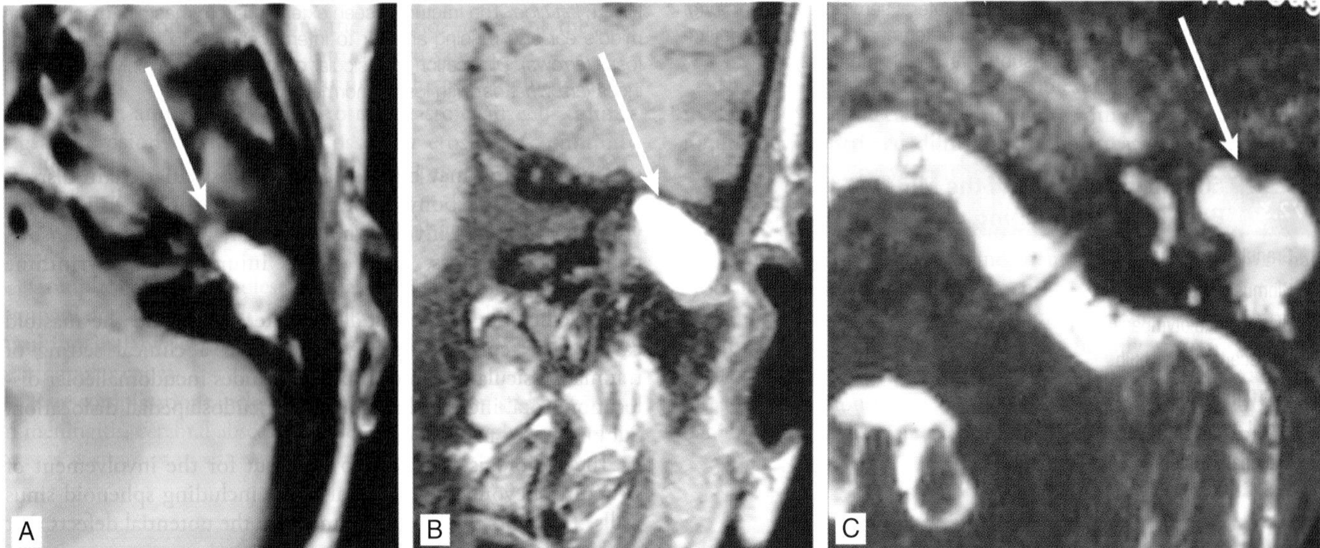

Figure 72.23 (A–C) Cholesterol granuloma (CG). Same patient as Fig. 72.22. Axial and coronal T1 and axial T2W images show high signal tissue filling (*arrows*) the cavity—typical of CG.

pulsatile tinnitus, including vascular tumor, an arteriovenous malformation, and congenital or acquired vascular abnormalities. Systematic evaluation is necessary to diagnose glomus tumors. See Table 72.3 for list of contrast enhancing lesions at middle ear.

Glomus tympanicum appears as a small soft-tissue mass overlying the cochlear promontory with avid enhancement, particularly on post-contrast T1W images. They lack bony erosion with a preserved tympanic cavity and intact ossicular chain (Fig. 72.24).

Glomus jugulo-tympanicum appears as an infiltrative mass and is an extension of glomus tumor arising in jugular fossa into the hypotympanum and middle ear cavity due to erosion of the jugular plate and floor of middle ear (Fig. 72.24). The imaging findings are similar to glomus jugulare and manifest as avid enhancing infiltrating lesion mass with blood products and flow voids (salt and pepper appearance on MR images). CT and MR imaging are necessary to delineate the extent and explore synchronous lesions in the neck and skull base (Fig. 72.25).

Facial Nerve Schwannoma

Schwannomas arising from the facial nerve are rare and typically occur in the third to fourth decade. They are generally asymptomatic and infrequently present with facial palsy, hemifacial spasm, and sensorineural hearing loss. Facial schwannomas can be isolated or associated with neurofibromatosis.

On HRCT (Fig. 72.26), there is smooth widening of the bony facial nerve canal by the thickened facial nerve; on MRI, the lesion show, enhancing tubular mass on fat saturated T1W imaging.

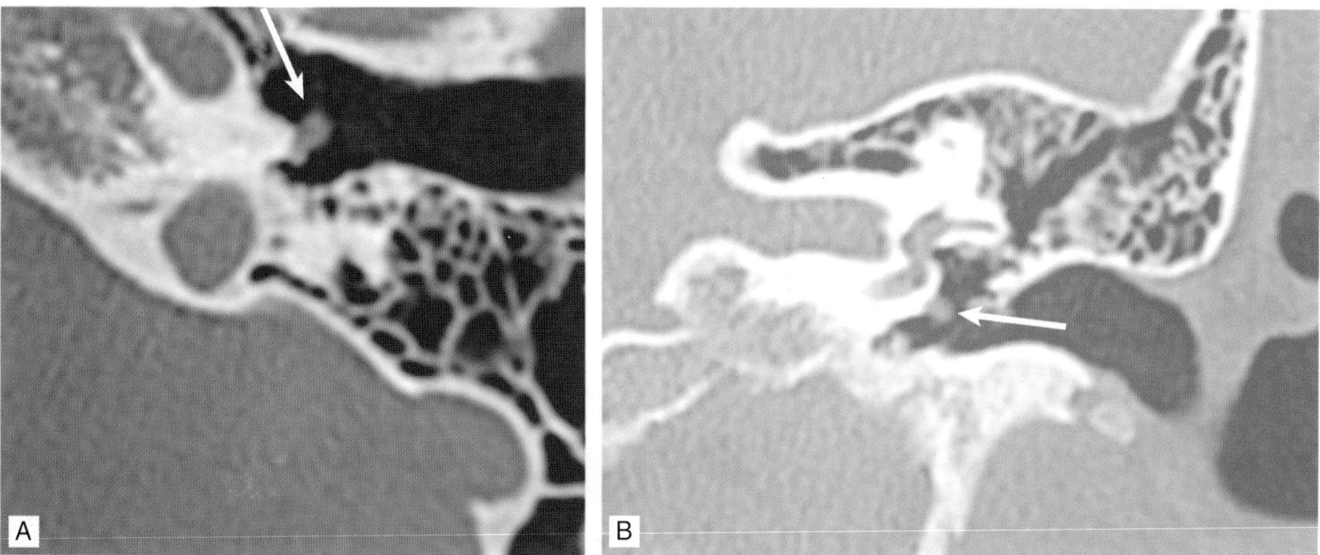

Figure 72.24 (A and B) Glomus tympanicum. Axial and Coronal HRCT, *left side*. Small nodular soft tissue density overlying cochlear promontory (*arrow*). (Courtesy: Dr B Sivasubramanian, Coimbatore.)

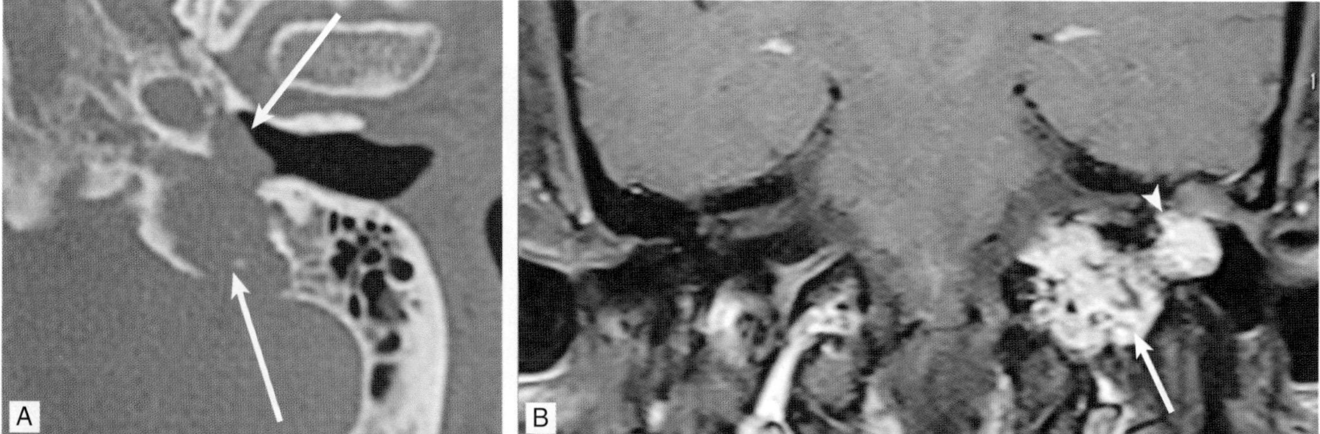

Figure 72.25 (A and B) Glomus jugulotympanicum. (A) Axial HRCT, *left side*. Soft tissue eroding the jugular fossa margins, few tiny bony fragments at margins and extending to hypo/mesotympanum (*long arrows*); (B) coronal T1W MRI with contrast (different patient)—enhancing mass lesion at left jugular fossa region with flow void areas (pepper) infiltrating into the left middle ear region.

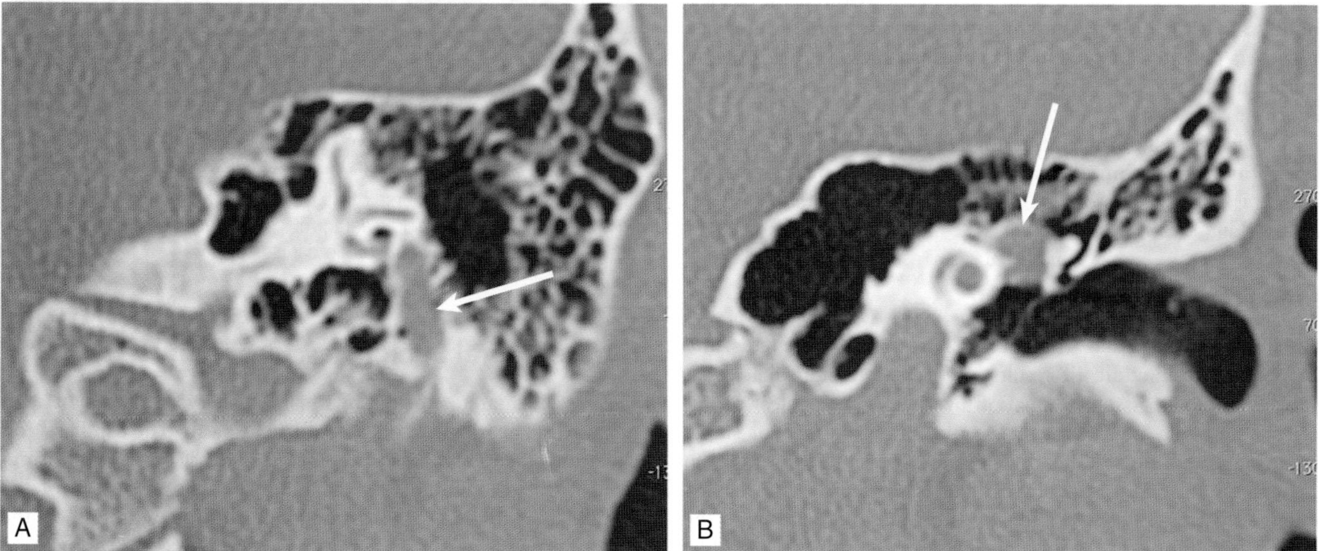

Figure 72.26 (A and B) Facial nerve schwannoma. Coronal HRCT, *left side*. Smooth expansion of the mastoid and tympanic facial nerve canal segments (*arrows*). (Courtesy: Dr B Sivasubramanian, Coimbatore.)

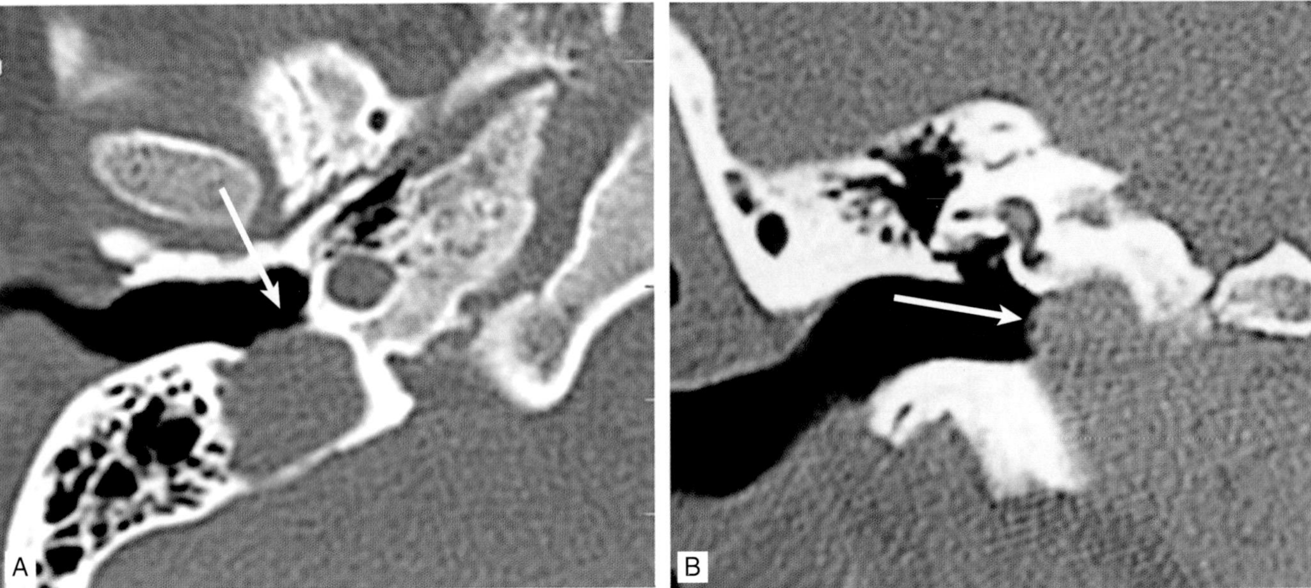

Figure 72.27 Dehiscent jugular bulb. Axial and coronal HRCT, *right side*. There is dehiscence of bony plate separating the jugular bulb bulging into middle ear (*arrows*).

Dehiscent Jugular Bulb (Fig. 72.27)

Jugular bulb dehiscence is the most common vascular anomaly related to the middle ear and occurs due to loss of cortical covering over the jugular bulb. As a result, the jugular vein bulges into the hypotympanum and appears as a bluish retro tympanic mass on otoscopy. They are often associated with high riding jugular bulb and may present with pulsatile tinnitus. A jugular bulb is considered "high riding" when the jugular dome extends above the floor of the internal auditory canal.

Aberrant ICA

This is a developmental vascular malformation, in which the ICA is coursing through the middle ear cavity. The inferior tympanic canaliculus, which enlarges to accommodate the aberrant course of ICA, resembles the carotid canal in both size and location. The aberrant ICA may be dehiscent or may be covered by cortical bone so that the otoscopic examination can sometime be normal; however, patient can present with reddish mass with history of pulsatile tinnitus. Vertical part of carotid canal is absent due to the aberrant course.

On HRCT abnormal posterior course of the ICA is noted, projecting into the middle ear cavity; the caliber of the aberrant course is narrow. This can be associated with persistent stapedial artery (Fig. 72.28).

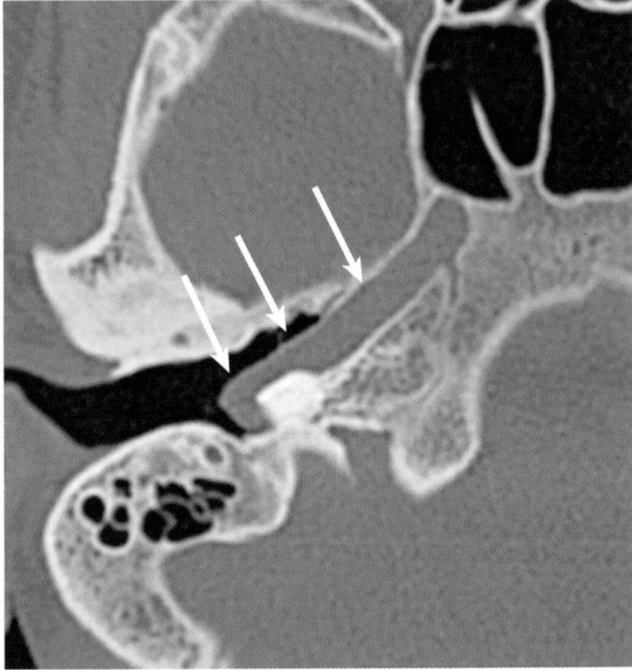

Figure 72.28 Aberrant course of internal carotid artery (ICA). Axial HRCT, *right side*. ICA entering middle ear forming a lateral bulge and narrow caliber before reaching the right carotid canal.

Persistent Stapedial Artery

An embryonic stapedial artery normally regresses in the fetus, and its persistence in adult life results in a persistent stapedial artery. It appears as soft tissue attenuation overlying the cochlear promontory and may pass through the obturator foramen of stapes resulting in conductive hearing loss and pulsatile tinnitus. On HRCT, the anterior tympanic segment of the facial nerve may be enlarged with a tiny vessel coursing from the oval window to the cochlear promontory. As the stapedial artery supplies the middle meningeal artery, the foramen spinosum that normally contains the middle meningeal artery is either hypoplastic or absent.

Intratemporal Benign Vascular Tumors

Venous vascular malformations of facial nerve can present with facial palsy, hearing loss, and hemifacial spasm. The capillary and cavernous hemangiomas may coexist with vascular malformations on histology. On CT, they appear as an expansion of the geniculate ganglion or proximal labyrinthine segment of the facial nerve with a honeycomb-like appearance and bony spicules. They demonstrate avid enhancement on post-contrast T1W images.

TABLE 72.4 Petrous Apex Lesions

Petrous Apex Lesions
Asymmetric pneumatization/retained fluid (variant)
Asymmetric signal (aeration and fatty marrow (variant)
Petrous apicitis (Gradenigo syndrome)
Mucocele
Cholesterol granuloma
Trigeminal nerve tumors (Schwannoma/perineural spread)
Chondrosarcoma
Chordoma
Metastases

Malignant Tumors of the Middle Ear

SCCA, metastasis, perineural spread of malignancy along the facial nerve, and endolymphatic sac tumor may involve the middle ear. Soft tissue mass with bone and ossicular chain destruction should raise the possibility of malignancy, including SCCA and metastasis. Smooth widening and enhancement of the facial nerve canal, raise concern for perineural spread (PN) of malignancy. This is often seen with adenoid cystic and squamous cell carcinomas and occasionally with melanoma and lymphoma.

In children, Langerhans cell histiocytosis can present as bone erosive lesion with soft tissue component affecting middle/external ear structures.

Lesions Involving the Petrous Apex

Petrous apex lesions are often symptomatic due to proximity to cranial nerves (fifth and sixth cranial nerves), cavernous sinus, and ICA. The normal variations of petrous apex due to asymmetric pneumatization, fluid or bone marrow may be mistaken for pathologies. Common variants and pathologies affecting petrous apex is described in Table 72.4.

Inner Ear Pathologies

Clinical Considerations

Sensorineural hearing loss is a key clinical feature of inner ear disease. In addition, tinnitus, dizziness, and headache can also be presenting symptoms. CT and MR imaging are complementary in the imaging of inner ear disease. Inner ear interpretation can be challenging even for the experienced radiologists.

Congenital Anomalies of the Inner Ear

Congenital inner ear anomalies are one of the crucial causes of sensorineural hearing loss in children. The etiologies of inner ear anomalies include congenital infections (TORCH (T)oxoplasmosis, (O)ther Agents, (R)ubella (C)ytomegalovirus, and (H)erpes Simplex), fetal isotretinoin or thalidomide exposure, and various syndromic and nonsyndromic genetic causes, including Alport, Pendred, Waardenburg, CHARGE coloboma, heart defects, atresia of choanae, retardation of growth, genital and ear abnormalities, and branchio-oto-renal syndromes. Recent studies suggest that otic capsule develop between the 3rd and 25th week of gestation. The severity of inner ear malformations ranges from mild dysplasias to complete labyrinthine aplasia; this depends on the developmental stage at which the embryogenic insult occurs. The early developmental insult results in complete labyrinthine aplasia, whereas delayed insult at 20 weeks results in semicircular canal abnormalities.

TABLE 72.5 Imaging Findings in Congenital Malformations of the Inner Ear

Malformation	Imaging findings
Complete labyrinthine aplasia	■ Complete absence of cochlea, vestibule and semicircular canals. ■ Facial nerve, if present, runs an aberrant course.
Rudimentary otocyst	Small rounded millimetric cyst in place of cochlea and vestibule.
Cochlear aplasia	Lack of cochlear development. There are two subtypes: ■ Cochlear aplasia with dilated vestibule, Dilated vestibular structures are posterolateral to the internal auditory canal. ■ Cochlear aplasia with normal labyrinth.
Common cavity	■ Single rounded cavity representing cochlea and vestibule. ■ Internal auditory canal opens in the center of common cavity.
Cochlear hypoplasia	Four different subtypes: ■ Defective internal architecture—type 1 and 2. ■ Relative preserved internal architecture—type 3 and 4.
Incomplete partition of cochlea	Three different subtypes: ■ Incomplete partition type I—figure of eight appearance. ■ Incomplete partition type 2—fusion of apical and middle turns of cochlea. Usually associated dilated vestibule and enlarged vestibular aqueduct. ■ Incomplete partition type 3—lack of cochlear modiolus with dilated cochlea, enlarged internal auditory canal, and preserved external contour of cochlea.
Enlarged vestibular aqueduct	■ Dilated vestibular aqueduct >1.5 mm in mid-segment. ■ Usually associated with dilated vestibule with small bony island.
Cochlear aperture anomalies	■ Cochlear aperture hypoplasia—cochlear aperture of <1.4 mm ■ Cochlear aperture aplasia—absent cochlear aperture, replaced by bone. Usually associated with small internal auditory canal and vestibulocochlear nerve aplasia or hypoplasia

The most recent classification scheme of inner ear malformations by Sennaroglu et al. [6] is described in Table 72.5.

Cochleovestibular Malformations

Complete labyrinthine aplasia (Michel deformity), the most severe and extremely rare malformation, is characterized by the complete absence of the labyrinthine structures.

Rudimentary otocyst is characterized by a tiny, few millimeter-sized, oval or round cavity in the otic capsule with an absent internal auditory canal.

Cochlear aplasia occurs due to a lack of cochlear development resulting in the absence of cochlea and anterior displaced

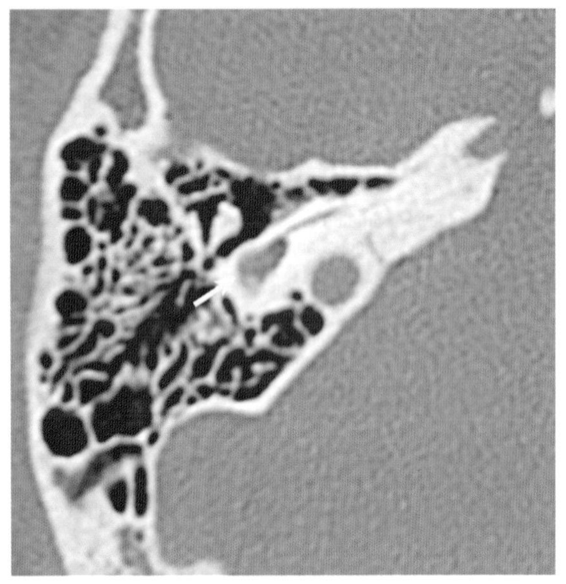

Figure 72.29 Cochlear aplasia with dilated vestibule. Right temporal bone HRCT image shows absent cochlea with dilated vestibule.

labyrinthine segment of the facial nerve with normal or dilated vestibule (Fig. 72.29).

The common cavity malformation manifests as a cystic cavity with no identifiable internal architecture and a lack of cochlear and vestibular differentiation.

Cystic cochleovestibular malformation (Type I incomplete partition—Fig. 72.30) presents as a cystic cochlea with aplasia or hypoplasia of the modiolus and interscalar septum along with dilated vestibule, forming the characteristic "figure of eight appearance."

Type II incomplete partition, most commonly encountered cochlear malformation (>50%), occurs due to the fusion of middle and apical turns forming a cystic apex due to defect in the osseous spiral lamina and the apical interscalar septum. Mondini deformity is characterized by the triad of the cystic apex, dilated vestibule, and an enlarged vestibular aqueduct (Fig. 72.31).

Type III incomplete partition (X-linked gusher) has a partial interscalar septum with the lack of normal modiolus resulting in direct communication between a bulbous internal auditory canal and dilated cochlea.

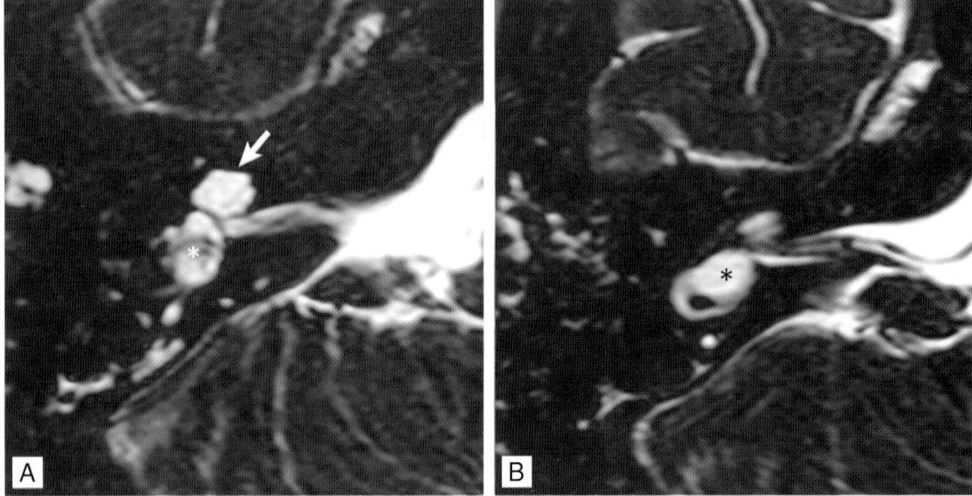

Figure 72.30 (A and B) Incomplete malformation type I—right temporal bone CISS images show malformed cochlea (*arrow* in A) and dilated vestibule (*asterisks* in A and B) with characteristic figure of 8 appearance.

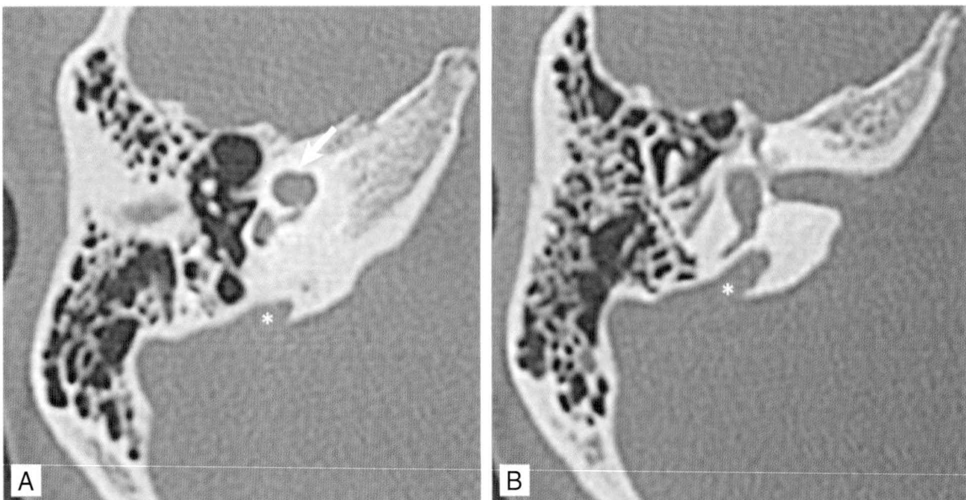

Figure 72.31 (A and B) Incomplete malformation type II—right temporal bone CT images show fusion of apical and mid turn of cochlea with the absence of interscalar septum (*arrow* in A) and dilated vestibular aqueduct (*asterisks* in A and B).

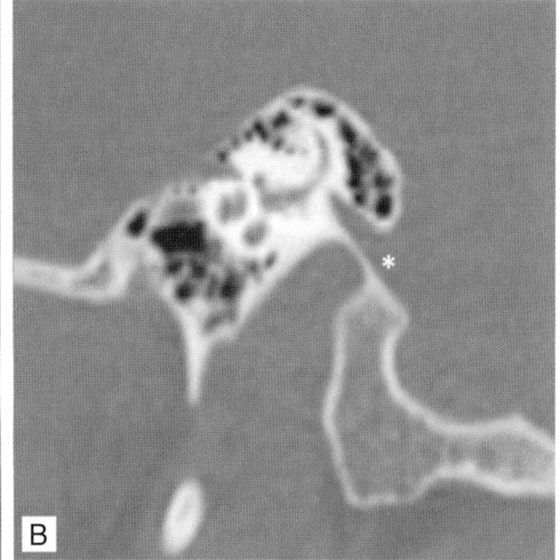

Figure 72.32 (A and B) Enlarged vestibular aqueduct—left temporal bone CT images show isolated dilated vestibular aqueduct (*asterisks* in A and B).

Vestibular Aqueduct (VA) Abnormalities

Enlarged vestibular aqueduct syndrome occurs due to vestibular aqueduct dilatation secondary to the endolymphatic duct and sac enlargement. It is one of the commonly missed diagnoses in temporal bone CT reporting.

It is a typical radiological abnormality encountered in most patients with early sensorineural hearing loss. On CT, the dilated vestibular aqueduct manifests as an enlarged VA measuring >1.5 mm in its mid-segment (Fig. 72.32). On MRI, the vestibular aqueduct is said to be dilated when the diameter is more than the ascending segment of the posterior SCC. They result in high-frequency hearing loss and can be an isolated abnormality or seen in association with cystic cochlear apex, enlarged vestibules, and abnormal semicircular canals. Pendred syndrome, CHARGE syndrome, and congenital viral infections are associated with enlarged vestibular aqueducts.

Semicircular Canal Anomalies

The semicircular canal development starts between 6 and 8 weeks of gestational age, to complete between 19 and 22 weeks. The superior semicircular canal develops initially, followed by the posterior and lateral semicircular canal. Hence, hypoplasia most commonly involves the lateral semicircular canal (Fig. 72.33). The malformed semicircular canals are often broad and short but may also be narrow. The semicircular canal dysplasia involving the vestibule and the lateral SCC presents as a broad cystic space with absent or small intervening bone island and enlarged vestibule. The lateral SCC dysplasia may be associated with cochlear malformations depending on the stage of inner ear development and embryonic arrest. Semicircular canal aplasia is often associated with CHARGE syndrome.

Superior SCC dehiscence [7] occurs due to thinning or defect of the arcuate eminence overlying the superior semicircular canal, resulting in formation of "third window" (Fig. 72.34).

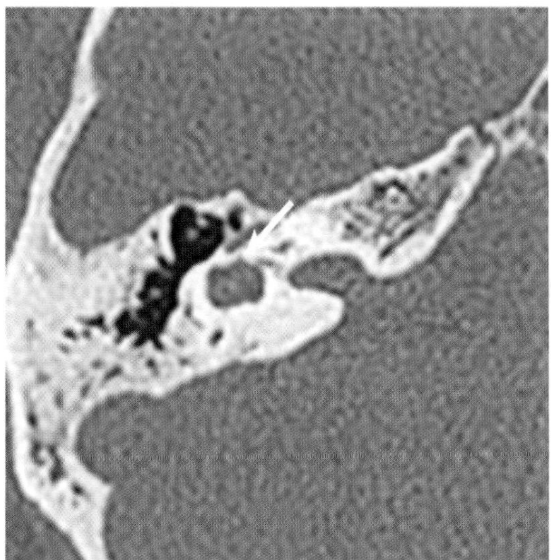

Figure 72.33 Lateral semicircular canal dysplasia—right temporal bone CT image shows fusion of vestibule and lateral semicircular canal with the absence of normal intervening bone island (*arrow*).

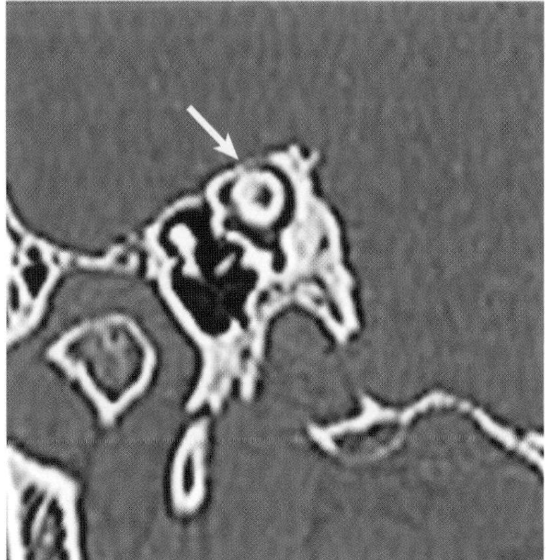

Figure 72.34 Superior semicircular canal dehiscence—right temporal bone CT image in Poschl's view shows dehiscence of the superior semicircular canal (*arrow*).

The third window abnormalities typically present with noise-induced vertigo, also called Tullio's phenomenon. Although SCC dehiscence has a genetic and syndromic association, it is also seen in the elderly, suggesting an acquired etiology. Similar dehiscence of the posterior SCC may be seen with a high-riding jugular bulb and fibrous dysplasia of the temporal bone. Surgical exploration through a middle cranial fossa approach with canal plugging is associated with long-term symptom control.

Congenital Internal Auditory Canal Anomalies

The internal auditory canal may be atretic with a nonvisualized internal auditory canal or stenotic, with a diameter of less than 2 mm. The duplication of the internal auditory canal is a rare anomaly associated with the bony septum resulting in two separate canals, the anterosuperior canal continuous with the labyrinthine segment of the facial nerve and the posteroinferior canal continuous with cochlea and the vestibule (Fig. 72.35). The duplication of the internal auditory canal is commonly isolated but rarely associated with Klippel–Feil syndrome and pontine tegmental cap dysplasia.

Cochlear Nerve Anomalies

The internal auditory canal atresia or stenosis may suggest an associated cochlear nerve anomaly and mandates a high-resolution T2W MRI for optimal cochlear nerve assessment. Various subtypes of cochlear nerve malformations are based on aplasia or hypoplasia of the nerve (Fig. 72.36) and its association with inner ear anomalies.

Genetic and Syndromic Association of Inner Ear Anomalies

Hereditary causes account for approximately 50% of congenital sensorineural hearing loss and syndromic associations. Cochlear hypoplasia and semicircular canal aplasia are seen in CHARGE syndrome. Cochlear hypoplasia is also associated with the branchio-oto-renal syndrome, Waardenburg syndrome, and Down's syndrome. The type II incomplete partition is associated with Pendred syndrome (SLC26A mutations) and type III incomplete partition with X-linked deafness (POU3F4 mutations).

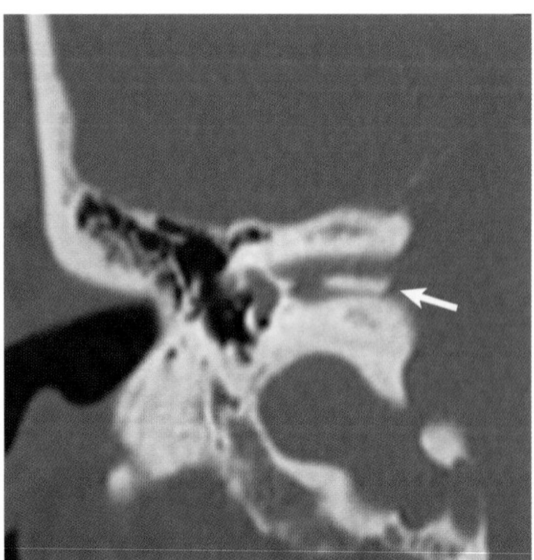

Figure 72.35 Duplication of internal auditory canal—right temporal bone CT image shows bony bar (*arrow*) separating the superior and inferior compartments of the internal auditory canal.

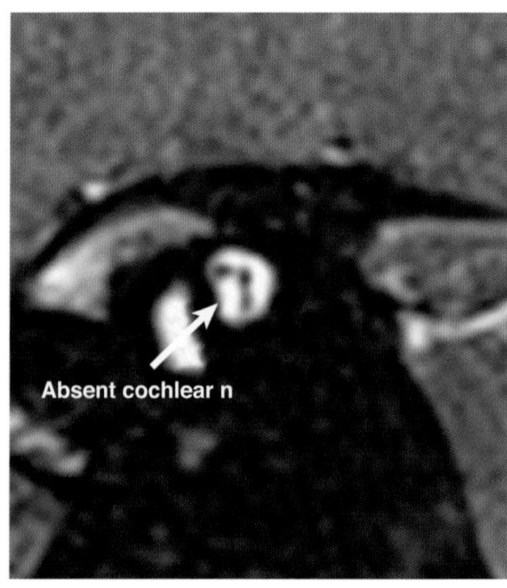

Figure 72.36 High-resolution T2 oblique sagittal view shows absence of cochlear division of VIII cranial nerve (n – nerve) at the anteroinferior compartment of IAC.

Other congenital syndromes commonly associated with the inner ear malformations include Apert syndrome, Treacher Collins syndrome, and Pierre Robin sequence.

Labyrinthine Disorders

Labyrinthitis

Labyrinthitis refers to inflammation of the inner ear involving one or more compartments of the membranous labyrinth. It is either due to inner ear infection secondary to the bacterial, fungal, viral, and protozoal invasion of labyrinthine structures or noninfective inflammation secondary to autoimmune disorders and vasculitis.

Based on the origin, it is classified into hematogenic, meningogenic, and otogenic labyrinthitis. Typically, otogenic labyrinthitis is unilateral and secondary to the spread of infections or toxins to the inner ear through the round or the oval window. Meningogenic labyrinthitis is common in the pediatric population. It is usually bilateral and occurs due to infection spread through the cochlear aqueduct and internal auditory canal.

Radiologically, labyrinthitis is classified into three stages: acute, fibrous, and osseous (labyrinthitis ossificans) stages.

- The acute phase is due to purulent infection that presents with an intense enhancement of the labyrinthine structures on post-contrast T1W images
- The intermediate fibrous stage is characterized by fibrous replacement leading to hypointense signal on T2W images with mild enhancement on post-contrast T1W images
- The late osseous stage manifests with ossific deposition in the inner ear with loss of normal bright fluid signal on T2W images and hyperdense replacement of inner ear on CT. CT allows for an optimal assessment of the location and extent of the ossification before cochlear implantation

Labyrinthitis Ossificans

Labyrinthitis ossificans also develops secondary to chronic middle and inner ear infections, temporal bone fractures, and bacterial meningitis. Fibroblastic proliferation, which eventually differentiates into osteoblasts, appears on imaging as initial fibrosis and progresses to ossific deposits in the membranous labyrinth. MR imaging with high-resolution T2W and post-contrast T1W sequences is optimal for diagnosing labyrinthitis in the initial stages. In comparison, the high-resolution CT is best for evaluating the extent and location of osseous replacement and dense sclerosis of labyrinthine structures later in the disease process (Fig. 72.37).

The salient imaging findings include cochlear stenosis, fibrous and ossific deposition in the cochlea. Rarely, labyrinthitis ossificans is also associated with obliteration of semicircular canals. Round window stenosis secondary to osseous deposits may lead to difficult and suboptimal cochlear implant placement.

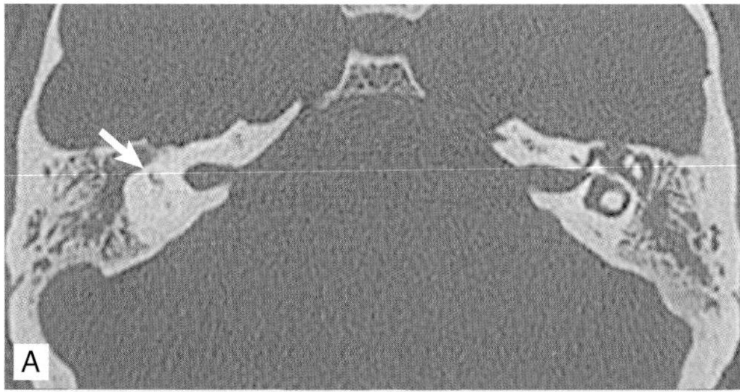

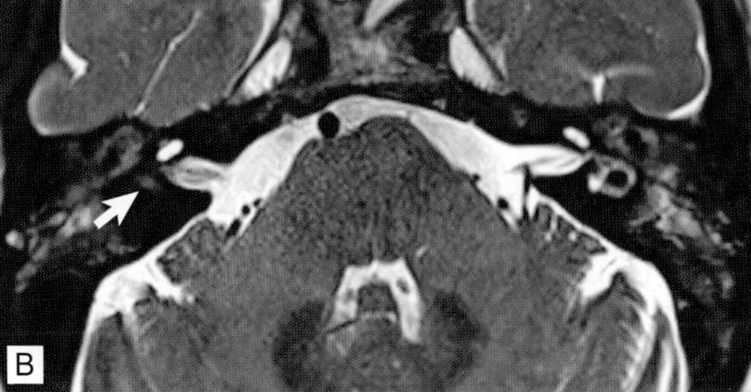

Figure 72.37 (A and B) Labyrinthitis ossificans—CT and MR images of the temporal bone shows dense sclerosis and osseous replacement of the vestibule (*arrow* in A) on CT with loss of normal fluid signal (*arrow* in B) on CISS images.

Otosclerosis (Otospongiosis)

Otosclerosis is autosomal dominant osteodystrophy that occurs due to spongy vascular bone replacing the normal dense endochondral bone. It commonly occurs in the second to fourth decades of life, usually bilateral (85%), and shows female preponderance.

Otosclerosis is of two types: the common fenestral and the rare retrofenestral type.

- Fenestral otosclerosis typically involves the fissula ante fenestrum (which is a small fold of connective tissue anterior to the oval window) and gradually progresses to involve the round window, oval window, and cochlear turns with late pericochlear involvement (Fig. 72.38). HRCT of the temporal bone is the imaging technique of choice that demonstrates bone rarefaction anterior to the oval window. The disease progression may lead to otosclerotic plaque formation, which may cause round window stenosis, stapes fixation, and rarely torsional subluxation of the incus. The grading of the extent and location of otosclerosis is by Symon and Fanning classification
- Retrofenestral otosclerosis is a rare subtype, typically bilateral, symmetrical, and almost always associated with the fenestral otosclerosis. It appears with a typical hypodense pericochlear hypodense double ring sign (aka fourth ring of valvassori). MR imaging may reveal hypointense signal on T1W with mild-to-moderate enhancement on post-contrast T1W images

The differential diagnoses include osteogenesis imperfecta, and rarely fibrous dysplasia, and Paget's disease.

Meniere's Disease

Meniere's disease is a clinical entity presenting with spontaneous episodes of vertigo, sensorineural hearing loss, and tinnitus that presents adults with a peak incidence in the fourth to fifth decade. Endolymphatic hydrops (Eh) occurs due to the distension of endolymphatic compartments causing secondary compression of perilymphatic structures. This can be demonstrated by high resolution MRI imaging, mainly using 3T with delayed post IV Gadolinium

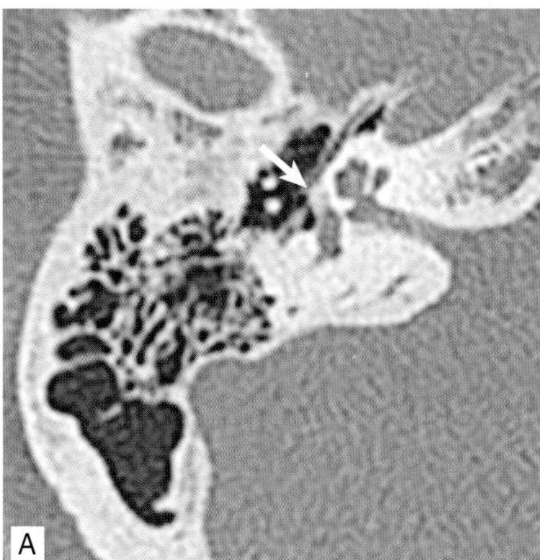

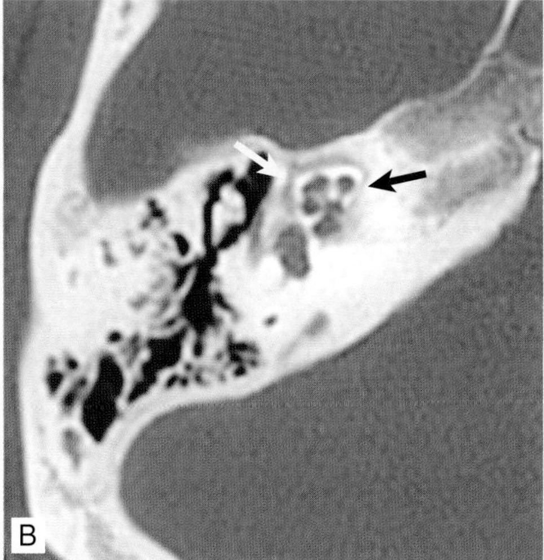

Figure 72.38 (A and B) Otosclerosis (otospongiosis). Fenestral otosclerosis—right temporal bone CT shows bone rarefaction with hypodensity in right fissula ante fenestrum (*arrow* in A). Retrofenestral otosclerosis—right temporal bone CT shows pericochlear hypodense ring sign (*arrow* in B).

(Gd) contrast FLAIR (fluid attenuated inversion recovery) sequence; post-contrast enhancement is seen best on 4 hour delayed imaging at the perilymphatic space. This enhanced space is compressed or obliterated in Eh. On HRCT, absent visualization of vestibular aqueduct predicts hydrops in more than 90% of subjects. Similarly, the cochlear hydrops shows dilatation of the scala media with partial or complete obliteration of the scala vestibuli.

Intralabyrinthine Schwannomas

Schwannomas typically arise from the vestibular ganglion near the fundus of the internal auditory canal and frequently extend into the cerebellopontine angle. Rarely, they may arise from the terminal ends of the eighth cranial nerve in the vestibule, cochlea, and semicircular canals. The intralabyrinthine schwannomas (Fig. 72.39) include

- intracochlear (confined to the cochlea);
- transmodiolar (cochlear origin with IAC extension through modiolus);
- intravestibular (confined to vestibule ± semicircular canals);
- transmacular (vestibular origin with IAC extension through macula cribrosa);
- vestibulocochlear (confined to vestibule and cochlea) and
- transotic (labyrinthine schwannomas with IAC and middle ear extension) subtypes.

On MR imaging, they are hypointense or replace the typical bright fluid signal on high-resolution T2W images with intense enhancement on post-contrast T1W images.

Bell's Palsy

Bell's palsy typically presents acute onset of infranuclear facial palsy, accounting for approximately 70% of facial nerve paralysis. It is likely due to reactivation of the herpes simplex infection in the geniculate ganglion resulting in the inflammatory edema and likely ischemia of the labyrinthine segment in the tight fallopian canal. MR imaging characteristically demonstrates enhancement of the canalicular and labyrinthine segments of the facial nerve (Fig. 72.40) in many patients. Similar imaging findings may be seen in Ramsay hunt syndrome (herpes zoster oticus) due to reactivation of varicella-zoster infection in the geniculate ganglion along with vesicular eruption in the external ear. Thickening and enhancement of the tympanic segment of the facial nerve raise concern for neoplastic etiology.

Any atypical presentation, including insidious onset, delayed recovery, progressive facial palsy, and recurrent Bell's palsy, necessitates further evaluation to rule out other inflammatory or neoplastic etiology along the course of the nerve.

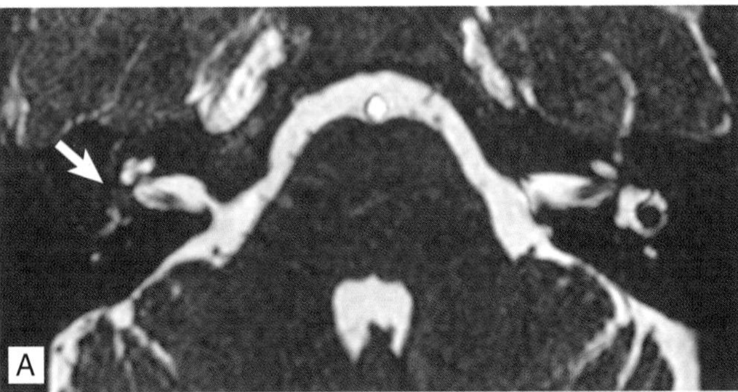

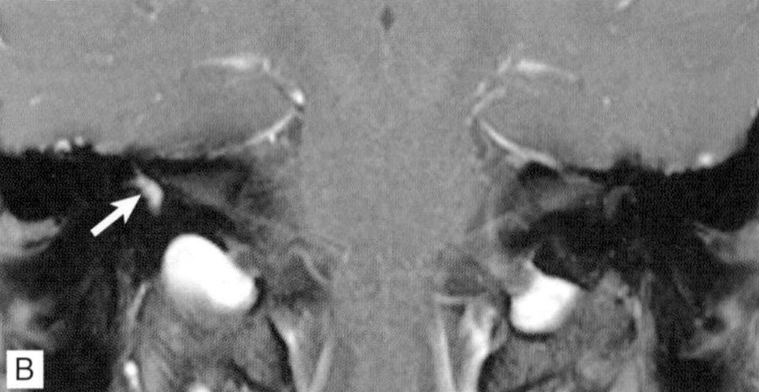

Figure 72.39 Labyrinthine schwannoma—axial CISS and coronal T1 post-contrast images of temporal bone show loss of normal fluid signal in the vestibule (*arrow* in A) and small enhancing mass in the vestibule (*arrow* in B).

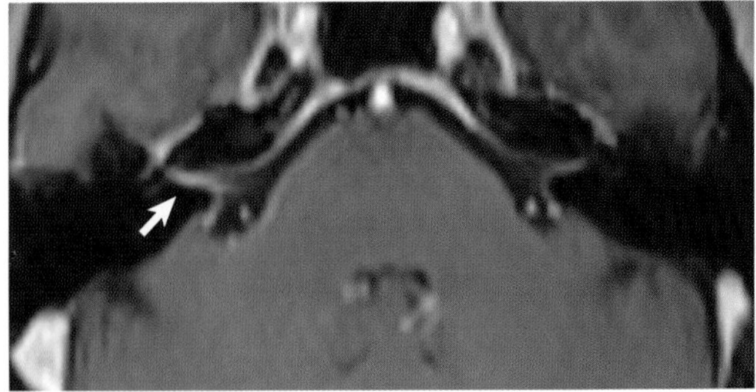

Figure 72.40 Bell's palsy—axial post-contrast T1 image shows asymmetric increased enhancement of the cisternal segment of right facial nerve (*arrow*).

Precochlear Implant Imaging

The presurgical mapping is essential for planning the route of cochlear implant electrode placement. CT and MRI provide critical information about the anatomical variations and imaging findings that may complicate surgical access and lead to iatrogenic complications.

Simple mastoidectomy with a posterior tympanotomy is considered the classical approach that may be associated with round window enlargement or separate "cochleostomy," aimed to access the scala tympani for electrode placement. Suprameatal approach, transcanal approach, middle cranial fossa approach with apical turn cochleostomy are some of the alternative routes, but less commonly used. In cases with chronic suppurative otitis media, unstable mastoid cavities with recurrent otorrhea, partially ossified cochleae, tympanosclerosis, and some inner ear dysplasias, an alternative to the classic route may be considered.

Both CT and MRI are needed for patient selection, side selection, and anatomical assessment. The common anatomical variations to be assessed include:

1. *Vascular anatomy*
   Sigmoid sinus—anteriorly/laterally placed (Fig. 72.41)
   Jugular bulb—high riding/dehiscent
   Carotid canal—dehiscent/aberrant course
2. *Facial nerve*
   Aberrant course—anterior course with decreased facial recess width
   Dehiscence of the intratympanic portion
3. *Mastoid and tympanic cavity*
   Degree of the middle ear and mastoid pneumatization/mastoiditis
   Ossicular chain status
   Chronic middle ear disease

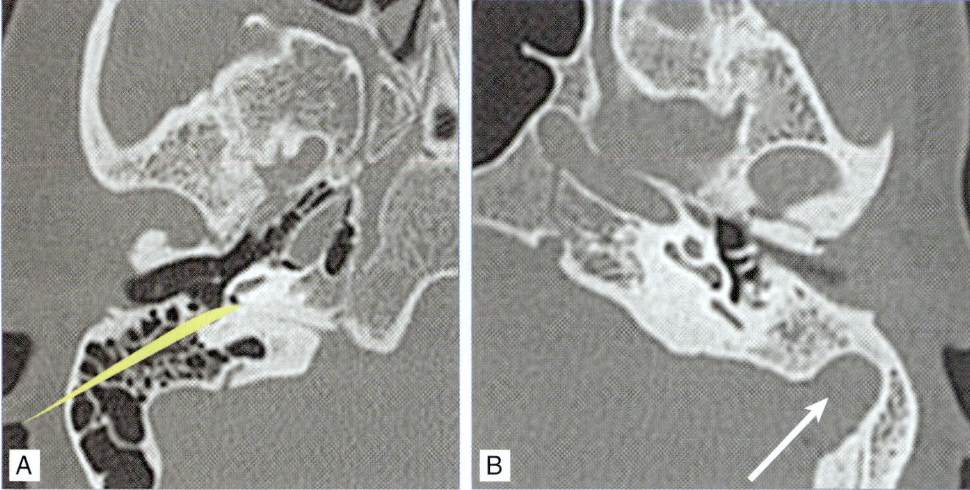

Figure 72.41 (A and B) Precochlear implantation. *Yellow line* in the first image depicting the course of electrode insertion from mastoid margin to the round window niche. *Arrow* in the second image shows anterolateral projection of the sigmoid sinus with thinning of the overlying bony plate, a variation that affecting the surgical plan of electrode insertion in this path.

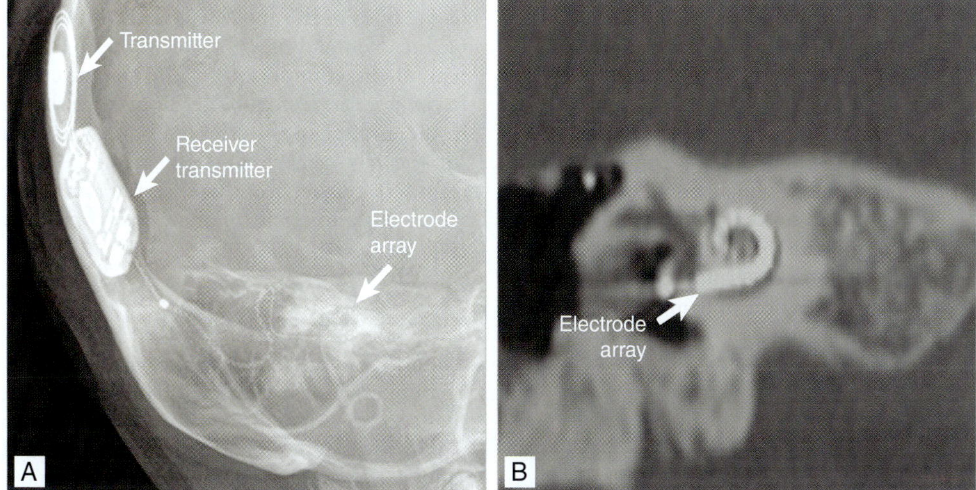

Figure 72.42 Cochlear implant. Radiograph (A) shows the parts of cochlear implant with electrodes located within the cochlea. Coronal CT image (B) shows tiny electrodes located in array noted within the cochlea; the number and exact location within the cochlear turns are important for hearing rehabilitation.

4. *Inner ear disease*

   Cochlear anomalies

   Other inner ear anomalies—vestibular/SCC dysplasia, dilated vestibular aqueduct syndrome, narrow internal auditory meatus (IAM)

5. *Nerve assessment*

   Cochlear or vestibulocochlear nerve hypoplasia or aplasia.

Post-implant assessment usually includes a radiographic evaluation (Fig. 72.42) with CT or cone beam CT that is utilized as a problem-solving tool in doubtful/complicated cases. The assessment includes careful evaluation of the location and number of electrodes within the cochlea, course of the wire, electrode displacement/fractures and associated complications [1–13].

Suggested Readings

- AF Juliano, DT Ginat, G Moonis, Imaging review of the temporal bone: part I, Anatomy and inflammatory and neoplastic processes, Radiology 269 (1) (2013 Oct) 17–33.
- SK Mukherji, consulting editor. Update on temporal bone imaging with emphasis on clinical and surgical perspectives, Neuroimag Clin 29 (1) (2019 Feb 1) xv.
- BM Allanson, TH Low, JR Clark, R Gupta, Squamous cell carcinoma of the external auditory canal and temporal bone: an update, Head Neck Pathol 12 (3) (2018) 407–418.
- JT Castle, Cholesteatoma Pearls: practical points and update. Head Neck Pathol 12 (3) (2018) 419–429.
- YY Kurihara, A Fujikawa, N Tachizawa, M Takaya, H Ikeda, J Starkey, Temporal bone trauma: typical CT and MRI appearances and important points for evaluation, Radiographics 40 (2020) 1148–1162.
- P Touska, SEJ Connor, Imaging of the temporal bone, Clin Radiol 75 (9) (2020 Sept 1) 658–674.

73 Skull Base

MOHANNAD IBRAHIM, HEMANT A. PARMAR, SURESH K. MUKHERJI

Introduction

Skull base comprises a complex area between the neurocranium and head and neck region, which is not always well accessible to clinicians for inspection. Advances in imaging over last few decades now allow radiologists to identify normal anatomy of the skull base in precise details. Imaging also helps to identify imaging characteristics of different pathology, staging of neoplasms, define extent of tumor spread, plan surgical approach, and evaluate tumor recurrence. Radiologists interpreting imaging studies in patients with skull base lesions need to be familiar with anatomy of this region and utilize correct imaging protocols.

In this chapter, we will outline the basic but critical anatomy of the skull base. We will discuss important and commonly used imaging techniques, protocols, and highlight some of the newer emerging tools. We will then focus on the various pathologies of the skull base. Discussion of the skull base lesions in this chapter is based on the nature of the lesions: congenital, benign neoplastic, malignant neoplastic, or infectious/inflammatory lesions. Tables of various lesions involving anterior, middle, or posterior skull base are also provided for easy reference.

Skull Base Anatomy

The floor of the cranial cavity separates the brain from the face and neck structures. It is divided by the sphenoid ridge anteriorly and the petrous ridge posteriorly into three distinct depressions, the anterior cranial fossa (ACF), middle cranial fossa (MCF), and posterior cranial fossa (PCF) (Fig. 73.1).

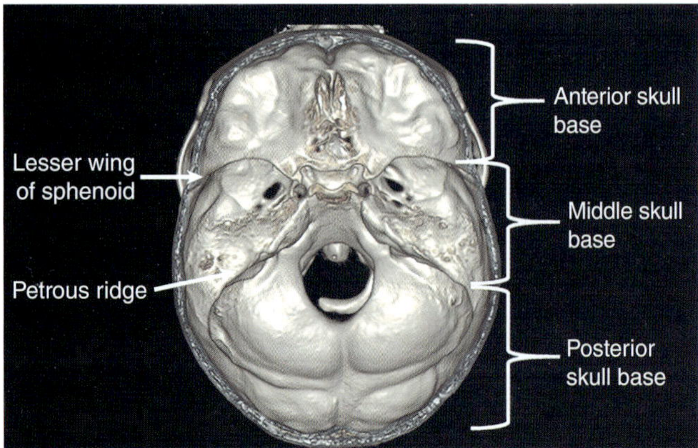

Figure 73.1 Endocranium view of the skull base. 3-D CT of the skull base showing subdivision into anterior (A), middle (M), and posterior (P) cranial fossa. The lesser wing of sphenoid with anterior clinoid process separates anterior from middle cranial fossa. The petrous ridge shows the approximate position of the tentorium cerebelli which divides middle from posterior cranial fossa.

Anterior Cranial Fossa

The ACF is a depression along the floor of the anterior cranial base that houses the orbitofrontal gyri of the frontal lobes, olfactory bulbs, and olfactory tracts. The ACF extends anteriorly from the posterior walls of the frontal sinuses and posteriorly to the sphenoidal limbus (the anterior margin of the chiasmatic groove) and the lesser sphenoid wings. The majority of the floor of the anterior fossa is formed by the orbital plates of the frontal bone. Between them is the thin cribriform pate of the ethmoid bone. The frontal crest, an osseous ridge in the midline frontal bone, along with the crista galli, situated in the midline of the ethmoid bone, acts as an attachment site for the falx cerebri. On either side of the crista galli is the cribriform plate, forming the floor of the olfactory groove, which has numerous foramina that transmit vessels and nerves (Fig. 73.2A,B).

Middle Cranial Fossa

The MCF is butterfly shaped with a central narrow part that accommodates the pituitary gland along with two lateral parts that accommodate the temporal lobes of the brain. The central part of the MCF contains the sella turcica (Latin for Turkish saddle) that holds and support the pituitary gland. The sella turcica consists of the tuberculum sellae, pituitary fossa, and dorsum sellae (Fig. 73.3A). It is bordered anteriorly by the chiasmatic groove and surrounded by the anterior and posterior clinoid processes on each side. The anterior clinoid processes arise from the lesser sphenoidal wings and project posterolaterally. The posterior clinoid processes are superolateral bony projections that serve as attachment points for the tentorium cerebelli which forms the superior boundary of the PCF.

There are many foramina that transmit vascular structures and nerves into and out of the MCF. The optic canals are situated anteriorly and superiorly transmitting the optic nerves and ophthalmic arteries into the orbits. The superior orbital fissures are located immediately inferior to the optic canals. Each of the superior orbital fissure transmits the oculomotor nerve (CN III), trochlear nerve (CN IV), ophthalmic branch of the trigeminal nerve (CN V1), the abducens nerve (CN VI), ophthalmic veins, and sympathetic tracts. The foramen rotundum transmits the maxillary branch of the trigeminal nerve (CN V2) into the pterygopalatine fossa (Fig. 73.3B). The foramen ovale and foramen spinosum both open into the infratemporal fossa transmitting the mandibular branch of the trigeminal nerve (CN V3) and accessory meningeal artery, respectively (Fig. 73.3C).

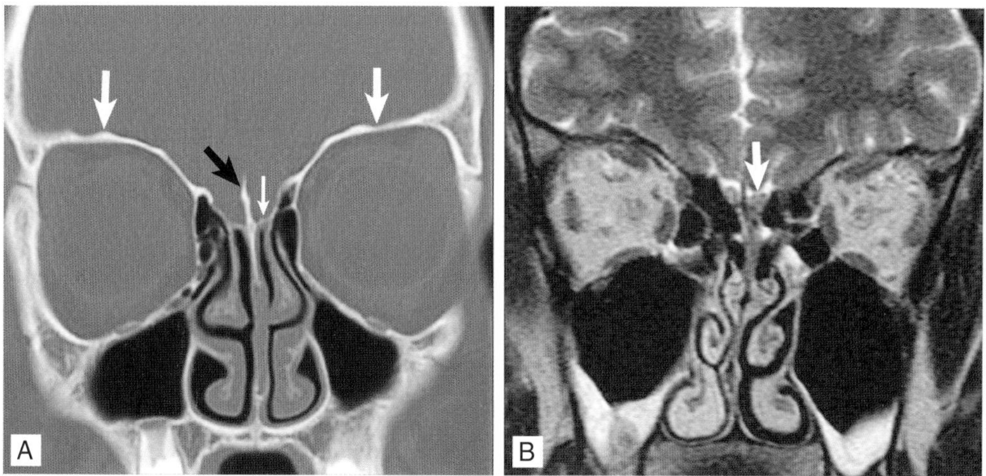

Figure 73.2 Normal anatomy—anterior skull base. (A) Coronal CT of the anterior skull base show crista galli (*black arrow*) with cribriform plates (*small white arrow*) on either side and orbital plates of frontal bone (*large white arrows*). (B) Coronal T2-weighted MRI through the same level show normal position of the olfactory bulb (*arrow*).

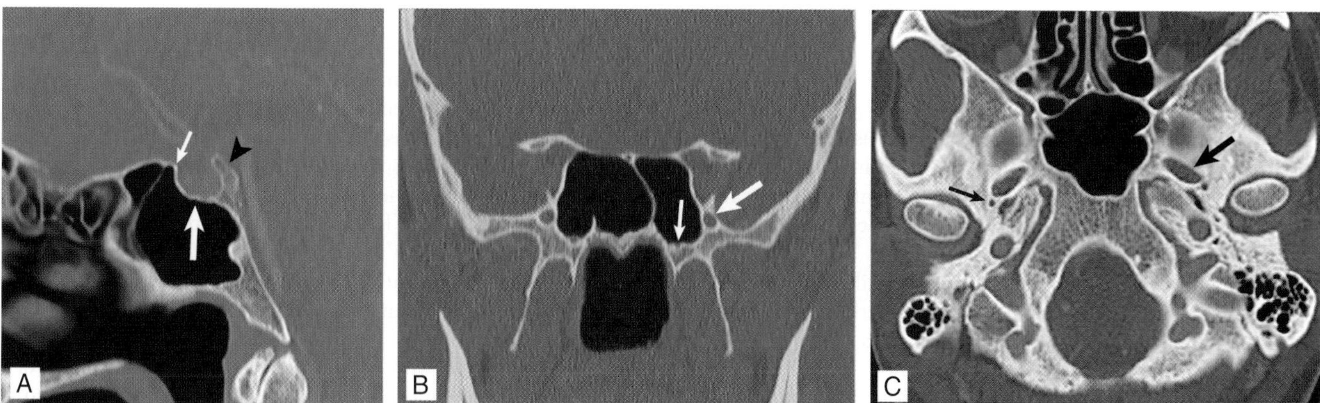

Figure 73.3 Normal anatomy—middle skull base. (A) Sagittal CT through the midline of middle cranial fossa shows depression of sella turcica (*large white arrow*) which bounded anteriorly by tuberculum sella (*small white arrow*) and posteriorly by dorsum sella (*black arrowhead*). (B) Coronal CT through the middle cranial fossa foramen rotundum (*large arrow*) and Vidian canal which is inferior and medial (*small arrow*). (C) Axial CT at the level of floor of middle cranial fossa show larger foramen ovale (*large arrow*) and smaller foramen spinosum (*small arrow*).

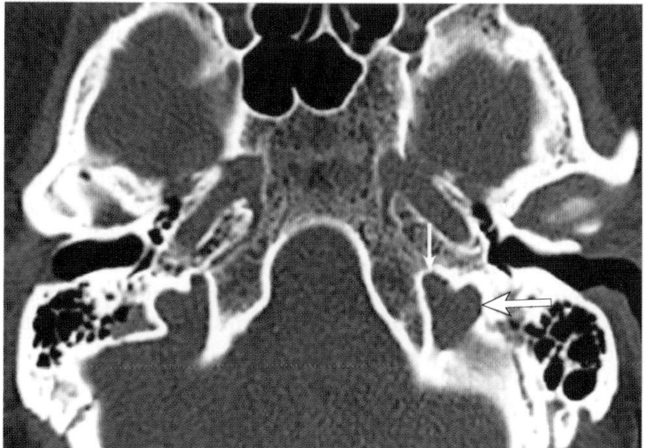

Figure 73.4 Normal anatomy—posterior skull base. Axial CT through the posterior cranial fossa shows jugular foramen that is divided by jugular spike into smaller pars nervosa anteriorly (*small arrow*) and larger pars vascularis posteriorly (*large arrow*).

Posterior Cranial Fossa

The PCF is the most posterior and deepest of the cranial fossae, accommodating the brainstem and cerebellum. Along with the brainstem and cerebellum, the PCF also accommodates the vertebrobasilar arteries, cranial nerves, and dural venous sinuses. The dorsum sellae and the two petrous ridges are the anteromedial and anterolateral boundaries, respectively, separating the MCF and the PCF.

The foramen magnum, the largest opening in the floor of the fossa, is located centrally in the PCF. It transmits the medulla oblongata along with the vertebral arteries, dural veins, and the anterior and posterior spinal arteries. The jugular foramina are situated on either side of the foramen magnum. Each jugular foramen is divided into anterior part (pars nervosa) that transmits the glossopharyngeal nerve and inferior petrosal sinus. The larger posterior part (pars vascularis) transmits vagus nerve, spinal accessory nerve, sigmoid sinus continuing into internal jugular vein and meningeal branches of the ascending pharyngeal and occipital arteries (Fig. 73.4). Immediately superior and medial to the jugular fossa is the hypoglossal canal, which transmits the hypoglossal nerve.

Embryologic Development

The skull base, also known as the chondrocranium, is formed mostly through endochondral ossification, in contrast to the neurocranium or the cranial vault that is formed by intramembranous ossification [1]. The formation of the chondrocranium is almost complete by the eight week [1], which is then ensued by endochondral ossification between 12 and 17 weeks [1,2], that progress from posterior to anterior in a well-defined pattern [2].

The notochord, a defining structure in the development of the neural plate, has an intimate relationship with the central skull base [1]. It develops between the third and fourth weeks of gestation and is a major regulator of embryonic patterning. The notochord develops along a tract that extends from Rathke's pouch to the buccopharyngeal membrane and further caudally in the vertebral column (Fig. 73.5). The notochord regresses as the axial skeleton develops, eventually contributing to the formation of the nucleus pulposus of the intervertebral disks. Regression of the notochord can sometimes be variable, particularly at the ends of the axial skeleton at the skull base and sacrococcygeal regions, which results in the persistence of a variety of vestigial notochordal remnants.

Imaging Technique

CT scan and MRI are the primary modalities used to evaluate the anterior skull base and these complement each other. For example, benign fibro-osseous lesions are fairly commonly seen at the skull base. They can appear like an aggressive lesion on MRI, but CT is often diagnostic.

CT provides excellent bony anatomic detail and is useful for evaluating the bony margins surrounding the lesion to characterize aggressive or benign growth pattern [3]. CT is useful to evaluate subtle changes in the fat planes around various skull base foramina. CT (without or with intrathecal contrast) is also useful in evaluation of cerebrospinal fluid (CSF) leaks (more details in section of CSF leak). Most of the skull base CT is obtained by helical acquisition technique using submillimeter slice thickness

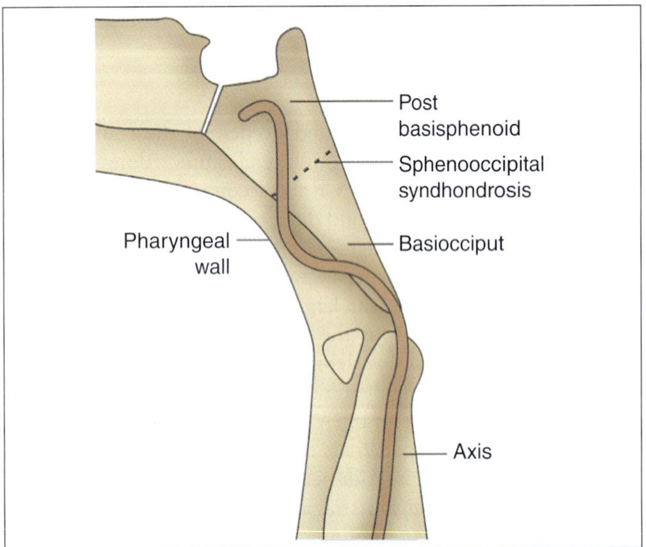

Figure 73.5 Embryology of the notochord. Midplane sagittal section of the skull base demonstrating the position of the notochord within the skull base.

and covering entire skull base. The raw data can be processed to provide reconstructions in any imaging plane from a single acquisition. Although orthogonal axes are most commonly used (axial, sagittal, and coronal), oblique planes can be used to correct for head tilt or provide optimal visualization of a specific structure. CT source data can also be subjected to sharpening algorithms (with more targeted field of view) to enhance osseous details.

MRI provides excellent soft tissue detail and most of the lesions involving skull base require different imaging protocol compared to that of brain. MRI protocol is based on the suspected abnormality, the available imaging equipment, and local imaging expertise. Most of the skull base protocols require smaller field of view with thinner (3 mm or less) slice thickness. Most commonly followed protocol includes T1- and T2-weighted sequences in axial and coronal planes followed by post-contrast enhanced T1-weighted sequence in multiple planes. Due to its intrinsic bright signal, fat provides excellent contrast with low-intensity structures, such as nerves and vessels on pre-contrast T1-weighted sequence [3,4]. This is helpful to check replacement of normal fat around the skull base foramina in cases with suspected perineural spread (PNS) of tumor. MRI, especially T2-weighted sequence, is helpful to separate mucosal thickening and retained secretions in the paranasal sinuses from tumor [3]. Replacement of normal marrow in osseous structures is also well evaluated by T1-weighted MRI scan (particularly helpful when there are no cortical erosive changes seen on CT). Fat suppression technique is another chosen technique for evaluation of skull base lesions that can be applied for T2 and post-contrast enhanced T1-weighted technique. This is especially helpful in evaluation of areas with intrinsic high T1 signal. However, caution should be exercised when using fat suppression as susceptibility artifacts from the bone and air can extend into important soft tissues and obscure it. It may be a good idea to obtain post-contrast enhanced images without and with fat suppression to minimize this problem. A newer generation of fat free sequences can provide non-saturated and fat saturated T1- and T2-weighted images based on chemical shift imaging with in-phase/out-of-phase cycling of fat and water. Finally, MRI is also helpful for evaluation of dural, pial, or brain parenchymal enhancement in case of intracranial extension of skull base disease process.

Diffusion-weighted imaging (DWI) is well recognized for its ability to characterize abscesses and head and neck tumors, and to differentiate cholesteatoma from granulation tissue. Other emerging applications for DWI include staging of neoplasms and differentiating tumor recurrence from post-treatment changes [5].

Another emerging MRI technique is perfusion imaging that can be used to characterize metastatic lymph nodes and to differentiate tumor recurrence from posttreatment changes. Among the different techniques of performing perfusion imaging such as dynamic susceptibility contrast (DSC), dynamic contrast-enhanced (DCE), and arterial spin labeling (ASL) available today, DCE perfusion has been studied the most for skull base applications due to the significant susceptibility artifact arising from the DSC technique and relatively long acquisition time with ASL technique [5].

High-resolution fluid-sensitive balanced steady-state free precession sequences, called by different propriety names by vendors such as FIESTA (fast imaging employing steady state acquisition, CISS (constructive interference in steady state) are extremely useful sequences obtained using thin-slice acquisitions (less than 1 mm) and can be reconstructed in different planes. This allows to image cisternal segments of the cranial nerves and their relationship to adjacent structures/lesions [6], which may not be readily seen on routine sequences.

Although not commonly utilized, conventional angiography remains an important tool for confirming the diagnosis of suspected vascular lesions such as carotid-cavernous fistula (often performed after CT or MR angiogram). It can also serve as a therapeutic option in many cases, either on its own or for presurgical embolization.

PET/CT is now a routine component of clinical practice for staging head and neck cancers and evaluation of tumor recurrent at many institutions. Nuclear medicine studies, such as Indium-111 labeled octreotide single-photon emission CT (SPECT) scan can also help confirm whether a tumor has a neuroendocrine origin, such as in glomus tumors/paragangliomas.

Pathology

Lesions of the skull base can be challenging to group and classify due to a wide array of pathology that may be encountered. Some of these pathologies can be unique to part of the skull base (e.g., esthesioneuroblastoma in the ACF or paraganglioma in the PCF), compared to other pathologies that can be seen throughout the skull base (i.e., infectious process or congenital lesions). General categorical classifications of pathologies of the skull base include grouping the lesions as congenital, neoplastic, infectious, or others. Such pathologic processes can be seen in the ACF (Table 73.1), MCF (Table 73.2), or the PCF (Table 73.3). Modern imaging techniques have increased the radiologist's ability in characterizing skull base lesions and determine a diagnosis.

TABLE 73.1 Anterior Skull Base Lesions

Neoplasm	■ Squamous cell carcinoma ■ Sinonasal adenocarcinoma ■ Adenoid cystic carcinoma ■ Sinonasal undifferentiated carcinoma ■ Sinonasal lymphoma ■ Sinonasal melanoma ■ Esthesioneuroblastoma ■ Metastatic lesions ■ Meningioma ■ Mesenchymal tumors (solitary fibrous tumor-hemangiopericytoma)
Congenital	■ Sincipital encephalocele ■ Dermoid/epidermoid cyst ■ Nasal sinus tract
Infection/other	■ Sinonasal empyema/Potts puffy tumor ■ Mucocele ■ Fibro-osseous lesions/fibrous dysplasia ■ Sinonasal osteoma

TABLE 73.2 Middle Skull Base Lesions

Neoplasm	■ Chordoma ■ Chondrosarcoma ■ Ecchordosis physaliphora ■ Schwannoma ■ Skull base metastasis ■ Non-Hodgkin lymphoma ■ Plasmacytoma ■ Meningioma ■ Mesenchymal tumors (solitary fibrous tumor-hemangiopericytoma)
Congenital	■ Arachnoid granulation ■ Encephalocele ■ Craniopharyngeal canal
Infection/other	■ Sinonasal empyema ■ Mucocele ■ Skull base osteomyelitis ■ Benign fibro-osseous lesions/fibrous dysplasia ■ Neurosarcoidosis

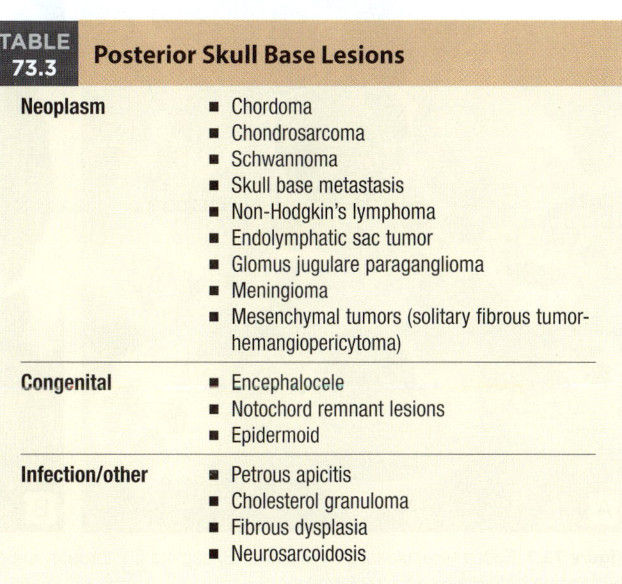

TABLE 73.3 Posterior Skull Base Lesions

Neoplasm	■ Chordoma ■ Chondrosarcoma ■ Schwannoma ■ Skull base metastasis ■ Non-Hodgkin's lymphoma ■ Endolymphatic sac tumor ■ Glomus jugulare paraganglioma ■ Meningioma ■ Mesenchymal tumors (solitary fibrous tumor-hemangiopericytoma)
Congenital	■ Encephalocele ■ Notochord remnant lesions ■ Epidermoid
Infection/other	■ Petrous apicitis ■ Cholesterol granuloma ■ Fibrous dysplasia ■ Neurosarcoidosis

Congenital Lesions

Notochord Remnants

There is a wide spectrum of anatomical variants and developmental defects related to the notochord development within the skull base [1,7]. Notochord-related lesions may be benign or malignant with variable locations, either submucosal in the nasopharynx, intraosseous/transosseous lesions, or intracranial lesions in the epidural, subdural, or subarachnoid spaces. Therefore, such lesions can often present a diagnostic dilemma with complex clinical presentation. Some of these lesions are benign "do not touch" lesions and mostly have no clinical significance. Clinical complications have been rarely reported in some of these benign embryonic remnants such as CSF leak [7], meningitis, otitis media related to compression of the Eustachian tube, or even neck pain and stiffness.

Canalis Basilaris Medianus

The canalis basilaris medianus **(CBM),** also known as chordal canal, or clival canal, refers to variety of midline canals, most commonly in the basioccipital region [7,8]. The CBM is thought to represent a vestigial notochord remnant. However, some studies of the canal contents have found no notochordal remnants but only venous channels emanating from the basilar plexus toward the vertebral venous plexus or veins located at the inferior aspect of the skull base [8] (Fig. 73.6).

Fossa Navicularis Magna

Fossa navicularis, or fossa navicularis magna, is a variant osseous depression that is oval shaped or round on the ventral surface of the basioccipital clivus, located superior to the pharyngeal

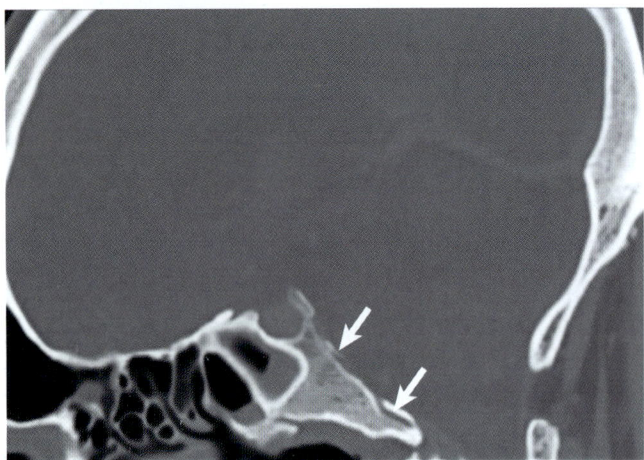

Figure 73.6 Median basal canal. Sagittal CT through the midline shows a small linear channel at the tip of the bony clivus suggestive of median basal canal (*arrows*).

tubercle [1,7]. This anatomic variant is thought to represent the persistent cephalic end of the notochord. Although sometimes confusing, but this is typically a larger defect compared to the smaller and linear CBM (Fig. 73.7A,B).

Tornwaldt Cyst

Tornwaldt cyst is an incidental midline mucosal cyst of the nasopharynx, typically seen in the adult patients [9]. The lesion is developmental and mostly asymptomatic, though it can present with halitosis or middle ear symptoms [1]. Tornwaldt cyst represents a communication between notochord remnants and the pharyngeal endoderm, with gradual accumulation of fluid within the cyst related to occlusion of the orifice of the pharyngeal bursa.

Tornwaldt cyst presents as well-circumscribed, submucosal lesion in the midline nasopharynx in between the longus colli muscles. A typical Tornwaldt cyst measures 2–10 mm in size, however it can be large measuring few centimeters in diameter [9]. On CT it appears as well-circumscribed, nonenhancing hypodense lesion. A protein-rich cyst may appear hyperdense. The MR signal characteristics depend on the protein content ranging from isointense to hyperintense on T1W images, and hyperintense on T2W images [9] (Fig. 73.8A,B).

Ecchordosis Physaliphora

Ecchordosis physaliphora (EP) is an ectopic notochordal remnant, located anywhere from the skull base to the sacrum, but characteristically presenting as retroclival, intradural lesion [10]. Unlike chordomas that are often symptomatic due to brainstem or cranial nerve compression, patients with EP and benign notochord cell tumor (BNCT) (discussed later) are usually asymptomatic. EP lesions are typically less than 2 cm in size [10]. There is controversy in differentiating large EP and intradural chordoma. Some authors used giant or symptomatic EP to describe intradural, extraosseous physaliphorous cell growth [11], while others suggested using the term intradural chordoma [10].

Assessment of EP is limited on CT scan due to its near CSF density and artifacts within the posterior fossa. Occasionally a pathognomonic osseous stalk can be seen at the base of the lesion, or it could appear as smoothly corticated osseous defect extending within the clivus [10] (Fig. 73.9A). EP lesions can sometimes hard to be seen. They are typically T1 hypointense, T2 hyperintense, and have no enhancement with gadolinium (Fig. 73.9B,C). A distinct pedicle, the hallmark of EP, is commonly seen and is typically T2 hypointense [10].

Craniopharyngeal Canal

Persistent craniopharyngeal canal, also known as the hypophyseal canal, is a rare congenital osseous defect extending through the central skull base from the floor of the sella to the nasopharyngeal roof. Craniopharyngeal canals can be asymptomatic incidental canals (type 1), or associated with ectopic adenohypophysis (type 2) [1,12]. Type 3 craniopharyngeal canals are associated with cephaloceles (type 3A), tumors (type 3B), or both (type 3C), including pituitary adenoma, craniopharyngioma, dermoid, teratoma, and glioma [1,12].

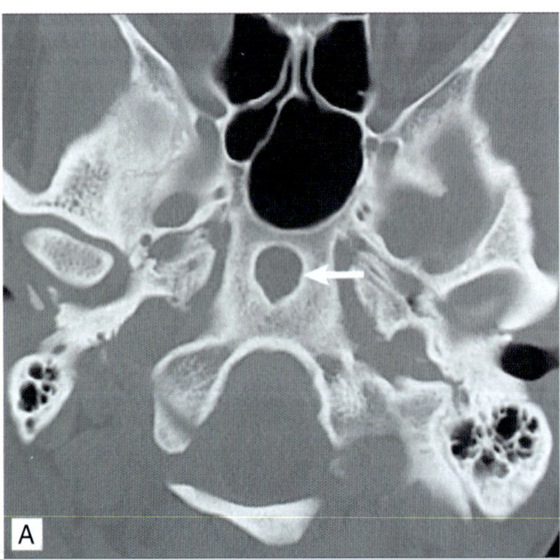

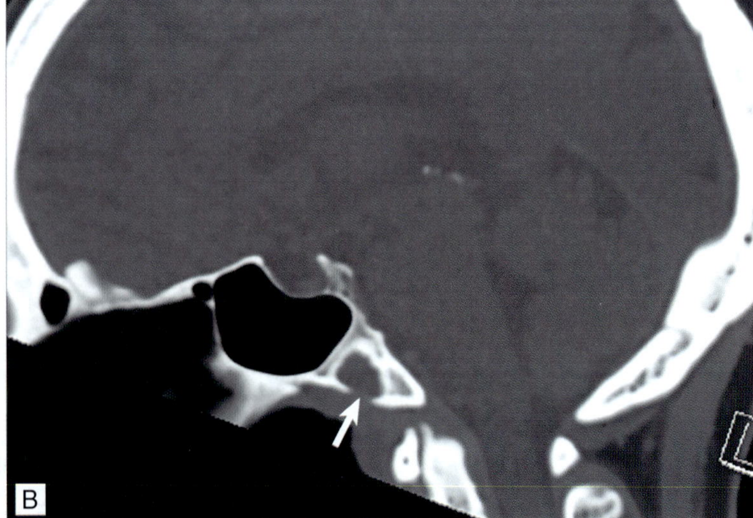

Figure 73.7 Fossa navicularis. (A) Axial and (B) sagittal CT through the central skull base level shows a well-defined, oval lytic lesion involving the clivus suggestive of fossa navicularis (*arrows*).

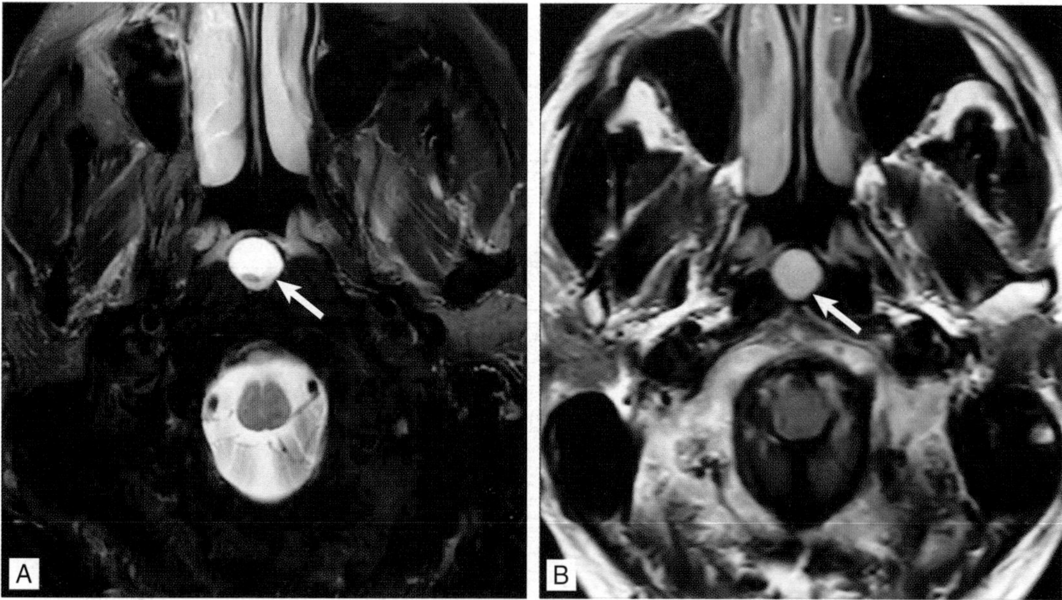

Figure 73.8 Tornwaldt cyst. (A) Axial T2 and (B) axial T1-weighted MRI at the level of nasopharynx show a well-defined oval lesion at the midline posterior nasopharyngeal mucosal space (*arrows*). The lesion was hyperintense on both sequences.

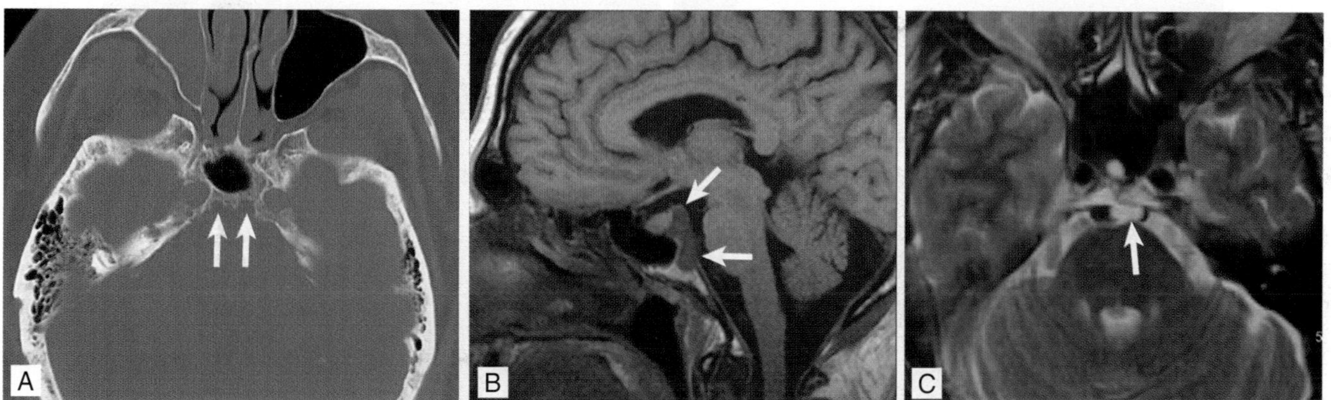

Figure 73.9 Ecchordosis physaliphora: (A) Axial CT image show a well-defined lytic lesion of the basisphenoid (*arrows*). This lesion was hypointense on sagittal T1 (B) and hyperintense on axial T2- weighted MRI images (C) (*arrows*). It was stable over multiple MRI exams over 10 years and was presumed for ecchordosis. Since it was an incidental finding, there was no pathology available for this lesion.

Encephalocele

Encephaloceles are uncommon lesions characterized by herniation of the meninges and cerebral tissues through a cranial osseous defect [1]. Congenital encephalocele represents a form of neural tube defect secondary to failure of fusion during embryogenesis. However, there is no clear-cut explanation for most of the neural tube maldevelopment leading to such defect. The majority of encephaloceles in adults are either posttraumatic or iatrogenic, related mostly to idiopathic intracranial hypertension.

Most of the encephaloceles are midline, either occipital (75%) or sincipital (15%) in location, and the rest are basal (10%) or parietal encephaloceles [13]. Atretic cephalocele contains dura, fibrous tissue, and degenerated brain. Most encephaloceles are sporadic without underlying genetic abnormality. Earlier descriptions of the encephalocele were based on the herniated tract of the encephalocele; however, later classification systems described the encephalocele depending on many aspects such as the content or the site of the cranial defect, the location of the encephalocele, or whether the encephalocele is occult or overt (Table 73.4).

Osseous pits related to arachnoid granulations are common incidental findings [14], most often located in the greater wing of the sphenoid bone or the posterior wall of the temporal bone. An empty or partially empty sella is commonly seen in association with these pits, suggesting that altered CSF dynamics have a role in their development [14,15]. The rare temporal lobe encephaloceles, type II lateral sphenoid cephalocele, involve only the greater sphenoid wing without extension into the sphenoid sinus. It can occasionally exist in asymptomatic patients or present with headache, meningitis, or cranial neuropathy; however, it can present a diagnostic challenge during imaging work-up for epilepsy [14]. The more medially located, type I lateral sphenoid cephalocele herniates into a pneumatized lateral recess of the sphenoid sinus and typically presenting with CSF leak or headache [14].

The radiographic features of encephaloceles depend on their contents, ranging from purely cystic lesions (meningocele) or

TABLE 73.4 Types of Encephalocele

1. According to Etiology
   - Congenital
   - Acquired
2. Location
   - Sincipital encephalocele
     a. Frontoethmoidal (nasoethmoidal, naso-frontal, nasoobrital)
     b. Interfrontal
   - Occipital or suboccipital encephalocele
   - Basal
     a. Transsphenoidal
     b. Transethmoidal
     c. Intranasal
     d. Sphenoorbital
     e. Transtemporal
   - Cranial vault
3. According to content
   - Meningocele
   - Encephalocele
   - Meningoencephalocele
   - Meningoencephalocystocele
4. Encephalocele as part of complex syndrome
   - Chiari III
   - Knobloch syndrome
   - Morning glory syndrome
   - Walker–Warburg syndrome
5. According to clinical presentation
   - Overt
   - Occult
     - Intranasal
     - Intraorbital
     - Intratemporal
     - Intradiploic

brain matter and meninges in case of meningoencephalocele (Fig. 73.10A,B). Ultrasound may demonstrate purely cystic, hypoechoic mass or may contain echoes related to herniated brain tissue. High-resolution CT is typically used to display the osseous defects and characterize the bone anatomy (Fig. 73.10C,D). The contents of the cephalocele are best defined with MRI, which aids in determining the prognosis and surgical planning.

High-resolution MRI, preferably coronal 3 mm T1W images, with matching fat-suppressed T2W images, and gadolinium-enhanced T1W spin-echo sequences, is often recommended to determine the contents of the soft tissue within the nasal cavity or sinus air cell, to distinguish between a meningocele and meningoencephalocele.

CSF Leak

CSF rhinorrhea or otorrhea occurs due to osteodural disruption between subarachnoid space and pneumatized structure. Any clinically suspected CSF leak should first be confirmed with testing for beta-2 transferrin, a protein specific to CSF. The presence

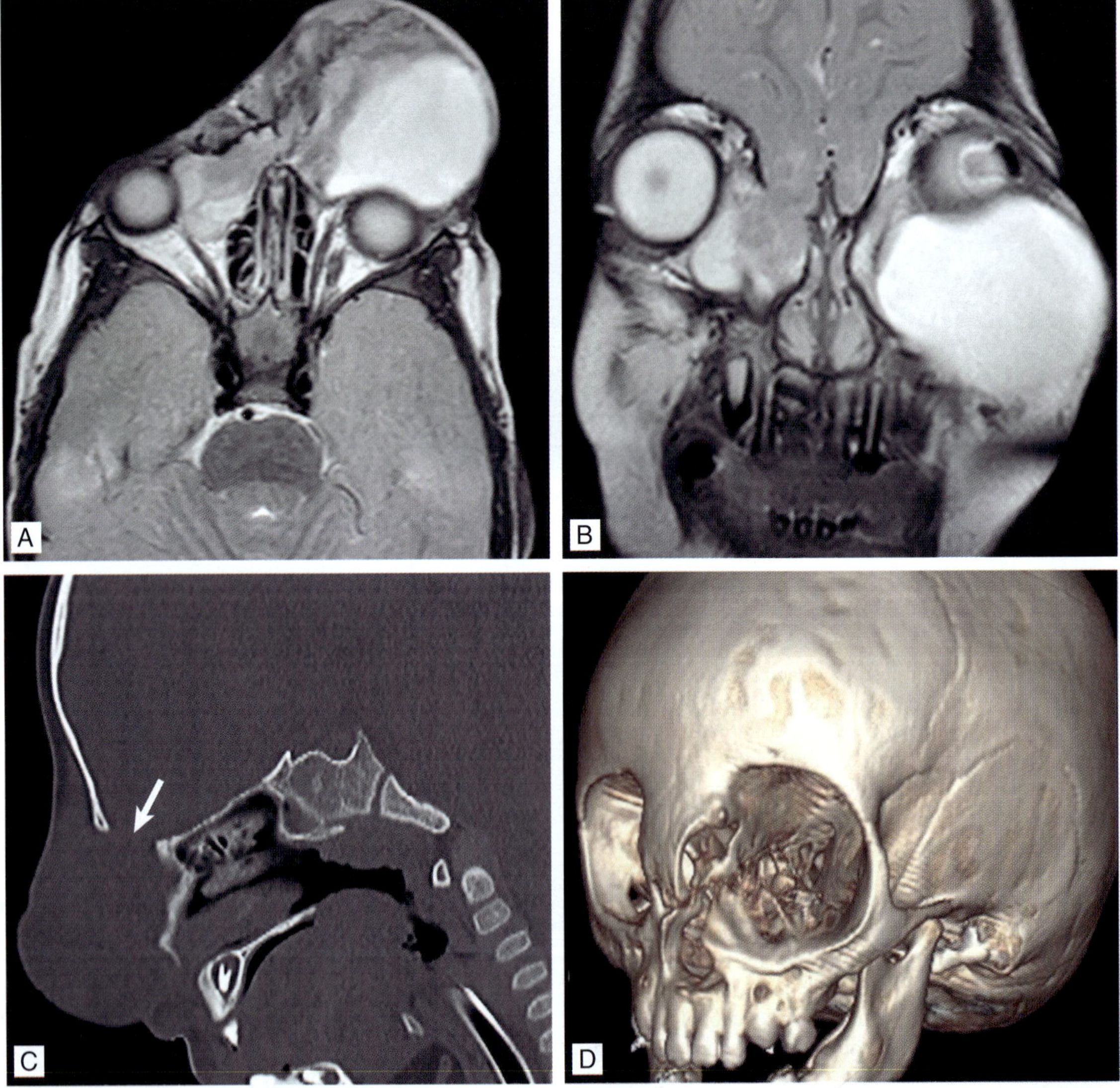

Figure 73.10 Frontonasal meningoencephalocele. (A) Axial and (B) coronal T2-weighted MRI shows a large frontonasal meningoencephalocele in an infant, with a large meningeal component on the left. (C) Sagittal CT shows a large osseous defect at the level of primitive foramen cecum (*arrow*). (D) 3-D rendered CT image shows marked enlargement and remodeling of the left bony orbit.

of β-trace protein (β-TP) in CSF is an alternative and cheaper method to test for CSF leak [16].

CSF leaks can be classified as acquired or congenital. The acquired CSF leak is further classified as traumatic, nontraumatic, or spontaneous [15]. Spontaneous CSF leak is considered to result from multifactorial process and is mostly associated with idiopathic intracranial hypertension [14,15]. This process occurs most commonly in areas of structural weakness in the ethmoid roof, sphenoid sinus, and temporal bone related to underlying anatomic predisposition and thinning of the cranial base [15]. The cribriform plate is the commonest site of spontaneous CSF fistulas [15]. CSF leak in the sphenoid sinus region is typically located in the parasellar region or the lateral recess of the sphenoid sinus, classically in middle aged female, and is probably related to arachnoid granulations [14,15]. CSF leak in the temporal region, typically seen in the seventh decade of life, is most frequently present in the tegmen tympani and mastoideum, likely associated with arachnoid granulations [15].

High-resolution unenhanced CT scan of the sinonasal and skull base region is the initial recommended imaging modality for patients with suspected CSF leak. Coronal and sagittal reformatted images are very helpful to assess the site of CSF leak. The presence of an osseous defect with an opacified air cell and olfactory recess/nasal cavity below the defect are findings that predict a CSF leak (Fig. 73.11A). The presence of a single osseous defect in patients with positive beta-2 transferrin will negate the need for a cisternogram [17]. CT cisternogram can be helpful to determine the culprit site of CSF leak in the presence of multiple osseous defects [17] (Fig. 73.11B).

Dermoid and Epidermoid Cysts

Dermoid and epidermoid cysts are uncommon congenital lesions related to inclusion of ectodermal elements during neural tube closure. Epidermoid cysts, comprising 0.2–1.8% of primary intracranial tumors, are four to nine times as common as dermoid cysts. They can present in a variety of intracranial locations or as intraosseous lesions associated with the sutures or the skull [12,18]. The majority of epidermoid cysts are intradural (90%), most frequently in the cerebellopontine angle cistern (40–50%), with 10% of the cysts being extradural in the skull or in the spine [18]. Dermoid cysts tend to occur in the midline at the anterior fontanelle, frontonasal region, or sellar/parasellar region. Nasal dermal sinuses with dermoid and epidermoid cysts occur at multiple locations from the foramen cecum to the columella Additionally, dermoid cysts can occur in the skull base along the craniopharyngeal canal [12].

Epidermoids have a thin capsule of stratified squamous epithelium, with internal components filled with desquamated epithelial keratin and cholesterol crystals, which accounts for their unique imaging characteristics (Fig. 73.12A,B). Dermoids have a similar stratified squamous epithelium, but contain epidermal appendages in addition to the ectodermal elements such as hair follicles, sweat glands, and sebaceous glands (Fig. 73.13A,B). Dermoids or epidermoids are ectodermal and do not contain adipose tissue, as lipocytes are mesodermal in origin.

The content of the lesion will determine its CT attenuation. Epidermoid cysts have fluid attenuation, compared to dermoid cysts that have fatty attenuation (Fig. 73.13A,B). Calcification may be present in the cyst wall. Enhancement is uncommon, and typically appears as a thin peripheral rim. Very rarely epidermoid cyst may demonstrate hyperdensity, which is probably related to saponification, microcalcification, and blood products [18]. This most often occurs when present in the posterior fossa, although the reason is uncertain.

Similarly, the signal intensity on MR imaging depends on the contents of the cyst, with fluid signal intensity (hypointense or isointense on T1 weighted and hyperintense on T2 weighted) in epidermoid, with often heterogeneous hyperintense signal on FLAIR images. Epidermoids typically have bright signal intensity on isotropic diffusion-weighted MR images. Dermoids have more complex signal intensity (hyperintense on T1 weighted due to cholesterol components and variable hypointense or hyperintense signal on T2 weighted) (Fig. 73.13A,B). Cyst rupture is the most

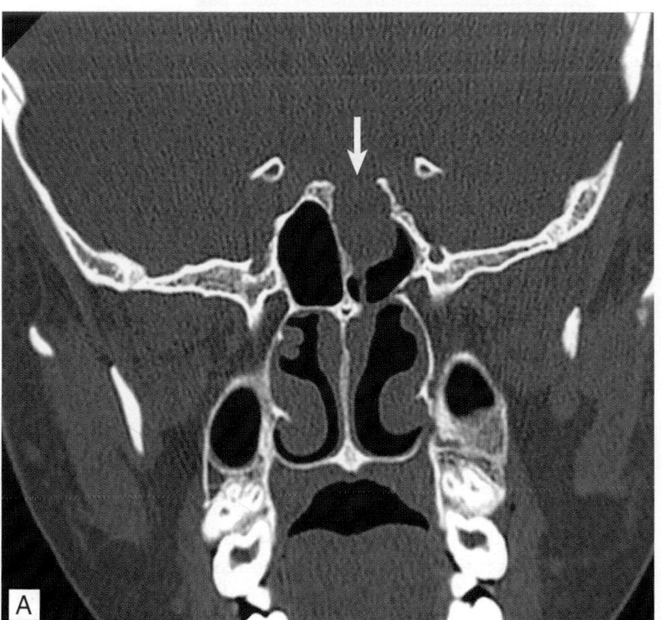

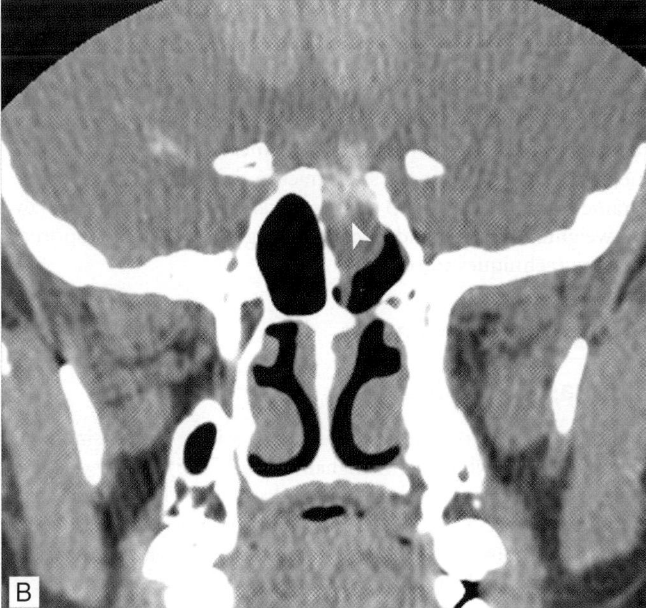

Figure 73.11 Traumatic CSF leak. (A) Coronal CT images in a bone window algorithm show a larger osseous defect at the level of roof of the left sphenoid sinus (*arrow*). (B) After CT cisternogram, there was clear CSF leak through the defect over the left sphenoid sinus (*arrowhead*).

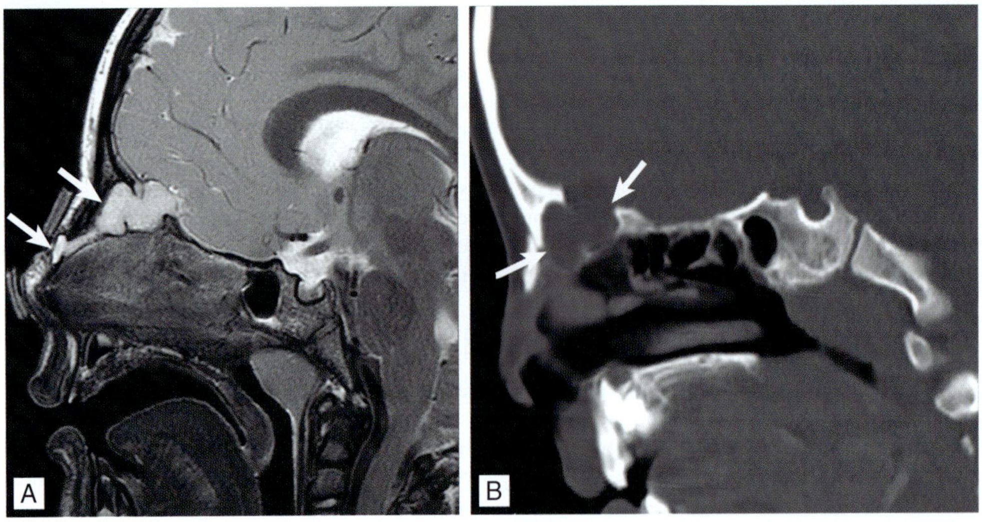

Figure 73.12 Epidermoid of anterior skull base. Sagittal T2-weighted MRI shows a well-defined T2 hyperintense lesion extending from the tip of the nose to the anterior skull base near the level of foramen cecum (*arrows*). There was remodeling the bony margins on sagittal CT image (*arrows*).

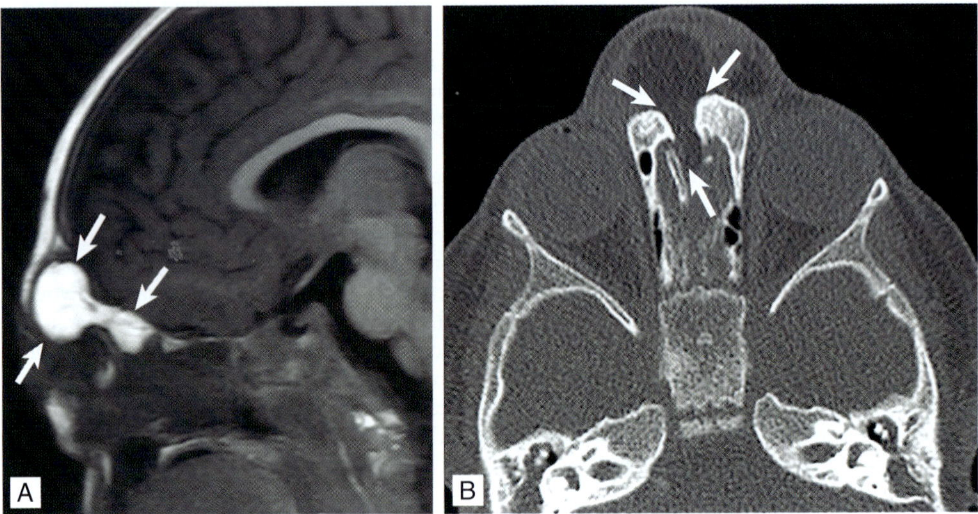

Figure 73.13 Dermoid of anterior skull base. Sagittal T1-weighted MRI shows a large well-defined T1 hyperintense lesion at the level of anterior skull base/glabella consistent with dermoid (*arrows*). Axial CT image shows osseous defect with thin stalk extending toward the crista galli (*arrows*).

common complication and appears as T1 hyperintense droplets in the subarachnoid spaces. To better delineate the ectodermal elements associated with nasal sinus tract in the prenasal space or the foramen cecum, thin (2–3 mm) sagittal T1-weighted or heavily T2-weighted images and preferably sagittal DWI are optimal imaging techniques to consider.

Malignant Neoplasms

Sinonasal Neoplasms

There is a variety of neoplastic processes arising in the sinonasal region, most of which are malignant (Table 73.5). Many of these lesions can involve the skull base and present with neurological complications. CT and MRI are complementary modalities in evaluating sinonasal lesions. CT scan is essential to assess the osseous structures and should be performed with thin, 1 mm, slices with coronal and sagittal reformations. CT typically demonstrates heterogeneously enhancing, poorly defined mass, and is particularly effective in delineating the extent of osseous changes and the pattern of bone invasion. Intralesional calcifications are seen in certain pathologies, such as olfactory neuroblastoma, adenocarcinoma, inverted papilloma, cartilaginous tumors, or fibro-osseous lesions such as fibrous dysplasia (FD), osteoma, and osteosarcoma [19]. Characteristic osseous changes can help predict the tumor histology. Extensive osseous destruction is typically seen in high-grade malignancies (Fig. 73.14A), compared to permeative changes associated with small round cell tumors. The slow growth

TABLE 73.5 Types of Sinonasal Malignancies

- Squamous cell carcinoma
- Sinonasal adenocarcinoma
- Adenoid cystic carcinoma
- Sinonasal undifferentiated carcinoma (SNUC)
- Sinonasal lymphoma
- Sinonasal melanoma
- Esthesioneuroblastoma

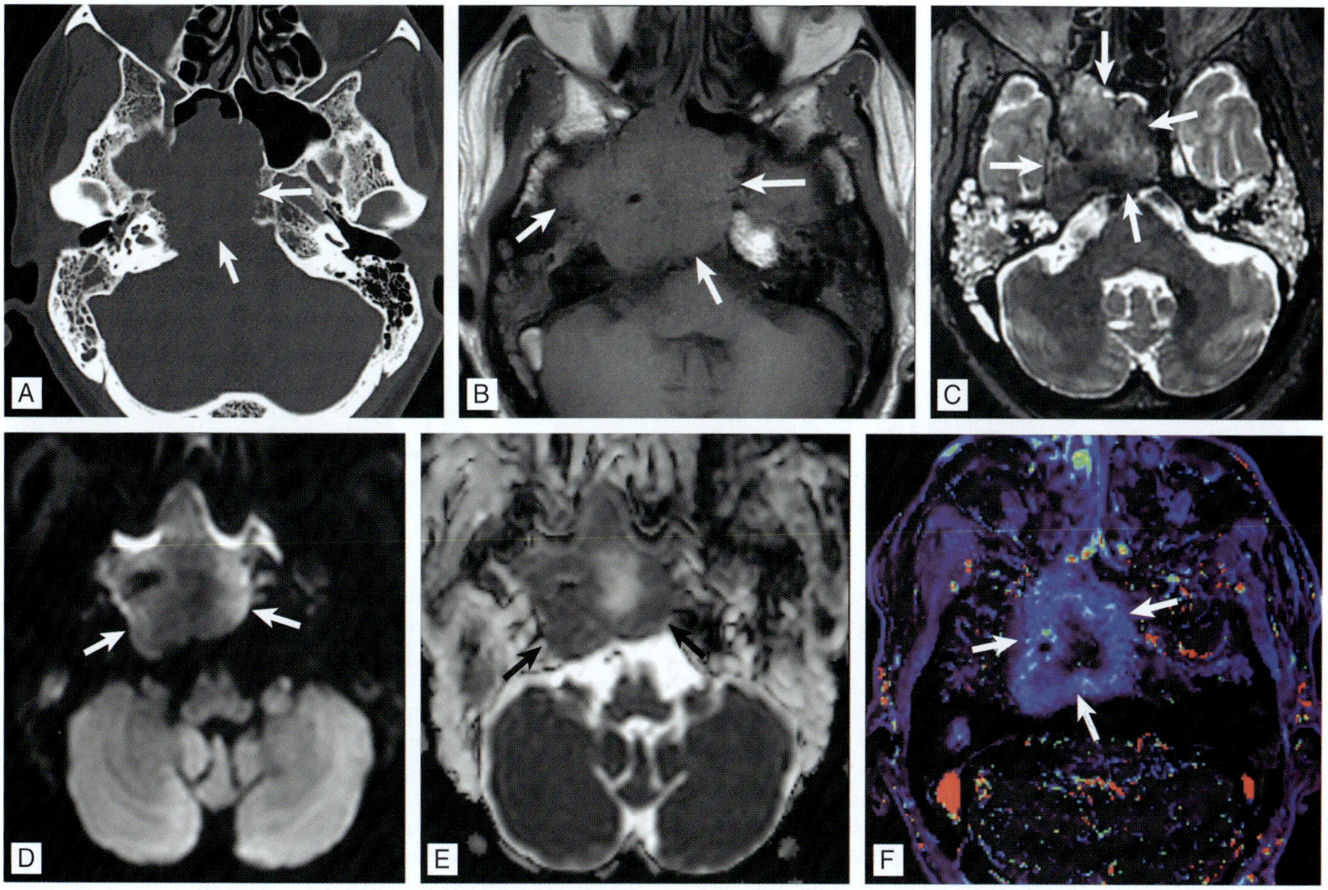

Figure 73.14 Squamous cell carcinoma. (A) Axial CT image at the level of central skull base shows a large, destructive mass that was Epstein-Barr virus–related nasopharyngeal cancer invading the skull base (*arrows*). The lesion was isointense on axial T1 (B), relatively hypointense on T2-weighted MRI (C) (*arrows*). The lesion had mild diffusion hyperintensity (D), with low signal on corresponding apparent diffusion coefficient images (E), particularly at the periphery of the mass (*arrows*). (F) MR perfusion show increased perfusion at the periphery of the lesion (*arrows*), corresponding to the area of reduced diffusion signal and suggestive of more cellular component of the mass.

associated with low-grade malignancies and benign lesions may result in bony remodeling.

MRI provides better characterization of the soft tissue components of the tumor and helps in differentiating the tumor from adjacent retained secretions. While tumor's signal intensity can slightly vary based on their components, however the MR imaging characteristics are generally nonspecific with relative hypointense/isointense T1 signal and hyperintense T2 signal [19,20] (Fig. 73.14B). Mucinous or cartilaginous tumors may demonstrate marked T2 hyperintensity, compared to tumors with calcification or highly cellular tumors that demonstrate T2 isointensity or hypointensity (Fig. 73.14C). Intratumoral T1 hyperintensity indicates the presence of methemoglobin, melanin, protein, and sometimes intralesional mineralization or calcification [19,20].

DWI and the value of diffusion coefficient (apparent diffusion coefficient [ADC] maps) can serve as useful imaging biomarkers [20] (Fig. 73.14D). Low-ADC lesions typically indicate hypercellularity, desiccated secretions, or hemorrhage, whereas high-ADC lesions indicate hypocellularity, "hydrated" mucus, or fluid/necrosis (Fig. 73.14E). A relatively low ADC values (0.87–1.10 × 10^{-3} mm^2/s) is typically seen in malignant sinonasal tumors, compared to a higher ADC values of benign sinonasal lesions (1.35–1.78 × 10^{-3} mm^2/s) [20]. MR perfusion can often show areas of increased perfusion (Fig. 73.14F). Lesions that cause dural invasion and perineural spread (PNS) are best characterized using contrast-enhanced MRI. Intracranial involvement is typically seen as an area of dural thickening >5 mm, pial enhancement, or the presence of focal dural nodules, in contrast to linear dural enhancement alone which is not a conclusive sign of dural invasion [20].

Esthesioneuroblastoma

Olfactory neuroblastoma or esthesioneuroblastoma is an important type of sinonasal malignant tumor. It is a rare neuroectodermal tumor arising of the olfactory epithelium [3,20]. There is bimodal age distribution in the second and sixth decades of life, with no recognized gender predilection. Esthesioneuroblastomas are slowly growing lesions, mostly seen at advanced stage as large lesions in the ACF and sinonasal region [3,20,21].

The CT imaging features are nonspecific, with smaller, intranasal, lesions appearing as polypoid soft tissue lesion that widens the olfactory recess [21]. Large esthesioneuroblastoma results in osseous destruction, or less frequently bony remodeling, and appears relatively isodense with intralesional focal calcifications, and scattered necrosis [20,21]. MRI signal characteristics can be variable but mostly heterogeneously T1 and T2 isointense, with variable enhancement [20] (Fig. 73.15A–C). Peritumoral cysts can be seen in larger lesions with intracranial extension; however, this is not pathognomonic for esthesioneuroblastoma [20]. Cervical and retropharyngeal nodal metastases are present in 10–44% of cases at diagnosis, with relatively poor prognosis [20]. PET-CT

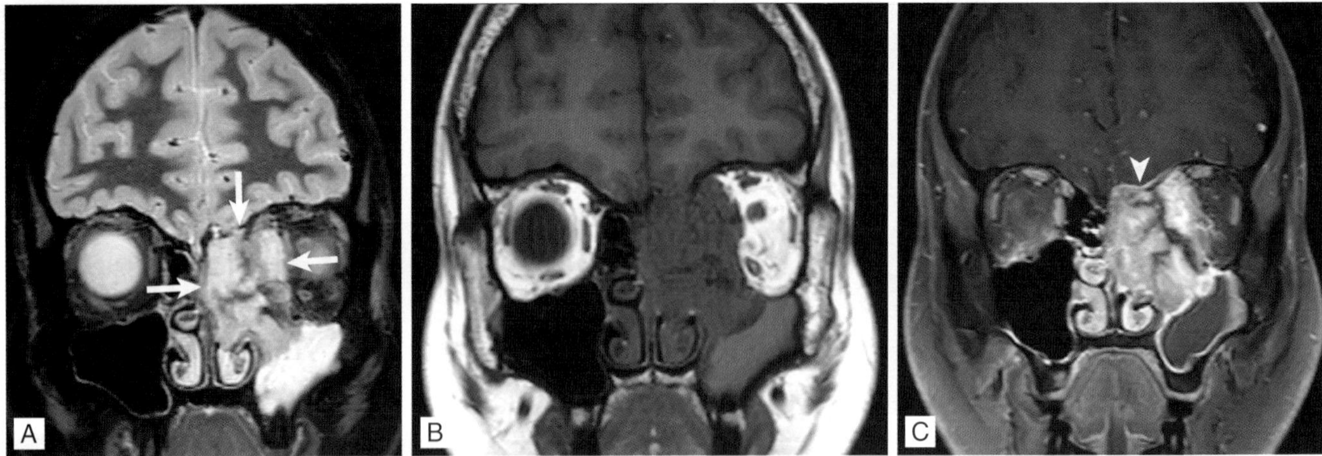

Figure 73.15 Esthesioneuroblastoma. Coronal T2 (A), T1 (B), and contrast-enhanced T1-weighted MRI shows an aggressive mass occupying the left nasal cavity and invading the left orbit (*arrows*). There was mild enhancement of the dura in the left anterior skull base (*arrowhead*), without parenchymal invasion.

and meta-iodobenzlyguanidine (MIBG) scans are useful adjunct to conventional imaging in the initial staging and restaging of esthesioneuroblastoma.

Chordoma

Chordoma is uncommon locally invasive tumor of the axial skeleton that originates from the embryonic remnants of the primitive notochord [22,23]. It can be histologically indistinguishable from EP, except by identifying infiltrative growth pattern along the margins of the chordoma. Chordomas are found along the axial skeleton with relatively even distribution among three locations, either the spheno-occipital (30–35%), sacrococcygeal (30–50%), or vertebral body (15–30%) [22]. Within the clivus, chordoma is classically centrally located, intraosseous and extraosseous lesion that projects posteriorly indenting the pons with "thumb sign" or thumbing of the pons appearance. BNCT is a poorly recognized entity, usually asymptomatic and discovered incidentally on imaging of the head or spine. The majority of BNCTs are intraosseous lesions with 50% of the lesions involving the skull base. Apart from the characteristic location of these lesions (intraosseous vs intra/extraosseous), the imaging findings can be confusing.

Chordomas are typically well-circumscribed expansile lesion and show variable osteolysis (Fig. 73.16A), sometimes with marginal sclerosis. Irregular intratumoral calcifications can be seen, thought to represent sequestra of normal bone, with intralesional hemorrhage or necrosis [22,24]. Chordomas are T1 hypo- or isointense and mostly T2 hyperintense [22,24] (Fig. 73.16B). Intralesional heterogeneity with small foci of T1 hyperintensity can be seen related to intratumoral hemorrhage or mucus pool. Susceptibility weighted imaging (SWI) or gradient recalled echo (GRE) images will demonstrate variable blooming artifact related to the intralesional hemorrhage. There is heterogeneous enhancement following the administration of gadolinium with a honeycomb appearance corresponding to low T1 signal areas within the tumor [22,24] (Fig. 73.16C). Greater intralesional enhancement has been associated with poorer prognosis [25]. All BNCTs demonstrate mild osteosclerosis without associated osteolytic changes, and are typically T1 hypo- or isointense with hyperintense T2 signal, usually without enhancement or restricted diffusion [24].

Chondrosarcoma

Chondrosarcomas of the skull base are rare tumors most commonly located off the midline compared to chordomas that are usually midline [23,26]. Clinical presentation is usually due to mass effect, either on the adjacent brainstem and brain, or cranial neuropathy. Chondrosarcomas probably arise from embryonal

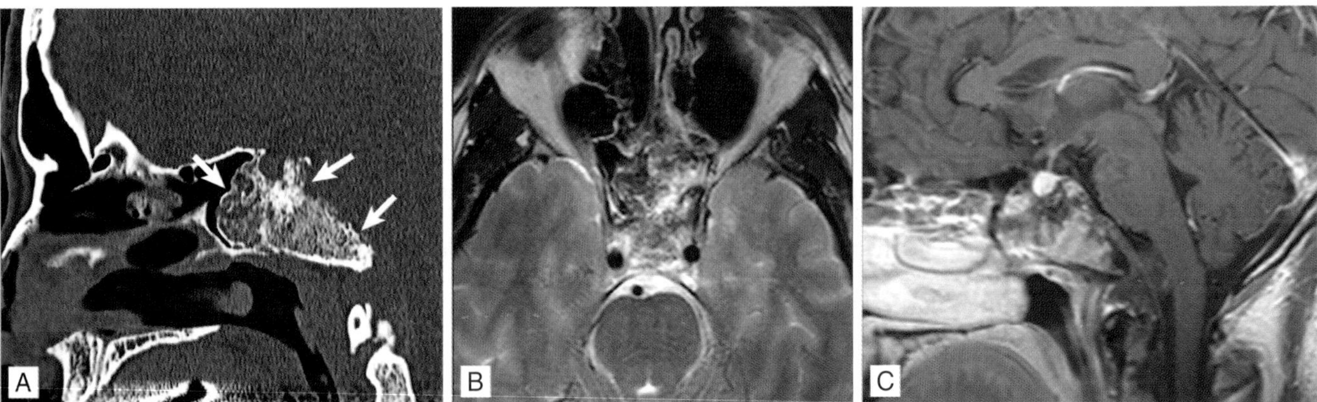

Figure 73.16 Chordoma. Sagittal CT (A) through the midline show large irregularly marginated and mixed lytic and sclerotic lesion of the bony clivus (*arrows*). The lesion has heterogeneous appearance on axial T2-weighted (B) and enhancement on post-contrast enhanced T1 sequence (C), respectively.

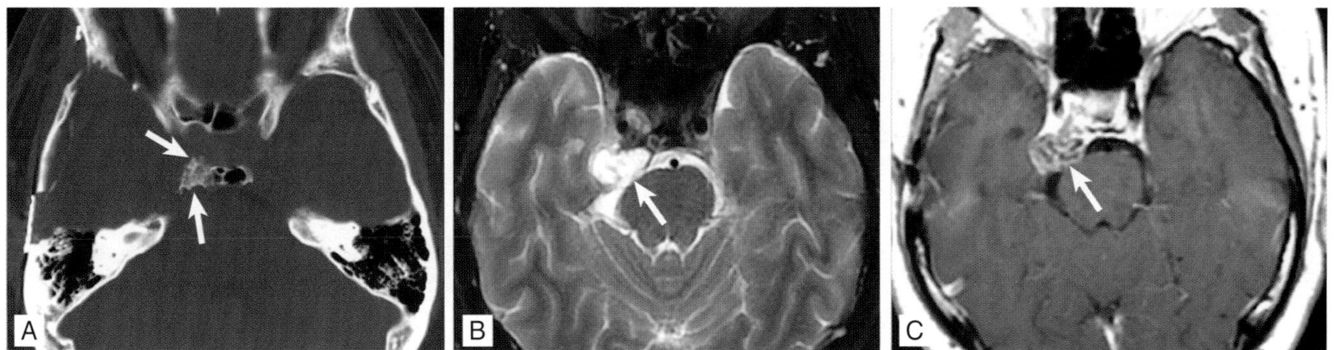

Figure 73.17 Chondrosarcoma. (A) Axial CT image shows a lytic mass centered near the right petro-clival fissure (*arrows*). The lesion has intralesion calcifications. The lesion is markedly hyperintense on axial T2 (B) and show "stippled" type of enhancement post-contrast enhanced T1-weighted MRI (C).

rest cells, most commonly at the petro-occipital synchondrosis or at the sphenoethmoidal junction and sella turcica [26,27]. Rare cases of chondrosarcoma have been reported arising from the choroid plexus, or dura matter [28], presumably from heterotopic cartilaginous rests or metaplasia.

Just like many other pathologies of the skull base, CT and MRI are complementary in imaging of chondrosarcoma. CT scan can characterize the relationship to the skull base structures, and exquisitely depicts intralesional calcification with osteolytic changes of the contiguous skull base [26,27] (Fig. 73.17A). There is typically minimal-to-moderate contrast enhancement. MRI can better characterize the extent of the lesion and relationship to neural structures [26]. MRI will demonstrate T1 hypointensity and T2 hyperintensity with heterogeneous enhancement (Fig. 73.17B–C). Hypointense or heterogeneous T2 signal is likely caused by matrix mineralization, intralesional hemorrhage, and fibrocartilaginous elements [27]. There are no reliable imaging characteristics to differentiate chondrosarcoma from chordoma, apart from their location.

Plasmacytoma

Plasmacytoma is a rare solitary tumor of neoplastic monoclonal plasma cells, most commonly occurs in bone (~70%), and less frequently presents as extramedullary lesion (~30%). It is typically associated with latent systemic disease with minimal or no systemic features. Involvement of the skull base is a rare entity mostly seen in the sphenoclival and petrous apex regions [29]. It is part of a larger differential diagnosis that includes chordoma, nasopharyngeal carcinoma, metastatic carcinoma, lymphoma, and multiple myeloma. CT scan can demonstrate osteolytic lesion or soft tissue mass (Fig. 73.18A). MRI features are nonspecific with T1 isointensity and T2 hyperintensity with heterogeneous enhancement [29,30] (Fig. 73.18B).

Perineural Spread

PNS is an important imaging feature of head and neck malignancies, with significant impact on management and prognosis. It is important to realize that PNS differs from perineural invasion, with the former is a radiological finding, compared to later which is a histological finding of tumor cell infiltration [3,30]. PNS can be seen in any of the head and neck malignancies, with adenoid cystic carcinomas of the salivary glands is the most notorious for producing PNS [3,30]. Mucosal and cutaneous squamous cell carcinomas are the most frequent malignancies associated with PNS, mostly due to its common incidence (Fig. 73.19A).

Typical imaging findings of PNS on CT scan include foraminal enlargement with or without destruction, and abnormal

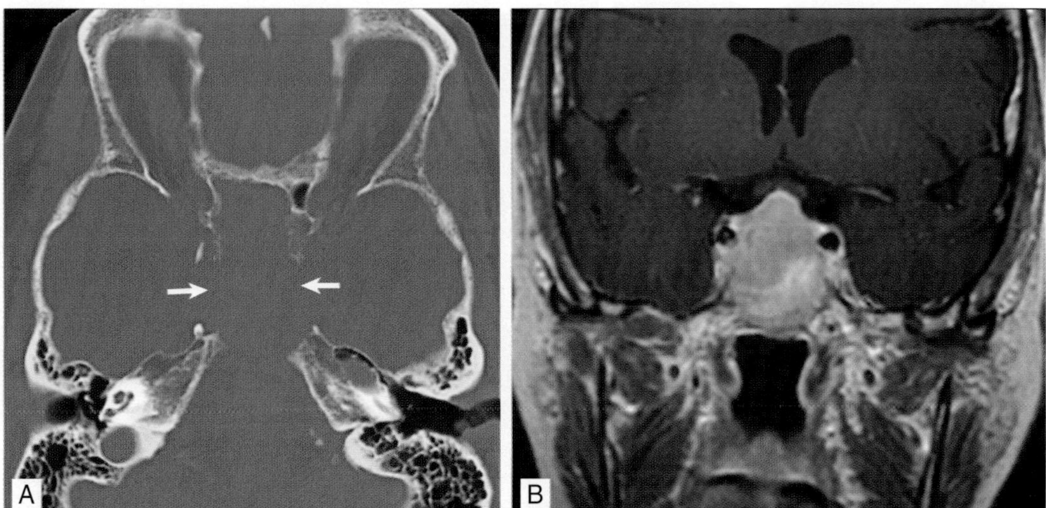

Figure 73.18 Plasmacytoma. (A) Axial CT at the level of central skull base and sphenoid sinus show a large aggressive lytic lesion involving the bony clivus (*arrows*). The lesion is iso to mildly hypointense on coronal T2-weighted MRI (not shown) and show moderate to avid post-contrast enhancement (B). The pituitary gland was elevated by this mass, but was separate.

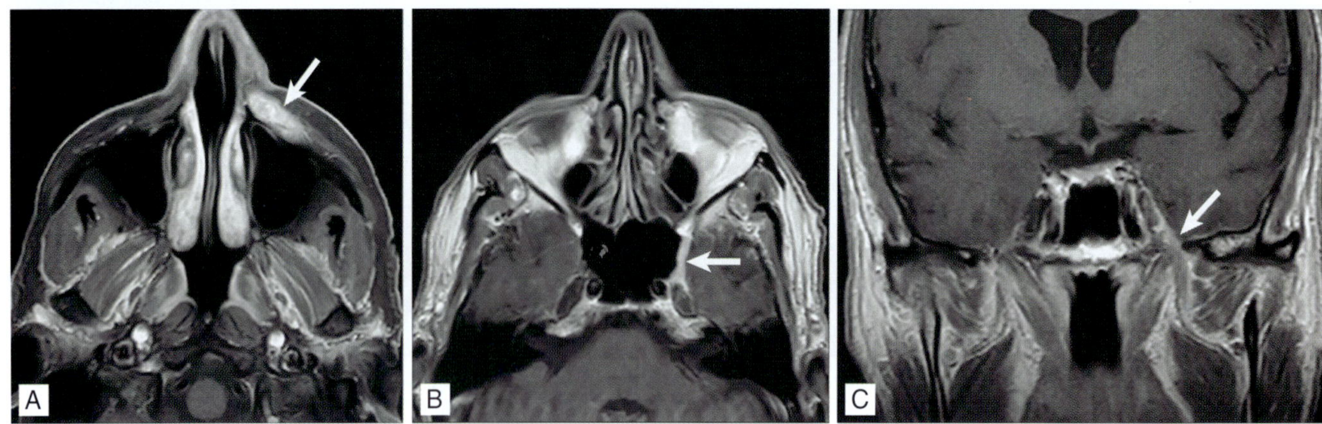

Figure 73.19 Perineural spread of squamous cell carcinoma. (A) Axial and coronal (B, C) post-contrast enhanced T1-weighted MRI shows an enhancing mass anterior to the left maxillary sinus which was proven for squamous cell carcinoma (*arrow*). On further inspection, there is retrograde extension of tumor though the second (V2) division of left trigeminal nerve with mild asymmetric enhancement of the left Meckel cave (*arrow*). Antegrade extension of cancer along the third (V3) division of left trigeminal nerve (*arrow* in C) is also seen.

enhancement within the foramen or canal [3,30]. MRI is superior to CT for evaluation of PNS, demonstrating nerve thickening, loss of the fat surrounding the nerve, and abnormal neural contrast enhancement (Fig. 73.19B–C).

Benign Neoplasms

Schwannoma

Intracranial schwannomas are common benign tumors, mostly sporadic, with few syndromic associations seen in neurofibromatosis type II and schwannomatosis syndrome. Schwannomas are most frequently encountered in middle-aged and elderly adults with recognized female predilection [31]. Clinical presentation depends on the nerve involved and the location of involvement. Larger tumors can result in symptoms related to mass effect on the surrounding structures. Any cranial nerve can be involved, though involvement of the sensory nerves is more common compared to the uncommon involvement of the pure motor nerves. The vast majority of intracranial schwannomas arises from the vestibular division of the vestibulocochlear cranial nerve, and less frequently in the trigeminal, facial, and glossopharyngeal nerves [31] (Figs. 73.20A–B and 73.21A–B).

The slow growth of intracranial schwannomas results in its typical imaging features with well-defined margins (Fig. 73.20A) and smooth expansion of osseous foramina, with deformation of the brain in large lesions. CT demonstrates isodense or hypodense lesion, with variable enhancement [31]. Intralesional cystic changes can be seen as prominent hypodense areas. MRI characteristics of individual schwannomas are typically related to its composition and the nerve of origin. Schwannomas typically have hyperintense or isointense T2 signal [23,30]. The presence of heterogeneous T2 hyperintense signal is attributed to the tumor's composition with regions of compactly arranged cells (Antoni type A) which demonstrate slightly darker T2 signal, adjacent to distinct loosely arranged cells (Antoni type B) which have brighter T2 signal [32] (Figs. 73.20A and 73.21B). The target sign typically seen in peripheral neurogenic tumors is essentially never seen at imaging

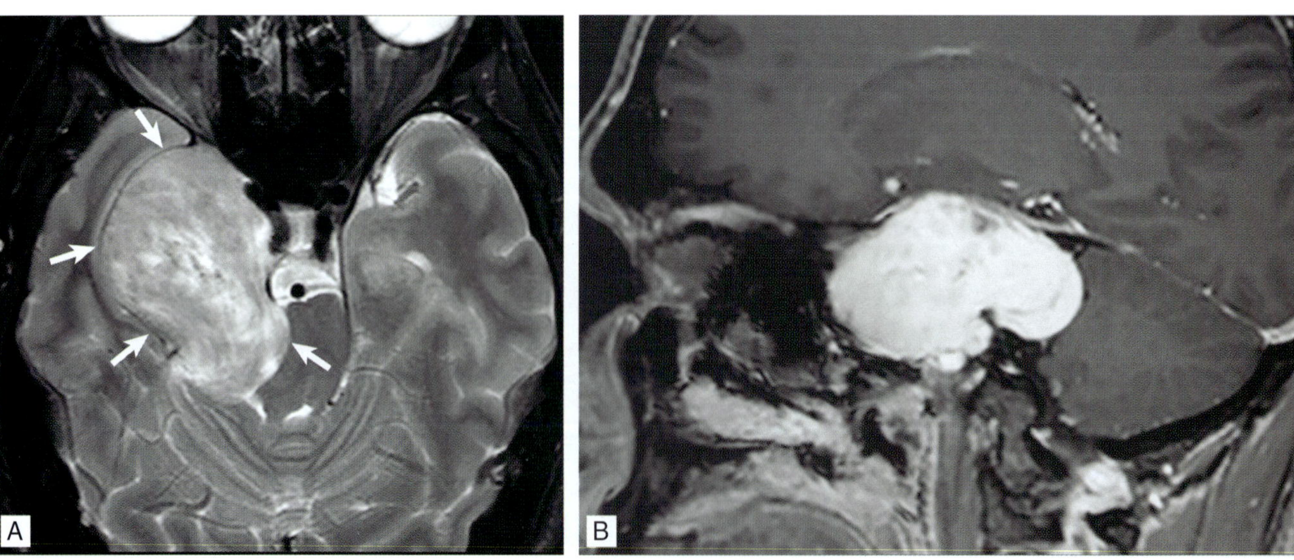

Figure 73.20 Trigeminal nerve schwannoma. (A) Axial T2 and (B) sagittal post-contrast enhanced T1-weighted MRI shows large and well-defined soft tissue mass at the level of right middle cranial fossa along the course of the trigeminal nerve extending toward right Meckel cave (*arrows*). The lesion is hyperintense with mild heterogeneity on T2 image and shows avid post-contrast enhancement.

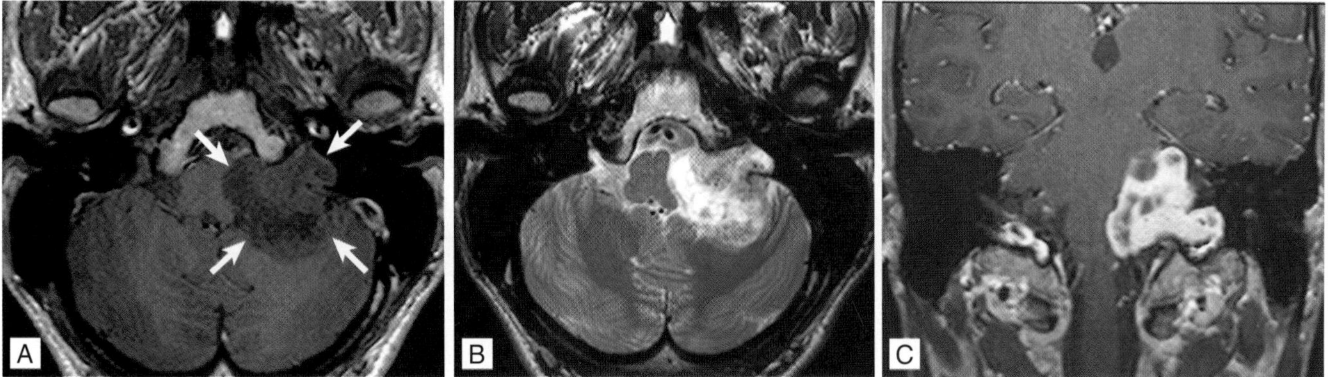

Figure 73.21 Jugular foramen schwannoma. (A) Axial T1, (B) axial T2, and (C) coronal post-contrast enhanced T1-weighted MRI shows a large well-defined soft tissue mass at the level of left jugular foramen extending into the left carotid space (*arrows*). The lesion is hypointense on T1, hyperintense with mild heterogeneity on T2 image and show marked post-contrast enhancement.

of intracranial schwannomas [31]. On T1-weighted images, these lesions have isointense or hypointense signal and demonstrate avid, mostly heterogeneous, enhancement after contrast material administration, with or without cystic changes [23–30] (Fig. 73.20B). Larger lesions commonly have heterogeneous enhancement, cystic spaces, and intralesional hemorrhage, and sometimes peritumoral cysts [23,30] (Fig. 73.21C).

Meningioma

Meningiomas are nonglial neoplasm that originates from the meningocytes or arachnoid cap cells of the meninges. Meningiomas are common primary intradural lesions, located anywhere that meninges are present, or can rarely present as primary extradural or ectopic extracranial lesions related to rest cells [33]. The majority of meningiomas have typical radiologic appearance with benign course; however there is a wide array of histological variants resulting in variable imaging features with, uncommonly, an aggressive biological behavior. Meningiomas are more common in female, with a female-to-male ratio of approximately 2:1. Many small meningiomas are entirely asymptomatic. Meningiomas may also become symptomatic due to mass effect, particularly lesions at the skull base as they involve the sphenoid ridge, juxtasellar or olfactory groove/planum sphenoidale region (Fig. 73.22A–B). Based on the WHO classification for CNS tumors, meningiomas are graded into benign grade I (70%), atypical grade II (30%), or anaplastic grade III (~1%) lesions [33].

Noncontrast CT typically demonstrate slightly hyperdense lesion compared to normal brain (60%), while the rest are relatively isodense [34,35], or rarely hypodense [34]. Up to one-third of the lesions have intralesional calcification. The majority of meningiomas demonstrate homogeneously contrast enhancement (Figs. 73.22C and 73.23A), with malignant or cystic variants demonstrate more heterogeneity/less intense enhancement. Bony hyperostosis is typically seen associated with skull base meningioma [35]. This is different than intraosseous meningioma, a rare meningioma subtype, that represents primary extradural meningioma with osteoblastic changes [35] or less frequently osteolytic changes [36] (Fig. 73.23B). Osteolytic and destructive changes are typically seen in higher grade tumors.

Signal changes on T1-weighted images are not particularly useful in discriminating pathologic subtype of meningiomas, with the majority of the lesions being isointense or hypointense [34, 37]. Signal intensity on T2-weighted images has a higher correlation with the histopathologic findings [37]. Predominantly fibroblastic or transitional meningiomas typically demonstrate T2 hypointense signal compared to the cortex (Fig. 73.22A), compared to syncytial or angioblastic meningiomas that are typically T2 hyperintense [37]. The appearance of meningiomas on DWI images is variable; however, the ADC value has no significance in determining histological behavior or in differentiating histopathological subtypes of meningiomas [38]. Dural tail is most commonly seen in meningiomas (60–72%), though it is not pathognomonic and can be seen with a variety of intraaxial and extraaxial pathologies

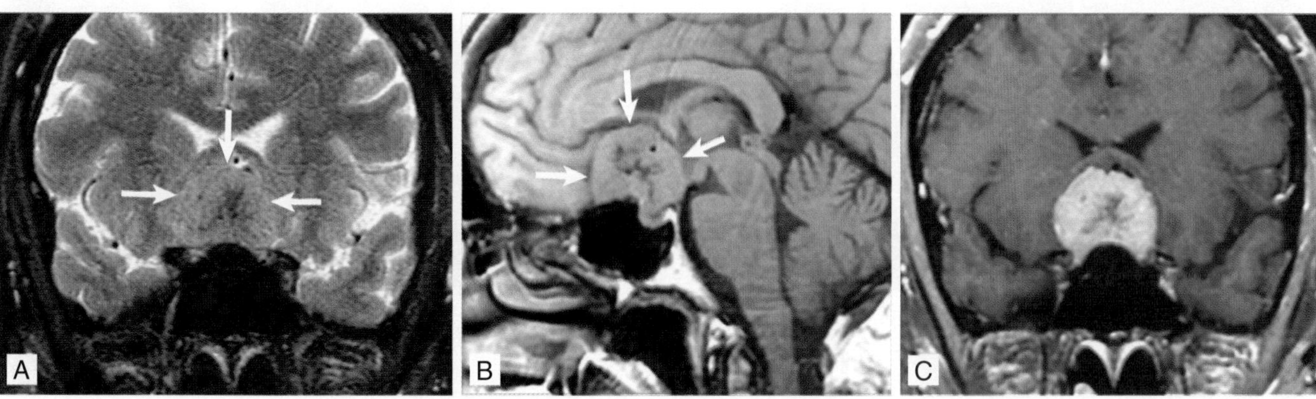

Figure 73.22 Planum sphenoidale meningioma. (A) Coronal T2, (B) sagittal T1, and (C) coronal post-contrast enhanced T1-weighted MRI show a large, well-defined, extraaxial soft tissue mass at the level of planum sphenoidale/anterior skull base (*arrows*). The lesion is isointense on T1, iso to mildly hyperintense on T2 and shows marked post-contrast enhancement.

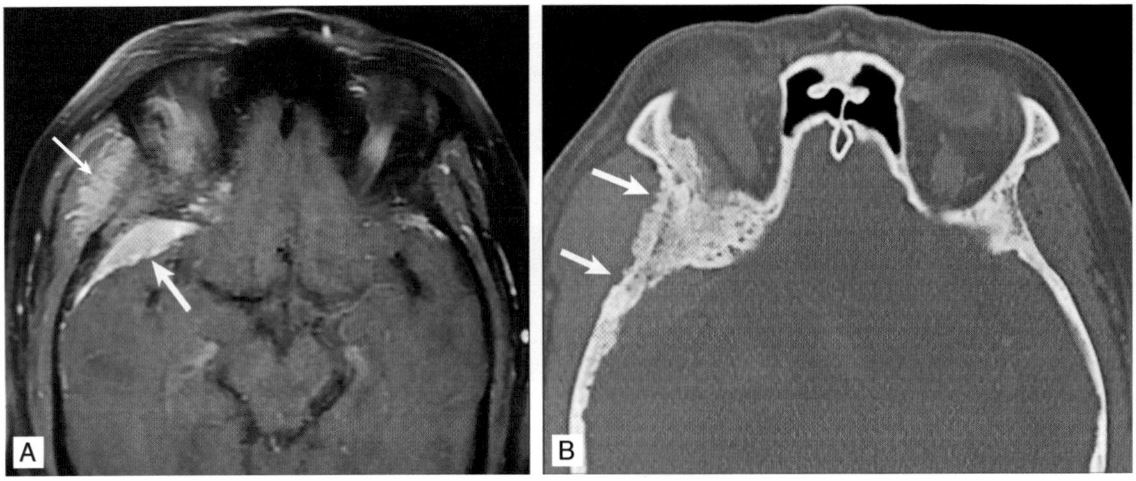

Figure 73.23 Intraosseous meningioma. (A) Axial post-contrast enhanced T1-weighted MRI shows a large, extra-axial soft tissue mass along the right greater wing of sphenoid bone (*large arrow*) with extension in the overlying right masticator space (*small arrow*). (B) Axial CT through the same level shows expansion and sclerosis suggesting intraosseous extension (*arrows*).

[39]. A variable amount of vasogenic edema in the adjacent brain parenchyma is seen in up to 75% of the lesions [35].

Some meningioma variants can vary dramatically in their imaging appearance. A burnt-out meningioma, typically psammomatous meningioma or osseous metaplastic subtype, describes a meningioma that is completely calcified/ossified. Cystic meningioma is uncommon variant characterized by intratumoral cyst formation, peritumoral cysts, or reactive intraparenchymal cysts [35]. Cystic meningiomas should not be confused with the rare microcystic meningiomas, a distinct variant, in which the cysts are microscopic. Microcystic meningiomas are typically hypodense on CT scan with bony hyperostosis. The lesion is fluid isointense on T1- and T2-weighted images with avid enhancement, related to its abundant vascularity.

Benign Fibro-osseous Lesions

A multitude of fibro-osseous lesions can involve the skull base, including FD, ossifying fibroma, or Paget disease. Contrary to Paget disease that mostly involves the calvarium, FD is a disease of the medullary cavity, involving the maxillofacial, skull base, and calvarial osseous structures [40]. FD is seen in children and young adults, compared to late presentation of Paget disease that is typically seen after the fifth decade of life [30]. Ossifying fibroma represent an aggressive monostotic form of FD [30]. FD is related to localized defect in osteoblastic differentiation and maturation, with replacement of normal marrow with large fibrous stroma and islands of immature woven bone. The underlying cause of FD is not fully understood, though it is probably caused by de novo mutation in a *GNAS1* gene [41].

Craniofacial involvement in FD occurs in 50% of the patients, with variable radiographic appearance. Plain radiographs demonstrate bony expansion with displacement of the outer table and relative sparing of the inner table, in contrast to Paget disease that typically involve the inner table [40]. The affected bones in FD appear either sclerotic or demonstrate bubbly cystic changes. It commonly crosses the sutures, and results in obliteration of the paranasal sinuses. CT scan will demonstrate a thin cortical outline with loss of the normal corticomedullary differentiation in the affected bones [40], with homogeneous pagetoid, or ground glass appearance (56%), homogeneous sclerotic pattern (23%), or a cystic variety (21%) (Fig. 73.24A). Histologic correlates have shown an equal

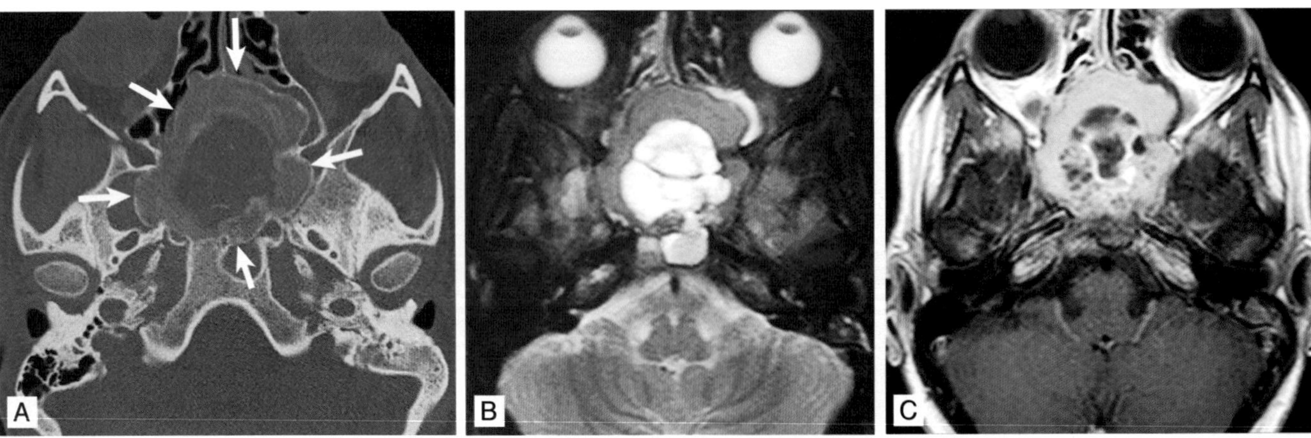

Figure 73.24 Fibrous dysplasia. (A) Axial CT mage at the level of central skull base shows a well-defined expansile lesion involving the sphenoid sinuses and basisphenoid (*arrows*). The lesion has well-defined margins and "hazy" internal matrix, which is highly suggestive for fibrous dysplasia. The lesion has heterogeneous appearance on axial T2 (B) and post-contrast enhanced T1-weighted MRI (C), mimicking a more aggressive lesion.

TABLE 73.6 Petrous Apex Lesions

- Asymmetric marrow/asymmetric pneumatization
- Cholesterol granuloma
- Congenital cholesteatoma
- Mucocele of the petrous apex
- Petrous apex cephalocele
- Petrous apicitis
- Malignant tumors: skull base chondrosarcoma, chordoma, or metastasis

mixture of fibrous tissue and woven trabecular bone in pagetoid lesions, compared to predominance of osseous elements in sclerotic type and fibrous elements in cystic variety [41]. The MRI features of FD can be sometimes confusing and resemble that of tumors, in contrast with the distinctive features of FD seen on radiography and CT (Fig. 73.24B,C). The signal intensity on T1- and T2-weighted images and the degree of contrast enhancement depend on the underlying histologic changes and the amounts of bony trabeculae, cellularity, or collagen [41]. FD lesions show well-defined borders with intermediate-to-low signal intensity on T1 and intermediate-to-high intensity on T2-weighted images [41]. A lower T2 signal is typically associated with higher bony trabeculae, whereas higher T2 signal is associated with fewer bony trabeculae. A cystic variant of FD lesions will appear T2 hyperintense. FD lesions typically demonstrate some degree of enhancement following gadolinium administration.

Cholesterol Granuloma

Cholesterol granuloma is the most common cystic lesion of the petrous apex, though it can occur in the mastoid segment or the middle ear [42,43]. On otoscopy, it may appear as a "blue lesion" [42], hence the name blue-domed cyst [43]. The cyst is filled with viscous brown fluid and cholesterol crystals, with granulation tissues, which are often contained within a thick fibrous capsule that lacks a true epithelial lining. The exact pathogenesis of cholesterol granuloma is unknown. It is probably related to Eustachian tube dysfunction causing inadequate ventilation of petrous apex air cells, which results in negative pressure, mucosal congestion, and repeated hemorrhage [43]. There is a foreign-body reaction that is typically seen related to local tissue breakdown and cholesterol formation. A newer theory suggests that hyperplastic mucosa leads to invasion of the underlying bone and exposure of bone marrow [44], which might hemorrhage resulting in subsequent cyst formation.

There are multiple pathological processes that involve the petrous apex (Table 73.6). Petrous apex effusion or trapped fluid, a "leave me alone" lesion, is a common incidental finding on routine imaging studies [45], probably related to middle ear infection resulting in obstruction of the air cell track pathways, with subsequent trapping of fluid in the petrous apex [45]. Cholesterol granuloma is pathologically different compared to mucocele, a rare entity at the petrous apex, which is characterized by an obstructed air cell containing respiratory epithelium. Congenital cholesteatoma of the petrous apex is uncommon, related to aberrant ectoderm trapped during embryogenesis. This is more common compared to the rare acquired cholesteatoma. Cholesteatoma contains keratinized, desquamated epithelial collection, without cholesterol or lipids.

Cholesterol granuloma on CT scan appears expansile, well-marginated lesion with thin overlying bone, reflecting its slow growth [42,43] (Fig. 73.25A). The lesion is isodense to brain, and sometimes demonstrates a peripheral rim of enhancement. There may be osseous dehiscence when the lesion is large. On MR images, the cholesterol granuloma will be hyperintense on T1- and T2-weighted images and may contain low signal linear areas compatible with septations [42] (Fig. 73.25B,C). This is likely related to the lesion's contents with paramagnetic effect of extracellular methemoglobin from blood breakdown products. Faint peripheral enhancement may be seen. In contrast to cholesterol granuloma, trapped fluid in the petrous apex appears hypo- or isointense on T1 and hyperintense on T2-weighted images, with no enhancement with gadolinium [45]. MRI appearance of petrous apex cholesteatoma is distinctive with CSF isointense collection on T1- and T2-weighted images, along with hyperintense signal on FLAIR and diffusion weighted images [42,43].

Glomus Tumors

Paraganglioma of the skull base typically occurs in the jugular fossa (glomus jugulare) or arising from the tympanic plexus in the middle ear cavity (glomus tympanicum). The majority of the lesions present in adults with pulsatile tinnitus, hearing loss, or multiple cranial neuropathies depending on the lesion's size. Only 3% of all head-neck paragangliomas secrete catecholamines.

CT typically demonstrates irregularly erosive changes of the jugular fossa [46] (Fig. 73.26A). Erosion of the caroticojugular spine between the carotid canal and jugular fossa (Phelp sign) and jugular spine can be seen as the tumor enlarges, differentiating paraganglioma from jugular fossa pseudolesions. Tumor can extend within the petrous bone, encasing the ossicular chain, though destruction of the ossicular chain is not typical [46]. Angiographic appearance is typically of a hypervascular lesion, with enlarged

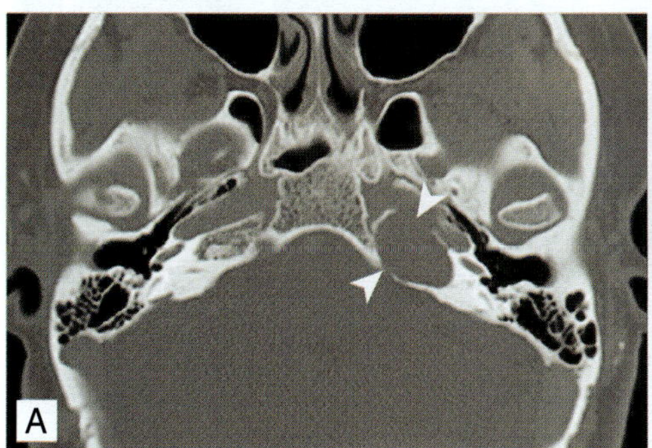

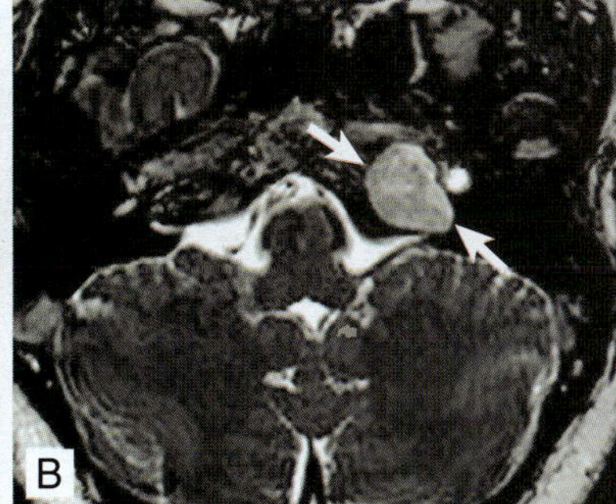

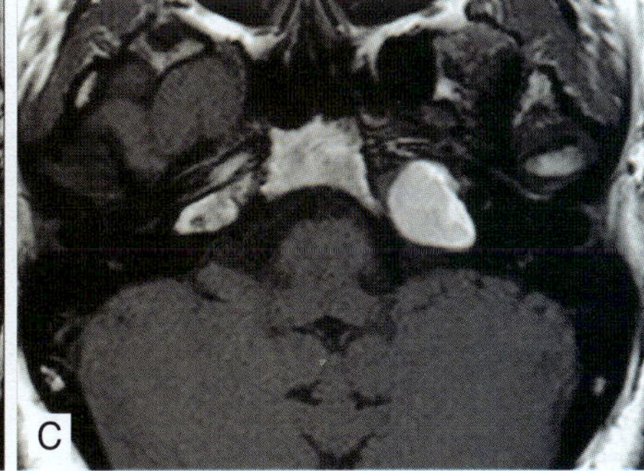

Figure 73.25 Petrous apex cholesterol granuloma. (A) Axial CT image show a well-defined, lytic lesion of the left petrous temporal bone with bony remodeling along the margins (*arrows*). (B) Axial T2 and (C) axial T1-weighted MRI shows hyperintense signal from the lesion. There was no enhancement noted (not shown).

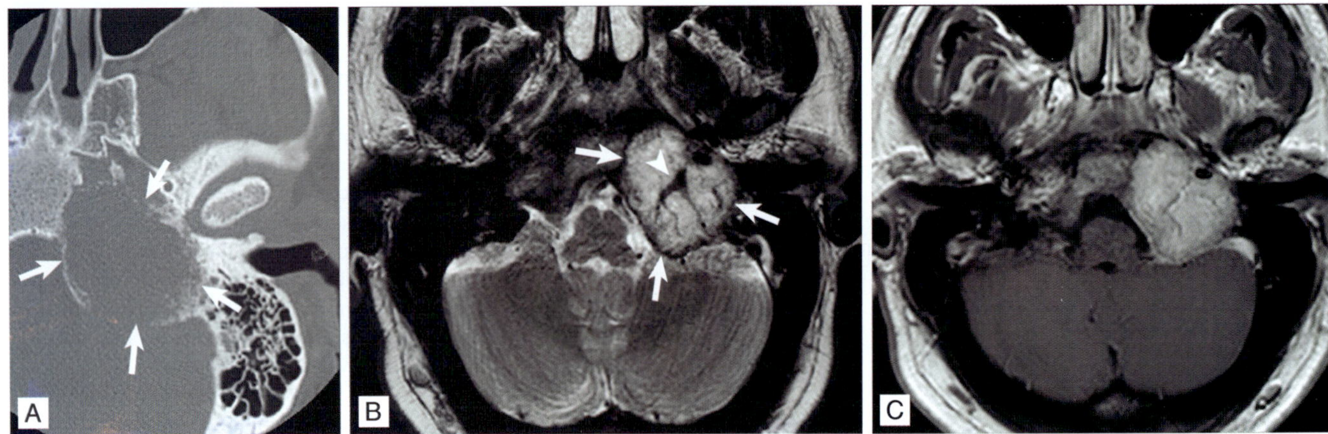

Figure 73.26 Glomus jugulare: [A] Axial CT image show a large mass with permeative bony destruction at the level of left jugular foramen (*arrows*). The lesion is hyperintense on T2 - weighted MRI [B] and reveals marked post-contrast enhancement [C] with prominent flow voids (*arrowhead*) within the lesion.

arterial feeders, mostly the ascending pharyngeal artery, along with early draining veins [46]. Preoperative embolization, typically 1–2 days prior to surgery, can be supportive in patient management.

Glomus tumors are typically T1 hypointense and T2 hyperintense with marked enhancement following gadolinium [46] (Fig. 73.26B,C). The so-called "salt and pepper" appearance is typically seen with lesions greater than 2 cm, with the salt representing blood products from slow flow or intralesional hemorrhage, and the pepper representing flow voids due to high vascularity. This appearance is not pathognomonic for glomus tumors and can be encountered in other hypervascular lesions (e.g. renal metastases). Avid fluorodeoxyglucose (FDG) uptake can be seen on 18FDG PET scan, creating confusion with more aggressive or malignant lesions. Indium-111 labeled octreotide SPECT scan will demonstrate tumoral uptake due to the presence of somatostatin receptors, which is seen in tumors greater than 1.5 cm in diameter [47].

Endolymphatic Sac Tumors

Endolymphatic sac tumors (ELSTs) are very rare tumors of the petrous temporal bone, located in the region of the vestibular aqueduct. ELSTs are most often associated with von Hippel–Lindau disease (VHL), with the presence of bilateral involvement in 30% of VHL patients. CT demonstrates locally aggressive lesion with erosion of petrous bone in an infiltrative or "moth-eaten" pattern with intralesional calcification and intense enhancement [48] (Fig. 73.27A). MRI demonstrates a hypervascular tumor with T1 hyperintensity, with heterogeneous T2 signal and avid enhancement in the noncystic component of the tumor (Fig. 73.27B,C). Tumors larger than 2 cm usually have intralesional flow voids [48].

Infectious and Inflammatory Processes

Infectious Osteomyelitis

Skull base osteomyelitis (SBO) is uncommon but potentially serious, most commonly seen in older diabetic or immunocompromised patients [49]. It typically arises as a complication of sinusitis, ear infection, or can be odontogenic in origin. It results in osseous destruction of the skull base and involves the skull base foramina, causing cranial neuropathies. Intracranial extension can result in epidural abscess, subdural empyema, meningitis, or even cerebritis and cerebral abscess formation. *Staphylococcus aureus* and *Pseudomonas aeruginosa* were the two most common causative pathogens [49].

Radiologic features of SBO may be similar to those of the neoplastic processes, presenting a diagnostic dilemma. CT changes during early stage can be normal or with nonspecific osseous demineralization, along with soft tissue swelling and obliteration of the fat planes. Osseous destruction and bony

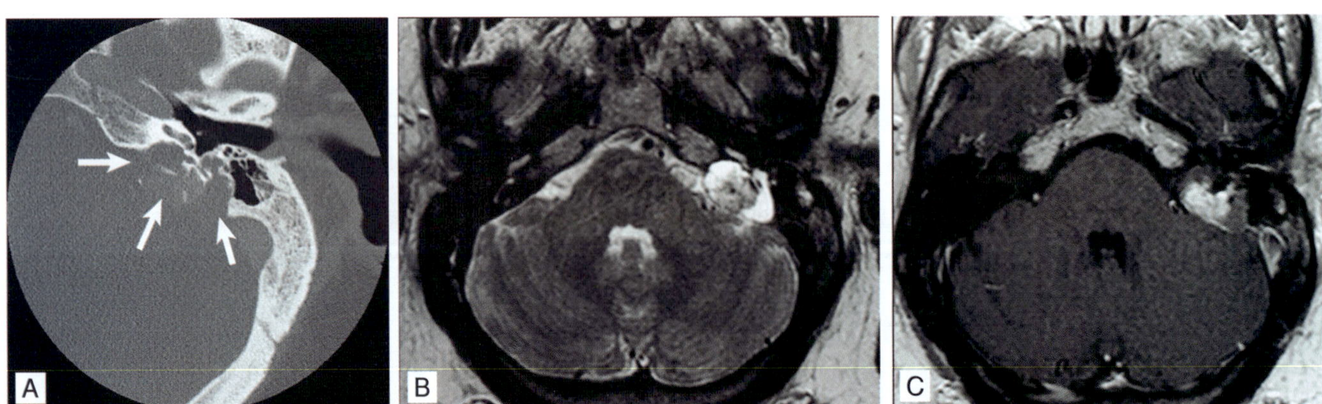

Figure 73.27 Endolymphatic sac tumor. (A) Axial CT show a large expansile and lytic abnormality along the posterior aspect of the left petrous temporal bone (*arrows*). This lesion is heterogeneous on axial T2-weighted MRI (B) and show moderate post-contrast enhancement (C).

sequestration are relatively late phenomena (Fig. 73.28A,B). Bone SPECT scintigraphy and MRI are more sensitive in detecting early osseous changes and determining the extent of the disease [50]. MRI is superior in the evaluation of disease spread to the soft tissues and involvement of the fat planes, dural and cranial nerve involvement, or intracranial complication [50] (Fig. 73.29A–D). The most consistent imaging findings on MRI are T1 hypointensity of the marrow with gadolinium enhancement. Diffusivity values on ADC maps are typically higher compared to those of malignant lesions [51]. Ischemic coagulative necrosis is a distinctive MR finding of angioinvasive fungal osteomyelitis, that is characterized by lack of enhancement with relatively low T2 signal of the involved soft tissues (Fig. 73.30A–C). Tc99 m methylene diphosphonate (MDP) bone SPECT scintigraphy and Tc-99m hexamethylpropyleneamine oxime (HMPAO) labeled white blood cell are sensitive but poorly specific techniques that are rarely used in the assessment of SBO [50].

Potts puffy tumor is a rare clinical complication of acute frontal sinusitis. It is characterized by osteomyelitis of the frontal bone with subgaleal collection and subperiosteal abscess formation [13]. CT scan will demonstrate opacification of the frontal sinuses with swelling of the overlying scalp [13] and sometimes bony sequestration. Intracranial involvement is better evaluated on MRI with thickening and enhancement of the dura, epidural abscess or subdural empyema, and sometimes cerebritis or focal cerebral abscess [13] (Fig. 73.31A–C).

Noninfectious Inflammatory Process

Hypertrophic pachymeningitis is uncommon condition characterized by localized or diffuse inflammatory thickening of the dura. On imaging, it presents as a localized, multifocal, or diffuse dural thickening, and sometimes has a mass-like tumefactive appearance [52]. Early reports were described in relation to tuberculosis or syphilis; however, hypertrophic pachymeningitis has diverse etiology (Table 73.7). Its presentation is nonspecific with progressive cranial nerve palsies, headaches, and cerebellar dysfunction [52], and rarely with seizure. A thickened, hyperdense dura is typically seen on nonenhanced CT scans, involving the tentorium, falx, and retroclival region, with marked enhancement on contrast administration [52]. The thickened dura will appear hypointense on T1- and T2-weighted images with avid enhancement following gadolinium administration [52].

Neurosarcoidosis: Involvement of the central nervous system is relatively common among patients with systemic sarcoidosis [53]. It typically presents with a wide array of manifestations, with lesions potentially involving the leptomeninges, pachymeninges, pituitary gland, and cerebral or spinal parenchyma (Fig. 73.32A–D). Focal or diffuse pachymeningeal thickening may be observed, with isointense signal on T1, hypointense signal on T2-weighted images, and moderate-to-intense contrast enhancement [53]. Simultaneous dural and leptomeningeal involvement is uncommonly observed [53].

Erdheim–Chester disease: Erdheim–Chester disease is a rare non-Langerhans cell, multisystemic histiocytosis, most commonly presenting as multifocal sclerotic lesions, with or without widespread manifestations. Neurologic involvement can be seen in up to half of the cases. Infiltration can involve the intraaxial and extraaxial compartments of the CNS, which can be symptomatic or asymptomatic [54]. The imaging features of intracranial lesions can have infiltrative pattern, widespread or focal meningeal pattern, or composite pattern of infiltrative and meningeal lesions [54].

IgG4-related disease: Immunoglobulin G4 (IgG4) related disease is a fibroinflammatory condition that can affect nearly any organ system. It was recognized as a systemic disease in 2003, characterized by fibro-inflammatory lesions rich in IgG4-positive plasma cells and often elevated serum IgG4 concentrations [55]. Central nervous system (CNS) involvement is uncommon, with hypopituitarism secondary to IgG4-related hypophysitis and pachymeningitis being the most common manifestations. MRI will demonstrate localized or less often diffuse dural thickening (Fig. 73.33). Tumefactive hypertrophic pachymeningitis is uncommon mass–like thickening of the dura [52].

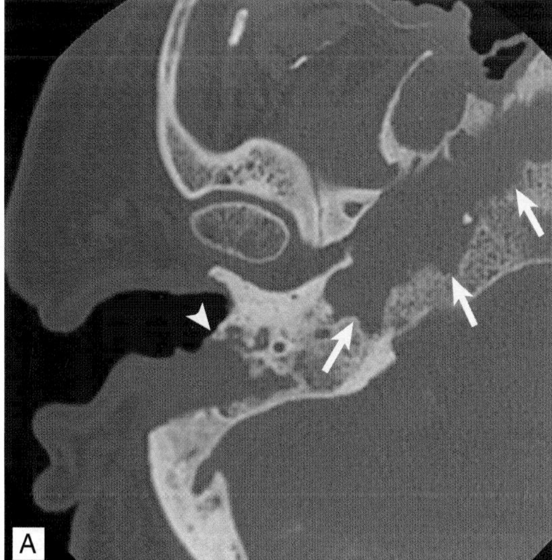

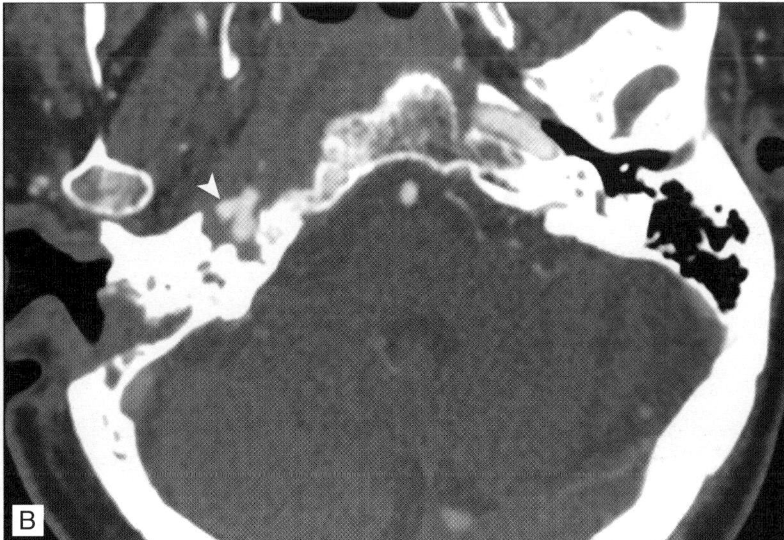

Figure 73.28 Skull base osteomyelitis. (A) Axial CT through the right petrous apex and skull base show an ill-defined lytic abnormality involving the right petrous apex, right basisphenoid level (*arrows*). Postsurgical changes are noted in the right mastoid bone (*arrowhead*). (B) CT angiogram show focal outpouching from the petrous segment of the right internal carotid artery suggestive for pseudoaneurysm (*arrowhead*), a complication from skull base osteomyelitis.

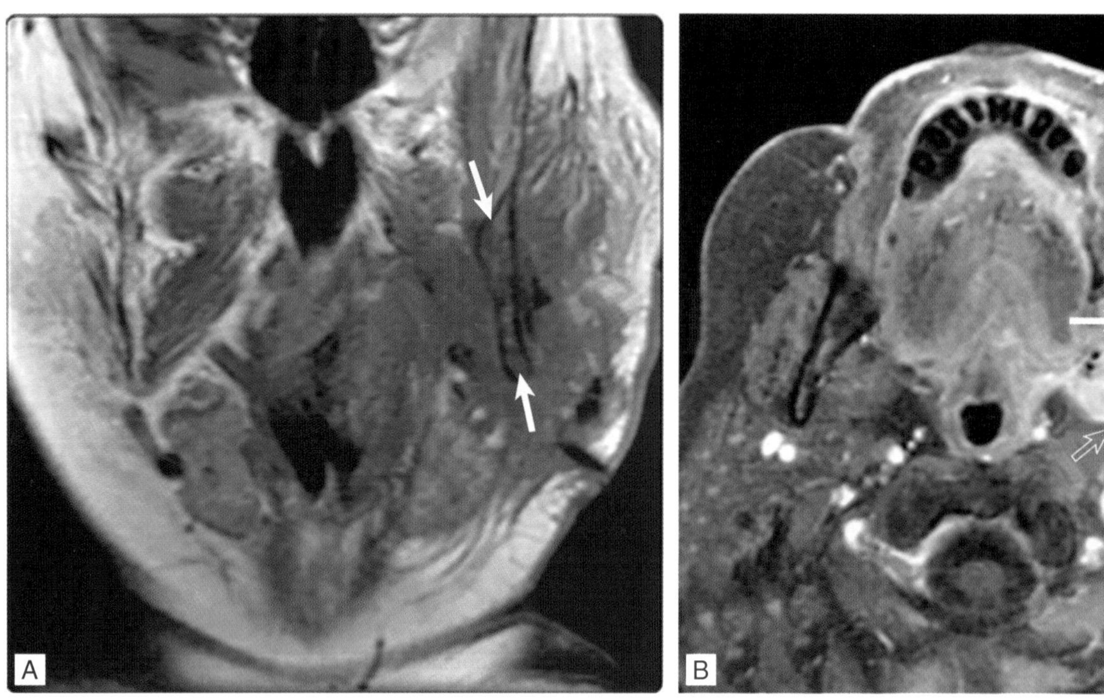

Figure 74.14 (A) Coronal T1WI MR shows 79-year-old with recurrent masticator space abscess 12 weeks after initial diagnosis and previous drainage. Normal high-signal marrow fat has been completely replaced in the left mandible consistent with osteomyelitis (*arrows*). (B) Axial T1Wi C+ fat-saturated MR in the same patient reveals diffuse enhancement of the left marrow space (*arrow*) with masticator space enhancement (phlegmon) (*open arrow*) and small lateral compartment abscess (*curved arrow*). (Adapted from: LM Koenig, D Tamimi, et al. Diagnostic imaging: oral and maxillofacial, second ed., Elsevier; 2017.)

density presentation, and periosteal reaction that is more prominent. Sequestra will have low-signal intensity on T1 and STIR and the surrounding tissue will have high-signal intensity on T2 and STIR (Fig. 74.14). Nuclear medicine imaging using three-phase bone scintigraphy with Tc-99m-labeled methyl disphosphonate can be useful in diagnosing early osteomyelitis. ^{18}F-Fluorodeoxyglucose positron emission tomography (FDG-PET) can be used in cases of chronic osteomyelitis [12] (Fig. 74.15).

b) ***Periodontal inflammation***: This is inflammation of the supporting structures of teeth. Periodontal disease starts with gingivitis (a clinical diagnosis) which may progress to periodontal bone loss. The bone loss may be mild, moderate, or severe and may affect the furcation area (Fig. 74.16). Severe bone loss can result in tooth loss, thus prevention through good oral hygiene practices and early diagnosis of gingivitis and periodontitis is important. The biggest consideration for a general radiologist is to make the distinction between bone loss due to periodontal disease and that due to malignancy.

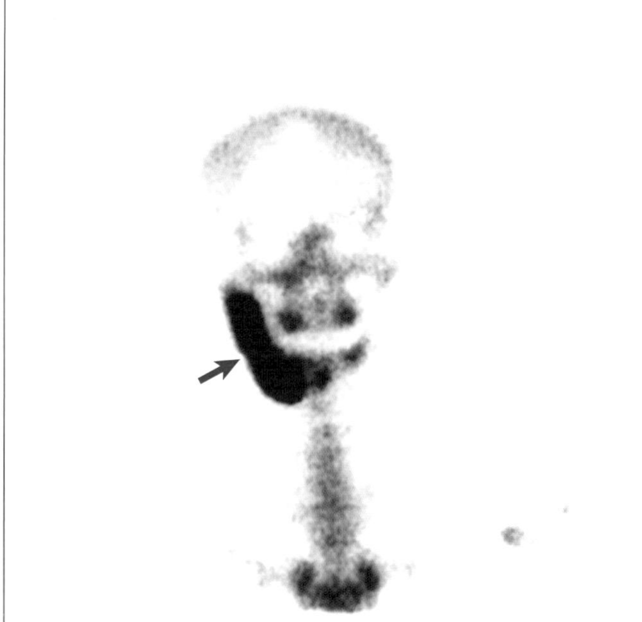

Figure 74.15 Anterior Tc-99m bone scan of a patient with osteomyelitis of the right mandible shows profound uptake of the tracer. (Adapted from: LM Koenig, D Tamimi, et al. Diagnostic imaging: oral and maxillofacial, second ed., Elsevier; 2017.)

Benign Odontogenic Lesions

The inflammatory benign lesions of the jaws arise from embryonic histologic structures that give rise to dental tissues. These are either ectodermal or ectomesenchymal cells. The ectodermal cells give rise to tooth enamel and the ectomesenchymal cells give rise to dentin, cementum, and the dental papilla that is the origin of the periodontium [13,14]. Benign odontogenic lesions can be divided into cysts and tumors. The cysts can be inflammatory or noninflammatory. One of the inflammatory cysts, the radicular cyst was covered previously in the previous section. It is important to note that because of the nature of the oral cavity with its flora, caries/pulp necrosis process, and numerous dental procedures, any noninflammatory cyst can become secondarily infected, and one should look for signs of that inflammation (marked sclerosis of the borders). It should also be noted that, very rarely, some benign odontogenic lesions can undergo malignant

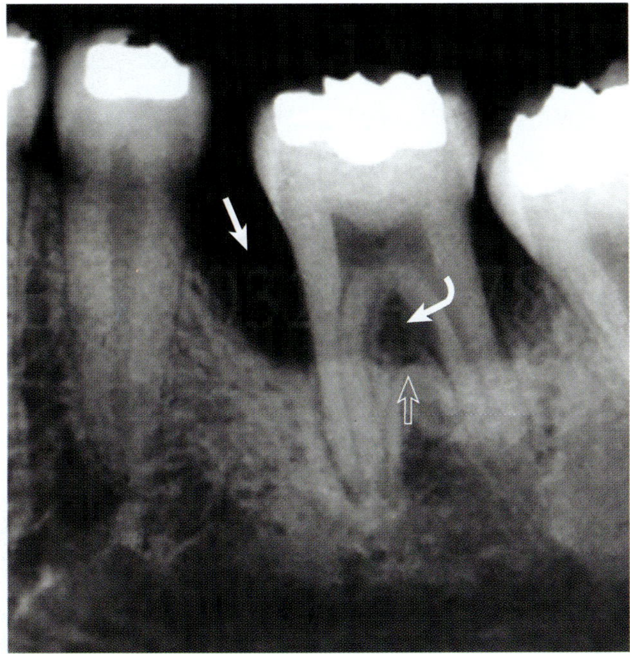

Figure 74.16 Intraoral periapical radiograph of the mandibular left first molar shows moderate periodontal bone loss (*open arrow*) with root furcation involvement (*curved arrrow*). (Adapted from: LM Koenig, D Tamimi, et al. Diagnostic imaging: oral and maxillofacial, second ed., Elsevier; 2017.)

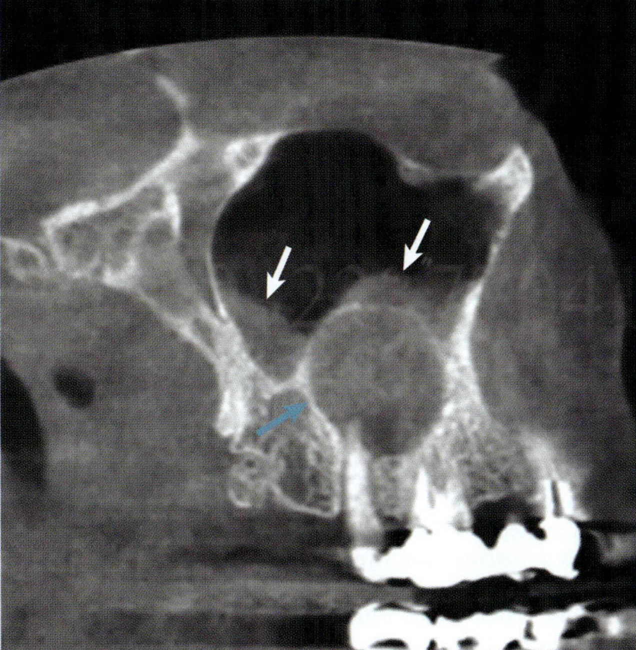

Figure 74.17 Sagittal CBCT shows a large radicular cyst lifting the floor of the maxillary sinus (*blue arrow*) and occupying the inferior third of the sinus. Note the inflammatory changes within the sinus (*white arrows*) which may be secondary to the odontogenic inflammation. (Adapted from: LM Koenig, D Tamimi, et al. Diagnostic imaging: oral and maxillofacial, second ed., Elsevier; 2017.)

transformation and the borders of a seemingly benign lesion should be evaluated carefully for a discontinuity.

Because there are so many lesions in this category, it is often confusing to try to remember them all. Rather than list these entities according to histologic classification, which is the classic way of presenting them, this section will review them in a manner that makes sense to the radiologist and that is according to their appearance (low density, mixed density, or high density), location, and relation to teeth (periapical, pericoronal, inter-radicular, and intraosseous) as seen on osseous (CT/CBCT) imaging [15].

Low-Density Lesions

Periapical

Radicular Cyst: This is an inflammatory cyst that was covered in the previous section. The etiology is pulp necrosis, so look for large carious lesions, restorations/root canal therapy, or fractures of the crown (Fig. 74.17). If these are not present, consider the differential diagnosis of periapical osseous dysplasia (see the Fibro-osseous Lesions section later) or other benign odontogenic cysts/tumors.

Pericoronal

Dentigerous (Follicular) Cysts: These are the second most common cysts following the radicular cysts. They are well-defined, well-corticated, and unilocular lesions that surround the crown of an unerupted tooth and attach to the tooth at the CEJ. When small, it is difficult to differentiate this entity from a normal dental follicle. A follicle space that is asymmetric or larger than 3 mm should raise the suspicion for cystic degeneration. This lesion can displace the associated tooth dramatically and resorb the adjacent tooth roots (Fig. 74.18). In long-standing cases, the cyst may detach from the CEJ and migrate more apically, making differentiating it from an odontogenic keratocyst (OKC) and other benign lesions difficult. The cyst can be secondarily infected, which may present clinically as pain and sclerosis of the adjacent bone radiographically. In rare cases, the epithelium may convert to other benign entities, such as an OKC and unicystic ameloblastoma, or, even more rarely, to squamous cell carcinoma or mucoepidermoid carcinoma. The borders of the lesion should

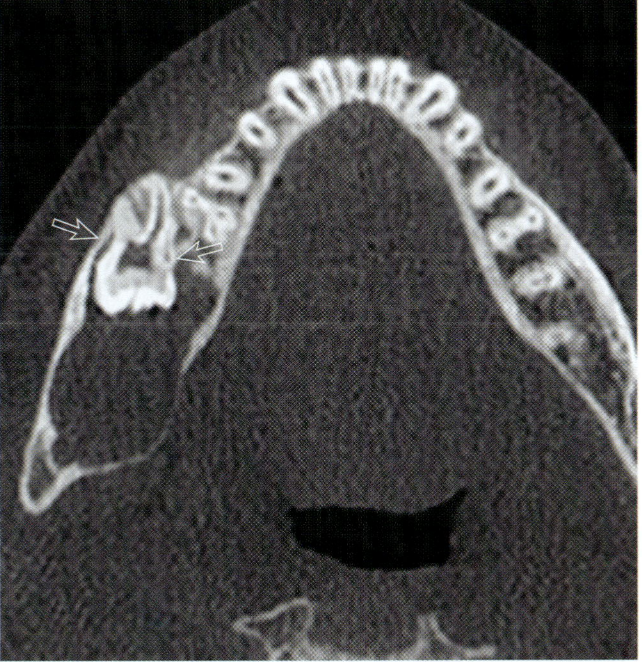

Figure 74.18 Axial CBCT shows a buccally displaced second molar with a well-defined unilocular low-density dentigerous cyst. The cyst attached to the cementoenamel junction of the tooth (*arrows*), a hallmark of this cyst. (Adapted from: LM Koenig, D Tamimi, et al. Diagnostic imaging: oral and maxillofacial, second ed., Elsevier; 2017.)

be carefully inspected to rule out secondary infection and other neoplasia. On T1-weighted MR imaging, dentigerous cysts are homogenous isointense and on T2-weighted imaging they are homogenous or heterogenous hyperintense. They may show rim enhancement on postgadolinium sequences [16].

Odontogenic Keratocyst: This is a well-defined, corticated entity that tends to occur more commonly in the mandible. This may occur pericoronally or within the alveolar bone independent of the tooth structure. One of its pathognomonic features is "growing in the length of the bone," which describes its appearance as being longer in the anteroposterior dimension that the mediolateral dimension as the mediolateral expansion is minimal. It can resorb and displace teeth and displaces the inferior alveolar nerve canal inferiorly. These lesions are largely low attenuating and unilocular, but can have thin and curved septations that mimic the soap bubble appearance of an ameloblastoma (Fig. 74.19). Multiple OKCs can be seen in basal cell nevus (Fig. 74.20) syndrome. The MR imaging appearance is different from a dentigerous cyst because of the high keratin content within its lumen. The T1-weighted imaging appearance is heterogenous hypointense or mildly hyperintense. On T2-weighted imaging, they are heterogenous or homogenous hyperintense. Focal inflammation and ulceration can result in rim enhancement. Histologically, this lesion can have peripheral soft tissue intramedullary extension called "daughter cysts" which contribute to the high recurrence rate. Mandatory periodic radiographic monitoring annually for 5 years postexcision then every 2–3 years is recommended [1,5,15,17].

Ameloblastoma: This odontogenic tumor arises from the enamel epithelium, an ectodermal layer of cells responsible for the formation of enamel. It is a benign but locally aggressive lesion and is the second most common odontogenic tumor (after odontomas). It can occur pericoronally or within the alveolus, and may present unilocularly (also called "unicystic ameloblastoma") or multilocularly. Unicystic ameloblastomas occur in younger age groups and present pericoronally. It can be difficult to differentiate from a dentigerous cyst, but with T1-weighted imaging, enhancement of mural nodules confirms the diagnosis of unicystic ameloblastoma. The multilocular lesions have a "soap-bubble" or "honey-comb" appearance. This may displace and resorb teeth and cause considerable expansion of the jaws that is evident clinically. The inferior alveolar nerve canal can be displaced, eroded, or may disappear within the lesion. Radiographic characterization

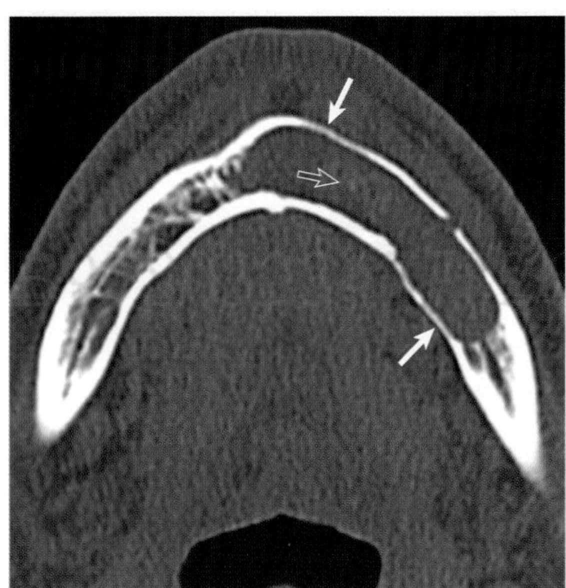

Figure 74.19 Axial bone CT shows an OKC "growing in the length of the bone": the AP growth is greater than the mediolateral growth. There is slight expansion and thinning of the cortices (*white arrows*) when compared with the AP dimension. This is characteristic of this lesion. (Adapted from: LM Koenig, D Tamimi, et al. Diagnostic imaging: oral and maxillofacial, second ed., Elsevier; 2017.)

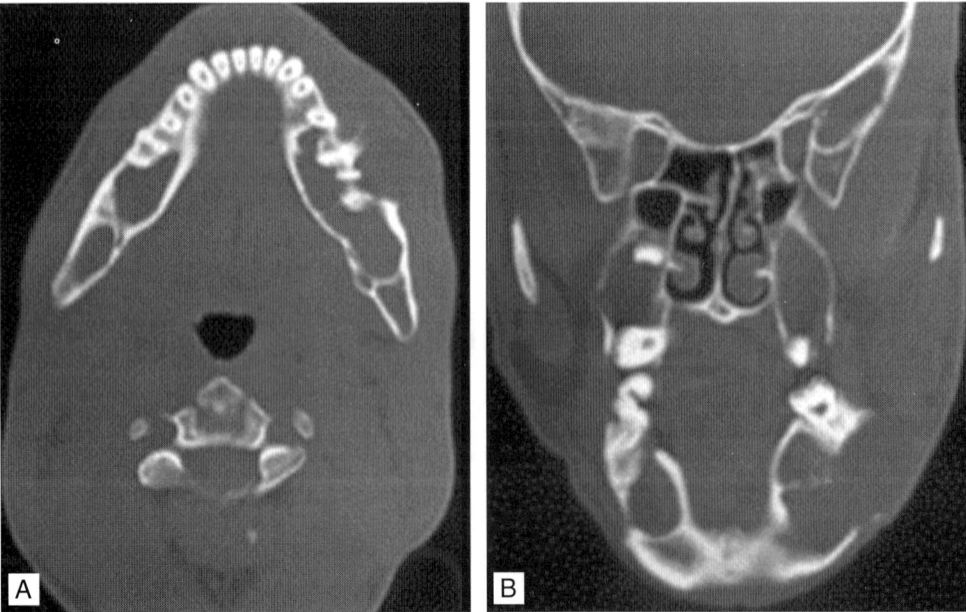

Figure 74.20 Axial (A) and coronal (B) images of the maxilla and mandible show multiple multilocular hypoattenuating lesions suggestive of odontogenic keratocysts in basal cell nevus syndrome. (Adapted from: WC Scarfe, S Toghyani, B Azevedo, Imaging of benign odontogenic lesions, Radiol Clin North Am 56 (1) (2018) 45–62.)

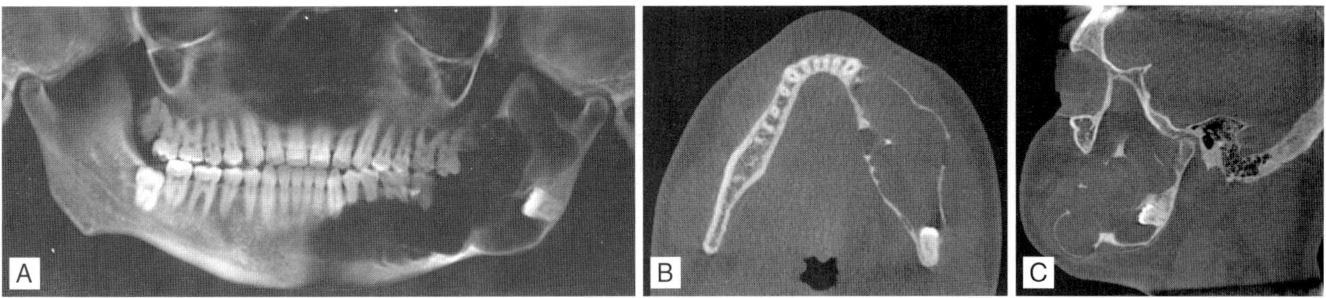

Figure 74.21 CBCT reformatted dental panoramic (A), axial view of the mandible at the level of the midroot (B) and sagittal view (C) of an ameloblastoma in the left ramus of a 34-year-old show a well-defined multilocular expansile lesion with scalloped borders developing pericoronal to the mandibular third molar. Thinning and erosion of the buccal and lingual cortical plates and knife-edge root resorption on the adjacent teeth is noted. The cortices of the inferior alveolar canal are not traceable within the lesion. (Adapted from: WC Scarfe, S Toghyani, B Azevedo, Imaging of benign odontogenic lesions, Radiol Clin North Am 56 (1) (2018) 45–62.)

can assist in choosing the correct treatment technique in relation to the variant (unicystic or multilocular), size, location, and involvement of the surrounding anatomy (Fig. 74.21). Contrast-enhanced CT shows irregular peripheral enhancement, septation, and solid and cystic mural nodule components within the lesion. T1-weighted MR shows a low to intermedial signal lesion, and on T2-weighted images the signal is intermediate to high. Contrast-enhanced T1-weighted imaging reveals a hyperintense signal in the solid components. Recurrence of this lesion is high [1,5,14,15].

Ameloblastic Fibroma/Fibroodontoma: Radiographically, an ameloblastic fibroma looks very similar to an ameloblastoma, except that it occurs in childhood and adolescence (if it looks like an ameloblastoma and it is in a child, then consider ameloblastic fibroma). It is a rare mixed ectodermal and ectomesenchymal lesion. It is well-defined, corticated low-density lesion that most commonly occurs in the posterior mandible (Fig. 74.22). Sometimes, tooth density structures occur within the stroma, giving a mixed attenuation appearance. This changes the diagnosis to ameloblastic fibroodontoma, but the management is similar. Malignant transformation occurs in about 10% of pediatric cases [1,5,15,22].

Inter-Radicular: Any odontogenic lesions (within the exception of the dentigerous cyst and the unicystic ameloblastoma) and non-odontogenic lesions (Table 74.2) can occur inter-radicularly. Listed below are a few lesions that occur exclusively inter-radicularly.

Mandibular Infected Cyst (Buccal Bifurcation Cyst): This is a rare inflammatory odontogenic cyst that occurs in the buccal aspect of the mandibular first or second molars in the pediatric population. This presents clinically as swelling, pain, and local suppuration. Radiographically, it is a well-defined and corticated unilocular low-density lesion that may resorb or displace the involved tooth or delay its eruption. Its presence on the buccal aspect of the tooth furcation causes the tooth roots to tip lingually sometime thinning or going through the lingual cortex of the mandible, a hallmark presentation of this lesion (Fig. 74.23). This is best visualized on CT or CBCT axial cross sections [1,5,15].

Lateral Periodontal Cyst: This is a noninflammatory developmental cyst that presents radiographically as a small, well-defined unilocular low-density lesion associated with the proximal surfaces of the teeth. The most common location is the mandibular lateral incisor to second premolar regions. A botryoid cyst is a

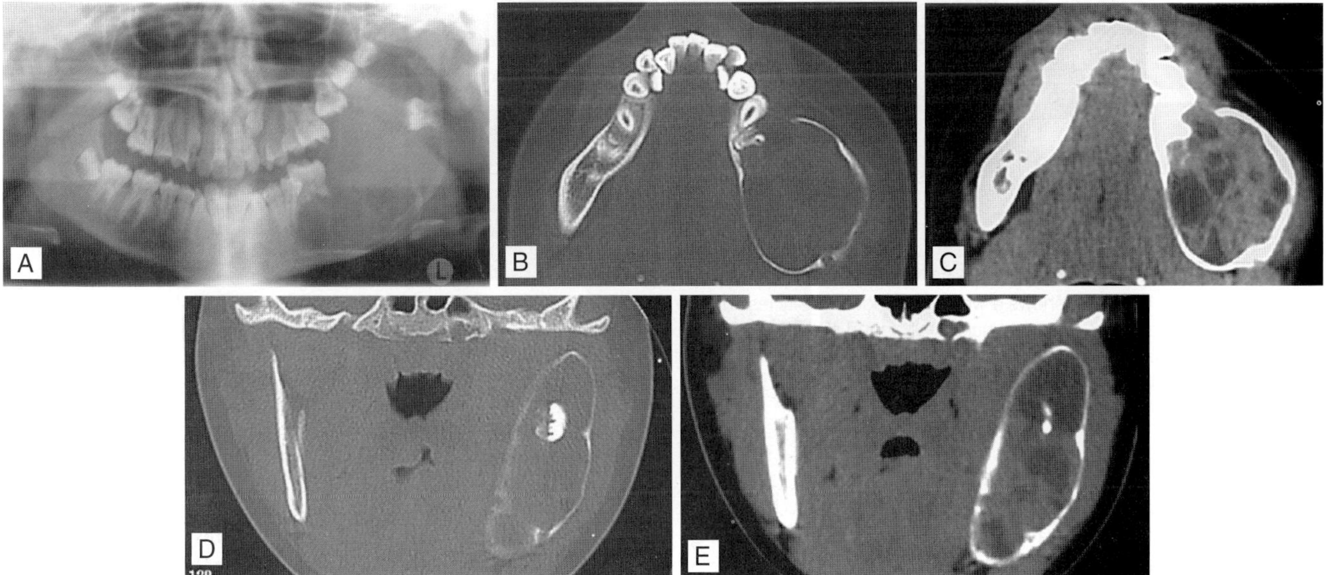

Figure 74.22 Conventional panoramic radiography (A) axial bone (B) and soft-tissue (C) window and coronal bone (D) and soft-tissue (E) CT images of a 14-year-old girl with an asymptomatic large multilocular expansion of the left mandible involving the body, angle, and ramus. Soft-tissue images show heterogenous contents consistent with ameloblastic fibroma. (Adapted from: WC Scarfe, S Toghyani, B Azevedo, Imaging of benign odontogenic lesions, Radiol Clin North Am 56 (1) (2018) 45–62.)

Odontogenic Myxoma: This is a rare benign odontogenic tumor of ectodermal origin. It occurs mostly in the posterior mandible. Radiographically, it is a multilocular low-density lesion with well-developed locules and scalloped borders which may be corticated or noncorticated. The septations are thin and can be arranged at right angles in a "step ladder" or "tennis racquet" appearance (pathognomonic feature). The septae can be coarse or curved. The lesion tends to scallop between the roots (Fig. 74.26). It has a high recurrence rate and should be followed up post-op [1,5,15].

Glandular Odontogenic Cyst: These are rare aggressive cysts of ectodermal origin. They are most common in the anterior mandible and maxilla. They are low-density multilocular cysts with scalloped cortical margins and can cause expansion and perforation of the cortices of the alveolar process and displacement of the teeth. Recurrence is high [1,5,15].

High-Density Lesions

Periapical

Periapical Sclerosing Osteitis: This is a sequela of dental inflammation as described in the previous section on infection. This is a hyperattenuating area of bone associated with the apex of a necrosing or necrotic tooth. This high-density area is a bone reaction to chronic low-grade inflammation. The tooth is nonvital and requires root canal therapy in most cases.

Idiopathic Osteosclerosis: This is a dense bone island located either at the apex of a tooth or anywhere in the jaws. This is isodense to cortical bone and blends into the adjacent cortical outline of the bone without expanding it (Fig. 74.27). An associated tooth is vital. No intervention is needed for this finding [1,5].

Odontoma: This is the most common benign odontogenic tumor in the jaws. The lesion stems from both ectodermal and ectomesenchymal cells and forms mature enamel, dentin, cementum, and pulp. These may be arranged to resemble a "bag of teeth," small teeth in low-density sac (compound odontomas) or may be haphazardly arranged to appear as an amorphous high-density mass surrounded by a low-density rim (complex odontomas) (Fig. 74.28). These lesions are asymptomatic and are often discovered when a tooth fails to erupt if they present pericoronally. This lesion is self-limiting and does not cause gross expansion [1,5,15].

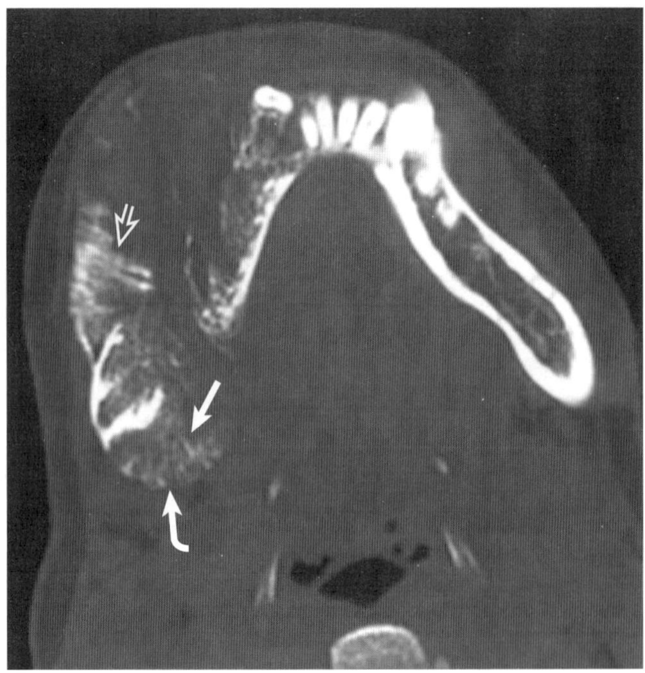

Figure 74.26 Axial bone CT shows an odontogenic myxoma with straight septa (*open arrow*) and radiating wisps of bone (*arrow*) at the periphery of the lesion. The thin corticated margin (*curved arrow*) can be discerned and helps us differentiate from an osteosarcoma. (Adapted from: LM Koenig, D Tamimi, et al., Diagnostic imaging: oral and maxillofacial, second ed., Elsevier; 2017. Courtesy: S. Kalathingal.)

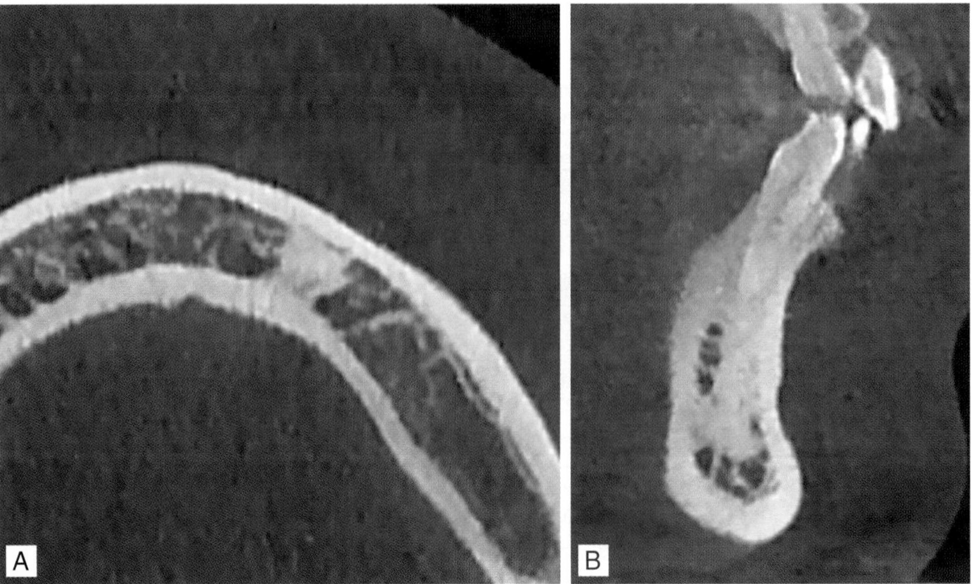

Figure 74.27 Axial (A) and cross-sectional (B) CBCT images of the mandibular left canine show a hyperdense area of bone that blends into the lingual cortex of the mandible without expanding it. This is a common finding in the jaws (idiopathic osteosclerosis or dense bone) and requires no intervention. (Adapted from: LM Koenig, D Tamimi, et al., Diagnostic imaging: oral and maxillofacial, second ed., Elsevier; 2017.)

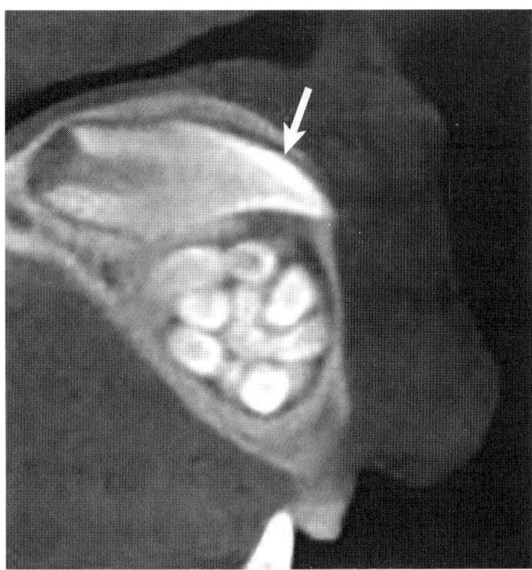

Figure 74.28 CBCT cross section shows a compound odontoma presenting pericoronal to the maxillary central incisor (*arrow*) and appearing as a bag of teeth. (Adapted from: LM Koenig, D Tamimi, et al., Diagnostic imaging: oral and maxillofacial, second ed., Elsevier; 2017.)

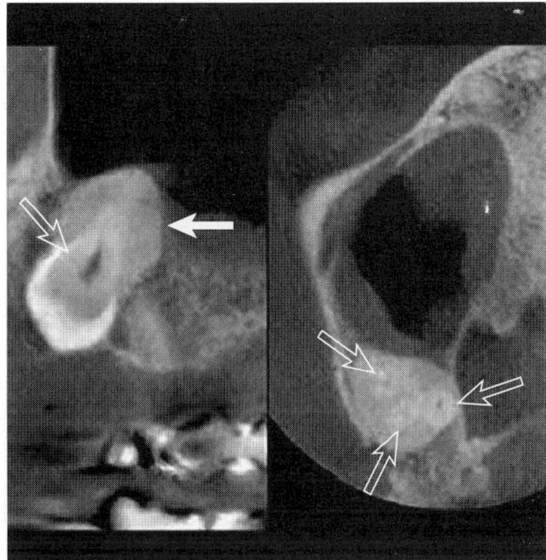

Figure 74.29 CBCT shows an impacted third molar with hypercementosis (*white arrow*). Note the normal higher density dentin outline can be seen within the lower density cementum (*open arrows*). (Adapted from: LM Koenig, D Tamimi, et al., Diagnostic imaging: oral and maxillofacial, second ed., Elsevier; 2017.)

Hypercementosis: The cementum surrounding the roots of the teeth may respond to external stimuli such as chronic infection or occlusal trauma by producing a non-neoplastic proliferation of the cementum, resulting in an irregular and sometimes bulbous root outline that is contained within the PDL and lamina dura (**Fig.** 74.29). This condition can occur in florid osseous dysplasia and Paget disease as well [1,5,15].

Cementoblastoma: This is a rare ectomesenchymal neoplasm of cementum that presents as a solitary round hyperattenuating structure that is attached to the root of a tooth, most commonly the mandibular molars. It is surrounded by a low-density rim and exhibits a sunburst pattern within the high-density mass [1,5,15] (Fig. 74.30).

Pericoronal

Odontomas: As previously noted, these lesions can occur around or close to the crown of a developing tooth and may impede its eruption. These pericoronal presentations occur more commonly in the anterior maxilla.

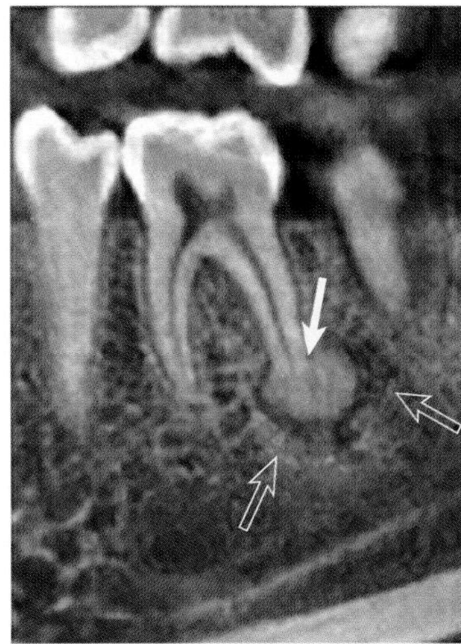

Figure 74.30 Sagittally reformatted CBCT shows a cementoblastoma (*open arrows*) on the distal root of the mandibular left first molar. There is root resorption and attachment to the root (*white arrow*). (Adapted from: LM Koenig, D Tamimi, et al., Diagnostic imaging: oral and maxillofacial, second ed., Elsevier; 2017.)

Inter-Radicular

Tooth Roots: Extraction of teeth is sometimes incomplete and a portion of the root is left behind. If the radiologist comes across these root tips, they should be evaluated for widening of the PDL space or development of infection surrounding it. If the root shows no signs of pathology, it is generally left alone.

Supernumerary Teeth: Extra teeth can develop anywhere in the arches. The most common type of supernumerary is the mesiodens, which is a small peg-shaped tooth that occurs in the midline between or palatal to the maxillary central incisors. If they do not cause impaction of the other teeth, complicate esthetics or orthodontic treatment and do not have associated pathology, they are generally left alone [1,5].

Mixed Density Lesions

Periapical: Other that complex odontomas, no odontogenic conditions appear as periapical mixed attenuating lesions. When faced with such a lesion in this location, one should consider a fibroosseous lesion (these are described in the Fibroosseous section later).

Pericoronal

Calcifying Epithelial Odontogenic Tumor: These are rare neoplasms that can occur at any age, but are most commonly seen in middle-age. It is more common in men. Painless jaw expansion is often the only clinical symptom. It occurs more frequently in the posterior mandible, with half of them associated with an impacted tooth. It is well defined and expansile with a cyst-like cortex, and it may be unilocular or multilocular with numerous scattered radiopaque foci or varying size and density (Fig. 74.31). The calcifications come very close to the crown of the associated tooth [1,5,15].

Adenomatoid Odontogenic Tumor: This is a rare nonaggressive tumor of mixed ectodermal and ectomesenchymal origin that mostly occurs in the second decade of life. Most of these tumors

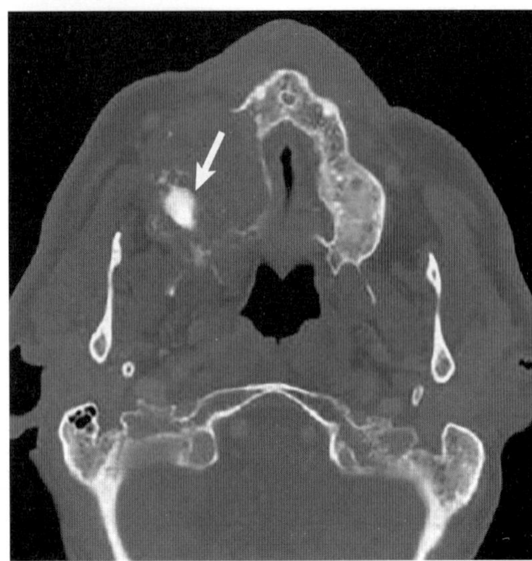

Figure 74.31 Axial bone CT shows a calcifying epithelial odontogenic tumor presenting as a large, expansile, mixed density lesion in the right maxilla. There is a large focus of calcification noted in the lesion in addition to multiple small flecks of calcification. (Adapted from: LM Koenig, D Tamimi, et al., Diagnostic imaging: oral and maxillofacial, second ed., Elsevier; 2017.)

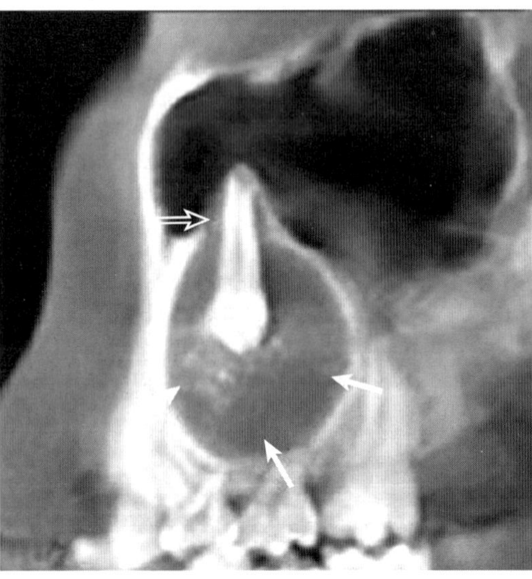

Figure 74.32 Sagittal CBCT shows an adenomatoid odontogenic tumor associated with a maxillary premolar (*block arrow*). The corticated boundary of the lesion is attached to the midroot of the tooth. There are multiple small calcified fleck noted within the lesion (*white arrow*). (Adapted from: LM Koenig, D Tamimi, et al., Diagnostic imaging: oral and maxillofacial, second ed., Elsevier; 2017. Courtesy: M. Noujeim DDS.)

develop surrounding the crown of an unerupted tooth and impede its eruption. About 75% of these tumors occur in the maxilla, especially in the area of the incisors, canines, and premolars. It is well defined with a corticated border with varying degrees of internal calcifications that can resemble small pebbles or appear as dense clusters of ill-defined opacities [1,5,15] (Fig. 74.32).

Ameloblastic Fibroodontoma: These lesions were covered previously in the discussion of ameloblastic fibroma, which is technically the same tumor without the calcified dental material.

Calcifying Cystic Odontogenic Tumor: This was previously classified as a cyst and called "calcifying odontogenic cyst." This is a rare tumor that is slow growing and that has a wide age distribution, with peaks at the second and seventh decades of life. Most occur anterior to the first molar. The periphery can vary from well defined and corticated to ill defined and irregular. The internal aspect may be completely radiolucent, or may show small flecks of calcified material that may coalesce and form larger solid masses. It is expansile but not-aggressive [1,5,15].

Radiation and Medication-Related Osteonecrosis of the Jaws

Osteonecrosis generally refers to the bone devitalization and subsequent lytic alterations. Histologically, bone necrosis is characterized by the lack of osteocytes inside the lacuna. Balance between osteoclastic and osteoblastic activities result in continuous bone turnover. In the jaws, osteonecrosis is a pathological consequence of some antiresorptive medications or previous radiotherapy (osteoradionecrosis [ORN]) which disturb this balance. Additionally, oral cavity situation and teeth can affect the changed bone homeostasis negatively [18].

Osteonecrosis is frequently a result of altered vascularity causing avascular (aseptic) necrosis at few sites like femoral head. However, ORN and medication-related osteonecrosis of the jaws (MRONJ) are different pathologies than avascular necrosis. Furthermore, despite the similarity in their treatment-associated causation, MRONJ, and ORN are different pathologies. They are characterized by distinct but often overlapping radiographic and clinical features and are treated differently [18].

Osteoradionecrosis of the Jaws

ORN is described as a region of irradiated and exposed bone which fails to heal for at least 3 months after radiation therapy (Fig. 74.33A–C) and in the absence of recurrent or residual tumor after other causes of osteonecrosis are excluded [19,20]. The pathogenesis of ORN is not yet clear. Commonly accepted theory is radiation produces microvascular alterations that generate hypovascularity, hypoxia, and hypocellularity disrupting bone homeostasis and causing to a chronic, nonhealing wound [19].

ORN may occur any time after radiotherapy, and usually expresses 6–12 months after radiation therapy. Yet, the time to onset varies from months to years. Mandible is affected more than the maxilla likely owing to its relatively lower vascular supply [18]. Even though any regions of the jaws are susceptible, the posterior mandible is more frequently affected than other regions as it is often in the direct field of the radiation therapy due to the vicinity of primary and metastatic lesions in lymph nodes being treated [5,20]. Although not common, maxillary osteonecrosis can occur frequently secondary to radiotherapy for nasopharyngeal cancer [18].

Total radiation dose, therapeutic field size, distance between the tumor and bone, simultaneous chemotherapy, dental appliance and denture trauma, tooth extraction, surgical procedures of the irradiated region, alcohol abuse, smoking, and poor oral hygiene modulate ORN risk. A determining factor is the total radiation dose. ORN is unlikely to develop if the patient receives radiation dose less than 60 Gy and is rare at doses less than 50 Gy. For doses exceeding 66 Gy, the risk for ORN is increased 11-fold [18].

Staging of the Osteoradionecrosis of the Jaws: There is no universal staging system for ORN and present staging systems of ORN considers the degree of the osseous necrotic alterations, hyperbaric oxygen therapy response, and clinical and radiological factors [18,19,21]. This chapter uses the staging system suggested by "Støre and Boysen" [21], which is an efficient tool for the ra-

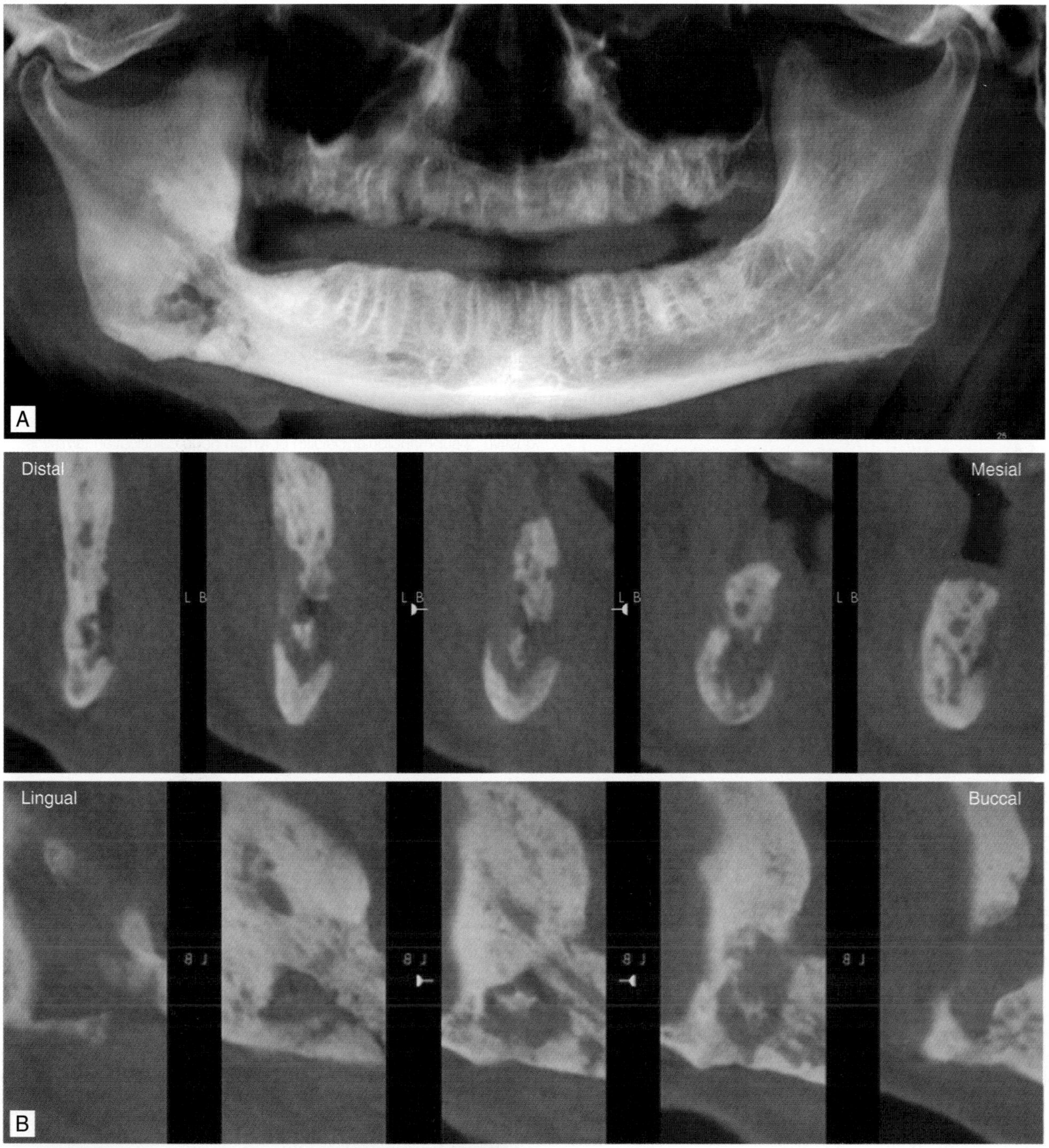

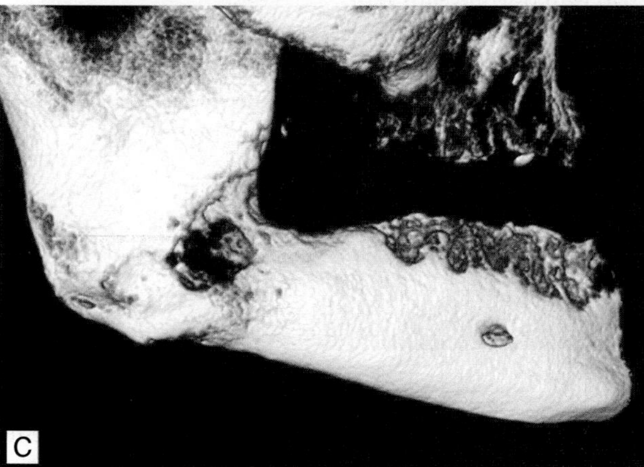

Figure 74.33 Osteoradionecrosis. (A) CBCT panoramic reconstruction of a patient with history of radiation therapy for salivary gland cancer showing irregular lytic changes in the right posterior mandible extending to partially interrupt the cortical margins of the mandibular canal. The bone between the area of the right mandibular first molar and the mid-height of the ramus is remarkably sclerotic with the presence of an irregular in shape low-density area at the level of the angle of mandible. (B) CBCT cross-sectional views showing the lesion interrupting both buccal and lingual cortices with no expansion. The sclerotic bone around the low-density area presents with multiple small round low-density regions with some detached bone fragments. The lesion is situated inferior to the mandibular canal. No periosteal reaction noted. (C) CBCT 3D reconstruction sagittal view showing the extent and effect of the lesion on surrounding structures (Case courtesy: Dr. M. Noujeim).

TABLE 74.3 Støre and Boysen's Classification of Osteoradionecrosis (ORN) [21]

Stage	Criteria
0	Only mucosa defect
1	Radiologically detectable necrotic bone with intact mucosa
2	Positive radiographic findings with intraoral exposed bone
3	Clinically exposed necrotic bone, confirmed by imaging, infection, and skin fistula

Adapted and modified from: G Støre, M Boysen, Mandibular osteoradionecrosis: clinical behaviour and diagnostic aspects, Clin Otolaryngol Allied Sci 25 (5) (2000) 378–384 [21] and SM Mallya, S Tetradis, Imaging of radiation- and medication-related osteonecrosis. Radiol Clin North Am 56 (1) (2018) 77–89. doi:10.1016/j.rcl.2017.08.006 [18].

diologist to score the disease status for the referring clinician (Table 74.3).

Imaging Goals and Protocols: Generally, small to medium field of view (FOV) CBCT or CT is sufficient to visualize the area of interest. Scan FOV must involve the unaffected contralateral side to compare due to the significant variation of the trabecular bone architecture and density in the jaws. MDCT must be the technique of choice if evaluation of the adjacent soft tissues needed (i.e., soft-tissue mass suggestive of recurrent malignancy, superimposed cellulitis, and osteomyelitis). The FOV of MDCT should include the area from frontal sinus to mandible. Axial images parallel to the dental occlusal plane should be acquired and evaluated applying soft-tissue and bone windows. Sinus walls and mandibular canal can be better seen in the coronal and sagittal reconstruction images [5,18].

Radiological Characteristics of Osteoradionecrosis: The first changes of ORN manifest as subtle regions of altered trabecular structure and rarefaction [18]. The altered bone can present with poorly defined, noncorticated border, with the presence of sclerosis and ill-defined, irregular areas of bone resorption. An early change observed in the mandibular cortex is a clearly defined bone resorption region. In the maxilla, portions of the maxillary sinus cortical walls might be missing [20]. Markedly, in the irradiated alveolar processes of the jaws, the most commonly developing alteration is a uniform but irregular widening of the PDL space surrounding the teeth. Moreover, the observed widening does not have a distinct epicenter and there is no bone loss. This is a frequent finding and does not require management in the lack of adjacent bone destruction [18,20].

Radiologic detection of ORN depends on the detection of sequestra which is a dead bone and positive patient history (Fig. 74.34A and B). Radiographically, sequestra may be seen as

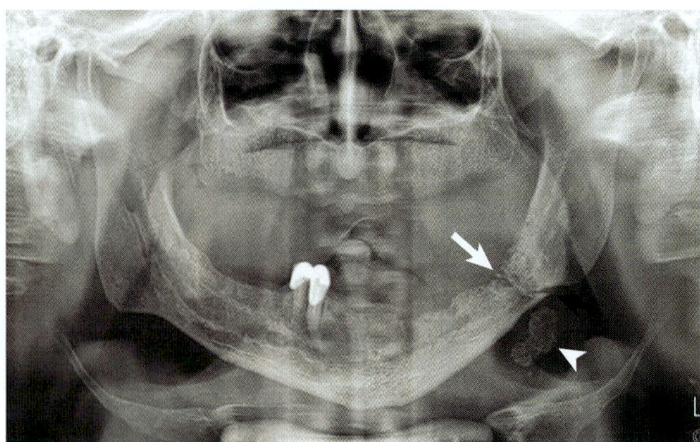

Figure 74.35 Panoramic radiograph showing osteoradionecrosis and pathologic fracture (*white arrow*) in the left mandibular posterior region in a patient with a history of radiotherapy due to squamous cell carcinoma. Note the step defect in the fracture line (*arrow*) and radiopaque entity suggestive of submandibular sialolith or lymph node calcification (*arrowhead*) inferior to the fracture region (Case courtesy: Dr. B. Kan).

patchy, low-density area with dense islands of necrotic bone, contrasted against the low-density lytic alterations. *Contrary to osteomyelitis, generally, there is no/minimal periosteal bone reaction in most of the patients.* The existence of a pathologic fracture suggests ORN (Fig. 74.35) [20]. However, radiographic expression of ORN is not specific, and therefore must be distinguished from recurrent malignancy, osteomyelitis, and other bone necrosis [18]. If recurrent malignancy is suspected, MRI and CT can be utilized to identify an accompanying soft-tissue mass. Differentiating ORN from sclerotic pathologies (i.e., chronic osteomyelitis) is easier due to the history of radiotherapy [20].

MRI has the ability to detect early ORN-induced bone marrow changes before being clinically visible. These changes are seen as decreased bone marrow signal on T1-weighted images and increased bone marrow signal on T2-weighted images. Cortical destruction and surrounding soft-tissue changes can also be detected with MRI [18,22].

Medication-Related Osteonecrosis of the Jaws

MRONJ is an osteonecrosis related to antiangiogenic or antiresorptive therapy [23]. Certain medications such as bisphosphonates and receptor activator of nuclear factor-κB ligand inhibitors (i.e., Denosumab) can produce chemical insult in the bone, changing the osteoclastic and osteoblastic balance activity, generating the disease. Similar to radiation therapy, most of the imaging characteristics (i.e., nonhealing, exposed bone) in MRONJ overlap with osteomyelitis [20].

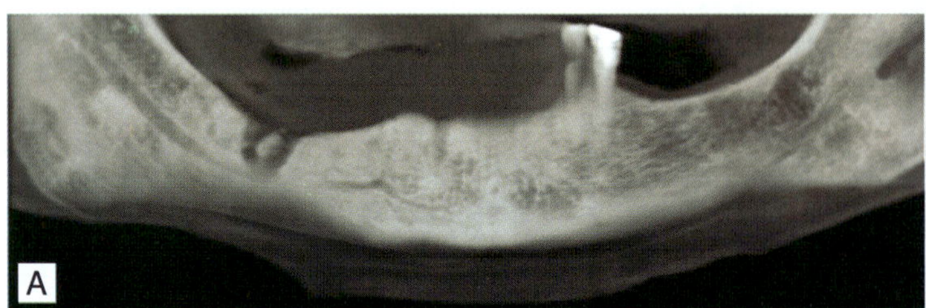

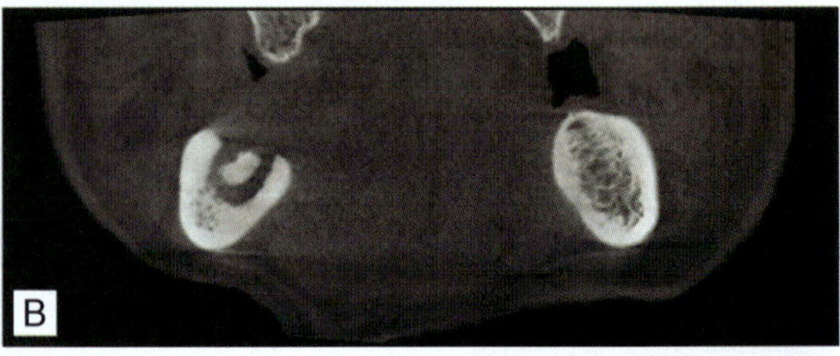

Figure 74.34 (A) CBCT panoramic reconstruction of a patient with history of radiation therapy showing lytic changes with the presence of sequestra at the center in the right posterior mandible extending to partially interrupt the cortical margins of the mandibular canal. The bone between the area of the right mandibular canine and second molar is significantly sclerotic. (B) Coronal CBCT view of the same patient showing sequestra surrounded by the lytic area in the right posterior mandible. Note the significant sclerosis of the trabecular bone comparing to the left side (Case courtesy: Dr. K. Orhan).

TABLE 74.4 Staging of Medication-Related Osteonecrosis of the Jaws (MRONJ) [18,23]

Stage	Necrotic or Exposed Bone	History and Clinical Findings
At risk	No clinical evidence	
Stage 0	No clinical evidence	Nonspecific radiologic and clinical findings
Stage 1	Necrotic and exposed bone or fistulae that probes to bone	Asymptomatic, no infection
Stage 2	Necrotic and exposed bone or fistulae that probes to bone	Erythema, pain and infection in exposed bone region with or without purulent drainage
Stage 3	Necrotic and exposed bone or fistulae that probes to bone	Infection, pain, and one or more of the following: ▪ Necrotic and exposed bone extending further than alveolar bone with the presence of pathologic fracture ▪ Oroantral or oronasal communication, extraoral fistula ▪ Lytic alterations extending to the floor of the maxillary sinus or inferior border of the mandible

Adapted and modified from: SL Ruggiero, TB Dodson, J Fantasia, et al., American Association of Oral and Maxillofacial Surgeons position paper on medication-related osteonecrosis of the jaw–2014 update, J Oral Maxillofac Surg 72 (10) (2014) 1938–1956 [23] and SM Mallya, S Tetradis, Imaging of radiation- and medication-related osteonecrosis, Radiol Clin North Am 56 (1) (2018) 77–89 [18].

To clarify its difference from other causes of exposed bone, the American Academy of Oral and Maxillofacial Surgery has established a diagnostic criterion to differentiate MRONJ-related bone exposure from other cause of exposed bone [23].

The diagnostic criteria for MRONJ are [23]:

- Previous or current antiangiogenic or antiresorptive treatment
- Exposed bone or bone which may be probed through an extraoral or intraoral fistula(e) persisted more than 8 weeks
- No clear metastatic disease or history of radiotherapy to the jaws

The American Academy of Oral and Maxillofacial Surgery has also developed a staging system for preclinical and clinical MRONJ (Table 74.4) [23].

Imaging Goals and Protocols: Despite nonspecific imaging findings associated with the clinically exposed bone, imaging can show detachment, sequestra, increased sclerosis, thickening of lamina dura and PDL space widening (Fig. 74.36A) [20]. MDCT and CBCT protocols are the same with ORN. Regular examinations of asymptomatic cases give a baseline to watch future subtle

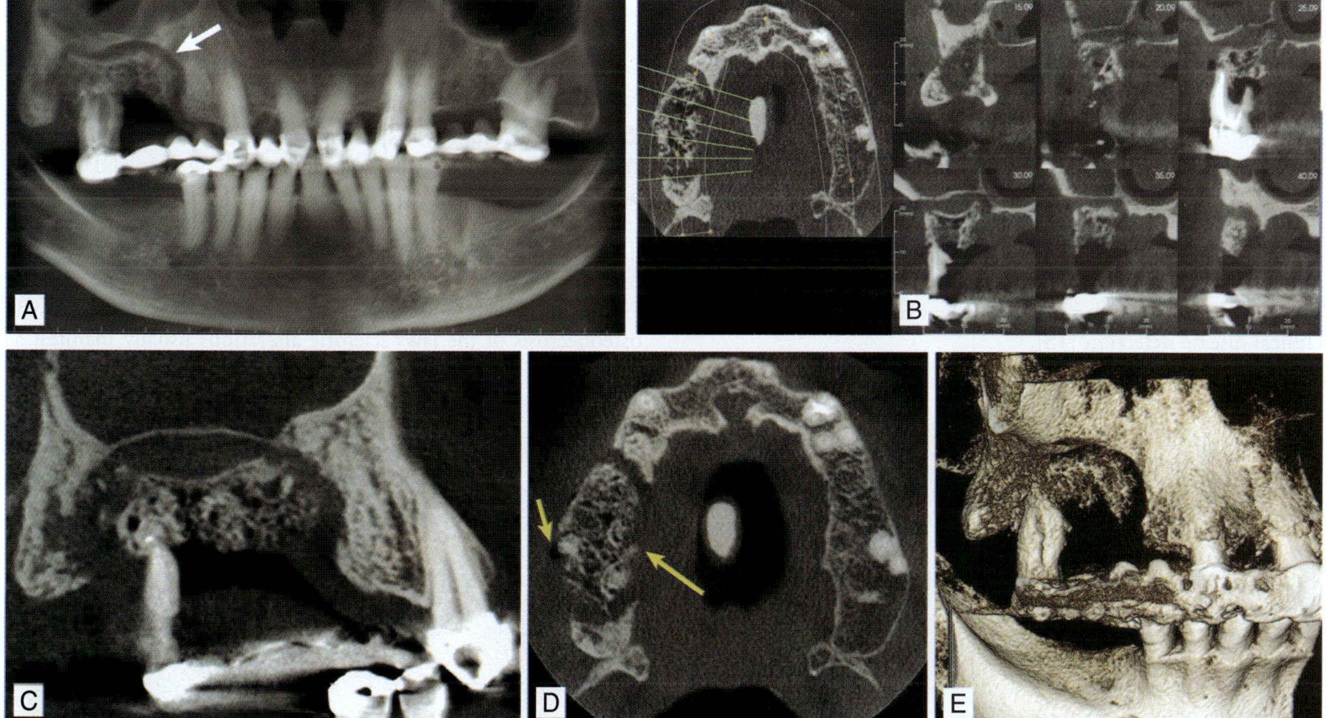

Figure 74.36 (A) CBCT panoramic reconstruction of a patient with history of bisphosphonates treatment showing a well-defined, low-density area with a tunnel like appearance (*arrow*) in the right maxillary posterior region extending from area of missing #15 posteriorly to the area of missing #18 through the maxillary alveolar bone above the apical region of #16. (B) CBCT cross-sectional views taken from right posterior maxilla showing buccal and palatal interruptions making the bony area below the low density similar to an island (bone sequestrum). The trabecular structure of the sequestrum is sclerotic with large bone marrow spaces. Note the presence of sinus reaction and possible sinus floor interruption. (C–E) CBCT sagittal (C), axial (D), and 3D reconstruction (E) views showing extension of the lesion with destruction of the buccal and lingual cortices (*arrows*) (Case courtesy: Dr. M. Noujeim).

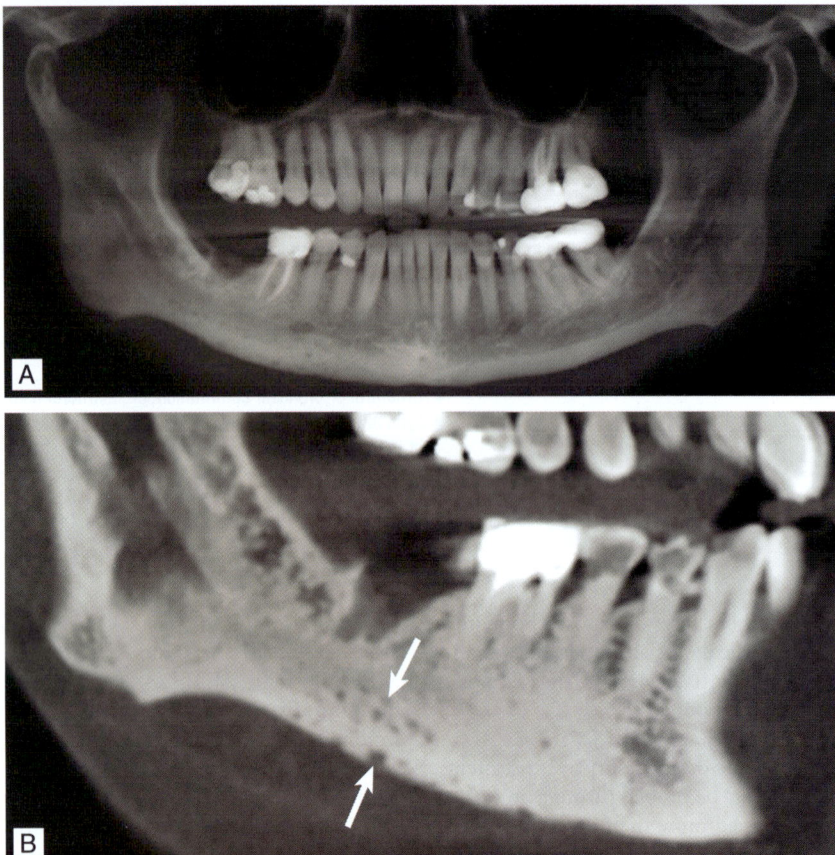

Figure 74.37 (A) CBCT panoramic reconstruction of a patient with history of Denosumab use for the treatment of osteoporosis showing diffuse sclerotic bone area in the right mandible mainly between the canine and third molar teeth with the presence of multiple small punctate low-density areas within the thickened and sclerotic bone (B) CBCT sagittal view of the same patient showing remarkable sclerosis extending from the alveolar crest to reach the basal cortex with multiple small punctate low-density areas (*arrows*) (Case courtesy: Dr. M. Noujeim).

alterations which can allow detection of early necrotic bone alterations. When clinical findings indicate the presence of MRONJ (stages 1–3), 3D imaging (i.e., CT or CBCT) should be performed to examine the extension of the alterations as well as the possibility of complications like interruption of the maxillary sinus and nasal cavity or pathologic fracture (Fig. 74.36B–E). MRI can show early trabecular bone changes which may result in preclinical disease detection [18].

Radiological Characteristics of Medication-Related Osteonecrosis of the Jaws: Radiologic findings show lytic and sclerotic bone changes (Fig. 74.37). Early lytic changes are seen as altered trabecular bone density and structure, following by patchy bone destruction and cortical interruption. The lytic alterations may progress to pathological fracture. Surgical defects and nonhealing extraction sockets must be detected (Fig. 74.38A and B). In the osteonecrosis of the jaws sclerotic alterations usually manifest as

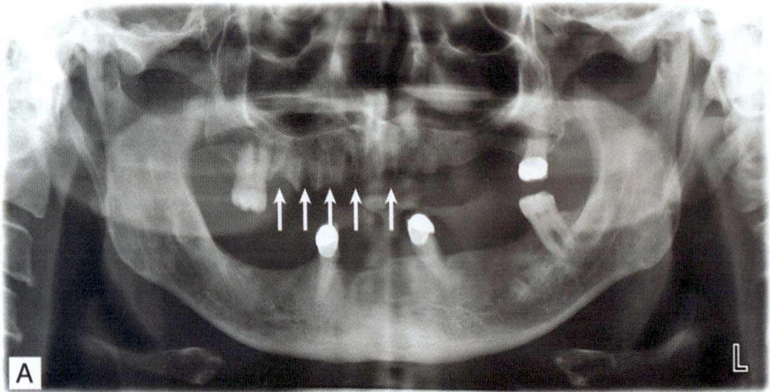

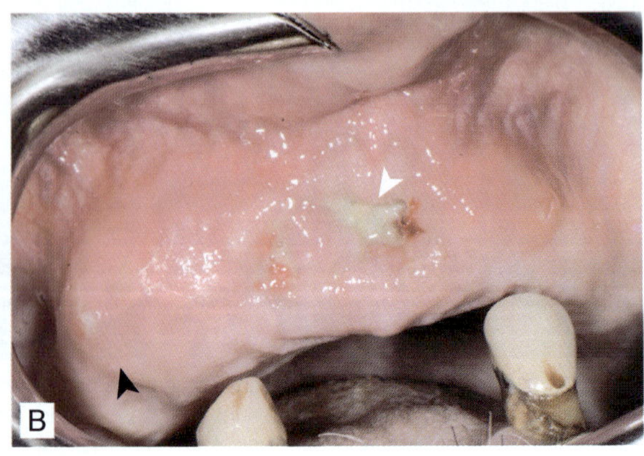

Figure 74.38 (A and B) Panoramic radiograph of a patient on a bisphosphate treatment with multiple extraction sockets (*arrows*) in the anterior maxilla and right maxillary premolar-molar region (A). Intraoral picture of the same patient with the development of MRONJ following extractions. Note the exposed bone (*white arrowhead*), swelling (*black arrowhead*) and redness (B) (Case courtesy: Dr. B. Kan).

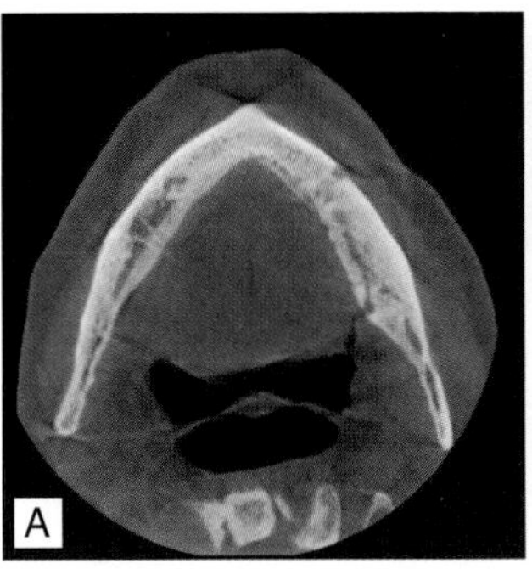

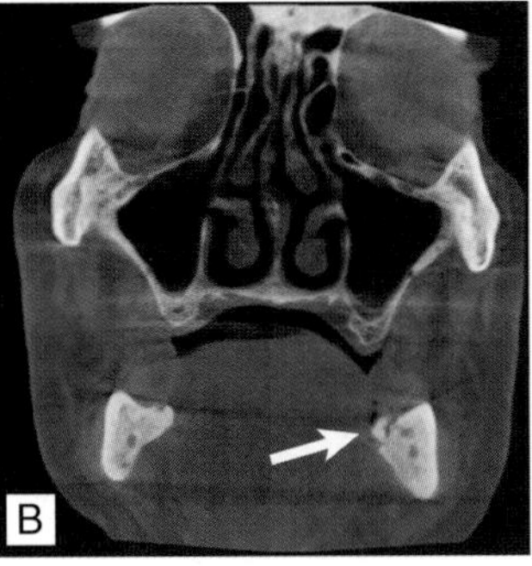

Figure 74.39 Axial (A), coronal (B), views showing MRONJ in the body of the left mandible. Note increased sclerosis of the area with the presence of partially detached bone (*arrow*) which possibly will proceed to sequestra. (Case courtesy: Dr. U Seki).

limited to extensive diffuse osteosclerosis, with the presence of periosteal reaction. When the necrotic changes progress and combine, sequestrate are formed [18].

Even though MRONJ and ORN have similar radiographic features, generally in MRONJ, increased cortical and trabecular bone density with associated significant periosteal reaction due to the inhibition of osteoclastic activity predominate (Fig. 74.39). In contrast, rarefaction, cortical interruption, and trabecular density loss as a result of increased osteoclastic and decreased osteoblastic activity dominate the ORN. Lytic lesions of MRONJ must be distinguished from the metastatic lesion and recurrent malignancy. Both malignant lesion and MRONJ can produce periosteal new bone formation. However, in metastatic malignancy, the periosteal reaction is irregular with radiating spicules of new bone perpendicular to the cortex. On the contrary, in MRONJ, the periosteal reaction is more organized, and paralleling the cortex. Assuming that large number of MRONJ patients are treated for metastatic pathology, this differentiation is very important [18].

Fibroosseous and Other Bone Lesions of the Jaws

Fibroosseous Lesions

Fibroosseous lesions of the jaws can be very problematic for radiologists that are not used to looking at conditions of the jaws. They range in appearance, location, and demographic distribution. Without adequate training, it would be difficult to recognize that these lesions belong to the same group of lesions. Their pathophysiology ranges from simple dysplasia to reactive lesions to formal neoplasms. The management of these lesions also varies greatly and differ from other lesions that they mimic, so reaching a correct diagnosis is important to plan the clinical course of the treatment [1,5,24].

Periapical Osseous Dysplasia: This type of dysplasia was recently renamed after being previously called "periapical cemental or cementoosseous dysplasia." As they are considered, "do not touch" lesions, biopsies of these areas are not advised as the risk of infection is high. They tend to occur in middle-aged African women but can occur in other populations as well. There are no signs or symptoms associated with the teeth and they are vital (no pulpal necrosis), an important diagnostic point to consider when differentiating them from periapical inflammation. They most commonly occur at the apices of the mandible anterior teeth, but can occur anywhere. Lesions limited to a few teeth are called focal osseous dysplasia. When more than two quadrants are involved, the term "florid osseous dysplasia" is used. Large lesions can displace the inferior alveolar canal inferiorly and the floor of the maxillary sinus superiorly. In these cases, the homogenous high-density foci are surrounded by wide areas of well-defined, noncorticated low densities. The concern with these lesions is secondary infection, either due to caries from an associated tooth or surgery, such as biopsy. Osteomyelitis develops easily in these lesions due to poor vascularity.

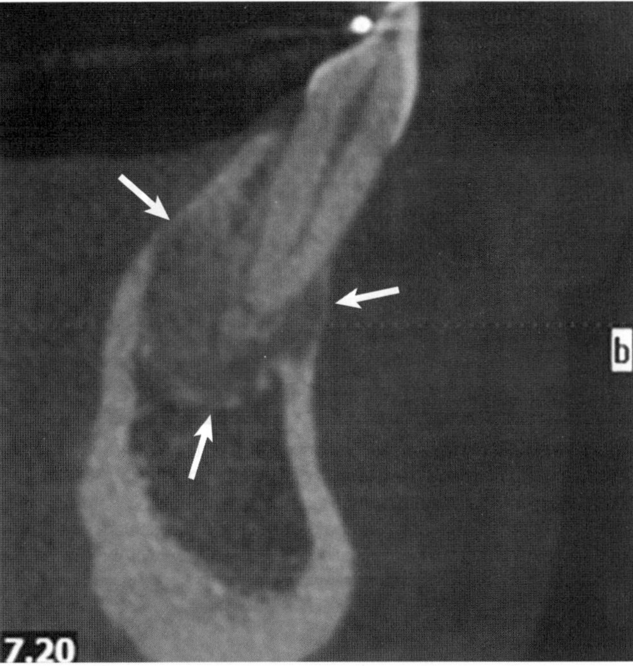

Figure 74.40 Cone beam CT cross section of a mandibular incisor shows a mixed density stage periapical osseous dysplasia with preservation of the peripheral lucent rim of varying thickness and definition (*arrows*). Portions of the buccal and lingual cortical plates are thinned. (Adapted from: M Ahmad, L Gaalaas, Fibro-osseous and other lesions of bone in the jaws, Radiol Clin North Am 56 (1) (2018) 91–104.)

Radiographically, periapical osseous dysplasia goes through three stages. In all three stages, the teeth are not resorbed or displaced. Larger lesions may expand and thin the alveolar cortices. The stages are:

1. Early: completely radiolucent, usually oval, round or lobular, and stays limited to the apices. This is the stage when they are most commonly mistaken for periapical inflammatory lesions.
2. Mixed stage: mixed density lesions with homogenous opacity with irregular margins (Fig. 74.40).
3. Late stage: completely radiopaque with homogenous density and with a thin low-density line between the border and the opacity [25].

Fibrous Dysplasia: This is a developmental condition that behaves similar to a tumor is its expansion and displacement of structures. It replaces the normal medullary bone with a combination of fibrous tissue and abnormal bone. It can affect one bone (monostotic) or multiple bones (polyostotic). The polyostotic type usually occurs in children under the age of 10 in McCune–Albright syndrome [26]. Mandibular lesions are mostly monostotic. Maxillary lesions are often polyostotic, extending into the adjacent bones. The course of this process becomes slow or static after the completion of skeletal grown, but may reactivate with pregnancy or the use of oral contraceptive.

apposition of bone that leads to distortion and weakening of the bone. It occurs in middle-age or older individuals, twice as often in males. It can affect multiple bones, with the jaw bone being less likely to be affects that other bones. The maxilla is more likely to be affected than the mandible. It has three radiographic stages

1. the radiolucent (resorptive) stage,
2. the granular stage, and
3. radiopaque stage (Fig. 74.46).

Tooth hypercementosis can be seen in association with this entity [1,5,24,30].

Simple (Idiopathic) Bone Cavity: This is a common condition with no known cause. It tends to occur in the first two decades of life and is asymptomatic. It most commonly occurs in the mandible, especially the posterior aspect. It is a well-defined low-density lesion that may be septated, corticated, or noncorticated, and tends to scallop between the roots of the teeth (Fig. 74.47). Expansion of the cortices is rare. Occasionally, simple bone cavities can occur in cases of fibrous dysplasia and florid osseous dysplasia [1,5,24,31].

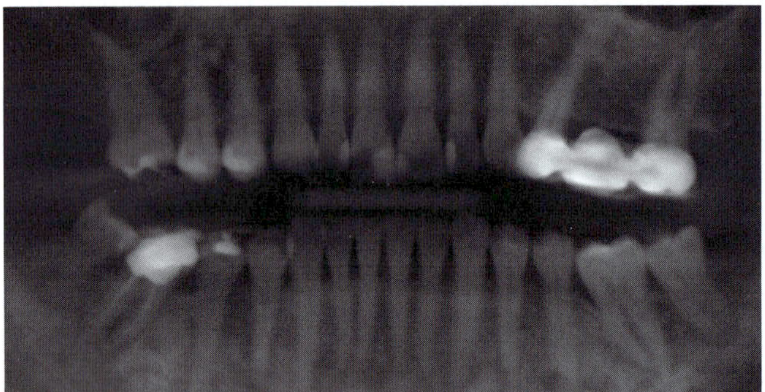

Figure 74.46 Reconstructed panoramic radiograph of a middle-aged male with Paget disease of bone shows irregular and heterogenous regions of calcification of the medullary bone present bilaterally. (Adapted from: M Ahmad, L Gaalaas, Fibro-osseous and other lesions of bone in the jaws, Radiol Clin North Am 56 (1) (2018) 91–104.)

Radiographic Analysis of the TMJs

Anatomy of the TMJs

The temporomandibular joint (TMJ) is among the most complex and poorly understood joints in the body. The complexity of this diarthrodial joint leads to much controversy regarding its diagnosis and treatment. To further complicate matters, there are two TMJs that work together to move a single piece of bone, the mandible, and create multidirectional and multifunctional movements. An understanding of the radiographic anatomy of the TMJ will help the radiologist become more familiar with identifying and diagnosing TMJ dysfunction. This review will cover the intracapsular components of the TMJs, which are generally visible and diagnosable on radiographic imaging.

To evaluate the TMJs correctly, one must obtain the correct cross sections. These images should be axially corrected sagittal and coronal oblique images of the TMJs along the long axes of the condyles and perpendicular to them (Fig. 74.48). This is true whether the imaging is CT, CBCT, or MRI. CT and CBCT imaging will show the osseous components of the TMJs as well as any resulting changes in the facial skeleton. MRI will give information about the soft-tissue condition, such as disc position and condition in the closed and open mouth positions, the presence of joint effusion and bone marrow edema, as well as the osseous contours and bone marrow homogeneity. It is important that the imaging be performed with the teeth in maximum intercuspation as a baseline image. This allows for the evaluation of spatial relation of the condyle and fossa on CT/CBCT and the relation of the disc to the osseous components on MRI [32].

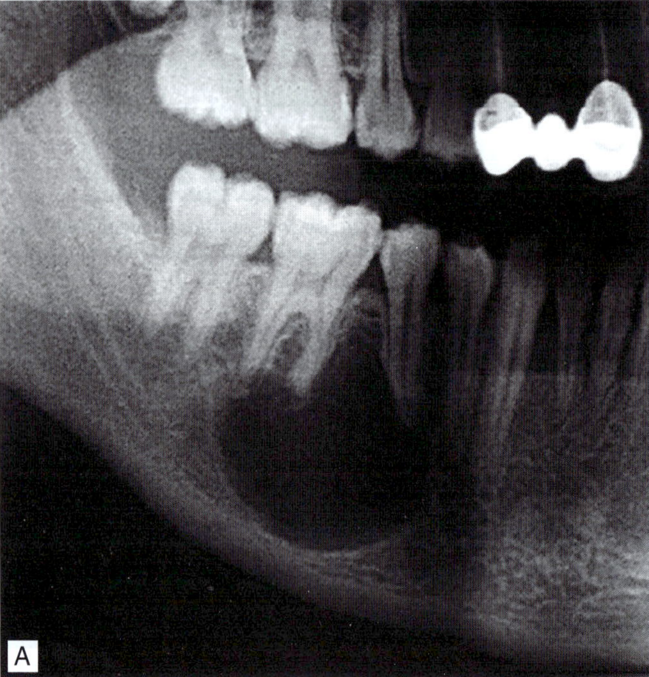

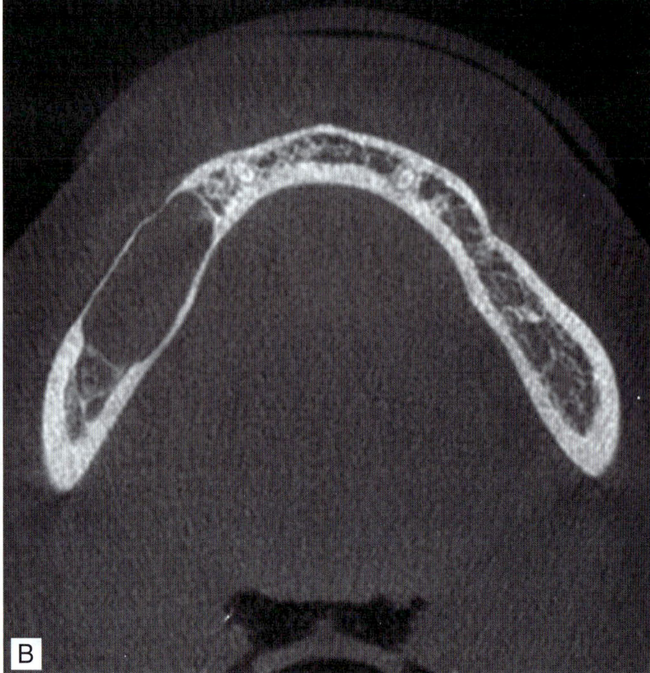

Figure 74.47 (A) Cropped panoramic radiograph of a 17-year-old male with a simple bone cavity in the right mandible. Inferiorly, the lesion seems thinly corticated and noncorticated superiorly. The lesion is scalloping between the teeth roots with no tooth displacement or resorption. (B) Axial CBCT shows thinning of the buccal and lingual cortices with minimal expansion. (Adapted from: M Ahmad, L Gaalaas, Fibro-osseous and other lesions of bone in the jaws, Radiol Clin North Am 56 (1) (2018) 91–104.)

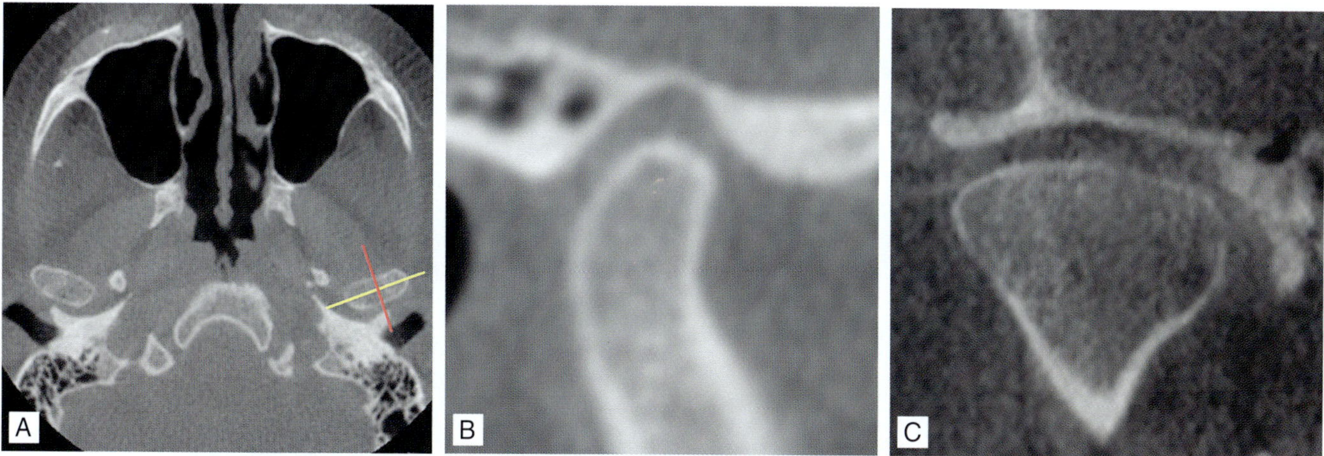

Figure 74.48 (A) CBCT axial view with schematic plane lines to show the orientation of the axially corrected, (B) sagittal oblique (same plane as the red line on (A)), and (C) coronal oblique (same plane as the yellow line on (A)) cross sections. These cross sections are correct and appropriate for the evaluation of the anatomy and spatial relations of the osseous structures. (Adapted from: D Tamimi, E Jalali, D Hatcher, Temporomandibular joint imaging, Radiol Clin North Am 56 (1) (2018) 157–175.)

Osseous Components

Condyle: The condyle should have a rounded articular surface with the posterior height of contour lower than the anterior height of contour (Fig. 74.49). This is an important diagnostic point, as it enables the reviewer to distinguish whether a small condyle is due to a condylar hypoplasia (where the contours are normal but the condyle is small or short) from end stage degenerative joint disease (where the condyle is small and short, but the articular surface is flattened and the heights of contour are approximately at the same level). The articular cortex between these heights of contour is eggshell thin. Flattening of the articular surface indicates functional remodeling and thickening of this cortex indicates subchondral sclerosis, both of which are results of increased biomechanical loading. The articular cortices should be continuous, rounded, and thin. Breaks in the cortices may indicate active degenerative joint disease, rheumatoid arthritis or, rarely, malignancy. The bone marrow spaces should be homogenous on CT and MRI.

Fossa: The articular surface of the glenoid fossa is the roof of the fossa, the posterior slope of the eminence and the crest of the eminence. The posterior slope of the eminence should be smooth and rounded and the crest of the eminence is normally broad and rounded. The roof of the fossa can vary in thickness.

Spatial Relations: When MRI is not available, evaluating the condylar relation to the fossa on CT or CBCT can be useful provided the teeth are in maximum intercuspation on the scan and the correct cross sections are used. It is a good exercise to envision the outlines of a disc in between the osseous components (Fig. 74.50). If the space is narrowed to a point where the components of a disc cannot fit in the space, or the condyle is posteriorly, medially, laterally, or superiorly positioned in the fossa, the disc is most likely displaced, but this cannot be verified without soft-tissue imaging and clinical evaluation.

Soft-Tissue Components

The intracapsular soft-tissue structures that are evaluated on MRI are the disc, the attachments and the synovial fluid-filled joint compartments. In the closed mouth position and on the sagittal oblique view (Fig. 74.51), the disc is biconcave with the thick posterior band of the disc positioned at the 12 o'clock position to the condyle, the intermediate zone positioned

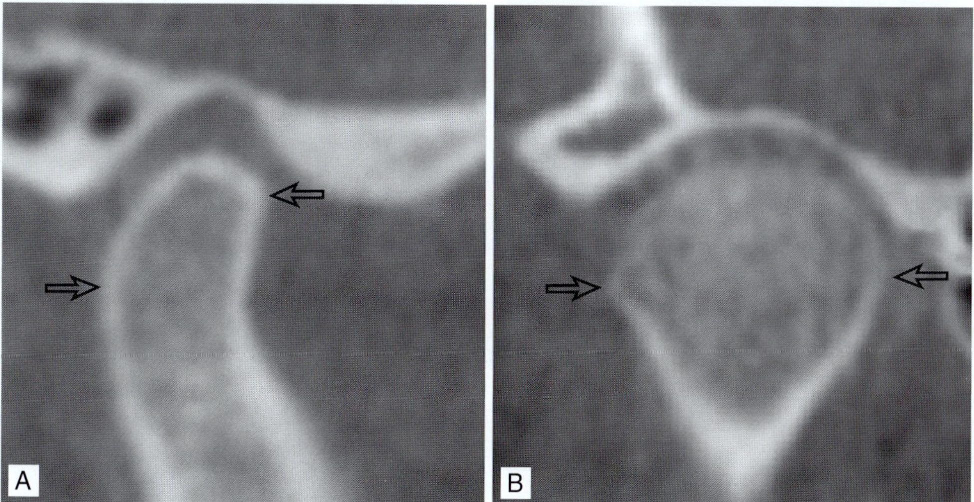

Figure 74.49 CBCT axially corrected (A) sagittal oblique and (B) coronal oblique cross sections show the position of the condylar heights of contours (*arrows*) in relation to one another in a normal condyle. (Adapted from: D Tamimi, E Jalali, D Hatcher, Temporomandibular joint imaging, Radiol Clin North Am 56 (1) (2018) 157–175.)

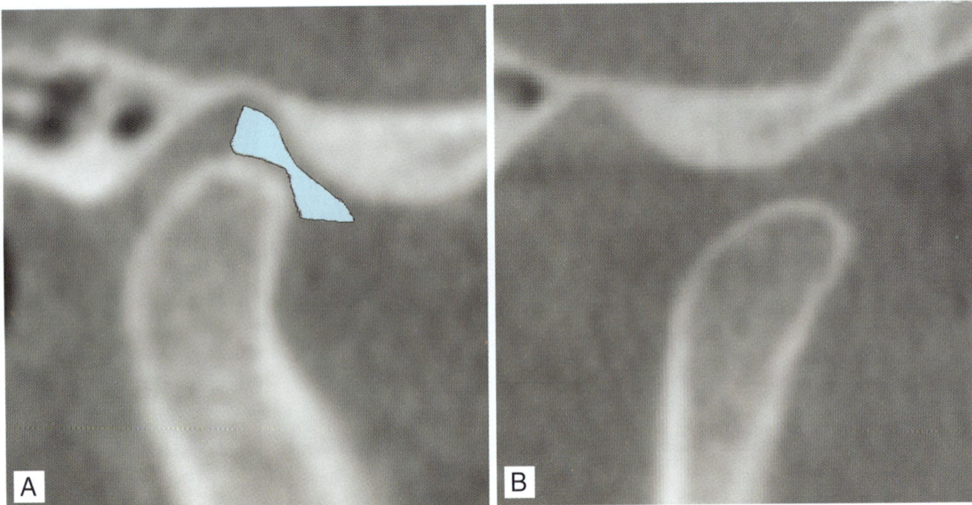

Figure 74.50 CBCT axially corrected sagittal cross sections in (A) closed and (B) open mouth positions show the normal spatial relations of the osseous structures. (A) A normal-shaped biconcave disc can be imagined in the joint space by the examiner, indicating that the spatial relations are within normal limits (the disc cannot be visualized or diagnosed without MRI). (B) The condyle translates to a point inferior and slightly anterior to the crest of the eminence (range of motion within normal limits). (Adapted from: D Tamimi, E Jalali, D Hatcher, Temporomandibular joint imaging, Radiol Clin North Am 56 (1) (2018) 157–175.)

between the heights of maximum curvature of the condyle and the posterior slope of the eminence, and the anterior band positioned anterior to the condyle. On the coronal oblique view, the disc resembles a crescent moon that tapes toward the poles and attaches to the lateral aspects of the condylar neck through the medial and lateral collateral ligaments (Fig. 74.52). The disc also attached to the condyle through the condylar posterior attachment (inferior lamina). The disc is attached to the fossa through the temporal posterior attachment (superior lamina). There are two joint compartments between the disc and the osseous surfaces: the superior and inferior joint compartments. A mild amount of joint effusion visualized on T2-weighted or STIR MRI is within normal limits, but larger fluid collections can be pathologic and symptomatic [33–35].

In the open mouth position the condyle should translate to a point inferior to the crest of the eminence. As is does this, the disc should move along with it, with the normal open mouth relation being the junction between the anterior band and the intermediate zone being interposed between the articular surfaces of the TMJ (Fig. 74.53). In the case of disc displacement with reduction, the disc/articular surface relation should be normal in the open mouth position.

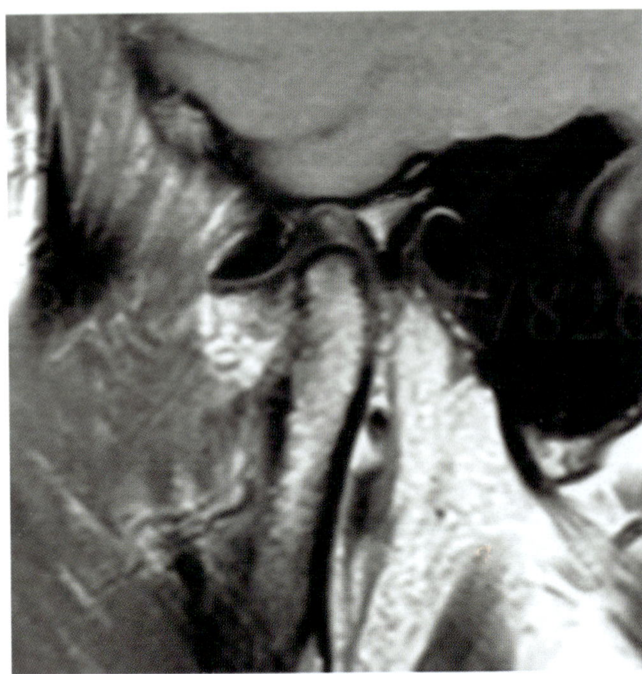

Figure 74.51 MRI axially corrected sagittal oblique cross section shows the normal anatomic relations of the disc with the osseous structures. (Adapted from: D Tamimi, DC Hatcher. Specialty imaging: temporomandibular joint. Salt Lake City, UT: Elsevier; 2016.)

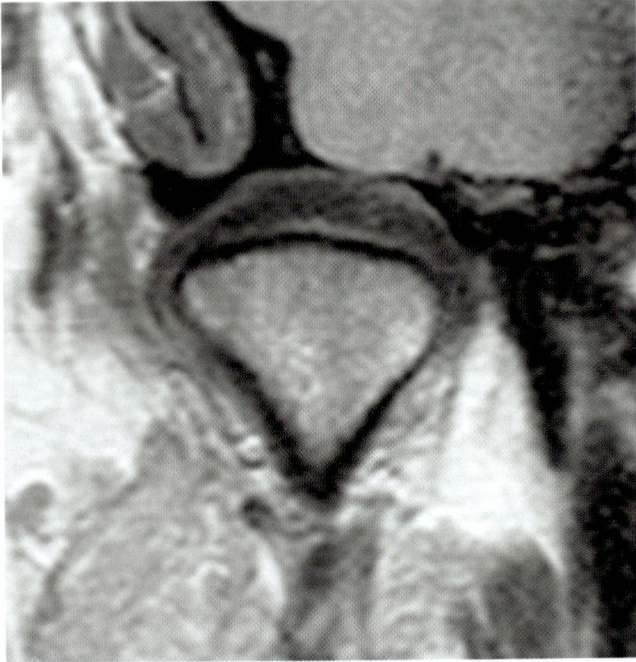

Figure 74.52 MRI axially corrected coronal oblique cross section shows the normal anatomic relations of the disc with the osseous structures. (Adapted from: D Tamimi, DC Hatcher. Specialty imaging: temporomandibular joint. Salt Lake City, UT: Elsevier; 2016.)

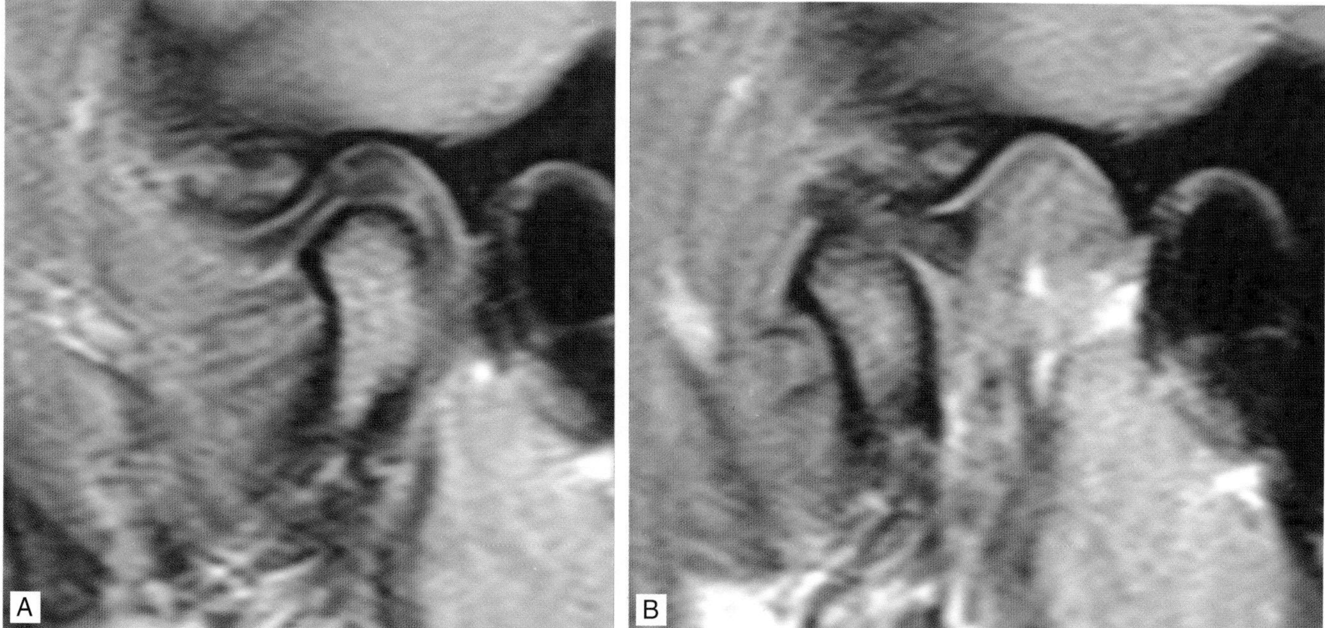

Figure 74.53 T1 MRI axially corrected cross sections shows the normal range of motion of the condyle and the disc. (A) indicates the closed mouth position. In the open mouth position (B), the part of the disc interposed between the condyle and the eminence is the junction between the anterior band and intermediate zones of the disc.

TMJ Imaging of Pathology

Internal Derangement and Degenerative Joint Disease

Soft-Tissue Changes: The TMJ is designed to withstand high multidirectional biomechanical forces. When the biomechanical demands exceed the biomechanical threshold of the disc, a loss of structural integrity of the disc and attachments occurs [32]. This leads to a gradual slipping (displacement) of the posterior band of the disc from the normal 11–12 o'clock position. If the biomechanical insult continues and increases, further damage can occur to these soft tissues and further displacement can occur. If the normal disc–condyle relation is restored in the open mouth position, this is called "disc displacement with reduction"; if it does not, then this is called "disc displacement without reduction" [32,36–38] (Fig. 74.54). TMJ discs can become displaced in multiple directions, such as the anterior, anteromedial, and anterolateral rotational and sideways (pure medial or lateral) (Fig. 74.55). Some authors advocate the presence of posterior disc displacement, but it is this author's opinion that this is most likely a false-positive appearance created by the formation of a "pseudodisc," a thickening and fibrosis of the posterior attachment area that give a morphologically thick low signal similar to that of the disc [7]. Obtaining axially corrected sagittal oblique and coronal oblique cross sections is crucial for the correct evaluation and diagnosis of the direction of a disc displacement [32,36,37].

Osseous Changes: The soft-tissue changes described previously precede the osseous changes seen in degenerative joint disease in both adults (DJD) and children (progressive condylar resorption/idiopathic condylar resorption). The morphology of the condyles at the end stage of the degenerative change is different for adults and children, but the process of destruction is similar. When the biomechanical threshold of the fibrocartilage and the articular surfaces is met, morphologic changes occur to the articular surfaces to adapt and to distribute these forces over a large surface area. These changes include thickening and sclerosis of the articular cortex and flattening of the articular surfaces (formation of congruent articulations). When the biomechanical threshold is exceeded, cortical breakdown (erosion) occurs (Fig. 74.56). The erosions destroy the articular surface and reduce its volume, and when the forces are alleviated or

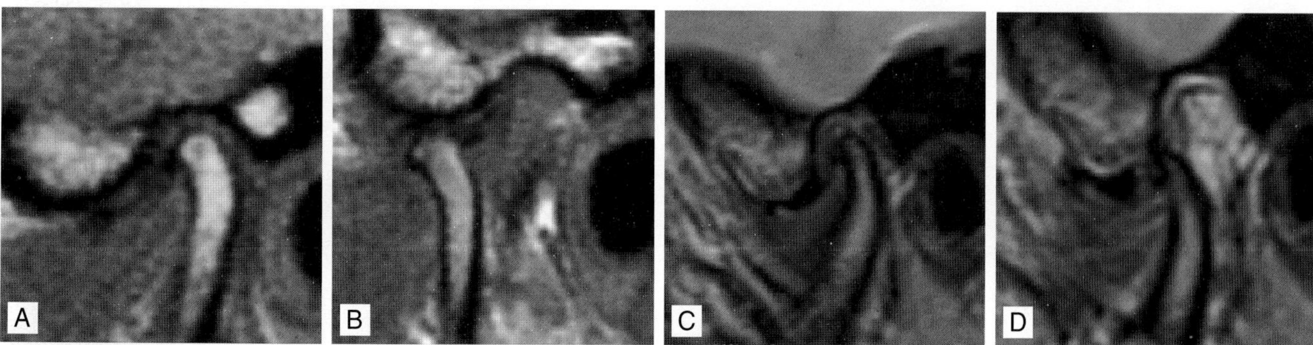

Figure 74.54 MR images show (A, B) disc displacement with reduction and (C, D) disc displacement without reduction. (A) T1WI shows a biconcave disc that has maintained its anteroposterior dimension positioned anterior to the condyle. (B) T1WI in the same patient shows recapture of the disc by the condyle and translation of the condyle to normal range of motion. (C) T2WI shows a disc that is anteriorly displaced and appears morphologically altered. (D) T2WI in the same patient show lack of recapture of the disc by the condyle and limitation of condylar range of motion. (Adapted from: D Tamimi, E Jalali, D Hatcher, Temporomandibular joint imaging, Radiol Clin North Am 56 (1) (2018) 157–175.)

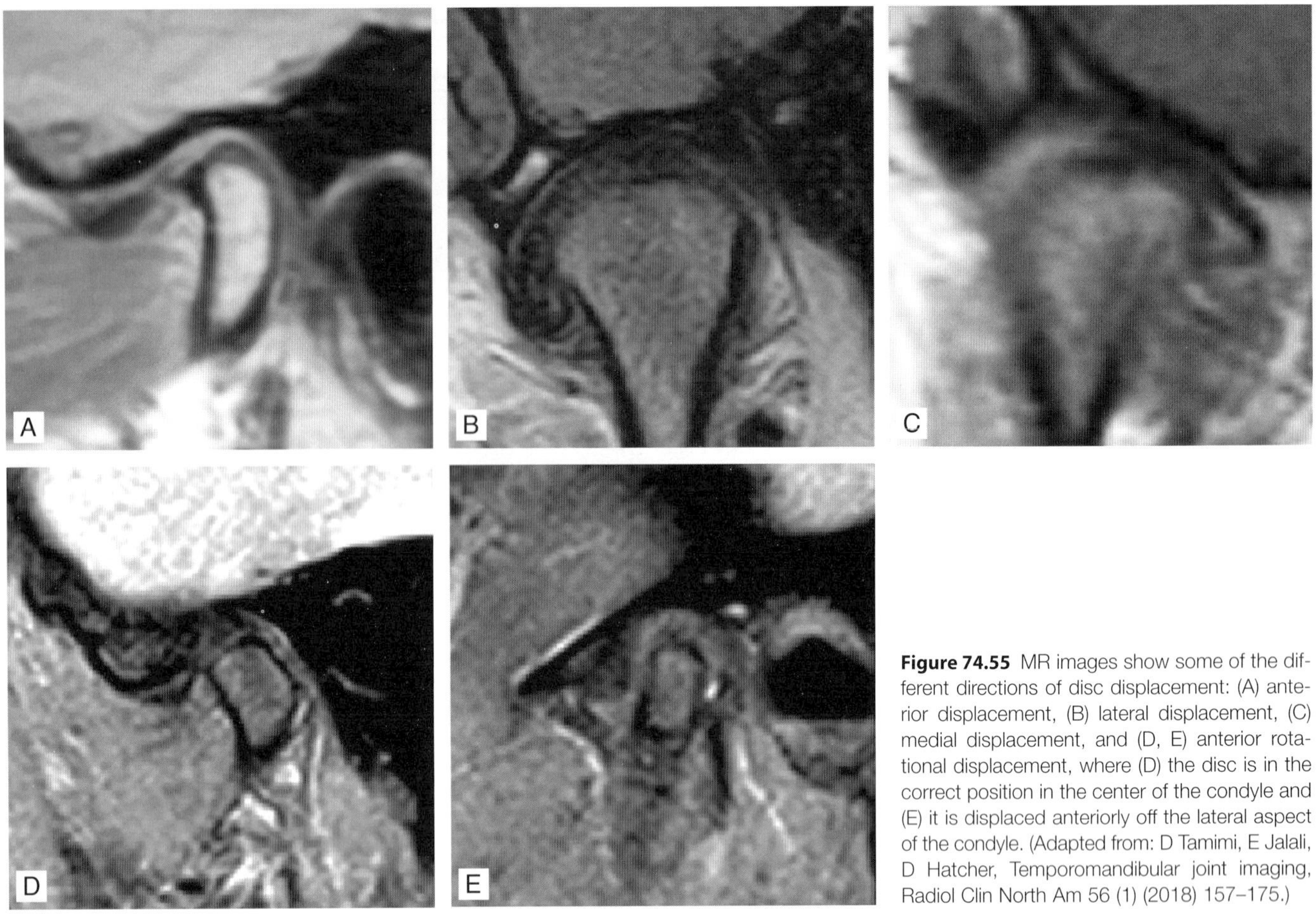

Figure 74.55 MR images show some of the different directions of disc displacement: (A) anterior displacement, (B) lateral displacement, (C) medial displacement, and (D, E) anterior rotational displacement, where (D) the disc is in the correct position in the center of the condyle and (E) it is displaced anteriorly off the lateral aspect of the condyle. (Adapted from: D Tamimi, E Jalali, D Hatcher, Temporomandibular joint imaging, Radiol Clin North Am 56 (1) (2018) 157–175.)

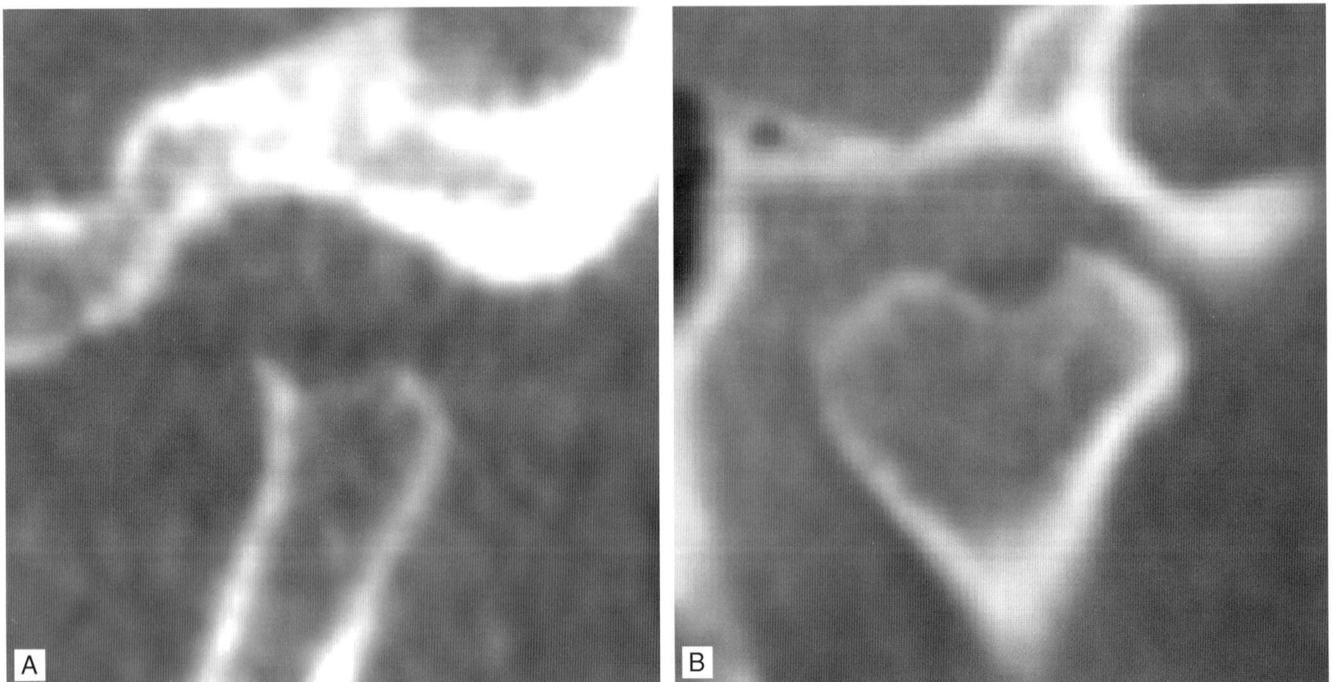

Figure 74.56 Axially corrected sagittal (A) and coronal (B) CBCT cross sections show erosion and volume loss on the articular surface of the condyle, indicating active degenerative changes. (Adapted from: D Tamimi, E Jalali, D Hatcher, Temporomandibular joint imaging, Radiol Clin North Am 56 (1) (2018) 157–175.)

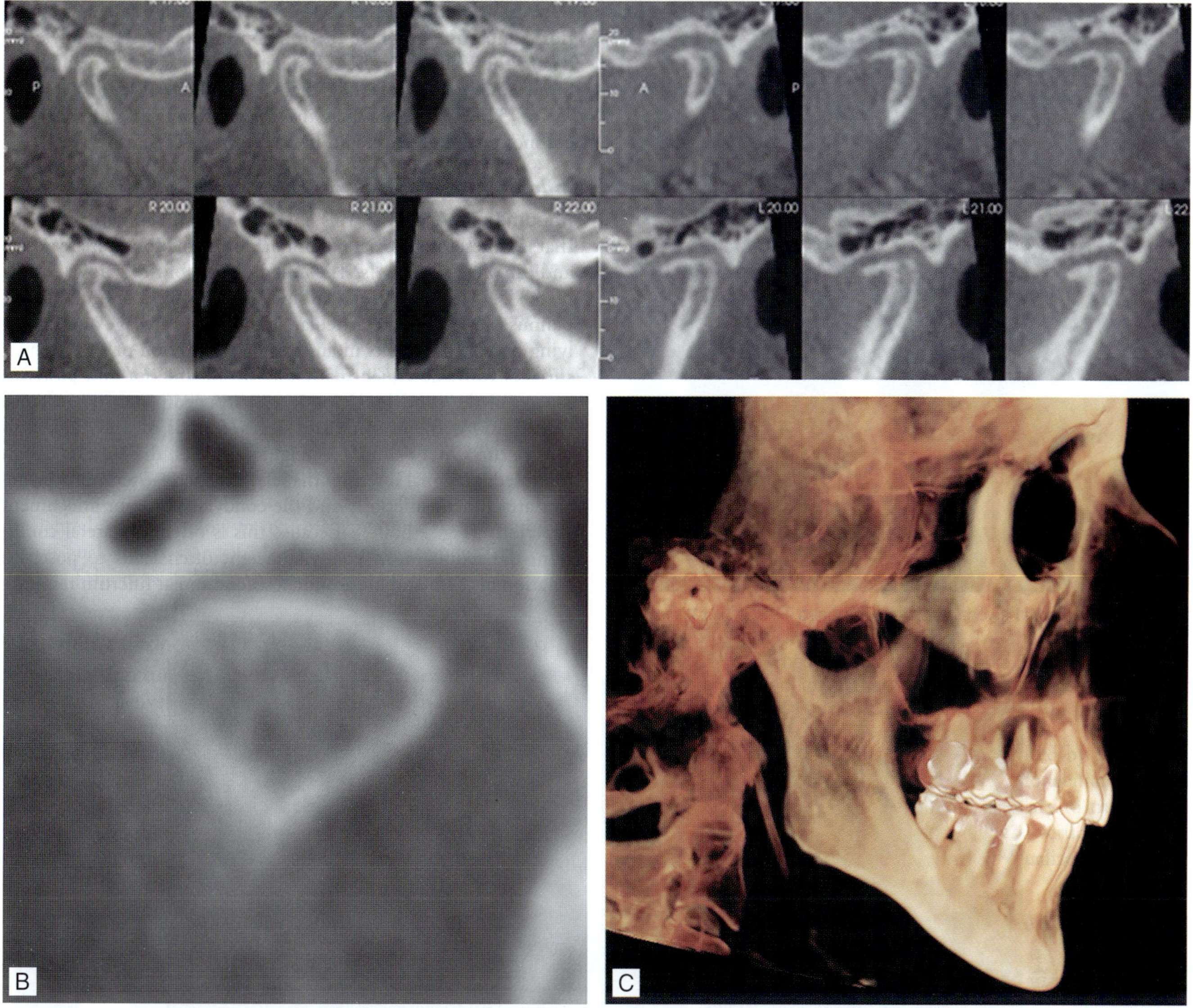

Figure 74.57 CBCT reformations show the effect of end-stage degenerative changes on the condylar dimensions and the facial skeleton. (A) Serial sagittal cross sections show reduction of condylar height and the formation of an osteophyte anteriorly on each condyle. (B) The coronal view shows a reduction of the condylar height. (C) Lateral 3D rendering shows the effect of the reduction of condylar height bilaterally on the mandible: posterior rotation of the mandible, small mandible, and a steep mandibular plane. This can result in a convex facial profile. (Adapted from: D Tamimi, E Jalali, D Hatcher, Temporomandibular joint imaging, Radiol Clin North Am 56 (1) (2018) 157–175.)

when the body adapts to their presence, the articular surfaces start to repair and recorticate. The lost bone, however, cannot be rebuilt, hence resulting in reduction of condylar height and volume with corticated surfaces and condylar heights of contour that have changed in relation to the fossa, while the repair process is complete. In adult DJD, it is common to see osteophytes as a method of increasing surface area for load distribution (Fig. 74.57A). Subchondral bone cysts can also be seen in adult DJD [32–35]. In both adults and children, changes to the mandibular and facial morphology can be expected, but it is more severe if the degenerative joint disease occurs in a growing individual as the growth plates of the condyles are affected (Fig. 74.57C).

Range of Motion: Condylar hypermobility is characterized by a condyle that moves more than 2-mm anterior and superior to the crest of the eminence. This occurs when there is elongation of the posterior attachments and the sphenomandibular and stylomandibular ligaments. This may be seen in some early cases of internal derangement of the joint, or in cases of Ehlers–Danlos syndrome [39]. It can manifest as subluxation of the condyle, where the condyle can return to the closed position, or dislocation, where the condyle cannot return and the patient is in an open lock (Fig. 74.58). Condylar restriction is characterized by a condyle that remains posterior and superior to the crest of the eminence. It can occur with internal derangement. Disc displacement with reduction usually has a normal range of motion, but an acute closed lock is usually experienced in the acute phase of disc displacement without reduction. As the condition becomes more chronic, range of motion may be restored. Disc adhesions can occur due to trauma or due to disc displacement (Fig. 74.59). Synovitis can lead to fibrin deposition and hence decrease in lubrication that results in the stiction effect (two solid objects pressed against each other but not sliding), reduced disc mobility and further increase in fibrin depositions and formation of fibrous adhesions. This most commonly occurs in the superior joint compartment (where the

Figure 74.63 CBCT panoramic reformat of the right half of the mandible shows anterior positioning of the condylar process. The condylar cortex traverses the ramus. There is an acute angle between the condylar process and the coronoid process giving the "scissors sign" typical of a neonatal fracture after forceps delivery. (Adapted from: D Tamimi, E Jalali, D Hatcher, Temporomandibular joint imaging, Radiol Clin North Am 56 (1) (2018) 157–175.)

oblique view) to duplication of the condyle (one condyle in front of the other) in the sagittal oblique view [32,36,37] (Fig. 74.65).

Ankylosis: This can be fibrous or bony and is usually secondary to an insult to the joint. Trauma is the most common cause, followed by inflammatory arthritides, previous joint surgery, and infection. These present clinically as marked limitation of opening, with bony ankylosis being more severe. On bone CT, a fibrous ankylosis maintains a soft-tissue separation between the irregular articular surfaces. Bony ankylosis fuses the condyle to the fossa at varying degrees [32,36,37] (Fig. 74.66).

Benign Neoplasia

Osteochondroma This is a benign, cartilage-capped, exophytic lesion arising from bone. It can arise from the condyle and from the coronoid process. It can present as a pedunculated mass of mixed density attached to the condyle that often extends from the anterior or anteromedial surface of the condyle at the attachment of the lateral pterygoid muscle and can grow in the direction of the muscle fibers (Fig. 74.67). When it is small, it is difficult to distinguish from osteophytes caused by degenerative joint disease. When large, it can displace the condyle in the fossa and displace the mandible inferiorly and contralaterally, resulting in an ipsilateral posterior open bite and a contralateral cross bite [32,36,37].

Osteoma: This is a benign slow-growing bone-forming tumor characterized by proliferation of either compact or cancellous bone. It usually originates from the surfaces of the condyle that are covered with periosteum (nonarticular surfaces). It appears as a pedunculated, homogenous, well-defined high-density mass. It

TABLE 74.5 A Classification for Severity of Condylar Fractures

Type	Fracture Position	Condylar Position
Type I	Neck	Slight displacement of the condyle; angle between the condyle and the axis of the ramus between 10° and 45°
Type II	Neck	Angle from 45° to 90°, resulting in tearing of the medial portion of the capsule
Type III	Neck/subcondylar	Fragments not in contact; displaced medially and forward
Type IV	Neck/subcondylar	Condyle articulates on or in a forward position with regard to the articular eminence
Type V	Vertical or oblique through the condyle	Fragment can be displaced or within the fossa

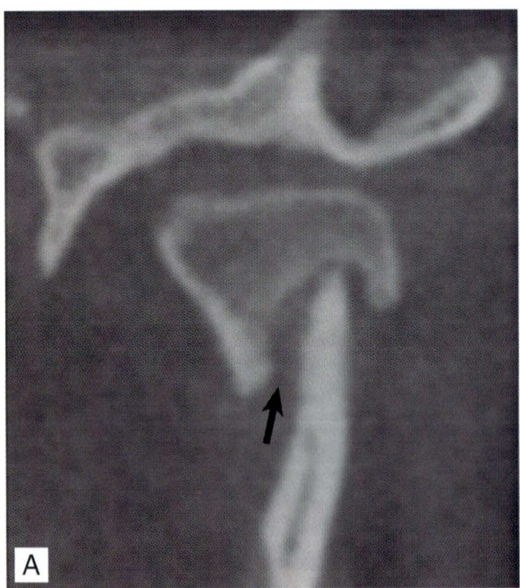

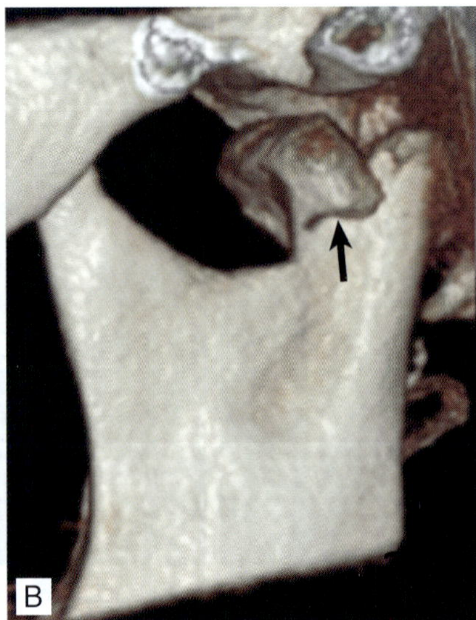

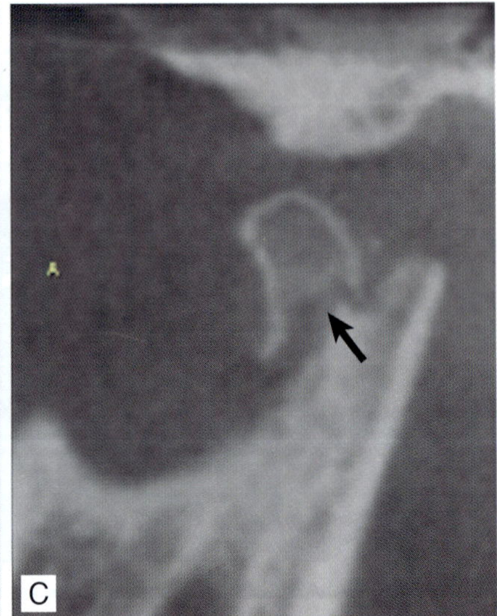

Figure 74.64 CBCT coronal (A), surface rendering (B), and sagittal (C) show condylar neck fracture (*arrow*) with limited anterior displacement due to the lodging of the fragment into the neck. (Adapted from: R Alimohammadi, Imaging of dentoalveolar and jaw trauma, Radiol Clin North Am 56 (1) (2018) 105–124.)

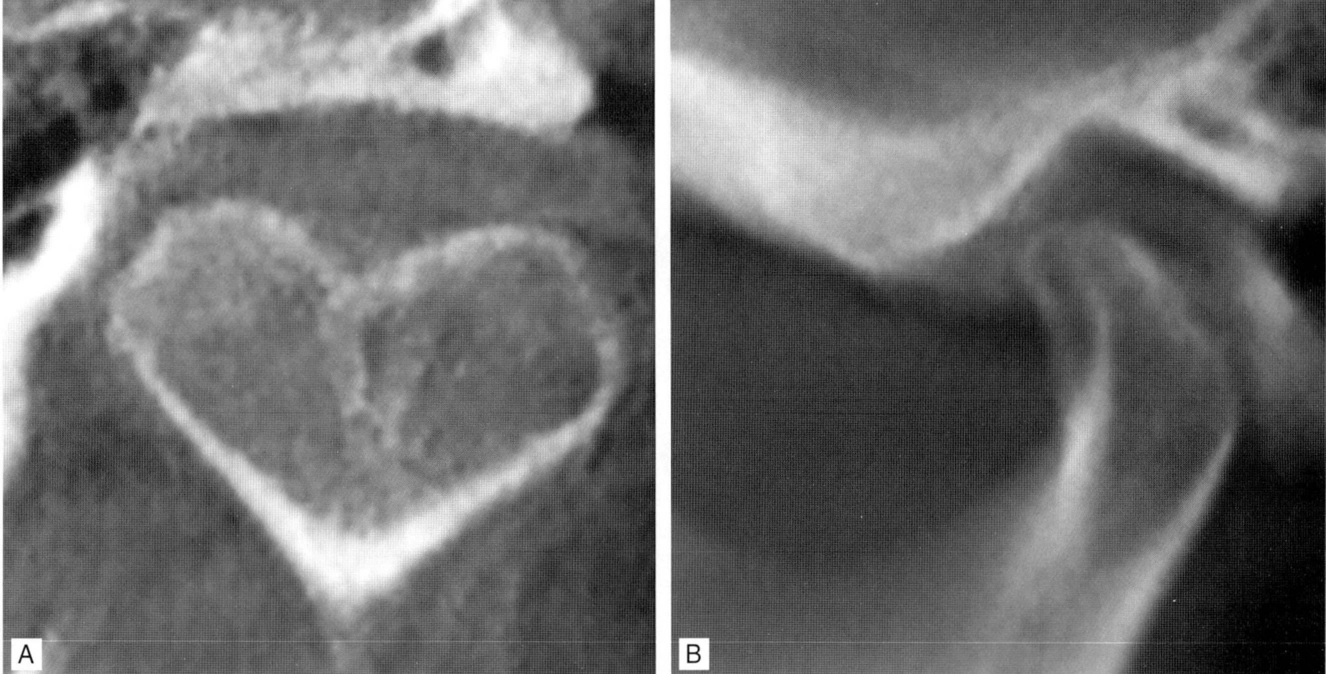

Figure 74.65 CBCT (A) coronal oblique and (B) sagittal oblique cross sections show a bifid condyle. Image (A) shows the typical appearance of a deep groove in the superior aspect of the condyle. Image (B) shows the radiographic appearance of "one condyle in front of the other" that can be seen on panoramic plain film imaging and CBCT reformations. (Adapted from: D Tamimi, E Jalali, D Hatcher, Temporomandibular joint imaging, Radiol Clin North Am 56 (1) (2018) 157–175.)

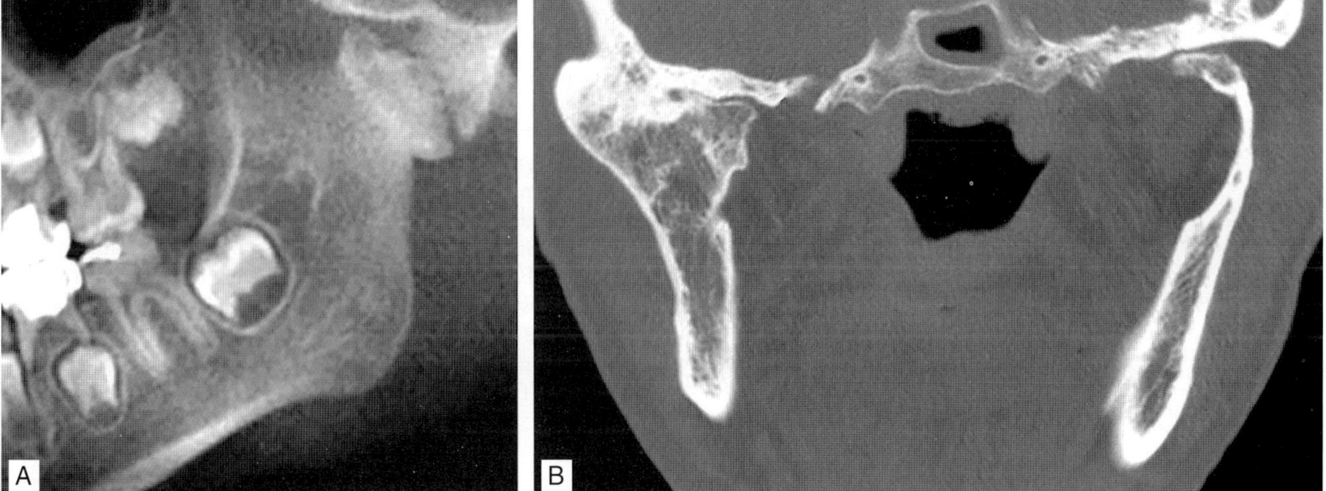

Figure 74.66 (A) CBCT sagittal oblique view shows abnormal remodeling of the left condyle and fossa following trauma. There is maintenance of a thin low-density band between the temporal and mandibular components, suggestive of a fibrous union, not a bony one. (B) Coronal bone CT shows gross enlargement of the right condyle and bony fusion with the temporal bone. (Adapted from: D Tamimi, E Jalali, D Hatcher, Temporomandibular joint imaging, Radiol Clin North Am 56 (1) (2018) 157–175.)

may be compact or cancellous and the bone pattern is normal (Fig. 74.68). This lesion can also cause displacement of the condyle and mandible if it is large enough [32,36,37].

Malignant Neoplasia

Chondrosarcoma: This is a malignant tumor that more commonly occurs in the skull base in the head and neck. It can occur centrally within the condylar or temporal bone, parosteally or in the soft tissues of the TMJs. On bone CT, a nonenhancing mass with flocculent calcifications around the condyle and the joint space that may or may not destroy the bone is observed. The joint space is widened, and the condyle may appear enlarged or lengthened. There can be a ringlet pattern of calcification in and around the condyle. Periosteal reaction may or may not be present. On T2WI, it shows a high-signal intensity and the hypointense foci signifying calcification may not be as prominent as the calcified appearance on CT. With contrast, a heterogeneously enhancing mass with whorls of intensifying lines within the tumor are often seen [32,36,37] (Fig. 74.69).

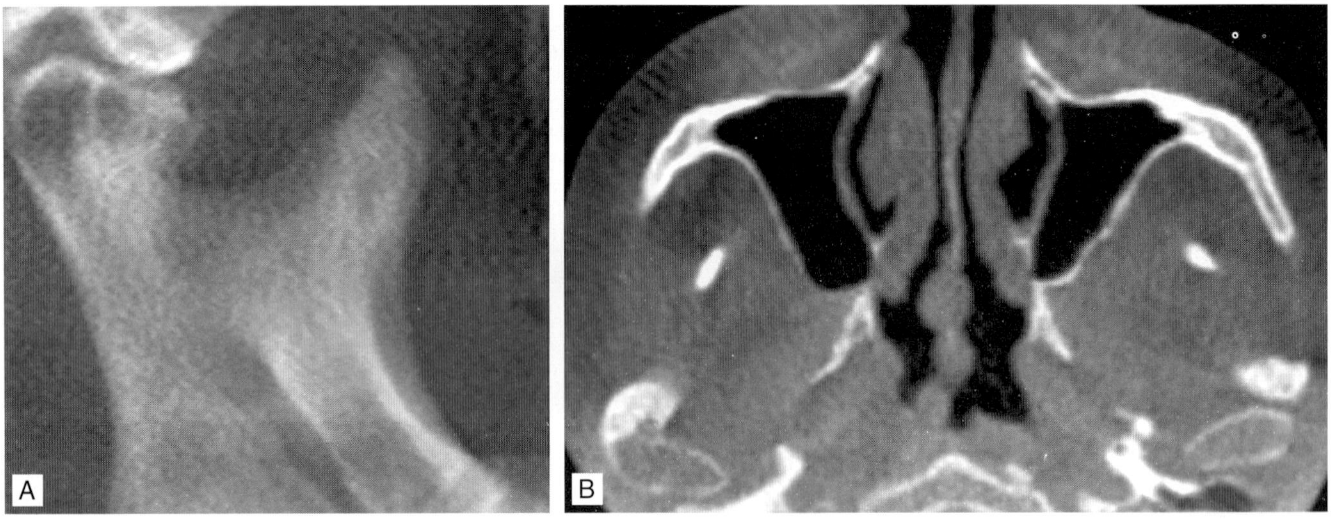

Figure 74.67 (A) CBCT panoramic reformat shows how an osteochondroma can mimic an osteophyte. The normal condylar outline is seen but it is inferiorly displaced by the lesion. The fossa contours are within normal limits. (B) Axial view shows orientation of the lesion with fibers of the lateral pterygoid muscle fibers. (Adapted from: D Tamimi, E Jalali, D Hatcher, Temporomandibular joint imaging, Radiol Clin North Am 56 (1) (2018) 157–175.)

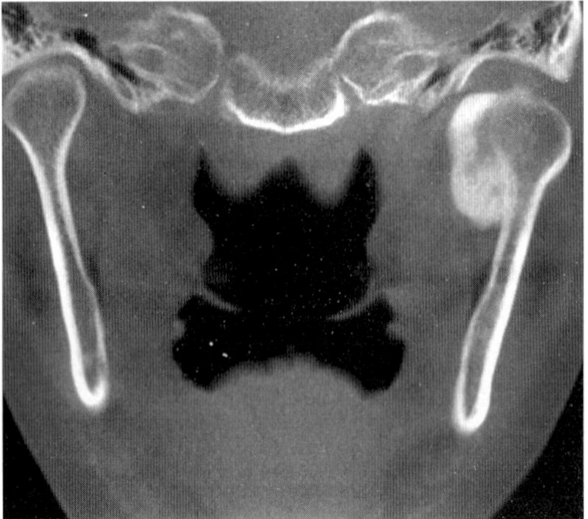

Figure 74.68 Coronal CBCT shows a large pedunculated high-density mass arising from the neck of the condyle, suggestive of an osteoma. (Adapted from: D Tamimi, E Jalali, D Hatcher, Temporomandibular joint imaging, Radiol Clin North Am 56 (1) (2018) 157–175.)

Osteosarcoma and Others: This has been discussed earlier under Effect of Malignancies on the Dentomaxillofacial complex.

Miscellaneous Conditions

Synovial Chondromatosis: Synovial chondromatosis can be primary (unrelated to DJD) or secondary to DJD. In the primary form, there is development of cartilaginous nodules within the subsynovial connective tissue that subsequently detach, ossify, and form loose articular bodies in the joint space. This is not a neoplastic entity but has a mass effect in widening the joint space, remodeling the surrounding bone and displacing the condyle. On bone CT, multiple calcified nodules can be seen surrounding the condyle with widening of the joint space. On T1-weighted imaging, the tissue planes between the mass and the surrounding soft tissues can be defined. Multiple hypointense loose articular bodies may be observed. On T2-weighted imaging the joint space in which these nodules reside is hyperintense due to fluid accumulation. Contrast-enhanced T1 MR imaging shows an enhancing synovium (Fig. 74.70).

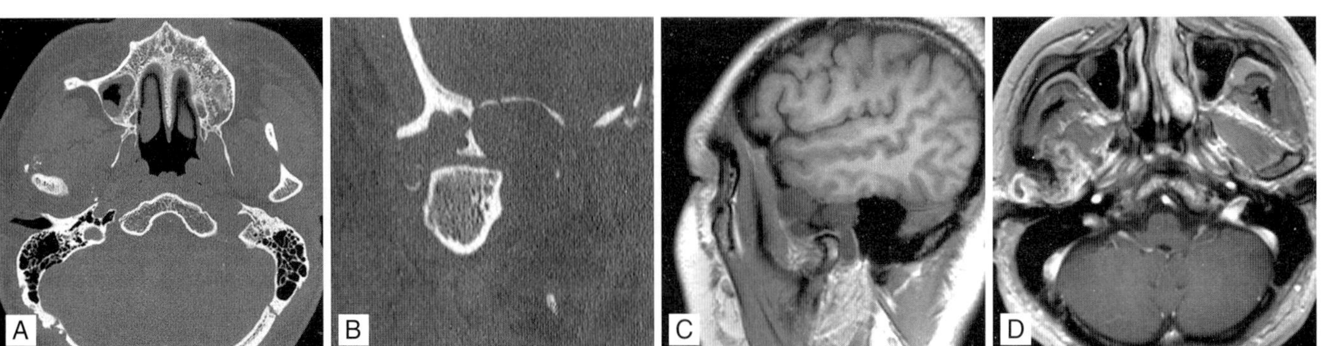

Figure 74.69 Chondrosarcoma: (A) Bone CT shows increased sclerosis of the right condyle and the presence of small calcifications lateral to the condyle. (B) Coronal view shows ring-like calcifications lateral to the condyle and destruction of the glenoid fossa. (C) Sagittal MR T1WI shows a lobulated mass extending into the middle cranial fossa. (D) Axial contrast-enhanced T1WI shows extensive solid enhancement of the lesion, indicating that is not inflammatory. (Adapted from: D Tamimi, E Jalali, D Hatcher, Temporomandibular joint imaging, Radiol Clin North Am 56 (1) (2018) 157–175.)

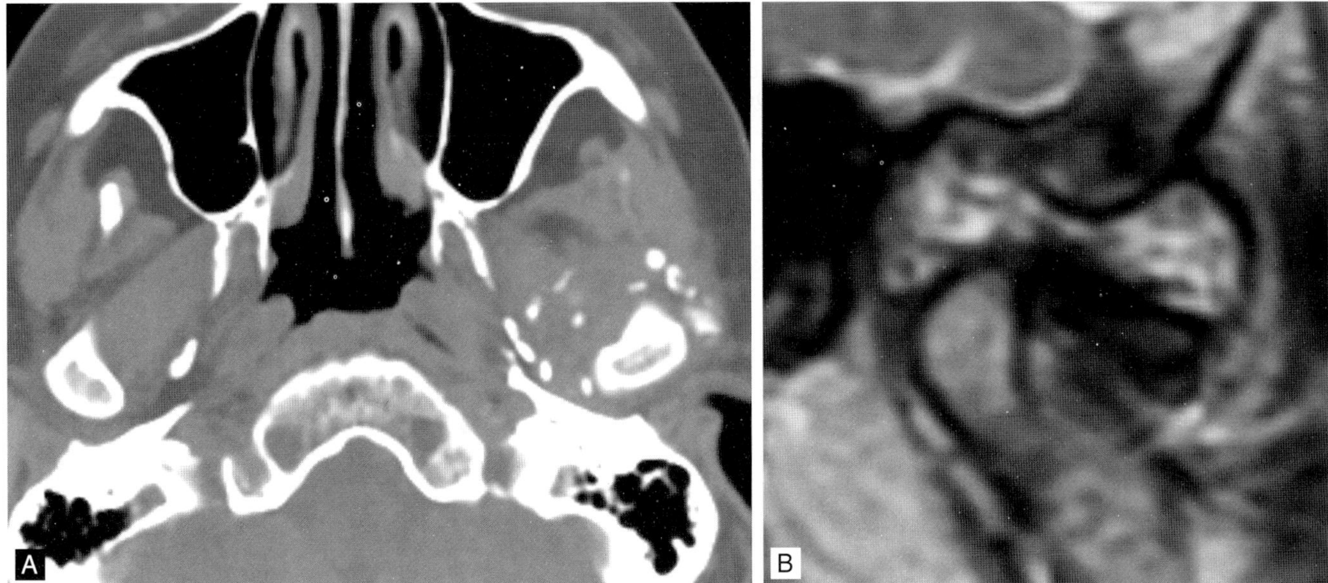

Figure 74.70 (A) Noncontrast-enhanced CT in a patient with synovial chondromatosis shows multiple small loos calcified articular bodies surrounding the left condyle. (B) Sagittal oblique T2WI MR shows high-signal mass with small low-density bodies within. (Adapted from: D Tamimi, E Jalali, D Hatcher, Temporomandibular joint imaging, Radiol Clin North Am 56 (1) (2018) 157–175.)

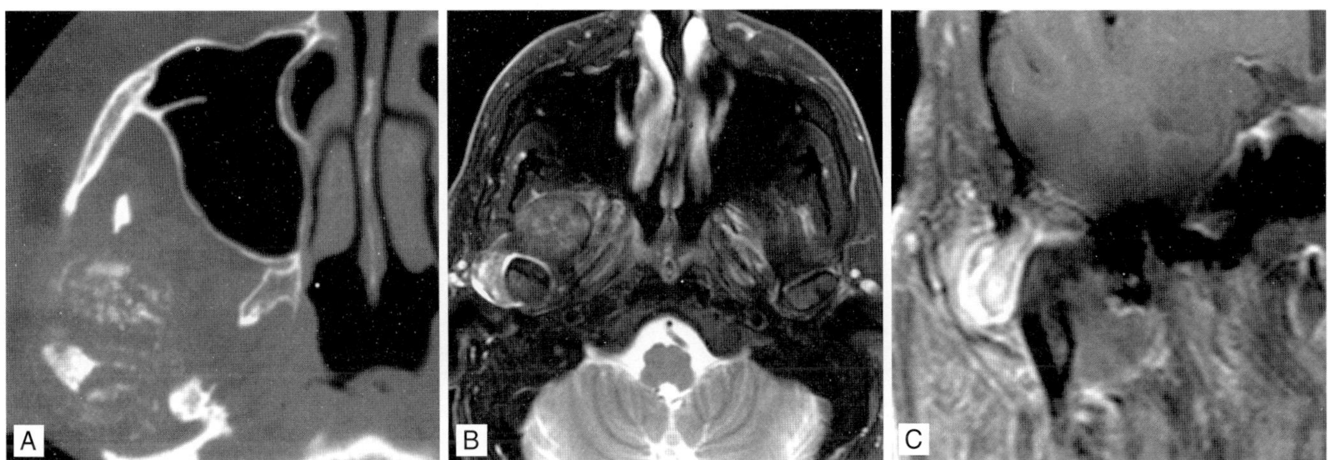

Figure 74.71 (A) Axial bone CT of a patient with CPPDD disease shows a large erosive defect in the medial aspect of the condyle and fine granular soft-tissue calcifications surrounding the condyle. (B) Axial MR T2WI FS shows a heterogenous but predominantly low-signal intensity lesion anterior to the condyle. Joint effusion is noted. (C) Coronal contrast-enhanced T1WI FS in the same patient shows enhancement of the inferolateral mass.

In the form secondary to DJD, there is production of 1 or more cartilaginous or osseous fragments along with irritation and metaplasia of the synovial membrane following unrelated breakdown of the articular surfaces caused by DJD. There are signs of advanced DJD (congruent articulation, osteophyte formation, joint space narrowing, and possible subchondral bone cyst formation). This form of synovial chondromatosis does not produce a mass effect, a point that is useful in distinguishing the two entities [32,36,37].

Calcium Pyrophosphate Dehydrate Deposition Disease: This is a metabolic disease in which calcium pyrophosphate crystals as deposited in the synovial fluid, resulting in calcification of the articular cartilage and leading to acute arthritis in some patients. Tumoral calcium pyrophosphate dehydrate deposition disease (CPPDD) is the most prevalent type in the TMJs. It differs from gout, in which uric acid crystals are precipitated, therefore it is called pseudogout. On bone CT, early CPPDD presents as fine, cloud-like calcifications with even distribution in the joint space, often encircling the condyle. Late CPPDD presents as a chunky, diffusely calcified mass that may have a ground glass appearance. There can be associated bone remodeling and mass effect that may mimic malignancy because of extensive bone destruction, which makes it difficult to distinguish from chondrosarcoma. On MR imaging T1W shows a low-signal to intermediate-signal lesion because of the soft-tissue mass in the joint space. Expansion of the joint capsule can be seen. Contrast enhancement yields a heterogeneously enhancing mass [32,36,37] (Fig. 74.71).

Suggested Readings

- LJ Koenig, D Tamimi, G Petrikowski, SE Perschbacher, A Ruprecht, BW Benson, et al., Diagnostic Imaging: Oral and Maxillofacial, second ed., Elsevier, Philadelphia, 2017.
- SMLE Mallya, White and Pharoah's Oral Radiology Principles and Interpretation, eighth ed., Elsevier, St Louis, 2019.
- D Tamimi, Oral and Maxillofacial Radiology, Radiol Clin North Am 56 (1) (2018).
- WM Scarfe, C Angelopolous, Maxillofacial Cone Beam Computed Tomography. Springer; 2018, Switzerland.
- O Langland, R Langlais, Principles of Dental Imaging. Williams & Wilkins; 1997, Baltimore, Maryland, USA.

75 Benign Brain Lesions and Epilepsy

MICHAEL TRAN DUONG, JOEL M. STEIN, VIVEK GUPTA

Introduction

The human brain, with an estimated 86 billion neurons [1], enables sensation, motion, emotion, memory, cognition, and consciousness, presenting great challenges to understanding its structure, function, and dysfunction. The brain's complexity both empowers and impedes the pursuit toward the Greek aphorism "to know thyself." Sealed in the cranial vault and guarded by the blood–brain barrier, the secrets of the brain have been slow to unravel. In his 1817 article, "An Essay on the Shaking Palsy," James Parkinson thanked "those who humanely employ **anatomical examination** in detecting the causes and nature of disease… To such research, the healing art is already much indebted for the enlargement of its power of lessening the evils of suffering humanity" [2].

For much of the history of medicine, such "anatomical examination" required pathological dissection or surgical vivisection. However, with the advent of successively more sophisticated imaging techniques, exploration of the brain today heavily relies on biomedical imaging technology, not only for diagnosis and management of neurological disorders, but also for advancement of the frontiers of neurobiology [3].

75.1 Review of Structural and Functional Anatomy

The following is an overview of structural and functional anatomy of the brain and central nervous system (CNS) (Figs. 75.1–75.6).

Cerebral Hemispheres

The cerebral cortex, containing about 20 billion neurons [1], refers to the thin, highly convoluted layer of gray matter encapsulating the white matter. Only a relatively small portion of the cortex is involved in the specific functions of receiving sensory input from the special senses or projecting motor outputs to the spinal cord. Over 80% of the cortex, known as the association cortex, is involved in more general information processing for higher cortical functions of cognition, language, and reasoning. Converging evidence from many different investigative approaches is beginning to reveal that the organization of human brain involves specialization of spatial function and integration of these regions into task-defined networks [4]. Cortical regions and subcortical nuclei act as processing modules, each with a distinct cytoarchitecture and connectivity profile specialized to process and relay-specific categories and hierarchies of input information [4]. Thus, each perceptual, executive, and motor task engages a subset of these modules into a network determined by input type (visual, auditory, and somatosensory, etc.) and output target (i.e., pattern recognition, motor response, etc.). Hence, the cortical regions may be construed as serial and parallel processors, while white matter tracts are cables for information flow across the network [4,5].

The cerebrum (forebrain or telencephalon) (Figs. 75.1–75.6) is divided into two hemispheres by the interhemispheric fissure, and each hemisphere is subdivided into four main lobes [5].

- *The frontal lobe governs executive and articulatory functions*
- *The parietal lobe processes sensory and visuospatial information* [6]
- *The temporal lobe regulates language, emotions, and memories*
- *The occipital lobe processes visual input*
- *The insular cortex, as the least understood lobe, may be involved in visceral sensorimotor, language, cognitive, and socioemotional functions*

Fissures and sulci separate these lobes anatomically. The sylvian fissure separates the temporal lobe from the frontal and parietal lobes on the lateral cerebral surface. The insula lies in the depth of the sylvian fissure, covered by frontal, temporal, and parietal opercula ("lids"). The central sulcus divides the frontal and parietal lobes on the superior and lateral surface. The parieto-occipital fissure separates the parietal and occipital lobes on the medial surface. However, it must be noted that these lobes are neither embryologically, nor functionally separate entities, and many distant areas of the cortex show greater connectivity than neighboring regions [4]. A detailed account of functional cortical specialization organization into networks is beyond the scope of this chapter [5].

Basal Ganglia

The basal ganglia, gray matter nuclei deep to the cerebral cortex, relay dopaminergic signaling from the substantia nigra to the thalamus and motor cortex through direct (cortex–putamen–globus pallidus interna–thalamus–cortex) and indirect (cortex–putamen–globus pallidus externa–subthalamic nucleus–globus pallidus interna–thalamus-cortex) pathways (Fig. 75.5) [5]. The structures in the basal ganglia include the caudate nucleus, putamen, globus pallidus, claustrum, and surrounding white matter tracts divided into internal and external

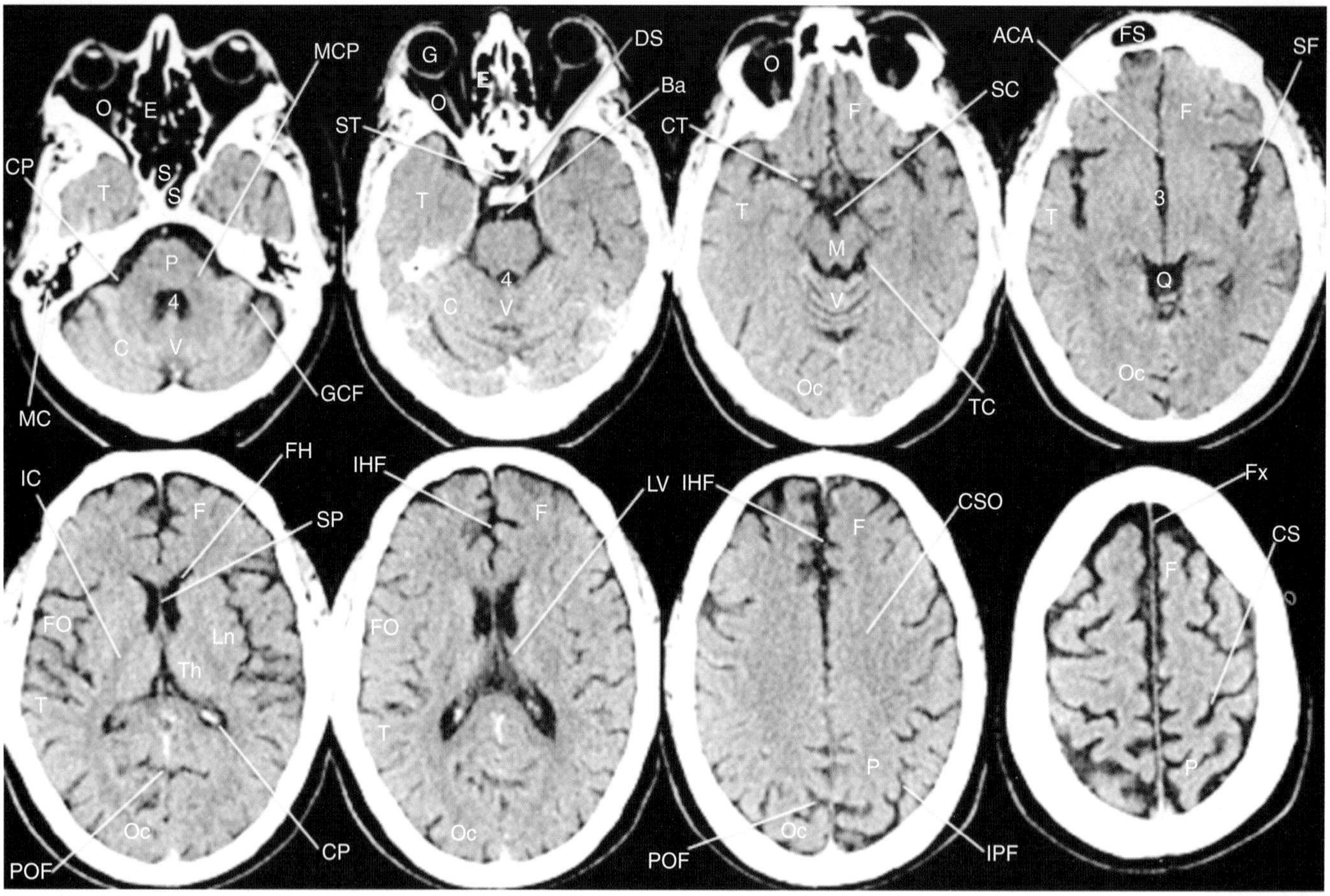

Figure 75.1 Normal craniocaudal cross-sectional brain anatomy on CT. *MCP*, middle cerebellar peduncle; *CP*, cerebellopontine angle; *P*, pons; *4*, 4th ventricle; *C*, cerebellar hemisphere; *V*, vermis; *GCF*, great cerebellar fissure; *O*, orbit; *G*, globe (eyeball); *E*, ethmoid cells; *S*, sphenoid sinus; *MC*, mastoid cells; *DS*, dorsum sellae; *ST*, sella turcica; *Ba*, basilar artery; *SC*, suprasellar cistern; *CT*, carotid artery terminus; *M*, midbrain; *T*, temporal lobe; *F*, frontal lobe; *Oc*, occipital lobe; *FS*, frontal sinus; *ACA*, anterior cerebral artery; *SF*, sylvian fissure; *3*, 3rd ventricle; *Q*, quadrigeminal cistern; *FH*, frontal horn; *SP*, septum pellucidum; *LN*, lentiform nucleus; *Th*, thalamus; *CP*, choroid plexus; *POF*, parieto-occipital fissure; *LV*, body of lateral ventricle; *P*, parietal lobe; *IPF*, intraparietal fissure; *CSO*, centrum semiovale; *IHF*, interhemispheric fissure; *CS*, central sulcus; *Fx*, falx cerebri.

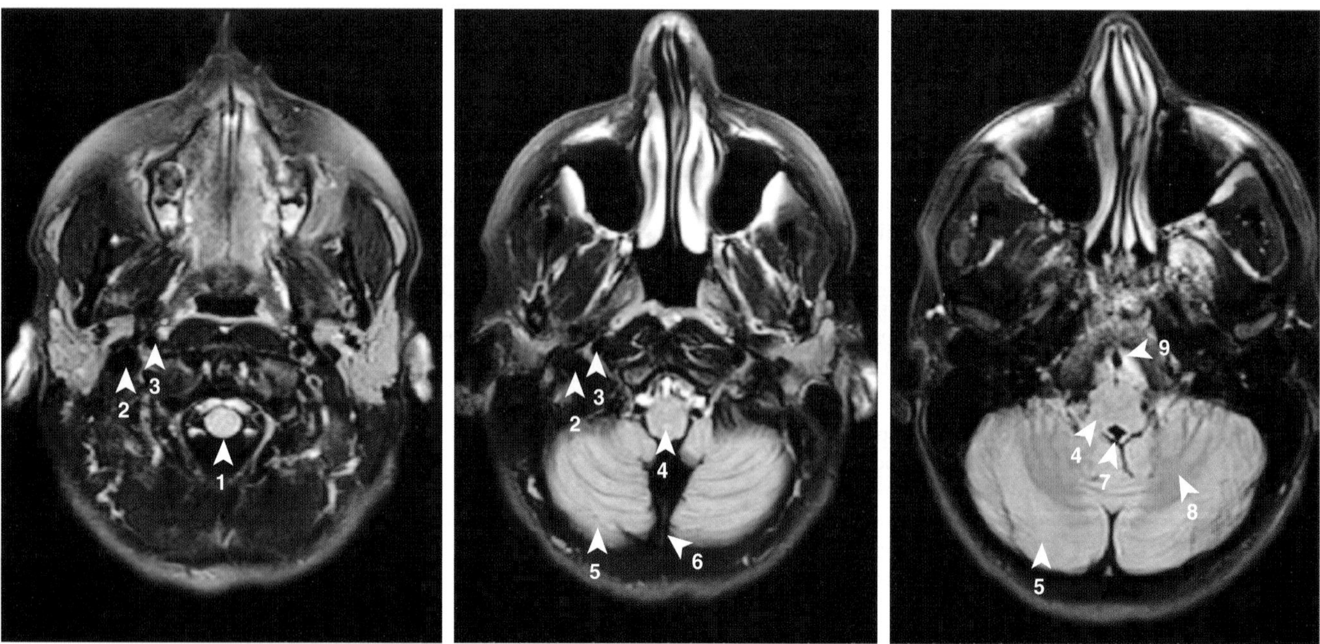

Figure 75.2 Cross sections of the upper cervical spinal cord to medulla and cerebellum. Cervical spinal cord (1). Internal jugular vein (2) and internal carotid artery (3). Medulla (4). Cerebellar gray matter with tonsils abutting medulla (5). Falx cerebelli (6). Fourth ventricle (7). Cerebellar white matter (8). Basilar artery (9).

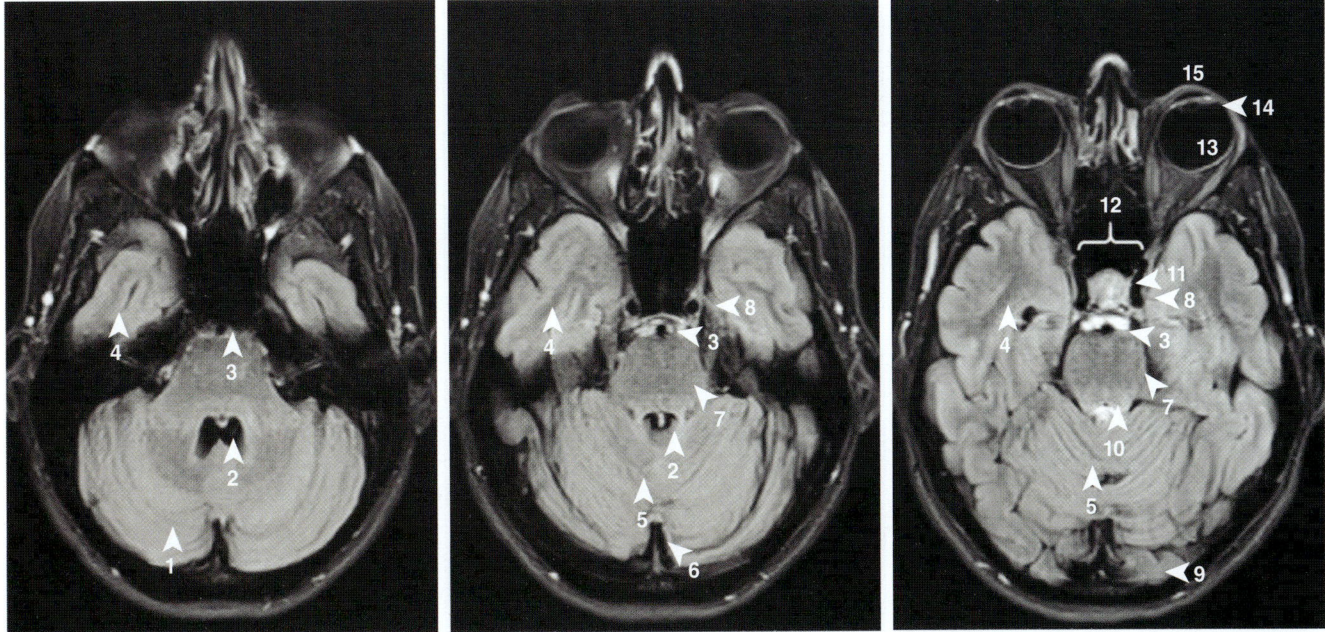

Figure 75.3 Cross sections of the medulla to the pons. Cerebellar gray matter (1). Fourth ventricle (2). Basilar artery (3). Temporal lobe (4). Cerebellar vermis (5). Falx cerebelli (6). Pons (7). Internal carotid artery (cavernous section) (8). Occipital lobe (9). Cerebral aqueduct of Sylvius (10). Pituitary gland (11). Cavernous sinus (12). Globe (vitreous humor) (13). Lens (14). Anterior chamber (aqueous humor, cornea) (15).

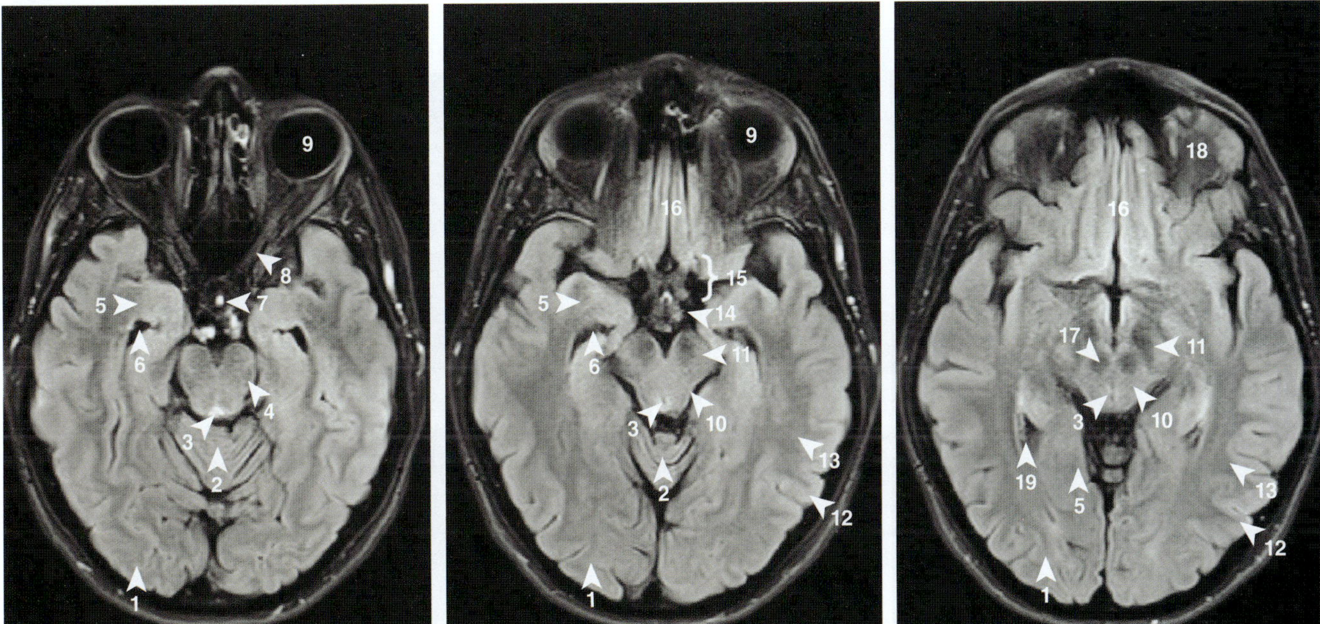

Figure 75.4 Cross sections of the pontomesencephalic junction and basal cisterns (suprasellar and interpeduncular cisterns in G) to the midbrain. Occipital lobe (1). Cerebellar vermis (2). Cerebral aqueduct of Sylvius (3). Pontomesencephalic junction (4). Medial temporal lobe (5). Temporal horn of the lateral ventricles adjacent to the hippocampus and medial temporal lobe (6). Pituitary stalk (7). Optic nerve (8). Globe (9). Midbrain (10). Cerebral peduncles (containing corticospinal tracts) (11). Cortical gray matter (12). Subcortical/juxtacortical white matter (13). Mammillary bodies (14). Optic chiasm (15). Olfactory bulbs and cortex (16). Red nucleus (17). Orbitofrontal cortex (18). Atrium of the lateral ventricles (19).

capsules. Other nomenclature associated with basal ganglia nuclei include lentiform nucleus (globus pallidus and putamen flanked by internal and external capsules) and corpus striatum (caudate nucleus and putamen). The basal ganglia are responsible primarily for motor control but also play a role in motor learning, executive function, and emotional states [4]. Disorders of the basal ganglia are characterized by hypokinesia with rigidity and tremor ***(Parkinson disease, corticobasal degeneration)*** as well as hyperkinetic involuntary movements in ***essential tremor*** and choreoathetosis ***(Huntington disease)*** [5,7]. The basal ganglia are supplied by lenticulostriate vessels from the middle and to a lesser extent anterior cerebral arteries [8,9].

Thalamus and Hypothalamus

The thalamus (meaning "chamber" in Greek) relays sensory input to cortical association areas, except for olfactory input which relays

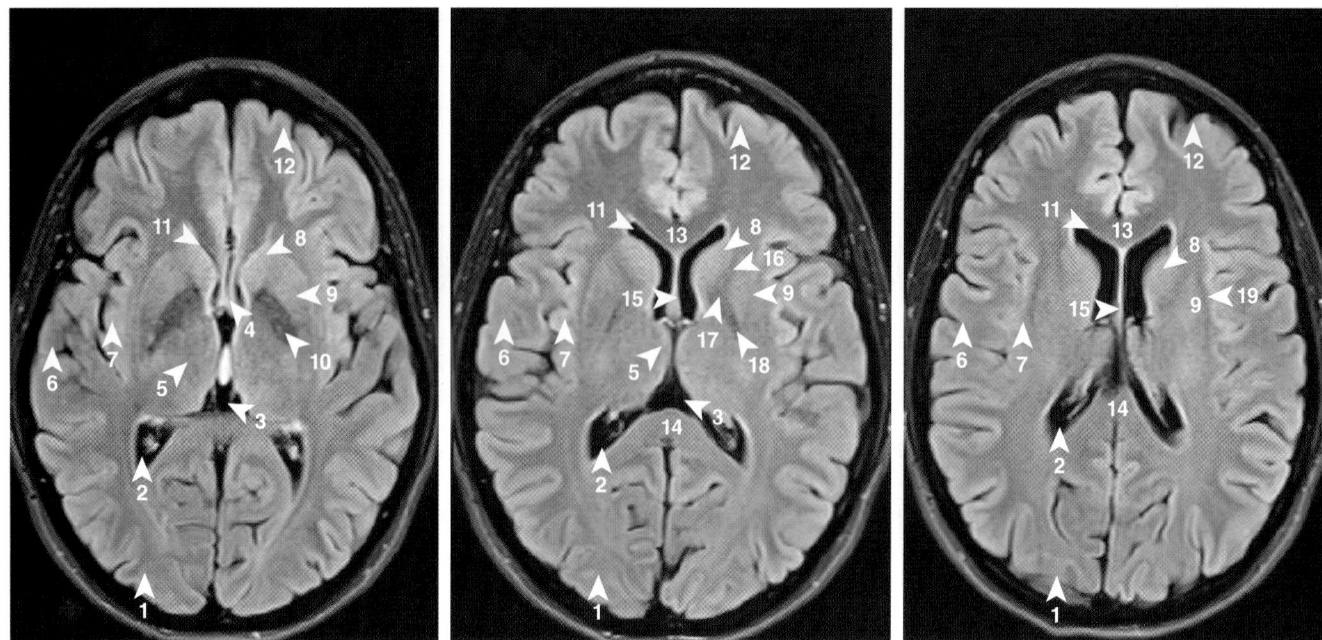

Figure 75.5 Cross sections of the basal ganglia and thalami to the lateral ventricles. Occipital lobe (1). Atrium of the lateral ventricles (2). Third ventricle (3). Fornix (4). Thalamus (5). Temporal lobe (6). Insular cortex (7). Head of the caudate (8). Putamen (9). Globus pallidus (10). Frontal horn of the lateral ventricles (11). Frontal lobe (12). Genu (13) and splenium of the corpus callosum (14). Septum pellucidum (15). Anterior limb (16), genu (17), and posterior limb of the internal capsule (18) (posterior limb contains motor fibers of corticospinal tract). External capsule (19). Note: globus pallidus + putamen = lentiform nucleus. Putamen + caudate nucleus = striatum.

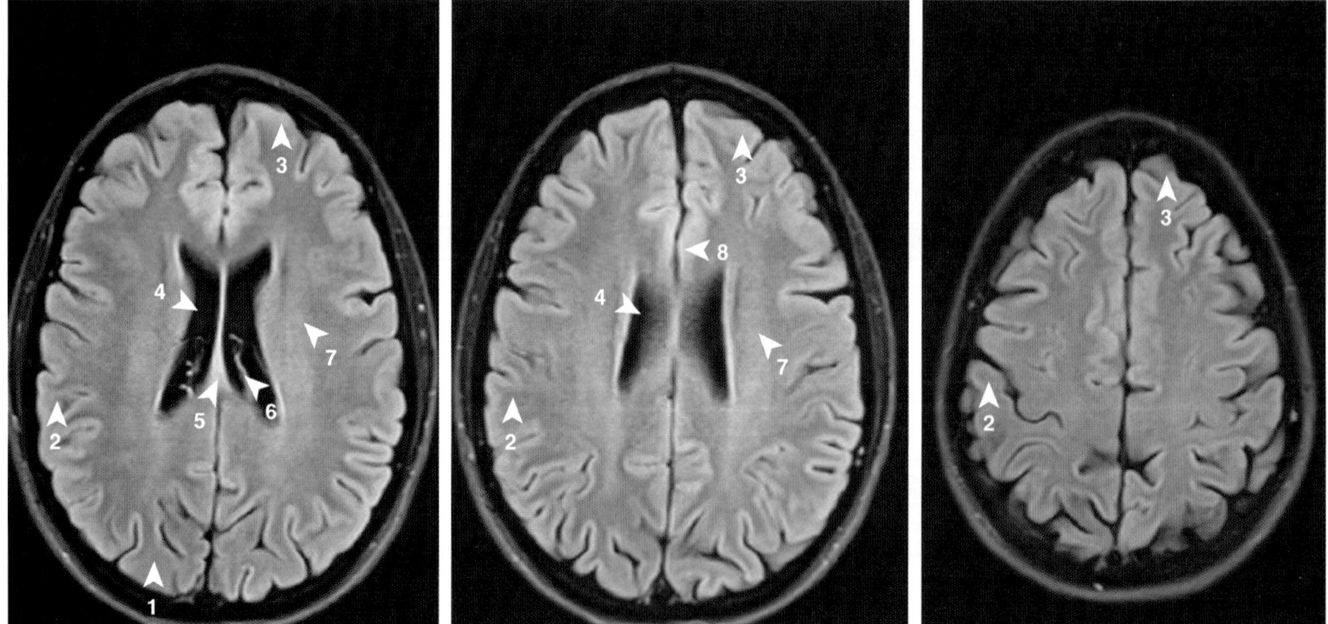

Figure 75.6 Cross sections of the lateral ventricles to the superior cortex. Parieto-occipital region (1). Parietal lobe (2). Frontal lobe (3). Lateral ventricle (4). Septum pellucidum (5). Choroid plexus of the ventricles (6). Corona radiata, the afferent projection fibers to the cortex (7). Cingulate gyrus (8).

directly to the entorhinal cortex (Fig. 75.5) [5]. It is a paired paramedian ovoid structure located above the midbrain, immediately medial to the posterior limb of the internal capsule. It extends anteriorly to the foramen of Monro and medially to the third ventricle. In addition to being a relay station for sensory techniques, it receives motor connections from the cerebellum and basal ganglia en route to the cortex. The thalamus also has key connections with the limbic system, assigning it an important role in emotions and memory. There are several thalamic nuclei, each receiving input from specific sensory techniques and relaying to distinct cortical regions. For example, the ventroposterolateral (VPL) nucleus receives pain and temperature information from anterolateral spinothalamic fibers and position and vibration sense from the dorsal column-medial lemniscal pathway; it then outputs this information to the somatosensory cortex [4]. The ventroposteromedial nucleus receives facial sensory information from the trigeminothalamic tracts and afferent taste sensation from the solitary tracts (which sends data to the gustatory cortex) [4]. The lateral geniculate nucleus receives visual information from the optic tracts and relays information to the primary visual cortex along the calcarine fissure [4]. Likewise, the medial geniculate nucleus receives auditory information from the cochlear nerve nucleus and relays to the primary auditory cortex in the temporal lobe (Heschl's and superior temporal gyri). The ventral anterior and ventral lateral are the motor nuclei of the thalamus, whereas the anterior and lateral dorsal nuclei are part of the limbic system [5,7]. The thalamus is supplied by several branches arising from the posterior communicating and posterior cerebral arteries [9].

The hypothalamus (meaning "under chamber" in Greek) is similarly comprised of several small nuclei located anteriorly and inferiorly to the floor of the third ventricle and is separated from the thalamus by the hypothalamic sulcus in the wall of the third ventricle [10]. These nuclei govern several important functions including generation of the circadian rhythms through melatonin secretion (suprachiasmatic nucleus), stimulation of the anterior pituitary (arcuate nucleus) and posterior pituitary gland (supraoptic and paraventricular nuclei), regulation of hunger and satiety (lateral and ventromedial nuclei), and control of body temperature (anterior and posterior nuclei). The hypothalamus is functionally connected directly to the posterior pituitary gland through the infundibulum and indirectly to the anterior pituitary gland through local venous connections known as the hypothalamic–hypophyseal portal system [5,10].

Limbic Structures

The hippocampus, named after its shape and meaning "seahorse" in Greek, plays an essential role in short-term memory and memory consolidation (Fig. 75.4) [4,11]. The amygdala regulates emotions, particularly fear conditioning. The limbic system is comprised of the medial temporal lobe (the amygdala, hippocampus, entorhinal and parahippocampal cortex), fornix, mammillary bodies, anterior thalamic nuclei, and cingulate cortex. This system is impaired in a variety of disorders, such as *Alzheimer disease (AD), Limbic-predominant Age-related TDP-43 Encephalopathy (LATE), mesial temporal sclerosis (MTS)* and *Kluver–Bucy syndrome. Thiamine (B1) deficiency* causes mammillary body degeneration resulting in *Wernicke–Korsakoff syndrome* [4–6].

Neuroendocrine Structures

The pituitary gland is the master regulator of the endocrine system (Figs. 75.3 and 75.4). It is located in the sella turcica (Latin for "Turkish seat") and secretes several hormones and hormone-releasing factors. This gland, along with the circumventricular organs (subfornical organ, organum vasculosum, and area postrema), is one of the few regions of the brain without a blood–brain barrier, thereby allowing for chemoregulation and hormone secretion. The area postrema of the medulla (chemotactic trigger zone) regulates vomiting due to noxious toxin ingestion [4]. The pineal gland, a common site for benign calcification, was used as an important radiographic landmark before the advent of CT and MR imaging [3]. Furthermore, pineal masses may compress the midbrain and superior colliculi, leading to ***Parinaud syndrome,*** which is marked clinically by vertical gaze palsy, eyelid retraction, and convergence-retraction nystagmus [5,6,12].

Brainstem

The brainstem is a complex highway of white matter tracts interspersed with gray matter nuclei. It is divided from superior to inferior into the midbrain, pons, and medulla (Figs. 75.2–75.4). The anterior midbrain is defined by the cerebral peduncles, two large fiber bundles [4,5]. Medially, the paired oculomotor nerves emerge from the interpeduncular fossa. The posterior midbrain consists of the quadrageminal plate, formed by two paired structures: superior colliculi and inferior colliculi. Immediately below the inferior colliculi, the paired trochlear nerves cross and exit the dorsal surface of the midbrain and traverse the perimesencephalic cistern [12]. The pons is characterized by a ventral "belly" or basis pontis containing the corticospinal, corticobulbar, and corticopontine tracts and a dorsal pontine tegmentum which includes the reticular formation, central tegmental tracts, and medial to lateral: the medial lemniscus, trigeminothalamic tract, and spinothalamic tract. The paired trigeminal nerves emerge from the anterolateral surface of the pontine belly and course through the prepontine cistern to reach Meckel's cave, a dural recess containing the Gasserian (trigeminal) ganglion. The medial longitudinal fasciculus lies paramedially on the dorsal pontine surface and is flanked by the abducens nucleus [13–15]. The medial longitudinal fasciculus is critical for conjugate gaze and damage due to demyelination or infarct results in internuclear ophthalmoplegia. Facial colliculi mark the location of the motor fibers of the seventh nerve passing over the abducens nuclei along the floor of the fourth ventricle in the lower pontine tegmentum. Along the ventral (anterior) medulla are paired protrusion called the pyramids, which contain motor fibers (corticospinal and corticobulbar—the pyramidal tracts). The pyramids are separated by a median fissure that continues along the spinal cord, briefly interrupted where the pyramidal tracts decussate (cross the midline) at the spinomedullary junction. Lateral to the pyramids, separated by ventrolateral sulci, are the olivary bodies, containing superior and inferior olivary nuclei. Posterior to the olives are the dorsolateral sulci. The hypoglossal nerves (cranial nerve 12) exit the medulla in the ventrolateral sulci while the roots of cranial nerves 9, 10, and 11 exit through the dorsolateral sulci. Dorsally, the gracile and cuneate tubercles mark the location of the corresponding nuclei [5,12].

Cerebellum

The cerebellum ("little brain") is responsible for coordination of movement. Structurally, it can be visualized by two paired lobes of white matter core and projections covered by thin convolutions of cortex called folia (Figs. 75.1–75.3). The motor and premotor cerebral cortex relay information about planned movements to the cerebellar cortex, while somatosensory, visual, and vestibular systems input into the cerebellar cortex to allow for the assessment of progressing motor task status [4]. After processing this complex information, the cerebellar cortex sends its output back to the cerebral cortex through the deep cerebellar nuclei. Midline cerebellar vermis damage (as in chronic alcoholism) causes truncal ataxia, while lesions of cerebellar hemispheres lead to dysmetria (impaired finger-to-nose/heal-to-shin testing), limb ataxia, intention tremor, and dysdiadochokinesia [4,6]. Recent evidence has also implicated the cerebellum in a few nonmotor functions, including cognition. The deep cerebellar white matter core contains four pairs of nuclei, located lateral to medial: the dentate, emboliform, globose, and fastigial nuclei. Of these, the dentate nucleus is the most clinically relevant as it relays the motor control output from the cerebellar hemispheres [5].

Sensory Pathways

Spinothalamic (anterolateral) tract: This tract includes pain and temperature fibers. Sensory input from the dorsal root ganglia travels through Lissauer's tract from the spinal cord, crosses through the anterior white commissure to the contralateral anterolateral pathway, ascends to synapse in the VPL nucleus of the thalamus, and projects through the corona radiata to somatosensory cortex [4]. ***Syringomyelia*** can affect this more centrally located tract in the spinal cord, causing bilateral cape-like dissociated sensory loss but sparing fine touch and proprioception [5,6].

Dorsal column-medial lemniscal tract: This tract includes vibration and proprioception fibers. Sensory input travels through dorsal columns, to gracile or cuneate fasciculi and nuclei, crosses in the dorsal medulla, ascends in the medial lemniscus to the VPL nucleus of the thalamus, and projects through the corona radiata to somatosensory cortex [4]. These tracts are affected in ***tabes dorsalis***, a form of tertiary neurosyphilis and ***subacute combined degeneration caused by B12 deficiency***, which leads to loss of proprioception and vibration perception and a positive Romberg sign [6]. These tracts are supplied by the posterior spinal arteries and therefore spared in anterior cord syndrome secondary to anterior spinal artery occlusion [5].

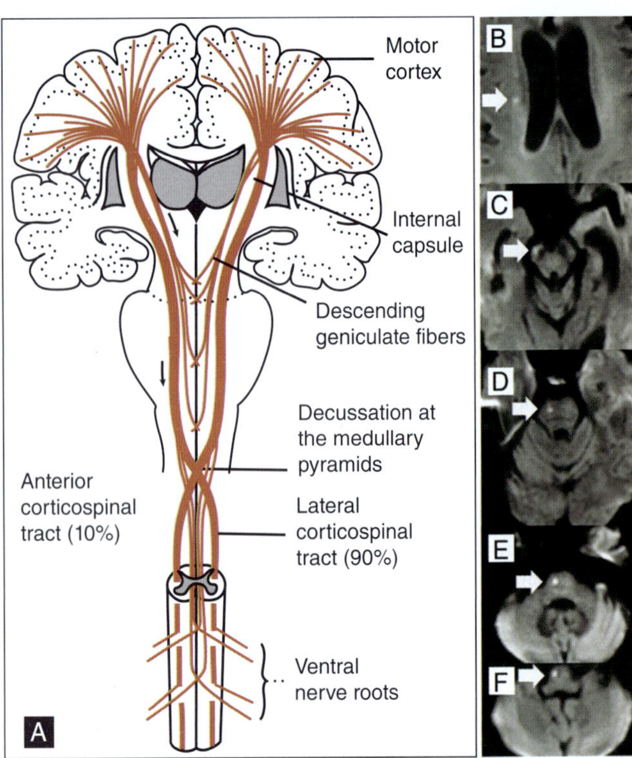

Figure 75.7 Schematic anatomy of the corticospinal tracts (A) (Adapted from Henry Gray, Gray's Anatomy, 1918). Acute Wallerian degeneration manifesting as long segment restricted diffusion (*arrow*) in the corticospinal tract: corona radiata (B), cerebral peduncle (C), pons (D), and medulla (E, F).

Motor Pathways

Corticospinal tracts: These tracts serve as descending pathways for voluntary motor control. These fibers originate from the pyramidal cells of the primary motor cortex and travel through the posterior limb of the internal capsule, cerebral peduncle, and pontine belly to the medullary pyramid, where 90% of the fibers decussate to the contralateral side and descend in the lateral corticospinal tracts. Only about 10% of fibers remain ipsilateral in the anterior corticospinal tract (Fig. 75.7A) [4]. Motor tracts are affected in ***amyotrophic lateral sclerosis***, ***corticobasal degeneration***, and ***vitamin B12 deficiency***. ***Wallerian degeneration*** is often seen distally in motor tracts when there is injury either to the pyramidal cells in the primary motor cortex (i.e., cortical infarction, tumor or amyotrophic lateral sclerosis), or to the more proximal descending axons (i.e., lacunar infarct in the coronal radiata or internal capsule) (Fig. 75.7B–F) [5,6].

Cerebellar Networks

Pontocerebellar tracts originate in the pons, cross the midline, and enter the cerebellum through the middle cerebellar peduncle (brachium pontis), which brings the input of the corticopontine fibers into the contralateral cerebellar cortex [4]. ***Ventral and dorsal spinocerebellar tracts*** bring sensory input from the spinal cord through the brainstem to the ipsilateral cerebellum through the superior and inferior cerebellar peduncles. These tracts are affected in ***vitamin B12 deficiency*** and ***spinocerebellar ataxia*** [6]. The cerebellar output to cerebral cortex is carried although the superior cerebellar peduncle (brachium conjunctivum) into thalamic ventral anterior and ventral lateral nuclei after decussating in midbrain. The dentate nucleus, projecting to the contralateral red nucleus through the superior cerebellar peduncle, also decussates in the midbrain [5]. The red nucleus sends projections to the ipsilateral inferior olivary nucleus through the central tegmental tract, while the inferior olivary nucleus then projects back to the contralateral dentate nucleus through the inferior cerebellar peduncle. Interruptions of this pathway, also known as the "triangle of Guillain and Mollaret," result in *hypertrophic olivary degeneration*, a type of trans-synaptic degeneration [16].

Language Networks

The initial cortical processing of speech occurs in Heschl's gyrus, along the superior temporal surface. The information then projects to the cortex flanking the posterior half of the superior temporal sulcus for phonological processing and representation. From here, language processing is carried along two distinct pathways, the ventral conceptual-semantic network and the dorsal articulatory pathway [4]. The dorsal articulatory pathway comprises the traditionally described strongly left dominant language network, which posteriorly includes Wernicke's area at the lateral parietotemporal junction. This region projects anteriorly through arcuate and superior longitudinal fasciculi onto the inferior frontal gyrus (Broca area) and superiorly onto the dorsolateral prefrontal cortex in the middle frontal gyrus, immediately in front of the precentral sulcus. The more recently understood ventral stream is relatively less left hemispheric dominant. This stream includes the posterior middle and inferior temporal gyri, which serve as lexical interface between phonological and semantic processing, and the anterior middle frontal gyrus and inferior frontal gyrus, which serve as part of the syntactical network [6]. Language networks are classically disrupted in middle cerebral artery infarcts and posterior temporal lobe and inferolateral frontal lobe tumors [17,18].

Olfactory System

The olfactory system is comprised of numerous free nerve endings in the nasal mucosa that pass through the cribriform plate as the ***olfactory nerves*** and synapse in the olfactory bulb on each side. The nerve fibers then travel from the olfactory bulbs through the olfactory tracts located immediately below the gyrus rectus to reach the ipsilateral primary olfactory (piriform) cortex [4]. Olfaction is the only sensory technique that remains uncrossed in reaching the brain [19,22]. The olfactory nerve is considered the first of the 12 paired cranial nerves that pass through skull base foramina. However, like the optic nerve it is not a peripheral nerve but rather part of the CNS and connects to the cerebrum instead of the brainstem.

Visual System

Axons of the retinal ganglion cells converge at the optic disks and exit each globe as the ***optic nerves***. Considered the second cranial nerve (CN II), the optic nerve is again embryologically part of the CNS and structurally a tract, surrounded by a CSF-containing meningeal sheath and myelinated by oligodendroglia instead of Schwann cells [4]. The optic nerve is frequently involved in CNS demyelinating disorders such as ***multiple sclerosis (MS) and neuromyelitis optica*** [6,19]. The arrangement of optic nerve fibers preserves the spatial orientation of light hitting different parts of the retina (visual somatotopy). The optic nerves enter the cranium through the optic canal, meet at the optic chiasm, and continue as the optic tracts. *Fibers from the nasal (medial) portion of each retina cross to the contralateral side at the chiasm so that each optic tract carries fibers from the nasal half of the contralateral retina and the temporal half of the ipsilateral retina.* The tracts project to the lateral geniculate nuclei of the thalamus and superior colliculi (located in the tectum or roof of the midbrain and mediating conjugate eye movements such as convergence and saccades) and to the calcarine cortex (also known as the primary visual cortex) through the optic radiations. The so-called direct pathway, representing the lower visual field, projects to the cortex on the superior bank of the calcarine fissure. The indirect pathway, representing the upper visual field and better known as Meyer's loop, makes a "U" turn in the temporal lobe before terminating in the cortex on the lower bank of the calcarine cortex [5,20].

Auditory System

Auditory information is carried by the cochlear nerve (also known as the auditory or acoustic nerve and part of the ***vestibulocochlear nerve***, CN VIII). Cochlear nerve cell bodies are located in the spiral ganglion along the modiolus of the cochlea. The cochlear nerve passes through the internal auditory canal, immediately below the facial nerve and anterior to the superior and inferior divisions of the vestibular nerve, to synapse in the cochlear nucleus of the upper medulla. Most auditory input crosses into the contralateral superior olivary complex. From here, the lateral lemniscus ascends through the brainstem into the inferior colliculi and thereafter projects to the primary auditory cortex through the medial geniculate nucleus of the thalamus [4]. *Many neurons in the auditory pathways cross at every level of the auditory system. Thus, each auditory cortex receives input from both ears* [5,21].

Additional Sensory and Motor Cranial Nerves

The oculomotor nucleus is located in the midbrain ventral to the cerebral aqueduct and receives afferent input from cerebral cortex, cerebellum, pons, and medulla [12]. It consists of subnuclei innervating ipsilateral inferior rectus, inferior oblique and medial rectus, contralateral superior rectus, and both levator palpebrae superioris muscles. The nerve fibers travel anteriorly to exit the

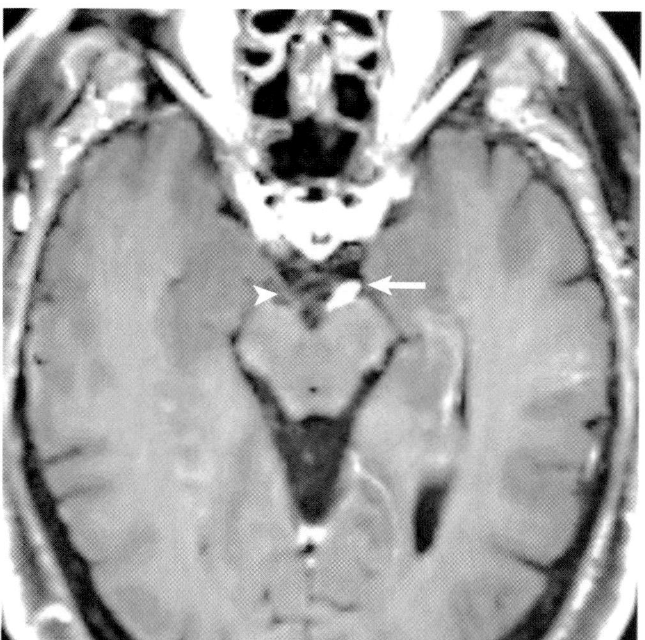

Figure 75.8 Focal inflammatory enhancement of the left oculomotor nerve at the root exit zone (*arrow*) in a 10-year-old boy with ophthalmoplegic migraine. Note the normal appearance and course of the right oculomotor nerve (*arrowhead*).

midbrain in the interpeduncular cistern [4]. These fibers merge with the preganglionic parasympathetic fibers from the Edinger–Westphal nucleus to form the ***oculomotor nerve*** (CN III). The nerve then courses anteriorly between the superior cerebellar and posterior cerebral arteries in the suprasellar cistern, immediately below the posterior communicating artery to the cavernous sinus along with ***trochlear nerve*** (CN IV) [5]. *Note that the cavernous sinus contains the cranial nerves III, IV, V_1, V_2, and VI* [35]. Inflammation or focal demyelination of the oculomotor nerve typically occurs near the root exit zone in the interpeduncular fossa and can be seen in ophthalmoplegic migraine, a type of cranial neuralgia presenting with headache and diplopia in children and young adults (Fig. 75.8). Compression by a ruptured or less commonly unruptured posterior communicating artery aneurysm is a well-known cause of acute, often partial, third cranial nerve palsy. This presents as ipsilateral pupillary dilatation (Fig. 75.9) [19,22].

The trochlear nerve nucleus is situated near the midline, ventral to the cerebral aqueduct, while the fibers pass dorsally around the cerebral aqueduct. Decussating in the superior medullary velum, the trochlear nerve exits the dorsal surface of the midbrain, below the inferior colliculus. It then wraps anteriorly in the ambient cistern near the free edge of the tentorium and reaches the cavernous sinus immediately below the oculomotor nerve [4]. In the cavernous sinus, the trochlear nerve runs along the lateral wall immediately below the third nerve. Due to its very small caliber, the trochlear nerve is not consistently identified on 3 Tesla (T) MRI but can often be seen on high-resolution 7 T MRI (Fig. 75.10). Isolated trochlear nerve palsies can rarely result from compression by lesions of the quadrigeminal plate and ambient cisterns [19,22,24].

The ***abducens nerve (CN VI)*** innervates the lateral rectus muscle and abducts the ipsilateral eye. The sixth cranial nerve nucleus is located under the facial colliculus in the floor of the fourth ventricle. The seventh ***facial nerve (CN VII)*** motor nucleus is anterolateral to the sixth nerve nucleus in the lower

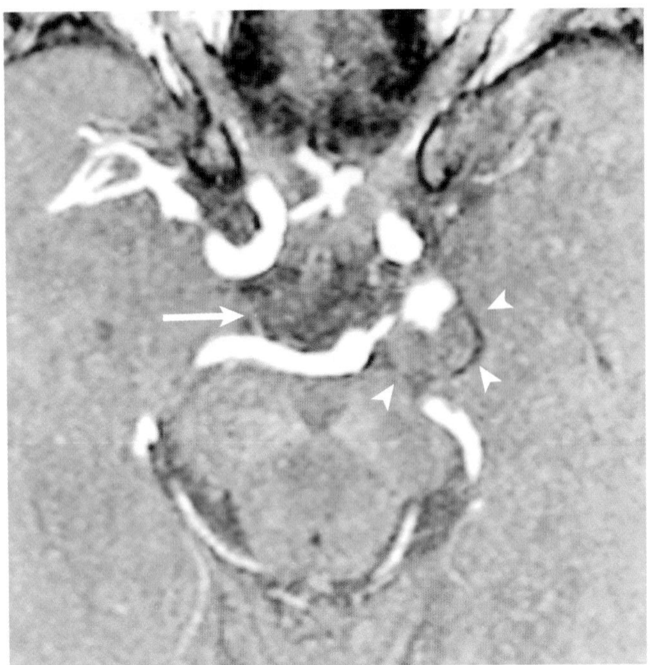

Figure 75.9 Partial oculomotor palsy resulting from a partially thrombosed aneurysm of the left posterior communicating artery (*arrowheads*) seen on a time-of-flight MRA. The right oculomotor nerve (*arrow*) can be seen emerging below the posterior cerebral artery.

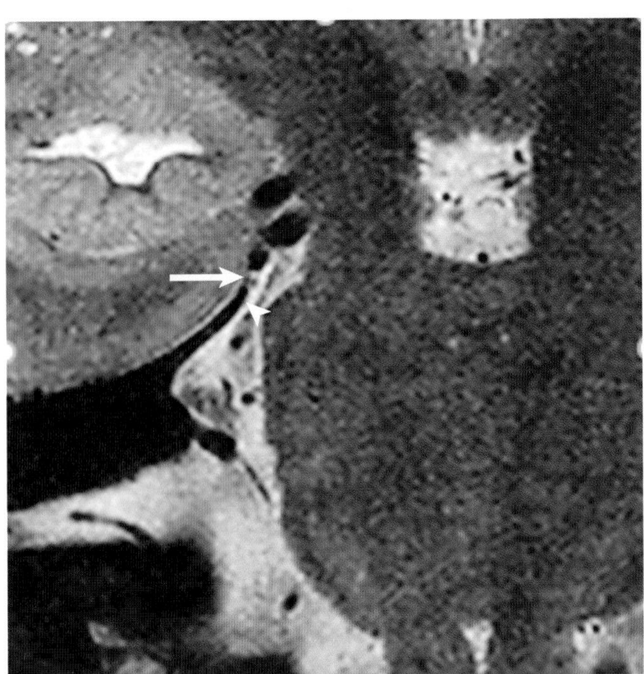

Figure 75.10 Right trochlear nerve (*arrow*) in the ambient cistern adjacent to the free edge of the tentorium (*arrowhead*) seen on a coronal T2-weighted 7 Tesla MR image. The superior cerebellar artery, posterior cerebral artery and basal vein of Rosenthal can be visualized in caudocranial order immediately above the nerve in the ambient cistern.

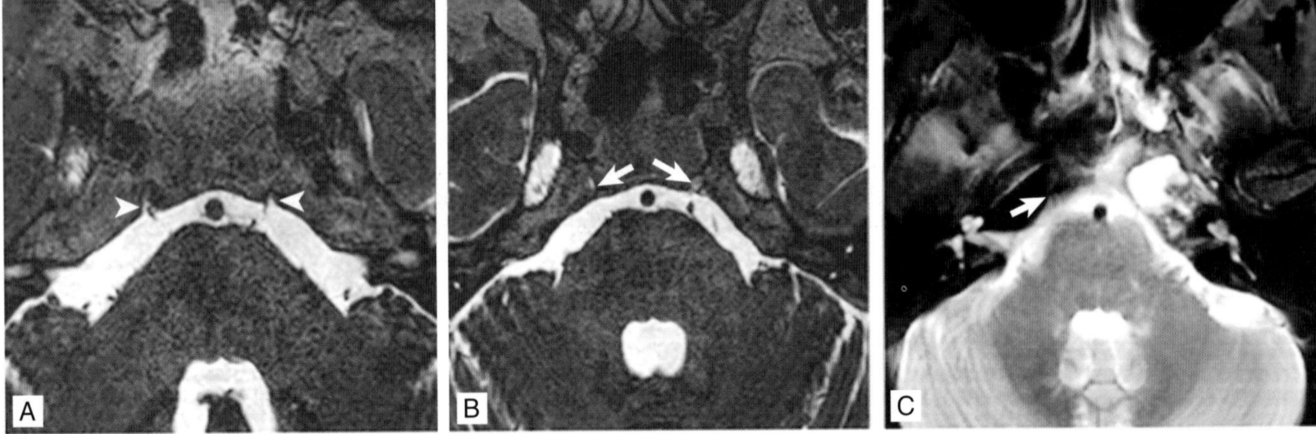

Figure 75.11 Abducens nerve (*arrowheads*) entering (A) and traversing (B) through the Dorello's canal at the petroclival synchondrosis (*arrows*). Left petrous apex granuloma (C) expanding the petrous apex and obliterating the left Dorello's canal; compare with normal right intracranial opening of the right Dorello's canal (*arrow*). (Courtesy: Dr. Amit Agarwal, Mayo Clinic, Florida.)

pontine tegmentum. *Fibers leaving the seventh nerve motor nucleus course posteromedially in the pons to pass around the sixth nerve nucleus in the facial colliculus* [4,24]. The sixth nerve fibers pass anteriorly near the midline in the pontine belly and exit at the level of the pontomedullary junction. The sixth nerve then courses through the prepontine cistern and enters a small fibrous canal along the surface of the petrous apex, known as Dorello's canal (Fig. 75.11). In Dorello's canal, the sixth nerve is vulnerable to trauma and compression by increased intracranial pressure and petrous apex lesions. *Proximity of the trigeminal and abducens nerves can result in facial pain or dysesthesia in petrous apex lesions.* The sixth nerve then enters the cavernous sinus, where it runs between the carotid artery and the trigeminal nerve branches [5]. The sixth nerve enters the orbit through the superior orbital fissure along with V1, oculomotor and trochlear nerves [19,22].

The ***glossopharyngeal nerve*** (CN IX) is primarily a sensory nerve to the pharynx and posterior one-third of the tongue. It has two ganglia (superior and inferior) located near the jugular foramen [4,24]. The nerve leaves the medulla along with the vagus nerve in the retro-olivary sulcus and exits through the jugular foramen through the pars nervosa (Fig. 75.12) to run in the cervical carotid sheath. It receives contributions from the spinal trigeminal nucleus, the nucleus solitarius, the nucleus ambiguous, and the inferior salivatory nucleus [5,19,22].

The ***vagus nerve*** (CN X) is a mixed sensory and motor nerve with general sensory afferent (external ear, tympanic membrane, and

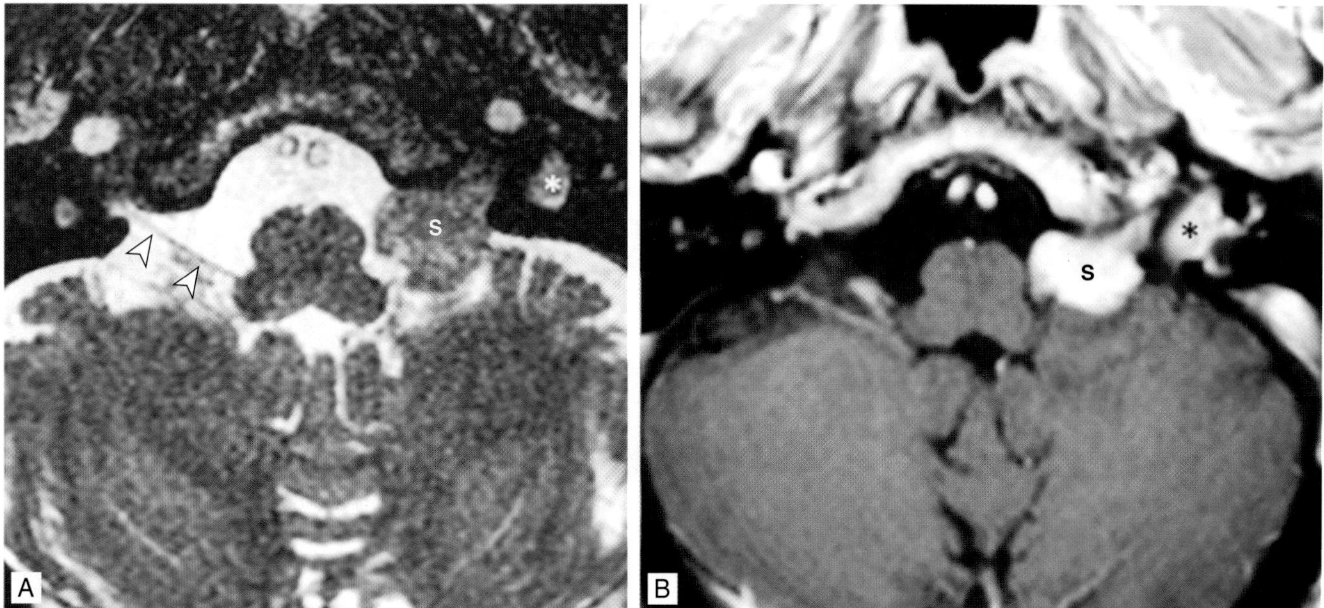

Figure 75.12 Axial T2 (A) and gadolinium-enhanced T1-weighted MR images (B) depicting schwannoma of the left glossopharyngeal nerve. Note the normal course of the right glossopharyngeal nerve (*arrowheads* in A) from the retro-olivary sulcus to the pars nervosa of the jugular foramen. The schwannoma (S) can be seen extending in the pars nervosa medial and anterior to the jugular bulb (*asterisk*).

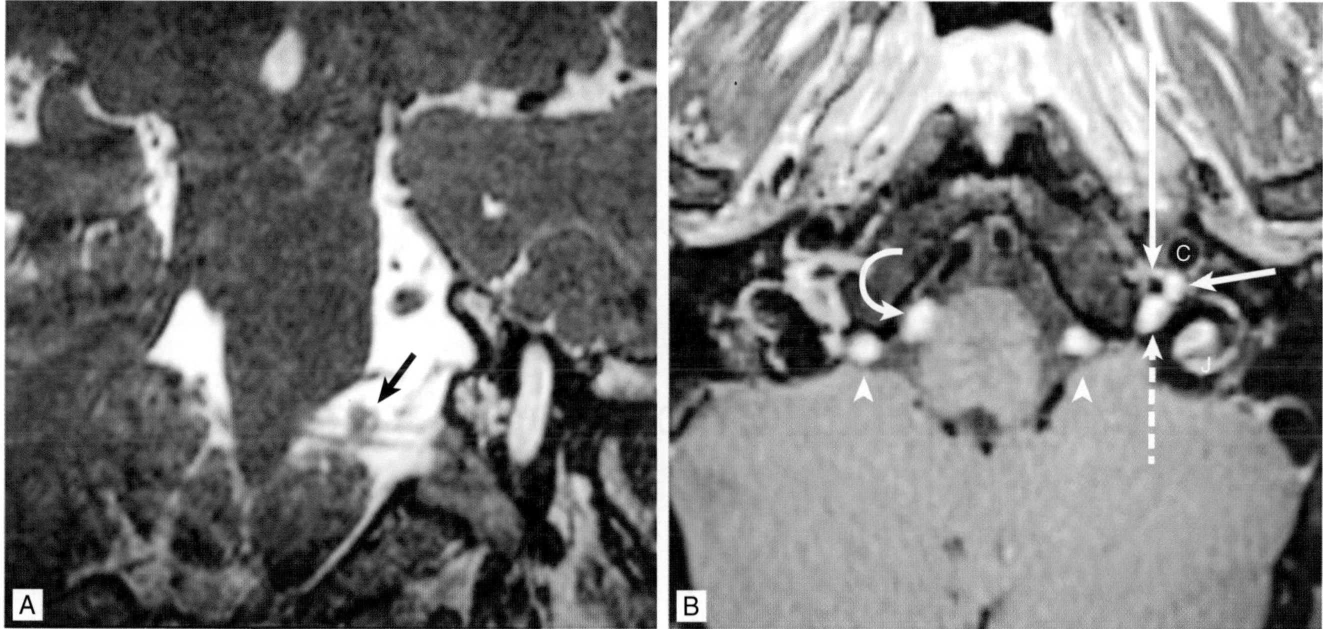

Figure 75.13 A patient with neurofibromatosis type II. Oblique coronal reformatted T2 MR image (A) showing the vagus nerve coursing immediately below a schwannoma (*arrow*) affecting the glossopharyngeal nerve in the lateral medullary cistern. Axial black blood T1-weighted MR (B) image depicting small schwannomas of the left glossopharyngeal nerve (*arrow*) and vagus nerve in the jugular foramen (*dotted arrow*). Schwannomas of bilateral intradural spinal accessory (*arrowheads*) nerves and right hypoglossal nerve (*curved arrow*) can also be seen. Long thin arrow: inferior petrosal sinus. Internal carotid artery (labeled C); jugular bulb (labeled J).

infratentorial dura), general visceral afferent (mucous membranes of the pharynx, larynx, trachea, esophagus, and gut to the splenic flexure of the colon), special visceral afferent (taste from epiglottis), special visceral efferent (muscles of larynx, pharynx, proximal esophagus levator veli palatine, and palatoglossus muscle), and general visceral efferent (preganglionic parasympathetic fibers to heart and abdominal organs) components [5,24]. *It is the major motor nerve to the pharynx and larynx, thus serving critical functions in swallowing and speech. Also, it is the major source of parasympathetic innervation to the heart and abdominal organs* [4]. Like CN IX, it has both a superior and inferior ganglion (called the nodose ganglion), which are located on the vagus nerve at the level of the jugular foramen. The vagus nerve exits the medulla immediately below the glossopharyngeal nerve and passes posteromedial to the glossopharyngeal nerve and posterior to the inferior petrosal sinus in the jugular foramen through the pars vasculosa (Fig. 75.13) [19,22,23].

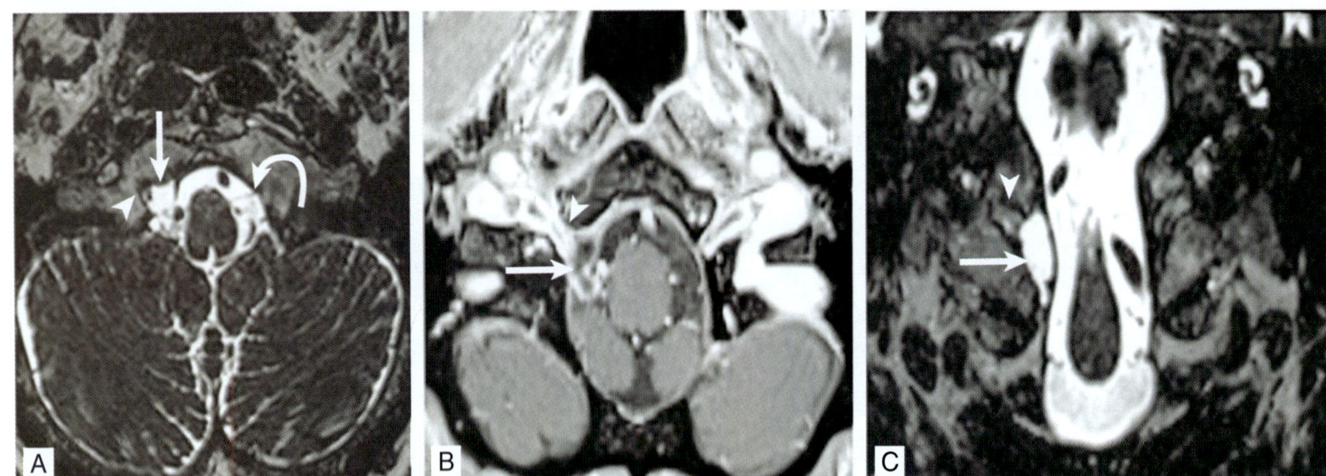

Figure 75.14 Axial T2 (A) and gadolinium-enhanced T1 (B); and coronal T2 (C) images showing a craniovertebral junction synovial cyst (*arrows*) encroaching upon the right hypoglossal nerve entering the hypoglossal canal (*arrowheads*) leading to hypoglossal nerve palsy. Note the normal left hypoglossal nerve entering the hypoglossal canal (*curved arrow*).

The ***spinal accessory nerve*** (CN XI) is a pure motor nerve, innervating the sternocleidomastoid muscle and the superior component of the trapezius. CN XI arises from the spinal accessory nucleus, located in the high cervical cord from C1 to C5 [4]. The rootlets form a common trunk running superiorly to enter the skull through the foramen magnum and exit through the jugular foramen with CN IX and X (Fig. 75.13). Injury to this nerve typically occurs in the foramen magnum, jugular foramen, or in the carotid sheath [19,22,24].

Due to their proximity in the jugular foramen, CNs IX, X, and XI may be simultaneously involved in lesions of the posterior skull base such as metastasis, meningioma, jugular paraganglioma, and schwannoma [6].

The ***hypoglossal nerve*** (CN XII) is a pure motor nerve [5,6]. Hypoglossal nuclei are located in the posterior medulla, just anterior to the floor of the fourth ventricle. The hypoglossal nerve leaves the medulla in the ventrolateral sulcus between the pyramid and olive. The nerve then travels in the perimedullary cistern and exits through the hypoglossal canal in the skull base. The main function is to innervate the extrinsic and intrinsic muscles of the tongue. Its lesions cause hemiatrophy with fatty replacement, so-called "fatty atrophy" of the tongue. Hypoglossal nerve dysfunction may occur secondary to brainstem stroke, tumors involving the nerve and skull base, basilar meningitis, carotid dissection, trauma, inflammatory demyelinating neuropathy, and motor neuron disease. Synovial cysts, arising from the craniovertebral junction and extending into the hypoglossal canal (Fig. 75.14), are a recently recognized cause of hypoglossal nerve palsy [19,22,24].

75.2 Brief Introduction to Neuroimaging Techniques

Computed tomography (CT) and ***magnetic resonance imaging (MRI)*** are now the techniques of choice for imaging most suspected lesions of the brain. This and the following chapter are mainly devoted to their use in investigating intracranial pathology.

Arteriography (CTA, MRA) and ***digital subtraction angiography (DSA):*** Modern technology has allowed the spatial resolution of computed tomography angiography (CTA) and magnetic resonance angiography (MRA) to become comparable to that of the "gold-standard" DSA [25]. CTA and MRA also provide additional information not available on DSA, such as status of the vessel wall and relation of vessels to adjacent intracranial structures. Therefore, noninvasive imaging, with the additional benefits of increased access and ease of acquisition, has become the preferred method for evaluating vascular lesions such as vaso-occlusive disease and aneurysms. DSA is usually reserved for definitive diagnosis of select vascular lesions (i.e., dural arteriovenous fistula) and for endovascular procedures [26].

CT and MRI Image Display

CT and MRI utilize a ray grayscale for depiction of cross-sectional anatomy in which the pixel brightness is proportional to either the x-ray attenuation coefficient or nuclear magnetic resonance (NMR) signal intensity of each corresponding tissue voxel (volume element). The ray grayscale intensity range, that is, the "window" (W) and the central intensity level (L) can be arbitrarily adjusted to optimize visualization. Standardizing W and L is of crucial importance in CT; the range of imaging options and signal variation in MRI mitigates against rigorous standardization although the basic principles still apply. Fig. 75.15 shows the relative density on the Hounsfield unit (HU) scale of the normal body tissues at CT. This HU is a universal ad hoc scale with air at -1000 HU and water at 0 HU as reference points. *The cerebral white matter ranges between 25 and 35 HU, gray matter between 35 and 40 HU, and acute clotted blood between 60 and 70 HU.* To

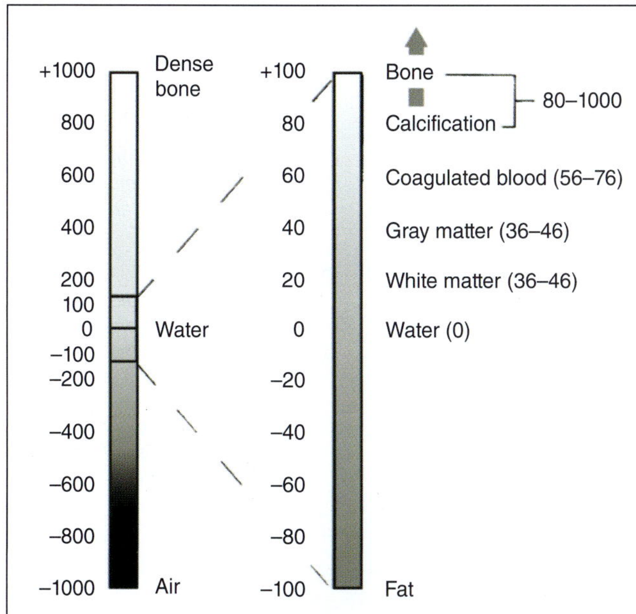

Figure 75.15 Hounsfield (HU) CT scale. The full scale extends below 0 HU to −1000 HU (the true zero of this scale, i.e., the attenuation of air). Head scans are obtained routinely at a window level (L) of 34–40 HU and a window width (W) of 0–80 HU.

optimize the visualization of brain on routine CT, L is typically chosen at 35 HU and W is spread over 80 HU to maximize gray and white matter contrast with tolerable perceived noise. The W can be narrowed arbitrarily to increase gray–white contrast, that is, in the detection of acute ischemic stroke but at the cost of greater perceived noise. Likewise, for optimal detection of extradural or subdural hemorrhage, the L is typically raised to 50–60 HU and W widened to 130–150 HU. Although tissue contrast in MRI depends mainly upon proton density and T1 and T2 relaxation times, other mechanisms also come into play, and absolute values show considerable variation according to acquisition technique and equipment used. Therefore, the default MR image display relies primarily on intrinsic tissue MR signal and contrast [3,26].

Contrast Enhancement

The signal arising from many normal structures and pathological conditions can be augmented using intravenous contrast material [3]. In CT, such enhancement is obtained by administration of a water-soluble iodinated compound; its relatively high atomic number (53), considerably increases the intravoxel electron density and leads to increased attenuation of the x-ray beam [26]. In MRI, this signal augmentation is commonly obtained with gadolinium-containing compounds, which lead to paramagnetic T1 shortening of nearby protons and signal increase on T1-weighted (T1w) MRI. These contrast agents do not penetrate the normal blood–brain barrier.

A variety of brain conditions, including a majority of inflammatory and many neoplastic lesions, leads to the blood–brain barrier disruption, which then allows contrast agents to enter into the extracellular compartment of the brain as well as pathological tissue. A much smaller amount of gadolinium is required to achieve enhancement on MRI compared with the concentration of iodine needed to achieve a similar result on CT. Therefore, contrast-enhanced MRI is much more sensitive than contrast-enhanced CT. Blood vessels, aneurysms, and vascular malformation enhance with contrast. This is the same for vascular structures such as choroid plexus [3]. Since gray matter contains considerably more blood than white matter, contrast between gray and white matter is accentuated by intravenous contrast agent administration.

Generally, dura including the falx and tentorium normally demonstrate thin enhancement on volumetric or 3D T1-weighted MRI, particularly at 3T and higher field strengths. Leptomeningeal enhancement follows the surface contours of the gyri, sulci, and basal cisterns. In contrast, dural enhancement does not. *Leptomeningeal enhancement typically results from infection (meningitis), inflammatory disorders such as sarcoidosis, leptomeningeal carcinomatosis, lymphomatosis, and conditions leading to gadolinium leakage through the leptomeninges such as acute arterial infarctions [27]. Dural or pachymeningeal enhancement may be seen with craniospinal hypotension, infections, metastasis, and pachymeningitis (idiopathic- or sarcoidosis-induced, granulomatous polyangiitis, and IgG4 disease, etc.)* [28–30].

Outside CTA for the detection of vascular lesions (Fig. 75.16) or CT perfusion for characterizing ischemia, contrast is rarely utilized in brain CT imaging, as gadolinium-enhanced T1-weighted MRI is vastly superior for most other applications. Due to signal loss caused by susceptibility arising from its strong paramagnetic properties, gadolinium can also be used as a negative contrast agent on T2*-weighted MRI, that is, dynamic susceptibility contrast (DSC) MR perfusion imaging [3,26].

Aneurysms and vascular structures are best imaged immediately after contrast injection when blood concentrations of iodine are highest. Enhancement of lesions due to blood–brain barrier breakdown usually peaks 10–15 minutes after contrast injection [26].

Administration of intrathecal contrast allows performance of cisternography and myelography by CT and MRI. *Although nonionic iodinated agents are routinely used for CT myelography and cisternography, safety of gadolinium-based agents is not yet established for MR applications and such usage remains off-label* [26,31].

Field Strength

Routine clinical MRI is performed at magnetic field strengths of 1.5 and 3T. Broadly speaking, while 1.5T MR is adequate for imaging of most routine brain conditions, 3T is superior for MRA and high-resolution MRI of cortex and hippocampus in epilepsy [11]. Higher field strength also accentuates T2* or susceptibility-weighted contrast and therefore, is also superior for susceptibility-weighted imaging (SWI), DSC perfusion, and blood oxygen level-dependent (BOLD) fMRI. Increasing the magnetic field strength increases the proportion of magnetized protons, thus improving the signal-to-noise ratio and allowing for greater spatial resolution with shorter scan duration. Hence, higher field strength scanners, especially 7T or higher, can better resolve finer anatomical details, particularly those of the hippocampus and cerebral cortex. However, ultrahigh field strength also leads to increased signal inhomogeneity due to magnet (B0) and radiofrequency (B1) field distortions and reduced contrast on T1-weighted sequences caused by prolongation of T1 at higher fields. Further, ultrahigh-resolution imaging is also more susceptible to both subject and physiologic motion artifacts [31].

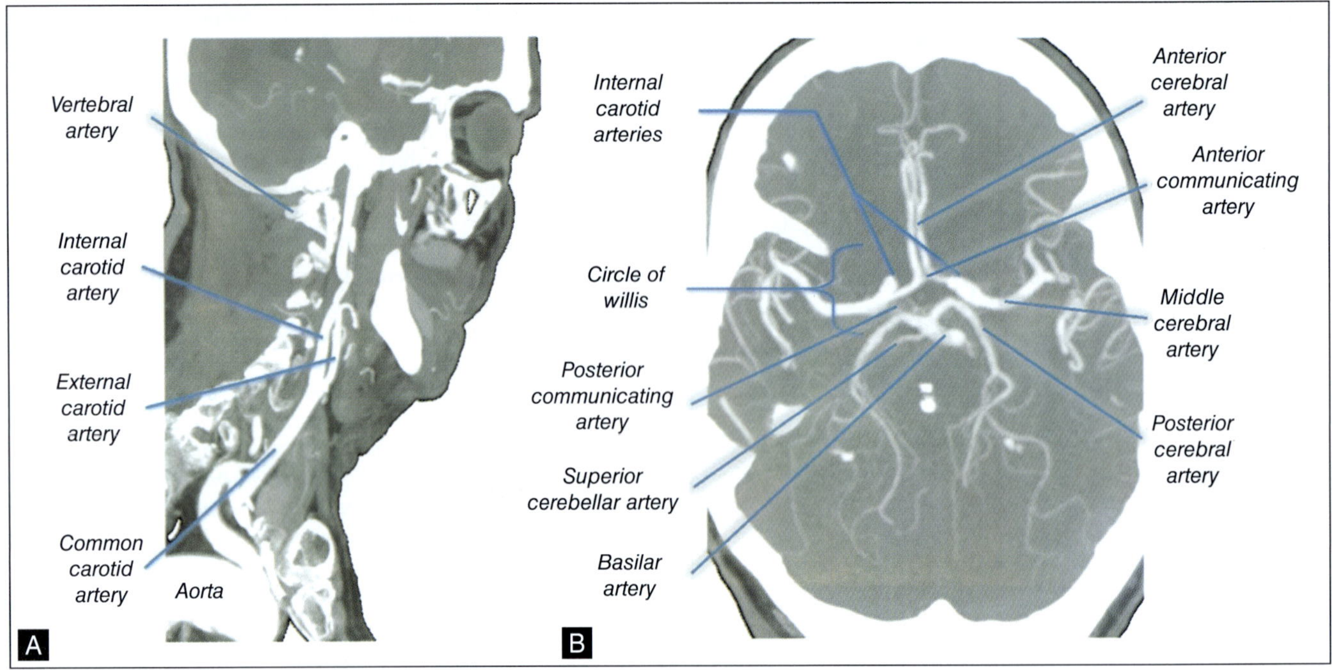

Figure 75.16 Cerebrovascular anatomy on CT angiography (CTA) in sagittal (A) and axial (B) views.

MRI Protocols

Protocol choice in MRI is much wider than in CT. Most modern units no longer use conventional *spin-echo* sequences but instead use one or more of the newer fast scanning techniques. In practice, this generally entails the use of ***gradient-recalled echo (GRE)*** imaging for three-dimensional (3D) or volumetric acquisitions and *fast spin-echo (FSE)* for multislice (2D) acquisitions [3]. Also, FSE techniques are used mainly to demonstrate proton density and T2-weighted contrast. T1-weighted contrast is best displayed by inversion recovery (IR) or magnetization-prepared GRE techniques [39]. FSE acquisitions can be used to acquire dual echoes by generating proton density and T2-weighted images from each excitation as in conventional spin-echo techniques. In the head, GRE techniques are used mainly for volumetric acquisitions with T1-weighted contrast and usually with some form of tissue magnetization preparation, of which the simplest is IR preparation. IR-prepared GRE (MPRAGE, BRAVO, IR-SPGR, etc.) is highly valuable in accentuating gray–white matter contrast, thereby allowing better detection of subtle cortical abnormalities such as focal cortical dysplasia (FCD) and more accurate segmentation of gray and white matter for volumetric analysis and voxel-based morphometry.

Fluid-attenuated inversion recovery (FLAIR) depends on conventional T2-weighted contrast and produces heavily T2-weighted CSF-nulled images by coupling an inversion pulse followed by a long inversion time with a long echo time [3]. FLAIR can enhance detection of lesions with conventional T2-weighted spin-echo sequences and retain sensitivity of T1 relaxation, thus allowing enhancement with gadolinium-based contrast agents. Contrast-enhanced FLAIR has exquisite sensitivity in detecting subtle changes in CSF composition and therefore, is ideally suited for evaluating leptomeningeal disease [28]. **T2* GRE, particularly SWI**, is sensitive to T2* signal decay caused by iron deposition and is routinely used to detect cerebral microbleeds seen in ***amyloid angiopathy*** and ***amyloid-related imaging abnormalities*** and chronic hypertension, superficial siderosis due to leptomeningeal hemosiderin deposition, and abnormal brain iron accumulation in neurodegenerative conditions such as ***multisystem atrophy and neuroferritinopathy*** [13]. More recently, fast spin-echo based MR techniques with variable flip angle evolution such as sampling perfection with application-optimized contrasts (**SPACE and CUBE**) have become available for 3D volumetric imaging for a variety of T1 and T2 image contrasts [32,33].

The routine MR brain examination in most centers remains a sagittal scout image or 3D T1-weighted GRE acquisition followed by an axial diffusion-weighted imaging (DWI), T2*-weighted GRE or SWI, and FSE T2 and FLAIR acquisition. Postcontrast T1-weighted imaging is performed with 2D T1 SE or FSE in axial and coronal planes or with a single sagittal 3D T1-weighted GRE or SPACE/CUBE, reformatted in axial and coronal planes as necessary [32,33]. Acquisition in the coronal plane is preferred in special situations, such as for hippocampal assessment in patients with epilepsy and dementia [11], detailed imaging of the pituitary gland and skull base [34] or better localization of lesions shown on other sequences. 3D magnetization-prepared GRE is preferred when specialized postprocessing is required, such as volumetry, morphometry, or surface rendering or registration. High-resolution 3D GRE or FSE imaging with submillimeter voxels, such as constructive interference steady state, fast imaging employing steady-state acquisition and SPACE are ideally suited for imaging of cranial nerves [35], vessel wall [36], membranous labyrinth [37], and the scolex in neurocysticercosis [38]. Two-dimensional, thin-slice, high inplane-resolution techniques can also be used for imaging small structures such as the pituitary gland, cranial nerves or internal auditory meatuses.

Perfusion-weighted imaging can be produced by analyzing the signal change over time in region of interest after the administration of a bolus of intravenous contrast medium on both CT and MRI. Perfusion can also be assessed with techniques such as BOLD or arterial spin tagging [3,13]. Both T1 (dynamic contrast enhancement) and T2* (DSC) contrast properties of gadolinium-based agents can be exploited to achieve perfusion weighting. Highly accelerated T2* imaging for DSC and BOLD can be performed using echo-planar imaging. BOLD imaging has become routine in

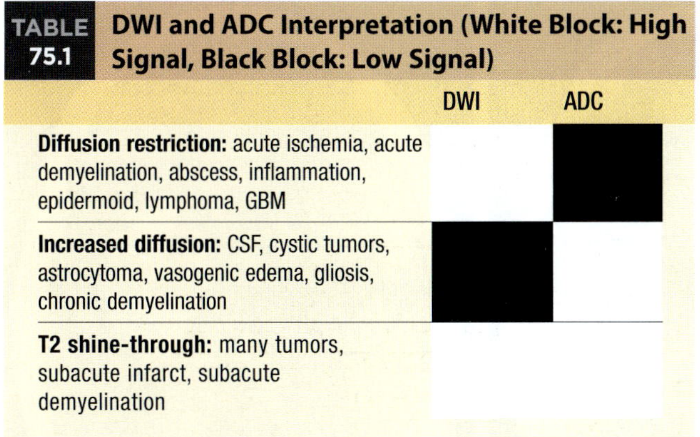

TABLE 75.1 DWI and ADC Interpretation (White Block: High Signal, Black Block: Low Signal)

	DWI	ADC
Diffusion restriction: acute ischemia, acute demyelination, abscess, inflammation, epidermoid, lymphoma, GBM	□	■
Increased diffusion: CSF, cystic tumors, astrocytoma, vasogenic edema, gliosis, chronic demyelination	■	□
T2 shine-through: many tumors, subacute infarct, subacute demyelination	□	□

task-activation studies for presurgical functional brain mapping in tumors and epilepsy [31].

MR Techniques Using Tissue Properties Other Than Magnetic Relaxivity

DWI and ***diffusion tensor imaging*** are achieved using strong magnetic gradients, typically with echo-planar imaging in routine clinical use [3,39]. Such strong gradients can lead to signal loss by incoherent phase shifts and consequent signal loss in tissues with rapid diffusion of water molecules, that is, the contrast depends on the diffusion coefficient of water. Diffusion behavior in brain is anisotropic, especially in white matter, and is greatest along the direction of the white matter tracts. Anisotropy is typically characterized by an elliptical diffusion tensor, the direction of which defines the longitudinal orientation of white matter tracts. Scalar DWI was initially used mainly in the evaluation of acute stroke but has also found widespread clinical applications in characterization of disease processes. Interpretation of DWI and apparent diffusion coefficient (ADC) is summarized in Table 75.1. Diffusion tensor-based mapping of white matter tracts or tractography has become routine in surgical planning to prevent injury to critical motor and language networks [3,26].

Magnetic resonance spectroscopy integrates data from MRI and NMR. NMR can detect tissue metabolites such as N-acetylaspartate (NAA, a neuronal marker), choline (cell membrane), creatine (metabolism), lipids (necrosis), and lactate (anaerobic glycolysis), based on subtle variations in resonances of protons based on their specific molecular environments. *Typically, tumors present with decreased NAA and elevated choline and lactate. Abscess typically shows decreased NAA and choline and elevated lactate, amino acid, and lipid peaks* [40]. *Detection of elevated lactate can also be useful in the diagnosis of mitochondrial encephalopathies such as Leigh's disease, myoclonic epilepsy with ragged-red fibers and mitochondrial encephalomyopathy, lactic acidosis, and stroke-like episodes.* Similarly, detection of elevated glycine and NAA can characterize leukoencephalopathies due to nonketotic hyperglycinemia and Canavan disease, respectively [26].

Magnetization transfer contrast imaging exploits contrast from reduction in relaxed T1 magnetization induced by a broad-spectrum off-resonance prepulse [3]. This prepulse saturates the tightly bound water fraction in normal tissues and causes signal loss on T1-weighted imaging. In pathological tissues, this fraction of water bound to macromolecules/membranes is reduced, resulting in less reduction of relaxed T1 magnetization. Magnetization transfer contrast is typically used to increase conspicuity of plaques in MS and corticospinal tract degeneration in amyotrophic lateral sclerosis [26].

Positron Emission Tomography

Positron emission tomography (PET) imaging is based upon positron-emitting radionuclide tracers such as ^{18}F (i.e., ^{18}F-fluorodeoxyglucose) and ^{11}C isotopes (i.e., ^{11}C-acetate or ^{11}C-raclopride). The tracer, differentially taken up by the tissues, decays by emitting positrons [41]. The positrons collide with electrons to produce two antiparallel gamma rays, are detected as a coincidence by a circular array of detectors and are mapped onto a CT or MR image [41]. Based upon differences in glucose metabolism and molecular biosynthesis, PET can help differentiate tumors from non-neoplastic conditions including post-treatment changes in the brain. *PET, using ^{18}F-fluorodeoxyglucose, and amyloid and tau binding agents (i.e., ^{18}F-florbetaben, ^{18}F-flortaucipir), is of considerable value in the diagnosis of Alzheimer's disease and other neurodegenerative disorders, optimization of their clinical management and prognostication of outcomes in patients with mild cognitive impairment* [42,43].

75.3 Basic Pattern Recognition

Knowledge of brain anatomy is essential to identifying structural changes caused by intracranial disease. Even though a wide variety of pathological conditions can affect the brain, from the neuroimaging standpoint their appearances can be classified into a few essential patterns. Interpretation of brain images begins by identifying these basic patterns to broadly define the nature of the disease process. Thereafter, searching for progressively more specific or characteristic features helps narrow down the list of possibilities. *Generating a final diagnosis or a narrow list of possibilities also requires the consideration of key features of clinical history, physical exam, laboratory findings, and change of imaging features over time.* For example, a subacute infarct can be radiographically indistinguishable from a tumor, and a history of abrupt onset of symptoms can be the principal distinguishing criterion. Similarly, a rapidly growing ring-enhancing intra-axial lesion in a patient with bacteremia is more likely to be an abscess than metastasis. Many a times, radiological interpretation serves as a guide to more tailored history and physical exam, strategies for high-yield laboratory tests, and further radiological imaging and tissue biopsy, if necessary [14,15]. That said, typical patterns in lesion locations and imaging characteristics allow an accurate detection and differential diagnosis in most cases by radiologists or even increasingly by automated methods [44–50].

Extra-Axial Versus Intra-Axial

Radiographic characterization of an intracranial disease begins with determining whether it is intra-axial or extra-axial in location. Intra-axial processes are within the substance of the brain, while extra-axial processes occur outside the brain and pia mater [13,14]. Classic patterns of extra-axial and intra-axial pathology

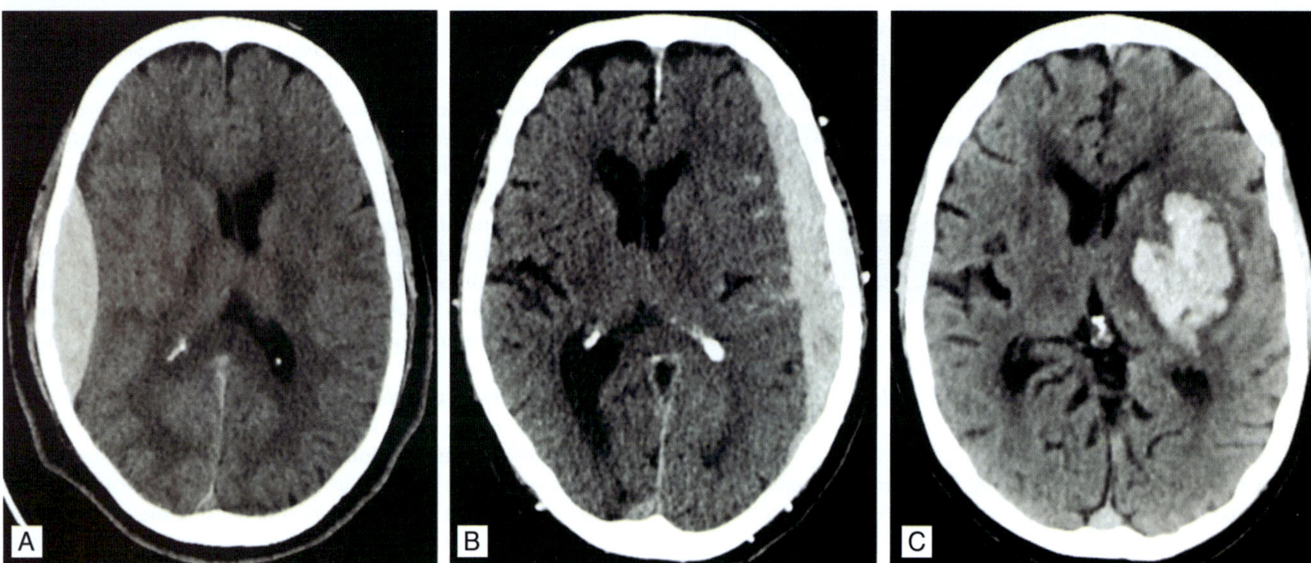

Figure 75.17 Extra-axial and intra-axial acute hematomas appearing hyperdense on CT. Biconvex epidural hematoma (A), crescentic subdural hematoma (B), and lobular parenchymal hematoma (C). The extra-axial epidural and subdural hematomas push the adjacent brain to the left or right. The intra-axial parenchymal hematoma is completely surrounded by brain tissue with low-density edema.

TABLE 75.2 Common Characteristics of Intracranial Extra-Axial Hemorrhage

Characteristic	Epidural Hematoma	Subdural Hematoma	Subarachnoid Hemorrhage
Population	Children, adults	Infants, elderly	Any
Incidence	Uncommon	Common	Common
Clinical presentation	Lucid interval followed by unconsciousness	In older adults: fall with gradual decline In children: non-accidental injury	Trauma, thunderclap headache, sudden onset of symptoms
Etiology	Trauma with skull fracture, lacerated middle meningeal artery	Trauma causing tearing of bridging cortical veins	Traumatic vessel injury, hemorrhagic contusions, aneurysm rupture
Location	Between skull and dura, most commonly supratentorial	Between dura and arachnoid, most commonly supratentorial	Between arachnoid and pia, in cisterns, layering along the sylvian fissures or other sulci
Shape	Biconvex (lentiform)	Crescentic or curvilinear	Focal curvilinear in sulci
Cross suture lines	Usually no, but can cross, for example, the sagittal suture with a fracture at the vertex	Can cross	
Cross falx or tentorium	Can cross	Usually no, but can have unconnected hematomas	

are exemplified by hematomas, which can occur in each location (Fig. 75.17). Extra-axial hematomas may occur in the epidural, subdural, or subarachnoid compartments; it is worth knowing classic features that differentiate these different types of hematomas (Table 75.2) and also considering other processes that occur in the different extra-axial compartments.

A. ***Epidural*** processes which occur between the skull and dura: these processes include hematoma, abscess, and tumors of the skull such as metastasis and myeloma that may extend intracranially. *Epidural lesions typically appear biconvex (lens shaped) and usually do not extend beyond sutures where the dura is tightly adherent to the skull.*

B. ***Subdural*** processes which occur between the dura and the arachnoid: these lesions include hematoma, empyema and hygroma. *These lesions classically appear crescentic, cross suture lines, and follow dural reflections such as the falx and tentorium.* Meningiomas and many other dural-based intracranial masses also occur in this space although rarely described as belonging to this compartment.

C. ***Subarachnoid*** processes which occur between the arachnoid and pia in spaces typically containing CSF (sulci, cisterns such as the suprasellar and cerebellopontine angle cisterns, and fissures such as the interhemispheric and sylvian fissures): the typical pathologies of this compartment include subarachnoid hemorrhage, suprasellar and pineal tumors, arachnoid cysts, aneurysms and nerve sheath tumors.

Intraventricular lesions are considered extra-axial processes. The imaging features of extra-axial processes may include: peripheral location; incomplete confinement by the normal brain; effacement, compression, and displacement rather than brain infiltration; sharp interface between brain and lesion; broad dural base and obtuse angle at the lesion edge; contrast enhancement of the adjacent dura, the so-called "dural tail" sign [51]; involvement of two adjacent intracranial compartments; extension across the midline (exceptions include intra-axial lesions affecting commissures such as corpus callosum and third ventricle); and adjacent skull involvement. *Meningioma is not only the most common extra-axial mass but is also the most frequent intracranial tumor* [13]. With few exceptions such as metastasis, lymphoma, gliosarcomas, and malignant meningiomas, most intracranial tumors remain confined to their space of origin over time, that is, maintain their intra- or extra-axial localization. In large intracranial masses, intra- versus extra-axial determination can be challenging.

Intra-axial processes occur within the brain parenchyma and include infarcts and hemorrhages, traumatic contusions, gliomas, metastasis, cysts, abscess, demyelination, neurodegeneration, vascular malformations, etc. [13]. Intra-axial disease processes frequently lead to disruption of the blood–brain barrier and produce expansion of the extracellular compartment in the surrounding brain by fluid leakage from the capillary bed known as "**vasogenic edema.**" Vasogenic edema primarily affects the white matter and is characterized by hypodensity on CT and T2 hyperintensity on MRI, which follows the distribution of white matter tracts and subcortical U fibers. Although vasogenic edema is primarily seen surrounding intra-axial lesions, it is often also associated with extra-axial tumors and subdural empyemas [40]. Many intra-axial processes such as cerebritis and infiltrative gliomas are ill-circumscribed and blend imperceptibly; conversely, circumscribed gliomas, metastasis, demyelination, and abscesses have more distinct margins. In malignant gliomas, the infiltrative tumor can be impossible to distinguish from vasogenic edema. Rarely, an intra-axial mass can have "exophytic" growth into extra-axial space and be indistinguishable from primary extra-axial tumors.

Location of the intra-axial lesions can help narrow down the differential diagnosis. For example:

- In MS there is preponderance of periventricular and callosal lesions
- Progressive multifocal leukoencephalopathy typically affects subcortical white matter
- Isolated focal gyriform cortical involvement may be seen in arterial infarcts, certain intracortical tumors such as dysembryoplastic neuroepithelial tumor (DNET), seizures, or encephalitis
- Traumatic brain contusions usually occur in cortex along the external surfaces, with the majority in frontobasal, temporal pole, and posteroinferior temporal locations
- Midline posterior fossa masses either arise in the fourth ventricle (ependymoma, epidermoid) or cerebellar vermis (medulloblastoma)
- A slowly growing infiltrative mass in the pons is characteristic of a midline glioma
- Bilateral paramedian cortical and subcortical hemorrhages are quite characteristic of venous infarcts due to sagittal sinus thrombosis
- Similarly, bilateral thalamic enlargement may be due to vein of Galen/straight sinus thrombosis or rarely bithalamic glioma or lymphoma or bilateral arterial infarction due to occlusion of the basilar artery summit or the artery of Percheron [7,8,14]

Mass Effect

Characteristically, hemorrhage, inflammatory processes, and tumors lead to increase in local tissue volume due to their intrinsic expansile nature as well as induction of vasogenic edema in the adjacent brain. Many other processes such as brain infarcts and traumatic contusions also lead to the development of the brain edema during their evolution, thus creating mass effect [15]. In the closed compartment of the cranium, mass effect not only leads to displacement and distortion of surrounding structures but also compression and decreased tissue compliance. This leads to reduced perfusion and venous congestion when severe. The primary source of mass effect could be within the brain (intra-axial) or ventricles (intra-ventricular) or outside the brain (extra-axial) in the meninges, CSF spaces, and skull. Although intra-axial mass lesions lead to compression and effacement of the CSF spaces (sulci and cisterns) in all directions, extra-axial masses lead to asymmetric expansion and effacement of these compartments.

Mass effect, midline shift, and ***herniation*** are essential features to assess in all brain images. Intracranial mass effect describes how a lesion displaces and compresses the adjacent structures. Lesions with mass effect can also cause ***midline shift*** or displacement of hemispheres across the midline, breaking the symmetry of the brain across the midsagittal plane. The term "herniation" is used to describe the displacement of brain structures in certain distinct locations, such as cerebellar ***tonsillar herniation*** below the foramen magnum and ***central herniation*** of the brainstem, which obliterates the perimesencephalic and perimedullary cisterns [4].

Transtentorial herniation occurs when the midbrain is displaced and compressed in the tentorial hiatus by the medial and downward displacement of the uncus and parahippocampal gyrus (Fig. 75.18A, B). *As a result of severe crowding and compression against the tentorial free edge, uncal or transtentorial herniation can be complicated by posterior cerebral artery infarction, oculomotor nerve dysfunction leading to fixed dilated pupil and ipsilateral hemiparesis from compression of the cerebral peduncle against the tentorial free edge.* ***Duret hemorrhage*** (Fig. 75.18C) can also occur in the midbrain or pons from venous compression in the setting of transtentorial herniation [12,14]. ***Ascending transtentorial herniation*** is sometimes used to describe upward displacement of the cerebellar vermis through the tentorial hiatus in posterior fossa mass lesions [13].

Subfalcine herniation occurs when the cingulate gyrus is displaced across the midline below the free edge of the falx cerebri and can later progress to additional structures including the corpus callosum and subcortical nuclei. One clinical complication of subfalcine herniation is lower limb hemiparesis due to compression of the anterior cerebral artery branches supplying the paracentral lobule [4,6].

Volume Loss

Brain tissue volume loss characterizes neurodegenerative processes and is typically accompanied by astrocytic **gliosis** in late stages of inflammatory disease, infarcts, intra-axial hematomas, and trauma [14]. Astrocytic gliosis is hypodense on CT and hyperintense on T2-weighted MRI. *Diffuse or regional brain volume loss or cerebral* ***atrophy****, in the absence of an antecedent process such as trauma, infarct*

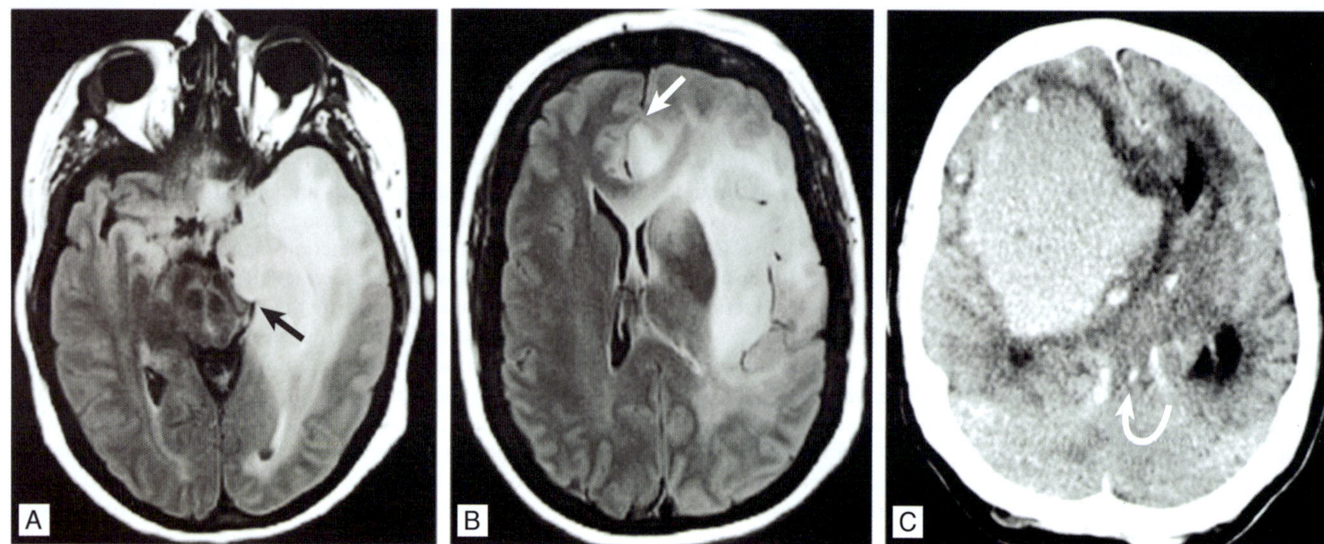

Figure 75.18 Transtentorial and subfalcine herniation on axial T2/FLAIR MRI (A, B). High-grade glioma with mass effect causes uncal and parahippocampal gyrus herniating below the free edge of tentorium cerebelli and compressing the midbrain (*black arrow*) and subfalcine herniation below the free edge of falx cerebri (*white arrow*). Duret hemorrhage (*curved arrow*) in midbrain complicating transtentorial herniation caused by large right intracerebral hematoma (C).

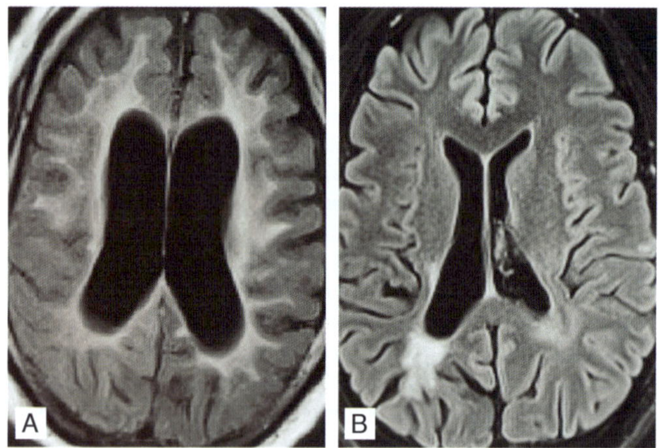

Figure 75.19 Hydrocephalus ex vacuo and cortical atrophy on FLAIR MRI can be bilateral (A) for example due to diffuse adrenoleukodystrophy or unilateral (B) (right) due to periventricular multiple sclerosis, causing right lateral ventricle expansion.

or inflammation, is a typical feature of aging and neurodegeneration. Distinct patterns of regional or lobar cortical atrophy in patients with cognitive decline or behavioral disturbances serve as markers of neurodegenerative conditions, such as *Alzheimer disease* (AD) and *frontotemporal dementia* (FTD) [4,42]. Distinct variants of AD include posterior cortical atrophy or logopenic variant primary progressive aphasia. Additional forms of neurodegeneration with etiologies distinct from Alzheimer pathology include *vascular contributions to cognitive impairment and dementia* (i.e., sequelae of atherosclerosis, small vessel ischemic disease, and infarcts), *Lewy body disease, LATE, FTD, corticobasal syndrome,* and *progressive supranuclear palsy* [55]. ***Encephalomalacia*** (brain softening) refers to end-stage astrocytic gliosis and cavitation ensuing from neural tissue loss from infection, ischemia, and hemorrhage, etc. Demyelinating diseases and blunt head trauma can also lead to diffuse brain atrophy [6]. Because the skull forms a rigid closed compartment, CSF spaces (ventricles, sulci, and cisterns) expand to make up brain volume loss. Ventricular enlargement of this type is called **ex vacuo dilatation** or **hydrocephalus ex vacuo** (Fig. 75.19) and should be distinguished from hydrocephalus caused by a blockage of CSF circulation or resorption [15].

TABLE 75.3 Neurological Diseases by Gray/White Matter Localization

Predominantly Cortical Gray Matter	Predominantly White Matter
Malformations of cortical development: focal cortical dysplasia, heterotopia, double cortex, lissencephaly	■ Microvascular ischemia or Binswanger disease ■ Microangiopathy: Susac syndrome
Neurodegenerative conditions: AD and FTD	Prototypical demyelination: multiple sclerosis and neuromyelitis optica
Mesial temporal sclerosis	Rare/uncommon demyelination: osmotic demyelination and Marchiafavi–Bignami disease
Cortically based neoplasms: dysembryoplastic neuroectodermal tumor and ganglioglioma	Inherited metabolic: adrenoleukodystrophy and metachromatic leukodystrophy
Acute hypoxemic–ischemic and hypoglycemic injury	Viral and postviral demyelination: acute disseminated encephalomyelitis and progressive multifocal leukoencephalopathy

Metastases and abscesses tend to occur at the junction of gray and white matter (Fig. 75.20) [13].

Gray Matter Versus White Matter and Cortical Versus Subcortical

Many diseases predominantly affect the cortical gray matter while certain disease processes are relatively restricted to white matter (Table 75.3 and Fig. 75.20) [13–15].

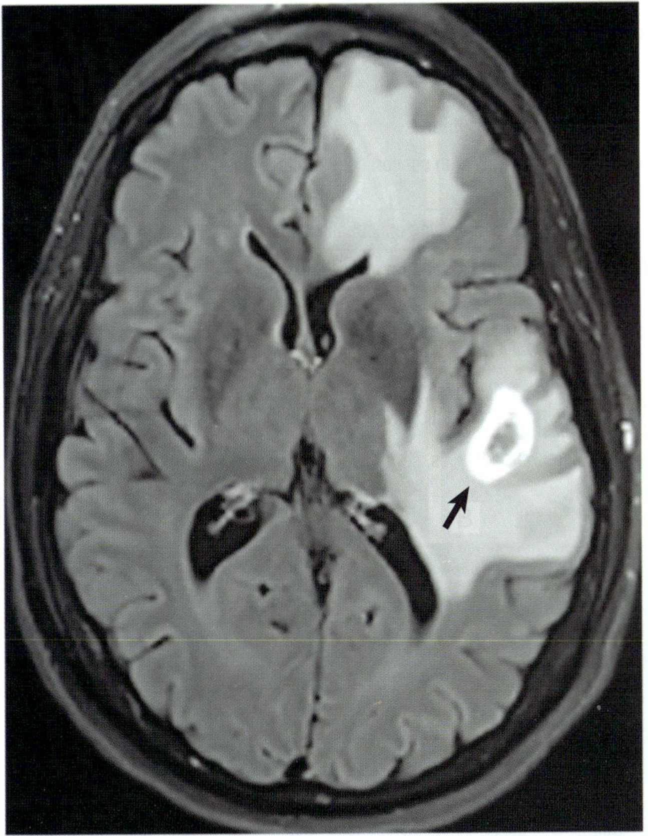

Figure 75.20 Juxtacortical metastases (*arrow*) on postcontrast FLAIR MRI appearing as ring-enhancing metastasis at the border of gray and white matter with surrounding FLAIR hyperintense vasogenic edema in the left anterior temporal lobe. Vasogenic edema is also seen in the left frontal lobe due to another metastatic lesion not included in this image.

However, many disease processes, such as infarcts, contusions, and infiltrative gliomas, can affect both gray and white matter. MS demonstrates white matter disease early in its course and later onset of gray matter atrophy after repeated periods of relapses or progression [52,53].

Some pathologies are generally localized to subcortical structures like the basal ganglia and thalami. Some processes are usually unilateral (although can also be bilateral), whereas others predominantly involve bilateral subcortical structures (Fig. 75.21 and Table 75.4) [7].

Some pathologies have unique cortical and subcortical features. *Creutzfeldt–Jakob disease* causes hyperintensity on DWI and hypointensity on ADC (diffusion restriction) and T2 hyperintensity of both the cortex ("*cortical ribboning*") and basal ganglia (Fig. 75.22) [6,7]. Diffusion restriction in acute *hypoxic ischemic encephalopathy* can occur in gray matter throughout the brain. Infarcts, tumors, and many additional pathologies can also span both cortical and subcortical locations [7].

Focal Versus Multiple Versus Diffuse

Many lesions are generally ***focal*** (single or solitary), such as most primary brain tumors and hypertensive hemorrhage. Other lesions are typically **multiple**, such as small vessel ischemic disease, MS, neurocysticercosis, toxoplasmosis, etc. [13]. Metastases are usually multiple but could be solitary. Bacterial abscesses tend to be solitary but could be multiple. Infarcts and lymphoma can be single or multiple. Glioblastoma can appear focal or multifocal/multicentric on imaging but may in fact be more diffuse histologically. High-grade primary brain tumors and metastatic disease can also disseminate in the CSF space. A leukodystrophy would be an example of a disease process affecting white matter fairly diffusely [15].

Homogeneous Versus Heterogeneous and Cystic Versus Solid

Homogeneous signal denotes lesions with relatively uniform MR signal and density. Meningiomas are typically homogenous on both CT and MRI, whereas glioblastomas are typically heterogenous. ***Heterogeneous*** signal occurs in lesions that have mixed tissue elements, necrosis, hemorrhage, calcification, or cystic change. Heterogeneity is best assessed on MRI (Fig. 75.23) [13].

Cystic brain lesions are fluid-filled sacs that may contain CSF, pus, serous, or serosanguinous fluid. Besides true cysts, the

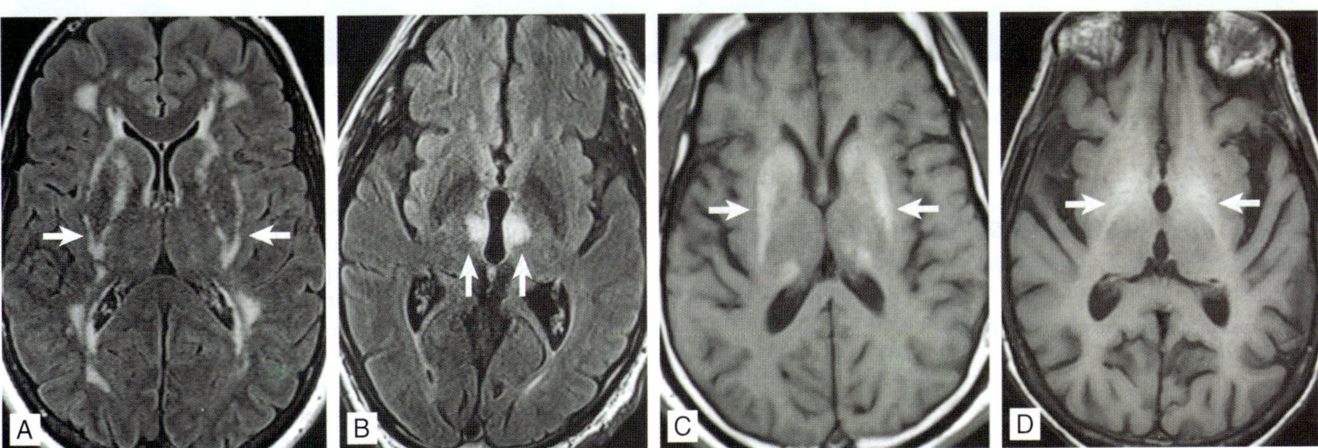

Figure 75.21 Bilateral subcortical lesions (*arrows*). CADASIL can show FLAIR hyperintensity of the lentiform nucleus due to lenticulostriate arteries vasculopathy (A). Artery of Percheron supplies both thalami from a single posterior cerebral artery, so infarct causes bilateral thalamic FLAIR hyperintensities (B). Calcinosis of the striatum in Fahr disease appears T1 hyperintense (C). Manganese in the globi pallidi is T1 hyperintense (D).

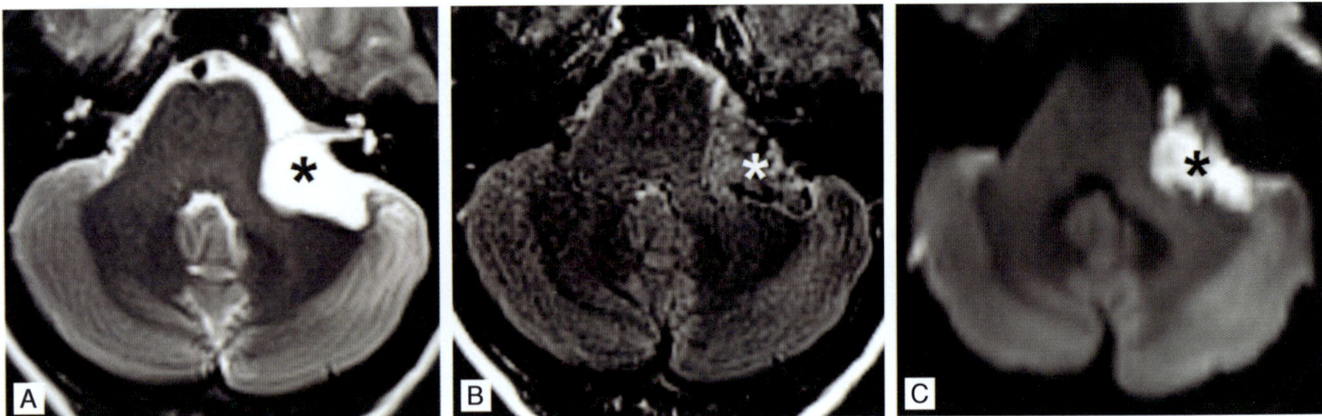

Figure 75.32 Epidermoid cyst. Axial MR images show mass effect from a left cerebellopontine angle cistern epidermoid cyst (*asterisk*). The cyst is bright on T2-weighted imaging (A) but does not lose signal like CSF on FLAIR (B) and is notable bright on diffusion-weighted imaging (C) due to diffusion restriction.

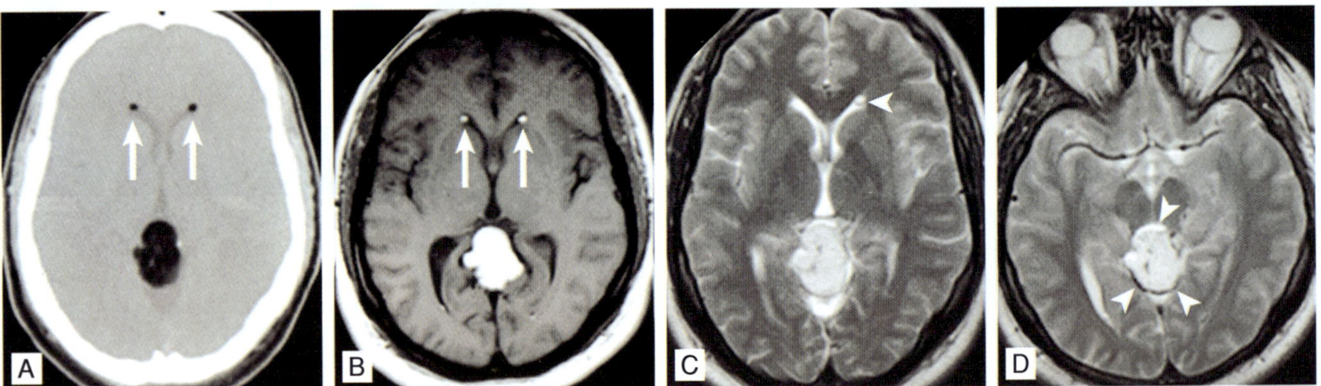

Figure 75.33 Ruptured dermoid in quadrigeminal plate cistern with scattered intraventricular fat droplets. Axial CT (A), axial-unenhanced T1-weighted (B), and axial T2-weighted (C and D) MR sections with demonstrate a mass with fat density (A) and high T1 signal (B) and intraventricular fat droplets (*arrows*). Chemical shift artifact due to fat causes bright and dark borders along the anterior and posterior margins of the primary mass and the intraventricular droplets (C and D: *arrowheads*).

ventricles. The exact site of origin is often difficult to determine as these lesions can extend around blood vessels and nerves as they grow in the subarachnoid space. The margins may be irregular although sharp, and there is no true invasion of adjacent brain [3].

On ***CT***, the cysts usually have low density, that of CSF or slightly higher, depending on the contents. Calcification is unusual but flecks of calcification have occasionally been noted in the capsule. They may be difficult to differentiate from arachnoid cysts [3,14].

MRI signal characteristics and appearances depend on relative proportions of cholesterol (short T1) and keratin (long T1) within the cyst. They are usually isointense or slightly hyperintense to CSF on T1 and bright like CSF on T2-weighted images. On heavily T2-weighted and FLAIR MR images, their internal keratinized matrix can often be appreciated (Fig. 75.32). On T2/FLAIR, their signal typically does not fully suppress due to proteinaceous contents, unlike the signal of arachnoid cysts, which does suppress like that of CSF. Diffusion-weighted sequences may also be helpful in differentiating epidermoid cysts from arachnoid cysts. *Since arachnoid cysts have free water diffusion, they completely lose their T2 signal on DWI. Epidermoid cysts have more restricted diffusion due to the presence of epithelial debris; hence, their T2 signal is partially retained, and they typically appear hyper- or isointense to the brain on DWI.* Epidermoids often expand the cisterns from which they arise and distort adjacent brain structures creating lobulated or scalloped margins (Fig. 75.32). Although extra-axial origin remains apparent, the larger lesions may invaginate deeply and falsely appear to invade the parenchyma. Surgical resection of such epidermoids is, therefore, often incomplete. There is complete lack of enhancement except for along the margin on occasion [54].

Dermoid Cyst

Dermoid cysts are more complex than epidermoids and more slow-growing. As rare entities, they arise from entrapment of embryonic ectoderm into the neural tube in early gestation and typically occur near the midline. Their wall contains full-width dermis, which may contain hair and sebaceous glands, and an outer layer of connective tissue and capsule. The cyst may contain matted hair and glandular secretions as well as desquamated keratinized epithelium. These lesions usually present in the third decade of life with chronic headache and other nonspecific symptoms [3]. Occasionally, they may be associated with seizures, focal neurologic deficits, and aseptic meningitis. Gradual enlargement may occur from glandular secretions and epithelial debris accumulation. Rupture of dermoid cysts spontaneously or iatrogenically at surgery can result in severe chemical meningitis that can be complicated by vasospasm and infarction. They can present in children in the midline at the base of the brain or near the fourth ventricle. The latter may show an occipital skin dimple with a stalk leading through bone and can become infected [54,56]. Arc-like calcification, occurring in the capsule, is seen in 20% of cases [54].

TABLE 75.6 Comparison of Epidermoid and Dermoid Cysts

	Epidermoid	Dermoid
Pathology	Ectodermal inclusion cyst with keratin and cholesterol but no dermal structures and rarely rupture	Ectodermal inclusion cyst with keratin, cholesterol, and dermal structures (hair, sebaceous glands) and may rupture
Location	Off-midline Cerebellopontine angle cistern > parasellar > middle cranial fossa > diploic space	Midline Intracranial: parasellar > frontobasal Infratentorial: vermis > fourth ventricle
CT	NECT: low density (like CSF) with uncommon calcification CECT: occasionally enhancing peripherally	NECT: low density (like fat) with common calcification CECT: no enhancement
MRI	Often isointense with CSF	T1 hyperintense, T2 hypo- to hyperintense

On ***CT***, dermoid cysts are well-circumscribed fat density masses without contrast enhancement and are usually more rounded than epidermoids (Fig. 75.33). They are seen in the posterior fossa near the midline or above the floor of the anterior fossa, but they can occur over the convexity and elsewhere. Capsular calcification occurs more commonly than with epidermoids [3]. Rupture of a cyst may occur, with escape of the fatty contents into the CSF, resulting in chemical meningitis followed by arachnoid scarring and hydrocephalus; rupture into the ventricle has also been reported, and this has been recognized at CT by a fat–fluid level [14,54].

On ***MRI***, dermoids show high signal on T1-weighted images due to the presence of fat and vary from hypo- to hyperintense on T2-weighted images. Chemical shift artifact is frequently visible, indicating the presence of fat on T2-weighted images. There is typically no contrast enhancement or vasogenic edema in the surrounding brain. Serpiginous hypointensities may be seen if containing hair. Mural calcification can sometimes be identified on MR [3,56]. On both CT and MR images, fat density and high T1 signal droplets may be seen scattered throughout the subarachnoid space, often remote from the lesion or in the ventricular system if rupture has taken place. Dermoids without fat or calcification may be indistinguishable from epidermoids or arachnoid cysts; the presence of material other than fat within a lesion is also useful in distinguishing dermoids from intracranial lipomas. See Table 75.6 for further comparison of epidermoid and dermoid cysts [54].

Neuroendocrine Diseases

Pituitary Apoplexy

This condition results from ischemia or hemorrhage of the pituitary gland, typically due to a previously undiagnosed pituitary adenoma (Fig. 75.34). Additional causes and predisposing associations include hypertension, trauma, and medications (anticoagulation, hormones). The classic clinical presentation involves acute headache, visual field defects due to compression of the optic chiasm, and diplopia if involving the cavernous sinus [60,61]. Long-term symptoms include endocrine dysfunction secondary to hypopituitarism and adrenal insufficiency. MRI, particularly DWI and GRE, reveals infarct and/or hemorrhage [61–63].

Sheehan Syndrome

This is a rare but potentially life-threatening condition associated with postpartum hemorrhage and/or hypovolemic shock, which triggers ischemic necrosis of the pituitary gland. Neuroendocrine sequelae include failure of lactation and rapidly developing panhypopituitarism. Variable pituitary gland enlargement with abnormal signal due to patchy central ischemic necrosis and hemorrhage and an abnormal lack of enhancement in the central portions of the gland (Fig. 75.35) are the typical radiologic findings of acute Sheehan's syndrome.

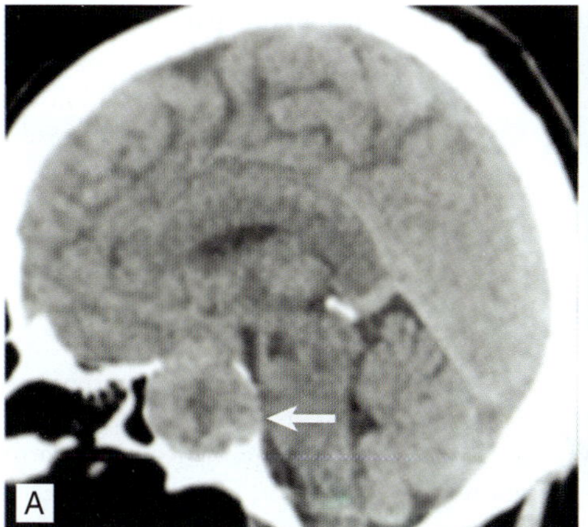

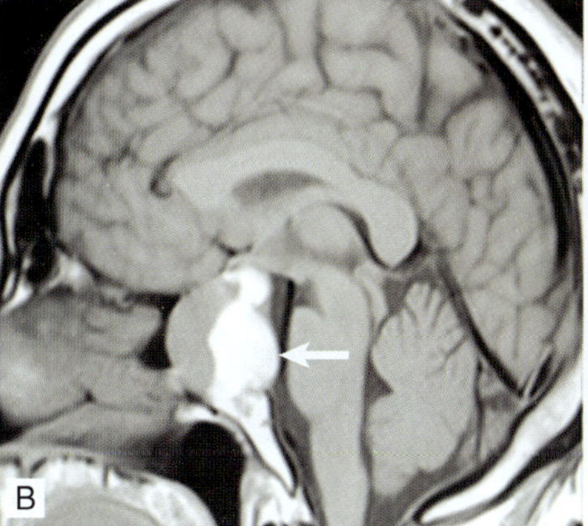

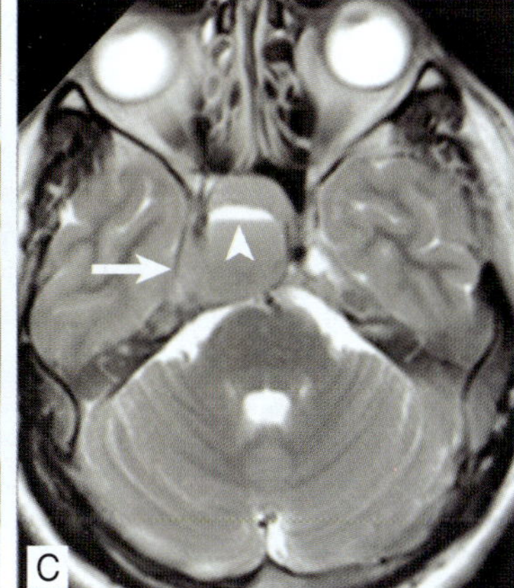

Figure 75.34 Pituitary apoplexy. CT showing a markedly expanded sella due to large pituitary adenoma (A, *arrow*) extending into the suprasellar cistern in a patient who presented with acute onset headache, visual field defects, and right abducens palsy. On sagittal T1-unenhanced MRI, the sellar/suprasellar mass shows large subacute hemorrhage appearing as high signal T1 (B, *arrow*) and a fluid level with mixed high and low signal on axial T2 MR (C, *arrowhead*), indicating the presence of deoxyhemoglobin and methemoglobin in the subacute hemorrhage. Involvement of the right cavernous sinus accounts for the right abducens palsy (C, *arrow*).

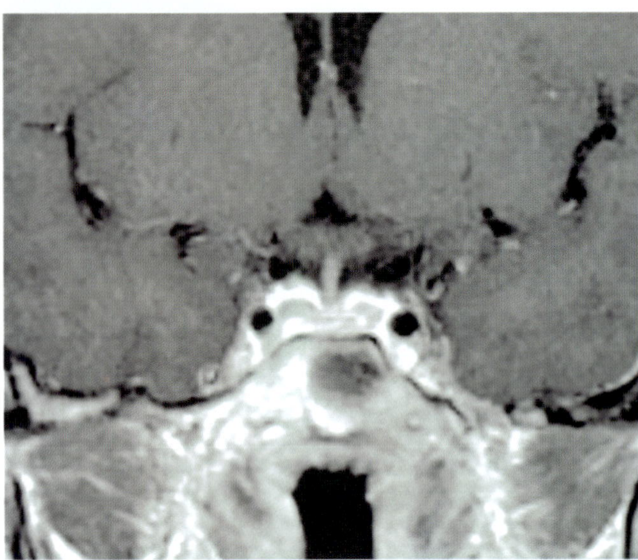

Figure 75.35 Sheehan syndrome. Postpartum necrosis of the pituitary gland appearing as lack of central enhancement on coronal-enhanced T1-weighted MRI.

In chronic stage, there is marked glandular atrophy with an empty appearing sella [62,64]. Commonly on the differential diagnosis is peripartum/postpartum lymphocytic hypophysitis [64,65].

Empty Sella

The "***empty sella syndrome***" rarely causes neuroendocrine sequelae (Fig. 75.36). An empty sella may be classified as primary or secondary.

- *Primary empty sella* is caused by herniation of suprasellar arachnoid and CSF into the sella through the normal opening in the diaphragm sellae for passage of the infundibulum. The pituitary gland is compressed against the back and floor of the sella causing much or most of the sella to be occupied by CSF. An empty sella may be asymptomatic and an incidental finding at imaging or autopsy for other causes. However, an empty sella should be recognized as evidence of elevated intracranial pressure that can cause headaches (*idiopathic intracranial hypertension,* aka pseudotumor cerebri), particularly in middle-aged women and associated with obesity [67]. Visual field defects can occur due to prolapse of the optic nerve or chiasmal tissue into the empty sella. The sella itself is often enlarged, presumably from pulsating CSF, and this, together with the clinical findings, can lead to an erroneous diagnosis of pituitary cyst [66]
- *Secondary empty sella* may occur after hypophysectomy or tumor removal, spontaneous pituitary infarction (i.e., Sheehan syndrome), radiation therapy, immune checkpoint inhibitor-associated hypophysitis or infectious/autoimmune etiologies [3,62,67]

Vascular Lesions

Vascular Compression of Cranial Nerves by Dolichoectatic Arteries

Dolichoectasia is the dilation and kinking of a tortuous vessel due to abnormal vessel shape and flow, which can lead to compression of cranial nerves and brain parenchyma. Direct observations at surgery led to the theory that tortuous vessels compressing the trigeminal nerve root exit zones can be a cause of trigeminal neuralgia. The compression is usually due to a tortuous branch of the superior cerebellar artery. Advances in MRA and high-resolution imaging have made noninvasive detection possible [3,8,13].

It is also now well recognized that hemifacial spasm can also be due to tortuous arteries arching into the pontomedullary junction and impinging on the facial nerve exit zone. The arteries implicated are either the vertebral artery, the anterior inferior cerebellar artery or the posterior inferior cerebellar artery. Other cranial nerves which may be affected by vascular compression include the vestibulocochlear nerve, giving rise to tinnitus and vertigo, and the glossopharyngeal nerve, leading to glossopharyngeal neuralgia. It is thought that dolichoectasia of the vertebrobasilar system may also cause tension in small-caliber arteries (such as pontine perforator arteries), thereby decreasing flow to the brainstem and potentially causing stroke or basilar migraine [3,8].

Arteriovenous Malformation

Arteriovenous malformations (AVMs) are abnormal intra-axial connections between cerebral arteries and veins without a capillary bed and involve the brain parenchyma and

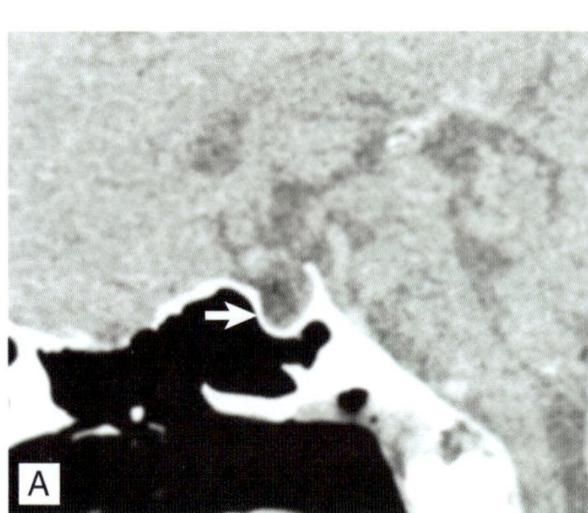

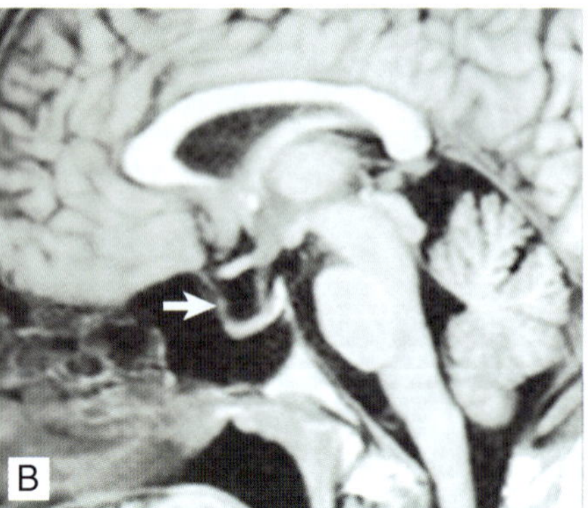

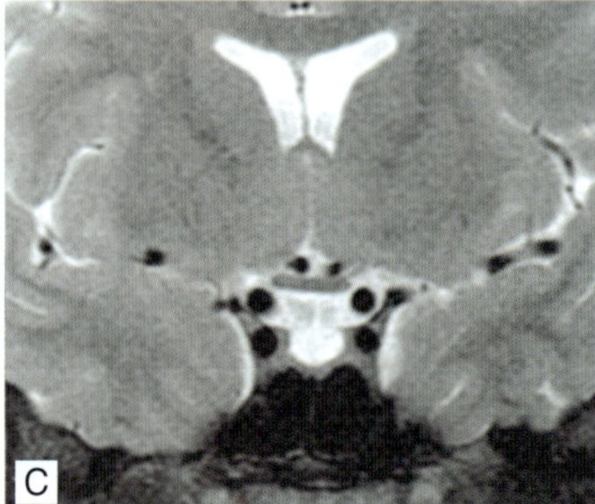

Figure 75.36 Empty sella in a patient with pseudotumor cerebri. Sagittal CT reformat (A, *arrow*) showing moderately expanded fluid dense sella without visible pituitary gland. Sagittal T1 (B, *arrow*) and coronal T2 (C) MRI shows the normal pituitary gland flattened against the sellar floor by intrasellar herniation of the suprasellar cistern.

overlying meninges. Sometimes incidentally found, they may present with acute intraparenchymal or subarachnoid hemorrhage. Other manifestations include headache and seizures [68,69].

Patients presenting with hemorrhage will usually show an intracerebral hematoma recognizable by its characteristic density; blood may also be seen in the basal cisterns, ventricles, or sulci.

Patients without subarachnoid hemorrhage will show no obvious lesion in 10–20% of unenhanced CT scans; this happens when the lesion is relatively small and superficial. However, a noncontrast CT scan may show characteristic serpiginous high-density structures suggestive of thrombosed enlarged vessels or hypertrophied veins. Characteristic ring-like or curvilinear and serpiginous calcification may also be shown. The appearance of the vessels in a large AVM will vary depending on the angle relative to the tomographic sections. Usually, tubular or vermiform densities may be recognized when sectioned longitudinally and rounded or ovoid densities when sectioned transversely [3].

CT low-density and T2 MR hyperintensity in brain parenchyma adjacent to the malformation can represent posthemorrhagic cysts or chronic ischemic gliosis, which along with dilated vessels in the vicinity can give rise to a mottled appearance [69].

After contrast injection, characteristic tortuous vascular structures are more easily recognized. Large lesions may penetrate deeply into the brain like wedges although the majority remain superficial. Most AVMs produce little mass effect unless there has also been a large hemorrhage. Nevertheless, it is possible to mistake the appearance for that of gliomas or infarcts, and the differential diagnosis should expand when appearances are not characteristic [3].

Although the diagnosis of AVMs is often established on CT and MR, most cases will require DSA before surgery or endovascular embolization to define the detailed anatomy of feeding and draining vessels [8].

CT shows an irregular hyperdense intraparenchymal lesion with calcification in about 30% of cases. Unless there is evidence of thrombosis or hemorrhage, the AVMs show homogeneous intense enhancement in the arterial phase of the intravenous bolus [3]. When superficial, they can resemble meningiomas but without edema or mass effect [69].

MRI shows characteristic round, tubular or punctate low signal areas due to vascular **flow voids**, especially on T2-weighted images. Large arteries and draining veins usually appear as signal voids although may be hyperintense on T1-weighted images due to flow-related enhancement. There may be regional brain atrophy or occasionally some local mass effect. Intracerebral hematoma may be shown in or adjacent to the malformation, usually clearly evident on MR with variable signal or edema depending on acuity. Frequently, there are areas of low signal on T2-weighted images, secondary to hemosiderin tissue deposition. Calcification can also manifest as low signal although more apparent on CT. High signal on T2/FLAIR may be seen in the adjacent brain due to gliosis (Fig. 75.37) [8]. Refer to Spetzler–Martin grading scale for AVMs in Table 75.7, which correlates to clinical outcomes [70,71].

Arteriovenous fistulas (AVFs) occur most commonly in the dura mater, frequently near or in the wall of a dural venous sinus. Dural AVFs, unlike AVMs, are direct arteriovenous shunts without an intervening nidus and are supplied primarily by the meningeal arteries and dural branches of the external and internal carotid arteries [3]. The drainage occurs usually through the dural venous sinuses (Fig 75.38) and occasionally through other superficial veins in the dura, orbit or scalp. Occasionally, dural AVFs drain or reflux intradurally into the cortical veins, causing enlarged tortuous cerebral veins to be visible (Fig. 75.39). Such AVFs carry high risk of rupture and intracranial hemorrhage [69].

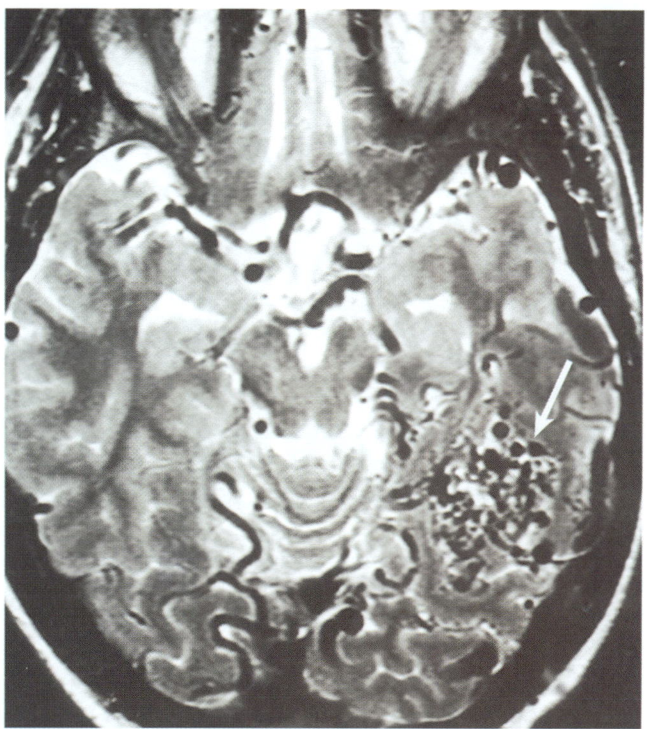

Figure 75.37 An arteriovenous malformation (AVM, *arrow*) mainly in the left temporal lobe appears as dilated tortuous vessels on T2-weighted MRI.

TABLE 75.7 Spetzler–Martin AVM Grading Scale (Lower Score Is Better Outcome) [70,71]

Trait	Points
Size	
<3 cm	1
3.1–6.0 cm	2
>6 cm	3
Location	
Noneloquent	0
Eloquent*	1
Deep venous drainage	
Not present	0
Present	1
AVM total score	1–5

*Eloquent areas include sensorimotor, language and visual cortex, thalamus, hypothalamus, internal capsule, brainstem, cerebellar peduncles, and deep cerebellar nuclei.

It is often difficult to detect dural AVFs on routine CT and MRI due to their proximity to the bony vault or skull base but enlarged draining cortical veins may be seen in some cases (Fig. 75.39) [8,69].

Dural AVFs are acquired lesions, often idiopathic but thought to be induced by previous known or unknown sinus thrombosis.

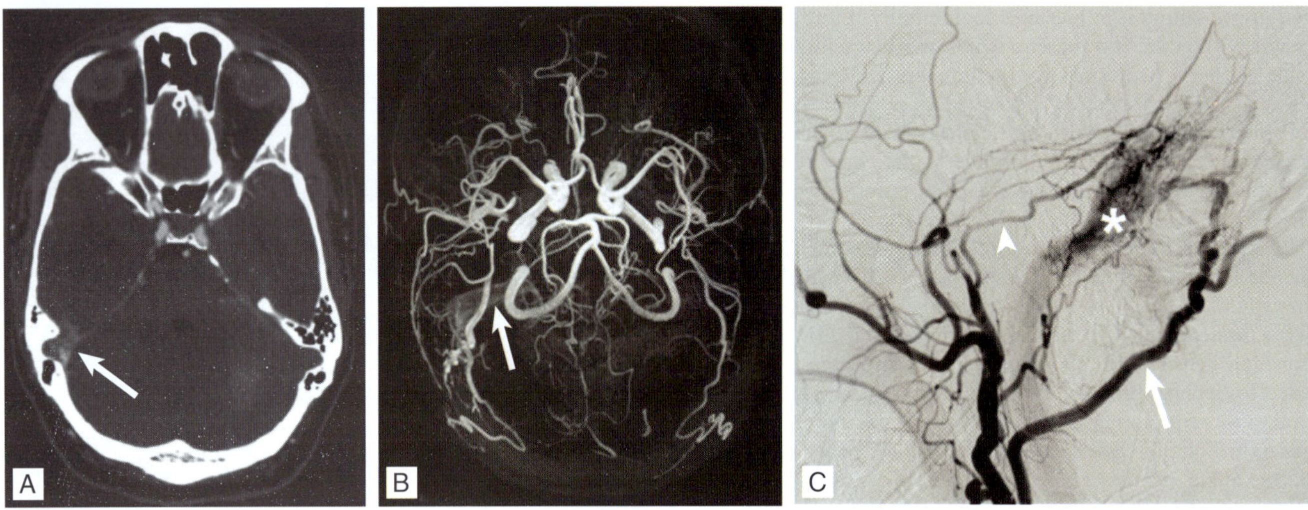

Figure 75.38 Dural arteriovenous fistula causing pulsatile tinnitus. CT angiogram (A) shows abnormal vessels along the right lateral tentorium and abnormal drainage into the sigmoid sinus (*arrow*) in the arterial phase. Maximum intensity projection image from time-of-flight MR angiogram (B) shows high flow in the right sigmoid sinus (*arrow*) and prominent vessels and external artery carotid branches extending to the fistula at the right lateral tentorium. Conventional angiogram (C) shows occipital (*arrow*) and middle meningeal artery (*arrowhead*) branch feeders to the fistula (*asterisk*).

More generally, AVFs may be acquired from trauma (for example, caroticocavernous fistula) or surgery. In the pediatric period, a cerebral AVF involving a persistent median prosencephalic vein (vein of Galen malformation) can present dramatically with cardiac failure or hydrocephalus [3,69].

Cerebral Cavernous Malformations

Cerebral cavernous malformations, ***cavernous angiomas,*** or ***cavernomas*** are vascular hamartomatous lesions comprised of sinusoidal spaces without intervening brain parenchyma. When occurring in familial syndromes caused by mutations in cerebral cavernous malformation 1, 2, or 3 genes, they are usually multiple [8,68]. Cavernomas are frequently asymptomatic and found incidentally on imaging. Seizures, headache, and hemorrhage are their most frequent clinical presentation when found in the cerebral hemispheres, whereas cavernomas of the brainstem typically present with focal neurological deficits. They commonly appear as small circumscribed intra-axial "popcorn"-like lesions with mixture of hypointense and hyperintense intralesional foci on T1- and T2-weighted MRI depending upon the presence of and stages of intralesional hemorrhages. Due to hemosiderin, lesions appear to bloom on susceptibility; cavernomas generally appear larger on T2* GRE or SWI than on T1 MRI or CT [3]. Very small cavernomas, therefore, may only be visualized on T2* GRE or SWI images. On CT, cavernomas are typically hyperdense with varying degrees of calcification. Sometimes, recent hemorrhage may be

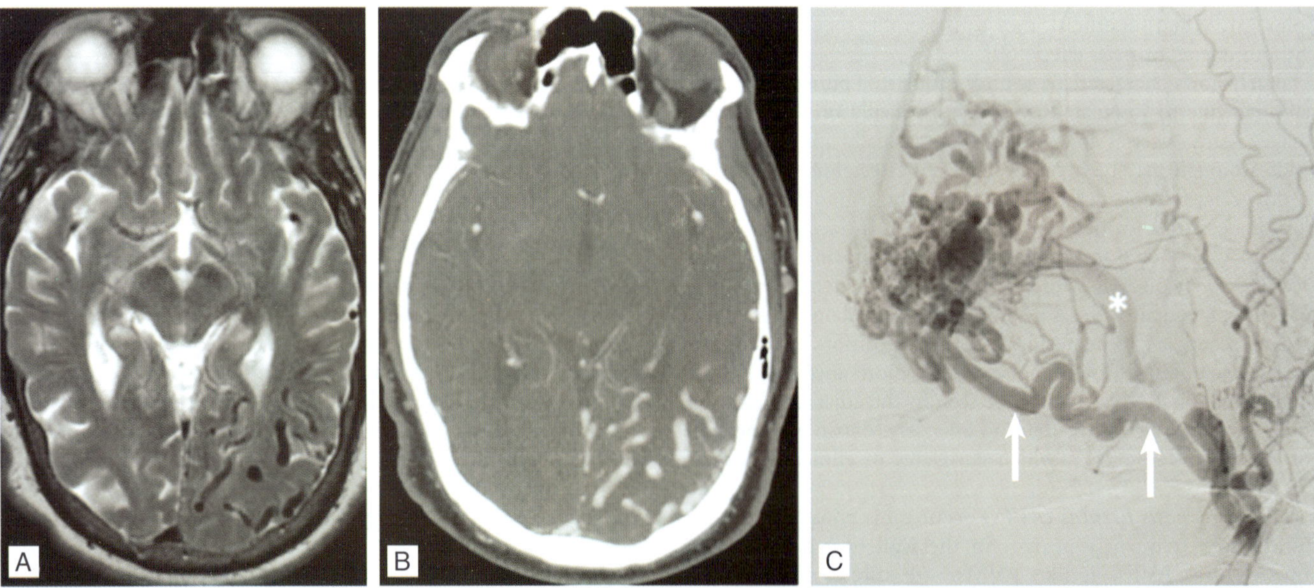

Figure 75.39 Dural AVF causing headache and pulsatile tinnitus. Axial T2 MRI (A) and contrast-enhanced CT (B) show dilated cortical veins in the left occipital lobe. Left external carotid DSA (C) shows a dural AVF of the transverse sinus (*asterisk*) supplied by a massively enlarged occipital artery (*arrows*) with venous reflux into occipital cortical veins. Cortical venous reflux significantly increases the risk of intracranial hemorrhage in dural AVF.

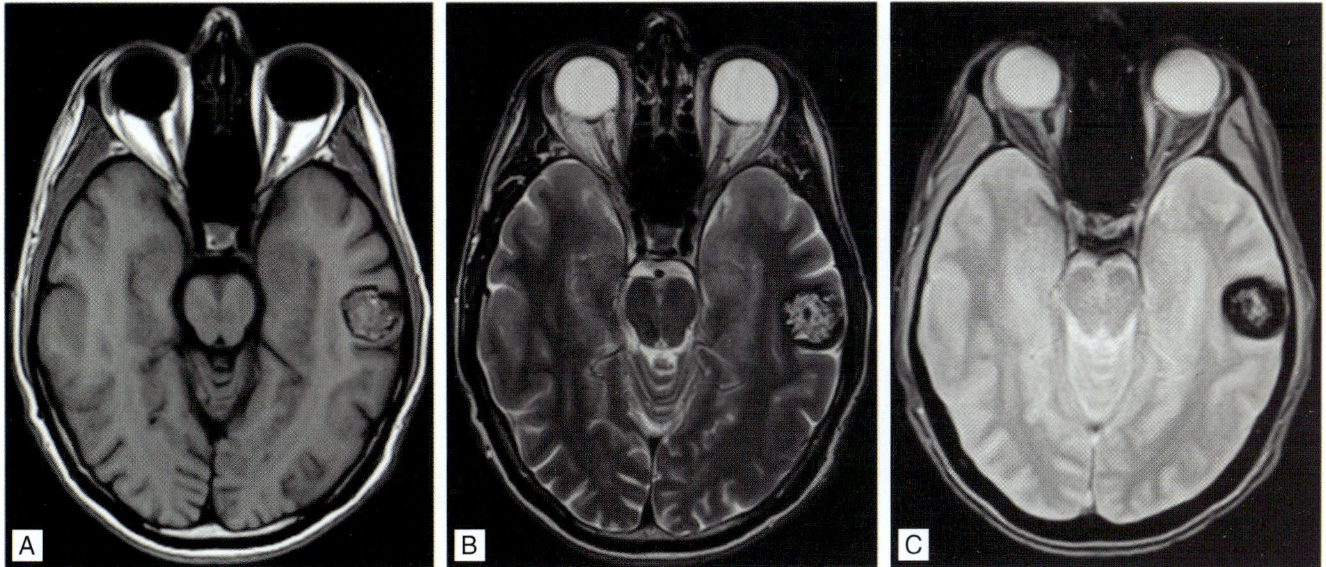

Figure 75.40 Cavernous malformation. T1-weighted (A) and T2-weighted MR (B) images show a round left lateral temporal cavernous malformation with typical heterogenous, "popcorn-like" areas of high and low internal signal and a low signal rim. A sequence sensitive to the magnetic effects of blood products shows even more pronounced low signal related to the malformation (C). There is no surrounding edema to indicate recent hemorrhage.

visible within or in the vicinity of the lesion. Rarely, underlying cavernomas may present only as an intracerebral, cerebellar or brainstem hematoma and may not be visualized on imaging. Cavernomas are characteristically invisible on DSA [8] (Fig. 75.40).

Capillary telangiectasia is a benign, asymptomatic, and small (few millimeters to 2 cm) intraparenchymal vascular lesion composed of dilated endothelium-lined capillary type vessels. Brain capillary telangiectasias most frequently occur in the pons but may also be encountered in the medulla, basal ganglia, and cerebral hemispheres. They are usually solitary but can be multiple in *hereditary hemorrhagic telangiectasia (Osler–Weber–Rendu syndrome), ataxia–telangiectasia, and Sturge–Weber syndrome* [3,8]. Capillary telangiectasias, usually hypointense or isointense on T1-weighted MR and slightly hyperintense on T2-weighted MR, can appear variable but typically show faint feathery or cloud-like enhancement in otherwise normal appearing brain parenchyma without mass effect [72]. Capillary telangiectasias also show susceptibility-related signal loss on T2* GRE and SWI due to higher levels of deoxyhemoglobin in the blood of their dilated capillary bed (Fig. 75.41) [8,69].

Developmental Venous Anomalies

Developmental venous anomalies or venous angiomas are simply aberrant venous drainage and are not pathological entities. On MRI, they appear as a curvilinear structure representing a large intraparenchymal draining vein onto which numerous smaller veins converge. They are often incidental findings but may be associated with cavernomas, parenchymal hemorrhage, or focal gliosis (Fig. 75.42).

See Table 75.8 for comparisons of vascular malformations [3,8,69].

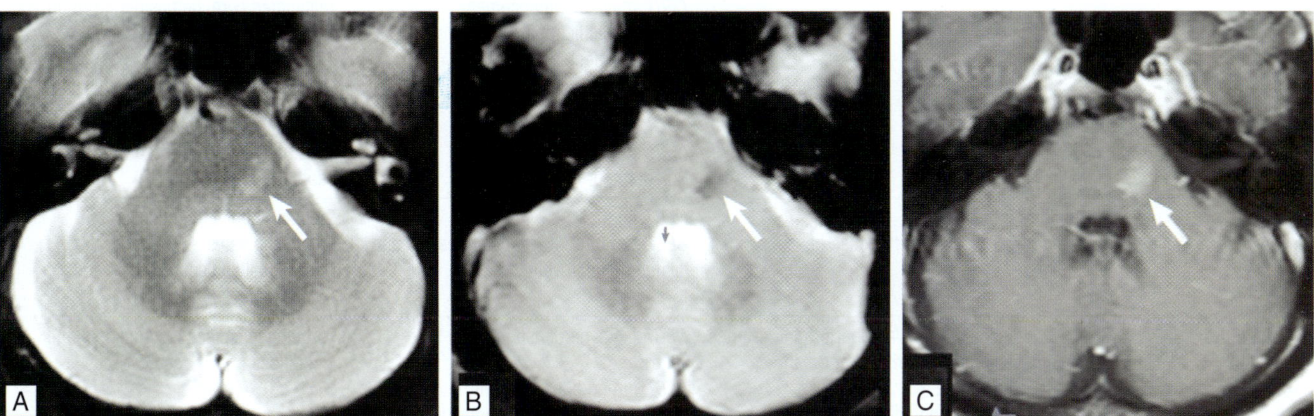

Figure 75.41 Pontine capillary telangiectasia (*white arrow*). Characteristic feathery or cloud-like hyperintensity on T2 (A), signal dropout on T2* GRE (B) and enhancement on T1 (C) MRI. Note the absence of mass effect in this incidentally identified lesion.

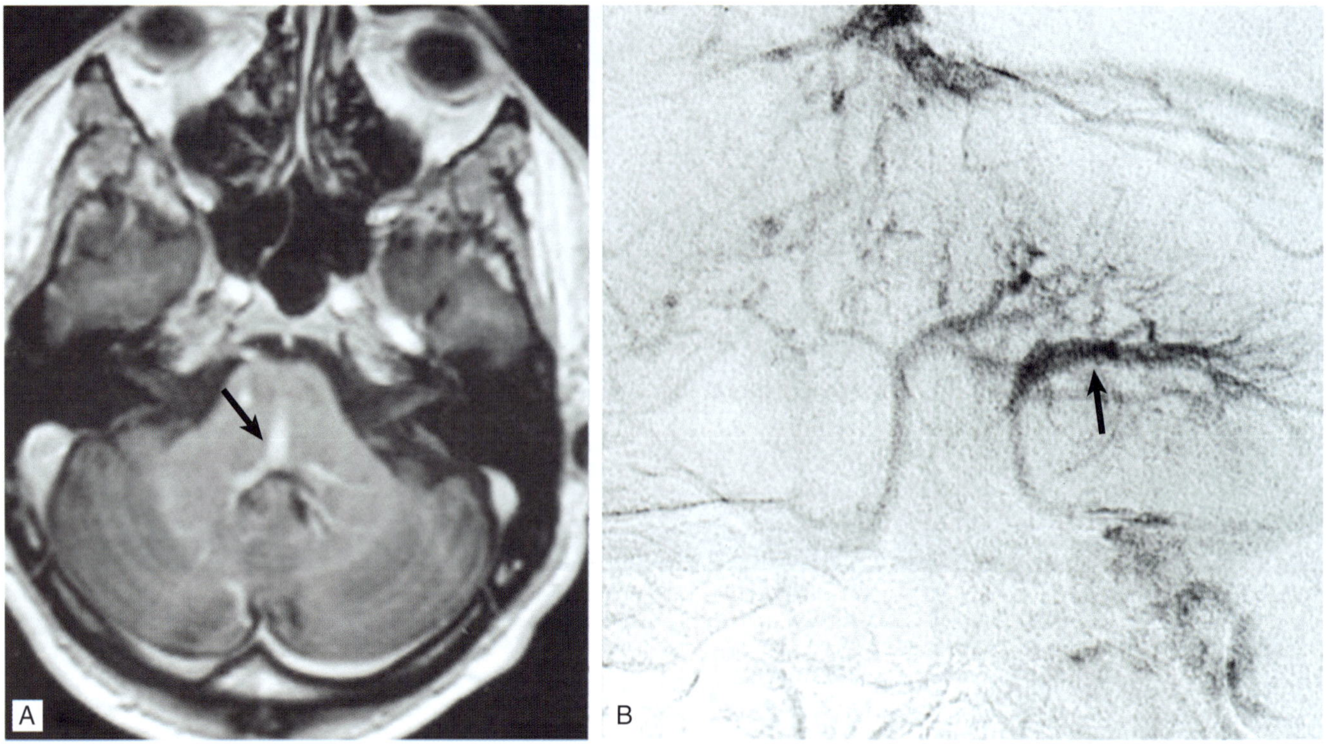

A

B

Figure 75.42 Axial MR (A) shows transpontine developmental venous anomaly (*arrow*). Digital subtraction angiogram venous phase (B) shows anomalous venous anatomy (*arrow*).

TABLE 75.8 Comparison of Intracranial Vascular Malformations

Malformation	DSA	CT	MRI
AVM, intracerebral, patent vessels	Enlarged vessels with arteriovenous shunting and early drainage Minimal mass effect	*NECT*: iso/hyperdense *CECT*: serpiginous enhancement Possible edema, mass effect, calcification	Flow voids, gliosis (T2 hyperintense), hemorrhage MRA: vessel nidus
AVM, thrombosed	Generally normal Mass effect, slow flow, and subtle shunting	Calcification and variable enhancement	Mixed signal
Dural AVF	Enlarged dural arteries with shunting Dural sinus stenosis or thrombosis	Generally normal Enlarged intradural veins	Generally normal Enlarged intradural veins MRA: enlarged dural arteries shunting into a venous sinus
CCM	Generally normal	*NECT*: iso/hyperdense *CECT*: minimal enhancement Variable calcification No mass effect	"Popcorn"-like, mixed signal with reticulated core, hemosiderin rim on T2 T2*GRE/SWI: blooming Often multiple lesions
Capillary telangiectasia	Often normal	*NECT*: normal *CECT*: focal enhancement No edema or mass effect	Iso to hyperintense on T2 and hypointense on T2*GRE or SWI Feathery enhancement
DVA	Normal arterial phase Enlarged medullary veins ("Medusa head")	*NECT:* normal *CECT*: tuft of periventricular vessels and dilated draining vein	Stellate, tubular, and convergent enhancing veins Occasionally adjacent gliosis and hemorrhage
Vein of Galen malformation	Enlarged choroidal and thalamoperforating arteries Aneurysmal enlargement of vein of Galen Accessory sinus seen Straight sinus atresia and altered flow	*NECT*: iso/hyperdense mass in third ventricle *CECT*: strong enhancement Often obstructive hydrocephalus and encephalomalacia	Turbulence causes mixed signal and signal loss

AVF, arteriovenous fistula; *AVM*, arteriovenous malformation; *CCM*, cerebral cavernous malformation; *DVA*, developmental venous anomaly.

CNS Infections

Abscess and Cerebritis

Abscess may be pyogenic, tuberculous, fungal, or parasitic. *Pyogenic abscesses* are collections of granulocytic exudate and are most frequently encountered in adults under 40 and children between 4 and 7. The male-to-female ratio is greater than 2:1 [40,73,74]. Common presentations include headache, altered mental status, and focal neurologic deficits that precede headaches by days to weeks. Abscess may occur secondary to local spread from paranasal sinus or mastoid infection; abscess can also occur secondary to hematogenous spread from endocarditis, suppurative chest diseases such as bronchiectasis and lung abscesses, or intra-abdominal sepsis. Intravenous drug use and immunocompromised status are also major predisposing factors in the development of brain abscesses [6,40].

Cerebritis precedes abscess formation whereby microbes cause localized inflammation leading to vasogenic edema, vascular congestion, petechial hemorrhage, and inflammatory exudate. Cerebritis and abscesses may occur anywhere in the brain [75]. Temporal lobe and cerebellar involvement can result as complications of suppurative otitis media and mastoiditis. Subdural and epidural abscess can also occur from skull osteomyelitis and septic thrombophlebitis of draining emissary veins (which lack valves) in paranasal infections. Post-traumatic or postsurgical dural tears involving the skull base can also lead to subdural empyemas and brain abscesses (Fig. 75.43). CT may provide more direct evidence by showing bone defects or opaque sinuses and air cells. In children, congenital malformations such as meningomyeloceles, encephaloceles, ectodermal defects, and right to left cardiac shunt diseases can predispose to intracranial abscess formation [40].

On imaging, *cerebritis is poorly localized and shows mass effect due to vasogenic edema and variable nodular to ring-like contrast enhancement. As the cerebritis progresses, an abscess develops once there is a central, liquefied necrotic zone surrounded by a collagen capsule and gliosis.* The capsule, which matures in about 2 weeks, is often less well formed on the side closer to the ventricle and tends to be thinner and more uniform than the capsule of a cystic/necrotic tumor [40]. Abscesses can be unilocular or multilocular. Those resulting from hematogenous spread tend to occur at gray–white matter junction, usually in the frontal or parietal lobes. Complications include ***satellite abscess*** formation, ***ventriculitis, choroid plexitis,*** and purulent ***leptomeningitis*** [27,76]. *Ventriculitis* or extension of inflammation to the ventricles is a poor prognostic sign.

CT shows focal hypodensity in most cases, and CECT demonstrates the abscess capsule as a thin-walled regular ring of enhancement [40,77]. Occasionally the lesion is multilocular. The capsule may sometimes be seen as a ring of increased density before enhancement, but this is not a universal feature of abscesses. Vasogenic edema may be the most prominent feature, and edema and mass effect in proximity to opacified paranasal sinuses or mastoid air cells should prompt careful evaluation of the intervening bone and further imaging with MRI. Gas may be present adjacent to or within an abscess and usually indicates that the cavity has been surgically accessed. In rare cases, gas is present preoperatively, where it may indicate the presence of either gas-forming organisms or, more commonly, a fistulous connection with the scalp or paranasal sinuses [40,75].

MRI better demonstrates abscess than CT, with notable T2/FLAIR hyperintense and T1 hypointense lesions. Appearance varies by stage. The central zone of liquefying necrosis in a mature abscess is slightly hyperintense to CSF on T1-weighted images and isointense

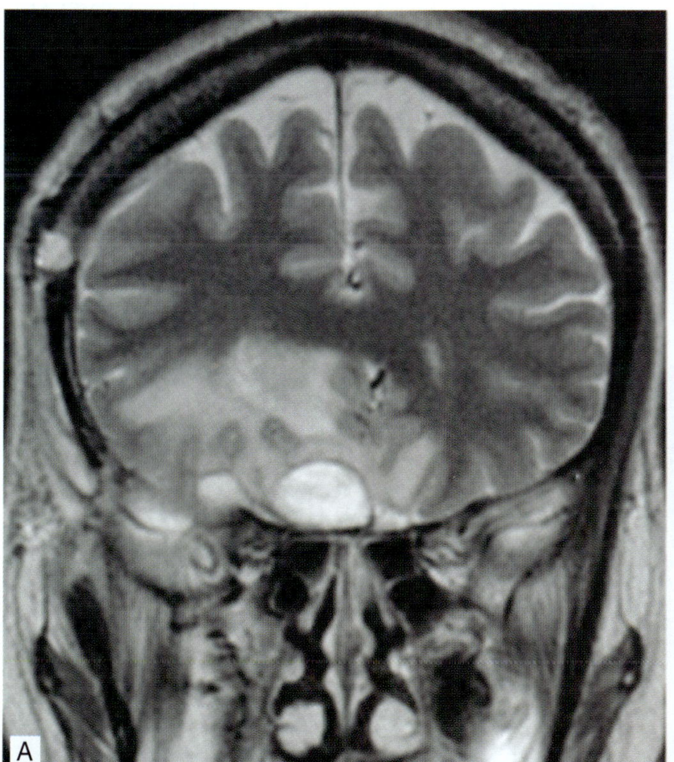

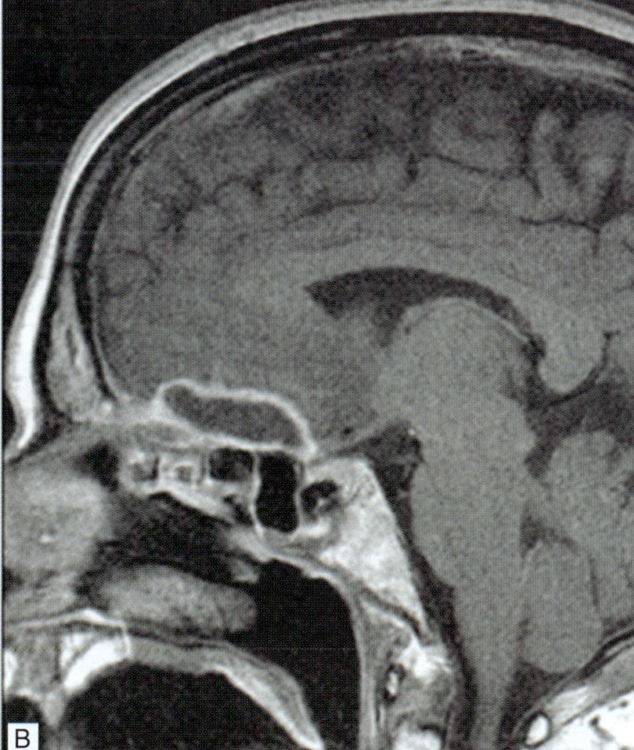

Figure 75.43 Orbitofrontal subdural empyema complicating fracture of the right ethmoid roof. Loculated subfrontal extra-axial hyperintense fluid collection on coronal T2 MR (A) along with reactive vasogenic edema in the adjacent brain. The collection shows typical peripheral enhancement on sagittal T1 MR (B).

to CSF on T2-weighted images with hyperintense surrounding vasogenic edema on T2 MRI. On unenhanced images, collagenous capsules are commonly T1-iso/hyperintense and T2-hypointense to parenchyma, likely attributable to paramagnetic-free radicals [40,75]. As with CT, the abscess capsule enhances intensely on MRI; therefore, intravenous contrast is important in recognizing whether the abscess cavity is unilocular or multilocular, which has surgical implications [74]. Even after successful abscess drainage, enhancement of the capsule may persist for weeks to months.

Although the sensitivity of MRI is greater than CT in detecting an abscess, the radiological differential of a ring-enhancing lesion includes glioma, metastasis, lymphoma, septic and aseptic infarcts, subacute hematoma, thrombosed aneurysm, and MS plaques (refer to Table 75.5 ***MAGIC DR***).

DWI can assist in differentiating an abscess from a liquefied/cystic tumor. Pyogenic abscesses demonstrate restricted diffusion, leading to bright signal on DWI with a low ADC; this is presumably due to viscosity of the cavity contents (Fig. 75.44). Conversely, necrotic tumors typically have *increased free water diffusion* with increased ADC [79,80].

Magnetic resonance spectroscopy of abscess may portray decreased NAA and choline/creatine ratio with elevated lactate, amino acids, and lipids. Comparatively, tumors show elevated choline/creatine (see Table 75.9).

Ventriculitis is an uncommon but serious complication of brain abscess located near the ependymal surface. It may follow spontaneous or iatrogenic abscess rupture into the ventricles and may sometimes result from leptomeningitis or shunt infection. It is characterized on CT or MRI by linear contrast enhancement outlining the ventricular wall. Ventriculomegaly, septation, adhesions, and trapping of the ventricles may also be seen. Other associated features may include transependymal CSF transudation manifesting as increased periventricular T2 signal and abnormally swollen choroid plexi indicative of a choroid plexitis. In chronic ventriculitis, parenchymal periventricular calcification may be present, particularly seen in neonatal ventriculitis and classically seen in **TORCH** infections (***Toxoplasma*, other, rubella, cytomegalovirus, HIV, HSV**) [27,77].

Meningitis

Meningitis can occur in several extra-axial locations: leptomeningitis of pia and arachnoid or pachymeningitis of the dura. A potential complication of meningitis is ventriculitis of the ependyma and CSF in the subarachnoid space. Leptomeningitis is often associated with parenchymal inflammation known as *meningoencephalitis* [78]. Clinical presentation includes fever, altered mental status, nuchal rigidity, and *Kernig/Brudzinsky* signs. As with cerebral abscesses, meningitis can be classified as acute (pyogenic or bacterial vs viral or aseptic) or chronic (pyogenic fungal or parasitic) [81,82]. Imaging is usually not indicated except for detecting complications such as hydrocephalus, venous thrombosis, or infarction. Acute meningitis is usually occult on CT and MR imaging; however, contrast-enhanced T2/FLAIR can often show leptomeningeal or sulcal hyperintensity reflecting leptomeningeal inflammation [27,28,77] (Fig. 75.45).

TABLE 75.9 Summary of MRS Characteristics of CNS Infections [27]

Decreased Neuron Metabolites	Increased Inflammation
■ *N*-acetyl-aspartate (2.0 ppm)	■ Lactate (1.3 ppm)
■ Creatine (3.0 ppm)	■ Lipids (0.9–1.3 ppm)
■ Choline (3.2 ppm	**Elevated and Specific to Infection**
	■ Valine, leucine, isoleucine (0.9 ppm)
	■ Succinate (2.4 ppm)
	■ Acetate (1.9 ppm)

Viral Meningitis

This is usually a self-limiting infection. The most common pathogen is an enterovirus such as echovirus, coxsackievirus (both A and B), and nonparalytic poliovirus. In most cases, CT and MRI are normal, unless associated with viral encephalitis. Sulcal/leptomeningeal enhancement (particularly on enhanced T2/FLAIR) and parenchymal edema may be seen on MRI [27,83].

Pyogenic Meningitis

Causative organisms will vary according to the age of the patient [27,81,82].

- Newborns 0–6 months: group B streptococci, *E. coli*, *Listeria*
- Older children: *Strep. pneumoniae*, *N. meningitidis*, *H. influenzae* type B in unvaccinated
- Young adults: *N. meningitidis* > *Strep. pneumoniae*
- Older adults: *Strep. pneumoniae*, *Listeria*

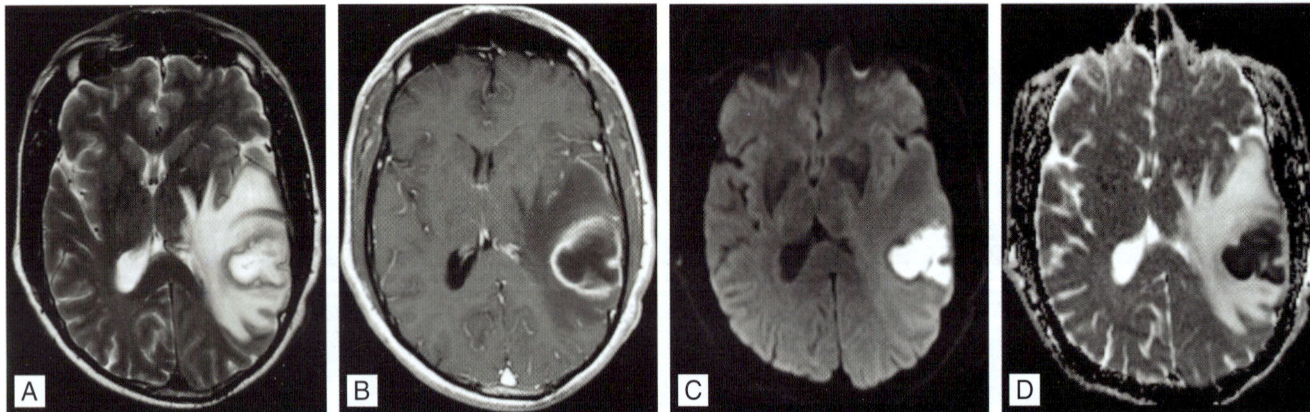

Figure 75.44 Pyogenic cerebral abscess. T2-weighted (A) and postcontrast T1-weighted axial MR (B) images show a left parietotemporal collection with a well-defined enhancing rim and prominent surrounding edema. Diffusion-weighted image (C) and ADC maps (D) show diffusion restriction of the abscess contents.

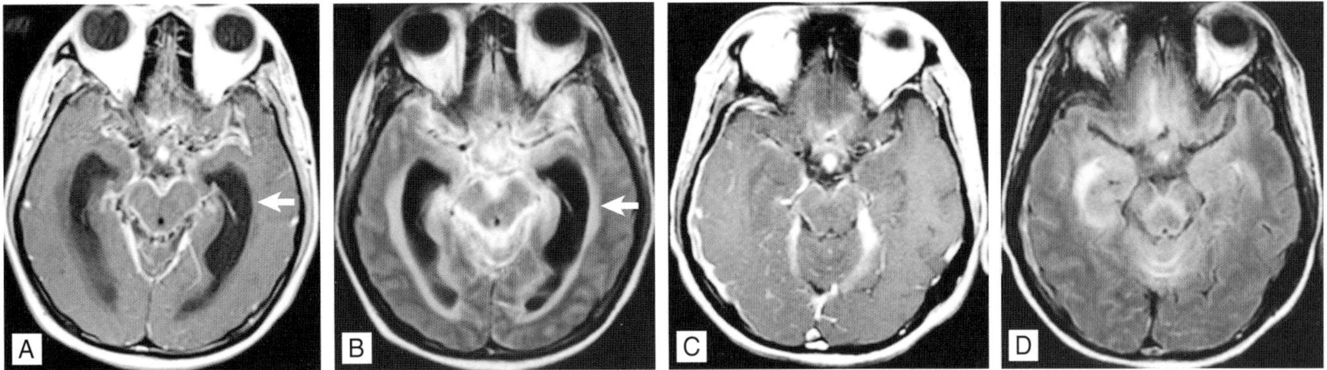

Figure 75.45 Pyogenic meningitis due to pneumococcus. Contrast-enhanced T1W axial MR image (A) shows diffuse leptomeningeal enhancement of the midbrain, medial temporal lobe, and sylvian fissures. Axial T2 FLAIR (B) shows diffuse hyperintensity of CSF in basal cisterns owing to lack of CSF suppression resulting from increased CSF protein and cellularity. Markedly dilated temporal horns with surrounding T2 hyperintensity from transependymal CSF flow are indicative of acute obstructive hydrocephalus (*arrows*, A, B). Significant resolution of the above abnormalities (C and D) after antibiotic therapy and ventriculostomy (not shown) can be seen on the same MR sequences 3 weeks later.

In untreated or partially treated pyogenic meningitis, there may be obliteration of subarachnoid (or basal) cisterns, cerebral sulci, and cerebellar sulci due to inflammatory exudate and edema. Cisternal or leptomeningeal enhancing exudates are appreciated better on contrast-enhanced MRI than CT [40].

Communicating hydrocephalus is the most common complication of meningitis, resulting not only from interrupted CSF flow but also from impaired CSF resorption by arachnoid villi due to inflammation and plugging by cellular and macromolecular debris floating in the CSF. Leptomeningeal–ependymal fibrosis may be a later complication resulting in irreversible communicating-obstructive hydrocephalus. Subdural effusions (infected or sterile) are sometimes seen with acute meningitis. Most common are sterile hygromas, likely secondary to irritation of dura or subdural veins [81,83].

Subdural Abscess (Empyema)

Paranasal sinusitis is the most common cause of subdural empyema [27]. The cerebral convexities and interhemispheric fissure are the most common locations; on CT, these are seen as crescentic or lentiform collections of variable hypodensity with marked enhancement of margins and occasionally the contents (Fig. 75.46). The outer enhancing rim represents hyperemic dura, and the inner enhancing membrane represents inflammatory granulation tissue on the leptomeningeal surface. Hypodensity of the adjacent brain

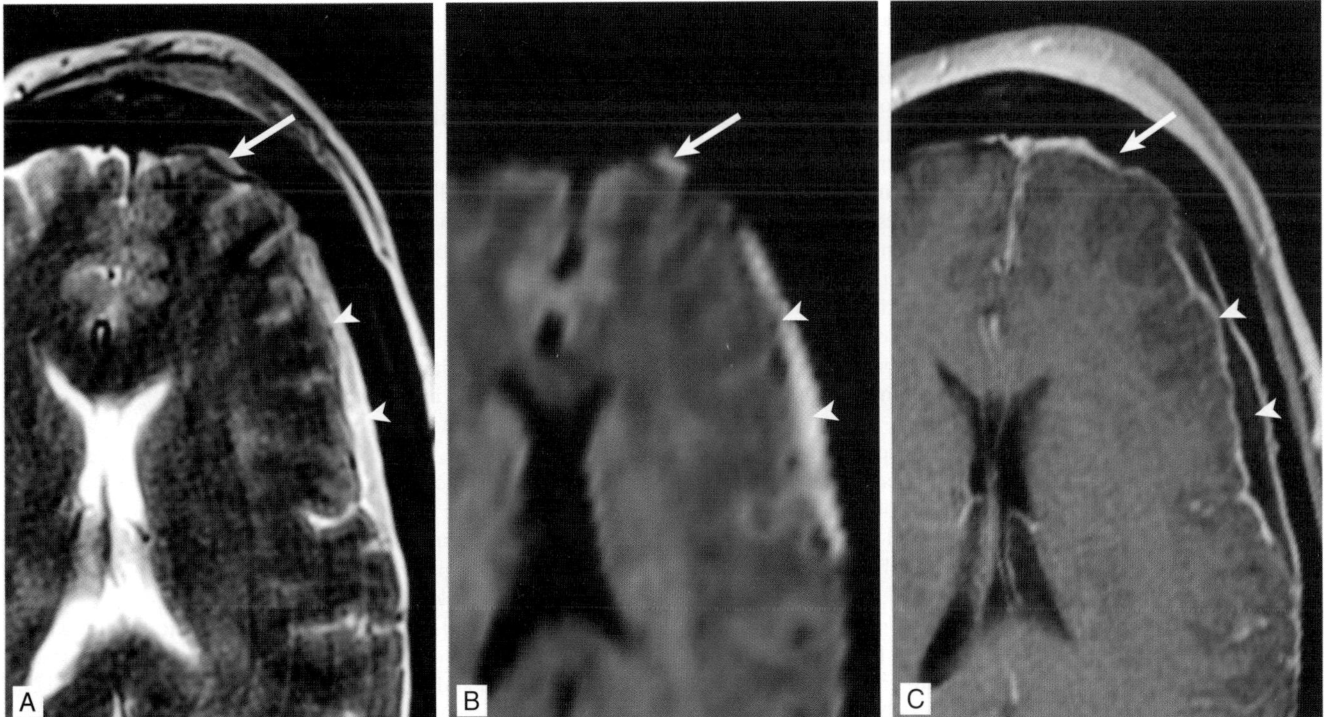

Figure 75.46 Epidural abscess and subdural empyema complicating sinusitis. Axial T2-weighted (A), diffusion-weighted (B), and postcontrast T1-weighted MR (C) images show a small left frontal epidural collection (*arrows* in A, B, C) and a more lateral subdural collection with diffusion restriction and adjacent meningeal enhancement (*arrowheads* in A, B, C). There is also involvement of the left frontal scalp.

may result from reactive vasogenic edema or from secondary thrombophlebitis of the subdural bridging veins, which can lead to venous infarction. MRI may be useful in differentiating sterile from infected subdural collection, as the former is more likely to be isointense to CSF on T1, whereas the latter is often more hyperintense due to proteinaceous contents [40,73]. Similar to brain abscess, DWI is extremely valuable in differentiating infected (empyema) from reactive subdural (hygroma) collections. The enhancing internal and external inflammatory membranes are easily appreciated with MRI. When subdural empyemas are adjacent to the tentorium, coronal sections may be indicated to show whether the lesion is supra- or infratentorial. They are readily detected by coronal MRI, especially T2, where the collection is variably hyperintense with respect to normal brain.

Epidural Abscess

When associated with meningitis, these are usually a result of direct extension from an external source such as skull osteomyelitis, frontal sinusitis and petromastoiditis, but they also occur after surgery or penetrating trauma [6,74]. On CT and MRI, the fluid collection is usually of slightly higher density and signal intensity than CSF, and the involved dura is markedly thickened and enhances. The underlying brain is usually normal as the dura resists intracranial dissemination of infection, but with advanced cases, retrograde thrombophlebitis may occur [27,40].

Tuberculosis

CNS infection with *Mycobacterium tuberculosis* occurs more often in immunocompromised patients, that is, patients with HIV and alcohol or IV drug abuse. Spread is often hematogenous, and intracranial manifestations include *meningitis* (most common manifestation), *cerebritis*, and *tuberculomas* [27].

Tuberculous meningitis primarily affects the basal meninges, resulting in thick proliferative arachnoiditis and meningeal exudate. This may lead to communicating or even obstructive hydrocephalus. Traversing arteries and veins may become involved, resulting in infarctions [84].

On *CT*, the basal cisterns appear obliterated by iso/hyperdense exudates. Thick enhancement of basal leptomeninges extending into ambient, sylvian, pontine, and chiasmatic cisterns can be seen with rare extension over cerebral and cerebellar hemispheres. Hydrocephalus is present in many patients at diagnosis [85].

MRI is more sensitive in detecting the presence of cisternal and leptomeningeal exudates and adjacent parenchymal granulomas. Infarcts due to vasculitis are most frequently seen in the basal ganglia due to involvement of the perforating arteries but may also occur in the cerebral cortex, pons, and cerebellum [86]. The imaging differential of tuberculosis (TB) meningitis includes late pyogenic, carcinomatous and fungal meningitis, and neurosarcoidosis [28,84].

Granulomatous basal meningitis is an uncommon presentation of tubercular meningitis. Diffuse granulomatous involvement of the basal meninges may result in visual disturbances by compression of the optic nerve/chiasm. On CT and MRI, there is dense basal meningeal enhancement with irregularly enhancing nodular masses.

Chronic tuberculous pachymeningitis results from focal or diffuse involvement of the dura, more frequently affecting the cavernous sinus, floor of the middle cranial fossa, cerebral convexities, falx, and tentorium. The dura becomes plaque-like, thickened, and often calcified, appearing hyperdense on CT and iso- to hypointense on T1 and T2 MRI, with marked contrast enhancement [77].

Parenchymal Tuberculosis

Parenchymal TB can be isolated or associated with TB meningitis, with the spectrum including cerebritis, TB granuloma (tuberculoma), abscess, and miliary TB [77].

Intracranial tuberculomas have variable quantity, size, and location (Fig. 75.47). Tuberculomas may be accompanied by meningitis [77]. The intraparenchymal tuberculous nidus begins as focal cerebritis and is hypodense on ***CT*** and hyperintense on T2-weighted ***MRI***; there may not be T1 signal change or enhancement. Then, cerebritis progresses to a focal noncaseating granuloma, which is isodense or mildly hyperdense on ***CT***, surrounded by perilesional low-density edema [3]. CECT shows dense nodular enhancement. On ***MRI***, these solid granulomas are slightly hypo- to isointense on T1 MR and iso- to slightly hyperintense on T2 MR with nodular enhancement [77].

As caseation occurs, the granuloma reverts to isodense or slightly hypodense signal on ***CT***. On ***MRI***, the caseating granuloma remains T1 iso/hypointense but becomes T2 hypointense. The lesion will show ring-enhancement and perilesional edema on both CT and MRI. The radiological differential of such ring-enhancing lesions includes abscess, neurocysticercosis, glioma, metastases, lymphoma, and other granulomatous processes such as sarcoid (Fig. 75.47) [27,77].

In ***miliary tuberculosis***, multiple enhancing small (<5 mm) granulomas are seen scattered throughout the brain, some of which may become calcified in the long term.

TB abscesses are rare. Usually on imaging, a single supratentorial abscess is seen at the gray–white matter interface, which has a hyperdense rim and low-density center on CT. On MRI, the abscess wall is slightly T1-hyperintense and T2-hypointense, whereas central contents are T1 hypointense and T2 hyperintense [3]. There is irregular dense wall enhancement and significant perilesional edema. TB abscesses typically occur in elderly and immunocompromised hosts; these are larger than TB granulomas, show restricted diffusion and may be indistinguishable from pyogenic abscess. However, they are more often multiloculated with thicker peripheral enhancement [6,77].

Fungal Infection

Fungal infection of the CNS is rarely seen in healthy people. In such cases, it usually spreads hematogenously from a primary focus in the lungs; a chest plain film may show evidence of a primary fungal or opportunistic infection. Most fungal infections occur in immunocompromised patients with leukemia, lymphoma, malignancy, HIV, or prolonged use of steroids or immunosuppressive drugs. Due to the intimate relation between immunosuppression, malignancy, and fungal infection, the differential diagnosis must also include tumor [3,27,77].

The most common cerebral fungal infections are candidiasis and cryptococcosis, occurring through hematogenous spread. They can give rise to granulomatous meningitis as well as parenchymal abscesses or granulomas. Mucormycosis and aspergillosis may complicate neutropenia, diabetes, or acute leukemia; these infections often begin with sinusitis or otitis and spread intracranially through the skull base [3,77].

Unique to fungal abscesses, ***MRI*** characteristically shows intracavitary lesions with contrast enhancement and diffusion restriction in the walls and without restriction in the abscess core [77].

Cryptococcosis

This is the *most common CNS fungal infection*, particularly affecting patients with HIV [77]. *Cryptococcus*, a ubiquitous encapsulated

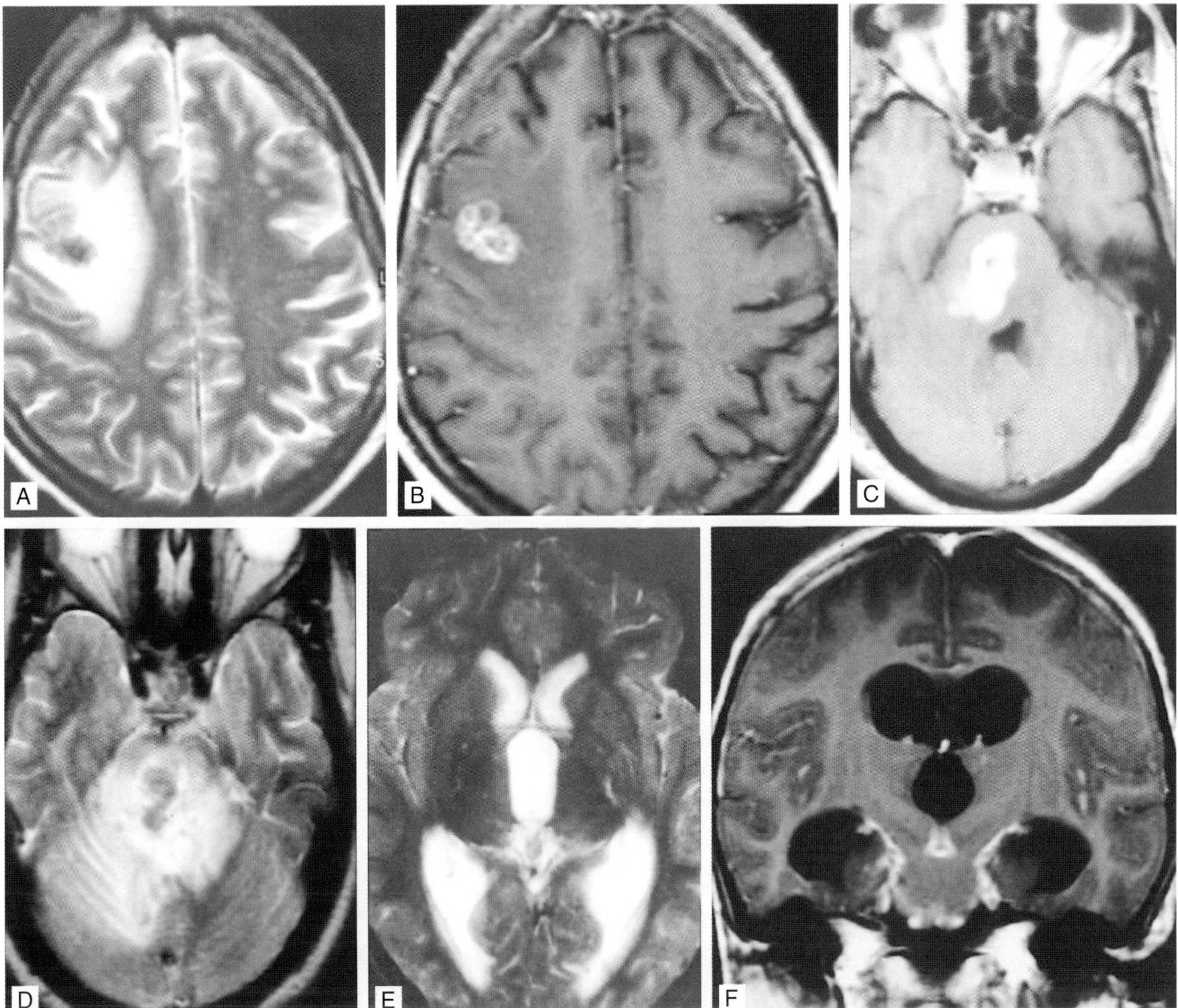

Figure 75.47 Tuberculoma. Axial T2 MRI (A) showing a hypointense caseating tuberculous granuloma in the right frontal lobe in association with vasogenic edema. The lesion is situated at the gray–white matter junction and on the postcontrast T1 axial image (B) has a multiloculated ring-enhancing appearance. Irregular enhancing tuberculoma within the pons on postcontrast axial T1 MRI (C). The lesion is of relatively low signal on the T2 axial image (D) and there shows extensive vasogenic edema and some modest mass effect with distortion of the 4th ventricle. Axial T2-weighted MR (E) demonstrates hydrocephalus. On the coronal T1 postcontrast image (F), there is leptomeningeal thickening and enhancement in the ambient cistern and aqueduct.

yeast found in the soil, enters the body through inhalation. Imaging findings in patients with CNS cryptococcosis are variable and in patients who have meningitis are often negative. *The most common finding is a communicating or obstructive hydrocephalus*, which occurs more often in immunocompetent (25%) than immunocompromised patients (9%); this is likely dependent on adequate immune response. Leptomeningeal enhancement is uncommonly seen (Fig. 75.48). The treatment includes amphotericin, fluconazole, flucytosine, and serial lumbar punctures to reduce intracranial pressure [6].

CT demonstrates low-density nonenhancing lesions in the basal ganglia; on ***MRI***, these are seen as hyperintense on T2 and hypointense on T1, often with a punctate appearance in the early stages and with a tendency to coalescence with progression. Pathologically, these lesions represent dilated perivascular spaces, which become distended with mucoid material from the yeast. Although these cryptococcomas can be associated with slight mass effect, they are not usually associated with edema or enhancement although leptomeningeal enhancement can occur [3]. Miliary cryptococcal granulomas may also occur in immunocompromised patients but occur less commonly than the pattern of basal ganglia cryptococcomas. Immunocompetent patients more commonly present with enhancing cryptococcomas [77].

Candidiasis

The yeast *Candida albicans* is normally present as part of the gastrointestinal flora. It can disseminate through hematogenous spread in immunocompromised patients or those with indwelling catheters or other devices. The most commonly involved organs with disseminated disease are the kidney and the brain, with CNS involvement in up to 50%. CNS candidiasis can give rise to a spectrum of radiological appearances including meningitis,

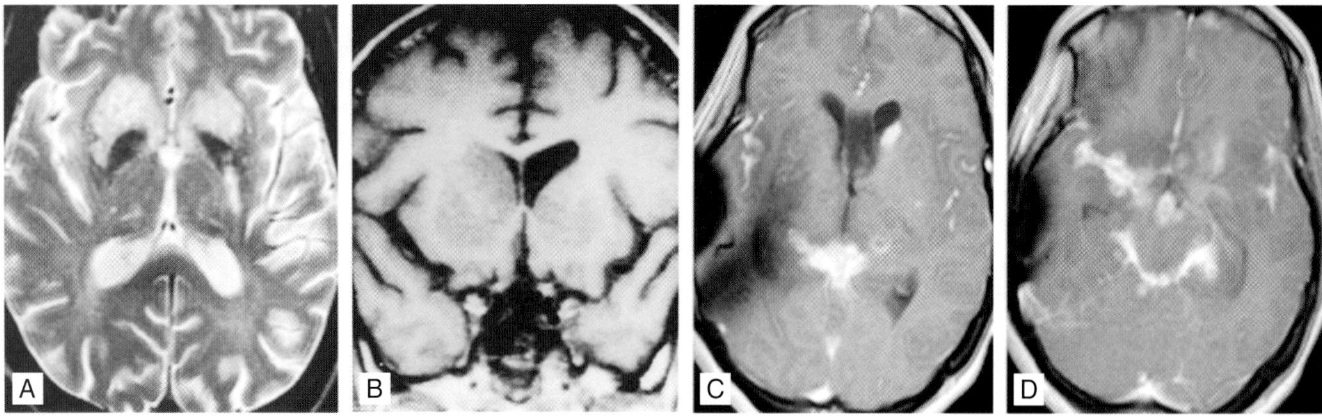

Figure 75.48 Cryptococcosis. Bilateral basal ganglia cryptococcomas, which have a slightly punctuate appearance on the T2 MRI (A). Lesions are slightly T1 hypointense and exert some mass effect on the right frontal horn (B). In a patient with HIV and stable CD4:CD8 ratio, cryptococcal meningitis and hydrocephalus status postshunt placement, T1 MRI postcontrast shows leptomeningeal enhancement of the basal cisterns and caudate lesion (C and D). Artifacts related to a ventricular shunt valve (low signal over the right calvarium) and cavum septum pellucidum are also seen.

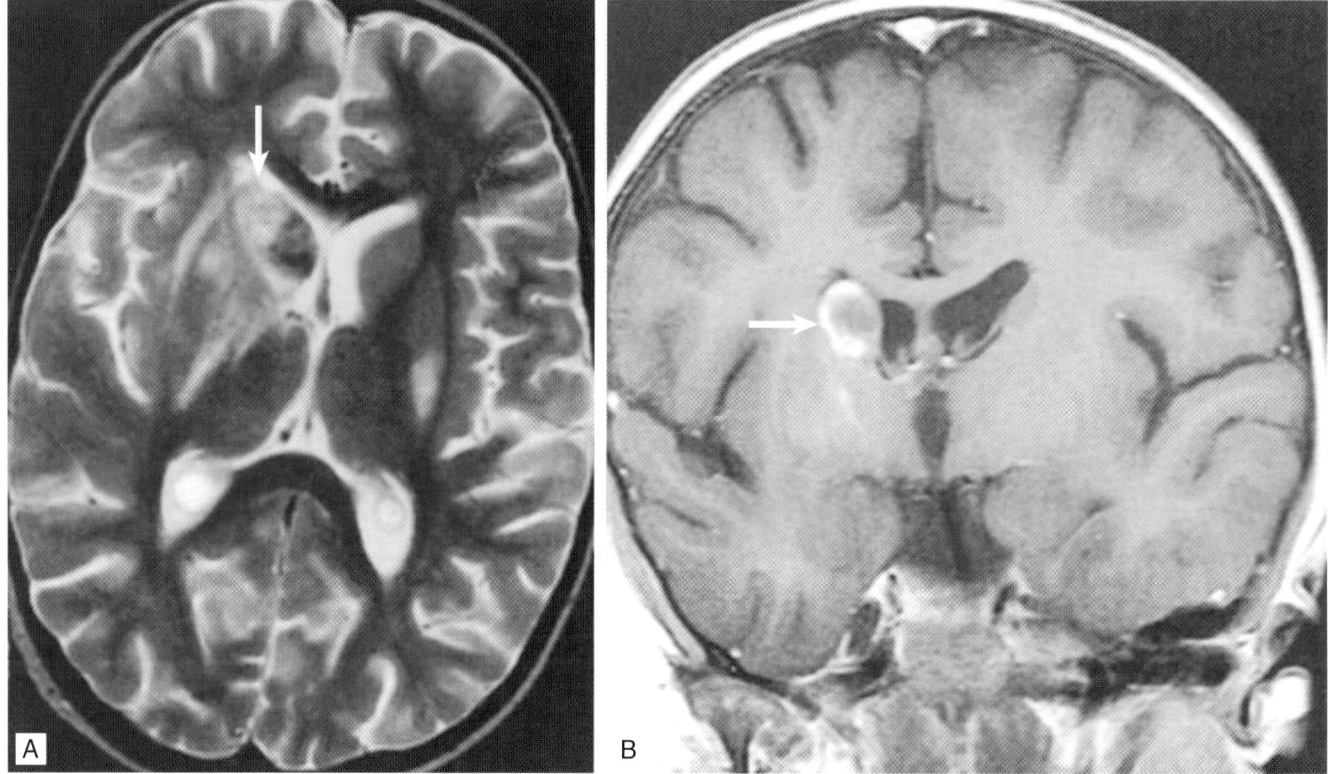

Figure 75.49 *Candida* abscess. Axial T2-weighted (A) and coronal T1-weighted (B) MR images show a small enhancing abscess (*arrow*) near the right frontal horn.

meningoencephalitis, microabscess, abscess and granuloma formation, and ependymitis. Mycotic aneurysms from vascular invasion with endarteritis have also been described. On ***CT***, the microabscesses and granulomas typically show enhancement [3]. On ***MRI***, a target appearance is common on T2 images with a well-delineated hyperintense area surrounded by a hyperintense rim (Fig. 75.49) [77].

Aspergillosis

Aspergillus is a ubiquitous mold that can cause intracranial infection including granuloma formation, encephalitis, abscess, or a vasculitis with resultant infarction (which may be hemorrhagic) [73,77]. Imaging findings include cortical and subcortical lesions that appear hypodense on CT but hyperintense on T2-weighted and FLAIR MR. Basal ganglia and thalamic involvement can occur. Mycotic aneurysms may also occur, and patients may present with subarachnoid hemorrhage. Brain abscesses have nonspecific imaging appearances on MRI, including ring enhancement and edema (Fig. 75.50) [3].

In diabetic and immunocompromised patients (i.e., chemotherapy and bone marrow transplant), invasive aspergillus sinonasal infections can rapidly spread to the brain through the skull base (Fig. 75.51). The fungus can invade the arteries (angioinvasion) and may lead to infarctions (Fig 75.51D) [40].

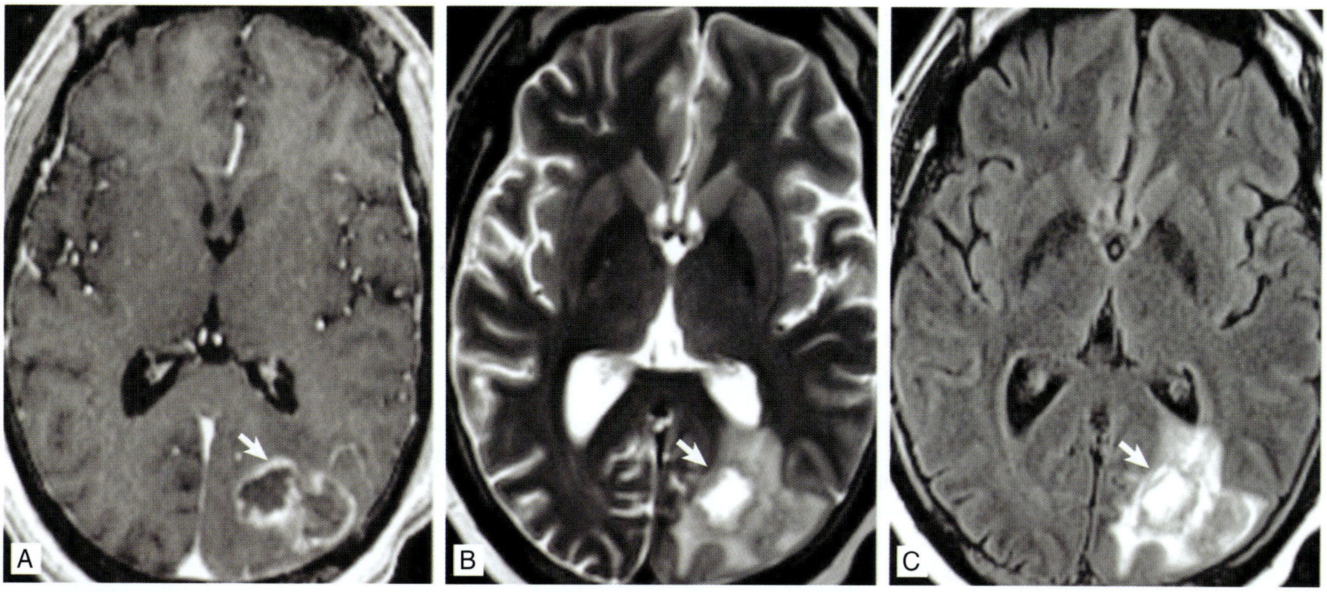

Figure 75.50 Aspergilloma of the left occipital lobe in an immunosuppressed patient with graft versus host disease presenting with right inferior quadrantanopia. Postcontrast T1-weighted (A), T2-weighted (B), and FLAIR (C) images show a ring-enhancing abscess (*arrow*) and surrounding vasogenic edema.

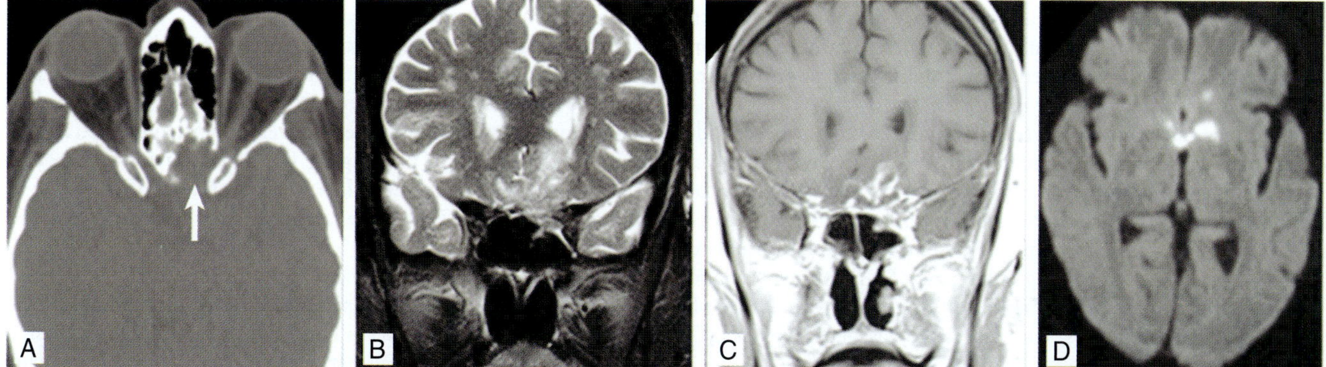

Figure 75.51 Invasive aspergillus infection spreading from the sphenoid sinus into brain through planum sphenoidale. Axial CT (A) shows left sphenoid sinus disease with bone destruction (*arrow*). Coronal T2 (B) and enhanced T1 (C) show invasion of the brain parenchyma. Basal ganglia infarcts are present on axial DWI (D) due to angioinvasion of small perforating branches of the anterior cerebral artery.

Mucormycosis

This group of fungi (including *Mucor*, *Rhizopus*, *Absidia*) is also ubiquitous in nature. Diabetic patients are at an increased risk for rhinocerebral mucormycosis and account for approximately 70% of cases. The diagnosis is aided by tissue biopsy and signs of necrosis. *The molds have a propensity for vasculature; hence, radiological findings include arteritis, ischemia, hemorrhagic infarction, and aneurysms.* Intracranial granulomas are rare. Meningitis is uncommon in the hematogenous form of this infection but more common in direct spread with resulting rhinocerebral or skull base involvement [73,77]. During the COVID-19 pandemic, patients in some parts of the world showed a predisposition to acute invasive mucor sinusitis associated with intracranial involvement [87]. Depending on severity, immediate treatment with amphotericin or posaconazole and surgical debridement are necessary for infection control [6].

CT findings include low-density lesions on NECT, which may show associated edema and hemorrhage, and ring enhancement after contrast. On ***MRI***, brain involvement associated with sinonasal mucormycosis is radiographically similar to that seen with aspergillosis. Signal may be variable when infection is associated with hemorrhage. Angioinvasion can result in both necrosis of the sinonasal mucosa (which will lack normal enhancement) and brain infarction [3,40].

Spirochete Infection

Several spirochete bacterial infections will be discussed, including neuroborreliosis and neurosyphilis.

Lyme Disease (Neuroborreliosis)

Neuroborreliosis is the neurological manifestation of Lyme disease (*Borrelia burgdorferi* infection), which occurs in about 20% of cases and can result in variable clinical presentations. Common neurological presentations include numbness, pain, weakness, cranial nerve palsies (most commonly facial palsy), visual disturbances, and meningitis [6]. Rarer presentations include encephalopathy and polyneuropathy. The definitive diagnosis is by serology or culture.

CT is relatively insensitive; rarely, there may be white matter hypodensities. On ***MRI***, T2 hyperintense lesions in periventricular and subcortical white matter, basal ganglia, and brainstem are seen, likely due to focal granulomas or vasculitis which can mimic demyelination. There may also be contrast enhancement of the meninges in the acute phase on MRI. Delayed imaging may show contrast leakage into CSF, enhancing the basal cisterns. Parenchymal lesions may or may not show enhancement [27]. Cranial nerve enhancement including that of the facial nerve in the internal auditory canal can be readily seen on high-resolution-enhanced T1-weighted MRI [77].

Neurosyphilis

This sexually transmitted disease is caused by spirochete *Treponema pallidum*, which penetrates intact mucous membranes. CNS involvement occurs as a late, usually tertiary stage, but patients with secondary syphilis can also develop meningeal involvement. Immunocompromised patients with HIV and neurosyphilis usually develop neurological symptoms earlier, within 3–18 months. Aseptic syphilitic meningitis, the most common manifestation, occurs within 2 years of infection while chronic encephalitis and tabes dorsalis do not seem to be a feature in patients with HIV [6].

Tertiary syphilis develops after a long latent phase of 6–40 years, with neurosyphilis occurring in approximately 8% of untreated patients.

- In meningovascular syphilis, there is invasion of the intracranial vessels and meninges, resulting in meningeal thickening and arteritis with consequent infarction. Infarction often affects the middle cerebral artery territory or small vessels, with a predilection for the basal ganglia. These infarcted areas on CT and MRI show underlying vasculitis and abnormalities affecting multiple vascular territories
- Gummas can occur in the brain but are rare and arise secondary to a leptomeningeal inflammatory reaction with involvement of local blood vessels; thus, they are usually found near the cerebral convexities adherent to both dura and brain parenchyma [3,6]. On ***CT***, gummas present as well-circumscribed homogeneous areas or ring-enhancing soft-tissue masses, and on ***MRI***, gummas are hyperintense on T1 and hypointense on T2-weighted sequences, with associated vasogenic edema [27]

Parasitic Infections

Various parasitic infections that can involve the brain (producing cysts, granulomas, or abscesses) or meninges are listed below. The incidence of parasitic infections of the nervous system varies greatly based on geographic regions [77] (Table 75.10).

TABLE 75.10 Parasitic Infections

Protozoal	Metazoal
Toxoplasmosis	Cestode/tapeworm
Amoebiasis	Neurocystercercosis, echinococcus, coenurosis
Malaria	Trematode/fluke
Trypanosomiasis	Paragonimiasis, schistosomiasis
Chagas disease	Nematode/roundworm
	Trichinosis, *Loa loa*

Toxoplasmosis

Toxoplasma gondii is an obligate intracellular parasite. The definitive hosts are cats, wherein the entire life cycle can be completed. Other mammals, birds, or reptiles can become infected. Human infection is usually through the fecal oral route. Brain infections can occur in adults, children, and congenital settings associated with immature or compromised immune systems. Toxoplasma infections in immunocompetent humans is mostly subclinical [77].

The congenital type can cause extensive brain damage secondary to necrotizing encephalomyelitis and chorioretinitis; this leads to hydrocephalus, microcephaly, and blindness. The infection runs its course early in fetal development, and there is usually little progression of imaging findings after birth. On ***CT***, there is gross ventricular dilatation dependent on severity of tissue destruction [77]. There is also extensive basal ganglia and subcortical calcification [6].

The adult form is the leading opportunistic infection and major cause of CNS disease in HIV patients in developed countries, particularly when peripheral CD4 counts fall below 200. Toxoplasma encephalitis is subacute in onset, presenting with fever, headache, focal neurological deficits, and altered sensorium [6]. Occasionally, the encephalitis can also present with neuropsychiatric disorders and dementia. Characteristically, multiple, variably sized, enhancing ring lesions on MR are seen in basal ganglia and at the

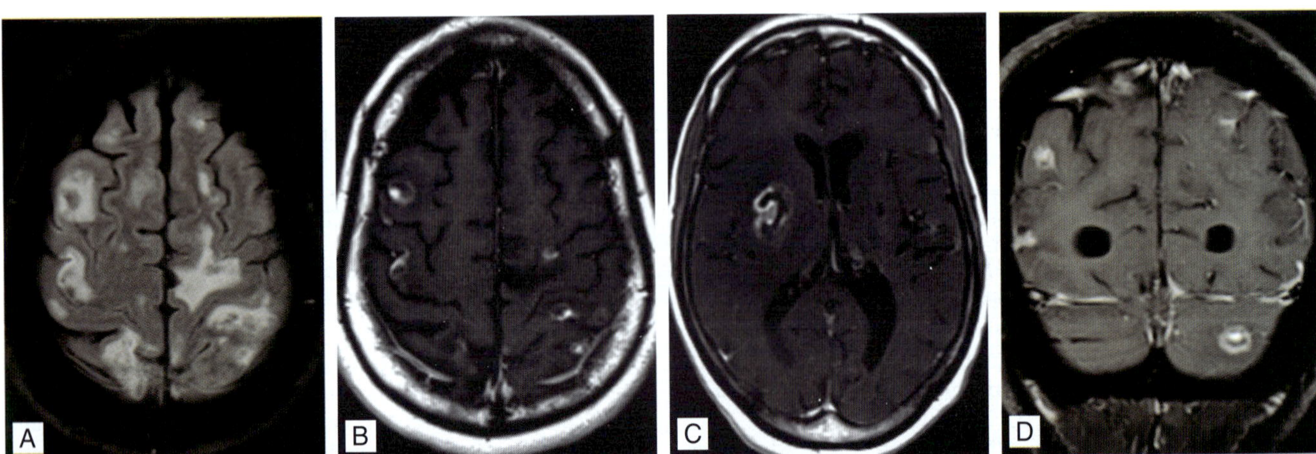

Figure 75.52 Toxoplasmosis in a patient with HIV. Axial fat-saturated FLAIR (A) and postcontrast T1-weighted (B) images show edema surrounding multifocal enhancing lesions. Additional axial and coronal images (C and D) show more examples of supratentorial and infratentorial lesions with characteristic "eccentric target" signs, enhancing rims with eccentric nodules.

gray–white matter junction. The disease can be fatal without prompt detection and antimicrobial treatment. On ***CT***, toxoplasmosis in adults shows multiple foci of slight hypodensity in the thalamus, basal ganglia or subcortical areas and is best identified as ring or nodular enhancing foci postcontrast (although some will not enhance). There is usually mass effect and local vasogenic edema. ***MRI*** is more sensitive and specific than CT and may permit earlier biopsy and/or treatment. The typical appearance is that of multifocal ring-enhancing lesions with surrounding edema (Fig. 75.52). These may show an "***eccentric target***" sign, a nodular focus of enhancement along one aspect of the enhancing ring [77].

Amoebiasis

Amoebic abscess of the brain is rare and is usually a late, fatal hematogenous complication of intestinal, hepatic or pulmonary infection with *Entamoeba histolytica*. There is usually a single abscess in the subcortical or basal ganglia region [3].

Infections of the CNS with other types of amoebae (*Naegleria fowleri*; *Acanthamoeba*) have also been described. ***Naegleria fowleri*** produces a *primary amoebic meningoencephalitis*. Although extremely rare, it is acquired by otherwise healthy individuals from swimming in contaminated water and is most often fatal within a few days, even with immediate amphotericin treatment. ***Acanthamoeba***, in contrast, affects immunocompromised individuals and produces a granulomatous amoebic encephalitis that is also fatal although the course is more prolonged [88].

Malaria

Cerebral malaria occurs only in tertian malaria due to *Plasmodium falciparum* and has a high mortality rate. The main macroscopic abnormalities in the brain are edema, vascular congestion, and petechial hemorrhages [6,27].

Neurocysticercosis

Taenia solium is a tapeworm whose definitive host is humans. Animals, including pigs, are intermediate hosts and harbor the cysts after ingesting eggs excreted in human feces. The eggs release the embryos in the intestine of the animal; they penetrate the intestinal wall and are carried to all organs, including brain and muscles. Here the larvae develop a cystic wall (Fig. 75.53). Eating undercooked meat containing these larval cysts can result in intestinal tapeworm infestation [6].

Humans acquire the disease of cysticercosis as intermediate hosts by ingesting food or water contaminated by eggs found in the feces of a person harboring an intestinal tapeworm. The disease is widespread in South Asia and Latin America, where it accounts for a high proportion of brain involvement. Cysticercosis can affect travelers to endemic regions or through contact with immigrants or visitors carrying intestinal tapeworms [6].

Plain radiographs can reveal "rice-grain or cigar-shaped" calcifications, most commonly seen in intramuscular cysts [3]. Disease of the nervous system most frequently occurs due to inflammatory response to intraparenchymal cysts, eventually leading to gliosis and calcification. Seizures and headaches are the most common clinical presentations in parenchymal neurocysticercosis. The less common extraparenchymal form manifests as mass effect in cisterns or ventricular obstruction by larval cysts. Hydrocephalus may develop from cysts obstructing the ventricles or basal cisterns; these cysts may then form racemose (grapelike) clusters (Fig. 75.54). Therefore, the imaging appearance of neurocysticercosis depends on the number, size, and distribution of the cysts as well as their stage of evolution. Their number can vary from single cysts to hundreds [77].

With live parenchymal cysts (vesicular stage), patients are typically asymptomatic; on CT, they appear as small, round 1–2 cm low-density thin-walled lesions, often with an eccentric hyperdense dot representing the scolex. Cysts with degenerating parasite represent the symptomatic stages (colloidal vesicular or granular-nodular) and result in surrounding edema or gliosis once inflammation sets in; subsequently, cysts develop thicker walls that strongly enhance with ring or nodular contrast enhancement. In the chronic stage (calcified nodular), they may develop punctate calcification [77].

MRI demonstrates the early stages of neurocysticercosis better than CT. Round live intraparenchymal cysts with scolex, degenerating cysts with ring or nodular wall enhancement and perilesional edema are more readily visualized (Fig. 75.53). A "***dot in a hole***" sign may appear as a hypointense scolex within a hyperintense cyst on T2 and constructive interference steady state MRI [38]. Complex extra-parenchymal cysts can form by segmentation of the cysticercus and sprouting of new cysts. With time, there is degeneration of the scolices forming variably sized cyst clusters; this leads to expansion of cisterns (racemose neurocysticercosis) and possible extension into surrounding brain (Fig. 75.54). The cyst wall may be difficult to visualize. Intraventricular cysts may be difficult to recognize because their signal may be similar to that of CSF although slight differences in signal on T2/FLAIR often permit detection. Rarely, leptomeningeal inflammatory reaction can lead to arachnoiditis and cranial nerve palsy and may be seen as contrast enhancement on MRI [77].

Echinococcosis (Hydatid Disease)

This is produced by the larval stage of the dog tapeworm. The eggs are ingested by sheep, who form the usual intermediate host. Humans can become the intermediate host through contact with infected dogs or by ingesting contaminated food [6]. The embryos pass through the portal system to the liver and move onward to the lungs and general circulation. Cerebral hydatid cysts are

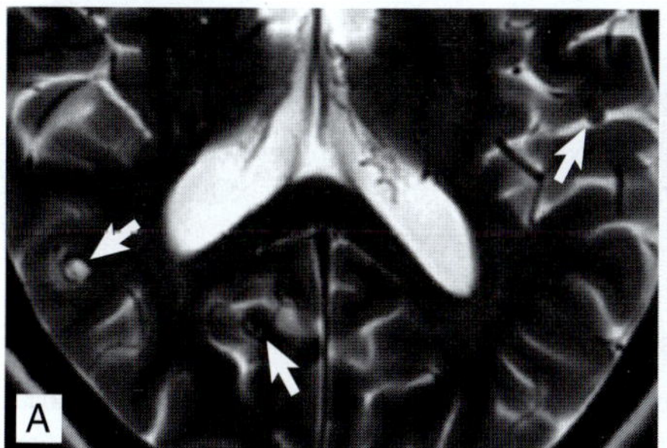

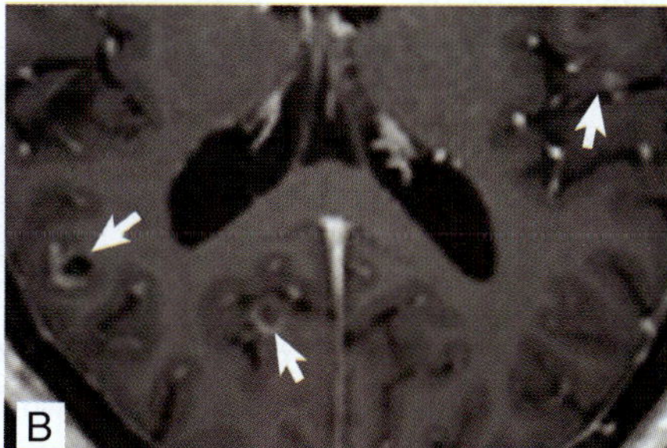

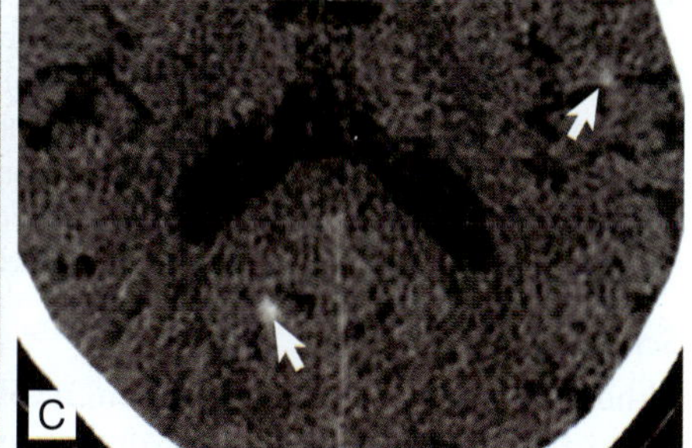

Figure 75.53 Neurocysticercosis. Axial T2-weighted (A) and postcontrast T1-weighted MR (B) images show scattered cystic and nodular enhancing foci (*arrows*), two of which show calcification on CT (C).

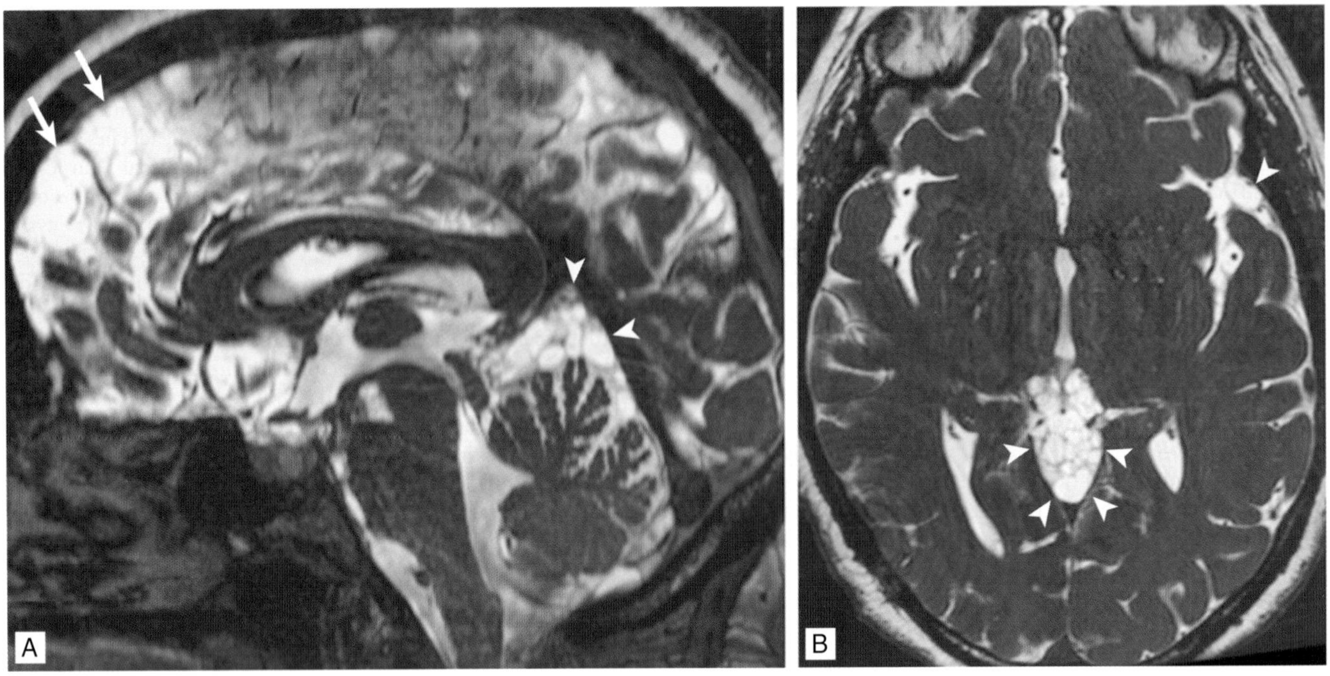

Figure 75.54 Racemose neurocysticercosis. Sagittal (A) and axial (B) heavily T2-weighted high-resolution SPACE MRI show scattered and clustered cysts along the anterior interhemispheric fissure (*arrows*) and in the supracerebellar cistern and left sylvian fissure (*arrowheads*).

usually solitary and unilocular. They commonly lie in the watershed zone of the middle cerebral artery, especially in the parietal lobe, and can reach a large size, often over 6 cm in diameter (Fig. 75.55). ***CT*** reveals a large cystic lesion located subcortically in the brain. Depending on lesion size, there may be mass effect but no enhancement after contrast and no surrounding edema or adjacent calcification [3]. In rare cases, daughter cysts may develop. ***MRI*** can also visualize the cyst well [77,89].

Coenurosis

This is an infection by another dog tapeworm, *Taenia multiceps*, which has occasionally infected humans. The cysts are similar to hydatid cysts but smaller in size [3]. In the brain, they are usually single, but racemose clustered cysts have been described in the ventricles or basal cisterns [77,89].

Paragonimiasis

This infection is caused by the lung fluke, *Paragonimus westermanii*, and may affect other organs, notably the brain. Human infection is caused by eating poorly cooked crustacea infected by the larval stage of the parasite. The disease was endemic in East Asia, although now becoming less frequent [3]. The organism gives rise to a large granuloma, usually in the temporal or parieto-occipital regions, which may later heal with marginal calcification [89].

CT and MRI of the acute stage show a large nonspecific irregular low-density and T1 hypointense and T2 hyperintense area within the affected lobe, with some mass effect. Marginal ring enhancement occurs after intravenous contrast administration, suggesting a multiloculated abscess or tumor. Later, in the chronic stage, the characteristic marginal calcification may be demonstrated [77,89].

Schistosomiasis

Although human infection is common, involvement of the brain is very rarely seen and is always secondary to infection elsewhere in the body. When it occurs, it gives rise to multiple small granulomas, which can involve the brain, spinal cord or meninges [27].

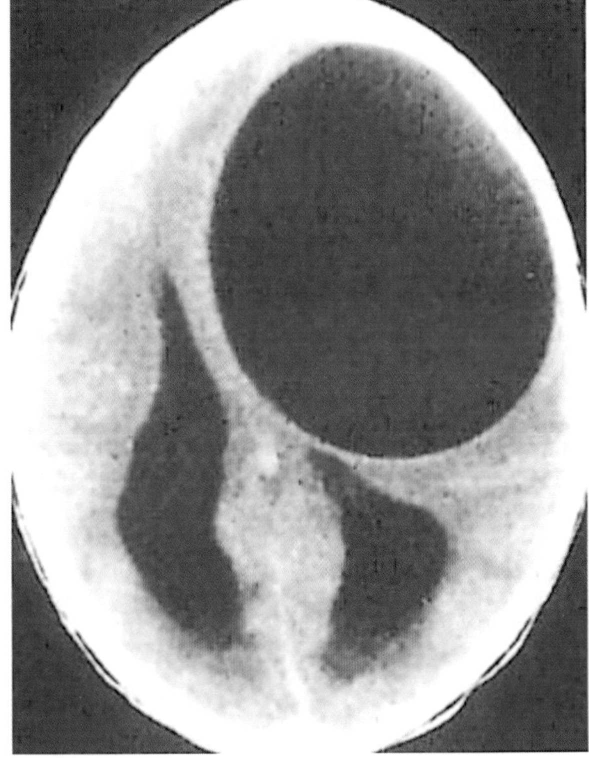

Figure 75.55 Large echinococcal hydatid cyst in the left frontal lobe of CSF density on CT with no capsular enhancement or adjacent edema.

Nematode Infections

These are roundworms that can invade the brain. *Loa loa*, a filarial worm, is prevalent in West Africa and can cause multiple small cerebral granulomas. Similar lesions may occur in trichinosis, which is caused by *Trichinella spiralis* and has a worldwide distribution [89].

Viral Infection

Acute Lymphocytic Meningitis

This is a common response to many different viral infections. The diagnosis is based on clinical findings and CSF laboratory values. Brain imaging is typically not necessary but may be obtained before lumbar puncture when there are focal neurologic findings, papilledema, or seizures and/or to exclude other etiologies or complications. *Parenchymatous viral disease* may be classified as nonspecific or specific [27].

Viral Encephalitis

Specific viral infections cause viral encephalitis and may be due to several types (Table 75.11). The best known of the enteroviruses is poliovirus, responsible for acute anterior poliomyelitis. *Arboviruses spread by mosquitoes are responsible for the St Louis, Eastern and Western equine, Japanese B, and Murray Valley encephalitides. Ticks spread Russian spring–summer and Central European encephalitis* [6].

Changes on both ***CT*** and ***MRI*** can be focal or multifocal and may involve one or both cerebral hemispheres, depending on the severity and type of infection. MRI is more sensitive than CT. CT shows areas of reduced density in the white matter, while MRI shows areas of higher signal on T2-weighted images. Abnormalities may be evanescent and fluctuate over a few days. Among the paramyxoviruses, measles can cause subacute sclerosing panencephalitis as well as postinfectious encephalitis [90].

TABLE 75.11 RNA and DNA Viruses

RNA Viruses	DNA Viruses
Enteroviruses	Herpes simplex viruses (HSV1, HSV2)
Arboviruses (arthropod-borne)	Cytomegalovirus (CMV)
Rabies virus	Herpes zoster (VZV)
Paramyxoviruses	Papovaviruses (JC virus, PML)
Retroviruses (HIV)	Unidentified viruses (encephalitis lethargica; uveomeningoencephalitis)
Coronaviruses (SARS CoV-2)	

Human Immunodeficiency Virus (HIV), Severe Acute Respiratory Syndrome Coronavirus 2 (SARS-CoV-2), John Cunningham (JC) Virus, Progressive Multifocal Leukoencephalopathy (PML)

Subacute Sclerosing Panencephalitis

This occurs in children or young adults several years after a known episode of measles (a paramyxovirus). The precise mechanism of this delayed or prolonged process is still poorly understood but is presumably related to a chronic immune-mediated brain injury. The disease runs a protracted course associated with severe impairment [90].

CT may show low attenuation in the white matter while ***MRI*** demonstrates hyperintensity on T2-weighted images involving the periventricular and subcortical white matter. The changes on MRI tend to begin in the subcortical white matter and progress into periventricular white matter including splenium of the corpus callosum; this can be accompanied by diffuse cerebral atrophy. Leptomeningeal and parenchymal contrast enhancement may also be seen [40,90].

Herpes simplex virus 1 (HSV1) encephalitis typically presents as an acute illness with fever, headache, altered sensorium, and seizures and carries a high mortality unless promptly identified and treated. *The infection predominantly involves the medial temporal lobes, often extending to the orbitofrontal cortex, insula, and cingulate gyrus.* Based on the severity of the infection, hemorrhagic necrosis and considerable mass effect can result. The changes are bilateral but may appear predominantly unilateral in the acute phase; therefore, this may lead to a false diagnosis of tumor at imaging. Suspicion of herpes encephalitis may be confirmed by CSF PCR testing and presumptive antiviral therapy is warranted ahead of confirmation [6].

CT shows low density in the affected temporal lobe(s) and in the adjacent posterior frontal region, usually with mass effect. The changes may be minimal in the first 2–3 days despite severe neurological impairment and should be carefully evaluated. Although hemorrhage rarely shows a gross hematoma, it may give rise to patchy areas of slightly increased density [3,90].

More sensitive to parenchymal changes, ***MRI*** usually shows lesions to be more extensive than seen at CT and identifies lesions at an earlier stage due to high signal on T2/FLAIR and DWI images (Fig. 75.56). Subacute hemorrhage may cause increased signal on T1-weighted images and usually implies extensive necrosis [90]. MRI may also show periventricular signal change not apparent at CT.

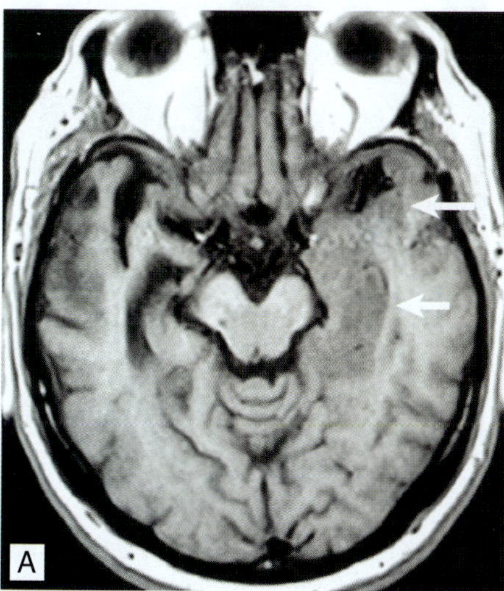

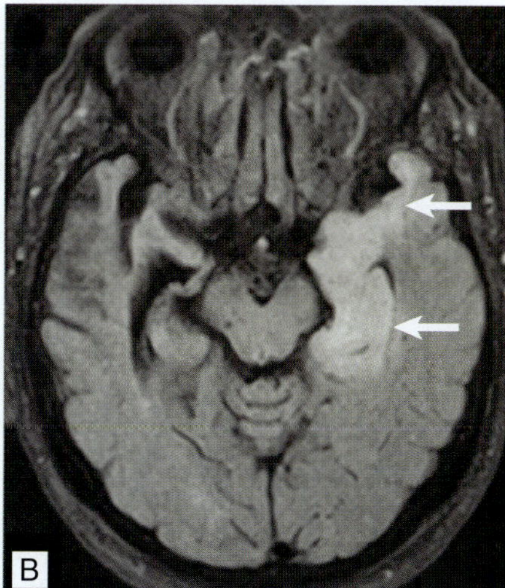

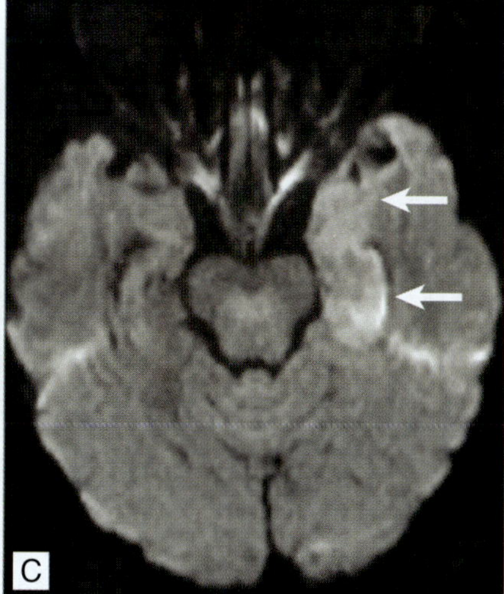

Figure 75.56 Herpes encephalitis on MRI. Axial T1 (A) and FLAIR (B) MR showing parenchymal signal changes and swelling in the left medial temporal lobe (*arrows*). DWI (C) showing corresponding restricted diffusion in a patient with CSF PCR confirmed HSV1 encephalitis.

After contrast injection, variable patchy or gyral enhancement may be seen. In the chronic stage, there may be residual gliosis with associated local atrophy in the affected regions [40].

Herpes Simplex Virus 2 (HSV2)

This may affect neonates and infants, as it is acquired either transplacentally or at birth. Intrauterine infection of the fetal brain may give rise to microcephaly and intracranial calcification (in periventricular regions, white and gray matter). This may be recognized both at simple x-ray and at CT [40,90].

Cytomegalovirus

Cytomegalovirus infection is widespread but does not normally involve the CNS except in patients with compromised immunity, as with HIV, or where immunity is undeveloped, as in the fetus. The fetus is infected from a carrier mother across the placental barrier [40,90].

X-ray of an affected infant may show microcephaly and calcification; these bilateral, symmetric, stippled lesions mainly localize to the subependymal and periventricular regions. Other causes of intracranial calcification in neonates are rubella and toxoplasmosis [3]. ***CT*** and ***MRI*** show dilated ventricles due to atrophy and paraventricular and cortical calcifications [90].

Arboviral Encephalitis

Arboviruses are arthropod-borne infections, often transmitted by mosquitoes. One example is ***Eastern equine encephalitis***, caused by a togavirus. This has a 1-week viral prodrome of fever, headache, nausea, vomiting, and fatigue followed by acute paresthesias, meningismus, and somnolence. On ***MRI***, ***Eastern equine encephalitis*** *is unique for the "****parentheses sign,****" the presence of linear T2/FLAIR hyperintense lesions of the bilateral internal and external capsules.* Typical T2/FLAIR hyperintensities of the thalami, basal ganglia, and upper brainstem reflect edema and ischemia (Fig. 75.57A, B). Leptomeningeal enhancement is uncommon [7].

The differential diagnosis includes ***flavivirus encephalitis*** (i.e., West Nile virus), which has similar clinical presentation and mosquito transmission. Radiographically, T2/FLAIR demonstrates hyperintensities of the bilateral red nuclei, posteromedial thalami, and globi pallidi (Fig. 75.57C) [7,40,90].

Progressive Multifocal Leukoencephalopathy

Progressive multifocal leukoencephalopathy (PML) is due to the John Cunningham virus (a papovavirus) and occurs only in special pathological circumstances (i.e., patients with HIV compromised immunity, leukemia, or those with MS or rheumatoid arthritis (RA) receiving immunosuppressive therapy). The prototypical PML-associated medication is **natalizumab**, which targets infiltrating T-lymphocytes in MS by blocking their interactions with the α4-integrin of the blood–brain barrier. Fingolimod and dimethyl fumarate are also associated. Methotrexate is linked to PML in RA patients. Newer generation MS treatments have lower risk of PML [6].

Multifocal demyelinating lesions occur and spread in the hemispheres, often asymmetrically. PML can cause a variety of progressive symptoms including motor deficits, ataxia, altered mental status, and dementia and carries a poor prognosis, particularly with HIV [90]. The treatment involves restoring immune function when possible, although this can be complicated by an ***immune reconstitution inflammatory syndrome***. Highly active antiretroviral therapy for HIV improves survival, and patients with natalizumab-related disease fare better than other groups.

Although ***CT*** and ***MRI*** both show white matter lesions well, MRI is more sensitive and portrays more widespread brain involvement. There is increased signal on T2-weighted and FLAIR images and less conspicuous reduced signal on T1-weighted images (Fig. 75.58). Rarely, necrosis and mass effect may occur [40,90].

HIV Encephalopathy

CNS infections are a common complication of HIV and manifest clinically as meningitis, focal lesion, or generalized abnormalities. ***Meningitis*** most commonly arises from *Cryptococcus neoformans* but can also arise from mycobacteria or herpes [6,90].

Focal lesions are mainly due to infections giving rise to abscesses and granulomas. Although the most common organism responsible is *Toxoplasma gondii*, other organisms seen are mycobacteria and fungi, that is, cryptococcus, *Aspergillus fumigatus* and

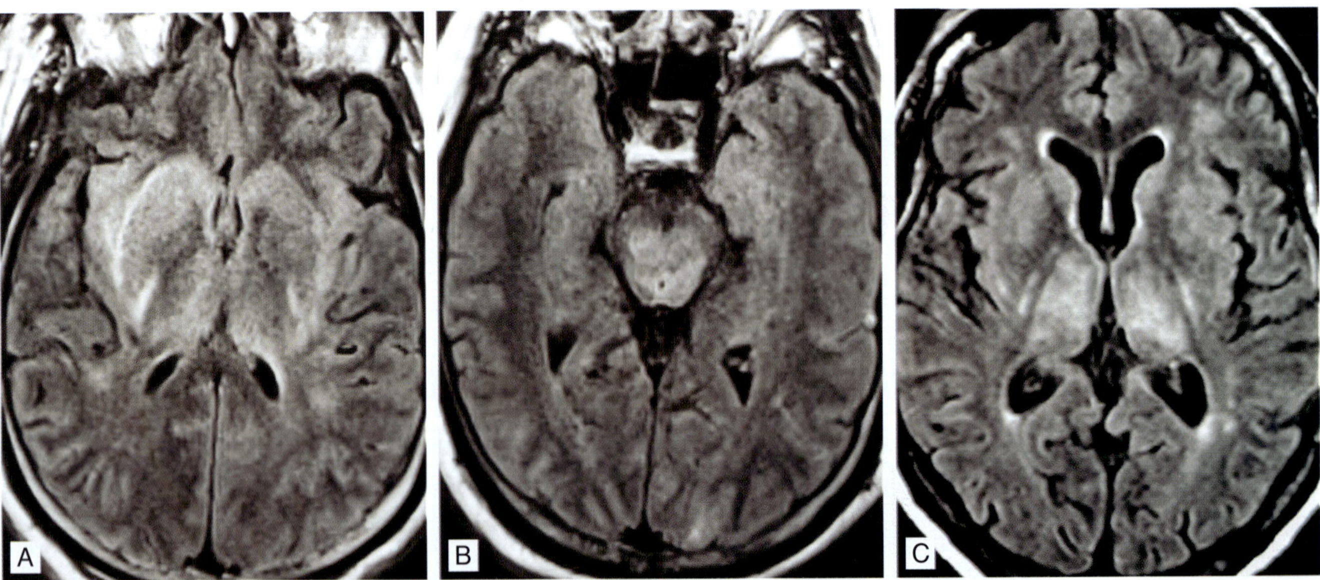

Figure 75.57 Arboviral encephalitis on FLAIR MRI. Eastern equine encephalitis seen as linear hyperintensities of the external and internal capsules ("parentheses sign") (A) and as midbrain lesions (B). West Nile encephalitis with bilateral thalamic and basal ganglia involvement (C).

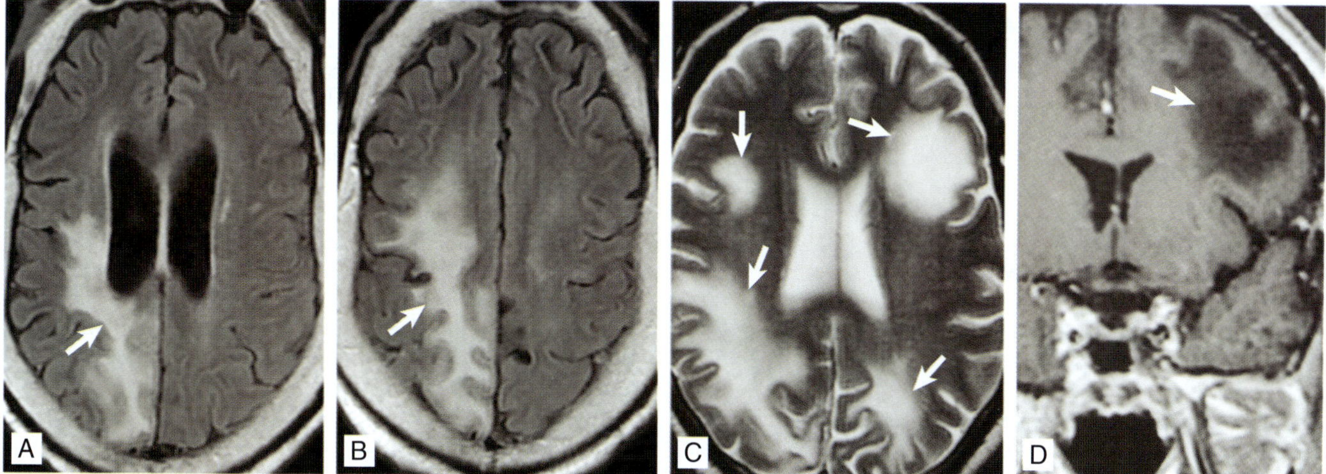

Figure 75.58 PML can extend throughout juxtacortical and periventricular white matter, as seen on posterior FLAIR lesions (A, B, *arrows*) and T2 hyperintense (C, *arrows*) and coronal T1 hypointense (D, *arrows*) lesions without enhancement or mass effect.

Candida albicans. Focal brain lesions can be neoplastic as well as inflammatory. For example, herpes viruses can cause brain tumors: Epstein–Barr virus causes CNS lymphoma and human herpesvirus 8 causes Kaposi's sarcoma of the brain in rare instances [90].

More *generalized changes* are seen with viruses such as cytomegalovirus, herpes simplex, and the John Cunningham papovavirus responsible for PML. HIV itself has been found in patients' brains at autopsy and is considered responsible for direct cytopathic effect leading to encephalopathy, atrophy, and HIV-associated dementia.

CT and ***MRI*** can identify focal lesions such as abscesses due to toxoplasmosis or cryptococcus. The appearances seen in PML and in lymphoma have been described above. In some cases, brain biopsy may be necessary to distinguish between abscess and neoplasm [3]. However, *toxoplasmosis is the most common cause of focal lesions in HIV patients*, and treatment with pyrimethamine and sulfadiazine may be trialed before resorting to brain biopsy [90].

Nonspecific changes such as brain atrophy with cortical atrophy and ventricular dilatation are readily identified by CT or MRI [91]. The latter can also demonstrate nonspecific white matter signal changes on FLAIR MR images in patients who are HIV positive and in a majority of cases with established AIDS (Fig. 75.59). They are thought in most cases to be due to a direct HIV infection [40,91].

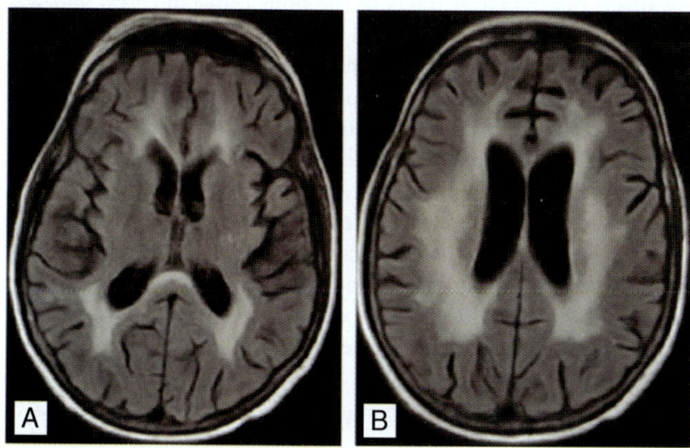

Figure 75.59 Nonspecific periventricular white matter changes in HIV encephalopathy on FLAIR MR (A, B).

Coronavirus Disease 2019 (COVID-19)

Although unsettled, an estimated 10–30% of coronavirus disease 2019 (COVID-19) patients infected with severe acute respiratory syndrome coronavirus 2 present with neurologic deficits including headaches, anosmia, seizures, and strokes. Although the neuropathogenesis of COVID-19 is still being illuminated, these diverse neurological manifestations may result from viral neural tropism, blood barrier dysfunction, hypercoagulability and/or innate immune system hyperactivation (aka cytokine storm) [92,93]. For critically ill patients, treatments such as prednisone, remdesivir, molnupiravir, and/or nirmatrelvir/ritonavir may improve outcomes such as decreased hospital stay duration or increased survival.

On ***CT*** and ***MRI***, patients with COVID-19 and focal deficits or impaired consciousness may be found to have infarcts, hematomas, encephalitis, posterior reversible encephalopathy syndrome (PRES) and toxic leukoencephalopathy. Possible abnormalities of the cranial nerves, including the olfactory bulbs, may be associated with clinical anosmia [92–94].

Demyelinating Diseases

Here, we discuss conditions of differing etiologies which have in common predominant involvement of the white matter. White matter diseases have been classified as *dysmyelinating*, where there is abnormal formation or maintenance of myelin, and *demyelinating*, where there is destruction of normally formed myelin [52,53,95]. Dysmyelinating diseases, including leukodystrophies and metabolic disorders, are discussed in a separate chapter. Here, we focus on demyelinating disorders in Table 75.12.

"Secondary" demyelination includes inflammatory and postinflammatory lesions from neoplastic, vascular, toxic, and other disorders. Some of these have already been discussed (disseminated encephalomyelitis, progressive multifocal encephalopathy, and Reye syndrome) or will be discussed in the section on inflammatory diseases.

Normal white matter is less dense than gray matter on CT, but demyelination accentuates this difference. MRI is more sensitive for white matter changes, which typically manifest as hyperintense areas on T2-weighted and especially FLAIR images. Compared with gray matter, normally myelinated white matter is hypointense on T2/FLAIR and hyperintense on T1-weighted images. This pattern is reversed at birth but established in a well-characterized temporal and spatial pattern as normal myelination proceeds

TABLE 75.12 The Differential Diagnosis for Demyelinating Disorders

Multiple sclerosis (MS)
Neuromyelitis optica (NMO)
Schilder disease
Osmotic demyelination
Marchiafava–Bignami disease
Secondary to other disorders (ADEM, PML, etc.)

during early development. White matter changes in specific pathological conditions are described below, but it should be noted that white matter changes are commonly seen incidentally due to chronic small vessel disease and normal aging [52,53].

Other causes of generalized low attenuation of white matter at CT and altered signal at MRI include *uremic or hepatic encephalopathy* and *hypertensive crises*; *malignant disease* and *muscular dystrophy* are other rare causes. *Vasogenic edema* from diverse causes can also produce focal or more generalized low density as can radiation damage [6,52].

Multiple Sclerosis

This is one of the most common neurological disorders and is characterized by disseminated plaques of demyelination and gliosis throughout the neuraxis [95,96]. Commonly infected sites include:

1. Periventricular and subcortical white matter
2. Optic pathways
3. Brainstem
4. Cerebellar white matter and peduncles
5. Spinal cord.

Although the exact target and pathogenesis remains unknown, MS is an autoimmune disease with increased levels of antibodies to glial antigens (i.e., CSF oligoclonal bands) in affected patients. Primarily, young adults (especially females) are affected, with an increased incidence in the colder wet temperate zones of the northern hemisphere and in those with lower vitamin D levels. Underlying genetic factors likely contribute and there may be inciting infectious agent.

MRI is far more sensitive than CT in revealing MS plaques with accuracy of nearly 100%. Acute lesions coincide with new-onset neurologic deficits, show marked gadolinium contrast enhancement, and demonstrate infiltrating and resident immune cell activity. Chronic, inactive lesions do not enhance [52,53].

Lesions of the corpus callosum radiating outward perpendicularly are classically denoted "*Dawson's fingers.*" The characteristic appearance includes hyperintense lesions on T2-weighted and FLAIR images that may develop central hypointense components ("**black holes**") on T1-weighted images [53,96]. These lesions are most numerous posteriorly while plaques are also prominent in the subcortical and juxtacortical white matter. MRI can image lesions in the spinal cord as well as the brainstem and cerebellum. Multiple cerebral lesions are demonstrated in over half the patients presenting with a single episode of optic neuritis or with clinically isolated brainstem or cord lesions. Figs. 75.60 and 75.61 demonstrate temporal changes in MS.

Classic cases show no mass effect or surrounding edema. Occasionally mass effect and edema are encountered, which can simulate tumor, particularly with a single large lesion. This is called ***tumefactive MS*** (Fig. 75.62) [53,95]. ***Optic neuritis*** is a stand-alone clinical entity associated with eye pain and vision loss [6,19]. It occurs in 20% of patients with MS and responds to steroids (Fig. 75.63).

It should be noted that MRI lesions are nonspecific and must be considered in the clinical context. MRI is so sensitive that it shows similar periventricular lesions in around 25% of elderly patients. These may represent ischemic lesions, which are particularly notable in patients with multiinfarct dementia. Similar lesions have also been noted after radiotherapy and in encephalomyelitis [95].

Despite the classification of MS as a predominantly white matter disease, pathology and MRI studies have increasingly documented cortical and deep gray matter involvement, with both lesions and atrophy contributing to disability and cognitive dysfunction [6,52,96].

Neuromyelitis Optica

The clinical presentation of neuromyelitis optica (NMO) includes optic neuritis with transverse myelitis and additional demyelination. It is often misdiagnosed as MS due to clinical and radiographic overlap. The presence of serum autoantibodies can support NMO diagnosis and distinguish between subtypes. Antibodies react to astrocyte aquaporin-4 channels, myelin oligodendrocyte glycoprotein and node of Ranvier protein, neurofascin. Demyelination can occur throughout the brain, optic nerve and spinal cord (Fig. 75.64) [52,53,95].

Schilder's Disease (Myelinoclastic Diffuse Sclerosis)

This condition, affecting children and young adults, shows histological lesions that are similar to MS plaques but are more extensive. Clinically, the course is continuous and progressive, even fulminant, rather than intermittent and relapsing. Lumbar puncture can differentiate Schilder's disease from MS and autoantibody demyelinating disorders (i.e., NMO) [97]. The main lesions extend through the corpus callosum into both parieto-occipital regions. On ***CT***, bilateral low-attenuation areas are shown in both parieto-occipital regions, which enlarge progressively but not symmetrically. Contrast enhancement is uncommon. ***MRI*** demonstrates white matter lesions better than CT, and their true extent is more clearly reflected [98].

Osmotic Demyelination Syndrome

This condition (formerly "central pontine myelinolysis") primarily affects dense matter tracts of the pons (50% of cases) and was classically described with rapid correction of hyponatremia in chronic alcoholism and malnutrition. However, it may be encountered with other illnesses, including Wernicke encephalopathy, neoplasia, hyperemesis gravidarum, hypokalemia, and liver/kidney disease. Although potentially fatal, recovery can occur with varying degrees of neurological deficit [6,99]. ***CT*** may demonstrate low density in the affected pons, usually only when the disease is well advanced. ***MRI*** is more sensitive and reveals more extensive change. There is T1 and T2 hyperintensity in the pons that can be more widespread, extending into midbrain, thalami and even subcortical white matter [7,99].

Marchiafava–Bignami Disease

This is rare condition also seen with alcoholism and malnutrition in which absence of B complex vitamins is associated with

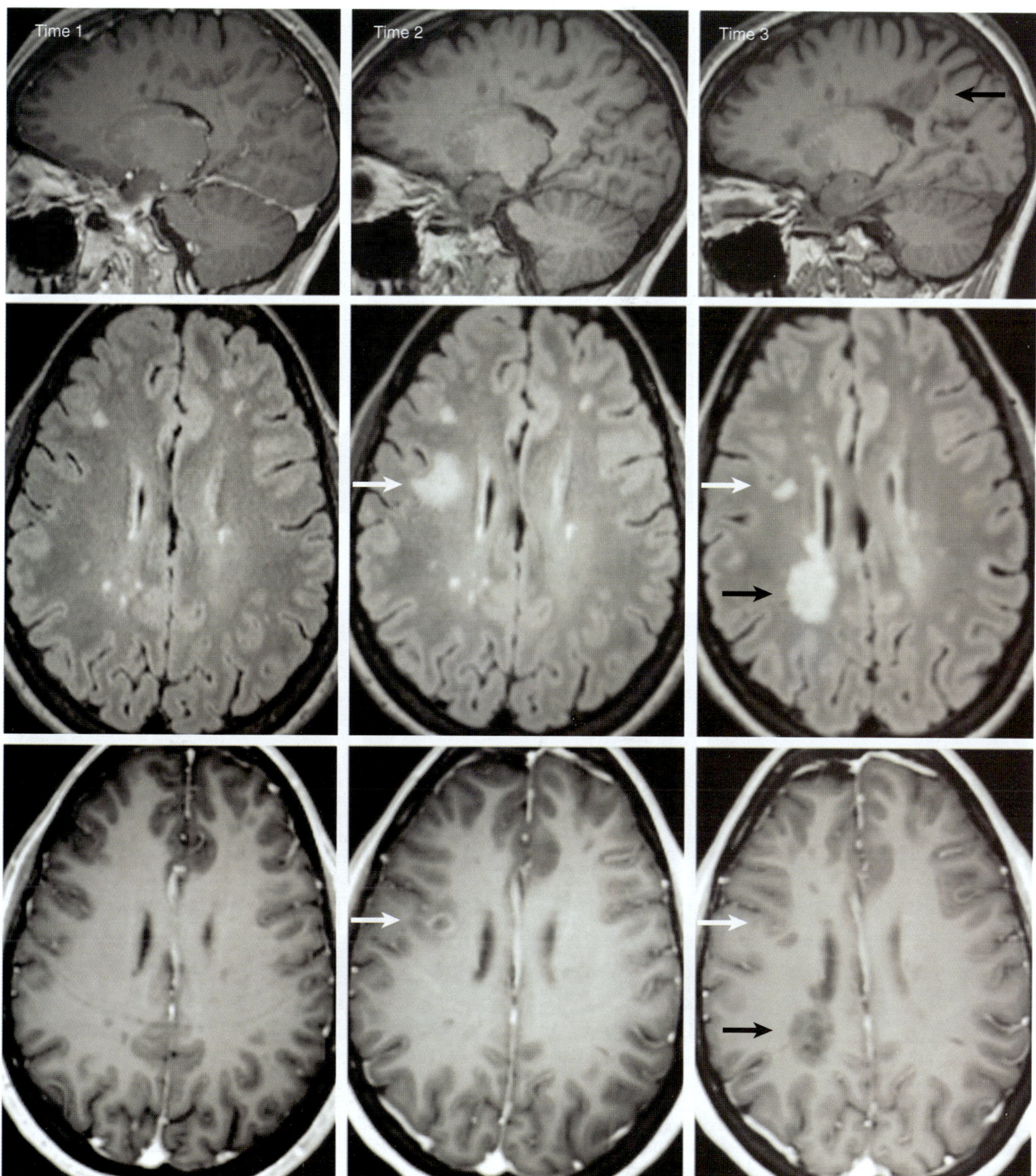

Figure 75.60 Multiple sclerosis. Time 1 is the left column, time 2 is the middle column, time 3 is the right column. The top row depicts pericallosal "Dawson's finger" lesions on T1 images. The middle row shows FLAIR hyperintense lesions. The bottom row shows T1 postcontrast images. At time 2, an active ring-enhancing lesion appears in the right corona radiata (*white arrow*) that becomes inactive by time 3. At time 3, a new but nonenhancing periventricular lesion arises (*black arrow*).

demyelination and necrosis in the corpus callosum. Other central white matter tracts may also be involved. Notably, chronic cyanide intoxication can produce similar lesions [100].

Viral-associated demyelinating disease includes acute disseminated encephalomyelitis (ADEM) and Reye syndrome.

Acute Disseminated Encephalomyelitis (ADEM)

ADEM is also known as *acute disseminated leukoencephalitis* or *postinfectious encephalitis*. The condition may be a complication of many viral diseases within weeks after onset, particularly the

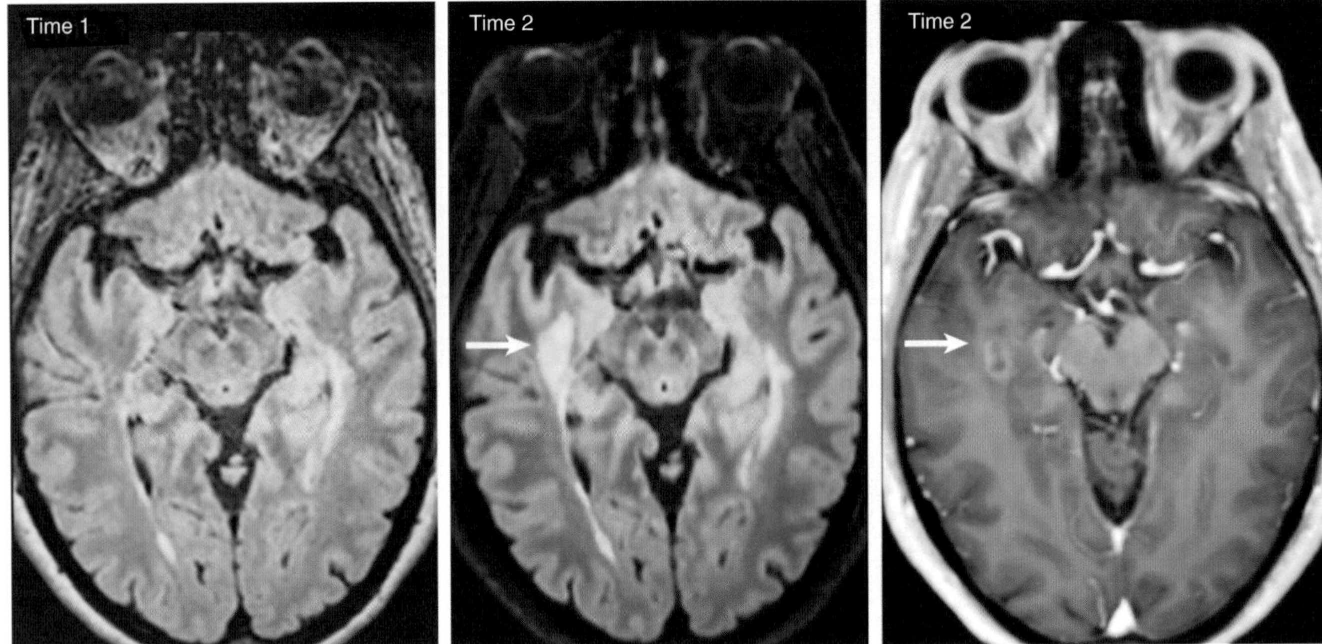

Figure 75.61 Temporal changes in active multiple sclerosis (MS). Between axial FLAIR MR images at time point 1 and time point 2, an active MS lesion (*arrow*) arises and shows corresponding rim enhancement postcontrast T1-weighted MRI.

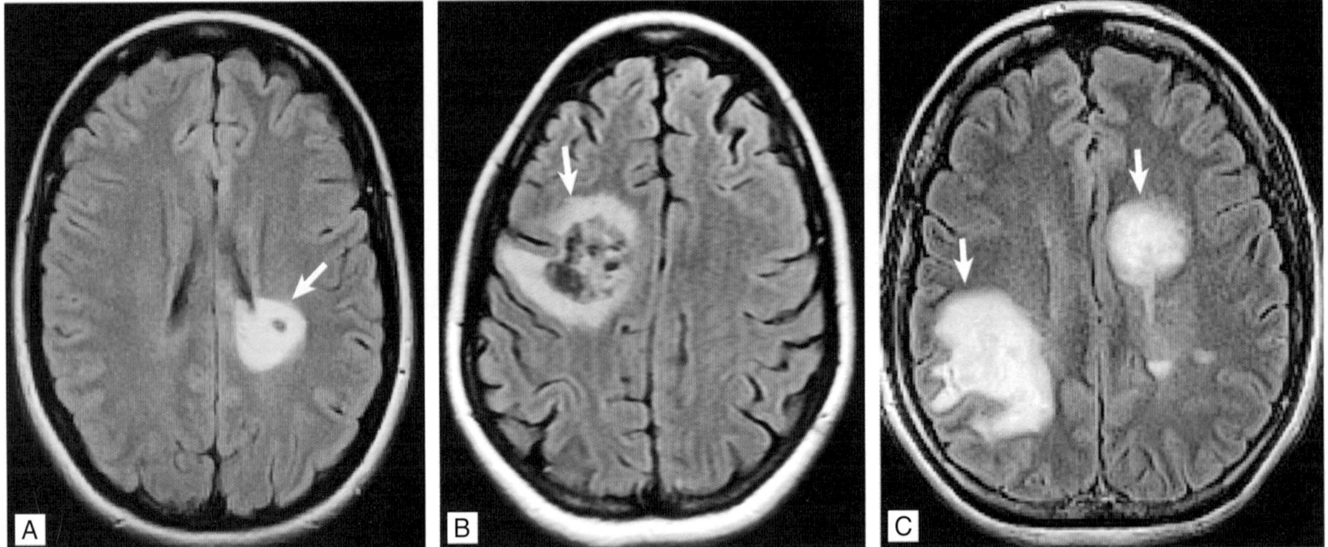

Figure 75.62 Tumefactive MS appearing as heterogeneous lesions with mass effect on FLAIR MRI (A–C, *arrows*).

exanthemas such as measles, chickenpox, rubella, and smallpox [52,53,95]. The basic mechanism is thought to be immunoallergic, and the characteristic histological features consist of lymphocytic and plasma-cell infiltrates around the venules of the neural parenchyma, with perivenous foci of demyelination. Clinically, most cases present with seizures or focal neurological signs and recover within 2–3 weeks although 10–20% may suffer permanent damage [13,52,53,95].

CT may show no changes, but more severe cases may show areas of patchily reduced density reflecting vasogenic edema in white matter. ***MRI*** is more sensitive than CT in demonstrating areas of edema and demyelination in white matter and may show changes more extensively than CT, or even when CT is negative (Fig. 75.65). As in other forms of encephalitis, the main change is increased signal on T2-weighted and FLAIR images with multifocal lesions. The brainstem is often involved, sometimes selectively, and the spinal cord may also be affected. *Unlike MS, another demyelinating disorder on the differential diagnosis, ADEM often involves deep gray structures.*

Reye Syndrome

This condition predominantly affects children below the age of 16 years but can affect adults as well. The patients are recovering from an illness of viral or presumed viral etiology when they develop both hepatitis and encephalitis. About one-third of patients may die within a few days from raised intracranial pressure. Liver function is severely affected, and half the patients have enlarged livers. Toxic agents, particularly salicylates, have been

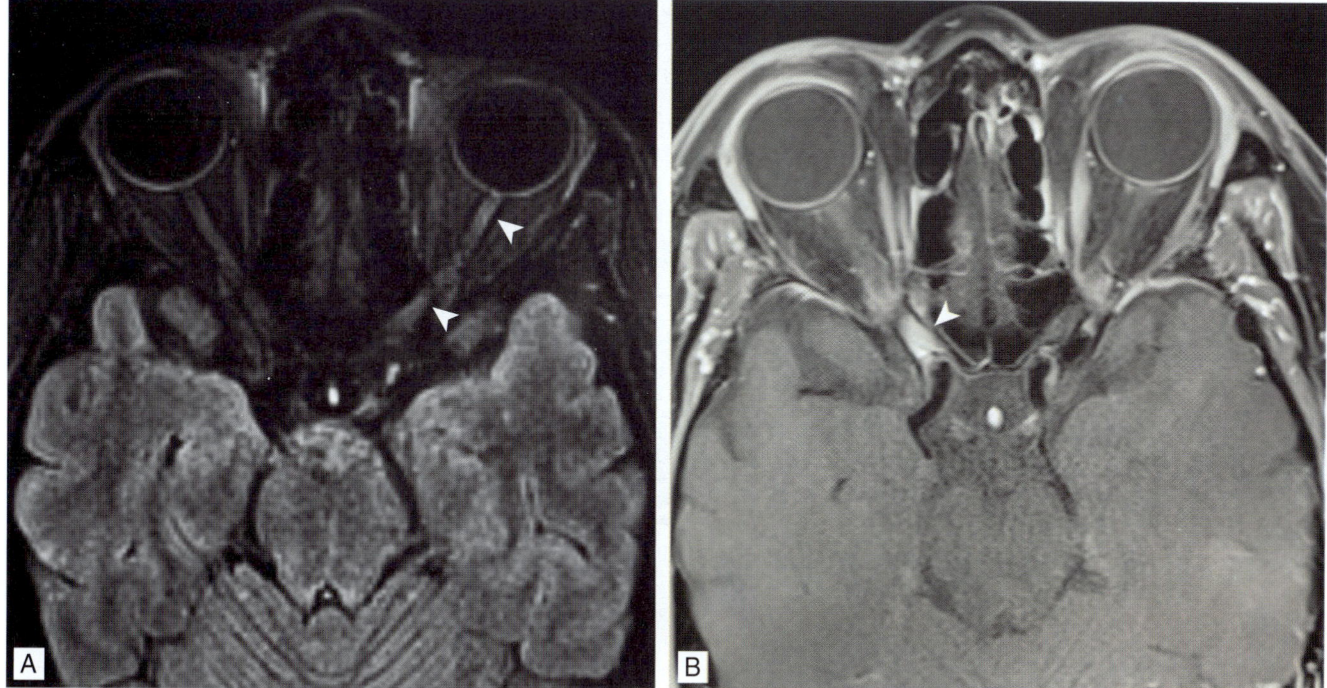

Figure 75.63 Optic neuritis in a patient with recurrent color vision loss. FLAIR hyperintensity of the left orbital and canalicular optic nerve segments (A, *arrowheads*) correlates to recurrent left visual deficits. Enhancement of the right optic nerve (B, *arrowhead*) corresponds to new onset of right-sided symptoms.

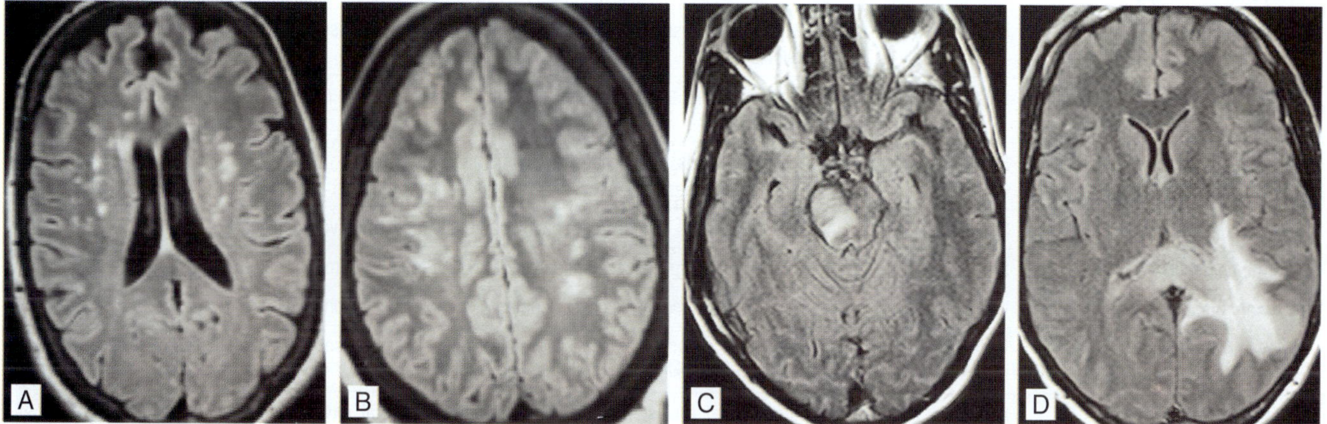

Figure 75.64 Neuromyelitis optica can have diverse presentations including scattered subcortical demyelinating lesions (A, B), focal lesions (C, right midbrain), and large infiltrative lesions on FLAIR MRI (D).

associated with the syndrome, and the interaction of toxin and virus has been postulated as the cause.

CT or ***MRI*** in the acute phase shows widespread cerebral edema with compression of the ventricles. Patients who recover may show enlargement of the ventricles and sulci and diminished attenuation of cerebral white matter. T2/FLAIR hyperintensities, edema, and diffusion restriction often localize to the bilateral thalamus, midbrain, and medial temporal lobes [101].

Neuroinflammatory Lesions

Vasculitis

Although protean in its clinical and imaging manifestations, cerebral vasculitis, the inflammation of cerebral blood vessel walls, can be categorized based on the size of affected vessels (Table 75.13). Several different vasculitides are surveyed as follows [8,29].

Imaging: Vascular imaging, including ***CTA, MRA, and DSA,*** are commonly used to assess cerebrovascular disease. Ultrasound can evaluate large arteries. In suspected vasculitis, vessel wall MRI is increasingly recommended [102]. Although vessel wall imaging can be technically demanding, imaging has improved due to: careful optimization of spatial resolution, acquisition of 2D/3D images, weighting of multiple tissues, and suppression of luminal blood and CSF signal. Field strengths of at least 3T are recommended, with isotropic voxel dimensions of 0.4–0.7 mm range for 3D acquisitions. Typical protocols incorporate time-of-flight MRA, pre- and postcontrast T1-weighted sequences as well as T2-weighted sequences. Sequences that suppress fat are needed for giant cell arteritis since the temporal artery is located close to

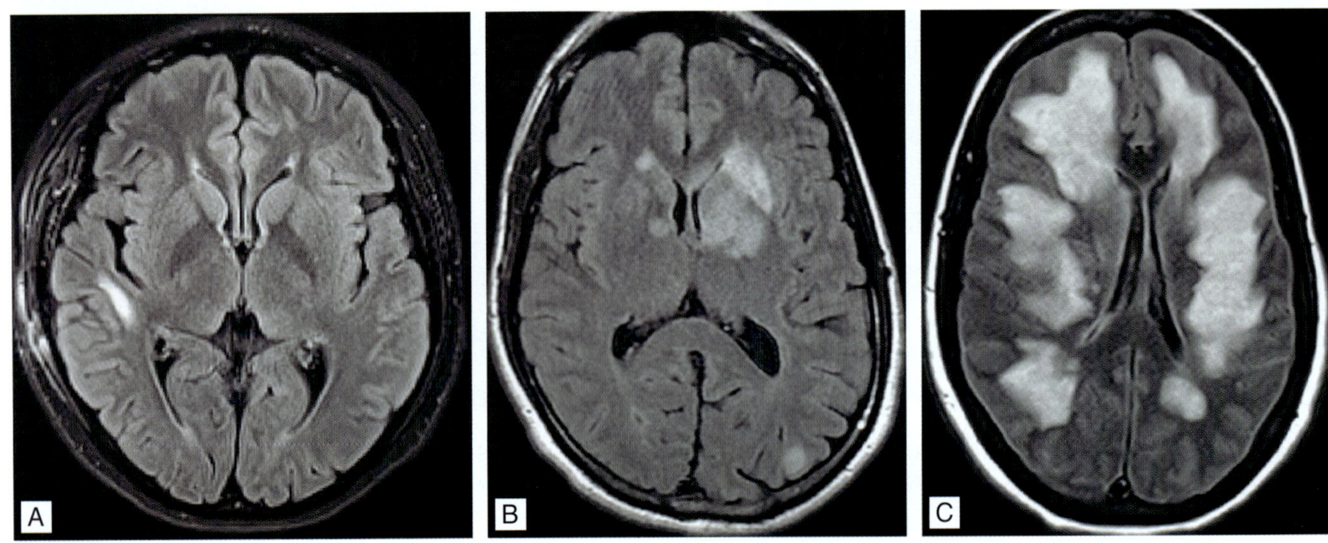

Figure 75.65 Acute disseminated encephalomyelitis (ADEM) often involves nonspecific white matter and deep gray matter on FLAIR MRI (A–C).

TABLE 75.13 Summary of Intracranial Vasculitis Findings

Vasculitic Disease	Affected Vessel Size	Clinical and Imaging Findings
Takayasu arteritis	Large	Thickening, dilation, and focal stenosis of common carotid arteries and aorta.
Giant cell arteritis	Large	Thickening and enhancement of temporal artery wall. *Halo sign* on color duplex ultrasound.
Polyarteritis nodosa	Medium	Aneurysm, stenosis, and occlusion of intracranial carotid arteries.
Kawasaki disease	Medium	Children with systemic vasculitis, nonspecific subdural effusions, infarcts, atrophy, or reversible callosal lesions.
Granulomatosis with polyangiitis	Small	Leptomeningeal enhancement. Soft-tissue nasal mass with obliteration of nasal septum/ turbinates.
Eosinophilic granulomatosis with polyangiitis	Small	Cerebral infarcts, hemorrhage, and optic neuropathy.
Microscopic polyangiitis	Small	Cerebral infarcts, hemorrhage, pachymeningitis, and small vessel disease.
Immunoglobulin A vasculitis	Small	Children with hypertensive encephalopathy and focal ischemia or hemorrhages.
Primary angiitis of the CNS	Variable	Discrete or diffuse MR lesions. Segmental stenosis/occlusion on DSA.
Moyamoya disease	Variable	Stenosis or occlusion of distal internal carotid arteries. Vessels with signal voids near basal ganglia and *ivy sign* on leptomeningeal collateral vessels.
Neuro-Behçet disease	Variable	Parenchymal: brainstem/basal ganglia. Nonparenchymal: cavernous sinus thrombosis.
Cogan disease	Variable	Ischemia, obliteration, narrowing, and enhancement of vestibular labyrinth.

the scalp. Additionally, spin echo sequences can yield blood signal suppression.

Importantly, there are common conditions that can mimic vasculitis and should be considered in reviewing vessel wall MRI [102]. It is important to separate atherosclerotic plaques from vasculitis. Furthermore, slow flow due to lower velocity of blood proximal to the vessel wall can lead to incomplete signal suppression and can appear as wall thickening/enhancement. Slow flow artifacts can occur at branch points, with retrograde flow near occlusions and within aneurysms. Vasa vasorum, the network of small vessels that feed large vessel walls, can appear as concentric wall thickening/enhancement, especially in patients with existing intracranial vascular disease. Veins running close to arteries, thromboembolism, and thrombectomy can also influence the appearance of cerebral arteries. Despite the utility of vessel imaging, biopsy of vessel walls remains the gold standard for the diagnosis of vasculitis [29], although vessel wall MRI can assist with localization of biopsy targets [103].

Takayasu Arteritis

This vasculitis affects the aorta and its branches (carotid and vertebral arteries), leading to the presentation as "pulseless" arteritis. It is seen in young adults in Asia, Latin America, the Mediterranean, and southern Africa. Vessel stenosis, occlusion, and aneurysms cause stroke and hypertensive encephalopathy [29]. Sensitive markers for early disease include the intimal–medial thickness measured on ***ultrasound***, hyperattenuation of vessel walls with thickening and calcification on nonenhanced ***CT*** or thickening and perivascular hyperintensities on T2-weighted ***MRI***. In acute phases, enhancement is seen in and around vessel walls. During advanced stages, occlusion of aortic branches and bypass collaterals may be noted on ***CTA***, ***MRA,*** or ***DSA*** [104].

Giant Cell Arteritis

This chronic granulomatous disease is noted for the giant cells seen on biopsy of the superficial temporal or occipital artery. It affects older patients, who may present with unilateral headache, jaw claudication, polymyalgia rheumatic, and vision loss [6]. A "**halo sign**" on ultrasound is seen due to hypoechoic temporal arterial wall with turbulent flow [29]. The vessel appears thickened and enhancing on ***MRI*** with segment inflammation on ^{18}F-FDG uptake [104].

Polyarteritis Nodosa

This disorder causes necrotizing vasculitis most commonly in the kidneys although the CNS is involved in 10% of cases. Aneurysms, wall thickening, stenosis, and occlusion of the carotids can lead to ischemia [8,29,104].

Kawasaki Disease

Children with a constellation of symptoms such as fever resistant to antipyretics, lymphadenopathy, and inflammation of the conjunctiva and mucous membranes with "*strawberry tongue*" may have this rare vasculitis linked to coronary aneurysms and cerebrovascular disease [6]. On ***MRI***, up to 30% of patients may have subdural effusions, infarcts, atrophy, and reversible T2 hyperintensities of the splenium of the corpus callosum [29]. Initial treatment includes high dose aspirin and immunoglobulin. Strikingly, the severe acute respiratory syndrome coronavirus 2 illness COVID-19 was linked to a "Kawasaki-like" disease [105].

Granulomatosis With Polyangiitis

This necrotizing vasculitis presents with cytoplasmic antineutrophilic antibodies (c-ANCA) and granulomatous vasculitis of the nasal cavity, sinuses and mastoid air spaces [6]. ***MRI*** and ***CT*** may reveal nasal granulomas and mucosal thickening with possible destruction of the nasal septum, turbinates or even the hard palate. The granuloma may have a "ground glass" appearance, and enhancement of the granuloma and the leptomeninges can be appreciated [29,104,106].

Eosinophilic Granulomatosis With Polyangiitis

This necrotizing vasculitis is linked to eosinophilia, perinuclear-ANCA, asthma, and allergic rhinitis. In later stages, the CNS may be affected with optic neuropathy, ischemia, and hemorrhage [29,104].

Microscopic Polyangiitis

Microscopic polyangiitis is a necrotizing small-vessel vasculitis with perinuclear-ANCA, glomerulonephritis, and dermatologic lesions. Neurological manifestations include neuropathy, pachymeningitis, infarcts, hemorrhage, and possible small-vessel disease [29,104,106].

Immunoglobulin A Vasculitis

Associated with Henoch–Schönlein purpura, this condition is caused by deposits of immunoglobulin A, a secretory antibody expressed at mucous membranes. Commonly seen in children, immunoglobulin A vasculitis may present with palpable purpura, joint disease, abdominal pain, and glomerulonephritis. CNS involvement often occurs secondary to hypertensive or uremic encephalopathy although cerebral ischemia and hemorrhage have been noted [29].

Primary Angiitis of the CNS

Primary angiitis of the CNS or primary CNS vasculitis affects small- and medium-sized CNS vessels. Patients may present with various nonspecific symptoms, including headache, cranial nerve involvement, and cognitive/psychiatric manifestations [6]. Leptomeningeal and brain biopsies provide a definitive diagnosis although noninvasive imaging can be supportive. ***MRI*** shows ischemic and hemorrhagic white matter lesions that may enhance. ***MRA*** may portray anomalies in the distal carotid artery and proximal anterior/middle cerebral arteries (Fig. 75.66). ***DSA*** can illustrate vessel stenosis and abnormalities in vessels, their collaterals and blood flow [29,106].

Neuro-Behçet Disease

Prevalence of neurological symptoms varies between 5% and 50% in patients with Behçet disease. This is more common in people of Mediterranean heritage and is noted for genital ulcers, aphthous stomatitis, uveitis, positive pathergy skin test, vasculitis and involvement of the eyes, joints, and gastrointestinal tract. Neurologic symptoms include brainstem disease, stroke-like episodes, seizures, and intracranial hypertension (headaches, vomiting, bilateral papilledema). ***MRI*** commonly reveals nonspecific changes, characterized by hyperintensity on T2-weighted images. Areas involved commonly include the brainstem, cranial nerves, optic chiasm, hypothalamus, followed by thalamus and basal ganglia (Fig. 75.67) [7]. The parenchymal form (80% of cases) appears as patchy, confluent areas, especially in the brainstem and/or basal ganglia, while the nonparenchymal form (20%) is associated with cavernous sinus thrombosis, which can present as multiple cranial neuropathies [29,107].

Cogan Disease

This is a rare multisystem disorder with features of interstitial keratitis and vestibulocochlear abnormalities. Patients present with myriad neuropsychiatric symptoms, from headache, neuropathy, stroke to psychosis. Imaging may show obliteration or stenosis of the vestibular labyrinth with possible enhancement of the membranous labyrinth [108]. Vasculitis occurs in roughly 15% of patients [109].

Drug/Radiation-Induced Vasculitis

Drugs of abuse, especially cocaine and heroin, as well as radiation, can induce vasospasm and vasculitis. Cocaine-induced vessel abnormalities can lead to infarct, leukoencephalopathy, hemorrhage, and *moyamoya-like syndrome* due to collateral vessel development. Heroin is more associated with spongiform leukoencephalopathy [104,106].

Secondary Cerebral Vasculitis Associated With Inflammatory Diseases

Systemic inflammation can lead to cerebral vasculitis; such conditions include: *systemic lupus erythematosus, RA, Sjögren syndrome, scleroderma, and antiphospholipid syndrome* [106]. CNS infections can also lead to vasculitic complications. Particularly, tuberculous meningitis and meningovascular syphilis are associated with basilar vasculitis. Vasculitis is also linked to HIV, varicella zoster, fungus, and neurocysticercosis [27,104,106].

Additional Neuroinflammatory Diseases

There are additional neuroinflammatory diseases that involve the brain parenchyma, which may involve vessels. These include:

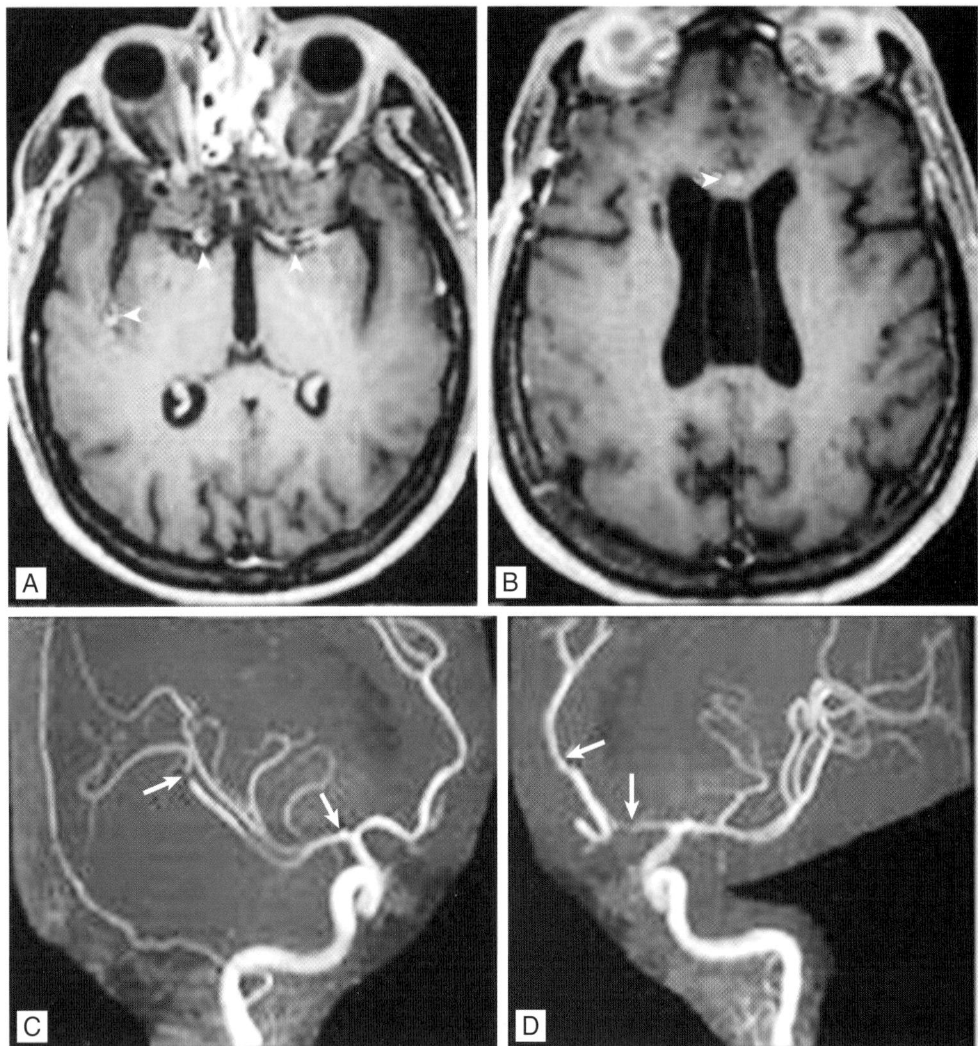

Figure 75.66 Primary CNS angiitis. Contrast-enhanced black blood T1 MRI (A, B) shows circumferential enhancement in the walls of multiple intracranial arteries (*arrowheads*). Maximal intensity 3D projection images of time-of-flight MRA (C, D) show corresponding focal luminal narrowings (*arrows*). These findings are not specific to primary CNS vasculitis and can be seen in a variety of secondary causes of CNS vasculitis.

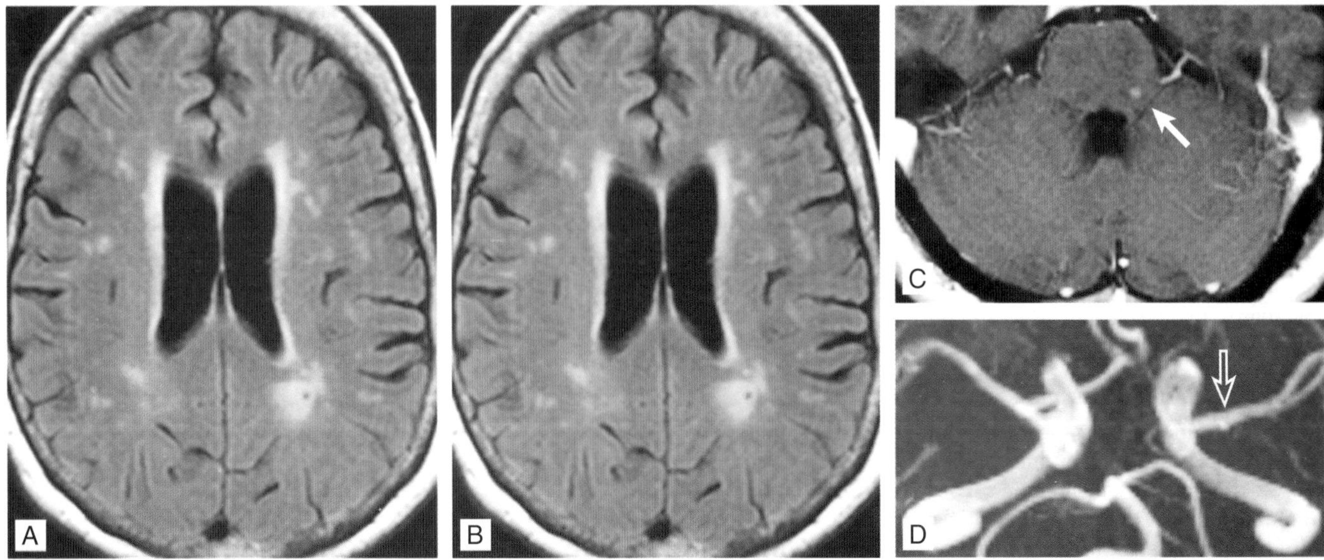

Figure 75.67 Neuro-Behçet disease on MR. Bithalamic (A) and subcortical white matter FLAIR hyperintensities (B). Mildly enhancing focus in right dorsolateral pons (C, *arrow*) on T1 postcontrast MRI. Focal beading in left proximal middle cerebral artery (D, *open arrow*) consistent with vasculitis on 3D time of flight (TOF) MRA.

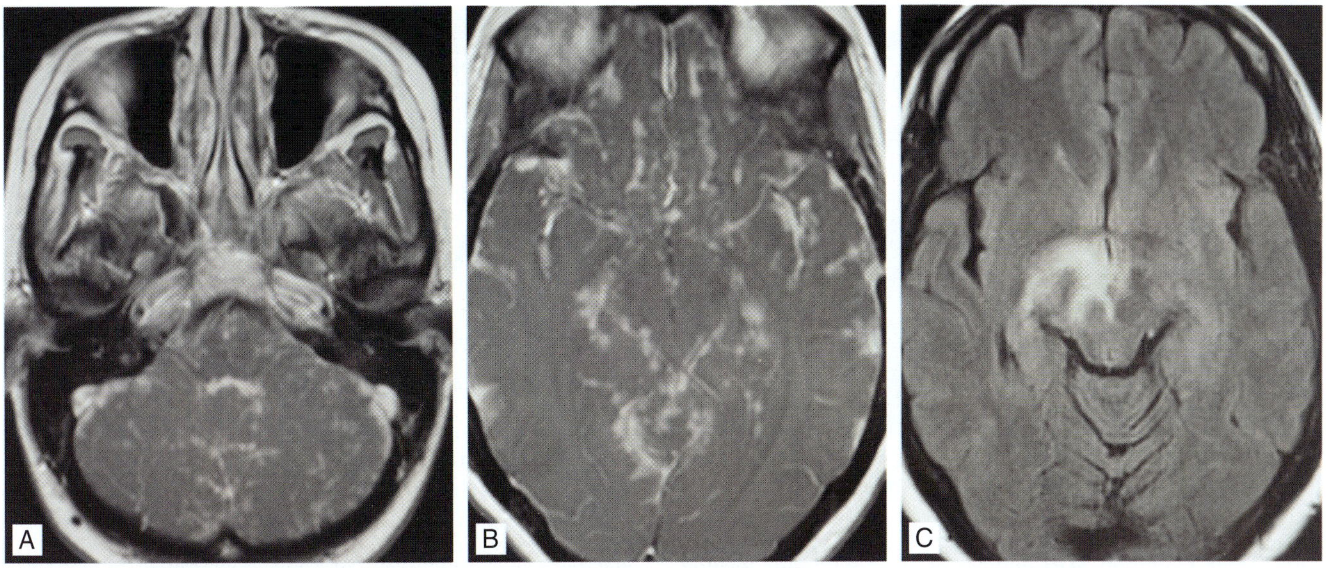

Figure 75.68 Neurosarcoidosis. Postcontrast T1-weighted MRI reveals leptomeningeal and peripheral cortical enhancement of the cerebellum (A) and edema with effacement of the basal cisterns (B). FLAIR hyperintensities of the brainstem and adjacent optic pathway (C).

neurosarcoidosis, PRES, Susac syndrome, radiation-associated disorders and amyloid-related imaging abnormalities.

Neurosarcoidosis

Sarcoidosis involvement of the CNS occurs in around 15% of affected patients. It can manifest as a basal leptomeningitis or intracerebral granulomas or both. Clinically, patients with chronic leptomeningitis may present with hydrocephalus while those with granulomas present with focal signs, depending on the site of lesion [110,112,113].

Neurosarcoidosis is a great mimicker of other identities. ***CT*** may demonstrate communicating hydrocephalus associated with enhancing hyperdensities in the basal cisterns, an appearance which is nonspecific. Granulomas are also hyperdense and enhance with contrast medium. They may be multiple and small, resembling metastases but without surrounding edema [3]. A single large lesion is occasionally seen and may simulate a neoplasm [112,113].

MRI visualizes a variety of changes, but they are also generally nonspecific. The most common abnormalities are areas of T2/FLAIR hyperintensity in cerebral white matter, usually located more superficially than the lesions of MS although periventricular lesions do occur. Surface granulomas may be shown, especially adjacent to the major cisterns. Deeper lesions involving the brainstem and basal ganglia typically enhance. Acute episodes can demonstrate leptomeningeal enhancement and edema (Fig. 75.68) [110,112,113].).

Posterior Reversible Encephalopathy Syndrome

PRES (also known as *reversible posterior leukoencephalopathy syndrome*) can present with headaches or seizures. Risk factors include immunosuppression, organ transplant, autoimmune disease, chemotherapy, eclampsia, sepsis, hemodialysis, renal disease, and hypertension [111]. Since lesions typically occur posteriorly, clinical manifestations include visual deficits including homonymous hemianopia and visual neglect. However, the inflammatory lesions of PRES may occur throughout the white matter, affecting basal ganglia and cerebral hemispheres, especially along vascular border zones. Cortical and subcortical T2/FLAIR hyperintensities are seen, with or without enhancement (Fig. 75.69) [111].

Susac Syndrome

Susac syndrome (*retinocochleocerebral vasculopathy*) is a very rare inflammatory microangiopathy noted for a *clinical triad of encephalopathy, retinal artery occlusions and sensorineural hearing*

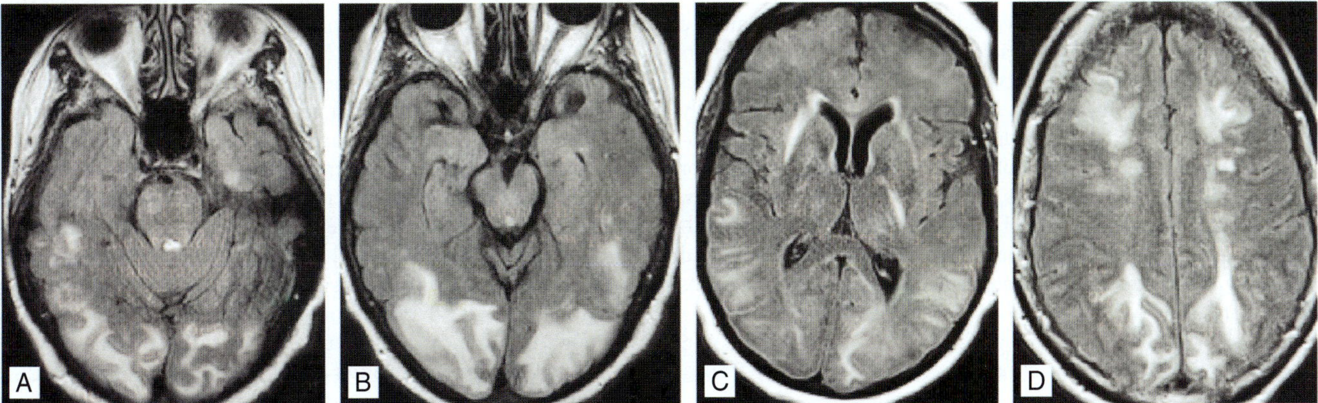

Figure 75.69 PRES on FLAIR MRI. Lesions are generally found in posterior juxtacortical white matter (A, B) although they may be seen more diffusely in the basal ganglia, along white matter tracts (C), and along cerebral watershed areas (D).

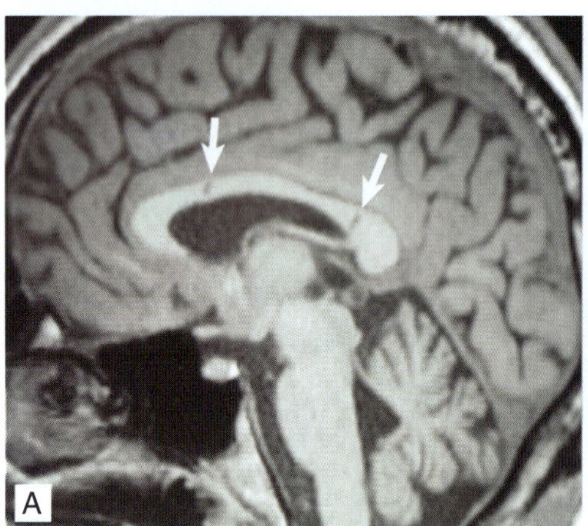

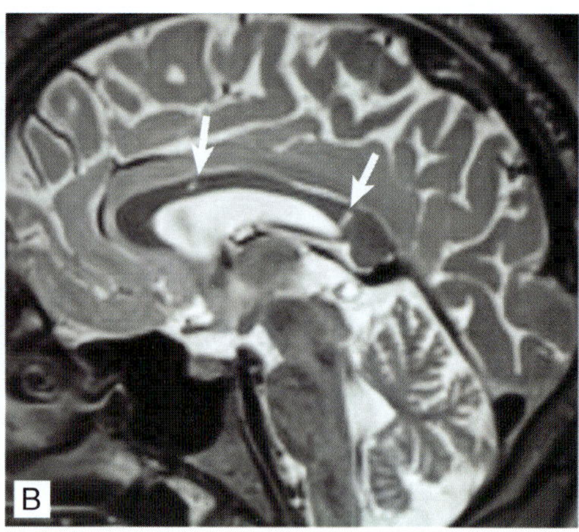

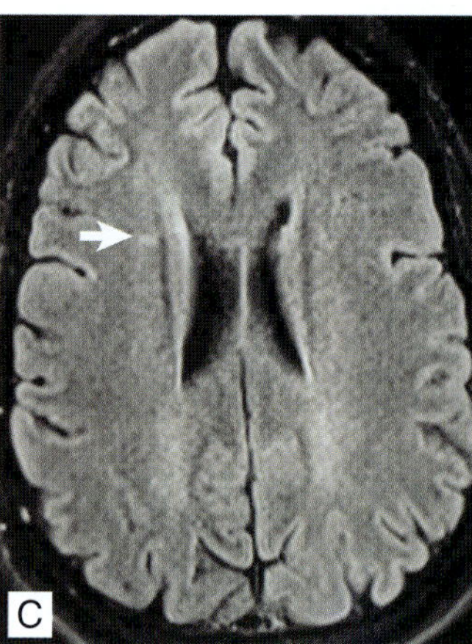

Figure 75.70 Susac syndrome on MRI. A patient with headaches, paresthesias, visual deficits, and tinnitus was found to have nonenhancing T1 hypointense (A, *arrows*) and T2 (B, *arrows*) and FLAIR hyperintense linear lesions in the right anterior and posterior corpus callosums (C, *arrow*).

impairment. Common ***MRI*** findings of Susac syndrome include linear or punctate, noncontrast enhancing, T1 hypointense ("black hole") and T2 and FLAIR hyperintense white matter lesions around central corpus callosum, often mimicking MS and ADEM (Fig. 75.70) [114]. Relatively unique to Susac syndrome are gray matter lesions and leptomeningeal enhancement.

Radiation and Drug-Related Inflammation

Radiation used in the treatment of malignant tumors can produce harmful effects, that is, occlusion of small vessels and resulting infarction. In the acute stage, there are changes in the white matter that are difficult to distinguish from tumor at both ***CT*** and ***MRI*** [13]. Radiation damage and inflammation is often delayed, leading to a common diagnostic dilemma between tumor recurrence/progression and radiation-therapy-related changes (radiation necrosis, pseudoprogression). In this situation, MRI perfusion imaging and PET may be helpful in showing *hyperperfusion or hypermetabolism, respectively, in tumor recurrence and hypoperfusion or hypometabolism in radiation necrosis* [3]. Radiation changes will eventually progress to local atrophy although white matter low density on CT and signal change on MRI will persist. Radiation can cause necrosis of irradiated tissue surrounding a tumor, leading to stroke. Moreover, certain immunomodulators and antibodies (i.e., anti-amyloid) lead to direct vs. indirect neuroinflammation (i.e., amyloid-related imaging abnormalities) [13].

Stroke-Like Migraine Attacks After Radiation Therapy Syndrome

Stroke-like migraine attacks after radiation therapy syndrome is a rare, delayed complication of radiation therapy for brain tumors (occurrence is generally 1–5 years after radiation but can be decades after). The clinical presentation includes migraines with generally reversible neurologic deficits including hemisensory loss and hemiparesis. Symptoms typically resolve within 1 month. Evidence for treatment is unclear, but patients may benefit from anticonvulsants, aspirin, and/or corticosteroids [115]. On ***MRI***, characteristic findings are areas of gyral enhancement with cortical thickening and edema, which are transient, unilateral, and in the region of previous treatment [115].

Epilepsy

Epilepsy is a neurologic disorder manifested by recurrent seizures, which are transient disturbances of sensory or motor function, alterations in consciousness, or convulsions caused by abnormal electrical activity in the brain [6,117]. Like strokes, seizures have typical symptoms allowing neurologists to diagnose epilepsy clinically. ***Electroencephalography (EEG)*** is used to confirm the diagnosis based on patterns of abnormal electrical activity and, in conjunction with clinical features, to characterize seizure types and locations of seizure onset. Generalized seizures involve both hemispheres simultaneously. Focal seizures arise in one part of the brain although they may generalize. In most cases, epilepsy can be effectively treated with medication. The primary role of imaging in epilepsy is to identify structural alterations causing focal seizures in medication refractory cases, so that patients can be treated appropriately with resective surgery or newer therapies including laser ablation and neuromodulation [116].

High-quality and high-resolution ***MRI*** is important for identifying subtle lesions that may cause seizures [6,117]. Whenever possible, epilepsy protocol studies should be performed at 3T rather than 1.5T; 7T MRI is even being used at some centers. A typical protocol should include high resolution whole brain 3D T1-weighted images and thin section coronal T2-weighted, FLAIR and T1-weighted images through the temporal lobes. *PET, single photon emission computed tomography, and magnetoencephalography* are functional imaging techniques that complement MRI and EEG in localizing seizure onset. Functional MRI may also be performed.

In a vast majority of cases of focal or localization-related epilepsy, cortical or juxtacortical structural abnormalities provide the locus for seizure generation. The role of surgery in medication-refractory epilepsy is to resect or disconnect the epileptogenic lesion. Surgical treatment of epilepsy heavily relies upon identification of a structural lesion on MRI. The epileptogenic lesions are often quite subtle; therefore, the MR protocol needs to be tailored for highest possible resolution and gray–white matter contrast. The epileptogenicity of the structural lesion seen on MRI must be established by scalp or intracranial EEG before proceeding to surgery. ***Functional MRI*** may also be performed to determine the dominant cerebral hemisphere for language and memory and motor mapping before surgical resection [116,117].

There are a variety of epilepsy syndromes, particularly affecting pediatric patients. In many of these, imaging will be normal although in some cases there are characteristic features or widespread structural abnormalities [117].

Tuberous sclerosis is one of the phakomatoses (or neurocutaneous disorders) and is caused by mutations in the *TSC1* or *TSC2* genes. Tuberous sclerosis was classically described as

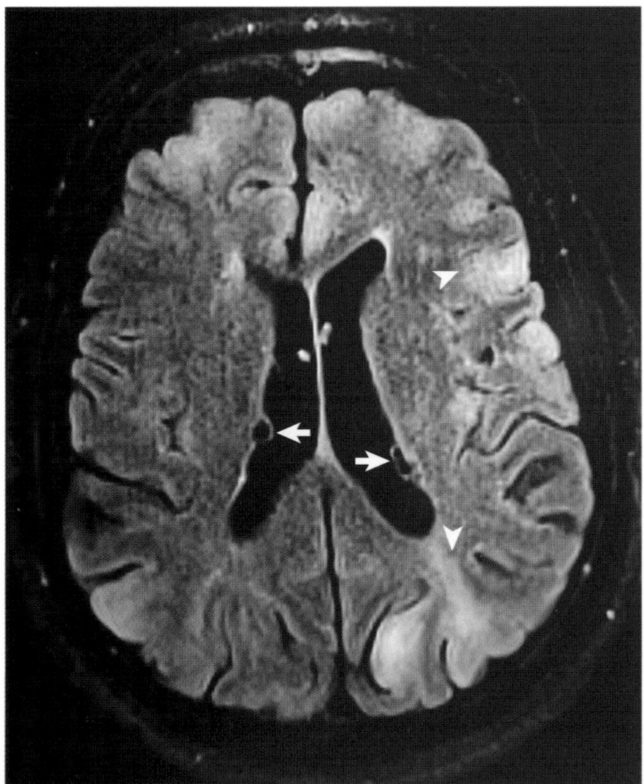

Figure 75.71 Tuberous sclerosis. Subependymal nodules are noted (*arrows*) with FLAIR hyperintense cortical tubers (*arrowheads*).

presenting in childhood with the triad of (1) seizures, (2) intellectual disability, and (3) adenoma sebaceum (a misnomer for facial angiofibromas), but one or more of these features may be absent. Typical brain imaging findings are "***cortical/subcortical tubers***" (triangular areas of signal alteration serving as epileptogenic foci) and ***subependymal hamartomas*** (nodules along the ventricles). Both types of lesions often calcify and may enhance (Fig. 75.71) [118].

Hypothalamic hamartoma is another cause of childhood seizures with classic imaging and clinical findings. These non-neoplastic lesions follow gray matter signal and are found along the floor of the third ventricle at the tuber cinereum, the part of the hypothalamus between the optic chiasm and the mammillary bodies (Fig. 75.72). They are associated with gelastic seizures typified by uncontrollable laughter [10,121].

Temporal lobe epilepsy is the most common type of epilepsy and MTS is the most common cause of epilepsy in patients who underwent surgery [119]. MTS affects the hippocampus, a curved structure in the medial temporal lobe important for memory. Imaging findings of MTS are best seen on MRI [117], particularly on high-resolution coronal images [122]; ***MRI*** demonstrates hippocampal (1) volume loss, (2) abnormal signal, and (3) loss of normal laminated internal architecture (Fig. 75.73). MTS may be associated with atrophy of the ipsilateral mammillary body or fornix, as these structures are connected as part of the medial limbic (or *Papez*) circuit. MTS can be unilateral or bilateral and may be associated with other epileptogenic lesions (a scenario called "dual pathology"). Hence it is imperative always to look for multiple abnormalities and avoid satisfaction of search.

Several low-grade tumors, tending to arise in the temporal lobes and affect younger patients, have epilepsy as their primary symptom [6,13,117]. These **long-term epilepsy-associated tumors** include **ganglioglioma**, **DNET,** and **pleomorphic xanthoastrocytoma**. Gangliogliomas may be solid with variable enhancement or cystic with a mural enhancing nodule (Fig. 75.74). DNETs have a very characteristic "*bubbly*" appearance (Fig. 75.75). Pleomorphic xanthoastrocytomas usually demonstrate a solid enhancing nodule often associated with a cyst and usually peripherally located, sometimes with leptomeningeal involvement or scalloping of the calvarium. **Oligodendrogliomas** are another tumor type often associated with seizures. These are more commonly seen in young to middle-aged adults, with ill-defined margins, often cortical infiltration and expansion, and variable calcification and enhancement. Glioblastoma is the most common adult primary brain tumor and metastases are the most common tumor; these and other tumors can also cause seizures although typically not as their primary symptoms [6].

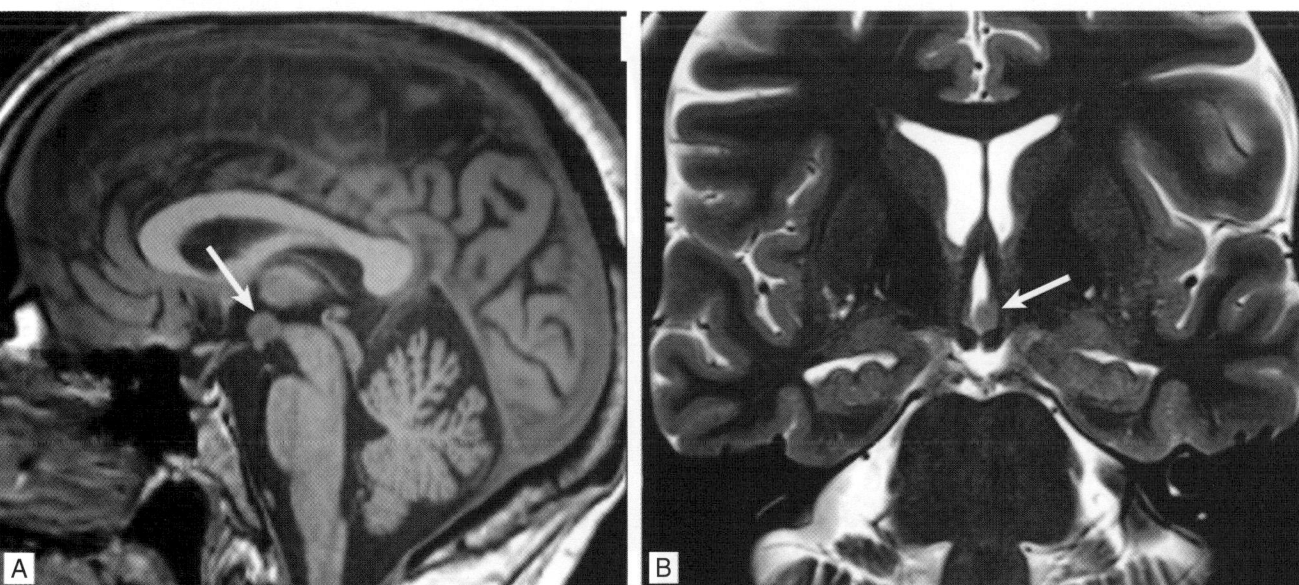

Figure 75.72 Sagittal T1-weighted (A) and coronal T2-weighted (B) images show a nodule (*arrow*) following gray matter signal reflecting a hypothalamic hamartoma along the floor of the third ventricle adjacent to the mammillary bodies.

76

Metabolic and Degenerative Diseases

MOHIT AGARWAL, AMOGH N. HEGDE, RYAN B. PETERSON, ILYA M. NASRALLAH

Introduction

This chapter discusses two distinct classes of central nervous system (CNS) disorders that have certain similarities yet are fundamentally different. Although the clinical course of toxic/metabolic disorders is usually rapidly progressive requiring prompt diagnosis and specific treatment, neurodegenerative disorders have an indolent course with a relative lack of the availability of specific treatment. The imaging manifestations of these two classes of diseases are also distinct, with symmetric involvement of deep gray structures and cortical gray matter often seen in metabolic disorders while loss of gray matter volume commonly seen in the neurodegenerative conditions. The apparent similarities of these disorders stem from the conspicuously overlapping clinical picture where symptoms of altered mentation, cognitive decline, delirium, confusion, etc. are common. The idea of these disorders being similar may also come from the "black box" reputation of these conditions, where an air of mystery surrounds the diagnosis. Thorough combing of lab tests and clinical history usually clears the air in the metabolic group of disorders, but such fortitude is elusive in the neurodegenerative conditions, especially if the underlying neuropathology is other than Alzheimer's disease (AD). In the next few pages, we will discuss these disorders and an approach to their diagnosis using a combined clinical, lab, and imaging pattern approach.

Metabolic Disorders

Metabolic brain disorders (Table 76.1) usually result from abnormal levels of substances that at normal levels are required for optimal functioning of the human body. Normal constituents of the blood such as glucose, copper, ammonia, calcium, lactate, ketones, etc., when raised or lowered to abnormal levels can affect the metabolically active and high energy requiring regions of the brain, which include the basal ganglia and the cerebral cortex. In this section, we will discuss these disorders and outline an approach to diagnose these conditions.

Wilson's Disease (Hepatolenticular Degeneration)

Wilson's disease is a genetic disorder of autosomal recessive inheritance due to variations in the copper-transporting gene *ATP7B* which leads to intracellular accumulation of copper in the brain, liver, and cornea secondary to abnormal ceruloplasmin metabolism. Clinical onset is often slow and staggered with variable symptoms like dysarthria, dystonia, tremors, ataxia, parkinsonian symptoms, and psychiatric problems. Kayser–Fleischer rings in the cornea are characteristic of the disease and liver cirrhosis may develop in the later stages. In the brain, basal ganglia, thalami, midbrain, dentate nuclei of the cerebellum, and cortical and subcortical regions of mainly the frontal lobes are mainly involved [1,2].

The affected structures in the brain show swelling in the initial phase of the disease, with development of atrophy in subsequent late phases. Typically, the putamen and caudate nuclei are involved with T2 prolongation in these nuclei. The "face of the panda" sign, originally described by Hitoshi et al. in 1991, refers to the increased signal intensity of the tegmentum, hypointensity of the superior colliculus, and preservation of the signal intensity of the red nucleus and the lateral portion of the pars reticulata of the substantia nigra (Fig. 76.1) [3]. Other T2W MRI features include abnormal hyperintensity in the globus pallidus, ventral nucleus of the thalamus, periaqueductal gray matter, and the dentate nuclei. "Face of the panda cub" sign has been recently described to depict involvement of the dorsal pons around the fourth ventricle area [4]. The abnormal signal in the putamina and caudate can be homogeneous, affect the periphery of the nuclei, or can be concentric due to associated accumulation of iron. In the acute phase of the disease, the T2W signal abnormalities are associated with restricted diffusion, although as necrosis ensues, the DWI abnormality is that of T2-shine through. Due to the paramagnetic effects of copper, T1W hyperintensity may be seen in the basal ganglia on MRI exams [1,2,5–7]. There is no contrast enhancement. Improvement in MRI findings correlates with clinical recovery [8–11].

TABLE 76.1 Metabolic and Toxic Disorders

Metabolic disorders—*due to intrinsic metabolites*

- Wilson's disease
- Hepatic encephalopathy
- Hypoglycemic encephalopathy
- Hyperglycemic encephalopathy
- Uremic encephalopathy
- Parathyroid disorders
- Fahr disease

Toxic disorders—*due to extrinsic toxins*

- Alcoholic encephalopathy
- CO poisoning
- Methanol poisoning
- Recreational drugs
- Chemotherapeutic agents
- Radiation toxicity

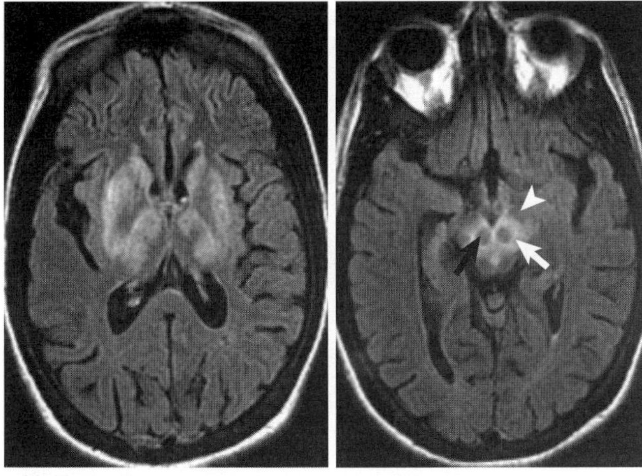

Figure 76.1 Wilson's disease. A 22-year-old female with recurrent dystonia and dysphasia shows abnormal hyperintensity within the caudate nuclei, putamina, and thalami bilaterally on axial FLAIR MRI image of the brain (left). "Face of the giant panda" sign is seen on axial FLAIR MRI image of the brain through the midbrain on the right with normal signal within the red nuclei (*black arrow*) and the substantia nigra (*arrowhead*) and abnormal hyperintense signal in the tegmentum (*white arrow*).

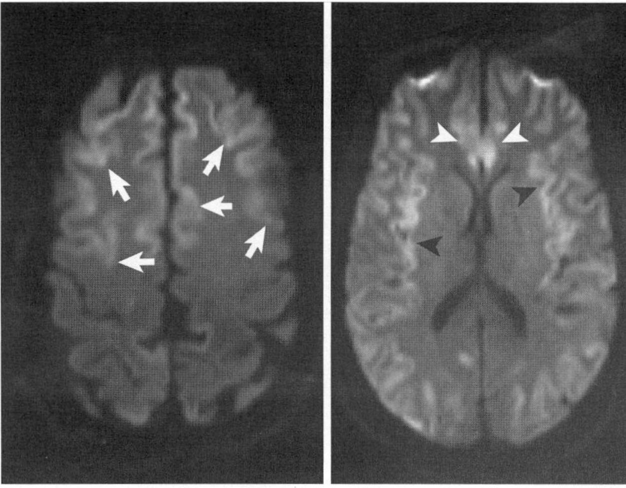

Figure 76.2 Acute hepatic encephalopathy. Patient with altered mental status, elevated liver enzymes, and increased ammonia levels. Axial diffusion-weighted MRI images demonstrate diffuse gyriform cortical restricted diffusion (*white arrows*). Involvement of the insular cortices (*black arrowheads*), and cingulate gyri (*white arrowheads*) is seen in acute hepatic encephalopathy, especially if it is associated with hyperammonemia.

Teaching Point

Slow onset movement disorders or vague neuropsychiatric symptoms with involvement of the basal ganglia may be seen in Wilson's disease, Pantothenate kinase associated neurodegeneration/Neurodegeneration with brain iron accumulation (PKAN/NBIA), chronic hepatic encephalopathy (Mn toxicity, TPN, etc.), and chronic sequel of CO poisoning or HIE.

Hepatic Encephalopathy

Hepatic encephalopathy (HE) is usually seen in the setting of liver cirrhosis with spontaneous or iatrogenic (transjugular intrahepatic portosystemic shunt surgery) portosystemic shunts. In this setting, nitrogenous wastes bypass liver metabolism with resultant neurotoxicity which is responsible for the imaging manifestations of [12]. Clinically, HE may present with altered mental status ranging from mild cognitive disturbances to coma or with motor disturbances (rigidity, tremors, movement, and speech disturbances) [13].

Acute HE is a life-threatening condition with high morbidity and mortality secondary to hyperammonemia. Besides hepatic insufficiency, inherited abnormalities of the urea cycle, citrullinemia, hematologic disorders, and certain drugs (valproate) may also cause hyperammonemia. The imaging findings are reversible and resolve with specific therapy [8,10,14–16]. The neuronal injury is that from combined cytotoxic and vasogenic edema leading to restricted diffusion and long TR signal abnormalities, respectively. This is the likely underlying mechanism for the imaging findings in the acute phase of HE, where bilateral symmetric T2W/FLAIR hyperintensity and restricted diffusion are seen in the insular cortices, cingulate gyri, and basal ganglia (Fig. 76.2). There is no contrast enhancement [17–19]. MR spectroscopy (MRS) reveals increased glutamine levels and elevated glutamine/creatinine ratio. Myoinositol and choline peaks are reduced on MRS [20]. These imaging findings are also associated with diffuse brain edema, which if severe may lead to brain herniation and death.

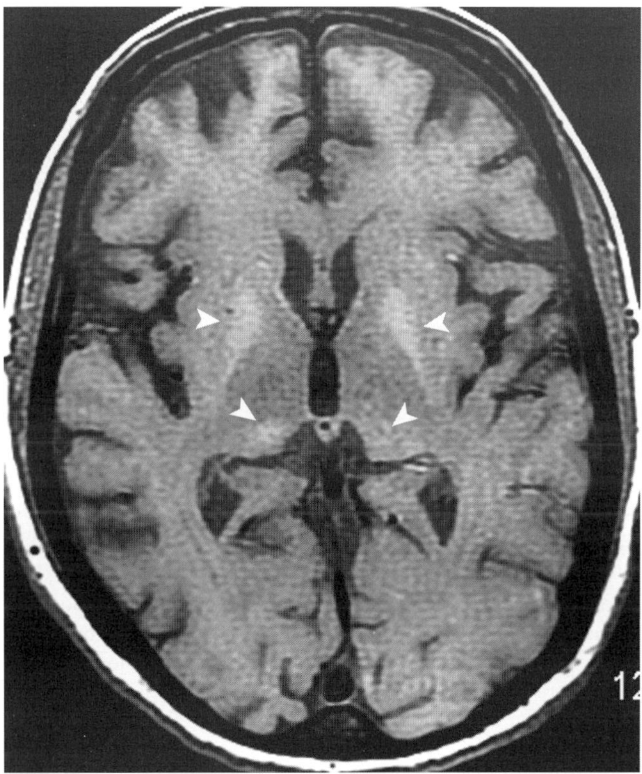

Figure 76.3 Chronic hepatic encephalopathy. T1W axial MRI image in a patient with chronic liver dysfunction. T1W hyperintense appearance of the deep gray structures (*arrowheads*) is due to the accumulation of manganese.

Chronic presentation of HE is predominantly due to the accumulation of manganese and often manifest as motor disturbances with parkinsonian features. Increased T1W signal is noted in the basal ganglia on MRI [13], particularly the globus pallidus and substantia nigra, due to the paramagnetic effects of manganese (Fig. 76.3). Similar T1W hyperintensity in the hypothalamus and the pituitary is less common. Diffuse brain atrophy, especially of the cerebellum, is also a common imaging finding seen in patients

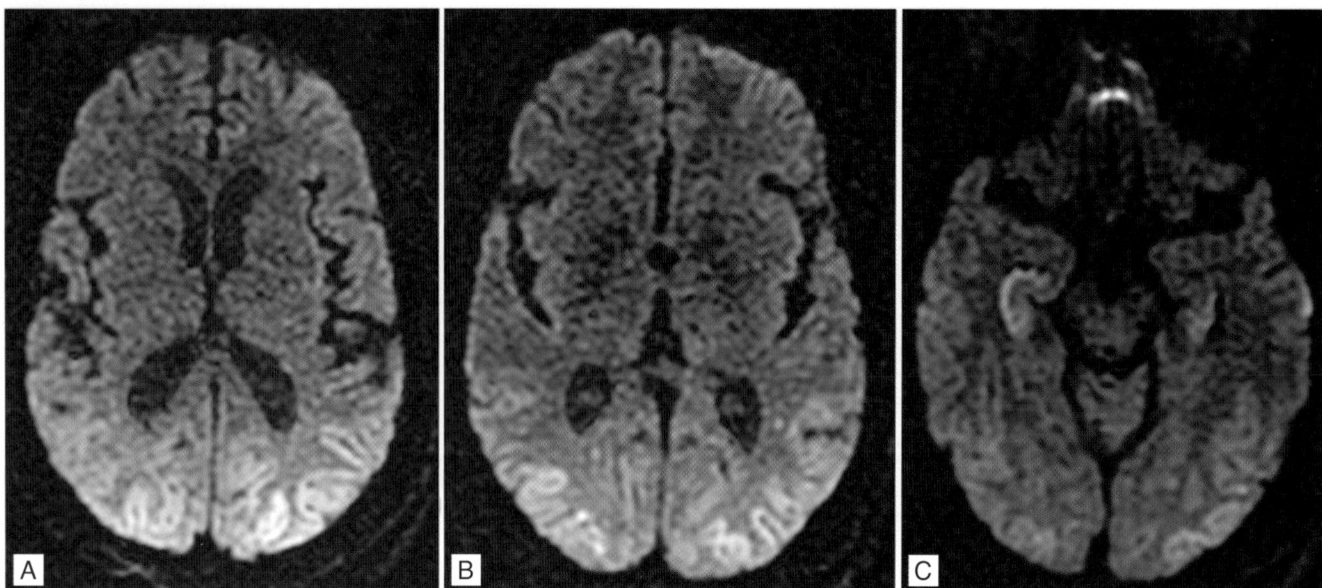

Figure 76.4 Hypoglycemic encephalopathy. Axial DWI MRI images show abnormal cortical reduced diffusivity in the parietal and occipital regions (A) and (B) and the hippocampi (C). The basal ganglia can also be involved in hypoglycemic encephalopathy (not seen here) but sparing of the thalami is common.

with chronic HE. The basal ganglia abnormalities revert after liver transplantation [12,17,19].

Besides chronic HE, bilateral pallidal T1W hyperintensity may be seen in

- conditions related to hypermagnesemia (total parenteral nutrition, occupational exposure, portal vein thrombosis, or congenital portal-systemic bypass without intrinsic hepatocellular disease)
- conditions unrelated to increased brain manganese levels (e.g., nonketotic hyperglycemic episodes, hypoxic–ischemic encephalopathy, basal ganglia calcification, neurofibromatosis type I, and Japanese encephalitis)

In the latter group, unrelated to manganese deposition, the signal abnormality may not be symmetric or restricted to the globus pallidus involvement [13].

Teaching Point

In an acute setting with severe altered mental status, bilateral symmetric involvement of insular cortices, cingulate gyri, and basal ganglia correlated with clinical findings and blood work up can help differentiate ischemic from metabolic (hypoglycemic, acute hepatic, and uremic) encephalopathy. If the presentation is chronic, prion disease is a consideration with similar pattern of imaging.

Hypoglycemic Encephalopathy

Hypoglycemic encephalopathy may result from sudden decrease in serum glucose to as low as 50mg/dl. This may be caused due to an overdose of insulin or oral hypoglycemic agents in diabetic patients or can be due to conditions like insulinoma, adrenal insufficiency, hepatic insufficiency, etc. Clinical presentation is acute, typically as seizures, focal neurologic deficits, and coma [21]. An important clinical consideration is that patients can present with stroke-like symptoms, where the radiologist can play an important role in suggesting the diagnosis in the emergency setting, potentially saving a life from timely and accurate management [22].

The brain uses glucose as its principal energy substrate. The energy substrate supply–demand deficit created by hypoglycemia leads to failure of the ATPase pump and release of aspartate which causes neuronal necrosis. Tissue necrosis manifests as restricted diffusion and increased T2W/FLAIR signal on MRI in the high energy requiring areas like basal ganglia, the cerebral cortices, and the hippocampi (Fig. 76.4). The thalami, brainstem, and cerebellum are usually spared. Sparing of the thalamus can help in differentiation from hypoxic ischemic injury, where thalamus is usually affected. Imaging changes are bilateral and somewhat symmetric [22–27]. There is no associated hemorrhage, and no contrast enhancement is usually seen.

Persistence of restricted diffusion on follow-up DWI MRI and the extent of DWI abnormality are poor prognostic indicators and herald tissue infarction and long-term neurologic deficits.

A milder reversible form of the condition affecting the white matter is also described. In the milder form, DWI and long TR signal abnormalities of bilateral periventricular and deep white matter (including internal capsule) may be present. Similar signal abnormalities may also be seen in the splenium of the corpus callosum, termed as transient splenial lesion or cytotoxic lesion of the splenium corpus callosum (CLOCC) or the boomerang sign [28] separately or associated with aforementioned deep white matter changes. Resolution of the signal changes indicates favorable long-term prognosis.

Hypoxic Ischemic Encephalopathy

Hypoxic ischemic encephalopathy (HIE) may show near similar imaging manifestations and may be difficult to differentiate from hypoglycemic encephalopathy based on imaging alone, since the mechanisms for imaging manifestations are somewhat similar. A significant circulatory or respiratory failure event from causes including cardiac arrest, drowning, or asphyxiation would be present. In adults, mild HIE may affect only the watershed zones.

Severe HIE characteristically affects the gray matter structures, including the cerebral cortex, basal ganglia, and hippocampi in a

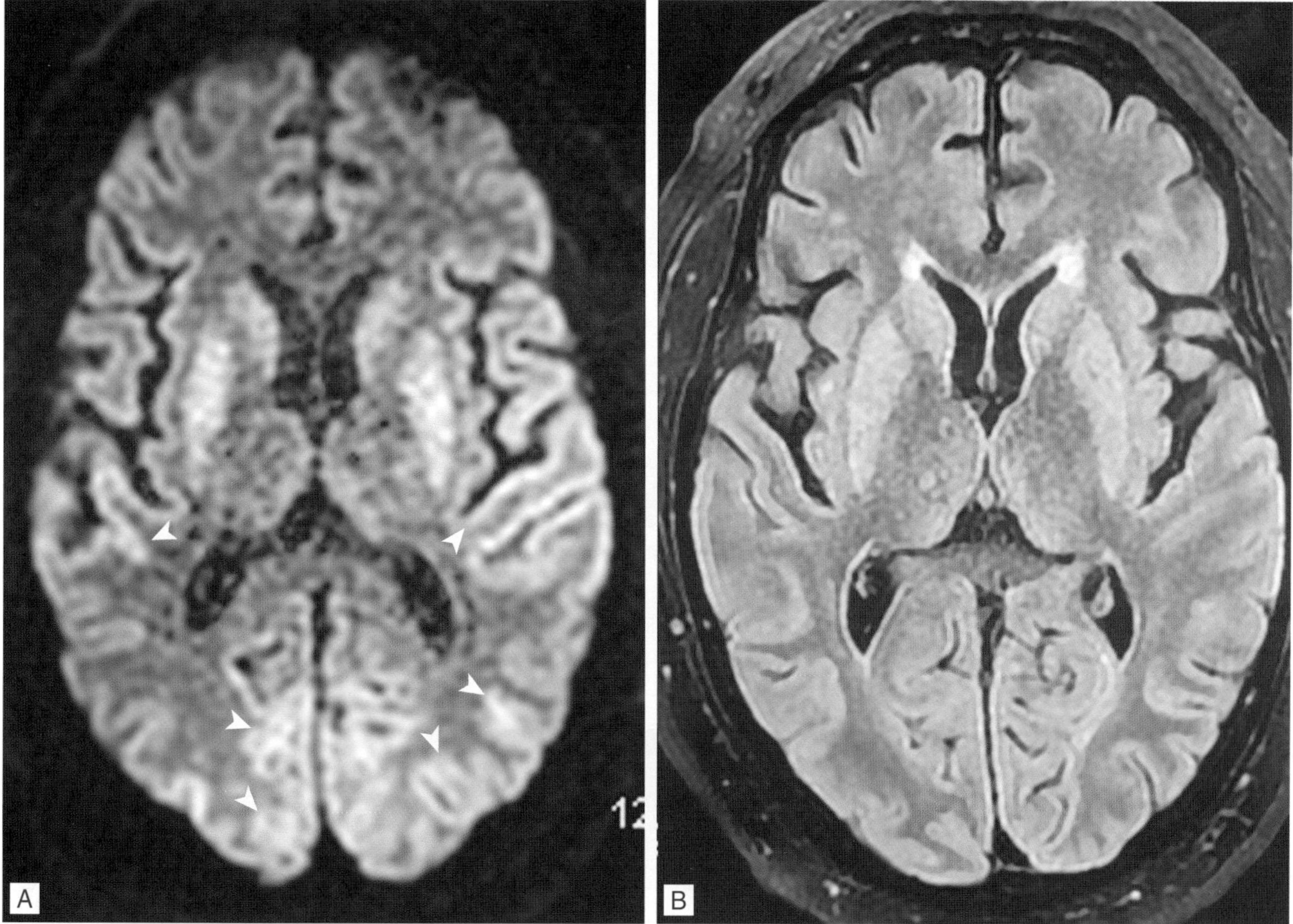

Figure 76.5 Hypoxic ischemic encephalopathy. A 55-year-old male with cardiac arrest. Axial DWI (*left*) and FLAIR (*right*) MRI images show reduced diffusivity and abnormal hyperintense signal in the deep gray structures (basal ganglia and thalami). There are associated areas of gyral swelling and abnormal signal in the cerebral cortices (*arrowheads*).

pattern similar to hypoglycemic encephalopathy. A differentiating feature may be the involvement of thalamus which is commonly involved in HIE but is consistently spared in hypoglycemic encephalopathy. (Fig. 76.5). In HIE, the "white cerebellum sign" and "reversal sign" are used to describe the sparing of the posterior fossa structures relative to the supratentorial parenchyma and sparing of the white matter relative to the gray matter on CT scans (Fig. 76.6). These findings in severe HIE usually indicate a poor prognosis [29,30].

Postictal changes may also present with mental obtundation after a prolonged episode of generalized tonic–clonic seizures, typically status epilepticus. On MRI, swelling and T2W /FLAIR hyperintensities and DWI restriction involving bilateral mesial temporal cortices/hippocampi are present. However, other areas of the cerebral cortices, subcortical white matter, corpus callosum, pulvinar region of the thalamus, and basal ganglia may show these changes [31–34]. Usually, the changes are reversible and resolve completely on follow-up imaging.

Teaching Point

In patients with unexplained coma, determination of blood serum sugar levels can help differentiate hypoglycemic encephalopathy, a potentially reversible condition from other causes such as HIE or acute cerebral infarction.

Hyperglycemic Encephalopathy

Metabolic disorders associated with hyperglycemia can broadly be classified into two categories, the first category occurring in younger patients with absolute insulin deficiency, characterized by ketosis and metabolic acidosis; known as **diabetic ketoacidosis** and the second category occurring in older patients with relative insulin deficiency, characterized by hyperosmolality without ketosis, and comparatively higher levels of serum glucose; known as **hyperosmolar hyperglycemic state (HHS).** Patients may present with drowsiness, lethargy, stupor or seizures with background polyuria, polydipsia, breathing abnormalities, and other constitutional symptoms.

The imaging findings in diabetic ketoacidosis are nonspecific and are seen in the form of diffuse cerebral edema, posterior reversible encephalopathy syndrome (PRES), CLOCC, and osmotic demyelination [26–28]. In HHS, parieto-occipital regions are commonly involved with areas of cortical hyperintensity and subcortical white matter *hypointensity* on T2W and FLAIR images [29]. This imaging finding is commonly associated with seizures. Imaging findings of PRES, CLOCC, and osmotic demyelination can also be seen with HHS [35–40].

By far the most dramatic and widely known clinical scenario in HHS or *nonketotic hyperglycemia* (NKH) is the occurrence of hemichorea–hemiballismus. The *characteristic imaging finding in this*

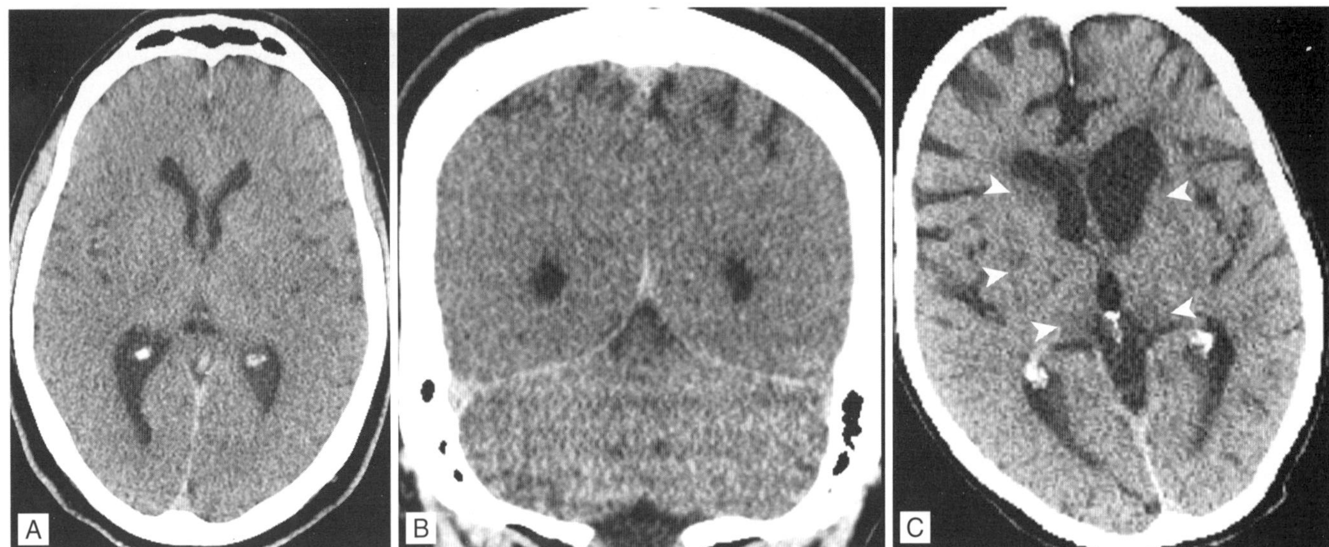

Figure 76.6 Hypoxic ischemic encephalopathy. Axial brain CT (A) in a patient with cardiac arrhythmia and arrest. Note the diffuse mottled appearance of the brain with loss of gray–white differentiation. The deep gray structures are not distinctly visible. Coronal brain algorithm CT (B) in the same patient shows diffuse hypodense appearance of the cerebrum with respect to the cerebellum (white cerebellum). Axial brain CT in another patient (C) with HIE shows hypodense appearance of the deep gray structures (*arrowheads*) with respect to the white matter (reversal sign). There is a pre-existing left corpus striatum infarct on the left with ex-vacuo dilatation of the left frontal horn in (C).

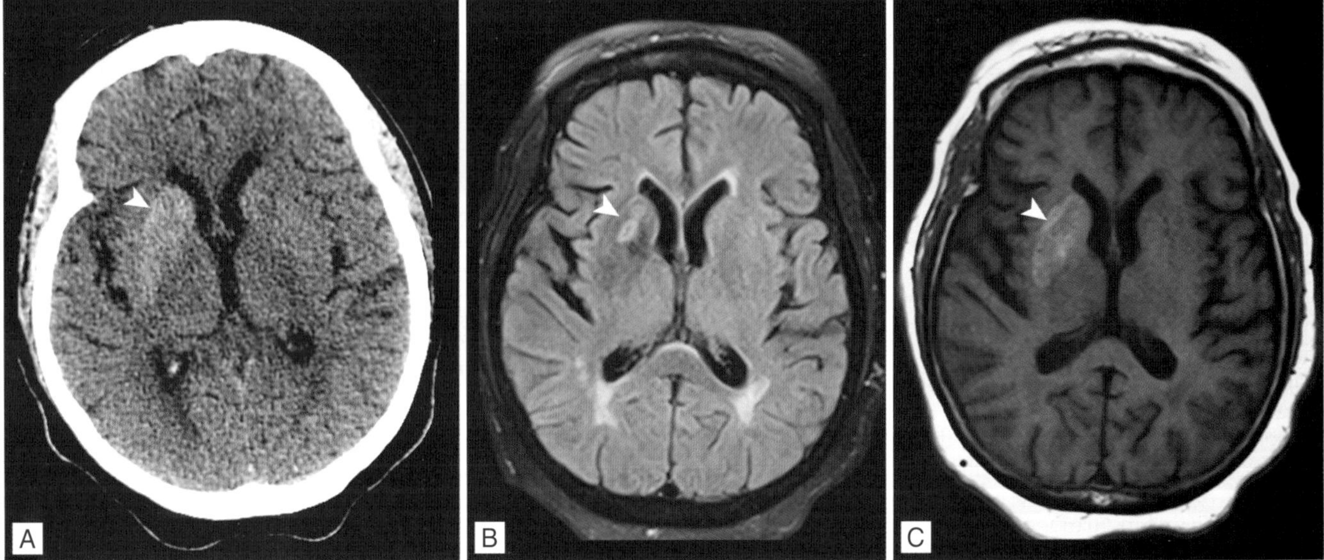

Figure 76.7 Nonketotic hyperglycemia. Diabetic patient presenting with hemichorea hemiballismus and elevated blood glucose. Axial noncontrasted CT of the head (*left image*) demonstrates unilateral asymmetric hyperattenuation of the right corpus striatum (*white arrowhead*). Axial FLAIR MRI (*middle image*) shows corresponding hypointensity. Axial T1-weighted sequence (*right image*) demonstrates associated T1 shortening/increased signal (*white arrowhead*) in the corpus striatum. Findings compatible with nonketotic hyperglycemic hemichorea.

clinical scenario is hyperattenuation of the basal ganglia (commonly caudate and putamen) contralateral to the chorea on CT, and T1W and T2W hyperintensity on MRI (Fig. 76.7). Low signal is noted on GRE/SWI images in the basal ganglia contralateral to the side of symptoms, which may not be apparent on initial imaging but may be seen on follow-up [41–45]. However, imaging findings may be present in the absence of hemichorea–hemiballismus. Findings may sometimes be bilateral. There is no contrast enhancement. Some of the proposed mechanisms for the T1W hyperintensity include hyperviscosity secondary to hyperglycemia, increased sensitivity of dopaminergic receptors and GABA depletion in the striatum [42,46,47].

Teaching Point

Typical imaging changes of hyperdensity or T1W hyperintensity in the basal ganglia may be present in patients with HHS/nonketotic hyperglycemia even without concurrent hemichorea–hemiballismus.

Uremic Encephalopathy

Acute or chronic renal failure causes accumulation of uremic compounds that are neurotoxic and lead to neurologic manifestations

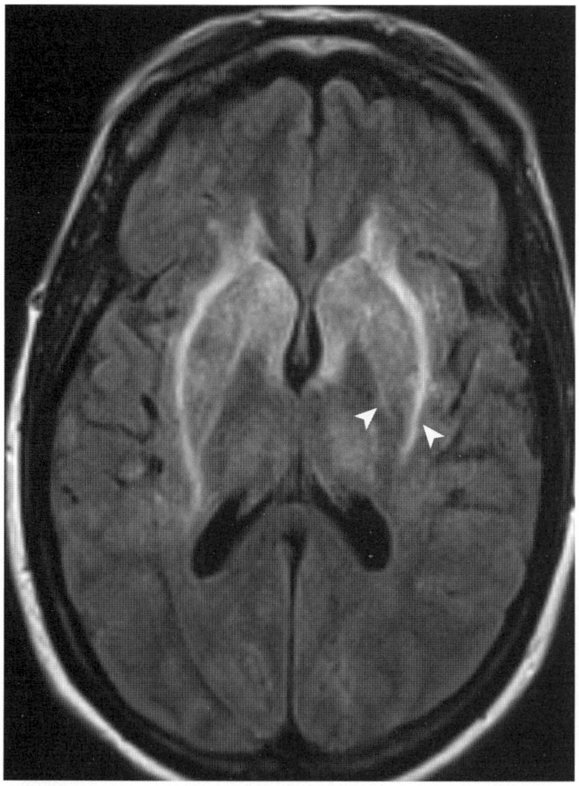

Figure 76.8 Uremic encephalopathy. Axial FLAIR MRI image of the brain in a 47-year-old female with renal failure shows symmetric putaminal hyperintensity with "lentiform fork" sign of hyperintense signal delineating the medial and lateral margins of the putamen (*arrowheads*).

that include confusion, seizures, movements disorders like tremors, asterixis, and myoclonus, etc. The mechanisms of the neurotoxicity are multifactorial, including hormonal disturbances, oxidative stress, imbalance of excitatory and inhibitory neurotransmitters, and disturbance of the intermediary metabolism [48]. EEG abnormalities are frequent in uremic encephalopathy (UE), characterized by disappearance of normal basic rhythm, appearance of theta waves and diminished reactivity to afferent stimulation [40].

On MRI, bilateral symmetrical involvement of the basal ganglia, and cortical and subcortical white matter may be present. Imaging manifestations of UE may be nonspecific and overlap those of could resemble PRES with presenting as bilateral symmetric cortical/subcortical parieto-occipital hyperintensities. *Lentiform fork sign* (Fig. 76.8) *is a characteristic imaging appearance, where T2W/FLAIR hyperintense rim-like regions marginate the lentiform nucleus/putamen.* These hyperintense regions involve the internal, external, and extreme capsules. Less commonly, symmetric confluent hyperintensities involve the centrum semiovale. Diffusion restriction may be present, particularly in the globus pallidus is but this is often inconsistent and indicates worse prognosis. Findings are largely reversible and improve after the initiation of dialysis [48–50].

Osmotic Demyelination

Osmotic demyelination may involve the pons (central pontine myelinolysis) or extrapontine structures (extrapontine myelinolysis). Extrapontine myelinolysis commonly occurs in conjunction with central pontine myelinolysis; however, it also may be seen in isolation. Osmotic demyelination is associated with electrolyte imbalances (in particular, rapid overcorrection of hyponatremia—increase in sodium level more than 12 mmol/L per day) which possibly leads to osmotic imbalance and myelin damage. Chronic alcoholics and malnourished patients are particularly susceptible to this osmotic imbalance, but other predispositions include prolonged use of diuretics, liver failure, organ transplantation, particularly liver transplantation with cyclosporine use, and extensive burns. The clinical manifestations are variable and include spastic hemiparesis, pseudobulbar palsy, decreased levels of consciousness, and coma [51].

Oligodendroglial cells are most susceptible to osmotic stresses, and the distribution of changes at MR imaging parallels the distribution of these cells in the central pons, thalamus, putamen, lateral geniculate bodies, and other extrapontine sites [52]. Abnormal T2W hyperintensity and T1W hypointensity are seen in the affected areas at MR imaging. *In central pontine myelinolysis, a symmetric trident-shaped or bat wing-shaped area of increased signal intensity in the central pons is characteristically seen on T2W and FLAIR MR images* (Fig. 76.9). The ventrolateral pons and the

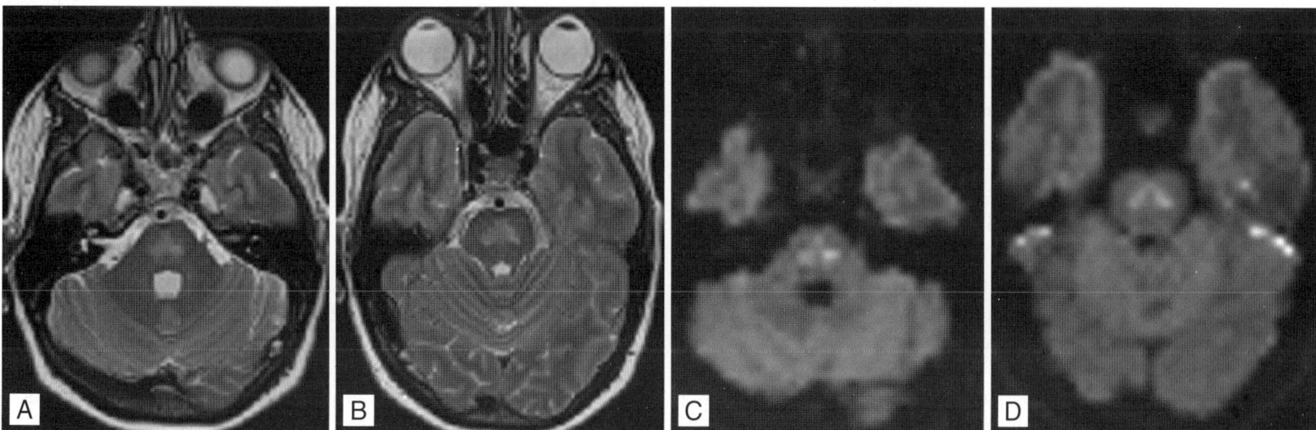

Figure 76.9 Osmotic demyelination (pontine myelinolysis). Axial T2W MRI images (A and B) and DWI MRI images (C and D) show abnormal signal within the central pons in a "trident" (A and C) or "triangular" (B and D) configuration. DWI changes may precede changes on T2W and FLAIR images. Note the sparing of the peripheral pons which is a differentiating feature from pontine changes seen in chronic cerebrovascular ischemic disease which tends to involve the lateral/peripheral areas.

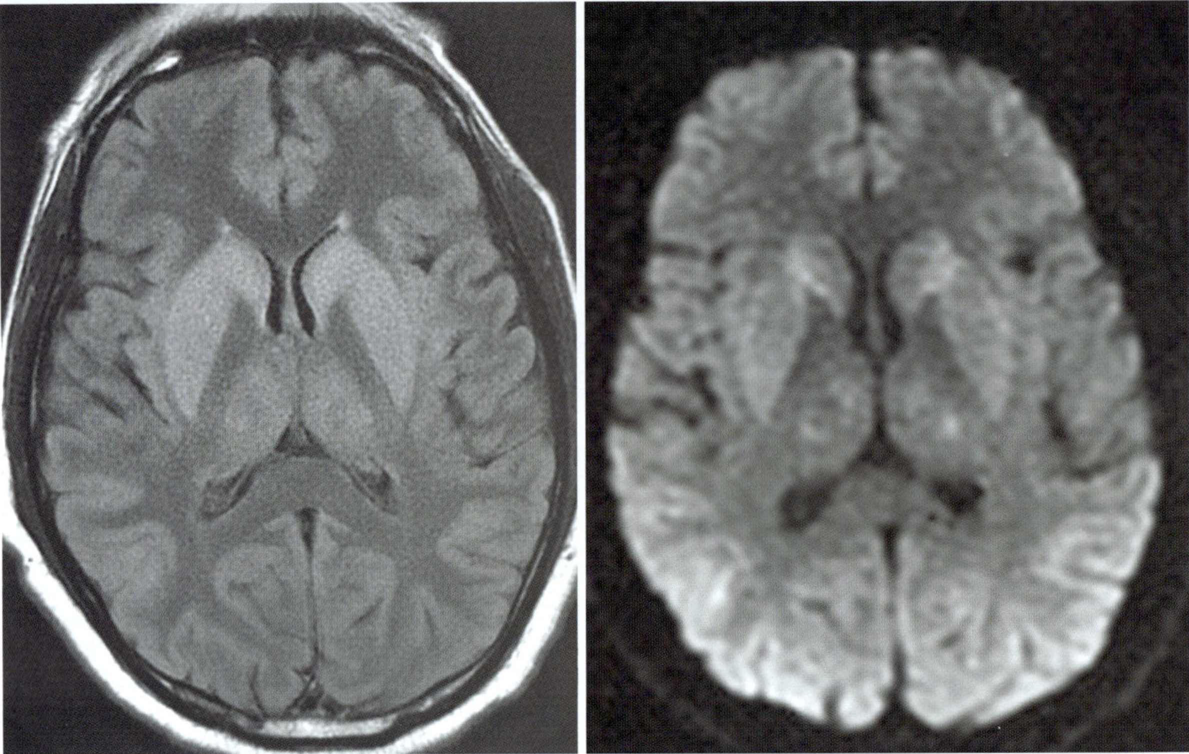

Figure 76.10 Extrapontine osmotic demyelination in a patient with rapid correction of hyponatremia. Axial FLAIR (*left*) and DWI (*right*) MRI images show abnormal symmetric hyperintense signal in the bilateral basal ganglia and to a lesser extent in the thalami.

pontine portion of the corticospinal tracts are typically spared [51]. Extrapontine myelinolysis manifests as areas of T2 prolongation in the globus pallidus, putamen, thalamus, and cerebellum (Fig. 76.10) [21]. The lesions may sometimes show restricted diffusion at diffusion-weighted MR imaging in the early stages of the disease process, although this is not typical. The imaging findings always follow the clinical manifestation with a lag of nearly 2 weeks or more. Serial measurements of serum sodium levels may be helpful for the diagnosis.

Parathyroid Disorders

Decreased and increased levels of parathormone can affect the brain due to alteration in the blood calcium levels [53]. Clinical presentation is variable with psychiatric and cognitive symptoms, reversible myopathy, neuromuscular irritability, paresthesias, and tetany.

There is calcium deposition in the basal ganglia including the globus pallidus, putamen, and the caudate nuclei. Calcium deposition may also be seen in thalami, dentate nuclei of the cerebellum, and the subcortical white matter. The abnormality is best seen as hyperdensity on CT or blooming hypointensity on SWI/GRE MRI images [10,11,14,54,55]. T1W hyperintensity and T2W hypointensity may be seen in the involved structures. Other radiological sequala of the disease like Brown tumors may be seen in the bones in hyperparathyroidism. Salt and pepper appearance of the bones of the skull due to bone resorption is seen in primary hyperparathyroidism and diffuse thickening of the skull and arterial calcifications are seen in secondary hyperparathyroidism [11].

Fahr Disease

Fahr disease (also known as bilateral strio-pallido-dentate calcinosis) is a rare neurodegenerative disease. Patients present with a gradual onset of nonspecific symptoms such as headache, vertigo, movement disorders, syncope, and seizures, dementia, and orthostatic hypotension. Intracranial calcification similar in pattern to that seen in parathyroid disorders is seen in a rare idiopathic neurodegenerative disorder known as Fahr disease.

Dense bilateral symmetric calcium deposits are seen in the basal ganglia, thalami, dentate nuclei, and subcortical white matter (Fig. 76.11), without the serum abnormalities of altered hormone or calcium levels. Nonspecific neurological symptoms of headache, ataxia, tremor, and dystonia may be seen. Imaging findings are indistinguishable from disorders of calcium metabolism, hypoparathyroidism, and pseudohypoparathyroidism and a serological work up of calcium and phosphorus and parathormone levels may be necessary to further narrow down the diagnosis [10,11,14,54–56].

Toxic Disorders

Although metabolic disorders result from abnormal levels of substances that are normally present in the human body, the term toxic encephalopathy is usually applied to brain affliction caused by extrinsic substances. These substances interfere with metabolic brain pathways and brain perfusion, and thus produce clinical and imaging manifestations that mimic the metabolic encephalopathies. Specific lab tests and clinical history proves useful in

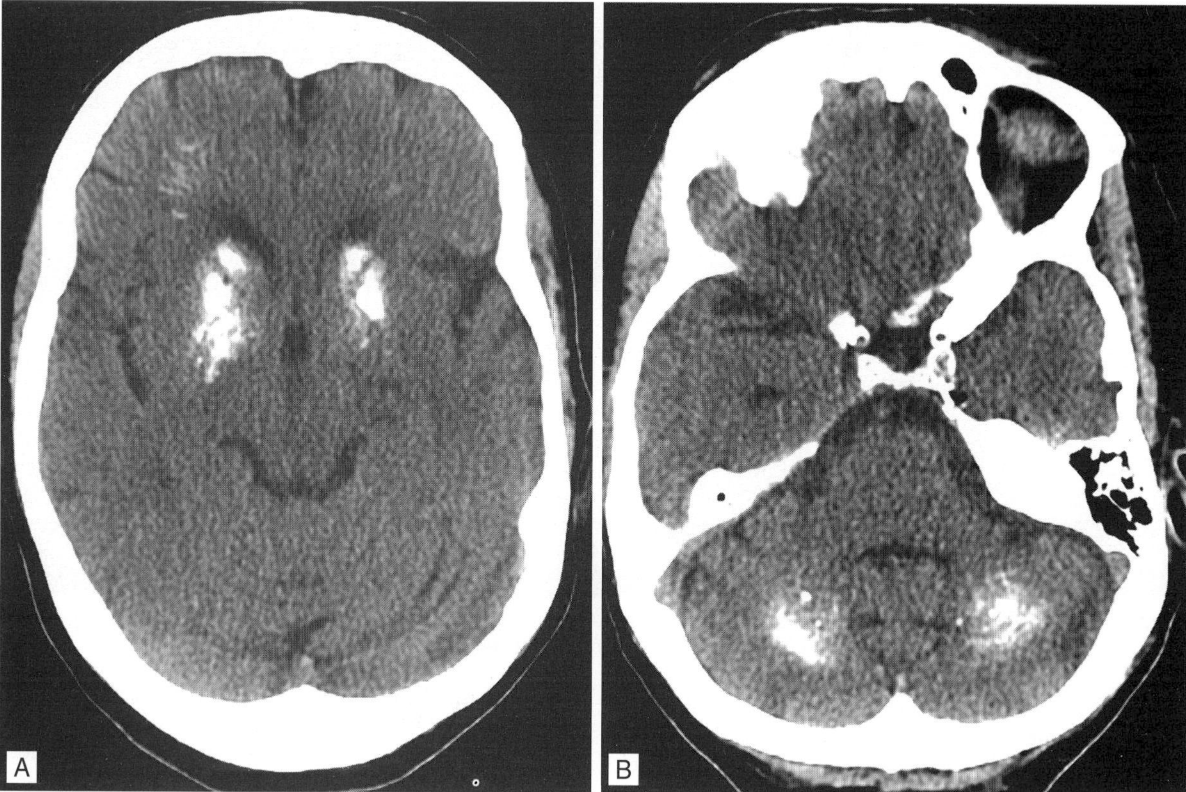

Figure 76.11 Fahr disease. Middle-aged male presenting with psychosis. Axial noncontrasted CT of the head demonstrates marked intraparenchymal calcifications in the corpus striatum, (A) periventricular white matter, and dentate nuclei (B) most compatible with Fahr's disease.

teasing out these toxic disorders and arriving at an accurate diagnosis.

Alcoholic Encephalopathy

Alcohol easily crosses the blood–brain barrier and affects many neurotransmitter systems. Alcohol can affect the brain by direct toxicity caused by upregulation of N-methyl-D-aspartate (NMDA) receptors, which increase the susceptibility to cytotoxic effects of glutamate. Dysfunction of synaptic connectivity, decreased expression of myelin protein encoding genes, and initiation of immune-mediated response to the brain tissue result in neuronal loss and white matter damage. Besides the direct toxic effects, alcohol affects the brain by causing nutritional deficiencies, the most important of which is thiamine (Vitamin B1), leading to Wernicke's encephalopathy (WE). Alcoholism can also affect the brain by its effects on the liver [57].

Rapid and large volume consumption of alcohol can cause acute toxicity, clinically presenting as seizures or unconsciousness. MRI features in these cases are nonspecific, with subcortical and deep white matter cytotoxic edema, imaging findings of osmotic demyelination, CLOCC, etc. [58–60]. A significant proportion of patients presenting with osmotic demyelination have a history of alcoholism. There may be diffuse cerebral edema [58–60].

Chronic alcohol intake causes brain atrophy, which begins in the superior vermis. As the direct toxic effects of alcohol progress in the brain, diffuse cerebellar atrophy may be seen, which differs from that in cerebellar degeneration by the sparing of pons. With further progression, there is atrophy of the frontal regions and finally there may be diffuse brain atrophy. The brain volume loss is due to involvement of both the gray and the white matter [58–61].

WE is caused by the deleterious effects of chronic alcoholism on thiamine intake, absorption, and cellular utilization. Malabsorption of thiamine due to gastrointestinal or hematologic neoplasms, chronic dialysis, bowel obstruction, hyperemesis gravidarum, or prolonged parenteral therapy without vitamin supplementation are other nonalcoholic causes of WE. *The classic clinical triad of WE is ocular dysfunction (in the form of ophthalmoplegia, nystagmus, conjugate gaze palsy), ataxia, and confusion.* However, the triad is not consistently present at clinical onset, and the symptoms may be confusing.

The regions of the brain commonly affected in typical WE are around the ventricles where the blood–brain barrier is deficient, namely the hypothalamus, mammillary bodies, periaqueductal gray, and the dorsomedial nuclei of the thalamus around the third ventricle. The affected regions demonstrate hyperintensity on T2W and FLAIR images (Fig. 76.12). True restricted diffusion can be seen due to cytotoxic edema or there may be T2-shine through due to vasogenic edema. There may be associated enhancement due to the disruption of blood–brain barrier. Enhancement can differentiate alcoholic WE from nonalcoholic WE. Symmetric alterations of the cerebellum, cranial nerve nuclei, red nuclei, caudate, splenium, and cerebral cortex are not typical and more often seen in nonalcoholism-related WE. Some of these features overlap with metronidazole-induced neurotoxicity.

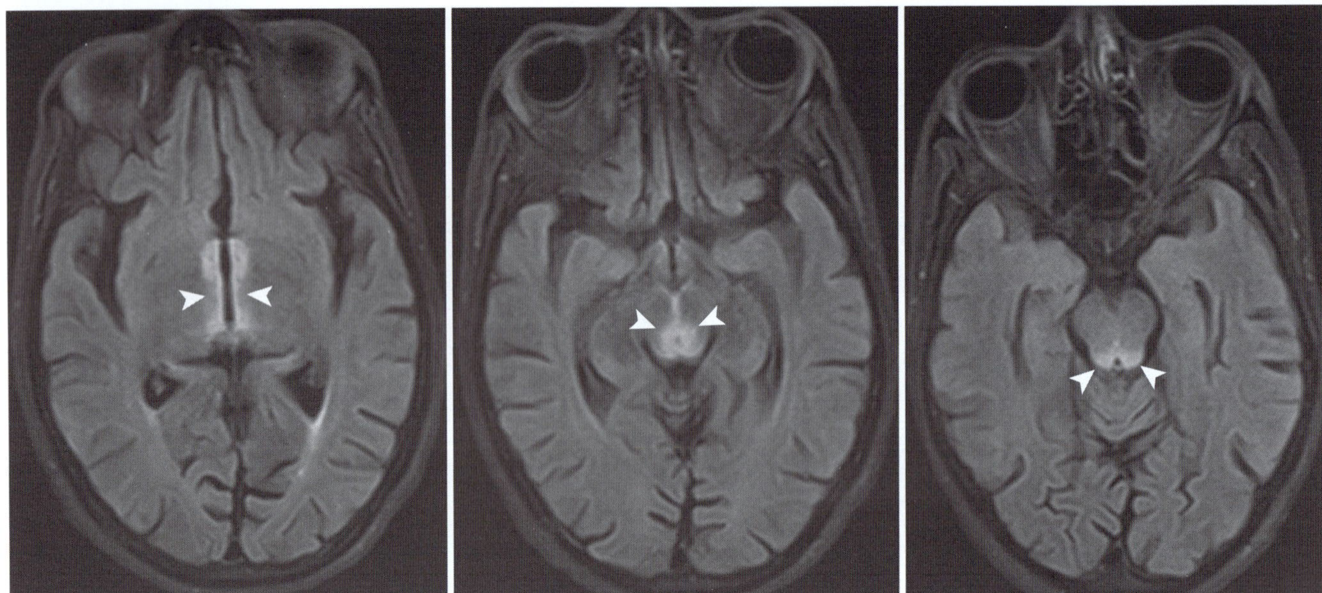

Figure 76.12 Wernicke encephalopathy. Man with history of alcohol abuse presents with ocular dysfunction. Axial FLAIR MRI images show abnormal hyperintense signal in the hypothalamus, around the third ventricle and in the periaqueductal regions (*arrowheads*).

WE represents a medical emergency, and treatment consists of intravenous replacement of thiamine [62]. Signal changes are reversible after successful treatment with thiamine. If left untreated, WE can progress to Wernicke–Korsakoff psychosis, which is an amnestic syndrome characterized by anterograde amnesia and confabulation [60,63–65].

A relatively rare disorder associated with chronic alcoholism is **Marchiafava–Bignami disease**. The corpus callosum is primarily affected in this disorder. In the acute form, the patients present with seizures, which may progress to coma and death within a few days. The entire corpus callosum is involved in acute cases. In the chronic form, the corpus callosum is involved in an anteroposterior configuration with the involvement of the genu in the early stages that progresses to involve the body, with relative sparing of the splenium. There is selective involvement of the middle layers of the corpus callosum, with sparing of the periphery. T2W and FLAIR sequences best demonstrate the abnormality. DWI hyperintensity and contrast enhancement may be seen in the acute phase. Corpus callosum atrophy can be seen in the chronic phase [61,65,66].

Carbon Monoxide Poisoning

Carbon monoxide (CO) poisoning is the most common cause of accidental poisoning in America. CO poisoning is a form of anoxic–ischemic encephalopathy due to impaired ability of the erythrocytes to transport oxygen. In the acute stages, the clinical presentation is with vomiting, headaches, visual disturbances, and altered mental status. Classical features of cherry red lips with peripheral cyanosis and retinal hemorrhages are rarely present [67]. Serum carboxyhemoglobin levels may be an important parameter to confirm the diagnosis. The chronic sequela of this condition includes memory deficits, dementia, mood disturbances, and parkinsonism.

CO has a propensity to affect the globus pallidus due to the high mitochondrial activity in these structures. The characteristic imaging feature of CO poisoning is globus pallidus necrosis (Fig. 76.13), seen as symmetric hypodensities on CT and hyperintensity on T2W/FLAIR MRI. Restricted diffusion may be seen in the acute phases and there may be associated hemorrhage. Rim enhancement is seen in the acute stages of the process. Other areas of involvement include the cerebral white matter, centrum semiovale, medial temporal lobes, and the hippocampi. Delayed leukoencephalopathy/encephalomalacia, lamellar necrosis, T1W hyperintensity of the globus pallidus, and diffuse atrophy may be seen in the chronic stages [68–72].

Methanol Poisoning

Methanol is a constituent of many liquids and poisoning from this toxin may occur from intentional or accidental ingestion of these liquids. Common among these are antifreeze, inadequately distilled ethanol, paint remover, and photocopying fluid. Methanol is metabolized to formic acid which is toxic to the optic nerves and the putamen. There is severe anion gap metabolic acidosis with patients presenting with altered mental status and a comatose state. Methanol poisoning, in particular, may manifest with optic neuritis as its initial symptom. Prognosis is poor with high mortality.

Imaging shows selective involvement of the putamina with relative sparing of the globi pallidi (commonly involved in CO poisoning). Optic nerve T2W/FLAIR hyperintensity/necrosis may be seen. Hemorrhagic necrosis is a common feature and white matter edema may be an additional feature of methanol poisoning [73–76].

Teaching Point
Respiratory toxins like CO, methanol, and cyanide tend to cause bilateral MR imaging abnormalities in the lentiform nuclei, sometimes with white matter involvement.

Toxicity From Recreational Drugs

Many recreational drugs in common use, including cocaine, methamphetamine, heroin, 3,4-Methyl enedioxy methamphetamine (MDMA), and cannabis, have frequent adverse effects on the brain. The mechanism of neurotoxicity is commonly vascular with many of these agents inducing vasoconstriction and vasculitis.

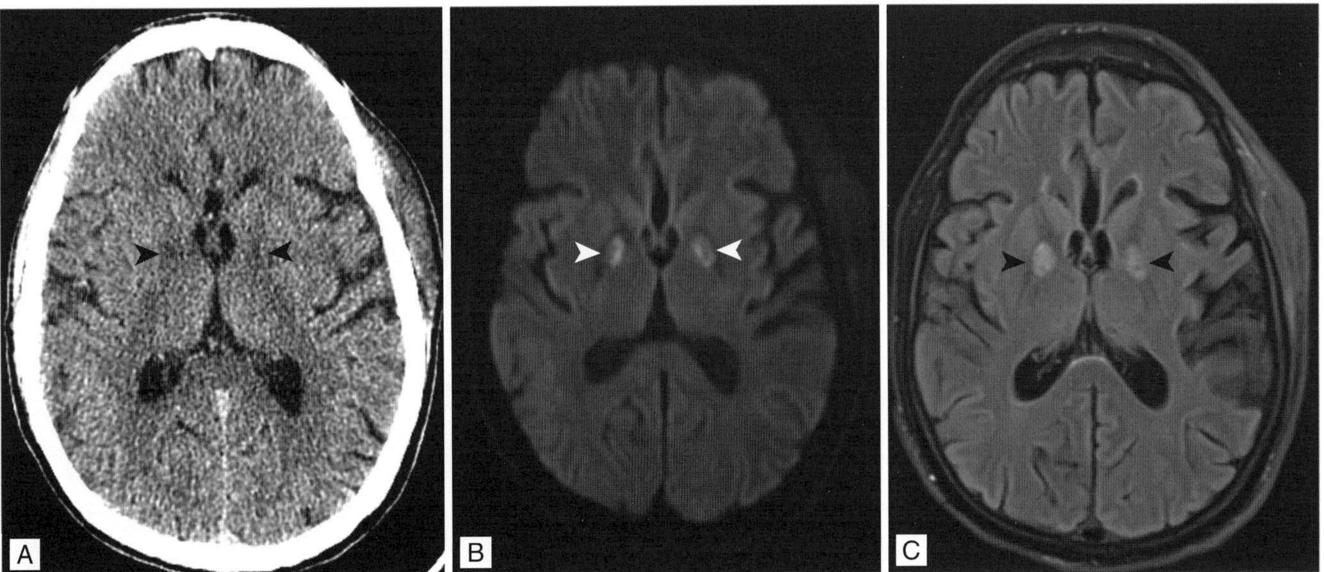

Figure 76.13 Carbon monoxide poisoning. Homeless man found down and altered in a car repair shop in winter. Axial noncontrast CT of the head (A) shows focal hypoattenuation in bilateral globi pallidi. Axial diffusion-weighted MRI image (B) and FLAIR image (C) demonstrate focal restricted diffusion and increased signal respectively in the same location. Globi pallidi are the most affected in the anoxic injury caused by CO poisoning (*arrowheads*).

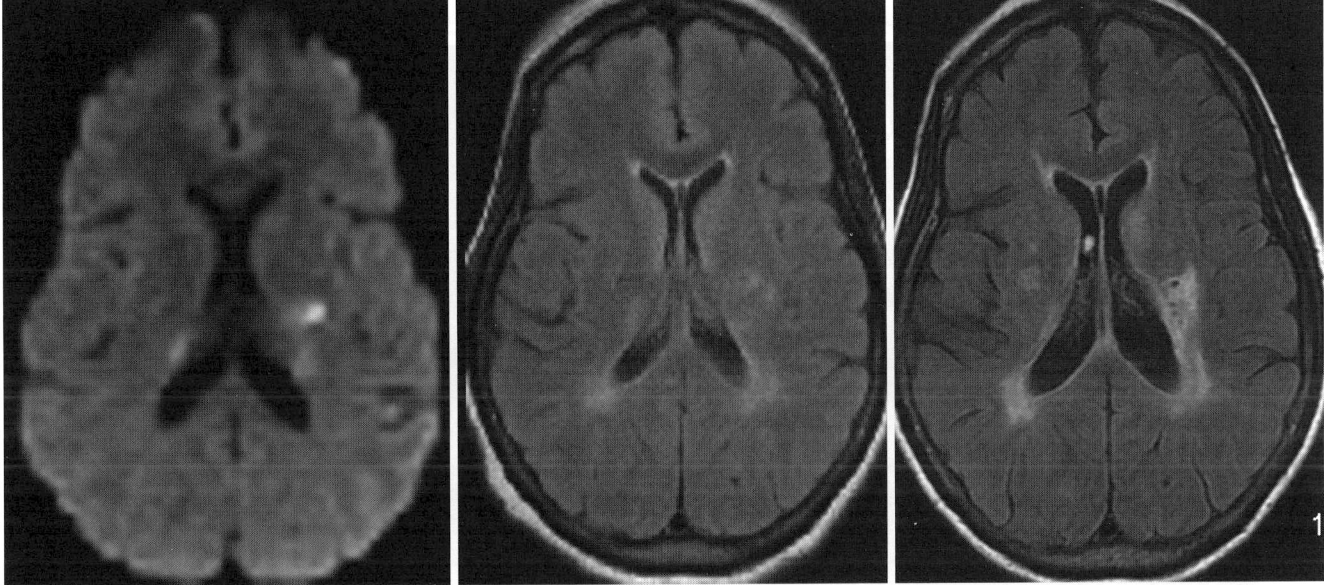

Figure 76.14 Cocaine abuse: bilateral corona radiata infarcts on axial DWI MRI image (*left*) in a 30-year-old presenting to the emergency room with stroke-like symptoms with history of cocaine use and no other vascular risk factors. Abnormal hyperintense white matter changes indicative of previous ischemic changes on axial FLAIR MRI image (*center*). Axial FLAIR MRI image (*right*) 2 years later in the same patient with continued cocaine use shows worsened white matter changes and interval volume loss consistent with continued chronic ischemic white matter changes. Most sequela of drug use on the brain are due to their effects on the cerebral vasculature.

The resultant lesions therefore are commonly vascular with areas of ischemic/infarcts (Fig. 76.14), subarachnoid or parenchymal hemorrhage, hypoxic–ischemic brain injury, and pseudoaneurysms. Inhalation of heroin vapors termed as "chasing the dragon" results in specific form spongiform leukoencephalopathy in the cerebral and cerebellar white matter and the corticospinal and solitary tracts (Fig. 76.15). MRI shows symmetric high signal on T2-weighted and FLAIR sequences in the cerebellum and the posterior limb of the internal capsule, with sparing of the anterior limb [77].

The basal ganglia are commonly involved although any region in the brain can be affected. History of illicit drug use and lab tests for the presence of toxins in the blood and urine are useful indicators to the diagnosis. Frequently, a single drug is difficult to implicate since polysubstance abuse is common [8,11,15,78–80].

Teaching Point

In young patients with unexplained neurovascular abnormalities on imaging like territorial or watershed infarcts, vascular occlusions, aneurysms or, intracranial hemorrhages, possibility of drug intoxication should be considered.

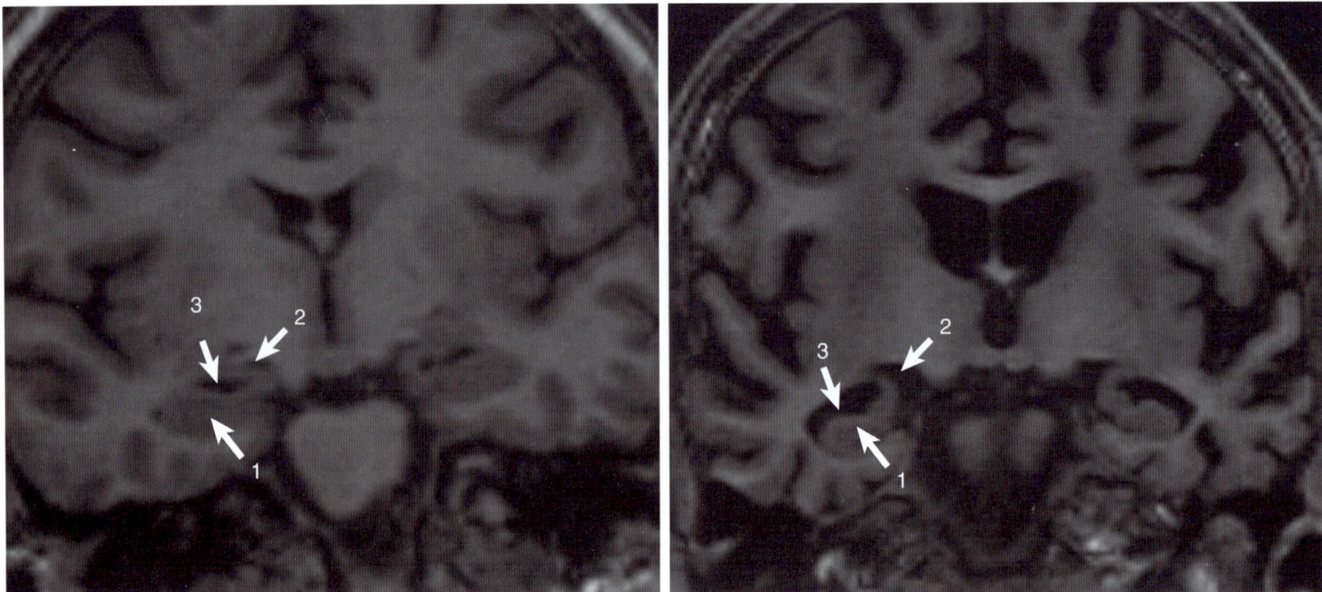

Figure 76.23 Visual assessment of hippocampal atrophy. Coronal T1W MRI images through the hippocampus in a normal patient (*left*) and in a patient with mild hippocampal atrophy (*right*). Visual determination of hippocampal atrophy requires assessment of the height of the hippocampus (1), width of the choroidal fissure (2), and the width of the temporal horn (3). Note the maintained height of the hippocampus and nearly collapsed choroidal fissure and temporal horn on the left image versus decreased hippocampal height and increased width of the choroidal fissure and temporal horn on the right image.

segmentation software [94]. Hypometabolism of the involved structures can be imaged by ^{18}F-FDG PET (Figs. 76.24 and 76.25), which can demonstrate typical lateral temporoparietal, posterior cingulate/precuneus, and medial temporal lobe hypometabolism in AD. PET can also be used to directly evaluate for the presence of amyloid-beta neuritic plaques or tau neurofibrillary tangles, providing noninvasive, in vivo evidence of the presence of this neuropathology, although these tests have lower sensitivity for early-stage deposits.

Although AD typically presents with an amnestic syndrome, there are atypical clinical presentations. The logopenic variant of PPA, which has predominant language symptoms, and posterior cortical atrophy (PCA), which has predominant visuospatial symptoms, are usually caused by underlying AD neuropathology [104,108,131]. These syndromes have early neurodegeneration and tau aggregation in regions associated with language and visual function, respectively, which is unusual for AD. However, the presence of tau neurofibrillary tangles and amyloid deposition in these atypical forms are shared with typical presentations of AD.

Teaching Point
AD is the most common neurodegenerative disease of the elderly, associated with amyloid and tau aggregation and typically an amnestic presentation.

Atypical AD

Logopenic Variant Primary Progressive Aphasia: Logopenic progressive aphasia (LvPPA) is most frequently due to AD neuropathology and is the most common atypical presentation of early onset AD. The core clinical features of LvPPA are impaired single-word retrieval and impaired repetition of sentences and phrases in spontaneous speech

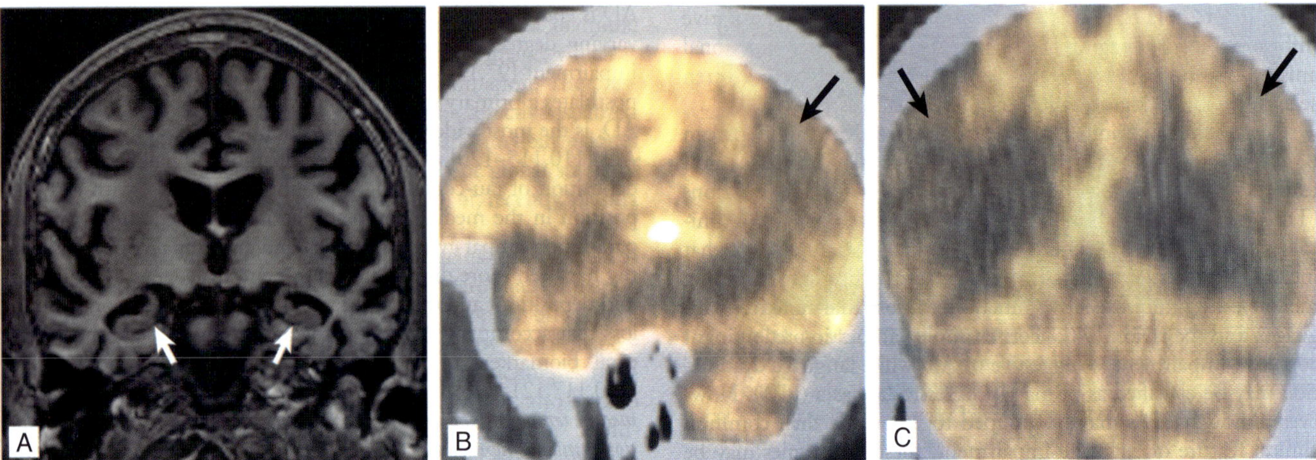

Figure 76.24 Alzheimer's disease. Coronal thin slice T1W MRI image (A) through the temporal lobes shows medial temporal lobe and bilateral hippocampal (*white arrows*) atrophy with ex vacuo dilated temporal horns. Sagittal (B) and coronal (C) ^{18}F-FDG-PET images of the brain show bilateral parietal (*black arrows*) and temporal lobe hypometabolism. Hippocampal volume loss and parietal and temporal lobe hypometabolism are features of Alzheimer's disease.

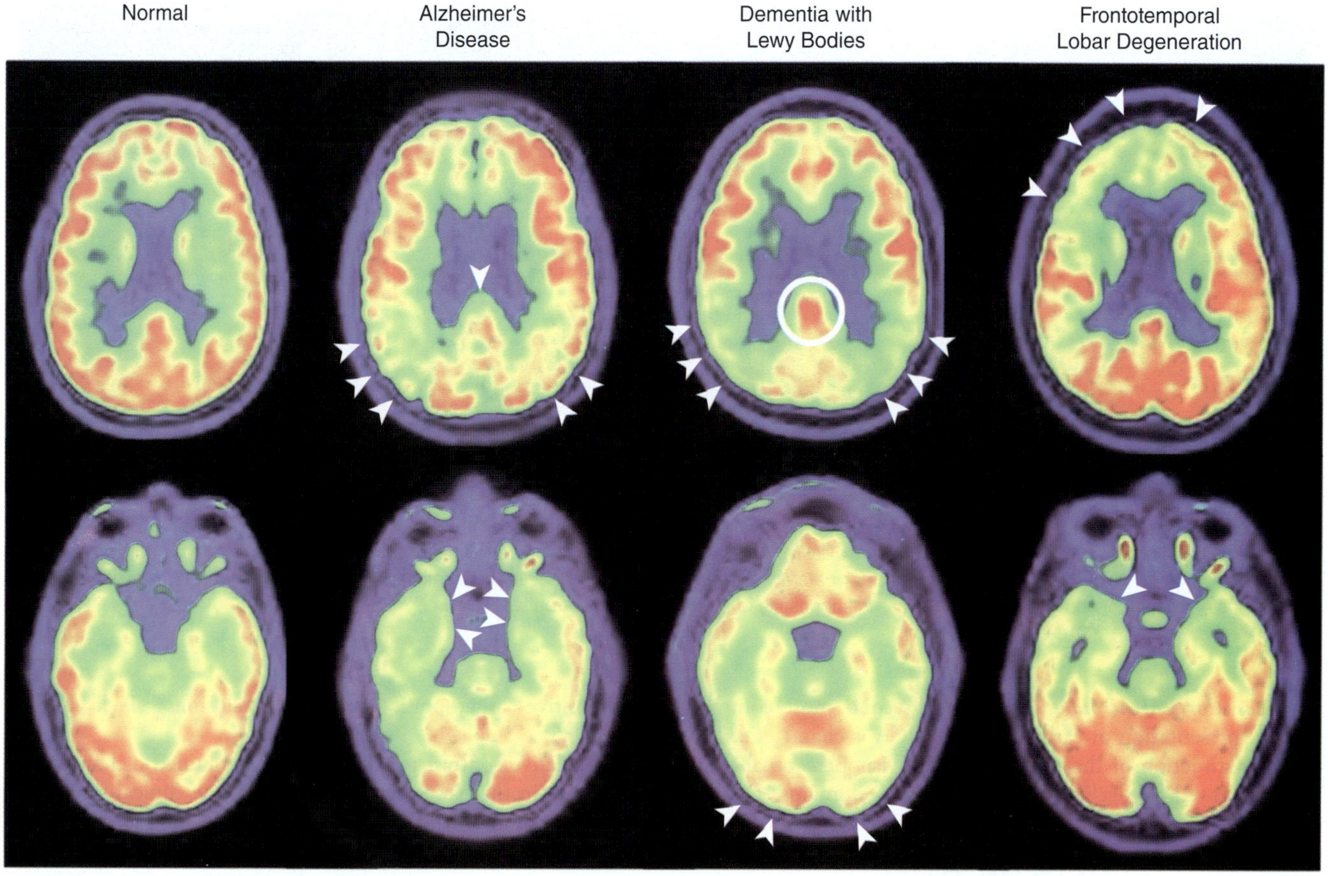

Normal | Alzheimer's Disease | Dementia with Lewy Bodies | Frontotemporal Lobar Degeneration

Figure 76.25 ^{18}F-FDG PET of the brain for neurodegenerative disease. Normal brain shows diffuse high uptake in gray matter (*red*). In Alzheimer's disease, there is hypometabolism in parietal and temporal cortex, including medial temporal structures, as well as the posterior cingulate cortex (*arrowheads*). In Dementia with Lewy bodies, there is similar temporoparietal hypometabolism, but also occipital hypometabolism (*arrowheads*, *bottom*) but preserved posterior cingulate cortex metabolism (*circled*). In frontotemporal lobar degeneration, there is variable frontal and temporal hypometabolism. In this case, there is right greater than left, frontal more than anterior temporal lobe hypometabolism.

and confrontation naming [99–102]. LvPPA has a high rate of amyloid/tau pathology upon PET imaging and autopsy [100,105,108]. *There is atrophy centered at the left temporoparietal junction involving the left inferior parietal and superior temporal regions* (Fig. 76.26) *including the supramarginal and angular gyri;* ^{18}F-FDG PET shows left-greater-than-right temporoparietal hypometabolism [100,105,108]. There is frequent hippocampal volume loss.

Teaching Point

LvPPA is usually an atypical presentation of AD with deficiencies in word retrieval and repetition. Left inferior parietal, superior temporal, and temporoparietal junction neurodegeneration, with frequent hippocampal involvement are typical of LvPPA.

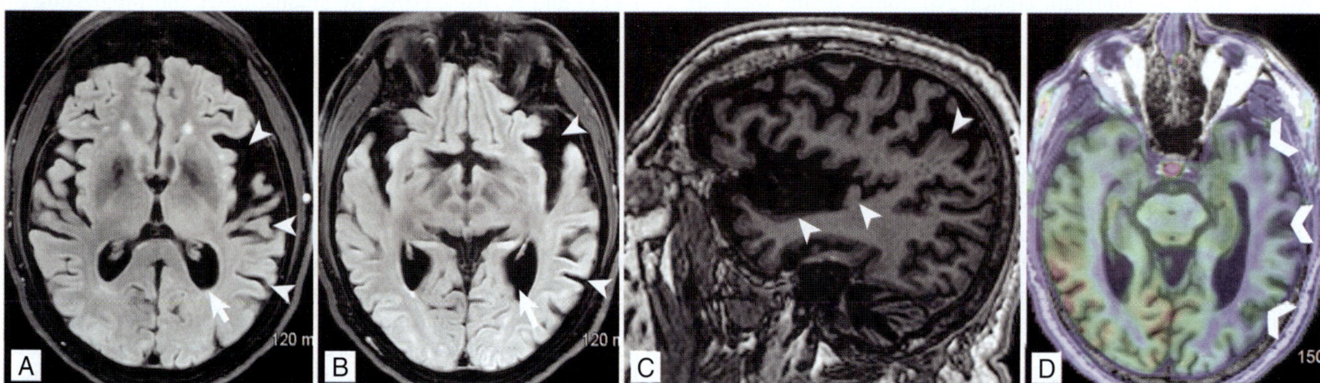

Figure 76.26 Elderly female with 2-year history of word finding difficulty and memory decline. Impaired sentence repetition on neuropsychological testing. Axial FLAIR images (A and B) and sagittal T1W image (C) show left predominant superior temporal, inferior parietal, and temporoparietal volume loss with asymmetric prominence of the left sylvian fissure (*arrowheads*). Mild left ventricle dilatation is ex vacuo due to left-sided volume loss (*arrow*). Axial ASL MRI (D), shown as a color overlay on T1 MRI, demonstrates hypoperfusion (likely hypometabolism related) in the areas showing atrophy (*chevrons*).

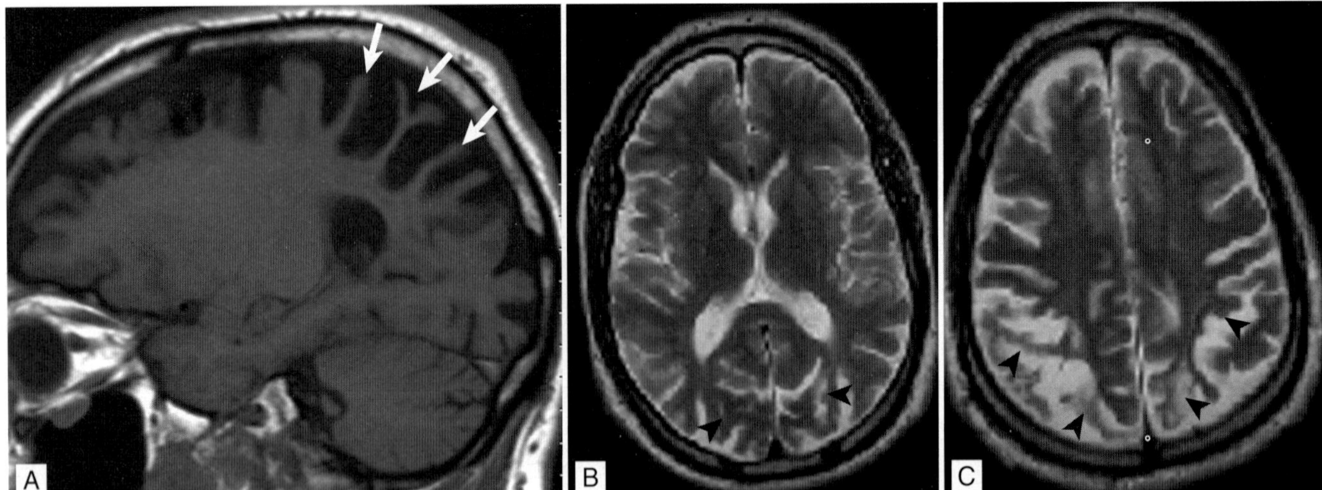

Figure 76.27 Sagittal T1W MRI image (A) shows marked posterior parietal and occipital lobe atrophy with knife-like gyri (*arrows*). Profound bilateral parietal and occipital lobe atrophy also noted on T2W axial MRI images (B and C) shown by arrowheads. The patient had a history of difficulty reading and trouble climbing stairs. He had been operated for cataract 2 years ago without benefit and continued progression of symptoms. This pattern of bilateral posterior parietal and occipital volume loss is suggestive of posterior cortical atrophy.

Posterior Cortical Atrophy: PCA is the second most common atypical presentation of early onset AD. PCA is characterized by initial dysfunction of the visuospatial and visuoperceptual functions, followed by decline in other cognitive domains. Defined syndromically, the causative neuropathological processes are heterogeneous, however AD with amyloidopathy and tauopathy is the most common [111,131,132]. Other far less frequent pathologies include DLB, corticobasal degeneration (CBD), or prion-associated disease processes. There is involvement of bilateral occipitoparietal areas in PCA, evident on structural imaging, ^{18}F-FDG PET, and ASL (Fig. 76.27) [131–133].

Frontotemporal Lobar Degeneration

FTLD is a genetically, neuropathologically, and phenotypically heterogeneous group of neurodegenerative disorders that typically feature progressive deterioration of behavior or language and are usually associated with neurodegeneration in the frontal and/or temporal lobes. FTLD collectively is most prevalent in the 45–64-year age group with comparable prevalence to AD for early-onset neurodegenerative dementia. FTLD includes six subtypes based on anatomic, genetic, and neuropathologic criteria. Three predominant clinical syndromes define these six subtypes.

The most common is a behavioral/dysexecutive disorder known as the behavioral variant frontotemporal degeneration (bvFTD). Language disorders associated with FTLD include two variants of PPA, the semantic variant (SV) and progressive nonfluent/agrammatic aphasia (PNFA). Certain motor disorders with common genetic, syndromic, or pathophysiologic features are classified as FTLD including progressive supranuclear palsy (PSP), CBD, and motor neuron disease (MND) [97,111–114,134,135]. Genetic cases of FTLD are most frequently associated with mutations in progranulin (*GRN*), microtubule-associated protein tau (*MAPT*), and *C9ORF72* genes [134–138]. On a neuropathological basis, these FTD variants most frequently demonstrate either a tauopathy or a Transactive response DNA binding protein of 43 kDa (TDP-43) proteinopathy as an underlying pathophysiological process, although other proteinopathy variants are also known. The previous term of "Pick's disease" previously used interchangeably with bvFTD is now reserved for patients showing tau-positive argyrophilic neuronal inclusions (Pick bodies) [134,135].

In relative contrast to AD, where the volumetric changes predominate in the parietotemporal regions, the clinical syndromes in FTD commonly demonstrate focal gray matter volumetric changes in bilateral dorsolateral and medial frontal, and insular regions [111,113,114,136,138]. Besides these shared areas of abnormalities, specific regions of damage are found in each variant (Fig. 76.28).

Teaching Point
FTLD is a heterogeneous group of neurodegenerative disorders with six primary subtypes; behavioral variant FTD, semantic variant PPA, progressive nonfluent aphasia, motor neuron disease, progressive supranuclear palsy and corticobasal degeneration. TDP-43 proteinopathy and tauopathy are usually the underlying neuropathology.

Behavioral Variant FTD: BvFTD is the most common form of FTLD and is characterized by gradual onset and progression of behavior, executive function, and/or personality changes with relative sparing of memory and visuospatial functions. The characteristic pattern of volume loss seen in bvFTD is involvement of the frontal and temporal lobes; while most commonly symmetric, the neurodegenerative pattern may be asymmetric [111,134–137,139,140].

MRI may show much more severe cortical atrophy in bvFTD compared with AD, resulting in a "*knife-edge*" *gyri on structural MRI* and 76.29). Hypoperfusion and hypometabolism of the frontal and temporal lobes seen on ASL/^{18}F-FDG PET with relative sparing of the parietal lobes contrasts to the posterior-predominant pattern in AD (Fig. 76.30). Amyloid PET imaging may also help differentiate FTD from AD, since FTD typically shows no or very little amyloid binding [111,134–137,139,140]. Although some forms of bvFTD are caused by tauopathy, the first- and second-generation tau PET tracers have low affinity for the prevalent isoforms in this disease.

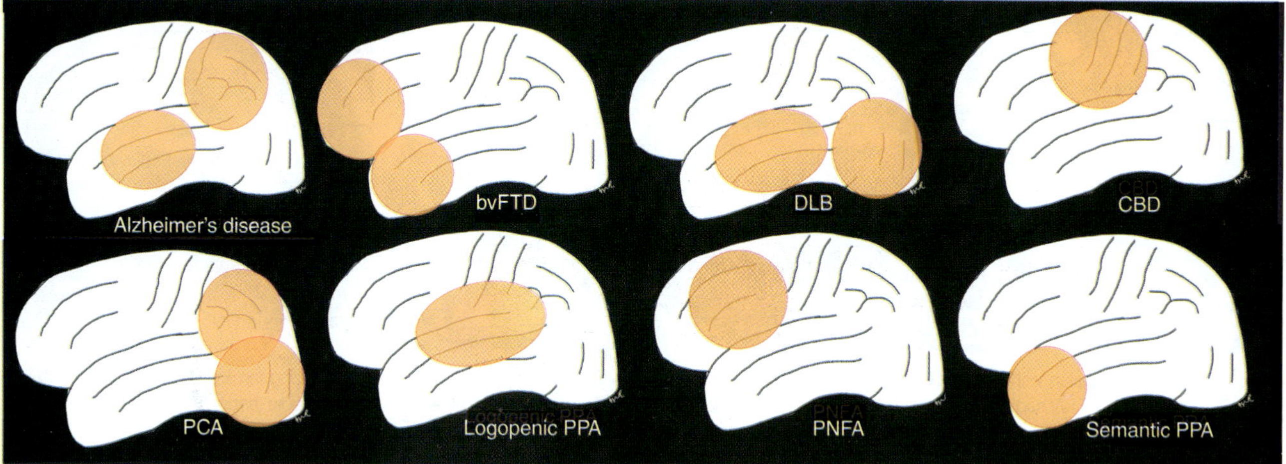

Figure 76.28 Patterns of neurodegenerative disorders. *bvFTD*, Behavioral variant frontotemporal degeneration; *CBD*, Corticobasal degeneration; *DLB*, Dementia with Lewy bodies; *PCA*, Posterior cortical atrophy; *PNFA*, Progressive nonfluent aphasia; *PPA*, Primary progressive aphasia.

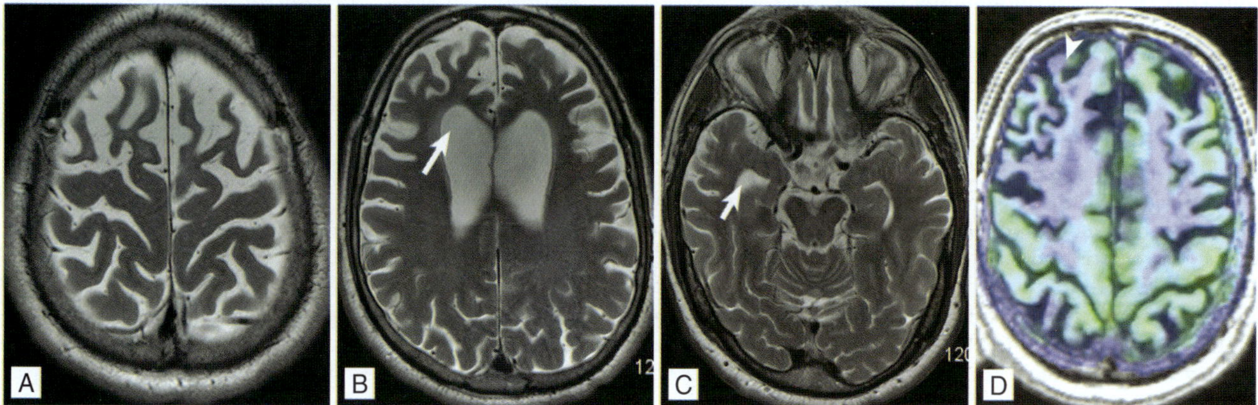

Figure 76.29 A 60-year-old male patient with history of inappropriate behavior, history of financial mismanagement. Bifrontal and bitemporal atrophy on T2W MRI images (A, B, and C) is more pronounced on the right evident by increased sulcal prominence and asymmetric ex vacuo prominence of the frontal and temporal horns (*arrows*). ASL MRI image (D), overlaid in color on T1 MRI, shows bifrontal hypoperfusion (likely due to hypometabolism) which is also more pronounced on the right (*arrowhead*). The pattern of brain atrophy is suggestive of behavioral variant of frontotemporal lobar degeneration. Note the thinned knife-edge gyri on image A indicative of marked atrophy.

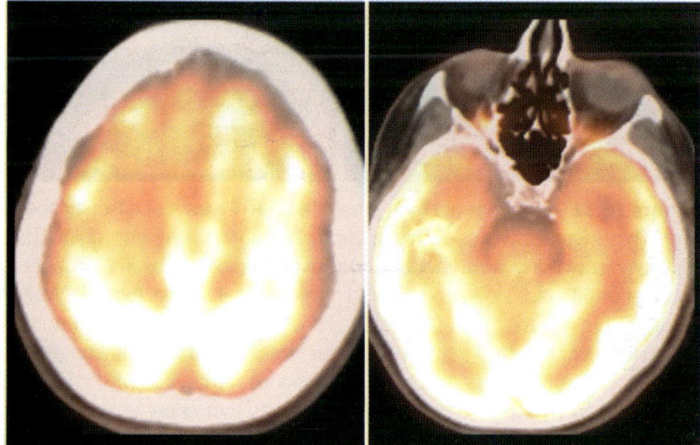

Figure 76.30 Selected axial ^{18}F-FDG-PET images of the brain in a patient with behavioral variant FTD show bifrontal and bitemporal hypometabolism, with greater involvement of the right side.

Semantic Variant Primary Progressive Aphasia: The core clinical features of svPPA are anomia and single-word comprehension deficits. The volumetric changes in svPPA affect the ventral and lateral portions of the anterior temporal lobes. Although bilateral anterior temporal lobes are affected, the majority of patients demonstrate a left asymmetric pattern, matching the left dominant pattern of language localization in the human brain. The anterior temporal lobe volume loss or hypometabolism on ^{18}F-FDG PET may be striking is usually disproportionate to other brain regions (Figs. 76.28 and 76.31). A common volumetric MRI feature of svPPA is asymmetric hippocampal volume loss, seen on the side of temporal lobe atrophy. Genetic causes are infrequent in svPPA and TDP-43 (Tar DNA-binding protein of 43 kDa) proteinopathy is the most common underlying neuropathology [107,141–144].

Teaching Point

Bilateral frontotemporal volume loss and hypometabolism is a feature of bvFTD. Behavioral, executive function, and personality symptoms are common with relative sparing of memory.

Teaching Point

Anomia and single-word comprehension deficits are core features of svPPA. Left anterior temporal pole and left asymmetric anterior hippocampal volume loss are imaging features of svPPA.

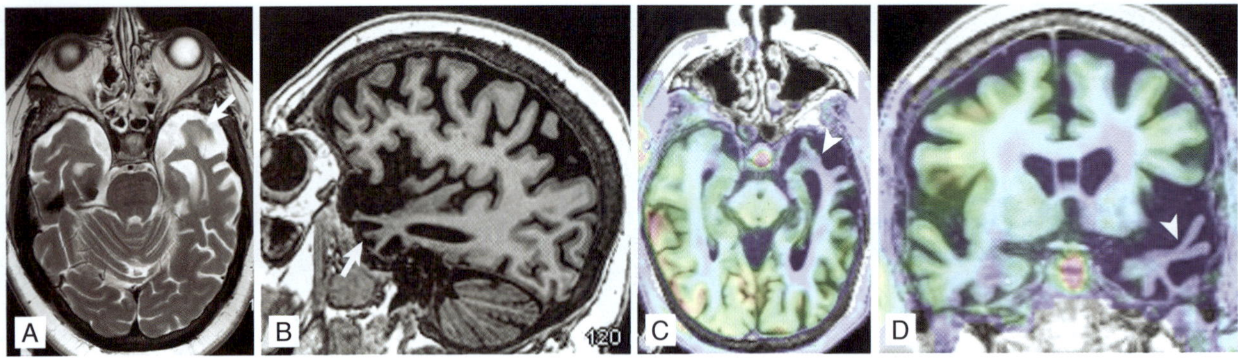

Figure 76.31 Septuagenarian with difficulty in understanding words and following conversations. She has trouble recognizing familiar faces (prosopagnosia). Axial T2W MRI image (A) and T1W sagittal image (B) show atrophy of the left temporal lobe especially of the anterior temporal pole (*arrows*). ASL MRI images, as color overlays on T1 MRI (C) and (D), show anterior temporal pole hypoperfusion (*arrowhead*), likely related to hypometabolism. The left temporal pole is considered an important area for semantic language processing in right-handed individuals. This imaging appearance is suggestive of semantic variant of primary progressive aphasia especially in this clinical context.

Progressive Nonfluent/Agrammatic Variant Aphasia: PNFA is a second phenotype of PPA that is within the FTLD spectrum. On a neuropathological basis, PNFA is usually associated with the accumulation of tau proteins [99,101,102,135,137,145]. Later in the course of disease, patients with PNFA may develop features of PSP and CBD, which are also associated with underlying tauopathy.

Neurodegeneration in PNFA is most commonly seen in the left inferior frontal region. The abnormality extends beyond the pars opercularis and pars triangularis to involve the anterior insula, left prefrontal regions, supplementary motor area, and superior portions of the left anterior temporal lobe [99,101–103,135–137,146]. Hypometabolism or hypoperfusion may be seen in these regions on ^{18}F-FDG PET or ASL, respectively (Figs. 76.28 and 76.32).

Teaching Point

Left inferior frontal lobe and perisylvian neurodegeneration is typical for PNFA. PNFA is usually due to a tauopathy, and cases may develop PSP or CBS later in disease.

Frontotemporal Dementia-motor Neuron Disease: There is a strong link between FTD and ALS, which is a neurodegenerative MND. Either FTD or ALS may present initially, with some cases progressing to both. Most FTD-MND patients show an underlying TDP-43 proteinopathy [134,135,147]. Associated FTD is more common in bulbar onset ALS compared with limb onset ALS. FTD-MND may be associated with frontotemporal neurodegeneration. Abnormal hyperintensity is noted along the corticospinal tracts on T2W and FLAIR MRI (Fig. 76.33). Additionally, gyriform hypointensity may be present along the motor cortices on susceptibility-weighted imaging (SWI/GRE) [148,149].

Progressive Supranuclear Palsy and Corticobasal Degeneration: PSP and CBD are two neurodegenerative syndromes associated with cognitive impairment and parkinsonism that most commonly demonstrate a tauopathy as the underlying neuropathology. In fact, syndromic overlap can occur between these syndromes and PNFA, another tauopathy. As these syndromes result in damage to the nigrostriatal dopamine pathway, ^{123}I-FP-CIT (3-fluoropropyl)-2β-carboxymethoxy-3β-(4-iodophenyl) nortropane SPECT, which measures the dopamine reuptake transporter

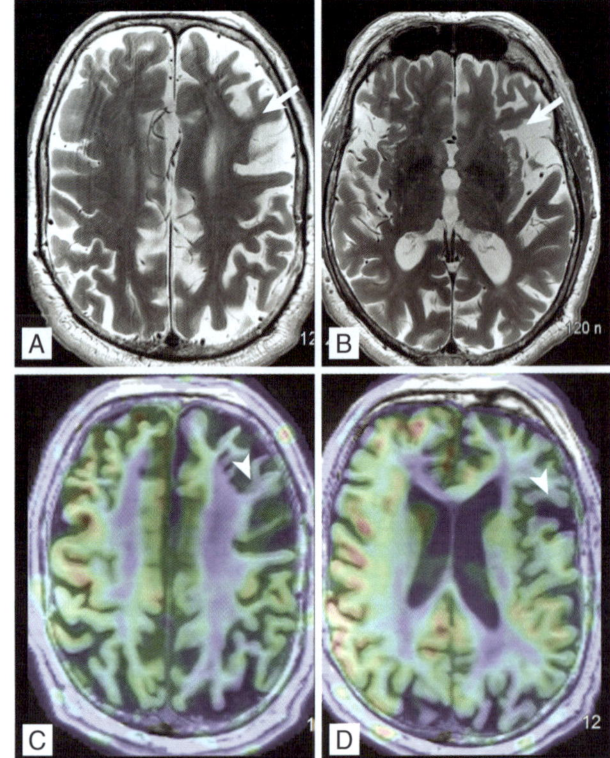

Figure 76.32 A 75-year-old man presented with 2 years of difficulty speaking. There was slowness to his speech. There was mild limb rigidity, and difficulty in walking with frequent falls. On neurological exam, his speech was effortful and slow and lacked grammatical style. Axial T2W MRI images through the brain (A and B) show left inferior frontal and anterior perisylvian volume loss (*arrows*). The left lateral ventricle is asymmetrically dilated due to the left hemispheric volume loss. Axial ASL MRI images (C and D) show hypoperfusion in the same areas that show volume loss on structural MRI (*arrowheads*). Findings are suggestive of the nonfluent variant of primary progressive aphasia (PNFA). The motor symptoms of limb rigidity and ataxia are due to the common association with corticobasal degeneration and progressive supranuclear palsy.

that is normally highly expressed in nigrostriatal axon terminals in the striatum, may show abnormal reduced uptake in the basal ganglia in PSP and CBD.

Characteristic volume loss is noted in the brainstem in PSP [134–136,150], which is most prominent in the midbrain. The

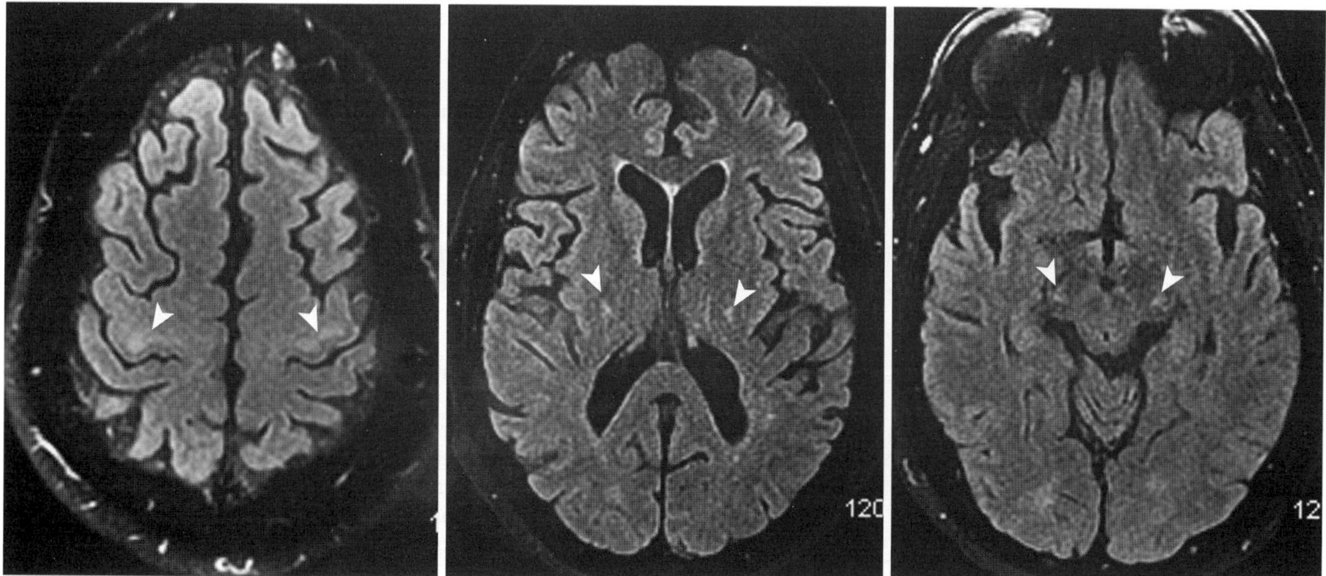

Figure 76.33 Amyotrophic lateral sclerosis. Axial FLAIR MRI images through the brain show abnormal hyperintense signal bilaterally along the entire corticospinal tract from the precentral gyrus, through the posterior limb of the internal capsule to the brainstem (*arrowheads*). Word of caution–mild FLAIR and DWI hyperintensity of the normal corticospinal tracts should not be confused with disease in normal asymptomatic individuals.

classic imaging sign of PSP is the "hummingbird" appearance of the brainstem on midsagittal images. Although a classic sign for PSP, the hummingbird sign (Fig. 76.34) is subjective and should be used with caution since advanced brain volume loss for other reasons could have a similar appearance. Quantification may assist in the diagnosis, with midbrain area of <70 mm^2 on midsagittal image or an anteroposterior diameter of the midbrain of less than 17 mm on axial T2W images suggestive of midbrain atrophy [151–157]. PSP also demonstrates volume loss within the superior cerebellar peduncles. Putamen, pallidal, thalamic, and frontal lobe atrophy may be present, however these are often challenging to detect visually [151–157]. Midbrain, deep gray, and cortical hypometabolism may be seen on ^{18}F-FDG PET.

CBD is a relatively rare dementia syndrome classically characterized by unilateral or asymmetric signs of parkinsonian rigidity, myoclonus, and apraxia. Asymmetric progressive limb dystonia and alien

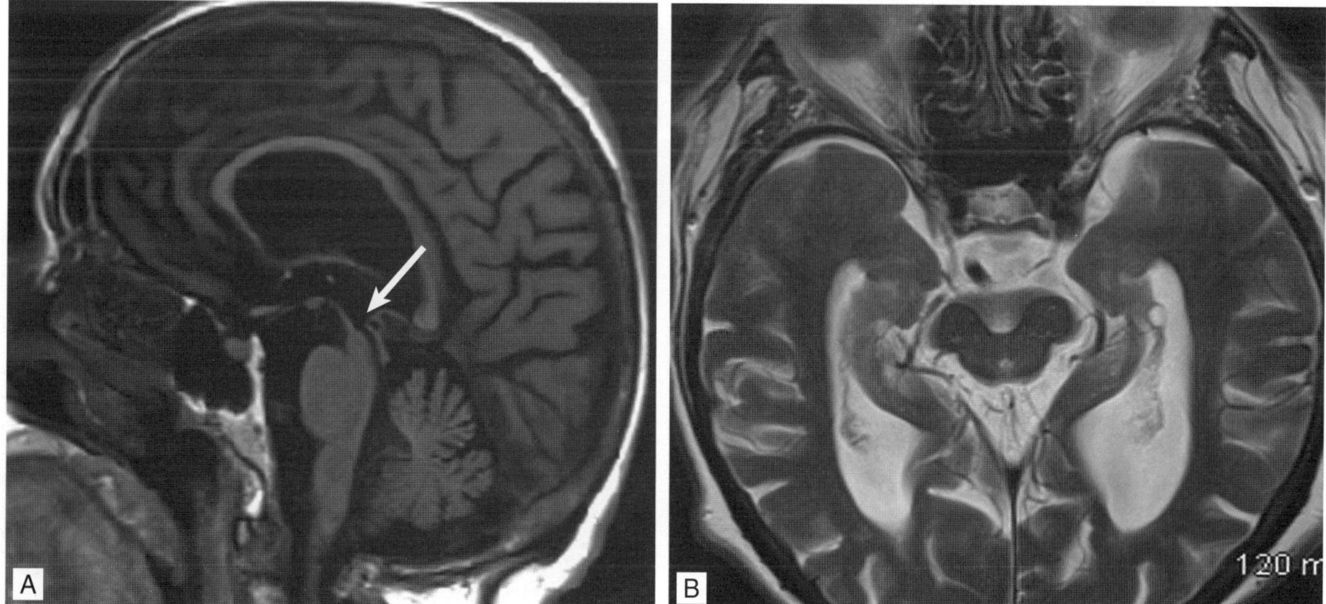

Figure 76.34 A 75-year-old woman presented with decline in general health and cognition for the past several years. The patient was progressively socially withdrawn and had difficulty talking, swallowing, and walking. There was upward gaze palsy and patient had frequent falls due to the inability to look downward. On neurological exam, the patient had axial rigidity, bradykinesia, mask-like face, and a positive glabellar tap. Sagittal T1W MRI image (A) shows marked atrophy of the midbrain tegmentum, giving it the typical "humming-bird" appearance (*arrow*) described with progressive supranuclear palsy. Axial T2W MRI image (B) also shows atrophy of the midbrain. Midbrain anteroposterior diameter of less than 17 mm in the midline is one of the objective signs of progressive supranuclear palsy.

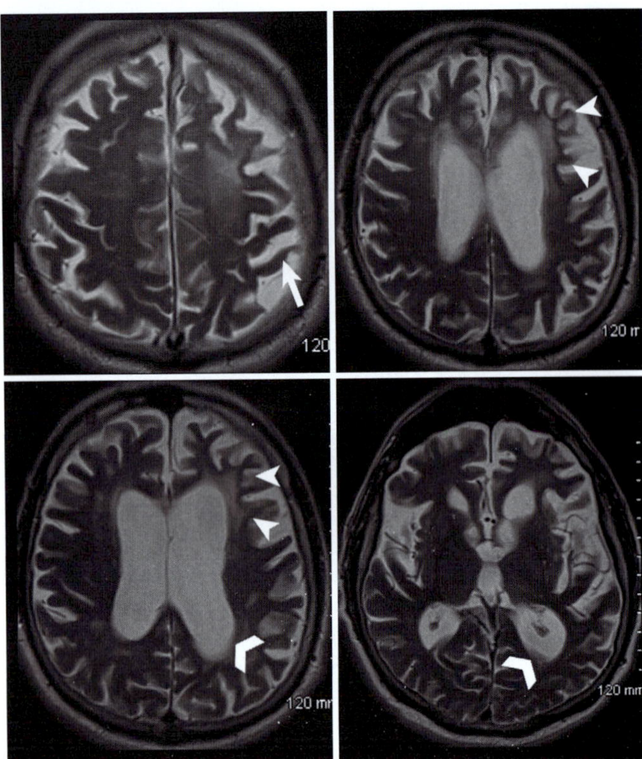

Figure 76.35 A 71-year-old man presented with 2 years of difficulty using his right hand. The patient felt like the hand acted on its own and he was "alien" to his own hand. He had difficulty walking and was recently having trouble getting the words out with agrammatism. On neurological exam, he had a shuffling unsteady gait, masked facial expression, and right limb apraxia. Axial T2W MRI images show asymmetric marked atrophy of the peri-Rolandic cortices (*arrow*). There is associated prefrontal, inferior frontal, and anterior perisylvian volume loss (*arrowheads*). Gyral thinning and cortical volume loss are associated with subcortical white matter T2W hyperintensity (not a necessary feature). Left-sided volume loss is also suggested by the dilated left lateral ventricle (*chevrons*). CTA of the head and neck (not shown) did not show flow-significant narrowing of the anterior circulation. The pattern of volume loss along with the provided history is suggestive of corticobasal degeneration. Dopamine uptake (DAT) scan in these patients (not performed for this patient) can show asymmetric decreased striatal uptake on the side of the abnormality.

limb phenomenon are clinical features of CBD. On gross examination, the brain is atrophied asymmetrically in the posterior frontal and parietal lobes in a perirolandic pattern that is otherwise uncommon in primary neurodegenerative diseases (Fig. 76.35). As with other parkinsonian syndromes, the more affected hemisphere is contralateral to the side of the most severe motor symptoms. Other identified imaging features include unilateral putamen atrophy and increased hypointensity of the globus pallidi and the putamina on T2W and GRE/SWI images. Associated unilateral cerebral peduncle atrophy may also be seen [151,155–158].

Teaching Point

The brainstem hummingbird sign may be suggestive of PSP but is nonspecific. Objective measurements of the brainstem are more useful. Movement disorder with asymmetric contralateral sensorimotor and premotor volume loss are features of CBD. Asymmetric progressive limb dystonia and alien limb phenomenon are the clinical features.

Dementia With Lewy Bodies

Although FTD is the second most common form of early-onset neurodegenerative dementia, DLB is the second most common form of neurodegenerative dementia after age 65. The core clinical features of DLB include recurrent visual hallucinations, fluctuating cognition, motor parkinsonism, and REM sleep behavior disorder. DLB is associated with less severe but somewhat more diffuse cerebral atrophy than AD with relative absence of medial temporal lobe atrophy, which is a feature useful in differentiating DLB from AD, where medial temporal lobe atrophy is typical [159–168]. Further, there is greater involvement of the posterior parietal and parieto-occipital regions in DLB in contrast to typical AD (Fig. 76.28), where there is greater involvement of the temporoparietal areas. Atrophy within the striatal structures and brainstem is also seen in DLB. ASL and ^{18}F-FDG PET studies show hypometabolism in posterior parietal and occipital regions (Fig. 76.25) with preservation of normal uptake in the medial temporal lobe and posterior cingulate gyrus. Sparing of the posterior cingulate but hypometabolism in surrounding cortex gives rise to the "cingulate island sign" of DLB (Fig. 76.25). However, DLB is frequently associated with AD copathology, and a combined pattern of neurodegeneration may then be present. ^{123}I-FP-CIT SPECT scan, used for imaging the dopaminergic pathway, may be useful in the workup of patients with DLB, who show decreased uptake of the tracer in the striatum as seen in other parkinsonian diseases (Fig. 76.36) [159–168]. Polysomnography is also an important aspect of the work up of these patients, where increased REM sleep without atonia (REM sleep behavior disorder) may help to diagnose DLB. Finally, ^{123}I-MIBG (meta-Iodobenzylguanidine) iodine 123-radiolabeled 2β-carbomethoxy-3β-(4-iodophenyl)-*N*-(3-fluoropropyl) nortropane) myocardial scintigraphy shows poor uptake which indicates reduced postganglionic sympathetic cardiac innervation, a feature of DLB [159–168].

Teaching Point

Cognitive fluctuations, parkinsonism, visual hallucinations, and REM sleep behavior disorder are the core clinical features of DLB. Parieto-occipital neurodegeneration with hippocampal sparing pattern of volume loss may help in suggesting the diagnosis. Polysomnography and ^{123}I-MIBG cardiac scintigraphy are other useful biomarkers.

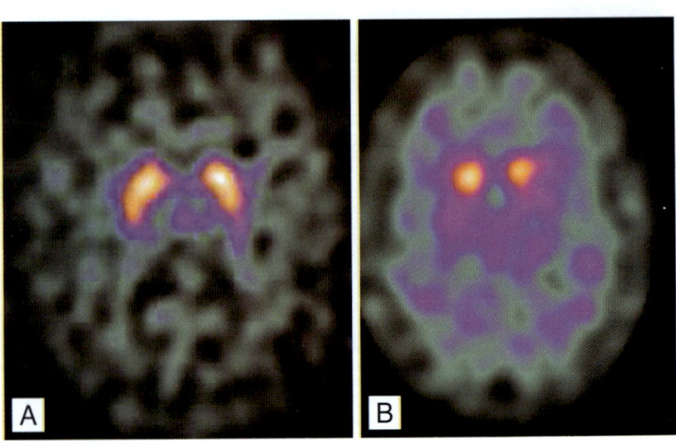

Figure 76.36 Dopamine uptake (DAT) scan. Axial dopamine uptake SPECT images (A and B) show the normal (A) and abnormal (B) configurations of the striatal uptake. Normal striatal uptake looks like a "comma" (A) while reduced uptake which can be seen in Parkinson disease, DLB and CBS looks like "period/full-stop" (B). The reduced uptake can be symmetric or asymmetric.

Limbic-Predominant Age-Associated TDP-43 Encephalopathy

Limbic-predominant age-associated TDP-43 encephalopathy (LATE) is a newly described neurodegenerative disease affecting older adults. Patients with LATE present with an amnestic syndrome that mimics AD, although LATE-neuropathologic change is characterized by TDP-43 proteinopathy with or without hippocampal sclerosis [169,170]. LATE differs from the TDP-43 proteinopathies of frontotemporal degeneration in the age of presentation since FTD disorders affect relatively younger individuals and LATE is a disease of "oldest of old." Coexistent amyloid and tau proteinopathies can be seen (although not necessary) and it is believed that LATE may lower the threshold for developing dementia due to amyloidopathy or tauopathy [169,170]. Amygdala, hippocampus, and the middle frontal gyrus are involved in a hierarchical fashion [169–172] and structural MRI changes constitute of marked hippocampal atrophy to a greater degree than generally seen with AD (Fig. 76.37). Hippocampal atrophy may be unilateral or bilateral and is seen progressing in a rostral-caudal gradient. Other findings on MRI are atrophy of the amygdala, mesial temporal, inferior frontal, and insular regions [169–172]. Amyloid PET may be positive due to coexistent pathology, in which case distinction from AD may be difficult since the clinical syndrome mimics AD. Negative amyloid PET in a patient with marked hippocampal atrophy and an AD-like clinical syndrome however makes a strong argument in favor of LATE.

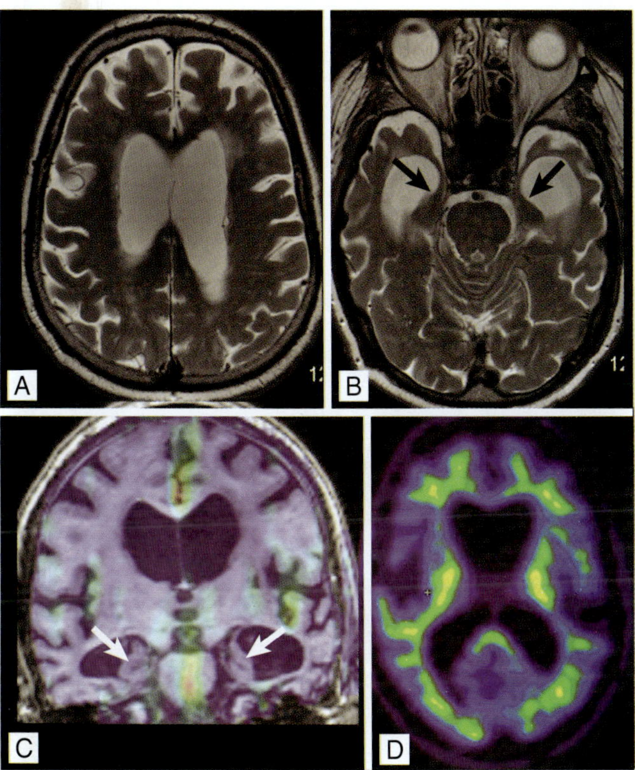

Figure 76.37 An 82-year-old right-handed female with history of forgetting names and conversations. On neuropsychological testing she showed impairments in new learning, and delayed recall with no benefit from cueing suggesting an encoding-based memory deficit. There was borderline clock drawing, impaired object naming and sematic fluency. Axial T2W MRI images (A and B) show marked medial temporal lobe atrophy (*black arrows*) with prominence of the temporal horns. Selected image more superiorly (A) was unremarkable for parietal or frontal lobe atrophy or asymmetry. Coronal ASL MRI image (C) shows marked bilateral hippocampal atrophy (*white arrows*) and hypoperfusion. The history and MRI findings were very suggestive of underlying AD pathologic change which prompted an amyloid PET scan (D). No cortical amyloid uptake was seen (amyloid negative scan) which led to the change of the diagnosis to limbic-predominant age-associated TDP-43 proteinopathy (LATE). There is a great overlap of the clinical profile of LATE with AD.

Teaching Point

Hippocampal atrophy in the "oldest old" with an Alzheimer's type clinical syndrome, especially in the absence of a positive amyloid PET should raise the possibility of LATE.

Movement Disorders

Parkinson Disease (PD)

PD is the most common neurodegenerative movement disorder, and the second most common neurodegenerative disorder after AD, characterized by loss of dopaminergic nigrostriatal neurons which project to the striatum [173]. The underlying pathological process is the death of dopaminergic neurons within the substantia nigra pars compacta due to intraneuronal aggregation of alpha-synuclein [158,174]. The loss of dopaminergic drive leads to motor symptoms such as rigidity, resting tremor, bradykinesia, and gait abnormalities; and nonmotor symptoms such as autonomic dysfunction, hyposmia, depression, fatigue, and cognitive impairment.

Anatomic MRI changes in PD are nonspecific and MRI is not used in the diagnosis of PD. The absence of the "swallow tail sign" on SWI (Fig. 76.38) has however been described in PD and other parkinsonian disorders. The substantia nigra pars compacta

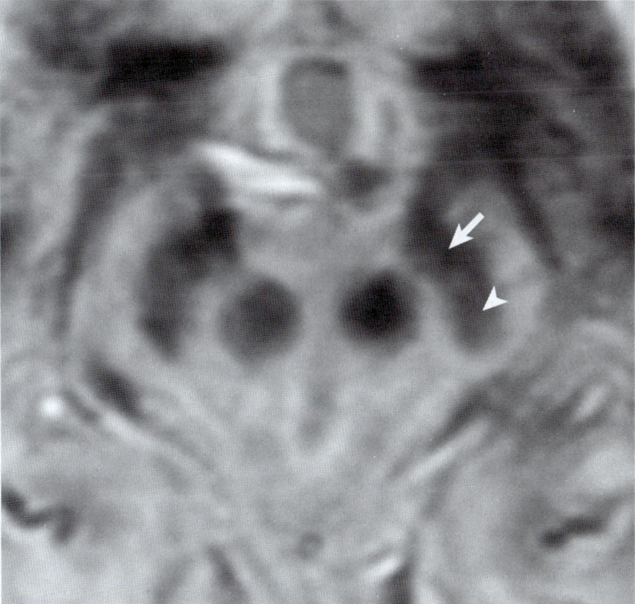

Figure 76.38 Swallow tail. Axial-focused SWI MRI image through the midbrain shows a normal "swallow tail," which is seen as a thin stripe of hyperintensity (*arrowhead*) along the posterolateral aspect of the dark band of substantia nigra (*arrow*). This is formed by the normal nigrosome-1 within the substantia nigra. Loss of the normal swallow tail is an imaging sign of Parkinson disease.

contain iron deposits, which result in hypointensity on SWI; the "swallow tail" is thought to be due to the presence of noniron containing neurons in the dorsolateral substantia nigra which split this hypointensity, cells which are usually lost in PD. The use of molecular imaging in for detection of functioning of presynaptic dopamine transporters is widespread. Commercially known as the DaTscan, reduced striatal uptake on ^{123}I-FP-CIT SPECT scan is a feature of PD (Fig. 76.36), although also seen in other parkinsonian syndromes including DLB, PSP, and CBS. ^{123}I-FP-CIT (iodine 123-radiolabeled 2β-carbomethoxy-3β-(4-iodophenyl)-*N*-(3-fluoropropyl) nortropane) SPECT may be of value in differentiating PD from drug-induced or vascular parkinsonism which have normal striatal uptake [151,167,175]. A fluorinated form of levodopa, F-DOPA is also used as a radiotracer in PD and utilizes the PET technique. F-DOPA crosses the blood–brain barrier and reaches the dopaminergic cells, where it can be used as a surrogate for dopamine precursor for the assessment of presynaptic dopaminergic integrity and reflects the disturbances in PD [176].

Parkinson Disease Dementia

In chronic cases of PD, there is widespread neurodegeneration frequently associated with cognitive decline and often dementia. Underlying this later stage disease, there may be atrophy of the temporal, parietal, and frontal lobes. Deep structures such as thalamus and basal ganglia also show atrophy in Parkinson disease dementia (PDD) compared with nondemented PD patients. The pattern of atrophy seen with PDD is not specific, and standard clinical neuroimaging frequently shows no clear correlate of PD/PDD neurodegeneration [155,173,177–180].

Teaching Point

Reduced striatal uptake on 123I-FP-CIT SPECT is a feature common to all neurodegenerative parkinsonian conditions, including PD, DLB, MSA, PSP, and CBS. Typical PD frequently does not show abnormality on standard neuroimaging, but other parkinsonian syndromes may have regional neurodegenerative patterns that can distinguish them.

Amyotrophic Lateral Sclerosis (ALS)

ALS is characterized by motor neuron degeneration due to protein aggregates formed by TDP-43, which disrupt cytoskeletal architecture, axonal trafficking, and mitochondrial function. The motor neuron axonal dysfunction progresses retrogradely to cell body death in the motor cortex. Clinically, the disease manifests as loss of motor functions of the body, ultimately being fatal due to loss of vital motor functions such as respiration [181].

The diagnosis is clinical. MRI performed in patients with ALS shows T2/FLAIR hyperintensity anywhere long the corticospinal tracts or diffusely involving the entire tract (Fig. 76.33) [182]. Due to the density of fibers in the corticospinal tract, mild hyperintense T2/FLAIR signal is normally seen along these tracts and should not be confused with pathology. Hyperintense signal in the corticospinal tracts that persist on proton density sequences adds specificity to this finding. Hypointense signal in the gray matter of the precentral gyri on T2W and GRE/SWI images can be seen but also lacks specificity, since this finding is seen commonly in elderly individuals. Advanced imaging techniques such as DTI may show reduced fractional anisotropy and increased mean diffusivity in the corticospinal tract before the anatomic MRI findings are evident [183].

Hereditary Ataxias

Hereditary ataxias are a heterogeneous group of slowly progressive neurodegenerative disorders, characterized by gait abnormalities, limb ataxia, oculomotor abnormalities, and dysarthria [184,185]. Noncerebellar features such as choreiform movements, parkinsonism, peripheral neuropathy, and cognitive impairment can also be seen [185,186]. Spinocerebellar ataxias (SCA) are dominantly inherited, and their list is continuously growing, with more than 45 types numbered in order of discovery, known to date; of which SCA3 (Machado–Joseph disease) and SCA6 are the most common [185]. Friedreich's ataxia is the most common recessive ataxia [185].

Three distinct patterns of cerebellar degeneration and atrophy can be seen in hereditary ataxias. Predominant atrophy of the cerebellar cortex with relative preservation of brainstem, spinal cord, and cerebral cortex is seen in SCA6; while accompanying atrophy of the brainstem, particularly the pons (olivopontocerebellar atrophy) is seen in SCA1, SCA2, and SCA3 (Fig. 76.39). This pattern of atrophy is also seen on MSA-C described later, although MSA-C affects more older population compared with SCA. The third pattern of atrophy is predominant atrophy of the spinal cord, with relative preservation of brainstem and cerebellum; seen in Friedreich's ataxia [186–188].

Multiple System Atrophy

Multiple system atrophy (MSA) is an uncommon neurodegenerative parkinsonian disorder with autonomic, cerebellar, and pyramidal tract dysfunction. The clinical course in MSA is more rapid compared with PD. Depending on the predominance of cerebellar or parkinsonian symptoms, the disorder is subdivided into MSA-C and MSA-P subtypes. There is greater involvement of the pons,

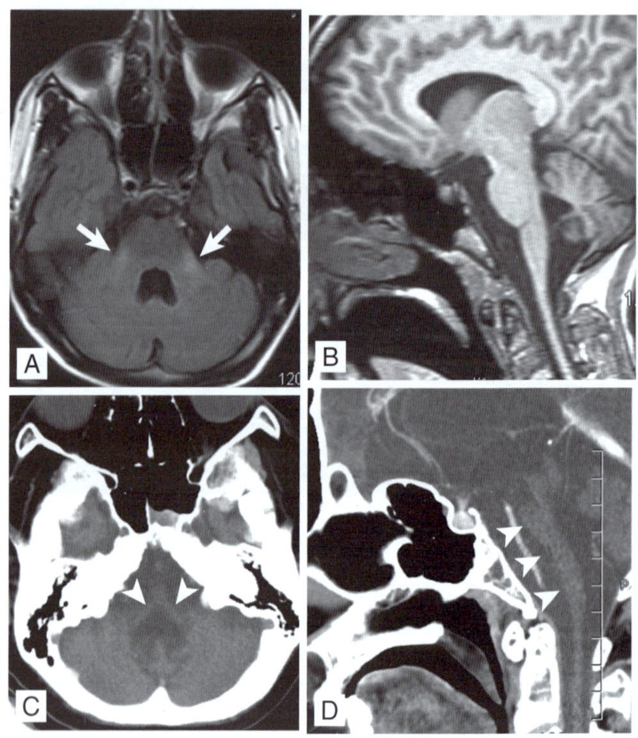

Figure 76.39 Spinocerebellar ataxia. Axial FLAIR MRI image (A) and sagittal T1W MRI image (B) of a patient with ataxia at 14 years of age. Hyperintensity noted in bilateral brachium pontis (*arrows* in A) and mild cerebellar atrophy in (B). Axial and sagittal postcontrast soft-tissue algorithm CT images (C and D) 4 years later show marked progression of the cerebellar atrophy with interval marked atrophy of the brainstem and the cerebellar peduncles (*arrowheads*).

cerebellum, and the middle cerebellar peduncles in MSA-C while putaminal volume loss outweighs pontocerebellar atrophy in MSA-P [151,155,158,191]. T2/SWI hypointensity can be seen in the posterior putamen in MSA-P. A thin stripe of hyperintensity has also been described on the lateral aspect of the putamen on T2W images. In MSA-C, there is often cruciform T2/FLAIR hyperintensity within the pons, termed the "hot-cross bun" sign (Fig. 76.40). Middle cerebellar peduncle atrophy is typical and may be associated with abnormal T2/FLAIR signal within the peduncle [151,155,158,191].

Teaching Point

MSA is clinically associated with parkinsonism and autonomic dysfunction and faster progression compared with PD. MSA may predominately affect either the cerebellum or striatum.

Huntington's Disease

Huntington's disease (HD) is a neurodegenerative disease with autosomal dominant inheritance which is characterized by gradually progressive psychiatric, cognitive, and motor symptoms. The disease has a devastating course with patient demise in one to two decades after the onset of symptoms [190]. The diagnosis is clinical and is based on motor symptoms criteria, with the imaging findings mostly of academic importance [190]. The neuropathology of HD predominantly affects the striatum, beginning in the dorsal caudate and progressing ventrally to the putamen. On imaging, this is seen as atrophy of the involved structures (Fig. 76.41), with the volume loss correlating with disease severity. Increased diffusivity is seen in the basal ganglia on DTI analysis [191,192]. Hypometabolism may be noted in the caudate nuclei on ^{18}F-FDG PET [193], although PET is rarely performed for HD.

Neurodegeneration With Brain Iron Accumulation (NBIA)

NBIA is a heterogeneous group of genetic neurodegenerative disorders characterized by abnormal accumulation of iron in the basal ganglia. Movement disorders, parkinsonian symptoms, dystonia, and cognitive decline constitute the common clinical features of NBIA. By far the most well-known and the most common entity in this group is the Pantothenate kinase associated neurodegeneration (PKAN) [194–196]. The other lesser known and less common entities are phospholipase A2-associated neurodegeneration, mitochondrial membrane protein-associated neurodegeneration, beta-propeller protein-associated neurodegeneration, neuroferritinopathies, and aceruloplasminemia [194–196]. The characteristic imaging finding in the PKAN is the "eye-of-the-tiger sign" (Fig. 76.42) which is profound hypointensity of the globus pallidus with an anteromedial region of hyperintensity on T2W images. Hypointensity of the substantia nigra is also seen. The next most common form, phospholipase A2-associated neurodegeneration shows cerebellar and cerebral atrophy with hypointense basal ganglia on T2*-sensitive sequences due to iron accumulation [194–196].

Secondary Cognitive Impairment

Protein misfolding, abnormal protein aggregation, and prion-like propagation leading to neurodegeneration are the major pathway causing cognitive dysfunction and dementia in the preceding section. Clinical cognitive impairment and dementia are however not unique to these mechanisms. Vitamin deficiencies, brain tumors (Fig. 76.43), polysubstance abuse, etc. can

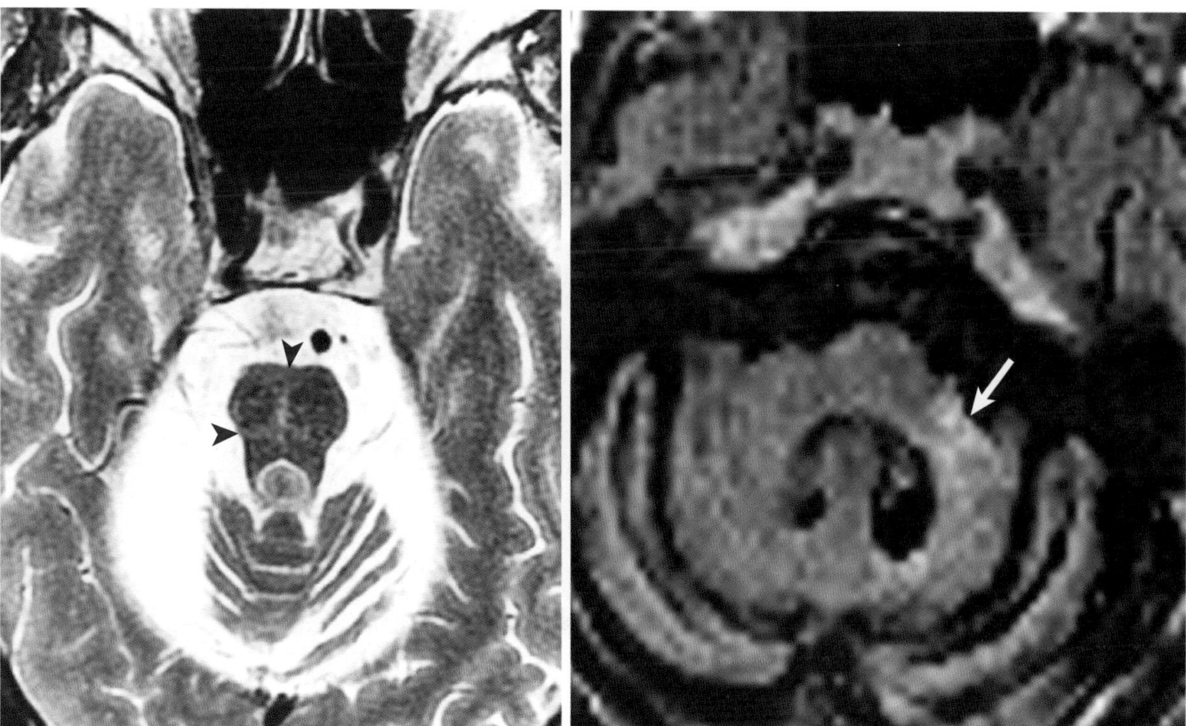

Figure 76.40 Multiple system atrophy. Elderly male with parkinsonian symptoms and cerebellar ataxia. Axial T2W (*left*) and FLAIR (*right*) MRI images through the posterior fossa show diffuse brainstem and cerebellar atrophy. Atrophy of bilateral middle cerebellar peduncles is also seen with abnormal hyperintense signal (*arrow* in B). Cruciform abnormal signal in the pons (hot-cross bun sign—*arrowheads*) is typical of the cerebellar type of multiple system atrophy (MSA-C) and is due to atrophy of the pontocerebellar fibers and preservation of the corticospinal tracts.

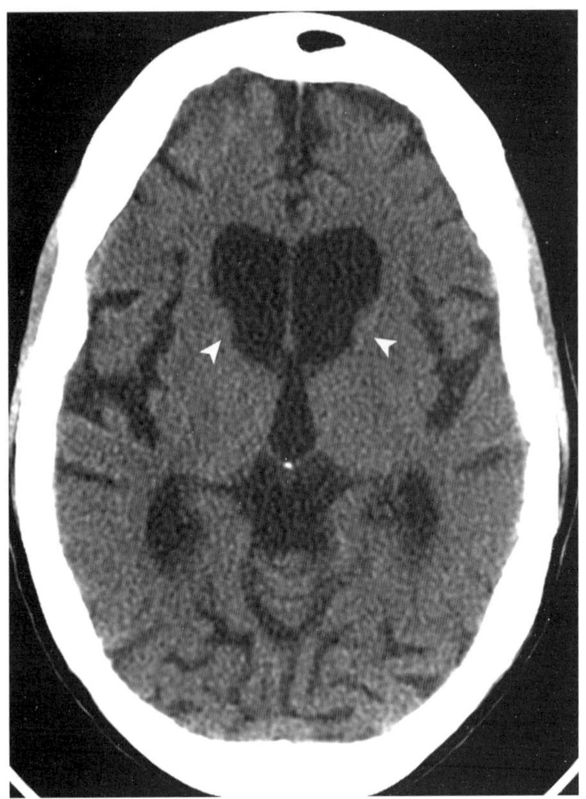

Figure 76.41 Adult male presenting with abnormal movements and progressive dementia. Axial noncontrasted CT of the head demonstrates age-advanced marked atrophy of the bilateral caudate heads (*white arrowheads*) with box-like configuration of the frontal horns of the lateral ventricles. Imaging findings support a diagnosis of Huntington's disease.

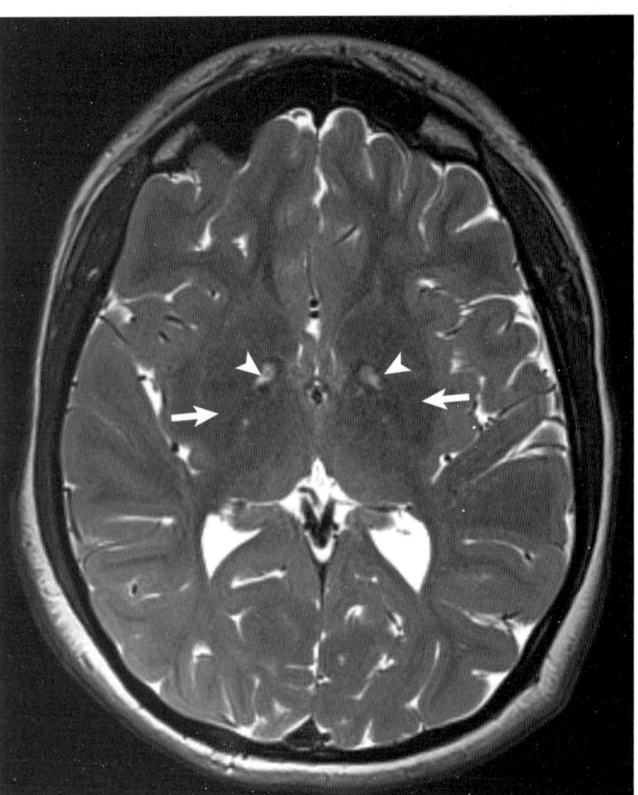

Figure 76.42 A 12-year-old with worsening seizures. Axial T2W MRI image through the globi pallidi shows hypointensity of the basal ganglia (*arrows*) with medial regions of hyperintensity (*arrowheads*) in a characteristic "eye-of-the-tiger" configuration typical for the pantothenate kinase-associated neurodegeneration (PKAN).

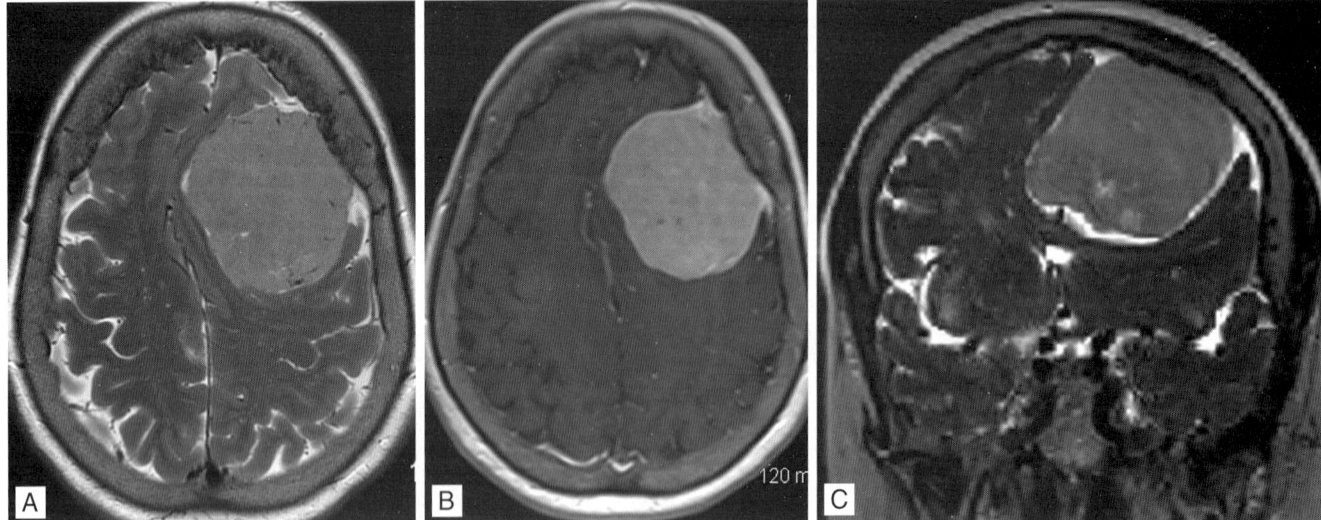

Figure 76.43 A 65-year-old female presents with progressive telegraphic speech for the past 1.5 years with lack of grammatical style and phonemic paraphasias. The diagnosis of nonfluent variant PPA was made in the clinic. MRI of the brain reveals a large avidly enhancing extra-axial mass in the left frontal lobe (A & B) consistent with a meningioma. Note the displacement of the brain region in the location of the frontal aslant tract on coronal T2W image (C), which is the white matter tract implicated in the pathogenesis of nfvPPA. The clinical features of dementia are caused by the involvement of the functional pathways by deposition of protein aggregates. Similar clinical features may be seen in other pathologies if the disease process mimics the involvement of the functional pathways.

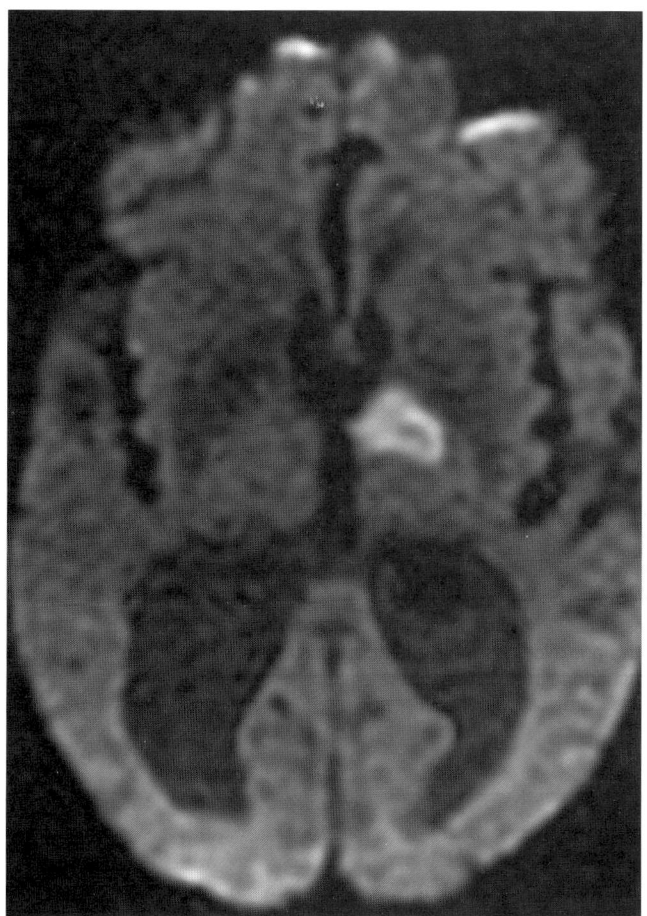

Figure 76.44 A 75-year-old male with a few days of word finding difficulty and semantic paraphasias. Axial DWI MRI image shows an infarct in the left dorsomedial thalamus. The dorsomedial thalamic nucleus has connections with the memory and language networks.

present with symptoms of dementia. Involvement of specific regions in the brain by infarct or tumor can manifest clinically as a dementia syndrome (Fig. 76.44). Chronic cerebrovascular ischemic disease and hemorrhages caused by cerebral amyloid angiopathy (CAA) can cause dementia by interruption of subcortical circuits. There is a far greater association of vascular disease and CAA with ageing than that of neurodegenerative diseases and these processes commonly overlap and co-exist [197–200]. In fact, the neurodegenerative effects of proteinopathies are accentuated by vascular disease, or by the presence of another proteinopathy (e.g., DLB pathology with AD) and this copathology can pose a challenge in differentiating the clinical and imaging effects of a single disease process (e.g., amyloid PET positivity in CAA and AD).

Vascular Contributions to Cognitive Impairment and Dementia

Cerebrovascular disease can have widespread effects on the brain. The most common consequence of uncontrolled vascular risk factors, such as hypertension, is a small vessel angiopathy, which disproportionately affects end artery distributions that are prevalent in cerebral white matter. Periventricular white matter is the most susceptible to these "small vessel ischemic changes" which result in the extremely common white matter hyperintensities seen on T2 FLAIR imaging (Fig. 76.45). A spectrum of vascular disorders, including hypertensive arteriopathy, amyloid angiopathy, or genetic causes (such as cerebral autosomal dominant arteriopathy with subcortical infarcts and leukoencephalopathy [CADASIL]), can thereby cause cognitive impairment by interruption of subcortical circuits and disruption of brain networks traversing the affected white matter regions [124,203–208]. There is a gradual slowing of cognitive function in small vessel disease and gait disturbances are common. On neuropsychological testing, these patients tend to perform worse on tests of executive function [124,201–206]. Although low-level pathology is common and not usually symptomatic, the likelihood that vascular

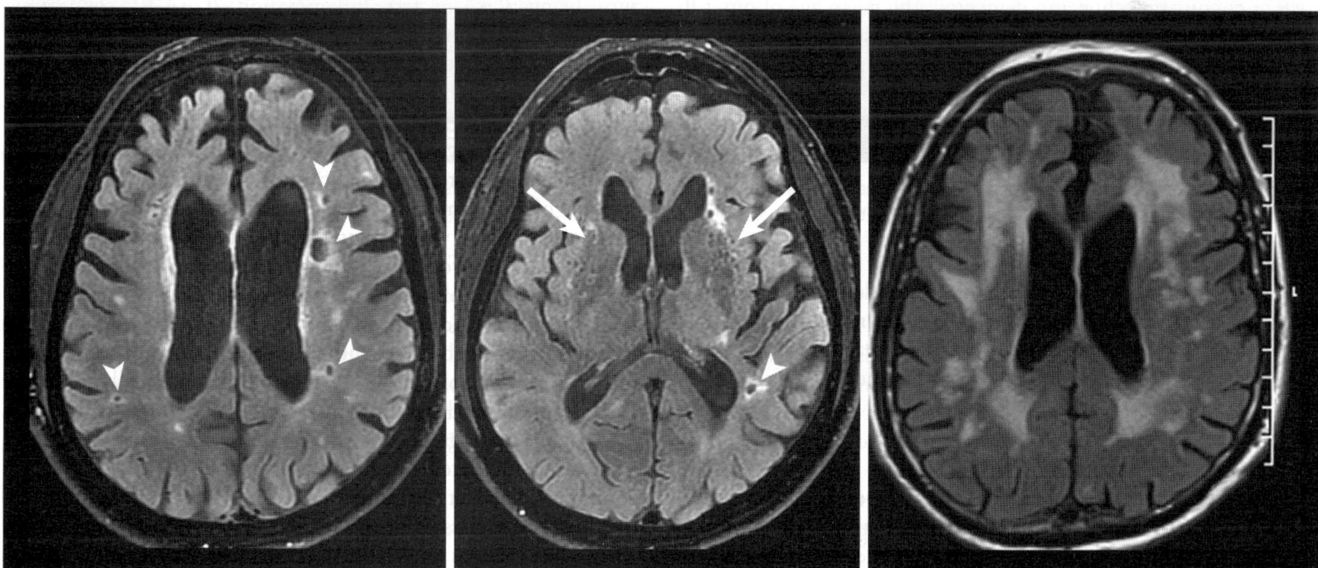

Figure 76.45 Stigmata of cerebrovascular ischemic disease. Axial FLAIR MRI images show multiple lacunar infarcts (*white arrowheads* in *left and middle images*), dilated perivascular spaces (*white arrows*) in the middle image (etat crible or widened peri-vascular spaces are considered a sequela of hypertension and cerebrovascular disease), and patchy/confluent FLAIR white matter hyperintensities in the right image.

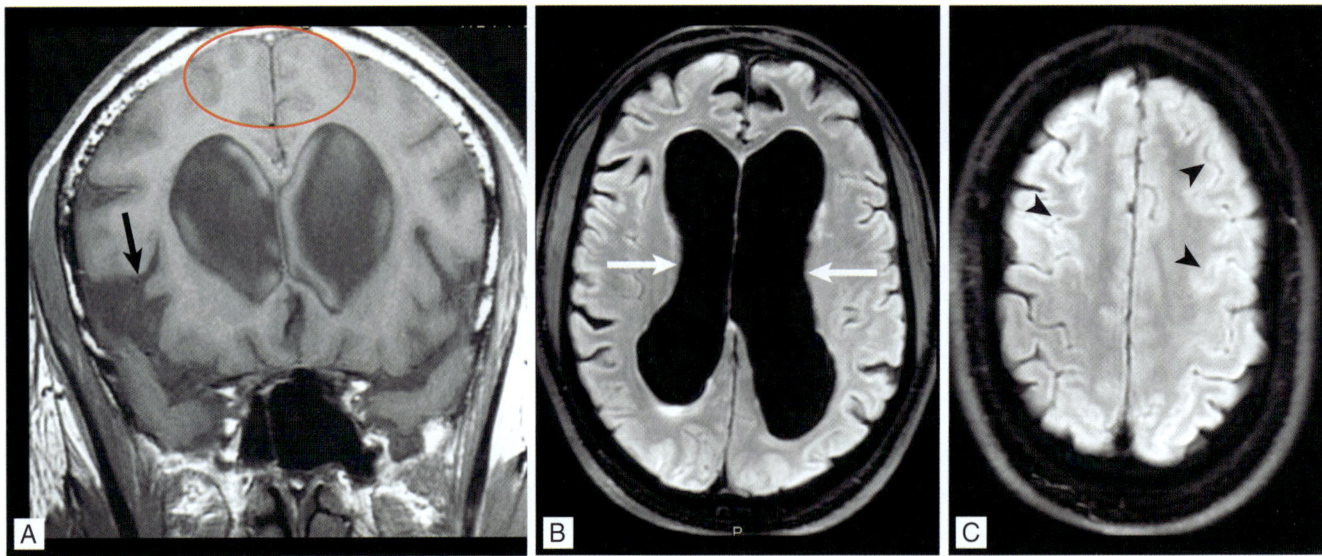

Figure 76.49 Normal pressure hydrocephalus. Disproportionately enlarged subarachnoid spaces as evidenced by effacement of the sulci at the vertex (*red circle* in A and *black arrowheads* in C) and widening of the sylvian fissures (*black arrow* in A) associated with ventriculomegaly that is out of proportion to the sulcal prominence (*white arrows* in B) are features that suggest normal pressure hydrocephalus (see the text for disproportionately enlarged subarachnoid space hydrocephalus).

sagittal images. Radionuclide cisternogram using ^{111}Indium- or ^{99m}Technetium-labled DTPA may show abnormal tracer reflux into the lateral ventricles and lack of tracer activity over the convexities 24–48 hours after intrathecal injection (Fig. 76.50). Improvement of ataxia after a high volume (30–50 mL) CSF tap is more frequently seen earlier in the course of disease and has a high positive predictive value for favorable postintervention results.

Creutzfeldt–Jakob Disease

CJD is a fatal prion neurodegenerative disease presenting with rapidly progressive dementia, myoclonus, and pyramidal, extrapyramidal, and cerebellar signs. The most common form of CJD is sporadic, followed by the familial form, the least common form being infectious (variant CJD) or iatrogenic. The underlying neuropathology in CJD is spongiform degeneration and gliosis. DWI MRI has high sensitivity and specificity in the detection of abnormal areas (Fig. 76.51). The characteristic imaging finding in CJD is DWI/FLAIR hyperintensity of the basal ganglia, thalami, and the cerebral cortices [219–222]. Within the thalamus, symmetric involvement of the pulvinar (pulvinar sign) and the dorsomedial nuclei (hockey-stick sign) is common in variant CJD but can also be seen in sporadic CJD. Involvement of the cerebral cortices is usually bilateral but asymmetric. Cerebellar involvement may be seen. Cortical atrophy may be associated with the signal abnormalities [219–222]. Enhancement is uncommon. Supportive diagnosis may be made with CSF sampling RT-QuIC CSF

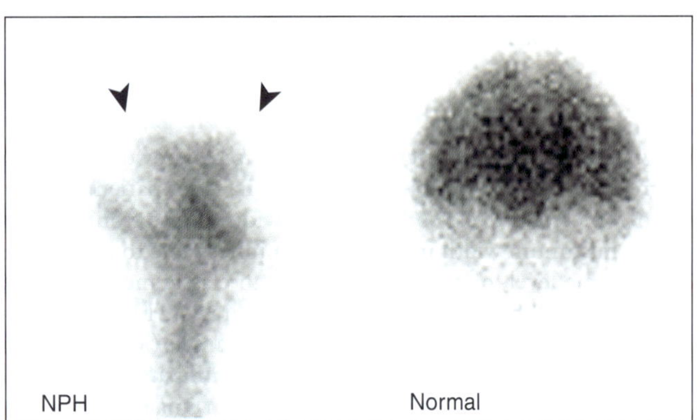

Figure 76.50 Radionuclide cisternogram. Anterior planar images of the head. On the left, there is reflux of tracer into the lateral ventricles 4 hours after lumbar injection (*arrowheads*). Tracer does not reach the vertex by 48 hours, and imaging is suggestive of NPH. In a normal scan, tracer is seen at the vertex by 24 hours after injection (*right*) but is never seen in the ventricles.

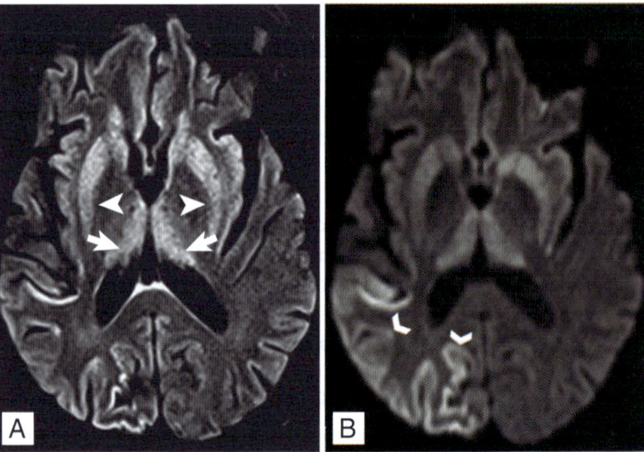

Figure 76.51 Patient presenting with rapidly progressive cognitive decline. Axial T2-FLAIR (A) and diffusion-weighted (B) MRI images demonstrate signal abnormality in the bilateral corpus striatum (*arrowheads*), dorsal thalamus and pulvinar (*white arrows*), and scattered cortical gyriform restricted diffusion (*chevrons*). The "hockey-stick" configuration of dorsomedial and pulvinar thalamic involvement is commonly described with Creutzfeldt–Jakob disease.

assay, but definitive diagnosis may require brain biopsy. Death occurs in a few months from the onset of clinical symptoms.

Chronic Traumatic Encephalopathy

Chronic traumatic encephalopathy (CTE) is a recently described entity of secondary neurodegeneration associated with repetitive neurotrauma seen in high impact sports, in war veterans, and in a subset of psychiatric patients. Incidence is highly variable as exposures and patient factors contribute to development of this neuropathology. The symptom onset is usually 8–10 years after retirement from active engagement in the inciting activity and is characterized by a constellation of symptoms of deteriorating memory, executive functioning, impulse control, and motor functioning [223–226]. The characteristic histologic lesions are perivascular hyperphosphorylated tau neurofibrillary tangles in the depths of the cerebral sulci [223–226]. On imaging, there is global brain volume loss, ventriculomegaly, callosal thinning, and medial temporal and hippocampal atrophy. Imaging signs of previous trauma in the form of multifocal encephalomalacia, chronic macro and microhemorrhages, and white matter abnormalities are commonly seen [223–226]. Association of CTE with other neurodegenerative disorders such as AD, PDD, and FTD has been shown and it is unclear whether pathological changes of CTE predispose the patients for these neurodegenerative conditions or the symptoms of CTE overlap with these neurodegenerative disorders [223–226].

Summary

In this chapter we discussed metabolic, toxic, and degenerative disorders of the brain. The metabolic and toxic disorders although, caused by endogenous and exogenous toxins, respectively, have a similar pattern of imaging abnormalities where excitotoxic brain injury disturbs the ionic flux and results in various patterns of cytotoxic, vasogenic, and intramyelinic edema.

The neurodegenerative conditions are usually caused by the accumulation of abnormal protein aggregates which ultimately lead to neuronal dysfunction and neuronal loss.

Assimilation of information from clinical history and examination, body fluid analysis, and knowledge of patterns of these abnormalities can help an astute radiologist to suggest possible diagnoses and help patient management.

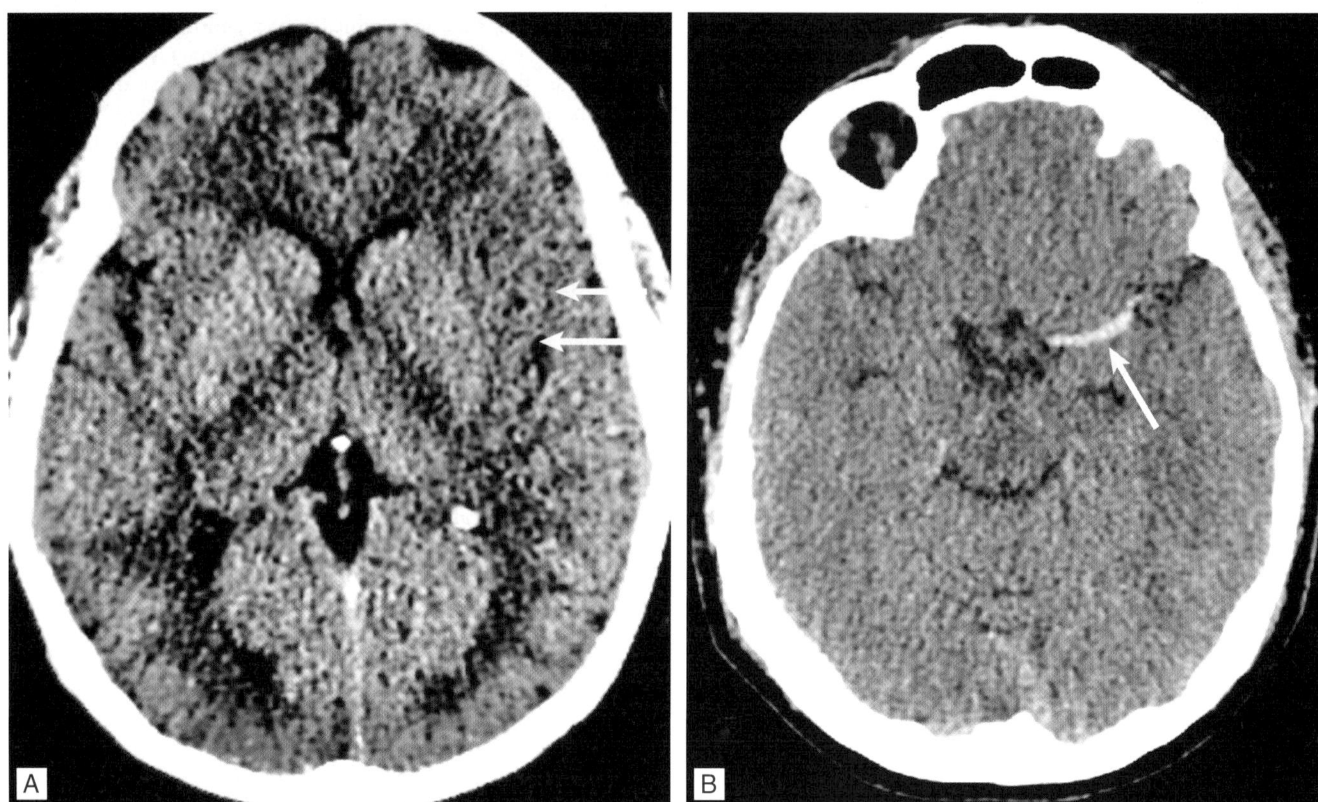

Figure 77.1 (A) Left insular ribbon sign (*arrows*). (B) Left hyperdense MCA (*arrow*).

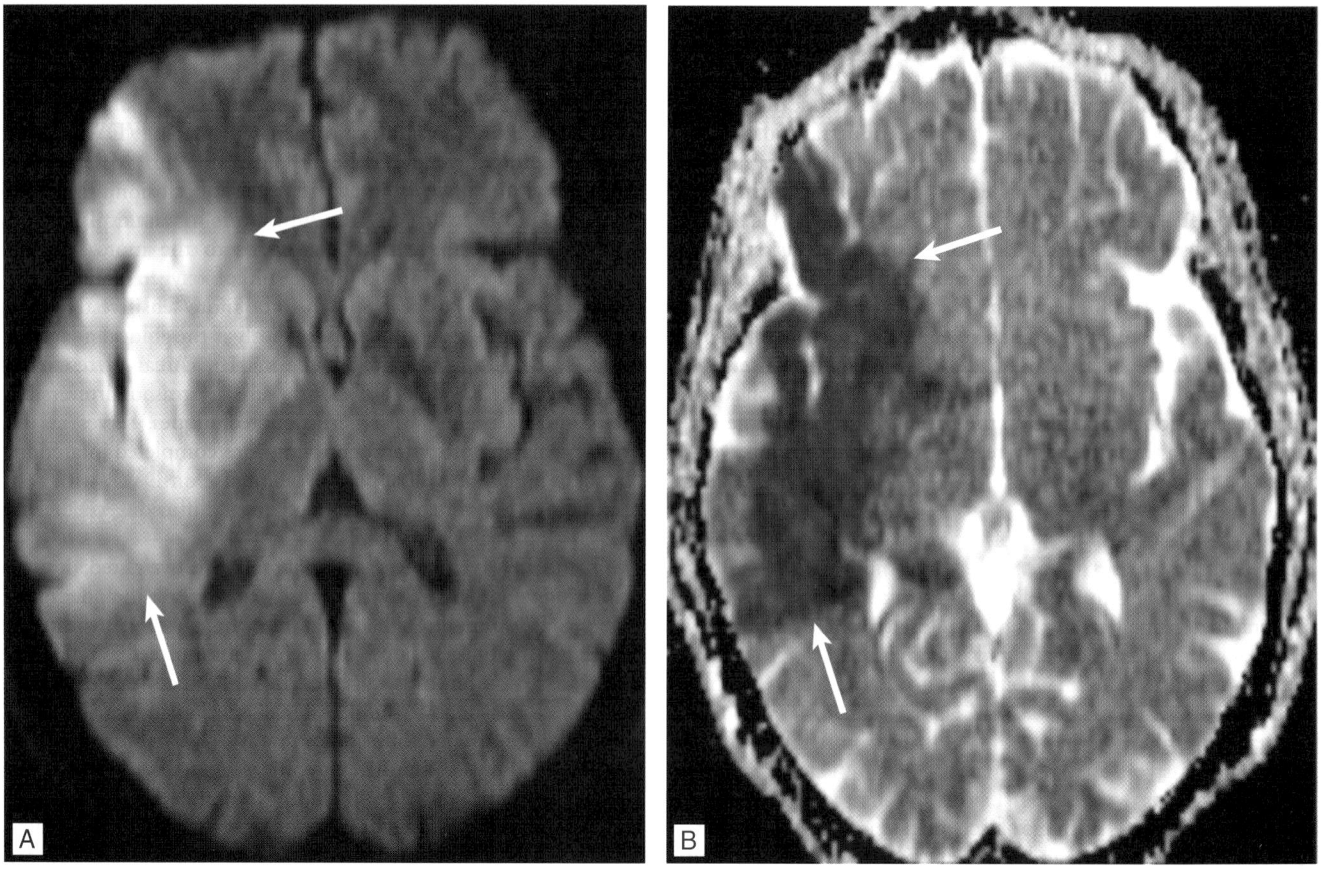

Figure 77.2 (A) Hyperintensity in the right MCA territory on DWI. (B) Corresponding hypointensity on ADC map. Arrows demarcate the infarction on diffusion weighted images.

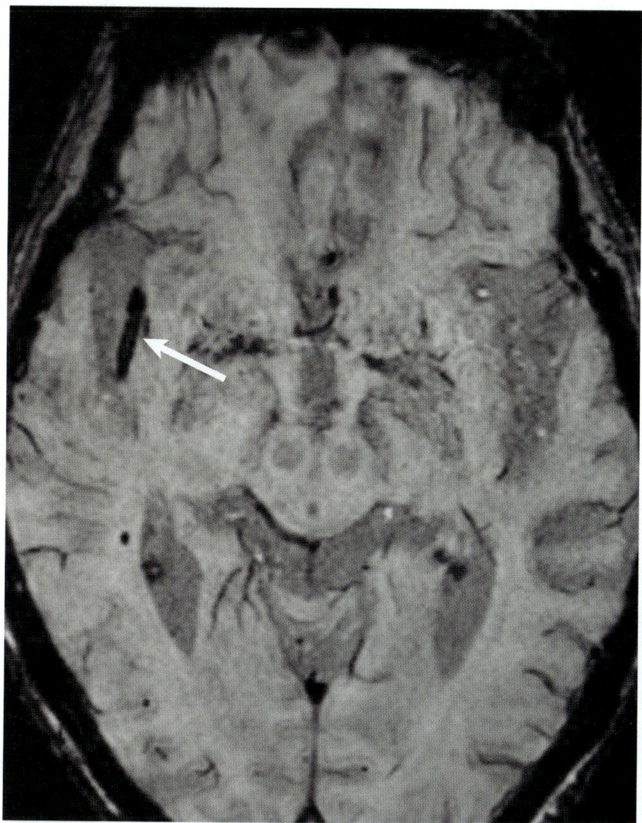

Figure 77.3 Right MCA thrombus showing hypointensity on susceptibility weighted image. Arrow denotes the susceptibility blooming from the MCA clot.

imaging (SWI) sequences are sensitive to the magnetic field disturbances caused by blood products such as deoxyhemoglobin and hemosiderin, resulting in loss of signal and hypointensity. These sequences are useful to identify areas of petechial parenchymal hemorrhage within the infarcted territory, which may not be visible on CT. They also often display areas of intravascular thrombus as prominent foci of hypointensity within the occluded vessel(s) (Fig. 77.3). *Slow flow in the arterial territory distal to a proximal occlusion may also manifest as hyperintensity on T2 FLAIR images (i.e., the ivy sign), and hypointensity on SWI due to higher concentrations of deoxyhemoglobin resulting from greater oxygen extraction* (Fig. 77.4).

Hemorrhagic transformation of infarctions is common, involving approximately half of cases. However, the majority (70–90%) of these are multifocal petechial hemorrhage, which is normally without significant mass effect or clinical sequelae [19–21]. A minority of cases will develop an intraparenchymal hematoma, which may cause mass effect and clinical deterioration. A 4-level grading scheme for CT was developed for the European Cooperative Acute Stroke Study (ECASS) II trial studying the risk of hemorrhage after tPA administration which divides petechial hemorrhage and intraparenchymal hematomas into subgroups based on the amount of infarcted territory involved (Table 77.1). That study found improved outcomes when tPA was given to patients with petechial hemorrhage, and worse outcomes when administered to patients with intraparenchymal hematomas [21].

Fogging and Pseudo-normalization

The normal evolution of ischemic infarction includes an acute to subacute phase of cerebral edema causing hypoattenuation on CT, hypointensity on T1 MRI, and hyperintensity on T2 MRI. As the edema begins to resolve and the necrotic brain is resorbed, the CT and MRI appearance of the infarcted territory may approximate the imaging appearance of normal tissue due to a combination of increased numbers of lipid-laden scavenging macrophages, petechial hemorrhage, and decreased water content [22–24]. This phenomenon of "fogging" usually occurs 2–3 weeks from stroke onset and may cause confusion in the setting of known infarction or cause a recent infarction to go undiagnosed. As the infarcted territory does not have an intact blood–brain barrier, gyriform or patchy enhancement will be seen if contrast is administered.

A similar phenomenon occurs with ADC values on diffusion imaging, wherein at approximately 1 week following stroke onset, ADC values become "pseudo-normalized" as increasing ADC signal intensity from necrotic tissue and edema reaches a similar level to that of normal surrounding brain parenchyma [25]. As the infarct continues to evolve, ADC signal intensity will continue to increase, reflecting progressively facilitated diffusion in the region of developing encephalomalacia.

Vascular Imaging

Ultrasonography (USG)

USG has a limited role in the initial diagnosis and management of acute ischemic stroke. Transcranial Doppler USG has been explored as a method of identifying vessel stenoses, occlusions, and microemboli in the setting of acute stroke [26–28]. USG has the advantage of real-time imaging, low cost, and the ability to investigate multiple structures, including intracranial and cervical vasculature, as well as the heart. However, USG is more operator-dependent than other imaging modalities, influenced by the technologist and their level of experience, and results may not be easily reproducible. In addition, the accuracy of the technique for detecting pathology at some locations is relatively poor, such as the vertebral and basilar arteries in the region of the skull base, where sensitivity of ultrasound for detecting arterial occlusion may be as low as 55% [27,28].

Sonothrombolysis has also been investigated as a potential method for clot lysis in the setting of acute thromboembolism, using pulsed-wave transcranial ultrasound to increase exposure of the intravascular thrombus to IV tPA. However, two large studies found no statistical benefit, and this technique is therefore not recommended by the American Stroke Association [29–31].

TABLE 77.1 ECASS-II Hemorrhagic Infarction Classification

Hemorrhage Classification	Description
Hemorrhagic infarction 1	Small petechiae along the margins of the infarct
Hemorrhagic infarction 2	Confluent petechiae within the infarcted area but no space-occupying effect
Parenchymal hemorrhage 1	Blood clots in ≤30% of the infarcted area with some/slight space-occupying effect
Parenchymal hemorrhage 2	Blood clots in >30% of the infarcted area with substantial space-occupying effect

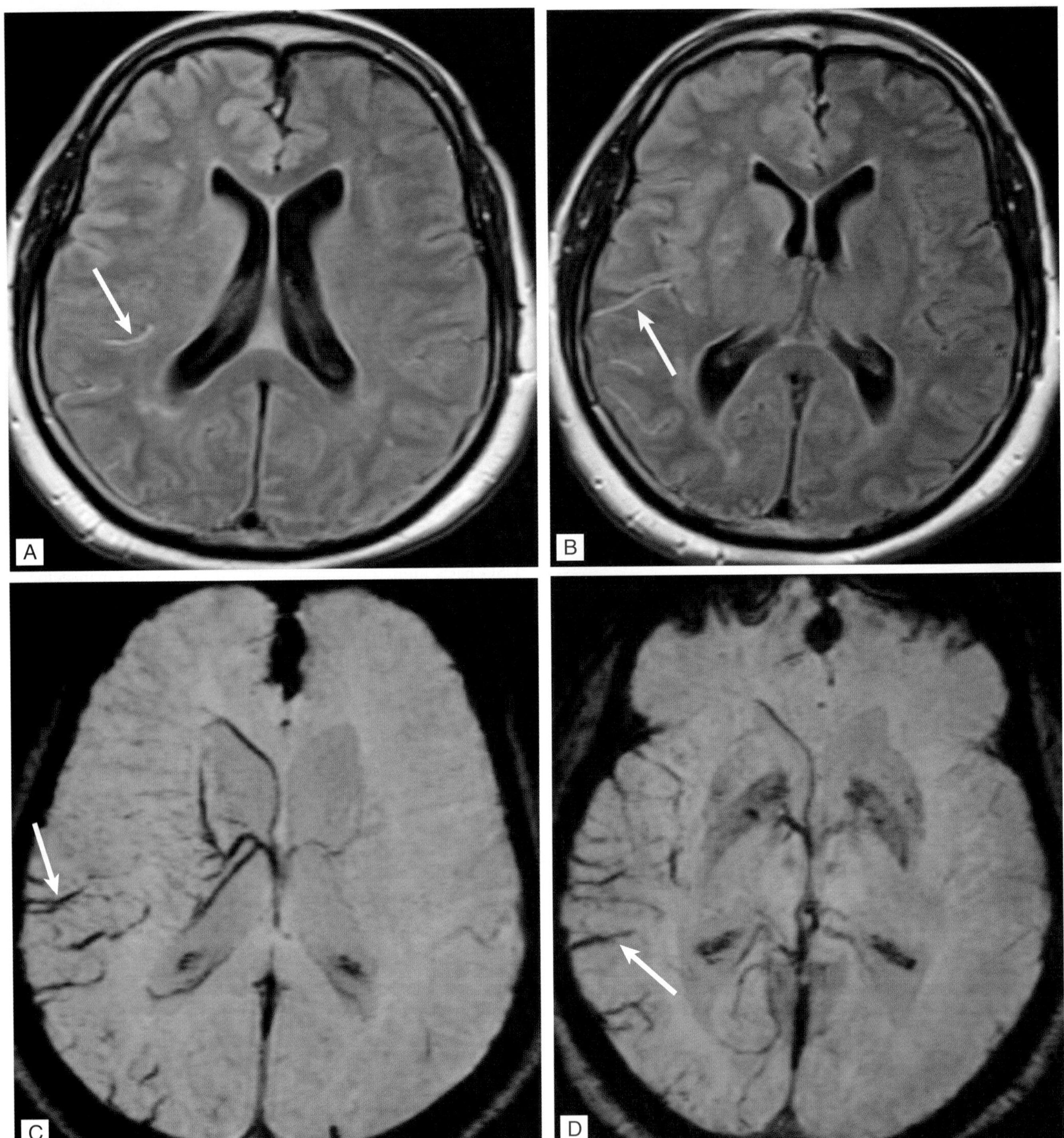

Figure 77.4 (A–D) Slow flow within distal right MCA cortical branches (*white arrows*) in the setting of a more proximal M1 segment occlusion with hyperintensity on FLAIR images and hypointensity on susceptibility weighted-images.

Computed Tomography Angiography

Computed tomography angiography (CTA) angiography is currently the workhorse for vascular imaging in acute ischemic stroke due to its speed, availability, and low cost compared to MRI. In addition, CTA provides reliable, high-resolution imaging of the entire vascular tree, from the aortic arch through the intracranial vessels, as well as provides the ability to perform functional perfusion imaging and assessment of collaterals.

An arterial occlusion will appear as an abrupt termination of a cervical or intracranial artery. The morphology of the occlusion on angiography may predict ease of revascularization. The "meniscus sign," described as a meniscoid appearance, or tram-track like appearance of antegrade side-wall contrast opacification at the proximal occlusion site is associated with higher first-pass successful recanalization [32]. There may be varying degrees of reconstitution of the more distal vascular territory

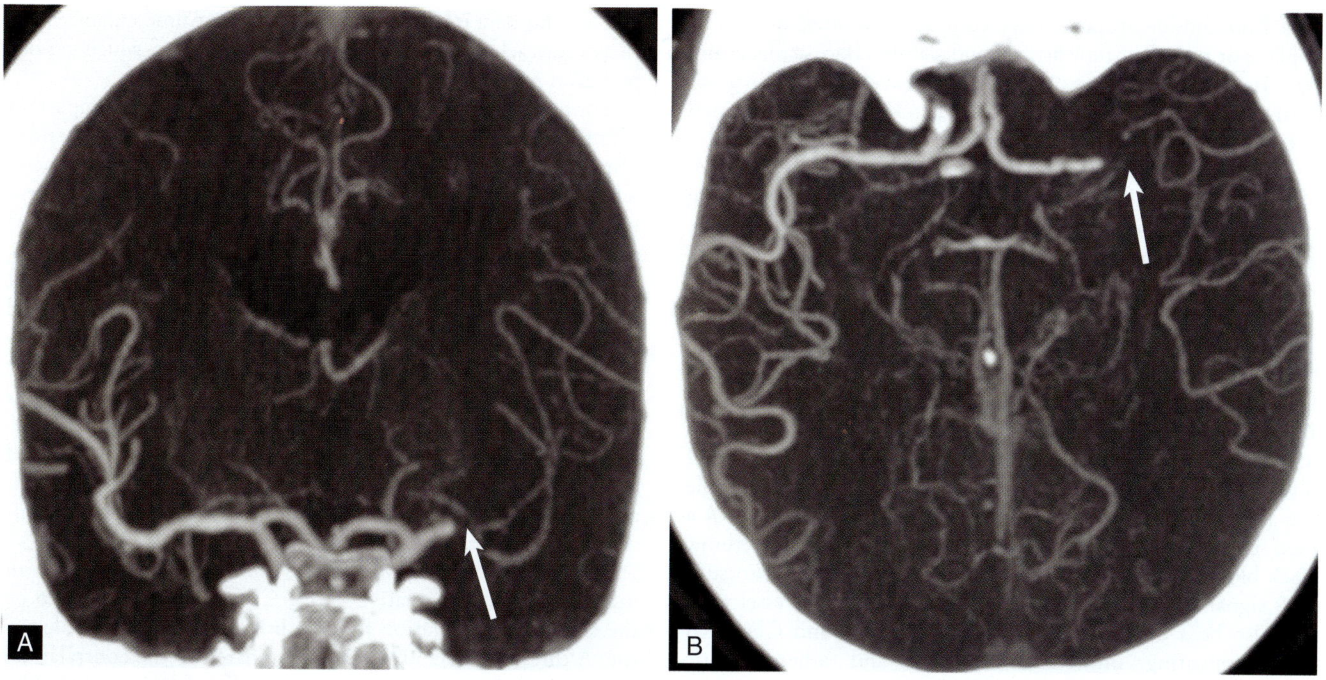

Figure 77.5 Cutoff of the left proximal M1 segment due to thromboembolism as seen in coronal (A) and axial (B) reformatted MIP images of CTA. Persistent filling of distal MCA branches via leptomeningeal collaterals. Arrow denotes the site of left MCA occlusion.

depending on the presence and degree of collateral flow. Rapidly identifying a vessel occlusion is critical in the management of acute ischemic stroke to target therapy. The ease of identification of a vessel stenosis or occlusion depends on multiple factors, including the size and location of the vessel in question, as well as the technical quality of the study. Occlusions of the cervical vessels or arteries of the circle of Willis are more readily identified, while occlusions of smaller, more distal segments of the anterior, middle, or posterior cerebral arteries may be more challenging to diagnose due to their small caliber and overlapping adjacent vessels. For this reason, it is critical to use multiple orthogonal planes as well as maximum intensity projection (MIP) images when interpreting these studies.

Technical problems may also drastically reduce the sensitivity of the study. Timing the scan too early or too late after the contrast bolus will result in either insufficient opacification of the arteries, or venous contrast contamination resulting in difficulty correctly identifying smaller arteries. Underlying health conditions such as congestive heart failure or central venous stenosis may contribute to errors in the timing of the contrast bolus.

Collateral flow to the territory beyond the occluded vessel has implications for management and outcome. Patients with good collateral flow, either via the circle of Willis or leptomeningeal collaterals, will have a slower progression to infarction in the affected territory. In a minority of cases where patients have very robust collaterals, they may be able to tolerate a proximal arterial stenosis without significant symptoms or resulting infarction. Patients with poor collaterals on the other hand will progress rapidly to tissue infarction. Not surprisingly then, patients with moderate/good collateral flow show the greatest benefit with endovascular thrombectomy [33–35].

Collateral flow can be assessed on CTA either using single-phase arterial imaging or multi-phase imaging (Fig. 77.5). A single-phase 4-point scale reported by Berkhemer et al. [34] categorizes collateral flow by percent filling of the occluded territory

TABLE 77.2 Collateral Grading by CTA

Grade	Description
0 – Absent collaterals	0% filling of occluded territory
1 – Poor collaterals	>0 to ≤50% filling of occluded territory
2 – Moderate collaterals	>50 to <100% filling of occluded territory
3 – Good collaterals	100% filling of occluded territory

(Table 77.2). A more complicated multi-phase 6-point scale developed by Menon et al. [36] also incorporates delay of filling of the occluded territory by collaterals, with better collateral flow showing little or no delay.

Collateral flow may also be assessed using perfusion imaging. *The Tmax parameter (a measure of the time to peak contrast opacification of the target tissue) will become prolonged in the vascular territory distal to an arterial occlusion.* More severe prolongation implies poorer collateral flow to the territory. A hypoperfusion intensity ratio (HIR), most commonly calculated as the volume of tissue with Tmax >10 seconds divided by the volume of tissue with Tmax >6 seconds, has been shown to correlate with quality of collateral flow, with lower HIR <0.5 associated with slower core infarct growth, smaller final infarct volume, and better functional outcomes [37–39].

Magnetic Resonance Angiography

Magnetic resonance angiography (MRA) is a useful modality in acute stroke imaging, with major benefits including the ability to image the vasculature without contrast or ionizing radiation, as well as being able to acquire diffusion weighted images during the same study. Time-of-flight (TOF) MRA is also not affected by the timing of contrast administration unlike bolus sensitive techniques such as CTA. On the other hand, MRA tends to suffer more from motion artifact compared to CTA, is often affected by in-plane or turbulent flow artifact and slab-interface artifacts and may also demonstrate loss of flow-related enhancement in regions of susceptibility artifact generated by hemorrhage or implanted metal devices such as endovascular stents or coils.

Contrast enhanced (CE) MRA is also sometimes performed when feasible and benefits from fewer artifacts, including motion and flow artifacts. In particular, areas of slow flow due to a severe proximal stenosis may appear occluded on TOF MRA, while filling with contrast will be apparent on CE MRA. CE MRA is often preferred when imaging the cervical vasculature, as TOF MRA often suffers from motion in the lower neck due to breathing and aortic pulsation, and turbulent flow/dephasing artifacts may overestimate stenosis at the carotid bifurcations. CE MRA also allows rapid imaging of the entire craniocervical vasculature from the aortic arch past the circle of Willis with a single bolus, whereas TOF MRA requires multiple slab acquisitions to cover the same territory, making CE MRA a good choice when considering a patient for thrombectomy. Black blood contrast enhanced MRA, a technique used to suppress signal within the lumen in order to image the vessel wall, may also be a useful adjunct to standard TOF and CE MRA when evaluating intracranial thrombi and atherosclerotic plaques, in particular intracranial plaques that do not cause stenosis [40].

Digital Subtraction Angiography

The gold standard for evaluation of the intracranial vasculature remains digital subtraction angiography (DSA). It provides unparalleled resolution of the vasculature as well as dynamic imaging through all phases of contrast injection, allowing for more sensitive evaluation of vessel stenoses or occlusions while also providing functional assessment of flow dynamics. However, as an interventional procedure, DSA carries a small risk of vessel injury or ischemic stroke (less than 1%) as well as entails greater costs compared to noninvasive imaging techniques. Consequently, DSA is primarily reserved for cases where an intervention is planned such as thrombectomy, or in a problem-solving capacity in instances where CTA/MRA are not conclusive (e.g., differentiating critical vessel stenosis versus complete occlusion) [41]. Collateral flow can also be assessed with DSA. However, a full assessment may be difficult as only a single vessel can be studied at a time, thereby limiting evaluation of collaterals between posterior and anterior circulations, as well as between cerebral hemispheres. Consequently, as multi-vessel angiography is not routinely performed in the setting of acute ischemic stroke in order to save time, collateral assessment may be more reliable with CTA methods [42].

Penumbra Imaging

The "penumbra" refers to brain tissue in the territory distal to an arterial occlusion that has not yet infarcted but is at risk of doing so due to decreased perfusion. This tissue is still salvageable but may go on to infarction if not rapidly reperfused. Identification and quantification of the ischemic penumbra is important in selecting patients who present in a delayed fashion (currently 6–24 hours from LKW) for endovascular reperfusion.

CT Perfusion

CT perfusion imaging uses a dynamic contrast enhanced acquisition to image the brain during intravenous contrast injection, capturing images throughout the contrast inflow and washout phases. This data is used to construct contrast time-enhancement curves for each voxel in the imaged volume, from which various perfusion parameters can be derived.

For imaging of acute ischemic stroke, the two most important parameters are "time to maximum of the residue function" (Tmax), and cerebral blood flow (CBF). The Tmax parameter reflects the contrast bolus delay between a chosen arterial input function (AIF, usually a large feeding artery such as the MCA) and the target tissue. Tmax has largely supplanted time-to-peak (TTP) for measurement of bolus delay on CT perfusion, however these measurements estimate the same phenomenon. A prolonged Tmax suggests slower flow of blood to the target tissue, which may be caused by a proximal arterial stenosis, or perfusion via collateral vessels taking a longer time to reach the target tissue. *Tmax >6 seconds has been reported as the threshold best correlating to salvageable penumbra* [43]. The DEFUSE 3 trial, which helped establish criteria for thrombectomy up to 16 hours after onset, also used the 6 second threshold for selecting patients, and this value is most often used clinically [8].

CBF represents blood flow within the target tissue in mL/100 g/min. The relative CBF (rCBF) has been found to be the closest approximation for core infarct, or unsalvageable tissue. A threshold of ≤30% rCBF (compared to the contralateral hemisphere) is used to determine core infarction [44]. The combination of Tmax and rCBF give accurate measurements of core infarction and at-risk penumbra, which are used clinically to determine the course of action in stroke management. A large mismatch between the core and penumbra (ratio of penumbra to core of ≥1.8 in the DEFUSE 3 study) is a prerequisite for endovascular therapy in the extended time window (Fig. 77.6) [8].

Additional parameters are commonly calculated in CT perfusion studies, including cerebral blood volume (CBV), and mean transit time (MTT). Decreased CBV has also been used in the past as a proxy for core infarct and usually closely tracks CBF, although CBF has been reported to better match diffusion abnormality on MRI [44]. MTT represents a measure of the average time for an erythrocyte to transit a volume of tissue and may be used as a marker of vasodilation. Autoregulation leads to vasodilation in oligemic and ischemic tissues, reducing the speed of transit through capillary beds to allow for maximal oxygen extraction. Areas of prolonged MTT will often overlap with areas of prolonged Tmax.

Key Point

Current guidelines in perfusion imaging define core infarction as ≤30% rCBF, and ischemic penumbra as Tmax >6 seconds. Perfusion imaging is a critical tool in decision making for stroke patients who are potential thrombectomy candidates in the extended window, 6–24 hours from last known well.

MR Perfusion

The same perfusion principles apply to MR perfusion as in CT perfusion regarding calculation of time-contrast curves for voxels of brain tissue and the resulting main derived perfusion parameters, however there are multiple methods by which to acquire the images.

The most commonly used method in stroke imaging is dynamic susceptibility contrast (DSC) perfusion, wherein a gadolinium-based contrast agent is injected intravenously and a T2 or T2*

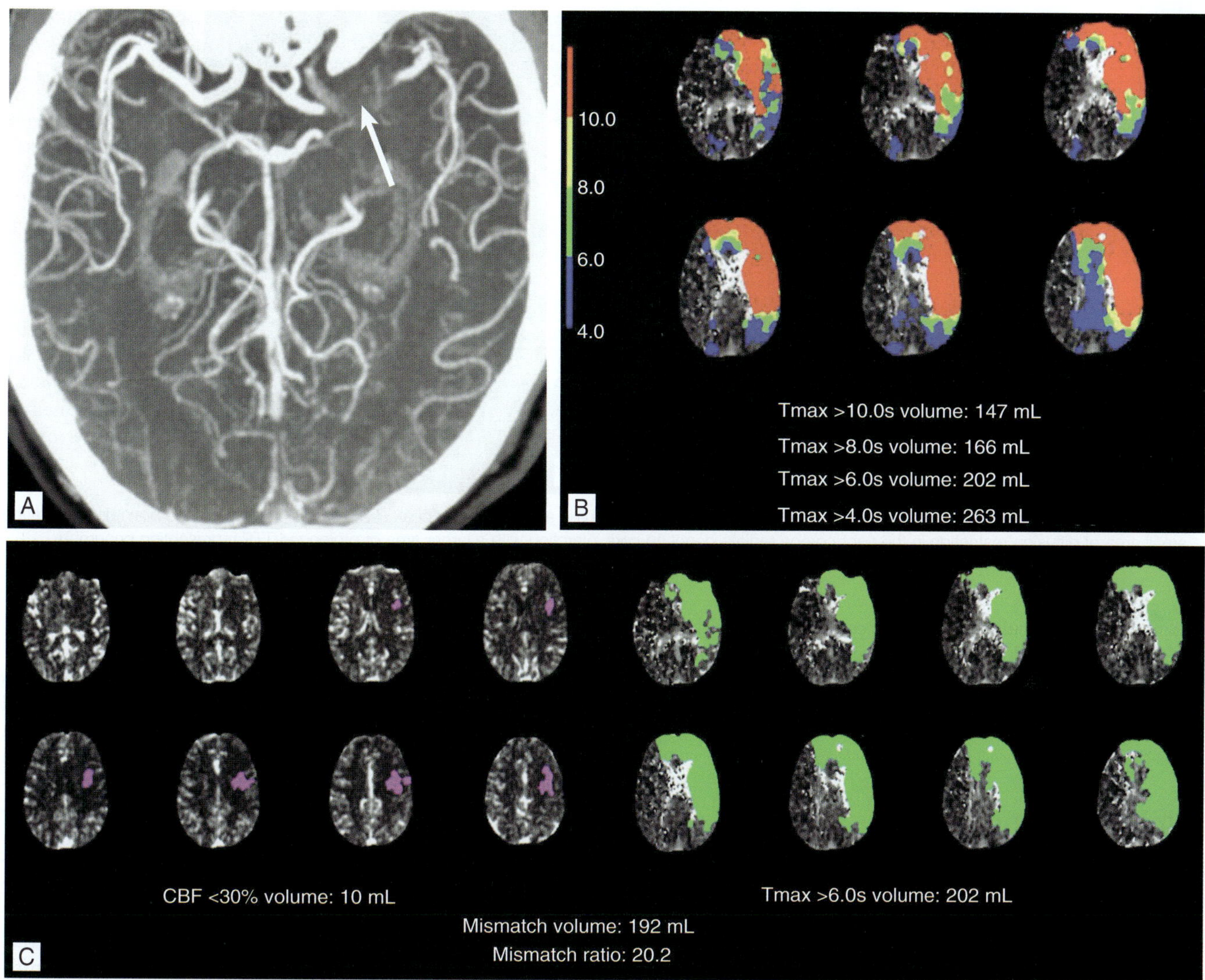

Figure 77.6 A patient with left hemispheric stroke in the delayed window (A) and left ICA occlusion (*arrow*). CT perfusion demonstrates a large area of prolonged Tmax (>10 seconds) with a hypoperfusion intensity ratio of 0.7 denoting poor collateral flow and likely rapid growth of the infarct core (B). Mismatch maps (C) showing a small core infarction in the left MCA territory (*purple*), and a large volume of ischemic, at-risk penumbra involving the left MCA and bilateral ACA territories (*green*).

weighted sequence is performed continuously throughout the wash-in and wash-out phases. The paramagnetic effects of the intravascular gadolinium cause susceptibility artifact and signal loss proportional to the concentration of contrast. The time-intensity curves are then used to derive perfusion parameters in a fashion similar to CT perfusion (Fig. 77.7).

Arterial spin labeled (ASL) perfusion imaging is a noncontrast method for acquiring perfusion images. The ASL technique utilizes magnetic labeling of upstream blood to quantify flow into the tissue of interest. In the case of brain imaging, this means labeling blood in the cervical vessels and acquiring signal from the labeled blood as it reaches the brain. This technique is attractive as it is simple to implement, non-invasive, and gives quantitative CBF values. ASL is often used when imaging pediatric patients as it does not require intravenous contrast and can be repeated multiple times if initial imaging is suboptimal. The technique is limited, however, as other perfusion parameters including Tmax, CBV, and MTT cannot be derived from ASL data using current clinically available techniques [45].

A third MR perfusion technique, dynamic contrast-enhanced (DCE) perfusion, is similar in technique to DSC perfusion, but utilizes a T1 weighted sequence during acquisition instead of a T2 or T2* weighted sequence. This approach uses increases in signal intensity rather than signal loss to construct the time-intensity curve and calculate perfusion parameters. The DCE technique brings an added ability to quantify vessel permeability, a measure that has been used in neuro-oncologic imaging [46]. DCE is not commonly employed in stroke imaging.

Automation

As imaging of penumbra has become an integral part of ischemic stroke management during the extended time window (>6 hours from stroke onset), methods to standardize and automate calculation of perfusion parameters have become more commonplace. The perfusion thresholds used in the DEFUSE 3 trial have become the basis for automated clinical decision-support tools, such as RAPID (iSchemaView), the tool used by the DEFUSE 3 investigators. The RAPID platform uses algorithms to automatically process source CT perfusion data, generate maps of the critical perfusion

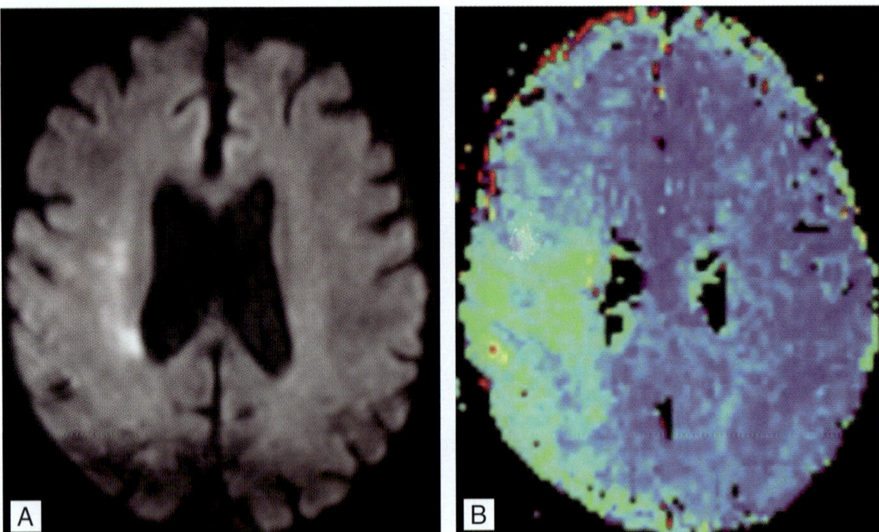

Figure 77.7 MRI perfusion with core-penumbra mismatch. (A) Diffusion weighted and (B) time to peak (TTP) perfusion image of the brain demonstrating a small area of diffusion restriction in the right corona radiata denoting core infarction with a larger area of prolonged TTP representing penumbra.

parameters, and calculate volumes of core infarction and penumbra. These automated tools also automatically alert members of the stroke team to the perfusion imaging and offer immediate access to the results, thereby helping to reduce the time needed to determine if a patient is eligible for thrombectomy.

Clinical Scenarios

Large Vessel Occlusion and Thromboembolism

Acute thromboembolic infarction results from the occlusion of a cerebral artery by embolic thrombus from a more proximal or central vessel, commonly the heart or carotid arteries. A large vessel occlusion (LVO), or occlusion of the proximal intracranial anterior or posterior circulation, accounts for approximately 24–46% of acute ischemic strokes. Major risk factors include hypertension, diabetes mellitus, arrhythmias, and smoking, among others. Less frequently, emboli may arise from deep veins in the setting of a patent foramen ovale, resulting in the so-called "paradoxical embolus." The MCA is the most common vessel for an embolus to occlude [47].

Acute Ischemic Stroke Management

In the setting of acute ischemic stroke, the earlier an intervention can be safely performed, the higher the chance of a good clinical outcome [3,4,48]. Imaging plays a central role in multiple critical decision points in the management of acute ischemic stroke. First, the decision to give IV tPA must be made. Early IV tPA administration has been shown to increase odds of good outcome when given less than 3 hours from stroke onset, and up to 4.5 hours in select patients [31,49]. Unenhanced head CT is therefore performed prior to its administration to exclude acute intracranial hemorrhage, major established infarction, or other contraindications to its use (e.g., evidence of a vascular malformation).

ASPECTS

The Alberta Stroke Programme Early CT Score (ASPECTS) was developed to help with the rapid estimation of core infarct volume on unenhanced CT in patients experiencing a middle cerebral artery stroke [50]. Previously, the definition of a "major infarction" was loosely defined as "greater than one-third the volume of the MCA territory", which is difficult for radiologists to accurately estimate. To help standardize this estimation and improve inter-reader reliability, the ASPECTS divides the MCA territory into 10 sections: C = Caudate nucleus; L = Lentiform nuclei; IC = Internal capsule; M1 = Anterior-inferior MCA cortex; M2 = MCA cortex lateral to the insular ribbon; M3 = Posterior-inferior insular cortex; M4 = Anterior-superior MCA cortex; M5 = Lateral-superior MCA cortex; M6 = Posterior-superior MCA cortex (Fig. 77.8).

The ASPECTS is calculated by assigning 1 point for each of the 10 sections and subtracting a point for each section that shows early ischemic changes, such as edema or hypoattenuation. Therefore, a higher score denotes a smaller infarction with a score of 10 meaning no evidence of infarction. An ASPECTS of 7 or less is associated with a significantly increased risk of functional dependence or death, and correlates well with the "1/3 MCA territory rule" in predicting risk of symptomatic hemorrhage [50].

Vascular Imaging and Indications for Thrombectomy

Following unenhanced CT, IV tPA is immediately administered if there are no contraindications identified. At this time, vessel imaging should be performed with either CTA or MRA. Depending on the time since stroke onset or last-known-well (LKW), imaging may or may not be performed with perfusion. Prior to 6 hours from onset, if a large vessel occlusion is identified on vessel imaging and there are no contraindications, evidence supports interventional thrombectomy regardless of perfusion imaging [4–6,31,51–54].

If more than 6 hours have passed since stroke onset, recent data have shown that patients may still benefit from intervention with thrombectomy, up to 24 hours after LKW [7,8,55]. These findings have significantly increased the number of patients who may be candidates for intervention, as patients who have unwitnessed stroke onset or who wake from sleep with a neurologic deficit (and therefore, onset time is not known) can still be eligible if certain criteria are met.

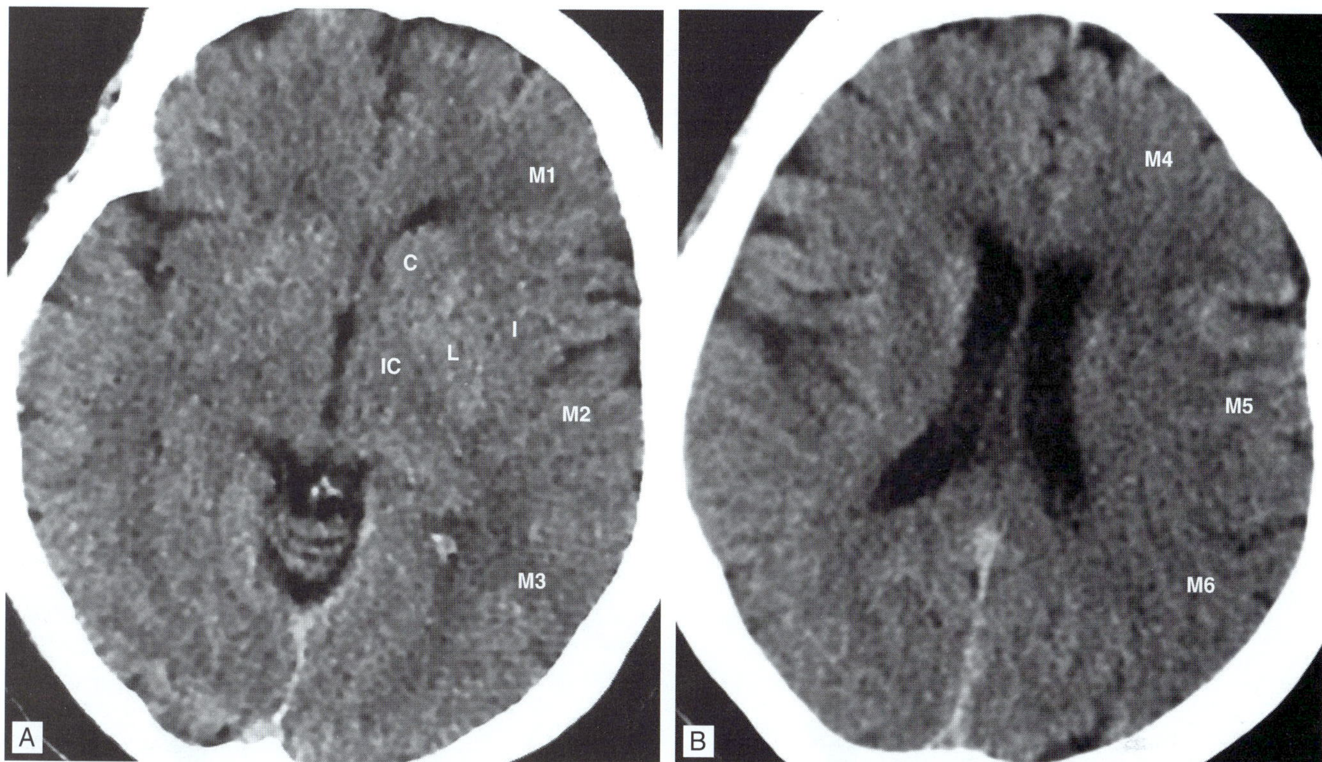

Figure 77.8 ASPECTS score [50] in axial CT images A & B at different levels. *C* = Caudate nucleus; *I* = insular ribbon; *IC* = Internal capsule; *L* = Lentiform nuclei; *M1* = Anterior-inferior MCA cortex; *M2* = MCA cortex lateral to the insular ribbon; *M3* = Posterior-inferior insular cortex; *M4* = Anterior-superior MCA cortex; *M5* = Lateral-superior MCA cortex; *M6* = Posterior-superior MCA cortex.

The criteria for thrombectomy in the extended 6 to 24-hour window relies heavily on imaging. The main goal of imaging in this setting is establishing the presence of a small volume, or core of completed infarction, with a large area of at-risk brain tissue (i.e., the penumbra). The penumbra can either be assessed directly with quantitative perfusion imaging, or by identifying a mismatch between the clinical stroke symptoms (NIH Stroke Scale) and the core infarct volume on imaging (either by diffusion weighted MRI or perfusion imaging). A high NIH Stroke Scale score, denoting a severe clinical deficit(s), in the setting of a small core infarct on imaging, implies the presence of a large penumbra of ischemic, but viable, brain tissue. As previously discussed, the specific protocol an institution uses to assess these parameters with imaging varies, and the use of either CTA or diffusion weighted MR, with or without perfusion imaging, are both reasonable options [31].

Once the decision has been made to proceed with thrombectomy, every effort is taken to perform the procedure and reperfuse the ischemic penumbra as quickly as possible. Multiple devices may be utilized for thrombectomy, the most common currently used include direct aspiration and stent retriever systems. A combination of techniques may also be used depending on the particulars of the case. Direct aspiration involves navigating an aspiration catheter to the site of thrombus (with or without the assistance of a microcatheter) and suctioning the thrombus into the catheter for retrieval [56,57]. Stent retrievers involve deploying a modified metallic mesh stent across the thrombus, which after allowing time for clot integration, is then removed from the body (Fig. 77.9).

Grading Reperfusion

The most widely used method for grading reperfusion on DSA after thrombectomy is the modified Thrombolysis in Cerebral Infarction (mTICI) scale, which has superseded prior grading scales such as AOL and TIMI [58–60]. The scale is based on real-time intraoperative arteriography of the territory distal to the occluded segment, immediately following thrombectomy (Table 77.3). Grades 2b, 2c and 3 have shown higher rates of good outcome and less infarct growth compared to Grades 1 and 2a [58,61].

Imaging Findings Post-Thrombectomy

Follow up imaging studies are routinely performed after thrombectomy to assess final infarct volume, monitor edema and mass effect resulting from the infarction, and to assess for potential complications, including subarachnoid hemorrhage and hemorrhagic conversion. If additional vascular imaging is performed in the post-thrombectomy setting, sequelae of the procedure may be evident, including focal spasm of the arteries adjacent to the original occlusion and/or vessel wall enhancement on contrast enhanced black blood MRI. Focal postprocedural vasospasm may be difficult to differentiate from residual thrombus. However, comparison with intraoperative DSA images is often helpful in this setting as spasm is often present immediately following thrombectomy and evident on DSA imaging.

Monitoring edema of the infarcted territory is also important, as up to 10% of patients will manifest a so-called *"malignant infarction" wherein severe edema and mass effect leads to neurologic deterioration, usually between days 2 and 5 after stroke onset* [62]. In this setting, decompressive craniectomy may be performed in select patients, preferentially within 48 hours of stroke onset [31,62].

Postintervention imaging at approximately 24 hours is recommended, in part to exclude hemorrhage prior to initiation of antithrombotic treatment for secondary prevention. CT imaging after thrombectomy often will demonstrate hyperdensity within infarcted tissue due to bloodbrain barrier breakdown and parenchyma contrast staining. This may pose a diagnostic dilemma as contrast

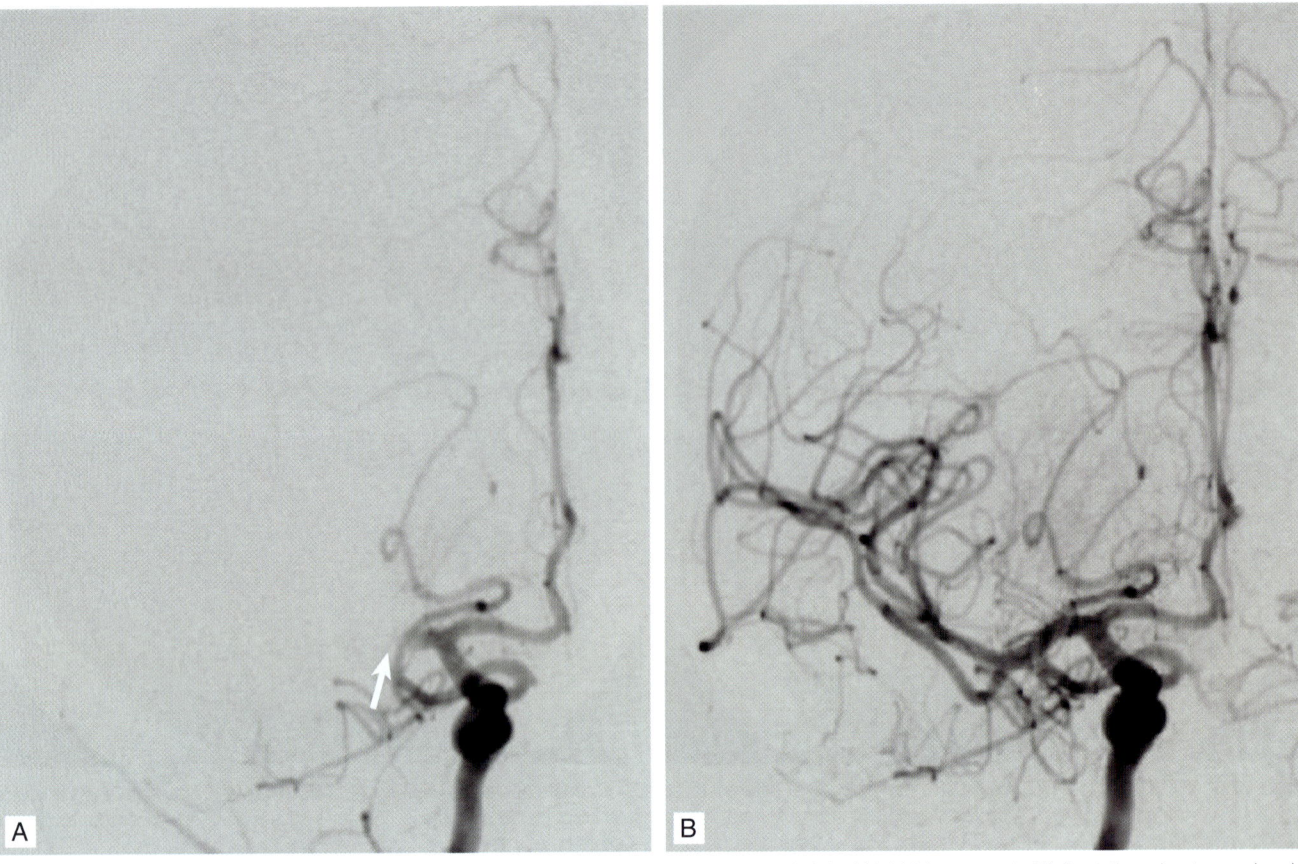

Figure 77.9 (A) Pre-thrombectomy DSA image showing occlusion (*arrow*) of the proximal right M1 MCA segment. (B) Post-thrombectomy showing recanalization of the previously occluded segment.

TABLE 77.3 Modified TICI Scale for Reperfusion Grading After Thrombectomy

mTICI Grade	DSA Findings
Grade 0	No perfusion
Grade 1	Antegrade perfusion beyond the initial occlusion, but limited distal filling and slow perfusion
Grade 2a	Antegrade reperfusion of less than half of the occluded target artery previously ischemic territory (e.g., in 1 major division of the MCA and its territory)
Grade 2b	Antegrade reperfusion of more than half of the previously occluded target artery ischemic territory (e.g., in 2 major divisions of the MCA and their territories)
Grade 2c	Near-complete perfusion except for slow flow in a few distal cortical vessels or presence of small distal cortical emboli
Grade 3	Complete antegrade reperfusion of the previously occluded target artery ischemic territory, with absence of visualized occlusion in all distal branches

staining may mimic and/or obscure true hemorrhage. Dual-energy CT may be used in this setting to create virtual non-contrast images and/or iodine map images, allowing simple separation of contrast from acute blood products (Fig. 77.10) [63].

Cervical Imaging

Atherosclerosis

Imaging of atherosclerotic disease involves using ultrasound, CT, MRI, or DSA to image the vessel lumen and determine if there is stenosis. The degree of luminal stenosis alone can predict risk of neurologic ischemic events as reported in the seminal NASCET trial in 1991, wherein those patients with a history of a hemispheric TIA or nondisabling stroke as well as ipsilateral carotid stenosis of 70–99% benefitted from endarterectomy [64,65]. The NASCET criteria and method of stenosis measurement is still used to stratify patients for surgical management, although recommendations have evolved to include asymptomatic patients with stenosis ≥75%, or symptomatic patients with stenosis ≥50% [66,67]. The NASCET style measurement was initially described on catheter directed carotid angiograms, however the same method is now used for CTA and MRA Eq. (77.1). The measurement is performed as follows:

$$\text{Percent stenosis} = 100 \times (1 - [\text{minimum residual lumen diameter (MRL)}/\text{distal lumen diameter (DL)}]),$$

where MRL is measured on the view or plane showing the smallest diameter, and DL is the lumen diameter at the next normal appearing arterial segment [66].

Cross sectional imaging and advanced techniques have opened many new areas of study beyond simply evaluating luminal diameter. CT, MRI and ultrasound all have an advantage over DSA in that the vessel wall and associated atherosclerotic plaque can be

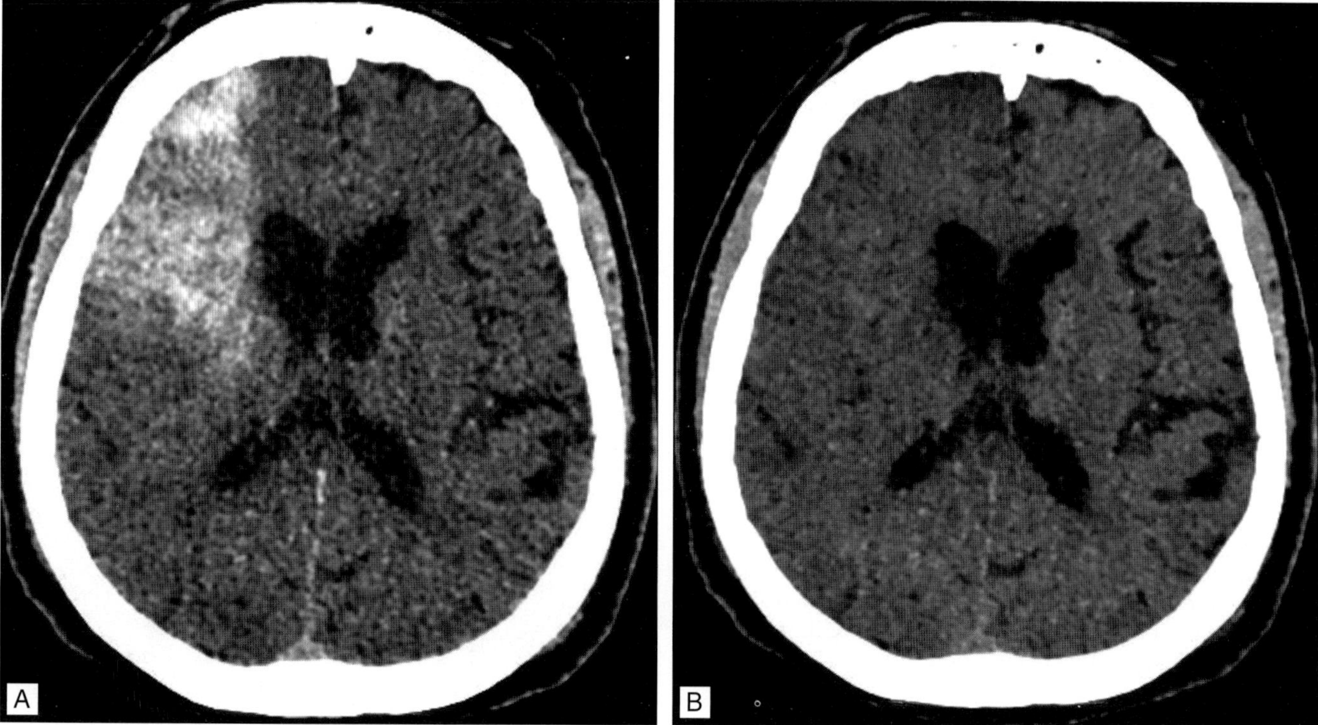

Figure 77.10 Dual energy axial noncontrast (A) and virtual monoenergetic 190 keV (B) images in a patient 2 hours post thrombectomy in the right middle cerebral artery. Standard noncontrast images show extensive parenchymal hyperattenuation in the right anterior MCA distribution. Virtual monoenergetic images at 190 keV show complete suppression of the hyperattenuation, indicating contrast staining rather than hemorrhage.

directly imaged in addition to the lumen. Plaque composition has been shown to affect risk of rupture and thrombosis, and both CT and MRI can be used to evaluate plaque composition. Plaques with certain features, including a thin fibrous cap, lipid-rich necrotic core, and/or intraplaque hemorrhage represent unstable lesions vulnerable to rupture [68–71]. CT Hounsfield unit thresholds have been used to characterize fibrous, calcified, lipid, and hemorrhagic components of carotid plaques. *Prior investigations have suggested an increased risk of subsequent rupture in plaques demonstrating lower attenuation (≤25 HU) suggestive of fatty composition, while calcified lesions had a significantly decreased risk of neurologic events* [71–74].

MRI is also very useful in differentiating fibrous cap from lipid core in atherosclerotic plaques. The fibrous cap will demonstrate avid enhancement on postcontrast T1 weighted images, whereas the avascular lipid core will not enhance [75,76].

The morphology of the plaque also has implications for stroke risk. Irregular or ulcerated surfaces are considered risk factors for TIA and stroke, as these may expose the pro-thrombotic lipid core of the plaque to the vessel lumen [72].

Key Point

Cross-sectional imaging in atherosclerosis has allowed evaluation of many parameters beyond luminal diameter, including plaque composition and morphology, allowing better risk stratification.

Dissection

Arterial dissection of a cervical artery is the most common cause of stroke in young and middle aged adults [77,78]. Dissection occurs when a defect in the intima allows flowing blood to enter between the layers of the arterial wall, often leading to compression and narrowing of the vessel lumen. The blood within the vessel wall may thrombose due to the exposed, thrombogenic adventitial and medial layers, resulting in intramural hematoma. This thrombogenicity may cause acute thrombus to form in the true lumen, resulting in occlusion of the dissected vessel, and, or embolization of clot to distal vascular territories. The latter is the most common cause of ischemic stroke in the setting of dissection [79].

Dissection may be spontaneous or result from direct vessel trauma. 80% of patients present with headache or neck pain, and 67% with neurologic symptoms of TIA or stroke [80]. Headache and neck pain may precede onset of neurologic symptoms, potentially serving as a warning sign [81]. Horner's syndrome and other cranial nerve palsies ipsilateral to the dissection have also been described in up to 25% of patients with extracranial ICA dissection, possibly due to stretching of nerves adjacent to the carotid or interruption of blood supply to the nerves [80,82].

CTA and MRA are most commonly used when dissection is suspected. Cervical artery dissection rarely manifests with a clearly visible intimal flap or patent false lumen as is often seen in aortic dissection [83]. The classic appearance of ICA dissection is a tapered, eccentric occlusion or stenosis just distal to the carotid bulb, appearing similar to a flame on coronal or sagittal views, known as the "flame sign." However, any intimal irregularity with or without associated luminal narrowing may be suggestive of dissection. A dissection that extends towards the vessel adventitia may form an associated pseudoaneurysm, which may also act as a nidus for distal thromboembolism [83]. Vertebral dissection most often manifests as irregular focal narrowing of the vessel or abrupt occlusion. This can be difficult to differentiate from atherosclerotic occlusion or thromboembolism, and in these cases patient history and demographics are helpful, for example, a young person or a history of recent neck trauma would be more suggestive of vertebral artery dissection.

With MRI, one can directly visualize intramural hematomas associated with the dissection. When dissection is a consideration, the MRA protocol should include an axial precontrast T1 sequence with fat suppression. This allows the intrinsically T1 hyperintense blood products in the vessel wall to stand out against the dark intraluminal blood and suppressed perivascular fat, appearing as a crescent of high T1 signal (Fig. 77.11).

DSA is also helpful in evaluation of dissection, both in diagnosis and potentially treatment. Carotid dissection again classically appears as a tapered occlusion or stenosis, sometimes with a long distal segment of severe stenosis with a tiny patent true lumen known as the "string sign." If the stenosis is able to be traversed with a microcatheter, stenting may optionally be performed to restore normal vessel caliber [84].

Key Point

Headache and/or neck pain with ipsilateral cranial nerve palsies may be a sign of carotid dissection. Fat-suppressed T1 weighted MRI may be used to directly visualize intramural hematoma in the setting of dissection.

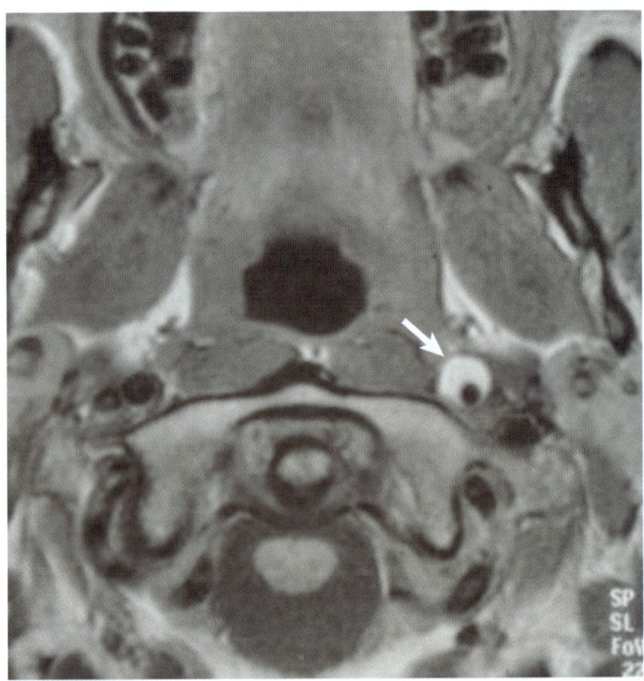

Figure 77.11 Left ICA dissection with a crescent of T1 hyperintensity surrounding the vessel lumen related to intramural hematoma (*arrow*).

Fibromuscular Dysplasia

Fibromuscular dysplasia (FMD) is an idiopathic arteriopathy with a strong female predilection resulting in concentric hypertrophy of smooth muscle resulting in irregular segments of stenosis and dilation. The cervical vessels are the second most common site of involvement with FMD, after the renal arteries [83,85]. Most lesions occur in the mid-to-distal cervical internal carotid and vertebral arteries; the vertebral arteries are less commonly involved than the ICA's. The proximal ICA and carotid bifurcation is nearly always spared, helping to distinguish this entity from atherosclerotic disease. Bilateral involvement is common, being present in 60–85% of cases.

On imaging, FMD manifests as irregular, segmental stenoses and dilations, resulting in a "string-of-beads" appearance (Fig. 77.12). On DSA, this should be distinguished from the "standing wave" phenomenon commonly seen as an artifact of contrast power injection.

FMD may cause hemodynamic compromise leading to stroke or TIA either through severe narrowing of the vessel, or spontaneous dissection of the affected segment [86]. Medical management is

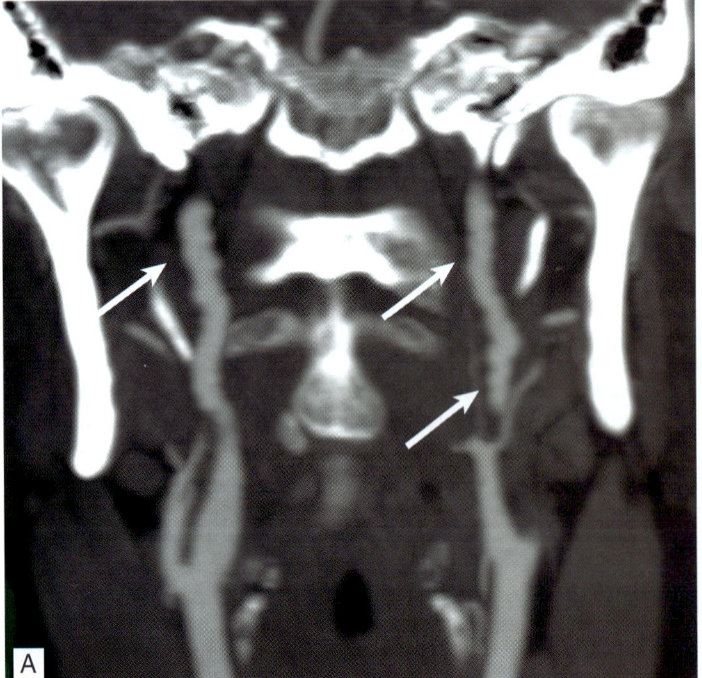

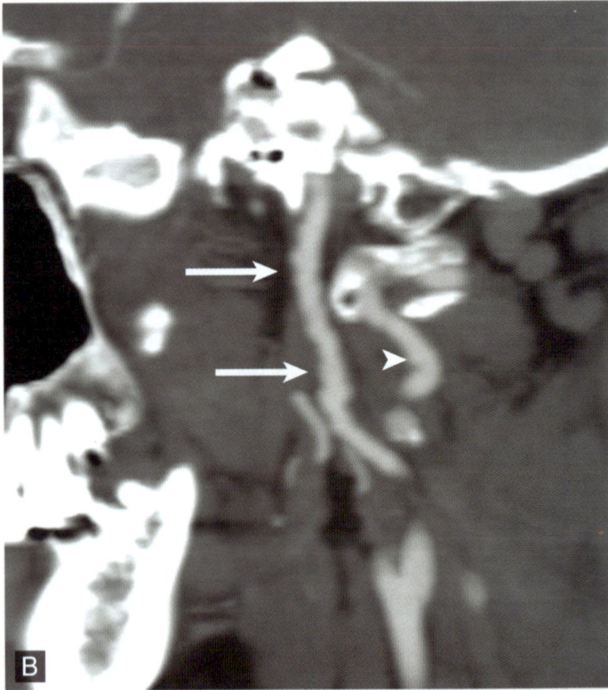

Figure 77.12 Coronal (A) and sagittal (B) reformatted maximum intensity projection CTA images of the neck showing string-of-beads appearance (*arrows*) of the bilateral cervical internal carotid arteries (A). Sagittal image (B) shows involvement of the left ICA (*arrows*) as well as the adjacent left vertebral artery (*arrowhead*).

generally preferred in patients with FMD, including antihypertensive and antiplatelet therapy. In some severe cases, endovascular angioplasty may be offered as a surgical treatment [87].

Key Point
FMD is most common in women, and the distal cervical arteries are commonly involved, second only to the renal arteries.

Carotid Web

A carotid web manifests radiologically as a shelf-like linear filling defect projecting into the carotid lumen at the posterior wall of the proximal internal carotid artery (Fig. 77.13). These lesions all show the classic location and appearance, are often bilateral, and have been found histopathologically to reflect fibrous intimal thickening resulting from an intimal variant of FMD [88]. Carotid webs should be distinguished from ulcerated atheromatous plaques or dissection flaps, lesions which may occur in the same location. Stasis and turbulence of blood flow just distal to the flap is thought to induce thrombus formation which may lead to TIA or ischemic stroke [88]. Carotid webs have been found to be associated with "cryptogenic strokes," particularly in young African American women [89]. Endarterectomy may be performed in symptomatic patients.

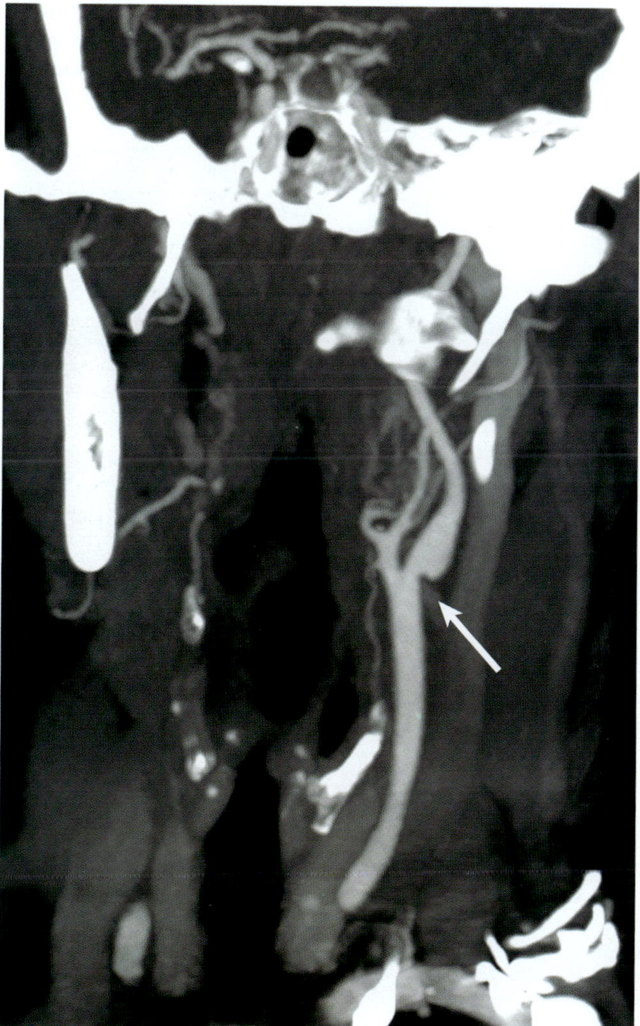

Figure 77.13 Coronal reformatted CTA of the neck with a shelf-like filling defect (*arrow*) projecting from the intima of the left carotid bulb, consistent with a web.

Small Vessel Ischemic Disease

Small vessel ischemic disease (SVID), commonly referring to a combination of white matter gliotic changes otherwise known as leukoaraiosis, and/or lacunar infarctions, is often seen involving the white matter and deep gray structures of older patients. The proposed mechanism of these changes is narrowing or occlusion of small perforating arteries primarily due to chronic hypertension, however other cardiac risk factors may also play a role [90,91]. Leukoaraiosis results from small vessel narrowing resulting in chronic ischemia and gliosis of the white matter, while a true lacunar infarction results from a small perforating artery occlusion. Lacunar infarctions are often clinically silent, however changes of SVID is associated with an increased risk of symptomatic stroke [92].

Leukoaraiosis manifests as patchy, symmetric white matter hypoattenuation or T2 hyperintensity most commonly involving the periventricular white matter of the lateral ventricles, the hemispheric subcortical white matter, and the central pontine white matter. Lacunar infarctions most commonly involve the basal ganglia, thalami, corona radiata, and pons, and may demonstrate central encephalomalacia with attenuation/signal equal to that of CSF.

A common diagnostic dilemma in CT imaging is distinguishing an acute or subacute lacunar infarction from a chronic infarction in the setting of new onset neurologic symptoms. As these lesions are small, features such as edema in acute lesions or encephalomalacia in chronic lesions are often difficult or impossible to distinguish. In these cases, prior imaging can be helpful for lesion aging. However, MRI with diffusion weighted images is ultimately most useful to assess acuity.

Intrinsic Disease of the Intracranial Arteries

Intracranial Atherosclerosis

Intracranial atherosclerotic disease (ICAD) is one of the most common causes of stroke worldwide, and the most common cause in patients of Asian descent [93]. These lesions typically involve proximal intracranial arteries resulting in vessel stenosis or occlusion and are associated with a high risk of recurrent stroke. Medical therapy was the mainstay of ICAD management, however as many patients continued to develop disabling strokes despite medical management, an interest arose in angioplasty and stenting for severe lesions. However, the Stenting and Aggressive Medical Management for Preventing Recurrent Stroke in Intracranial Stenosis Trial (SAMPRIS) in 2011 established the superiority of aggressive medical management in the treatment of intracranial atherosclerotic lesions, both due to the increased risk of early stroke in the interventional arm, and a lower than expected risk of stroke with aggressive medical therapy [94]. Aggressive medical management, as defined in the SAMMPRIS trial, involves dual antiplatelet therapy with aspirin and clopidogrel, management of primary stroke risk factors including hypertension and elevated LDL, management of secondary risk factors including diabetes, smoking, and obesity.

Imaging of intracranial atherosclerotic plaques remains largely focused on the degree of stenosis, however plaque imaging techniques similar to those used in the cervical arteries have been used to image intracranial lesions as well, potentially providing additional risk stratification for stroke. In particular, plaques imaged with contrast enhanced black blood MRI sequences showing plaque enhancement, arterial positive remodeling, and plaque surface irregularity are associated with stroke events in the corresponding territory [93,95].

> **Key Point**
> Intracranial atherosclerosis is treated medically rather than with interventional techniques.

Vasculitis

Stroke may also manifest as a complication of vasculitis or other intrinsic vasculopathies resulting in arterial narrowing or occlusion. CNS vasculitis is generally divided into two categories: primary angiitis of the CNS (confined to the CNS without involvement of other areas), and secondary. Secondary causes of CNS vasculitis include a wide range of diseases such as Takayasu arteritis, sarcoidosis, polyarteritis nodosa, systemic lupus erythematosus, and many others, with the primary diagnosis relying on combination of patient history, imaging, and various biomarkers from blood or CSF analysis [96,97].

Vascular imaging by DSA, CTA, or MRA in severe cases will classically show multifocal segmental narrowing of small and medium sized vessels, occlusions, and occasionally pseudoaneurysms. MRA and DSA are considered the most sensitive modalities, however sensitivity and specificity remain poor [98,99]. CT and MRI may show complications of vessel stenoses, including territorial or watershed infarctions, parenchymal hemorrhages, and nonspecific leukoencephalopathy.

Black blood vessel wall MRI is very helpful in the evaluation of CNS vasculitis, particularly in distinguishing vasculitis from other causes of vessel narrowing. Active vasculitic lesions will show avid vessel wall enhancement most often in a smooth, concentric fashion, as opposed to the heterogeneous and eccentric enhancement that may be seen with atherosclerotic disease.

Other potential causes of narrowing, including reversible cerebral vasoconstriction syndrome (RCVS) and Moyamoya disease may show no enhancement or mild enhancement, although research in this area is ongoing [100].

Reversible Cerebral Vasoconstriction Syndrome

Reversible cerebral vasoconstriction syndrome (RCVS) is a clinical and imaging syndrome characterized by sudden onset severe headache with segmental intracranial vasoconstriction that resolves by 3 months [101]. While most commonly a benign process, some cases may result in intracranial hemorrhage or stroke. Women are more frequently affected, and patients typically range from 20 to 50 years old. More than half of RCVS cases are associated with use of vasoactive drugs or the postpartum state, although many other potential triggers have also been proposed.

DSA remains the gold standard for evaluation of RCVS, however noninvasive CTA and MRA are commonly used. The classic appearance on imaging is of multi-territorial segmental vasoconstriction resulting in a beaded appearance of medium-to-large arteries (Fig. 77.14). Affected segments are interspersed with normal appearing segments [102]. Imaging may be normal early in the disease, possibly due to a distal-to-proximal progression of

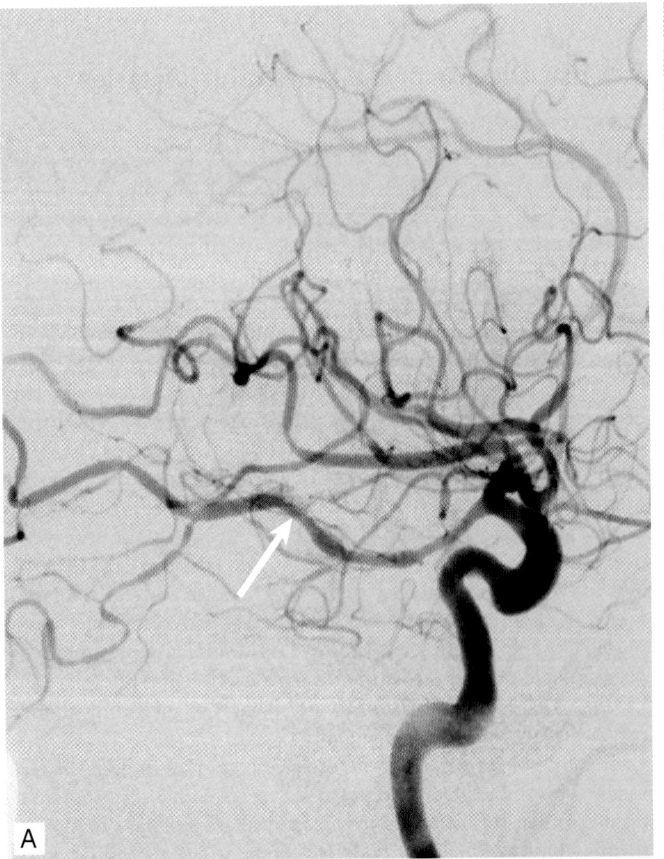

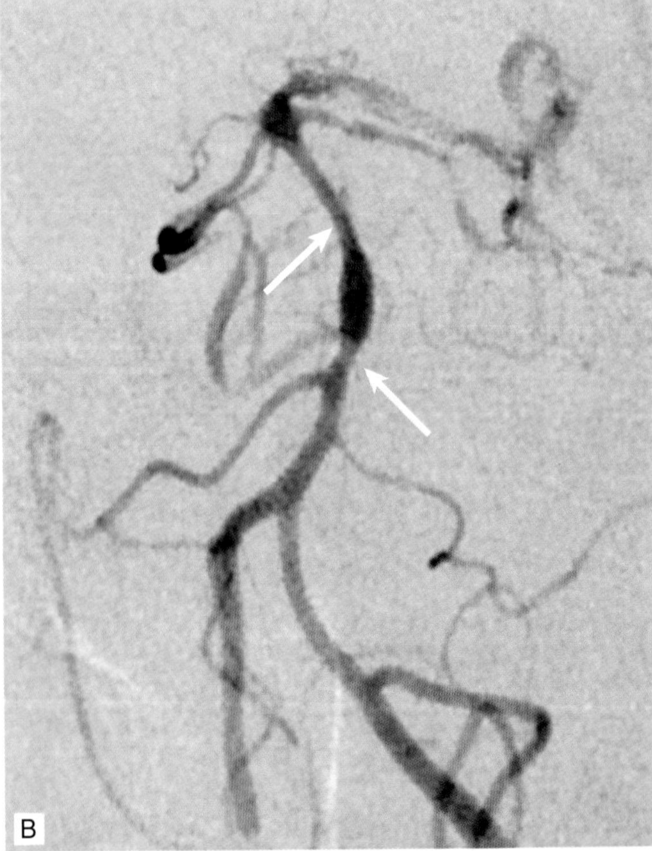

Figure 77.14 Lateral and PA DSA images showing multifocal vasoconstriction (*arrows*) resulting in a beaded appearance compatible with RCVS in a patient with acute onset headache and left extremity weakness.

affected vascular segments with later involvement of larger vessels that are more easily visualized [102].

Imaging with CT or MRI may reveal watershed infarcts due to restricted blood flow, most often bilateral, as well as subarachnoid hemorrhage.

Black blood vessel wall MRI may show significant thickening of the vessel walls in affected segments, however only a minority will display enhancement. Abnormalities are also typically transient, resolving over a few months, in contradistinction to CNS vasculitis [100,102].

Key Point
RCVS most commonly affects young to middle-aged women, and while usually benign, can result in hemorrhagic or ischemic stroke.

Moyamoya Disease

Moyamoya disease is an idiopathic, progressive stenosis of the carotid terminus leading to development of a network of abnormal collateral vessels at the base of the brain [103]. While the term "Moyamoya disease" is reserved for idiopathic cases, "Moyamoya syndrome" or "Moyamoya" phenomenon may be used to describe an array of conditions leading to a similar pathological appearance, including atherosclerotic stenosis, sickle cell vasculopathy, radiation-induced vasculopathy, and others.

Vascular imaging will show severe stenosis or occlusion of the carotid terminus, usually bilaterally with enlarged, abnormal collateral vessels in the parasellar region, perimesencephalic cisterns, and within the basal ganglia. The angiographic appearance of these collateral vessels produced the name "Moyamoya", translated from Japanese as "hazy, as a puff of smoke" (Fig. 77.15) [103].

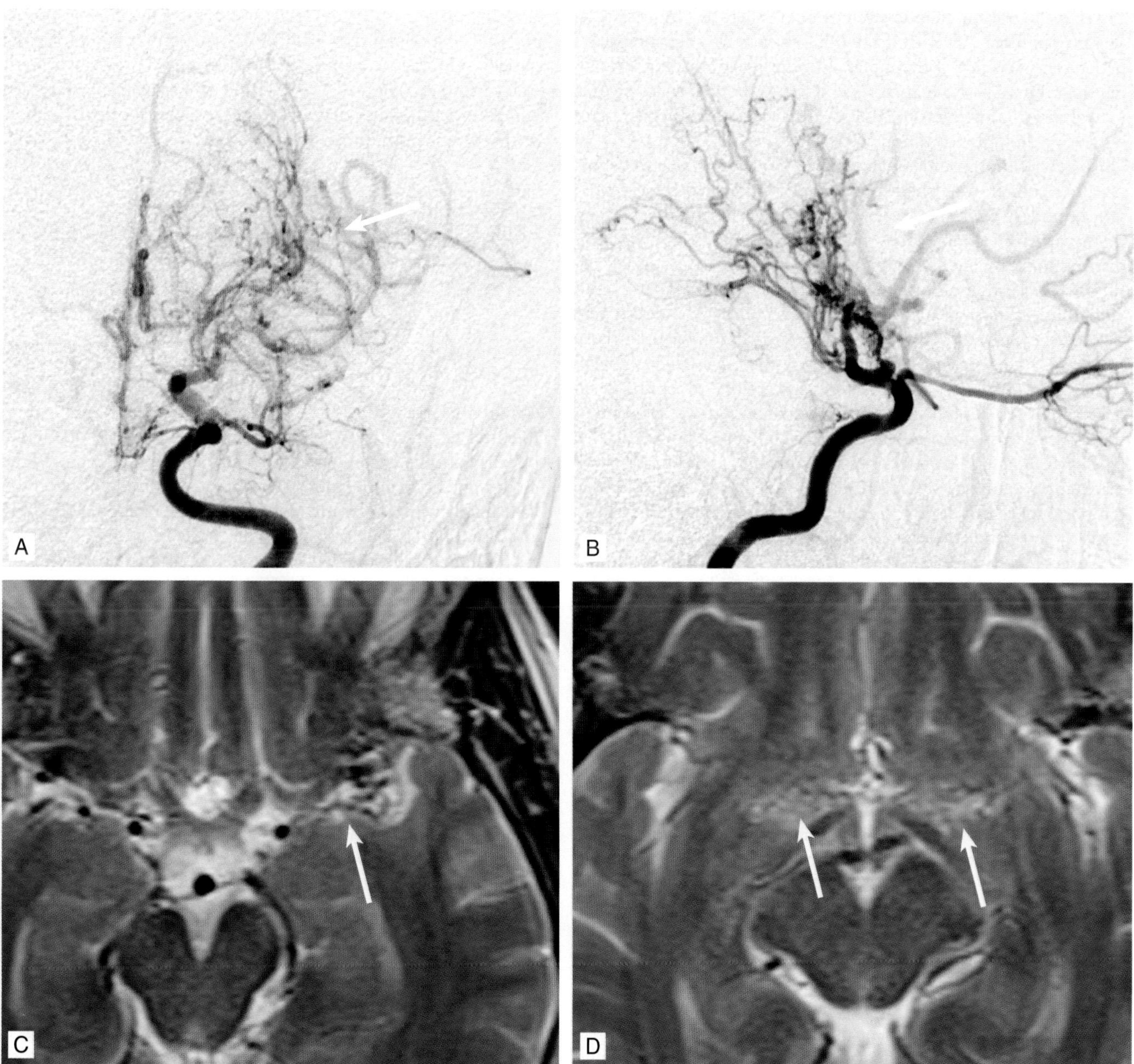

Figure 77.15 Moyamoya syndrome. (A) AP and (B) Lateral DSA views of the left internal carotid demonstrating chronic occlusion of the carotid terminus. Adjacent extensive opacification of tortuous collateral vessels (*arrows*). (C, D) Axial T2 spin echo MRI images in a different patient with Moyamoya show prominent flow voids from dilated lenticulostriate vessels along the expected course of the left MCA (A) and in the bilateral suprasellar cistern (B).

Parenchymal imaging may show multifocal territorial or watershed infarctions of the anterior circulation. The "ivy sign" of engorged leptomeningeal collateral vessels manifesting as hyperintensity within the sulci on T2 FLAIR or T1 postcontrast images is also a classic finding [104,105].

Only a minority of patients with Moyamoya will show vessel wall thickening or enhancement on black blood vessel wall imaging, however those cases which do show enhancement or thickening are associated with ischemic events [106].

Global Ischemic and Hypoxemic Injuries

Global ischemic and hypoxemic events can result in devastating neurologic injury, depending on the degree and duration of the insult, as well as a patient's individual physiology. Common etiologies include cardiac arrest, trauma, or asphyxiation. Generically termed "hypoxic-ischemic injury" (HII) or the clinical correlate "hypoxic-ischemic encephalopathy" (HIE), injuries may present radiologically with many different patterns depending on patient age, severity of the injury, and timing of imaging following the injury. HII in infants and children is more likely to be due to asphyxiation, whereas in adults, cardiac arrest or cerebrovascular disease are more common [107].

In older children and adults, mild to moderate global ischemia usually results in watershed zone infarcts. Watershed zones represent boundary regions between major vascular territories, such as in the anterior frontal lobes between ACA and MCA vascular distributions, or in the occipital lobes between MCA and PCA supply. The exact location of watershed zones varies between individuals due to normal anatomic variations in the size and distribution of the cerebral vessels. As the watershed zones are farthest from the large afferent arteries supplying the brain, they are relatively hypo-perfused and therefore susceptible to episodes of decreased cerebral perfusion. Watershed infarctions are most commonly seen involving the white matter and cortex bordering the ACA, MCA, and PCA territories in a roughly parallel parasagittal orientation, however PCA/MCA watershed infarctions in the temporal lobes can also be seen, again reflecting anatomic variation in the cerebral vessels.

Severe HII in adults primarily affects the gray matter structures including the basal ganglia, thalami, cerebellum, hippocampi and cortex, particularly the pre- and postcentral gyri. These gray matter structures are more metabolically active due to synaptic activity than white matter, and are more susceptible to the effects of neuronal excitotoxicity [107].

Imaging of HII can be particularly difficult, as early post-injury studies may be completely normal, or show only the subtlest of abnormalities. Furthermore, abnormalities are often symmetric, which may mask subtle parenchymal changes. Fogging and pseudo-normalization of CT and MRI may also mask even severe injuries if a study is acquired 1–3 weeks post-injury. Consequently, history is often very helpful to alert the radiologist to the possibility of a HII.

CT imaging may initially demonstrate hypoattenuation in involved structures secondary to edema, which may manifest as blurring of the border between gray and white matter in a diffuse or patchy manner. In severe cases, global cerebral edema may be present, with narrowing of the sulci and Sylvian fissures, decreased ventricular size, and effacement of the basal cisterns. The injured basal ganglia may become edematous and enlarged symmetrically. These changes may produce the "reversal sign," or an inversion of the normal attenuation relationship between gray and white matter as a result of diffuse gray matter edema. The deep gray structures, brainstem and cerebellum in some cases may appear relatively spared, producing the "white cerebellum" sign [108]. The cause of this apparent sparing is poorly understood and may reflect any combination of preferential maintenance of blood flow to the posterior circulation, postischemic hypervascularity, distention of deep medullary veins, petechial hemorrhage, or other potential explanations.

MRI will show restricted diffusion of injured structures acutely, and later edema. Cortical laminar necrosis of injured cortex may develop in the subacute to chronic period, manifesting as gyriform CT hyperattenuation and associated T1 hyperintensity.

Delayed changes may also be seen in the weeks and months after injury in those patients who survive the initial insult. Post anoxic leukoencephalopathy is a delayed white matter injury occurring in 2–3% of patients suffering hypoxic-ischemic events, manifesting as either progressive neurologic decline or an acute decline after 2–3 weeks of clinical stability [107]. On MRI, diffusion images will show diffuse white matter diffusion restriction and T2 hyperintensity [109]. The majority (75%) of these patients go on to complete or near-complete recovery over the following 6–12 months [107]. Patients surviving hypoxic-ischemic injuries may also develop progressive global cerebral atrophy in the weeks and months after the event. Also see chapter 76.

Key Point

Imaging findings in HII are heterogeneous, and depend on patient age, severity and length of insult, and other factors. History is very helpful in identifying subtle cases.

Fat and Air Emboli

Cerebral fat embolism (CFE) typically occurs 24–48 hours after fractures of large, lower extremity long bones such as the femur, but may also be encountered following small bone fractures and, or orthopedic manipulations. The classic syndrome of fat embolism involves multiple other organ systems, including the lungs and skin, with major criteria for diagnosis including a petechial rash, respiratory insufficiency, and abnormal mental status [110].

Initial unenhanced head CT often appears on remarkable, however diffuse edema may be present in severe cases, as well as scattered areas of hypoattenuation and, or hemorrhage. On MRI, the classic "star field pattern" is produced on DWI with numerous small hyperintense foci throughout the cerebral hemispheres, deep gray structures, brainstem and cerebellum, with a predilection for the watershed zones. Susceptibility images (SWI) may show corresponding punctate hemorrhages (Fig. 77.16).

Cerebral air embolism (CAE) is a potentially catastrophic complication of vascular procedures. Cerebral arterial air may result from direct manipulation of the arterial system during surgery or catheterization, or by a paradoxical venous route via a patent foramen ovale [111]. Arterial air may occlude small arteries in the brain and cause diffuse ischemic injury, leading to cerebral edema and death. Larger air emboli may be visible on unenhanced head CT as tubular, serpiginous air densities within the brain parenchyma (Fig. 77.17).

Small amounts of cerebral venous air are often present on routine imaging, likely due to bubbles of air injected during IV contrast or medication administration floating retrograde to the larger cerebral venous structures including the cavernous sinuses and superior sagittal sinus. These small venous air emboli are generally of no clinical significance [112].

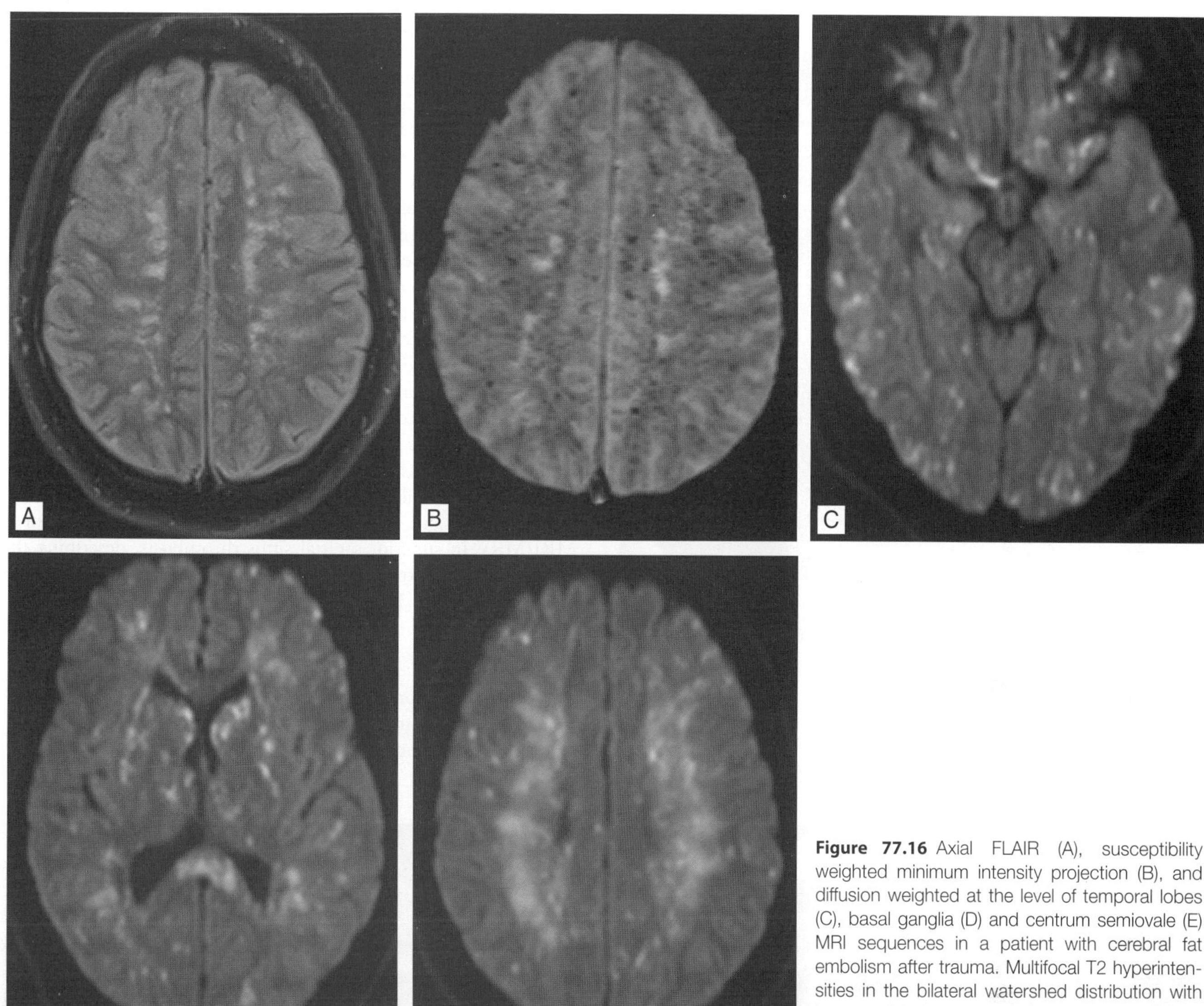

Figure 77.16 Axial FLAIR (A), susceptibility weighted minimum intensity projection (B), and diffusion weighted at the level of temporal lobes (C), basal ganglia (D) and centrum semiovale (E) MRI sequences in a patient with cerebral fat embolism after trauma. Multifocal T2 hyperintensities in the bilateral watershed distribution with innumerable foci of restricted diffusion bilaterally (starfield pattern) as well as diffuse punctate hemorrhages.

Venous Infarction

Although arterial pathology, such as arterial stenosis or occlusion, is the most common and widely recognized causes of interruption of blood flow to the brain leading to infarction, downstream venous occlusion may also precipitate acute ischemic stroke. Various venous pathologies—including traumatic or iatrogenic venous thrombus or occlusion, venous hypertension related to a dural arteriovenous fistula, or occlusion of a developmental venous anomaly—may interrupt or slow venous drainage from the upstream parenchyma [113]. Without a pathway for venous drainage, intravascular pressures rise and eventually equal that of the cerebral perfusion pressure, preventing arterial blood from flowing into the territory and leading to ischemia and infarction. Venous infarction is rare, accounting for only 0.5% of all stroke [114] and clinical presentations as well as underlying predisposing factors may vary greatly. However, when compared to arterial thromboembolism, affected individuals tend to be younger and present more often with headache and diffuse encephalopathy rather than with a painless focal neurologic deficit. Pregnancy, malignancy, steroid or oral contraceptive use, or any underlying prothrombotic condition are all known risk factors, among many others [114,115].

In addition to variability in clinical presentation, venous infarctions have a varied appearance on imaging, which can add to diagnostic difficulty. Parenchymal lesions will commonly cross arterial vascular boundaries and may be bilateral or symmetric if a midline venous structure is affected, such as the superior sagittal sinus or straight sinus. Hemorrhagic complications of venous infarctions are much more common compared to arterial infarctions, occurring in up to 40% of patients with cerebral venous thrombosis, presumably as a result of the underlying venous hypertension in the affected region [115].

The location of parenchymal changes corresponds to the causative thrombosed venous structure:

- Frontal and parietal paramedian lesions will be seen with superior sagittal sinus occlusion
- Temporal lesions with transverse sinus and vein of Labbe occlusion
- Bilateral thalamic lesions with straight sinus and vein of Galen occlusion

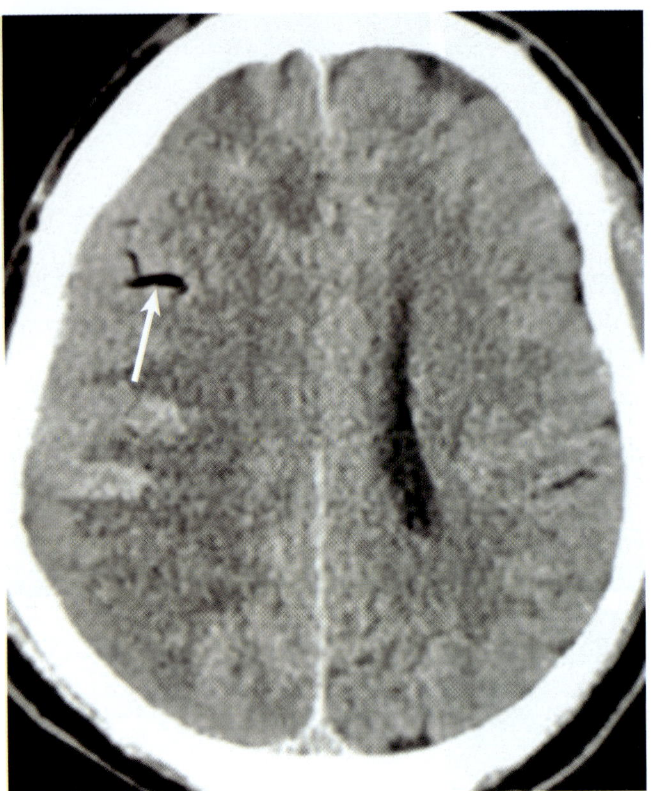

Figure 77.17 Air density in a distal right anterior MCA branch (*arrow*). Edema of the visible MCA territory parenchyma due to evolving infarction.

Parenchymal changes of venous infarction include edema, commonly with superimposed hemorrhage within the infarcted territory. Adjacent thrombosed venous structures will appear hyperattenuating on CT or show blooming artifact on susceptibility weighted MRI, described as the "cord sign" when involving cortical veins (Fig. 77.18).

MRI may show patchy restricted diffusion, often to a lesser degree and more heterogeneous than that encountered with arterial infarction [116]. Vascular congestion within the affected parenchyma may lead to heterogeneous parenchymal and leptomeningeal enhancement, as well as increased cerebral blood volume (CBV) on perfusion imaging [115,117].

Associated venous thrombus may be visible as blooming artifact on susceptibility weighted or T2* images, absence of the normal flow void on T2 weighted images, or as T1 hyperintensity along an adjacent cortical vein or dural sinus. CTV and contrast-enhanced MRV are also very helpful in these cases to delineate the degree of thrombus propagation as well as to monitor improvement if anticoagulation is initiated. The classically described "empty delta sign" may be seen on CTV or contrast-enhanced MRI/MRV in superior sagittal sinus thrombosis, describing the lack of central contrast filling of the triangular sinus, with peripheral enhancement [118].

Key Point

Venous infarctions tend to cross arterial territory boundaries and have a high incidence of hemorrhage compared to arterial infarctions.

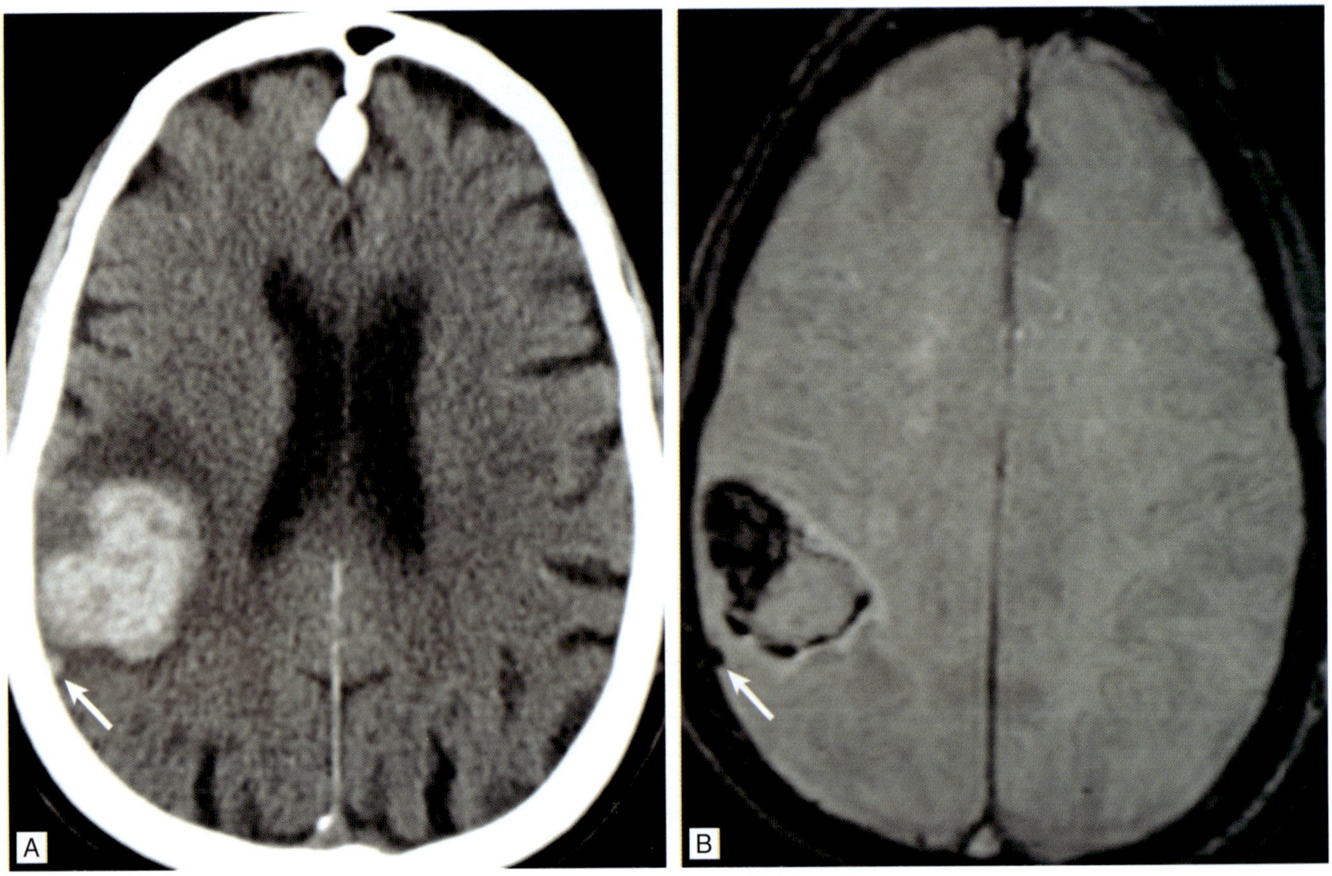

Figure 77.18 Right parietal hematoma with adjacent thrombosed cortical vein (*arrows*) showing hyperattenuation on CT (A) and blooming artifact on MRI (B).

TABLE 77.4 Modified Fisher Scale for Stratifying Risk of Vasospasm After Subarachnoid Hemorrhage

Grade	SAH	IVH	Risk of Vasospasm
0	None	None	Very low risk
1	Focal or diffuse thin layer	None	Low risk
2	Focal or diffuse thin layer	Present	Moderate risk
3	Focal or diffuse thick layer	None	High risk
4	Focal or diffuse thick layer	Present	Very high risk

Arterial Vasospasm

Cerebral arterial vasospasm may occur following an insult to the intracranial arteries, most commonly after aneurysmal subarachnoid hemorrhage where vasospasm may be encountered in up to 50–90% of cases on DSA [119]. Vasospasm following aneurysm rupture may begin a few days after hemorrhage and typically peaks around 1-week post ictus. Involvement may be focal or diffuse, and vary in severity from mild and asymptomatic to severe with resulting focal neurologic deficits and, or acute infarctions. A large volume of subarachnoid clot is the best predictor for spasm, and the modified Fisher scale may be used to stratify risk (Table 77.4). Other predictors of spasm include slow clearance of hemorrhage from the subarachnoid space, intraventricular hematoma, poor neurologic condition on admission, and other vascular risk factors such as history of smoking, diabetes, or hypertension [119]. Symptomatic vasospasm after aneurysm rupture may be treated with endovascular techniques including balloon angioplasty and/or infusion of vasodilators at the site of spasm, or nonendovascular therapies such as intrathecal nimodipine.

Modified Fisher Scale

Vascular imaging in suspected vasospasm cases is commonly performed with transcranial Doppler ultrasound (TCD), CTA, and DSA. TCD is used to detect increased flow velocities in the proximal branches of the circle of Willis. While TCD is more operator dependent than cross sectional imaging and may not detect areas of more distal spasm, evaluation is low cost and may be helpful for surveillance [119]. CTA is very useful in vasospasm evaluation, owing to wide availability, repeatability, and the ability to perform concurrent perfusion studies. CTA will show concentric focal, segmental, or diffuse narrowing of the affected intracranial arteries. The most severely involved arteries often correspond to areas of greatest subarachnoid clot, which tends to be centered around the circle of Willis due to the predilection of aneurysms to originate from this region. The degree of stenosis is evaluated in comparison with prespasm imaging, most often CTA performed on admission. Without comparison imaging, vasospasm can be difficult to differentiate from congenitally hypoplastic segments or pre-existing stenoses from atherosclerosis or other causes. Perfusion imaging is commonly used in conjunction with CTA to assess the functional effect of stenosis on the distal territory, helping to delineate areas of infarction or ischemic penumbra in severe cases. DSA is reserved for severe cases when intra-arterial therapy is being considered.

Conclusion

Acute ischemic stroke remains a large source of morbidity and mortality across the globe, and recent developments in diagnosis and management have increased access to life-saving therapies. Diagnostic imaging and image-guided interventions remain the bedrock of stroke management, and familiarity with new imaging techniques and workflows are required for swift and accurate decision making during time-sensitive stroke management.

Suggested Readings

- JL Saver, GC Fonarow, EE Smith, MJ Reeves, MV Grau-Sepulveda, W Pan, et al., Time to treatment with intravenous tissue plasminogen activator and outcome from acute ischemic stroke, JAMA 309 (23) (2013 Jun) 2480.
- M Goyal, AP Jadhav, A Bonafe, H Diener, V Mendes Pereira, E Levy, et al., Analysis of workflow and time to treatment and the effects on outcome in endovascular treatment of acute ischemic stroke: results from the SWIFT PRIME Randomized Controlled Trial, Radiology 279 (3) (2016 Jun) 888–897.
- RG Nogueira, AP Jadhav, DC Haussen, A Bonafe, RF Budzik, P Bhuva, et al., Thrombectomy 6 to 24 hours after stroke with a mismatch between deficit and infarct, N Engl J Med 378 (1) (2018 Jan) 11–21.
- American College of Radiology, ACR Appropriateness Criteria: Cerebrovascular Disease, American College of Radiology, 2016.
- BK Menon, CD d'Esterre, EM Qazi, M Almekhlafi, L Hahn, AM Demchuk, et al., Multiphase CT angiography: a new tool for the imaging triage of patients with acute ischemic stroke, Radiology 275 (2) (2015 May) 510–520.
- TG Jovin, A Chamorro, E Cobo, MA de Miquel, CA Molina, A Rovira, et al., Thrombectomy within 8 hours after symptom onset in ischemic stroke, N Engl J Med 372 (24) (2015 Jun) 2296–2306.
- C Virapongse, C Cazenave, R Quisling, M Sarwar, S Hunter, The empty delta sign: frequency and significance in 76 cases of dural sinus thrombosis, Radiology 162 (3) (1987 Mar) 779–785.

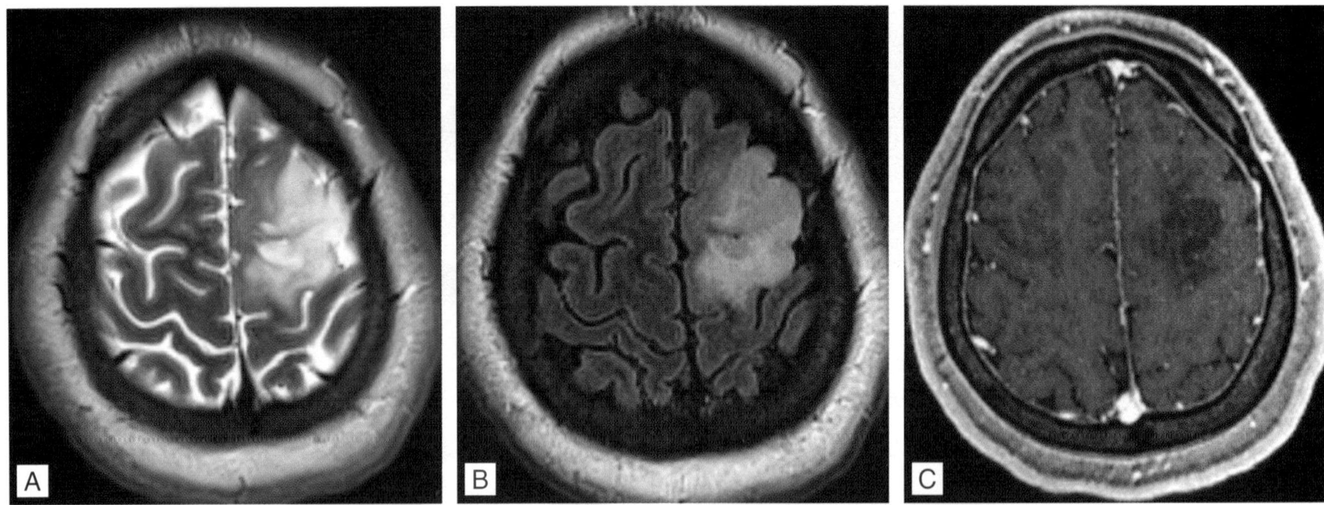

Figure 78.12 Oligodendroglioma (WHO grade 2). (A) Axial T2, (B) axial FLAIR, and (C) axial T1 postcontrast images demonstrate a nonenhancing mass in the left frontal lobe infiltrating and expanding the overlying cortex.

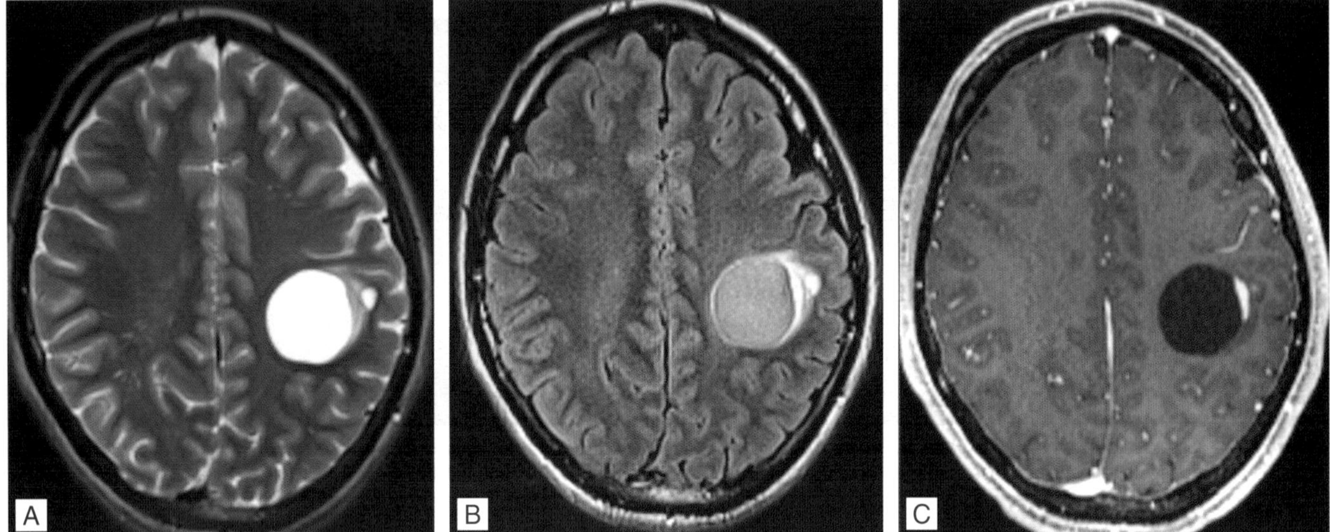

Figure 78.13 Pilocytic astrocytoma. (A) Axial T2, (B) axial FLAIR, and (C) axial T1 postcontrast images demonstrate a well-circumscribed, cystic mass with an enhancing mural nodule.

ages of 5 and 15 years. It has a strong association with NF1. PA typically presents as a cystic mass with enhancing mural nodule in the cerebellum or as an infiltrative lesion along the optic pathway that elongates and widens the optic nerve [28]. Involvement of optic nerves is a feature of neurofibromatosis type I. It is difficult to diagnose when in atypical locations as it can resemble more aggressive and infiltrative lesions.

On imaging, cystic lesion with enhancing mural nodule is more common than purely solid lesions (Fig. 78.13). About 10–20% lesions can show calcification. Cystic component shows fluid signal with enhancement of cyst wall in 50% cases. Solid mural nodule is hypointense on T1, hyperintense on T2 and shows intense enhancement. There is usually little or no surrounding edema. Infiltrative pattern is seen in optic pathway and hypothalamic lesions. The tumors involving the chiasm or hypothalamus are often large, lobulated, and well circumscribed at presentation and can be partially cystic.

Key Point
Pilocytic astrocytoma typically presents in children as an expansile cystic mass lesion with enhancing mural nodule in the cerebellum.

Pilomyxoid Astrocytoma

This neoplasm was previously considered just a "juvenile" variant of PA. It is now recognized as a distinct entity with unique clinical characteristics and histological appearance. It is an aggressive neoplasm usually seen in very young children with mean age at diagnosis being 18 months. It can occur anywhere along the neuraxis, however, these lesions have a strong predilection for the suprasellar region. Hypothalamus/optic chiasm is the most common location [30].

On imaging, majority of pilomyxoid astrocytomas (PMAs) are large, well-circumscribed, lobulated, homogeneously enhancing solid mass lesions. Some lesions may show minimal cystic component [30]. They can expand from midline into both temporal lobes. Imaging findings are somewhat similar to PA; however, PMAs are brighter on T2 due to higher proportion of myxoid matrix (Fig. 78.14). PMA may show intratumoral hemorrhage on T2* images, which is very rare in PA. The most prominent

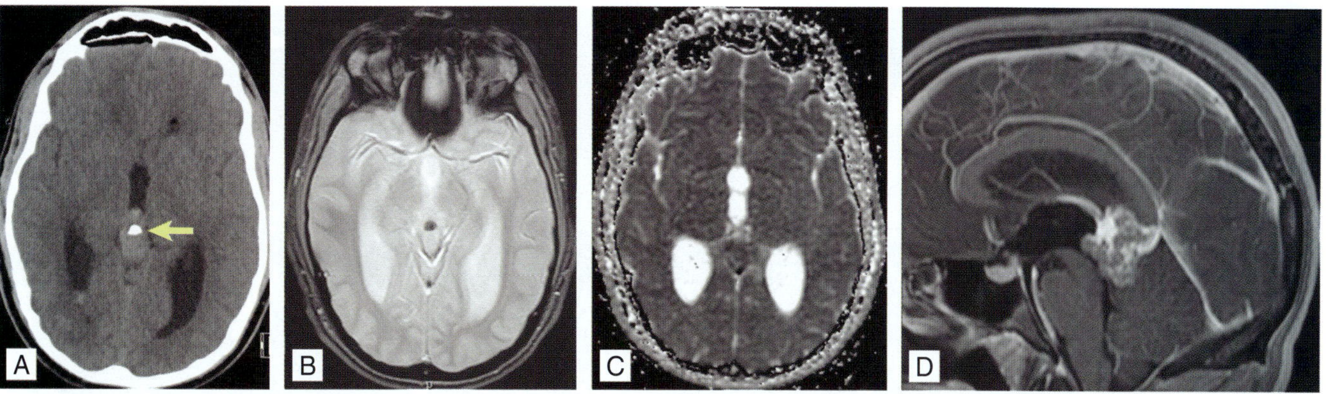

Figure 78.61 Germ cell tumor of the pineal region. (A) Axial CT, (B) axial gradient echo, (C) axial ADC, and (D) sagittal T1 postcontrast images demonstrate a solidly enhancing pineal-region mass with low ADC values indicative of high tumor cellularity. The mass surrounds the pineal calcifications, which suggest this represents a germ cell tumor (*yellow arrow*, "engulfed calcifications").

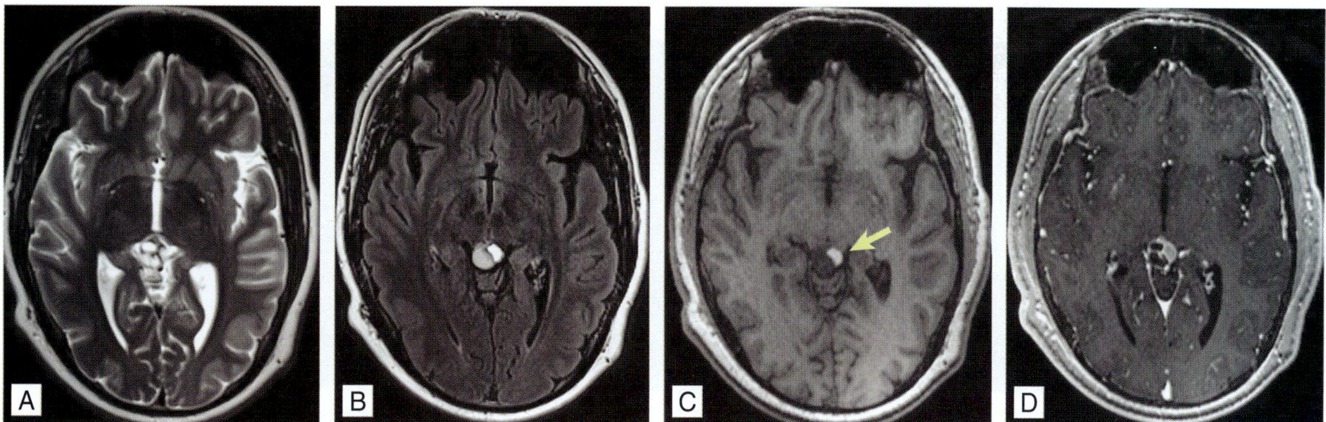

Figure 78.62 Teratoma of the pineal region. (A) Axial T2, (B) axial FLAIR, (C) axial T1 precontrast, and (D) axial T1 postcontrast images demonstrate a cystic pineal-region mass with a T1-hyperintense fatty component (*yellow arrow*) and enhancing septations.

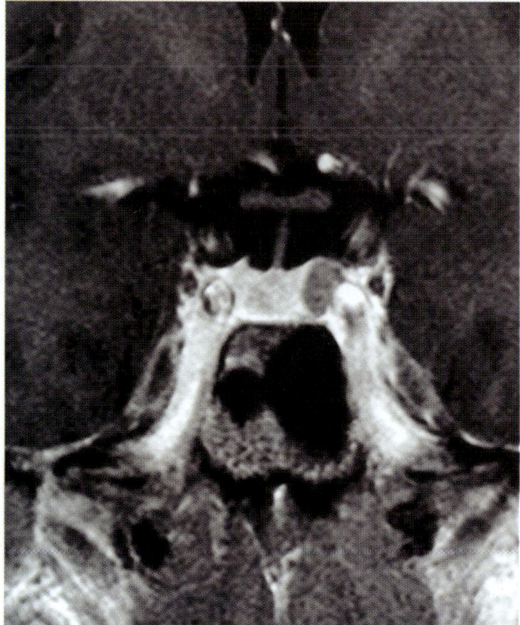

Figure 78.63 Pituitary microadenoma. (A) Coronal T1 postcontrast image demonstrates a rounded hypoenhancing nodule in the left aspect of the pituitary gland, causing slightly increased height of the pituitary gland on the left and deviation of the infundibulum to the right.

Key Point

Teratoma is usually an irregular heterogeneous solid enhancing mass containing fat, clumps of calcification, and cystic areas in a fetus or child. The presence of fat in the lesion can aid in the diagnosis.

Tumors of the Sellar Region

Pituitary Microadenoma

They are small pituitary tumors that are by definition less than 10 mm in size. They can be asymptomatic or can present with hormonal disturbances. Prolactinoma is the most common functioning adenoma presenting with amenorrhea, galactorrhea, and elevated prolactin levels. These lesions are isointense to pituitary on T1 and slightly hyperintense on T2. Dynamic contrast-enhanced pituitary MRI is also performed for a subset of these microadenomas, as they usually enhance slowly compared with the surrounding pituitary gland, therefore appear as well-defined, rounded, hypoenhancing lesions on early phases (Fig. 78.63) and show delayed enhancement compared with rest of the gland on dynamic contrast images. Pituitary gland may be enlarged and pituitary stalk can be deviated away from the adenoma.

Pituitary Macroadenoma

Pituitary adenomas larger than 10 mm are categorized as macroadenomas. It is the most common suprasellar mass in adults.

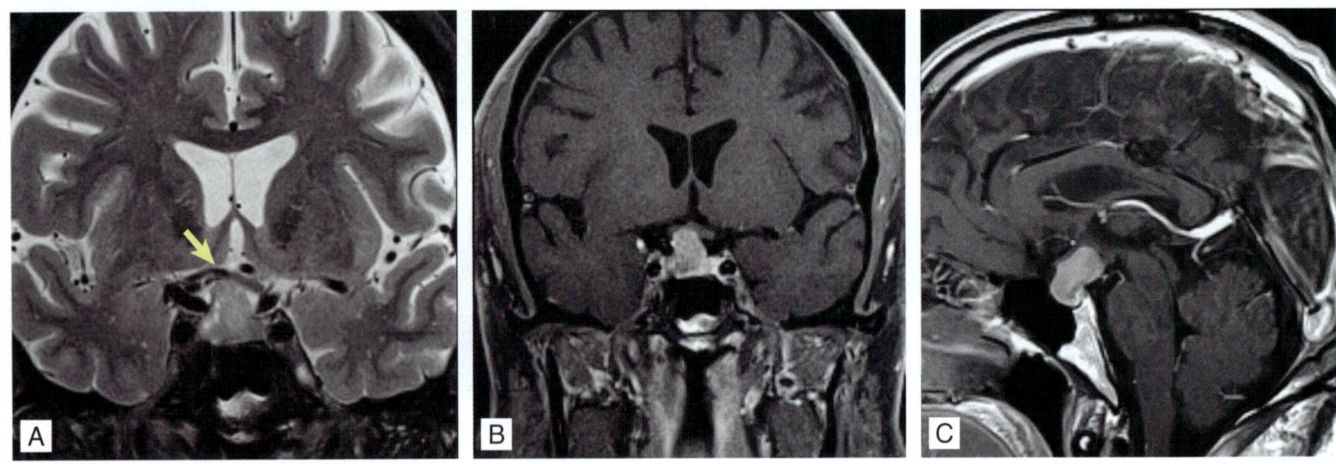

Figure 78.64 Pituitary macroadenoma. (A) Coronal T2, (B) coronal T1 postcontrast, and (C) sagittal T1 postcontrast images demonstrate a slightly hypoenhancing mass with intermediate T2 signal intensity arising in the sella, inseparable from the pituitary gland. The mass extends into the suprasellar cistern and exerts mass effect upon the optic chiasm (*yellow arrow*).

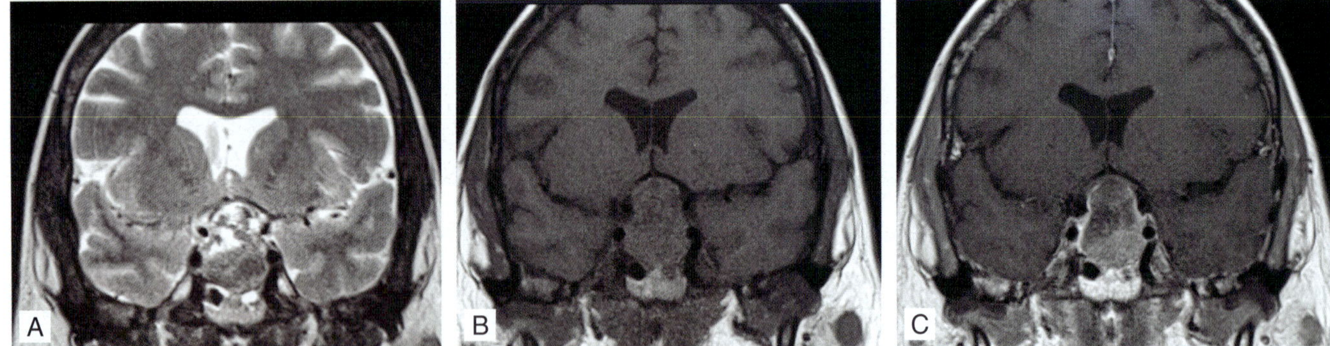

Figure 78.65 Pituitary apoplexy. (A) Coronal T2, (B) coronal T1 precontrast, and (C) coronal T1 postcontrast images demonstrate a large heterogenous sellar mass with suprasellar extension and compression of the optic chiasm. The presence of central nonenhancement and heterogenous cystic change on T2 represents necrosis within the macroadenoma, which may occur as an acute phenomenon necessitating urgent surgical intervention to preserve visual function.

Most of pituitary macroadenomas are nonfunctioning. Prolactinoma is the most common functioning adenoma. They can present with endocrine disturbance or compression of the optic chiasm resulting in bitemporal hemianopia (Fig. 78.64). They are usually sellar–suprasellar masses with waist at diaphragma sellae giving "snowman" or "figure of eight" appearance [108,109] (Fig. 78.64). Sella is usually enlarged in these cases.

On MRI, they usually show intermediate signal on T1 and T2W images with moderate to intense enhancement. Necrosis and hemorrhage may be seen. These tumors can invade cavernous sinuses. Knosp classification is commonly used to determine the likelihood of cavernous sinus invasion based on tumor extension past tangents drawn along the medial, central, and lateral aspects of the cavernous and supraclinoid ICA [110]. The differential diagnosis is meningioma which can cause narrowing of the flow void of cavernous ICA in addition to encasement. Meningiomas show stronger enhancement than pituitary macroadenomas, and pituitary gland can be identified separately in the case of meningiomas.

Pituitary Apoplexy

Pituitary apoplexy is a catastrophic acute clinical syndrome in which patients present with headache, visual deficit, opthalmoplegia, and altered mental status. It is caused by hemorrhagic or nonhemorrhagic necrosis usually in an existing pituitary macroadenoma. Pituitary gland is enlarged and shows peripheral enhancement with nonenhancing infarcted/necrotic center (Fig. 78.65). MRI may show T1 hyperintense signal due to blood products in cases with hemorrhagic infarction (Fig. 78.66). Urgent neurosurgical decompression is needed.

Craniopharyngioma

Craniopharyngiomas are suprasellar tumors arising from remnants of the craniopharyngeal duct or Rathke's pouch [111]. They are histologically benign, WHO grade 1 neoplasms, but these tumors are considered clinically aggressive due to their tendency to recur [112].

They are most frequent in children between 5 and 15 years of age and have a second peak in fifth to sixth decade. The adamantinomatous subtype which presents as a cystic mass in children is more common than the papillary subtype which presents as a solid mass in older adults. Clinically, they can present with headache, visual defect, or endocrine disturbances.

On CT, adamantinomatous subtype tumors are usually large, lobulated, multiloculated cystic lesions with small enhancing solid component and calcification. On MRI, cystic component shows isointense to hyperintense signal on T1 due to proteinaceous contents. They are usually hyperintense on T2 but may show variable signal. There is intense enhancement of the solid component (Fig. 78.67).

Papillary craniopharyngiomas are mostly solid and rarely show calcification. It is useful to radiologically differentiate adamantinomatous type from papillary type because prognosis may differ. T1 bright signal intensity, calcification on CT, and pediatric age range favor the adamantinomatous type over papillary type of craniopharyngiomas [112].

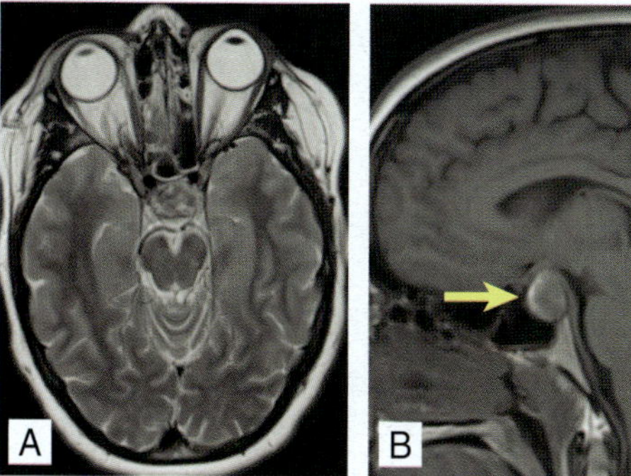

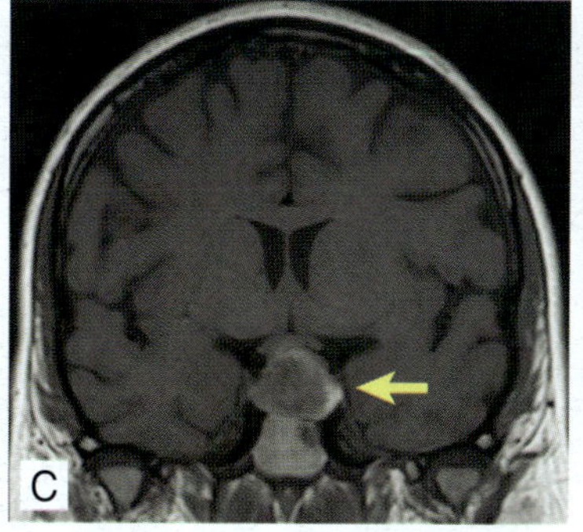

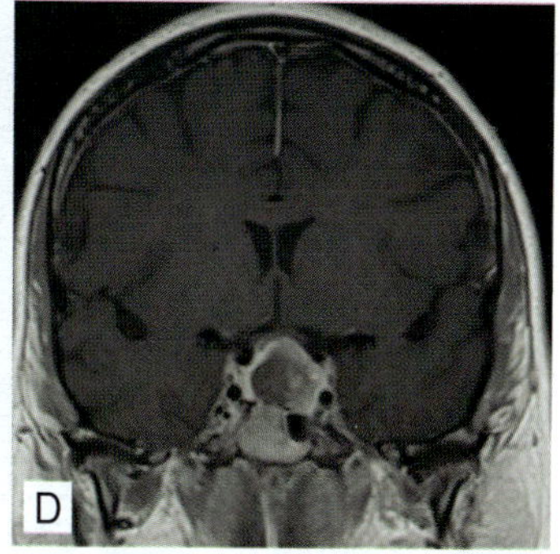

Figure 78.66 Pituitary apoplexy. (A) Axial T2, (B) sagittal T1 precontrast, (C) coronal T1 precontrast, and (D) coronal T1 postcontrast images demonstrate a large heterogenous sellar mass with suprasellar extension and compression of the optic chiasm. In addition to central necrosis, there is T1 hyperintense material within the mass (*yellow arrows*) representing hemorrhage.

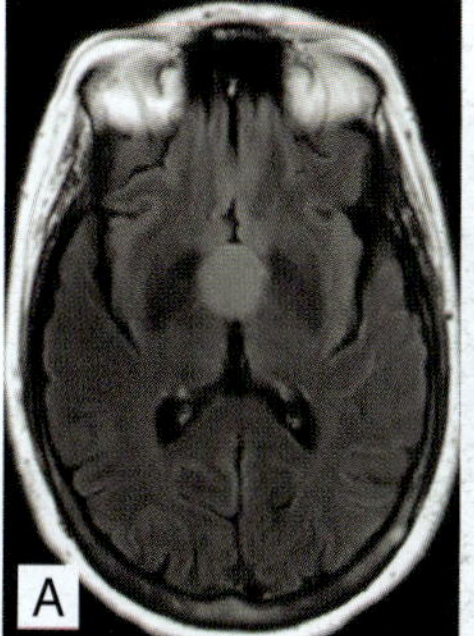

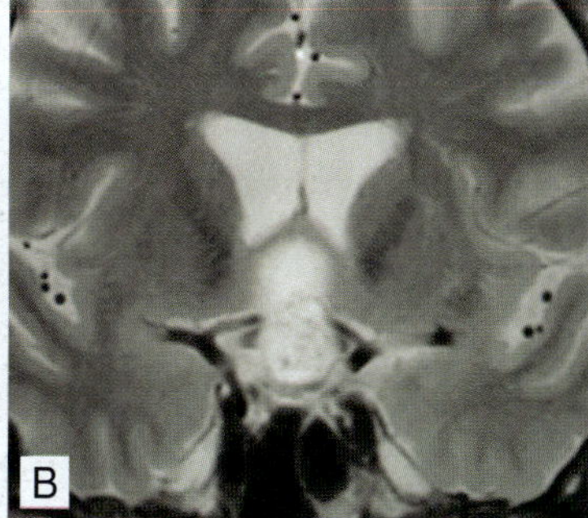

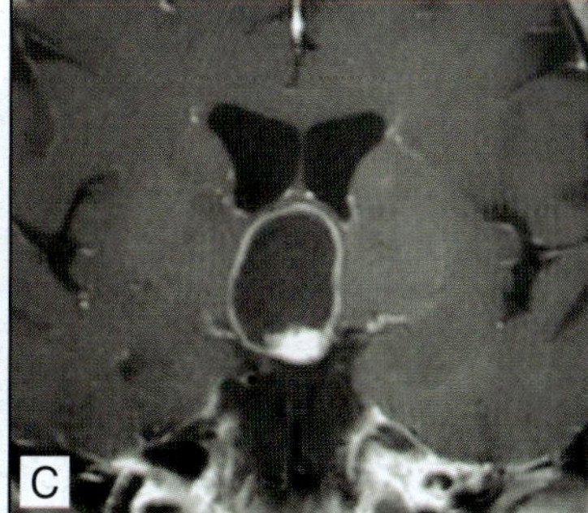

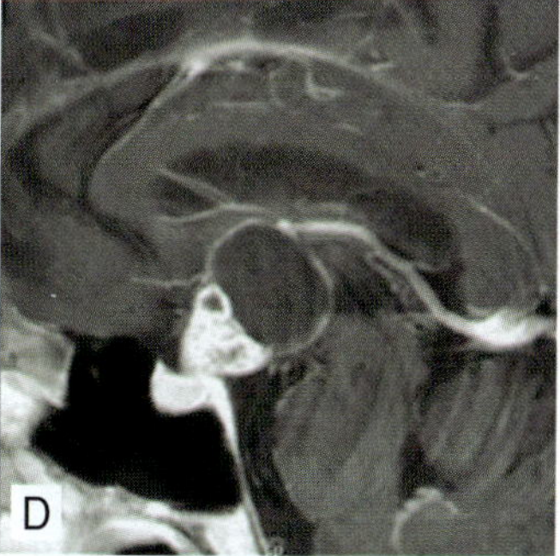

Figure 78.67 Craniopharyngioma. (A) Axial FLAIR, (B) coronal T2, (C) coronal T1 postcontrast, and (D) sagittal T1 postcontrast images demonstrate a mixed solid and cystic mass centered in the suprasellar cistern and appearing separate from the pituitary gland. The cystic component protruding into the anterior third ventricle contains complex proteinaceous material which does not suppress on FLAIR, and a thin enhancing rim.

Key Point

Typical craniopharyngioma is a large, lobulated, cystic suprasellar mass lesion with calcification and enhancing solid component in a child.

Metastatic Tumors

Brain metastases account for nearly 40% of intracrania l tumors in adults. *The most common primary tumors to metastasize intracranially include lung, breast, melanoma, kidney, and gastrointestinal tract.* Eighty percent of metastases are supratentorial in distribution, but infratentorial metastases still account for the most common intra-axial posterior fossa neoplasm. Hemorrhage can be seen in association with metastases from melanoma, renal cell carcinoma, choriocarcinoma, thyroid, lung, or breast primary tumors. Brain metastases are less common in children and can be seen in neuroblastoma, Wilms' tumor, rhabdomyosarcoma, and osteogenic sarcoma. Patients commonly present with headaches, seizures, mental status alterations, ataxia, nausea, vomiting, and visual disturbances. However, large number of patients can be asymptomatic at the time of imaging. Brain metastases commonly present as multiple lesions, however, nearly 50% are solitary at diagnosis.

MRI is more sensitive than CT in detecting small metastatic deposits, even if double-dose intravenous contrast and delayed imaging is performed with CT.

On imaging, cerebral metastases are usually well-defined lesions, typically located at the gray–white matter interface and they are associated with a disproportionately large amount of vasogenic edema considering their size, even with a very small superficial lesion (Fig. 78.68). Metastatic deposits can occur anywhere including cerebral white or gray matter, brainstem, cerebellum, and basal ganglia. Interestingly, cortical metastases are associated with very little vasogenic edema. On CT, metastases can be isodense, hypodense, or hyperdense, hyperdensity being a frequently encountered feature of melanoma secondaries. Calcification is very rare and is a point against the diagnosis of metastasis. However, it can occur and has been described in metastasis from bone sarcoma and colonic carcinoma. It may also be seen after radiation treatment. Larger metastases tend to become necrotic centrally and may appear cystic (Fig. 78.69). Contrast enhancement is an almost universal feature of brain metastases. Enhancement may be seen as a well-defined nodule within an area of surrounding edema, or, if the center is necrotic or cystic, as marginal or ring enhancement. Superficial nodules easily missed on the preenhancement scan may be more easily recognized after contrast enhancement.

On MRI metastases are iso to hypointense on T1, hyperintense on T2, and enhancement patterns are similar to those described for CT. T1 hyperintensity can be seen in hemorrhagic and melanoma metastases. Delayed sequences may show additional lesions.

MR spectroscopy shows reduced NAA and intratumoral choline peak with no choline elevation in the peritumoral edema. There is low peritumoral CBV on perfusion (Fig. 78.69). Lipid peak is seen in areas of tumor necrosis. FDG PET can only detect larger lesions, therefore contrast-enhanced MRI is the gold standard to rule out small metastases.

The presence of multiple discrete lesions within the brain should always suggest the diagnosis of metastases. Similar appearances may be seen with multiple small abscesses or granulomas, although the clinical features will often help to differentiate. In the posterior fossa multiple hemangioblastomas may have to be considered in the differential diagnosis.

Imaging of brain metastases is challenging due to difficulties in differentiating metastases from potential mimics such as primary brain tumors, lymphoma, and infection, detecting small metastases, and differentiating treatment response from tumor recurrence.

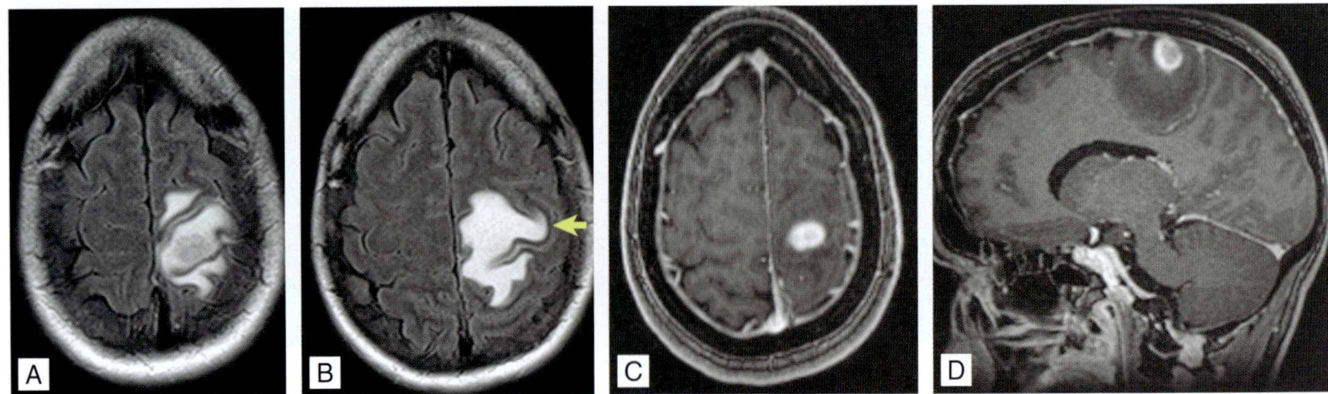

Figure 78.68 Metastasis. (A and B) Axial FLAIR, (C) axial T1 postcontrast, and (D) sagittal T1 postcontrast images demonstrate an enhancing mass in the posterior left frontal lobe. The surrounding FLAIR signal abnormality largely spares the overlying cortex (*yellow arrow*), suggesting this represents vasogenic edema. The large extent of surrounding vasogenic edema relative to the small size of the enhancing lesion is more typical of metastasis than a high-grade glioma.

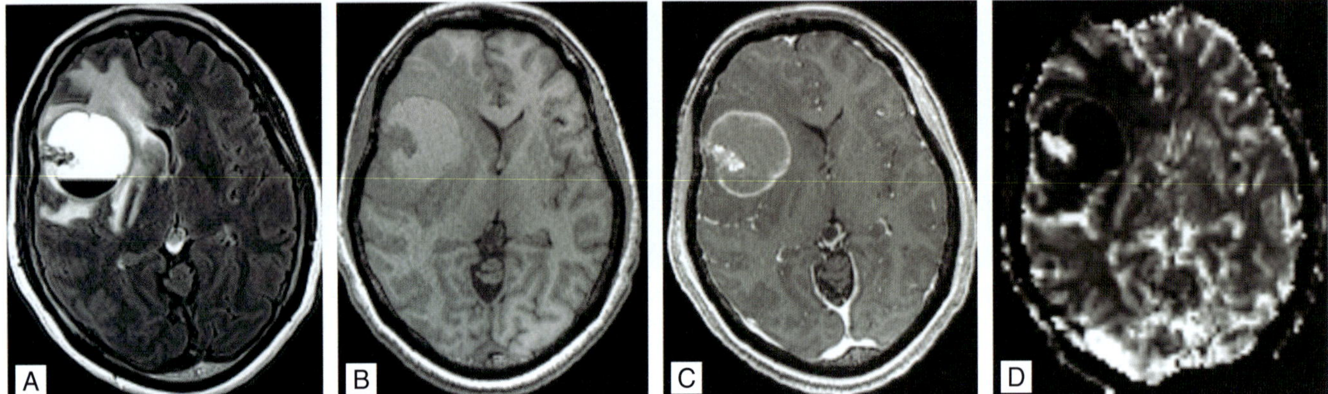

Figure 78.69 Metastasis (lung adenocarcinoma). (A) Axial FLAIR, (B) axial T1 precontrast, (C) axial T1 postcontrast, and (D) rCBV images demonstrate a hemorrhagic mass in the right frontal lobe with a nodular and rim enhancement. rCBV is markedly elevated in association with the nodular enhancement but is decreased in the peritumoral region, a feature more suggestive of metastasis than high-grade gliomas which unlike metastases often feature elevated peritumoral rCBV due to infiltration of glioma cells beyond the borders of the dominant enhancing component.

Therefore, MRI remains the technique of choice to identify brain metastases and monitor their response to treatment [113].

Treatment-Induced Pathologies, Tumors, and Assessment of Treatment Response

These days a wide range of treatment options and treatment protocols are available for brain tumors. This is making assessment of treatment-related changes and complications very challenging. Treatment-related complications/changes may include intracranial hemorrhage, ischemia, subdural and extradural collections, increased intracranial pressure, hydrocephalus, infection, CSF leak, chemotherapy-induced posterior reversible encephalopathy syndrome, toxic leukoencephalopathy, postradiation cavernoma, radiation necrosis, pseudoprogression, and pseudoresponse.

Radiation Necrosis

This is necrosis of brain tissue due to radiation treatment that can present as a space-occupying mass lesion with mass effect and sometimes neurological dysfunction (but this is not true tumor). Radionecrosis typically occurs months to years after radiation, but may be seen as early as a few weeks after and has been reported as late as 19 years after the completion of RT [114].

- On MRI, it appears as localized or diffuse white matter hyperintensity on T2 and FLAIR images with "Swiss-cheese" pattern of contrast enhancement [115]
- *MR perfusion shows low rCBV even in enhancing areas of radiation necrosis* (Fig. 78.70). MR spectroscopy shows depressed levels of choline, creatine, and NAA with elevated lipid/lactate. Radiation necrosis is hypometabolic on PET

Pseudoprogression

This is actually treatment-related change that simulates disease progression on imaging. This is commonly seen in gliomas treated with radiation and temozolomide. Pseudoprogression should be differentiated from true tumor progression as it represents a favorable treatment response (Table 78.4).

On imaging, pseudoprogression appears as increasing size and/or number of enhancing lesions (Fig. 78.71), increase in surrounding T2/FLAIR signal abnormality and mass effect due to increased chemotherapy-induced cytotoxicity and breakdown of the blood–brain barrier [116]. *However, MR perfusion does not show any increase in rCBV in pseudoprogression. rCBV remains stable or is reduced compared with pretreatment scans* [117]. *Also, diffusion can show high ADC values in pseudoprogression.*

18F-FET-PET (amino-acid analogue 18F-fluoroethyltyrosine) has higher specificity, and equally high sensitivity than MRI to differentiate between recurrent tumor and treatment effects. It is important not to switch therapy as pseudoprogression actually reflects positive response to therapy and is associated with longer progression-free interval. Tumors with hypermethylated MGMT promoter status have up to 91% incidence of pseudoprogression,

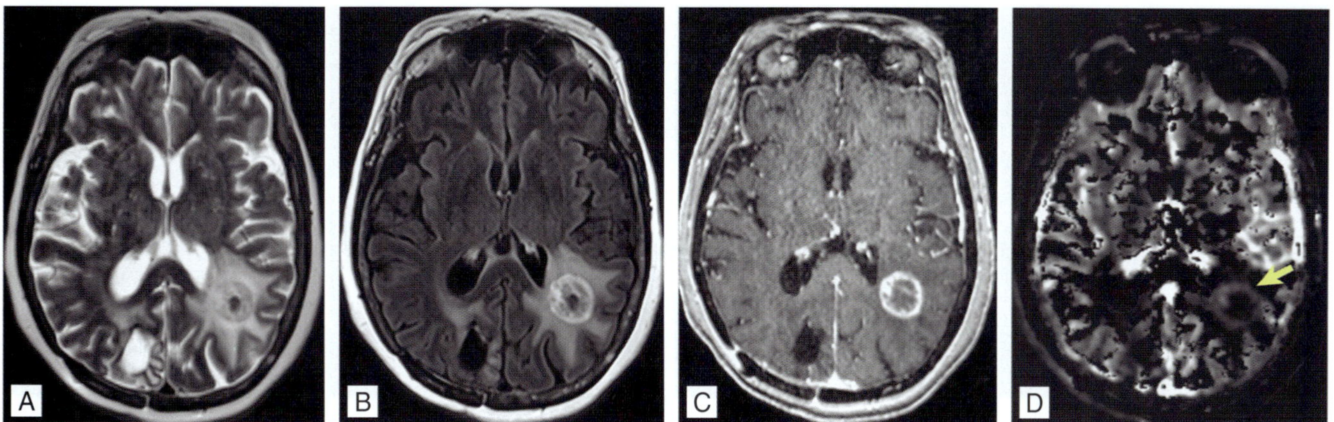

Figure 78.70 Radiation necrosis. (A) Axial T2, (B) axial FLAIR, (C) axial T1 postcontrast, and (D) axial DCE perfusion plasma volume (Vp) images demonstrate a heterogeneously enhancing mass in the left parietal lobe with surrounding vasogenic edema, at the site of stereotactic radiosurgery performed for non–small-cell lung cancer metastasis 9 months prior. There is only mild Vp elevation associated with the enhancing rim (*yellow arrow*). Surgical resection demonstrated necrotic tissue with no viable tumor cells.

TABLE 78.4 Pseudoprogression (PsP) Versus True Progression (TP)

- Conventional MRI alone is limited in differentiating PsP from TP.
- Progressive enhancement and edema in the lesions with stable or reduced rCBV suggests PsP.
- PsP represents favorable treatment response—Important *NOT* to discontinue or switch therapy.
- MGMT status is a useful marker—*PsP is more frequently seen* with a methylated promoter status.
- Patients with PsP are usually doing clinically well and improve on follow-up without any further treatment.

possibly reflecting the increased sensitivity of these tumors to chemoradiation [118]. These patients usually have a better performance status and improve on follow-up without any further treatment.

Pseudoresponse

This entity mimics treatment response on imaging, while the infiltrating tumor component actually remains stable or has even progressed. Pseudoresponse is seen most commonly after treatment with antiangiogenic drugs like bevacizumab, which act to inhibit vascular endothelial growth factor. On imaging, pseudoresponse

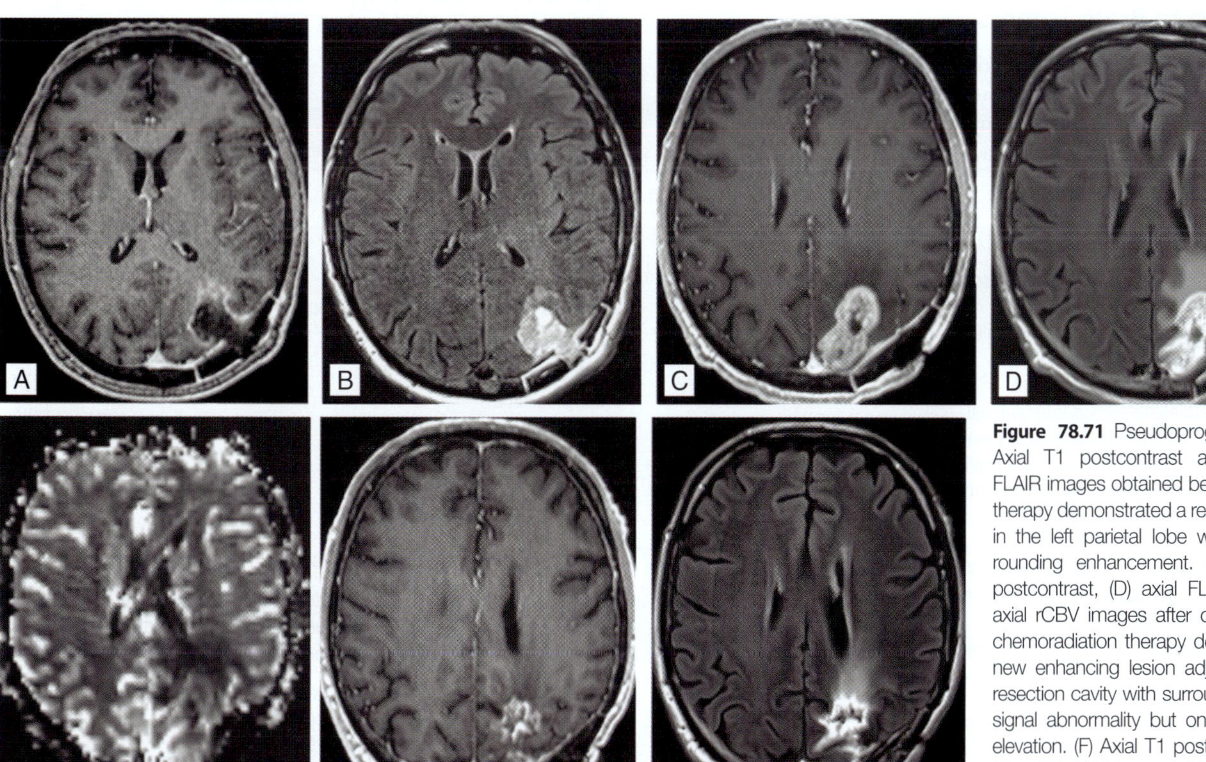

Figure 78.71 Pseudoprogression. (A) Axial T1 postcontrast and (B) axial FLAIR images obtained before radiation therapy demonstrated a resection cavity in the left parietal lobe with mild surrounding enhancement. (C) Axial T1 postcontrast, (D) axial FLAIR, and (E) axial rCBV images after completion of chemoradiation therapy demonstrate a new enhancing lesion adjacent to the resection cavity with surrounding FLAIR signal abnormality but only mild rCBV elevation. (F) Axial T1 postcontrast and (G) axial FLAIR images 18 months later demonstrate gradual decrease in size of the enhancing lesion with regression of the surrounding FLAIR abnormality.

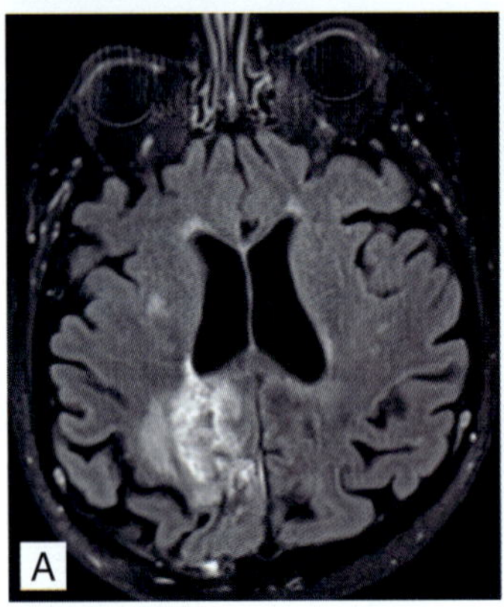

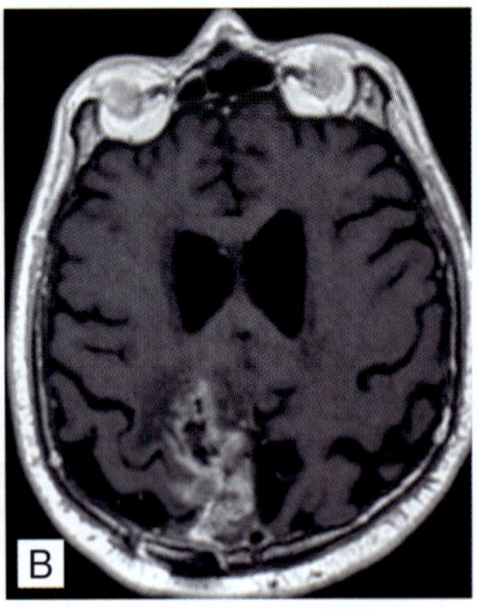

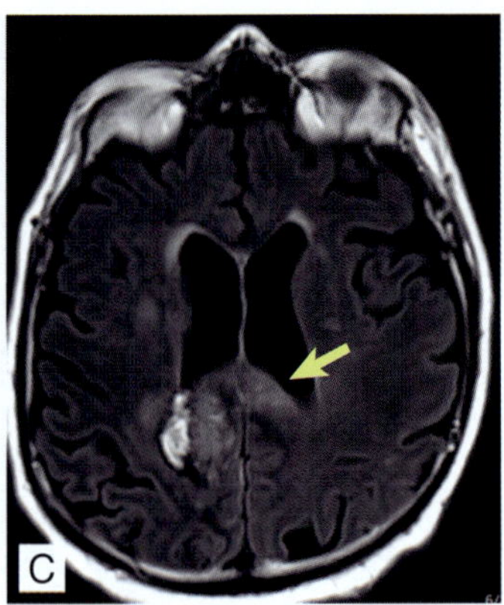

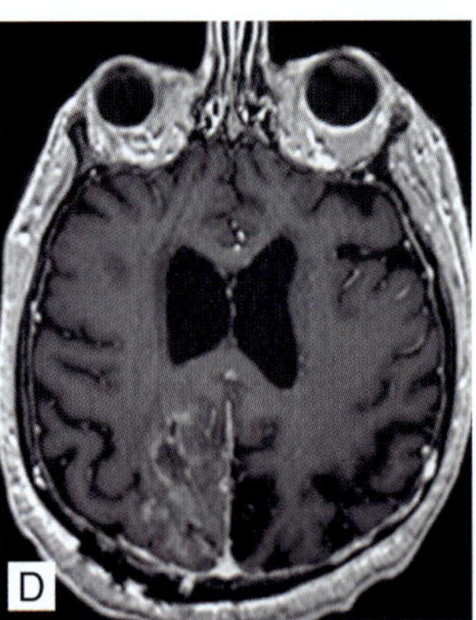

Figure 78.72 Pseudoresponse. (A) Axial FLAIR and (B) T1 postcontrast images demonstrate and enhancing mass in the right parietal lobe reflecting recurrent glioblastoma in this patient. (C) Axial FLAIR and (D) axial T1 postcontrast images obtained after the initiation of bevacizumab therapy demonstrate decrease in size and avidity of the enhancement. Although some aspects of the FLAIR abnormality have decreased (representing decrease in vasogenic edema), areas expansile FLAIR abnormality represent infiltrative tumor exhibiting progressive extension into the splenium of the corpus callosum (*yellow arrow*).

appears as rapid decrease in enhancing component of the tumor or reduction in edema, however, nonenhancing tumor appears larger (or unchanged) on T2 and FLAIR images (Fig. 78.72). MR perfusion is not very helpful as rCBV remains low with decreased enhancement.

MRS, MR perfusion, and DWI may help in differentiating pseudoprogression and pseudoresponse from true progression and true response, respectively. However, both phenomena appear to be best diagnosed through follow-up scans [119]. Timing of therapy, knowledge of tumor genetic markers, clinical course, and comparison of serial imaging are critical for the diagnosis.

Approach to Brain Tumors

A systematic approach can be followed on imaging for the detection and diagnosis of brain tumors depending on age of the patient, location of the lesion, multiplicity, conventional, and advanced imaging features. We should be looking to answer the following questions (Table 78.5).

TABLE 78.5 Approach to Brain Tumors

1. Age of the patient: Pediatric or Adult
2. Location: Where is the tumor?
   - Intra-axial versus extra-axial
   - Supratentorial versus infratentorial
3. Single or multiple: Is there more than one?
4. Is it causing complications? *H*ydrocephalus, *H*emorrhage, or *H*erniation?
5. Tumor versus pseudotumors/tumor mimics—Is it really neoplastic, could it be something else?
6. Conventional imaging features:
   - What is the size, signal intensity, and enhancement pattern?
   - Is there presence of calcification, fat, or hemorrhage?
7. Functional imaging:
   - Diffusion—Is there restricted or facilitated diffusion?
   - Perfusion—low or high rCBV?
   - Spectroscopy findings—peaks on MRS (choline, creatine, NAA, myoinositol, lipid, lactate, alanine)?

Tumors With Calcification

Oligodendroglioma
Subependymal giant cell astrocytoma
Ependymoma
Subependymoma
Choroid plexus papilloma
DNET
Ganglioglioma
Gangliocytoma
Central neurocytoma
Pineoblastoma/pineocytoma
Medulloblastoma
Embryonal tumor with multilayered rosettes (ETMR)
Atypical Teratoid/Rhabdoid Tumor (ATRT)
Olfactory neuroblastoma
Meningioma
Chordoma
Chondrosarcoma
Germinoma
Teratoma
Craniopharyngioma

Tumors With Cyst and Mural Nodule

Pilocytic astrocytoma
Hemangioblastoma
Ganglioglioma
Pleomorphic xanthoastrocytoma
Cystic metastasis

Tumors With Helpful MR Spectroscopy

Diffuse astrocytoma	Elevated choline, reduced NAA, elevated choline/creatine ratio, elevated myoinositol, and the absence of lactate
Glioblastoma	Elevated choline, reduced NAA, reduced myoinositol, and a lipid/lactate peak

Tumors With Helpful MR Spectroscopy—cont'd	
IDH mutant glioma	2-HG (hydroxyglutarate) MRS has high specificity for IDH mutant gliomas
Central neurocytoma	Glycine peak reported at 3.55 ppm
Medulloblastoma	Taurine peak at 3.4 ppm is characteristic
Meningioma	Alanine peak at 1.48 ppm is relatively specific for meningioma
Primary CNS lymphoma	Elevated choline, large lipid peak in the absence of necrosis seems to be a specific finding in PCNSL

Suggested Readings

- DN Louis, A Perry, G Reifenberger, A von Deimling, D Figarella-Branger, WK Cavenee, et al., The 2016 World Health Organization Classification of Tumors of the Central Nervous System: a summary, Acta Neuropathol 131 (6) (2016) 803–820.
- J Bai, J Varghese, R Jain, Adult glioma WHO classification update, genomics, and imaging. What the radiologists need to know, Top Magn Reson Imaging 29 (2) (2020) 71–82.
- J AlRayahi, M Zapotocky, V Ramaswamy, P Hanagandi, H Branson, W Mubarak, et al., Pediatric brain tumor genetics: what radiologists need to know, Radiographics 38 (7) (2018) 2102–2122.
- Z Rumboldt, M Castillo, B Huang, A Rossi, Brain Imaging with MRI and CT, Cambridge University Press, Cambridge, 2012, ISBN:1139576399.
- KK Koeller, GD Sandberg, Cerebral intraventricular neoplasms: radiologic-pathologic correlation, Radiographics 22 (2002) 1473–1505.
- LC Hygino da Cruz Jr, I Rodriguez, RC Domingues, EL Gasparetto, AG Sorensen, Pseudoprogression and pseudoresponse: imaging challenges in the assessment of posttreatment glioma, AJNR Am J Neuroradiol 32 (11) (2011) 1978–1985.

79

Spine

COLBEY W. FREEMAN AND JOHN H. WOO

Imaging Techniques of the Spine

Plain Radiographs

Although cross-sectional imaging has markedly increased in availability in recent decades, *plain radiographs are still widely used, particularly in low back pain in the setting of low-impact trauma, older age, osseous demineralization, or risk factors for osteoporosis.* Anteroposterior and lateral projections of the region of interest are standard with cone-down views of the lumbosacral junction also being common (Fig. 79.1). Supplementary oblique views are occasionally helpful to show the intervertebral foramina in the cervical region and the pars interarticularis in the lumbar region. Stability of the cervical or lumbar spine can be evaluated by lateral views in flexion and extension.

Computed Tomography (CT)

Modern CTs consist of a ring of x-ray detectors that receive radiation transmitted through a patient by one or more x-ray sources. Since its initial development, CT technology has undergone multiple generations of improvements culminating in a marked increase in scan speed made possible by wide fan x-ray beams, hundreds of x-ray detectors, helical acquisition with slip ring technology, and multiple x-ray sources. This has been aided by the development of multiple **reconstruction kernels**, such as soft-tissue and bone kernels, which manage the conversion of raw scanner data into an image. Each kernel emphasizes the visualization of specific structures and pathology. For example, a bone kernel will generate a sharper image, but with greater noise, which is ideal for visualizing osseous structures. A soft-tissue kernel sacrifices sharpness for a reduction in noise (Fig. 79.2).

Dual-energy CT acquisition, facilitated by multiple sources capable of producing beams of different kVp or sources that can switch between kVp settings, represents an emerging technology. It can facilitate further characterization of imaging findings on CT and has been used to detect iodinated contrast, create virtual noncontrast images from contrast-enhanced studies, and evaluate bone marrow edema-like signal associated with fractures. Dual-energy CT with high-energy monoenergetic reconstructed images may also assist in reducing artifacts from metallic hardware (Fig. 79.3).

CT is useful for the evaluation of bone, notably in the setting of trauma. *The high-spatial resolution of CT, combined with slices as thin as 0.5 mm, is an advantage and is superior to MRI for the imaging of bone trabeculae.* This resolution facilitates multiplanar reconstruction, and images can be generated in the axial, sagittal, and coronal planes. In addition, CT is more broadly available, more affordable than MRI, and provides significantly faster acquisition times, making it ideal for initial trauma evaluations. Visualization of spinal canal contents with CT can be limited by photon starvation and beam hardening artifacts from adjacent bone. The upper cervical cord is often discernible, but in most patients the lower cervical, thoracic, and lumbar intrathecal contents are not well-visualized without intrathecal contrast. CT remains an option to diagnose disc protrusions and degenerative disease of the lumbar and cervical spine when MRI is contraindicated or impossible. If

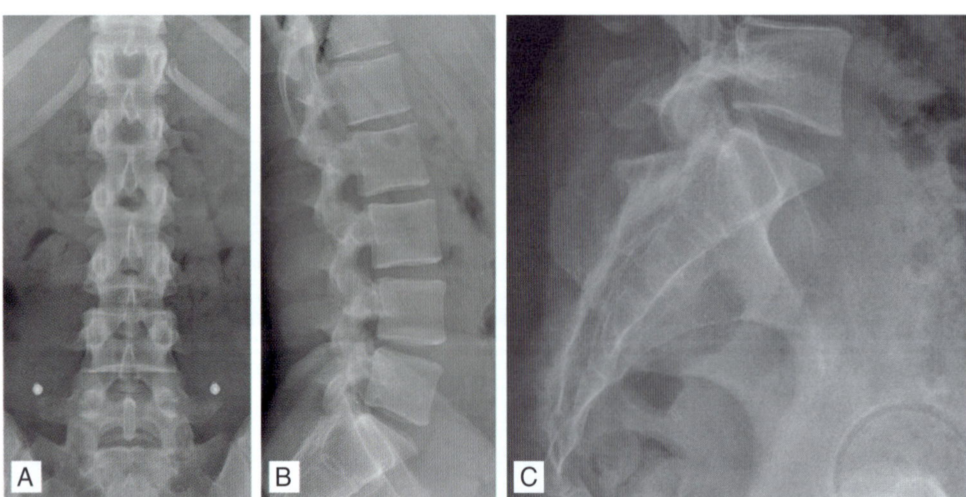

Figure 79.1 Normal 3-view radiograph series of the lumbar spine. Anteroposterior (A) and lateral (B) views, as well as a coned lateral view of the lumbosacral junction (C). The vertebral morphology and alignment can be assessed.

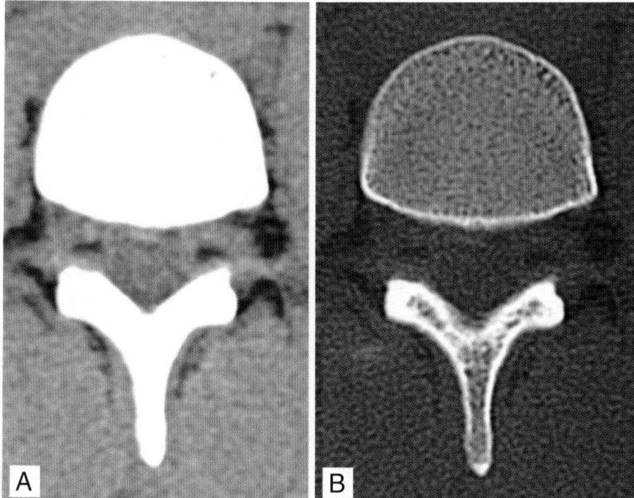

Figure 79.2 Normal axial CT of the lumbar spine at the level of the intervertebral foramina, using low-frequency (A) ("soft tissue") and high-frequency (B) ("bone") reconstruction kernels. Osseous integrity is generally assessed using the bone kernel image (B). Paraspinal or foraminal soft-tissue findings are better shown on the soft-tissue kernel image (A), with fat as a natural contrast agent. Intraspinal contents are often poorly depicted without intrathecal contrast.

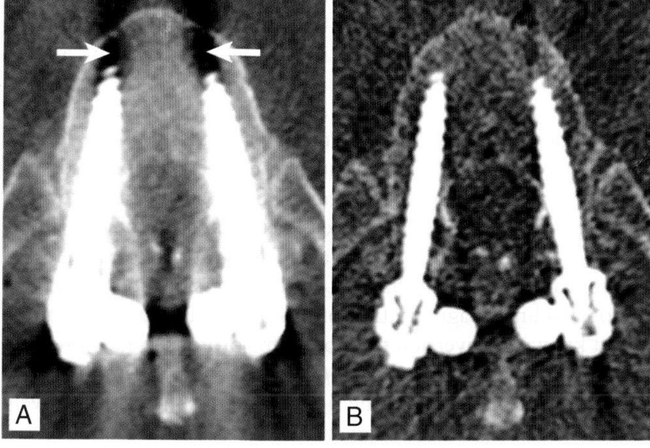

Figure 79.3 Metal artifact reduction using dual-energy CT and high-energy monoenergetic reconstruction. The axial image shows significant artifact (A, *arrows*) along the trajectory of the pedicle screws, which can be significantly reduced using this dual-energy technique (B).

MRI is contraindicated, CT with intravenous contrast may allow characterization of spinal infection or neoplasm.

Additional contrast in spine CT, particularly in the paraspinal soft tissues, can be provided by intravenous injection of iodinated contrast media. Intravenous, water-soluble iodinated contrast can be characterized by osmolality and ionicity. Older iodinated contrast agents were high-osmolality, ionic compounds and associated with higher risk of adverse reactions, whereas newer agents are low-osmolality and nonionic. The latter are associated with lower risk of both allergic-like reactions, which occur in fewer than 1% of patients [1], and physiologic reactions, such as headache, nausea, and vomiting. *Contrast-induced nephropathy is a controversial topic, but growing evidence suggests that low-osmolality agents delivered intravenously are associated with little to no risk of acute kidney injury* [2,3]. Injection of contrast typically occurs peripherally, with antecubital or forearm injections being preferred, ideally with 20-gauge or larger access and an injection rate of 3 mL/s.

Artifacts represent a broad topic, but recognition of these entities is an important part of reading CT:

- **Motion artifact**: Usually caused by gross patient motion, resulting in blurring or misalignment of images. This is particularly important in the evaluation of trauma, where motion can result in misaligned bone cortex and fractures can be mistakenly diagnosed.
- **Streak artifact**: Umbrella term for the artifacts created by beam hardening and photon starvation. Beam hardening occurs when low-energy x-rays are removed from a polychromatic beam by a dense surface or object, such as bone or surgical hardware, increasing the overall energy of the beam and decreasing the apparent attenuation of structures the "hardened" beam subsequently passes through. Photon starvation occurs when this interaction between the x-ray beam and the dense object results in insufficient photons reaching the detector and has a similar effect on imaging, decreasing the attenuation of voxels.
- **Volume averaging**: When a structure is smaller than the size of a given voxel, its attenuation will be averaged with other structures in the voxel, producing an attenuation somewhere between the attenuations of the two separate objects. This can be alleviated using thinner slice acquisition; using thin slices of less than 1 mm markedly reduces and nearly eliminates volume averaging artifacts.

Magnetic Resonance Imaging (MRI)

As MRI has become more affordable and widely available, it has superseded other modalities, such as myelography and CT, for many spinal pathologies. MRI does not produce ionizing radiation and instead relies on detection of nuclear magnetic resonance signal or "echoes" from hydrogen protons that have been placed in a strong external magnetic field and excited by radiofrequency pulses at resonance frequencies. With higher field strengths, more protons align parallel to the direction of the main magnetic field, allowing better spatial resolution and higher signal-to-noise ratio. However, this comes at the expense of increased deposition of energy in tissues, quantified by **specific absorption rate**. *MRI possesses superior soft-tissue contrast resolution to CT and has become the modality of choice for evaluating intervertebral discs, supporting ligaments, and neural structures of the spine, including the cord and nerve roots* (Figs. 79.4 and 79.5).

The fundamental MRI spine protocol includes T1- and T2-weighted sequences acquired in the axial and sagittal planes using fast or turbo spin-echo technique. Conventional spin-echo produces signal using an initial 90° radiofrequency pulse followed by a 180° pulse, both produced by a transmitter coil, to generate a signal/echo, which is detected by receiver coil. In fast or turbo spin-echo, the 90° pulse is followed by a series of 180° pulses that generate multiple echoes per 90° pulse and allow the collection of greater signal more rapidly than multiple separate excitations by multiple 90° pulses. The advent of fast spin-echo techniques with long echo-trains has dramatically shortened acquisition times and made MRI a more viable option in acute settings.

Additional sequences can serve as useful adjuncts to standard T1- and T2-weighted sequences in spine MRI. **Diffusion-weighted imaging (DWI)**, whereby MRI signal is highly sensitive to molecular diffusion of water, is a useful sequence for the identification and characterization of neoplastic and infectious processes, which may limit or "restrict" the diffusion of water, in the spinal cord and vertebrae. **In-and-out of phase sequences** are gradient-echo sequences that exploit slight differences in the precession frequencies of fat- and water-bound protons, which create constructive and destructive interference when in the same voxel,

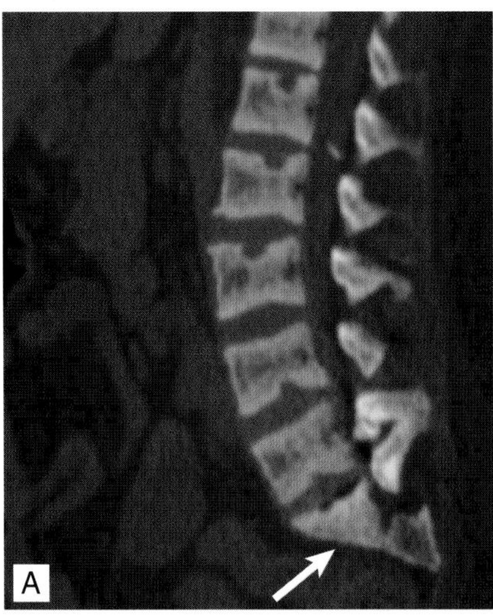

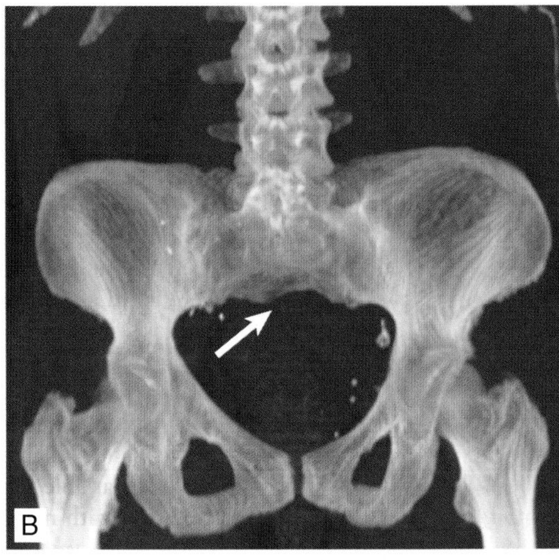

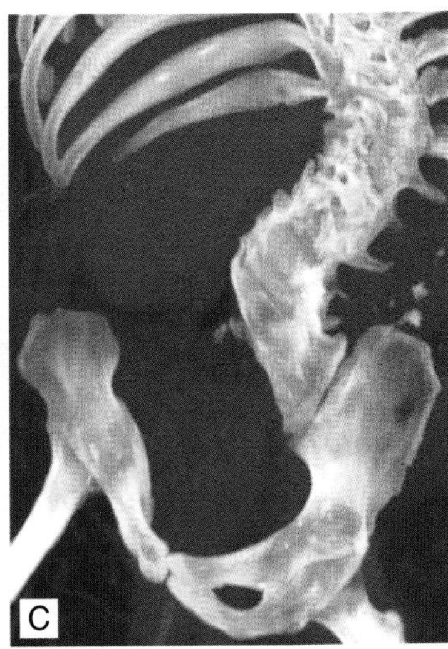

Figure 79.31 Caudal regression. Caudal regression is a spectrum of deficiency of the lumbar and sacral spine and coccyx. Sagittal CT (A) demonstrates a hypoplastic sacrum and absent coccyx (*white arrow*), confirmed on maximum-intensity-projection CT (B). On maximum-intensity projection of a CT (C), a different patient had more severe regression with absence of the right sacrum, a hypoplastic left sacrum, and, although poorly visualized on this image, multilevel lumbar spinal abnormalities, including absent laminae and spinous processes as well as hemivertebrae.

Pathophysiology

In children, infection typically begins as discitis from hematogenous spread and may spread to the vertebrae. In adults, infection may be the result of most commonly hematogenous spread, contiguous spread from infection originating outside the spine, or direct inoculation through instrumentation. The most common organism in tuberculosis-nonendemic countries is *Staphylococcus aureus*, which accounts for approximately 50% of cases [21,22]. Coagulase-negative *Staphylococcus*, *Streptococcus* species, *Escherichia coli*, *Pseudomonas aeruginosa*, and others can also cause **pyogenic discitis-osteomyelitis**. In endemic areas, tuberculous spondylodiscitis (**Pott's disease**) and fungal spondylodiscitis are important considerations. Antibiotics and, if needed, surgical debridement are standard treatment approaches.

Meningitis represents an inflammatory state of the meninges of the brain and spinal cord, from internal to external, the pia mater, arachnoid mater, and dura mater. Infectious meningitis is most commonly viral, typically caused by *Enteroviruses* [23], with Herpes family viruses being another contributor. Bacterial or pyogenic meningitis is less common, with the major pathogens including *Streptococcus pneumoniae*, Group B *Streptococcus*, *Neisseria meningitidis*, *Haemophilus influenzae*, and *Listeria monocytogenes* [24]. Again, tuberculous and fungal meningitis represent differential considerations in areas in which they are endemic. **Arachnoiditis** refers to inflammation of the arachnoid layer of the meninges, and may also be infectious or noninfectious in etiology.

Imaging Features

Radiographs are often normal in the early stages of discitis-osteomyelitis. As infection progresses, irregularity and/or lucency of the vertebral body endplates with narrowing of the intervertebral spaces can be seen (Fig. 79.32). In the chronic stage, these findings progress to endplate sclerosis, with vertebral deformation. *CT can better demonstrate endplate irregularity and erosion than radiography, but is still inferior to MRI of the spine with contrast, which according to ACR Appropriateness Criteria is the optimal imaging modality for suspected spinal infection* (Fig. 79.33) [12]. MRI without contrast may also be an adequate imaging study, particularly if the clinical suspicion for epidural or paraspinal infection is low. T2-weighted images demonstrate marrow edema-like endplate signal with abnormal high T2 signal in the discs. Fat-suppressed sequences such as STIR also show these edematous marrow changes well. On unenhanced T1-weighted images, this marrow edema corresponds to T1 hypointensity. On MRI with contrast, enhancement may be seen in the endplates and intervertebral disc. T2 hyperintensity and enhancement in the paraspinal soft tissues are highly suspicious for infection as opposed to its mimics, such as degenerative change. This includes the **"imaging psoas sign,"** abnormal T2 signal in the adjacent psoas muscle [25], a specific sign for infection. Epidural or paraspinal abscess is best visualized on MRI with contrast, but can still be visualized on noncontrast exams. If MRI cannot be obtained, CT with contrast can be performed. Radiography is unhelpful. On MRI, the inflammatory tissue will begin as **phlegmon** (Fig. 79.33), which has heterogeneous signal and enhancement throughout the tissue. As phlegmon matures into an abscess, it increases in central T2 signal and shows peripheral enhancement typical of an abscess (Fig. 79.34). The central fluid of the abscess will show restriction on DWI.

It can be challenging to differentiate between early spondylodiscitis and edematous Modic type I degenerative change, as both can show edematous marrow signal as well as abnormal disc and marrow enhancement. *In many cases, the presence of fluid in the disc space is the distinguishing feature, as discitis will often show T2 hyperintensity within the disc, whereas degenerative change usually will not.* Subtle blurring of the adjacent cortex is an important imaging feature that supports the diagnosis of infection, as is evidence of paraspinal or epidural involvement, including the "imaging psoas sign" mentioned earlier. The "**claw sign**" on DWI refers to well defined and linear areas of diffusion restriction in adjacent vertebral bodies in the shape of a "claw" (Fig. 79.35) [26]. This sign has a high negative predictive value for excluding infection.

Although they often resemble each other, tuberculous discitis-osteomyelitis can be differentiated from pyogenic infection through several features:

- The presence of associated lesions in other organs, especially the lung, urinary tract and other bones in tuberculosis.
- The tendency of untreated tuberculosis to induce less bone formation and to produce cold abscesses extending along muscle planes and beneath the anterior longitudinal ligament, eroding contiguous bone. This behavior represents "subligamentous spread."
- The tendency for pyogenic organisms to induce sclerotic bone reaction within the vertebral bodies and under the elevated

periosteum. The various organisms cause generally similar reactions, which require bacteriological study for distinction.
- The tendency of tuberculosis to be multifocal in the spine.
- The tendency of tuberculosis to cause deformity, especially gibbus deformity.
- Involvement of adjacent vertebral levels without involvement of the intervening disc is a classic appearance for Pott's disease

Paraspinal tuberculous abscesses in the thorax have classically been described as producing a "**paraspinal shadow**" on plain radiography (Fig. 79.36). The posteromedial pleura can be displaced laterally by many space-filling structures, including a fractured vertebral body, hematoma, or tumor, producing this shadow. However, in the tuberculosis-endemic areas, a tuberculous abscess must be considered.

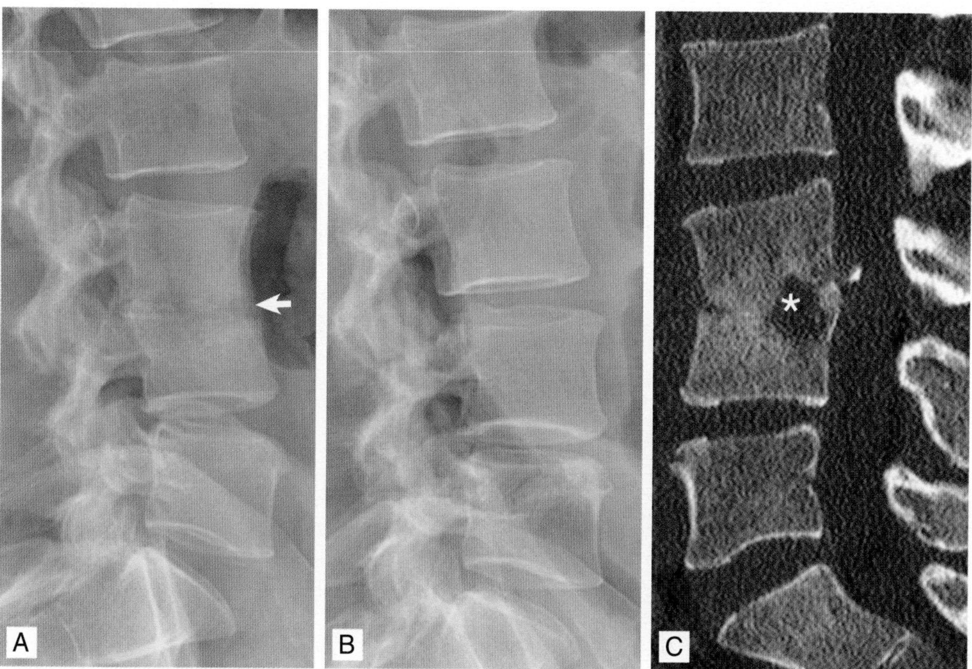

Figure 79.32 Discitis/osteomyelitis. Lateral radiograph (A) shows obliteration of the L3-4 disc (*white arrow*) with poorly defined endplates, a dramatic change from 3 months previous (B). Sagittal CT image (C) shows similar obliteration of the L3-4 disc, with eroded endplates, and a lucent area of osseous destruction (*asterisk*) centered at the disc.

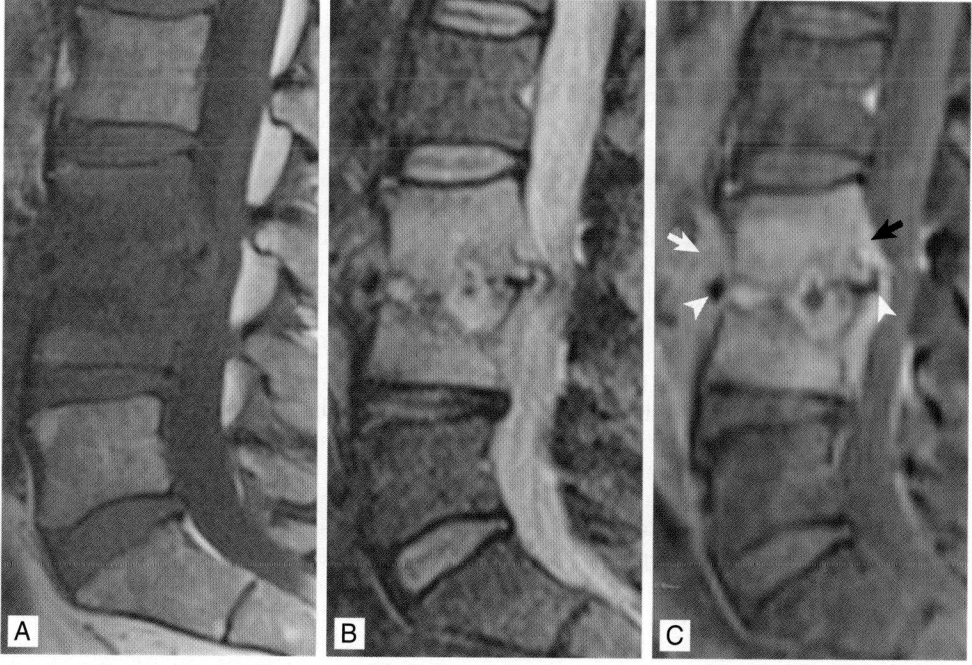

Figure 79.33 Discitis/osteomyelitis with paraspinal and epidural phlegmon on sagittal MRI. MRI of same case as Fig. 79.32. Sagittal T1-weighted image (A) and sagittal STIR image (B) show marrow edema in L3 and L4, loss of the cortex of the inferior L3 and superior L4 endplates, and abnormal anterior paraspinal as well as epidural tissue. The sagittal STIR image (B) also shows fluid signal in the disc. Sagittal fat-saturated postcontrast image (C) shows enhancement of the vertebrae and disc space. Solid enhancement of the anterior paraspinal (*white arrow*) and epidural (*black arrow*) tissues is consistent with phlegmon instead of abscess. Nonenhancing disc material (*white arrowheads*) is also shown.

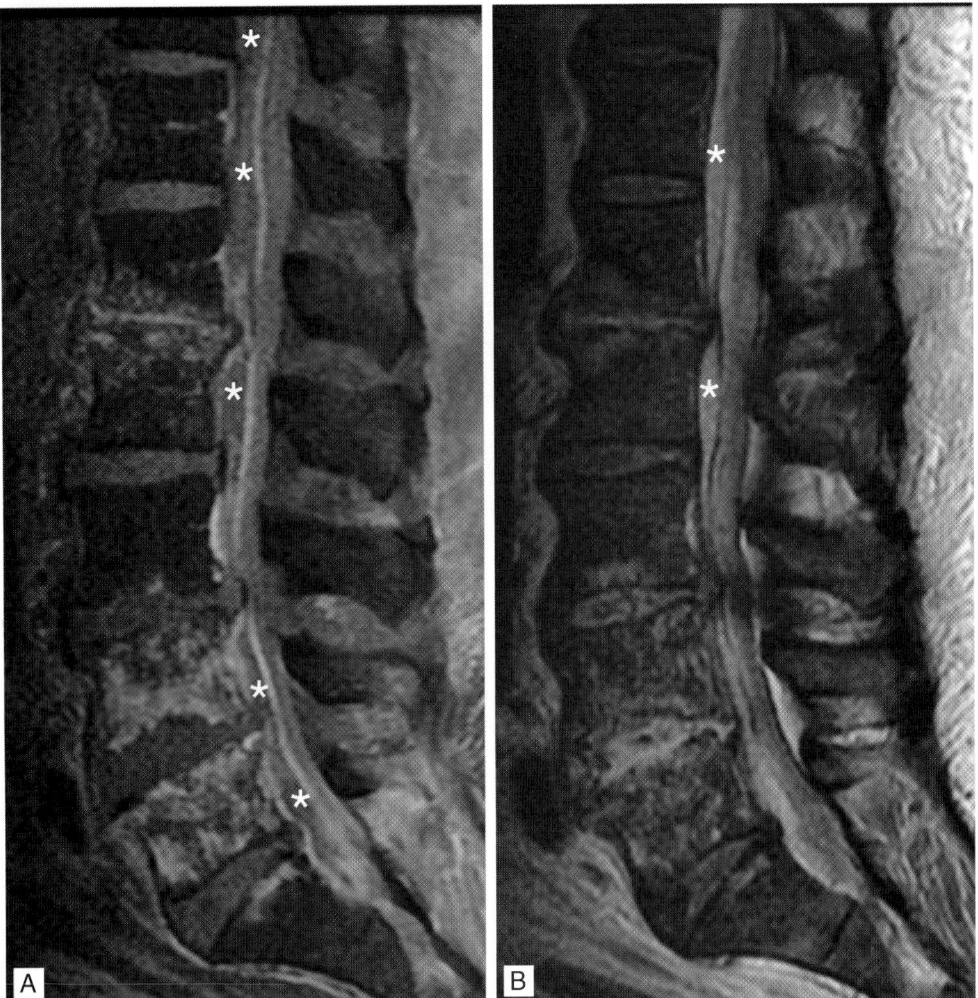

Figure 79.34 Epidural abscess. Sagittal fat-saturated postcontrast T1-weighted image (A) shows enhancement in the L1, L2, L4, and L5 vertebral bodies, and the sagittal T2-weighted image (B) shows fluid signal in the L1-2 and L4-5 discs, consistent with discitis/osteomyelitis at L1-2 and L4-5. There is a rim-enhancing epidural collection in the ventral spinal canal (*asterisks*) consistent with epidural abscess.

Spinal imaging is often not performed in cases of **infectious meningitis**, as even MRI with intravenous contrast may be normal, and in general, imaging findings of meningitis are nonspecific—many neoplastic or inflammatory diseases can have similar appearances. The findings of infectious meningitis on imaging, if present, vary based on whether the **leptomeninges (arachnoid and pia mater)** or the **pachymeninges (dura and arachnoid mater)** are involved and the category of infectious etiology. As in the brain, leptomeningeal changes, such as thickening or enhancement, closely follow the contour of the spinal cord, whereas pachymeningeal changes involve the more peripheral aspects of the spinal canal and may form mass-like areas with mass effect on the cord. The vector of infection also affects the appearance of meningitis on imaging. Viral and bacterial meningitides are more likely to cause smooth leptomeningeal enhancement involving the cord and nerve roots. Tuberculus and fungal etiologies, however, may cause more meningeal thickening and nodularity (Fig. 79.37). Meningitis is another potential cause of epidural abscess.

Arachnoiditis is best diagnosed by MRI, high-resolution axial T2-weighted fast spin-echo acquisitions usually being the most helpful. Chronic adhesive arachnoiditis results in adhesions between intradural roots and with the wall of the thecal sac, producing mass-like clumps, or incorporation of roots into the thecal wall creating an empty thecal sac (Fig. 79.38). It can be very extensive, however, with distortion and cavitation of the spinal cord. The organized adhesion may calcify or even ossify, producing **arachnoiditis ossificans**.

Direct parenchymal invasion and infection of spinal cord parenchyma, **infectious myelitis**, are mostly associated with viral etiologies (Fig. 79.39), but may also rarely be bacterial, fungal, or parasitic in nature. Among viral entities, the enteroviruses, which include poliovirus, typically infect the ventral cord, whereas herpesviruses, such as CMV, exhibit a preference for the white matter. Imaging findings are nonspecific, with T2 hyperintense cord signal, cord swelling, and enhancement.

What the Referring Physician Wants to Know

In patients suspected of bacterial vertebral osteomyelitis, MRI is the test of choice to confirm the diagnosis. Further tests (e.g., blood cultures, aspiration of infected fluid) may be needed to determine the causative organism and direct treatment, although empiric therapy may be started in patients with neurologic compromise, sepsis, or hemodynamic instability. When epidural abscess is present, emergent surgery may be indicated. Therefore, in addition to description of the infective process, referring physicians will be interested in the effect on neural structures, such as narrowing of the spinal canal by abscess. Adjacent soft-tissue manifestations, such as **psoas abscess**, should be described, as they may provide a target for aspiration and culture.

MRI is generally not indicated for routine follow-up of osteomyelitis, as some imaging findings, including edematous marrow signal and endplate erosion, may transiently worsen even with

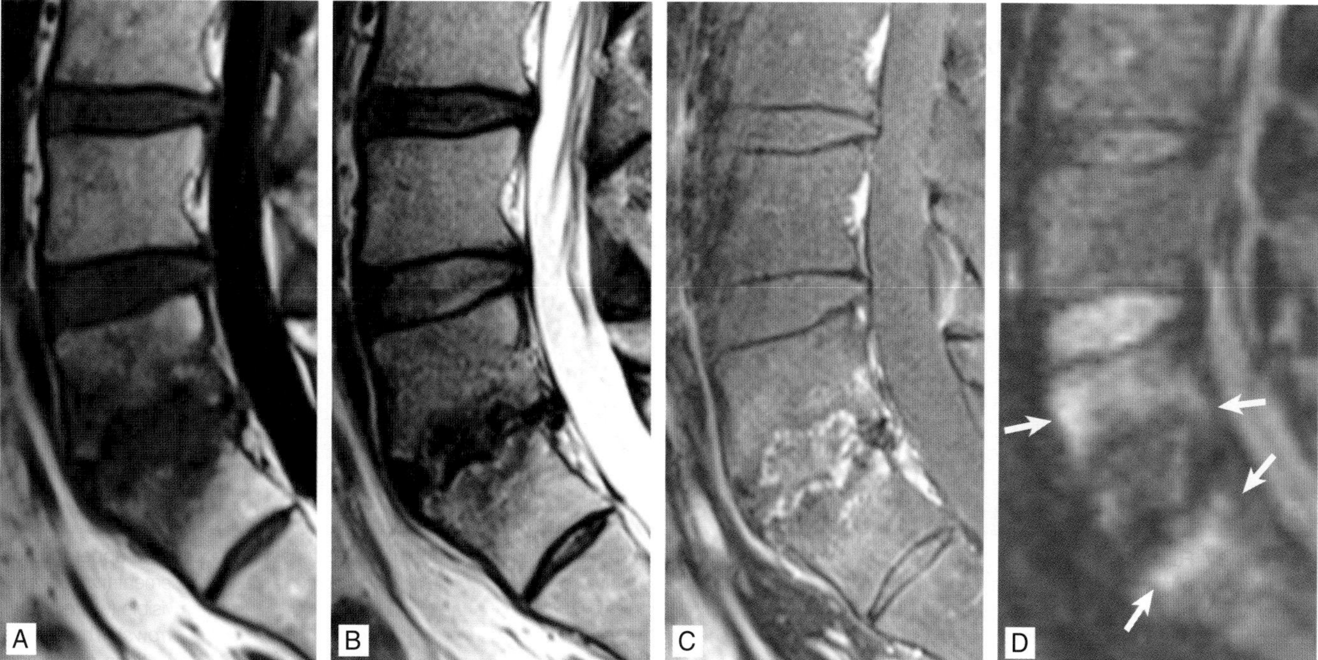

Figure 79.35 The "claw sign" on diffusion-weighted imaging (DWI). Sagittal T1-weighted image (A) shows edema in the endplates abutting the L5-S1 level, and some endplate irregularity. The sagittal T2-weighted image (B) does not show significant fluid in the disc, raising the possibility of degenerative marrow change, rather than discitis/osteomyelitis. The sagittal fat-saturated postcontrast image (C) shows enhancement in the endplates and mild enhancement in the disc, nonspecific. The sagittal diffusion-weighted image (D) shows hyperintense signal in the vertebral bodies in the shape of a "claw" opened anteriorly (*white arrows*). This sign suggests that the marrow changes do not reflect osteomyelitis.

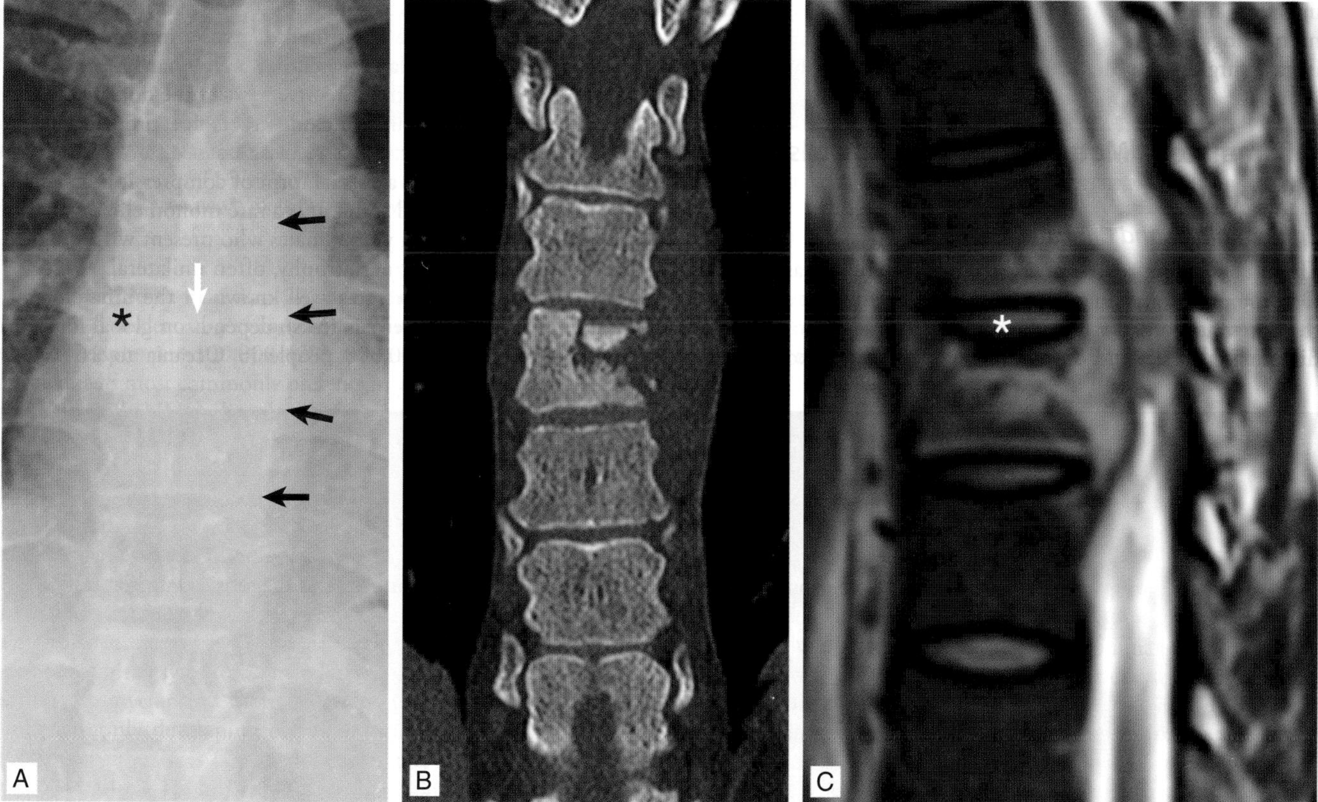

Figure 79.36 Tuberculosis of the spine (Pott's disease). Coned view of frontal chest x-ray (A) shows destruction of the left T7 pedicle and vertebral body (normal right T7 pedicle marked with *asterisk*), along with depression of the left superior T7 endplate (*white arrow*). Lateral displacement of the "paraspinal shadow" (*black arrows*) indicates paraspinal spread of infection (phlegmon). Coronal CT (B) confirms destruction of the left T7 vertebral body, depressed fracture of the superior endplate, and paraspinal soft-tissue mass. Sagittal off-midline T2-weighted image (C) shows the height loss at T7, with subligamentous epidural phlegmon extending superiorly and inferiorly. Note that the superiorly adjacent vertebral body of T6 is involved, with relative sparing of the intervening T6-7 disc space (*asterisk*), a pattern classic for this disease.

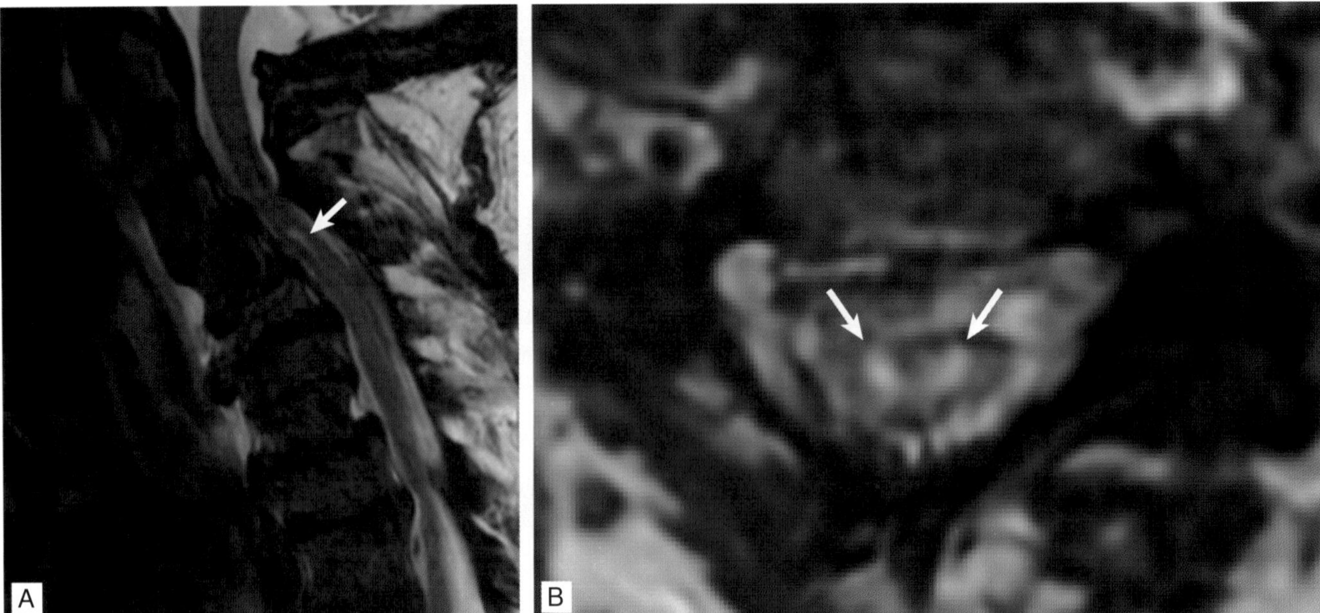

Figure 79.46 "Owl eye" sign. Sagittal T2-weighted image (A) demonstrates thin, linear T2 hyperintense signal in the cervical spinal cord (*white arrow*). Axial T2-weighted image (B) shows bilateral symmetric ovoid foci of T2 hyperintense signal (*white arrows*) in a patient with chronic compressive myelopathy.

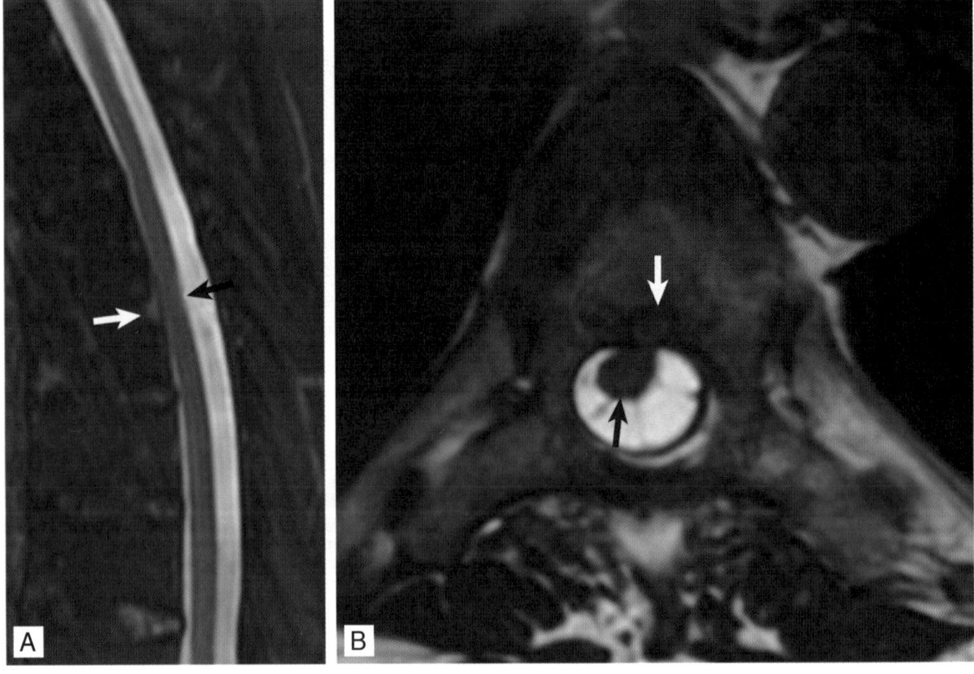

Figure 79.47 Anterior spinal cord herniation. Sagittal fat-saturated T2-weighted image (A) shows anterior cord displacement (*black arrow*) at a level where a well-defined defect (*white arrow*) is noted at the posterior margin of the vertebral body. Axial high-resolution MR myelographic (FIESTA-C) image (B) shows the spinal cord rotated to the right (*black arrow*), with complete loss of ventral cerebrospinal fluid, and cord parenchyma herniated ventrally into the dural defect (*white arrow*).

Pathophysiology

Intramedullary tumors are most commonly gliomas, arising from cells found within the spinal cord, such as the ependymal cells lining the central canal and astrocytes supporting the neurons and axons of the cord. Hemangioblastomas arise from vascular stromal cells and intervening blood vessels. Cavernomas comprise vessels without normal intervening brain parenchyma.

The intradural–extramedullary meningioma arises from arachnoid cap cells of the arachnoid villi. The myxopapillary ependymoma is a subtype of ependymoma. Both schwannomas and neurofibromas arise from Schwann cells.

Most extradural masses are metastatic in etiology. Osteoid osteomas, osteoblastomas, and giant cell tumors are osteogenic in origin with predilection for the neural arches. The chordoma specifically arises from notochord remnants.

Imaging Features

In the setting of suspected malignancy or mass, MRI with contrast is the most appropriate imaging study, with a noncontrast

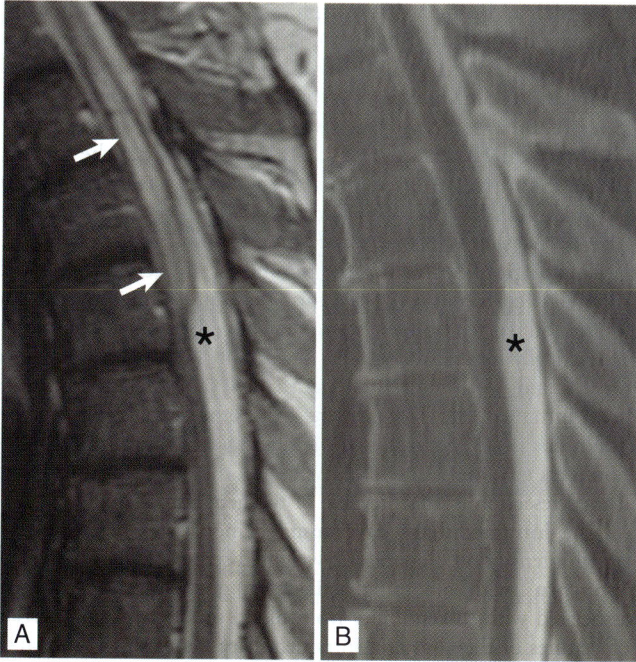

Figure 79.48 Dorsal arachnoid web. Sagittal T2-weighted image (A) of the thoracic spine shows a focal dorsal deflection of the spinal cord, with a smooth posterior contour, where the cerebrospinal fluid space (*asterisk*) resembles a scalpel blade, the so-called "scalpel sign." Note the syrinx (*white arrows*) within the cord superiorly. Sagittal CT myelogram image (B) shows a similar scalpel-like shape of the posterior cerebrospinal fluid space (*asterisk*).

MRI being an alternative if contrast cannot be used [12]. If MRI cannot be performed, CT with contrast is the next best option, although CT myelography may be needed to diagnose cord or cauda equina compression, particularly if urgent treatment is needed. Radiography has a limited role in evaluating these masses and may only show secondary osseous changes.

Localizing the spinal spatial compartment of a mass lesion is best done with MRI, with myelography or CT myelography as

TABLE 79.2 Common Causes of Myelopathy

Category	Typical Onset	Comment
Compressive		
Degenerative	Acute/subacute	Disc, osteophyte, ligaments
Neoplastic	Acute	Most commonly extradural (metastasis)
Infectious	Acute	Abscess, phlegmon
Traumatic	Acute	Hematoma, disc, fracture fragments
Other	Subacute	Arachnoid cyst, arachnoid web, Hirayama disease
Demyelinating	Acute	MS, NMO spectrum disorders, ADEM
Systemic disease	Acute	Sarcoid, systemic lupus erythematosus, Sjogren's
Infectious myelitis	Acute	Usually viral; bacterial/fungal/parasitic less common
Ischemic		
Arterial	Acute	Atherosclerotic, aortic dissection/surgery
Venous	Subacute	AVF/AVM
Postradiation	Acute	Months-to-years after treatment
Paraneoplastic	Subacute	Overlap with autoimmune myelitides
Metabolic	Subacute	B12, copper, or vit E deficiency Nitrous oxide/zinc toxicity
Traumatic (noncompressive)	Acute	Cord edema (central cord syndrome), cord hemorrhage
Idiopathic	Acute/subacute	
Myelomalacia	Chronic	End-stage cord damage/injury, myriad causes

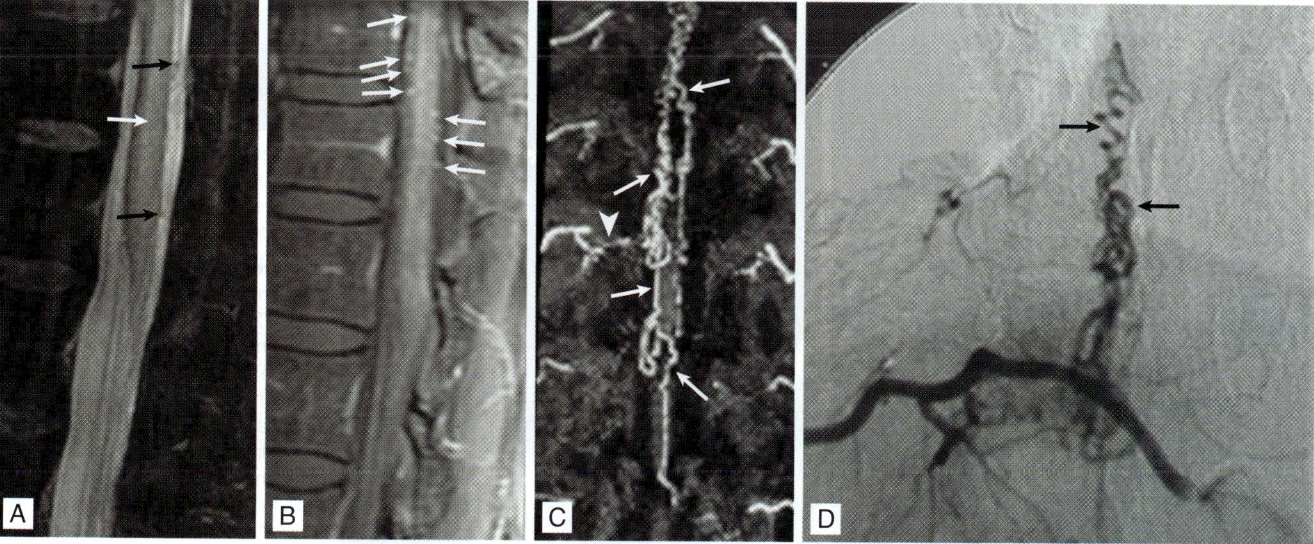

Figure 79.49 Dural arteriovenous fistula with myelopathy from venous hypertension. Magnified sagittal fat-saturated T2-weighted image (A) shows hyperintense signal in the conus medullaris (*white arrow*). The flow voids, small black rounded intradural signal foci around the cord (*black arrows*) are suggestive of an underlying vascular anomaly. Postcontrast fat-saturated T1-weighted image (B) confirms numerous enhancing vessels around the conus, indicating dilated perimedullary veins, and suggesting venous hypertension as the cause of myelopathy. A coronal maximum-intensity-projection image from an MR angiogram (C) confirms multiple dilated intradural vessels (*white arrows*) and also suggests the site of fistula at a right foramen (*white arrowhead*). Selective angiogram (D) at that level confirms multiple dilated perimedullary veins (*black arrows*).

80 Pediatric Brain and Spine

TUSHAR CHANDRA, PANKAJ WATAL, MANISH BAJAJ, LAURA HAYES

Introduction

Imaging of the pediatric brain has rapidly evolved over the last few decades. There have been significant strides in both the quality of imaging and the understanding of disease processes that involve the pediatric central nervous system (CNS) along with a paradigm shift toward identifying the genetic basis of various disorders. Understanding the embryology, growth, developmental as well as maturation of the pediatric brain provides a fundamental basis for assessing the pediatric brain abnormalities.

Embryology and Normal Prenatal Brain Development

Brain development begins in the third gestational week with dedifferentiation of neural progenitor cells. By the end of the embryonic period, the rudimentary structures of brain and CNS are established. The stages of brain development are as follows:

1. Dorsal induction
2. Ventral induction
3. Proliferation
4. Migration
5. Organization
6. Myelination

The first step in the human brain development is differentiation of the progenitor cells. The early CNS begins a simple neural plate in the dorsal midline of the embryo, which forms as thickening of the ectoderm. The neural plate folds to form a neural groove and the sides of the neural groove, known as the neural folds come together and join to form the neural tube. The neural tube is formed by the 20th day of gestation and begins to close in the early stages of neurulation. The brain forms at the rostral end of the neural tube and three distinct primary vesicles are formed by the fourth week of gestation.

- The three primary vesicles are the forebrain (prosencephalon), midbrain (mesencephalon), and hindbrain (rhombencephalon). The secondary vesicles arise from the primary vesicles
- The prosencephalon divides into telencephalon anteriorly and diencephalon posteriorly
- The rhombencephalon divides into anterior metencephalon and the posterior myelencephalon
- The mesencephalon remains a single vesicle
- The lateral ventricles develop in the prosencephalon, the third ventricle develops in the mesencephalon, and the fourth ventricle in the rhombencephalon

The telencephalon expands and differentiates to form the cerebral hemispheres by the 11th week of gestation, through a process of neuronal proliferation. Migration of the neuronal cells continues to about the 35th week. Through the process of operculization, the insular cortex and Sylvian fissures are formed. The lobes of the cerebral hemispheres and the sulci and gyri start forming and continue to the 35th week.

The diencephalon develops into thalamus, hypothalamus, epithalamus, globi pallidi, pineal gland, and neurohypophysis of the pituitary gland.

The cerebral commissures of the telencephalon begin to form and are the site of origin of the anterior commissure and the corpus callosum. The progression of formation of corpus callosum begins with the posterior aspect of genu, followed by the body, splenium, anterior genu, and rostrum during weeks 10–12 of gestation. The sequence of these events is somewhat controversial and has been challenged by some authors.

The mesencephalon forms the superior and inferior colliculi of the tectum, cerebral peduncles, optic lobes, and tegmentum.

The metencephalon portion of the rhombencephalon gives rise to the cerebellum and pons.

The myelencephalon portion of the rhombencephalon develops into the medulla oblongata and the rostral neural tube is contiguous with the myelencephalon and forms the spinal cord.

Although the brain continues to grow and myelinate after birth, structurally, the brain at birth is similar to the adult brain.

Brain Myelination

Assessment of myelination is an integral part of evaluation of the pediatric brain. Myelin is produced by the oligodendrocytes and contains approximately 70% lipid and 30% protein [1]. MRI allows for a reliable and quick estimation of the degree of myelination of the brain, which can be categorized as normal for age, delayed, or abnormal. This has greatly enhanced of our ability to evaluate pathologies that are associated with abnormalities of myelination, such as leukodystrophies and neurometabolic abnormalities.

It is important to understand that anatomical regions in the brain that are responsible for more primitive and basic functions myelinate earlier than anatomic structures that are responsible for more advanced functions. Brain myelination, therefore is a sequential process that occurs in an orderly and predictable course. *In general, brain myelination progresses from caudal to cephalad, dorsal to ventral, and from central to peripheral areas of the brain.* For example, the brainstem myelinates before the deep gray matter structures and the cerebellum, and the cerebral hemispheres myelinate even later. Furthermore, projection tracts within the brain generally myelinate before the association tracts.

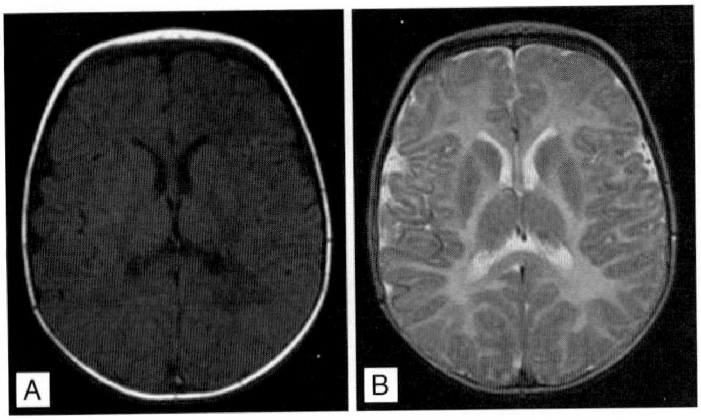

Figure 80.3 Pelizeas–Merzbacher disease. Axial T1W (A) and T2W (B) images demonstrate complete lack of myelination in this 5-year-old male.

nystagmus, often with extrapyramidal features such as dystonic postures and torsion spasms. On imaging, there is complete lack of myelin that can be seen on both T1- and T2-weighted sequences [5] (Fig. 80.3).

Other hypomyelinating leukodystrophies include:

- **Pelizaeus–Merzbacher-like disease**, also called hypomyelinating leukodystrophy type 2, which is autosomal recessive, but otherwise similar to Pelizaeus–Merzbacher disease
- **Pol III-related leukodystrophies** are autosomal recessive disorders characterize by mutations in POLR3A and POLR3B genes. In this disorder, apart from homogeneous hypomyelination, there are hyperintense signals in the globus pallidus and thalami on T2-weighted sequences and cerebellar atrophy
- **Hypomyelination with congenital cataracts** is another rare, autosomal recessive disorder that is caused by a mutation in FAM126A gene. Patients with this order presented with developmental delay and congenital or childhood cataracts. On imaging, there is heterogeneous hypomyelination with T2 hyperintense signal more increased in the periventricular white matter compared with the subcortical and deep white matter [6]
- **Hypomyelination with atrophy of basal ganglia and cerebellum** is a sporadic disorder characterized by mutation in the TUBB4A gene, which is characterized by homogeneous hypomyelination along with atrophy of the cerebellum, putamen, and caudate nucleus, as the name suggests [7]
- **Hypomyelination with brainstem and spinal cord involvement and leg spasticity** is characterized by muscle spasticity in the legs that worsens over time along with other symptoms such as nystagmus, hypertonia, and mild intellectual disability. This is caused by DARS gene mutation that affects amino acids. On imaging there is homogeneous hypomyelination involving the cerebrum, brainstem, cerebellum, and spinal cord. The pyramidal tracts and dorsal columns are primarily affected by this condition [8]

Metachromatic Leukodystrophy

This is one of the commoner hereditary leukodystrophies; clinical symptoms usually commence in infancy, although they can be delayed into adolescence or later. This is a lysosomal disorder caused by a deficiency of the enzyme arylsulfatase A. There is mental retardation or regression and other neurological signs, which are progressively fatal.

On MRI, the classical appearances confluent and symmetric hyperintense T2 signals that involve the periventricular and deep white matter related to sparing of the subcortical U fibers. There is relative sparing of the perivenular myelin leading to a tigroid pattern. In late stages that can be involvement of subcortical U fibers, corpus callosum, and descending pyramidal tracts with atrophy.

Globoid Leukodystrophy (Krabbe's Disease)

This is also a lysosomal disorder, characterized by a lack of the enzyme P-galactocerebrosidase. It presents in infancy with retardation and spasticity, and is usually fatal by the second year. Rarely, it presents in later childhood with a more chronic course and early visual failure.

On CT, symmetric hyperdensity can be seen in basal ganglia, thalami, cerebellum, and corona radiata. On MRI there is confluent, symmetric T2 hyperintense signal in the periventricular and deep white matter along with alternating hyperintense, hypointense, and hyperintense signals in the cerebellar white matter around the dentate nuclei. Furthermore, there can be enlargement and postcontrast enhancement of the cranial nerves as well as cauda equina nerve roots.

Adrenoleukodystrophy

This is an inherited X-linked peroxisomal disorders caused by ABCD1 mutation that results in accumulation of very long chain fatty acids in the white matter. The classic form of X-linked ALD primarily affects boys of 5–12 years age.

On MR imaging, there is involvement of the splenium of corpus callosum, peritrigonal periventricular and deep white matter, corticospinal tracts, and visual and auditory pathways. The classic imaging feature is confluent T2 hyperintense signal involving the periventricular and deep white matter in the peritrigonal regions with marked rim enhancement on postcontrast T1 images of the leading edge. Contrast enhancement represents perivascular inflammation at the margins of the demyelinating process (Fig. 80.4).

Alexander's Disease

This disease is inherited sporadically and is characterized histopathologically by the abundant presence of Rosenthal fibers in the affected brain. There are three clinical forms: infantile, juvenile, and adult. The infantile form is most common and these patients present with macrocephaly. There is a variable rate of progression and the disease is invariably fatal.

On MR imaging, that is characteristic T2 hyperintense signal that involves bifrontal white matter (Fig. 80.5). In early disease, intense postcontrast enhancement may be observed.

Organic Acidemias and Aminoacidopathies

This is a wide group of metabolic disorders caused by defects in the intermediate metabolic path results of amino acid, carbohydrate, and fatty acid oxidation. They present in infants and with improved methods of biochemical assay many different types have now been defined. The diagnosis is usually made biochemically but imaging may help by showing the degree of myelin damage or the effect of treatment on progression. This group of disorders includes conditions such as propionic acidemia, methylmalonic acidemia, multiple carboxylase deficiency, Canavan disease, glutaric aciduria, phenylketonuria, maple syrup urine disease, nonketotic hyperglycemia, homocystinuria, sulfite oxidase deficiency, etc. (Fig. 80.6).

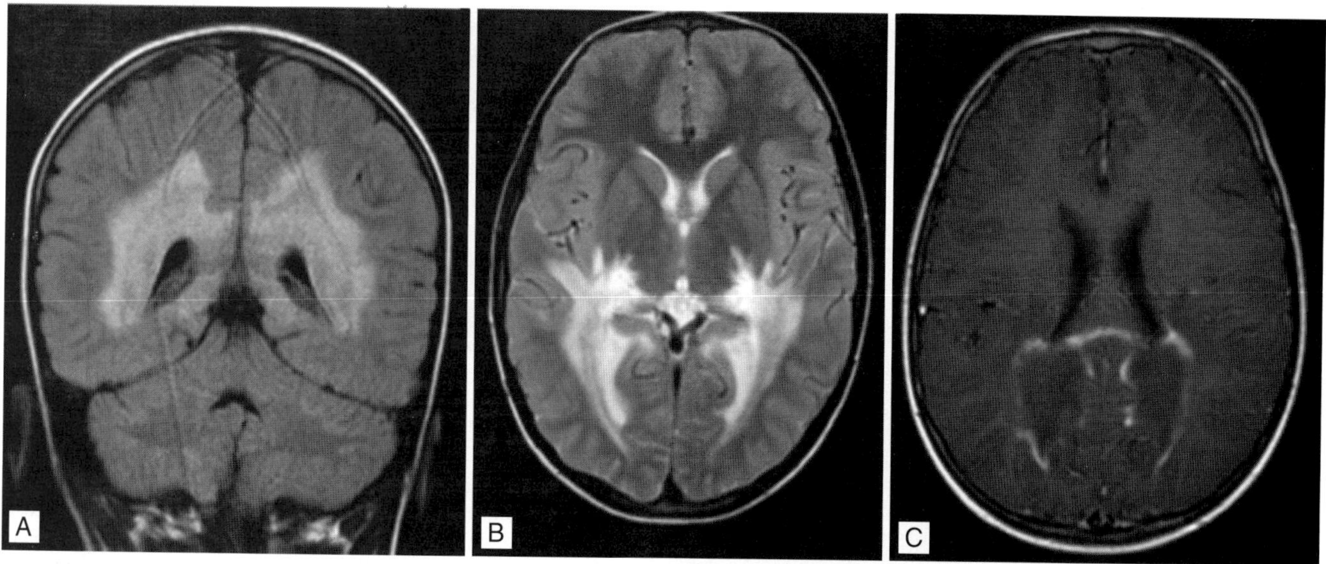

Figure 80.4 X-linked adrenoleukodystrophy. Coronal FLAIR (A) and axial FLAIR (B) images demonstrate confluent hyperintense signal in the peritrigonal white matter. Postcontrast T1 (C) image enhancement along the leading edge.

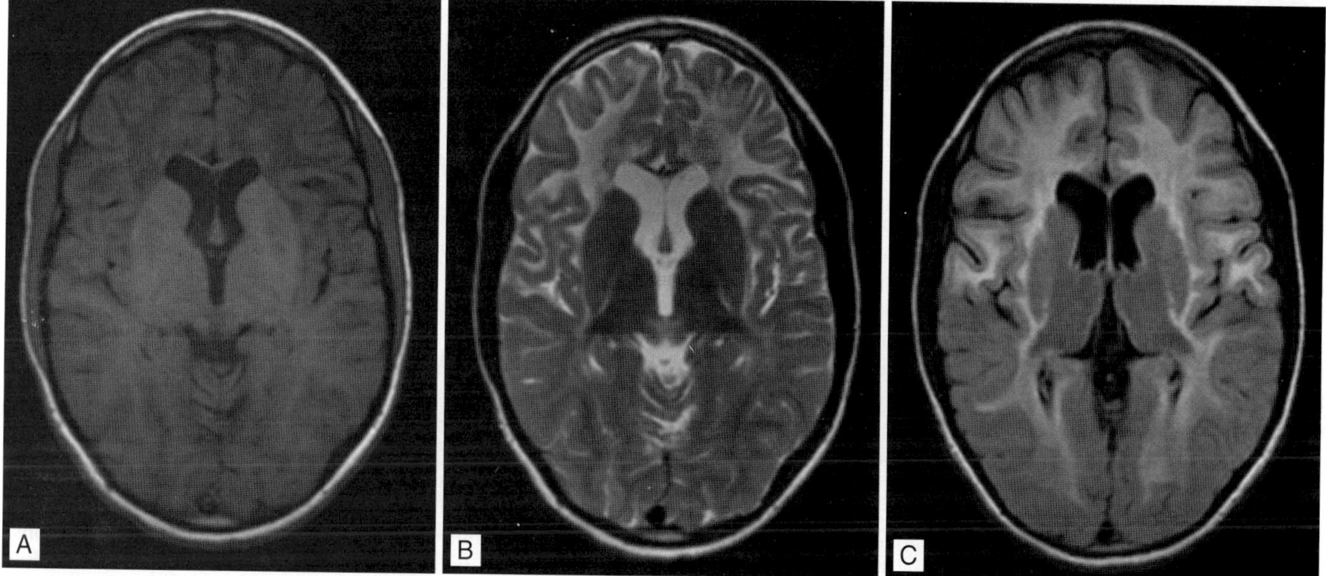

Figure 80.5 Alexander's disease. Axial T1(A), T2 (B), and FLAIR (C) images demonstrate confluent and symmetric T1 hypointense and T2/FLAIR hyperintense signal in the frontal white matter bilaterally.

Canavan Disease

This is an autosomal recessive disorder characterized by deficiency of aspartoacylase enzyme which results in increased N-acetyl aspartate (NAA) in the brain, causing spongiform degeneration of the white matter, globus pallidus, and thalami. Patients present with macrocephaly and hypotonia which is evident in the first few months of life.

On MRI there is involvement of the subcortical U fibers, thalamus, and globus pallidus with relative sparing of the internal capsules and putamen. The characteristic finding on MR spectroscopy is increase in NAA.

Phenylketonuria

This is an autosomal recessive disorder of amino acid metabolism caused by mutation in PAH gene, leading to the absence of phenylalanine hydroxylase which hydrolyses phenylalanine to tyrosine. Severe mental impairment may ensue if the condition is unrecognized and untreated, and there are alterations in the hemisphere myelin resembling leukodystrophy. On MRI, T2/FLAIR hyperintensity can be seen in periventricular or subcortical white matter.

Mitochondrial Disorders

This is a group of diseases that have in common a defect in mitochondria, with consequent deficiency of enzymes controlling oxidative phosphorylation and/or the respiratory chain. As the spermatozoa are deficient of mitochondria, these diseases have maternal inheritance. The affected persons are often short in stature. The histopathology includes subacute necrotizing encephalomyelopathy associated with proliferation of capillaries and glia and with spongiform degeneration. The distribution, reflected in

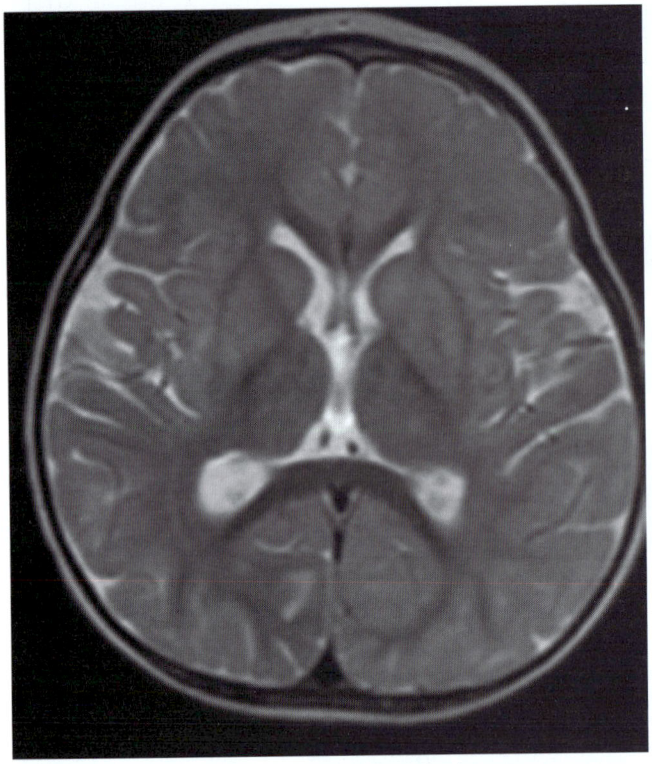

Figure 80.6 Propionic acidemia. Axial T2 image demonstrate symmetric T2 hyperintense signals involving bilateral basal ganglia.

the MRI appearances, includes symmetric necrosis in the basal ganglia, spongiform change with increase in T1 and T2 in the thalamus, brainstem, and/or hemispheric white matter. There is frequent involvement of muscles resulting in a proximal myopathy. Involvement of the CNS can result in varied clinical presentations, associated with elevation of the serum and cerebrospinal fluid (CSF) lactate.

- **Leigh's syndrome** or subacute necrotizing encephalomyelopathy is caused by mitochondrial DNA mutations. Typical MRI findings include symmetrical areas of T2 prolongation involving bilateral caudate nuclei and lentiform nuclei with less common involvement of the thalami, periaqueductal gray matter, tegmentum, red nuclei, and dentate nuclei (Fig. 80.7). The T2 hyperintense signals are thought to reflect spongiform changes and vacuolization of gray matter structures. As the disease progresses, global atrophy can be seen and basal ganglia can show volume loss. On MR spectroscopy, there is a characteristic lactate doublet at 1.3 ppm (Fig. 80.8)

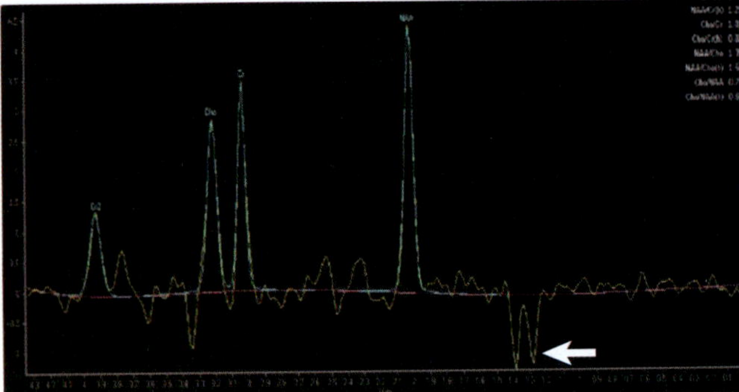

Figure 80.8 Leigh disease. MR spectroscopy demonstrates characteristic lipid-lactate inverse doublet at 1.33 ppm (*white arrow*).

- **Mitochondrial myopathy, encephalopathy, lactic acidosis, and stroke-like episode** is another progressive neurodegenerative disorder caused by mitochondrial DNA mutation. On MRI, the classical findings are acute stroke-like cortical lesions that crosses vascular territories and may appear, disappear, and then reappear elsewhere. As the disease becomes chronic, it may lead to brain atrophy
- **Myoclonic epilepsy with ragged red fibers** is another mitochondrial disorder that has a predilection for basal ganglia and can present with watershed ischemia/infarction
- **Kearnes–Sayre syndrome** is characterized by a triad of ataxia, ophthalmoplegia, and retinitis pigmentosa. There are calcifications in bilateral basal ganglia, caudate nucleus, and subcortical white matter. On MRI, there may be T1 and T2 hyperintense signal within the basal ganglia and cerebellar white matter

Hypoxic Ischemic Encephalopathy

HIE is one of the major causes of cerebral palsy and severe neurological deficits in the pediatric age group. Neonatal encephalopathy can result from a diverse number of underlying conditions. Encephalopathy due to hypoxic ischemic injury presents within

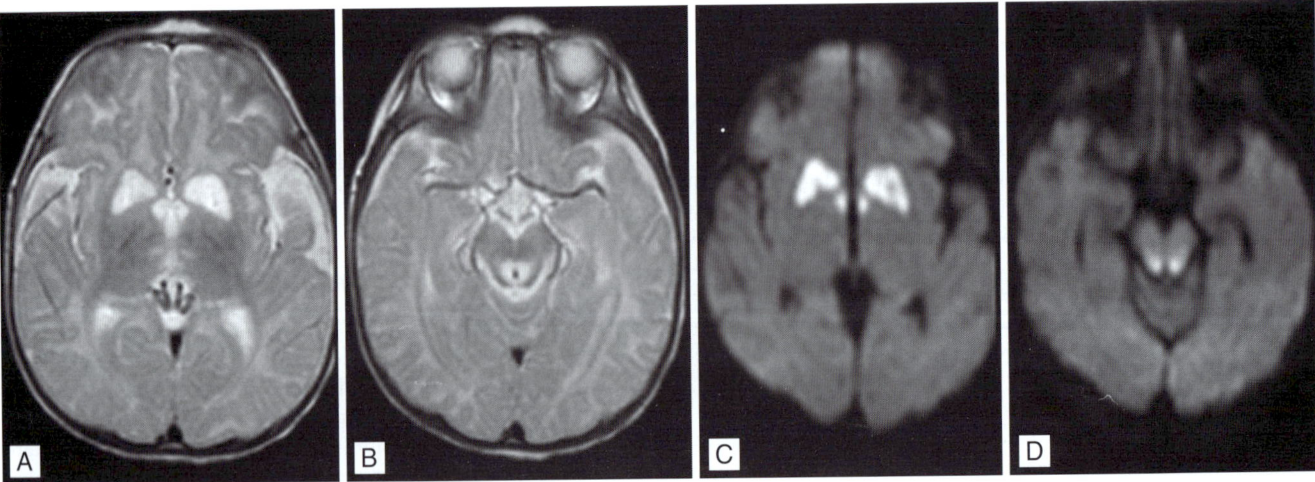

Figure 80.7 Leigh disease. Axial T2 (A and B) images demonstrate symmetric T2 hyperintense signals involving bilateral caudate nuclei and dorsal brainstem. DWI images (C and D) demonstrate restricted diffusion in those regions.

the first few hours after birth. If encephalopathy develops later (e.g., a few days after birth), infectious and metabolic causes should be considered. It is also important to remember that encephalopathy is a clinical term characterized by a low Apgar score and clinical signs such as bradycardia, poor respiratory effort, hypotonia, and absent or weak cry at birth [9].

In terms of imaging, while describing the anatomical findings, hypoxic ischemic injury is a more appropriate term to use than HIE. Perinatal asphyxia leading to hypoxia and hypercapnia is the underlying pathophysiological mechanism for HIE. Hypoxia with loss of cerebral autoregulation leads to decreased cerebral blood flow and through a cascade of abnormal pathogenic mechanisms. This causes acidosis, release of inflammatory mediators and excitatory neurotransmitters, free radical formation, and lipid peroxidation, eventually leading to neuronal death [9,10]. The reasons for imaging patients with suspected HIE include confirmation of the diagnosis, exclusion of other structural abnormalities and assessing the extent of the injury for predicting the neurodevelopmental outcome.

The patterns of injury depend on three primary factors:

1. Maturation of the brain (preterm vs term)
2. Duration of the insult
3. Severity of the insult

The vascular supply of the brain evolves as the brain matures. In the preterm neonate (<36 weeks), the penetrating arterioles terminate in the periventricular region and therefore in this age group, HIE results in injury to the periventricular white matter, resulting in periventricular leukomalacia.

In the term neonate (>36 weeks), the vascular border zone moves more peripherally in a more parasagittal location and HIE results in involvement of vascular watershed zones, with involvement of the cortex and the deep white matter. Severe and more prolonged injury results in greater involvement of deep gray matter structures such as the thalami and basal ganglia, cerebellum, and brainstem in both preterm as well as term infants. Furthermore, actively myelinating structures are more prone to hypoxic injury compared with other regions of the brain.

Ultrasound of the neonatal brain is the initial investigation that helps in the detection of germinal matrix hemorrhage and hydrocephalus. However, ultrasound is not the preferred technique for the detection of changes of HIE in the early stages. It is operator defendant and has low sensitivity for the detection of cortical and brainstem abnormalities. In the more chronic setting, ultrasound can be used for the detection of periventricular leukomalacia.

MRI is the most sensitive and specific technique for evaluation of suspected HIE. The most useful sequences on MR imaging are diffusion-weighted (DW) sequence and T1 sequence. DW sequence demonstrates the cytotoxic edema caused by neuronal death as restricted diffusion. If performed within 24 hours of hypoxic injury, DW sequence may be falsely negative. DW changes last for 10–12 days after hypoxic injury and thereafter pseudonormalization occurs [9]. T1 sequences are also useful for the detection of injury to the deep gray matter structures as well as the cortex. Deep gray matter injury is characterized by T1 hyperintense signal in the basal ganglia and thalamus. In the term neonate, this is accompanied by the absence of the normal T1 hyper intensity of the posterior limb of internal capsule (which should be present due to myelination in a normal term infant). T1 hyperintensity may also be seen along the cortex in cases with cortical injury. MR spectroscopy can be very useful in the evaluation of HIE. There is elevation of lactate with reduction of NAA (Figs. 80.9 and 80.10). An elevated lactate to creatine ratio on first day of life is a predictor of adverse outcome [11]. Caution must be used while interpreting MR spectroscopy findings in a preterm neonate as a high lactate and low NAA are normal findings in this age. The treatment of HIE is usually supportive and involves therapeutic hypothermia.

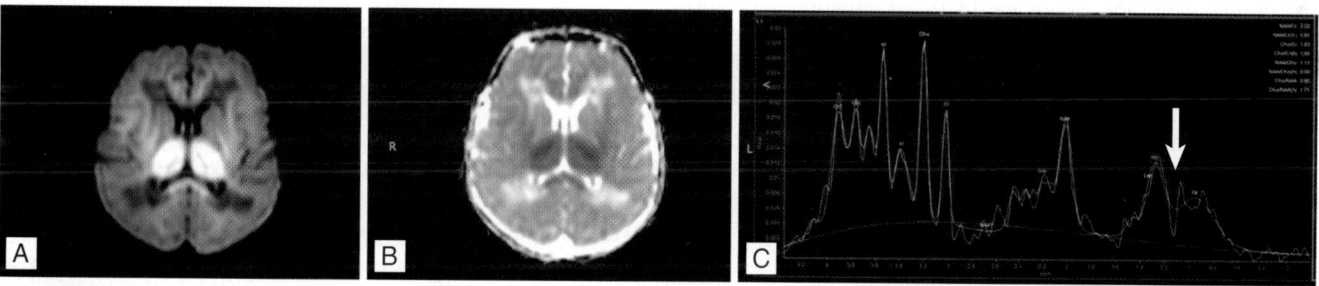

Figure 80.9 Hypoxic ischemic encephalopathy. Axial DWI (A) and ADC (B) images demonstrate restricted diffusion involving bilateral thalami and splenium of corpus callosum. MR spectroscopy (C) demonstrates elevated lipid-lactate (*white arrow*) and decreased NAA.

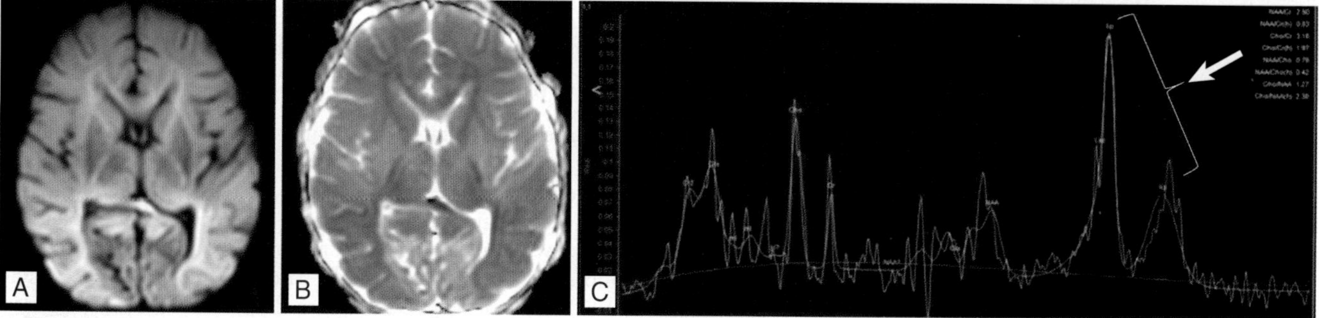

Figure 80.10 Severe hypoxic ischemic encephalopathy. Axial DWI (A) and ADC (B) images demonstrate extensive restricted diffusion involving bilateral deep gray matter, white matter, and the cortex. Note relative sparing of medial occipital lobes. MR spectroscopy (C) demonstrates elevated lipid-lactate (*white arrow*) and decreased NAA.

Congenital and Developmental Supratentorial Brain Anomalies

There is a wide array of congenital supratentorial brain abnormalities. Patients often present with seizures or developmental delay, and prognosis is variable. Congenital brain malformations are best demonstrated with MRI. It is important for the radiologist to identify the abnormalities to help prognosticate outcomes and assist in surgical planning in some cases.

Pertinent Embryology

Supratentorial brain development is a series of very complex, carefully orchestrated events that are beyond the scope of this chapter, and therefore a simplified review is included herein. The basic events that occur embryologically during development of the brain are neurulation, neuronal proliferation, and neuronal migration. The development of gyri and sulci takes place after the 11th week of gestation. Cortical neurons are formed in the embryonal germinal matrix which lies along the inner margins of the lateral ventricles. These neuroblasts migrate centrifugally out along the radial glial cells to the surface of the brain, where they form the cerebral cortex, the deeper layers being constituted first. Interruption of this process, which takes place primarily between the 11th and 15th fetal weeks, may give rise to various cortical anomalies including heterotopias, focal cortical dysplasias (FCDs), and lissencephaly.

Anomalies of the Cortex

Lissencephaly (from the Greek language meaning "smooth brain") is characterized by the absence of sulci and convolutions in the cortex, resembling the normal fetal brain before the seventh month of gestation (Fig. 80.11). Lissencephaly may be spontaneous or inherited. LIS1, DCX, and TUBA1A mutations are associated with the lissencephaly spectrum of disorders. Clinically these patients usually demonstrate developmental delay and seizures. Lissencephaly can involve the entire brain or only a portion of the hemispheres, most often in the parieto-occipital region. Some degree of pachygyria (meaning "thick brain") with abnormally broad and thick convolutions may also be present [12]. Subcortical band heterotopia, also called "double cortex" syndrome, is the mildest form of classic lissencephaly.

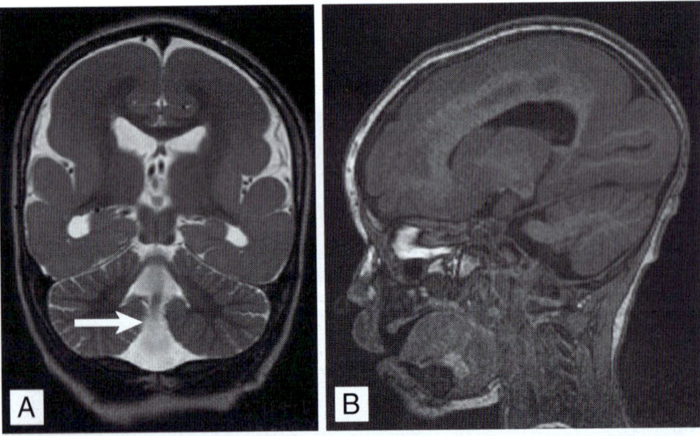

Figure 80.11 Lissencephaly. Axial T2 (A) and sagittal T1 (B) images demonstrate broad gyri with paucity of sulci resulting in smooth appearance of the brain. Note a small Dandy–Walker cyst communicating with the fourth ventricle in the posterior fossa (*arrow*).

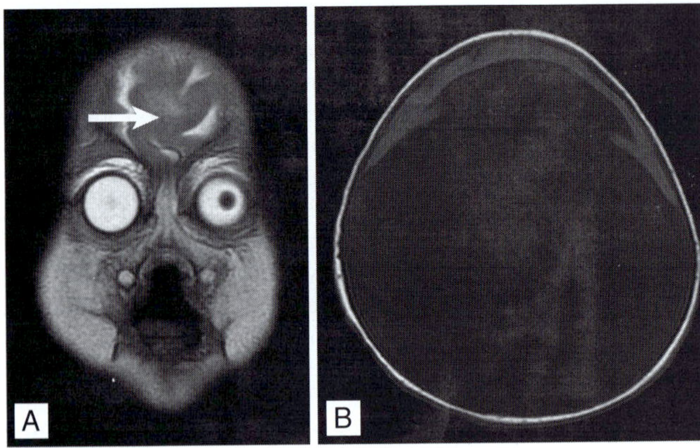

Figure 80.12 Holoprosencephaly. Coronal T2-weighted image (A) and axial T1-weighted image (B) demonstrate absent interhemispheric fissure (*arrow*) and fused frontal lobes in keeping with holoprosencephaly. A dilated monoventricle with a thin cortical mantle is present.

Holoprosencephaly (Fig. 80.12) is a complex craniocerebral and facial anomaly classified in grades of severity from alobar through semilobar to lobar, which is the least severe. It results from a failure of normal development of the forebrain (prosencephalon).

- The severe alobar form is incompatible with survival beyond infancy. The child has multiple craniofacial anomalies (cleft lip and palate, hypotelorism, anophthalmia, or cyclopia). Intracranially, the midline structures (falx, corpus callosum, septum pellucidum, and olfactory bulbs) are absent and the two hemispheres are replaced by a single large ventricle with a thin rim of cortical mantle. The thalami are fused, unlike hydranencephaly (Fig. 80.13), where they remain normal and the falx is present
- Semilobar holoprosencephaly (Fig. 80.14), the intermediate form, shows less severe facial deformity and the brain has a thicker mantle with recognizable occipital horns
- In the mildest (lobar) type there are well-formed lateral ventricles and a recognizable third ventricle, although the septum and Sylvian fissures are usually absent. The grosser forms may be suspected from the clinical appearance of the infant, but imaging is required in all varieties to delineate the intracranial anomalies

Heterotopias may be observed as an isolated phenomenon due to arrest of migrating neurons in the form of small masses of gray matter. They may form subependymal nodules protruding into the lateral ventricles similar to those seen in tuberous sclerosis or lie in the deep or subcortical white matter (Fig. 80.15). Gray matter heterotopias may be nodular or band-like.

White Matter Anomalies With Cortical Malformation

Hemimegalencephaly is a condition with unilateral enlargement of the skull. The asymmetrical skull is secondary to a congenital unilateral enlargement of the brain, and is associated with seizures, hemiplegia, and hemianopsia. There are migrational abnormalities with thickening of the gray matter and white matter with abnormal shallow sulci on the affected side (Figs. 80.16 and 80.17). The ventricle in the enlarged hemisphere is also enlarged.

Cobblestone lissencephaly, or cobblestone cortical malformation, is characterized by a nodular surface of the brain resembling a cobblestone street. The malformation is caused by defects

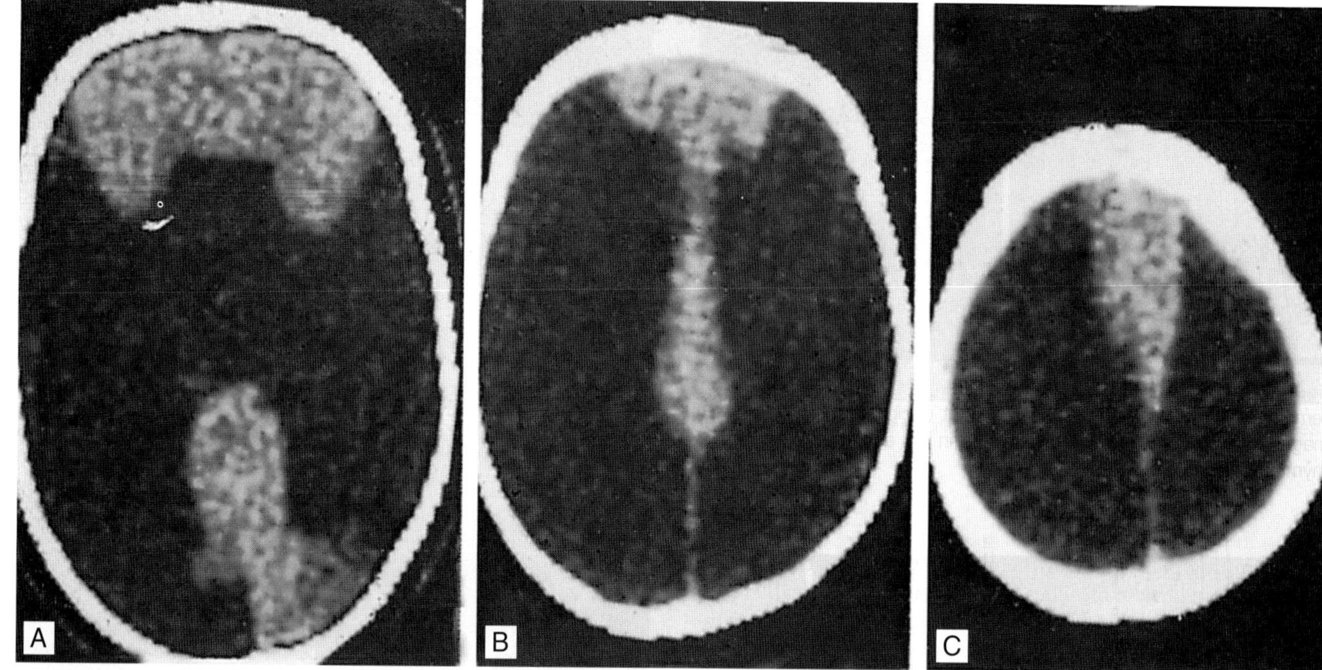

Figure 80.13 (A–C) Hydranencephaly.

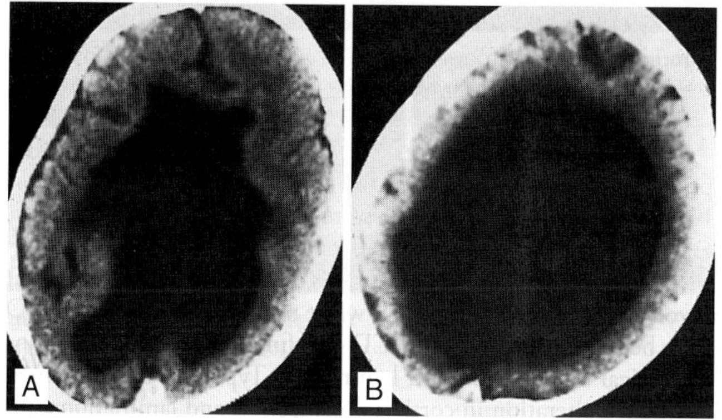

Figure 80.14 (A and B) Semilobar holoprosencephaly.

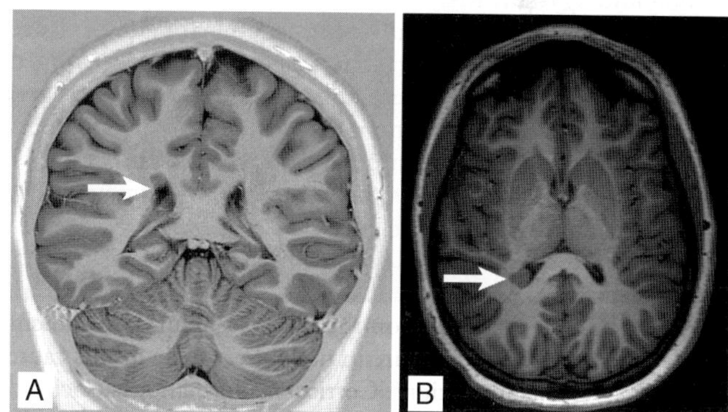

Figure 80.15 Heterotopia. Coronal T1 inversion recovery (A) and axial T1-weighted image (B) demonstrate a nodular focus of gray matter in the right parietal lobe, in keeping with a subependymal nodular gray matter heterotopia.

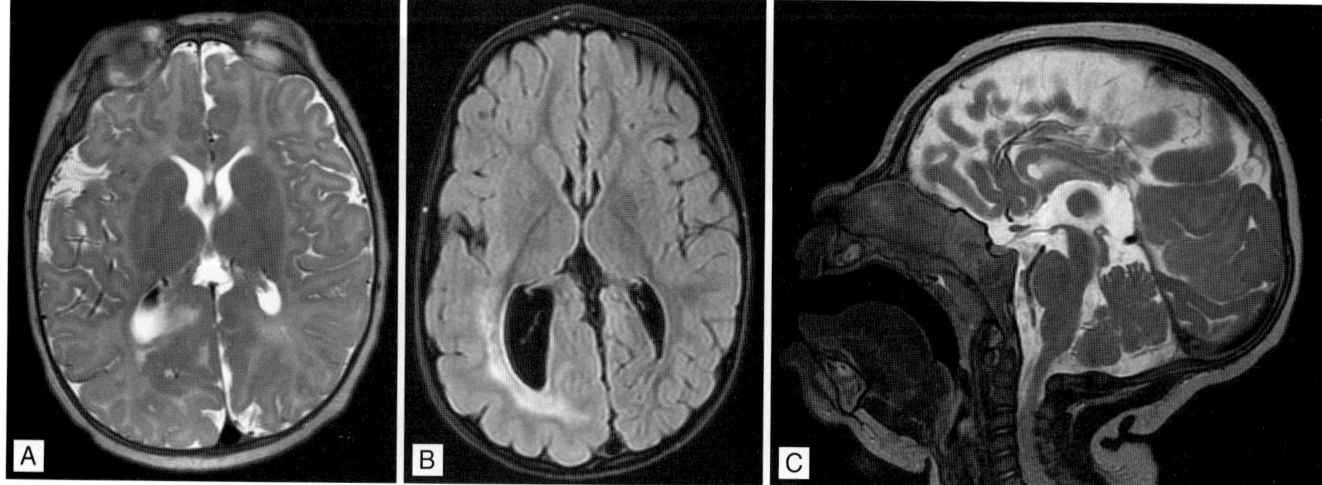

Figure 80.16 Hemimegalencephaly. Axial T2 (A), axial FLAIR (B), and sagittal T2 (C) images demonstrate an enlarged right occipital lobe with increased T2 signal in the periventricular white matter. The ventricle is enlarged in this affected area.

Evaluate the cerebellum and brainstem to look for signs of dysgenesis that can be associated with supratentorial malformations. For instance, rhombencephalosynapsis can be associated with other midline anomalies and a "Z-shaped" brainstem can be seen with dystroglycanopathies.

Indications for Surgical Referral

Hydrocephalus

Hydrocephalus is often associated with supratentorial brain malformations, often detected prenatally, and may require shunting.

Epilepsy Surgery

Patients with intractable epilepsy refractory to treatment and with focal, resectable lesions (such as FCD) often benefit from resection of the seizure focus. Conventional MR imaging can be coupled with diffusion-tensor imaging (DTI)/tractography and functional MRI to aid in surgical planning and attempt to avoid areas with eloquent functions such as language, vision, or motor areas.

Key Teaching Points

- There is a wide array of supratentorial brain malformations. These vary based on the timing of the insult during brain development
- The most common etiologies are genetic mutations and in utero infections
- MRI is the best imaging technique to evaluate for supratentorial brain malformations, preferably using volumetric 3D sequences
- Many malformations are detected on prenatal ultrasound studies, but others may be detected after birth when imaging is performed for seizures, atypical facies, abnormal head circumference, hypo/hypertonia, or developmental delay
- Brain malformations may be incidental findings when the brain is imaged for other reasons, such as head trauma. For example, asymptomatic callosal lipomas
- Pay close attention to the midline structures. If abnormal, look for other malformations as they are often associated

Congenital and Developmental Infratentorial Brain Anomalies

Congenital and developmental infratentorial lesions result from alteration in normal development of cerebellum and brainstem. Malformation, by definition, implies congenital anomaly of a single organ or body part caused by disruption of primary developmental program that is nonprogressive. MR imaging using both conventional and advanced techniques plays a pivotal role in delineating normal anatomy of posterior fossa and identifying and classifying malformations.

On the basis of neuroimaging pattern, malformations can be classified into:

1. Predominantly cerebellar malformations
2. Cerebellar and brainstem malformations
3. Predominantly brainstem malformations

Predominantly Cerebellar Malformations

Dandy–Walker Malformation

This results from more or less complete membranous obstruction to the foramina of Magendie and Luschka, which causes cystic dilatation of the fourth ventricle. There is hypoplasia or agenesis of cerebellar vermis, particularly the inferior portion, although superior portion may also be affected [16–18]. There is upward and counterclockwise rotation of hypoplastic vermis. The grossly dilated fourth ventricle extends upward to and above the tentorium and also backward to the occipital bone, which is thinned and bulging, expanding the posterior fossa. Cerebellar hemispheres are hypoplastic and displaced anterolaterally (Fig. 80.28). Most children present in infancy with symptoms of increased intracranial pressure consequent to hydrocephalus.

CT or MRI shows the anatomical features described and permits an immediate diagnosis. In the neonate or small infant, the diagnosis may be made by ultrasound. Differentials include other cystic posterior fossa malformations such as giant cisterna magna, posterior fossa arachnoid cyst, and Blake pouch cyst.

Mega Cisterna Magna

In this condition the cisterna magna appears abnormally large or dilated (>10 mm on midsagittal images) and the posterior fossa may be enlarged [18,19]. The fourth ventricle, cerebellum, and vermis, however, are seen to be normal. This is usually an incidental finding without any clinical relevance.

Posterior Fossa Arachnoid Cyst

Arachnoid cysts are usually unilocular, but septated cysts may occur. They may be retrocerebellar (located posterior or posteroinferior to vermis), supravermian (superior to vermis), anterior or lateral to hemispheres or brainstem. They can present in adults but more usually they present in infants or children, particularly if large enough to

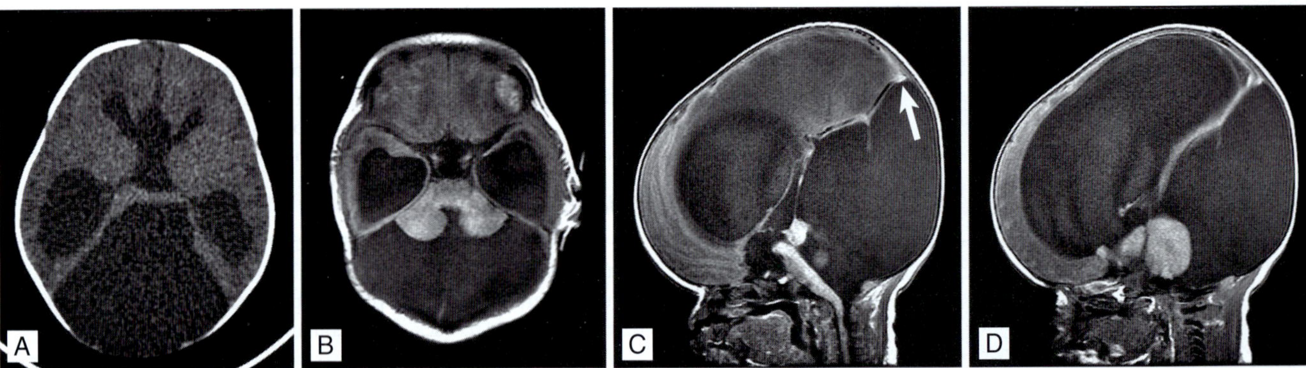

Figure 80.28 Dandy–Walker malformation. (A) CT scan and (B) T1 axial MR image shows large posterior fossa cyst in open communication with the fourth ventricle. (C) and (D) T1 Sagittal midline and a lateral image showing absent vermis and hypoplastic upturned hemispheres with elevation of torcular herophili (*arrow*) and large posterior fossa.

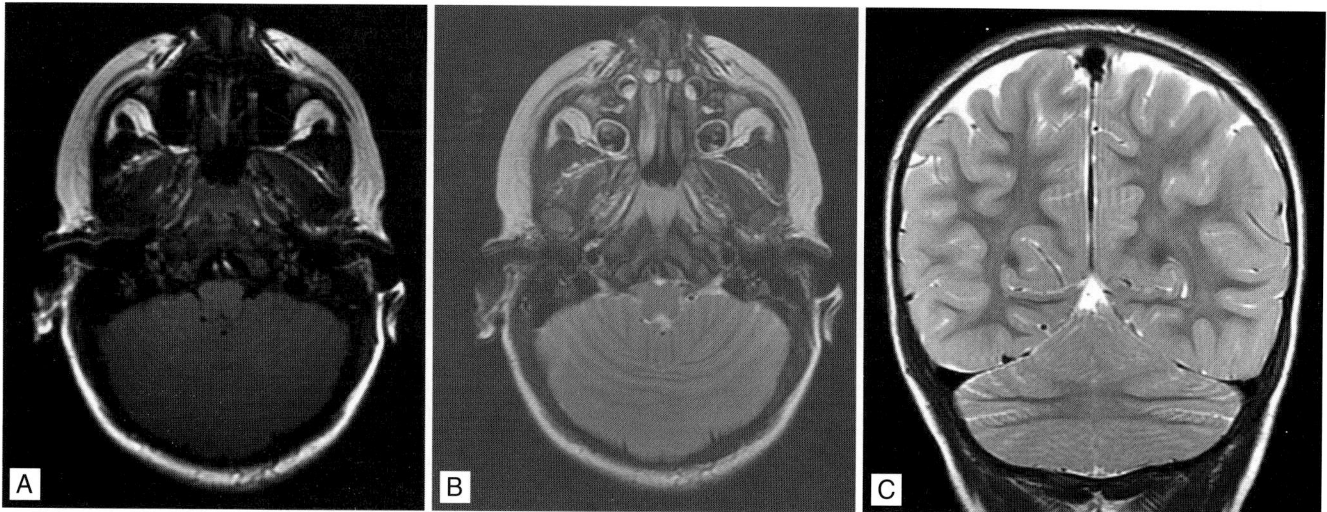

Figure 80.29 Rhombencephalosynapsis. (A) T1 axial and (B) T2 axial images showing continuation of cerebellar hemispheres across midline with the absence of vermis. (C) Coronal T2W image depicting the same finding.

produce a mass effect or obstructive hydrocephalus. On MRI, these are well-circumscribed extra-axial fluid collections following CSF on all pulse sequences. Lack of communication with ventricular system and subarachnoid spaces is characteristic [20,21].

Blake Pouch Cyst

This results from failure of regression of the Blake pouch due to nonfenestration of foramen of Magendie. Patients may be asymptomatic or show symptoms of raised intracranial pressure or macrocephaly. MRI reveals a retrocerebellar or infravermian cyst that represents a diverticulum of the fourth ventricle. It does not communicate with subarachnoid space and almost always results in tetraventricular hydrocephalus. Choroid plexus may curve under the vermis into the superior portion of the cyst, a characteristic feature, that can be seen best on sagittal T1 postcontrast MR images. Of note, the vermis is normally developed.

Rhombencephalosynapsis

This is believed to result from disruption in dorsoventral patterning in the rostral dorsal midline region of Rhombomere 1. The condition is sporadic with low recurrence risk. Clinical presentation is with truncal and/or limb ataxia, stereotypical head movements, and delayed motor development. Key findings on neuroimaging are agenesis/hypogenesis of vermis with continuous cerebellar hemispheres across midline. MRI shows horizontal folial pattern in the coronal images, whereas midline fusion of dentate nuclei and often superior cerebellar peduncles can be seen on axial and sagittal images (Fig. 80.29). The condition may be associated with hydrocephalus secondary to aqueductal stenosis and forebrain anomalies, such as absent septum pellucidum, dysgenetic corpus callosum, the absence of olfactory bulbs, and rarely holoprosencephaly.

Cerebellar and Brainstem Malformations

Pontocerebellar Hypoplasia

This is a diverse group of entities with characteristic findings of reduction in volume of both cerebellum and pons. There may be hypoplasia with superimposed atrophy of the cerebellum and significant reduction of pontine prominence (best appreciated on sagittal MR Images). Cerebellar cavitation (cysts) may be seen. Cerebellar hemispheric and vermian volume loss may be symmetric, but predominant hemispheric involvement with preserved vermis may result in a "dragonfly appearance." Ten subtypes with different phenotypes and pathogenesis have been described. Multiple genes including TSEN54, CASK (X-linked recessive inheritance), RELN, and VLDLR have been implicated in pathogenesis. Clinical presentation includes ataxia, nystagmus, microcephaly, cognitive impairment, seizures, deafness, retinopathy, and sometimes cataracts.

Alpha-Dystroglycanopathies

These refer to a group of congenital muscular dystrophies resulting from defective O-glycosylation, or rarely N-glycosylation of alpha-dystroglycan. Clinically, there is variable involvement of muscle (weakness, increased creatine kinase values), eye (microphthalmia, optic nerve hypoplasia, coloboma), and brain (seizures, intellectual impairment). Characteristic neuroimaging findings include pontocerebellar hypoplasia, cysts involving cerebellum, dysplasia of midbrain tectum, ventral cleft involving pons, and kinking of pontomesencephalic junction.

Tubulinopathies

These are a group of malformations resulting from mutations in genes encoding for microtubule formation and function. Posterior fossa involvement is in the form of pontocerebellar hypoplasia, dysplasia of the cerebellum, and midbrain tectum, with asymmetry of midbrain and pons. Cerebellar involvement is seen as diagonal folia seen on axial images, crossing the midline. Associated characteristic supratentorial imaging findings include dysmorphic basal ganglia with the absence of anterior limb of internal capsule, lissencephaly, and PMG. Clinical manifestations are wide including intellectual disability, cerebral palsy, microcephaly, and intractable seizures.

Joubert Syndrome

This is a malformation with classical imaging findings described as "molar-tooth" configuration of superior cerebellar peduncles that are thick, elongated, and horizontally oriented along with a deep interpeduncular fossa. It is consistently associated with hypoplasia and dysplasia of vermis. The fourth ventricle appears large and triangular with the apex pointing backward at its midportion, and

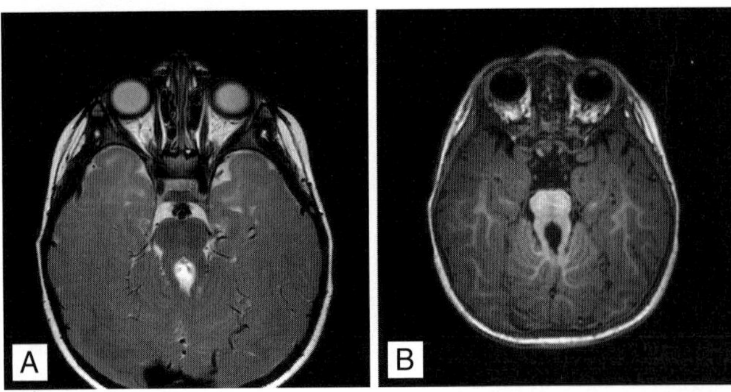

Figure 80.30 Joubert syndrome. (A) Axial T2W and axial T1W (B) images at the level of superior cerebellar peduncles demonstrating "molar-tooth" appearance.

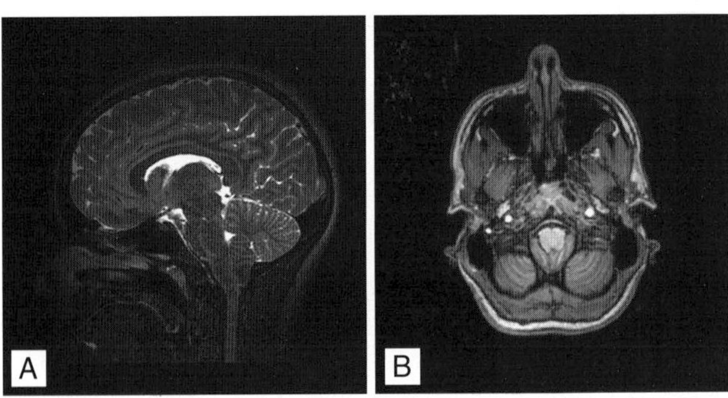

Figure 80.31 Chiari 1 malformation. (A) Sagittal T2 image showing tonsillar herniation below the foramen magnum. Axial T1W image (B) shows crowding at the level of foramen magnum.

large and "bat's wing" at a higher level (Fig. 80.30). Up to one-third of affected individuals may have supratentorial involvement in the form of callosal dysgenesis, hippocampal malrotation, cephaloceles, and ventriculomegaly. DTI and tractography may reveal the absence of decussation of superior cerebellar peduncle and corticospinal tracts. This condition is characterized clinically by ataxia, mental retardation, episodic hyperpnoea, and abnormal eye movements, and is due to total aplasia of the cerebellar vermis.

Predominant Brainstem Malformations

Pontine Tegmental Cap Dysplasia

This is a rare sporadic brainstem malformation with pathognomic conventional neuroimaging findings including flattening of ventral pons, "cap"-like vaulted pontine tegmentum, partial absent middle and inferior cerebellar peduncles, hypoplastic vermis, and molar-tooth configuration of pontomesencephalic junction along with the absence of inferior olivary prominence. Associations include duplicated internal auditory canals and hypoplastic cranial nerves. Clinical presentation is with hearing loss, facial paralysis, difficulty in swallowing, anesthesia in trigeminal nerve distribution and ataxia. Intellectual prognosis appears to correlate with imaging findings: mildly affected individuals have a rounded "cap"-like configuration of tectum while more severe developmental disability is seen with more angular "beak"-like brainstem protrusion.

Horizontal Gaze Palsy With Progressive Scoliosis

This is a rare disorder caused by mutation in ROBO3 gene with autosomal recessive inheritance. Pathognomic neuroimaging findings include butterfly-shaped medulla (due to the absence of gracile and cuneate nuclei prominence), and inferior olivary prominence. There is associated hypoplasia of pons with a dorsal midline cleft.

Brainstem Disconnection

Rostral and caudal brainstem segments in this abnormality are connected only by a thin cord of the tissue. Characteristic imaging findings are appreciated on sagittal images and supratentorial abnormalities are unusual. Clinical presentation is absent or weak suck and swallow at birth, central respiratory insufficiency, poor visual fixation, and hypo/hypertonia.

Chiari Malformations

These were originally described by Chiari in 1891 and 1896, and were graded types 1–4 according to degree of deformity.

Chiari Type 1: This is the least obvious clinically and may not be diagnosed until adult life. It consists of tonsillar herniation through the foramen magnum with or without varying degrees of elongation of the medulla oblongata and fourth ventricle (Fig. 80.31). There is associated crowding at the level of foramen magnum with paucity of CSF flow craniocaudally across the cervicomedullary junction, that can be assessed using cine flow MRI technique. Syringohydromyelia is associated with the condition in up to 70% of cases. The patients do not present clinically until adult life when the symptoms and signs of syringohydromyelia develop; less typically, symptoms suggesting involvement of the lower cranial or cervical nerves are seen, and very rarely patients present with hydrocephalus. Bony anomalies of the craniovertebral junction can be present, particularly assimilation of the atlas. Basilar invagination and dysplasias of the vault are other rare associations.

The diagnosis is best confirmed by MRI, which also shows the syrinx. Caution is required when interpreting sagittal images of the craniovertebral junction as partial volume effects result in visualization of 3–4 mm of cerebellar tissue apparently lying below the foramen magnum in 15–20% of normal individuals [21]. Coronal imaging is helpful in equivocal cases. Differential consideration is tonsillar descent in cases of intracranial hypotension.

Chiari Type 2: This presents in neonates or infants, virtually always with a thoracolumbar myelomeningocele. The associated brain deformities consist of caudal herniation of the medulla and vermis with a caudally displaced and elongated fourth ventricle, a small posterior fossa and low-lying torcula. A backward kink may be seen at the caudally displaced junction of cervical cord and medulla. Hydrocephalus may be due to associated aqueduct stenosis or to occlusion of the ambient cisterns. Associated malformations include hypoplasia or the absence of the falx and tentorium with interdigitation of the cerebral hemispheres; absence of the corpus callosum with forward pointing of the frontal horns; beaked tectum, medullar spur and kink, enlargement of the cerebellar vermis, and forward protrusion of the cerebellar hemispheres as pointed projections around the brainstem; gyral malformations, and other lesions. Many of these brain deformities can be identified by CT or MRI, and some by neonatal ultrasound. Skull x-ray may show a lacunar skull and forward bowing of the petrous bones and clivus.

Chiari Types 3 and 4 have major deformities with cerebellar hypoplasia and downward displacement of the brainstem and a high cervical or occipital encephalocele.

Imaging Techniques and Analysis

MR imaging on midline sag T1WI and T2WI is ideal for the evaluation of posterior fossa size, shape and size of vermis, morphology and size of the fourth ventricle and brainstem. The craniocaudal length of pons is roughly twice that of midbrain (third ventricle to ventral midbrain-pons junction) and medulla (obex to ventral pontomedullary junction). Parasagittal images provide good visualization of hemispheres and peduncles, whereas axial images are best for evaluating vermian morphology and size, dentate nuclei and superior and middle cerebellar peduncles. Coronal images show radiating folia and also help in the assessment of size, symmetry and contour of cerebellar peduncles.

Advanced imaging techniques such as DTI may provide detailed information on white matter tracts noninvasively in children with posterior fossa malformations. This has allowed clinicians to delve into depths of pathogenesis of certain posterior fossa malformations such as Joubert syndrome and pontine tegmental cap dysplasia.

Key Teaching Points

- The diagnosis of posterior fossa malformations as well as classification is based on neuroimaging findings
- MRI is the best technique for evaluation of posterior fossa and multiplanar evaluation on conventional sequences may help identify malformations
- Well-defined criteria for the diagnosis and classification are available for various malformations and should be used
- Advanced techniques such as DTI and tractography may provide additional information in understanding pathogenesis of cerebellar and brainstem malformations

Pediatric Brain Tumors

Introduction

Primary brain tumors constitute about one-third of all neoplasms in the pediatric population [22]. Neoplasms of the CNS are the most common type of solid tumors in children in the age group 0–19 years. The overall incidence of primary CNS tumors in the United States is approximately 6 per 100,000 across all pediatric age groups. The age groups 0–4 and 15–19 years show maximum incidence of primary CNS tumors within the pediatric population [2].

Approach to an Intracranial Mass

The fundamental imaging approach to a mass in the central neural axis is essentially similar in both adults and pediatric patients. Spatial localization of any intracranial mass and its relation to surrounding anatomical structures is the first key step in further characterization of a mass in the intracranial compartment. The determination of whether the mass is in intra-axial or extra-axial (extraparenchymal) location should be the first objective of any radiologist in such a scenario. The definitive imaging findings that point to extra-axial location of a mass are elucidated in Table 80.2.

The incidence of extra-axial lesions or masses in pediatric population is much lower than adults. The localization of a mass or lesion to extra-axial compartment in a pediatric patient considerably narrows the differential diagnosis. The characterization of an intraparenchymal mass in a child can be aided by precise anatomical location of the mass and age of the patient in combination with imaging appearance of the mass. The commonest site of an intra-axial primary CNS tumor in the pediatric age group is cerebellum. The commonest extra-axial location is pituitary region [23].

TABLE 80.2 High Yield Imaging Signs That Aid in Localization of an Extra-axial Mass

- Cerebrospinal fluid strip between the mass and the brain parenchyma, may be seen as dark cleft on the fluid-attenuated inversion recovery (FLAIR) imaging.
- Vascular structures interposed between the brain and mass, identified as flow voids on spin echo sequences.
- The presence of cortical mantle between the mass and underlying brain parenchyma especially white matter.

Adapted from: SW Atlas, ed. Magnetic Resonance Imaging of the Brain and Spine, fourth ed., Vol. 1 and 2, Lippincott Williams & Wilkins, 2008.

World Health Organization 2016 Classification of Tumors of Central Nervous System

The concept of tumor pathogenesis driven by genetic makeup of the neoplastic cell has been well known in the literature. For the first time since the introduction of World Health Organization (WHO) CNS tumor classification system, this concept was incorporated into the 2016 WHO classification of CNS tumors. The classification thus recommended use of molecular characteristics, in addition to histologic features of tumor tissue, to define CNS tumor entities. The aim is to create a classification system with homogeneous and sharply defined groups or subgroups. The classification introduced the term "integrated" diagnosis for CNS tumors based on a combination of both phenotypic and genotypic information. The classification also recommended deletion of certain nomenclature including primitive neuroectodermal tumor, gliomatosis cerebri, protoplasmic and fibrillary astrocytoma, and cellular ependymoma. Importantly, the classification does not recommend exclusive use of genetic information for definition of CNS tumor entities [24]. Expectedly, the 2016 classification led to the creation of loosely defined category of tumors, with designation not otherwise specified, that did not meet the narrow criteria prescribed in the new classification [24].

Consortium to inform molecular and practical approaches to CNS tumor taxonomy (cIMPACT-NOW or cIMPACT) updates: After the release of WHO 2016 CNS tumor classification, a group of expert neuropathologists and oncologists set up a formal working group, outside the realm of WHO. The aim of the group was to recommend updates and changes to CNS tumor classification in the time interval between WHO classification updates [25]. The cIMPACT updates that specifically apply to CNS tumors in the pediatric population are summarized in Table 80.3.

Gliomas

Gliomas represent the most common type of pediatric brain tumors. Based on clinicopathologic characteristics and long-term prognosis, these are classified into two broad categories—low-grade glioma and high-grade glioma [30]. High-grade gliomas in children show a higher rate and varied spectrum of mutations compared with low-grade gliomas [9]. Low-grade gliomas represent about 30% of all pediatric CNS tumors [30]. Common pathological subtypes of this group are detailed in Table 80.4.

TABLE 80.3 Summary of cIMPACT Updates as Applicable to Pediatric CNS Tumors

Update	Proposed Update
1	Use of the term NEC (not elsewhere classified) when the available pathologic information (molecular or histologic) is NOT enough to assign a specific WHO diagnosis. Not otherwise specified (NOS) term should be used exclusively when required pathologic information to assign a specific WHO diagnosis is NOT available. For example, embryonal tumor with multilayered rosettes that shows the absence of C19MC alteration on testing should be designated as ETMR, NEC [25]
2	The diagnostic entity *diffuse midline glioma, H3 K27M-mutant* diagnosis must be exclusively used for a CNS tumor that involves midline structures, is diffuse or infiltrating in appearance, a glioma, and positive for H3 K27M-mutation. Even though the H3 K27M-mutation is not exclusive to *diffuse midline glioma, H3 K27M-mutant* CNS tumor; however, this nomenclature should NOT be used for other pediatric tumors (pilocytic astrocytomas, diffuse astrocytomas, and gangliogliomas) that may sometimes bear H3 K27M-mutation such as [26]
4	Delineation of molecular alterations that can be used for further classification of IDH-wild type H3-wild type WHO grade II diffuse pediatric gliomas, with emphasis on integrated diagnosis. This would involve analysis of tumors for alterations in the BRAFV600E, MYB, or MYBL1, FGFR1 genes and/or genes resulting in activation of MAPK pathway [27]
5	Introduction of newly recognized CNS tumor diagnostic entities in pediatric population including CNS neuroblastoma, FOXR2-activated; Diffuse glioma, H3.3 G34-mutant, polymorphous low-grade neuroepithelial tumor of the young. Introduction of key principles related to CNS tumor classification, nomenclature, and grading, for example proposed classification for pediatric-type glial/glioneuronal tumors [28]
6	Molecular or genetic criteria used for the classification of supratentorial, posterior fossa, and spinal cord ependymomas and their clinical implications. For example, MYCN amplified spinal cord ependymomas is a distinctive subgroup with a poor outcome [29]

TABLE 80.4 Common Pathologic Subtypes of Pediatric Low-Grade Gliomas

- Pilocytic astrocytoma
- Ganglioglioma
- Pleomorphic xanthoastrocytoma
- Dysembryoplastic neuroepithelial tumor
- Diffuse astrocytoma (angiocentric type)

TABLE 80.5 Clinicopathologic Differences Between Pediatric and Adult Low-Grade Gliomas

Pediatric	Adult
Lower frequency of mutations	Higher mutation burden
Mutation profile is limited	Wide spectrum of mutation such as frequent IDH1 mutation and 1p/19q codeletion
Risk of malignant transformation is low	Risk of transformation to high-grade glioma higher

The most common molecular defect in pediatric low-grade gliomas is BRAF proto-oncogene mutation, either a BRAF V600E point mutation or *BRAF* fusion (*KIAA1549:BRAF* fusion). The common end result of these mutations is dysregulation of MAPK pathway [30]. The major differences between pediatric and adult low-grade gliomas are detailed in Table 80.5.

Pilocytic astrocytoma is the most common type of low-grade glioma reported in children. The most frequent site of involvement is the cerebellum and hypothalamus-chiasm followed by supratentorial structures. *The typical appearance is a circumscribed complex solid cystic mass with enhancing solid component* (Fig. 80.32). Usually, pilocytic astrocytoma in the hypothalamus-chiasm region present as predominantly solid,

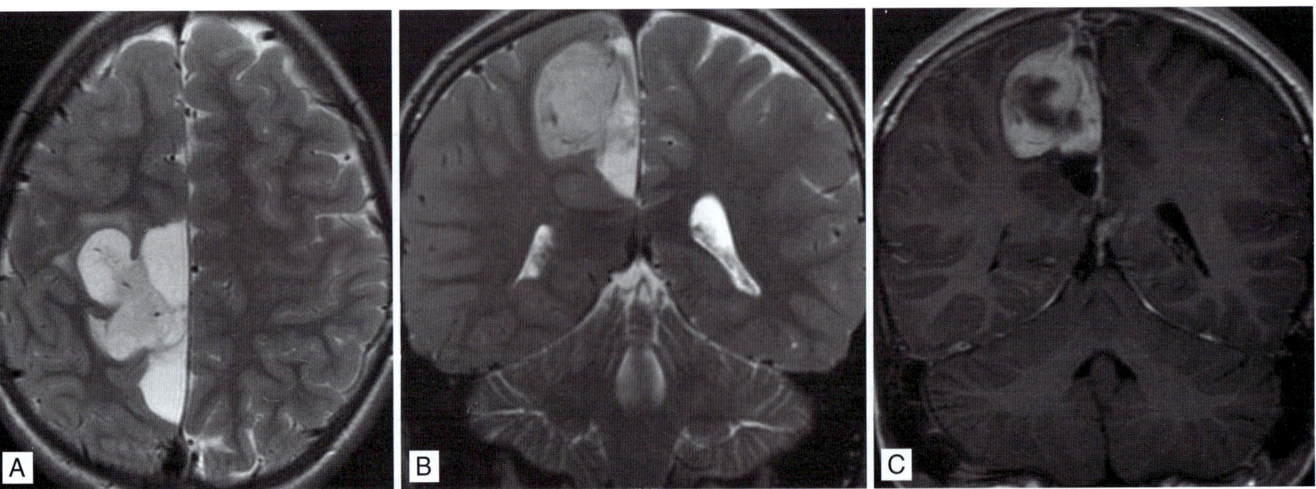

Figure 80.32 A 11-year-old male complained of left side weakness. Axial (A) and coronal T2 magnetic resonance (MR) image (B) demonstrated a large circumscribed solid cystic mass centered in paramedian frontal lobe. Coronal contrast-enhanced MR image (C) showed intense enhancement of solid component with internal areas of necrosis. This was later confirmed as pilocytic astrocytoma on histopathology.

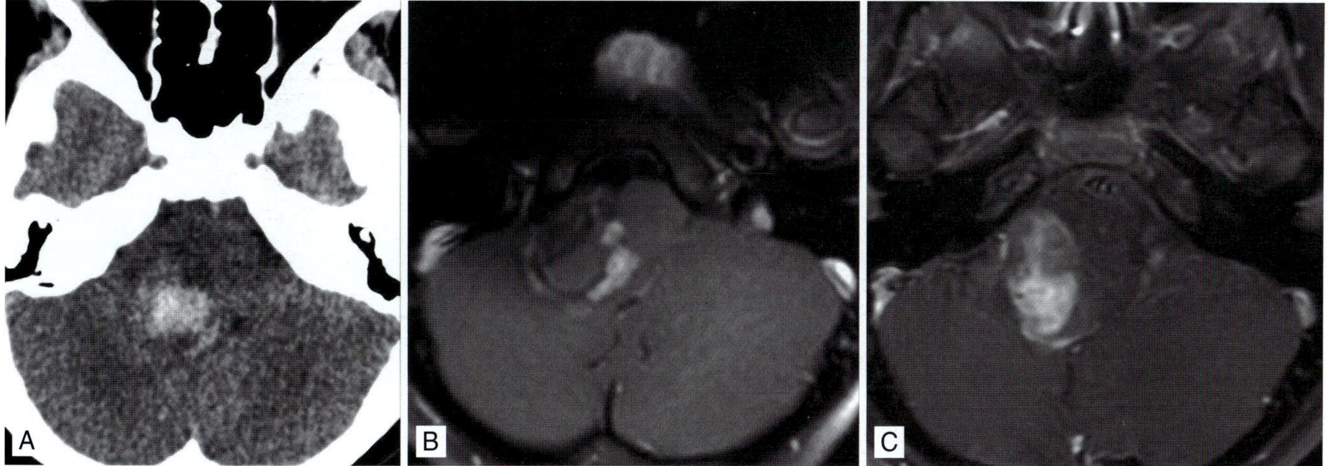

Figure 80.33 A 9-year-old female presented with severe headache and vomiting. Nonenhanced axial computed tomography image (A) showed focus of hemorrhage in right cerebellar hemisphere at the level of inferior cerebellar peduncle. Axial contrast-enhanced MR image (B) demonstrated a mass-like lesion with suspicious peripheral nodular enhancement. Follow-up axial contrast-enhanced MR image at 9 months (C) clearly revealed a mass lesion with significant contrast enhancement. Histopathological examination confirmed pilocytic astrocytoma.

TABLE 80.6 Atypical Imaging Features of Pilocytic Astrocytoma [33,34]

- Complex solid cystic mass, with significant internal necrosis within the solid component.
- Predominantly solid appearing mass with minimal or no cystic areas.
- The presence of calcification and hemorrhage (alternative entities should be considered).
- In some series up to half of PAs may present as infiltrative solid masses on imaging making distinction from high-grade gliomas challenging.

less sharply defined infiltrative mass with minimal to no contrast enhancement. Infrequently, pilocytic astrocytoma can have imaging features which may be mistaken for aggressive brain tumors (Fig. 80.33). These are detailed in Table 80.6 [31,32].

Diffusion-weighted imaging is critical in differentiating low-grade gliomas from other aggressive neoplasms. The ADC is uniformly high in all pilocytic astrocytoma correlating with large volume of extracellular matrix [31,32,35].

MR spectroscopy and perfusion MRI should be utilized cautiously in pilocytic astrocytoma. The data for pilocytic astrocytoma from these advanced imaging tools must be correlated with conventional imaging features [31,32]. The differential diagnostic entities for pilocytic astrocytoma are elucidated in Table 80.7.

Focal well-circumscribed gliomas based in the brainstem gliomas are usually low-grade gliomas. These are typically centered in the dorsal or dorsolateral brainstem with relative sparing of ventral such as tectal glioma (Fig. 80.35), posterior cervicomedullary pilocytic astrocytoma. They can show unusual exophytic growth pattern [32,36].

Ho et al. analyzed TSITC data from DSC perfusion in pediatric brain tumors reporting high positive predictive value of T1 dominant leakage pattern (continuing above baseline or high percent signal recovery pattern) for low-grade gliomas specifically pilocytic astrocytoma [22].

The oligodendroglioma entity in children is unique since these frequently show lack of IDH mutation and 1p/19q codeletion. This is unlike adults where IDH mutation and 1p/19q deletion form the basis for the diagnosis of oligodendroglioma [38].

TABLE 80.7 Differential Considerations for Pilocytic Astrocytoma [31,32]

Entity	Features
1. Pilomyxoid astrocytoma (WHO grade II) (Fig. 80.34)	▪ Chiasmatic hypothalamic region ▪ Solid and more infiltrative appearance ▪ Higher incidence of intratumoral hemorrhage, local recurrence, and CSF dissemination ▪ Relative homogenous contrast enhancement
2. Ganglioglioma or pleomorphic xanthoastrocytoma	▪ Suspected supratentorial pilocytic astrocytoma with intratumoral calcification or hemorrhage ▪ Absence of meningeal involvement
3. Hemangioblastoma	▪ Older child or teenager with cystic cerebellar mass ▪ Prominent flow voids ▪ Significantly high rCBV values on perfusion MRI
4. Medulloblastoma, ATRT, or ependymoma	▪ Suspected infratentorial pilocytic astrocytoma with intratumoral calcification or hemorrhage ▪ Age of child

Recent literature has shown that the frequency of surveillance imaging and overall duration of surveillance in cerebellar grade 1 astrocytomas can be reduced if complete resection can be achieved. Importantly the data for noncerebellar tumors were considered inadequate and authors suggested continuing with practice of 6 monthly follow-up imaging in this group [39]. When gross total resection of a pilocytic astrocytoma is not achieved, surveillance imaging has been recommended at defined intervals such as 6, 12, or 24 months. On follow-up imaging PAs may show spontaneous fluctuations in contrast enhancement in the absence of any recent therapy. In the absence of corresponding change in tumor dimensions, these random findings are not favored to represent tumor progression or regression [32]. Malignant transformation of a pilocytic astrocytoma is a very rare event

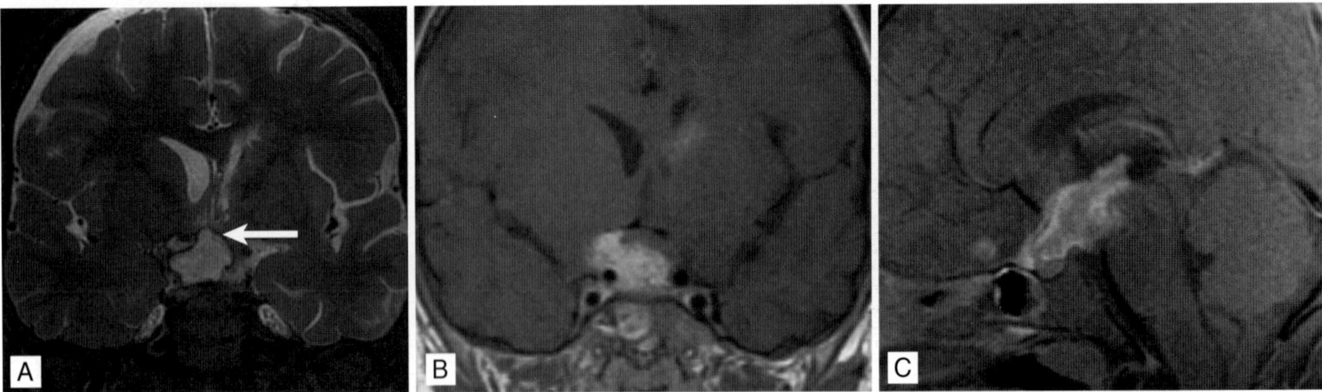

Figure 80.34 A 6-year-old male presented with severe headache, emesis, and altered mental status. Coronal T2 MR image (A) showed an irregular T2 hyperintense mass centered in suprasellar cistern and hypothalamic-chiasmatic region. Note the low signal along tumor periphery representing blood products (*white arrow*). Contrast-enhanced coronal and sagittal MR images demonstrated heterogeneous enhancement of the mass (B and C). Histopathologically proved case of pilomyxoid astrocytoma.

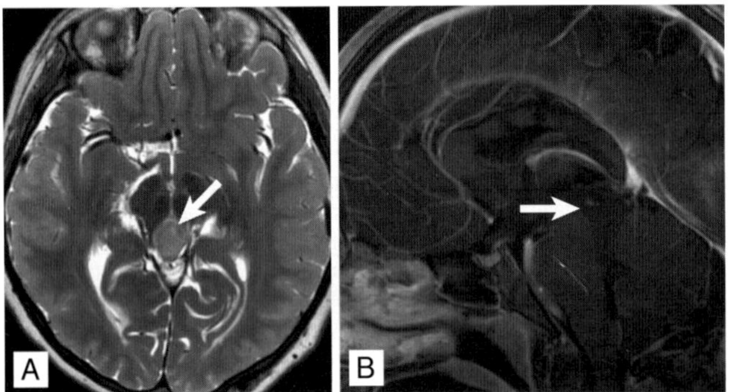

Figure 80.35 A 2-year-old male with increasing head circumference. Axial T2 MR image (A) showed partly exophytic mild T2 hyperintense expansile mass involving dorsal mid brain (*white arrow*). The mass protrudes into the quadrigeminal cistern. On contrast-enhanced sagittal MR image mass showed minimal to absent contrast enhancement (*white arrow* in B). Histopathologically proved low-grade glioma.

with few reported cases [34]. Dissemination of PA to other CNS sites is extremely rare with less than 100 reported cases in English language literature (Fig. 80.36) [39,35]. None of the documented patients demonstrated malignant transformation of the primary site. It is not clear if the dissemination leads to increased mortality. The most common associated risk factor reported in these patients is subtotal resection with residual tumor in the operative bed and location of primary tumor site close to CSF [39].

High-grade gliomas constitute about 15% of pediatric CNS tumors. The most common site of involvement is brainstem. This is in contradistinction to adults where most high-grade gliomas are seen in the supratentorial space [30,37]. WHO 2016 classification introduced a new entity diffuse midline glioma, a grade IV tumor (Fig. 80.37). The diagnosis is based on K27M mutation in H3 histone gene, irrespective of histopathology. The classification includes diffuse intrinsic pontine glioma as a subtype of diffuse midline gliomas, H3K27M mutant. About 60–80% of DIPG show this mutation [37]. Somatic mutations in histone gene

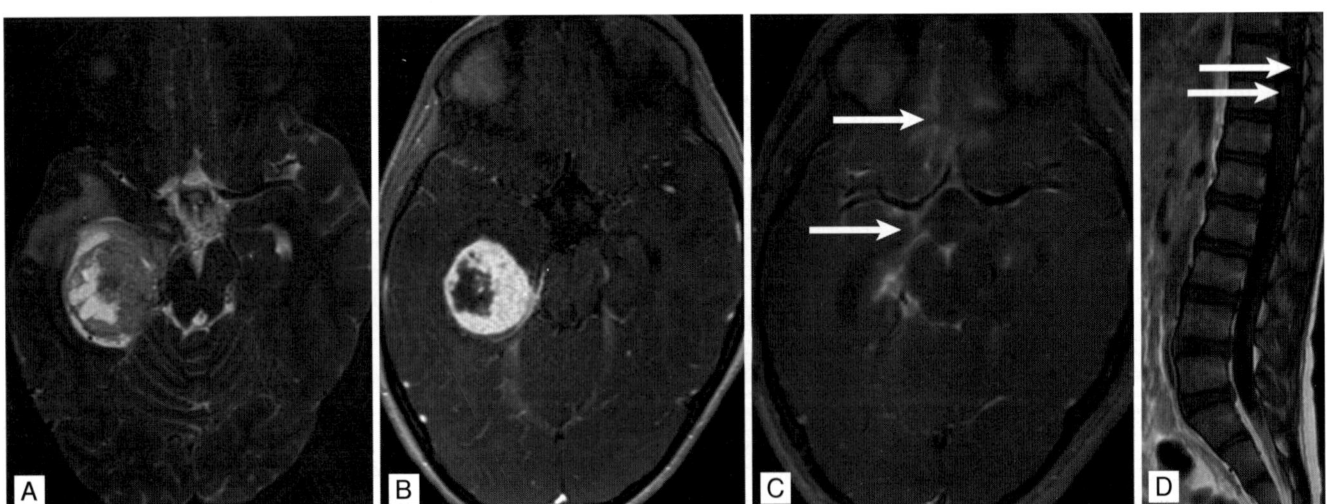

Figure 80.36 A 7-year-old male presented with seizures and vomiting. Axial T2 MR image showed a large heterogenous mass based in temporal region (A) with intense enhancement of solid component on axial contrast-enhanced MR image (B). Follow-up imaging 6 years later, contrast-enhanced axial MR image of brain and contrast-enhanced sagittal lumbar spine MR image (C and D) showed evidence of leptomeningeal metastatic dissemination (*white arrows*). The primary intracranial mass was a proved pilocytic astrocytoma on histopathology.

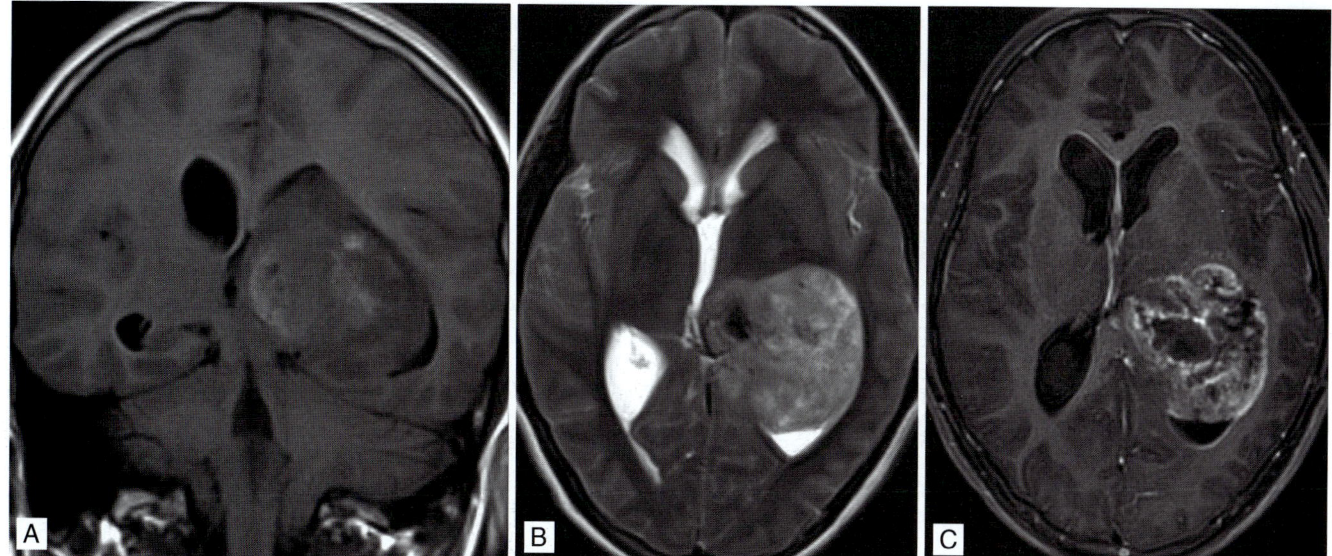

Figure 80.37 A 14-year old with headache, paresthesia, and vomiting. Coronal T1 MR image (A) showed a large heterogenous mass filling the left lateral ventricle. Axial T2 MR image (B) delineated the exophytic nature of mass originating from paramedian basal ganglia structures. Note the T2 hypointense focus representing blood product or calcification. Axial contrast-enhanced MR image (C) showed very heterogenous enhancement of the mass with numerous internal areas of necrosis. Histopathologic examination and molecular analysis confirmed high-grade glioma with H3K27M mutation.

complex are highly specific genetic alterations reported in pediatric high-grade gliomas. The most common types are K27M and G34R/V mutations in histone 3 variants with downstream consequence of dysregulation of glial differentiation [30,40].

Diffuse intrinsic pontine glioma is based in ventral pons with expansion and infiltration into adjacent structures like midbrain, medulla, brachium pontis. Contrast enhancement is minimal to none in most cases. Exophytic component in anterolateral aspect may be associated with basilar artery encasement. No significant differences in imaging feature have been reported between H3K27M mutant and wild type diffuse midline gliomas. Atypical imaging findings of heterogenous contrast enhancement with areas of necrosis and CSF spread to distant sites have been reported [40]. Noncontiguous involvement of supratentorial structures has also been reported. This may mimic gliomatosis on imaging [37]. Diffuse intrinsic pontine glioma is currently an imaging diagnosis with rare use of biopsy for histopathological proof except under clinical trial protocols [41]. Imaging findings may be used for guiding prognosis as mentioned in Table 80.8.

Embryonal Tumors

Medulloblastoma

Medulloblastoma is the most common primary CNS malignancy affecting pediatric population. The age group most affected is between 3 and 7 years of age. Medulloblastoma accounts for about 65% of all pediatric embryonal tumors [30,43,44].

In young children with medulloblastoma presence of falcine/tentorial calcification at an early age (specifically <3 years) should raise concern for underlying basal cell nevus (Gorlin) syndrome. Overall, less than 5% of medulloblastoma patients have underlying Gorlin syndrome. The inherent sensitivity of these patients to radiation makes it important to identify [43–45]. MRI surveillance is recommended for family members of children with medulloblastoma with extensive nodularity and desmoplastic/nodular subtypes of medulloblastoma (strong association with basal cell nevus syndrome) [43,44]. Table 80.9 details the differences between childhood and adult medulloblastomas.

Summary of WHO 2016 classification of CNS embryonal tumors is presented in Table 80.10.

The anatomic location and spatial relation (to surrounding structures) information of a medulloblastoma on imaging can be predictive of the medulloblastoma molecular subtype.

Wingless and Int-1 (WNT) type is the least common molecular subtype of medulloblastoma. The associated gene defect is an activating mutation in catenin beta 1 (CTNNB1) gene [43]. These tumors are characteristically centered in the paramedian posterior fossa (Fig. 80.38), away from vermis, either in the foramen of Luschka (lateral recess) or cerebellopontine angle cistern.

TABLE 80.8 Imaging Features With Prognostic Significance in Diffuse Intrinsic Pontine Glioma [42]

Increased Progression-Free Survival and Overall Survival	Reduced Progression-Free Survival and Overall Survival
Reduction in tumor volume by at least 25% compared with preradiotherapy imaging	The presence of enhancement within mass at baseline Progressive increase in enhancement on follow-up imaging

TABLE 80.9 Differences in Clinical Characteristics of Medulloblastoma Between Pediatric and Adult Patients [30,43,44]

Pediatric	Adults
Peak incidence 3–7 years	Less common; 20–40 years
Cerebellar vermis is the most common site (75% of pediatric medulloblastomas)	Cerebellar hemisphere is the commonest site (70% of adult medulloblastomas)
Well-defined enhancing mass; cystic changes less common	Ill-defined mass with frequent cystic changes

TABLE 80.10 WHO 2016 Classification of Central Nervous System (CNS) Embryonal Tumors [16,22]

Medulloblastoma, genetically defined Wingless and Int-1 (WNT)-activated Sonic hedgehog (SHH)-activated and TP53-mutant SHH-activated and TP53 wild-type Non-WNT/non-SHH (group 3 and group 4)	Medulloblastoma, histologically defined Classic Desmoplastic/nodular With extensive nodularity Large cell/anaplastic Medulloblastoma, not otherwise specified (NOS)
Atypical teratoid/rhabdoid tumor, genetically defined	
Embryonal tumor with multilayered rosettes (ETMR) or CNS primitive neuroectodermal tumor (PNET), genetically defined (previously ependymoblastoma (EBL), or embryonal tumor with abundant neuropil and true rosettes [ETANTR])	
CNS embryonal tumor, NOS (previously CNS PNET, **not** genetically defined including medulloepithelioma/CNS neuroblastoma/CNS ganglioneuroblastoma)	

The tumors may show variable extension to the fourth ventricle, foramen magnum or the foramen of Magendie [46–48]. A majority of these tumors reveal intratumoral blood degradation products [47,49]. Rarely, the tumor may associated with Turcot syndrome [43]. The clinical and pathological characteristics are detailed in Table 80.11.

Sonic hedgehog medulloblastoma is associated with inactivating gene mutations in PTCHD1 [patched-1] gene and SUFU gene and/or amplification of gene MYCN and GLI gene.

TABLE 80.11 Clinicopathologic Characteristics of Wingless and Int-1 (WNT) Type Medulloblastoma [43]

Gender	Female > male
Age	Children >3 years
Spatial location	Dorsolateral brainstem, level of middle cerebellar peduncle or fourth ventricle or inferior [46]
Histopathology	Classic [37]
Cerebrospinal fluid dissemination	Extremely rare
Prognosis	Excellent [30,40]. The presence of metastatic disease does not change the favorable outcome [30]

These are typically centered in the cerebellar cortex (Fig. 80.39). The tumors involving flocculus and nodulus may present as a mass in the cerebellopontine angle and fourth ventricle, respectively. Uncommonly this subtype may also present as multifocal cerebellar cortical nodules or masses (Fig. 80.40). The involvement of the midline structures such as vermis is highly uncommon, except in the first year of life [37,46,48]. Intense contrast enhancement is a characteristic imaging feature of vast majority of sonic hedgehog medulloblastomas [48,49]. These tumors may be associated with nevoid basal cell carcinoma syndrome [30]. The clinical and pathological characteristics are detailed in Table 80.12.

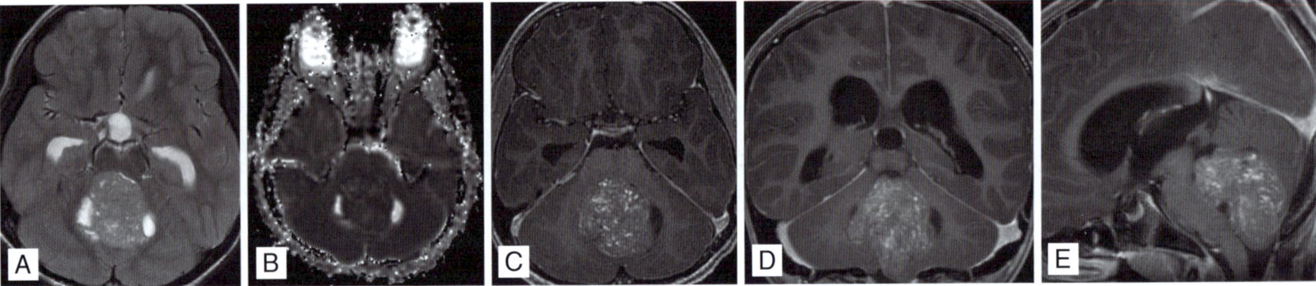

Figure 80.38 An 8-year-old female with headache and vomiting. Axial T2 MR image (A) showed a heterogenous relatively defined solid mass centered in the fourth ventricle near midline. ADC showed reduced values of the mass (B). Axial contrast-enhanced MR image (C) showed significant enhancement of the mass. Note the mass reaches up to foramen magnum with proximal hydrocephalus on coronal and sagittal contrast-enhanced MR images (D and E). Histopathologic examination confirmed WNT type medulloblastoma.

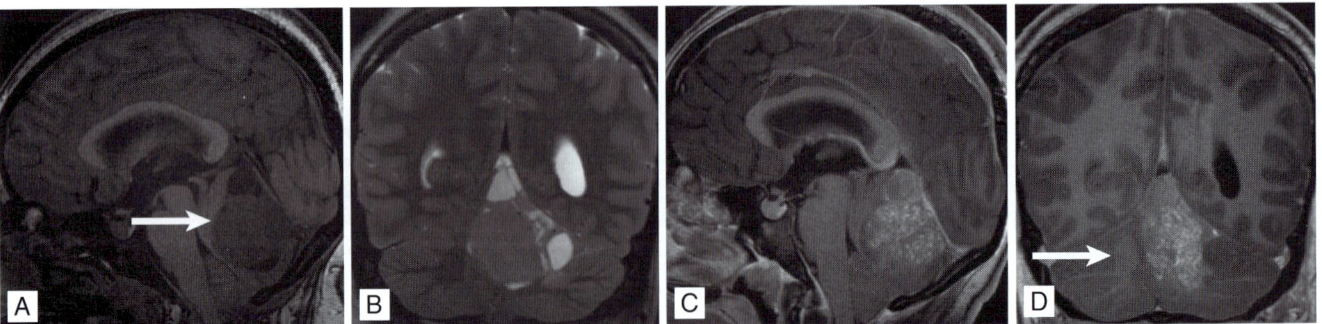

Figure 80.39 A 17-year-old female with vomiting and headache. Axial T1 (A) and T2 MR images (B) showed a circumscribed heterogenous mass based in the periphery of cerebellar hemisphere or cerebellar cortex. Note buckling of white matter and collapsed fourth ventricle (*white arrow*) displaced away from the mass (A and B). Sagittal and coronal contrast-enhanced MR images showed intense enhancement within the mass lesion (C and D). Note the additional mildly enhancing cortical nodular mass on coronal contrast-enhanced MR image (*white arrow* in D). Histopathologic examination confirmed SHH type medulloblastoma.

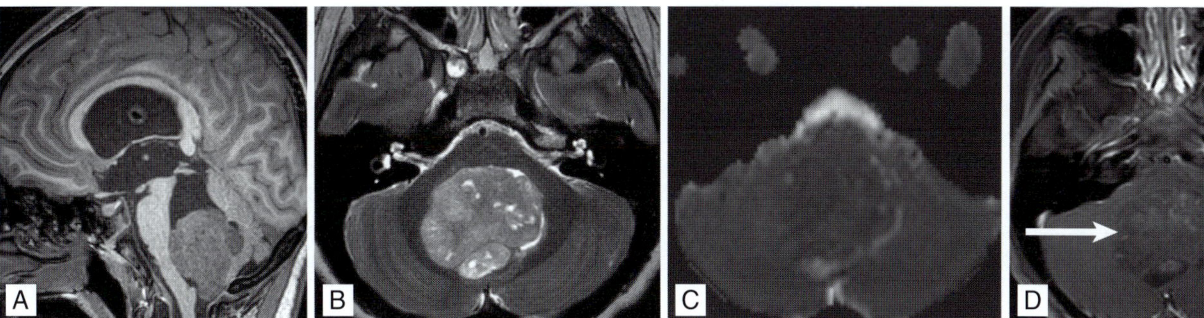

Figure 80.40 A 12-year-old male presented with headache and dizziness for 2 months. Sagittal T1 MR image (A) showed a circumscribed mass centered in the fourth ventricle extending to the foramen magnum. Axial T2 MR image (B) demonstrated the midline location of the mass. ADC showed mildly reduced diffusivity values within the mass (C). Axial contrast-enhanced MR image (D) showed minimal to mild patchy enhancement of the mass (*white arrow*). Histopathologic examination confirmed non-WNT non-SHH group 4 medulloblastoma.

TABLE 80.12 Clinicopathologic Characteristics of Sonic Hedgehog Type Medulloblastoma

Gender	Male = Female
Age	Children <3 years including infants, adolescent, young adults [50,51]
Spatial location	Cerebellar cortex (peripheral) >> midline-vermis (overall) Desmoplastic/nodular variant—cortex >> vermis [48] Medulloblastoma with extensive nodularity—vermis >> hemisphere
Histopathology	**TP53 wild type**—children <3 years—Medulloblastoma with extensive nodularity Children <3 years, adolescent, young adult—desmoplastic/nodular variant. **TP53 mutant**—children, large cell/anaplastic variant (high risk of relapse) [49]
Cerebrospinal fluid dissemination	Uncommon **except** TP53 mutant tumors Local recurrence in the tumor bed common [30]
Prognosis	**TP 53 wild type**—favorable especially Medulloblastoma with extensive nodularity and desmoplastic/nodular types **TP 53 mutant**—poor

TABLE 80.13 Clinicopathologic Characteristics of Group 3 Medulloblastoma

Gender	Male > Female
Age	Infants, children
Spatial location	Midline/fourth ventricle including vermis
Histopathology	Large cell/anaplastic (high relapse risk)
Cerebrospinal fluid dissemination	High incidence (40% at presentation)
Prognosis	Poor

TABLE 80.14 Clinicopathologic Characteristics of Group 4 Medulloblastoma

Gender	Male >> Female
Age	All age groups
Spatial location	Midline/fourth ventricle including vermis [50]
Histopathology	Classic; large cell/anaplastic pattern uncommon [49]
Cerebrospinal fluid dissemination	Frequent
Prognosis	Pediatric—intermediate Adult—worse

Group 3 and 4 subtypes are considered truly midline medulloblastoma [33]. Group 3 tumors are biologically aggressive with underlying MYC and OTX2 gene amplification. The primary mass is frequently not well circumscribed. Nearly 25% of these tumors present as a small primary mass (without hydrocephalus) with a larger metastatic lesion. A small but significant proportion of Group 3 tumors may show minimal to no contrast enhancement [30,37,48]. The clinical and pathological characteristics are detailed in Table 80.13.

Group 4 tumors also have an aggressive biologic course with associated molecular alterations such as MYCN and OTX2 gene amplification. The presence of prominent intralesional flow voids reflects high perfusion nature of the tumor [48]. Minimal contrast enhancement or complete lack thereof is a very characteristic imaging feature of group 4 subtype tumors [30,48,50]. The clinical and pathological characteristics are detailed in Table 80.14.

Uncommon imaging features of medulloblastoma include extension into the cerebellopontine angle cistern and porous acusticus, mimicking a vestibular schwannoma [44]. The presence of multiple intratumoral flow voids in adolescent or young adult patient should raise concern for other differential consideration such as a hemangioblastoma [44]. Rarely imaging features of medulloblastoma may mimic Lhermitte–Duclos disease (dysplastic cerebellar gangliocytoma). The presence of abnormally high choline levels on MR spectroscopy would favor the diagnosis of high-grade tumors such as embryonal tumors in these situations [52]. Imaging findings observed in histologically defined medulloblastoma variants are elucidated in Table 80.15.

The prevalence of leptomeningeal metastatic disease is about 20–35% and 30–50% of all medulloblastoma patients at the initial diagnosis and during follow-up surveillance, respectively [43,48,53]. Baseline imaging assessment for leptomeningeal

TABLE 80.15 Imaging Findings of Histologically Defined Medulloblastoma Subtypes

Classic	High ADC values
Large cell/anaplastic	Ring enhancement Leptomeningeal enhancement Intratumoral hemorrhage Low ADC values
Medulloblastoma with extensive nodularity (previously cerebellar neuroblastoma)	Enhancing multinodular mass with racemose appearance (pathologic correlation to reticulin-rich nodular areas with neuronal differentiation)
Desmoplastic/nodular	Focal abnormal leptomeningeal enhancement overlying mass (involvement of overlying dura or meninges)

TABLE 80.16 Imaging Patterns of Metastatic Disease in Non-WNT/Non-SHH Medulloblastoma Subtypes

Group 3	Group 4
Late metastatic disease common (distant sites in central nervous system without recurrence in treated primary site) [48]	
Local recurrence in a treated non-WNT/non-SHH medulloblastoma suspicious for radiation-induced tumor like high-grade glioma [30]	
Laminar metastatic pattern	Nodular metastatic disease Metastases in the anterior third ventricle or suprasellar region
Matching pattern (both subarachnoid space and ependymal metastases show diffusion restriction and contrast enhancement)	**Mismatching** pattern (ependymal metastases like primary tumor [restriction, no enhancement], in contrast to subarachnoid space metastatic disease [restriction and enhancement])

metastatic disease is important before surgical resection, for optimal disease staging. If not feasible, postoperative assessment within 72 hours or more than 2 weeks after surgery is recommended to avoid false-positive imaging findings related to operative procedure[53]. The most common location of spinal metastases is along the posterior surface of spinal cord. *Extraneural metastasis is rare in medulloblastoma, bone being the most common site followed by lymph nodes* [44]. A significant proportion of patients may develop metastatic disease in the peritoneal cavity through ventriculoperitoneal shunt [44]. Recurrent medulloblastoma is most common within first 2 years after completion of treatment [44]. The imaging patterns of metastatic disease in non-WNT/non-SHH subtypes of medulloblastoma are detailed in Table 80.16.

Posterior fossa syndrome is a clinical condition reported in up to one-third of patients after posterior fossa tumor surgery such as resection of medulloblastoma. Hypertrophic olivary degeneration is a MR imaging marker of posterior fossa syndrome, manifested as abnormal signal in inferior olivary nuclei (less commonly dentate nucleus and superior cerebellar peduncle) especially on Proton density imaging. These patients typically present with cerebellar mutism after few days of surgery [54,55]. Susceptibility weighted imaging may reveal significant asymmetry at the level of midbrain with loss of expected T2 hypointensity within the red nucleus (compared with substantia nigra) [56].

Atypical Teratoid Rhabdoid Tumor

Atypical teratoid rhabdoid tumor (ATRT) is a high-grade embryonal tumor commonly affecting children less than 4 years of age specifically within first year of life. The distinctive genetic alteration is loss of SMARCB1 (BAF47/hSNF5/INI1) tumor suppressor gene. An inherited germline deletion of the SMARCB1 tumor suppressor gene is associated with rhabdoid tumor predisposition syndrome (combination of ATRT and rhabdoid tumors outside CNS) [44,57]. A significant proportion of these tumors are based in the supratentorial space. The classical presentation is a markedly heterogenous intra-axial tumor in the posterior fossa in the infantile age showing combination of solid component, internal necrosis, calcification, and blood products (Fig. 80.41). Leptomeningeal metastatic disease is frequently observed as with other embryonal tumors [57]. The imaging findings specific for ATRT include presence of peripheral cysts, thick band-like wavy enhancement or involvement of the adjacent native dura,

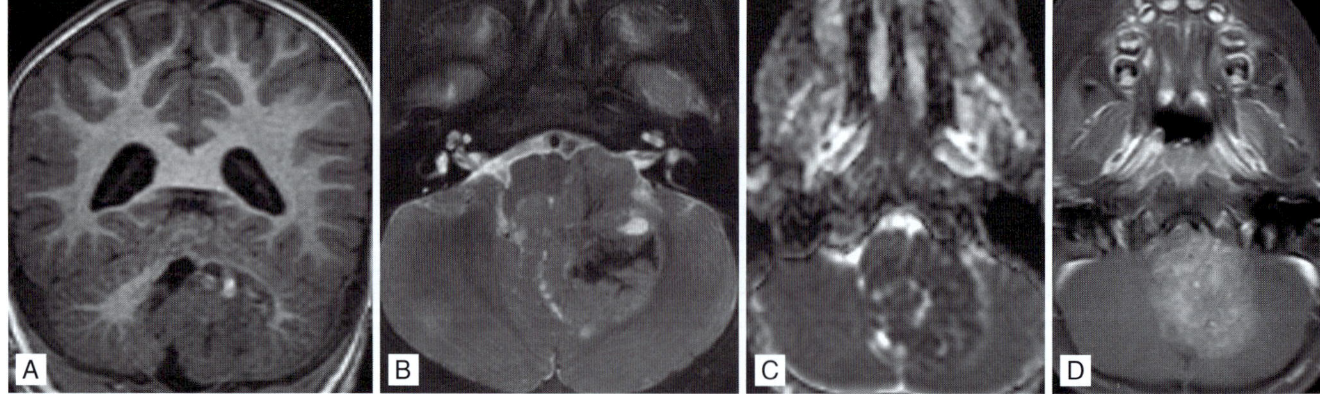

Figure 80.41 A 14-month-old boy complained of vomiting and head tilt. Coronal T1 (A) and T2 MR images (B) showed a markedly heterogenous solid mass centered in the left cerebellar hemisphere. The mass appears to protrude into the fourth ventricle and through the foramen of Luschka. The T1 hyperintense and T2 hypointense areas in the mass represent blood products. The mass showed reduced ADC values (C). Axial contrast-enhanced MR image (D) showed near homogenous enhancement of the mass. The age of the patient favors the diagnosis of atypical teratoid rhabdoid tumor (ATRT). The differential diagnosis includes medulloblastoma. Histopathologic examination confirmed ATRT.

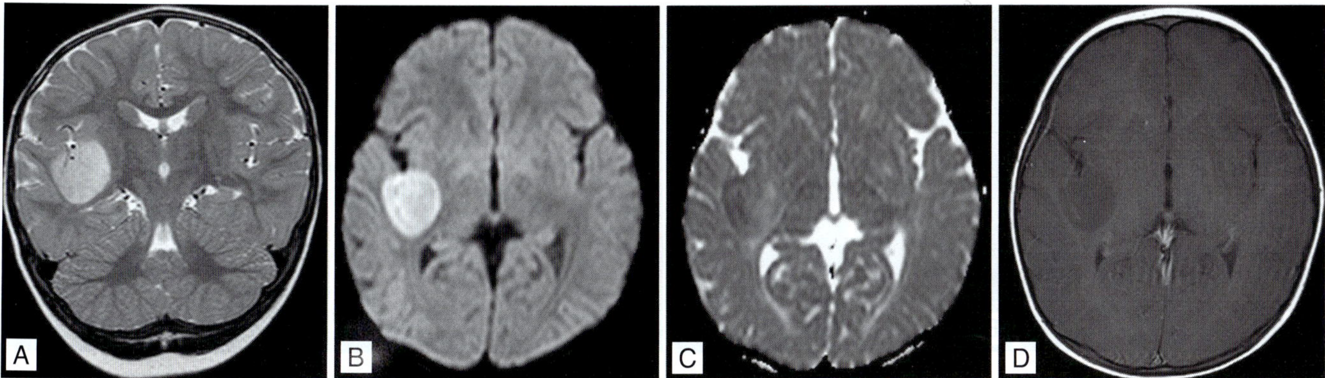

Figure 80.42 A 1-year-old-female patient presented with seizures. Coronal T2 MR image (A) demonstrated a large circumscribed homogenous hyperintense mass centered within the right frontotemporal lobe. The mass showed restricted diffusion (B and C) suggestive of hypercellularity and complete absence of enhancement on axial contrast-enhanced MR image (D). Given patient's age and features including significant restricted diffusion and lack of contrast enhancement, findings suggestive of ETMR which was histopathologically confirmed.

calvarium, or skull base by an intra-axial mass, however these may be seen only in a minority of patients [58]. Rare imaging presentation such as extra-axial location, cranial nerve origin, primary diffuse leptomeningeal disease have been reported [57].

Embryonal Tumor With Multilayered Rosettes

The diagnostic molecular defect in this tumor is amplification of a microRNA cluster at long arm of chromosome 19 (C19MC) and LIN28A overexpression. There is significant overlap of clinical and imaging features with other embryonal tumors, specifically AT/RT, such as predominantly affecting infants and children less than 4 years, heterogenous intra-axial hypercellular mass, and frequent metastatic spread along CSF. In contrast to other embryonal tumors, embryonal tumor with multilayered rosettes is usually well circumscribed with minimal to mild contrast enhancement (Fig. 80.42) [59]. Cerebral hemisphere is the most common site observed in majority of tumors (supratentorial > infratentorial > spinal) [37].

Ependymal Tumors

Ependymoma is an ependymal origin primary pediatric brain neoplasm typically reported in the age group of 1–5 years [37]. The majority (up to two-thirds) of ependymomas are based in the posterior fossa. The posterior fossa ependymomas typically present as an intraventricular mass. Calcification is a common feature of infratentorial ependymomas, in contrast to other posterior fossa tumors, seen in up to half of all such tumors. Infrequently, intratumoral hemorrhagic residue may be observed. Baseline imaging of the craniospinal axis is critical to search for the presence of leptomeningeal metastatic disease, since there is a definite risk of spread through CSF [60]. The cIMPACT group does not recommend use of histologic subtyping for the purpose of pathologic classification of classic ependymomas since they are of no clinical benefit [29]. MR imaging evaluation of precise location and extent of posterior fossa ependymomas is used to classify these tumors into two groups. These are further detailed in Table 80.17.

Supratentorial ependymomas represent about one-third of all intracranial ependymomas. These tumors are commonly extraventricular in location [63]. The WHO 2016 classification of supratentorial ependymomas is elucidated in Table 80.18 with associated clinical and imaging features.

Non-RELA/non-YAP1 ependymomas typically present as large predominantly solid tumors in midline, with internal necrotic

TABLE 80.17 Clinical and Imaging Features of Posterior Fossa Ependymomas [63]

Lateral Type (Posterior Fossa Type A) (Fig. 80.43)	Midfloor Type (Posterior Fossa Type B)
Young children	Older children, adolescents
Based in foramen of Luschka/ lateral recess ▪ absence of obex involvement ▪ lateral displacement of the brainstem (axial imaging plane)	Mass in midline within the fourth ventricle ▪ involvement of the obex ▪ anteroposterior brainstem displacement (sagittal plane)
Complete resection less feasible (extension into adjacent cisterns, encasement of neurovascular structures)	More amenable to complete surgical resection
Higher risk of residual tumor	Lower risk of residual tumor (better prognosis)

TABLE 80.18 WHO 2016 Classification of Supratentorial Ependymomas With Elucidation of Clinical and Imaging Features

RELA Fusion Ependymomas [63] (Fig. 80.44)	YAP1-MAMLD1 Ependymomas [64]
Specific translocation between RELA- and C11orf95-forming oncogenic fusion gene resulting in pathological activation of NFkB (nuclear factor k of B cells) signaling pathway (70%)	Fusion gene
Older children poorer outcomes [30]	Female patients less than 3 years of age
Predominantly cystic unilocular or multilocular lesion centered in the cerebral cortex with smooth peripheral enhancement	Large T2 isointense mass with prominent cystic component in an intra- or paraventricular location with heterogeneous contrast enhancement
Diffusion restriction demonstrated by reduced ADC values has been reported in the solid enhancing portion of supratentorial tumors	Multinodular appearance of the solid component, with often associated hemorrhage

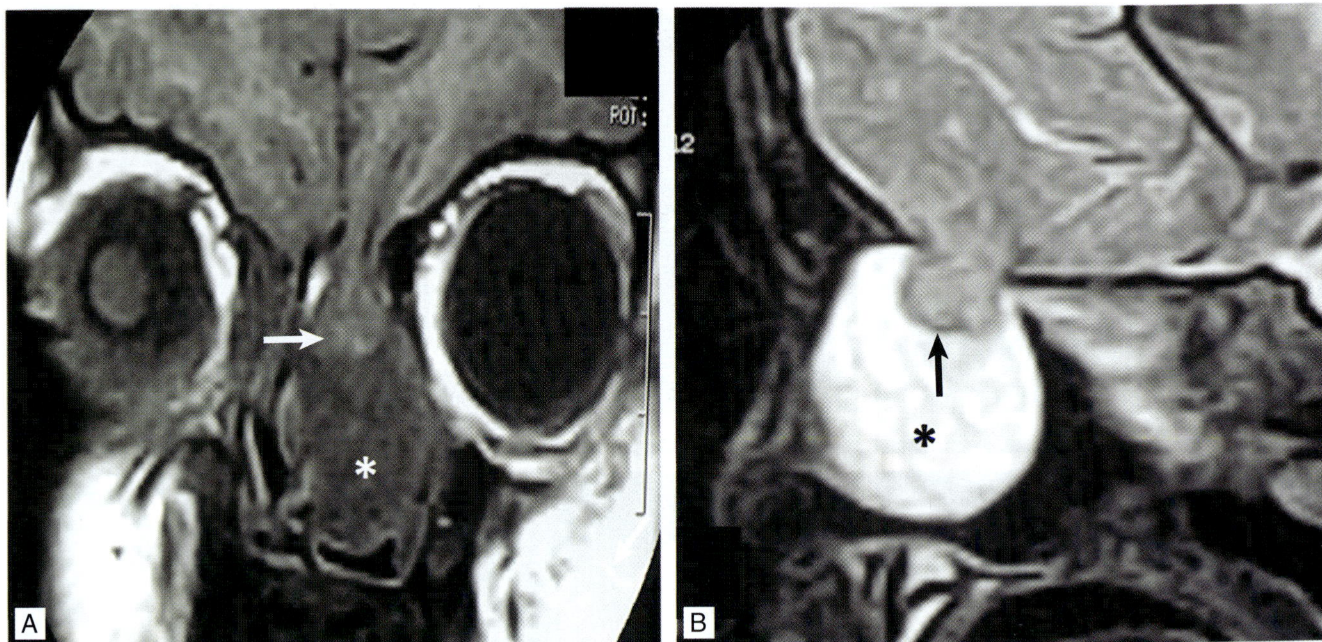

Figure 81.4 Coronal T1W (A) and parasagittal T2W (B) images of a left frontonasal meningoencephalocele with inferior herniation of the left gyrus rectus (*arrows*) within a large CSF-filled sac (*asterisk*).

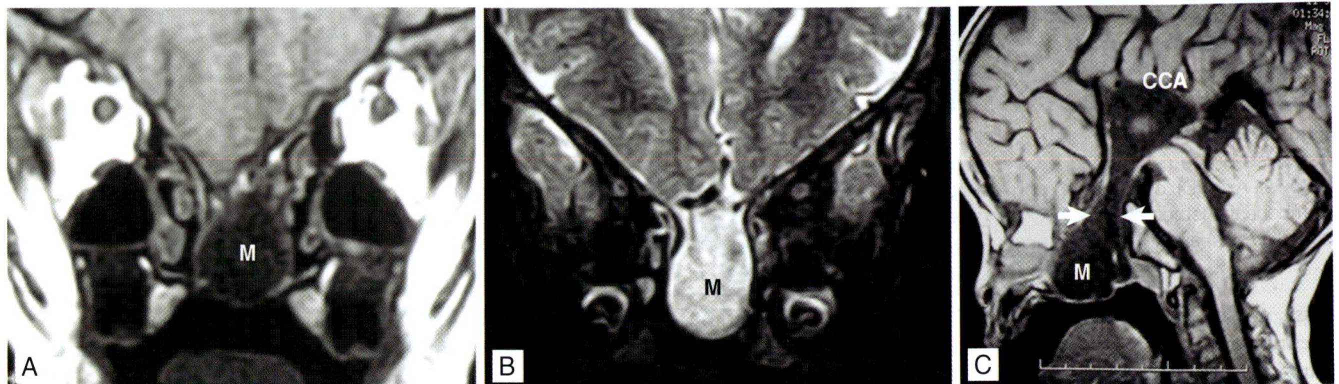

Figure 81.5 Coronal T1W (A), coronal T2W (B), and midline sagittal T1W (C) images of a large left paramidline trans-sphenoid meningocele (M) through a patent craniopharyngeal canal (*arrows*) with associated corpus callosum agenesis (CCA).

to primitive mesenchyme in the posterior choanal tissue. Juvenile nasopharyngeal angiofibromas are not malignant but can be locally aggressive and infiltrative. The lesions are densely enhancing with flow voids on MRI and enlarged feeding vessels on CTA/MRA. Potential spread patterns include:

- Pterygopalatine fossa (early and first: reliable diagnostic sign), sphenoid/maxillary/ethmoid sinuses, pterygomaxillary space to infratemporal fossa into the middle cranial fossa by erosion of the floor, infra/supraorbital fissures into orbit, and nasopharynx/nasal cavity/oral cavity
- Anterior bowing of posterior maxillary wall (Holman–Miller sign) is considered pathognomonic of this lesion. Remodeling of bony structures rather than destruction

  DSA is essential for preoperative embolization and tumor mapping (Fig. 81.6). Feeders can arise from external carotid artery (internal maxillary, ascending pharyngeal, palatine arteries) from contralateral ECA, or from internal carotid artery (Vidian artery and lateral mainstem trunk).

Paranasal Sinuses and Nasal Cavity (Table 81.3)

Congenital Pyriform Aperture Stenosis (CPAS)

Congenital nasal pyriform aperture stenosis is associated with medial deviation of anterior maxillary walls that impinge on the nasal lumen may be associated with thickening of the nasal processes (Fig. 81.7). Congenital pyriform aperture stenosis can be associated with abnormal maxillary dentition like solitary median maxillary central incisor syndrome [13,14].

Choanal Atresia

Ipsilateral or bilateral narrowing or complete obstruction of the posterior nasal cavity with membranous (rare, <10%) or partial/complete osseous pathology (>90%). Narrowing should be considered if the size of the posterior choanal opening in newborn is

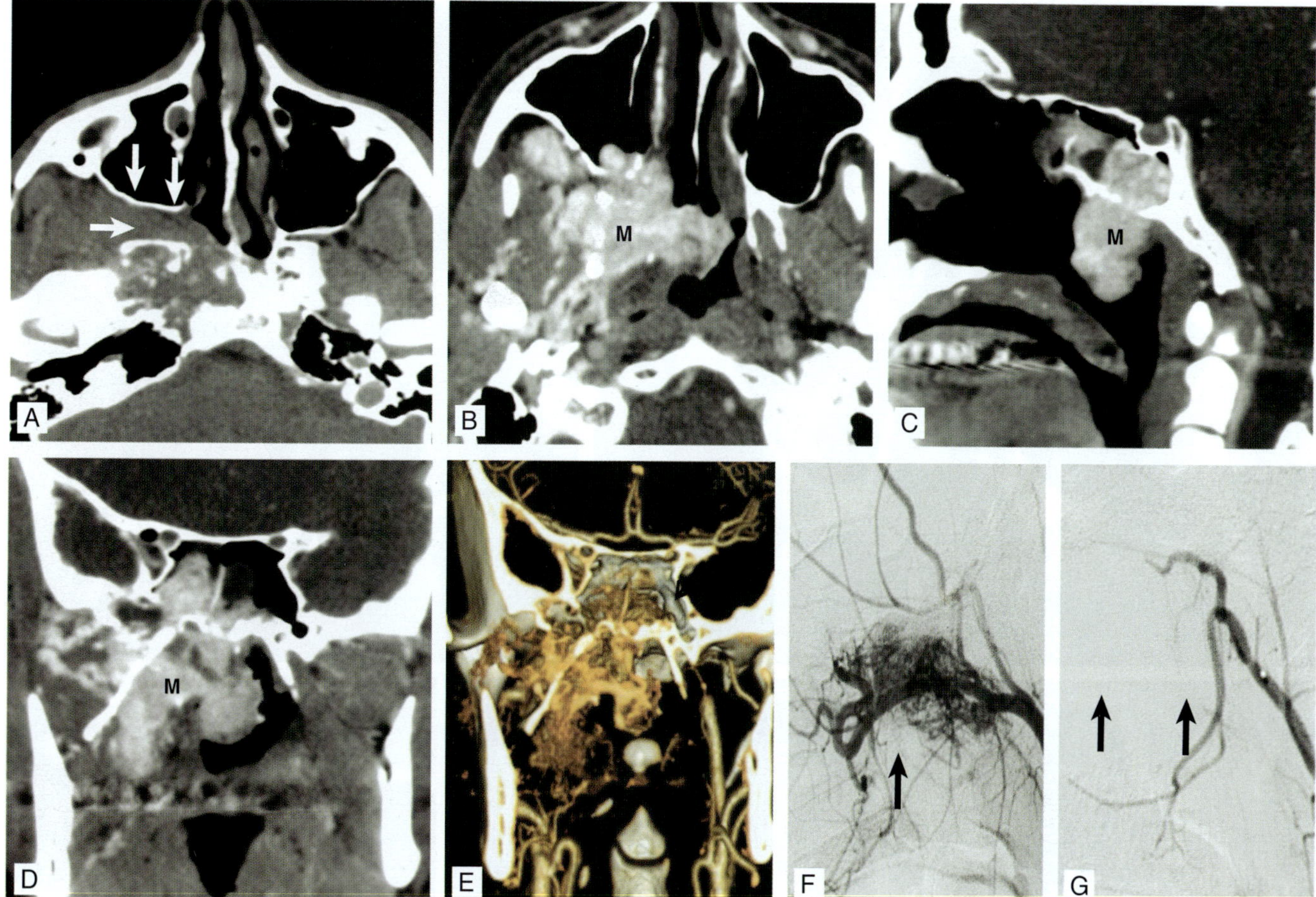

Figure 81.6 Juvenile nasopharyngeal angiofibroma (JNA): Noncontrast axial CT (A), axial/sagittal/coronal CECT (B–D), and 3D VRCT (E) show a large intensely enhancing polypoidal mass (M) centered on the right sphenopalatine foramen, widening the right pterygopalatine fossa (*short horizontal arrow*) with typical anterior bowing of the posterior maxillary sinus wall (*vertical arrows*): Holman–Miller sign. Pre-embolization (F) and successful postembolization (G) DSA images of the highly vascular tumor (*arrows*).

less than 0.37 cm and if the vomer bone thickness exceeds 0.34 cm [13]. Bilateral choanal atresia will present at birth with respiratory distress and inability to pass a nasogastric feeding tube. Unilateral choanal atresia can present in an older child. Characteristic CT findings are medial bowing of posterior maxilla, thickened posterior and inferior portions of the vomer, bone or soft-tissue membrane of varying thickness at the choana, and proximal accumulated secretions (Fig. 81.7).

Nasal Glioma

These are developmental sinonasal defects that extend through the fonticulus frontalis permitting inferior descent of dysplastic neural tissue into the prenasal space (between the nasal bones and cartilaginous nasal capsule). This may result in an encephalocele, which directly connects to the intracranial cavity, and nasal gliomas which is ectopic brain tissue. Nasal gliomas located in the region of the prenasal space are intranasal (40% of cases) and not clinically apparent unless large. Extra nasal gliomas are located in the region of the fonticulus frontalis (60% of cases) and prenasal space (40%). These lesions usually present as a midline skin-covered glabellar lesion [13,14].

Sagittal MR is helpful to show the lesion has no intracranial connection. Nasal gliomas typically have intermediate T1W signal, high T2W signal (due to gliotic change), and minimal

TABLE 81.3 Classification of Sinonasal Pathologies

Congenital Conditions	Inflammatory Conditions	Neoplastic and Tumor-Like Conditions
▪ Choanal atresia ▪ Congenital nasal pyriform aperture stenosis ▪ Nasal dermoid/nasal gliomas ▪ Cephaloceles ▪ Proboscis lateralis with partial or complete arrhinia	▪ Acute and chronic rhinosinusitis without/with complications (orbital/intracranial/soft tissue) ▪ Fungal and allergic rhinosinusitis ▪ Postinflammatory masses (cysts, polyps, mucoceles) ▪ Sinus inflammatory pathology in cystic fibrosis	▪ Benign: Fibro-osseous lesions (fibrous dysplasia and ossifying fibroma), bony tumors (giant cell tumor and aneurysmal bone cyst), juvenile angiofibroma of the nasopharynx), nasal pleomorphic adenoma, odontogenic cysts or tumors, hemangiomas and lobular capillary hemangioma (nasal pyogenic granuloma), hemangiopericytoma ▪ Malignant: Rhabdomyosarcoma, lymphoma, esthesioneuroblastoma, leukemia ▪ Nasopharyngeal carcinoma ▪ Metastatic neuroblastoma

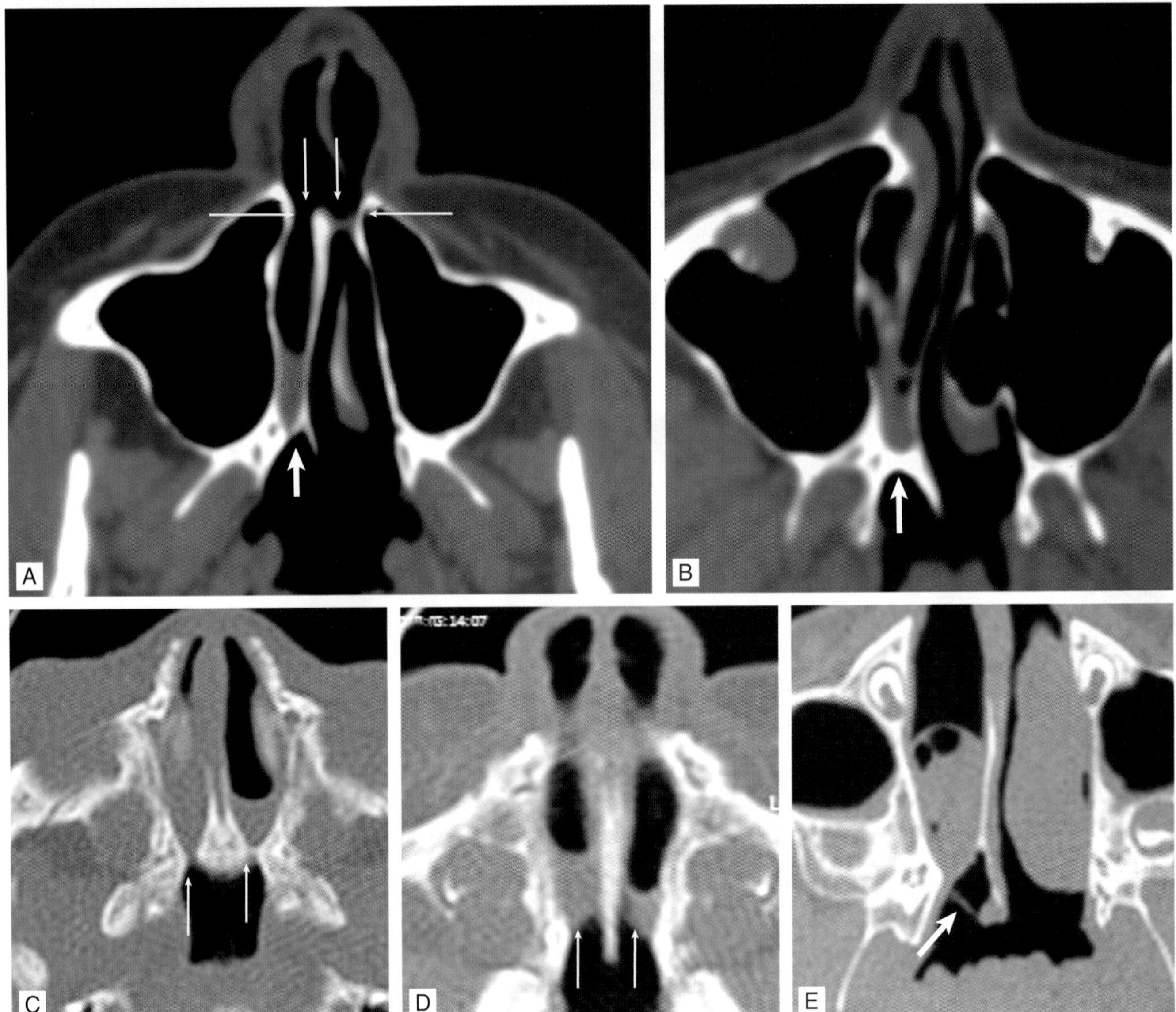

Figure 81.7 Congenital nasal pyriform aperture stenosis and choanal atresia. Axial (A) NCCT image showing marked bilateral narrowing of the pyriform aperture (*thin arrows*). Evidence of right-sided complete choanal atresia (A, B) with thick bony bar (*vertical thick arrows*) and proximal collection of secretions. Right membranous/left bony choanal atresia (*vertical arrows* in C), bilateral membranous choanal atresia (*vertical arrows* in D) in newborns with failed attempts to pass a nasogastric tube. Thin membrane with mild choanal atresia on the right side and proximal secretions in a 7-year-old girl (*thick oblique arrow* in E).

enhancement. CT demonstrates a widened foramen caecum. Encephaloceles may show a bifid and widened crista galli if there is a dysplastic rudimentary tract extending from the nasal glioma to the cranial vault (Fig. 81.8).

Trapped nonglial elements within the dural diverticulum that extends from the anterior cranial fossa to the prenasal space may result in teratomas, dermoid cysts (DCs), and epidermoids along the diverticulum tract. These lesions can be identified from the tip of the nose till the floor of the anterior cranial fossa.

Proboscis Lateralis With/Without Spectrum of Arrhinia

Rare craniofacial malformation due to developmental defect in the nasal placode resulting anomalies involving the nose, paranasal sinuses, orbits, and brain. These were characterized by Khoo into four groups based on severity proboscis malformation [15]. CT and MRI (Fig. 81.9) demonstrate the bony abnormalities and the soft-tissue trunk containing all tissues found in the nasal cavity including viable mucosa. MRI shows the status of the olfactory pathway and assesses for the presence of associated intracranial abnormalities which include corpus callosum agenesis and encephaloceles.

Cystic Fibrosis

Cystic fibrosis affects 1 in 3500 newborns and is characterized by sinonasal disease (nasal polyposis, chronic mucosal inflammation), bronchiectasis, pancreatic insufficiency, and focal biliary cirrhosis [16]. Imaging is indicated in patients who are unresponsive to conservative treatment. Imaging shows medial displacement of the lateral nasal walls, deossification of bony structures and opacification of the sinuses. Frontal and sphenoid sinuses may appear underdeveloped due to chronic obstruction. Hyperdensities on CT within the

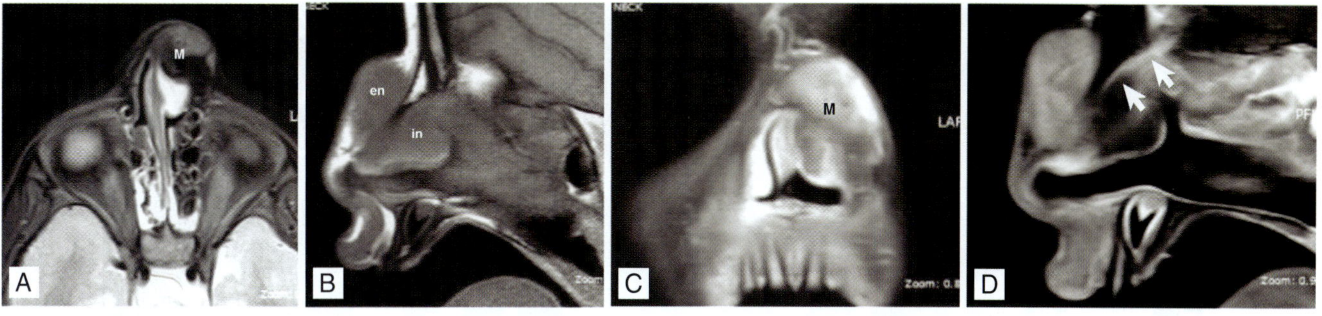

Figure 81.8 Nasal glial heterotopia (nasal glioma): STIR axial (A), sagittal T1W (B) images and postcontrast coronal (C), sagittal (D) postcontrast images showing lobulated partially enhancing complex signal intensity mass (M) at the glabella with an extra nasal (en) and intranasal (in) component. Small pedicle (*oblique arrows*) is seen extending up the foramen cecum (*oblique arrows* in D) without any intracranial extension.

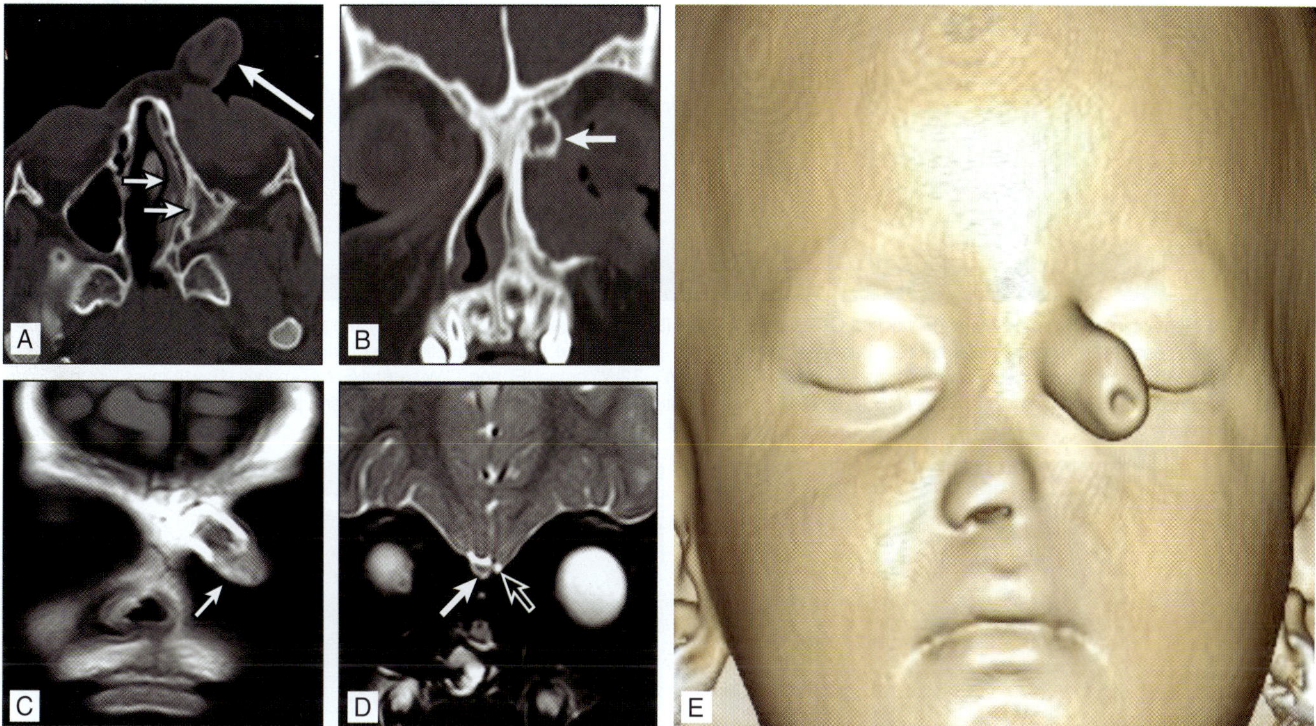

Figure 81.9 Proboscis lateralis: Axial HRCT image (A) in bone windows shows a tubular trunk-like process (*large white arrow*) arising from superomedial aspect of the left orbit with aplasia of ipsilateral nasal cavity and maxillary/ethmoid sinuses (*small arrows*). Coronal HRCT image (B) in bone windows shows well-formed bony canal in superomedial compartment of the left orbit (*horizontal arrow*). T1W coronal MR image (C) showing the left-sided proboscis (*oblique white arrow*). T2W coronal MR image (D) showing normal right olfactory bulb (*oblique white arrow*). Hypoplastic left olfactory groove with absent left olfactory bulb (*oblique black arrow*). Coronal 3D reformatted image of the patient (E) showing the tubular trunk-like process arising from medial canthus of the left orbit with absent left nasal cavity. (*Source:* S Vaid, D Shah, S Rawat, R Shukla, Proboscis lateralis with ipsilateral sinonasal and olfactory pathway aplasia, J Pediatr Surg 45 (2) (2010) 453–456.)

opacified sinuses due to inspissated secretions may mimic fungal disease. However, fungal pathology is uncommon in the pediatric age group. The chronic inflammation of cystic fibrosis can cause bone thickening and sclerosis of the sinus walls.

Capillary Hemangiomas and Lobular Capillary Hemangioma (Nasal Pyogenic Granulomas)

Sinonasal hemangiomas in the pediatric age group occur commonly in the nasal septum and nasal vestibule. Lobular capillary hemangiomas (previously referred to as nasal pyogenic granulomas) are benign lesions arising from skin, oral mucosa or nasal mucosa over the septum, nasal turbinates or roof of the nasal cavity. Imaging reveals a well-defined lobulated enhancing mass on both CT and MRI with avidly enhancing mass. Other vasoproliferative disorders with enhanced vascularity in the sinonasal region include hemangiopericytoma (Fig. 81.10) and glomangiopericytoma.

Leukemia

Extramedullary leukemic infiltration in the paranasal sinuses and nasal cavity is rare but important consideration in sinonasal soft-tissue masses. A combination of CT and MRI provides exact extent of the disease process, evidence of intracranial/intraorbital and intraoral extension as well as the lymph node involvement (Fig. 81.11). MRI also helps differentiate leukemic infiltrates from trapped sinus secretions and identifies perineural spread.

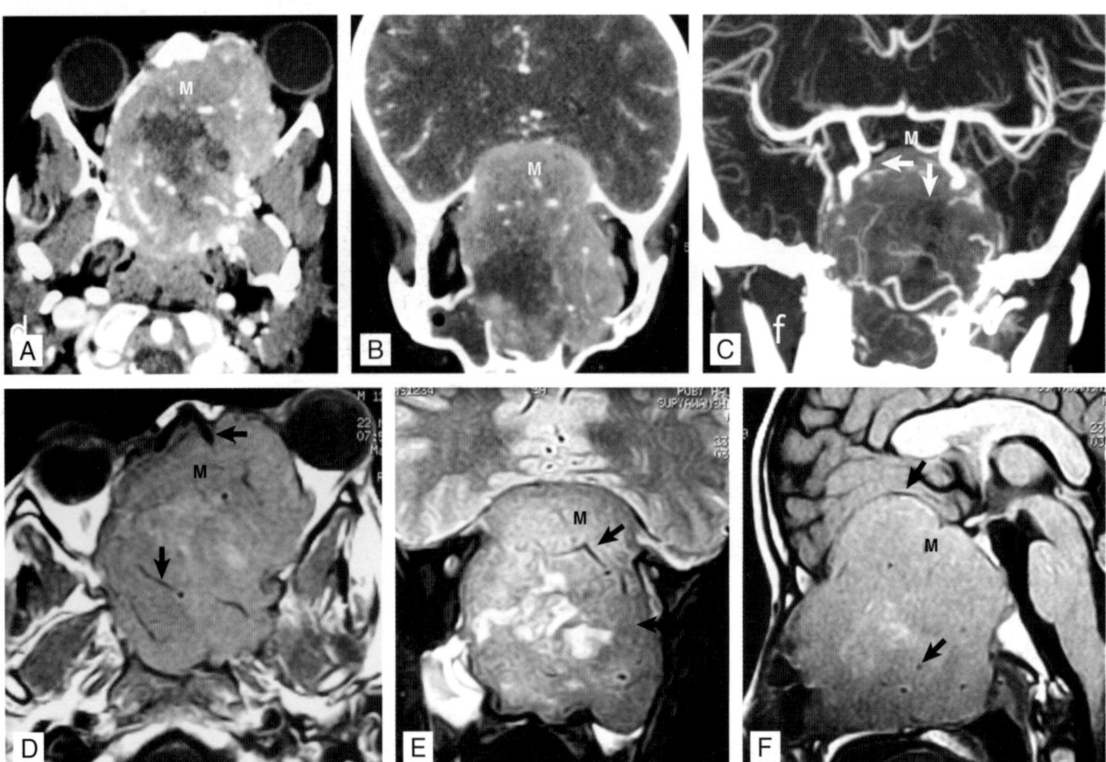

Figure 81.10 Hemangiopericytoma: Contrast-enhanced CT axial (A), coronal (B), and coronal CT angiography (C) images showing a large densely enhancing soft-tissue mass lesion (M) involving nasal cavities, paranasal sinuses, with anterior skull base destruction and bilateral orbital and intracranial extension. CT angiography shows multiple intralesional vessels. (*white arrows*). T1W axial (D), T2W coronal (E), and T1W sagittal (F) MR images show a mass which is isointense on T1W images and heterogeneously hyperintense on T2W images. Multiple flow voids indicate prominent intra- and perilesional vessels (*black arrows*).

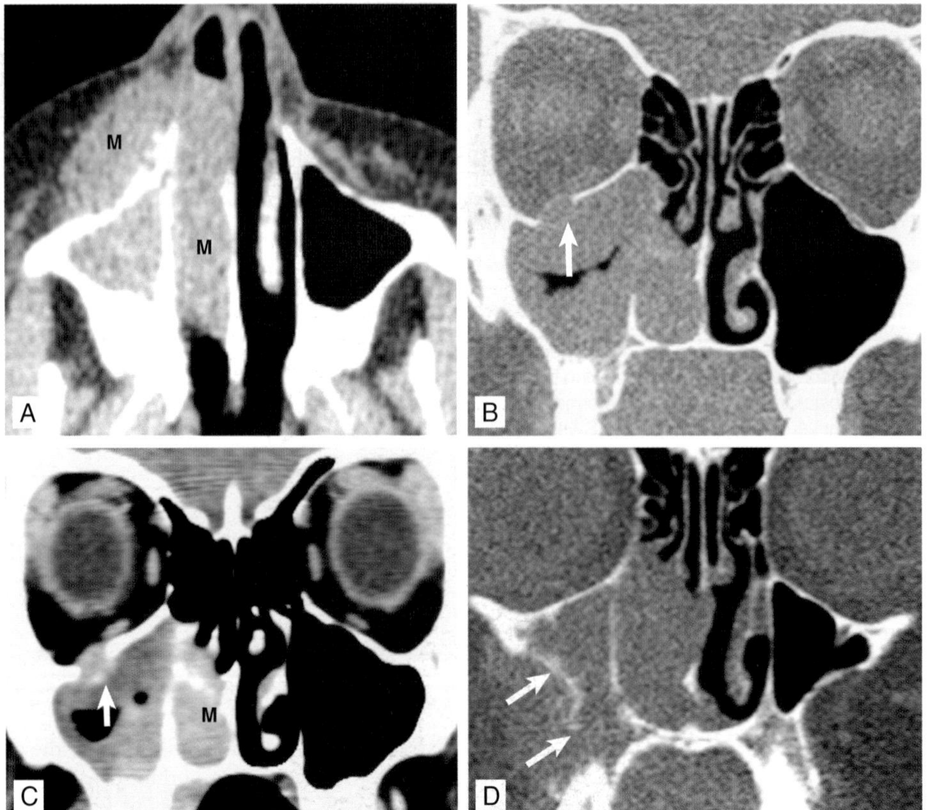

Figure 81.11 Leukemia: Postcontrast axial (A) and coronal (C) images showing an enhancing leukemic soft-tissue mass infiltrating the right maxillary sinus, nasal cavity, and the right premaxillary soft tissues. Perineural spread is evident on the right infraorbital nerve. Bone coronal HRCT images (B, D) show irregular permeative destruction of the walls of right maxillary sinus (*oblique arrows* in D) and bony canal for the right infraorbital nerve (*vertical arrows* in B, C).

TABLE 81.4 Classification of Temporal Bone Pathologies

Congenital Pathologies	Acquired Pathologies
Congenital aural dysplasia spectrum: External and middle ear with surrounding soft tissue/bone/temporo-mandibular joint abnormalities Syndromic and nonsyndromic ***Congenital inner ear abnormalities*** *[17]:* Labyrinthine aplasia (Michel deformity) Rudimentary otocyst Cochlear aplasia Common cavity Cochlear hypoplasia (Type I–IV) Incomplete partition defects: ▪ Incomplete partition Type 1 ▪ Incomplete partition Type 2 (with LVAS = Mondini deformity) ▪ Incomplete partition Type 3 (X-linked deafness; DFNX2) LVAS (large vestibular aqueduct syndrome) Cochlear aperture abnormalities ***Congenital Cranial Nerve VII (Facial)/VIII (Cochleovestibular; CVN) abnormalities*** *[18]:* Type 1: CVN aplasia—absent VIII nerve Type 2: CVN dysplasia ▪ UCVN (undivided VIII nerve) ▪ ACB (absent cochlear branch) ▪ HCB (hypoplastic cochlear branch) Type 1/2A (if associated abnormal labyrinth) Type 1/2B (if normal labyrinth)	***Infective/inflammatory:*** Necrotizing otitis externa Acute coalescent otitis media (with intracranial/extracranial complications) Chronic otitis media Congenital cholesteatomas Cholesterol granuloma Noncholesteatomatous ossicular erosions and postinflammatory ossicular fixations Labyrinthitis ossificans ***Neoplastic pathology:*** Rhabdomyosarcoma Lymphoma ***Trauma:*** Fractures, facial nerve injury, skull base trauma ***Miscellaneous:*** Osteogenesis imperfecta Third window pathologies Langerhans cell histiocytosis

TABLE 81.5 Classification of Pathologies

Developmental	Inflammatory	Neoplastic and Other Masses
Anophthalmia PHPV Coloboma, Staphyloma Optic nerve hypoplasia Norrie disease Coats disease Dacryocystocele	*Acute:* Orbital cellulitis Dacryocystitis *Chronic:* Orbital pseudotumor Graves orbitopathy Sarcoidosis Wegener's granulomatosis Optic neuritis Devic Disease LCH	*Benign:* Optic glioma Orbital hemangioma Inclusion cysts *Malignant:* Retinoblastoma Medulloepithelioma PNET Orbital rhabdomyosarcoma Leukemia Lymphoma Metastases (neuroblastoma)

Nasopharyngeal Carcinoma

NPC (Type III—undifferentiated type) is common in adolescent Asian and African-American children with a known association to EBV. Unlike other sinonasal malignancies, undifferentiated NPC presents first as a mass in the neck (commonly at Level V nodal station). CT and MRI used in conjunction can identify soft-tissue extent, bony destruction, invasion of neurovascular structures (internal carotid artery, cavernous sinus), and cranial nerves III, IV, V, and VI. NPC in the pediatric age group is an aggressive malignancy with poor survival rates despite intense multimodality therapy.

Pediatric Temporal Bone

Please refer to Chapter 72 and Table 81.4.

Orbit and Lacrimal Glands (Table 81.5 and Box 81.3)

Persistent Hyperplastic Primary Vitreous

Persistence of the embryonic hyaloid vascular system termed as persistent hyperplastic primary vitreous, results in fibrosis,

BOX 81.3 Pediatric Globe

- Infant globe occupies 20% of orbital cavity and reaches adult size by 13 years of age.
- Ultrasonography: Preliminary evaluation of pediatric orbital–lacrimal gland pathologies.
- CT: Trauma, subperiosteal abscesses (SPA), and localizing foreign bodies.
- MRI: Integrity of optic nerve, intracranial extension/structures, vascular malformations.

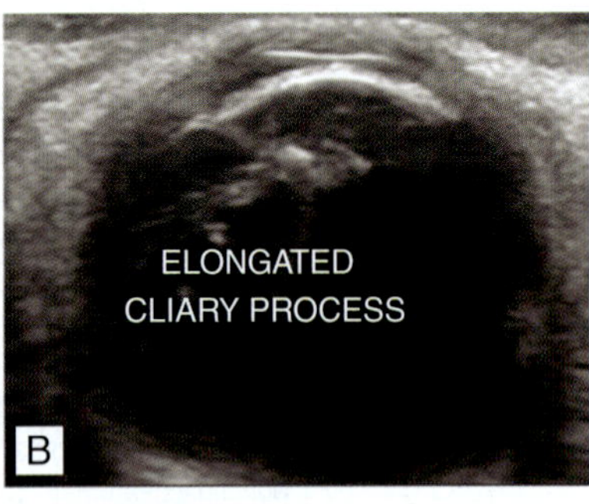

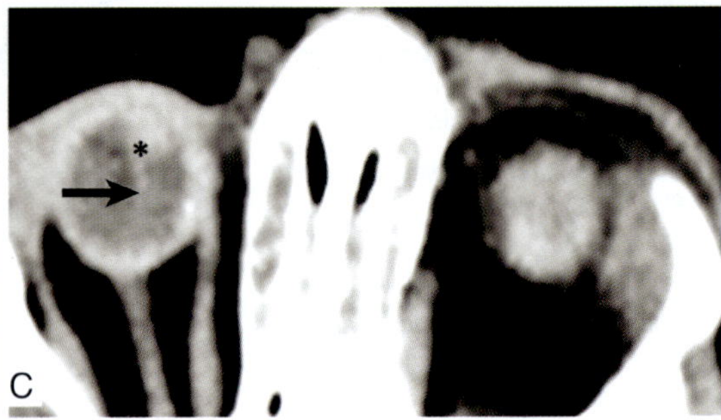

Figure 81.12 PHPV: Transverse grayscale ultrasound images (A, B) of the left orbit in a 14-month-old boy presenting with a white reflex in the left eye since birth reveals an echogenic band in the posterior chamber extending from the posterior surface of the lens to the optic disc (*oblique arrows*) without appreciable vascularity on color Doppler. Note completely collapsed anterior chamber, distorted, and echogenic lens (*horizontal arrow* in A) with elongated ciliary processes and hypertrophied optic disc (*asterisk*). Axial CECT (C) in another case shows a relatively hyperdense band (*arrow*) representing a hyaloid remnant that courses from the lens to the optic disc on right side, enhancing retrolental tissue (*asterisk*) corresponding to the primary vitreous. (Ultrasound images courtesy: Dr. Joban Babhulkar, Pune, India.)

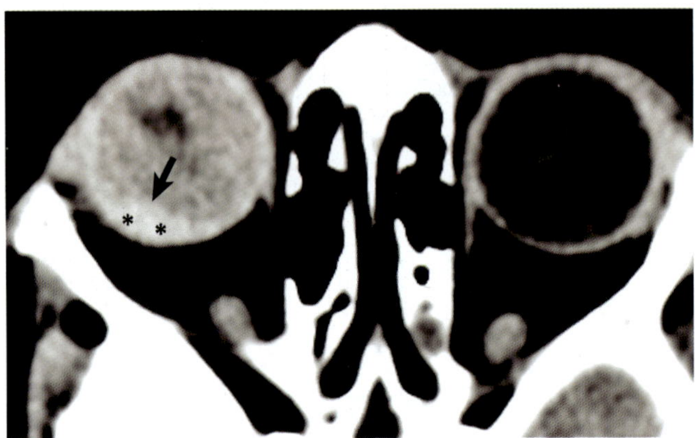

Figure 81.13 Coats disease. Axial contrast-enhanced CT of the orbit in a 6-year-old patient reveals intraocular high attenuation soft tissue presenting as a pseudomass (*asterisks*) along the posterior wall of right globe without any obvious calcifications. Note the associated retinal detachment (*arrow*).

traction to the ciliary process followed by retinal detachment. It clinically presents as unilateral/bilateral leukocoria affecting ventral or dorsal aspects of eyeball. USG reveals an echogenic band connecting optic nerve head with posterior surface of lens and Doppler identifies the arterial flow within. CT helps in assessing the proliferative ill-defined noncalcified soft tissue in vitreous body caused by retinal detachment (Fig. 81.12). MRI reveals the triangular shape T2W hypointense band as seen on USG.

Differential diagnosis: Retinoblastoma, retinopathy of prematurity, coats disease (Fig. 81.13). (Coats disease is characterized by progressive retinal detachment induced by subretinal exudative collection and is seen on CT or MRI as enhancing granulation tissue along the posterior margin of the globe.)

Orbital Cellulitis

Orbital cellulitis is common in children (>50% are below 4 years of age). It occurs subsequent to ethmoid sinusitis, orbital trauma, or obstructed nasolacrimal duct. Classified as periorbital (preseptal location) and orbital (postseptal location) cellulitis.

Preseptal cellulitis presents with edematous eyelid, inflamed lacrimal apparatus, and ocular adnexa. CT shows discontinuity in lamina papyracea, enhancement of periorbital tissues, intraorbital fat stranding, and identifies subperiosteal abscess (SPA) (Fig. 81.14). Contrast-enhanced MRI helps evaluate the extent of the SPA, intracranial complications, cavernous sinus involvement which are facilitated by the valveless ethmoidal veins which facilitate spread of ethmoid infection through the thin lamina papyracea leading to orbital cellulitis, SPA formation and superior ophthalmic vein thrombosis. Thrombophlebitis of superior ophthalmic vein is a common complication and can lead to cavernous sinus thrombosis [19]. This can be associated with reactive inflammation of extraocular muscles (EOMs) leading to limited eye movements and lateral displacement of the medial rectus muscle. If untreated this can lead to severe acute to subacute proptosis and decreased vision. CECT and CE-MRI can also help in guiding drainage of SPA.

Chandler Classification of Orbital Cellulitis

I. Preseptal cellulitis: Inflammation anterior to orbital septum with eyelid edema, nontender, visual loss, or impaired EOM motility (ophthalmoplegia)
II. Orbital cellulitis without abscess: diffuse postseptal edema of orbital fat
III. Orbital cellulitis with SPA: Proptosis, impaired vision, or limited EOM motility
IV. Orbital cellulitis with intraorbital abscess: Usually severe proptosis, reduced vision, and limited EOM motility
V. Cavernous sinus thrombosis secondary to orbital phlebitis: Bilateral or unilateral

Differential diagnosis: Inflammatory pseudotumor, orbital neoplasm.

Inflammatory Pseudotumor

Uncommon inflammatory process in pediatric population (about 7–16%) arises from an idiopathic nongranulomatous inflammatory process with variable degree of fibrosis and infiltration of lymphocytic cells mostly involving lacrimal gland and EOM.

CECT or CE MRI reveals homogenous contrast enhancement of the involved intra/extraconal soft tissues and the EOM [20].

Acute Proptosis

Causes of acute proptosis include trauma, infection (periorbital and postseptal cellulitis), vascular malformations, and neoplasms (Fig. 81.15). Neurofibromatosis II, retinoblastomas, and acute

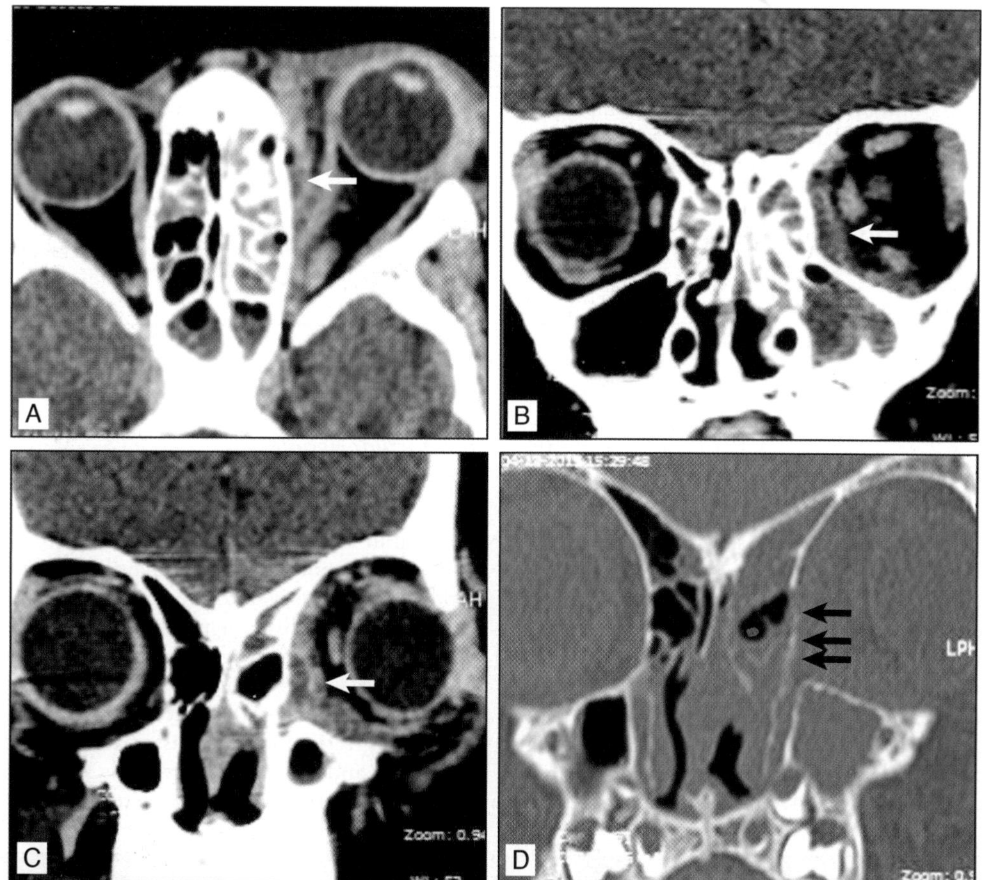

Figure 81.14 Orbital cellulitis with SPA. Axial (A) and coronal (B and C) images of the orbit show inflammatory changes in left ethmoid sinus and left orbit with a thin lenticular-shaped subperiosteal abscess (*white arrows*). Coronal CT image (D) in bone windows shows breach in the left lamina papyracea (*black arrows*) allowing spread of infection into the orbit (postseptal orbital cellulitis).

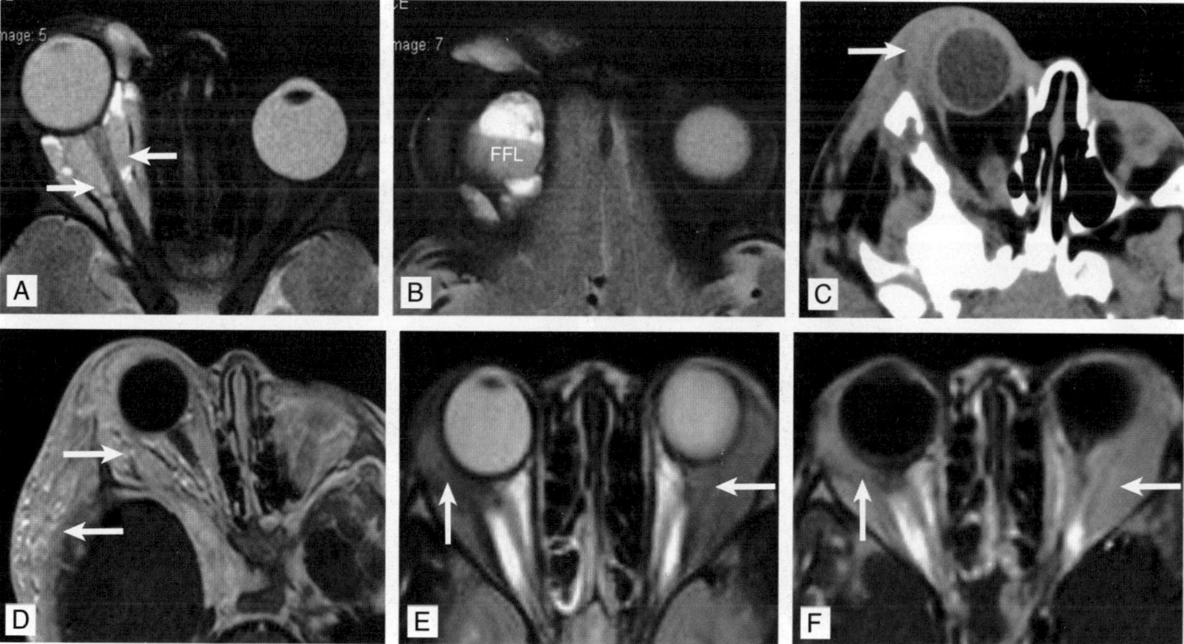

Figure 81.15 Spectrum of pathologies causing acute proptosis. Lymphatic malformation: Axial T2W FS (A and B) a 10-year-old girl with subacute to acute proptosis show a multiseptated retro-orbital intraconal lesion with fluid–fluid levels due to Hb breakdown products (FFL). Neurofibromatosis II: Axial CECT (C) of the orbit reveals mildly enhancing infiltrative plexiform neurofibroma on the right side (*arrows*). Insinuating around the structures of the superior orbit and into the temporal soft tissues. Acute myeloid leukemia (Type M3): Axial T2W (E) and contrast-enhanced image T1W FS (D, F) show smooth, homogenous T2W hypointense enhancing lesions in the intraconal and extraconal compartments of both orbits (*arrows*) due to acute infiltration caused by the myeloid tissue. (Courtesy: Dr. Anand Rahalkar, Pune India.)

lymphoblastic leukemia may also cause unilateral or bilateral acute proptosis in children [21]. Contrast-enhanced CT and MRI helps to assess the degree and extent of inflammation, abscess formation, the involvement of the intra/extraconal structures, compressive effect on structures in optic canal and ophthalmic fissures as well as presence of any intracranial vascular complications.

Orbital Neoplasms and Other Masses

Orbital tumors in the pediatric age group are mostly benign in nature, however, intraorbital masses need immediate attention to avoid irreversible deterioration in vision.

Dermoid Cysts and Epidermoid Inclusion Cysts

Dermoid Cysts (DCs) present mainly along embryonic fusion lines and consist of epithelium-lined cavities filled with skin appendage elements such as hair, fat, and sebaceous glands. Epidermoid cysts (ECs) consist of epithelial elements only and present as a cystic fluid-filled mass. ECs are slow growing, painless orbital lesions along frontozygomatic suture. Presentation depends on the location and vector of growth (outward or inward). These are soft fluctuant masses, generally not affecting vision, but may hinder the EOM movement. EC and DC are most commonly situated in the orbit (50%), however also occur in the floor of mouth (23%), neck (14%), and nose (13%), anterior midline neck, submandibular space, and sinonasal region.

Imaging Features: USG identifies the echo pattern and intrinsic vascularity of superficial DC (Fig. 81.16). CT demonstrates any sudden increase in the size, fat content, calcification, bony changes. EC shows uniform echogenicity with midlevel internal echoes and posterior acoustic enhancement if cystic. DCs show a more complex appearance due to associated lipomatous and calcific components. Cross-sectional imaging shows that DC to have heterogenous intensity due to the presence of fat and/or calcification). EC appear as hypodense lesions with predominantly cystic appearance. EC show diffusion restriction on MRI, and both lesions may show minimal peripheral marginal enhancement. These lesions may remodel the adjacent bony structures. Contrast-enhanced MRI is useful to identify intracranial extension and rare complications which may include meningitis or abscess.

Intraocular Neoplasms

Retinoblastoma (RB) is the most common intraocular neoplasm below 3 years of age. They are unilateral in 60% and bilateral in 40% of cases [22]. Retinoblastoma may be familial and may present earlier. RB may be bilateral or, "trilateral" (additional primary midline pineal tumor), and "quadrilateral" (second midline or paramidline sellar/parasellar tumor) variants due to embryogenic neuroectodermal origin. Nonfamilial cases usually present later and are often unilateral. White eye (leukocoria) is the most striking clinical sign for diagnosing retinoblastoma, associated with decreased vision, proptosis, and redness. Ultrasounds shows a posterior chamber lobulated calcified masses, heterogeneous in echo pattern,

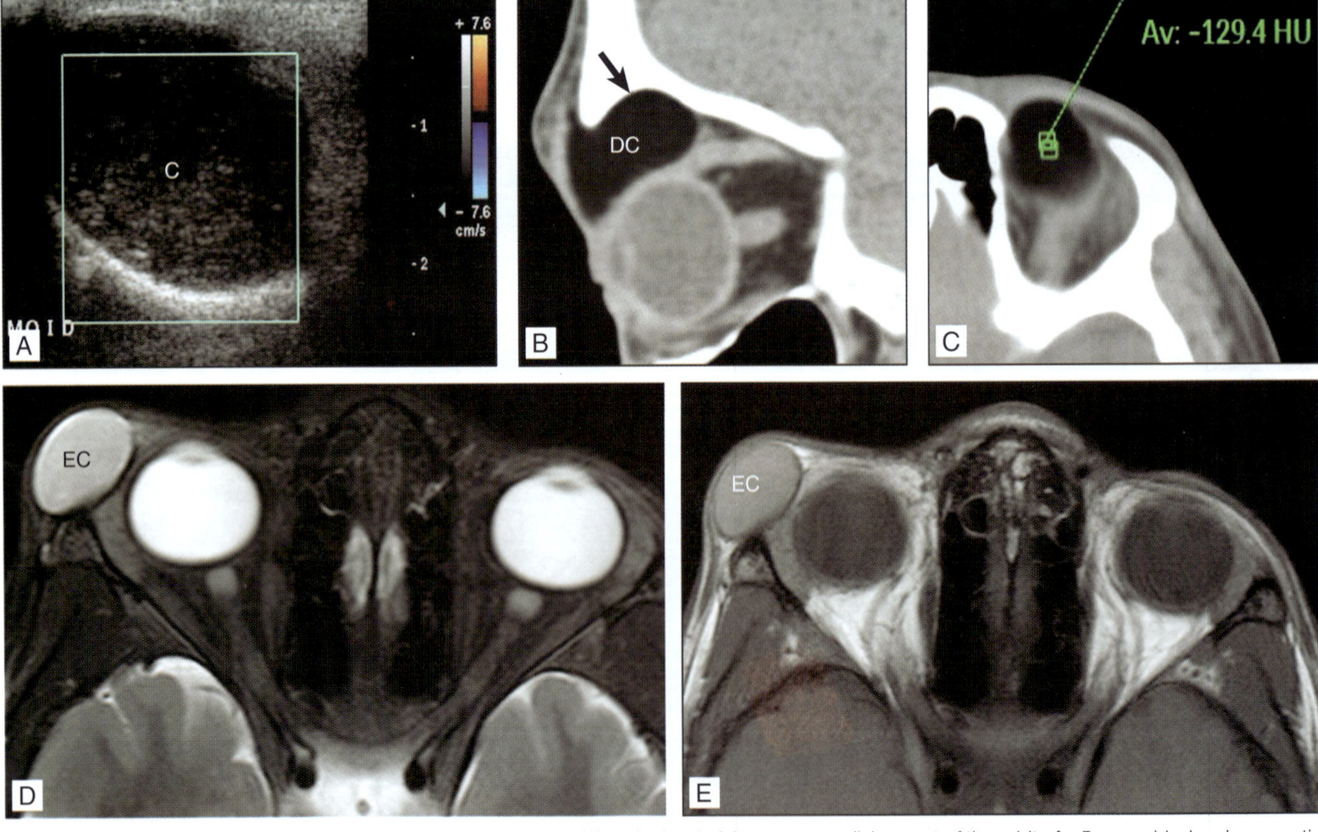

Figure 81.16 Dermoid cyst. Transverse ultrasound Doppler image (A) at the level of the superomedial aspect of the orbit of a 5-year-old, showing a cystic mass lesion (C) with midlevel internal echoes and absent internal vascularity. Sagittal (B) and axial (C) CT images of the orbit reveal the extraconal fat-containing dermoid cyst (DC) with mass effect on the globe. Note smooth scalloping and remodeling of the orbit roof (*arrows*). Epidermoid cyst. Axial T2W FS (D) and T1W (E) images show a well-defined ovoid mass lesion (EC) in the superior and lateral aspect of the right orbit, in relation to the frontozygomatic suture of the right orbit. (Images of epidermoid cyst courtesy: Dr. Foram Gala, Mumbai, India.)

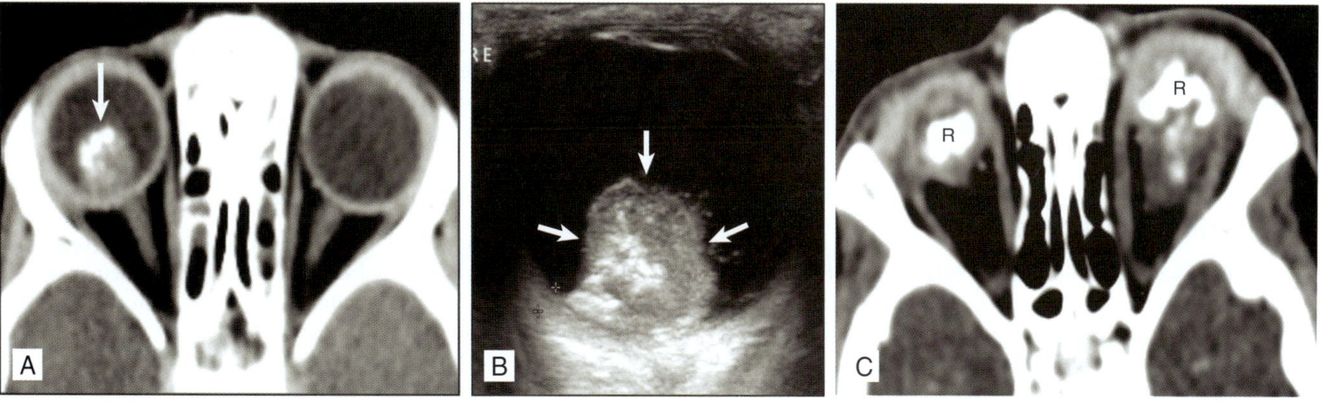

Figure 81.17 Retinoblastoma. Axial noncontrast CT image (A) shows a densely calcified intraocular mass in the center of the posterior chamber (*arrows*) indicating endophytic growth pattern of the retinoblastoma. Transverse ultrasound image of the orbit (B) demonstrates a polypoidal mass lesion in the posterior chamber (*arrows*) with irregular eccentric calcification. Axial noncontrast CT (C) shows bilateral intraocular retinoblastomas (R) in a 14-month-old child. Note the crumpled involuted globes on both sides with depletion of the vitreous material. On the left side the nodular partly calcified lesion tends to breach the posterior limits of the globe to encroach into the retrobulbar region along the course of the optic nerve (*arrows*). (CT image of bilateral retinoblastomas courtesy: Dr. Foram Gala, Mumbai, India.)

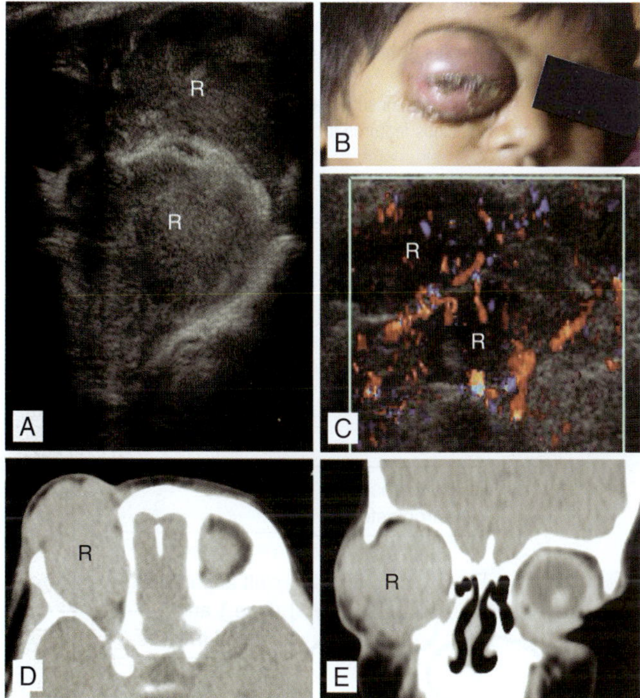

Figure 81.18 Retinoblastoma. Clinical photograph (B) of a 19-month-old girl child with an exophytic pattern of retinoblastoma involving the preseptal soft tissues of the right eye. Grayscale (A) and color Doppler (C) ultrasound of the same patient shows the aggressive, infiltrative nature of the solid tumor (R) distorting the morphology of the globe. Axial and coronal CT images (D, E) reveal significant intra- and extra-orbital spread of the tumor (R).

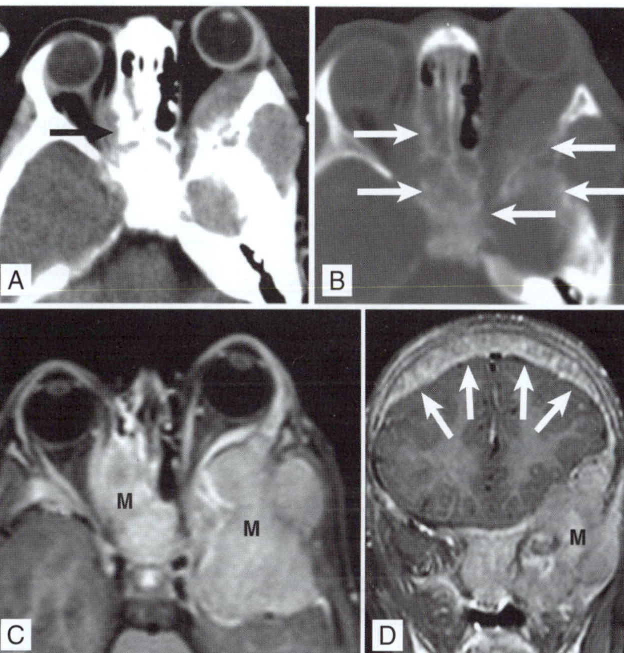

Figure 81.19 Metastatic neuroblastoma. Axial CECT image (A), bone window algorithm (B) shows classical permeative destruction with periosteal new bone formation (*arrows*) involving the left sphenoid bone and the cribriform plate. Note the encroachment into the contralateral orbit (*black arrow*). Axial T1W FS+C image (C) of the orbits shows large associated enhancing mass adjacent to the bone involvement (M) with resultant left side exophthalmos. Coronal T1W FSC image (D) shows the craniocaudal extension of the osseous metastatic deposit (M) with extensive calvarial deposits (*arrows*). (Courtesy: Department of Radiodiagnosis, BVMC, Pune, India.)

exhibiting posterior acoustic shadowing. Diffuse retinal thickening and micronodules are better visualized on USG. CECT and CE MRI show calcified intraocular masses, usually bilateral, in posterior chamber of the eyeball with variable degree of tumor calcification and moderately enhancing noncalcified tumors (Figs. 81.17 and 81.18). MRI is superior to CT for assessment of accompanying retinal detachment, optic nerve involvement as well as trilateral/quadrilateral pattern of disease. DW imaging reveals restriction due to cellular nature of this neoplasm.

Extraocular Neoplasms

Orbital NB metastases are often the only manifestation of the disease in patients below 2 years of age [23]. Tumor hemorrhage and ecchymosis result in acute proptosis in 8% of NB patients. CT reveals ill-defined hyperdense lesions along the posterolateral orbital wall with epidural neoplastic deposits that widen adjacent orbital sutures (Fig. 81.19). On MRI, NB deposits exhibit low T1W and inhomogeneous T2W signal intensity due to subtle intralesional hemorrhages or tissue necrosis. Contrast study reveals hypervascular lesions with nonenhancing foci due to intralesional hemorrhages. MIBG scans and PET-CT are useful in staging and disease monitoring.

Lacrimal Gland

Nasolacrimal Duct Mucocele

These can present as unilateral or bilateral, well-defined cystic masses along the medial can thus, due to obstruction of the distal duct by the Hasner membrane. The swelling usually presents very early (3–4 days after birth) and may undergo inflammation with cellulitis (dacryocystitis). CECT shows a thin imperceptible wall of nonenhancing cystic lesion unless infected. Chronic lesions scallop or remodel the bony margins. MRI can help differentiate the T2W hyperintense mucoceles from proximally situated lacrimal sacs.

Dacryocystitis

Obstruction to normal drainage of secretions from the lacrimal gland results in dacryocystocele formation. A superimposed infection is termed dacryocystitis with exacerbation of clinical symptoms. USG may reveal intracystic debris with perilesional vascularity. CT and MRI demonstrate heterogenous appearance with peripheral enhancement in the case of abscess formation.

Pediatric Neck Masses (Box 81.4)

Diagrammatic representation of the location of commonly encountered head, neck, and face lesions in the pediatric age group (Fig. 81.20).

Masses of Developmental Origin in Children

Common developmental masses in children include branchial cleft anomalies, thyroglossal duct cyst, congenital hemangioma, ectopic thyroid, vascular malformations, cervical thymic cyst, dermoid/epidermoid cyst, congenital muscular torticollis, neurenteric cyst, meningocele congenital midline cervical cleft, congenital cervical teratoma, epignathus, congenital benign granular cell tumor (epulis), hairy polyp (rare fat-containing lesion), and congenital goiter [24] (Box 81.5).

BOX 81.4 Approach to a Pediatric Neck Mass

- History: present at birth, accompanying pain/fever, any change in size over time.
- Examination: location, fixed/mobile, compressibility, texture (smooth or irregular), associated tenderness, raised temperature or erythema.
- USG and Doppler: initial technique of choice except in airway/infection-related emergencies.
- CT/MRI: in emergent situations/large mass with deep space extension/if the mass exhibits suspicious features for malignancy.

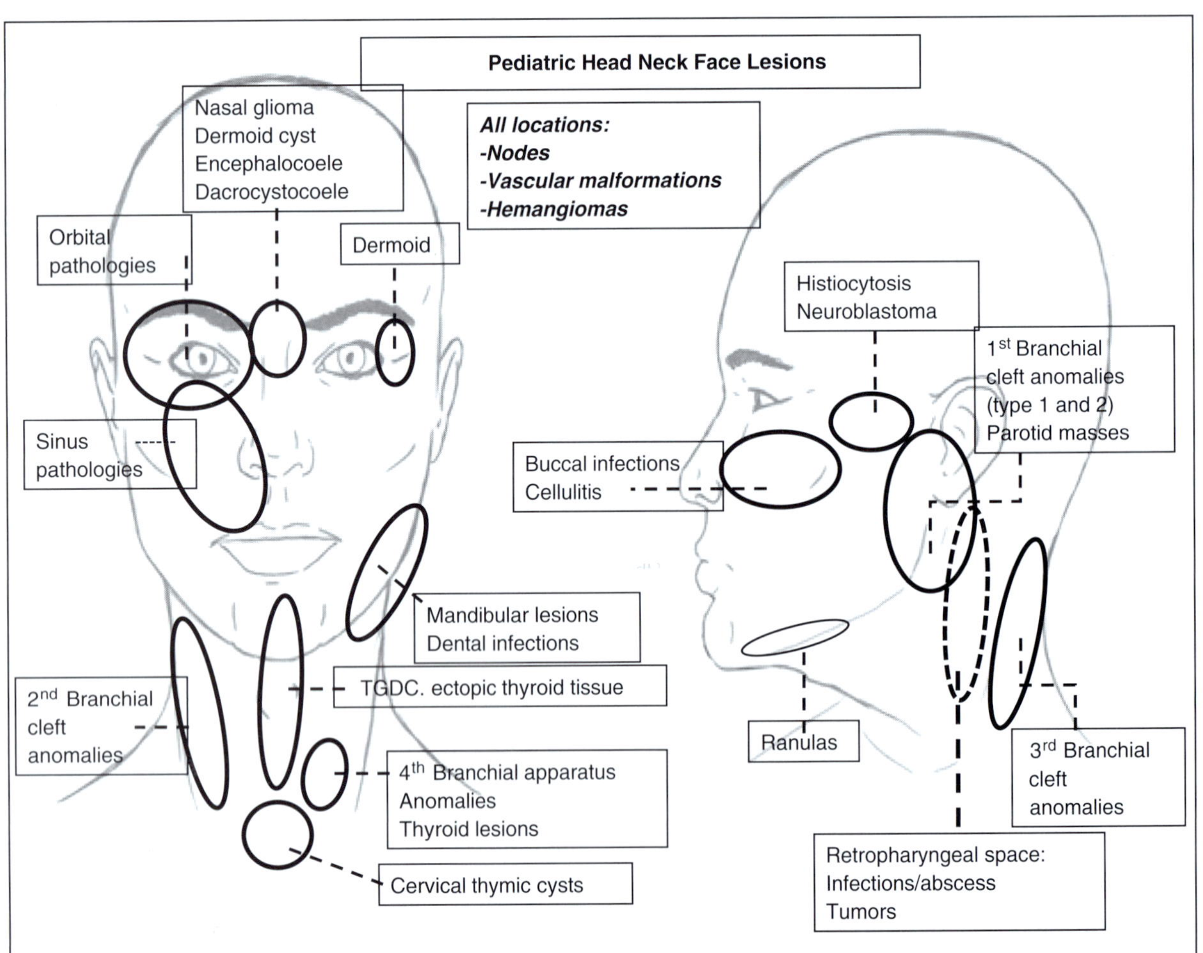

Figure 81.20 Diagrammatic representation of the location of commonly encountered head, neck, and face lesions in the pediatric age group. *TGDC*, thyroglossal duct cyst.

BOX 81.5 Key Features and Imaging Appearances of the Common Masses of Developmental Origin [25]

Branchial cleft anomalies (BCA)

Congenital malformations of the branchial apparatus (branchial arches, pharyngeal pouches, branchial grooves/membranes). Labeled as first, second, third, and fourth arch anomalies according to the pouch or cleft of origin and can present as fistulas, sinuses, and cysts.

Imaging:

1. *First BCAs* (Fig. 81.21):
   Can be cysts or sinuses and the location depends on the subtype:
   Work type I: periauricular.
   Work type II: periparotid in location.
   High index of suspicion in a patient with chronic, unexplained otorrhea or recurrent parotid gland abscesses. Surgery of the anomaly may be complicated in Wok Type II cases due to proximity to Cr Nv VII.
2. *Second BCAs* (Fig. 81.22):
   Can be cyst, sinus, or fistula.
   Typically seen as a cystic neck masses posterolateral to submandibular gland, lateral to carotid space, anterior (or anteromedial) to the sternocleidomastoid muscle.
   Bailey classification:
   Type I–IV (Type II: Most common, cystic remnant of cervical sinus of His) based on superficial to deep location from the subplatysmal soft tissues to the lateral pharyngeal wall.
   The second peak in demographics occurs in second or third decade: Consider a cystic metastatic squamous cell carcinoma node as a differential diagnosis in adults.
3. *Third BCAs* (Fig. 81.23):
   Can be cyst, sinus or fistula
   An ovoid/round cystic mass in the upper posterior cervical space/lower anterior neck.
   Less common in the pediatric age group.
   High index of suspicion if recurrent abscess in posterior neck.
4. *Fourth BCAs* (Fig. 81.24):
   Most are sinus tracts and fistulas coursing from the apex of the pyriform sinus to the upper aspect of the left thyroid lobe.
   Fourth BCAs will always be located in the left lower neck within or in close proximity to the left thyroid lobe.
   High index of suspicion if there are recurrent left-sided neck abscesses in children or recurrent focal thyroiditis/suppurative thyroiditis on the left side.

Thyroglossal duct cyst (TDC)

Most common congenital pediatric neck mass due to failure of involution of the thyroglossal duct (which extends from the foramen cecum at the base of the tongue to the pyramidal lobe of the thyroid gland).

Location: 50% at the level of the hyoid bone and the remaining 50% in the suprahyoid and infrahyoid region each. Suprahyoid/hyoid TDCs tend to be in the midline while the infrahyoid TDCs are mostly paramedian. The tract can have a small outpouching that hooks inferior and posterior to the hyoid bone.

Imaging (Fig. 81.25):

Goal: Confirm the presence of normal thyroid/ectopic thyroid tissue before planning surgery. Important to evaluate the posterior hyoid space [26] before surgery for complete resection of the central hyoid bone/abnormal tissue—additional component to the "Modified Sistrunk procedure" (the standard treatment for the TDC). Identify enhancing soft tissue/chunky nodular calcifications which could indicate a papillary carcinoma (seen in less than 1% of cases).

Findings:

USG: well-marginated hypo-anechoic oval/rounded lesion with posterior enhancement in relation to the hyoid bone in the anterior neck. Internal echoes indicate previous infections/hemorrhage/inspissated material high in protein content. CT/MRI: TDC may show peripheral enhancement after contrast administration if associated inflammation/infection or a high precontrast T1W signal due to high proteinaceous content.

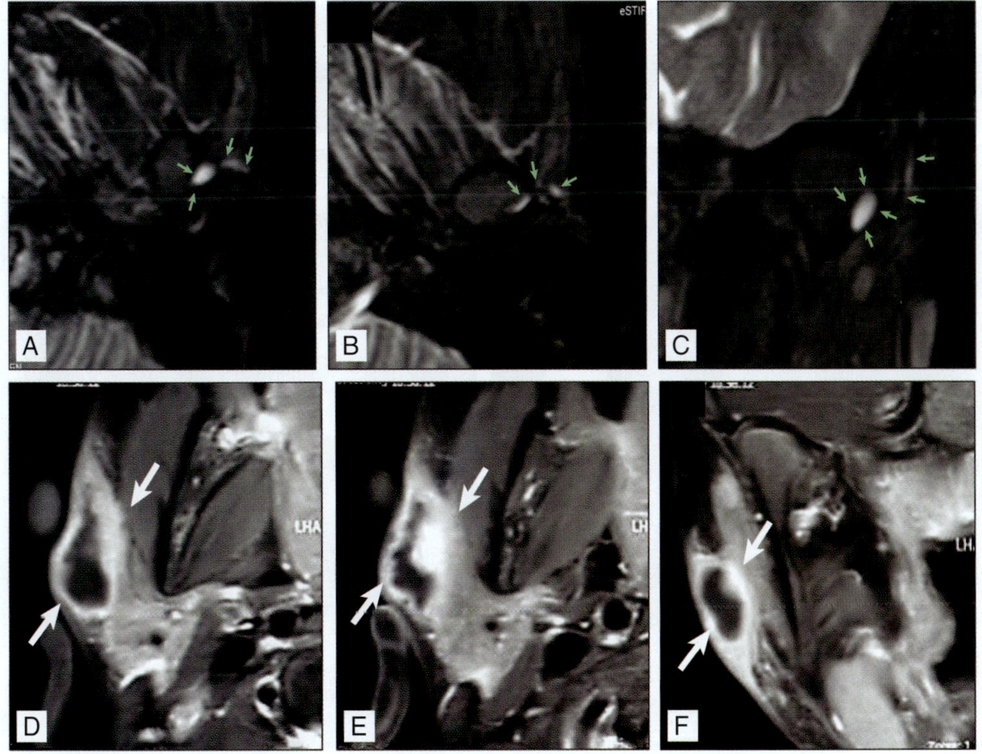

Figure 81.21 First BCA: STIR axial (A and B) and coronal (C) images show tubular hyperintense structure coursing parallel to the left external auditory canal (*small green arrows*) representing sinus tract of Work type I first BCA within the preauricular soft tissues. Postcontrast FS axial (D and E) and coronal (F) images show peripherally enhancing lesion in the right periparotid soft tissues (*arrows*) representing infected Work type II first BCA.

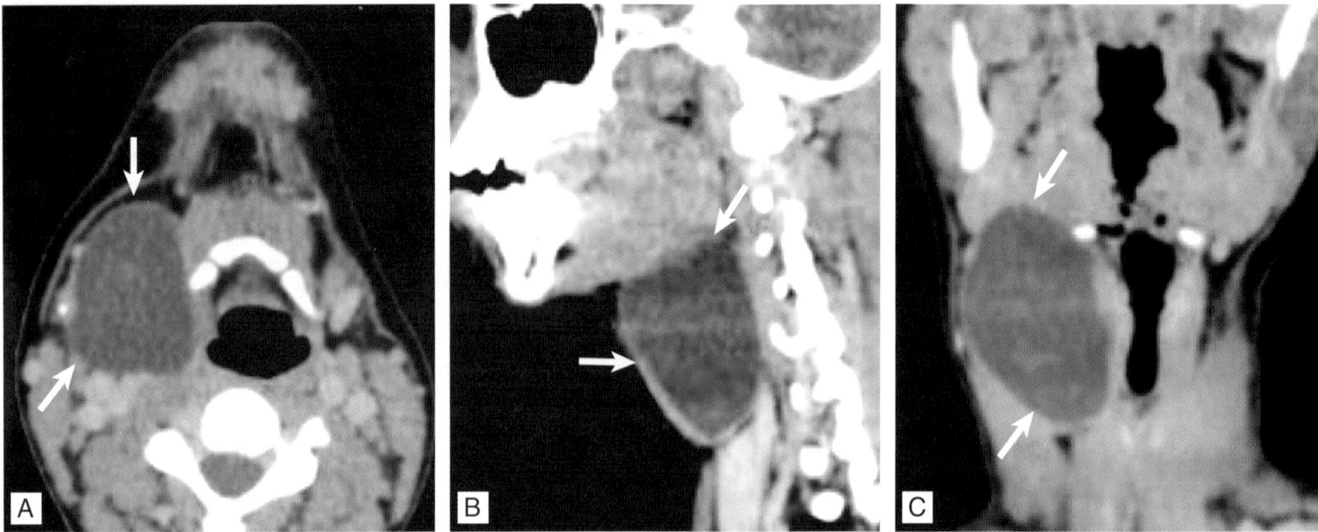

Figure 81.22 Second BCA: Postcontrast axial (A), coronal (B), and sagittal (C) CT images show well-defined nonenhancing cystic lesion (*arrows*) in the infrahyoid neck on the right side inferior to the right submandibular gland (SMG) and anterior to the right sternocleidomastoid muscle (SCM) representing Bailey's type II second BCA.

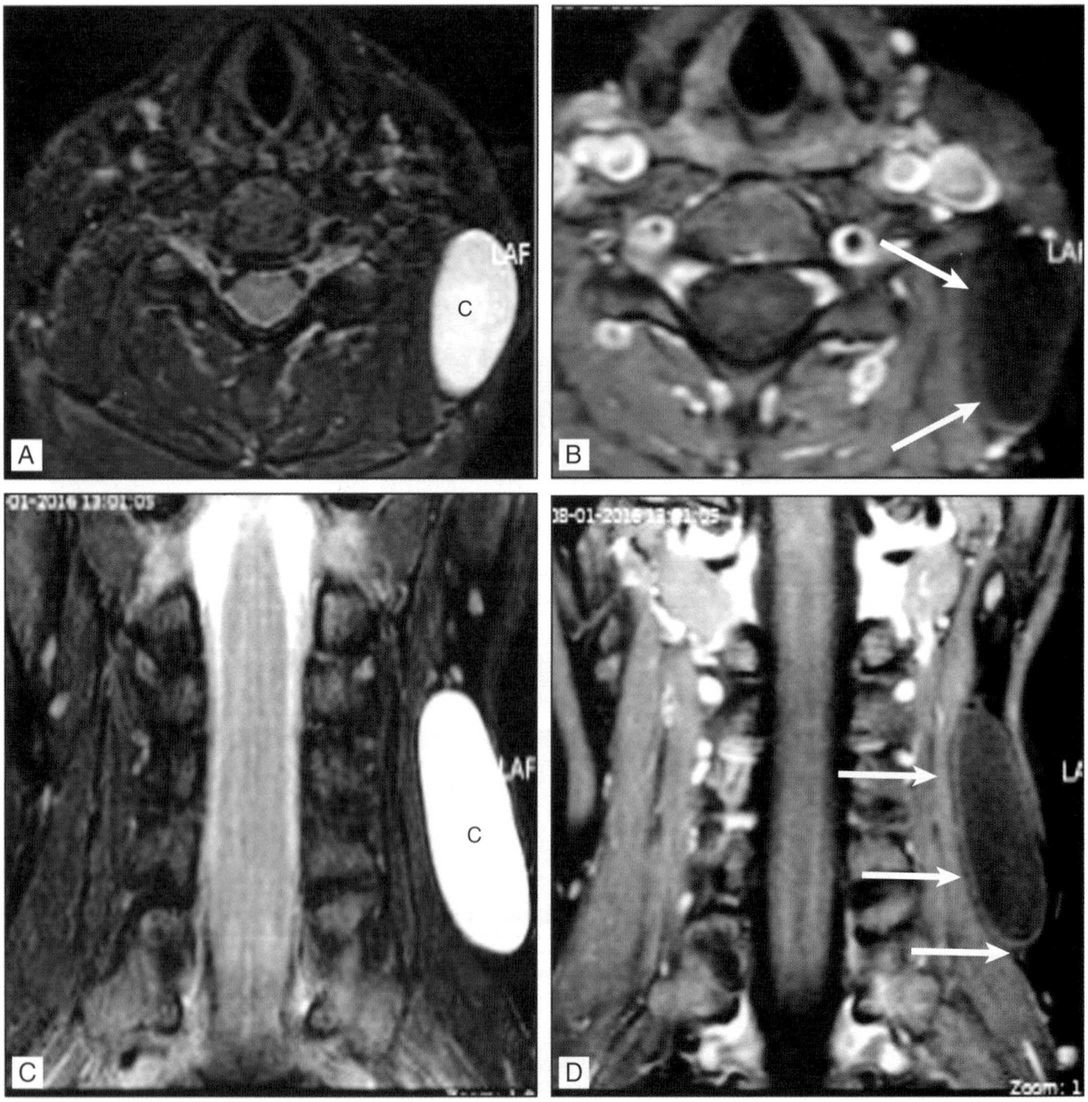

Figure 81.23 Third BCA: STIR axial (A) and coronal (C) images show well-defined tubular cystic hyperintense lesion (c) in the left posterior cervical space with thin marginal rim enhancement on postcontrast FS axial (B) and coronal (D) images (*arrows*).

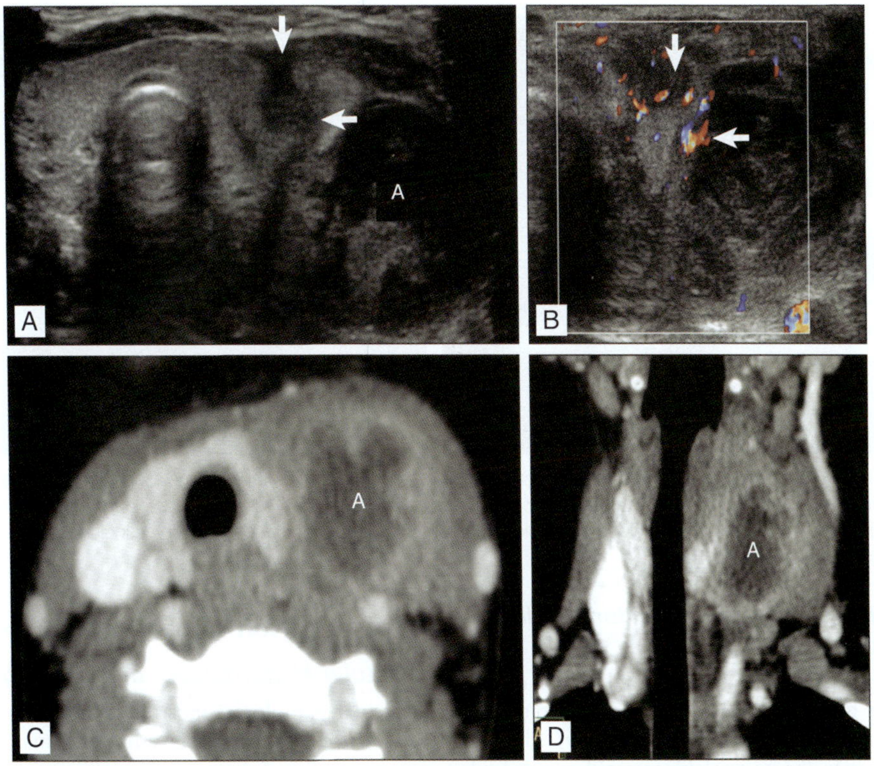

Figure 81.24 Fourth BCA: Transverse grayscale (A) image of the neck demonstrates irregular margins of left thyroid lobe with peripherally located hypoechoic lesions (*arrows*) representing focal thyroiditis. A large heterogenous mixed echoic complex lesion is seen abutting the left lobe (A) with scattered peripheral increased vascularity (*arrows*) on color Doppler (B). Postcontrast axial (C) and coronal (D) CT images show large well-defined enhancing lesion with focal areas of liquefaction (A) representing an abscess formation.

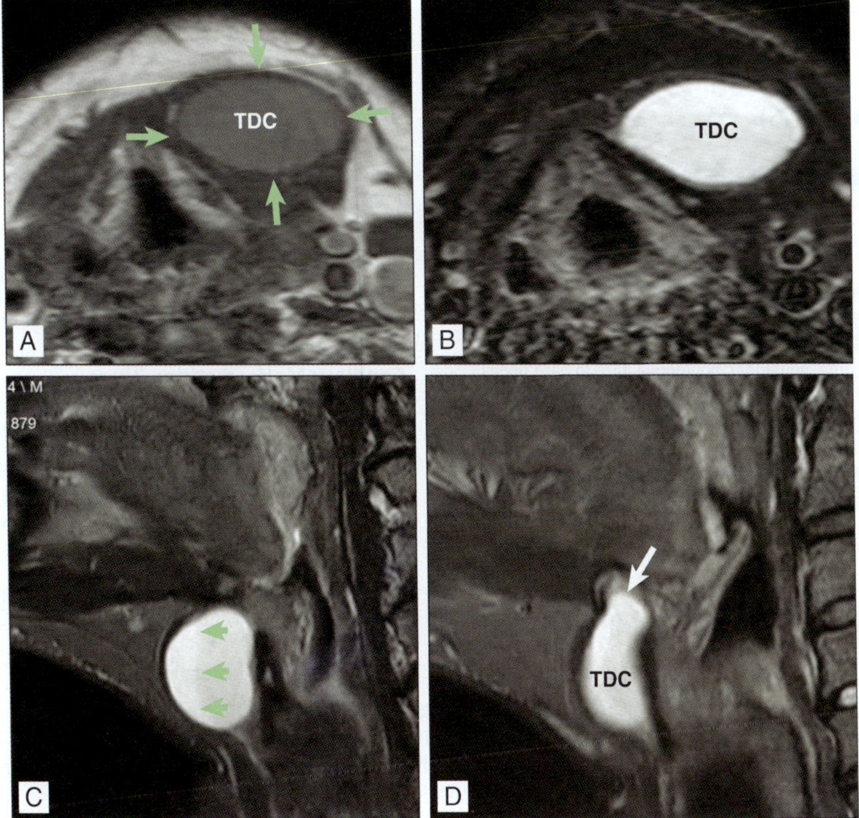

Figure 81.25 Thyroglossal duct cyst (TDC): T1W axial (A), STIR axial (B), and STIR sagittal (C, D) images show a well-defined oval-shaped infrahyoid cystic lesion (TDC) embedded in the left strap muscles with focal extension into the posterior hyoid space (*white arrow* in D). High T1W signal represents increased proteinaceous content of the fluid and *green arrows* in C show contained fluid level.

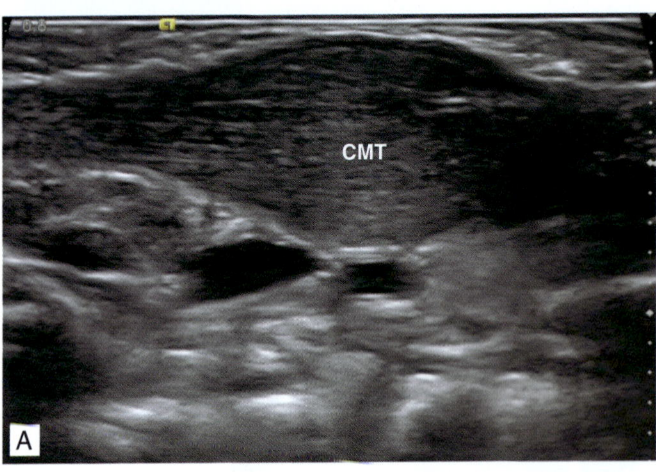

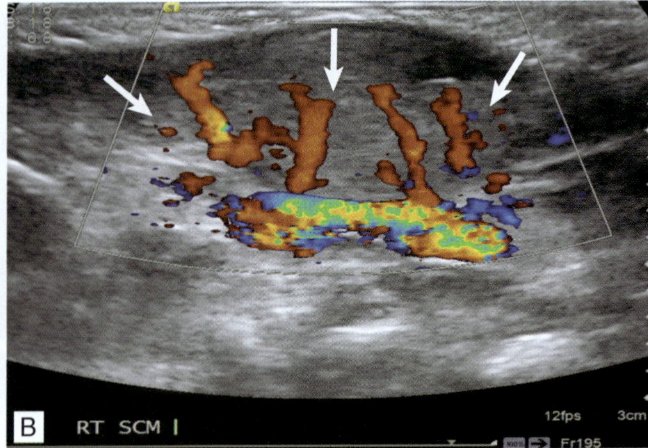

Figure 81.26 Congenital muscular torticollis. Longitudinal grayscale image of the neck (A) parallel to the longitudinal axis of the sternocleidomastoid muscle reveals diffuse fusiform thickening of the belly of the sternocleidomastoid muscle (CMT). Dynamic ultrasound revealed synchronous movement of the focal thickening with the normal uninvolved muscle fibers. Color Doppler (B) revealed increased intrinsic vascularity with a high resistance waveform (*arrows*). (Courtesy: Dr. Asif Momin, Mumbai, India.)

Congenital Muscular Torticollis (Sternocleidomastoid Pseudotumor of Infancy)

A congenital fibrotic process, generally unilateral (more on the right side and seen more in male babies) seen as a sequel to trauma during birth (breech presentation/forceps delivery) due to obstructed venous outflow in the sternocleidomastoid muscle leading to necrosis and fibrosis in the muscle fibers. Ultrasound shows fusiform enlargement and secondary shortening of the sternocleidomastoid muscle leading to torticollis (Fig. 81.26). Echogenicity may vary depending on the presence/absence of calcification. MRI shows a well-defined signal alteration within the normal muscle with increased signal on both T1 weighted and T2 sequences.

Masses of Lymph Nodal Origin in Children (Box 81.6 and Table 81.6)

BOX 81.6 Key Points

1. Up to 90% of healthy children in the age group of 4–8 years have palpable cervical nodes.
2. Assess the duration of the lymphadenopathy: acute (<2 weeks), subacute (2–6 weeks), and chronic (>6 weeks). Acute: likely reactive/infectious causes. Chronic: likely neoplastic or metabolic causes.
3. Indications for imaging: Large, nontender, nonmobile, firm to hard nodes. No response to empirical treatment with antibiotics (4–6 weeks course)/ increasing size and number of nodes. Accompanied by systemic symptoms.
4. Technique: USG/Doppler. Other techniques like CT, MRI, and PET-CT may be used depending on the clinical picture, information required for further management, and the appropriateness criteria (ACR).

Masses of Non-Nodal Origin in Children (Table 81.7)

Vascular Malformations and Hemangiomas

Vascular pathologies must be identified accurately as the diagnosis, further natural progression and management differs significantly in this diverse group of diseases. Vascular malformations differ from vasoproliferative lesions in that they do not exhibit mitosis and endothelial cell turnover and are endothelial cell glucose transporter 1 (GLUT1) isoform protein negative (International Society for the Study of Vascular Anomalies) [28].

Lymphatic Malformation: Lymphatic malformations (LM) are low flow malformations. The older terminology which should be avoided includes lymphangioma and cystic hygroma. May be unifocal or trans-spatial, unilocular or multilocular. Histologically, they may be microcystic or macrocystic. LM do not have a well-defined capsule and do not enhance unless infected or combined with a venous (venoLM [VLM]) or capillary (lymphocapillary) malformations. USG and MRI using short tau inversion recovery or fat-saturated T2W sequences are considered optimal to evaluate the internal fluid, fluid–fluid, or blood–fluid levels, and the extent of the lesion (Fig. 81.27). LVA may be associated with developmental venous anomaly and other intracranial vascular anomalies if located in periorbital location.

Capillary Malformation: There are two main types of capillary malformation. One is the classic “port-wine stain” associated with Sturge–Weber syndrome and the other is telangiectasia. The port-wine stain is the most common head and neck capillary malformation. These lesions are superficial and imaging is not routinely performed to evaluate these low flow vascular malformations unless there is concern for an associated intracranial anomaly.

TABLE 81.6 Causes of Abnormal Neck Nodes in Children [27]

Reactive/Infectious	Immunologic	Metabolic	Neoplastic
Viral: IM, HIV, CMV, HSV, rubella, varicella, measles Bacterial: Staphylococcal, tubercular and atypical nontubercular mycobacterial and Cat-scratch disease Fungal: Histoplasmosis/blastomycosis) Protozoal: Toxoplasmosis	Association with: Granulomatous disorders (sarcoidosis, Kimura disease) Rheumatoid disorders (SLE, JRA) Lymphoproliferative and histiocytic disorders (Kawasaki, Kikuchi-Fujimoto, Castleman disease, Rosai–Dorfman disease, Langerhans cell histiocytosis)	Storage disorders (amyloidosis, Gaucher's) Hypersensitivity to drugs	Lymphoma Leukemia Metastases

TABLE 81.7 Classification of Non-Nodal Masses

Vascular Pathology	Infections/ Inflammatory Pathology	Tumors and Tumor-Like Lesions
▪ Vascular malformations and hemangiomas ▪ Vasoproliferative disorders (lesions/ tumors of vascular origin) ▪ Jugular vein phlebectasia ▪ Lemierre syndrome	▪ Retropharyngeal and other neck space abscesses ▪ Abscesses in the neck secondary to mastoid infections ▪ Langerhans cell histiocytosis ▪ Acute/recurrent parotitis and parotid abscess ▪ Ranula	▪ Rhabdomyosarcomas and other sarcomas ▪ Leukemia and lymphoma ▪ Paragangliomas ▪ Dermoid and epidermoid cysts ▪ Lipomas ▪ Thyroid papillary carcinoma ▪ Parathyroid adenoma ▪ Neurogenic tumor

Venous Malformation: Venous malformations (VMs) are low flow malformation and were previously known as cavernous malformation and cavernous hemangioma. The characteristic finding of a pure VM is a well-defined lesion that involves the muscle and may be associated with phleboliths.

MRI using short tau inversion recovery or fat-saturated T2W is considered optimal to demonstrate the extent of the lesion, assess for skip lesions, and evaluate for airway involvement. Characteristically the lesions are very hyperintense on these sequences. Typical features include the presence of phleboliths, osseous remodeling in adjacent bone, and fat hypertrophy in adjacent soft tissues (Fig. 81.28). The degree of enhancement depends on the number and size of venous channels, the rate of venous blood flow within, and the presence of lymphatic tissue component (VLM) (Fig. 81.29). VMs and VLMs are easily differentiated from high-flow arteriovenous malformations using color Doppler, dynamic postcontrast CT, and MR imaging as well as DSA studies (Fig. 81.30).

Hemangioma

Congenital Hemangioma: The two subtypes include rapidly involuting congenital hemangioma, which involutes by 8–14 months and the noninvoluting congenital hemangioma. GLUT-1-negative status on immunohistochemistry differentiates this entity from the infantile hemangioma.

Infantile Hemangioma: Infantile hemangioma (capillary hemangioma) usually presents within 3 months of birth and with most resolving by 9 years of age. Two phases of development include the proliferative phase and the involuting phase. These hemangiomas are GLUT-1-positive on immunohistochemistry [26].

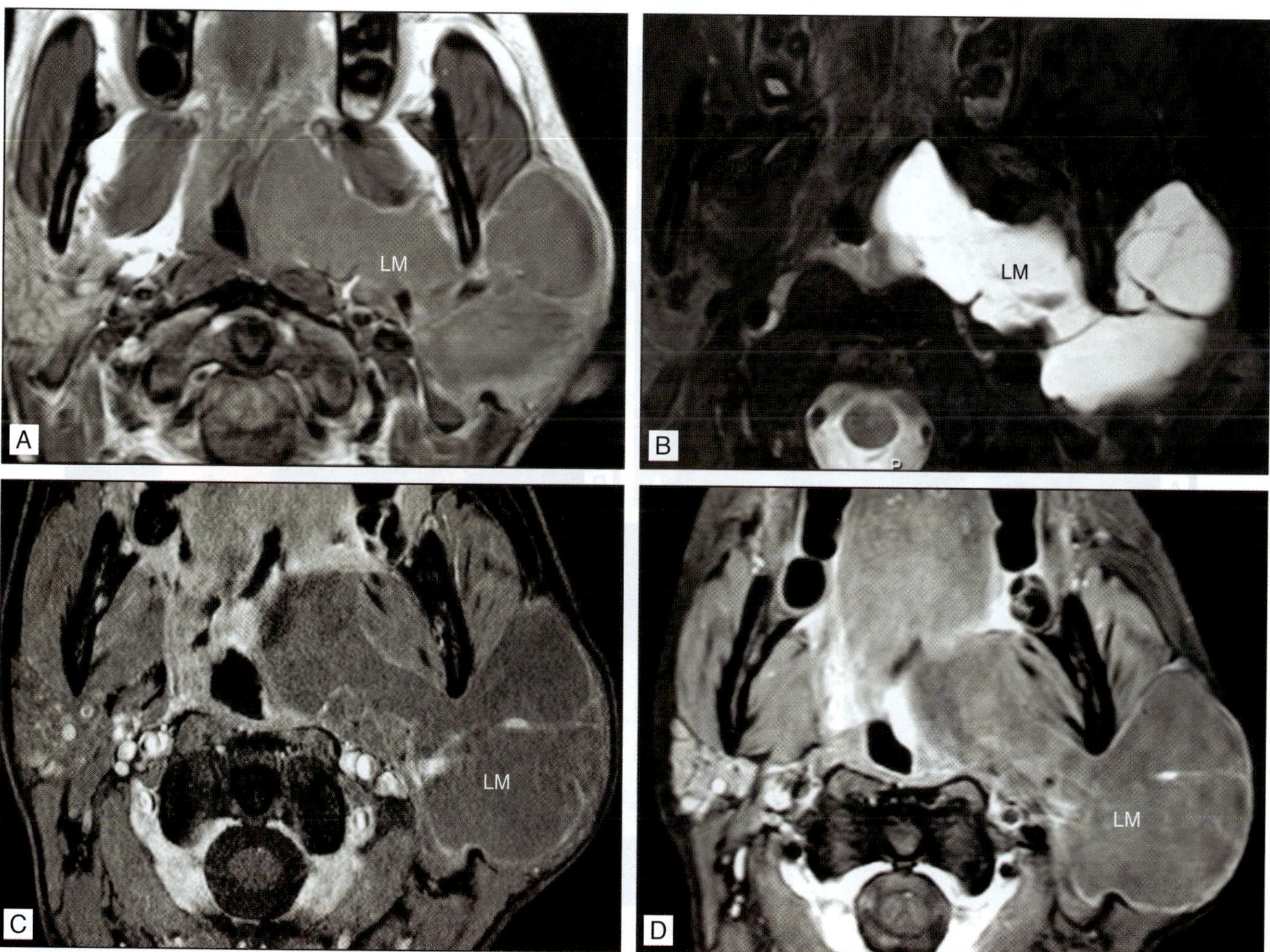

Figure 81.27 Lymphatic malformation (LM): T1W (A) and STIR (B) reveal a large LM involving entire left parotid gland (LM) conforming to the shape of the gland. Postcontrast FS axial (C and D) images show minimal enhancement of the margins and the thin internal septae.

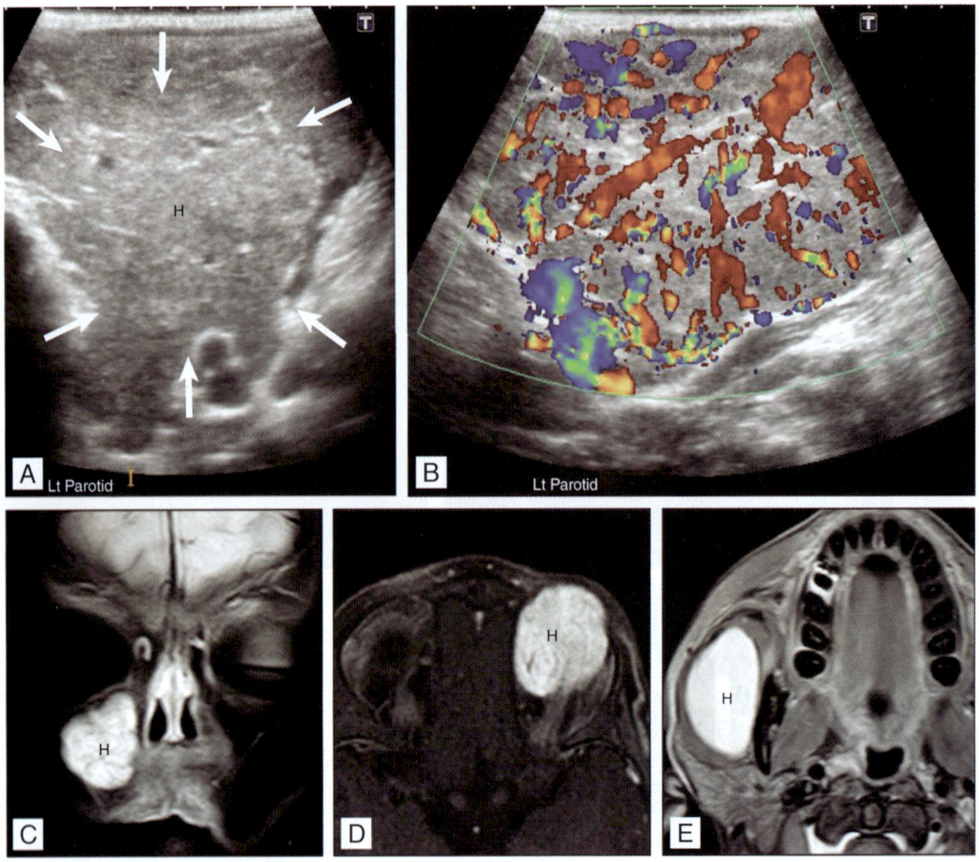

Figure 81.31 Hemangiomas at multiple sites: Transverse grayscale ultrasound (A) and longitudinal color Doppler image (B) shows a focal isohypoechoic appearance of a parotid gland hemangioma (H, *arrows*) with diffuse increase in the intrinsic vascularity. Right buccal space hemangioma (H) on coronal postcontrast FS MR (C). Left intraorbital hemangioma (H) on STIR axial MR (D). Right masticator space hemangioma (H) on axial postcontrast FS MR (E).

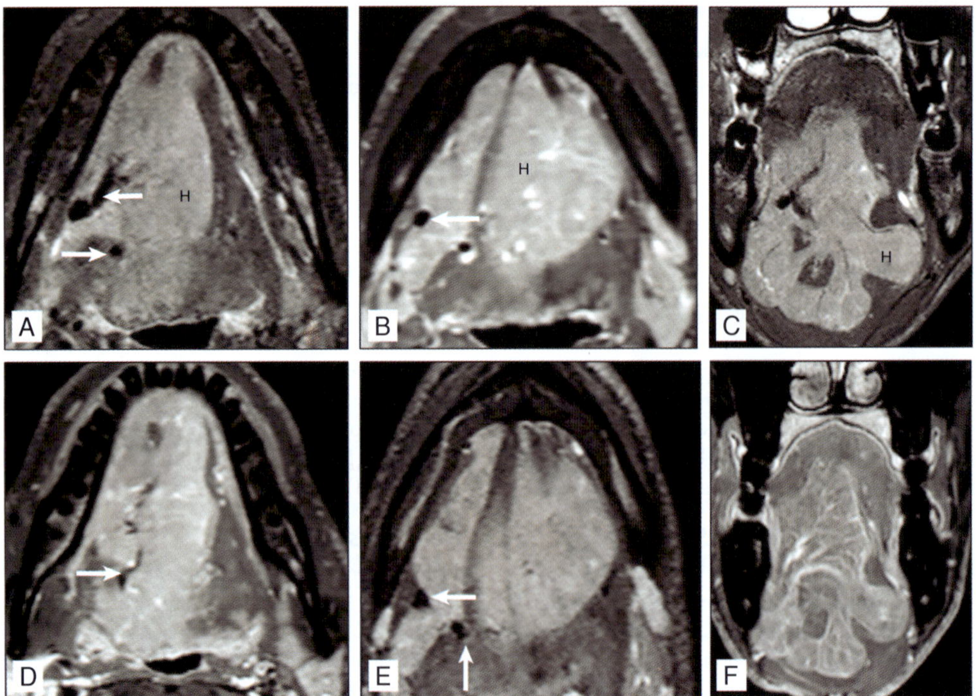

Figure 81.32 Hemangioma in oral cavity: STIR axial (A) and coronal (C) images and postcontrast FS axial (B) and coronal images (B, D, E & F) reveal a large hemangioma in the proliferative phase (H) with multiple intralesional enlarged vessels in image D and E (*arrows*), intense enhancement and infiltrating multiple oral cavity subsites.

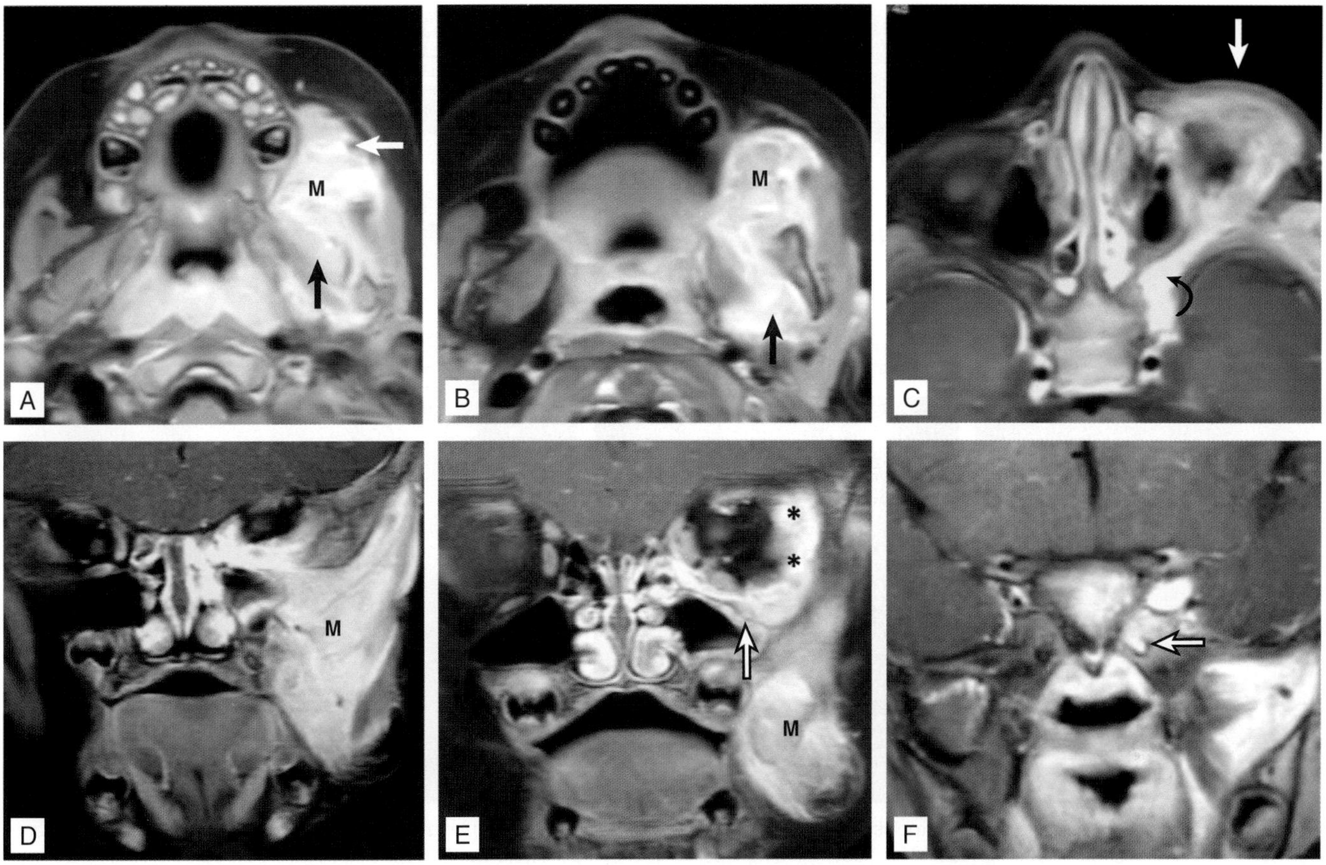

Figure 81.33 Soft-tissue sarcoma: Axial (A–C) and coronal (D–F) postcontrast FS MR images show a large infiltrative enhancing mass (M) in the left infra- and suprazygomatic masticator space (*vertical black arrows* in A and B) with intraorbital (*black asterisks* in E), left buccal space (*horizontal white arrow* in A) extension, and involvement of left-sided premaxillary soft tissues (*vertical white arrow* in C). Perineural spread is seen involving branches of the maxillary division of left trigeminal nerve (*curved black arrow* in C) with enhancing left infraorbital nerve (*vertical block arrow* in E), and left Vidian nerve (*horizontal block arrow* in F).

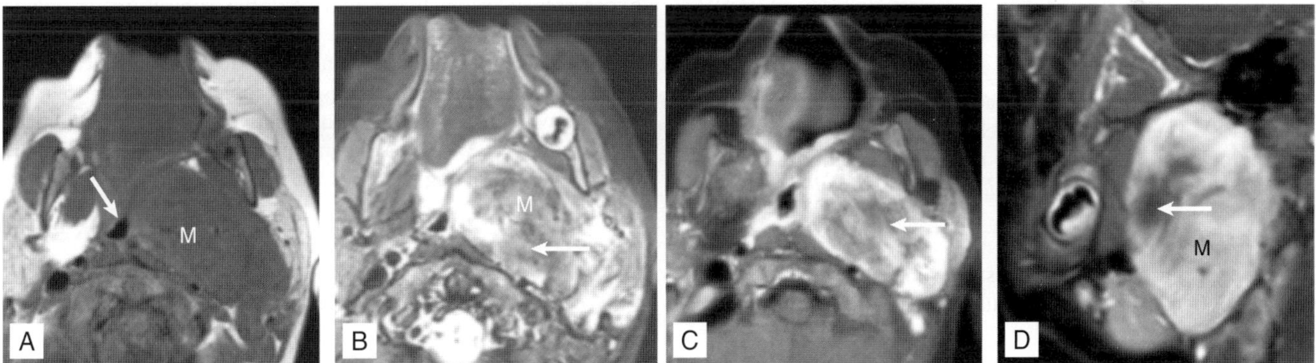

Figure 81.34 Infantile fibromatosis (desmoid type): Large lobulated left parapharyngeal space (*arrows*), causing marked indentation on the oropharynx and lateral oropharyngeal wall. It appears hypointense on T1W axial image (A), hyperintense on STIR axial image (B) with scattered hypointense components (*arrows*). Postcontrast FS axial and sagittal images (C–D) reveal dense heterogenous enhancement with large nonenhancing foci (*arrows*).

sheath with/without calcifications (Fig. 81.35). Metastatic cervical NB exhibit spiculated "hair on end" periosteal reaction in the orbit, skull base, temporal bone with associated enhancing soft-tissue mass. CT helps in bone evaluation and contrast-enhanced MRI identifies associated soft tissue, dural, and other intracranial pathology. Abdominal imaging (USG, CT, MRI) is essential to identify the primary pathology and is staged according to the International Neuroblastoma Staging System [29].

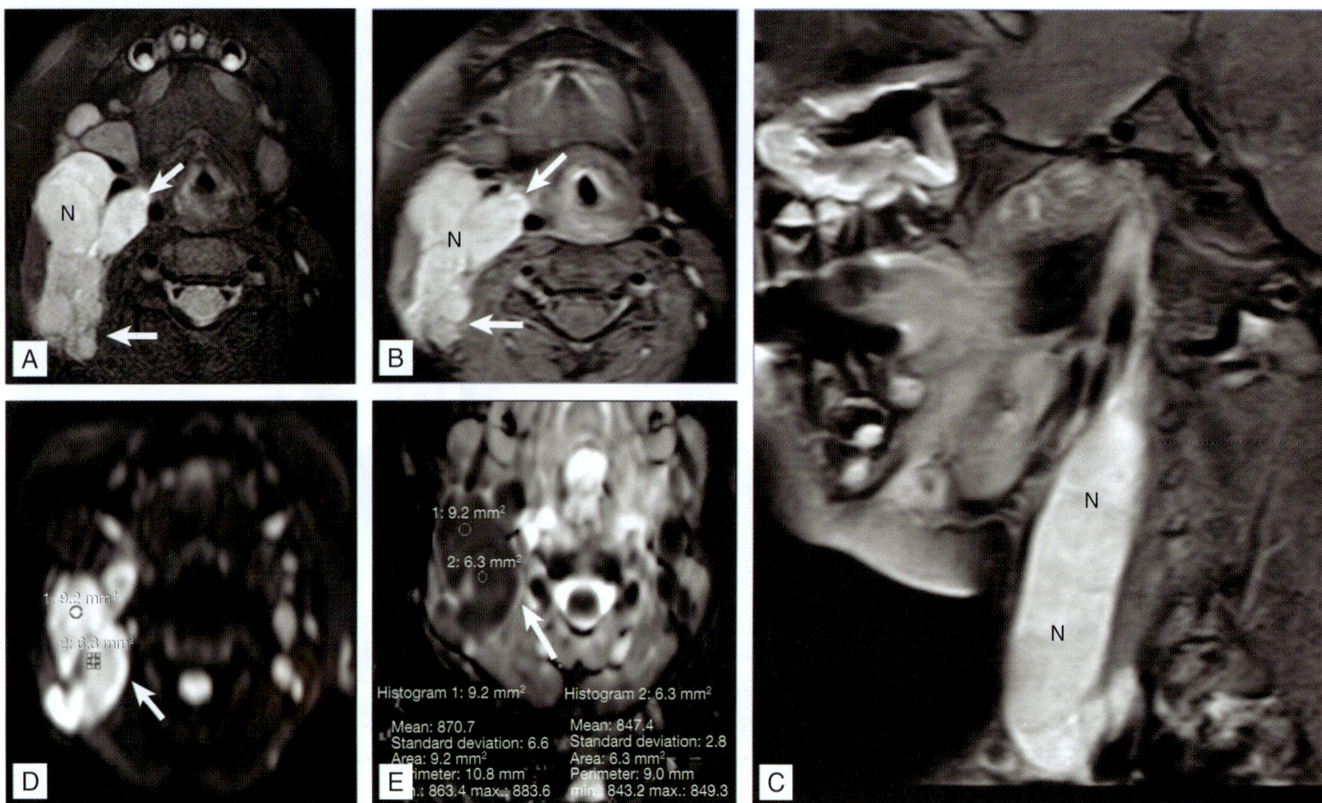

Figure 81.35 Cervical sympathetic chain neuroblastoma: STIR axial (A), postcontrast FS axial (B), and sagittal (C) images of a 2-year-old show a large well-defined tubular-shaped enhancing mass (N) infiltrating the right suprahyoid and infrahyoid carotid space insinuating between the vessels (*arrows*). Extensive bilateral multilevel reactive cervical lymphadenopathy is noted (*straight arrows*). The mass shows diffusion restriction (D) with hypointense appearance on ADC images (*arrows* in D and E) and low ADC values measuring 0.84–0.87 × 10^{-3} mm^2/s (E).

Imaging of Thyroid/Parathyroid and Salivary Glands

Thyroid Gland

Introduction

Most childhood thyroid disorders are treatable endocrine disorders (Table 81.8). The thyroid gland achieves adult size by 15 years of age. Thyroglossal duct cyst is one of the most common developmental anomalies in children (*see Developmental neck masses*).

Diffuse Thyroid Disease

Chronic Lymphocytic Thyroiditis: Autoimmune thyroid disease with lymphocytic infiltration results in endocrine abnormalities (Fig. 81.36) and may be associated with other autoimmune diseases, type I diabetes, Graves' disease [30], and neoplasms. On USG, the swollen thyroid gland is diffusely heterogeneous with hypervascular parenchyma and multiple subcentimeter hypoechoic nodules [31].

Painful Thyroid Gland: A painful, tender, asymmetrically enlarged thyroid gland can be caused by infection, leading to acute suppurative and subacute nonsuppurative thyroiditis (secondary to a fourth BCA). Ultrasonography detects the heterogeneous echogenicity, evolving focal abscesses [32], and inflammation in adjacent structures.

TABLE 81.8 Classification of Pediatric Thyroid Disorders

Infancy	Childhood and Adolescence
Congenital hypothyroidism Transient hypothyroidism Chronic lymphocytic thyroiditis Transient neonatal hyperthyroidism	Hypothyroidism: ■ Congenital ■ Acquired (dietary, postsurgical) Thyroiditis: Chronic lymphocytic thyroiditis, infiltrative (hemochromatosis, LCH) Hyperthyroidism: Graves' disease Infective: Acute or subacute thyroiditis

Ectopic Thyroid

Lingual thyroid accounts >90% of all ectopic thyroid tissue with female preponderance. It may cause dysphagia, dyspnea, and globus. Empty native thyroid bed is determined by USG neck and CECT or MRI can identify determine the presence of orthotopic thyroid tissue [33]. At times, ectopic thyroid tissue may be the only functioning tissue in the body (Fig. 81.37).

Parathyroid Gland

Parathyroid gland pathologies are uncommon in children. Familial causes include congenital absence of parathyroid gland or dysfunctional parathyroid gland. Multiple abnormal parathyroid glands may develop into single or multiple parathyroid adenomas. Adolescent primary hyperparathyroidism results from hyperplastic glands. Pediatric hypoparathyroidism is uncommon. A hypoechoic well-circumscribed lesion on sonography represents parathyroid adenoma. 4D CT determines the pattern of vascularity of these lesions in various phases of contrast enhancement [34]. An undetected ectopic parathyroid adenoma can be identified by a Tc-99m sestamibi scan.

Pediatric Salivary Glands

The salivary glands are best evaluated initially with ultrasonography. CT is useful in deep extension of salivary gland pathologies inaccessible to the USG probe. MRI additionally identifies perineural spread and skull base invasion. Conventional sialography has now been replaced by MR sialography (Table 81.9) [35].

Viral Sialadenitis

Mumps is a common cause for bilateral inflammation of parotid glands [36], submandibular, and sublingual glands being less commonly involved. USG reveals enlarged glands with diffuse heterogeneous echogenicity, entrapped secretions, and enlarged intraparotid nodes.

Juvenile Recurrent Parotitis

Juvenile recurrent parotitis is a commonly encountered nonobstructive, nonsuppurative parotid gland inflammatory disorder with

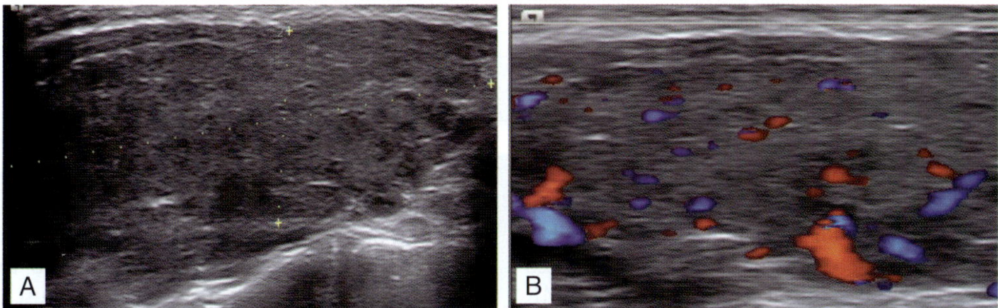

Figure 81.36 Chronic lymphocytic thyroiditis. Longitudinal grayscale ultrasound (A) reveals diffuse heterogenous mixed hypoechoic appearance of an enlarged thyroid gland with lobulated contour, numerous poorly defined hypoechoic foci with prominent intervening hyperechoic septae. Longitudinal color Doppler (B) examination reveals moderate increase in the intrinsic vascularity of the entire thyroid gland. Note: Important to exclude any dominant nodule that could have a potential to undergo malignant transformation. (Courtesy: Dr. Varsha Sarda, Nagpur, India.)

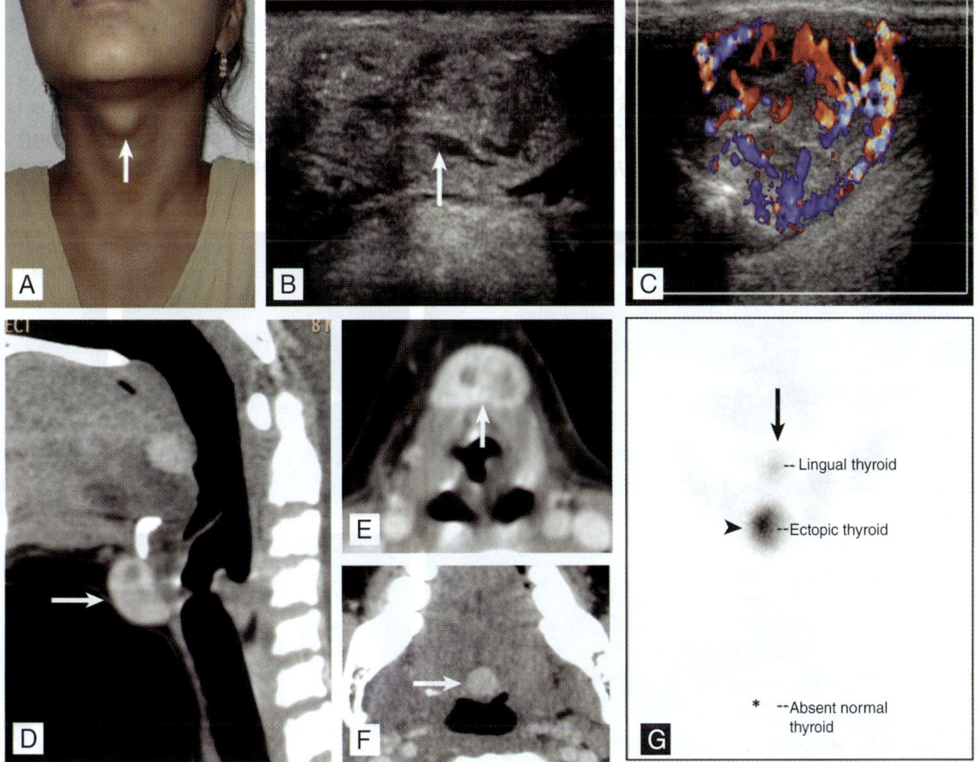

Figure 81.37 Dual ectopic thyroid: Clinical photograph (A) of a 14-year-old female with a midline neck swelling (*arrow*). Transverse grayscale ultrasound (B) and longitudinal color Doppler examination (C) reveal a lesion of heterogenous echogenicity with scattered hypoechoic foci (*arrow*) showing diffuse increase in the intrinsic vascularity. Postcontrast sagittal (D) and axial (E, F) images reveal a heterogeneously enhancing infrahyoid anterior midline lesion (*arrows* in D and E) representing ectopic thyroid tissue (within a likely thyroglossal duct cyst) and presence of a lingual thyroid (*arrow* in F). Technetium-99m pertechnetate thyroid scan (G) reveals uptake in the lingual thyroid (*arrow*) and ectopic thyroid tissue (*arrow head*) without any uptake within the normal thyroid bed (*asterisk*).

BOX 81.7 Differences Between Adult and Pediatric Upper Airway [40,41]

- The pediatric larynx is more anterior and superiorly located than the adult (epiglottis at C1 and inferior margin of the cricoids cartilage at C4 level).
- The infant larynx is one-third the size of the adult larynx with larger vocal processes of the arytenoids/larger cuneiform cartilages. Nasopharynx is narrower, and trachea is shorter in children with a larger tongue compared with the adjacent airway.
- More pliable cartilages/submucosal soft tissue/ligaments (conus elasticus): more prone to inflammatory edema and rapid airway obstruction.
- Infant larynx is omega-shaped, and the airway is narrowest at the level of the cricoid cartilage, unlike the adult larynx where the glottis is the narrowest portion.
- The lingual, palatine, and pharyngeal (adenoid) tonsils are more prominent in children leading to upper airway obstruction.
- Weaker intercostal muscles and diaphragms with narrower caliber of the trachea in children compared with adults predispose to rapid deterioration in respiratory function.

TABLE 81.10 Classification of Airway Obstructive Pathologies

Inflammatory	Neoplastic	Airway Foreign Body (AFB)
Croup, epiglottitis, exudative tracheitis, Relapsing polychondritis, Retropharyngeal cellulitis/abscess	*Intrinsic lesions:* Recurrent respiratory papillomatosis Laryngoceles Subglottic hemangiomas *Extrinsic compression by:* Lymph nodes, Bronchogenic/neurenteric cysts Neurogenic tumors (neuroblastoma) Sarcomas	*Partial or complete obstruction* *Type of foreign body:* Endogenous: mucus and bronchial casts Exogenous: food particles (peanuts, small plastic/metallic items

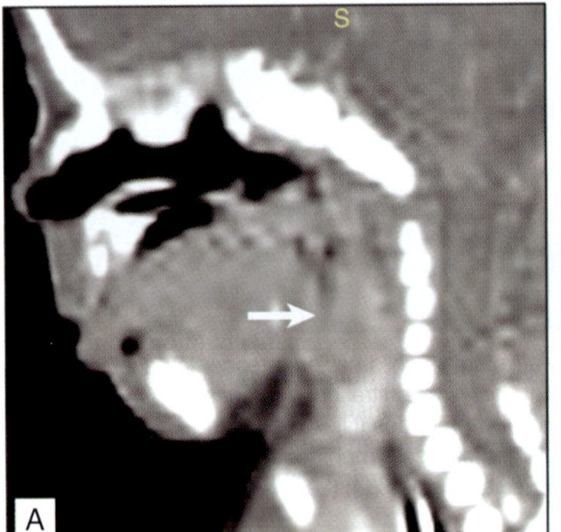

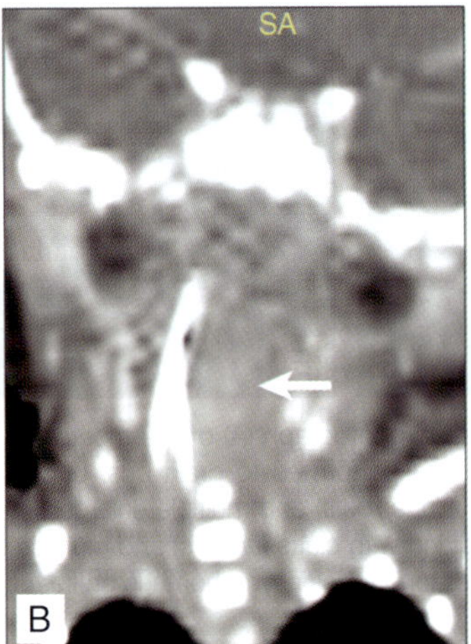

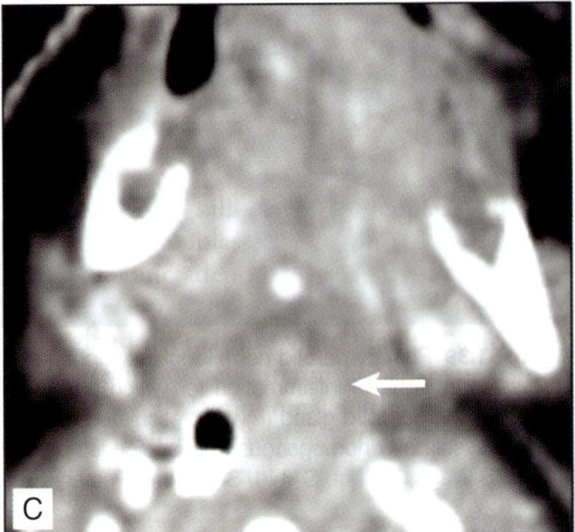

Figure 81.40 CHAOS: Sagittal (A), coronal (B), and axial (C) CECT images following intubation in an infant presenting with postnatal respiratory distress. Diffuse soft-tissue thickening (*arrows*) noted surrounding the obliterated and displaced cervical airway.

changes due to obstructive sleep apnea syndrome (OSA). This is seen as a result of soft-tissue hypertrophy around the upper airway: adenoidal/tonsillar hypertrophy, soft palate elongation/thickening, glossoptosis, and associated with generalized obesity. It is also seen as a result of specific craniofacial malformations and central neuromuscular disorders. Although the sleep study or the nocturnal polysomnography is the ideal test for diagnosing and grading the OSA, imaging does play a role in the assessment and management of this condition [44].

Lateral neck radiographs are useful in the evaluation of adenoidal and tonsillar hypertrophy causing airway narrowing. Thickness of the adenoid soft tissue can be measured on a lateral neck radiograph using a line drawn from the basiocciput to the maximum convexity of the adenoidal enlargement:

- Normal: 5–10 mm
- Mildly to moderately hypertrophied: 11–20 mm
- Severely hypertrophied: >20 mm

The adenoidal–nasopharyngeal ratio described in the earlier literature is no longer considered as a clinically useful parameter of airway obstruction. Soft-tissue shadows of the lingual and palatine tonsils can be observed indenting the airway on the lateral neck radiograph. However, no specific measurements are available as references. Video fluoroscopic studies are no longer considered useful in the work-up of OSA. Dynamic/cine MRI provides an accurate estimation of airway compromise during sleep state and additional useful information regarding the lateral pharyngeal walls' soft-tissue thickening at the level of the velopharynx that contributes to the airway narrowing. It also evaluates the degree of glossoptosis and airway compromise at the level of the base of the tongue and hyoid bone. It is especially useful to evaluate airway obstruction at multiple levels (Trisomy 21 and craniofacial anomalies). CT cephalometric measurements provide an estimation of craniofacial abnormalities, such as a low-placed hyoid bone in OSA cases and the presence of an elongated and thickened soft palate.

TABLE 81.11 Classification of Pediatric Emergencies

Inflammatory/Infective	Neoplastic	Other
Ludwig's angina Epiglottitis, laryngotracheobronchitis, pharyngotonsillitis, retropharyngeal abscess, acute sinusitis Orbital cellulitis Cervical lymphadenopathy Acute otitis/mastoiditis	Juvenile nasopharyngeal angiofibroma retinoblastoma	Foreign body aspiration traumatic; retinal hemorrhages due to child abuse Vascular malformations infantile fibromatosis

Pediatric Velopharyngeal Insufficiency

Velopharyngeal insufficiency occurs due to inadequate closure of the velopharynx and due to anatomical defects resulting in abnormal speech with typical nasal twang and inability to enunciate certain sounds [45]. Usually, it is diagnosed on physical examination, nasopharyngoscopy, and nasometry. Real-time phonation-linked cine MRI imaging helps to identify the type of velopharyngeal closure and structural and functional abnormalities of the levator veli palatini muscle. MR angiography can identify a medially buckled internal carotid artery at the level of the velopharynx.

Pediatric Head & Neck Emergencies

There are a variety of clinical indications for imaging a child in an emergency setting (Table 81.11), however, in most cases it is usually for symptoms of acute upper airway obstruction which is mostly as a result of acute infection or due to foreign body aspiration [46]. Imaging provides answers to the three critical questions in an emergency setting of upper airway obstruction:

1. Is there a mass obstructing in the airway?
2. Is there dynamic narrowing or a vascular compression of the airway?
3. Is there evidence of an infective etiology or associated vocal cord paralysis?

It is imperative to choose an imaging technique that can address the above questions as quickly as possible.

Vincent (Ludwig) Angina

A rapidly progressive trans-spatial necrotizing cellulitis of the upper neck soft tissues and oral cavity with potential to form multifocal abscesses compromising the airway and further spreading to deep/lower neck spaces and mediastinum. It is most commonly seen as a result of untreated odontogenic infection with patient typically presenting with throat pain and fever.

Contrast-enhanced CT is the technique of choice to assess the patency of the airway and to determine the source and extent of the abscesses/inflammatory edema (Fig. 81.41). It also helps in planning surgical approach to decompress the distended superficial and deep neck spaces.

Acute Tonsillitis and Adenoidal Hypertrophy

Enlarged tonsils and adenoid hypertrophy are treatable causes of airway obstruction in children and elective surgical procedures are undertaken for recurrent infections. Peritonsillar cellulitis, if untreated, can result in a tonsillar or peritonsillar abscess with patients typically presenting with fever and odynophagia. This is usually uncommon in children but can occur in an immune compromised patients. Peritonsillar inflammation and abscess may extend to the adjacent parapharyngeal or masticator space. Tonsillar and peritonsillar inflammation and infections occur as a result of beta-hemolytic streptococcal infection. Imaging is usually is not performed for uncomplicated cases being treated conservatively. Lateral neck soft-tissue radiograph is useful in assessing mass effect on the airway due to adenoidal hypertrophy. USG using an intraoral probe, CECT or CE-MRI is performed to assess unilateral or bilateral involvement and to identify the presence of an abscess. USG-guided abscess drainage may also be undertaken in co-operative patients.

Acute Epiglottitis

Epiglottitis is a potentially life-threatening condition in young children with edema of the epiglottis and aryepiglottic folds compromising the airway. Patients usually present with fever, stridor, and dysphagia. Lateral soft-tissue radiograph demonstrates a globular soft-tissue indentation on the air way of the pharynx. The "thumb-sign" (if seen) is a characteristic radiographic feature due to the edematous aryepiglottic folds and effaced glossoepiglottic space (Fig. 81.42). CT is indicated in cases of a diagnostic dilemma, to assist in emergent endoscopic assessment in restoring the airway and to evaluate other emergent neck conditions occurring concomitantly.

Acute Laryngotracheobronchitis

Infants usually present with low-grade fever, barking cough, stridor, hoarseness (elder children), secondary to a viral infection. Frontal soft-tissue radiograph shows widening of the hypopharynx with narrowed glottic region: the "steeple" sign or "inverted V" sign [47]. CT is indicated in cases of a diagnostic dilemma and shows the effaced airway of the larynx, trachea with symmetric straightening of the subglottic airway. CT can also identify foreign body impaction and a normal appearing epiglottis and aryepiglottic folds on cross-sectional imaging rules out possibility of clinical entities with similar presentations. Differential diagnosis: foreign body aspiration, epiglottitis.

Retropharyngeal Abscess

Affected children are usually acutely ill, febrile with neck pain. They have difficulty in swallowing, sore throat, drooling, stridor, and muffled voice. This is typically due to a bacterial infection of tonsils and pharynx, and less commonly, due to penetrating trauma. Patients initially have suppurative adenitis of the lateral

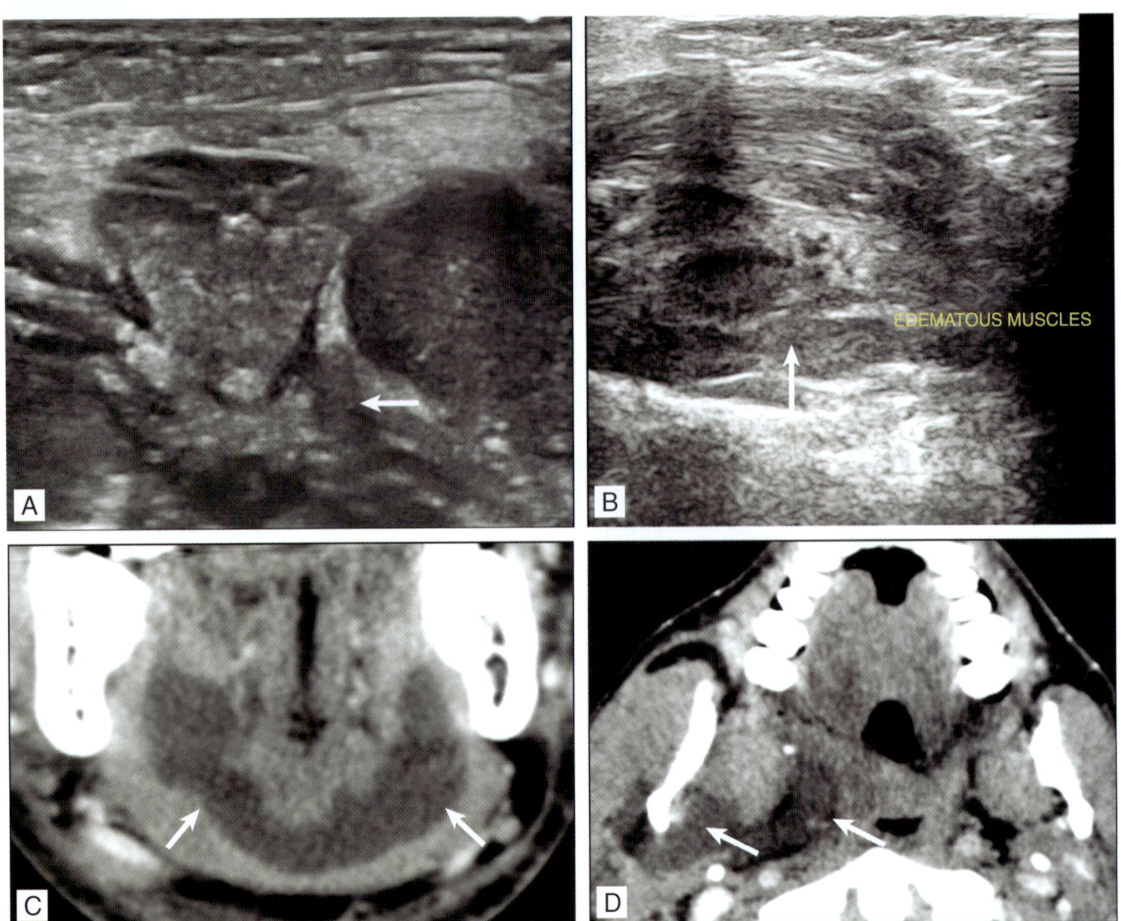

Figure 81.41 Vincent angina: Transverse (A) and longitudinal (B) grayscale ultrasound images reveal a well-circumscribed evolving abscess in the submandibular space, abutting the adjacent submandibular gland. Note the finger-like projection from the abscess that extends to the adjacent dentition (*arrow*) in transverse grayscale ultrasound. Reactive diffuse edema of the overlying mylohyoid muscle (*arrow*) in the longitudinal ultrasound image. Coronal (C) and axial (D) contrast-enhanced CT images reveal well-circumscribed hypodense fluid collection in the sublingual space (floor of mouth) on both sides (*arrows*). The axial image is obliquely rotated to reveal its origin from the right side mandibular alveolar arch or third molar tooth with extended fluid collection in right masticator/parapharyngeal space (*arrows*). (Ultrasound image courtesy: Dr. Ankit Shah, Mumbai, India.)

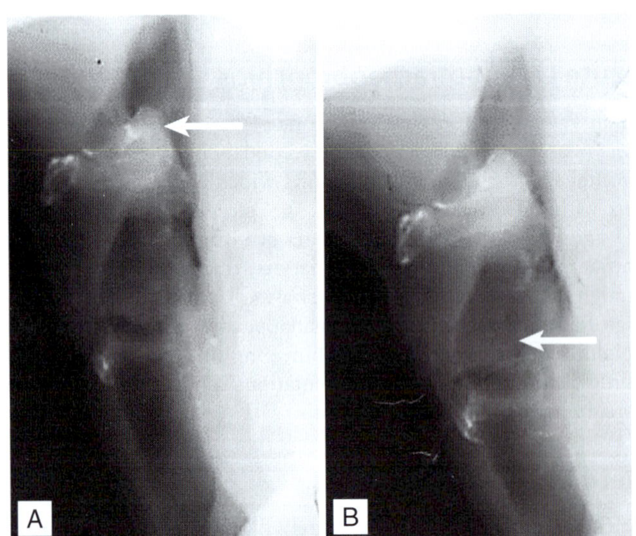

Figure 81.42 Acute epiglottitis: Lateral soft-tissue radiographs normal view (A) and magnified view (B) of the neck demonstrates the thickening of the epiglottis (*arrow* in A) represented as the "thumb-print" sign. Note the overdistended hypopharynx (*arrow* in B). (Courtesy: Dr. Mukund Rahalkar, Pune, India.)

retropharyngeal lymph node which may rupture into the retropharyngeal space causing a retropharyngeal abscess. The retropharyngeal space contains a slip of coronally oriented prevertebral fascia—the alar fascia which divides this space into an anteriorly situated true RPS. The alar fascia fuses anteriorly to the visceral fascia effectively cutting off the true RPS from the posteriorly situated "danger space" at approximately T3. The danger space extends inferiorly into the posterior mediastinum to the level of the diaphragm. Hence infections, abscesses, and tumors can extend through the danger space from the neck into the thorax and vice versa [48].

Contrast-enhanced CT is the imaging technique of choice as it defines the full extent of the collection due to the peripherally enhancing wall and pressure effect on the airway. A retropharyngeal abscess may also involve the adjacent vascular structures causing narrowing or pseudoaneurysm of the ICA, thrombosis of thrombophlebitis of the IJV, and mediastinitis (Fig. 81.43). Lateral neck radiographs are also used to demonstrate prevertebral space widening but can be misleading due to neck flexion, and phase of respiration. Plain radiographs also cannot differentiate RPS abscess from RPS edema. However, if CT is not easily available fluoroscopy of the sick child in lateral neck extension and during inspiration can demonstrate widening of the

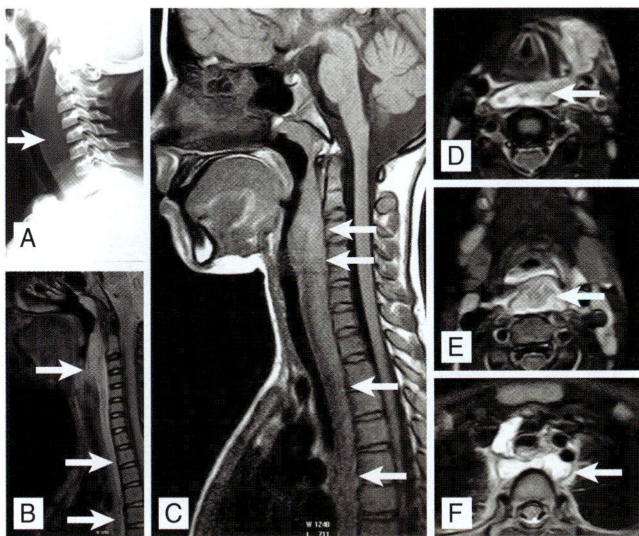

Figure 81.43 Retropharyngeal space abscess: Lateral neck soft-tissue radiograph (A) showing markedly widened prevertebral soft tissues (*arrow*). STIR sagittal (B) and axial (D–F) and T1W sagittal (C) images reveal a large retropharyngeal abscess (*arrows*) extending into the thorax along the danger space up to D7 level (*arrows*).

retropharyngeal soft tissues (more than 7 mm at C2 level and more than 14 mm at C6 level or more than half the width of the vertebral body from C1 to C4 levels).

Foreign Body Aspiration

Children usually present with breathlessness, low-grade fever, cough. A history of foreign body aspiration is available or can be elicited. Frontal and lateral radiographs of neck and thorax are helpful in assessing position of radio dense foreign bodies but have a low specificity (approximately 17%). Right mainstem bronchus is the most common site for an obstructed lower airway foreign body. Frontal radiographs can show asymmetric lung aeration, increased lucency on the side of obstruction due to hyperinflation with contralateral shift of the mediastinum. Noncontrast ultralow dose CT is useful in identifying radiolucent foreign bodies like fish bones [49].

Acute Suppurative Lymphadenitis

Suppurative lymphadenitis is the most common cause of acute painful neck masses in the pediatric age group (age 4–8 years) and is a common sequel of bacterial infections involving the upper respiratory tract with subsequent liquefaction and abscess formation within the draining lymph nodes. Imaging: High-resolution USG provides significant information with an added advantage of guided aspiration/tissue sampling. CT and MRI evaluate mass effect/encasement of adjacent structures and the degree of conglomeration.

Syndromes in Children With Head & Neck Manifestations

There is an extensive list of syndromic conditions presenting with clinical abnormalities in the head and neck which have been discussed exhaustively in the medical literature [50,51]. It is important to try and diagnose a specific syndrome based on typical findings (Tables 81.12 and 81.13) to enable identification of multisystemic anomalies. The diagnosis can guide further genetic testing and parental counseling.

TABLE 81.12 Clinico-radiological Manifestations of Commonly Encountered Syndromes

A. Syndromes With External Ear Abnormalities, Conductive Hearing Loss; Congenital Sensorineural Hearing Loss; Neck Cysts/Sinuses [50,51]	B. Syndromes With Abnormal Facial Skeleton: PNS, Mandible, Skull Vault
1. Pendred syndrome: Cochlear modiolar and interscalar septum deficiency, dilated vestibule/large vestibular aqueduct (LVAS), euthyroid goiter.	**1. Basal cell nevus syndrome (Gorlin syndrome):** multiple keratocystic odontogenic tumors.
2. Branchiootorenal syndrome (BOR): Branchial cleft cyst/fistula, EAC stenosis/atresia, dysplastic ossicles, "unwound cochlea" with offset middle/apical turns, posterior semicircular canal anomaly, LVAS, renal anomalies. **Branchiootic syndrome**: similar findings except for normal kidneys (Fig. 81.44).	**2. CHARGE:** Bony/membranous choanal atresia.
3. Waardenburg syndrome: Aplasia/hypoplasia of the posterior semicircular canal, LVAS, and hypoplastic cochlea/small deficient modiolus.	**3. Goldenhar syndrome**: Mandibular/zygomatic arch hypoplasia, hypoplasia of the muscles of mastication/facial muscles, Klippel–Feil anomaly.
4. CHARGE: ***C***oloboma, ***H***eart anomaly, ***A***tresia choanae, ***R***etardation: mental & somatic development, ***G***enital hypoplasia, ***E***ar abnormalities (Fig. 81.45).	**4. Treacher Collins syndrome:** Symmetric micrognathia, zygomatic/malar hypoplasia.
5. Goldenhar syndrome: microtia/anotia, EAC atresia/stenosis, middle ear hypoplasia and ossicular malformations, oval window atresia & VII nerve hypoplasia.	**5. Pierre Robin sequence (PRS):** Bilateral symmetric micrognathia, glossoptosis, and posterior U-shaped cleft palate.
6. Treacher Collins syndrome: EAC stenosis/atresia, hypoplastic/atretic middle ear, malformed/absent ossicles, oval window stenosis/atresia, facial nerve canal anomalies.	**6. McCune–Albright syndrome (MAS):** Polyostotic FD, endocrine dysfunction, and cutaneous hyperpigmentation;
7. Pierre Robin sequence (PRS): Stenotic/atretic EAC, middle ear and mastoid hypoplasia with malformed ossicles, small semicircular canal bone island/anlage	**7. Cherubism:** Familial, bilateral symmetrical expansile fibro-osseous jaw and maxillary involvement.
	8. Crouzons'syndrome and Apert's syndrome: middle cranial fossa and petrous apex deformities leading to Eustachian tube dysfunction and mastoid—middle ear pathology.

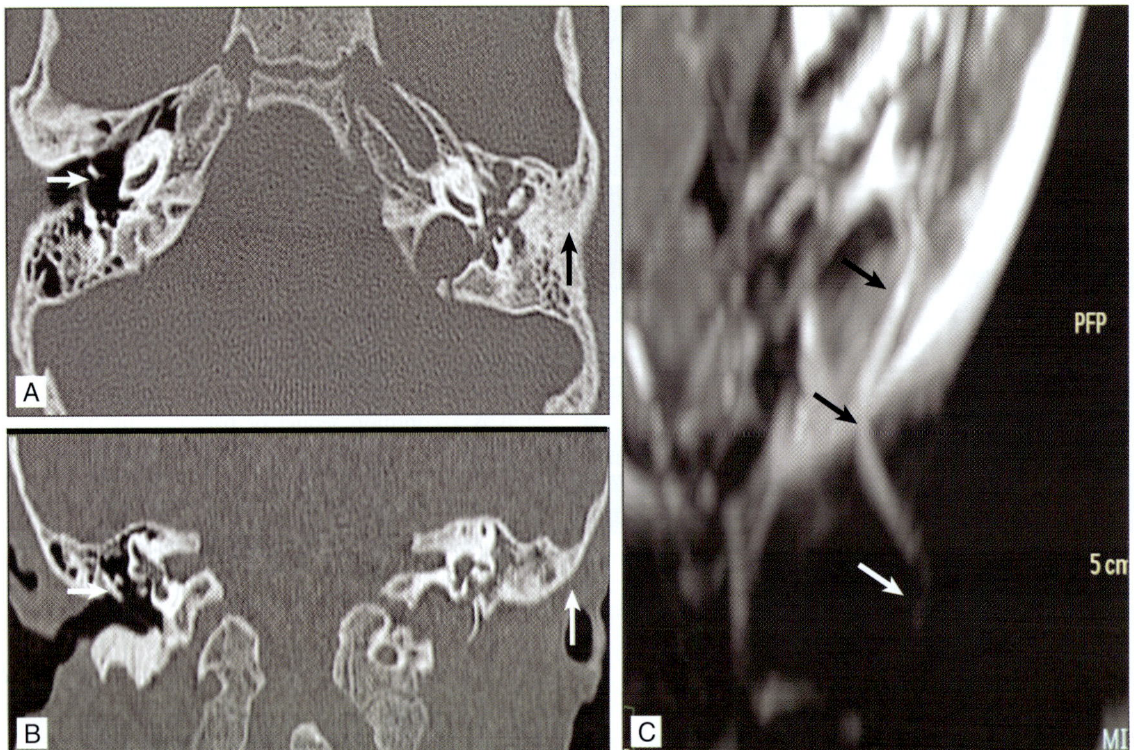

Figure 81.44 Branchiootic syndrome (BOS): Axial (A) and coronal (B) HRCT images of the temporal bone reveal left microtia and EAC atresia (*arrows*). Ossicular chain is dysmorphic and dysplastic on both sides (*arrows*) with small sized opacified left middle ear cavity (*horizontal white arrows*). Coronal reformatted heavily T2W MR sinogram (C) reveals a well-defined sinus tract (*oblique arrows*) extending from a small skin opening in the left lower neck to the lateral pharyngeal wall. USG examination revealed normal kidneys.

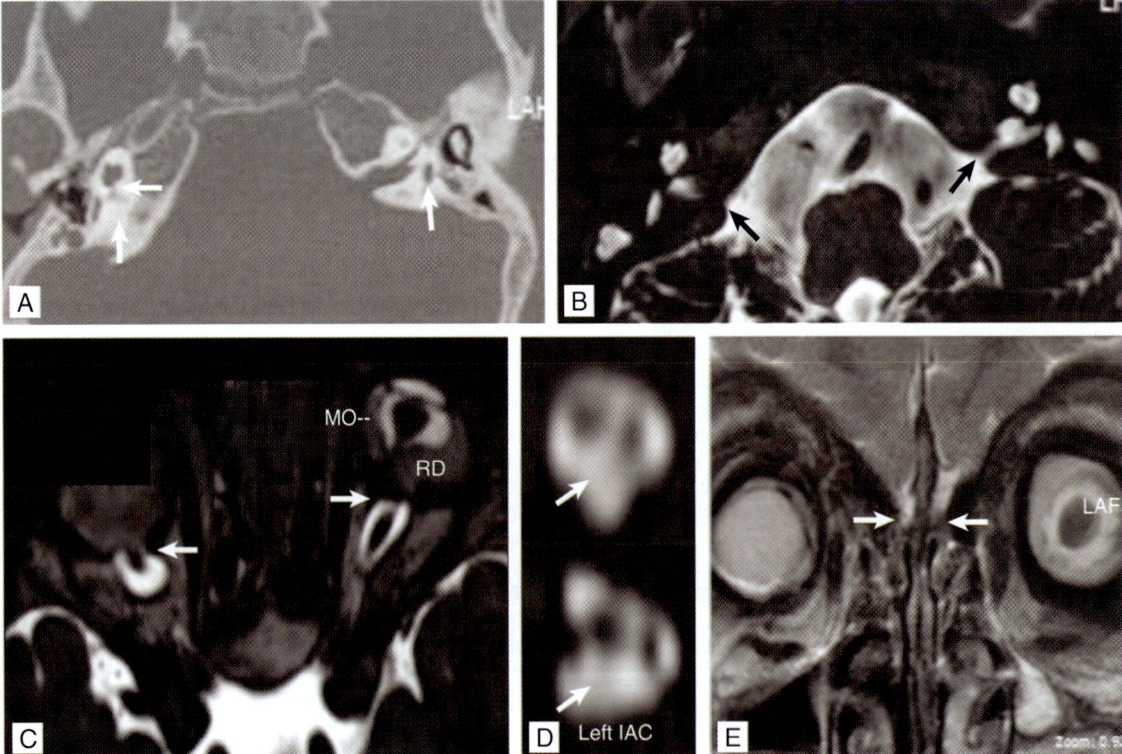

Figure 81.45 CHARGE syndrome: Axial HRCT (A) image reveals bilateral cochlear turn abnormalities with cochlear aperture stenosis, hypoplastic vestibules, and absent semicircular canals (*arrows*). CISS (DRIVE) T2W axial (B and C) and sagittal oblique IAC images (D) reveal bilateral Type 2A cochleo-vestibular nerve dysplasia with hypoplastic/absent cochlear branch of the eighth nerve bilaterally (*angulated arrows* in D). Bilateral globe deformities with small colobomas, left microphthalmos (MO), and left retinal detachment (RD) seen in (D). Coronal T2W image (E) reveals bilateral shallow olfactory fossae with hypoplasia/absence of the olfactory bulbs (*arrows*).

TABLE 81.13 Clinico-radiological Manifestations of Commonly Encountered Syndromes

A. Port-wine Stain, Visible Hemangioma, or Vascular Malformation	B. Orbital Abnormalities
1. **Sturge–Weber syndrome** 2. **PHACES syndrome:** Posterior fossa structural anomalies, *H*emangioma (segmental, infantile type, multiple), *A*rterial anomalies (agenesis, hypoplasia, and stenosis/occlusion of vessels, aneurysm, the aberrant origin of vessels), *C*ardiac defects (aortic coarctation/aneurysm/dysplasia, aberrant subclavian artery ± vascular ring, VSD), *E*ye (persistent hyperplasia primary vitreous, coloboma, morning glory disc anomaly, optic nerve hypoplasia, peripapillary staphyloma, microphthalmia, cataract, sclerocornea), and *S*ternal/supraumbilical raphe clefts and defects other midline anomalies (Fig. 81.46). A facial hemangioma and either one other major criterion or two minor criteria above must be present to qualify for the diagnosis of PHACES syndrome according to recent consensus statement released in 2009 [52]. 3. **Maffucci syndrome:** multiple enchondromas, bone deformities, and hemangiomas.	1. **Neurofibromatosis-1:** Lisch nodules (optic hamartomas), buphthalmos, "empty orbit" due to sphenoid wing dysplasia 2. **CHARGE:** colobomas 3. **Goldenhar syndrome:** colobomas 4. **Treacher Collins syndrome:** colobomas 5. **PHACES syndrome:** persistent hyperplasia primary vitreous, coloboma, morning glory disc anomaly, optic nerve hypoplasia, peripapillary staphyloma, microphthalmia, cataract, sclerocornea.

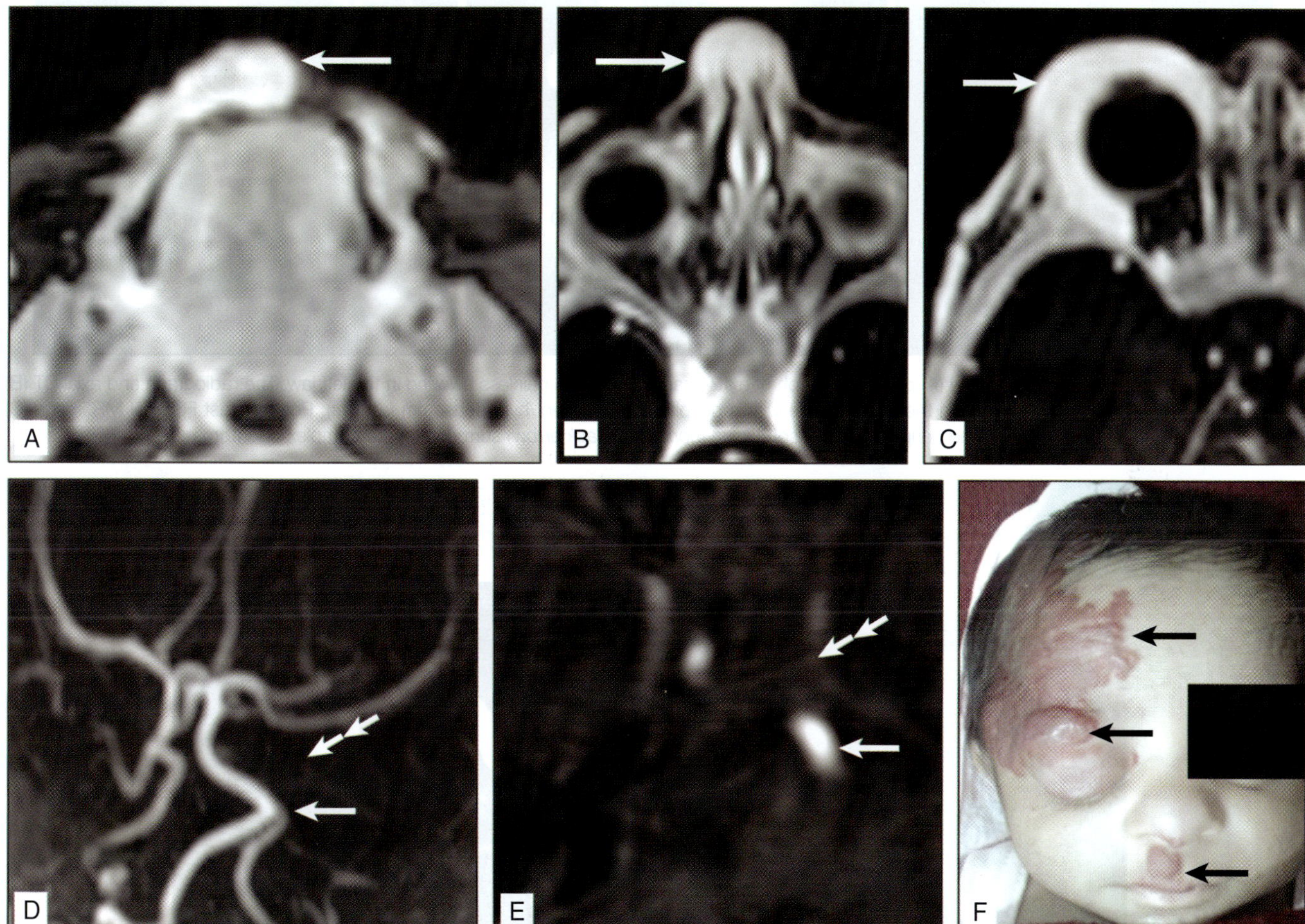

Figure 81.46 PHACE syndrome: Postcontrast FS axial MR images (A–C) reveal multiple densely enhancing lesions in the right lip, nasal ala, right periorbital and intraorbital region, and frontal scalp (*arrows*) indicating multifocal infantile HNF hemangiomatosis evident on clinical photograph (F). MR angiography images (D and E) reveal multiple craniovertebral arterial anomalies: hypoplastic left ICA (*oblique double arrow* in D and E). Vertebral arteries are hypertrophied (*horizontal arrows* in D and E) with luminal caliber equal to common carotid arteries.

82

Pediatric Congenital Heart Disease

JENA N. DEPETRIS, SANDEEP HEDGIRE, NANDINI M. MEYERSOHN

Introduction

Congenital heart disease (CHD) is perhaps one of the most complex topics within medicine, requiring imaging specialists to have highly subspecialized knowledge and to work within an interdisciplinary team to provide optimal care for these unique patients. There is a wide spectrum of pathologies that fall under the umbrella of CHD, and the goal of this chapter is to educate the reader on how to approach describing complex congenital cardiac anatomy and to identify the characteristic imaging features of these unique pathologies. Moreover, we will focus on the roles, advantages, and disadvantages of various imaging modalities and their diagnostic applications in CHD.

The overall incidence of all CHDs combined is approximately 1% of the population, with the most common defects being bicuspid aortic valve (BAV) and mitral valve prolapse [1]. With respect to symptomatic CHD, Table 82.1 summarizes the incidence of the most common pathologies both overall and diagnosed within the first month of life.

TABLE 82.1 Frequency of Symptomatic Congenital Heart Disease for All Groups and Within the First Month of Life

Frequency of Symptomatic Congenital Heart Disease	
Most common congenital anomalies (all ages; bicuspid aortic valve and MVP excluded)	
Ventricular septal defect (VSD)	30%
Atrial septal defect (ASD)	10%
Tetralogy of Fallot (TOF)	10%
Patent ductus arteriosus (PDA)	10%
Aortic coarctation	7%
Transposition of great arteries (TGA)	5%
First month of life (serious clinical problems; high mortality)	
Hypoplastic left heart syndrome (HLHS)	35%
Transposition of the great arteries (TGA)	25%
Aortic coarctation	20%
Multiple serious defects	15%
Pulmonary atresia/stenosis	10%
Tetralogy of Fallot (TOF) with pulmonic atresia or severe pulmonic stenosis	10%

Adapted from Harisinghani et al. [1].

Normal Fetal Circulation

Before discussing the immense complexity of CHD, it is critical to understand the fundamentals of normal fetal and adult circulation. Neonatal circulation (Fig. 82.1) is unique because it is inherently connected to and dependent upon the maternal placenta. Deoxygenated blood from the fetus travels toward the placenta in two umbilical arteries, while oxygenated nutrient-rich blood travels from the placenta through the single umbilical vein toward the right atrium of the fetal heart. From the right atrium, some blood may travel through the tricuspid valve into the right ventricle and the pulmonary artery, mimicking adult circulation patterns. However, since the fetal lungs are underdeveloped and not yet being used for oxygen exchange, the pulmonary arterial system has a relatively high resistance and the majority of the freshly oxygenated blood in the right atrium will be shunted across the *foramen ovale*, a normal defect in the fetal interatrial septum, into the left atrium, where it can continue through the mitral valve into the left ventricle and out into systemic circulation. Besides the

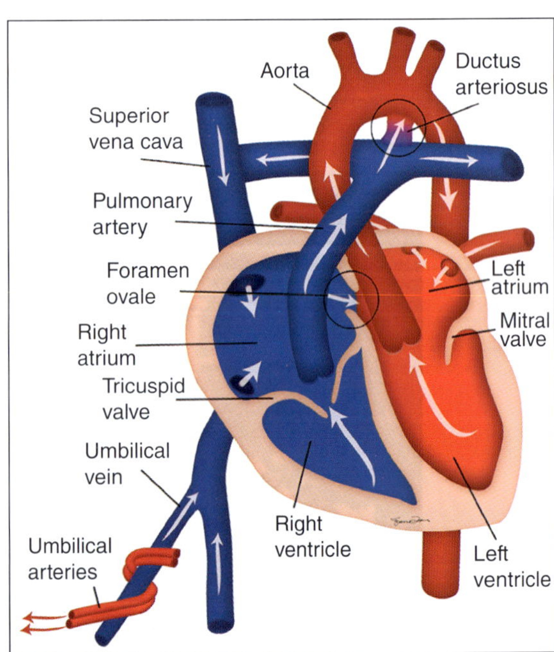

Figure 82.1 Normal fetal circulation, wherein oxygenated blood travels from the placenta toward the fetus in a single umbilical vein and bypasses the developing fetal lungs through two normal shunts, including the ***foramen ovale*** and the ***ductus arteriosus***, deoxygenated blood then travels from the fetus toward the placenta in two umbilical arteries. (Courtesy: Susanne Loomis.)

foramen ovale, there is another unique connection normally present in fetal circulation called the **ductus arteriosus**, which is a connection between the pulmonary arteries and the aorta that also serves to shunt blood away from the developing fetal lungs [2].

At the time of birth, a significant shift occurs in the circulation of the newborn child with a sudden drop in pulmonary vascular resistance occurring as the lungs fill with air. Under normal circumstances, this drastic pressure shift results in the closure of both the foramen ovale and ductus arteriosus. These small but important structures may occasionally stay patent in the postnatal period, and in the context of CHD can be vitally important for survival.

Role of Advanced Imaging

In a tertiary care setting, the diagnosis of CHD is often made during prenatal or early postnatal life, largely through clinical assessment and echocardiography. Plain chest radiography in early neonatal life can also be useful in the assessment of CHD, as many have classic radiologic signs, which will be discussed in the respective sections for each pathology. Radiography can be used to assess cardiac position and shape, sidedness of the aortic arch, lung volumes, and the presence of pulmonary edema or other signs of fluid overload.

However, with continuing advances in the surgical management of CHD resulting in a greater population of adults living with CHD, advanced imaging beyond conventional echocardiography and plain radiography has also become critically important in the pre- and postsurgical evaluation of CHD patients [3,4]. Increased availability and technical advances in multidetector ECG-gated computed tomography (CT) and magnetic resonance imaging (MRI) have rendered these noninvasive modalities valuable complementary tools for anatomic and functional assessment of CHD, particularly as these patients undergo sequentially or staged therapeutic interventions and live long into adulthood. The American College of Radiology (ACR) 2020 Appropriateness Criteria considers both cardiac MRI and cardiac CT more appropriate diagnostic tests in the evaluation of adult congenital heart disease (ACHD) compared with invasive coronary angiography and nuclear scintigraphy [5].

Given the complex anatomy, image acquisition protocols often need to be tailored on an individual patient level to sufficiently answer the diagnostic question while minimizing radiation doses for CT in accordance with the ALARA principle (as low as reasonably achievable) and optimizing scan times for MRI. The following sections will provide an overview of advanced imaging techniques and protocols, as well as their applications for CHD.

Cardiac CT

ECG-gated cardiac CT is a versatile imaging technique that allows for precise anatomic delineation, evaluation of vessel/shunt patency, and assessment of cardiac function. A standard image acquisition protocol begins with a precontrast scan, which is particularly helpful in identifying prior surgical repair and cardiac valves, where applicable. This is typically followed by a prospectively or retrospectively ECG-gated arterial phase acquisition and may also be followed by a subsequent delayed phase acquisition.

Requirements for a safe and diagnostic quality cardiac CT include adequate renal function (GFR >30) and intravenous access of the appropriate size to achieve a contrast injection rate adequate for optimal contrast opacification of smaller vessels in and around the heart. A normal heart rate and regular cardiac rhythm are ideal for optimizing image quality and minimizing radiation dose. However, utilization of arrhythmia rejection technology, modifications of image acquisition parameters, and post-acquisition image reconstruction can be used for troubleshooting in the setting of rapid or irregular heart rhythms, as are often present in CHD patients.

Advantages of cardiac CT include capabilities for isotropic multiplanar image reconstruction, excellent spatial resolution, and improved temporal resolution with advances in scanner technology. Faster image acquisition times compared to MRI allows for imaging of patients with claustrophobia or with non-MRI compatible metallic implants. These advantages come at the expense of radiation exposure, noting that dose reduction strategies and improvements in scanner technology have significantly improved per-scan radiation doses.

Cardiac MRI

Cardiac MRI is a highly utilized imaging technique in CHD due to its excellent soft-tissue resolution, precise anatomic delineation, and dynamic assessment of both qualitative and quantitative cardiac function without the use of ionizing radiation or iodinated contrast media. It remains the technique of choice for estimating myocardial mass and ventricular volumes, calculating ventricular ejection fractions, and detecting the presence of myocardial fibrosis. Furthermore, with the administration of intravenous gadolinium during an MR angiogram, evaluation of vessel, and shunt patency is possible. The combination of these imaging features and functional parameters often drives management decisions for CHD patients, and the 2018 American College of Cardiology/American Heart Association Guidelines for the Management of Adults with Congenital Heart Disease (ACHD) consequently recommends cardiac MR imaging for a variety of CHDs [6].

Recent advances in faster magnetic field gradients, image reconstruction techniques, and newer pulse sequences including 4D flow, T1/T2 mapping, free-breathing acquisitions, arrhythmia rejection technology, and strain imaging have further improved the utility of cardiac MRI in the CHD population. There is no single standard image acquisition protocol for cardiac MRI, as sequence selection is often tailored at the individual patient level for targeted clinical questions. With that said, broadly useful sequences include SSFP cine sequences, "black blood" double inversion recovery sequences, T1/T2 weighted sequences, MR angiography, delayed inversion recovery sequences to evaluate for late gadolinium enhancement (LGE), and velocity-encoded phase-contrast cine sequences.

Requirements for a high-quality cardiac MRI include adequate renal function (GFR >30), ability to sustain breath holds, and ability to lay flat for a prolonged period of time. As with cardiac CT, a normal heart rate and regular cardiac rhythm are ideal for optimal image quality.

Major limitations of cardiac MRI include long scan times, claustrophobia, and significant image artifacts related to metallic implants from prior surgeries, which are common in CHD patients. Pacemaker-dependent patients have traditionally not been subjected to MRI due to concerns for pacemaker malfunction, however, that practice is evolving as our understanding of device safety in settings of diagnostic magnetic fields continues to improve.

TABLE 82.2 Factors to Consider When Choosing CT Versus MRI as a Diagnostic Technique

Factors Favoring Choice of CT	Factors Favoring Choice of MRI
Indwelling metallic implants or devices (particularly if not MRI safe)	Concern for repeated radiation exposure
Claustrophobia	Flow or ventricular volume quantification assessment
Coronary assessment (anomalies and/or preoperative clearance)	Myocardial perfusion at rest and stress
Plan for re-do sternotomy	Myocardial fibrosis/scar assessment

Adapted from Babu-Narayan et al. [3].

TABLE 82.3 Morphologic Characteristics of the Cardiac Chambers

Chamber	Morphologic Characteristics
Right atrium	Coronary sinus drainage
	Crista terminalis
	Pyramidal or trapezoidal shaped atrial appendage
Right ventricle	Moderator band
	Septal papillary muscles
	Muscular infundibulum
	Tricuspid atrioventricular valve separated from the outflow valve by a muscular infundibulum
Left atrium	Variable atrial appendage morphology (more tubular or finger-like)
Left ventricle	Smooth upper septal surface
	Mitral atrioventricular valve in fibrous continuity with the outflow valve

Choosing Modalities

The choice of which technique to utilize in the evaluation of any CHD patient should be based on a balanced multidisciplinary discussion of the risks and benefits among cardiac radiologists, pediatric/adult cardiologists specializing in CHD, interventional cardiologists, electrophysiologists, and cardiac surgeons. Both cardiac CT and cardiac MRI can offer excellent anatomic assessment for CHD patients as previously discussed, but each has its own unique strengths, and therefore the decision, although complex at times, should ultimately be centered around the primary clinical question Table 82.2 summarizes key factors involved in deciding whether to choose CT or MRI for evaluating a CHD patient.

Special Considerations

Patients with CHD represent a unique population with a number of special considerations that factor into their management.

First of all, with continuous improvements in prenatal care and fetal anatomic assessment, the vast majority of CHD diagnoses are made in utero or early in infancy. Evaluation of a pediatric population from an imaging perspective can be uniquely challenging given concerns about large or repeated radiation doses in early life.

Secondly, pediatric patients are often unable to cooperate with breathing instructions during an imaging examination and the use of sedation or general anesthesia may need to be considered to acquire diagnostic images. Depending on the configuration of their congenital anatomy, these patients can be systemically cyanotic and/or hemodynamically unstable, which further complicates the clinical picture when considering the use of general anesthesia.

Given these special considerations, decisions on when and how to image these patients should be carefully considered and discussed among the various members of the multidisciplinary care team in conjunction with patients' families, with full understanding of the risks, benefits, and potential implications.

Segmental Approach to Congenital Heart Disease

Due to the inherent complexity of the CHD spectrum, a structured, segmental approach for describing the underlying anatomy is critical, not only for making a correct diagnosis but also for effectively communicating amongst various members of the multidisciplinary care team.

The first step is to become familiar with the characteristic morphologic features of the various cardiac chambers so that their position within a congenitally abnormal configuration can be correctly identified (Table 82.3). It is important to note that these characteristics are a guide to identifying the correct morphologic cardiac chambers, however definitive chamber identification may remain uncertain in highly complex cases (Table 82.4).

Following the identification of the morphologic cardiac chambers, a segmental approach is necessary for describing the anatomical configuration of these chambers, as well as inflow and outflow patterns. The widely used Van Praagh approach to the segmental classification of CHD, originally developed in Boston, Massachusetts in the 1960s [7], employs a three-letter notation signifying (1) the visceroatrial situs, (2) the orientation of the ventricular loop, and (3) the conotruncus (or origin and position of the great vessels). An additional important step is to identify the atrioventricular and ventriculoarterial concordance or discordance, although this is not represented in the three-letter notation system [8]. While this chapter will contain a detailed discussion of the various individual CHDs, a schematic representation of the segmental approach described by Van Praagh is included here for reference (Table 82.5).

Classification of Congenital Heart Disease

Cyanotic Congenital Heart Disease

Cyanotic CHD represents a complex spectrum of congenital abnormalities that result in varying degrees of cyanosis, which clinically presents as bluish discoloration of the skin (particularly perioral, periorbital, and digital), digital clubbing, end-organ damage, and failure to thrive. Systemic desaturation may occur as a result of blood flow being redirected away from the pulmonary arterial system and preventing adequate oxygenation, or mixing of oxygenated and deoxygenated blood (right-to-left shunting) before exiting into the systemic circulation.

TABLE 82.4 Segmental Approach to Congenital Heart Disease

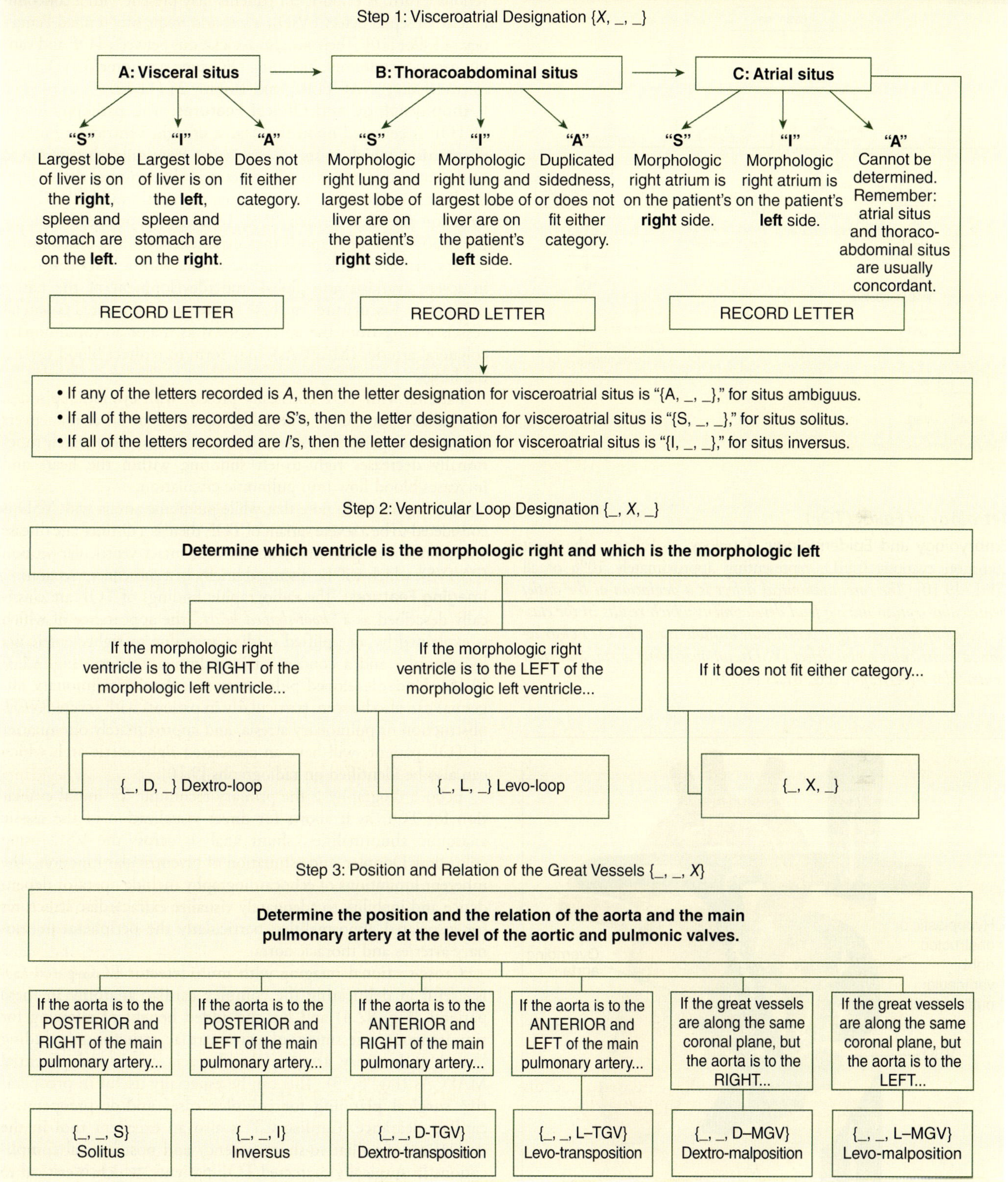

Step 1: Visceroatrial Designation {X, _, _}
A: Visceral situs
B: Thoracoabdominal situs
C: Atrial situs
"S"
Largest lobe of liver is on the right, spleen and stomach are on the left.
"I"
Largest lobe of liver is on the left, spleen and stomach are on the right.
"A"
Does not fit either category.
"S"
Morphologic right lung and largest lobe of liver are on the patient's right side.
"I"
Morphologic right lung and largest lobe of liver are on the patient's left side.
"A"
Duplicated sidedness, or does not fit either category.
"S"
Morphologic right atrium is on the patient's right side.
"I"
Morphologic right atrium is on the patient's left side.
"A"
Cannot be determined. Remember: atrial situs and thoraco-abdominal situs are usually concordant.
RECORD LETTER
RECORD LETTER
RECORD LETTER
• If any of the letters recorded is A, then the letter designation for visceroatrial situs is "{A, _, _}," for situs ambiguus.
• If all of the letters recorded are S's, then the letter designation for visceroatrial situs is "{S, _, _}," for situs solitus.
• If all of the letters recorded are I's, then the letter designation for visceroatrial situs is "{I, _, _}," for situs inversus.
Step 2: Ventricular Loop Designation {_, X, _}
Determine which ventricle is the morphologic right and which is the morphologic left
If the morphologic right ventricle is to the RIGHT of the morphologic left ventricle...
If the morphologic right ventricle is to the LEFT of the morphologic left ventricle...
If it does not fit either category...
{_, D, _} Dextro-loop
{_, L, _} Levo-loop
{_, X, _}
Step 3: Position and Relation of the Great Vessels {_, _, X}
Determine the position and the relation of the aorta and the main pulmonary artery at the level of the aortic and pulmonic valves.
If the aorta is to the POSTERIOR and RIGHT of the main pulmonary artery...
If the aorta is to the POSTERIOR and LEFT of the main pulmonary artery...
If the aorta is to the ANTERIOR and RIGHT of the main pulmonary artery...
If the aorta is to the ANTERIOR and LEFT of the main pulmonary artery...
If the great vessels are along the same coronal plane, but the aorta is to the RIGHT...
If the great vessels are along the same coronal plane, but the aorta is to the LEFT...
{_, _, S} Solitus
{_, _, I} Inversus
{_, _, D-TGV} Dextro-transposition
{_, _, L-TGV} Levo-transposition
{_, _, D-MGV} Dextro-malposition
{_, _, L-MGV} Levo-malposition

Adapted from Schallert et al. [7].

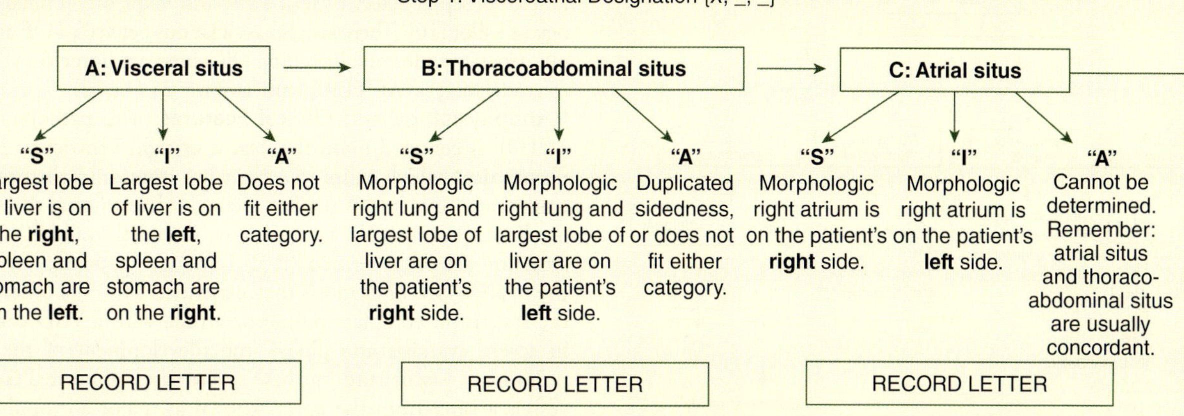

TABLE 82.5 Classification Schema of Congenital Heart Disease

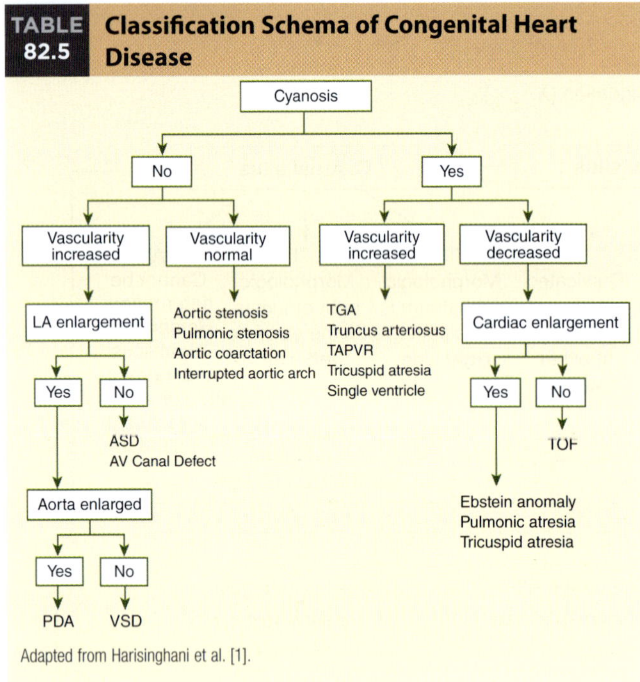

Adapted from Harisinghani et al. [1].

Tetralogy of Fallot (TOF)

Embryology and Epidemiology: Tetralogy of Fallot is the most common cyanotic CHD, representing approximately 10% of all CHD [9,10]. *The core anatomical defect is a deviation of the outlet ventricular septum during fetal development which results in the classic tetrad of findings: right ventricular outflow tract (RVOT) obstruction, a ventricular septal defect (VSD), an overriding aorta, and right ventricular hypertrophy* (Fig. 82.2) [4,9,10].

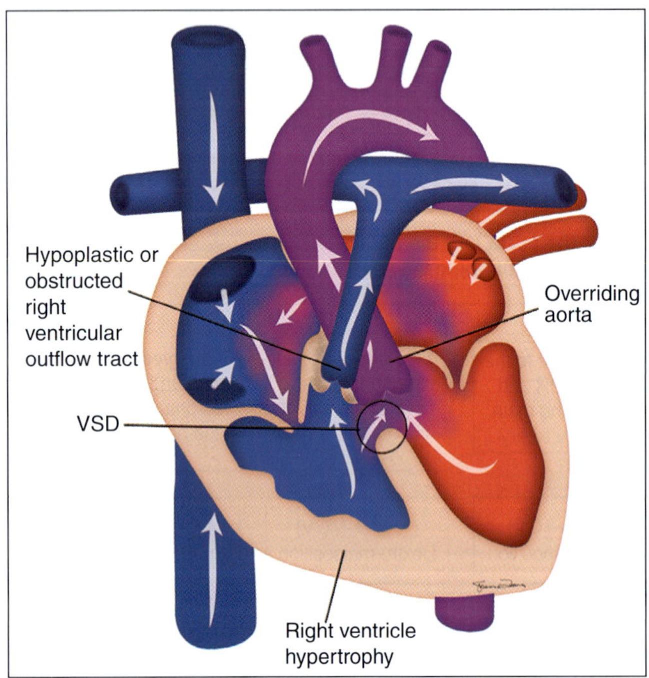

Figure 82.2 Schematic representation of Tetralogy of Fallot, demonstrating the classic tetrad of findings, including right ventricular outflow tract (RVOT) obstruction/hypoplasia, an overriding aorta, a ventricular septal defect (VSD), and right ventricular hypertrophy. (Courtesy: Susanne Loomis.)

TOF is commonly associated with other congenital anomalies, such as a right-sided aortic arch, BAV, or anomalous pulmonary venous return. A minority of patients may present with a concomitant atrial septal defect (ASD), a scenario frequently termed Pentalogy of Fallot [10]. There are also associations between TOF and various genetic syndromes, including DiGeorge syndrome (CATCH 22 microdeletion), VACTERL, and Trisomy 21 [11,12].

Pathophysiology and Clinical Features: The pathophysiology of TOF is centered upon the degree of right ventricular outflow obstruction, which exists on a spectrum from mild obstruction to complete atresia and is the key factor in determining the severity of clinical cyanosis. In fact, patients with only mild RVOT obstruction are often termed "Pink Tetralogy" patients, referencing the relative lack of cyanosis they experience. On the other end of the spectrum, complete pulmonic atresia with a VSD can result in severe cyanosis and global underdevelopment of the native pulmonary vasculature. In these severe cases, abnormal collateral vessels arising from the aorta, known as major aortopulmonary collateral arteries (MAPCAs), may form to redirect blood toward the lungs.

Patients with TOF classically present with cyanotic episodes, also called "Tet spells," relieved by squatting or other maneuvers that increase peripheral systemic vascular resistance, which functionally decreases right-to-left shunting within the heart and increases blood flow into pulmonic circulation.

It is important to note that while pulmonic atresia with VSD is considered to be a severe variant of TOF, there is a distinct rare disease entity known as pulmonary atresia with intact ventricular septum (PA/IVS), which will be discussed briefly in a subsequent section.

Imaging Features: The radiographic findings of TOF are classically described as a "*boot-shaped heart*," the appearance of which is explained by an uplifted cardiac apex due to right ventricular hypertrophy and a concave main pulmonary artery (Fig. 82.3) [9,10]. Underdeveloped pulmonary vasculature (pulmonary oligemia) can also be seen, particularly in patients with severe RVOT obstruction or pulmonary atresia, and approximately one-quarter of TOF patients will have an associated right aortic arch which can also be identified on radiographs [9,10].

Echocardiography is the primary technique for initial evaluation for TOF, as it allows for direct visualization of the classic anatomic abnormalities, shunt analysis across the VSD using color flow Doppler, and estimation of biventricular function. The inherent limitations of echocardiography include operator dependence and inability to adequately visualize extracardiac structures for associated abnormalities, particularly the peripheral pulmonary arteries and thoracic aorta.

Cross-sectional imaging with multidetector ECG-gated CT is useful in delineating the complex cardiac anatomy in these patients (Fig. 82.4) and has the added benefit of allowing for simultaneous assessment of extra-cardiac structures including branch pulmonary arteries, the thoracic aorta, and potential MAPCAs (Fig. 82.5). This can be especially useful in preoperative surgical planning for complex cases and/or preoperative cardiac clearance. Cardiac CT is also an excellent tool in the evaluation of palliative shunt patency and postsurgical complications in surgically corrected TOF patients, which is critical to their ongoing cardiovascular management.

MR imaging has the unique advantage of providing both detailed anatomical information and quantitative functional data without the use of ionizing radiation. MRI can be used to quantify ventricular volumes using steady-state free precession cine sequences and remains the gold standard for quantification of flow fractions and valvular regurgitation using phase-contrast imaging. For patients with TOF,

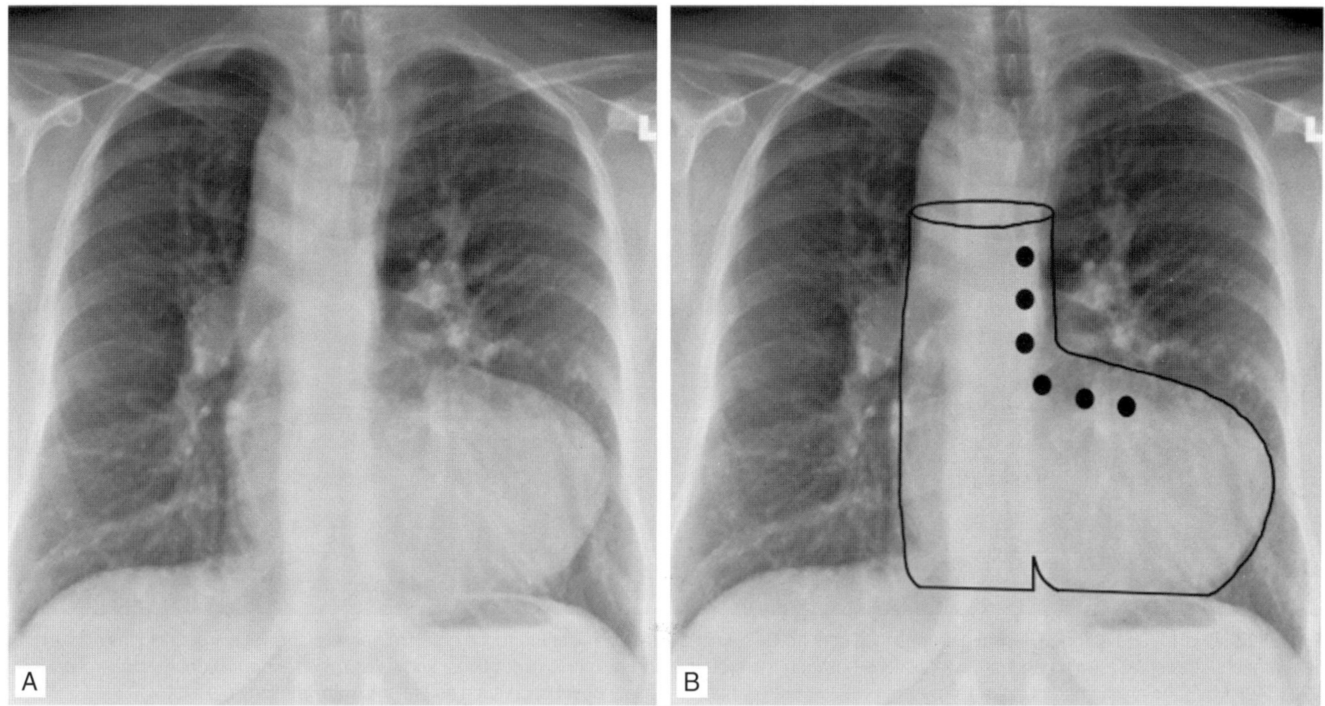

Figure 82.3 Frontal chest radiograph (A) demonstrating the classic *boot-shaped heart* (B) of Tetralogy of Fallot, which refers to the uplifted cardiac apex due to right ventricular hypertrophy and a concave main pulmonary artery.

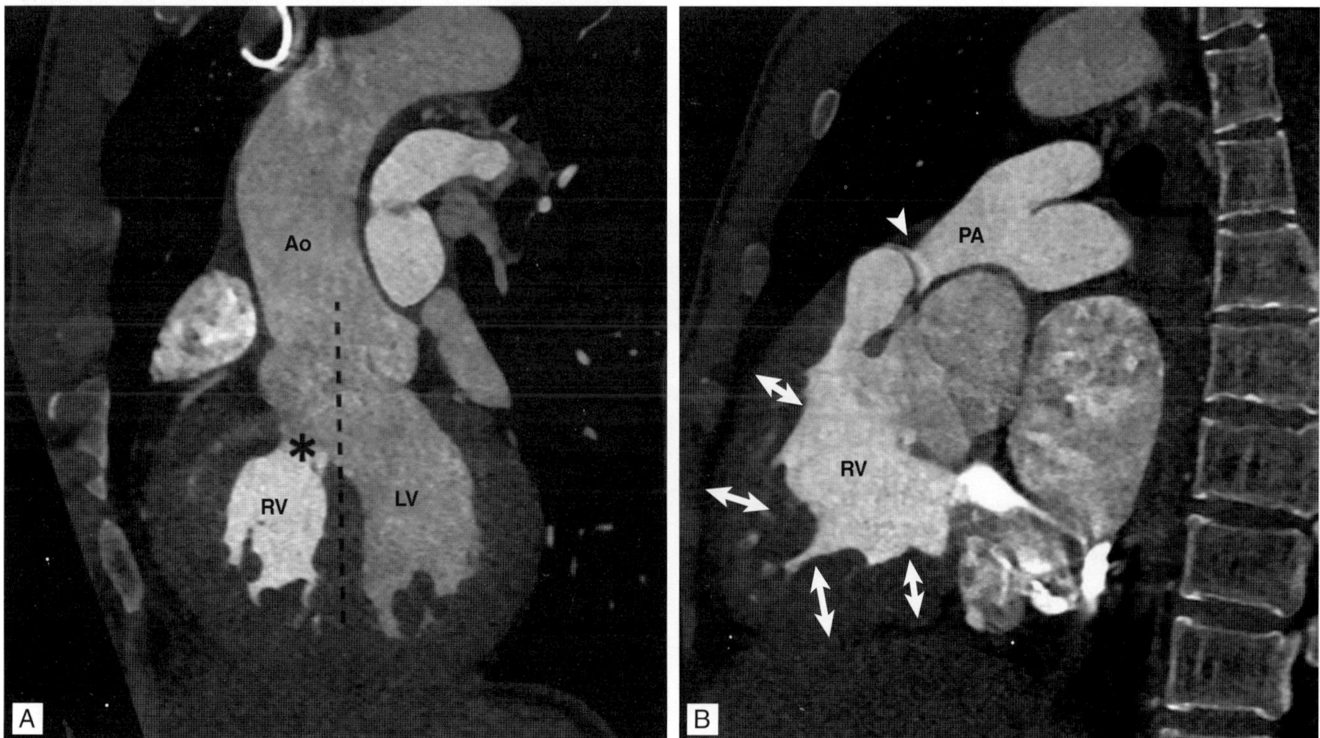

Figure 82.4 Oblique coronal (A) and sagittal (B) contrast-enhanced ECG-gated cardiac CT images demonstrate the four characteristic features of Tetralogy of Fallot, including an aorta that overrides the interventricular septum (dotted line), a ventricular septal defect (*asterisk*), right ventricular outflow obstruction/narrowing (*arrowhead*), and right ventricular hypertrophy (*double-headed arrows*). *Ao*, aorta; *LV*, left ventricle; *PA*, pulmonary artery; *RV*, right ventricle.

MRI is important in assessing the pulmonic valve/RVOT, as the degree of residual stenosis and/or pulmonic regurgitation often dictates management. The use of gadolinium-based contrast agents to assess for myocardial fibrosis or scarring is also important for assessing a patient's risk of ventricular arrhythmia.

The key imaging findings are summarized in Table 82.6 and the differential diagnosis of uncorrected TOF is shown in Table 82.7, which includes other cyanotic CHDs such as tricuspid atresia with transposition of the great arteries and double outlet right ventricle (DORV).

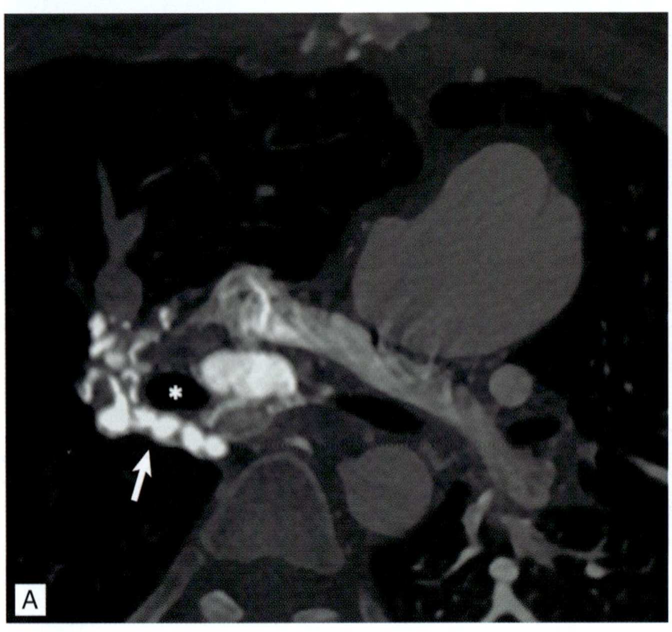

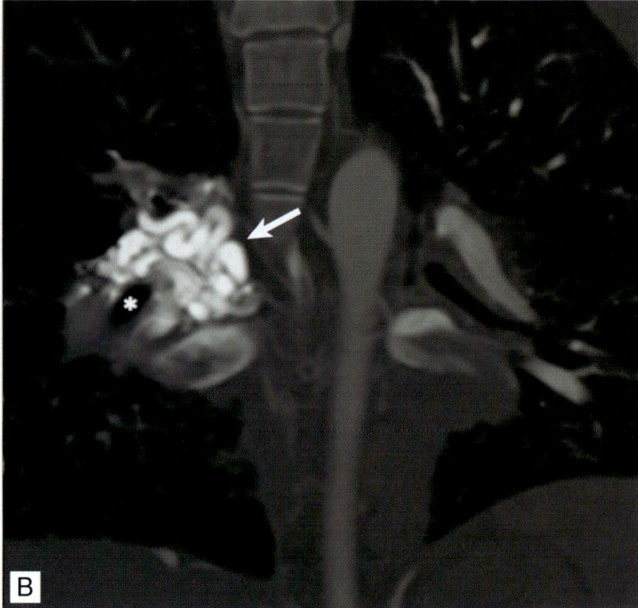

Figure 82.5 Axial (A) and coronal (B) contrast-enhanced caridac CT demonstrates prominent tortuous collateral vessels (*arrows*) surrounding the right main-stem bronchus (*asterisk*) forming aberrant connections between the systemic and pulmonic circulations, known as *major aortopulmonary collateral arteries (MAPCAs)*. MAPCAs are commonly found in patients with severe pulmonary outflow obstruction such as patients with Tetralogy of Fallot.

TABLE 82.6 Summary of the Key Imaging Features of Tetralogy of Fallot

Technique	Imaging Features
Chest radiograph	"Boot-shaped heart" Decreased (underdeveloped) pulmonary vascularity Small or concave pulmonary artery Possible right-sided aortic arch
Cardiac CT/MRI	Overriding aorta Ventricular septal defect Right ventricular outflow tract obstruction/pulmonary atresia Right ventricular hypertrophy Presence of major aortopulmonary collateral arteries (MAPCAs) Main or branch pulmonary artery stenoses Associated abnormalities of the thoracic aorta

TABLE 82.7 Differential Diagnosis for Uncorrected Tetralogy of Fallot

Pentalogy of Fallot (Tetralogy of Fallot + ASD)
Tricuspid atresia with ASD ± VSD/PDA ± transposition of the great arteries (TGA)
Double outlet right ventricle (DORV) with pulmonary stenosis

Treatment and Outcomes: The current mainstay of treatment for TOF involves primary surgical repair in infancy, consisting of VSD closure and relief of the right ventricular outflow obstruction in the form of pulmonic valvuloplasty or a transannular patch repair. Although no longer the preferred surgical approach, a transannular patch is occasionally required in settings of severe RVOT obstruction and is known to result in a large area of akinesis in the RVOT. Rarely in extreme cases, palliative shunts such as a Blalock–Thomas–Taussig shunt (subclavian artery to pulmonary artery shunt), Waterston shunt (ascending thoracic aorta to right pulmonary artery shunt), or a Pott shunt (descending thoracic aorta to left pulmonary artery shunt) may be used as a bridge to total surgical repair.

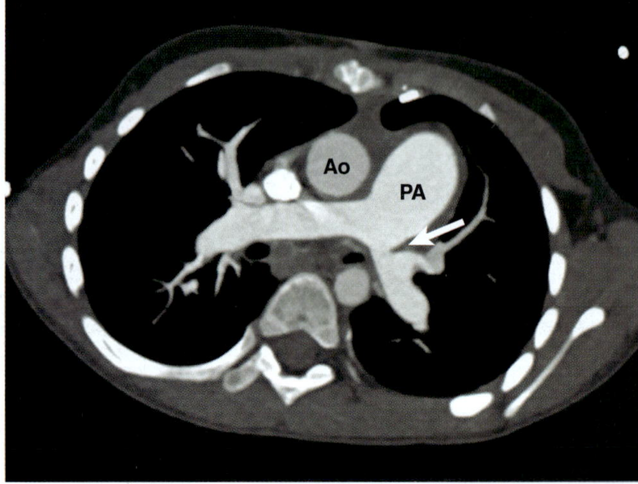

Figure 82.6 Axial contrast-enhanced ECG-gated cardiac CT demonstrates focal stenosis (*arrow*) of the proximal left main pulmonary artery, a frequent postsurgical complication seen in patients with Tetralogy of Fallot. *Ao*, aorta; *PA*, pulmonary artery.

The prognosis for patients with TOF is largely dependent on the age at which the abnormality is diagnosed and surgically corrected. While a majority of uncorrected TOF patients will have a life expectancy of less than 10 years, patients who undergo surgical repair early in life are now commonly able to live into adulthood, with the understanding that a degree of residual right ventricular dysfunction is common and reoperation in the future may be unavoidable. Common postsurgical complications for TOF patients in adolescence or adulthood include main or branch pulmonary artery stenoses (Fig. 82.6), RVOT transannular patch aneurysms, and right ventricular volume overload due to significant pulmonic regurgitation [4].

Transposition of the Great Arteries

Transposition of the Great Arteries (TGA) is a relatively common cyanotic CHD, representing approximately 5–7% of all CHD [9]. *The fundamental embryologic defect is abnormal conotruncal septal rotation resulting in ventriculoarterial discordance, and patients most commonly present with progressive cyanosis within the first 24 hours of life.* This disease entity can be subdivided into two types based on concurrent morphologic atrioventricular concordance (D-Type) or discordance (L-Type) which will be discussed separately, as their presentation, imaging features, and management are distinct.

Transposition of the Great Arteries, D-Type

Embryology and Epidemiology: TGA (D-Type) refers to the presence of ventriculoarterial discordance with atrioventricular concordance, a so called "uncorrected" transposition. In D-TGA, the morphologic right atrium connects to the morphologic right ventricle through the tricuspid valve with outflow into the aorta, while the morphologic left atrium connects to the morphologic left ventricle through the mitral valve with outflow into the main pulmonary artery (Fig. 82.7). In the D-TGA configuration, the aorta arises anteriorly and to the right of the main pulmonary artery (Fig. 82.8).

While D-TGA most commonly occurs in isolation, it can be associated with other congenital defects, including VSDs, aortic coarctation, and coronary artery anomalies. Extracardiac syndromic associations are rare.

Pathophysiology and Clinical Features: In order for patients with this type of congenital abnormality to survive, a shunt between the systemic and pulmonic circuits must be present to allow for mixing of oxygenated blood from the lungs with deoxygenated systemic blood [4,9]. As is typical of cyanotic CHDs, the degree of right-to-left shunting is the key factor in determining the degree of clinical cyanosis. *An anatomic shunt is usually present in the form of a patent foramen ovale (PFO) and/or patent ductus arteriosus (PDA)* [4].

Imaging Features: The classic radiographic findings of D-TGA are cardiomegaly with an *"egg-on a string" appearance* and increased pulmonary vasculature (Fig. 82.9), [9]. These findings on plain film radiography refer to the relatively narrow superior mediastinal contour which is a consequence of thymic hypoplasia, the underlying cause of which is unknown, and the orientation of the abnormally rotated transposed great vessels.

Echocardiography is usually the initial imaging technique, allowing for visualization of the abnormally positioned aorta and pulmonary arteries, as well as characterization of any intracardiac shunts with color flow Doppler. Echocardiography can also be useful in assessment of the AV and outflow valvular morphologies. While visualization of the coronary arteries is often possible, evaluation can become difficult or impossible in the setting of concurrent coronary anomalies, and additional imaging may be necessary for preoperative planning. The known limitations of operator dependence and suboptimal visualization of extra cardiac structures always apply, and advanced imaging does play an important adjunctive role.

Cardiac CT can provide additional anatomic and functional detail for problem-solving in particularly complex cases, as well as excellent visualization of the coronary arteries for detection and characterization of anomalies of coronary origins or course, which may be critical for preoperative planning. Cardiac CT is also a valuable tool in the assessment of surgically corrected D-TGA patients, with excellent visualization of the postoperative anatomy (i.e., size of interatrial septal defect, patency of surgical baffles, etc.) and high sensitivity for the detection of potential postsurgical complications.

Cardiac MRI is similarly useful in the assessment of surgically corrected D-TGA patients, with the added capability of quantitatively assessing the flow dynamics across intracardiac shunts, at anastomotic sites, and across the cardiac valves with phase-contrast

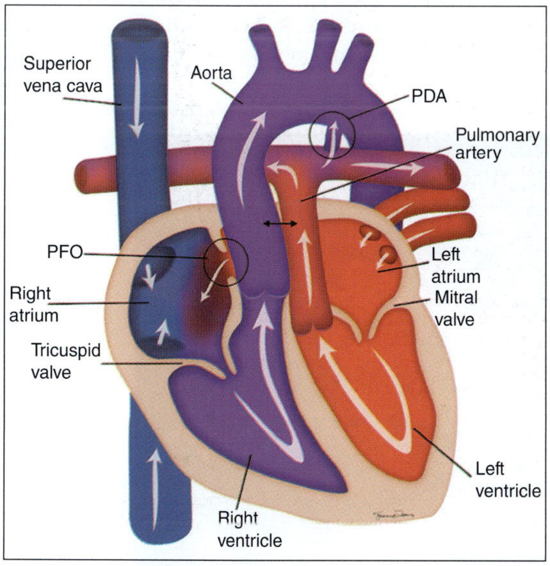

Figure 82.7 Schematic representation of D-type transposition of the great arteries (D-TGA), demonstrating the aorta arising from the right ventricle and the pulmonary artery arising from the left ventricle. This illustration also includes a patent foramen ovale (PFO) and a patent ductus arteriosus (PDA), at least one of which is required for survival by allowing mixing of oxygenated and deoxygenated blood. (Courtesy: Susanne Loomis.)

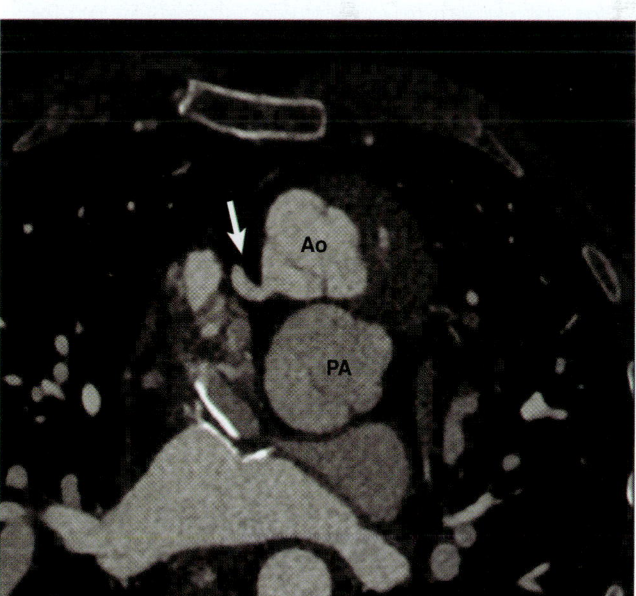

Figure 82.8 Axial contrast-enhanced ECG-gated cardiac CT demonstrates a patient with D-TGA, wherein the aorta (Ao) arises anteriorly and to the right relative to the pulmonary artery (PA). Note that in this patient, a coronary artery (*arrow*) is seen arising from the right aspect of the transposed aorta.

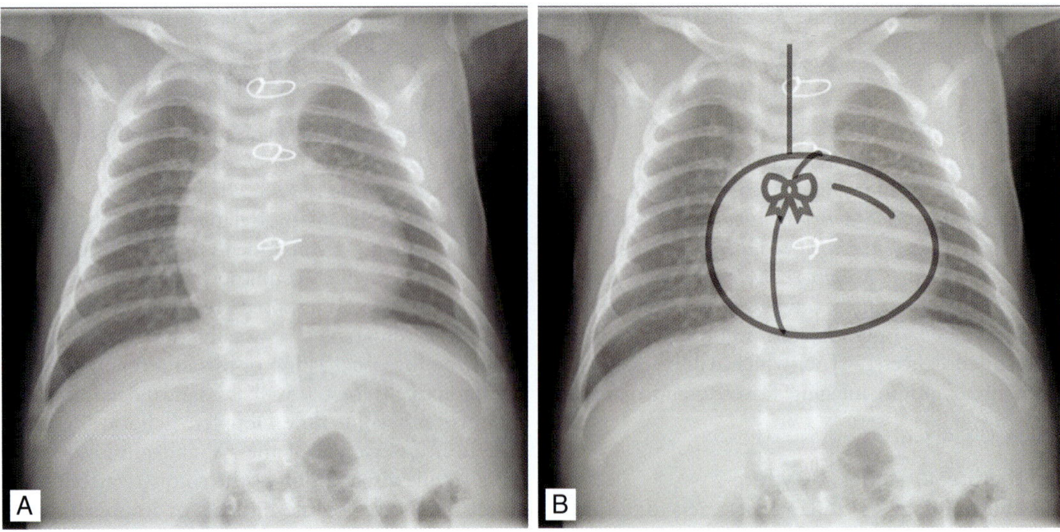

Figure 82.9 Frontal chest radiograph (A) demonstrating the classic *egg on a string appearance* (B) of Transposition of the great arteries, which refers to the relatively narrow superior mediastinal contour caused by thymic hypoplasia and the abnormal orientation of the transposed great vessels.

TABLE 82.8 Summary of the Key Imaging Features of D-Type Transposition of the Great Arteries

Technique	Imaging Features
Chest radiograph	"Egg on a string" appearance of the heart Increased pulmonary vascularity Cardiomegaly Thymic hypoplasia
Cardiac CT/MRI	Atrioventricular concordance[a] Ventriculoarterial discordance Aorta anterior and to the right of the pulmonary artery Patent foramen ovale (PFO) or patent ductus arteriosus (PDA)

[a]Note that atrioventricular concordance is the key feature distinguishing D-Type from L-Type transposition of the great arteries.

sequences. The imaging features of D-Type TGA are summarized in Table 82.8.

Treatment and Outcomes: While D-TGA will ultimately require surgical correction, palliative bridging therapies include neonatal prostaglandin therapy for maintaining patency of the ductus arteriosus and balloon atrial septostomy (BAS or Rashkind procedure) for enlarging the ASD to increase the degree of intracardiac shunting. Definitive surgical correction of D-TGA can be performed, usually in the first week of life, through either an atrial switch procedure such as a Mustard or Senning procedure (Fig. 82.10) or an arterial switch operation with coronary reimplantation such as the Jatene procedure (Fig. 82.11).

Current practice patterns favor the arterial switch operation with coronary reimplantation as the treatment of choice for D-TGA, given better long-term outcomes. Postoperative surveillance of surgically corrected D-TGA patients via the arterial switch operation focuses on monitoring for the development of

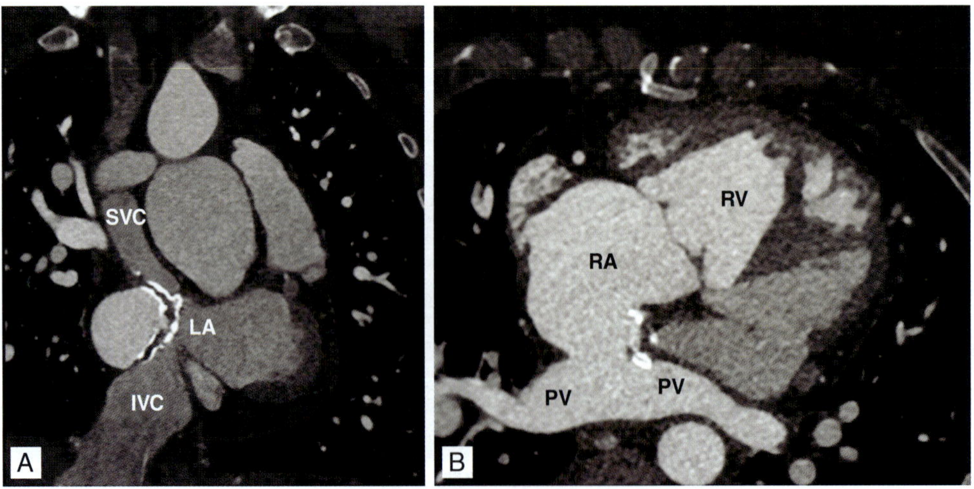

Figure 82.10 Oblique coronal (A) and axial (B) contrast-enhanced ECG-gated cardiac CT demonstrates the postoperative appearance of a patient with D-TGA who underwent an atrial switch operation, in which the pulmonary veins (PV) were baffled to the morphologic right atrium (RA) and the superior vena cava (SVC) and inferior vena cava (IVC) were baffled to the morphologic left atrium (LA). In this postoperative configuration, the right ventricle (RV) functions as the "systemic ventricle" and undergoes hypertrophy over time due to chronic exposure to systemic pressures, as seen in this patient.

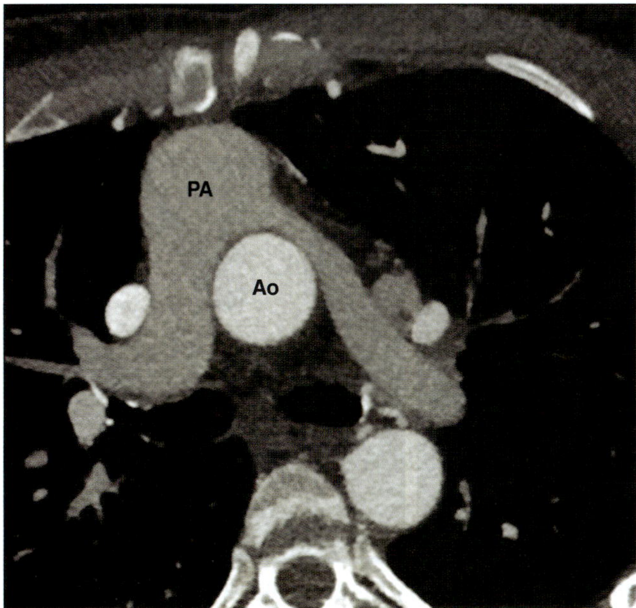

Figure 82.11 Axial contrast-enhanced ECG-gated cardiac CT demonstrates the postoperative appearance of a patient with D-TGA who underwent an arterial switch operation (Jatene procedure), in which the great arteries are surgically switched and the coronary arteries are reimplanted. This operation creates a characteristic postoperative appearance wherein the pulmonary arteries (PA) appear draped anteriorly over the aorta (Ao).

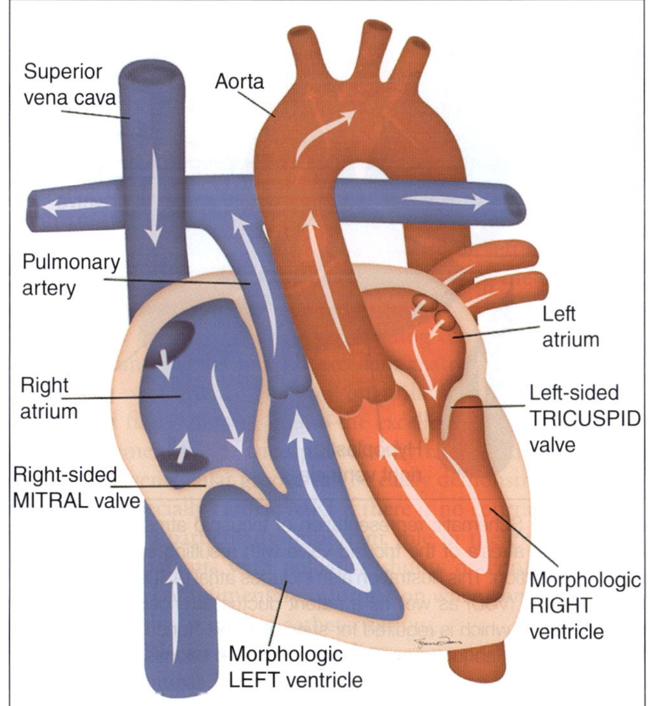

Figure 82.12 Schematic representation of L-Type Transposition of the Great Arteries (L-TGA), demonstrating the anatomic right atrium connecting to the morphologic left ventricle with outflow into the pulmonary artery and the anatomic left atrium connecting to the morphologic right ventricle with outflow into the aorta. (Courtesy: Susanne Loomis.)

neo-aortic root dilation, aortic regurgitation, left ventricular dysfunction, supravalvular (anastomotic) pulmonic stenosis, and coronary occlusion. By contrast, D-TGA patients who have undergone an atrial baffle switch (Mustard or Senning) procedure are at risk for developing dysfunction of the systemic (morphologic right) ventricle, which is the major source of morbidity and mortality, as well as baffle stenosis.

Transposition of the Great Arteries, L-Type

Embryology and Epidemiology: TGA (L-Type), in contrast, refers to the combination of *atrioventricular discordance and ventriculoarterial discordance*, a so-called "congenitally corrected" transposition. In L-TGA, the anatomic right atrium connects to the morphologic left ventricle via the mitral valve with outflow into the main pulmonary artery, while the anatomic left atrium connects to the morphologic right ventricle via the tricuspid valve with outflow into the aorta (Fig. 82.12). By comparison to the previously discussed subtype, in the L-TGA configuration, the aorta arises anteriorly and to the left of the pulmonary artery.

L-TGA can be associated with Ebstein anomaly as well as other congenital defects, including VSDs and pulmonic stenosis [1,3]. When these abnormalities are present, cyanosis may occur. Rarely L-TGA can be seen in combination with right ventricular hypoplasia, resulting in single ventricle physiology.

Pathophysiology and Clinical Features: In contrast with D-TGA, *patients with L-TGA are not dependent on intracardiac shunting and may be asymptomatic or present in adulthood.* In certain patients, however, significant tricuspid insufficiency and systemic ventricular dysfunction can occur, as the morphologic right ventricle faces higher left-sided (systemic) pressures [4].

Imaging Features: With the exception of the atrioventricular discordance, the imaging findings of L-TGA by radiography and echocardiography are often indistinguishable from D-TGA and are summarized in Table 82.9.

Echocardiography can be useful evaluating for coexisting VSDs and/or the presence of pulmonic stenosis in these patients.

Advanced imaging modalities, such as cardiac CT and cardiac MRI, are again valuable for anatomic delineation (Fig. 82.13) as well as detection of associated abnormalities if a definitive diagnosis cannot be made by echocardiography alone. These modalities

TABLE 82.9 Summary of the Key Imaging Features of L-Type Transposition of the Great Arteries

Technique	Imaging Features
Chest radiograph	"Egg on a string" appearance of the heart Increased pulmonary vascularity Cardiomegaly Thymic hypoplasia
Cardiac CT/MRI	Atrioventricular discordance[a] Ventriculoarterial discordance Aorta anterior and to the left of the pulmonary artery Hypertrophy of the morphologic (systemic) right ventricle Tricuspid insufficiency or Ebstein anomaly Ventricular septal defects

[a]Note that atrioventricular discordance is the key feature distinguishing L-Type from D-Type transposition of the great arteries.

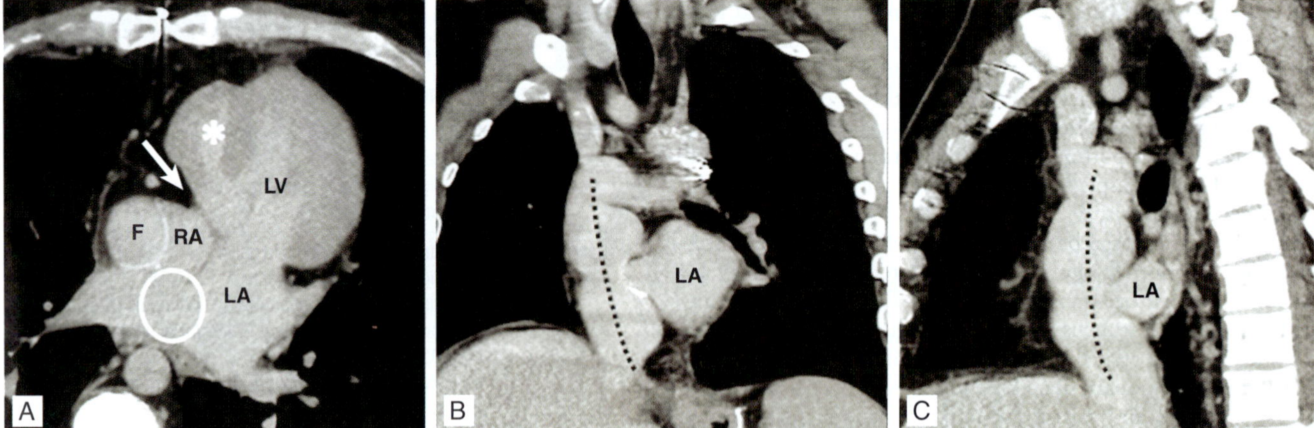

Figure 82.15 Axial (A), coronal (B), sagittal (C) contrast-enhanced ECG-gated cardiac CT demonstrates the postoperative appearance of a patient with tricuspid atresia who has undergone single ventricle palliation with a lateral tunnel Fontan shunt (F), seen on the axial image within the right atrium (RA). The tricuspid valve is atretic (*arrow*) and there is an underdeveloped nonopacified right ventricle (*white asterisk*) that does not participate in cardiac output. An atrial septal defect (*white circle*) allows some blood exchange between the right atrium (RA)/Fontan and the left atrium (LA), while the left ventricle (LV) functions as the "single ventricle" pumping blood into systemic circulation. Coronal (B) and sagittal (C) reformats demonstrate the lateral tunnel Fontan (dotted line) connecting the superior and inferior vena cava to the right pulmonary artery, also known as total cavo-pulmonary connection.

commonly in the form of a total cavo-pulmonary connection (TCPC), but can alternatively be seen in the form of a right atrium to pulmonary connection (AP).

Long-term survival and morbidity data for patients with Fontan circulation are promising, with reported survival rates of nearly 90% at age 30 years and approximately 60% at age 50 years, noting relatively low rates of cardiac transplantation overall [13]. The most common causes of death in these patients are cardiac failure and presumed arrhythmia-related sudden death.

Truncus Arteriosus

Embryology and Epidemiology: Truncus arteriosus is a rare cyanotic congenital heart defect, accounting for 1–4% of all CHD [10,14], in which *the aorta, pulmonary arteries, and coronary arteries all arise from a common trunk (the truncus arteriosus) that most commonly overrides an associated large VSD* (Fig. 82.16). The underlying cause is the failure of septation of the common truncus in the fetus, and arrangement of the cardiac chambers is otherwise anatomically normal in most cases. However, the common truncal valve is often abnormal in its development, with myxomatous valve leaflets arranged in a bicuspid, quadricuspid, or even pentacuspid morphology, often resulting in mixed valvular stenosis and insufficiency.

Truncus arteriosus is closely associated with right-sided aortic arch with mirror image branching and is commonly seen as part of DiGeorge syndrome (22q11.2 microdeletion) [1,10]. PDA and other anomalies of the aortic arch and branch pulmonary arteries can also be seen in association, some of which have been identified as independent risk factors for surgical mortality, including IAA. Truncus arteriosus can be subdivided into different types depending on the location or takeoff orientation of the pulmonary arteries, and there are multiple historical classification systems used to describe the heterogeneity of the branching pattern (Tables 82.12 and 82.13).

Pathophysiology and Clinical Features: The clinical presentation of truncus arteriosus is highly variable and is predominantly dependent upon the morphology of the truncus, the degree of truncal valve regurgitation, and the relative resistances in the pulmonary and systemic vascular systems. Patients will commonly present in early neonatal life with some degree of cyanosis, but

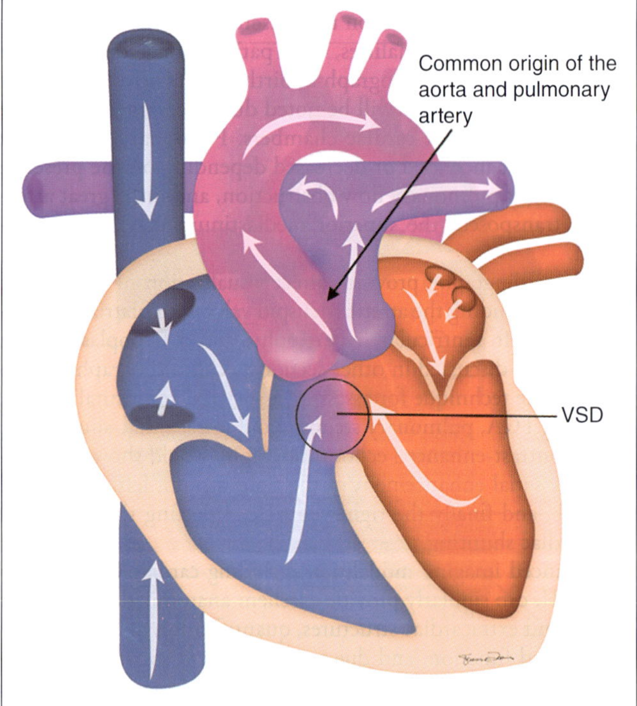

Figure 82.16 Schematic representation of truncus arteriosus, demonstrating a common origin of the aorta and pulmonary artery in the Collett and Edwards Type 1 (most common) configuration overriding a large ventricular septal defect (VSD). (Courtesy: Susanne Loomis.)

may experience shortness of breath and congestive heart failure to a much greater extent due to pulmonary overcirculation. From a physiologic standpoint, there is complete intracardiac mixing of oxygenated pulmonary and deoxygenated systemic venous blood across the VSD, which explains the systemic desaturation. Given that the pulmonary vascular system is frequently lower resistance when compared with the systemic circulation, blood flow within the truncus is preferentially directed into the pulmonary vasculature, causing symptoms of congestive heart failure. Chronically increased pulmonary flow predisposes to early pulmonary vascular obstructive disease.

As with many other CHDs, prenatal diagnosis is typically feasible with routine prenatal ultrasound screening. Targeted prenatal screening is commonly pursued in patients with a family history of conotruncal abnormalities, CHD, or DiGeorge syndrome. However, a postnatal presentation of truncus arteriosus is not uncommon. While prenatal diagnosis of truncus arteriosus has not been shown to have a survival benefit, it does allow for family counseling, proper delivery planning, and development of a postnatal care plan. Furthermore, a delay in diagnosis places patients at greater risk of developing progressive coronary steal phenomenon with decreasing pulmonary vascular resistance, as well as significant pulmonary arterial hypertension.

TABLE 82.12 Collett and Edwards Classification System for Truncus Arteriosus

Type 1 (most common)	Short main pulmonary artery from truncus
Type 2	Two separate pulmonary arteries from truncus (posterior origin)
Type 3 (least common)	Two separate pulmonary arteries from truncus (lateral origin)
Type 4 (pseudotruncus)	Now recognized as Pulmonary Atresia with VSD (severe Tetralogy of Fallot variant)

TABLE 82.13 Van Praagh Classification System for Truncus Arteriosus

Type A1	Origin of the pulmonary trunk from the truncal root
Type A2	Separate origin of the branch pulmonary arteries from the truncal root
Type A3	Absent left, right, or both pulmonary arteries with absent pulmonary artery originating from an arterial duct or collateral artery
Type A4	Associated with aortic coarctation or interruption of the aortic arch
A	Denotes presence of a ventricular septal defect (VSD)
B	Denotes rare occurrence of intact ventricular septum

Imaging Features: The radiographic findings of truncus arteriosus are similar to many other cyanotic CHDs, and include cardiomegaly, increased pulmonary vascularity, and a narrow superior mediastinum due to concurrent thymic agenesis. An associated right-sided aortic arch is also commonly present.

Echocardiography, as the first line technique, allows for definitive diagnosis in a majority of cases, with excellent delineation of the ventricular origin and branching pattern of the common arterial trunk, truncal valvular morphology, and function, associated VSDs, or other intracardiac abnormalities. Advanced imaging modalities, such as cardiac CT and MRI, may be helpful in characterization of truncal anatomy (Fig. 82.17) in complex cases where findings on echocardiography are equivocal, as well as evaluation of truncal valvular and biventricular function. These modalities are also particularly useful in assessing for postsurgical complications such as RV to PA conduit stenosis, truncal root dilation, or anastomotic pseudoaneurysm formation.

The imaging features for truncus arteriosus are highlighted in Table 82.14 and the differential diagnosis is summarized in Table 82.15, which includes other CHDs that allow for pulmonary-systemic mixing, including TGA, aortopulmonary window, and atrioventricular canal defects.

Treatment and Outcomes: Definitive surgical management for patients with truncus arteriosus involves closure of the VSD, resection of the main/branch pulmonary arteries from the common arterial trunk, and placement of a conduit reestablishing a con-

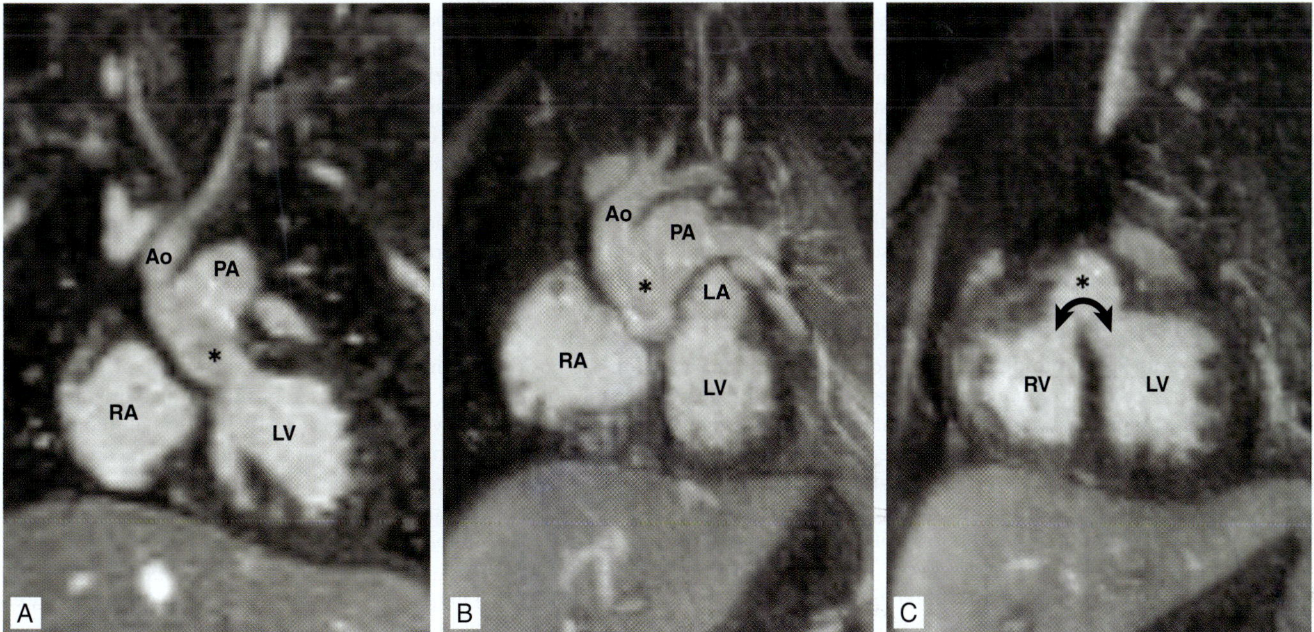

Figure 82.17 Coronal (A), sagittal (B), and short-axis (C) MR Angiogram images demonstrate a patient with uncorrected Collett and Edwards Type 1 configuration Truncus Arteriosus. The common truncal root (*asterisk*) gives rise to both the aorta (Ao) and pulmonary artery (PA) and overrides a large ventricular septal defect (*double-headed arrow*), thus receiving blood flow from both the right ventricle (RV) and left ventricle (LV). *LA*, left atrium; *RA*, right atrium.

TABLE 82.14 Summary of the Key Imaging Features of Truncus Arteriosus

Technique	Imaging Features
Chest radiograph	Increased pulmonary vascularity Cardiomegaly Narrow superior mediastinum/thymic agenesis Possible right-sided aortic arch (with mirror image branching)
Cardiac CT/MRI	Common arterial trunk Ventricular septal defect (VSD) Variable truncal valve function (regurgitation)

TABLE 82.15 Differential Diagnosis for Truncus Arteriosus

Transposition of the great arteries (TGA)
Aortopulmonary window
Atrioventricular canal defect

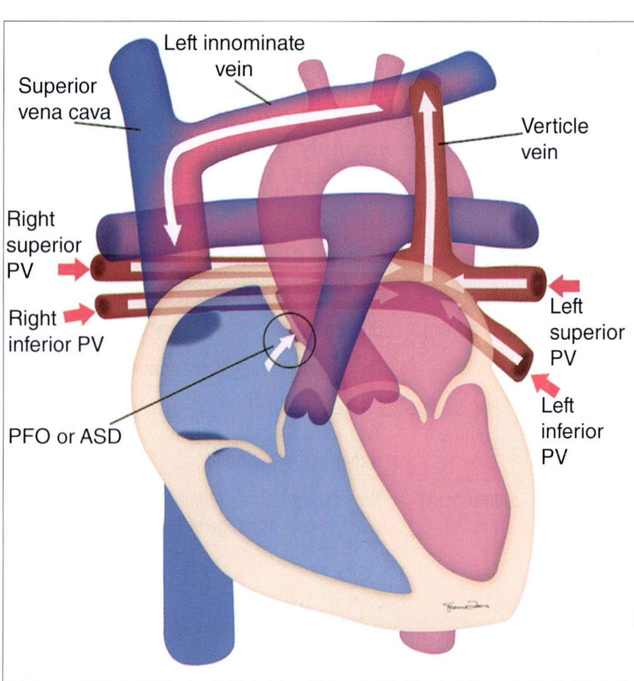

Figure 82.18 Schematic representation of total anomalous pulmonary venous return (TAPVR), supracardiac subtype (Type 1) wherein all the pulmonary veins (PV) drain above the level of the superior vena cava (SVC) into the left innominate vein through a "vertical vein." This illustration also includes an atrial level shunt in the form of a patent foramen ovale (PFO) or atrial septal defect (ASD), which is necessary for survival in patients with this congenital defect. (Courtesy: Susanne Loomis.)

nection between the right ventricle and the pulmonary arteries, typically early in neonatal life. Although this procedure is one of the more complicated neonatal surgeries, given the reactivity of the pulmonary vascular bed as well as the large ventriculotomy required, modern-day surgical outcomes in most centers are excellent. Truncus arteriosus patients often outgrow their original conduit with time and require reoperation in the future to resize the conduit. Additional potential reoperations or postsurgical interventions may involve the truncal valve or branch pulmonary arteries.

Before the era of surgical repair, mortality for truncus arteriosus was exceedingly high with a survival rate of only 15–30% at 1 year [15]. Even in the early days of surgical management where neonatal pulmonary artery banding was initially performed and followed by staged repair later in infancy, mortality was still double what it is with more modern techniques. Currently, despite still having one of the highest early mortality rates among all CHD surgeries, primary repair in the first few weeks of life is the favored approach. Notably, truncal valve manipulation in early life is avoided whenever possible as neonatal valve repair is also associated with an increase in mortality. Long-term outcomes ultimately depend on the adequacy of conduit function in restoring pulmonary arterial flow, pulmonary vascular resistance, and truncal valve competency.

Total Anomalous Pulmonary Venous Return (TAPVR)

Embryology and Epidemiology: Total anomalous pulmonary venous return (TAPVR) is a rare cyanotic congenital heart defect in which all the pulmonary veins drain anomalously into the right heart, forming a left-to-right shunt of oxygenated blood back to the lungs (Fig. 82.18). Similar to tricuspid atresia, TAPVR is incompatible with life in isolation, and thus an obligate coexisting right-to-left shunt, commonly in the form of a PFO or an ASD, is required for survival [9].

Surprisingly, despite continued technological advances in prenatal ultrasonography, TAPVR has one of the lowest prenatal detection rates for CHD, with detection as low as 2–10% [16]. The fetal pulmonary veins carry only a small percentage of blood from the developing lungs, and thus visualization by ultrasound can be challenging. If prenatal diagnosis is not made by screening ultrasound, the initial presenting symptoms of TAPVR can be difficult to distinguish from other cyanotic CHDs or neonatal respiratory diseases, including respiratory distress syndrome or persistent pulmonary hypertension.

Pathophysiology and Clinical Features: TAPVR can be classified into different subtypes based on the anatomic location of the pulmonary venous drainage (Table 82.16), with the most common morphology being the supracardiac type [9,17]. Physiologically, TAPVR may be classified as obstructive or nonobstructive depending on the degree of obstruction to pulmonary venous flow, which is most commonly seen in infracardiac TAPVR at the level of the diaphragmatic hiatus. Although this congenital heart defect usually occurs in isolation, it can be seen as a component of more complex CHD, particularly in heterotaxy syndromes. Notably, 50% of patients with asplenia will have CHD and the vast majority of those patients will have TAPVR [9].

Clinical presentation and radiographic findings depend heavily on the position of the venous drainage, the degree of pulmonary venous obstruction, and the degree of intracardiac mixing. Neonates with obstructive infracardiac TAPVR most commonly present with cyanosis in the first hours of life while neonates with nonobstructive supracardiac TAPVR are more likely to present with signs and symptoms of congestive heart failure within the first six weeks of life.

Imaging Features: In suspected cases, echocardiography with Doppler is generally able to identify the site of anomalous venous drainage, along with the presence of an atrial level shunt and right heart dilation.

The radiographic features, like the clinical symptoms, vary depending on the position of the pulmonary venous drainage.

TABLE 82.16 Classification System for Total Anomalous Pulmonary Venous Return [9,17]

Type I Supracardiac (55%)	Pulmonary veins drain at or above the level of the SVC, most commonly draining into the left innominate vein through a vertical vein (gives the classic **"snowman" appearance** on CXR)
Type II Cardiac (30%)	Pulmonary veins drain into the coronary sinus or right atrium
Type III Infracardiac (13%)	Pulmonary veins drain below the level of the diaphragm, most commonly into the hepatic veins or IVC (obstruction at the level of the diaphragm causes pulmonary edema)
Type IV Mixed	A combination of the types described above

Neonates with obstructive infracardiac TAPVR most commonly demonstrate florid pulmonary edema with pleural effusions on chest radiograph. Conversely, neonates with nonobstructive supracardiac TAPVR often demonstrate the classic *"snowman" appearance* on chest radiograph due to widening of the superior mediastinum from the dilated right-sided SVC and left-sided vertical vein (Fig. 82.19).

CT and MRI can provide valuable supplemental information in complex, mixed, or equivocal cases, and are particularly helpful for infracardiac variants which can be notoriously difficult to image by ultrasound. CT and MRI can also be useful for detecting pulmonary venous stenoses commonly seen in TAPVR repairs. The multiplanar reformatting and three-dimensional volume rendering capabilities of both CT and MRI can be exceptionally helpful for preoperative surgical planning, and cardiac MRI has the added benefit of flow analysis capabilities, allowing for detailed physiologic assessment.

Although cardiac MRI is the most common choice for advanced anatomic delineation of a majority of congenital pulmonary vein anomalies, in the setting of obstructed TAPVR, cardiac CT would be a better choice due to the shorter scan time in a more urgent clinical scenario.

The key imaging features for TAPVR are highlighted in Table 82.17 and the differential diagnosis is summarized in Table 82.18.

Treatment and Outcomes: Definitive surgical repair of TAPVR involves surgical reimplantation of the pulmonary venous drainage into the left atrium. This surgery is performed on an urgent basis for patients with obstructive TAPVR but can be pursued less urgently in nonobstructive TAPVR. Prostaglandin E1 infusion is typically initiated in neonates to maintain patency of the ductus arteriosus as an additional right-to-left shunt before surgical intervention. Additional closure of the ASD may be pursued at a later date.

The presence of preoperative pulmonary venous obstruction is associated with increased preoperative morbidity related to the development of pulmonary hypertension and the potential requirement for extracorporeal membrane oxygenation (ECMO). TAPVR found in association with heterotaxy syndromes is associated with the highest rates of postoperative morbidity, with patients often requiring repeated surgical interventions for the postoperative complication of pulmonary venous stenosis/obstruction (Fig. 82.20). Heterotaxy patients with TAPVR also experience postoperative mortality rates up to ~50% at three years, particularly if they have complex CHD with single ventricle

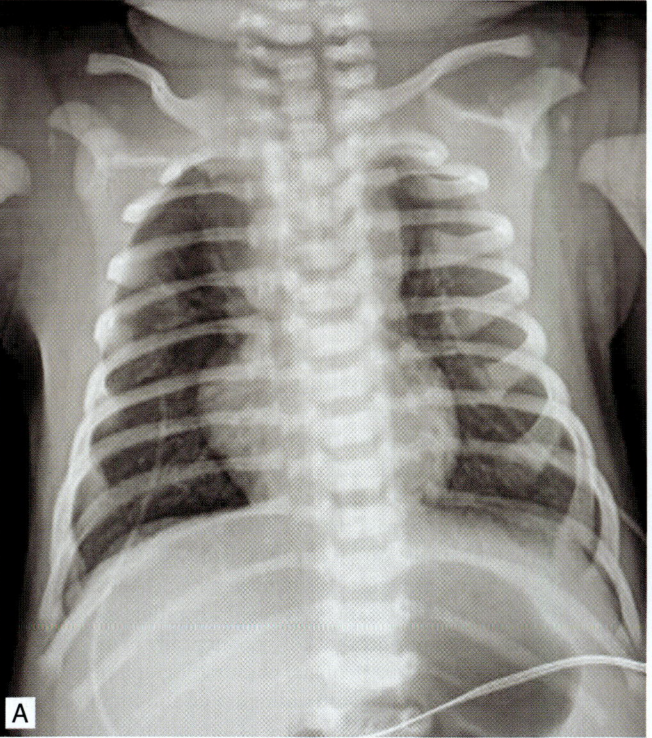

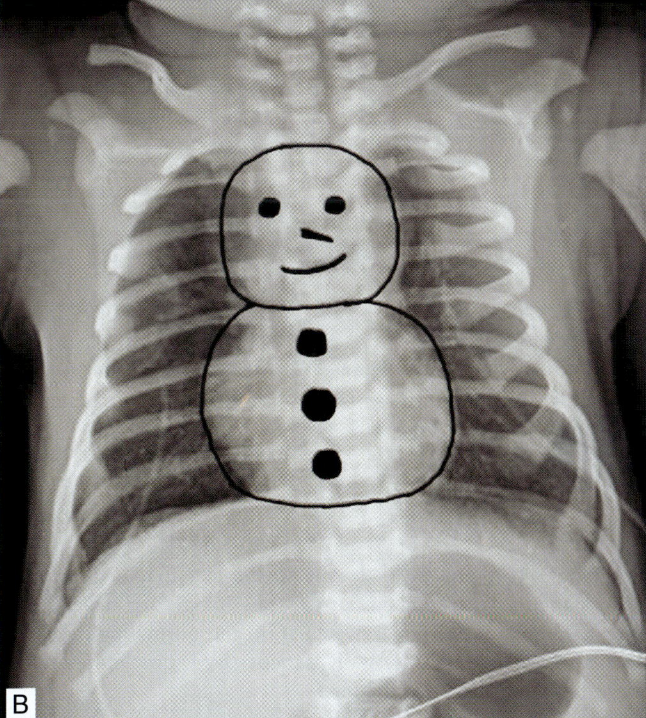

Figure 82.19 Frontal chest radiograph (A) demonstrating the classic *snowman appearance* (B) of supracardiac TAPVR, which is explained by the widening of the superior mediastinum resulting from dilation of the right-sided superior vena cava and total anomalous drainage of the pulmonary veins into a left-sided "vertical vein."

TABLE 82.17 Summary of the Key Imaging Features of Total Anomalous Pulmonary Venous Return

Technique	Imaging Features
Chest radiograph	"Snowman" appearance (supracardiac type) Florid pulmonary edema + bilateral pleural effusions (infracardiac type)
Cardiac CT/MRI	Anomalous (systemic) drainage of all pulmonary veins Patent foramen ovale (PFO) or Atrial septal defect (ASD) Pulmonary vein stenoses

TABLE 82.18 Differential Diagnosis for Total Anomalous Pulmonary Venous Return

Tetralogy of Fallot (TOF)
Transposition of the great arteries (TGA)
Truncus arteriosus (TA)
Respiratory distress syndrome (RDS)
Persistent pulmonary hypertension (PPHN)

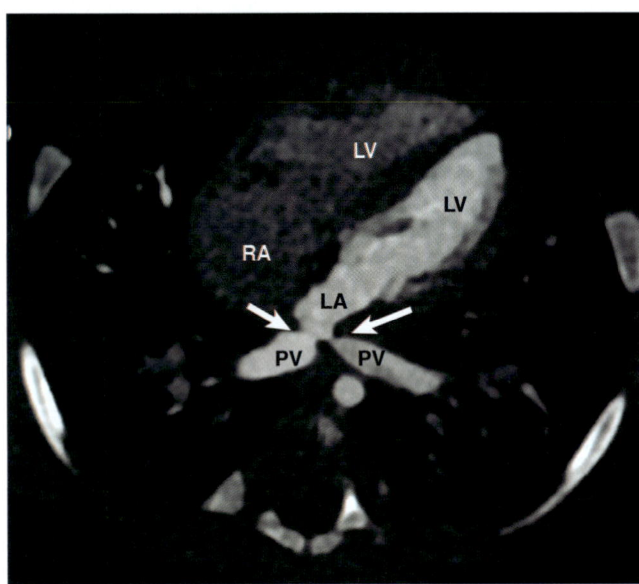

Figure 82.20 Axial contrast-enhanced ECG-gated cardiac CT demonstrating anastomotic pulmonary vein stenosis (*arrows*) as a complication of surgical pulmonary venous reimplantation in a patient born with TAPVR. *LA*, left atrium; *LV*, left ventricle; *PV*, pulmonary vein; *RA*, right atrium; *RV*, right ventricle..

physiology [16]. This is likely due to the fact that in the long term, patients with single ventricle physiology are dependent upon a compliant pulmonary vasculature and normal pulmonary vascular resistance, and TAPVR patients have developmentally abnormal pulmonary vasculature.

Hypoplastic Left Heart Syndrome

Embryology and Epidemiology: Hypoplastic left heart syndrome (HLHS) is a rare spectrum of cyanotic congenital heart

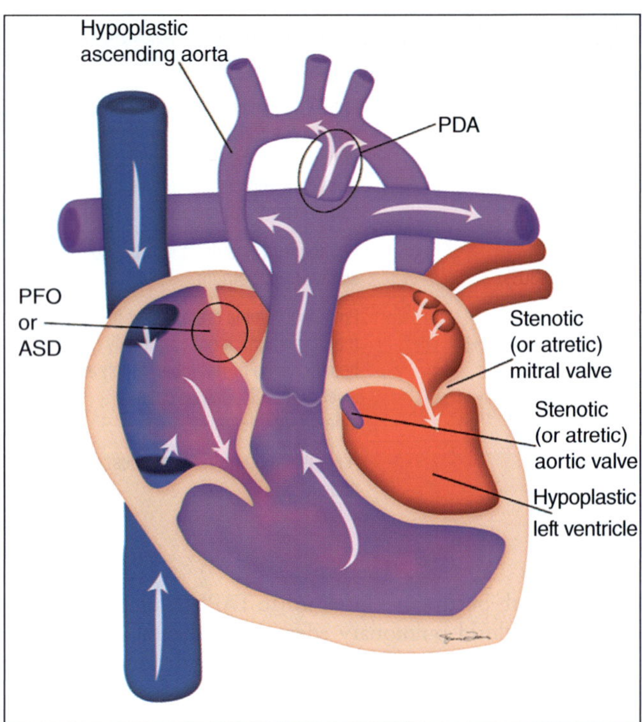

Figure 82.21 Schematic representation of hypoplastic left heart syndrome (HLHS), demonstrating underdeveloped of the left-sided heart structures, including mitral stenosis/atresia, hypoplastic left ventricle, aortic stenosis/atresia, and hypoplastic thoracic aora. This illustration also includes an atrial level shunt in the form of a patent foramen ovale (PFO) or atrial septal defect (ASD), as well as a patent ductus arteriosus (PDA), which are necessary for survival in patients with this congenital defect. (Courtesy: Susanne Loomis.)

abnormalities representing the fourth most common CHD to present in the first year of life and constituting 1.2–1.5% of all CHDs [1,10,18]. *HLHS is characterized by underdevelopment of the left-sided cardiac structures, including the left atrium, mitral valve, left ventricle, aortic valve, and aorta* (Fig. 82.21)(1,10). The pathogenesis of this CHD remains poorly understood, but may be attributable to abnormal cardiac partitioning during embryogenesis.

Approximately 25% of patients with HLHS will exhibit coexisting complex congenital heart defects, such as DORV, and other common associations include aortic coarctation, VSDs, and endocardial fibroelastosis (EFE) [10]. In addition, up to 25% of HLHS patients will exhibit a major extracardiac anomaly or genetic syndromes such as Turner, Noonan, Holt-Oram, or Smith-Lemli-Oplitz [10].

Pathophysiology and Clinical Features: HLHS is the most common of the "single ventricle defects" with a 2:1 male to female ratio [10]. Initial survival is dependent upon both an ASD and a PDA to allow for blood to bypass the underdeveloped left heart and return to systemic circulation [1,10]. Neonates with this congenital defect may be asymptomatic at birth, however, once the PDA closes in the first few days of life, patients will quickly progress to cyanosis, congestive heart failure, and shock if not surgically managed.

Imaging Features: Initial neonatal chest radiograph may be normal in patients with HLHS with radiographic abnormalities often developing within the first 2–3 days of life upon closure of the PDA. These features include increased pulmonary vascularity, severe pulmonary edema, and cardiomegaly—particularly dilation of the right-heart structures.

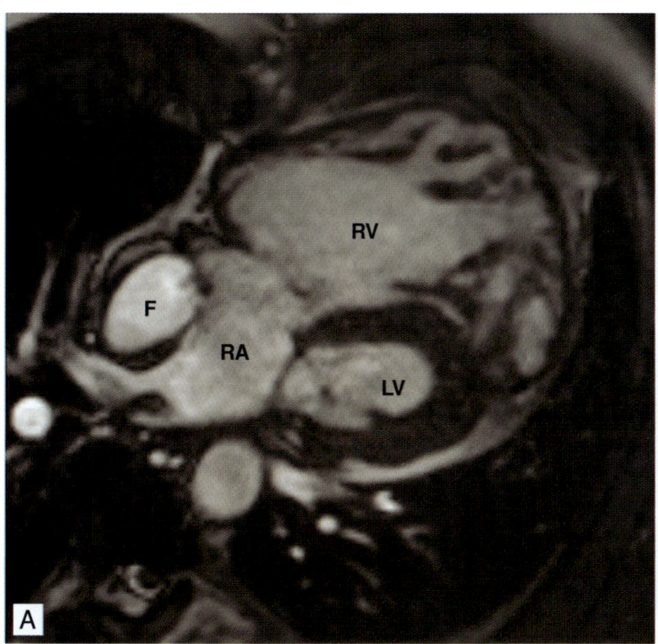

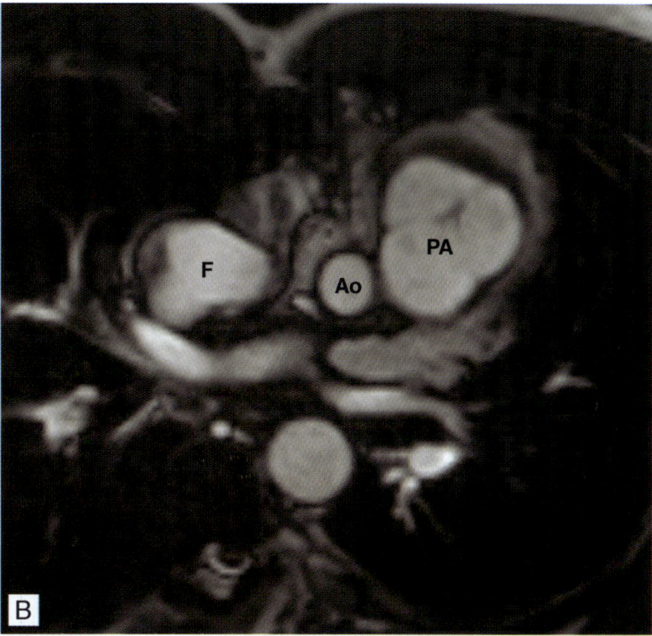

Figure 82.22 Two axial SSFP images at the level of the cardiac chambers (A) and great vessels (B) demonstrate the classic imaging findings of hypoplastic left heart syndrome, including an underdeveloped left ventricle (LV) and small-caliber hypoplastic aorta (Ao). This patient has undergone single ventricle palliation surgery with a lateral tunnel Fontan (F) seen adjacent to the right atrium (RA). Notice the compensatory hypertrophy of the right ventricle (RV), which functions as the single systemic ventricle in this patient, as well as the enlarged pulmonary artery (PA).

Echocardiography is often sufficient for initial diagnosis and preoperative planning, providing a clear visualization of the underdeveloped left-heart structures, identification of any coexisting abnormalities, such as aortic coarctation, and comprehensive noninvasive evaluation of relevant shunts and valvular competency.

Preoperative cardiac CT and MRI are usually only necessary in the case of unusually complex cardiac anatomy in the setting of multiple concomitant congenital abnormalities, but will clearly demonstrate the underdeveloped left-sided heart structures (Fig. 82.22). One potential preoperative use for cardiac MRI is for the detection of EFE. In patients with relatively mild left-sided hypoplasia and functioning mitral and aortic valves, the presence or absence of EFE can be a deciding factor in determining whether a single ventricle repair or double ventricle repair is the appropriate course of action.

Advanced imaging modalities have a more established role in the postoperative monitoring of HLHS patients who have undergone multistaged single ventricle repair (Fig. 82.23), providing useful information related to ventricular function, valvular competency, and overall cardiovascular anatomy. The key imaging features for HLHS are highlighted in Table 82.19 and the differential diagnosis is summarized in Table 82.20.

Treatment and Outcomes: Before the introduction of surgical techniques designed to palliate single ventricle pathologies, HLHS was a universally fatal disease. Today, the two main treatment strategies for surgical management of HLHS include a multistage Norwood repair (described in detail in the tricuspid atresia section) and cardiac transplantation. Despite nontrivial postsurgical and interstage mortality risk, long-term outcomes continue to improve and HLHS patients are now surviving into teenage and adult years.

Some HLHS patients will develop end-stage circulatory failure, and cardiac transplantation is the only available option for long-term survival.

TABLE 82.19 Summary of the Key Imaging Features of Hypoplastic Left Heart Syndrome

Technique	Imaging Features
Chest radiograph	Increased pulmonary vascularity Severe pulmonary edema Cardiomegaly (enlarged right heart structures) May be normal in the first 1–2 days of life
Cardiac CT/MRI	Hypoplastic left ventricle ± hypoplastic aorta Variable degree of aortic stenosis/atresia Variable degree of mitral stenosis/atresia Patent foramen ovale (PFO) or Atrial septal defect (ASD) Patent ductus arteriosus (PDA) Dilated right atrium and right ventricle Increased pulmonary vascularity and pulmonary edema

TABLE 82.20 Differential Diagnosis for Hypoplastic Left Heart Syndrome

Congenital aortic stenosis

Aortic coarctation/interrupted aortic arch

Unbalanced atrioventricular canal defect

Ebstein anomaly

Ebstein Anomaly

Embryology and Epidemiology: Ebstein anomaly refers to a congenital malformation characterized by *apical displacement of the septal and posteroinferior tricuspid valve leaflets* (Fig. 82.24), representing 0.3–1% of all CHD and accounting for nearly 40%

TABLE 82.21 Summary of the Key Imaging Features of Ebstein Anomaly

Technique	Imaging Features
Chest radiograph	Enlarged "box-shaped heart"–marked right atrial enlargement Decreased pulmonary vascularity
Cardiac CT/MRI	Apically displaced septal and posteroinferior tricuspid valve leaflets Atrialization of the right ventricle PFO or ASD Variable degree of tricuspid regurgitation Small caliber aorta and pulmonary artery

TABLE 82.22 Differential Diagnosis for Ebstein Anomaly

Tricuspid atresia
Atrial septal defects
Congenital pulmonary stenosis

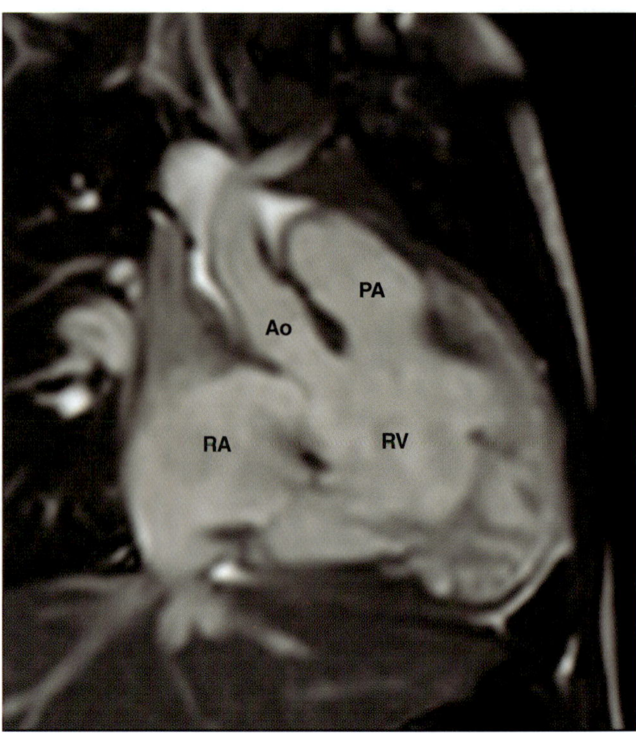

Figure 82.27 Oblique coronal SSFP image demonstrates a patient with double outlet right ventricle (DORV), wherein the aorta (Ao) and pulmonary arteries (PA) both arise from the morphologic right ventricle (RV). *RA*, right atrium.

Treatment and Outcomes: Management of Ebstein patients is variable, depending upon the severity of the defect and associated symptoms. Although many patients may be managed nonoperatively, patients with severe defects may require neonatal ECMO for temporization of cyanosis. While some patients can undergo surgical tricuspid valve repair, others with severely displaced and dysplastic tricuspid valves may ultimately require complete tricuspid valve closure with a Blalock–Thomas–Taussig or Bidirectional Glenn shunt to redirect and improve pulmonary blood flow. Given the predisposition to arrhythmias in these patients, pacemakers or catheter ablation therapy can be considered for long-term management [1,10].

Other Rare Cyanotic Congenital Heart Diseases

While this section focuses on the most common, high-yield cyanotic CHD pathologies, there are several additional more rare pathologies worth mentioning briefly, should they be encountered in clinical practice.

Pulmonary Atresia With Intact Ventricular Septum (PA/IVS): Pulmonary atresia with intact ventricular septum (PA/IVS) accounts for 3% of all CHD with a slight male predominance [14], wherein the development of the pulmonary valve is abnormal and results in complete obstruction of the RVOT. Patients with PA/IVS frequently have tricuspid regurgitation and a coexisting PFO or ASD, which serves to partially decompress the elevated right ventricular pressures. Other common associations include right ventricular hypoplasia, an underdeveloped or dysplastic (Ebstein anomaly) tricuspid valve, and ventriculocoronary fistulas. PA/IVS is a single ventricle physiology equivalent, and in early neonatal life, the appearance by plain radiograph may be identical to Ebstein anomaly, with massive cardiomegaly predominantly due to right atrial enlargement and decreased pulmonary vasculature. Importantly, if severe tricuspid regurgitation develops in utero, patients may present with intrauterine fetal hydrops or fetal demise.

Double Outlet Right Ventricle (DORV): DORV represents less than 1% of all CHD and reflects a type of ventriculoarterial discordance in which both the aorta and pulmonary artery effectively arise from the morphologic right ventricle, resulting in a functional single ventricle physiology (Fig. 82.27) [19]. There is vast morphologic heterogeneity within this particular disease pathology—the great arteries may be normally related to each other or transposed, a coexisting VSD is always present, and superimposed pulmonic stenosis is commonly associated. The unique combination of the various anatomic features determines the symptomatology and clinical course for any given patient, which may range from pulmonary overcirculation to transposition-liked physiology. Similarly, surgical treatment and consequently long-term prognosis for DORV is highly dependent on the morphologic subtype.

Double Inlet Left Ventricle (DILV): Double Inlet Left Ventricle (DILV) is present when greater than 50% of each atrioventricular connection is contiguous with a dominant left ventricle, and reflects one of the functional single ventricle CHDs. The right ventricle is commonly hypoplastic and if there is ventriculoarterial concordance, a VSD will be present so that blood can shunt left-to-right and exit into the pulmonary arteries for reoxygenation. DILV also represents a heterogeneous spectrum of diseases and is commonly associated with other defects including TGA, pulmonic stenosis/atresia, and aortic coarctation/obstruction. Similar to other cyanotic CHDs, the presence and severity of pulmonary outflow obstruction is the key factor in determining the degree of cyanosis versus congestive heart failure seen in the clinical presentation. Management is predominantly surgical, most often in the form of staged single ventricle palliation with a Fontan pathway. If there is significant pulmonic stenosis, this may additionally need to be addressed in the form of a Damus–Kaye–Stansel operation.

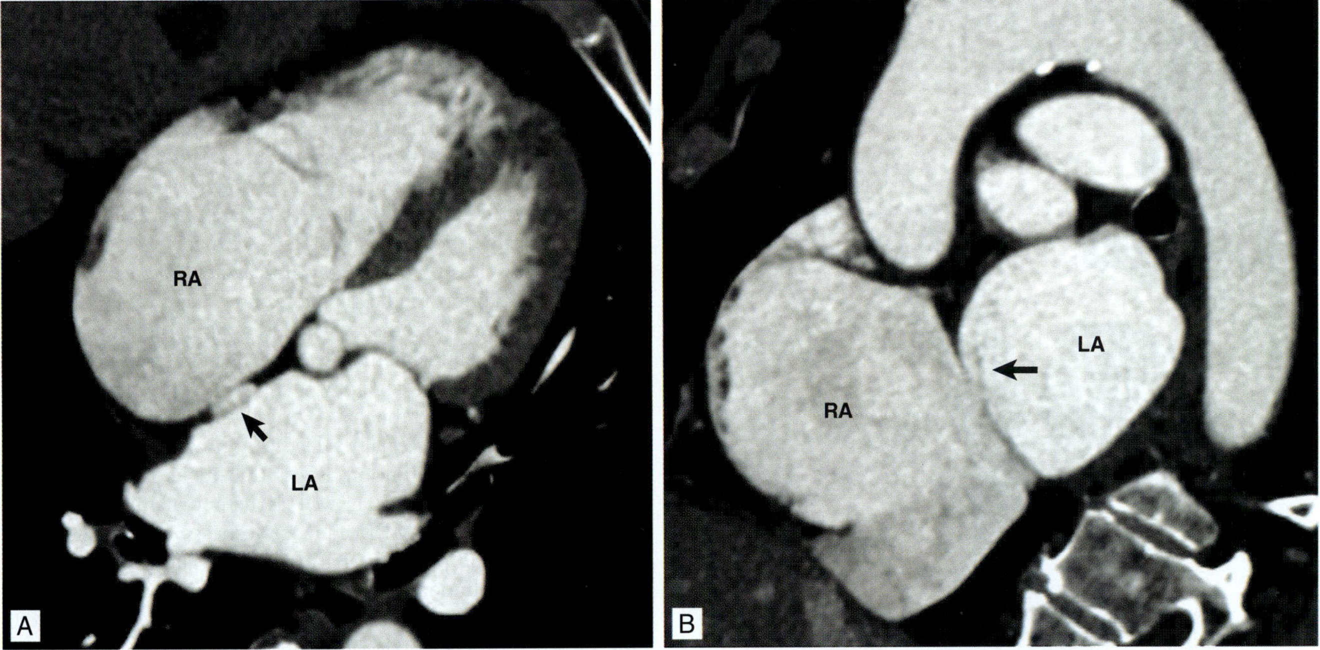

Figure 82.28 Four-chamber (A) and short-axis (B) contrast-enhanced ECG-gated cardiac CT demonstrates a channel-like tunnel in the interatrial septum with a flap valve appearance on short-axis (*arrows*), compatible with a small patent foramen ovale. *LA*, left atrium; *RA*, right atrium.

Acyanotic Congenital Heart Disease

Acyanotic CHD similarly represents a wide spectrum of pathologies which, despite the absence of cyanosis, can be clinically significant if severe. This category of CHD is made up of intracardiac left-to-right shunts, obstructive pathologies such as valvular stenoses or HLHS, and a mix of other congenital anomalies.

While many of these defects can also be detected with prenatal echocardiography, cardiac CT and MRI again can be valuable adjuncts in delineating anatomy and determining the functional significance of many of these pathologies. This section will contain detailed discussions of the clinical and imaging features of the various acyanotic CHDs, current strategies for management, and the role of advanced imaging in evaluating patients with each pathology.

Persistent Fetal Circulation

Two normal shunts from fetal circulation, the **foramen ovale** and **ductus arteriosus**, may fail to close in the early postnatal period. In patients without other underlying CHD, these findings may be incidentally discovered and asymptomatic. By contrast, in patients with cyanotic CHD, patency of these shunts can be crucial to survival.

Patent Foramen Ovale (PFO)

Embryology and Pathophysiology: *PFO refers to the failure of fusion of the primum and secundum atrial septa, typically resulting in a flap-valve opening in the interatrial septum.* This finding is most commonly incidental, reportedly found in approximately 25% of the adult population [20], but has also been identified as a potential source of cryptogenic stroke via paradoxical embolism across the shunt.

Imaging Features: PFO is commonly a radiographically occult diagnosis as the degree of shunting across the interatrial septum is usually clinically insignificant.

In the setting of high clinical suspicion for PFO, transesophageal echocardiography (TEE) is often the imaging technique of choice for investigation. A TEE "bubble study" involving the intravenous injection of agitated saline during a valsalva maneuver can detect even a small PFO, which is suggested by the early appearance of bubbles within the left atrium.

PFOs are commonly visualized on ECG-gated contrast-enhanced cardiac CT, often appearing as a flap valve or channel-like tunnel in the interatrial septum (Fig. 82.28). This appearance helps distinguish a PFO from an ostium secundum ASD, described in detail in a subsequent section. Cardiac MRI, though not a first-line study for evaluation of PFO, may also be able to demonstrate the defect if large or resulting in significant intracardiac shunting. The imaging features of PFO are summarized in Table 82.23.

Treatment and Outcomes: PFO frequently requires no treatment, particularly if small and discovered incidentally. In the setting of hemodynamically significant defects or stroke due to suspected paradoxical embolism, both an open surgical approach or percutaneous closure devices can be used for repair.

Patent Ductus Arteriosus (PDA)

Embryology and Epidemiology: *PDA refers to failure of closure of the ductus arteriosus, which is a normal connection between the aorta and pulmonary artery in fetal circulation* (Fig. 82.29). Isolated PDA is estimated to account for ~10% of all congenital heart anomalies (21) and the highest incidence of PDA occurs in premature infants [1].

TABLE 82.23 Summary of the Key Imaging Features of Isolated Patent Foramen Ovale

Technique	Imaging Features
Chest radiograph	Normal
Cardiac CT/MRI	Channel-like tunnel or flap valve in the interatrial septum Qp/Qs > 1.0 (if clinically significant)

Qp/Qs, pulmonary-systemic flow ratio.

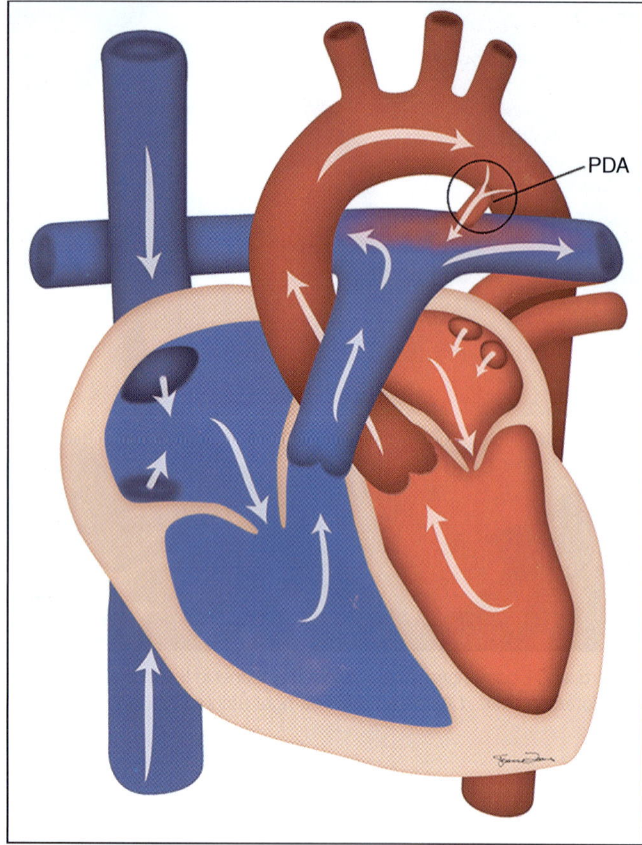

Figure 82.29 Schematic illustration of a patent ductus arteriosus with blood flow shunting left-to-right from the higher pressure aorta into the lower pressure pulmonary arteries. PDA, patent ductus arteriosus. (Courtesy: Susanne Loomis.)

Pathophysiology and Clinical Features: PDA can be detected on physical examination, classically described as a *continuous machine-like systolic and diastolic murmur*. While most PDAs are asymptomatic, the physiologic consequences of a PDA may vary depending on the size of the defect and the pressure differential between systemic and pulmonary circulation. Given higher systemic arterial pressures, initially, left-to-right shunting will occur across a PDA. If the degree of shunting is significant, this can result in pulmonary overcirculation and symptoms of congestive heart failure. If uncorrected, long-standing shunting can result in elevated pulmonary arterial pressures and reversal of the shunt to right-to-left, a phenomenon known as *Eisenmenger syndrome*.

Imaging Features: Small isolated PDAs are often radiographically occult, but larger defects may present with increased pulmonary vascularity as well as left atrial and ventricular enlargement on a chest radiograph. Additional radiographic features may vary if a PDA occurs in association with other CHDs, as is commonly the case.

The traditional initial noninvasive investigation for suspected PDA is transthoracic echocardiography with color Doppler, which may demonstrate a flow jet through a PDA into the pulmonary artery.

Cardiac MRI is an equally effective noninvasive technique for detecting clinically significant PDAs due to its ability to assess detailed vascular anatomy as well as hemodynamic evaluation. Velocity-encoded cine MRI sequences can assess relative flow in the aorta (Qs) and pulmonary arteries (Qp), allowing for the calculation of a pulmonary-systemic shunt fraction (Qp/Qs) which indicates shunt severity. For a PDA, a Qp/Qs ratio > 1.0 suggests the presence of a left-to-right shunt and Qp/Qs > 1.7 suggests shunting significant enough to warrant consideration of surgical repair [21].

While echocardiography and MRI are the imaging tools of choice, cardiac CT may also be useful in evaluating the presence of a PDA (Fig. 82.30), assessing size for consideration of percutaneous closure, and identifying sequela of resulting increased pulmonary arterial pressures, particularly in the setting of complex anatomy due to associated congenital abnormalities. Key imaging features of PDA are summarized in Table 82.24.

Treatment and Outcomes: In early neonatal life, closure of a PDA can often be achieved with the administration of indomethacin, which inhibits the vasodilator prostaglandin E (PGE) and promotes PDA closure. When this approach is unsuccessful, surgical PDA ligation may be performed with a lateral approach through a left thoracotomy. Depending on the morphology of the PDA, percutaneous catheter closure devices are also available as a

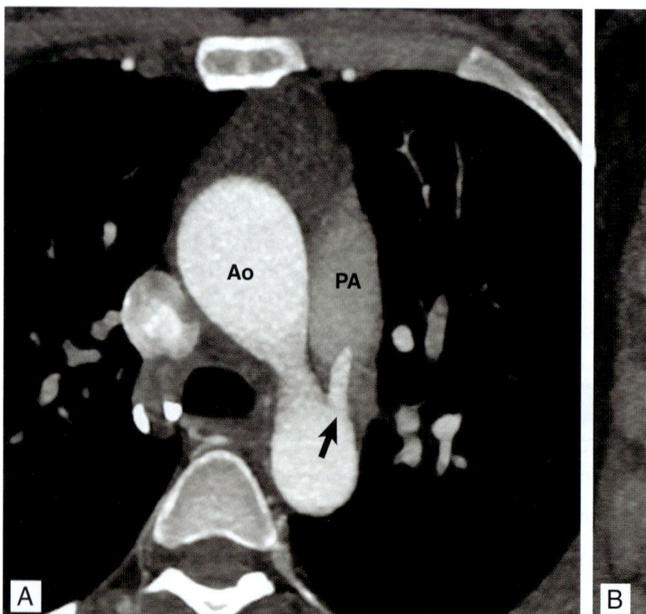

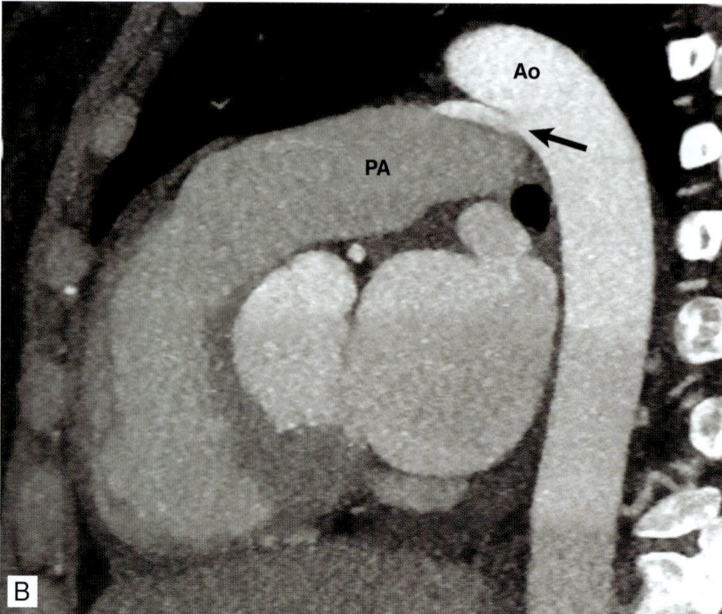

Figure 82.30 Axial (A) and sagittal (B) contrast-enhanced cardiac CT demonstrates a patent ductus arteriosus (*arrows*) with densely contrast opacified blood shunting left-to-right from the aorta (Ao) to the pulmonary arteries (PA).

TABLE 82.24 Summary of the Key Imaging Features of Isolated Patent Ductus Arteriosus

Technique	Imaging Features
Chest radiograph	May be normal Increased pulmonary vascularity Enlarged left atrium and left ventricle
Cardiac CT/MRI	Patent connection between aorta and pulmonary arteries Qp/Qs > 1.0 (if clinically significant)

Qp/Qs, pulmonary-systemic flow ratio.

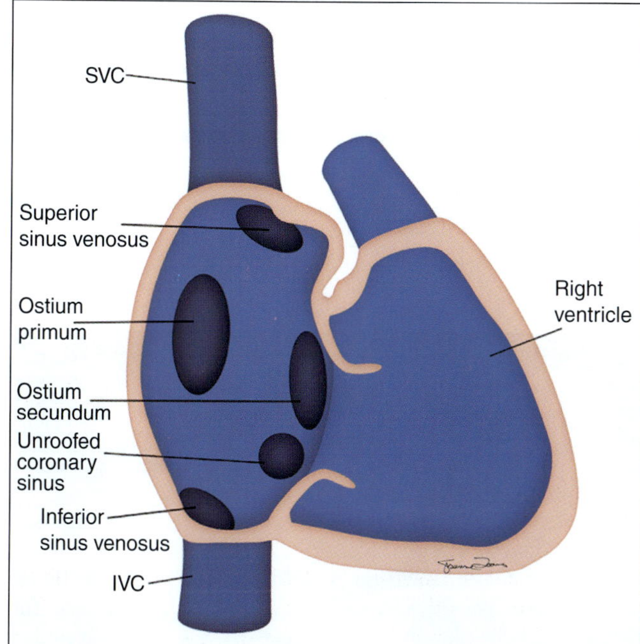

Figure 82.31 Schematic illustration of the interatrial septum demonstrating the location of various types of atrial septal defects (ASDs), including ostium primum, ostium secundum, superior and inferior sinus venosus, and unroofed coronary sinus defects. *IVC*, inferior vena cava; *SVC*, superior vena cava. (Courtesy: Susanne Loomis.)

minimally invasive option. If a PDA is small and incidentally discovered in adulthood, often no treatment is indicated.

Atrial Septal Defects (ASD)

Embryology and Epidemiology: *ASDs are a persistent opening or defect in the interatrial septum after birth allowing communication between the left and right atria* (Fig. 82.31) and are the most commonly encountered congenital heart abnormality overall [1,22,23]. They may be found in isolation, but are also a very common abnormality found in patients with other complexes CHDs, frequently playing a crucial role in patient survival in numerous cyanotic CHDs.

The interatrial septum begins to develop approximately 4 weeks after gestation with atrial septation occurring around the fifth–eighth gestational week [23–25]. The key embryological events of normal atrial septation are summarized below in Table 82.25.

TABLE 82.25 Summary of the Embryological Events Involved in Normal Atrial Septation [23–25]

Gestational Age	Embryological Event
~ Week 4	***Septum primum (SP)*** grows from the posterior edge of the common atrium (atrial roof) toward the endocardial cushions at the level of the atrioventricular canal
~ Week 4–6	Opening develops between the septum primum (SP) and the endocardial cushions, termed the ***ostium primum (OP)***
~ Week 6	Ostium primum (OP) defect closes as the septum primum fuses with the endocardial cushions, while a second opening simultaneously appears more posteriorly, termed the ***ostium secundum (OS)***
~ Week 7	A second septum, termed the ***septum secundum (SS)***, also grows from the atrial roof toward the endocardial cushions, to the right of the septum primum (SP)
By week 8	Opening develops in the septum secundum (SS), termed the ***foramen ovale (FO)***, which somewhat overlaps with the ostium secundum to form the interatrial connection necessary for shunting of oxygenated blood from the placenta toward systemic circulation, found in normal fetal circulation

Pathophysiology and Clinical Features: Depending on the size, ASDs may remain asymptomatic for years to decades. This is in part due to low atrial pressures, which often means that the degree of interatrial shunting is not clinically significant. Despite the initial lack of clinical symptoms, at least half of adolescents and adults with ASDs will develop symptoms [22]. If an ASD is large and unrepaired for many years, the chronic left-to-right shunting can result in patients presenting with dyspnea, fatigue, atrial fibrillation/flutter, right heart failure, or pulmonary hypertension. As with an uncorrected PDA, the resulting pulmonary hypertension may result in *Eisenmenger syndrome*, with reversal of the atrial level shunt to become right-to-left.

Imaging Features: Similar to a PFO, ASDs are often radiographically occult. If large or longstanding, there may be dilatation of the right heart chambers and pulmonary arterial enlargement. These findings, in combination with a slight rotation of the heart, can make the ascending aorta appear deceivingly small on plain radiograph, though it remains normal in caliber.

Transthoracic or TEE is the primary imaging technique of choice for initial diagnosis due to high sensitivity, easy accessibility, and low-cost relative to other imaging modalities. Similar to a PFO workup, a TEE “bubble study” can detect even a small ASD by the early appearance of bubbles within the left atrium. Echocardiography may be limited, however, in its ability to clearly visualize the location and size of the ASD.

ASDs are well-visualized on ECG-gated contrast-enhanced cardiac CT, with the appearance depending on the type of ASD (Fig. 82.31). The embryologic origin and imaging features of the various subtypes of ASDs are summarized in Table 82.26. Cardiac CT again provides a more thorough evaluation for coexisting congenital defects, such as anomalous pulmonary venous drainage, and can be particularly useful in assessing the size of the septal defect while also providing information about the surrounding septal rims, which is important for preprocedural planning, especially for percutaneous ASD closure devices. The relevant anatomic septal rims are summarized in Table 82.27.

TABLE 82.26 Description of Different Types of Atrial Septal Defects

Type	Location	Embryology	Associations
Ostium primum (15–35%)	Anterior interatrial septum near the atrioventricular valves (Fig. 82.32)	Septum primum fails to fuse with endocardial cushions	Associated with Down syndrome (Trisomy 21) Considered the mildest form of the endocardial cushion defect spectrum (discussed separately)
Ostium secundum (60–75%)	Mid interatrial septum near the fossa ovalis (Fig. 82.33)	Excessive resorption of the septum primum or deficient growth of the septum secundum causing a shortened valve of the foramen ovale	Holt–Oram syndrome
Superior sinus venosus (4–11%)	Posterior superior interatrial septum where the SVC joins the RA (Fig. 82.34)	Thought to result from lack of septation between the pulmonary veins and the SVC or RA	Strongly associated with right upper lobe partial anomalous pulmonary venous return (PAPVR)
Inferior sinus venosus (rare)	Posterior inferior interatrial septum where the IVC joins the RA (Fig. 82.35)	Thought to result from lack of septation between the pulmonary veins and the IVC or RA	Less common than superior sinus venosus defects but also associated with right-sided PAPVR
Unroofed coronary sinus (rare)	Posterior interatrial septum where the coronary sinus contacts the LA (Fig. 82.36)	Lack of septation between the inferior LA and the roof of the coronary sinus	Associated with a persistent left-sided SVC

IVC, inferior vena cava; *LA*, left atrium; *PAPVR*, partial anomalous pulmonary venous return; *RA*, right atrium; *SVC*, superior vena cava. [1,23,24,26–28].

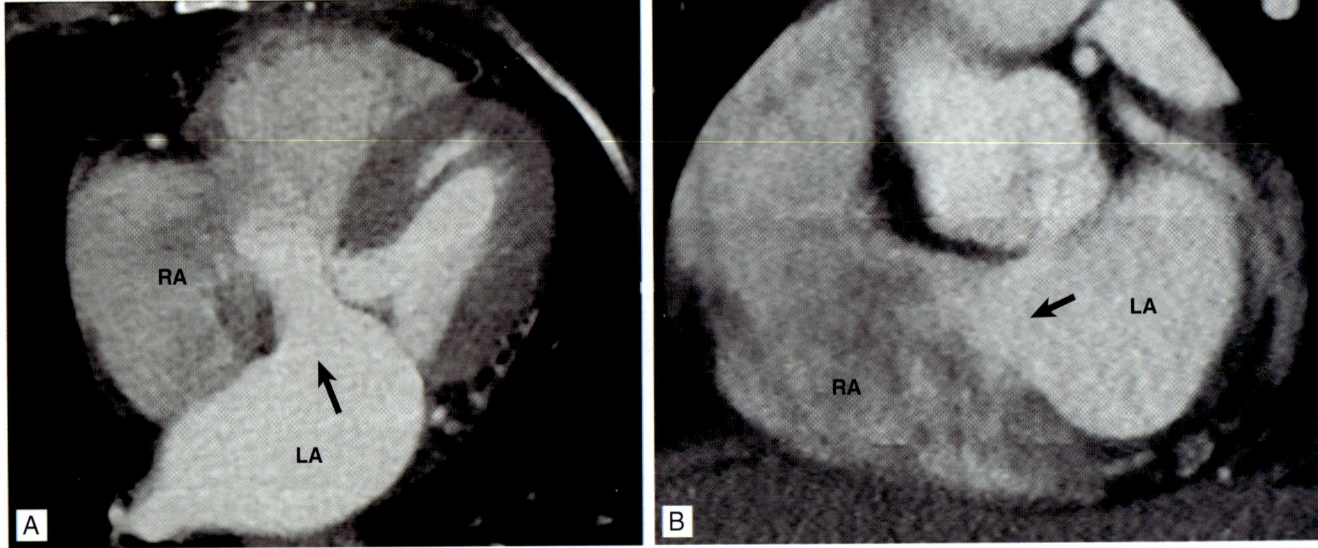

Figure 82.32 Four-chamber (A) and short-axis (B) contrast-enhanced ECG-gated cardiac CT demonstrates an ostium primum type atrial septal defect (*arrows*) with shunting of blood from the left atrium (LA) toward the right atrium (RA).

TABLE 82.27 Description of Atrial Septal Rims Relevant for Percutaneous Closure Devices [29]

Location	Rims	Definition
Superior	Superior vena cava (SVC) rim	Minimum distance between ASD and the superior vena cava
	Superior rim	Rim between the SVC and aortic rim
Anterior	Aortic rim	Minimum distance between ASD and the aortic wall
	Atrioventricular (AV) rim	Minimum distance between ASD and the atrioventricular (tricuspid and mitral) valves
Inferior	Inferior vena cava (IVC) rim	Minimum distance between ASD and the inferior vena cava
Posterior	Posterior rim	Minimum distance between ASD and the posterior atrial wall

ASD, atrial septal defect.

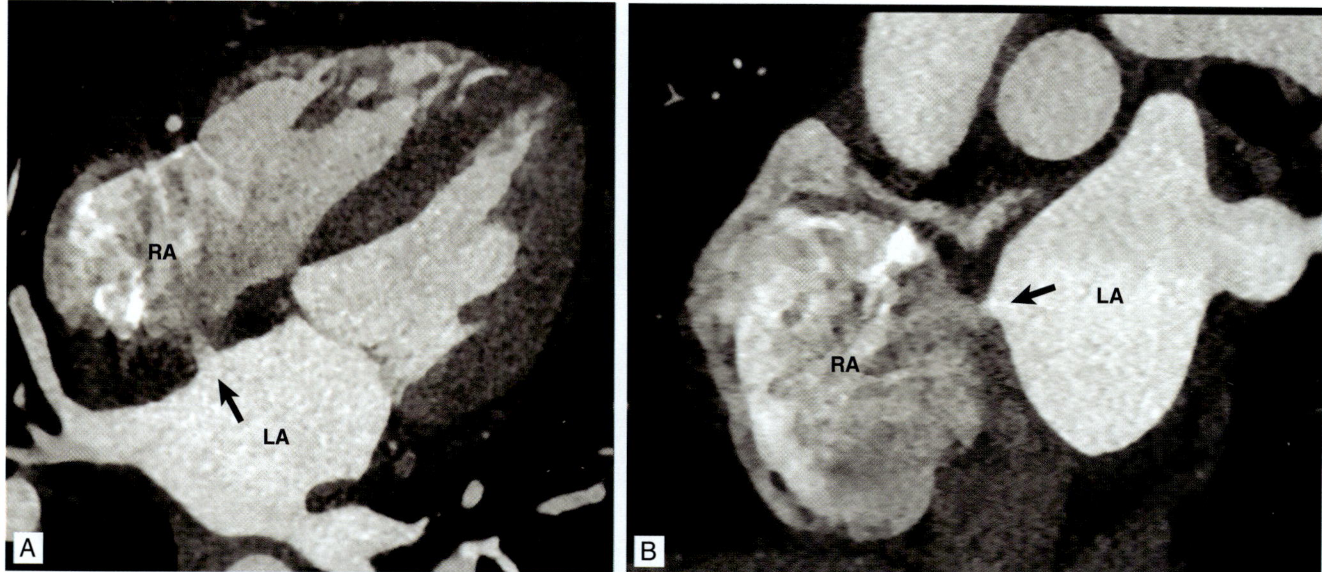

Figure 82.33 Four-chamber (A) and short-axis (B) contrast-enhanced ECG-gated cardiac CT demonstrates an ostium secundum type atrial septal defect (*arrows*) with shunting of blood from the left atrium (LA) toward the right atrium (RA). Notice the difference in appearance of this atrial septal defect compared with the appearance of a patent foramen ovale, despite being in a similar location.

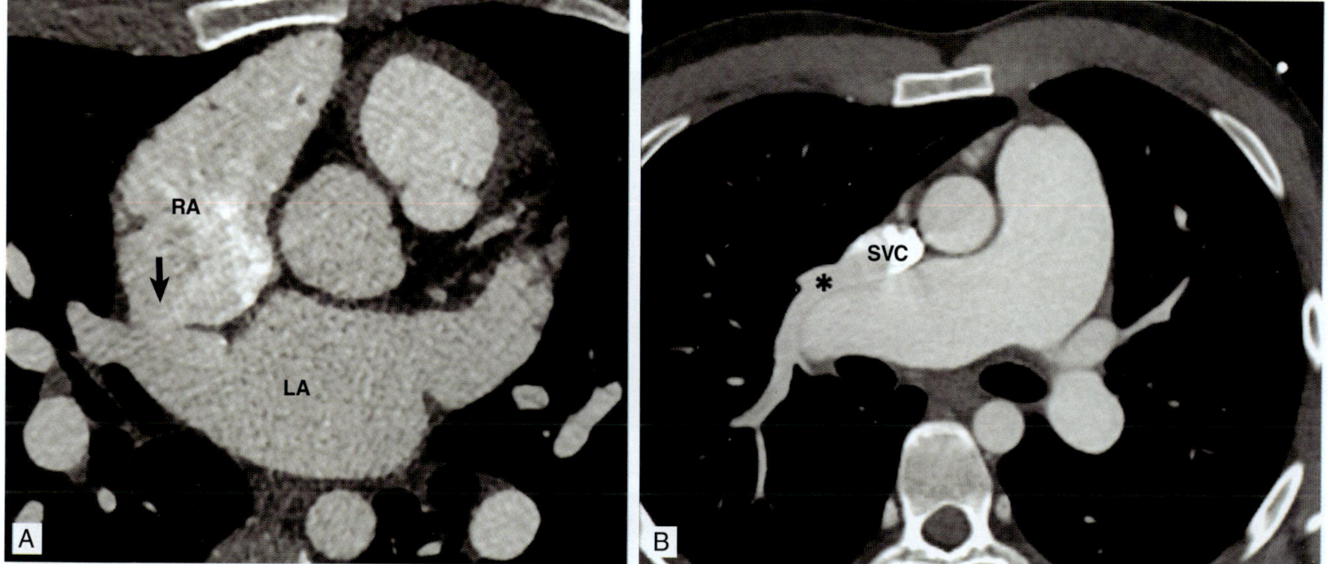

Figure 82.34 Axial (A) contrast-enhanced ECG-gated cardiac CT demonstrates a superior sinus venosus type atrial septal defect (*arrows*), which occurs along the posterior superior aspect of the interatrial septum where the superior vena cava (SVC) joins the right atrium (RA). An additional axial contrast-enhanced chest CT (B) demonstrates anomalous drainage of the right upper lobe pulmonary vein (*asterisk*) into the superior vena cava (SVC). Right upper lobe partial anomalous pulmonary venous return (PAPVR) is frequently associated with superior sinus venosus atrial septal defects. *LA*, left atrium; *RA*, right atrium.

Cardiac MRI is a useful adjunctive imaging technique for quantifying the degree of atrial shunting utilizing velocity encoding sequences, as described in an earlier section about PDA. SSFP cine and spin-echo sequences are often useful for localizing the ASD to set up the shunt quantification sequences appropriately. The imaging features of ASDs are summarized in Table 82.28.

Treatment and Outcomes: Isolated ASDs warrant surgical repair when patients become symptomatic. Depending on the size and location of the defect, this may be accomplished with percutaneous ASD closure device or open surgical closure.

Atrioventricular Canal (Endocardial Cushion) Defect

Embryology and Epidemiology: Atrioventricular canal defects (also commonly termed endocardial cushion defects) *result from*

TABLE 82.28 Summary of the Key Imaging Features of Isolated Atrial Septal Defect

Technique	Imaging Features
Chest radiograph	May be normal Enlarged pulmonary artery with increased pulmonary vascularity Enlarged right atrium and ventricle No left atrial enlargement (unless Eisenmenger syndrome develops)
Cardiac CT/MRI	Patent connection between the left and right atria Qp/Qs > 1.0 (if clinically significant)

Qp/Qs, pulmonary-systemic flow ratio.

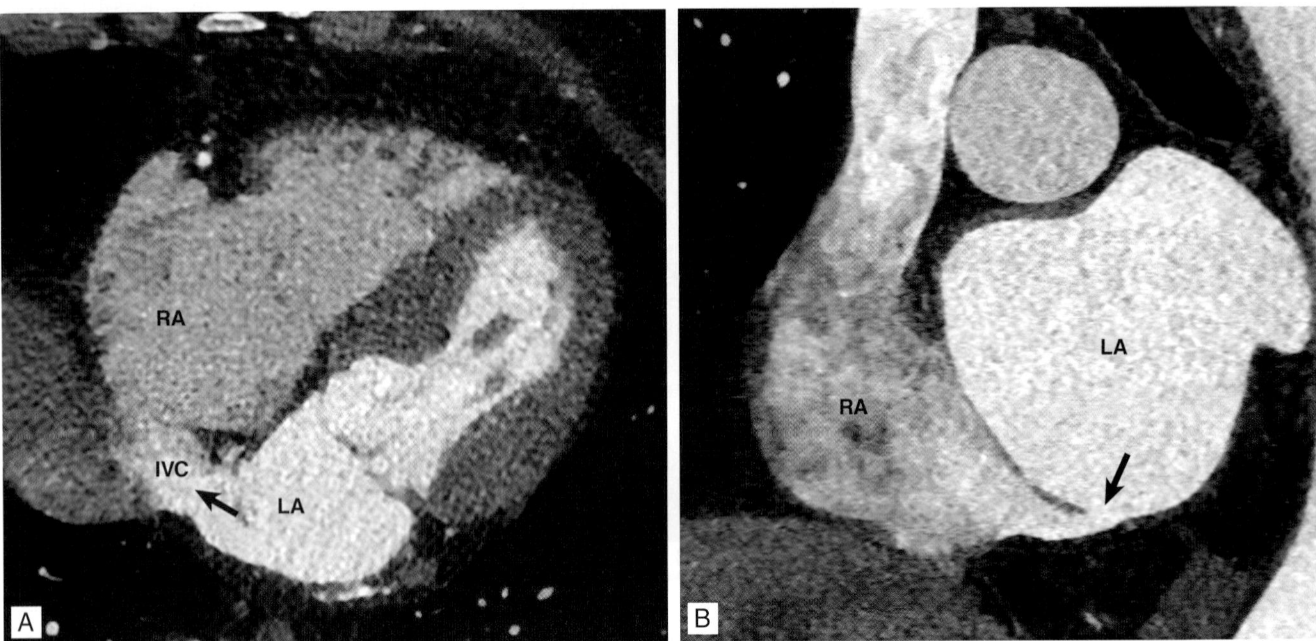

Figure 82.35 Four-chamber (A) and short-axis (B) contrast-enhanced ECG-gated cardiac CT demonstrates an inferior sinus venosus type atrial septal defect (*arrows*), which occurs along the posterior inferior aspect of the interatrial septum where the inferior vena cava (IVC) joins the right atrium (RA). *LA*, left atrium; *RA*, right atrium.

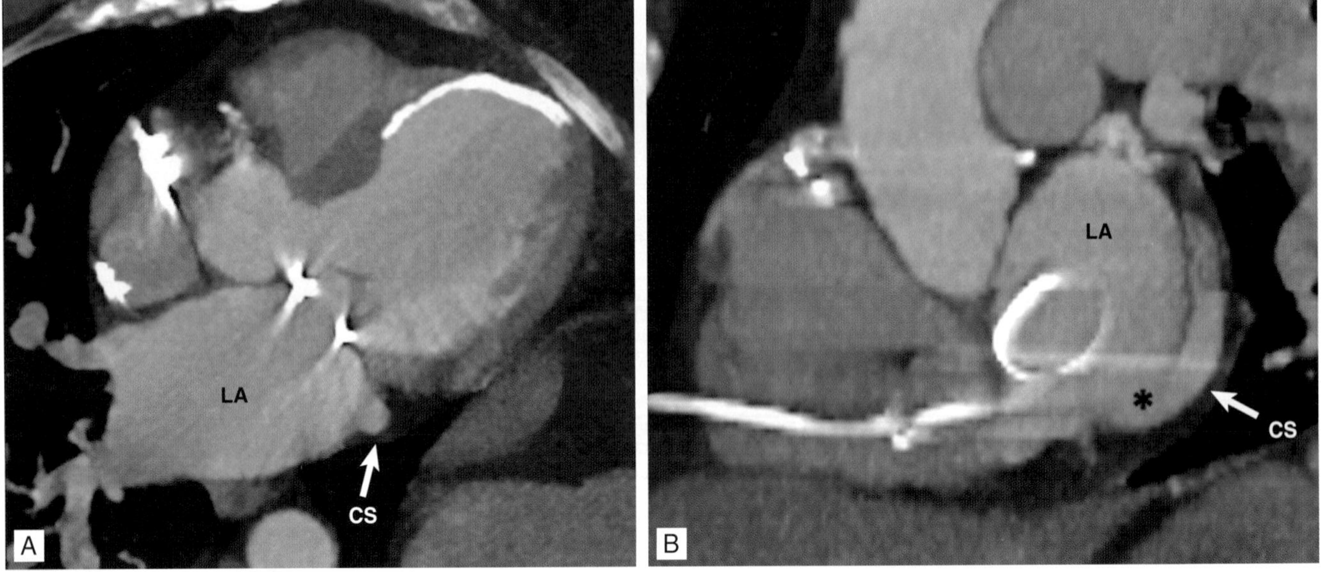

Figure 82.36 Oblique axial (A) and sagittal (B) contrast-enhanced ECG-gated cardiac CT demonstrates an unroofed coronary sinus defect (*asterisk*), which occurs along the margin of where the coronary sinus (CS) abuts the left atrium (LA).

abnormal formation or fusion of the endocardial cushions during embryological development [1,9] and account for approximately 2–7% of congenital heart defects [9,27]. This can range from an ostium primum ASD with mild abnormalities of the atrioventricular (tricuspid or mitral) valves to a single common atrioventricular valve with associated atrial and VSDs (Fig. 82.37), allowing for free communication of blood between the right and left heart [1,3,9,22,27].

There is a strong association with Trisomy 21 (Down syndrome)—up to 40% of patients with atrioventricular canal defects have Trisomy 21. [1]. This congenital heart defect may also be seen associated with other genetic disorders as well, including heterotaxy syndromes and Trisomy 18.

Pathophysiology and Clinical Features: While milder spectrum abnormalities may remain asymptomatic or resemble other ASDs in clinical presentation, severe or complete atrioventricular canal defects result in free communication of all four cardiac chambers with significant bidirectional shunting through the atrial and VSDs. These patients may present with florid congestive heart failure and/or pulmonary hypertension in infancy.

Imaging Features: Radiographic features of atrioventricular canal defects are often nonspecific and include cardiomegaly with increased pulmonary vascularity.

Although rarely performed now given modern advances in cross-sectional imaging, left ventricular angiography was once used for diagnosis and workup of this abnormality. On a lateral

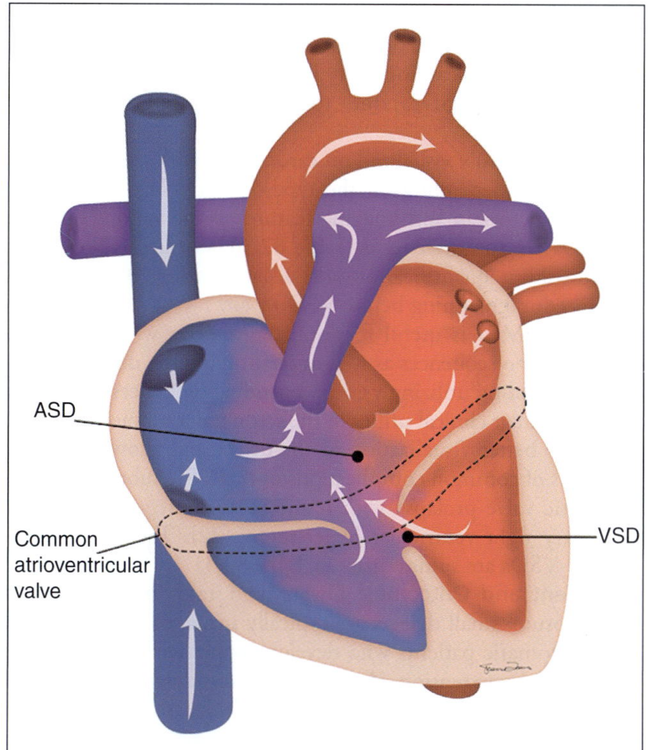

Figure 82.37 Schematic representation of an atrioventricular canal defect (also known as an endocardial cushion defect), demonstrating a common atrioventricular valve with associated atrial septal defect (ASD) and ventricular septal defect (VSD). (Courtesy: Susanne Loomis.)

oblique view during left ventriculography, this abnormality may result in a "*gooseneck sign*," explained by a concave interventricular septum below the mitral valve as well as narrowing and elongation of the left ventricular outflow tract [9].

Atrioventricular canal defects can be accurately diagnosed by echocardiography and will be most visible as a large central defect on a four-chamber view with free communication between the cardiac chambers on color Doppler images.

Cardiac CT and cardiac MRI are both excellent modalities for visualizing the atrioventricular defect (Fig. 82.38), can demonstrate the common atrioventricular valve in motion, and are useful adjuncts in determining complete cardiac and extracardiac anatomy in the setting of multiple congenital abnormalities. The imaging features of atrioventricular canal defects are summarized in Table 82.29.

Treatment and Outcomes: Treatment for this congenital abnormality is primarily surgical. The surgical approach will depend not only on the severity of the atrioventricular canal defect but also on the presence or absence of unilateral ventricular hypoplasia, which can occur in the setting of an asymmetric common atrioventricular valve favoring one side of the heart. Without two well-developed ventricles, these patients may require some version of single ventricle palliation to survive.

Ventricular Septal Defects (VSD)

Embryology and Epidemiology: *VSDs are a persistent opening or defect in the interventricular septum after birth allowing communication between the left and right ventricles* (Fig. 82.39) and are the second most common congenital heart abnormality in children, accounting for 20–40% of all congenital heart defects [1,22,24,27]. Embryologically, a VSD may occur due to maldevelopment of the muscular septum, malformation of the endocardial cushions, or

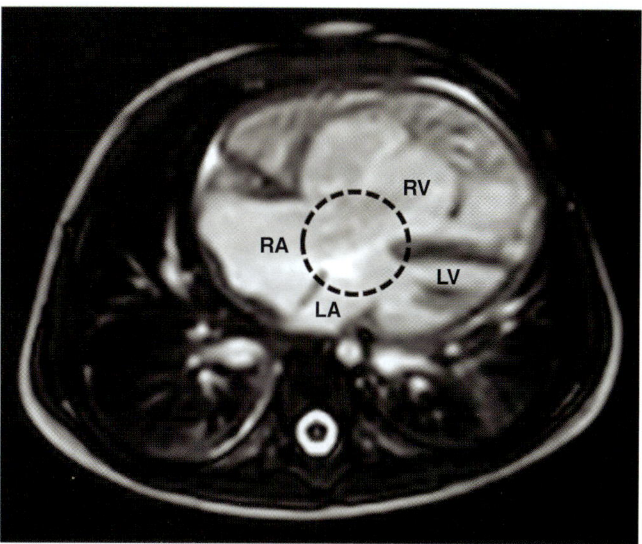

Figure 82.38 Four-chamber SSFP image demonstrates a patient with Down syndrome who has a complete atrioventricular canal defect (also known as endocardial cushion defect). Notice in this case that the right atrium (RA) and right ventricle (RV) are larger and more hypertrophied compared to the left atrium (LA) and left ventricle (LV), indicating that there is a right-dominant atrioventricular (AV) valve with more flow entering the right-sided chambers. Given the mobility of the AV valve, the leaflets are often not well seen by imaging, but the absence of the internal cardiac crux (*dotted circle*) gives a characteristic imaging appearance.

abnormal resorption of myocardial tissue in the interventricular septum. Interestingly, up to 75% of isolated VSDs will close spontaneously by age 10 [1].

The interventricular septum begins to develop around the same time as the interatrial septum, approximately 4 weeks after gestation with ventricular septation occurring during the fourth–seventh gestational week [27]. Notably, ventricular septation is closely related to the septation of the truncus and conus cordis, which develop into the future ventricular outflow tracts, and thus abnormalities of these processes commonly occur simultaneously [24].

Pathophysiology and Clinical Features: VSDs can be detected on physical examination, classically described as a *holosystolic murmur heard best at the left sternal border*, due to turbulent flow across the defect. Pathophysiologically, VSDs are similar to ASDs in that they allow for an abnormal intracardiac left-to-right shunt. While small VSDs can be asymptomatic and remain undetected until after birth, ventricular pressures are much higher than atrial pressures, and therefore even relatively small VSDs may present as

TABLE 82.29 Summary of the Key Imaging Features of Atrioventricular Canal Defects

Technique	Imaging Features
Chest radiograph	Cardiomegaly Increased pulmonary vascularity
Left ventriculography	"Gooseneck sign"
Cardiac CT/MRI	Common atrioventricular valve—may favor right or left heart Atrial and ventricular septal defects Possible underdevelopment of either side of the heart

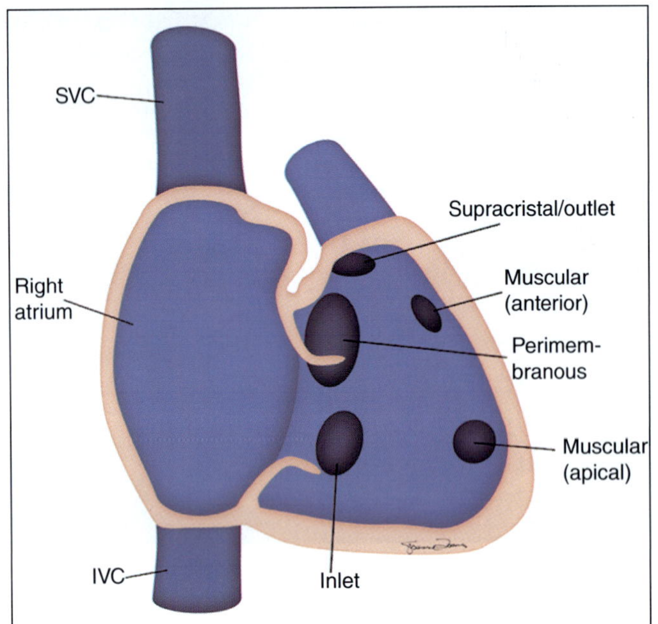

Figure 82.39 Schematic illustration of the interventricular septum demonstrating the location of various types of ventricular septal defects (VSDs), including inlet, perimembranous, supracristal/outlet, and muscular defects. *SVC*, superior vena cava; *IVC*, inferior vena cava. (Courtesy: Susanne Loomis.)

clinically symptomatic. Large VSDs can result in florid congestive heart failure within 2–3 months of birth [1]. Longstanding uncorrected VSDs can also eventually result in pulmonary arterial hypertension and *Eisenmenger syndrome*, with reversal of the ventricular level shunt to become right-to-left.

Imaging Features: Similar to other types of septal defects, small VSDs are often radiographically occult. If large or longstanding, cardiomegaly may be present, including left atrial dilation, and pulmonary arterial enlargement.

VSDs can usually be visualized with a four-chamber view on echocardiography, which remains the primary imaging technique for initial diagnosis as with many other congenital heart defects. Echocardiography may be limited in detecting smaller defects, though the use of color Doppler can increase sensitivity. In particular, echocardiography is less sensitive for the detection of supracristal VSDs, due to the commonly retrosternal location.

VSDs are easily visualized on cardiac CT, with the appearance and location depending on the type of VSD (Fig. 82.39). The embryologic origin and imaging features of the various subtypes of VSDs are summarized in Table 82.30. Cardiac CT can also provide shunt quantification and accurate sizing of defects for preprocedural planning before VSD repair.

Cardiac MRI is useful for localizing defects with SSFP cine and spin-echo sequences as well as quantifying the degree of ventricular shunting utilizing velocity encoding sequences. MRI may be of particular clinical utility in the setting of a supracristal VSD, providing better visualization of the defect and allowing for the diagnosis of common complications of this VSD subtype, including aortic valve prolapse with resultant aortic regurgitation and secondary right ventricular hypertrophy [22]. The imaging features of VSDs are summarized in Table 82.31.

Treatment and Outcomes: Given high rates of spontaneous VSD closure, small defects are typically managed conservatively. In symptomatic patients who develop congestive heart failure or pulmonary hypertension, closure can be considered in the form of a surgical patch or percutaneous closure device, depending on the size and location.

Partial Anomalous Pulmonary Venous Return: *Described in detail in the Chapter 26 on Diseases of Veins and Lymphatics.*

Congenital Pulmonary Stenosis

Embryology and Epidemiology: Congenital pulmonary stenosis refers to the *congenital narrowing of the pulmonary outflow tract which can be subvalvular, valvular, or supravalvular.* Valvular pulmonic stenosis is commonly an isolated abnormality and is reported to represent 10% of all CHD [30]. However congenital pulmonary stenosis at any level can be associated with certain genetic syndromes, including Williams syndrome, Noonan syndrome, and TOF [1,30,31].

TABLE 82.30 Description of Different Types of Ventricular Septal Defects

TYPES OF VENTRICULAR SEPTAL DEFECTS AND IMAGING FEATURES		
Type	**Location**	**Associations**
Perimembranous (70–80%)	Membranous interventricular septum Below the aortic valve and behind the septal leaflet of the tricuspid valve (Fig. 82.40)	Associated with aortic or tricuspid regurgitation due to proximity of the defect to these valve leaflets
Muscular (10–20%)	Muscular (trabecular) interventricular septum (Fig. 82.41)	Most frequently involves the apical two-thirds of the muscular septum
Inlet or atrioventricular (5–10%)	Inlet interventricular septum Extends from the tricuspid annulus to the attachments of the tricuspid valve leaflets	Associated with atrioventricular septal defects or anomalous insertion of the chordae tendinae
Outlet or supracristal (5–8%)	Outlet interventricular septum Above the crista muscle and below the aortic and pulmonic valves	Associated with truncus arteriosus, Tetralogy of Fallot, and double outlet right ventricle Aortic valve prolapse and aortic regurgitation are important complications

LV, left ventricle; *RV*, right ventricle [1,22,24,27].

TABLE 82.31 Summary of the Key Imaging Features of the Isolated Ventricular Septal Defect

Technique	Imaging Features
Chest radiograph	May be normal Enlarged pulmonary artery with increased pulmonary vasculairty Enlarged right heart + left atrial enlargement
Cardiac CT/MRI	Patent connection between the left and right ventricles Qp/Qs > 1.0 (if clinically significant)

Qp/Qs, pulmonary-systemic flow ratio.

Pathophysiology and Clinical Features: Congenital pulmonary stenosis is frequently asymptomatic and well-tolerated for many years. Valvular pulmonic stenosis can be detected on physical examination, classically described as a *midsystolic crescendo-decrescendo ejection murmur in the second intercostal space along the left sternal border*. In cases of severe or long-standing stenosis, patients may present with symptoms of right heart failure and other sequelae of elevated right heart pressures.

Congenital pulmonary stenosis can be morphologically classified based on the location of the stenosis, summarized below in Table 82.32.

Imaging Features: The radiographic features of congenital pulmonary stenosis are nonspecific, but may include dilated right

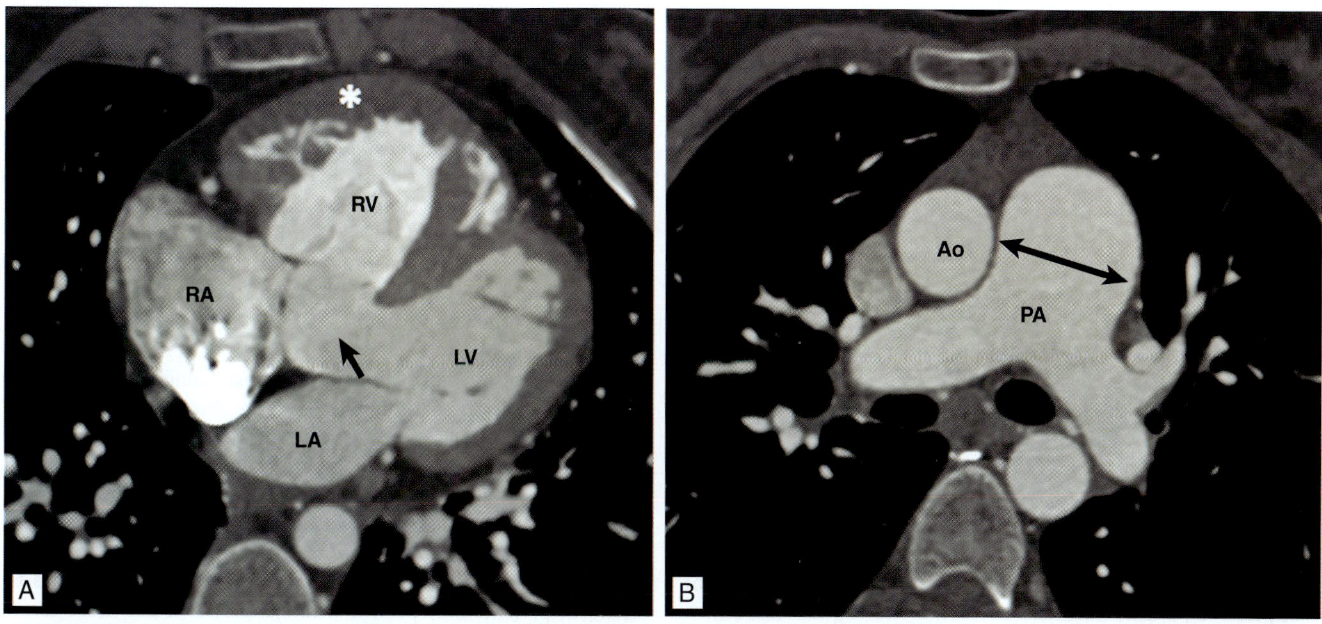

Figure 82.40 Four-chamber (A) and axial (B) contrast-enhanced ECG-gated cardiac CT images demonstrate a perimembranous ventricular septal defect (*arrow*), which occurs along the upper membranous portion of the interventricular septum allowing communication between the right ventricle (RV) and left ventricle (LV). This abnormality was detected in adulthood and there is obvious sequela of long-standing left-to-right shunting with elevated right heart pressures, including dilated right atrium (RA) compared with the left atrium (LA), hypertrophy of the right ventricular myometrium (*asterisk*) and a dilated main pulmonary artery (*double-headed arrow*). *Ao*, aorta; *PA*, pulmonary artery.

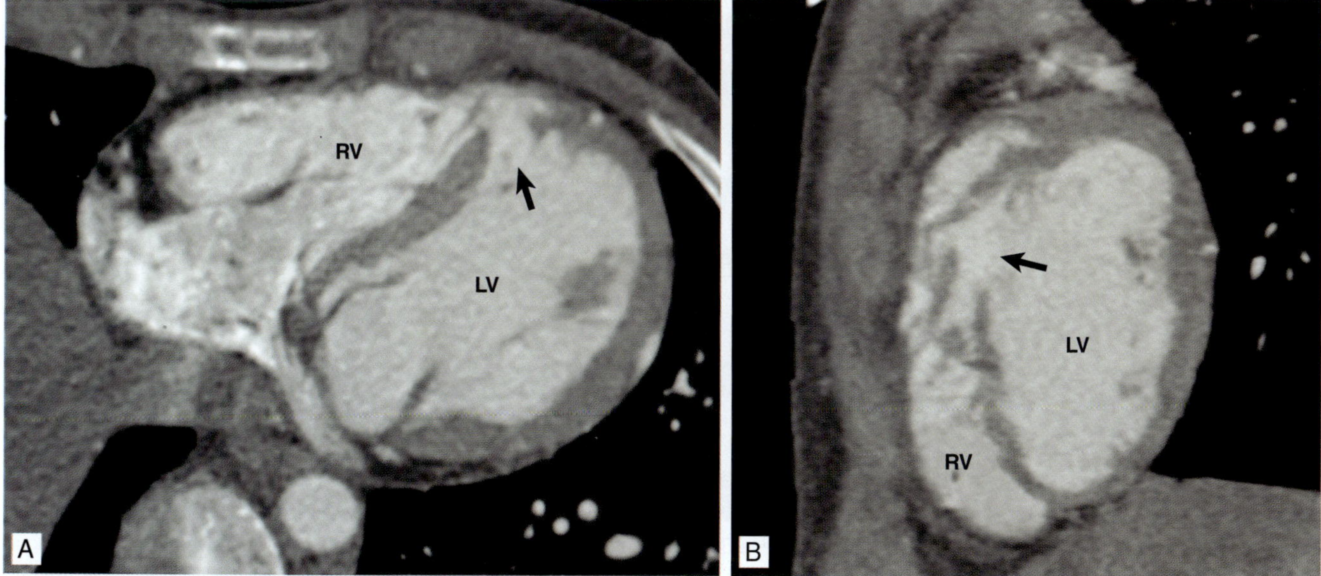

Figure 82.41 Axial (A) and short-axis (B) contrast-enhanced ECG-gated cardiac CT images demonstrate an apical muscular ventricular septal defect (*arrows*), which occurs along the lower muscular portion of the interventricular septum allowing communication between the right ventricle (RV) and left ventricle (LV).

TABLE 82.32 Description of Different Types of Congenital Pulmonary Stenosis [30,32]

Type	Location	Associations
Supravalvular (most common)	Above the level of the pulmonic valve	Associated with Williams syndrome
Valvular	At the level of the pulmonic valve Dome-shaped (40–60%): Mobile valve with 2–4 raphes and partial commissural fusion; small valve orifice Dysplastic (20–30%): Thickened, dysplastic, immobile cusps without commissural fusion Bicuspid/multicuspid (rare): Abnormal number of pulmonic valve leaflets/cusps	Associated with Noonan syndrome
Subvalvular	Below the level of the pulmonic valve	Associated with Tetralogy of Fallot

heart chambers, evidence of right ventricular hypertrophy, or pulmonary arterial enlargement. Occasionally, in patients with vavular pulmonic stenosis, a jet of pulmonary blood flow may be preferentially directed toward the left lung, resulting in asymmetric enlargement of the left pulmonary artery and increased left-sided pulmonary vascularity, a finding known as the *Chen sign* [32,33].

In the setting of valvular pulmonic stenosis, echocardiography may demonstrate abnormal motion (systolic doming) or dysplastic morphology of the pulmonic valve leaflets. In the setting of subvalvular or supravalvular pulmonary stenosis, color Doppler may aid in diagnosis by demonstrating increased flow velocities across the area of greatest narrowing. In severe cases, echocardiography will also demonstrate sequela of elevated right heart pressures including right heart chamber enlargement and possible right ventricular dysfunction.

Advanced cross-sectional imaging modalities including CT and MRI allow for three-dimensional visualization of stenotic segments (Fig. 82.42) as well as areas of poststenotic dilation. Cardiac MRI is useful in assessing the severity stenosis with the use of velocity encoded sequences to evaluate flow volumes, velocities, and pressure gradients across a narrowed segment. The imaging features of congenital pulmonary stenosis are summarized below in Table 82.33.

Treatment and Outcomes: Isolated congenital pulmonary stenosis, if severe and symptomatic, may be managed medically or treated with balloon valvuloplasty or valvulotomy to reduce the degree of stenosis. Severely dysplastic valves may alternatively be treated with surgical pulmonary valve replacement.

Congenital Aortic Stenosis

Embryology and Epidemiology: Congenital aortic stenosis refers to the *congenital narrowing of the systemic (aortic) outflow tract*. Valvular aortic stenosis is most commonly due to a congenitally BAV, which is the overall most common congenital heart defect [34,35]. While the entity of BAV will be discussed in detail separately, this section will focus broadly on subvalvular, valvular, and supravalvular aortic stenosis. Note that aortic coarctation and other abnormalities of the aortic arch will also be discussed separately.

Pathophysiology and Clinical Features: Congenital aortic stenosis is parallel in pathophysiology and clinical presentation to congenital pulmonary stenosis, but affecting the left heart chambers rather than the right. Patients are frequently asymptomatic and valvular aortic stenosis can be detected on physical examination, classically described as a *mid-systolic crescendo-decrescendo ejection murmur in the second intercostal space along the right sternal border with radiation to the right neck*. In cases of severe or long-standing stenosis, patients may present with symptoms of left heart failure and other sequelae of elevated left heart pressures.

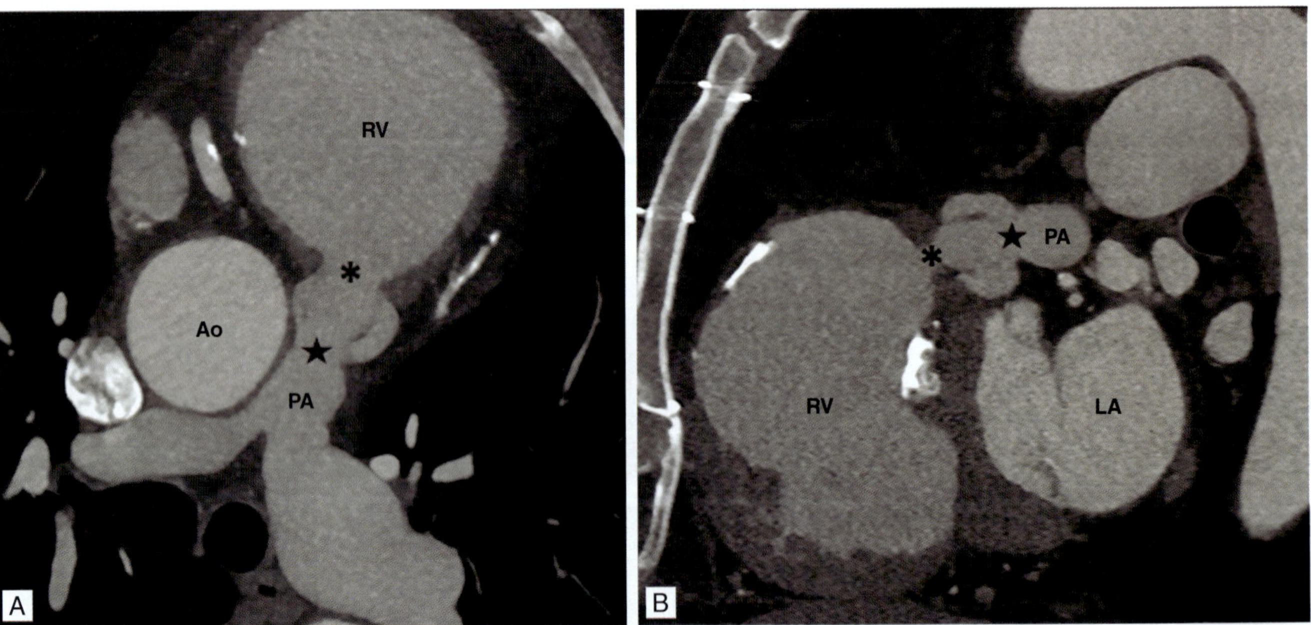

Figure 82.42 Oblique axial (A) and sagittal (B) contrast-enhanced ECG-gated cardiac CT images demonstrate both valvular and supravalvular pulmonic stenosis in a patient with Tetralogy of Fallot. There is focal narrowing at the level of the pulmonic valve (*asterisk*) followed by a second focal narrowing in the supravalvular proximal main pulmonary artery (*star*). *Ao*, aorta; *LA*, left atrium; *PA*, pulmonary artery; *RV*, right ventricle.

TABLE 82.33 Summary of the Key Imaging Features of Isolated Congenital Pulmonary Stenosis

Technique	Imaging Features
Chest radiograph	Enlarged right heart/right ventricular hypertrophy Enlarged main pulmonary artery or left pulmonary artery Possible asymmetric increased left-sided pulmonary vascularity (*Chen sign*)
Cardiac CT/MRI	Narrowing of the right ventricular outflow tract, pulmonic valve, or supravalvular proximal pulmonary artery +/ poststenotic dilation Abnormal pulmonary valve leaflets (if valvular pulmonary stenosis)

Congenital aortic stenosis can also be morphologically classified based on the location of the stenosis, summarized below in Table 82.34.

Imaging Features: The radiographic features of congenital aortic stenosis are also nonspecific, but may include dilated left heart chambers and poststenotic dilation of the ascending aorta, often seen only in valvular aortic stenosis.

In the setting of valvular aortic stenosis, echocardiography may demonstrate abnormal motion (systolic doming) or abnormal morphology of the aortic valve leaflets. In the setting of subvalvular or supravalvular aortic stenosis, color Doppler may aid in diagnosis by demonstrating increased flow velocities across the area of greatest narrowing. In supravalvular aortic stenosis, the ascending aorta take on an *hourglass appearance*, which refers to an area of focal severe narrowing with more diffuse narrowing of the adjacent aortic segments [36].

TABLE 82.34 Description of Different Types of Congenital Aortic Stenosis [1,36]

Type	Location	Subtype
Supravalvular (least common)	Above the level of the aortic valve	Localized: Focal or discrete narrowing of the proximal ascending aorta (also associated with Williams syndrome)
		Diffuse: Generalized underdevelopment or small caliber of the ascending aorta
Valvular (most common)	At the level of the aortic valve	Bicuspid Aortic Valve: Two functional leaflets or cusps of the aortic valve (associated with Turner syndrome and aortic coarctation)
		Unicommisural Aortic Valve: Single horseshoe-shaped valve leaflet
Subvalvular	Below the level of the aortic valve	Membranous: Discrete fibrous membrane narrowing the left ventricular outflow tract
		Hypertrophic: Muscular hypertrophy of the infundibulum narrowing the left ventricular outflow tract

Advanced cross-sectional imaging modalities including CT and MRI allow for three-dimensional visualization of stenotic segments (Fig. 82.43) as well as areas of poststenotic dilation and sequela of elevated left heart pressures. Cardiac CT and MRI may also be helpful in delineating discrete subaortic membranes or

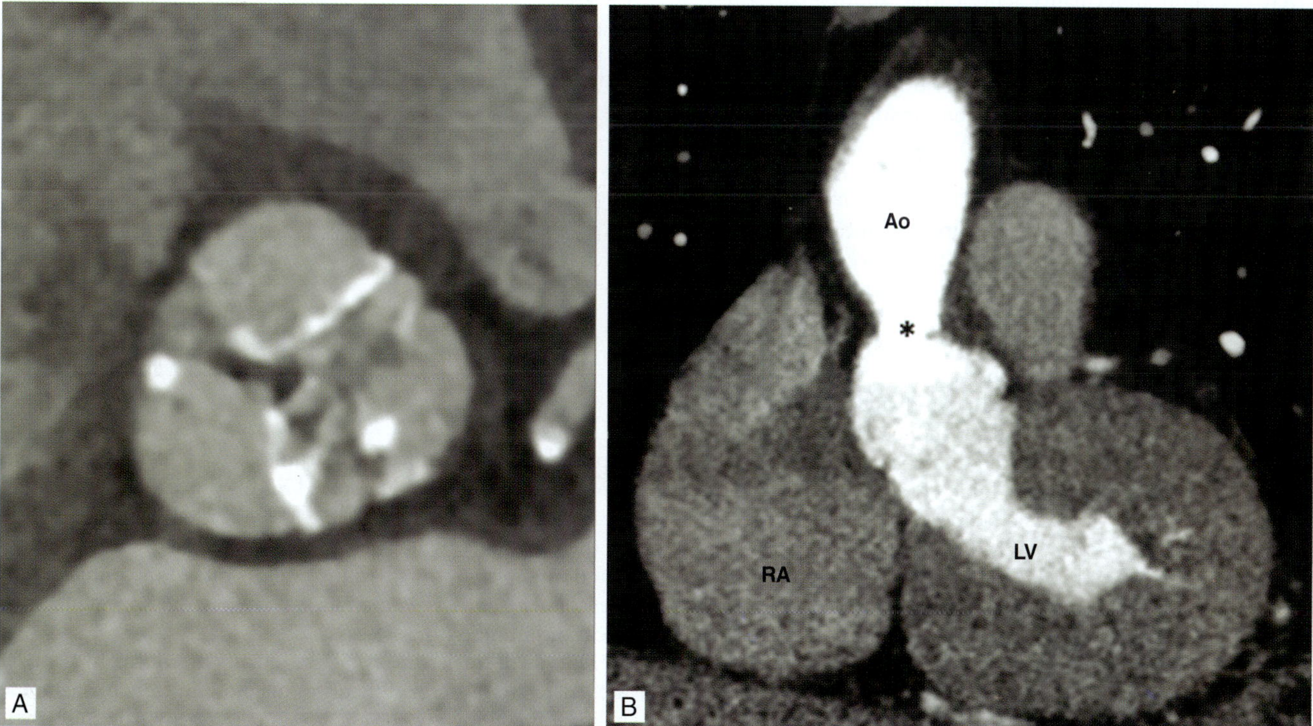

Figure 82.43 Short-axis (A) image from a contrast-enhanced ECG-gated cardiac CT demonstrates a calcified aortic valve in a patient with valvular aortic stenosis. Coronal (B) image from a contrast-enhanced ECG-gated cardiac CT in a separate patient with demonstrates focal narrowing of the supravalvular proximal ascending aorta (*asterisk*) with an ***hourglass appearance***, commonly seen in patients with Williams syndrome. *Ao*, aorta; *LV*, left ventricle; *RA*, right atrium.

TABLE 82.35 Summary of the Key Imaging Features of Isolated Congenital Aortic Stenosis

Technique	Imaging Features
Chest radiograph	Enlarged left heart/left ventricular hypertrophy Normal pulmonary vascularity Enlarged ascending aorta (valvular subtype only)
Cardiac CT/MRI	Narrowing of the left ventricular outflow tract, aortic valve, or supravalvular proximal ascending aorta +/ poststenotic dilation Abnormal aortic valve leaflets (valvular subtype only)

evaluating for restricted aortic valve leaflet motion. Calcifications of the aortic valve are easily depicted on cardiac CT, which are commonly seen in valvular aortic stenosis.

Cardiac MRI is useful in assessing the severity stenosis with the use of velocity encoded sequences to evaluate flow volumes, velocities, and pressure gradients across the narrowed segment. The imaging features of congenital aortic stenosis are summarized below in Table 82.35.

Treatment and Outcomes: Isolated congenital aortic stenosis, if severe and symptomatic, may be managed medically or treated with balloon valvuloplasty or valvulotomy to reduce the degree of stenosis. Severely dysplastic valves may alternatively be treated with aortic valve replacement. Patients with subvalvular or supravalvular aortic stenosis may require alternative surgical intervention, such as resection of a subaortic membrane or reconstruction of the ascending aorta depending on the severity of the defect.

Aortic Coarctation

Embryology and Epidemiology: Aortic coarctation is a relatively common abnormality representing approximately 4–8% of all CHDs (37–39) and is defined by *congenital narrowing of the aortic lumen*, commonly in a juxta ductal location at the aortic isthmus (near the ductus arteriosus). Coarcatation may occur as a sporadic defect or in combination with other congenital defects, most commonly BAV, VSDs, and PDA, and can be seen with increased frequency among patients with Turner syndrome [1,9,37].

Pathophysiology and Clinical Features: Clinical presentation of aortic coarctation depends largely on the degree of luminal aortic narrowing and may present with variable symptomatology. Coarctation may present in neonates as acute heart failure or may be diagnosed in an adult due to hypertension with differential upper and lower extremity blood pressures.

Aortic coarctation is classically subdivided into two types, preductal and postductal, based on the location of the narrowing relative to the position of the ductus arteriosus, depicted in Fig. 82.44 and summarized in Table 82.36.

Imaging Features: The classic radiographic sign of aortic coarctation is the *figure-of-three sign* with associated *rib notching* on a frontal chest radiograph (Fig. 82.45). The *figure-of-three sign* is explained by the appearance of focal narrowing in the proximal descending thoracic aorta and associated dilation of the left subclavian artery, giving a lobulated contour to the left superior mediastinum that resembles the number three. *Rib notching* is a phenomenon that occurs as a result of dilated tortuous collateral intercostal arteries which form deep grooves along the inferior margins of the posterior ribs, especially the third–eighth ribs, also known as the *Roesler sign* [9]. The first two intercostal arteries are

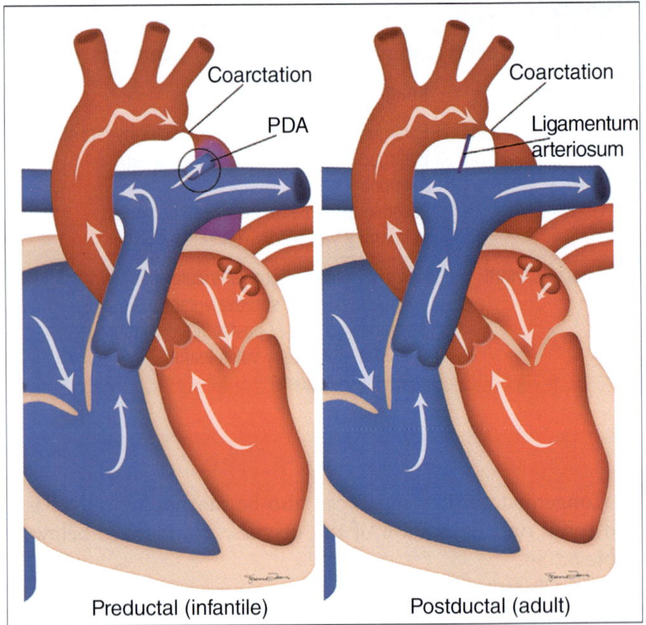

Figure 82.44 Schematic illustration of preductal (infantile) and postductal (adult) variants of aortic coarctation. Preductal coarcatation refers to narrowing of the proximal descending thoracic aorta proximal to the level of the ductus arteriosus, which commonly remains patent to allow for right-to-left shunting for compensatory systemic blood flow. Postductal coarctation refers to narrowing of the proximal descending thoracic aorta distal to the level of the ductus arteriosus, which often closes at birth to become the ligamentum arteriosum. (Courtesy: Susanne Loomis.)

TABLE 82.36 Description of Different Types of Aortic Coarctation [1,9,38,39]

Type	Location	Features
Preductal (infantile type)	Between left subclavian artery and ductus arteriosus	▪ Ductus arteriosus commonly remains patent ▪ Diffuse narrowing with tubular aortic hypoplasia ▪ More commonly associated with bicuspid aortic valve
Postductal (adult type)	At or distal to ductus arteriosus	▪ Ductus arteriosus often closed (ligamentum arteriosum) ▪ Localized, short segment of narrowing ▪ Extensive collateral vessel formation in the chest wall

supplied by the costocervical trunk instead of the descending thoracic aorta, and are thus spared in this process of rib notching.

A corresponding *reverse-figure-of-three sign* has been described in these patients, which refers to the lobulated contour of the anterior esophagus on a barium swallow due to the impression of the adjacent aortic coarctation, which has the appearance of a backward number three [9].

Due to normal patency of the ductus arteriosus in neonatal life, coarctation can be difficult to diagnose in early neonatal life. Echocardiography may be able to visualize the narrowed segment and quantify and gradient across this segment, however, limited acoustic windows limits the utility of echocardiography in clinical assessment.

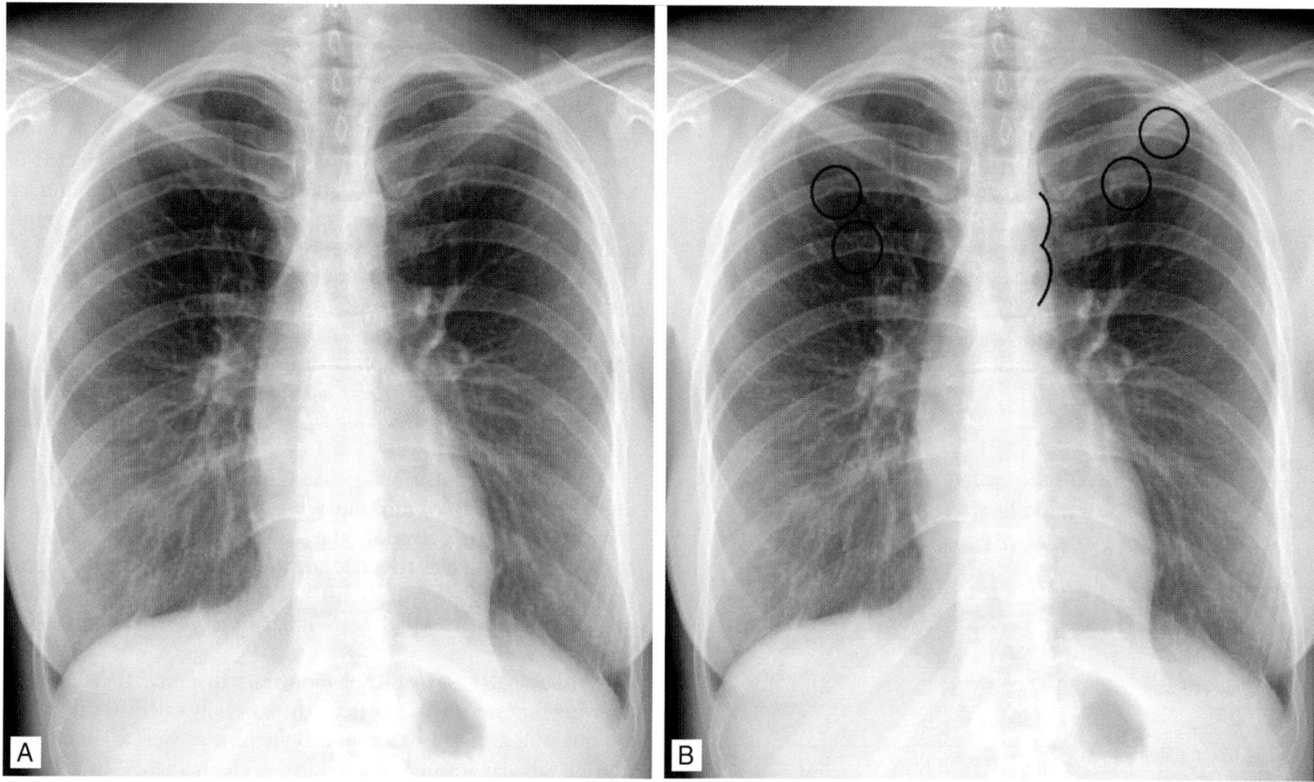

Figure 82.45 Frontal chest radiograph (A) demonstrating the classic ***figure-of-three sign*** (B) associated with aortic coarctation. There are also several bilateral areas of posterior rib notching (*circles*) caused by dilated tortuous collateral intercostal vessels.

Cross-sectional imaging modalities, especially CT and MR angiography, are capable of delineating not only the location and anatomy of a coarctation (Fig. 82.46), but can also provide a thorough evaluation of the extent of collateral vessels in the chest and abdomen. The imaging features of aortic coarctation are summarized below in Table 82.37.

Treatment and Outcomes: Treatment of aortic coarctation is primarily surgical, with the timing depending on the severity of clinical symptoms. Neonates with acute heart failure early in life will require intervention more urgently compared with patients who have milder symptoms. Coarctation repair can range from simple balloon angioplasty with stent placement to resection of the narrowed segment and primary end-to-end anastomosis. The left subclavian artery can also be ligated and used as a flap repair across the narrowed segment.

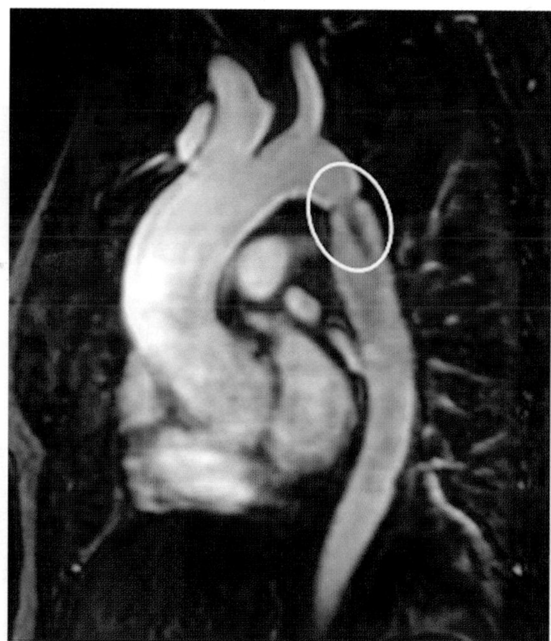

Figure 82.46 Oblique sagittal SSFP image from an MR Angiogram demonstrates focal aortic coarctation with an associated jet of dephasing artifact (*circle*) due to turbulent flow across the stenotic segment.

Bicuspid Aortic Valve

Embryology and Epidemiology: *BAV is the most common congenital heart abnormality, found in ~0.5–2% of the general population* [34,35] *and refers to an anomaly of the aortic valve wherein there are two functional valve leaflets, or cusps, instead of the normal three.* BAV is commonly associated with other CHDs, particularly aortic coarctation, atrial or VSDs, PDA, or HLHS, and is a common feature of the genetic disorder Turner's syndrome. In addition, coexisting thoracic aortopathy is found in approximately 40% of BAV patients [40].

Pathophysiology and Clinical Features: Patients with BAV often present in the third to fifth decade of life with symptoms of valvular dysfunction, commonly in the form of aortic stenosis or less commonly aortic insufficiency. Given the known associated predilection for developing associated ascending thoracic aortic aneurysms, patients with known BAV may undergo routine imaging surveillance to monitor ascending aortic diameters, as they are at risk for developing aortic complications, such as aortic dissection, earlier in life.

The widely used Sievers classification for BAV was proposed in 2007 and subclassifies BAVs based on the pattern of leaflet fusion

TABLE 82.37 Summary of the Key Imaging Features of Isolated Aortic Coarctation

Technique	Imaging Features
Chest radiograph	Figure-of-three sign Posterior rib notching (3rd–8th ribs) Normal pulmonary vascularity
Cardiac CT/MRI	Focal narrowing of the proximal descending thoracic aorta Dilated tortuous collateral intercostal arteries (postductal type) ± Patent ductus arteriosus

TABLE 82.38 Sievers Classification System for Bicuspid Aortic Valve [41]

	Type 0	Type 1	Type 2
Morphology			
Number of raphes	0	1	2
Subcategories (cusp fusion patterns)	AP	L-R	L-R
	Lateral	R-N	R-N
		L-N	

L, left coronary cusp; *N*, noncoronary cusp; *R*, right coronary cusp.

and the number of *raphes*, defined as the fusion of two underdeveloped cusps to form a commissure between two cusps [41]. Table 82.38 summarizes the Sievers classification and Fig. 82.47 provides a visual depiction of various valve morphologies on ECG-gated cardiac CT.

Imaging Features: Isolated BAV cannot be reliably detected on a chest radiograph, although associated findings such as a thoracic aortic aneurysm or aortic coarctation can be detected radiographically and can suggest the presence of an underlying BAV.

Transthoracic echocardiography can easily demonstrate a BAV morphology, best in the parasternal windows, while also providing information regarding valvular function and ascending thoracic aortic diameters. Sonographic features of a BAV include *systolic doming of the valve leaflets, possible diastolic leaflet prolapse, and an ellipsoid or "fish mouth" morphology of the valvular orifice in systole.*

Multiphase acquisition cardiac CT is also highly sensitive for the detection of BAV morphology and provides a larger field of view allowing for detection and assessment of associated aortic abnormalities, such as thoracic aortic aneurysm or aortic coarctation. Early leaflet calcification is a common finding, easily seen on CT, and there will be a similar *"fish mouth" valve orifice morphology.*

Cardiac MRI can easily demonstrate dynamic BAV motion, allowing for assessment, particularly of heavily calcified valves that are not well assessed by echocardiography, as well as quantification of valvular insufficiency and pressure gradients. In addition MRI can provide simultaneous assessment of ascending aortic diameters, and hemodynamic significance of an aortic coarctation when present. The imaging features of BAV are summarized below in Table 82.39.

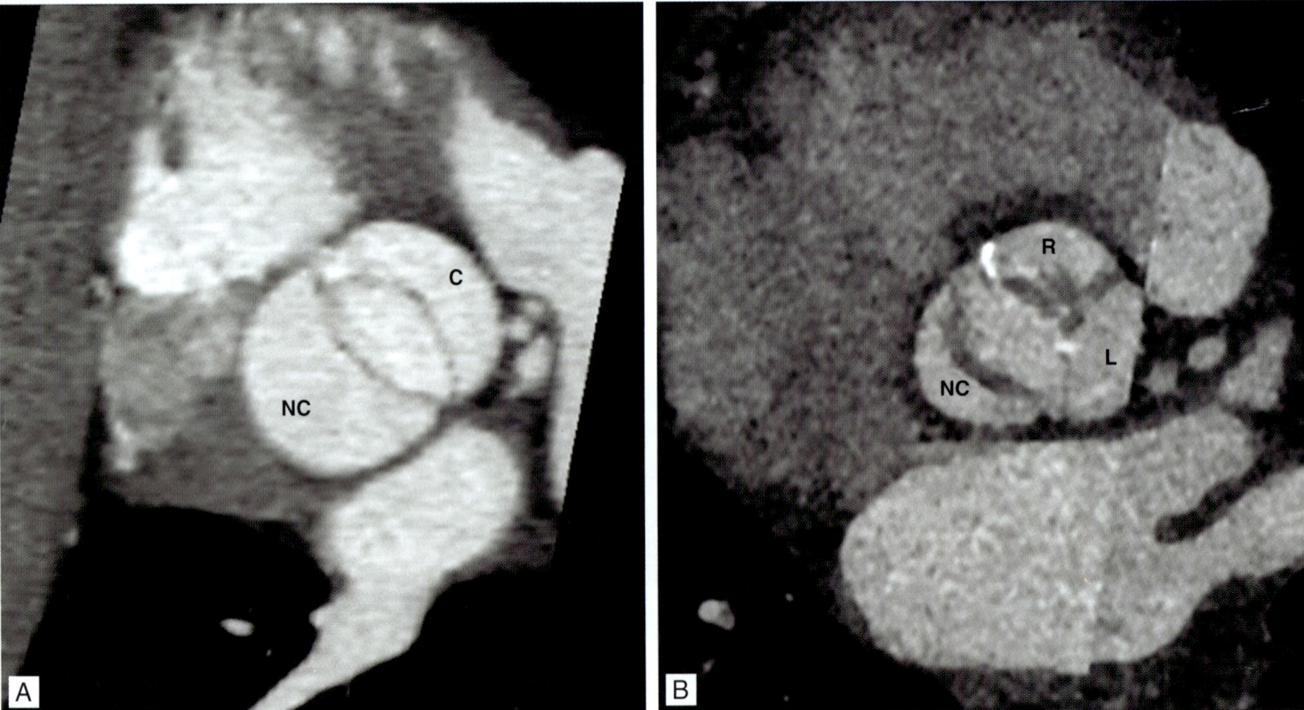

Figure 82.47 Multiple short-axis images from contrast-enhanced ECG-gated cardiac CT in two separate patients demonstrate multiple variants of bicuspid aortic valve morphology during systole. Image (A) demonstrates a Sievers Type 0 bicuspid aortic valve with a classic ***fish-mouth morphology*** of the aortic valve orifice. Image (B) demonstrates a Sievers Type 1 bicuspid aortic valve with a single raphe formed by fusion of the right and left coronary cusps. *C*, coronary cusp; *L*, left coronary cusp; *NC*, noncoronary cusp; *R*, right coronary cusp.

TABLE 82.39 Summary of the Key Imaging Features of Isolated Bicuspid Aortic Valve

Technique	Imaging Features
Chest radiograph	Normal chest radiograph Normal pulmonary vascularity
Cardiac CT/MRI	Calcified aortic valve leaflets with bicuspid morphology ± Restricted aortic leaflet motion ± Increased flow velocities across the aortic valve

Treatment and Outcomes: Patients with BAV may develop valvular dysfunction significant enough to warrant surgery in early to midadulthood. In addition, due to the risk of ascending aortic aneurysm and aortic complication, lifetime aortic surveillance is generally advised and The American Association for Thoracic Surgery 2018 consensus BAV guidelines recommend a surgical threshold for ascending aortic repair of 5.5 cm in patients without significant valvular dysfunction and 4.5 cm in patients with valvular dysfunction significant enough to warrant aortic valve repair [42].

Coronary Artery Variants and Anomalies

Background: Many complex CHD pathologies are associated with congenital anomalies of the coronary arteries, which represents *a wide spectrum of pathologies related to the origin and course of the coronary arteries with varying levels of clinical significance* Table 82.40 aims to summarize the most commonly encountered coronary artery anomalies in clinical practice.

Pathophysiology and Clinical Features: While the majority of coronary artery anomalies are asymptomatic, several of the above-described anomalies have significant clinical implications. For example, an anomalous left coronary artery arising from the right coronary cusp that takes an interarterial and intramural course is associated with myocardial infarction and sudden cardiac death. This is felt to be related to compression of the proximal left coronary artery as it travels in the wall of the aorta.

ALCAPA and ARCAPA are severe coronary anomalies that result in global myocardial ischemia due to reversal of flow within the anomalous coronary artery into the lower pressure pulmonary artery and resulting shunting across the myocardium from the contralateral coronary artery, or "coronary steal." Patients with these anomalies who present with symptoms early in childhood often die within the first few years of life due to extensive myocardial infarction and congestive heart failure.

Imaging Features: Anomalies of the coronary arteries are largely radiographically occult with the exception of nonspecific imaging features related to congestive heart failure. Although echocardiography can often identify abnormal coronary artery origins, cross-sectional imaging modalities such as cardiac CT and MRI are essential adjunctive imaging modalities for delineating coronary artery anomalies.

Cardiac CT can provide an excellent assessment of the origins and courses of anomalous coronary arteries utilizing contrast injection rates of 4–5 mL/second to optimize opacification of the coronary arteries. With the use of multiplanar reformatting and three-dimensional reconstruction capabilities, highly detailed evaluation of the coronary arteries can be performed with ease.

Cardiac MRI is particularly useful in assessing for signs of myocardial ischemia and/or infarction in patients with coronary artery anomalies. LGE sequences are highly sensitive for the detection of fibrosis or scar, and in combination with quantitative biventricular functional information, cardiac MRI can provide critical information to guide therapeutic intervention.

TABLE 82.40 Description of Different Types of Anomalous Coronary Arteries [1]

ANOMALOUS ORIGIN FROM THE AORTIC ROOT		
Description	**Type/Course**	**Clinical Significance**
Left coronary artery arising from the right coronary cusp (Fig. 82.48)	Interarterial (intramural)	Associated with myocardial infarction and sudden death, requires surgical intervention in the form of coronary artery unroofing
	Subpulmonic	Often clinically insignificant
Right coronary artery arising from the left coronary cusp	Retroaortic	May become relevant if the patient has aortic valve replacement as sutures along the valve annulus may inadvertently occlude the vessel along its retroaortic course
	Prepulmonic	Often clinically insignificant. May become relevant in patients undergoing pulmonic valve interventions
Left circumflex coronary artery arising from the right coronary cusp	Retroaortic	Also potentially relevant for patients undergoing aortic or mitral valve replacement
ANOMALOUS ORIGIN FROM THE PULMONARY ARTERY		
Description	**Acronym**	**Clinical Significance**
Left coronary artery arising from the pulmonary artery (Fig. 82.49)	ALCAPA (Bland–White–Garland syndrome)	Lower pressure in the pulmonary artery causes reversal of blood flow in the anomalous coronary artery and results in global coronary artery enlargement due to shunting from the normal coronary artery to the anomalous artery and possible global myocardial ischemia
Right coronary artery arising from the pulmonary artery	ARCAPA	

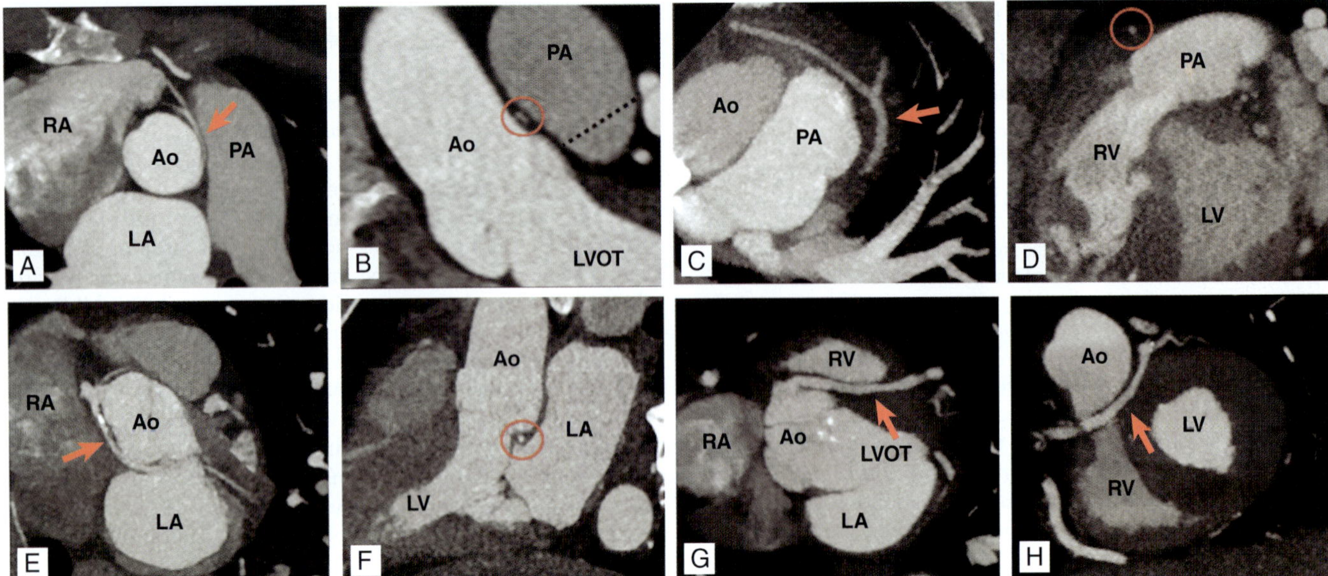

Figure 82.48 These images demonstrate multiple different examples of anomalous coronary arteries. Oblique axial (A) and oblique coronal (B) images of an anomalous right coronary artery (*red arrow and circle*) with an intraarterial, intramural course above the plane of the pulmonic valve (*dotted line*). Oblique axial (C) and oblique sagittal (D) images of an anomalous right coronary artery (*red circle*) originating from left coronary artery (*red arrow*) with a prepulmonic course. Oblique axial (E) and oblique sagittal, 3 chamber view (F) images of an anomalous left circumflex artery (*red arrow and circle*) with a retroaortic course. Oblique axial (G) and short-axis (H) images of an anomalous left main coronary artery (*red arrow*) originating from right sinus of Valsalva with a trasseptal course of left anterior descending coronary artery. *Ao*, aorta; *LA*, left artery; *LV*, left ventricle; *LVOT*, left ventricular outflow tract; *PA*, pulmonary artery; *RA*, right atrium; *RV*, right ventricle.

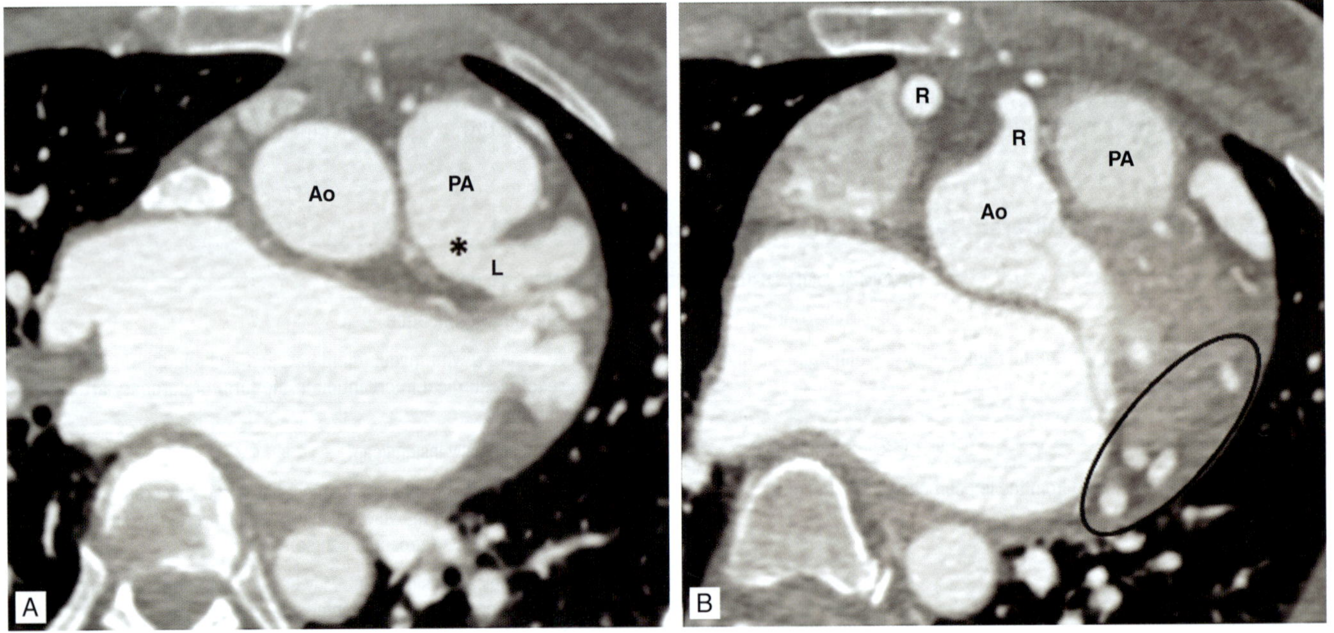

Figure 82.49 Two axial images from a contrast-enhanced ECG-gated cardiac CT demonstrating (A) the left coronary artery arising from the main pulmonary artery (*asterisk*) and (B) the right coronary artery arising normally from the aorta. Notice that both coronary arteries appear large in caliber with prominent collateral vessels in the myocardium (*circled*), which is a result of flow reversal in the left coronary artery and shunting physiology within the myocardium. *Ao*, aorta; *L*, left coronary artery; *PA*, pulmonary artery *R*, right coronary artery.

Treatment and Outcomes: While many coronary anomalies require no intervention, certain high-risk anomalies may be surgically repaired in the form of coronary artery unroofing, coronary artery bypass grafting, or coronary artery reimplantation. It should be noted that familiarity with the postoperative appearance of reimplanted coronary arteries is critical for radiologists to avoid misdiagnosis or misinterpretation for coronary artery aneurysms.

Other Rare Acyanotic Congenital Heart Diseases

While this section focuses on the most common, high-yield acyanotic CHD pathologies, there are several additional more rare pathologies worth mentioning briefly, should they be encountered in clinical practice.

Gerbode Defect: Gerbode defect is a left-to-right communication between the left ventricular outflow tract and the right atrium. This rare entity, which can be congenital or acquired, may

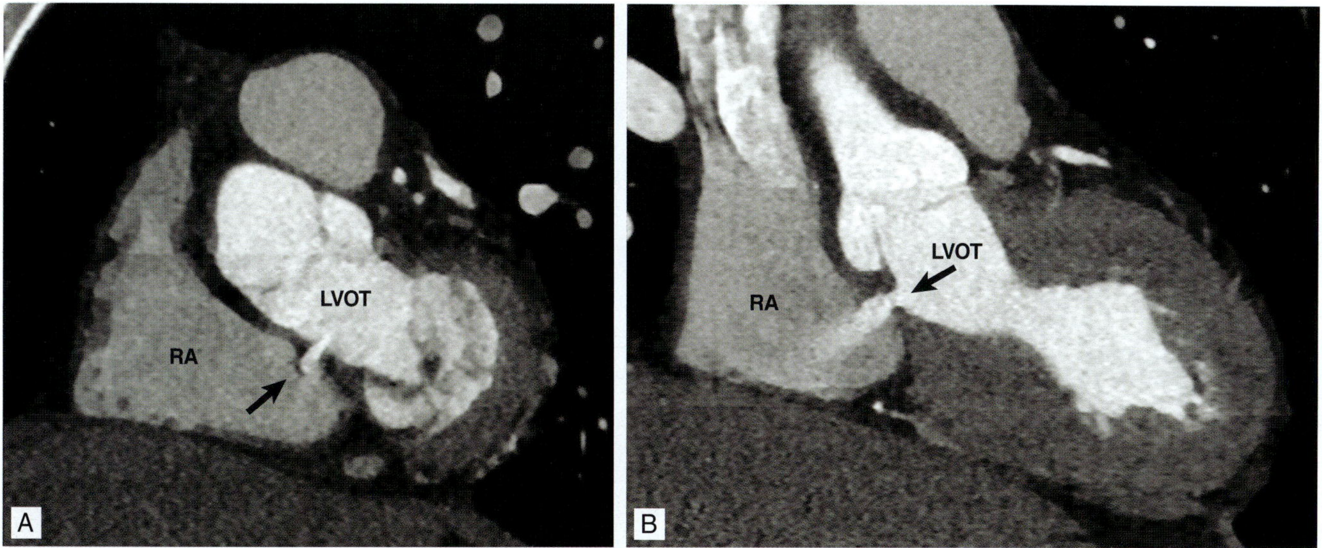

Figure 82.50 Short-axis (A) and oblique coronal (B) contrast-enhanced ECG-gated cardiac CT images demonstrate a shunt between the left ventricular outflow tract (LVOT) and the right atrium (RA), consistent with a Gerbode defect (*arrows*).

be subclassified into direct and indirect defects, where a *direct defect* represents a deficiency in the atrioventricular aspect of the membranous interventricular septum and an *indirect defect* describes a membranous VSD with associated perforation of the septal leaflet of the tricuspid valve, allowing for indirect shunting between the left ventricle and right atrium due to tricuspid regurgitation [43]. Similar to other congenital intracardiac shunts, the resulting left-to-right shunt across a Gerbode defect often causes enlargement of the right heart chambers and may present as right-sided congestive heart failure if severe. This rare congenital abnormality can easily be mistaken for a simple membranous VSD, particularly by echocardiography. Distinguishing features include atypical jet direction, persistent shunt flow during diastole, and lack of interventricular septal flattening [43]. Cardiac CT and MRI may prove particularly useful in delineating this defect, allowing for direct visualization of shunt flow into the right atrium (Fig. 82.50).

Cor Triatriatum: Cor triatriatum is a rare congenital anomaly defined by abnormal septation within the left or right atrium leading to obstruction of venous inflow to the corresponding ventricles. This anomaly exists along a spectrum from a complete imperforate membrane to a highly fenestrated membrane, which determines the degree of ventricular blood flow and thus clinical severity. Associated congenital heart defects are common, including ASDs, PDA, and anomalous pulmonary venous return [44]. The more common left-sided cor triatriatum, also known as *cor triatriatum sinistrum*, results from abnormal or incomplete incorporation of the pulmonary veins into the left atrium, and clinically mimics mitral stenosis. The more unusual right-sided cor triatriatum, also known as *cor triatriatum dextrum*, results from abnormal or incomplete incorporation of systemic venous return into the right atrium and clinically mimics tricuspid stenosis. The key imaging feature, irrespective of technique, is a thin fibrous membrane within one of the atrial chambers, which creates the appearance of a "third atrium" (Fig. 82.51). Clinical symptoms may include congestive heart failure, cyanosis, syncope, or sudden cardiac arrest, and complete cor triatriatum is almost universally fatal within the first two years of life if the membrane is not surgically resected [1,44–46].

Aortopulmonary Window: Aortopulmonary window is a rare congenital heart defect in which there is a direct communication between the aorta and main (or occasionally right) pulmonary artery. This entity can be distinguished from truncus arteriosus based on the presence of both aortic and pulmonic valves and is commonly associated with other congenital heart defects such as VSDs, PDA, or aortic coarctation [22]. Patients may present with congestive heart failure in early neonatal life and plain radioagraphic features are similar to those seen in PDA [1,22].

Interrupted Aortic Arch: IAA is an uncommon congenital anomaly wherein the ascending and descending thoracic aortas are separated from each other, either by a remnant fibrous band or with complete discontinuity. Common associations include VSDs, PDA, DiGeorge syndrome, and truncus arteriosus [47]. Imaging findings and clinical presentation are often similar to severe focal aortic coarctation, and this abnormality ultimately requires definitive surgical correction.

Overall Approach to CHD

- Due to the complexity of the CHD spectrum, a structured, segmental approach for describing the underlying anatomy is critical for making the correct diagnosis and effectively communicating amongst various members of the multidisciplinary care team.
- The choice of imaging technique to utilize in the evaluation of any CHD patient should be based on a balanced multidisciplinary discussion of risks and benefits and a clear understanding of the targeted clinical questions that need to be answered.
- While CHD is often diagnosed during prenatal or early postnatal life through clinical assessment and echocardiography, continuing advances in the surgical management of CHD have resulted in a growing population of adult CHD patients.
- Advanced imaging modalities such as cardiac CT and MRI may play an important role in the imaging evaluation of the CHD population, thus familiarity with the preoperative and postoperative appearances of various common CHDs is crucial to ensure high-quality patient care and appropriate clinical management.

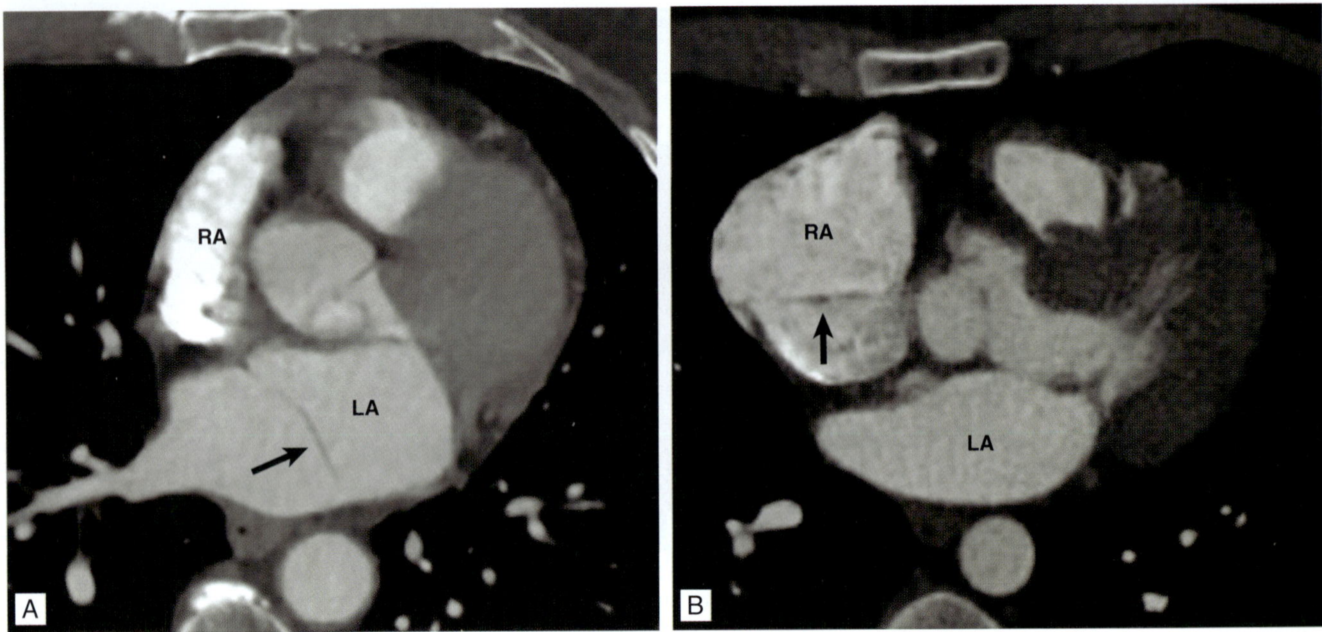

Figure 82.51 Multiple short-axis images from contrast-enhanced ECG-gated cardiac CTs demonstrate two examples of cor triatriatum with incomplete fibrous septations (*arrows*) identified within the (A) left atrium, termed ***cor triatriatum sinistrum*** and (B) right atrium, termed ***cor triatriatum dextrum***, respectively.

- Clinically, CHD can be subdivided into cyanotic and acyanotic heart diseases. Severity of cyanotic CHDs is dependent upon the amount of pulmonary blood flow and the degree of intracardiac mixing of oxygenated and deoxygenated blood (right-to-left shunting) before exiting into systemic circulation. Acyanotic heart diseases predominantly encompass left to right shunts and obstructive lesions.

Suggested Readings

- SV Babu-Narayan, G Giannakoulas, AM Valente, W Li, MA Gatzoulis, Imaging of congenital heart disease in adults, Eur Heart J 37 (15) (2016) 1182–1195. Available from: http://www.ncbi.nlm.nih.gov/pubmed/26424866.
- EK Schallert, GH Danton, R Kardon, DA. Young, Describing congenital heart disease by using three-part segmental notation, Radiographics 33 (2) (2013) E33–E46. Available from: https://pubs.rsna.org/doi/10.1148/rg.332125086.
- EC Ferguson, R Krishnamurthy, SAA. Oldham, Classic imaging signs of congenital cardiovascular abnormalities, Radiographics 27 (5) (2007) 1323–1334. Available from: https://pubs-rsna-org.ezp-prod1.hul.harvard.edu/doi/full/10.1148/rg.275065148.
- EJ Zucker, JL Koning, EY. Lee, Cyanotic congenital heart disease: essential primer for the practicing radiologist, Radiol Clin North Am 55 (4) (2017) 693–716. Available from: http://www.ncbi.nlm.nih.gov/pubmed/28601176.
- ZJ Wang, GP Reddy, MB Gotway, BM Yeh, CB. Higgins, Cardiovascular shunts: MR imaging evaluation, Radiographics 23 (Suppl 1) (2003) S181–S194. Available from: https://pubs.rsna.org/doi/10.1148/rg.23si035503.

83 Pediatric Chest

ESTHER PARK, BOJAN KOVACINA

Introduction

Pediatric chest radiology encompasses a vast spectrum of topics ranging from congenital and syndromic abnormalities to acquired diseases. A detailed discussion of this wide-ranging field is beyond the scope of this textbook, and this chapter will instead aim to give a broad overview of pediatric chest radiology. Particular attention will be given to chest radiography, as it is the most commonly used imaging technique for evaluating the respiratory system in children.

Congenital Thoracic Abnormalities

Congenital Tracheobronchial Abnormalities

Tracheal Agenesis

Tracheal agenesis is a rare anomaly characterized by complete tracheal agenesis or partial underdevelopment [1,2]. As such, this anomaly manifests clinically as severe respiratory distress immediately upon birth, lack of an audible cry, and failed intubation efforts. It is often associated with polyhydramnios in the antenatal period. Tracheal agenesis can be categorized into three main types [1]:

- Type 1. Absent upper trachea. Connection between the lower trachea and esophagus
- Type 2. Most common. Absent trachea. The main bronchi are connected to the esophagus via a common bronchus
- Type 3. The right and left main bronchi connect to the esophagus separately

Given the connections with the esophagus, intubation of the esophagus consequently improves lung ventilation.

Chest radiographic findings include the absence of the tracheal air column, abnormal position of the carina, and absent or decreased lung volumes [1,2]. The diagnosis may be confirmed by chest computed tomography (CT) or broncho-esophagoscopy. Though surgical approaches to maintain airway patency have been proposed, this condition is typically fatal.

Tracheal Bronchus

A tracheal bronchus is a branching anomaly that occurs when there is a direct tracheal origin of all or part of an upper lobe bronchus (Fig. 83.1) [3,4]. This anomaly most commonly occurs on the right, though it may also occur on the left or even bilaterally [3,4]. A tracheal bronchus may be described as supernumerary or displaced. In the setting of an otherwise normal segmental branching pattern to the upper lobe, the tracheal bronchus is supernumerary. However, if one or more of the normal upper lobe segmental bronchi are absent, the tracheal bronchus is considered to be displaced. Of note, when the entire right upper lobe is supplied by the tracheal bronchus, it is referred to as a bronchus suis. This anomaly is often asymptomatic but may also present with recurrent upper lobe infections or air trapping due to impaired drainage. Unintended blockage of a tracheal bronchus by a low-lying endotracheal tube may also cause partial or complete upper lobe collapse.

Tracheal Stenosis

Congenital tracheal stenosis is a rare anomaly that typically arises due to the presence of complete cartilaginous rings and the absence of the normal posterior membranous portion of the trachea [3]. There is resultant narrowing of the trachea, which can be focal (most common), generalized, or funnel shaped (Fig. 83.2A) [3]. Importantly, there is no associated tracheal wall

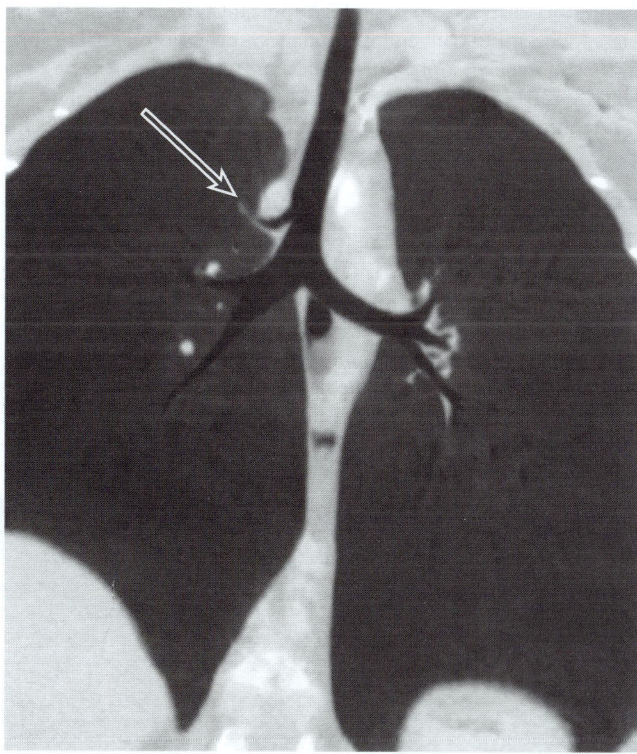

Figure 83.1 A 6-year-old male with a supernumerary tracheal bronchus. Coronal MinIP CECT image demonstrates this tracheal bronchus (*white block arrow*) arising 2 cm proximal to the carina. This had branches to the apical and anterior segments of the right upper lobe. There was otherwise normal segmental branching pattern, with a right upper lobe bronchus originating from the right mainstem bronchus and demonstrating normal trifurcation.

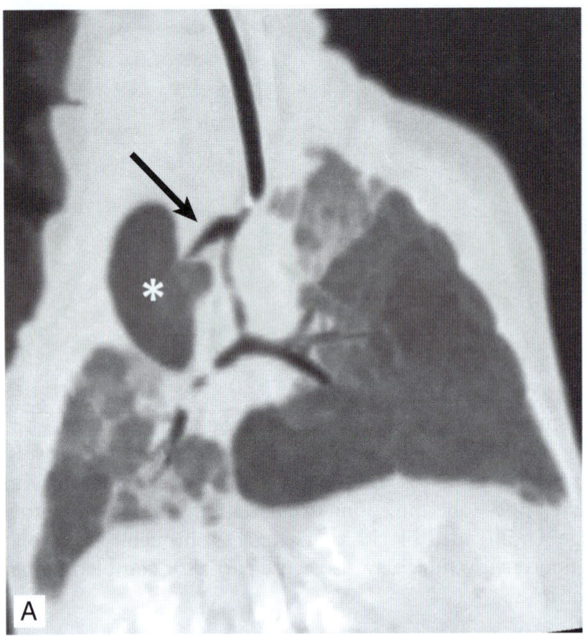

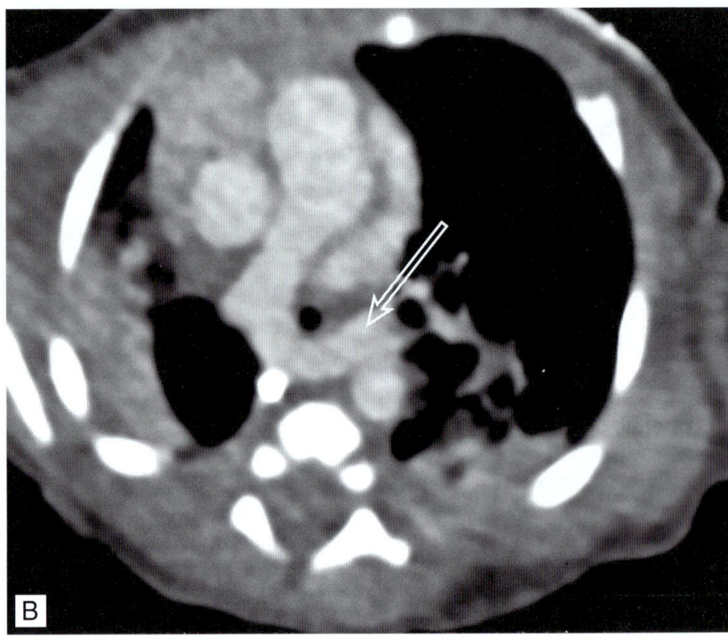

Figure 83.2 An 8-day-old female with congenital tracheal stenosis. (A) A coronal CECT minimum intensity projection image demonstrates significant narrowing of the trachea distal to the endotracheal tube (luminal diameter of 1 mm). There was also an incidentally noted azygous lobe (*asterisk*) supplied by a right tracheal bronchus (*black solid arrow*). (B) Axial CECT demonstrated a pulmonary sling with a left pulmonary artery (*white block arrow*) originating from the right pulmonary artery and traversing between the trachea and esophagus, an anomaly that has been associated with congenital tracheal stenosis.

thickening, which is often seen with acquired causes of tracheal stenosis. This condition manifests early in life with stridor and respiratory distress and has a high mortality rate. It is often associated with other congenital anomalies, such as bronchial or lung agenesis, tracheoesophageal fistula, and pulmonary artery sling (Fig. 83.2B) [3].

Acquired causes of tracheal stenosis are discussed in the dedicated airway section of this textbook.

Tracheobronchomalacia

This refers to a congenital (primary) or acquired (secondary) weakness of the airways [3,5]. While this condition can arise secondary to a number of conditions, including prior intubation, prior lung surgery, external masses causing compression, and chronic obstructive pulmonary disease, this section will focus on congenital tracheomalacia caused by abnormalities in the cartilaginous matrix. Clinically, tracheomalacia may present with an expiratory wheeze, stridor, or a barking cough. While a well-accepted standard for the diagnosis of tracheomalacia is bronchoscopy, paired inspiratory-dynamic expiratory CT is a comparable method for evaluating tracheomalacia. On imaging, a greater than 50% decrease in the cross-sectional area of the tracheal lumen in expiration is used to define tracheomalacia in the pediatric population (Fig. 83.3A,B) [5]. Tracheal collapse will also lead to inward bowing of the posterior membranous trachea, giving the appearance of the crescentic "frown" sign. Lateral fluoroscopy may also be used to assess for excessive tracheal collapsibility upon expiration.

Tracheoesophageal Fistula

The majority of this congenital anomaly occurs in the setting of esophageal atresia and a distal tracheoesophageal fistula [3]. These may present with respiratory distress during initial feeding attempts and inability to pass a feeding tube into the

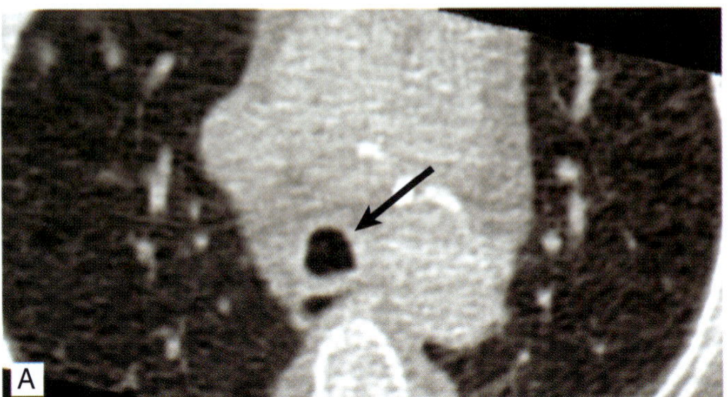

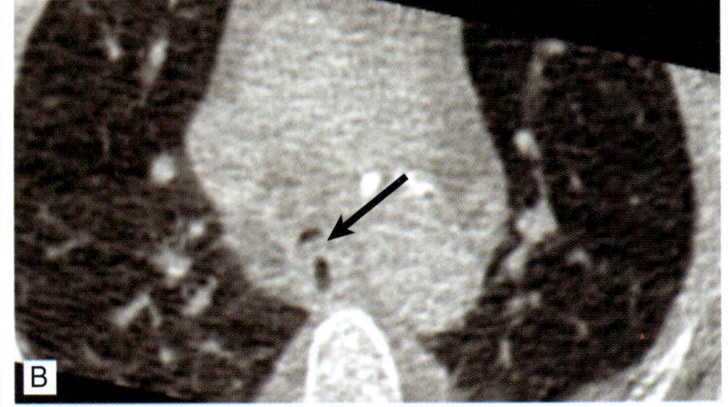

Figure 83.3 A 71-year-old female with severe tracheomalacia. Dynamic noncontrast axial chest CT images demonstrated severe collapse of the trachea and bilateral main bronchi (the latter not shown) on the expiratory images (*arrow* in B). (A) In inspiration, the tracheal (*arrow* in A) diameter was 11 mm. (B) In expiration, there was severe tracheal collapse, and the tracheal diameter reduced to 2 mm.

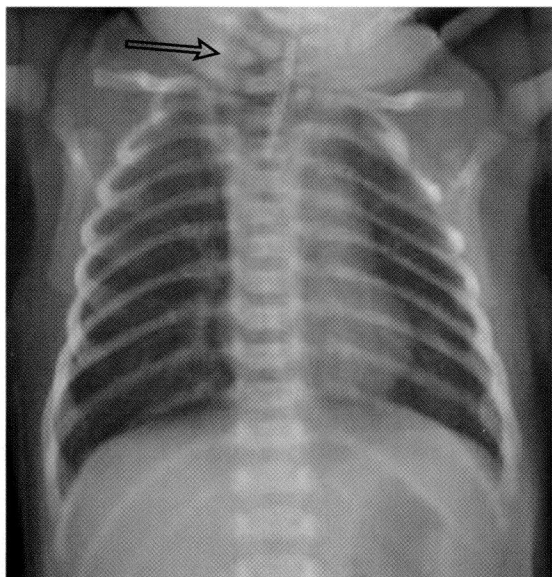

Figure 83.4 A 12-month-old male with a frontal chest radiograph demonstrated a feeding tube in an aerated pouch in the upper chest, consistent with known history of esophageal atresia. There is also a vertebral segmentation anomaly in the lower cervical spine (*black block arrow*), which is a component of the VACTERL constellation.

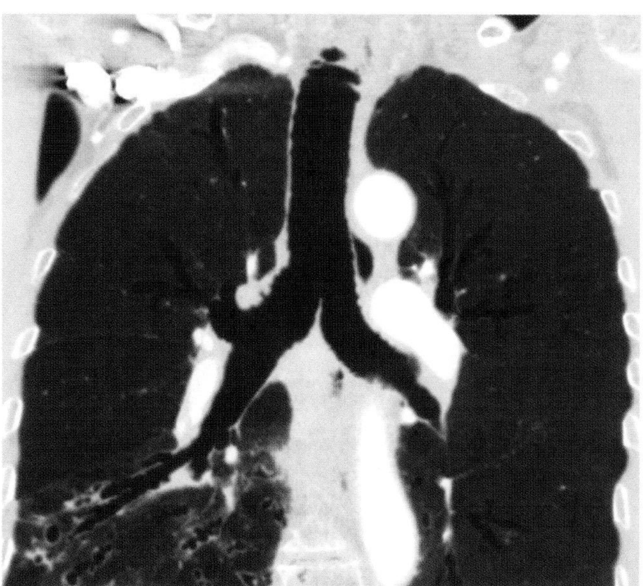

Figure 83.5 A 77-year-old male with history of congenital tracheobronchomegaly. A coronal minimum intensity projection CECT image demonstrates diffuse tracheal and central bronchial dilatation with irregular, corrugated appearance.

stomach (Fig. 83.4). Less frequently, they can also occur in the setting of a continuous esophagus (H-type), which may present with recurrent infections. An esophagogram can be used to demonstrate the fistulous connection in proximal and H-type tracheoesophageal fistulas. Congenital tracheoesophageal fistulas are strongly associated with other congenital anomalies, including those belonging to the VACTERL (**V**ertebral defects, **A**nal atresia, **C**ardiac defects, **T**racheo-**E**sophageal fistula, **R**enal anomalies, and **L**imb abnormalities) constellation (Fig. 83.4) [3].

Tracheobronchomegaly

Also known as Mounier–Kuhn syndrome, this refers to abnormal dilatation of the trachea and main bronchi [6]. It may be associated with tracheal diverticula and corrugated appearance of the central airways, thought to be related to weakening and redundancy of the elastic and muscular walls (Fig. 83.5). CT is a useful technique for diagnosis, particularly as dynamic inspiratory-expiratory imaging can be used to evaluate for possible concomitant tracheobronchomalacia, a condition that occurs with increased incidence in tracheobronchomegaly patients.

Accessory Cardiac Bronchus

This is a rare anomaly characterized by a supernumerary bronchus that arises from the bronchus intermedius medially [4]. The presence of cartilage in its walls differentiates it from a diverticulum. This anomaly is typically stump-like (Fig. 83.6), though less frequently it may supply a small lobule known as a cardiac lobe. This is typically asymptomatic and incidentally found on imaging. However, it can on rare occasion be associated with conditions such as chronic infections or inflammation and malignancy.

Bronchial Atresia

This is characterized by focal atresia at the lobar, segmental, or subsegmental level, resulting in mucoid impaction distal to the point of interruption and formation of a mucocele (Fig. 83.7) [4,7,8]. In the neonate, the affected segment may be atelectatic or fluid-filled, which gradually becomes air-filled. As collateral air drift increases, the lung distal to the atretic bronchus will become hyperinflated due to air trapping. There will also be decreased vascularity in the affected lung segments(s). While bronchial atresia can occur in any location of the lungs, the apicoposterior segment of the left upper lobe is the most commonly affected. These imaging findings can be demonstrated by both chest radiography and CT, with the tubular branching mass corresponding to the mucocele often referred to as the "finger in glove" sign.

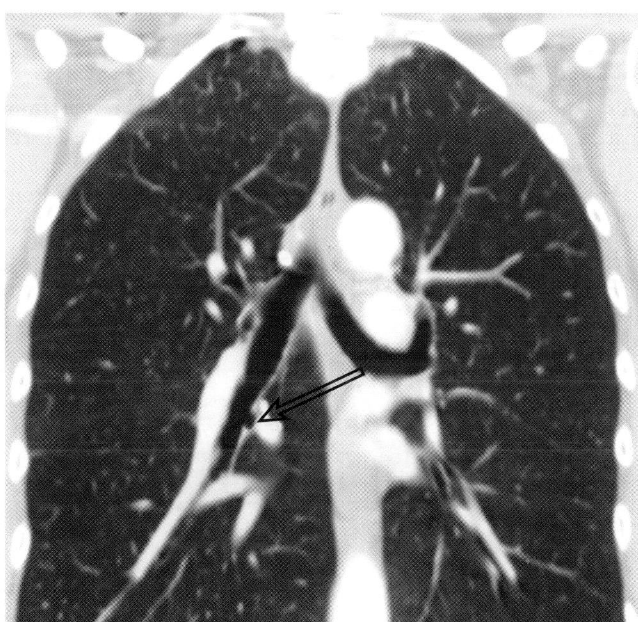

Figure 83.6 A 57-year-old female with an incidentally noted stump-like supernumerary bronchus arising from the bronchus intermedius medially (*black block arrow*) on this coronal CECT, consistent with an accessory cardiac bronchus.

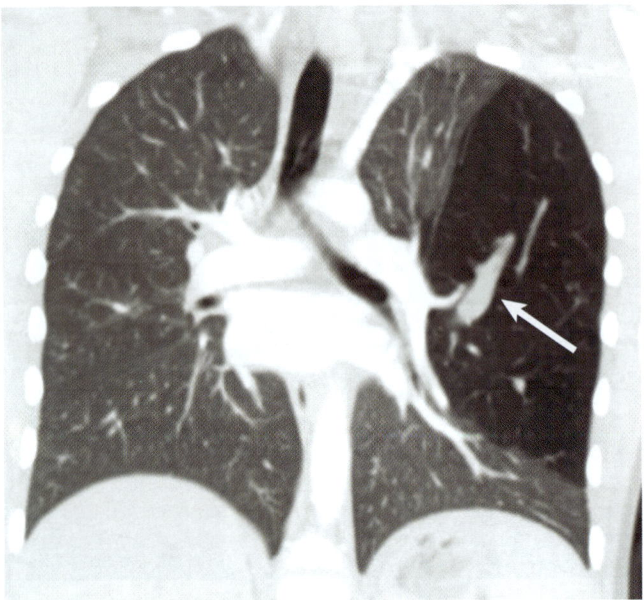

Figure 83.7 A 10-year-old female with bronchial atresia. A coronal CECT image demonstrates increased lucency involving the left upper lobe and lingula representing air trapping, with associated attenuation of pulmonary vascularity. There was also extensive mucus plugging within dilated bronchi distal to the atretic bronchus, one of which is seen on this image (*white arrow*).

Congenital Bronchiectasis

Also known as Williams–Campbell syndrome, this results from partial or complete congenital absence of cartilage in the subsegmental bronchi, typically fourth to sixth order (Fig. 83.8) [9]. The cartilages in the trachea, mainstem bronchi, and segmental bronchi are normal. This leads to diffuse bilateral bronchiectasis and airway collapse during expiration. As such, this presents as recurrent pneumonias and wheezing. Acquired forms of bronchiectasis are discussed in further detail in the dedicated airway section.

Congenital Lung Abnormalities

Pulmonary Underdevelopment

Also known as lung agenesis-hypoplasia complex, this describes a spectrum of abnormal lung formation ranging from agenesis to aplasia to hypoplasia [3,7,8]. The cause may be primary or secondary, the latter of which includes *in-utero* processes that impair development via decreased vascular perfusion or space-occupying masses such as diaphragmatic hernias. Of note, pulmonary underdevelopment often occurs with other multisystem congenital abnormalities.

Pulmonary agenesis occurs when there is complete absence of the lung, and there are no bronchi or vessels distal to the carina [3,7]. As such, there is mediastinal shift to the affected side and compensatory hyperinflation of the contralateral lung, which crosses the midline (Fig. 83.9). Pulmonary aplasia is also characterized by absent lung tissue and vasculature [3,7]. However, the presence of a rudimentary bronchial stump differentiates pulmonary aplasia from pulmonary agenesis. In the least severe form of this complex, pulmonary hypoplasia, bronchi and pulmonary vessels are present but reduced in number [3,7]. Its appearance on imaging therefore varies depending on the degree of hypoplasia (Fig. 83.10). Transpleural collateral arteries may be seen in pulmonary hypoplasia when the ipsilateral pulmonary artery is small.

Scimitar Syndrome

Also known as a hypogenetic lung syndrome, this refers to a syndrome in which part or all of the right lung is hypoplastic and demonstrates partial or complete anomalous pulmonary venous return [3,7,8]. The anomalous pulmonary vein most frequently drains the affected right lung into the suprahepatic inferior vena cava, though drainage into other systemic circulations, such as the portal vein, azygous vein, right atrium, or coronary sinus has also been described. The anomalous vein takes on the appearance of the scimitar Turkish sword along the right heart border on chest radiography (Fig. 83.11). The affected lung is typically hypovascularized and occasionally coexists with a sequestration receiving

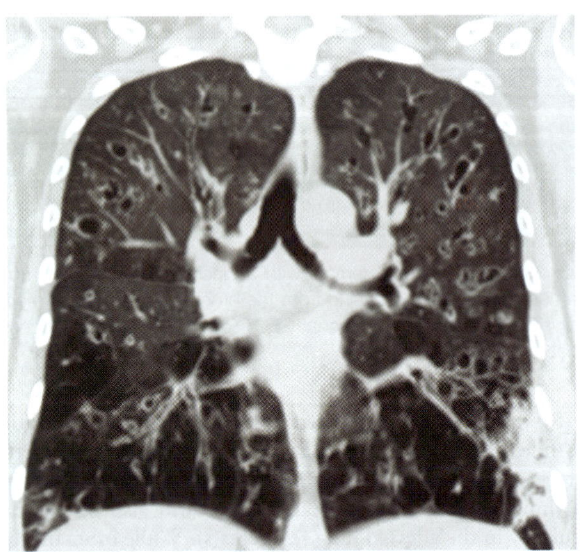

Figure 83.8 A 49-year-old female with history of congenital bronchiectasis. This coronal chest CT image demonstrates diffuse extensive cylindrical and varicose bronchiectasis with associated bronchial wall thickening and multifocal mucus plugging. The trachea and mainstem bronchi were normal in caliber.

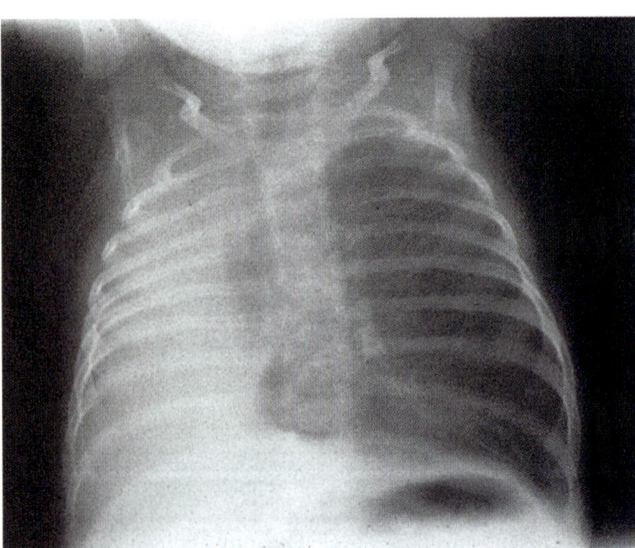

Figure 83.9 A chest radiograph in a neonate with agenesis of the right lung demonstrates opacification of the right hemithorax and crowding of the right ribs. There is compensatory hyperinflation of the left lung, which crosses the midline.

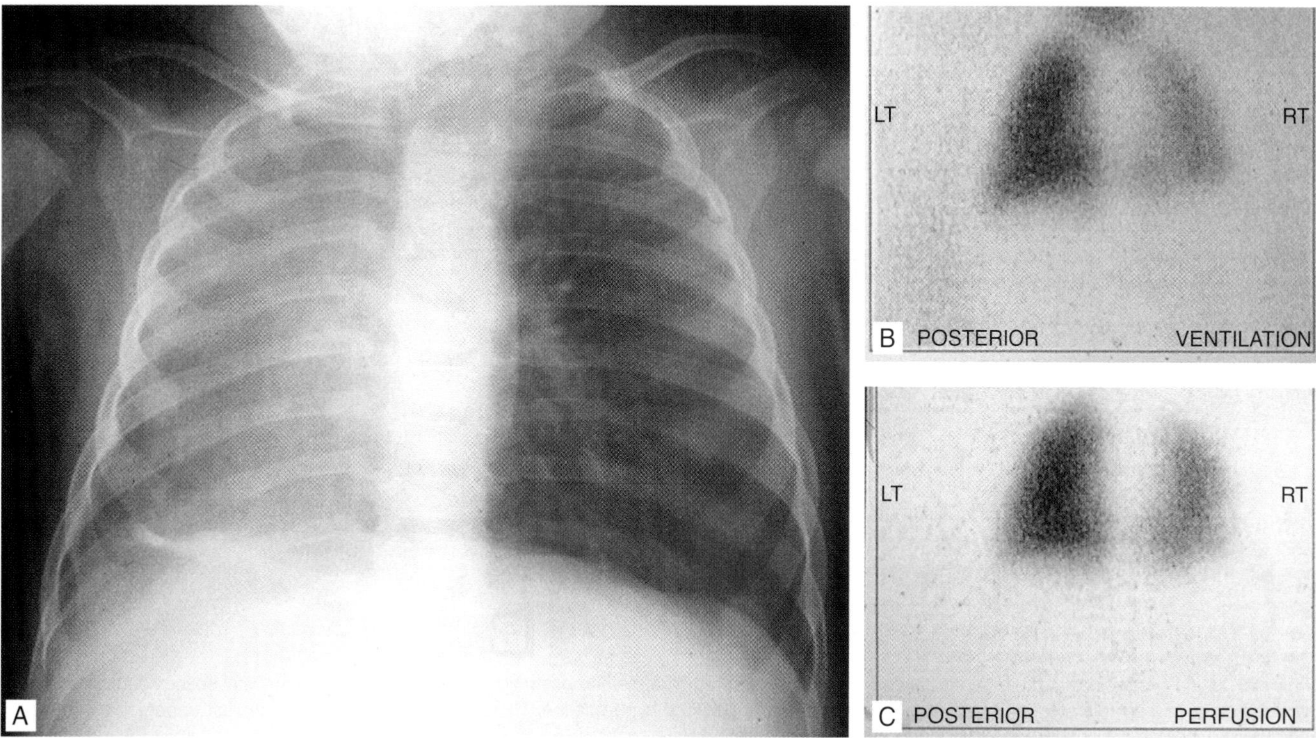

Figure 83.10 (A) A chest radiograph of a hypoplastic right lung demonstrates rightward mediastinal shift. (B, C) Posterior views of VQ scans show reduced ventilation and perfusion in the hypoplastic right lung.

a systemic arterial supply. Additional bronchial branching anomalies and lung lobation/segmentation anomalies may also coexist.

Congenital Lobar Overinflation

Also known as congenital lobar hyperinflation, this is due to narrowing of a bronchus, which results in air trapping and subsequent progressive overinflation of the affected lobe [3,7,8]. The narrowing can be related to intrinsic weakening or the absence of the bronchial cartilage. Alternatively, it can be due to extrinsic compression by enlarged vessels or masses. The term "congenital lobar emphysema," which this condition is also sometimes referred to as, is therefore a misnomer as the mechanism does not involve

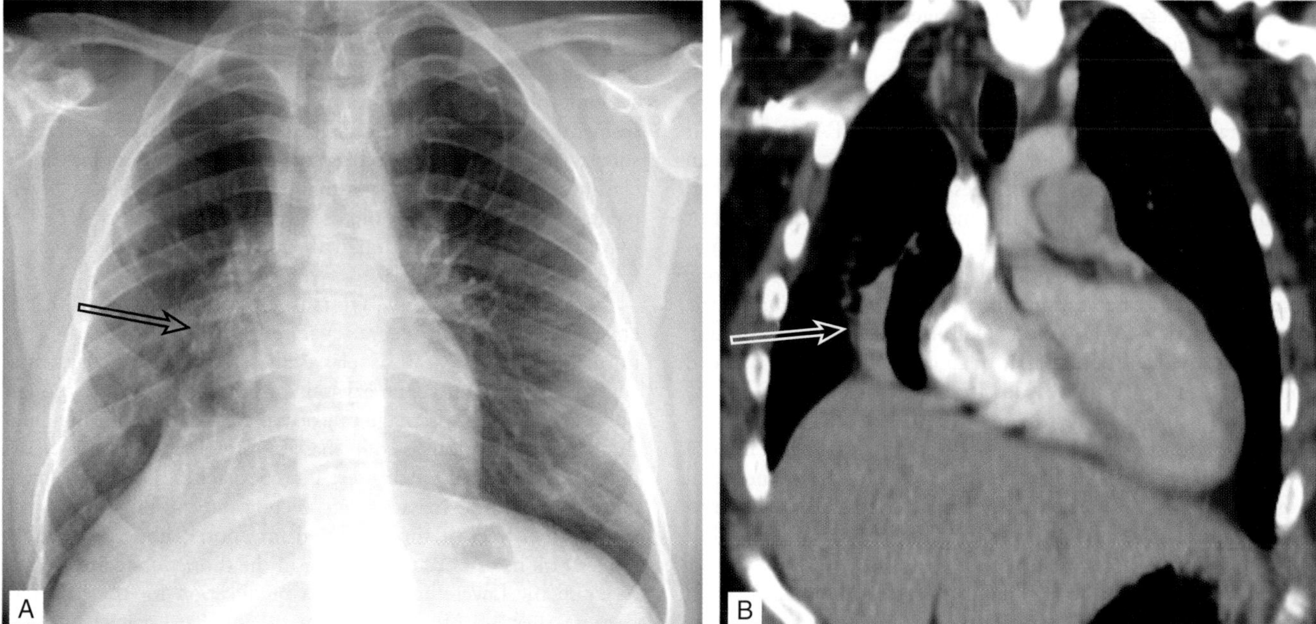

Figure 83.11 A frontal chest radiograph (A) demonstrates right hemithorax volume loss consistent with pulmonary hypoplasia and a curvilinear opacity along the right heart border (*black block arrow*) consistent with partial anomalous pulmonary venous return draining a portion of the right lung into an infradiaphragmatic systemic venous circulation. These findings are redemonstrated on a correlative coronal oblique chest CT (B), including the anomalous pulmonary vein (*white block arrow*). The constellation of findings are consistent with Scimitar syndrome.

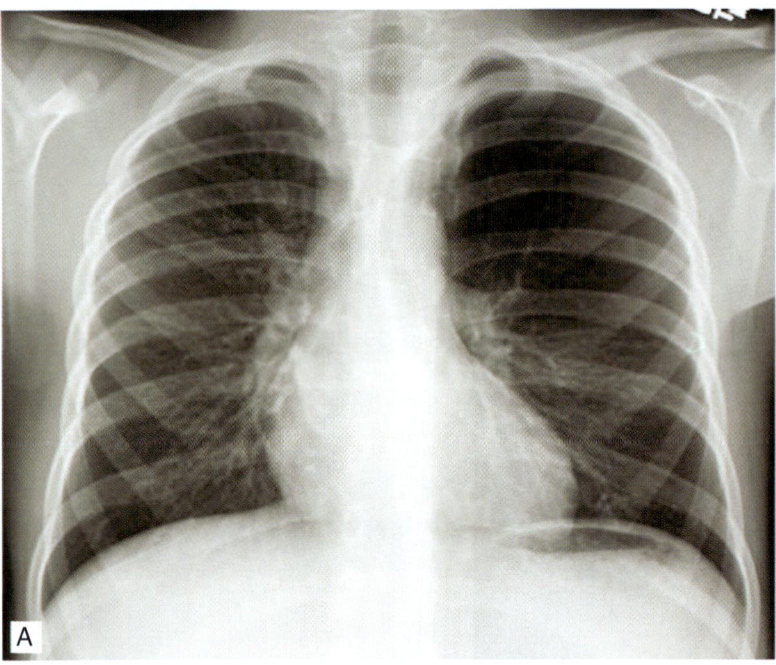

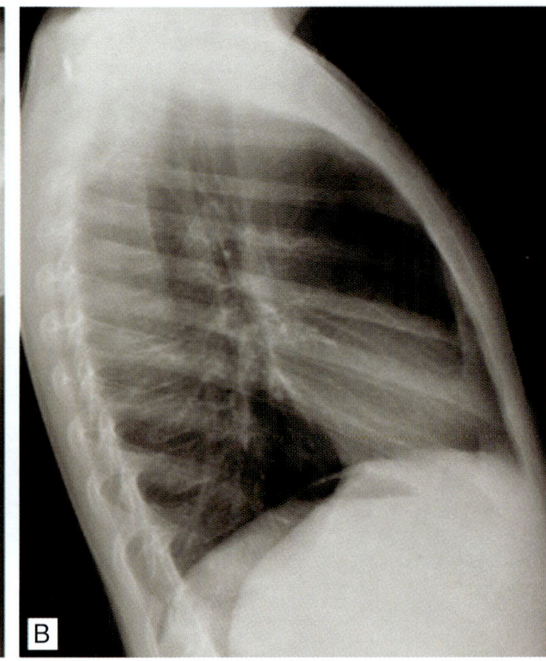

Figure 83.12 A 9-year-old male with (A) frontal and (B) lateral chest radiographs demonstrating mildly widened left intercostal spaces compared to the right and an increased retrosternal airspace consistent with left upper lobe hyperinflation. There is also hyperlucency of the left upper lobe with vessel attenuation. Findings are consistent with congenital lobar hyperinflation.

alveolar destruction. Though this condition can affect any lobe, it most frequently affects the left upper lobe and has a slight male predilection.

The imaging appearance of this condition varies over time [3,8]. In newborns, retained fetal lung fluid causes this to appear as an increased lobar opacity. As the fluid begins to clear and lung aeration increases, the affected lobe will become hyperexpanded and hyperlucent, causing shift and displacement of the nearby structures (Fig. 83.12). Symptomatic cases require surgical lobectomy, with conservative/expectant management reserved for those with no or minimal symptoms.

Congenital Pulmonary Airway Malformation

Congenital pulmonary airway malformations (CPAM) represent a heterogeneous group of lung masses communicating with an abnormal bronchial tree [3,7,8]. These were previously described as congenital cystic adenomatoid malformations (CCAM) but are now referred to as CPAMs because not all of these malformations contain cystic or adenomatoid components. When large, these can cause neonatal respiratory distress, compression on the adjacent structures, and contralateral mediastinal shift. Though CPAMs are typically unilateral, bilateral involvement has been reported. CPAMs can be divided into five main types [3,7,8].

- Type 0: Incompatible with life. All lobes are affected
- Type 1: Composed of large cysts (typically 2–10 cm in size) that may be surrounded by smaller cysts. During the neonatal period, the cystic portions may appear solid due to the presence of retained fetal lung fluid. However, as the fluid is cleared, this will become air filled (Fig. 83.13)
- Type 2: Composed of small cysts (typically less than 2 cm in size) (Fig, 83.14)
- Type 3: Composed of microcysts (less than 0.5 cm in size) and therefore appears solid. May demonstrate mild enhancement and contains adenomatous tissue
- Type 4: Composed of large, peripheral thin-walled cysts

Unlike pulmonary sequestrations, CPAMs demonstrate normal blood supply from the pulmonary arteries and normal pulmonary venous drainage [3,7,8]. While symptomatic CPAMs are universally treated by surgical resection, the treatment of asymptomatic CPAMs is more controversial. However, some argue that asymptomatic CPAMs should also be resected to avoid associated complications such as recurrent infections and a small risk of malignant transformation.

Pulmonary Sequestration

Pulmonary sequestrations are lung malformations that do not connect with the tracheobronchial tree [3,7,8]. They demonstrate a systemic blood supply, typically from the aorta, though origins from other systemic vessels such as mesenteric, intercostal, and subclavian arteries have also been described. Sequestrations can be classified into extralobar or intralobar types depending on their pleural investment. Of note, sequestrations can also occur as hybrid lesions in association with other lung anomalies such as CPAMs (Fig. 83.14).

Extralobar sequestrations contain abnormal lung tissue that is enveloped by its own pleura separate from the remainder of the normal lung [3,7,8]. It is classically drained by the systemic venous circulation via the azygous or hemiazygos veins, though pulmonary venous drainage can occasionally occur. On imaging, these typically appear as solid masses, though cystic components may also be present when there is a coexistent CPAM. The presence of air in these masses suggests communication with the gastrointestinal tract or superimposed infection. Though extralobar sequestrations can occur anywhere in the thorax, they most often occur in the lower thorax, with a predilection for the left side. Because they are often asymptomatic and have a lower rate of complications, their management is controversial but typically expectant.

Intralobar sequestrations consist of abnormal lung tissue that is enveloped by the visceral pleura of the affected lobe and drained

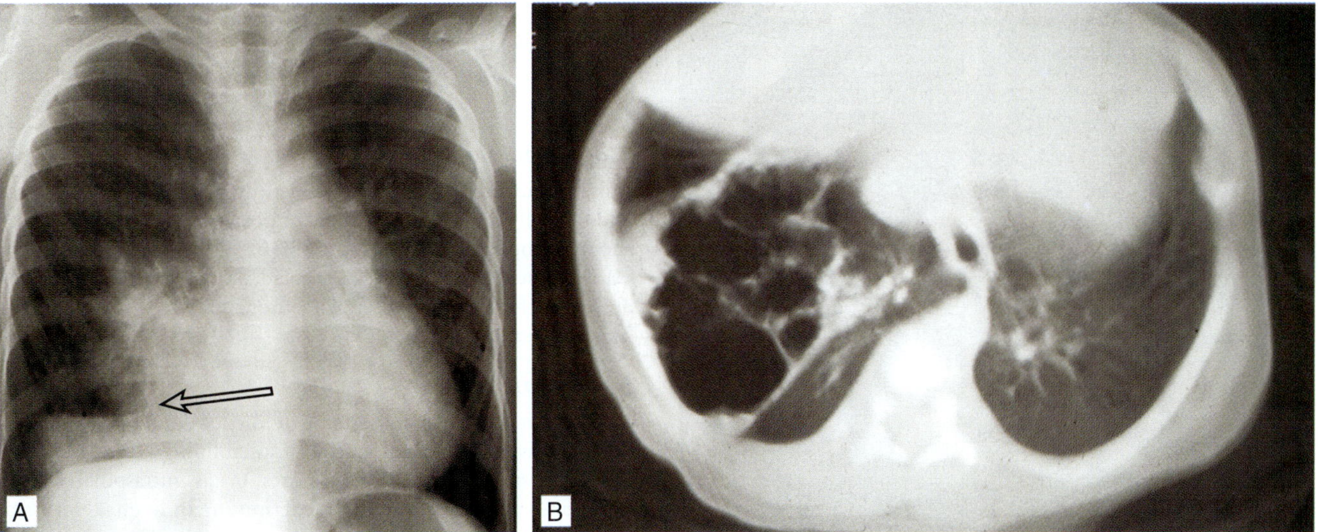

Figure 83.13 A chest radiograph (A) and axial chest CT (B) demonstrate a cystic type 1 congenital pulmonary airway malformation in the right lower lobe. There is an air-fluid level (*black block arrow*) on the chest radiograph due to superimposed infection.

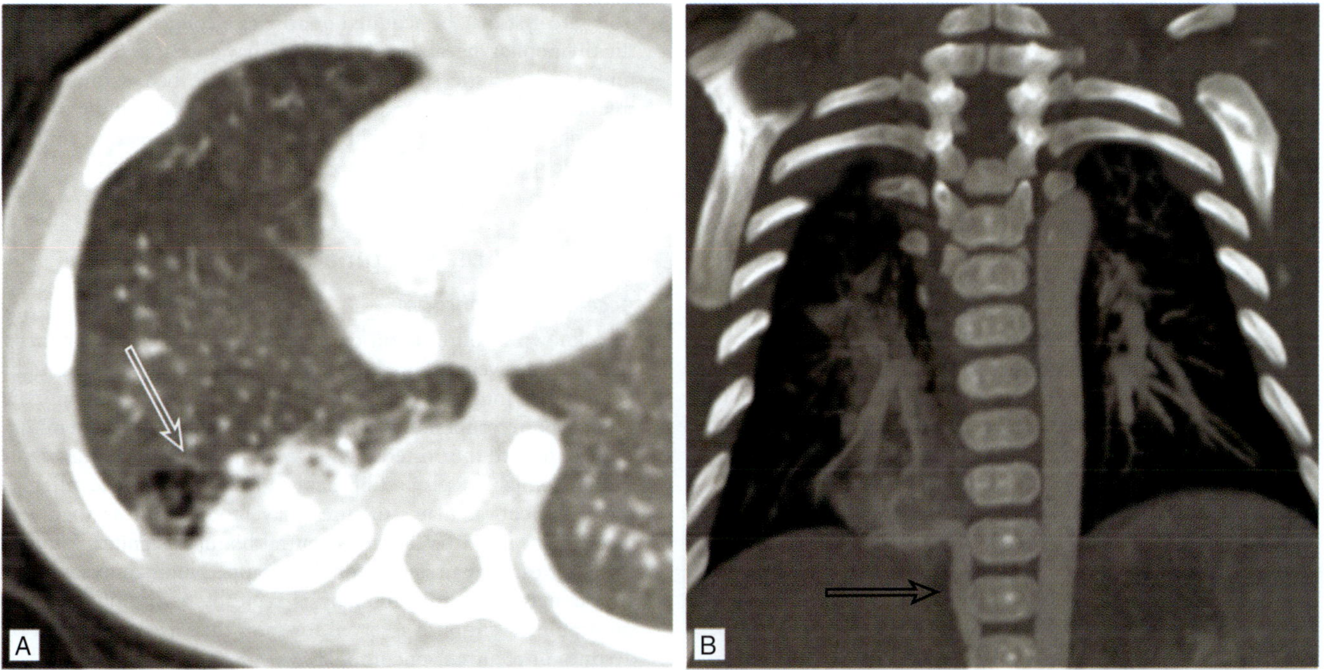

Figure 83.14 A 22-month-old male with (A) axial and (B) coronal maximum intensity projection CECT images demonstrating a mixed solid and cystic lesion in right lower lobe (*white block arrow*). There was a prominent systemic arterial feeding vessel (*black block arrow*) arising from the celiac axis (origin not shown). This was consistent with a pathology proven type 2 CPAM hybrid lesion with sequestration.

by the regional pulmonary veins [3,7,8]. They most often occur in the lower lobes, preferentially on the left side. Unlike extralobar sequestrations, they do not have their own separate pleural lining. Therefore, though intralobar sequestrations have been reported antenatally, not all of these masses are thought to be congenital. Some of these malformations are theorized to be results of recurrently infected or inflamed lung tissue parasitizing its own arterial supply from the aorta. Intralobar sequestrations receive collateral air drift from the adjacent normal lung tissue and therefore will appear aerated on imaging (once retained fetal lung fluid has cleared). The presence of air-fluid levels suggests superimposed infection. Because intralobar sequestrations are at risk for recurrent infections and have a small chance for malignant transformation, they typically undergo elective surgical resection.

Congenital Mediastinal Abnormalities

Bronchogenic Cyst

A bronchogenic cyst is a foregut malformation resulting from a tracheobronchial branching anomaly [3,7,8,10]. It is lined by respiratory epithelium and is attached to the tracheobronchial tree but does not communicate with the airways. Therefore, the

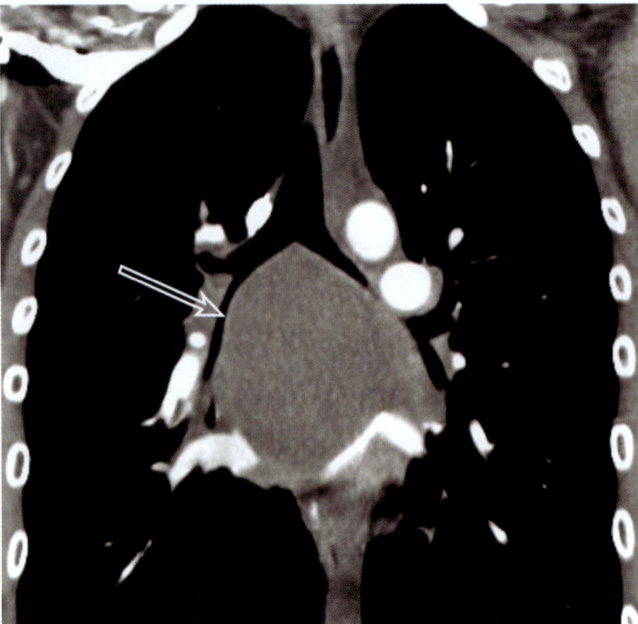

Figure 83.15 A 29-year-old female with a large, homogeneous thin-walled cystic subcarinal mass on a coronal CECT (*white block arrow*). There was no internal enhancement or mural nodularity. This was consistent with pathology proven bronchogenic cyst.

presence of an air-fluid level is abnormal and indicates superimposed infection or prior intervention (such as attempted cyst aspiration). While these cysts can arise anywhere in the thorax, they are most commonly found in the middle mediastinum (particularly in the right paratracheal or subcarinal regions) (Fig. 83.15). They may contain mucoid material, layering milk of calcium, or proteinaceous and hemorrhagic contents, in which case they may demonstrate an attenuation higher than simple water on CT. In these cases, MRI can confirm their cystic nature by demonstrating homogeneous hyperintensity on T2-weighted images and no internal enhancement. Cysts containing simple fluid will be hypointense on T1-weighted images, but complicated cysts may be hyperintense on the same sequence.

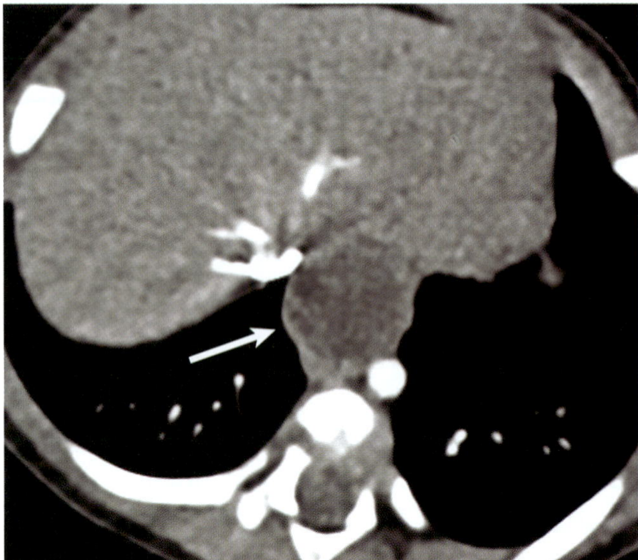

Figure 83.16 A 270-day-old male with a round, cystic paraesophageal lesion near the esophageal hiatus on this axial CECT (*white arrow*). This was consistent with a pathology proven esophageal duplication cyst.

Esophageal Duplication Cyst

This foregut duplication cyst is lined by gastrointestinal mucosa and typically found in the middle or posterior mediastinum along the paraesophageal region (Fig. 83.16) [10]. Those that contain ectopic gastric mucosa can secrete acid, and these cysts may ulcerate or perforate into the tracheobronchial tree with resultant hemoptysis.

Neurenteric Cyst

Neurenteric cysts are another type of foregut duplication cyst that are lined by mixed neural/gastrointestinal lining [10]. They present as posterior mediastinal masses or as intraspinal masses extending into the posterior mediastinum through a vertebral defect. The presence of vertebral anomalies in the setting of an intraspinal cyst is very suggestive of this diagnosis (Fig. 83.17).

Thymic Cyst

This rare cyst may be acquired or arise as a congenital remnant of the thymopharyngeal duct [10]. They may appear as unilocular or multilocular cystic structures in the thymic bed. Complicated thymic cysts may appear solid-like; however, they will be nonenhancing on CT and MRI. Ultrasound can also be used to confirm its cystic nature.

Congenital Diaphragmatic Abnormalities

Accessory Diaphragm

Also known as duplication of the diaphragm, this rare anomaly almost exclusively occurs on the right side and divides the right hemithorax into two parts [1]. This fibromuscular membrane extends posterosuperiorly from the anterior aspect of the hemidiaphragm toward the posterior chest wall. It exhibits a central hiatus through which vessels and bronchi can traverse, and crowding of these bronchovascular structures may be apparent as they pass through the hiatus. When this central hiatus is significantly narrowed, it can impair aeration of the trapped lung and cause it to appear mass-like. This anomaly is typically asymptomatic, and surgical intervention is reserved for cases that are complicated by dyspnea or recurrent pneumonias.

Congenital Diaphragmatic Hernias

Bochdalek hernias are congenital posterolateral hernias that may contain bowel, stomach, kidneys, liver, and/or spleen depending on its location [10,12]. They most frequently occur on the left side and are associated with significant morbidity and mortality due to associated pulmonary hypoplasia. Herniated bowel loops and stomach are also at risk for incarceration and strangulation. The imaging findings are dependent on the contents of the hernia. On radiography, it may initially appear as a posterior mass silhouetting the diaphragm, with associated contralateral mediastinal shift. However, if the hernia contains bowel, it will become air-filled over time as the infant begins to swallow (Fig. 83.18). If the majority of the bowel loops are located in the hernia, the abdomen will appear scaphoid, with paucity of air on abdominal radiographs.

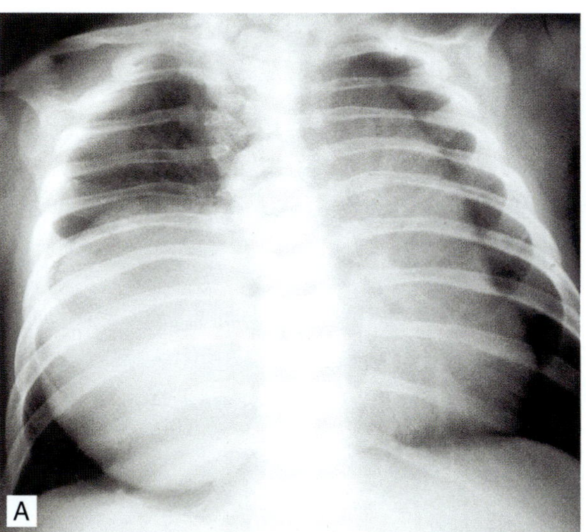

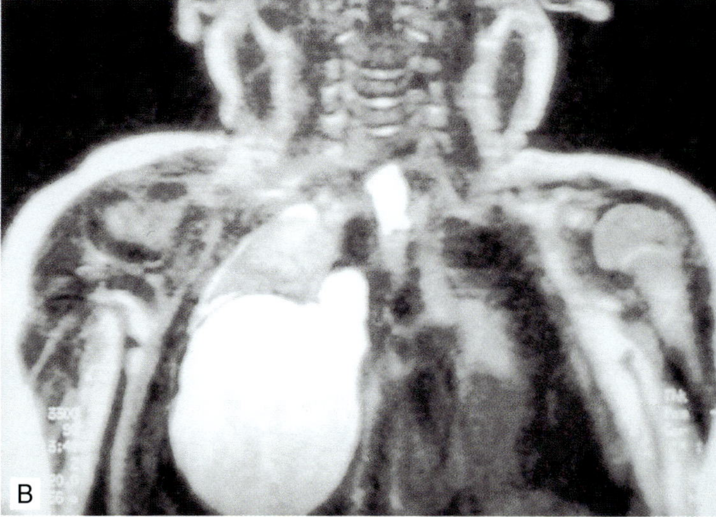

Figure 83.17 Neurenteric cyst (A) A chest radiograph demonstrates multiple segmentation anomalies of the thoracic vertebral bodies and a large round opacity in the right hemithorax. (B) A coronal T2-weighted spin-echo image demonstrates a hyperintense cystic mass arising from the cervicothoracic spine with consequent compressive atelectasis of the adjacent right upper lobe.

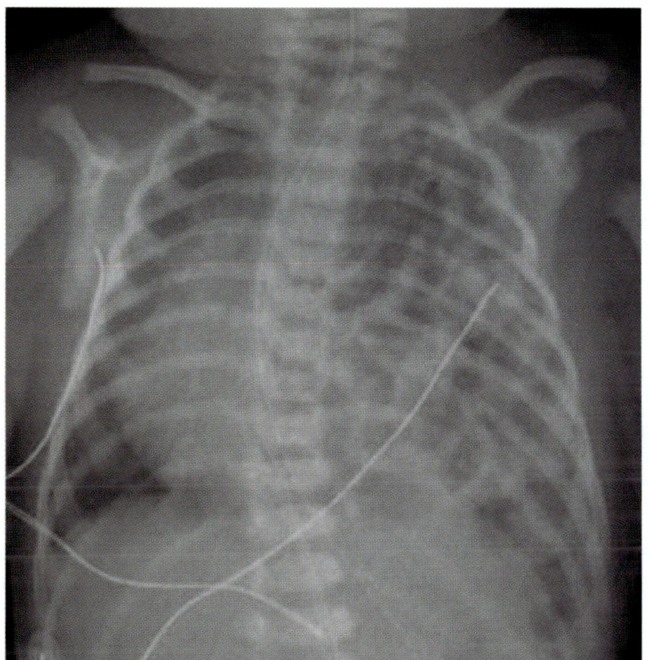

Figure 83.18 A 1-day-old male with a frontal chest radiograph demonstrating a left congenital diaphragmatic Bochdalek hernia containing multiple gas-filled bowel loops that fill almost the entire left hemithorax. There is associated mediastinal shift to the right.

Morgagni hernias refer to anterior diaphragmatic hernias occurring through a retrosternal diaphragmatic defect [12]. The majority of these occur on the right side (Fig. 83.19). They are associated with other congenital anomalies, such as congenital heart disease, intestinal malrotation, and Down syndrome.

Eventration

This refers to a focal or diffuse thinning of the diaphragm, most often occurring on the right, with resultant elevation of the affected portion (Fig. 83.20) [12]. This may be congenital (due to failed muscularization of the diaphragm) or develop later in life due to paralysis. While this is often asymptomatic, the diffuse form can cause respiratory insufficiency and require surgical plication.

Intrathoracic Neoplasms and Masses

There are numerous neoplasms and masses that occur in the thorax, which are discussed in detail in their respective chapters of the Respiratory System section. This chapter will therefore focus on intrathoracic neoplasms and masses that are more commonly seen in the pediatric population.

Mediastinal Masses

Normal Thymus

The thymus is a normal cause of superior mediastinal widening in the pediatric population and should not be confused as pathology (Fig. 83.21) [10,13]. It is particularly prominent in those under the age of five and can have a triangular shape, particularly on the right, giving rise to the "sail sign." The thymus gradually involutes over time, but processes such as stress and steroid administration may also cause involution. Thymic rebound hyperplasia after a period of stress can further be a source of confusion and make differentiation of physiologic thymic tissue from pathologic tissue difficult. In such cases, ultrasound or cross-sectional imaging, such as MRI, can be helpful by demonstrating the homogeneous appearance of physiologic tissue.

Germ Cell Tumor

These are anterior mediastinal masses arising from primitive germ cell rests [10,13]. The majority of the germ cell tumors in children are mature teratomas (Fig. 83.22). Immature, malignant teratomas also occur in the pediatric population at a lower frequency and are suggested by their invasive features. Both mature and immature teratomas classically demonstrate fat, fluid, and calcifications on imaging. However, some mature teratomas do not demonstrate fat or calcium, so the lack of these findings does not exclude a teratoma. Though older children tend to be asymptomatic, younger infants with mediastinal germ cell tumors may present with symptoms related to airway compression.

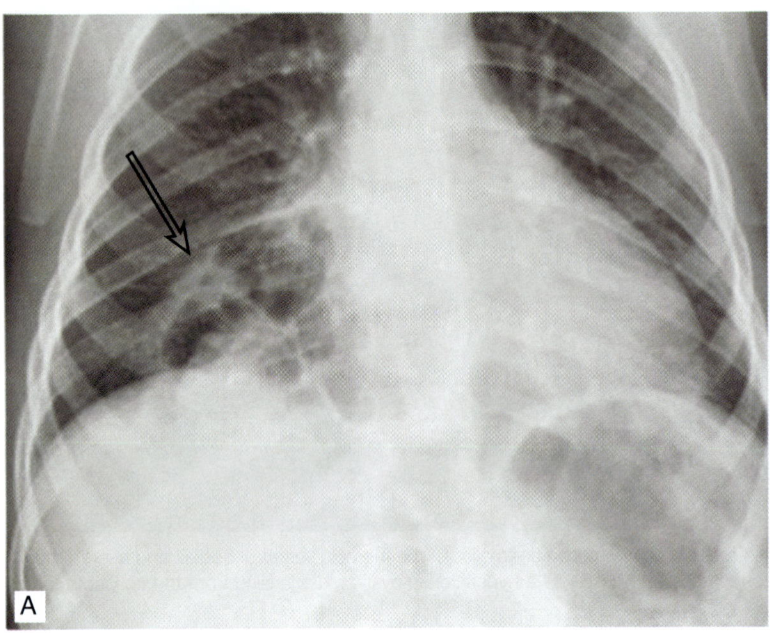

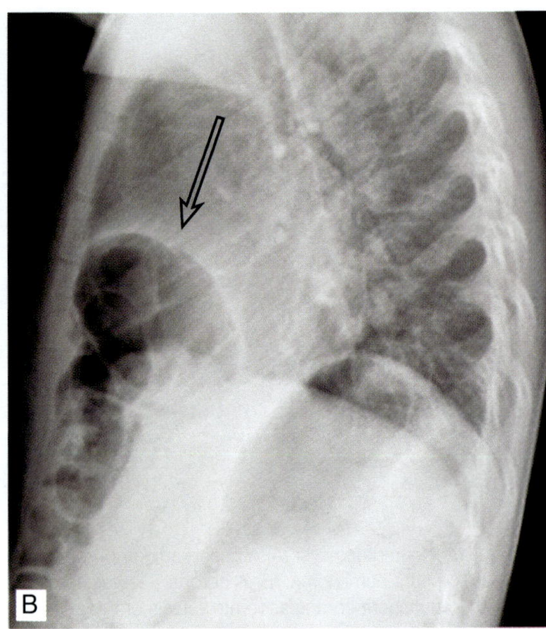

Figure 83.19 A 2-year-old male with a right anterior diaphragmatic Morgagni hernia containing colon (*black block arrow*), as shown on these frontal (A) and lateral (B) chest radiographs.

Lymphoma

Lymphoma is the most common abnormal anterior mediastinal mass in children [10,13]. The lymphomas that typically occur in the pediatric mediastinum are Hodgkin lymphoma and the lymphoblastic type of non-Hodgkin lymphoma (Fig. 83.23). On imaging, they may present as discrete lymphadenopathy or nodal conglomerates in the anterior mediastinum and/or hila. They are classically noncalcified, unless there is a history of prior treatment. Larger lymphomatous masses may demonstrate heterogeneous enhancement due to underlying necrosis. When sufficiently large, lymphoma can also displace and compress the adjacent airways and vessels. These features can help differentiate lymphoma from a prominent thymus.

Neurogenic Tumor

Neurogenic tumors, including neuroblastomas, ganglioneuroblastomas, ganglioneuromas, and peripheral nerve sheath tumors, make up the majority of posterior mediastinal masses in children [10,13]. Neuroblastomas are the most malignant of these tumors and can occur anywhere along the sympathetic chain. Approximately 20% of neuroblastomas occur in the mediastinum [13].

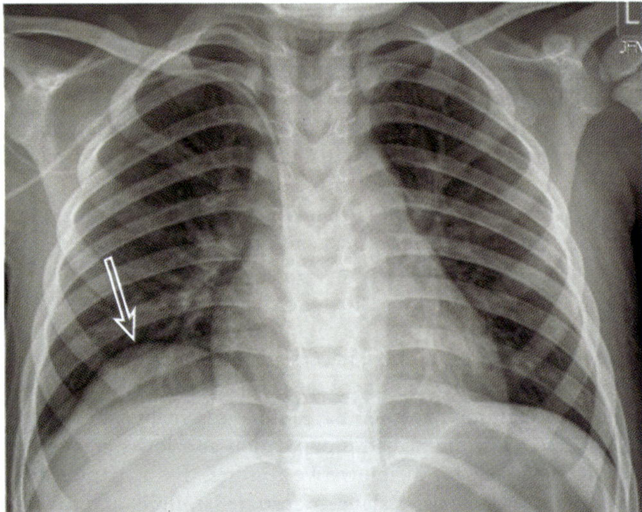

Figure 83.20 A 4-year-old male with abnormal smooth elevation of a portion of the right hemidiaphragm on this frontal chest radiograph, consistent with eventration of the right hemidiaphragm (*white block arrow*).

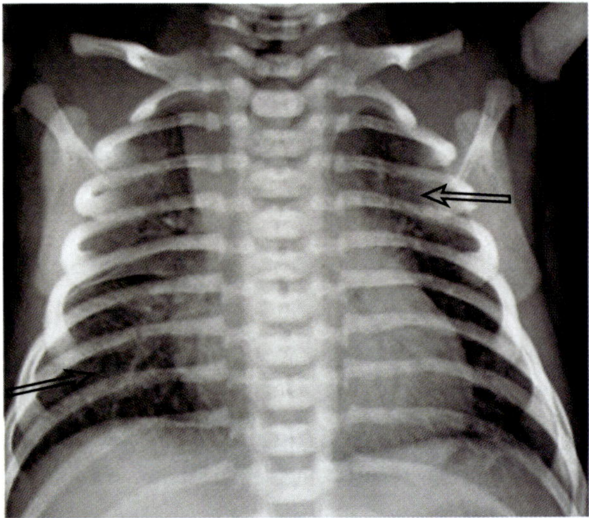

Figure 83.21 A 0-day-old with a frontal chest radiograph demonstrating apparent superior mediastinal widening, which represents the normal thymus in a patient of this age. There is also indistinctness of the pulmonary vasculature and diffuse bilateral hazy opacities (*black block arrows*), consistent with transient tachypnea of the newborn.

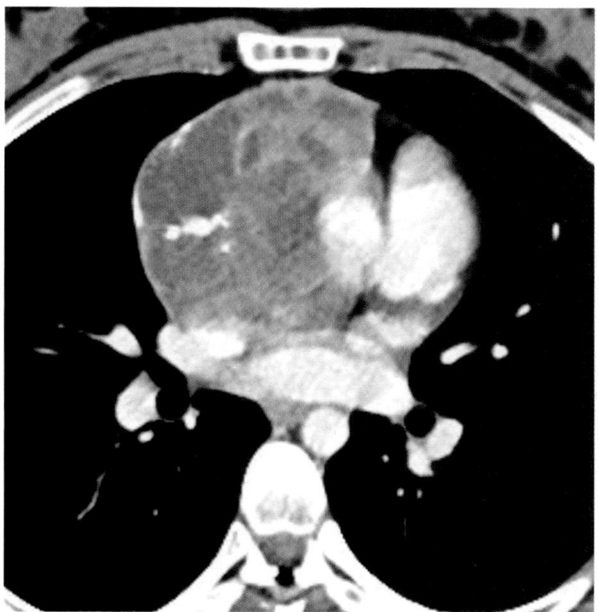

Figure 83.22 A 22-year-old female with a pathology proven mature teratoma. Axial CECT demonstrates a mediastinal complex cystic lesion with multiple septations and calcifications. This mass did not demonstrate fat, which emphasizes the important learning point that the absence of fat does not exclude a mature teratoma.

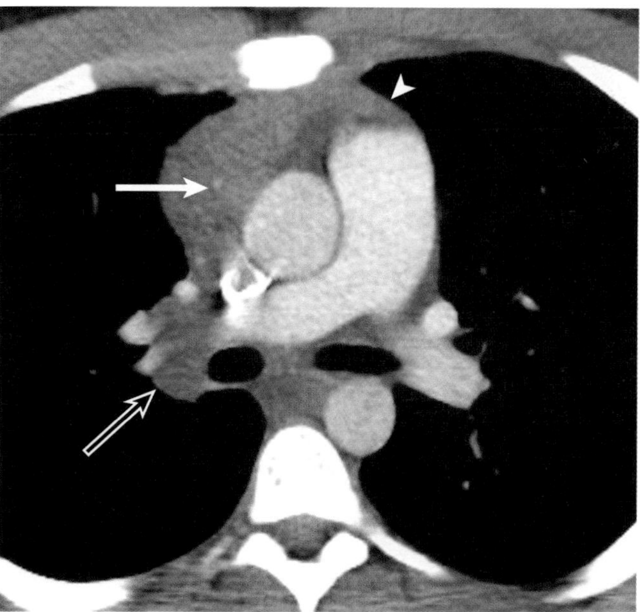

Figure 83.23 A 17-year-old male with Hodgkin lymphoma. Axial CECT demonstrated a homogeneous nodal conglomerate manifesting as an anterior mediastinal mass (*white arrowhead*). Mediastinal blood vessels were seen traversing through this mass (*white solid arrow*). Conglomerate right hilar lymphadenopathy (*white block arrow*) and multistation mediastinal lymphadenopathy (not shown) were also seen.

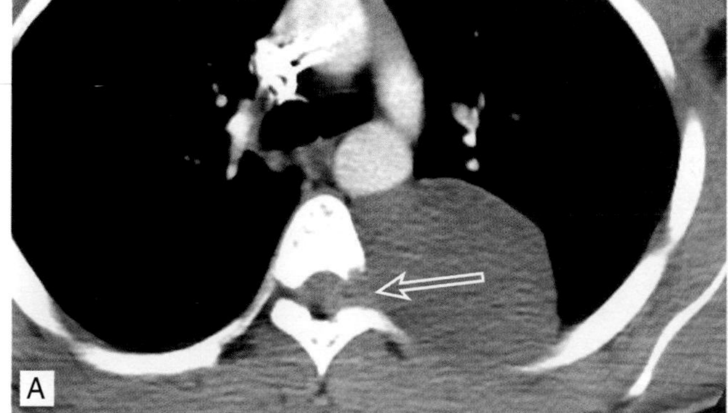

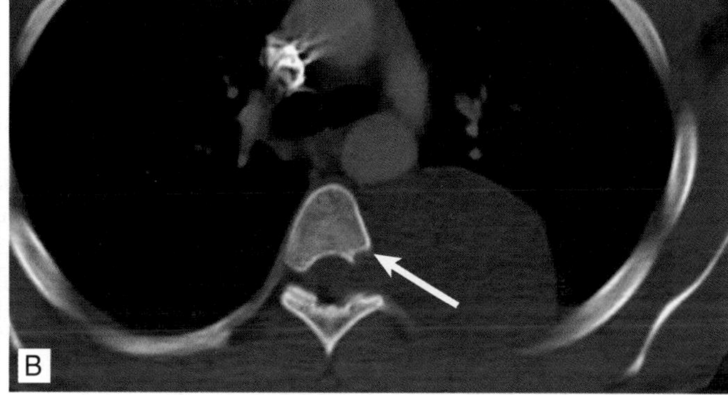

Figure 83.24 A 19-year-old male with neuroblastoma. (A) Axial CECT demonstrates a well-defined paravertebral soft tissue mass that extends into and widens the left T5-T6 neuroforamen (*white block arrow*). (B) This mass also erodes the adjacent vertebral body (*white solid arrow*).

These neurogenic tumors appear as solid masses with variable enhancement that may cause adjacent osseous destruction or scalloping (Fig. 83.24) [10,13]. The presence of calcification favors a sympathetic chain tumor, such as a neuroblastoma, over a peripheral nerve sheath tumor. On MRI, sympathetic chain tumors appear as paraspinal, heterogeneously enhancing sausage-shaped structures that are hyperintense on T2-weighted images. They may also demonstrate intraspinal extension with associated widening of the neuroforamina (Fig. 83.24). On the other hand, peripheral nerve sheath tumors classically demonstrate the "target" sign, characterized by a high peripheral signal intensity and intermediate central signal intensity on T2-weighted images.

Lung Neoplasms

Pleuropulmonary Blastoma

Pleuropulmonary blastoma (PPB) is a rare embryonal malignancy composed of primitive mesenchymal tissue that usually occurs before the age of 6 [14,15]. There is an association with other embryonal tumors, such as renal cystic nephroma. The three types of PPB are as follows:

- Type I: Multilocular cystic mass that is difficult to differentiate from type I CPAM by imaging
- Type II: Mixed cystic and solid mass
- Type III: Heterogeneously enhancing mass

These masses can cause contralateral mediastinal shift due to mass effect and respiratory distress. They are typically treated by surgical resection ± adjuvant chemoradiotherapy.

Recurrent Respiratory Papillomatosis

This is characterized by the growth of mucosal papillomas in the airways and is caused by human papilloma virus (HPV) types 6 and 11 acquired during vaginal birth [16]. Though the larynx is most commonly affected, this can spread to the lung parenchyma in a minority of cases and appears as multiple bilateral nodular and cavitary lesions (Fig. 83.25). Post-obstructive atelectasis and

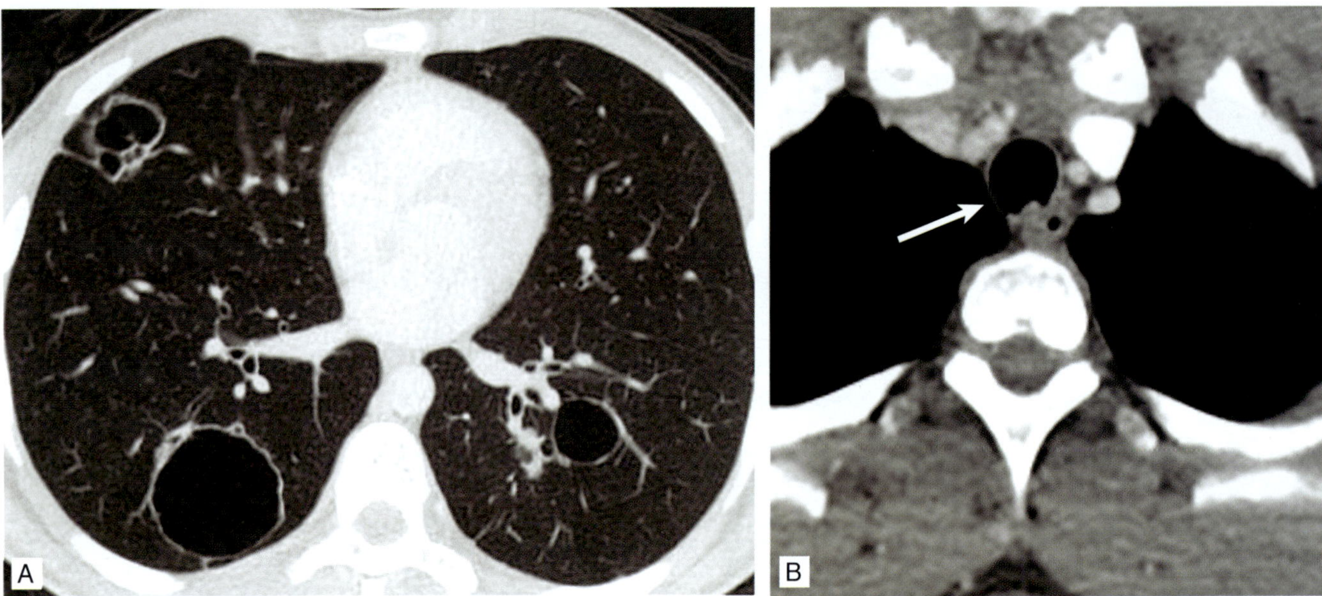

Figure 83.25 A 17-year-old male with respiratory papillomatosis. Axial CECT demonstrated (A) multiple bilateral cavitary nodules and (B) polypoid soft tissue lesions along the tracheal wall compatible with tracheal papillomas (*white arrow*).

bronchiectasis can also be seen. Complications include malignant transformation into squamous cell carcinoma (rare) and secondary infections.

Neonatal Chest

Meconium Aspiration Syndrome

Meconium aspiration syndrome (MAS) occurs due to aspiration of meconium-stained amniotic fluid before or during birth, typically in the setting of a stressor, such as hypoxia [17]. It more frequently affects term or postmature neonates and can be a significant cause of neonatal respiratory distress. The aspirated meconium causes small-airway obstruction and chemical pneumonitis, which on imaging manifests as segmental hyperinflation alternating with hazy or patchy areas of atelectasis, as well as coarse, asymmetric "rope-like" perihilar opacities (Fig. 83.26). Pleural effusions may also be seen. Pneumothorax is a relatively common complication (Fig. 83.26). Additional possible complications include pneumomediastinum, pulmonary interstitial emphysema (PIE), and persistent pulmonary hypertension.

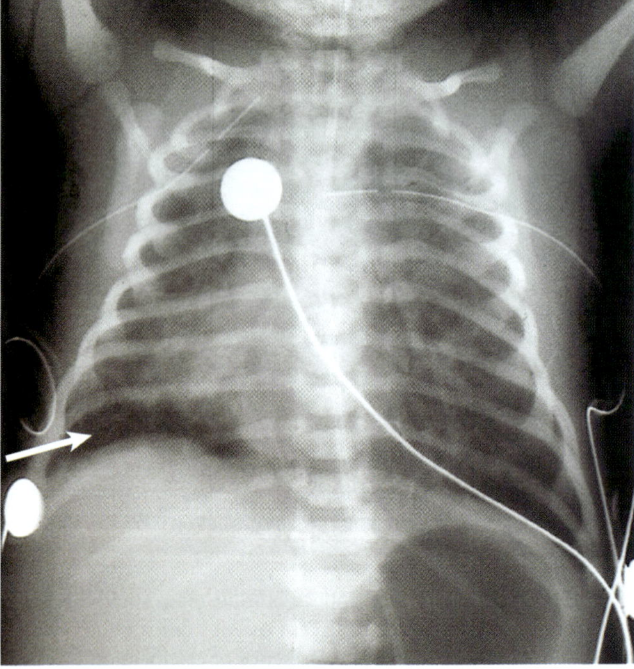

Figure 83.26 A chest radiograph demonstrates coarse, rope-like opacities throughout hyperinflated lungs compatible with meconium aspiration syndrome (MAS). Bilateral chest tubes were placed after the patient developed pneumothoraces, relatively common complications of MAS. A persistent right basilar pneumothorax remains (*white arrow*).

Transient Tachypnea of the Newborn

Also known as wet lung disease or transient respiratory distress, transient tachypnea of the newborn (TTN) occurs when there is delayed evacuation of fetal lung fluid [17]. This typically affects neonates born via caesarean section, during which they bypass the natural thoracic compression of vaginal delivery that would have otherwise facilitated fetal lung fluid clearance. Neonates born to diabetic mothers or those that required anesthesia are also more predisposed to developing this condition. Imaging findings in the first 6–24 h are similar to those found in pulmonary edema, including indistinctness of the pulmonary vasculature, airspace opacification, pleural effusions, and fissural thickening (Fig. 83.27). Lung volumes may be normal or increased. TTN usually takes a benign course that resolves by 2–3 days.

Surfactant Deficiency Disease

Surfactant deficiency disease (SDD) is also known as respiratory distress syndrome and sometimes inaccurately referred to as hyaline membrane disease [17]. This occurs due to surfactant deficiency, which consequently leads to alveolar collapse and decreased lung compliance. As immature type II pneumocytes cannot produce enough surfactant, this is primarily a disease of prematurity.

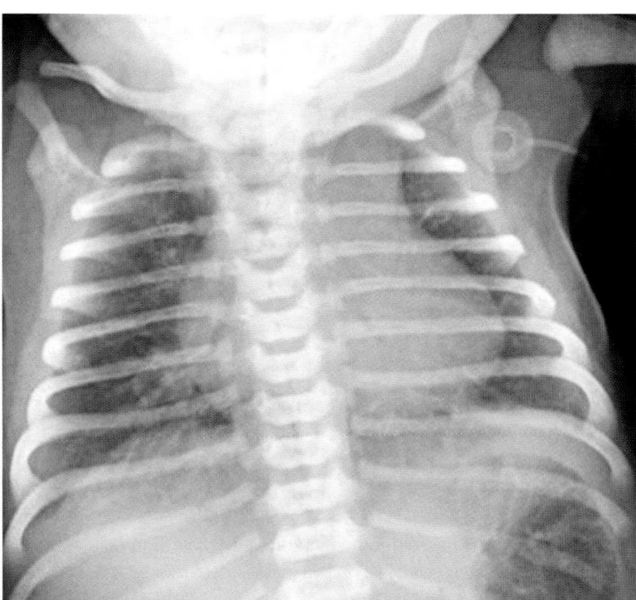

Figure 83.27 A 0-day-old female born via caesarean section presenting with respiratory distress. This frontal chest radiograph demonstrates low lung volumes and indistinctness of the pulmonary vasculature, compatible with transient tachypnea of the newborn.

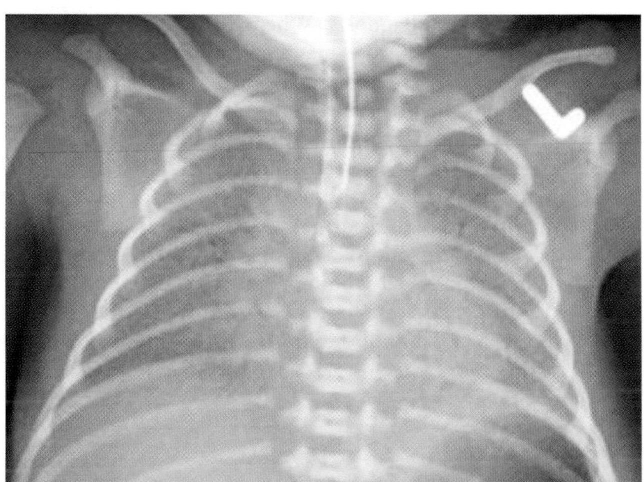

Figure 83.28 A 0-day-old premature male born at 26 weeks' gestation with surfactant deficiency disease. This frontal chest radiograph demonstrates low lung volumes and diffuse bilateral granular opacities, compatible with surfactant deficiency disease.

However, primary forms of SDD due to genetic mutations in surfactant and secondary forms of SDD (due to conditions such as MAS or infection that inactivate surfactant) may also occur. On imaging, low lung volumes are seen with bilateral granular opacities representative of the collapsed alveoli accompanied by air bronchograms representing the noncollapsed larger bronchi that are not dependent on surfactant for patency (Fig. 83.28). When severe, the granular opacities become more confluent and result in diffuse lung opacities.

Persistent Pulmonary Hypertension of the Newborn

Also known as persistent fetal circulation, this phenomenon occurs when there is persistent pulmonary hypertension and failure of the fetal shunts to close after birth [18]. Normally, there is high pulmonary vascular resistance in the fetal circulation causing the blood to bypass the lungs. With increased aeration of the lungs after birth, pulmonary vascular resistance normally decreases while systemic vascular resistance simultaneously increases. This leads to increased lung perfusion, as well as reversal of blood flow through fetal shunts (such as the ductus arteriosus) and their eventual closure. However, in conditions that cause hypoxia, such as MAS, SDD, or pulmonary hypoplasia, high pulmonary vascular resistance and pulmonary hypertension can persist. Chest radiographs are often reflective of the underlying etiology of the persistent pulmonary hypertension but can also be normal.

Neonatal Pneumonia

The majority of neonatal pneumonias are caused by bacteria and can have variable appearances that are difficult to distinguish from other neonatal conditions, such as MAS, TTN, and SDD [17,19]. Group B streptococcal (GBS) pneumonia is one of the most common neonatal pneumonias acquired during passage of a colonized vaginal canal, and it can have imaging findings similar to SDD. In GBS pneumonia, the lung volumes are also typically low, and bilateral diffuse granular opacities are seen. However, pleural effusions frequently accompany GBS infections but are uncommon in SDD.

Pulmonary Interstitial Emphysema

Pulmonary Interstitial Emphysema (PIE) is a part of the neonatal air leak syndrome, which includes multiple entities in which air collects in spaces outside the tracheobronchial tree (such as pneumomediastinum, pneumothorax, pneumopericardium, pneumoperitoneum, and PIE) [17]. In PIE, elevated alveolar pressures lead to alveolar perforation and leakage of air into the pulmonary interstitium. This typically occurs in premature or low birth weight patients with SDD and on ventilatory support. On chest radiographs, PIE will manifest as bubbly cystic or linear lucencies ranging from single lobar involvement to diffuse bilateral involvement (Fig. 83.29). In more advanced PIE, these cystic lucencies can develop into large cystic masses that can cause mediastinal shift. While PIE is usually asymptomatic, its early recognition can prompt switching from conventional positive pressure to high-frequency ventilation to avoid potential complications such as pneumothorax or pneumomediastinum.

Bronchopulmonary Dysplasia

Also known as chronic lung disease of prematurity, bronchopulmonary dysplasia (BPD) is currently defined as oxygen dependency for at least 28 days after birth in those born at less than 32 weeks of gestational age [20]. It is thought to be related to lung injury from long-term mechanical ventilation and oxygen toxicity. Abnormal chest radiograph findings are no longer part of the definition for BPD, and early chest radiographs may be normal. However, over time, diffuse hazy opacities will develop and eventually may progress into cystic changes, air trapping, and linear parenchymal bands (Fig. 83.30). These findings may improve with age and clinically have no significant long-term effects. However, some children may experience complications such as exercise intolerance or asthma. Wilson–Mikity syndrome is controversial but refers to the development of BPD despite no or minimal ventilatory support.

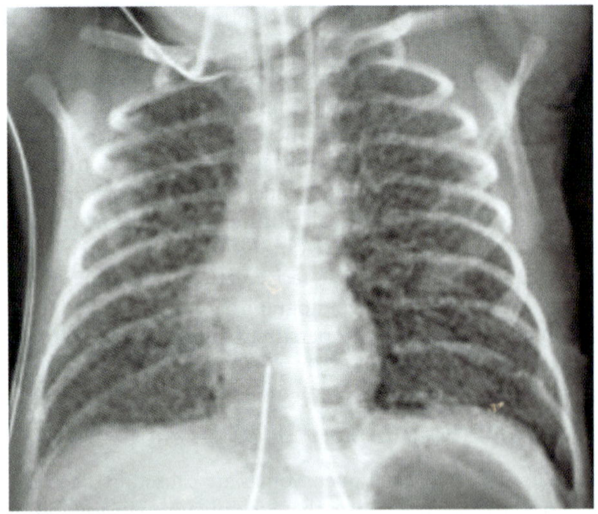

Figure 83.29 A 4-day-old intubated male with pulmonary interstitial emphysema. A frontal chest radiograph demonstrates diffuse tubular and linear lucencies throughout both lungs, in keeping with pulmonary interstitial emphysema. There is also a background of diffuse bilateral granular lung opacities consistent with underlying surfactant deficiency disease.

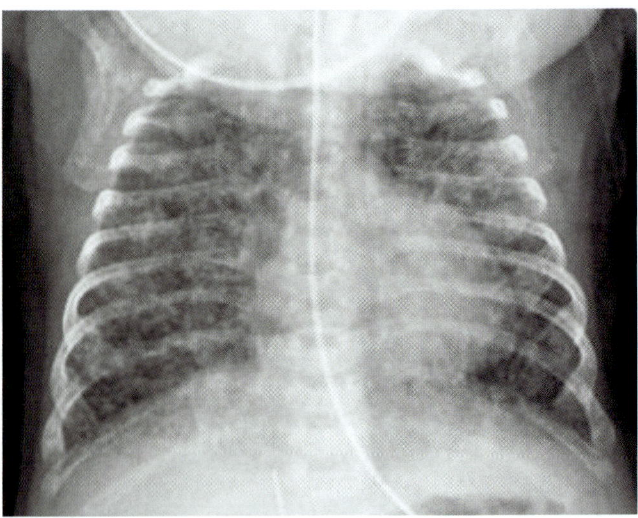

Figure 83.30 A 76-day-old formerly premature male with diffuse bilateral hazy and coarse lung opacities on this frontal chest radiograph, consistent with bronchopulmonary dysplasia.

Lung Pathologies in the Older Child

Foreign Body Aspiration

Foreign body aspiration is a common cause of acute respiratory distress in children, particularly in those younger than 3 years [21,22]. The aspirated foreign body can lodge in multiple locations along the airways, including the trachea. However, the bronchus is the most commonly affected site, with the right mainstem bronchus being favored due to its more vertical orientation.

Radiography can easily diagnose this entity when the foreign body is radiopaque [21,22]. However, not all foreign bodies are radiopaque, in which case ancillary findings may be used to suggest the diagnosis. When the foreign body causes complete obstruction, the imaging finding will be postobstructive atelectasis. However, if it causes incomplete obstruction, there may be hyperinflation and air trapping of the affected lung upon expiration (Fig. 83.31). On lateral decubitus radiographs with the affected side down, air trapping will cause the incompletely obstructed lung to appear more hyperlucent compared to the normally deflated adjacent nonobstructed lung. On inspiratory radiographs, the nonobstructed lung will have increased volume compared to the obstructed side, with associated mediastinal shift toward the affected side. However, it should be noted that in approximately

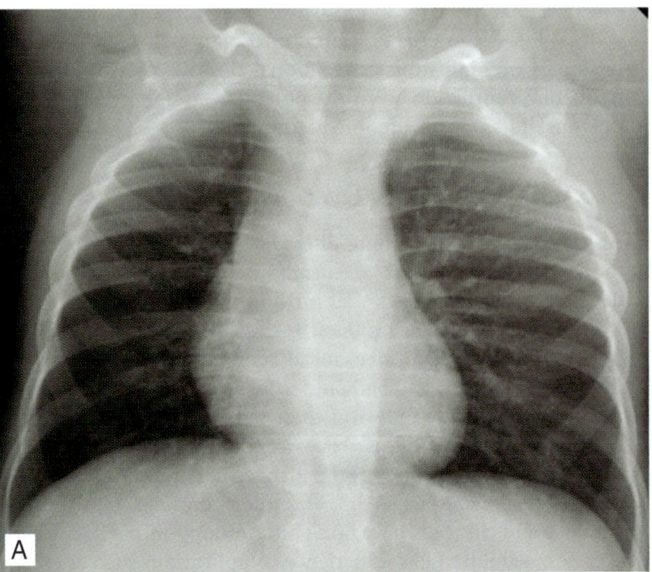

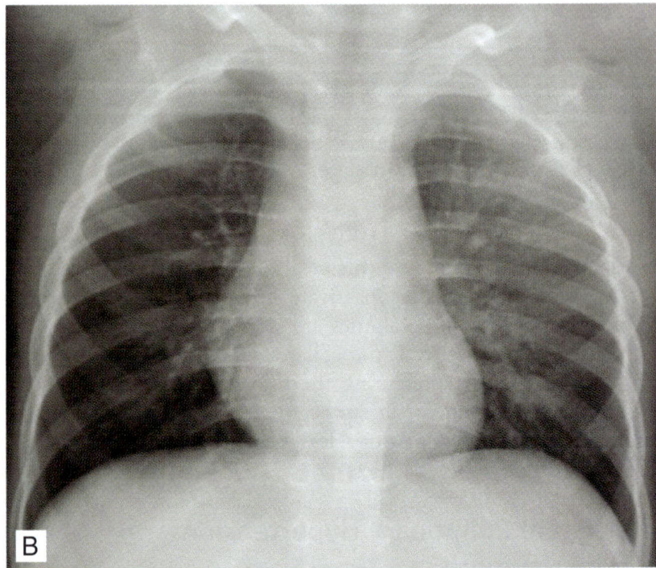

Figure 83.31 Foreign body in the right lung. Inspiratory (A) and expiratory (B) chest radiographs demonstrate appropriate loss of volume and increased density in the normal left lung upon expiration. However, the affected right lung remains hyperlucent and overinflated compared to the left upon expiration, compatible with air trapping secondary to a foreign body (not seen in the radiographs).

one-third of bronchial foreign body cases, the chest radiograph can be normal.

Bronchiolitis Obliterans

This results from bronchiolar inflammation that leads to fibrosis and subsequent stenosis or occlusion of the affected small airways [23,24]. A number of etiologies can serve as the inciting event, including but not limited to a respiratory viral infection, graft-versus-host-disease, and lung transplant allograft rejection. Chest radiograph may demonstrate a hyperlucent, underperfused lung that may have normal or decreased volumes. Expiratory air trapping and mosaic attenuation, hyperlucency, decreased pulmonary vasculature, bronchial wall thickening, and bronchiectasis may be seen on CT. Swyer–James–Macleod syndrome refers to a form of postinfectious bronchiolitis obliterans (typically a viral respiratory infection) affecting central larger bronchi. It most often manifests as unilateral involvement on chest radiographs. However, bilateral involvement can also occur.

Viral Pneumonia

Viruses cause more cases of lower respiratory tract infections than bacteria in the pediatric population, so it is important to be familiar with their appearance on imaging [19]. These infections typically affect the small airways and cause peribronchial edema, which often manifest as symmetric peribronchiolar coarse opacities radiating from the hila. Children have smaller airway diameters and incompletely formed collateral ventilation pathways compared to adults. The increased mucus production and reactive peribronchial edema may therefore lead to small airway occlusion, air trapping, and areas of subsegmental atelectasis. This accounts for the hyperlucent and hyperinflated lungs characteristic of viral pneumonias in pediatric patients.

Round Pneumonia

Younger children have inadequately formed collateral ventilation pathways, and therefore pneumonias may appear more "round" in younger children (particularly those caused by *Streptococcus pneumoniae*) (Fig. 83.32) [19]. This should not be confused with a mass, particularly in a child younger than 8 years of age. In the setting of infectious symptoms, a repeat chest radiograph to ensure clearance is the follow-up imaging of choice. A follow-up CT exposes the patient to unnecessary radiation and should be avoided, unless the round opacity is seen in an older child or a child without infectious symptoms.

Cystic Fibrosis

Cystic fibrosis is a multisystemic autosomal recessive genetic disease caused by mutations in the cystic fibrosis transmembrane conductance regulator (CFTR) protein [25]. In the respiratory system, this mutation causes increased viscosity of the mucus secretions resulting in airway obstruction and recurrent infections. Chest imaging demonstrates evidence of air trapping, and in advanced disease, there may be upper lobe predominant bronchiectasis, bronchial wall thickening, and parenchymal architectural distortion (Fig. 83.33). Mucous plugging can be seen, sometimes giving rise to the finger-in-glove appearance that can also be seen in allergic bronchopulmonary aspergillosis. Chronic inflammation can result in mediastinal/hilar lymphadenopathy and pulmonary hypertension manifesting as pulmonary artery enlargement.

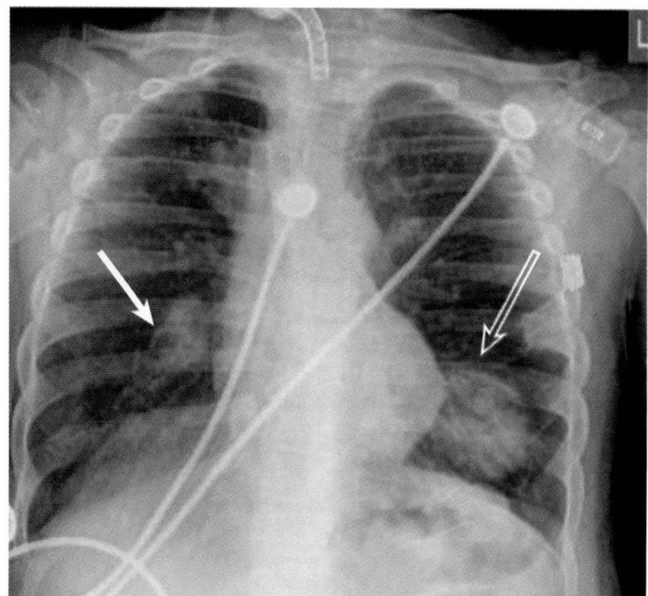

Figure 83.32 A 5-year-old male with multifocal round pneumonia. Front chest radiograph demonstrates a 4 cm rounded opacity in the left lower lung zone (*white block arrow*) and an additional smaller 2.7 cm rounded opacity in the right perihilar region (*white solid arrow*). Subsequent chest radiographs demonstrated resolution of these opacities, most consistent with multifocal round pneumonia.

Primary Ciliary Dyskinesia

This refers to a genetic disorder causing ciliary dysfunction with multisystemic consequences [26]. In the respiratory system, there is impaired clearance of mucous secretions. Imaging findings therefore include middle and lower lung zone predominant bronchiectasis, bronchial wall thickening, mucus plugging, centrilobular nodules, mosaic attenuation, and expiratory air trapping. Approximately half of the patients with primary ciliary dyskinesia also have Kartagener syndrome, which is characterized by a combination of bronchiectasis, sinusitis and/or polyposis, and situs inversus (Fig. 83.34).

Idiopathic Pulmonary Hemosiderosis

This is caused by recurrent alveolar capillary hemorrhage and most commonly occurs in children, although cases in adults can also occur [27]. While the pathogenesis is unclear, some have theorized that this may have an autoimmune or allergic etiology given associations with autoimmune disorders (such as celiac disease) and allergies to cow's milk, respectively. An association with black mold has also been demonstrated. Imaging findings in the acute phase are representative of pulmonary hemorrhage giving rise to perihilar ground glass opacities and/or consolidations (Fig. 83.35). A crazy-paving pattern with interlobular septal thickening may also represent. In the chronic phase, this progresses to lower lobe predominant fibrosis with reticular opacities, traction bronchiectasis and bronchiolectasis, and architectural distortion. In rare cases, this may be complicated by progressive massive fibrosis or hemothorax.

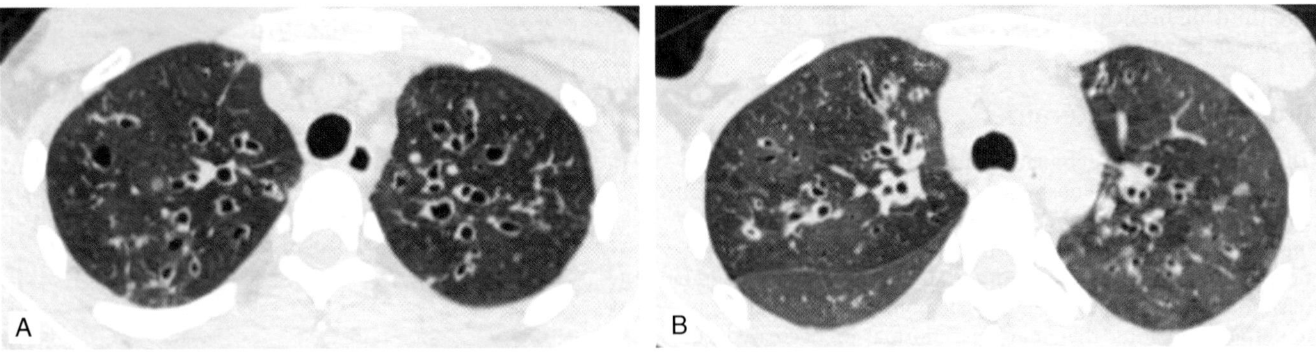

Figure 83.33 A 23-year-old male with history of cystic fibrosis. Axial chest CT images (A and B) demonstrate extensive, bilateral upper lobe predominant cylindrical bronchiectasis, bronchial wall thickening, and scattered foci of airway mucous plugging, in keeping with cystic fibrosis. There is diffuse mosaic attenuation in keeping with air-trapping, confirmed with expiratory phase images (B).

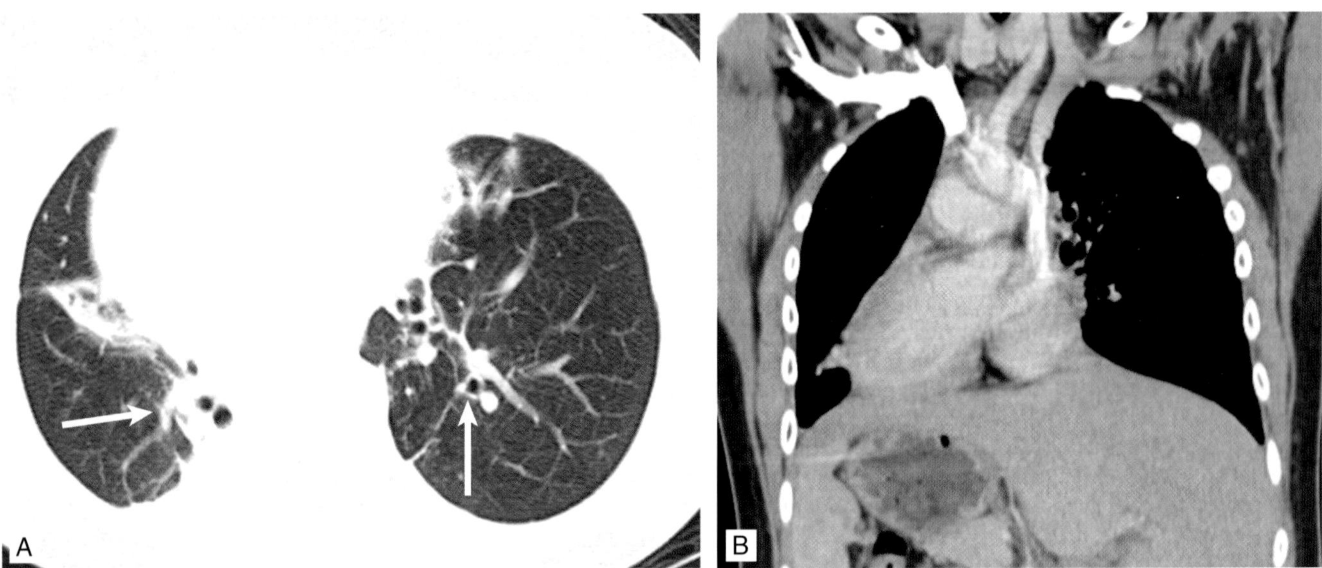

Figure 83.34 A 14-year-old female with history of primary ciliary dyskinesia (PCD). (A) Axial CECT images demonstrated middle and lower lung zone predominant bronchial wall thickening and bronchiectasis (*white arrows*) compatible with PCD. (B) Coronal CECT demonstrates dextrocardia and abdominal situs inversus, which are associated with PCD.

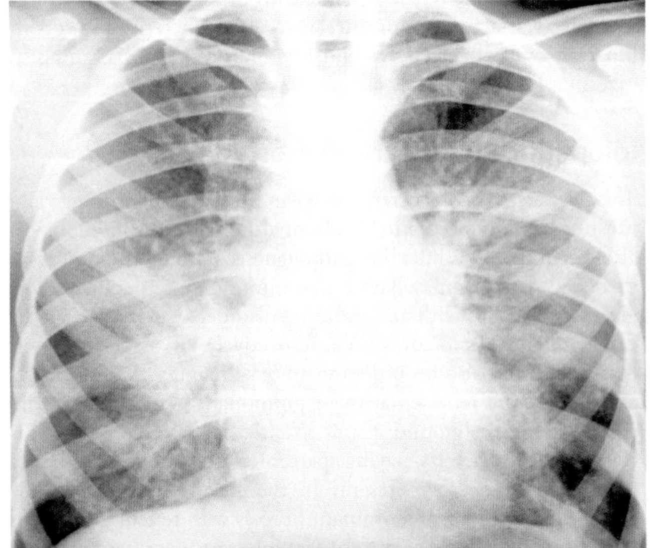

Figure 83.35 Idiopathic pulmonary hemosiderosis. A chest radiograph demonstrates patchy and reticulonodular perihilar opacities.

Pulmonary Alveolar Proteinosis

This results from accumulation of surfactant and lipoproteinaceous material in the alveoli and terminal bronchioles, which gives rise to the classic crazy-paving pattern of ground-glass opacities combined with interlobular/intralobular septal thickening on chest CT [28]. The typical appearance on chest radiographs includes predominantly symmetric and central opacities, with sparing of the apices and costophrenic angles (Fig. 83.36). The appearance can mimic pulmonary edema, though other features often associated with pulmonary edema (such as cardiomegaly or pleural effusions) can be absent. Less frequently, pulmonary alveolar proteinosis (PAP) can also manifest as extensive consolidations or as multifocal, asymmetric lung opacities.

Most cases of PAP occur in older children or adults and are autoimmune processes in which autoantibodies to granulocyte macrophage colony-stimulating factor (GM-CSF) are produced. GM-CSF is involved in alveolar macrophage signaling, and when this is disrupted, clearance of intraalveolar lipoproteinaceous material is disrupted. Congenital forms of PAP may also arise, although less frequently, due to surfactant deficiency. There are also multiple secondary causes of PAP, including hematologic

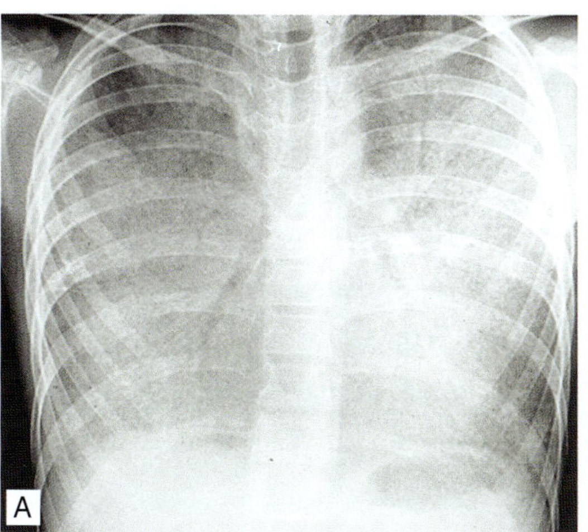

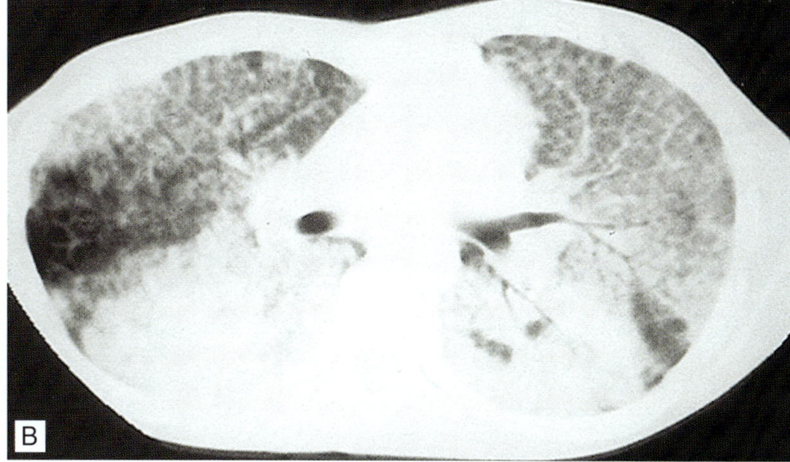

Figure 83.36 Pulmonary alveolar proteinosis. A chest radiograph (A) demonstrates extensive perihilar opacities. A correlative axial chest CT image (B) shows areas of interlobular septal thickening and ground glass opacities in a crazy paving pattern throughout the nondependent lungs and dense consolidations in the dependent lungs.

disorders, toxic inhalation exposure, autoimmune disorders, and other disease processes that interfere with alveolar macrophage function. Treatment is with bronchoalveolar lavage.

Sickle Cell Disease

Sickle cell disease is a multisystemic, autosomal recessive hereditary disease that causes abnormal hemoglobin formation [29]. Acute chest syndrome (ACS) is an important pulmonary manifestation of this disease in children and is the leading cause of death in these patients. ACS is characterized by chest pain, elevated white blood cell count, fever, and new (nonspecific) pulmonary opacities (Fig. 83.37). Whether the etiology of ACS is due to infection or infarction is up to debate, but one of the hypotheses holds that bone infarctions lead to splinting and subsequent atelectasis. Pneumonia is another pulmonary process that occurs more frequently in sickle cell disease, thought to be related to functional asplenia.

Figure 83.37 A 12-year-old male with history of sickle cell disease. Frontal chest radiograph demonstrated new scattered patchy and linear opacities in the lungs bilaterally, consistent with acute chest syndrome.

Langerhans Cell Histiocytosis

Langerhans cell histiocytosis (LCH) is characterized by proliferation of histiocytes and can involve one site or multiple sites [30]. The most common presentation is osseous lesions, but other organs including the lung, liver, and spleen can also be involved. While pulmonary LCH can be seen as a single organ disease in adult smokers, this is rare in children. Lung involvement in the pediatric population typically occurs in the setting of multisite disease. Chest imaging findings in LCH vary from normal chest radiographs to extensive cystic disease. The characteristic small nodules and irregular cysts typically have an upper lobe predominance. Spontaneous pneumothorax is a well-known potential complication of this disease.

Suggested Readings

- T Berrocal, C Madrid, S Novo, J Gutiérrez, A Arjonilla, N Gómez-León, Congenital anomalies of the tracheobronchial tree, lung, and mediastinum: embryology, radiology, and pathology, Radiographics 24 (1) (2004) e17.
- DR Biyyam, T Chapman, MR Ferguson, G Deutsch, MK Dighe, Congenital lung abnormalities: embryologic features, prenatal diagnosis, and postnatal radiologic-pathologic correlation, Radiographics 30 (6) (2010) 1721–1738.
- SH Ranganath, EY Lee, R Restrepo, RL Eisenberg, Mediastinal masses in children, Am J Roentgenol 198 (3) (2012) W197–216.
- JP Lichtenberger, DM Biko, BW Carter, MA Pavio, AR Huppmann, EM Chung, Primary lung tumors in children: radiologic-pathologic correlation from the radiologic pathology archives, Radiographics 38 (7) (2018) 2151–2172.
- MC Liszewski, EY Lee, Neonatal lung disorders: pattern recognition approach to diagnosis, Am J Roentgenol 210 (5) (2018) 964–975.

84

Pediatric Gastrointestinal Tract and Hepatobiliary System

PRIYA PATHAK, HASSAN ABOUGHALIA, GARVIT KHATRI, PUNEET BHARGAVA

Normal Embryology

The primitive gut is derived from the yolk sac initially as a cylinder of endodermal cells surrounded by mesoderm around the third intrauterine week. It subsequently differentiates into the foregut, midgut, and hindgut. This is followed by series of complex duodenal and colonic rotations, herniation of midgut into the umbilical cord, 270-degree rotation, eventual return to the peritoneal cavity, and fixation by the 12th week, such that *the duodenojejunal junction (DJJ) is positioned to the left of the superior mesenteric artery (SMA) and cecum in the right lower quadrant* (Fig. 84.1) [1]; this is further discussed in the malrotation section. Complete fixation also leads to the formation of a broad-based mesentery from the DJJ to the cecum. The terminal part of the hindgut, known as the primitive cloaca, is divided into ventral (urogenital sinus) and dorsal parts (rectum and proximal anal canal] by the urorectal septum formed around the seventh week. The cloaca is separated from the amniotic cavity by the cloacal membrane, which ruptures to form the urogenital and anal orifices in perineum at the end of seventh week [2].

The liver and pancreas form within the mesentery surrounding the primitive gut, the liver within the ventral mesogastrium or the ventral part of mesentery suspending the stomach, and the pancreas within the dorsal mesogastrium [3]. Hepatic diverticulum is derived from the ventral foregut, forming the liver and intrahepatic ducts from the anterior portion and the gallbladder and extrahepatic ducts from the posterior portion [4]. The pancreas is derived from two foregut endodermal buds. Ventral bud forms the head and uncinate process, and the dorsal bud forms the neck, body, and tail. The ventral bud rotates and unites with dorsal bud with integration of dorsal duct (also known as accessory duct of Santorini) and ventral duct (also known as main duct of Wirsung) around the seventh intrauterine week (Fig. 84.2) [5].

Imaging Techniques

- Radiographs, esophagography, upper gastrointestinal (GI) series, small bowel follow-through, contrast enema, and ultrasonography (USG) are the available modalities for the evaluation of congenital anomalies of the proximal and distal GI tract. Multidetector computed tomography (CT) has a specific role in the evaluation of complicated appendicitis, mesenteric abnormalities, liver neoplasms, and pancreatic disorders. Magnetic resonance imaging (MRI) is predominately indicated for assessment of anorectal malformations and biliary and pancreatic duct anomalies and for characterization of hepatic neoplasms
- *Supine abdominal radiography is the initial examination for evaluation of most patients with bowel disorders, with addition of left lateral decubitus and cross-table views to detect ectopic air in suspected cases.* Rectal air is best detected in prone views. Chest radiographs are indicated in cases with suspected esophageal anomalies
- A fluoroscopic upper GI examination delineates the anatomy of the esophagus, stomach, duodenum, and duodenojejunal junction. It involves monitoring of oral contrast bolus with image acquisition in various sequential, well-centered projections. The overall technique is essentially tailored to the individual patient, clinical manifestations, and preliminary findings. For example, in a patient with malrotation, steps such as imaging the first bolus through the duodenum and DJJ(because the latter gets obscured subsequently by opacification of jejunum), documentation of the DJJ in both frontal and lateral

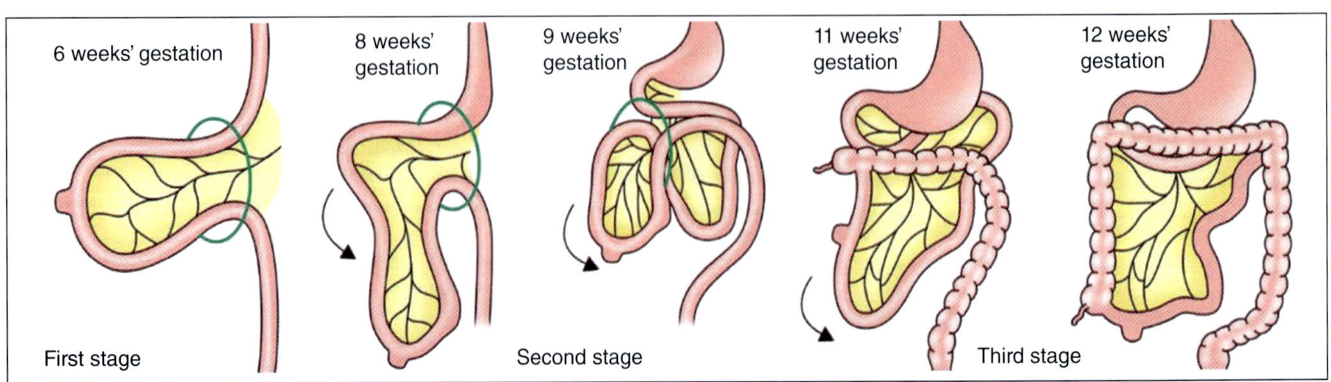

Figure 84.1 The sequence of normal intestinal rotation.

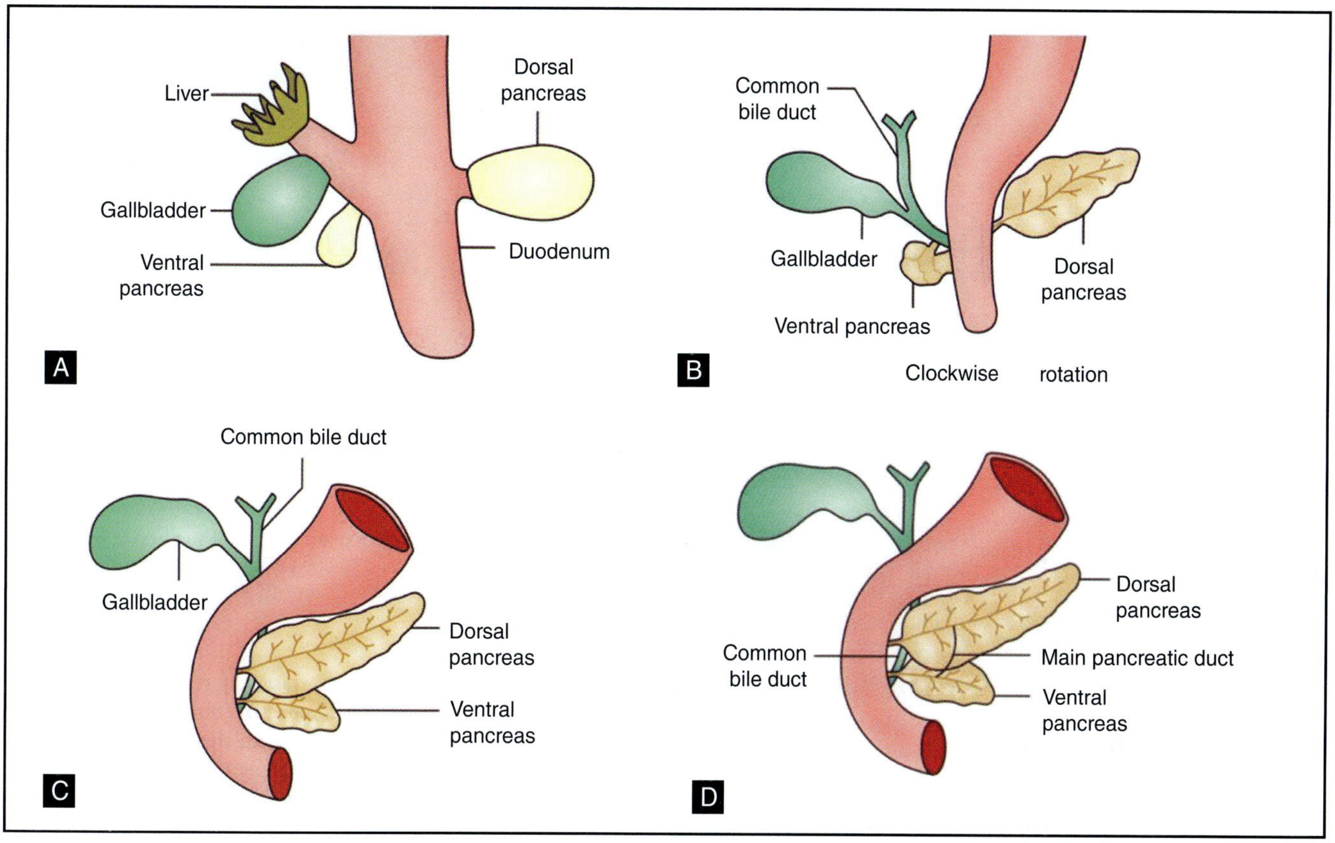

Figure 84.2 (A) Formation of the ventral and dorsal pancreatic bud. (B and C) showing development of the bud followed by 180 degree clockwise rotation of the ventral pancreatic duct. (D) The ventral duct unites with the hepatic duct to form the common bide duct and with the dorsal duct to form the main pancreatic duct.

projections, and combining a small bowel follow-through to assess cecal position increase the diagnostic accuracy [1]

- Contrast can be administered via a bottle, cups, syringes, orogastric, and nasogastric tubes depending on the patient's age and comfort. Neonates are imaged in a lying-down position. Contrast enema elucidates the anatomy of rectum, colon, and terminal ileum. It involves instillation of contrast into the rectum via a catheter and image acquisition in the frontal and lateral projections

In all cases, principles of *ALARA (as low as reasonably achievable)* should be followed to minimize radiation exposure by adhering to techniques such as intermittent fluoroscopy, last image capture, minimizing patient-image intensifier distance, magnification, and appropriate collimation [6].

Upper Gastrointestinal Tract Anomalies

Esophageal Atresia and Tracheoesophageal Fistula

A spectrum of congenital anomalies is characterized by malformations of the esophagus and tracheoesophageal separation caused by aberrant folding and separation of the primitive foregut. Approximately *15% to 30% of cases occur as a part of VACTERL syndrome* (vertebral anomaly, anorectal malformation, cardiac anomalies, tracheoesophageal fistula, renal anomalies, and limb deformities) [7–9]. Clinical presentations are cyanosis in early neonatal period, apnea, drooling, and respiratory difficulties [9]. The H type may present in young adults with recurrent lung infections [10]. It is classified into the following types [6,8] (Fig. 84.3):

- Type A: isolated esophageal atresia

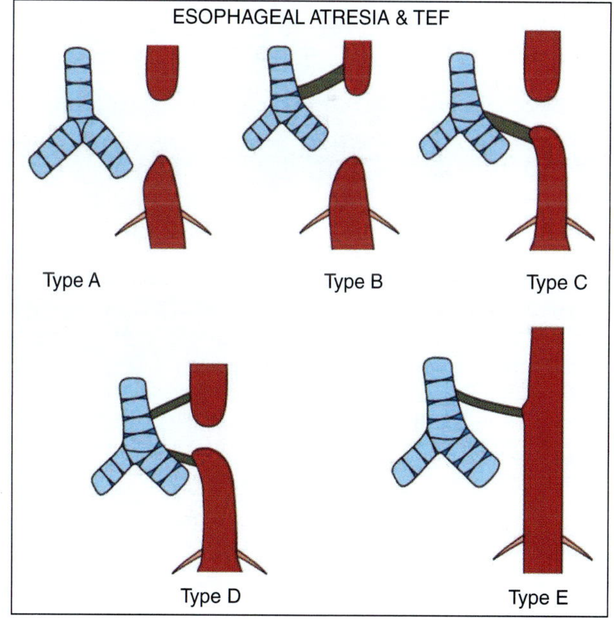

Figure 84.3 The types of tracheoesophageal anomalies.

- Type B: esophageal atresia with proximal tracheoesophageal fistula
- Type C: esophageal atresia with distal tracheoesophageal fistula
- Type D: esophageal atresia with both proximal and distal tracheoesophageal fistulas
- Type E: tracheoesophageal fistula without esophageal atresia

The diagnosis is usually indicated on antenatal USG by the absence of a gastric bubble and polyhydramnios. Postnatally, *it*

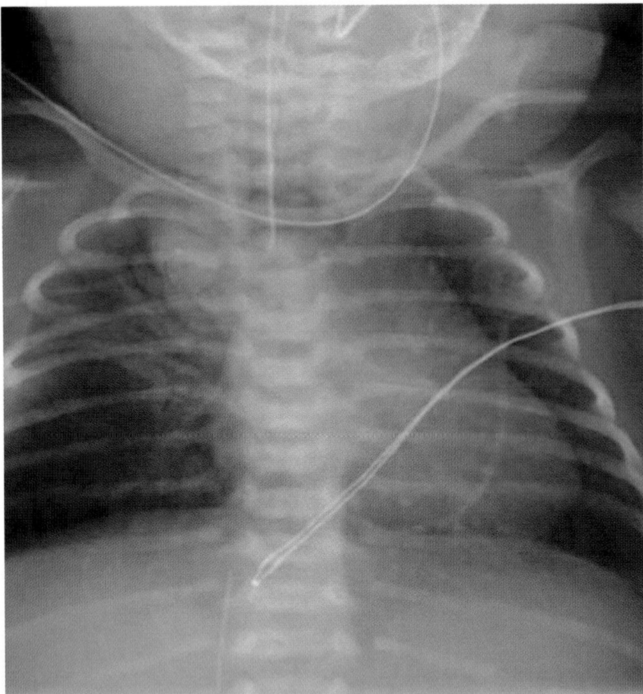

Figure 84.4 Chest radiograph from a 2-day-old boy with esophageal atresia shows a Replogle tube in the proximal esophageal pouch.

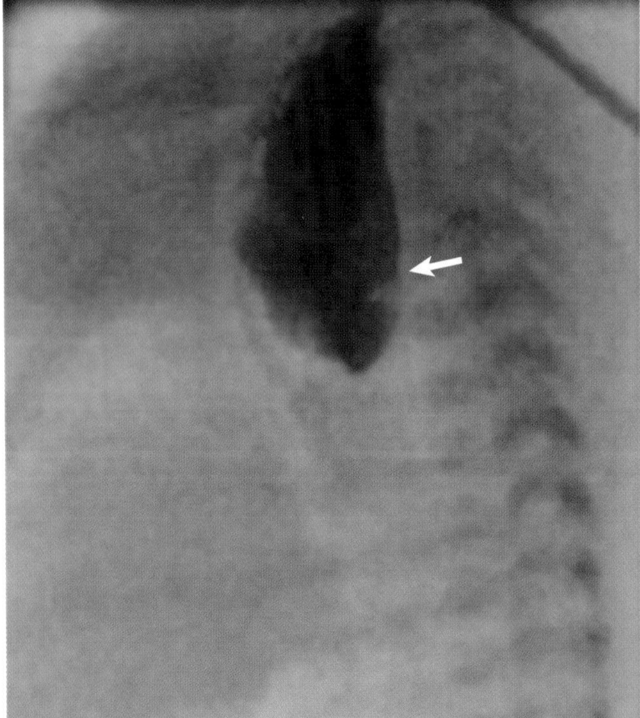

Figure 84.5 Esophagram from a 1-month-old boy with esophageal atresia (type A) demonstrates a contrast-filled dilated proximal esophageal pouch (*white arrow*).

presents with an air-filled and distended esophageal pouch on chest radiography (Figs. 84.4 and 84.5). Attempts to pass a nasoenteric tube leads to curling within the esophageal pouch. The abdomen is gasless in cases without tracheoesophageal fistula and demonstrates bowel gas with tracheoesophageal fistula [8,9].

H-type fistula is evaluated with an esophagogram as a part of presurgical planning [9]. Nonionic low-osmolality contrast media

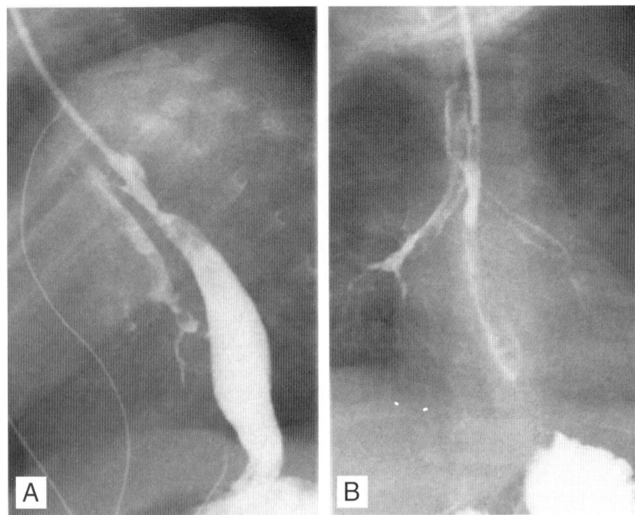

Figure 84.6 Contrast esophagogram (A) Lateral showing contrast opacification of the esophagus and trachea with delineation of the H shaped tracheo-esoheageal fistula (Type E), and (B) antero-posterior view showing the same findings.

is used because high-osmolar contrast may reach the lungs via the fistula and lead to pulmonary edema. The oblique fistulous tract is delineated in a prone position and with the pull-back technique, which involves placement of nasogastric tube in the stomach followed by stepwise contrast injection as the tube is withdrawn along the esophagus (Fig. 84.6). Postrepair complications are anastomotic leak and strictures, recurrent fistula, tracheomalacia, esophageal dysmotility, and gastroesophageal reflux [9].

Hypertrophic Pyloric Stenosis

Hypertrophic pyloric stenosis refers to thickening and elongation of the pyloric canal caused by abnormal hypertrophy of the pyloric musculature. Resultant failure of pyloric relaxation leads to gastric outlet obstruction. The disease commonly manifests between 2 weeks and 3 months of age with *characteristic higher incidence in first-born boys* [11]. Clinical presentations include projectile nonbilious vomiting, dehydration, and sometimes a palpable mass in the epigastrium. Implicated risk factors are male sex, prematurity, and postnatal erythromycin exposure, although the exact cause remains unclear [6].

Ultrasonography is the mainstay diagnostic examination. It involves assessment of

1. The pylorus with respect to overall appearance, thickness, and canal length, and
2. Real-time evaluation of gastric peristalsis and egress of contents through the pyloric canal

A high frequency probe is used with the patient placed in a supine position. Oblique positions displace gastric contents and may help in reduction of air artifacts. *The pyloric muscle is visualized as a hypoechoic layer present in between echogenic mucosa and serosa.* The hypertrophied pylorus resembles a cervix (*cervix sign*) (Fig. 84.7). The *antral nipple sign* refers to a nipplelike protrusion of echogenic pyloric mucosa into the gastric antrum (Fig. 84.8). *Upper limits of pylorus measurement can be remembered by "π"—3 mm for muscle thickness and 14 mm for canal length* [12,13]. These findings are accompanied by gastric hyperperistalsis and lack of egress of intraluminal contents through the pyloric canal. *Pylorospasm is the major differential consideration,* which can be excluded by a prolonged or repeat scan [6].

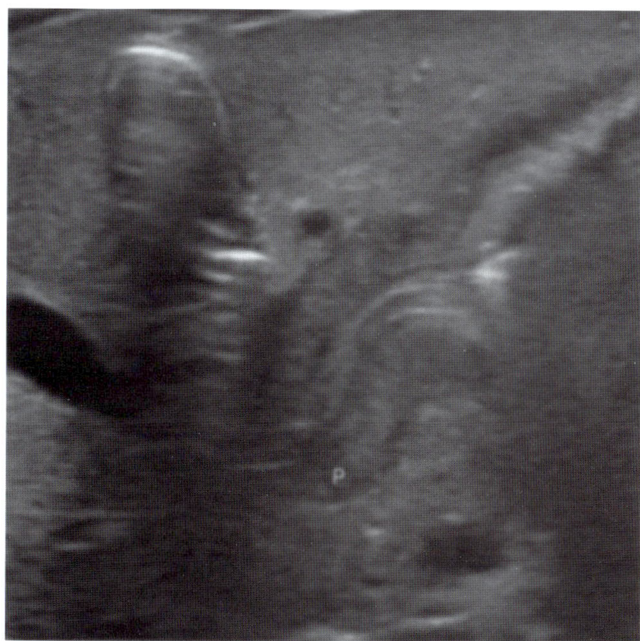

Figure 84.7 Longitudinal ultrasound image of the abdomen from a 4-week-old boy demonstrates the configuration of the pylorus (P) resembling a cervix (cervix sign) in hypertrophic pyloric stenosis.

Hypertrophic Pyloric Stenosis: Pearls to Remember

- Thickening and elongation of the pyloric canal caused by abnormal hypertrophy of pyloric musculature
- Manifests between 2 weeks and 3 months of life with a higher incidence in first-born boys
- Cervix and antral nipple signs on USG
- Upper limits of pylorus measurement are 3 mm muscle thickness and 14 mm canal length
- Pylorospasm is the differential consideration

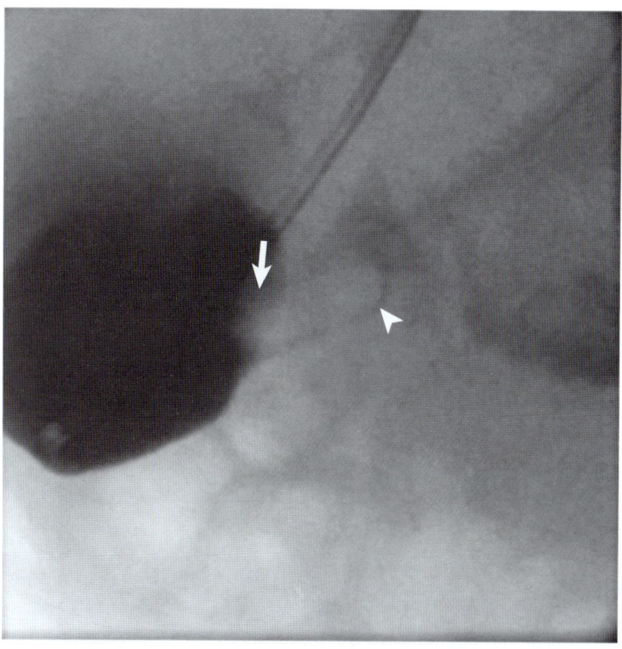

Figure 84.9 Upper gastrointestinal study from a 3-week-old boy demonstrates a thin stream of contrast into the duodenum (string sign, *white arrowhead*) and an extrinsic shoulder-like impression on the gastric antrum from the pyloric muscle (shoulder sign, *white arrow*) in hypertrophic pyloric stenosis.

Findings on upper GI series are passage of a thin stream of contrast through the pylorus (*string sign*) and shoulder-like extrinsic impression of pylorus on the gastric antrum *(shoulder sign)* (Fig. 84.9) [12].

Duodenal Obstruction

Causes of duodenal obstruction are duodenal atresia, duodenal web and stenosis, annular pancreas, preduodenal portal vein,

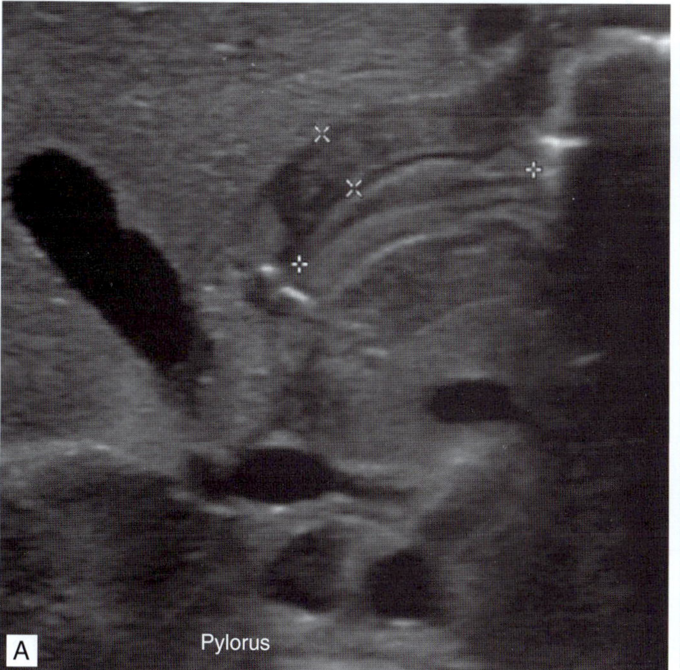

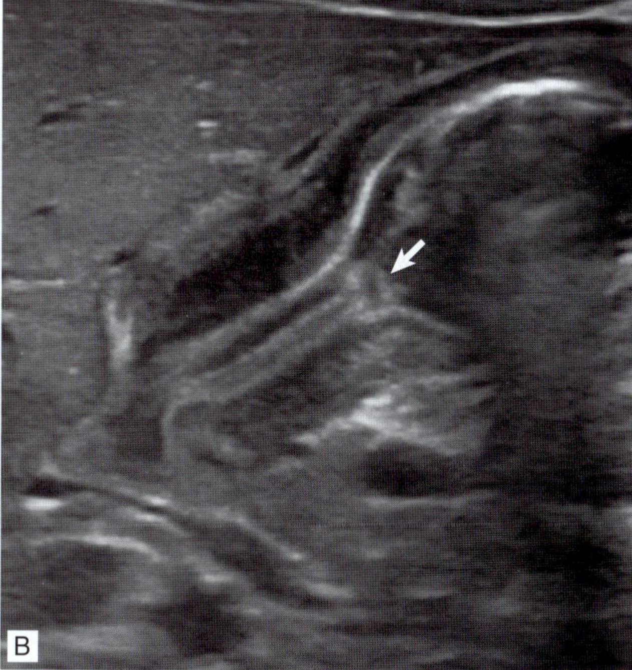

Figure 84.8 Longitudinal ultrasound image of the abdomen from a 5-week-old boy shows hypertrophic pyloric stenosis (A), with a nipplelike projection of pyloric mucosa into the gastric antrum (antral nipple sign) (*white arrow*) (B).

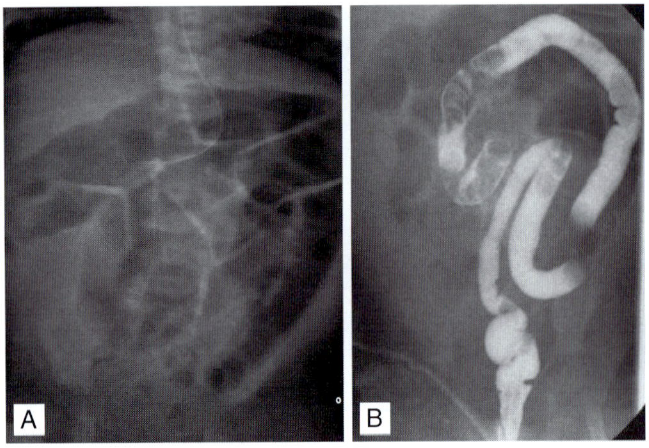

Figure 84.21 (A) Abdomen radiograph from an 8-day-old boy with meconium ileus shows multiple gas-filled distended bowel loop. (B) Subsequent contrast enema demonstrates diffuse microcolon with several meconium filling defects.

Hirschsprung Disease

Pathophysiology and Clinical Presentation

Hirschsprung disease is characterized by functional intestinal obstruction caused by arrested migration of ganglionic cells in the intramuscular and submucosal nerve plexus of the bowel wall. There is resultant failure of relaxation of the aganglionic segment with absent peristalsis. *The extent of involvement is variable from isolated anal involvement to aganglionosis of the entire colon, always extending from distal to proximal bowel in the direction opposite to neural crest migration.* Short segment disease involving the rectosigmoid colon is the most common [9]. Clinical presentations are failure to pass meconium in first 24 to 48 hours, bilious vomiting, and abdominal distension in neonates. Older children present with defecation issues and chronic constipation. *The condition is strongly associated with Down syndrome.* Complications are colonic perforation and enterocolitis [6].

Imaging Features

- Abdominal radiographs demonstrate findings of low obstruction with bowel dilation and air-fluid levels
- *Contrast enema is the diagnostic modality of choice. It demonstrates reversal of rectosigmoid ratio (ratio <1 on measurement of widest width of rectum to sigmoid colon), small irregular rectum, and rectal serrations or a sawtooth appearance caused by spasm* (Figs. 84.23 and 84.24) [6]. The site of caliber change or transition zone may be identified
- Total colonic Hirschsprung can present with a normal colon, microcolon, or a question mark–shaped colon with a rounded configuration of hepatic and splenic flexures and shortening [17]. Definitive diagnosis is made by rectal full-thickness biopsy

Hirschsprung Disease: Pearls to Remember

- Functional intestinal obstruction caused by arrested migration of ganglionic cells
- Short segment disease involving the rectosigmoid colon is the most common
- Low obstruction with bowel dilation and air-fluid levels on radiographs
- Reversal of rectosigmoid ratio (ratio <1 on measurement of widest width of rectum to sigmoid colon), small irregular rectum, and rectal serrations or sawtoothed appearance on contrast enema

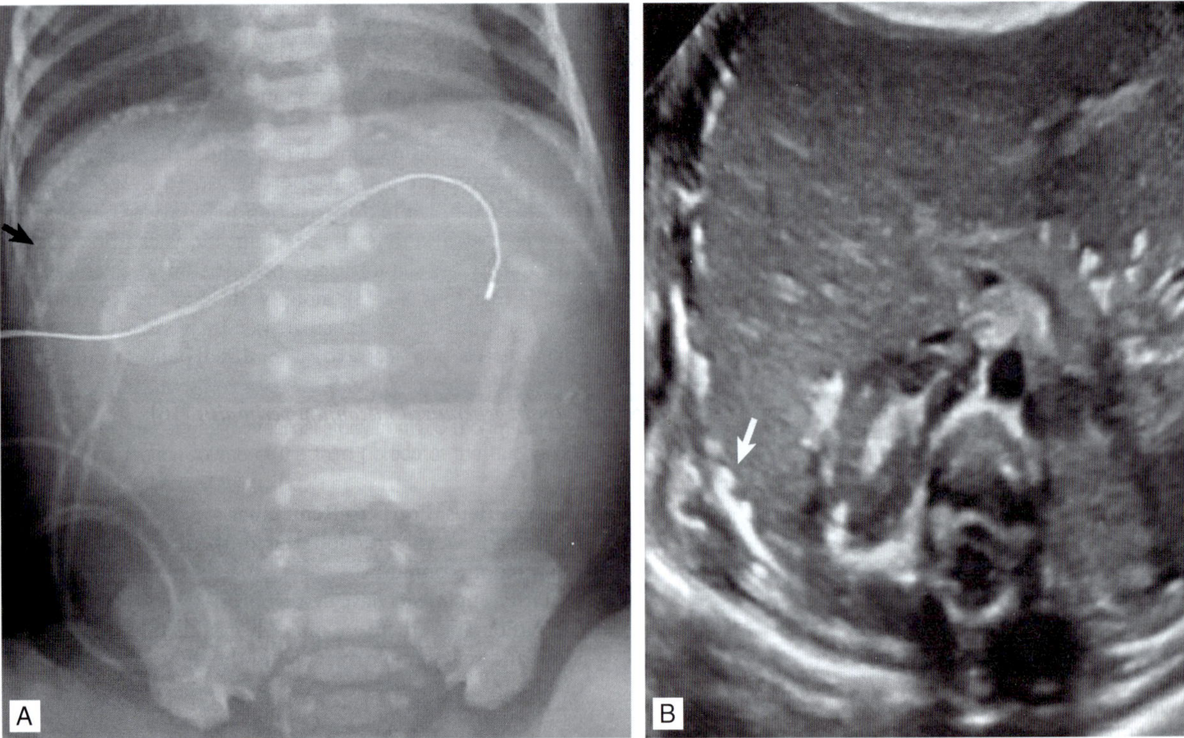

Figure 84.22 Abdomen radiograph demonstrates multiple calcifications in the right upper abdomen secondary to meconium peritonitis *(black arrow)* (A), visualized as echogenic foci on ultrasound abdomen (*white arrow*) (B).

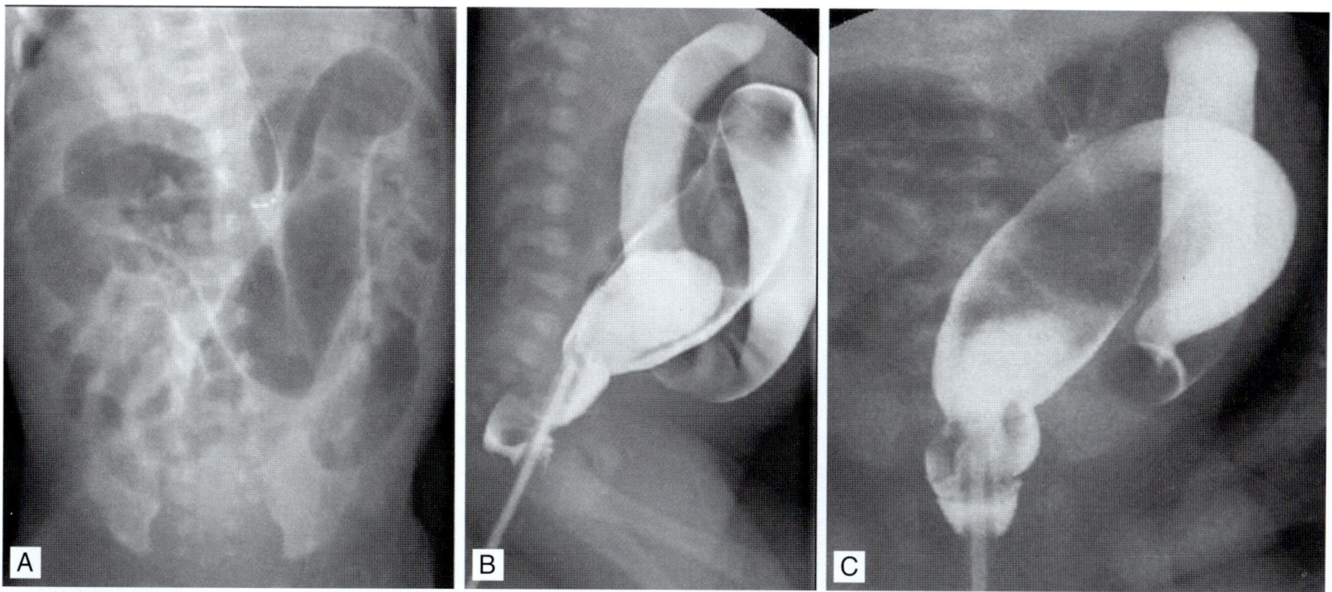

Figure 84.23 (A) Abdomen radiograph of a 1-month-old boy shows a distal obstructive bowel gas pattern with multiple dilated bowel loops. (B) Subsequent lateral and (C) antero-posterior contrast enema demonstrates reversal of rectosigmoid ratio due to Hirschsprung disease.

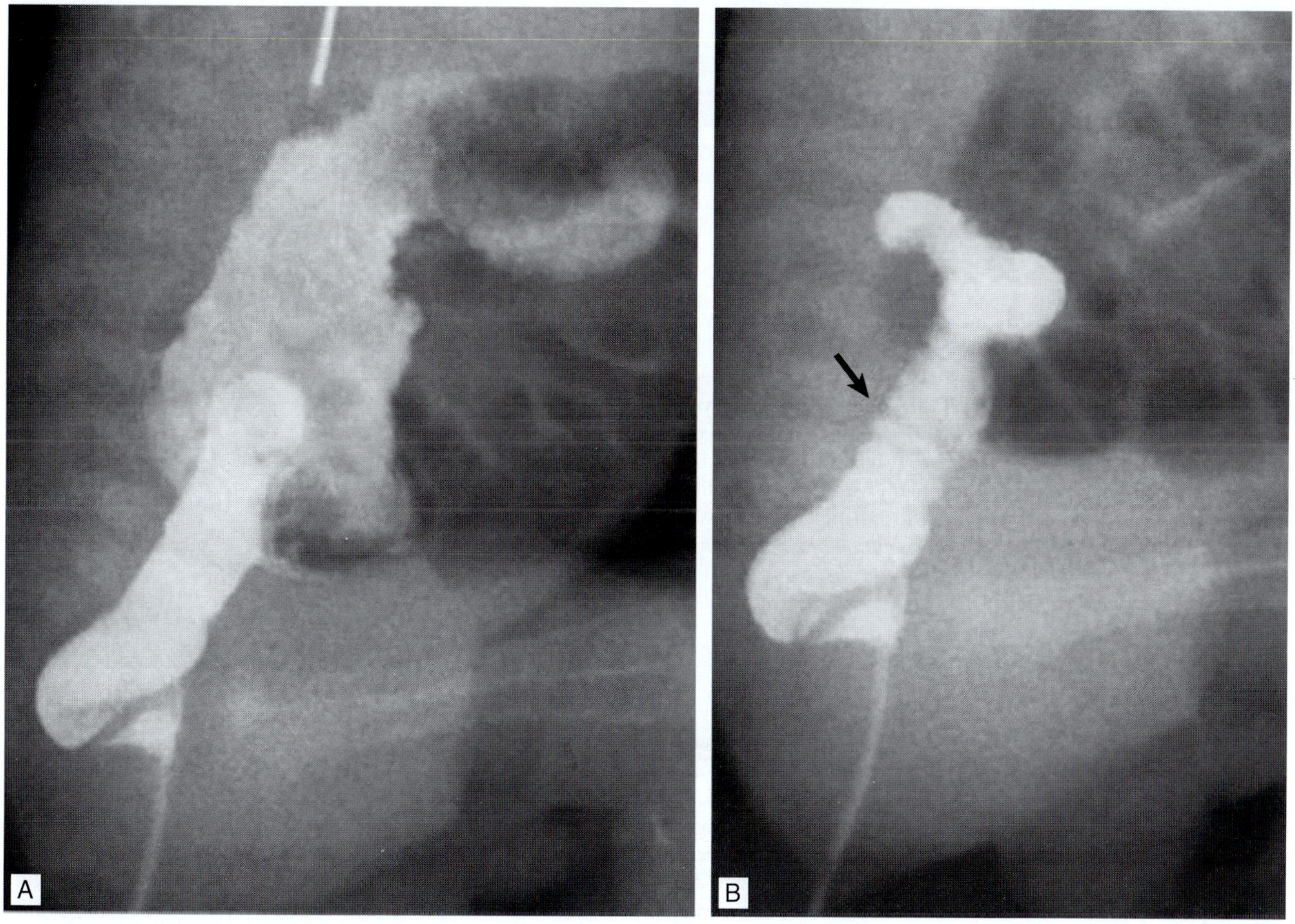

Figure 84.24 Contrast enema shows reversal of the rectosigmoid ratio in Hirschsprung disease (A). The transition zone is located in the distal sigmoid colon, which demonstrates a sawtooth pattern caused by spasm (*black arrow*) (B).

Small Left Colon Syndrome

Also known as *functional immaturity of the colon or meconium plug syndrome*, it is a self-limiting functional obstruction of left colon in neonates. The cause is proposed to be secondary to immaturity of ganglionic cells; however, the exact cause remains unclear. *Meconium plug is the consequence of obstruction rather than the cause, unlike meconium ileus.* Risk factors are neonates of mothers with diabetes and mothers administered magnesium sulfate during pregnancy. The typical clinical presentation is

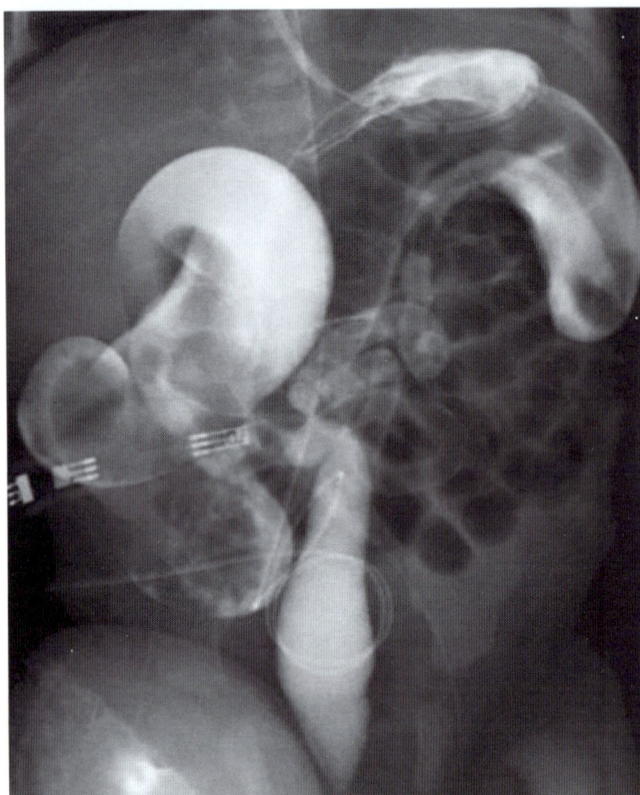

Figure 84.25 Contrast enema in a 2-day-old neonate with a history of maternal diabetes demonstrates small caliber of the left colon and relative dilation of the transverse and ascending colon caused by small left colon syndrome.

failure to pass meconium for more than 48 hours after birth [6,18].

Abdominal radiography demonstrates findings of low intestinal obstruction with multiple bowel dilation and air-fluid levels. Contrast enema shows a decreased caliber of the left colon, containing meconium filling defects. There is relative upstream dilation of the ascending and descending colon with a normal-caliber rectum (Fig. 84.25). Contrast enema is also therapeutic because it softens and clears the meconium. *Nonresolution of symptoms after enema warrants biopsy to exclude Hirschsprung disease, which is the major differential consideration* [18].

Anorectal Malformations

Anorectal malformations are myriad congenital anomalies involving the rectum and anal canal, commonly occurring in conjunction with varying combinations of urogenital tract anomalies. These are also associated with a multitude of cardiovascular (e.g., septal defects), GI (e.g., intestinal atresia and malrotation), musculoskeletal (e.g., sacral agenesis, tethered cord), urogenital (e.g., vesicoureteral reflux, renal agenesis), and chromosomal anomalies (e.g., trisomy 13, 18, and 21).

Ectopic anal orifice and fistula result secondary to abnormal development of cloaca and cloacal membrane during early embryonic weeks; abnormalities of a normally located anus occur secondary to disturbances in anal recanalization. The incidence is slightly higher in males [2].

Wingspread classification divides the malformation into low, intermediate, and high depending on the location of the rectal pouch with respect to the puborectalis sling (Table 84.1). The more recent Krikenbeck classification includes the fistula types and locations with respect to the rectum [2].

TABLE 84.1 Wingspread Classification

	Males	Females
Low	Anal stenosis and anocutaneous fistula	Anal stenosis, anal agenesis ± external fistula
Intermediate	Anal agenesis ± rectourethral bulbar fistula.	Anal agenesis ± rectovestibular or rectovaginal fistula
High	Rectal atresia, anorectal agenesis ± rectourethral or rectoprostatic fistula	Rectal atresia, cloacal malformations, anorectal agenesis ± rectovaginal fistula

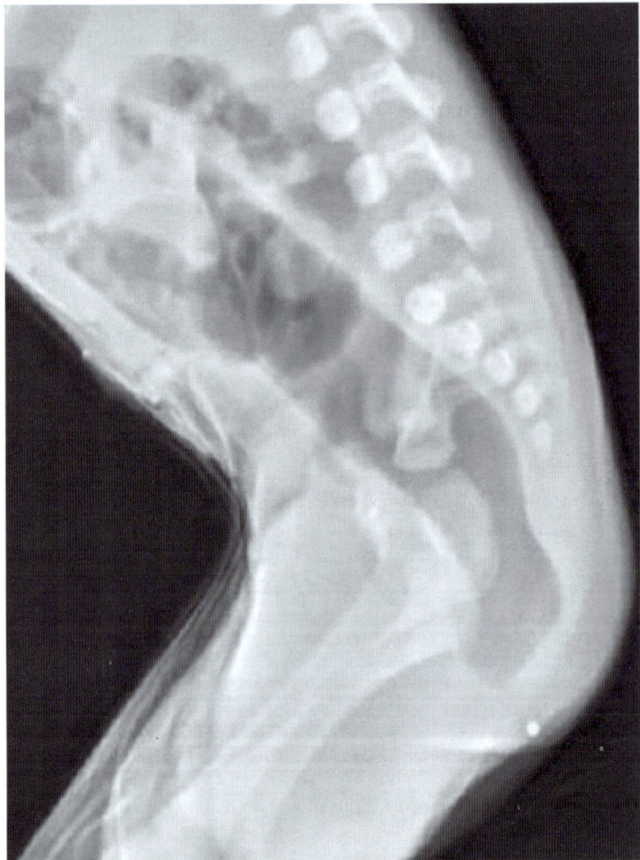

Figure 84.26 Invertogram in anorectal malformation demonstrates a blind-ending rectum located approximately 9 mm from the skin, as indicated by the radiopaque marker placed at the expected location of the anus.

These abnormalities are commonly clinically evident. Findings on abdominal radiography include low intestinal obstruction with multiple dilated loops, absence of rectal gas, air within the bladder, and pelvic calcifications caused by admixture of urine and meconium in cases with urinary fistula. Traditional methods to determine high versus low fistula such as radiographic invertogram (involving placement of a coin at the expected anus and measurement of distance between rectus bubble and the coin) (Fig. 84.26), cross-table lateral views, contrast fluoroscopy (Figs. 84.27 and 84.28), and USG can be used for initial evaluation; however, these have low diagnostic accuracy. Pelvic MRI is the mainstay for accurate localization of rectal

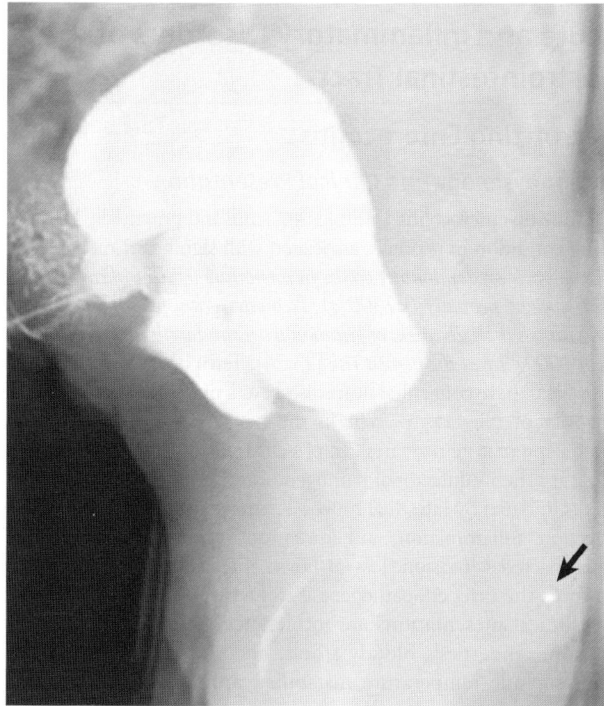

Figure 84.27 A 3-month-old girl with anorectal malformation. Contrast injection into the mucous fistula demonstrates the rectourethral fistula. The blind-ending rectum is located approximately 4 cm from the skin marker placed at the expected location of the anus (*black arrow*).

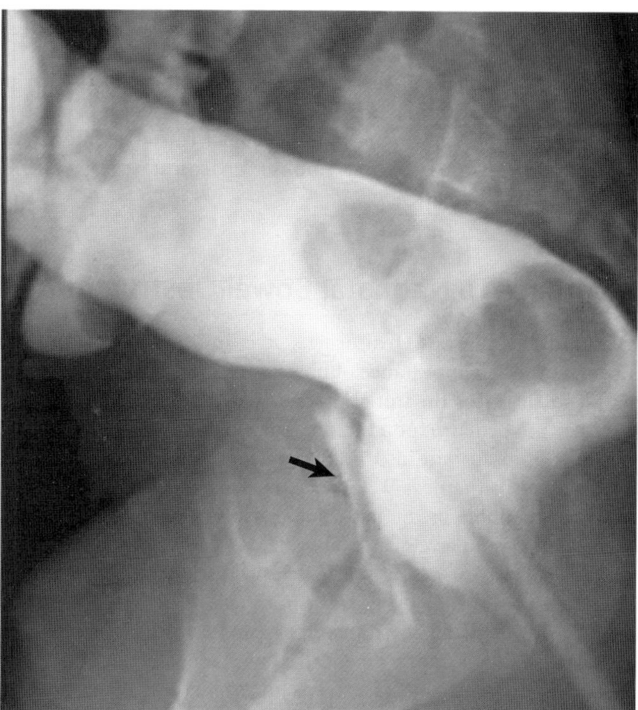

Figure 84.28 Contrast enema demonstrates rectovaginal fistula (*black arrow*) as a part of anorectal malformation.

pouch, and detailed assessment of pelvic floor and sphincter muscle anatomy (Fig. 84.29). Voiding cystourethrogram is performed to look for any accompanying urogenital abnormality or fistula in suspected cases [2,9].

Treatment of patients with anorectal malformations aims at maximizing continence while maintaining urinary and sexual functions. Attempted primary repair in the neonatal period can be pursued in patients with perineal fistula. Otherwise, a multistage correction is performed, which involves initial diverting colostomy followed by posterior sagittal anoplasty and fistula closure. Additional laparoscopic intervention may be required in the interim to remove certain types of fistulas, such as fistulas to the bladder neck or the prostate. Postoperative continence depends mainly on the type of fistula, the associated spine anomalies, the degree of sacral dysplasia, and the type of surgery [19]. After initial repair, pelvic MRI is the modality of choice to assess the need for further surgical intervention, to examine the sphincter muscle and rectum position, and to look for postoperative complications [20].

Colonic Atresia

Colonic atresia is caused by intrauterine ischemic insult to the developing bowel, similar to jejunoileal atresia. Although it leads

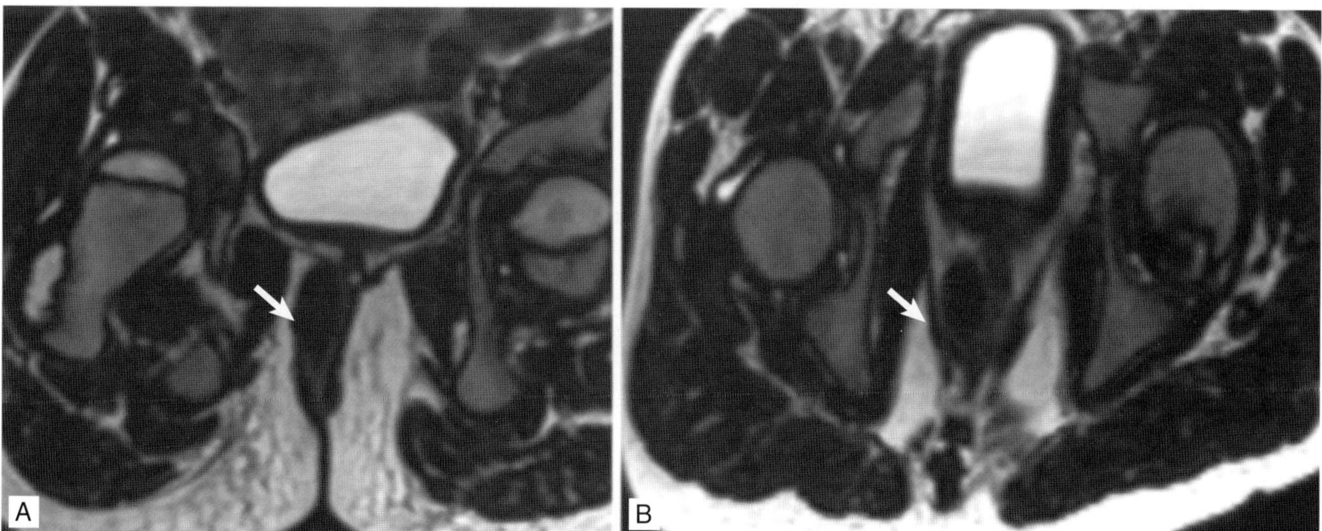

Figure 84.29 Coronal T2W MRI pelvis demonstrate malpositioned anorectal junction to the right of midline (*white arrow*) (A), with atrophy of right levator muscle in anorectal malformation (B) (*white arrow*) (B).

to low intestinal obstruction, the condition is so rare that it is usually excluded from the list of differential consideration in usual clinical scenarios. Three types are described: type I with an obstructive intraluminal membrane presenting with windsock sign on enema, type II (proximal), and III (distal) demonstrating abrupt termination of colonic opacification on enema caused by cordlike atresia [21].

Approach to Neonatal Bowel Obstruction

Before discussing bowel disorders, it is important to revise the normal expected appearance of bowel on a plain abdominal radiograph because it is the initial modality of choice for bowel assessment in the pediatric population. The small bowel is expected to be filled with air within 3 hours of delivery, and air reaches the rectum within the next 9 hours. Also, it is important to localize the gastric bubble in the left upper quadrant of the abdomen. A few [1,2] air-fluid levels can be normally seen. A normal bowel gas pattern consists of nearly symmetrical polygonal air spaces with thin walls. Instead of using strict numbers to highlight a dilated loop of bowel, using the transverse diameter of the vertebra as a reference point is more practical. Bowel loops are identified as dilated if bowel diameter exceeds the transverse diameter of a single vertebra [22].

When evaluating a neonate suspected of bowel obstruction, it is helpful to classify the bowel gas pattern on abdominal radiographs as high or low (Fig. 84.30). High obstruction presents with few dilated loops, whereas low obstruction demonstrates multiple dilated loops. Certain radiographic findings such as double bubble (duodenal atresia) and triple bubble (proximal jejunal atresia) are indicative of specific pathologies. Upper GI findings in patients with high obstruction can be broadly categorized into malrotation and other causes. High obstruction caused by pyloric stenosis is solely evaluated with USG in most cases. Patients undergo contrast enema in low obstructive pattern, with findings broadly categorized by the presence or absence of microcolon.

Acute and Inflammatory Disorders of the Gastrointestinal Tract

Necrotizing Enterocolitis

Pathophysiology and Clinical Presentation

Necrotizing enterocolitis (NEC) is an acute and potentially life-threatening condition in neonates associated with significant morbidity and mortality. *It predominantly occurs in premature (≤90% of cases) and low birth weight neonates (<1500 g). Neonates admitted in intensive care units, at less than 28 weeks of gestational age, and with birth weights of less than 1000g are at the highest risk* [23,24]. Term born neonates affected with NEC have congenital heart disease as a major risk factor [23]. The majority of the cases present in the first 2 weeks of life; however, severely premature neonates can present later in second to third weeks [23,25]. The multifactorial pathogenesis is believed to be a cascade of events initiated by intestinal mucosal damage secondary causes such as infection, inflammation, and immature immunity, leading to ischemia, bacterial invasion, loss of bowel integrity, and eventual sepsis; however, the exact etiopathogenesis still remains unclear.

Clinical presentations are intolerance to feed, abdominal distension, tenderness, bloody stools, and shock [23,26]. Systemic signs include temperature instability, apnea, bradycardia, metabolic acidosis, and coagulopathy [26].

Imaging Features

Serial abdominal radiographs are the mainstay modality for diagnosis and follow up. It includes supine view coupled with cross table or left lateral decubitus views to detect ectopic air.

- Early disease can present with normal bowel gas pattern or nonspecific focal or generalized gaseous bowel distension related to ileus (Fig. 84.31). *Ischemic bowel demonstrates more focal, asymmetrical dilation with a fixed configuration on serial examinations* (Fig. 84.32). Bowel distension can sometimes precede the clinical manifestations [23]
- Intramural gas or pneumatosis presents as bubbly, curvilinear lucencies along the bowel wall (Fig. 84.33). *In the setting of*

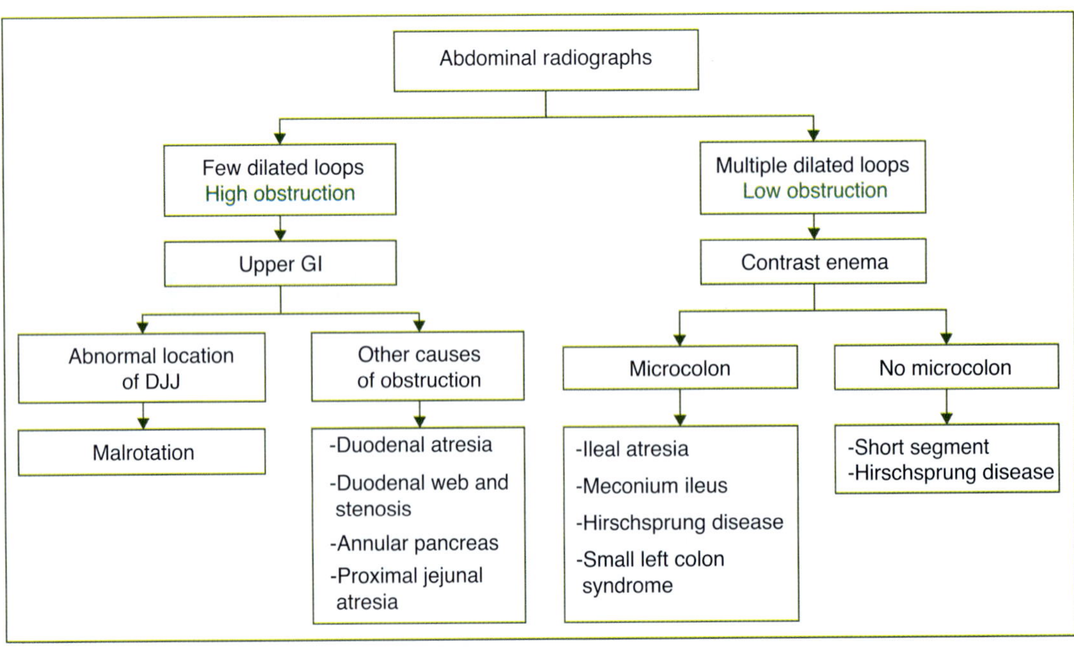

Figure 84.30 Approach to neonatal bowel obstruction.

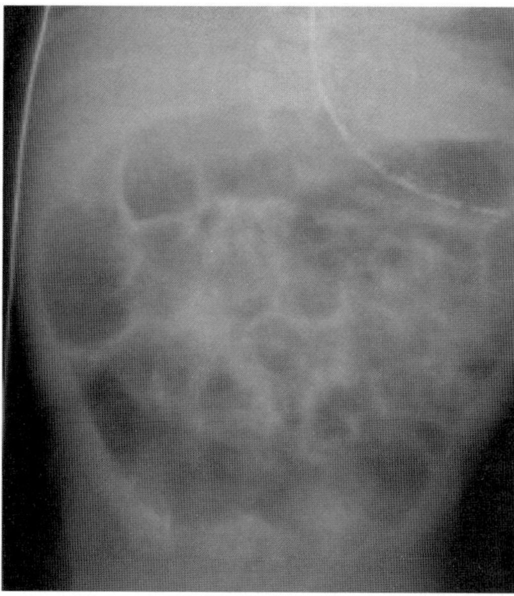

Figure 84.31 Supine abdomen radiograph from a 13-day-old boy shows diffuse gaseous distension of bowel in early necrotizing enterocolitis.

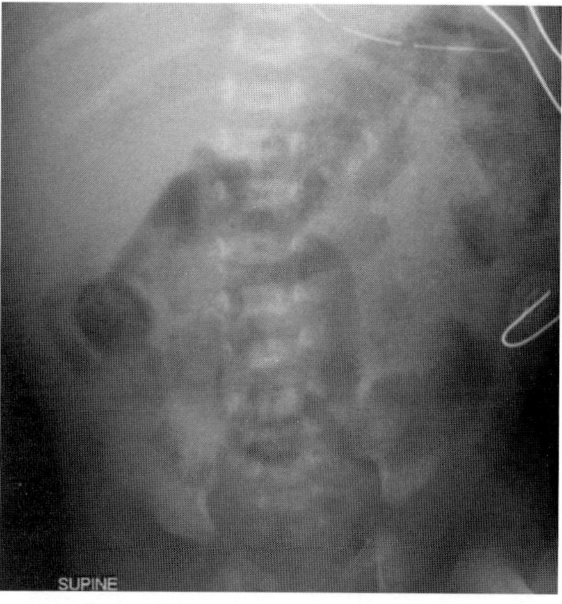

Figure 84.32 Supine abdomen radiograph from a 11-day-old boy shows mildly dilated, featureless, and fixed bowel loops in necrotizing enterocolitis.

appropriate clinical features, presence of intramural gas is essentially confirmatory of NEC [23,27]

- Portal vein gas is identified as branching linear lucencies overlying the liver (Fig. 84.34). Pneumoperitoneum indicates advanced disease and warrants immediate surgical intervention (Fig. 84.35)

Ultrasonography can be used in conjunction with radiographs to support the diagnosis. Findings are simple or complex ascites, decreased or loss of bowel peristalsis, bowel wall thickening, or thinning with alteration in color flow [23].

Modified Bells criteria guides the clinical management. It consists of three stages (stage I, suspected NEC; stage II, definite NEC; stage III, advanced NEC) and is based on a combination of clinical and imaging findings. Stages I and II are managed medically, whereas stage III disease requires surgical intervention [26].

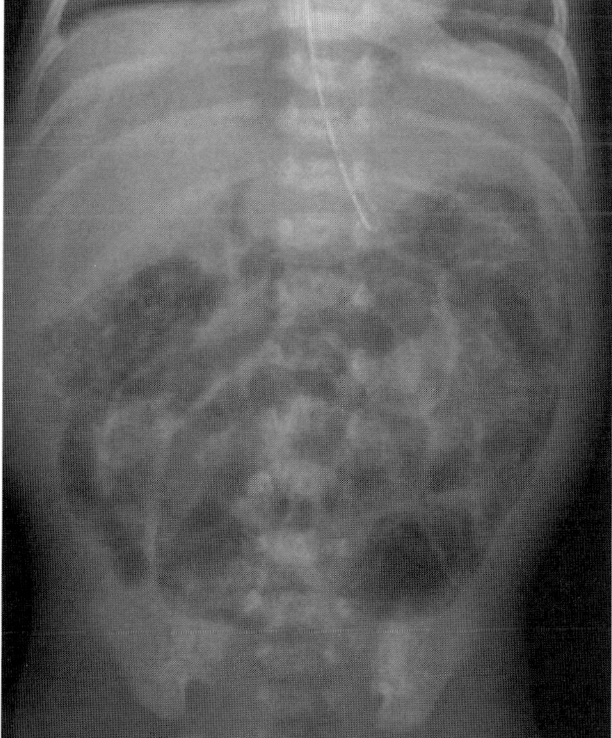

Figure 84.33 Supine abdomen radiograph from a 11-day-old girl with necrotizing enterocolitis shows mildly dilated featureless bowel loops with diffuse pneumatosis.

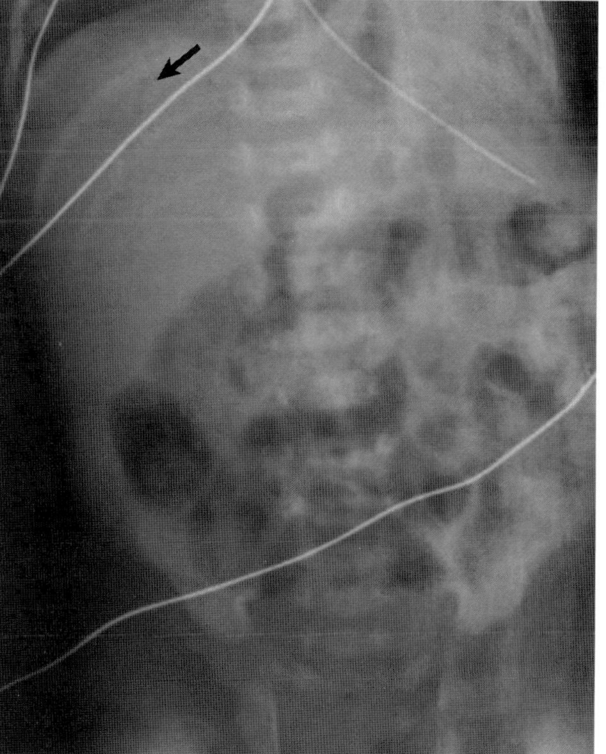

Figure 84.34 Left lateral decubitus radiograph demonstrates portal venous air in necrotizing enterocolitis (*black arrow*).

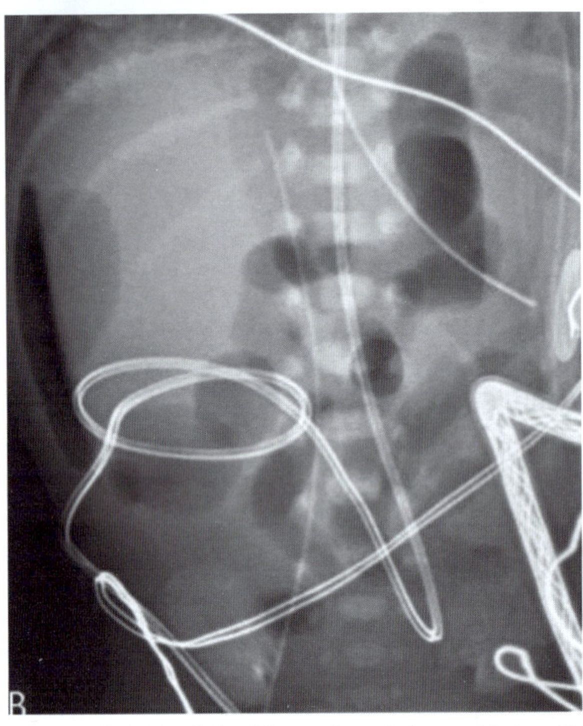

Figure 84.35 Left lateral decubitus radiograph from a 15-day-old boy demonstrates pneumoperitoneum caused by necrotizing enterocolitis. There are several distended and featureless bowel loops in the central abdomen.

Necrotizing Enterocolitis: Pearls to Remember

- Predominantly affects premature and low-birth-weight neonates
- *Serial abdominal radiography is the mainstay modality for diagnosis and follow up*
- Radiographic findings are focal or generalized gaseous bowel distension, fixed asymmetric loops, pneumatosis, portal venous gas, and pneumoperitoneum
- Sonographic findings are ascites, decreased or loss of peristalsis, bowel wall thickening, or thinning with altered color flow

Appendicitis

Pathophysiology and Clinical Presentation

Acute appendicitis is one of the most common surgical emergencies in children, characterized by inflammation of the vermiform appendix. The incidence is higher between 10 and 20 years of age with a slight male predominance. Clinical features are abdominal pain typically localized to the right lower quadrant, rebound tenderness, vomiting, fever, and leukocytosis [28].

The appendix is a blind-ending structure arising from the posteromedial aspect of the cecum. The length varies from 7.5 to 10 cm. Although the position of tip is variable, the base is relatively constant in position corresponding to the Mc Burney point. Pathogenesis of acute appendicitis involves luminal obstruction secondary to causes such as fecolith or lymphoid hypertrophy, which leads to progressive build-up of intraluminal secretions, edema, mucosa ulceration, and superimposed infection [29]. Continued inflammation causes venous compression and ischemia followed by perforation, periappendiceal phlegmon, and abscess formation.

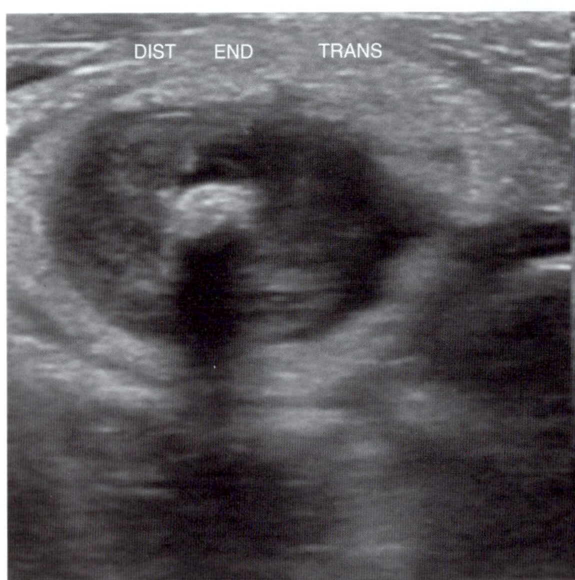

Figure 84.36 Transverse ultrasound image from a 12-year-old boy with acute appendicitis demonstrates dilated appendix with an appendicolith in the lumen.

Imaging Features

Ultrasonography is the mainstay diagnostic modality. It is performed with graded compression technique using a linear high-frequency transducer. Normal bowel loops are displaced by gentle probe pressure, with scanning performed in longitudinal and transverse planes.

Findings of acute appendicitis are categorized into two groups, direct and indirect signs.

- *Direct signs are appendiceal noncompressibility, diameter larger than 6 mm, wall thickness exceeding 3 mm, wall stratification and target appearance, wall hyperemia, and presence of appendicolith* (Figs. 84.36 and 84.37) [29–31]
- *Indirect signs are increased echogenicity of periappendiceal fat, periappendiceal fluid, abscess, and enlargement of mesenteric nodes* (see Fig. 84.37) [31]
- Heterogeneous periappendiceal fluid and collections without discrete identification of appendix are indicative of perforation (Fig. 84.38)

Computed tomography has a highly sensitive diagnostic accuracy; however, it involves radiation exposure. It is predominantly reserved for patients with equivocal sonographic findings and suspected perforation.

- An inflamed appendix demonstrates wall thickening, stratification and hyperenhancement, appendicolith, periappendiceal fat stranding, and mesenteric adenopathy (Fig. 84.39)
- *Documented upper limit of appendiceal diameter on CT is 10 mm; a diameter of 6 to 10 mm is considered equivocal in absence of additional findings. A possible explanation for this discrepancy between USG and CT is that USG images are acquired using a graded compression technique, which might alter the appendiceal diameter* [32]
- Cecal findings are apical thickening, the arrowhead sign, and the cecal bar sign. The *arrowhead sign* refers to a triangular configuration of enteric contrast near the appendiceal orifice caused by surrounding focal cecal thickening. *Cecal bar* refers to a barlike inflammatory soft tissue separating the cecum from the appendix [33]
- Extraluminal air, extraluminal appendicolith, phlegmon, complex rim enhancing periappendiceal and pelvic collections are features of perforation (Fig. 84.40). Bowel obstruction may result

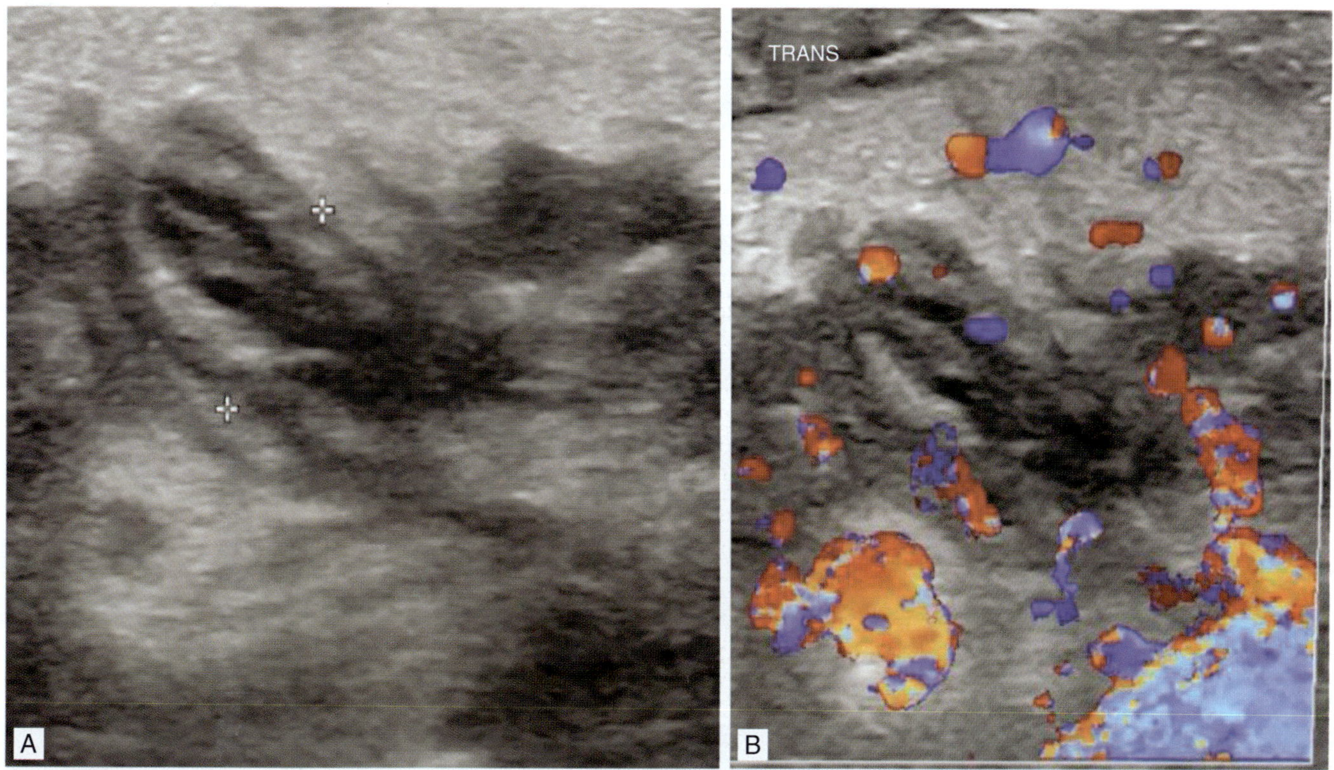

Figure 84.37 Longitudinal ultrasound image from a 10-year-old girl with acute appendicitis demonstrates dilated appendix with thickened wall (*calipers*) (A), periappendiceal echogenic fat, and wall hyperemia (B).

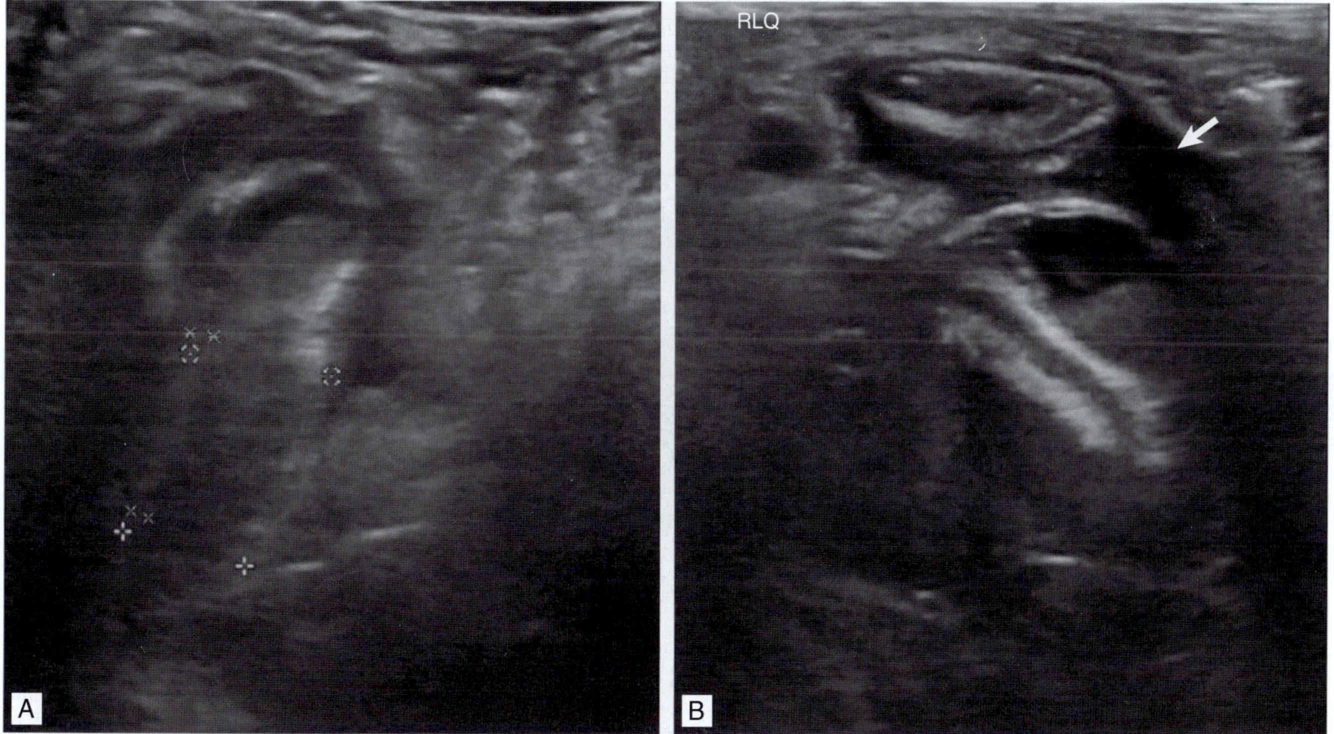

Figure 84.38 Longitudinal (A) and transverse ultrasound images (B) from a 13-year-old young woman with perforated appendicitis demonstrates complex periappendiceal fluid (*white arrow*) (B), with only the base of the appendix identified within the phlegmon (*calipers*) (A).

Magnetic resonance imaging is considered as reliable, radiation free alternative to CT for evaluation. However, its overall utility is limited in actual clinical practice because of factors such as availability, cost, increased scan time, and sedation requirements in pediatric population.

Radiographs are rarely done. They may demonstrate appendicolith, obscuration of the psoas margin, increased soft tissue density, or localized ileus in the right lower quadrant [29].

Differential diagnoses are mesenteric adenitis, epiploic appendagitis, omental infarction, and Crohn's disease [33].

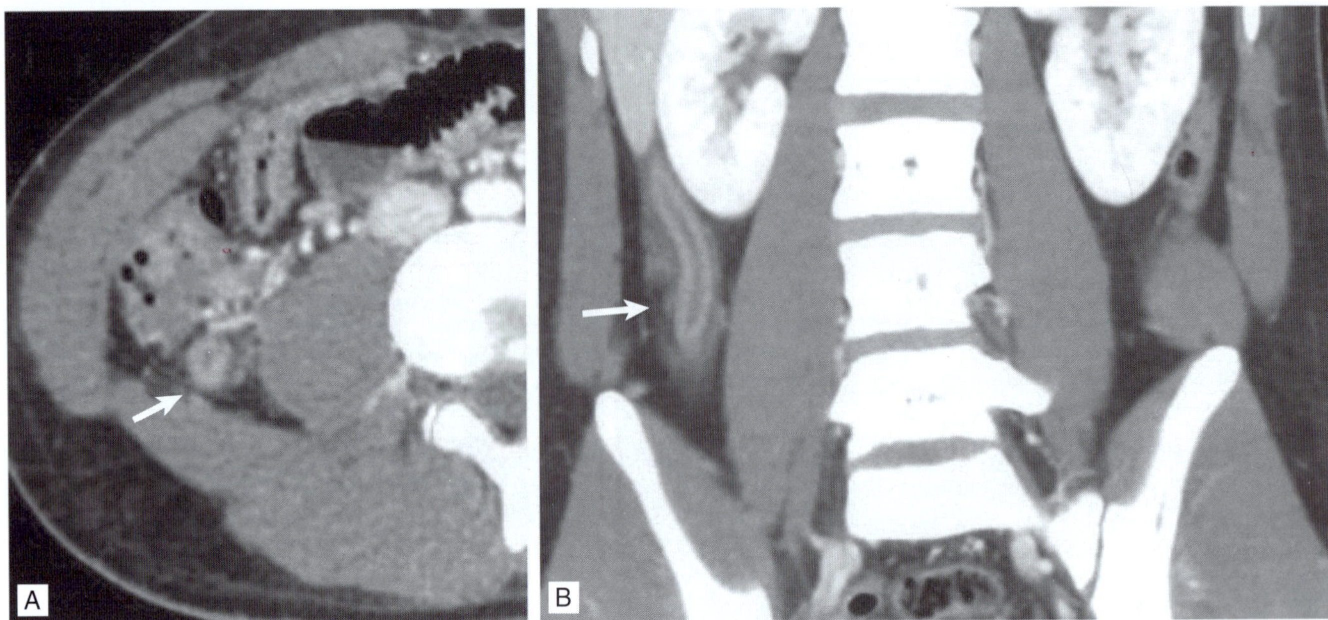

Figure 84.39 Contrast-enhanced axial (A) and coronal (B) computed tomography of the abdomen and pelvis from a 16-year-old young man with abdominal pain shows a dilated appendix with mural hyperenhancement and mild periappendiceal stranding caused by acute appendicitis (*white arrow*).

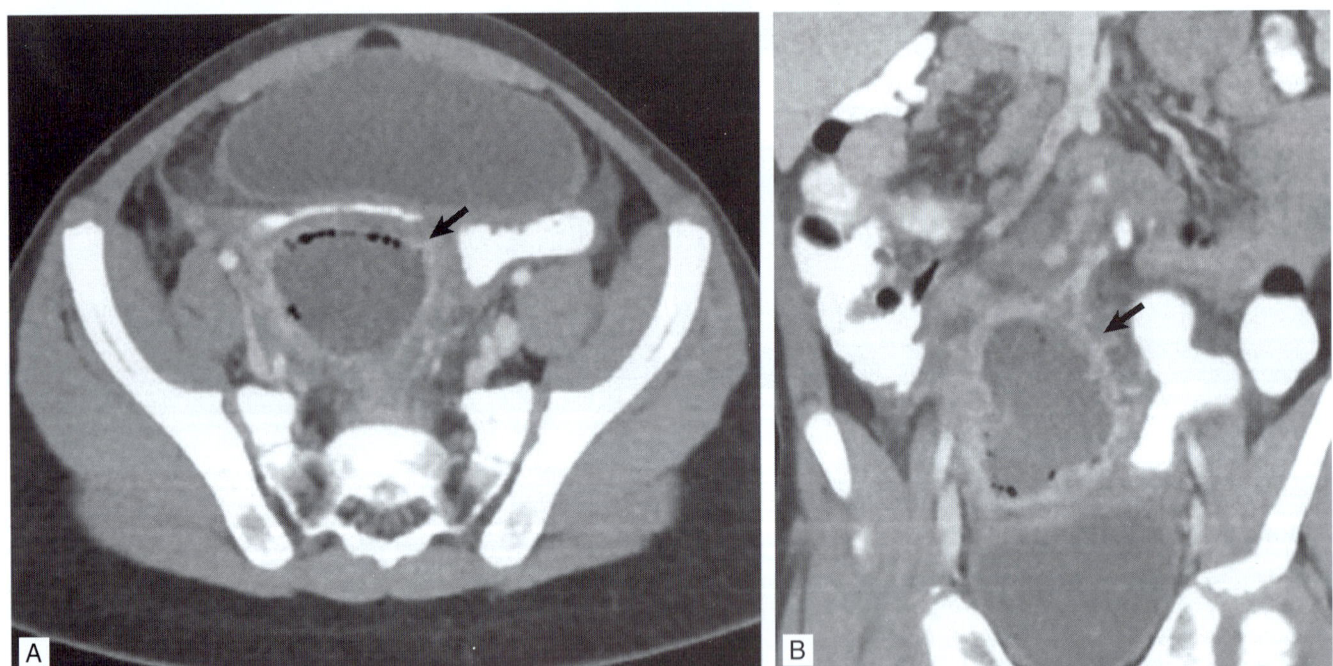

Figure 84.40 Contrast-enhanced axial (A) and coronal (B) computed tomography of the abdomen and pelvis from a 14-year-old boy with perforated appendicitis demonstrates rim enhancing abscess in the right lower quadrant (*black arrow*).

Acute Appendicitis: Pearls to Remember	
Direct Ultrasound Signs	**Indirect Ultrasound Signs**
Appendiceal noncompressibility Diameter >6 mm Wall thickness >3 mm Wall stratification and target appearance Wall hyperemia Appendicolith	Increased echogenicity of periappendiceal fat Periappendiceal fluid and abscess Enlargement of mesenteric nodes

Mesenteric Adenitis

Mesenteric adenitis is a self-limiting condition in children and adolescents characterized by inflammation and enlargement of the mesenteric nodes. Clinical presentation is nonspecific with symptoms such as generalized abdominal pain or pain localized to the right lower quadrant, fever, vomiting, and leukocytosis. The disease can clinically mimic acute disorders such as appendicitis, ovarian torsion, and intussusception [34,35].

It can be categorized into primary and secondary groups. Primary mesenteric adenitis has no identifiable intrabdominal process to account for the adenopathy. Secondary mesenteric adenitis is

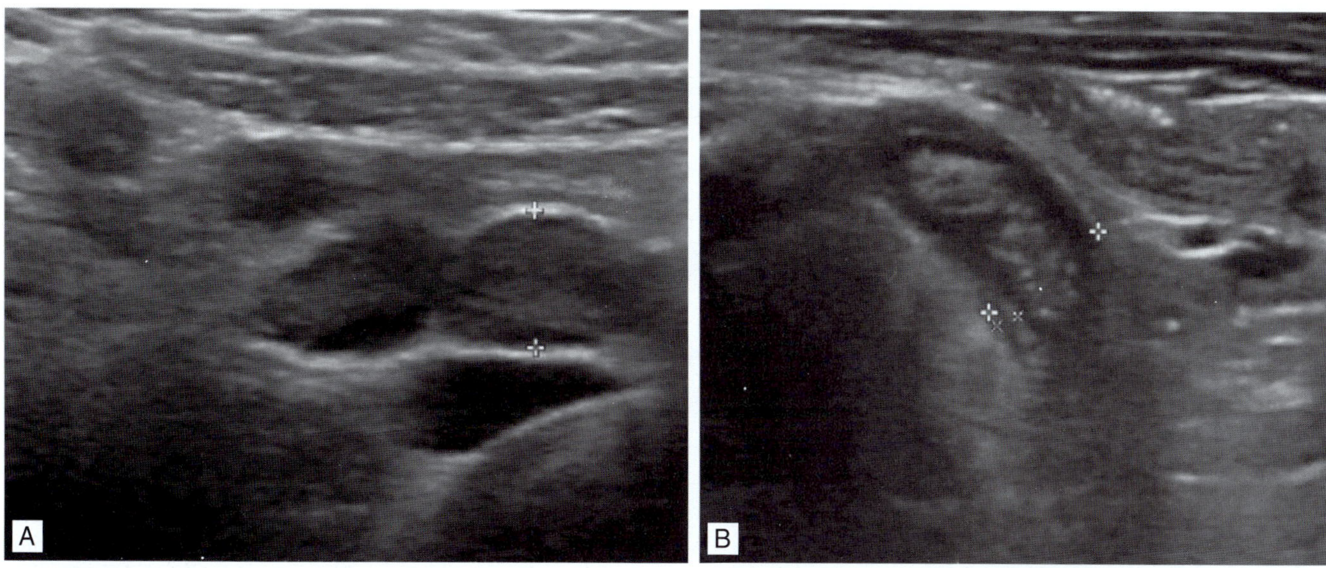

Figure 84.41 Transverse ultrasound of the right lower quadrant from a 15-year-old young man demonstrates a cluster of enlarged mesenteric nodes in mesenteric adenitis (*calipers*) (A). The appendix is normal (*calipers*) (B).

associated with an identifiable intraabdominal inflammatory cause [36]. Infections with *Yersinia* spp., staphylococcus, *Salmonella* spp., mycobacteria, and certain viruses are also implicated in the pathogenesis [34].

Enlargement of mesenteric nodes is a common incidental finding on USG in asymptomatic children. *Proposed sonographic criteria for diagnosis include a cluster of three or more mesenteric nodes with a short-axis diameter greater than 8 mm* [35] (Fig. 84.41). However, the diagnosis should only be made in combination with an appropriate clinical setting. USG also helps to exclude other acute disorders such as appendicitis and ovarian torsion, which can mimic the clinical symptoms.

Computed tomography is usually reserved as problem solving tool in older children. *Suggested CT criteria for diagnosis is a cluster of three or more nodes with short-axis diameter greater than 8 mm* (Fig. 84.42) [37].

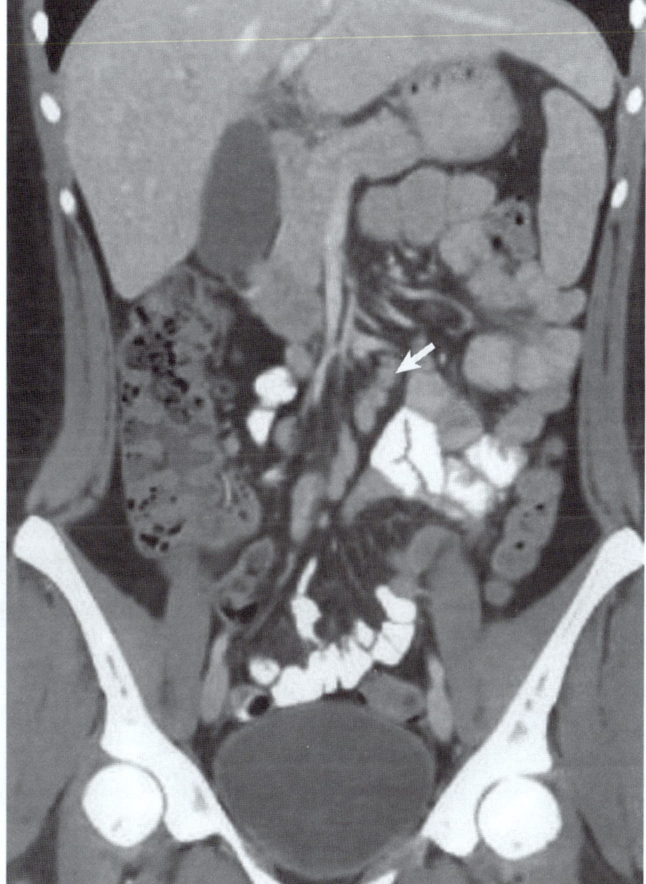

Figure 84.42 Contrast-enhanced coronal computed tomography of the abdomen and pelvis from a 12-year-old boy demonstrates a cluster of enlarged nodes in the mesenteric root in mesenteric adenitis (*white arrow*).

Meckel Diverticulum

Pathophysiology and Clinical Presentation

Meckel diverticulum is a congenital intestinal diverticulum located along the antimesenteric border of the ileum. It occurs secondary to incomplete obliteration of omphalomesenteric or vitelline duct [38] and is *the most common congenital anomaly of the GI tract* [39]. General features are classically remembered by the *rule of 2*:

- Occurring in about 2% of the population
- Usually located within 2 feet of the ileocecal valve
- About 2 inches in length
- Commonly presents before 2 years of age [40]

On histology, the diverticulum is lined by intestinal epithelium with occasional presence of heterotopic gastric or pancreatic tissue, which typically leads to GI bleeding [40]. It can be incidental or present with painless, sometimes massive rectal bleed in a previously healthy child, abdominal pain, and fever. Complications are GI hemorrhage *(most frequent)*, inflammation, perforation, bowel obstruction, and intussusception [12].

Imaging Features

- *Technetium-99m pertechnetate scintigraphy is the modality of choice for evaluation.* It detects the diverticulum secondary to radiotracer uptake in the ectopic gastric mucosa (Fig. 84.43).
- Meckel diverticulum can be incidentally detected on CT as a blind-ending pouch along the ileum. Contrast-enhanced CT helps in detection of Meckel diverticulitis presenting as a

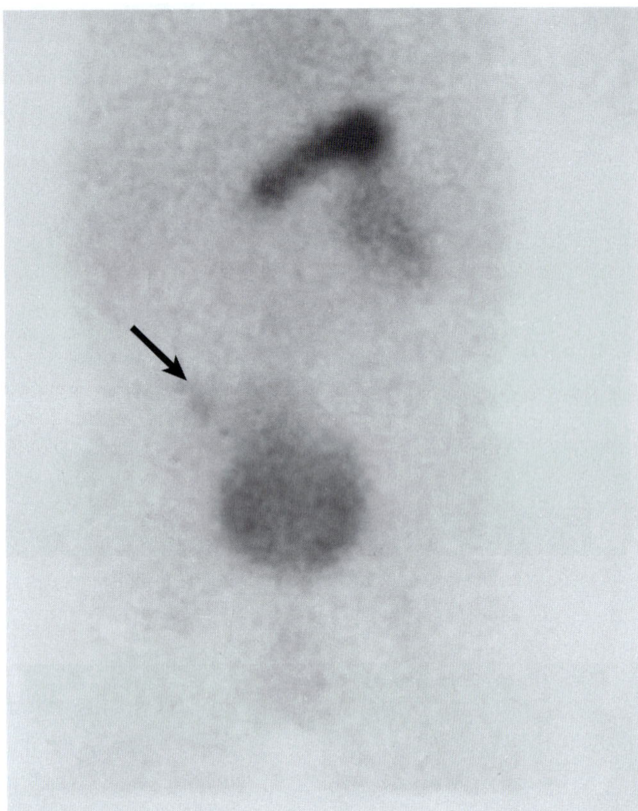

Figure 84.43 Technetium-99m pertechnetate scintigraphy from a 2-year-old boy demonstrates focal radiotracer uptake in the right lower quadrant, delineating ectopic gastric mucosa in Meckel diverticulum (*black arrow*).

dilated tubular, bling-ending structure along the ileum associated with perilesional fat stranding (Fig. 84.44). Perforation can lead to localized fluid collection, abscess, or pneumoperitoneum (Fig. 84.45) [39]

It is imperative to document a normal appendix in all cases to avoid false-positive results.

Intussusception

Pathophysiology and Clinical Presentation

Intussusception is the telescoping and pulling of a segment of bowel (known as *intussusceptum*) into distal segment or adjacent bowel lumen (known as *intussuscipiens*). *The most common presentation is between 3 and 12 months of age with a classic triad of colicky abdominal pain, currant jelly stool, and a palpable mass.* Other symptoms include lethargy and drawing up of the legs [12,41,42]. *The vast majority of intussusceptions are idiopathic and are commonly ileocolic or ileoileocolic.*

The cause is believed to be secondary to lymphoid hyperplasia in the ileum. Less commonly, it is associated with a pathological lead point secondary to myriad of focal and diffuse intestinal pathologies such as Meckel diverticulum, polyp, enteric cysts, tumors, Henoch-Schoenlein purpura, celiac disease, and cystic fibrosis. The cause in more diffuse intestinal disorders such as celiac disease is proposed secondary to altered peristalsis. Indwelling enteric catheter and certain surgical procedure involving bowel and retroperitoneal dissection are additional risk factors [43]. The major complications are bowel obstruction, ischemia, and perforations.

Imaging Features

- Abdominal radiography has low detection sensitivity and is mostly used as a screening tool for pneumoperitoneum and bowel obstruction. It may demonstrate a soft tissue opacity along the bowel with an air crescent or increased gas-filled small bowel loops in the right lower quadrant caused by cecum displacement and replacement by multiple ileal loops [13]
- USG is the mainstay diagnostic modality. A linear high-frequency transducer is used with scanning in transverse and longitudinal planes. *The transverse view demonstrates the target or donut sign with a bowel-in-bowel appearance, consisting of consecutive hypoechoic and echogenic layers. The pseudokidney sign is seen in the longitudinal view, with the fat-containing mesentery trapped within the intussusception mimicking the renal hilum and the edematous surrounding bowel resembling*

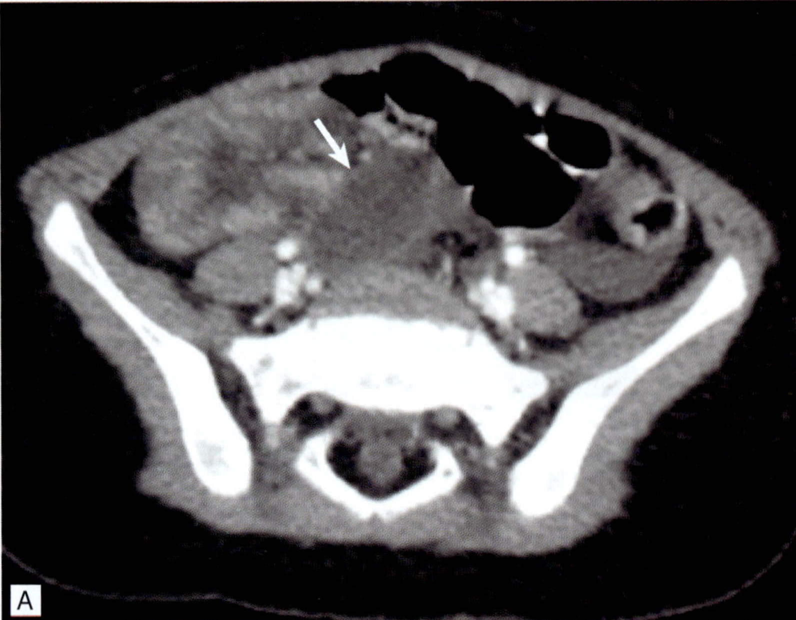

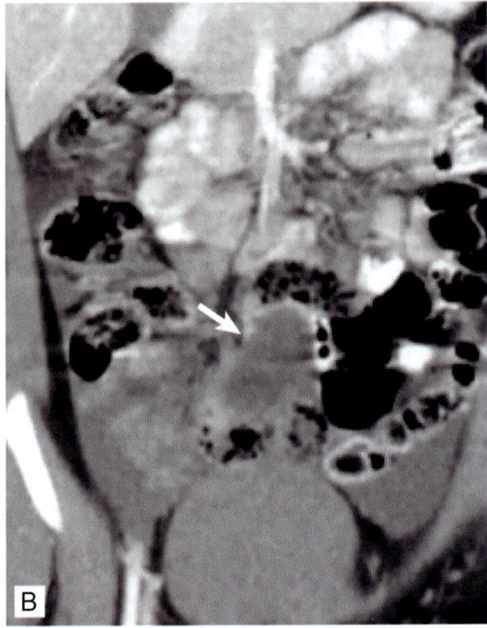

Figure 84.44 Contrast-enhanced axial (A) and coronal (B) computed tomography of the abdomen and pelvis from a 11-year-old boy with Meckel diverticulitis demonstrates a dilated blind-ending Meckel diverticulum in the central pelvis (*white arrow*), with mild surrounding stranding and free fluid.

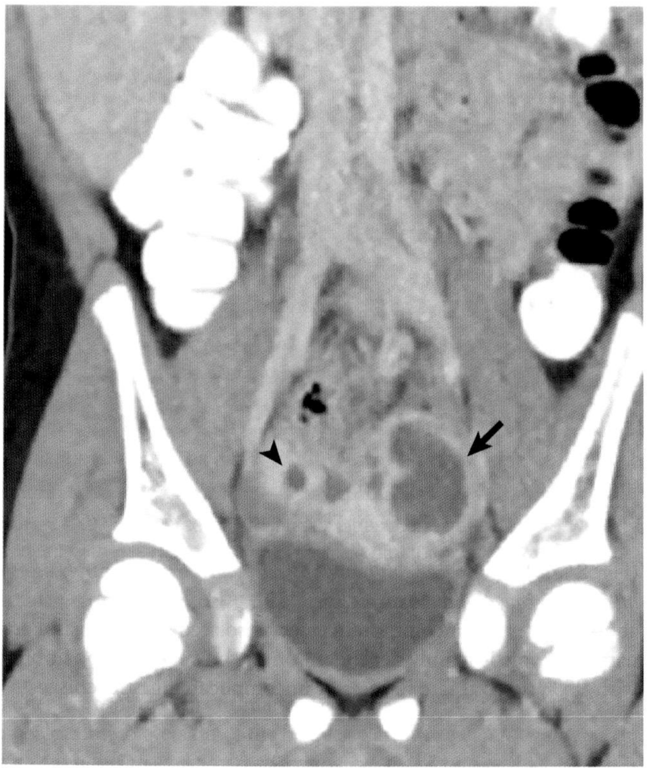

Figure 84.45 Contrast-enhanced coronal computed tomography of the abdomen and pelvis from a 9-year-old girl with perforated Meckel diverticulitis demonstrates multiple rim-enhancing abscesses in the pelvis (*black arrow, arrowhead*).

the renal cortex (Fig. 84.46). The bowel-in-bowel configuration may be simulated by echogenic stools, appendicitis, or Meckel diverticulum, leading to false-positive results [12,42]. *Findings such as interbowel fluid, fluid between the layers of intussusception, and absence of color flow are indicative of ischemia, irreducibility, and greater failure rates with enema reduction* [42]

Short-segment intussusception usually resolves spontaneously; however, the chances are low with the ileocolic type.

Radiologic management includes fluoroscopic air enema, liquid describing enema, and less commonly sonographic hydrostatic reduction.

- *Air enema is the most preferred because it is faster and associated with smaller perforations and lesser peritoneal contamination.* Pneumoperitoneum is an absolute procedural contraindication
- Hydrostatic enema is mostly reserved for cases with excessive gaseous distension of bowel or with a known pathological lead point [12]. A water-soluble near-isotonic or iso-osmolar contrast media is preferred [44]. Normal saline is used for sonographic guided hydrostatic enema reduction
- Overall, the rates of intussusception reduction using air enema are higher than those using contrast media with no significant difference in complication rates [45]

Air enema involves placement of a rectal catheter along with balloon inflation to keep it in position followed by air insufflation under fluoroscopy with pressure monitoring (pressure level not exceeding 120 mm Hg). Intussusception is identified as intraluminal soft tissue, commonly encountered within the transverse or ascending colon. Successful reduction leads to resolution of the intraluminal soft tissue and air reflux in the terminal ileal loops (Fig. 84.47). Repeat or delayed repeat (>2 hours) attempts after unsuccessful reduction allow for reduction in bowel wall and ileocecal valve edema. *Bowel perforation and tension pneumoperitoneum are the major procedural complication* [12,46].

Intussusception: Pearls to Remember

- Most common are idiopathic, ileocolic, or ileoileocolic
- Target or donut sign with bowel-in-bowel appearance is seen on transverse USG. Pseudokidney sign is seen on the longitudinal view
- Nonsurgical management includes fluoroscopic air enema, liquid enema, and sonographic hydrostatic reduction
- Air enema is faster and is associated with smaller perforations and lesser peritoneal contamination

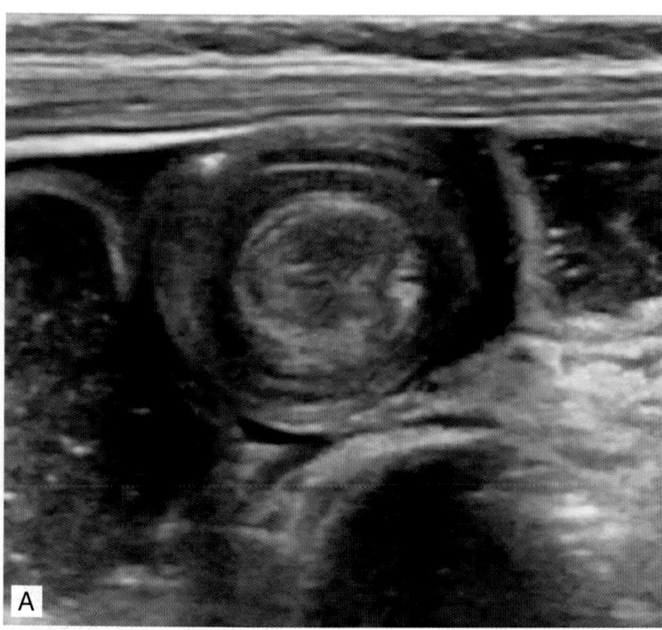

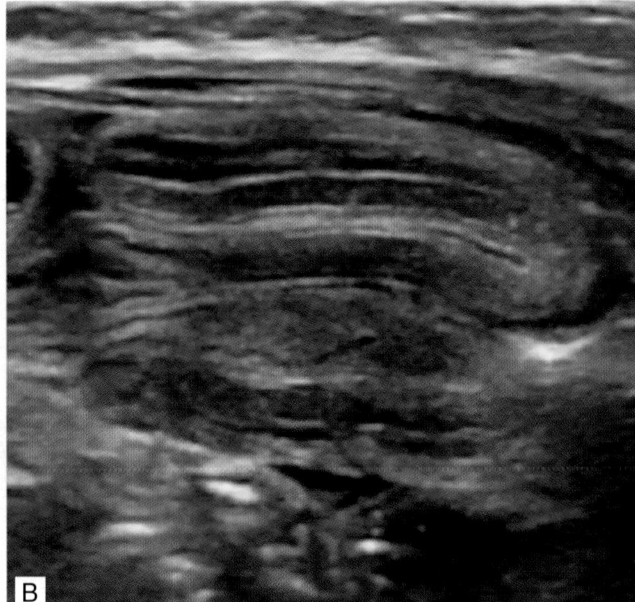

Figure 84.46 Ultrasound images of the right lower quadrant in a 4-month-old boy with ileocolic intussusception demonstrates the target or donut sign in transverse view (A) and pseudokidney sign in longitudinal view (B).

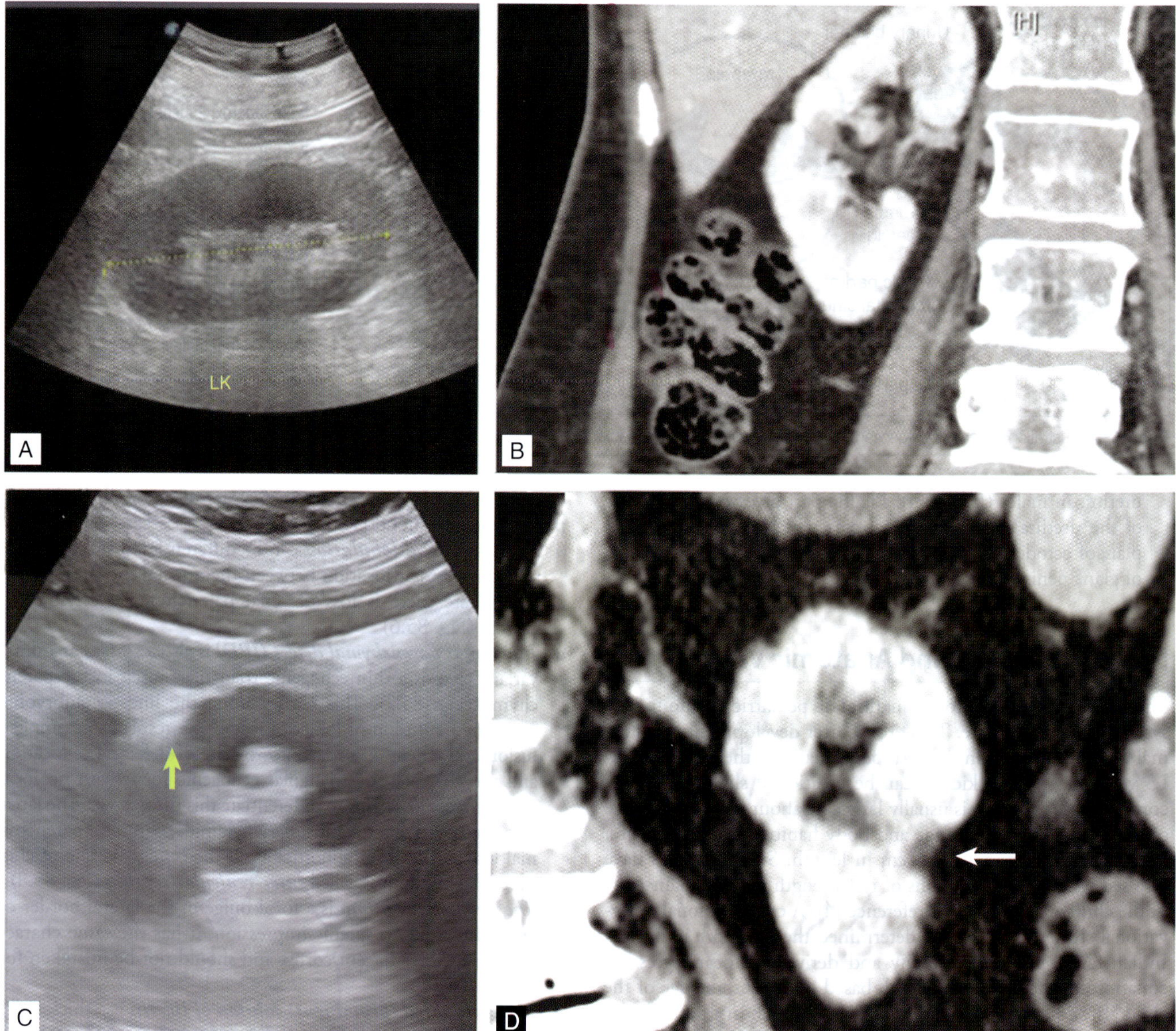

Figure 85.6 Persistent fetal lobulation versus parenchymal scar. (A) Sonogram and (B) CT coronal section showing lobulated contour of the kidney with parenchymal indentation in between the calyces. (C) Sonogram and (D) CT coronal section in another patient showing a left lower pole renal parenchymal scar overlying the region of medullary pyramid with loss of and resultant thinning of parenchyma.

either isoechoic or sometimes more echogenic compared to the adjacent cortex, but the renal outline is preserved. This can be mistaken for an intrarenal mass especially if the echogenicity is different (Fig. 85.9). In case of doubt, contrast enhanced computed tomography/magnetic resonance imaging (CT/MRI) will demonstrate density/signal characteristics and enhancement similar to the adjacent cortex, which helps in differentiating this from a focal lesion [13]

The renal pelvis can be completely within the renal sinus or partly outside the renal sinus called the *extrarenal pelvis*. Prominent extrarenal pelvis has to be differentiated from renal pelvis dilatation due to ureteropelvic junction (UPJ) obstruction; the latter usually shows some backpressure changes. Functional imaging like Lasix urography or dynamic renal scintigraphy would be helpful in this differentiation if there is a doubt.

Mild ureteral elongation and tortuosity, prominent mid segment of ureter, short kinks, and intraluminal mucosal folds in the proximal ureter are some fetal characteristics which can persist in newborns and infants and should not be mistaken for a pathology [3]. Mucosal folds disappear as the child grows whereas congenital ureteral valves can sometimes cause ureteric obstruction and should be included in the differential diagnosis of ureteric obstruction in children [14].

Another phenomenon in infants which should not be mistaken as pathological is focal bulge of inferolateral wall of urinary bladder, sometimes almost reaching up to the deep inguinal ring. This is called *bladder ears*, usually seen in infants less than 6 months of age and usually disappears in a fully distended bladder (Fig. 85.10). However, if there is herniation into the inguinal canal, it suggests a persistent processus vaginalis.

Urethra: Certain normal anatomical findings in voiding cystourethrogram of male posterior urethra can mimic disease. A shallow mucosal fold in the anterior wall of prostatic urethra called incisura is a common variant (Fig. 85.11). Thin folds can be seen as a filling defect in the posterior urethra below the level of verumontanum, simulating a posterior urethral valve. These are nonobstructing valves called plicae colliculi and do not cause obstruction or

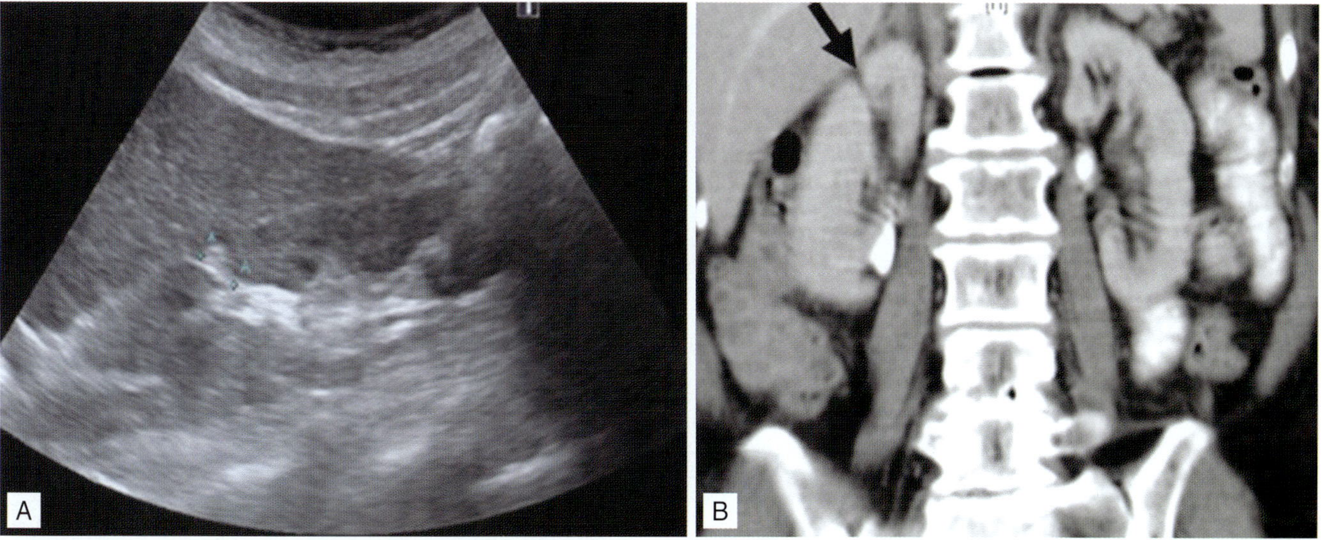

Figure 85.7 Junctional parenchymal defect. (A) Sonogram of right kidney showing a triangular echogenic notch in the parenchyma at the upper pole. (B) Coronal CT section of the same patient showing the junctional parenchymal defect (*arrow*).

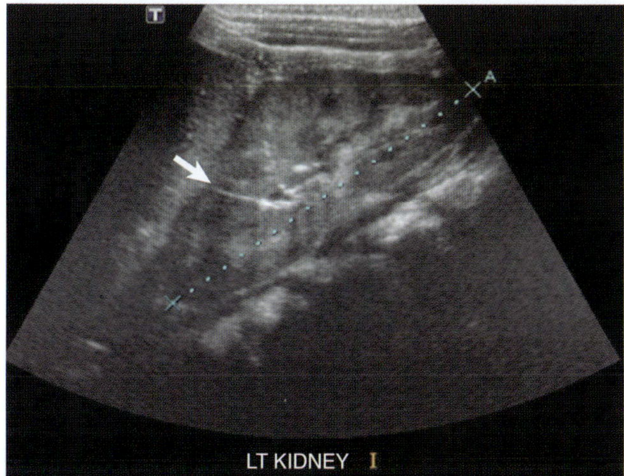

Figure 85.8 Inter-renicular septum. Sonogram through the left kidney in a 5-months-old child showing a linear echogenic focus (*arrow*) in the upper pole extending up to the hilum.

proximal dilatation (Fig. 85.12). Ectasia of posterior urethra is rarely seen as a normal variant without obstruction [15].

Diagnostic Procedures

Knowledge of various imaging techniques available, their techniques, indications, and limitations are of paramount importance in the radiological evaluation of a patient. In particular, for the pediatric age group, each examination has to be justified and chosen based on the age and clinical presentation weighing the risk versus benefit. Imaging techniques have to be optimized to produce images of diagnostic quality in a safe and comfortable environment to allay anxiety while the radiation is kept as low as reasonably achievable. Special attention to create a child-friendly environment like painting on the walls, toys, videos, and immobilization devices for very small children all go a long way in ensuring smooth conduct of examination of the child. The various imaging techniques available for evaluation of genitourinary tract pathologies in a child is discussed briefly.

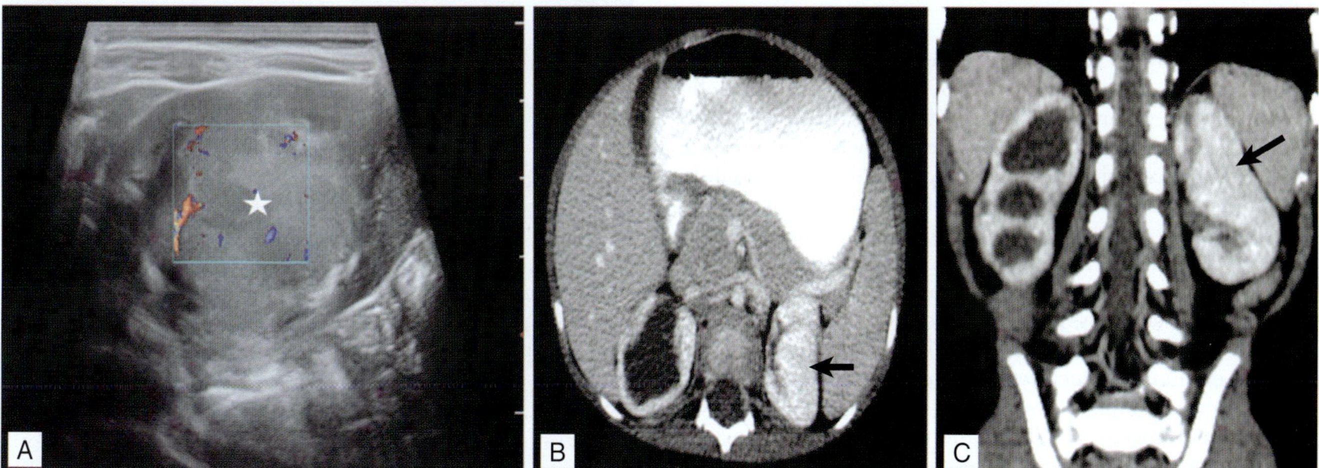

Figure 85.9 Prominent column of Bertin. (A) Ultrasonography of left kidney in a 2-year-old child shows a thick band of cortex (*asterisk*) causing splaying of the renal sinus which was initially mistaken for an intrarenal mass due to its increased echogenicity. (B & C) CECT scan of the abdomen, axial and coronal images shows hypertrophied parenchyma (*arrows*) with enhancement similar to the adjacent parenchyma and preserved renal outline in keeping with a prominent column of Bertin. Note the right hydronephrosis on CT.

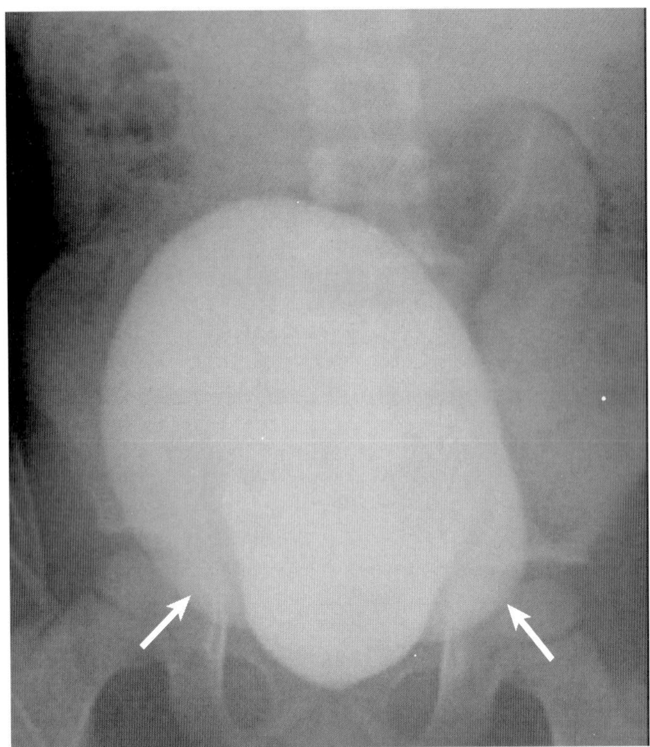

Figure 85.10 MCU in a 5-year-old child, full bladder image shows bilateral bladder ears (*arrows*).

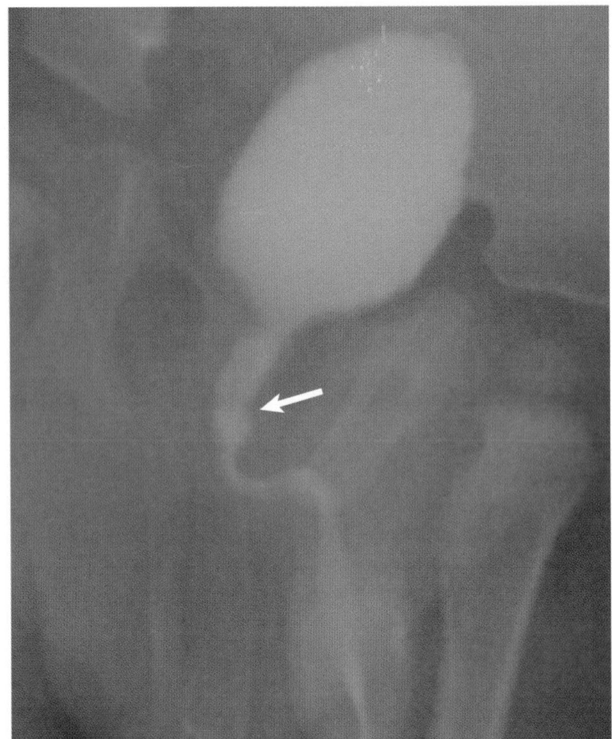

Figure 85.11 MCU in a 1-year-old child shows incisura—a shallow mucosal fold (*arrow*) in the anterior wall of prostatic urethra which is a normal variant.

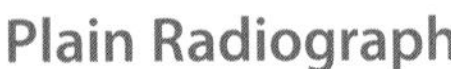

Plain Radiograph

Plain radiography has limited role in the evaluation of children with suspected genitourinary tract (GUT) pathologies. Abdominal radiographs of kidney, ureter, bladder (KUB) region provide information regarding urinary tract calculi, abnormal air in the GUT, pneumoperitoneum, pneumoretroperitoneum, retained foreign bodies, position of stents and bony abnormalities of spine and pelvis [16]. However, ionizing radiation exposure is a major limitation especially in children with chronic diseases warranting repeated imaging.

Ultrasonography

Ultrasonography (USG) is most widely used and is often the initial technique in the evaluation of pediatric GUT pathologies. It has the advantage of being widely available, affordable and lacks ionizing radiation. The technological advances in USG over the years has resulted in significant improvement in image quality. Use of appropriate probes and pediatric settings is important to obtain quality images. Using a linear high frequency probe (up to 12–15 MHz depending on the equipment) is recommended for neonates and focused examination of structures in older children. Low frequency curvilinear probe (frequency of 2.5–7.5 MHz) is useful while scanning older children and for examining structures at a depth. A small foot print sector probe is gaining popularity for scanning through narrow windows like intercostal spaces. The main indications include screening of a neonate with suspected congenital anomalies, antenatally detected hydronephrosis, renal cysts/mass, complicated urinary tract infections (UTI), hematuria, renal/ureteric colic, post void residue (PVR) evaluation, evaluation of internal gonads in disorders of sexual differentiation (DSD), testicular and scrotal pathologies like torsion, tumors, epididymo-orchitis, hydrocele, etc.

Contrast enhanced USG using microbubble contrast agents instilled into the bladder has been suggested as a radiation free alternative to look for vesicoureteric reflux (VUR). Some studies have reported almost similar diagnostic accuracy in comparison

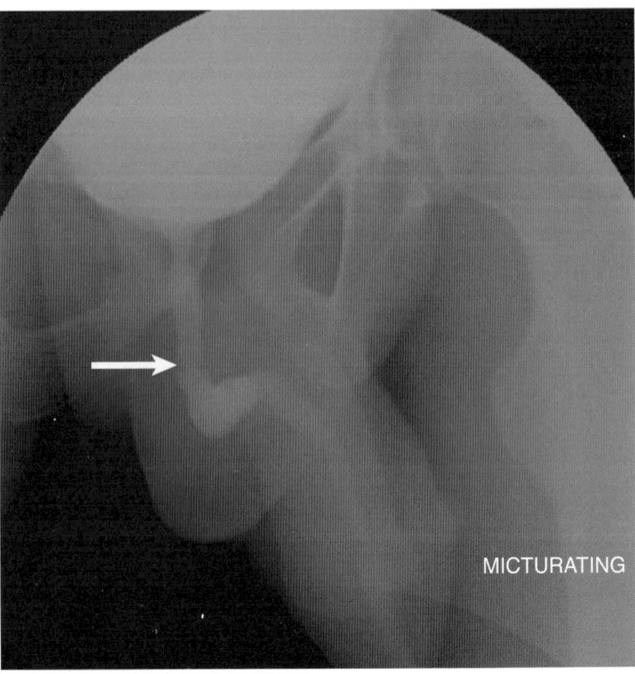

Figure 85.12 MCU in a male child showing a thin lucent filling defect (*arrow*) in the posterior urethra with no features of obstruction—representing a nonobstructing plicae colliculi.

to voiding cystourethrography (VCUG) for higher grades of VUR. However, the procedure is highly operator dependent [17].

Duplex sonography provides important hemodynamic information using both color and spectral display of blood flow in the organ and vessels. It plays an important role in the evaluation of pyelonephritis, epididymo-orchitis, testicular and ovarian torsion, evaluation of vasculature in renovascular pathologies and in post renal transplant settings.

Intravenous Urography

Intravenous urography enables both morphologic and functional evaluation of the kidney and upper urinary tract. It involves intravenous injection of a low osmolar iodinated contrast media and series of imaging done at specific intervals subsequently. Due to concerns related to radiation exposure and with advent of low dose CT and MR urography, the role of IVU is limited to a few specific indications in certain centers, which include congenital anomalies like UPJ obstruction, evaluation of hydroureteronephrosis, ectopic insertion of ureter, and GU tuberculosis. The protocol for IVU in children varies between centers. In our institution, we avoid tomogram images.

- A scout KUB is initially performed followed by IV contrast which is administered in the dose of 1 mL/kg body weight
- After IV injection of contrast, KUB images are taken at 3, 7, and 15 minutes interval
- Delayed images are performed if indicated after evaluation of these initial images
- Abdominal compression using a binder is also avoided in children
- Lasix urogram is performed in patients with suspected congenital UPJ obstruction. Injection Furosemide is given IV at a dose of 1 mg/kg (maximum 20 mg) after the 15-minute film and a post Furosemide image is performed 10–12 minutes after diuretic injection (Fig. 85.13)
- Full bladder and post void images are not routinely performed in a child to avoid unnecessary radiation

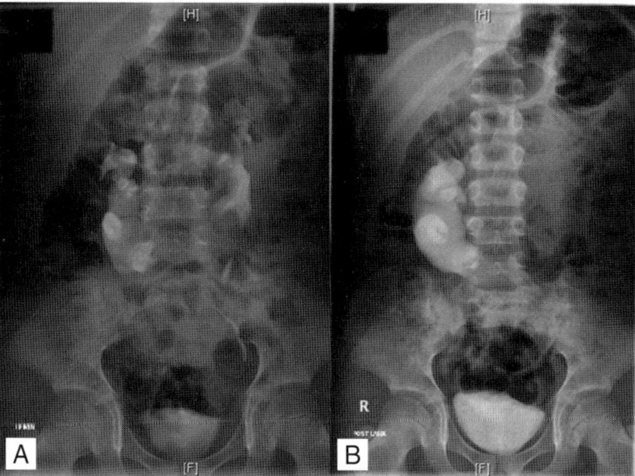

Figure 85.13 (A) IVU Lasix urogram in a 9-year-old boy with abdominal pain. 20-minute urogram shows horseshoe kidney and hydronephrosis of *right-side* moiety with disproportionate dilatation of renal pelvis. (B) Lasix urogram demonstrates ballooning of the renal pelvis suggestive of PUJ obstruction.

Micturating/Voiding Cystourethrogram (MCUG/VCUG)

Micturating cystourethrogram is the investigation of choice for evaluation of bladder, urethra, and VUR (Fig. 85.14). Retrograde urethrography (RGU) is not routinely performed in children. It is important to remember that overfilling or underfilling of the bladder should be avoided. The normal bladder capacity for age can be calculated using the formula:

$$\text{Bladder capacity (mL)} = [\text{Age in years} + 2] \times 30 \text{ mL.}$$

Fluoroscopic screening is done to look for reflux while filling the bladder. To increase the detection rate of VUR, some authors suggest a cyclic VCU approach [18] where the bladder is filled in cycles three times, with the child voiding around the catheter twice and the third time, catheter is removed when the child starts to void. Passive VUR occurs during the bladder-filling phase whereas active reflux occurs during micturition. Lateral and oblique views are essential to avoid missing mild reflux in the distal ureters which can be obscured by a filled bladder on AP films (Fig. 85.15). These views also help in visualization of bladder diverticula (Fig. 85.16). The micturition phase is carefully assessed for voiding dysfunction or structural abnormalities of the urethra like posterior urethral valves (PUV), stricture, fistula or congenital anomalies like duplication.

Genitography

Genitography is a fluoroscopic procedure which involves injection of a water-soluble contrast media into the perineal opening to opacify the urethra, bladder, and vagina in a case of persistent urogenital sinus (UGS). In persistent UGS, where there is failure of separation of urinary and genital tracts resulting in a single perineal opening in a female child, genitogram demonstrates the exact site of communication and rectourogenital

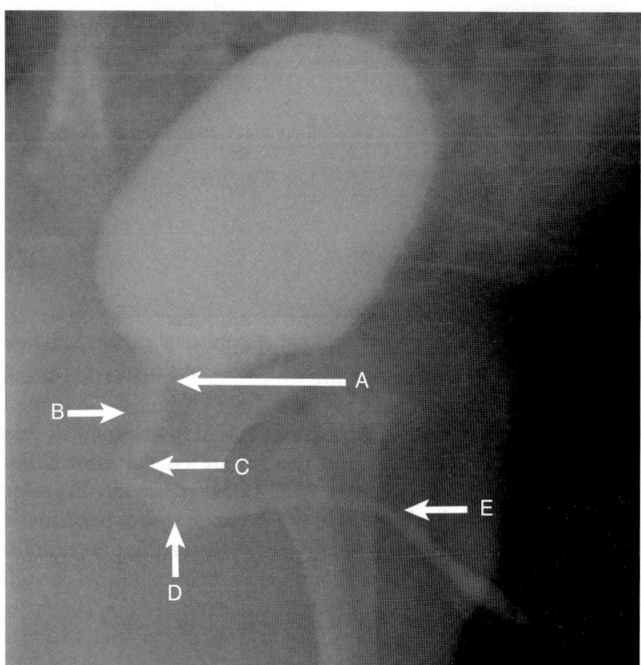

Figure 85.14 Normal MCU in an 8-months-old male child. (A) Bladder neck. (B) Verumontanum. (C) Membranous urethra. (D) Bulbar urethra. (E) Penile urethra.

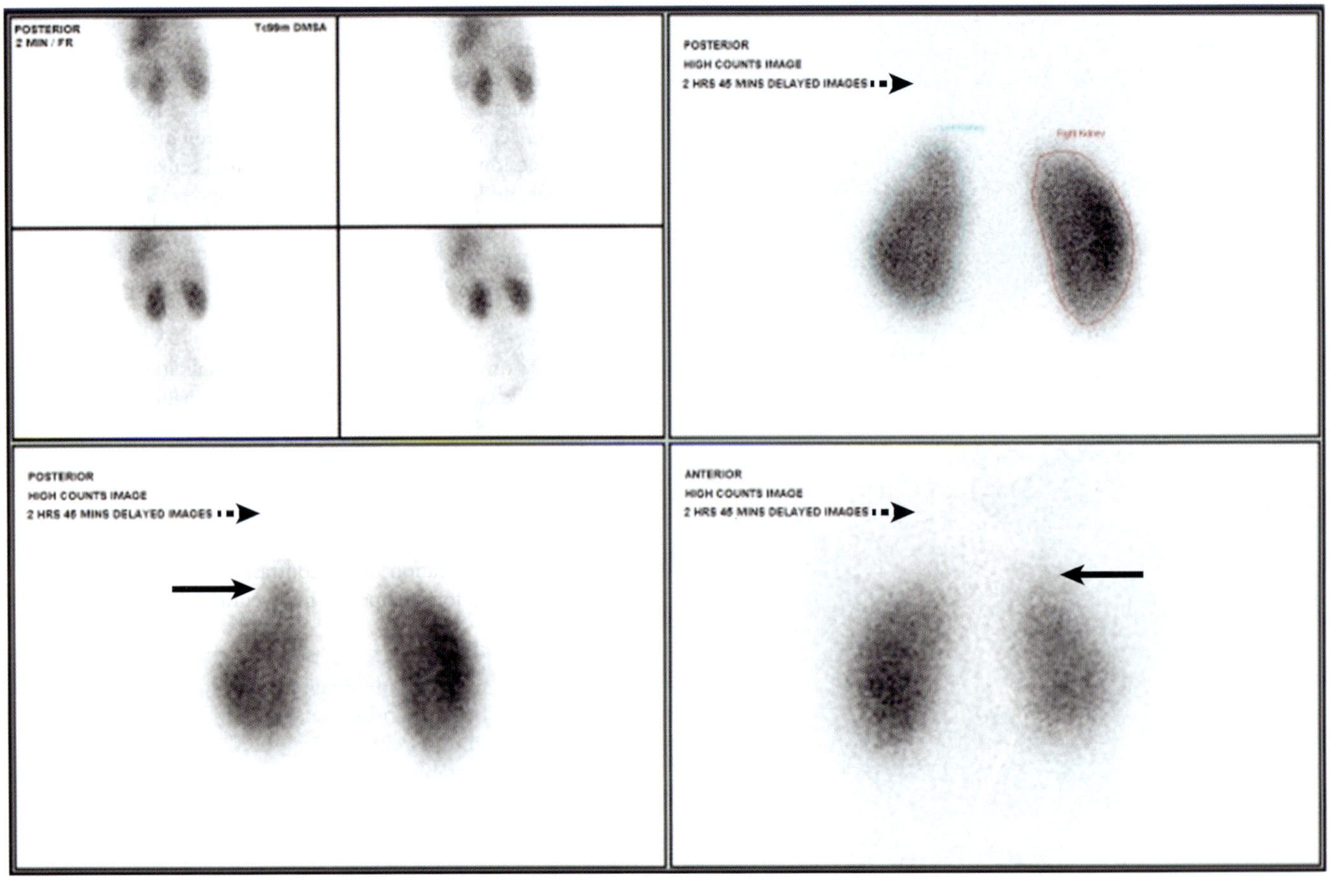

Figure 85.19 Tc99m DMSA scan in a 5-year-old girl with left VUR and recurrent UTI shows mildly impaired tracer uptake in the left renal parenchyma on the early images (left top column) and normal excretion. There is inhomogeneous tracer uptake in the cortex in the left kidney on the delayed images with a photon deficient area in the upper pole suggestive of a scar (*black arrow*).

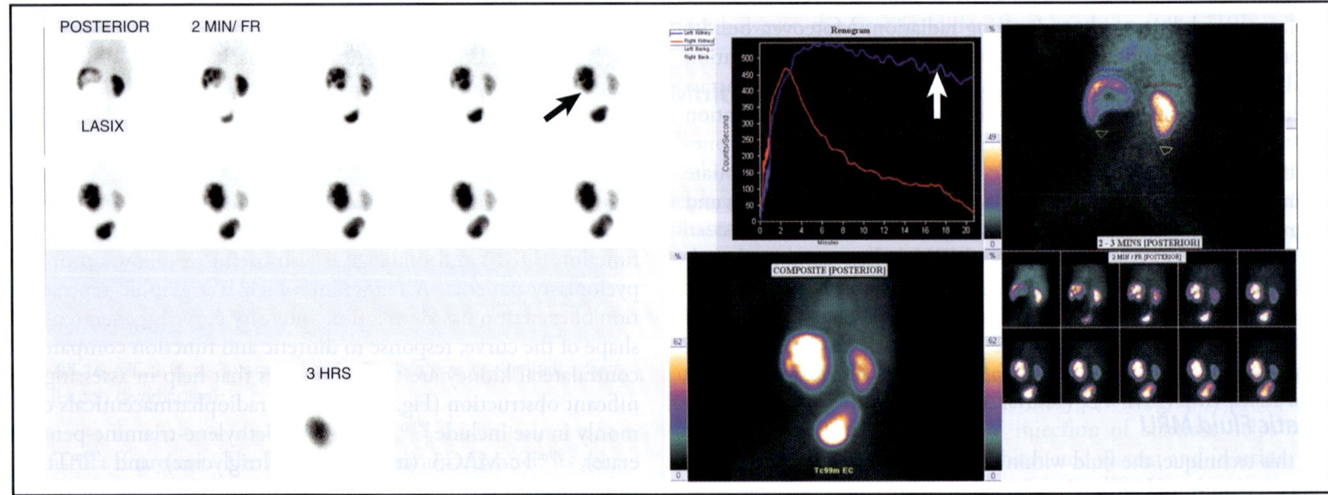

Figure 85.20 Tc 99m EC (L-Ethylenedicysteine) dynamic renal scintigraphy of a 5-months-old child with left PUJ obstruction shows an enlarged left kidney with slow tracer clearance into a dilated pelvicalyceal system (*black arrow*), delayed drainage and significant holdup on delayed image. Time activity curve shows obstructed drainage in the left kidney (*white arrow*) and normal drainage in the right kidney.

Videourodynamics (VUD)

Videourodynamic study is performed in children with neurogenic bladder and complex voiding dysfunction. The bladder and sphincter functions are assessed during the filling, storage, and micturition phases. A graphic recording of the various pressures (bladder pressure, rectal pressure, detrusor pressure), urine flow and electromyography of the sphincter is done along with voiding cystourethrography (VCUG) [3].

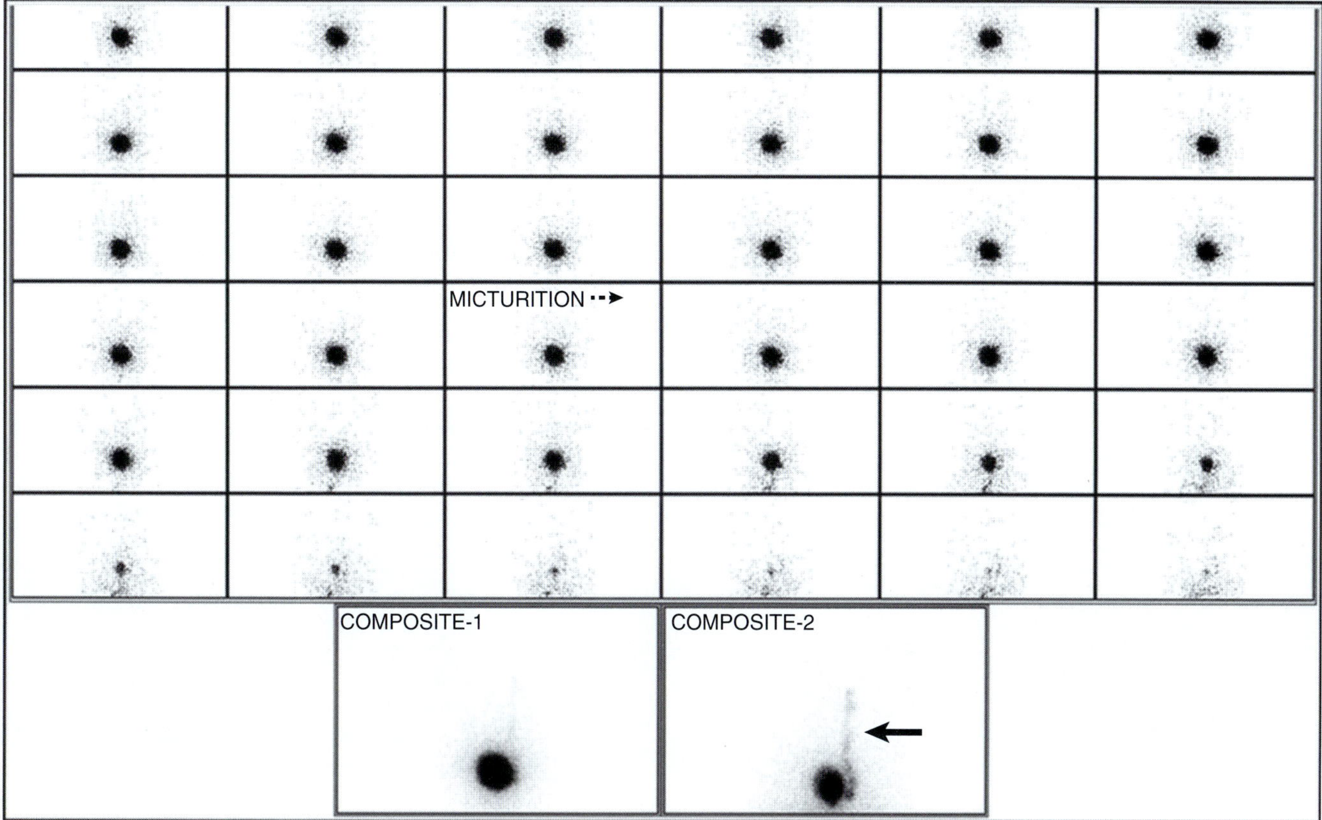

Figure 85.21 Direct isotope cystography showing right vesicoureteric reflux in the micturition phase (*black arrow*).

Developmental Anomalies of the Kidney and Urinary Tract

Renal Agenesis

Failure of ureteric bud to come in contact with the metanephric blastema results in failure of induction to form nephric vesicles and hence the development of the kidney. This is often associated with failure of development of the ipsilateral ureter and hemitrigone. In some cases, a blind ending ureter may be seen. Unilateral agenesis has a prevalence of 0.1% of live births and is more commonly seen in males with a male to female ration of 3:1. Agenesis of ipsilateral adrenal gland is seen in 10% of patients with unilateral renal agenesis [3].

The other anomalies associated with renal agenesis include agenesis of ejaculatory duct with resultant seminal vesicle obstruction/cyst, which is called Zinner syndrome. Uterine anomalies like bicornuate uterus with ipsilateral obstruction of hemivagina and renal agenesis constitute the OHVIRA (obstructed hemivagina and ipsilateral renal agenesis). Zinners syndrome has been proposed as a male counterpart of OHVIRA [26,27]. Renal agenesis can be associated with various other syndromes and chromosomal disorders including VACTERL association. This acronym stands for V—vertebral anomalies, A—anorectal malformation, C—cardiac defects, T—tracheal anomalies, E—esophageal anomalies, R—renal and radial ray anomalies, and L—limb anomalies. Another association includes the MURCS, which constitutes Müllerian aplasia, renal agenesis, and cervicothoracic somite dysplasia (Fig. 85.22).

Bilateral renal agenesis is very rare and incompatible with life. Severe oligohydramnios in this situation results in Potter's syndrome with abnormal facial features, small chest, and limb abnormalities. Death occurs due to pulmonary hypoplasia.

Supernumerary Kidneys

This is a rare anatomic variant where one or more kidneys are present in addition to the native kidneys. They have separate collecting systems with a complete or partially duplicated ureter. A distinct capsule and separate blood supply helps one to differentiate supernumerary kidney from a Duplex kidney [28]. Embryologically, it occurs due to division of the nephrogenic cord into two metanephric blastemas. The ureteric bud may or may not undergo division.

Abnormalities of Position and Rotation

Positional abnormalities occur when the normal migration and ascent of the developing kidney is disrupted.

- Congenital simple ectopia refers to the kidney lying outside of the renal fossa on the same side. This could be caudal abdominal ectopia when kidney is located below the normal position of D12-L3 vetebra, pelvic ectopia (if the kidney does not ascend above the pelvic brim) and rarely intrathoracic, if it is associated with a congenital diaphragmatic hernia
- Sometimes the kidney crosses over to the other side producing crossed renal ectopia, which can be fused or unfused. Lot of other urological abnormalities can be associated with renal ectopia, VUR being the commonest [29]
- If associated anomalies or syndromes are excluded and if there is a normal contralateral kidney and no hydronephrosis, an ectopic kidney may not require any further investigation

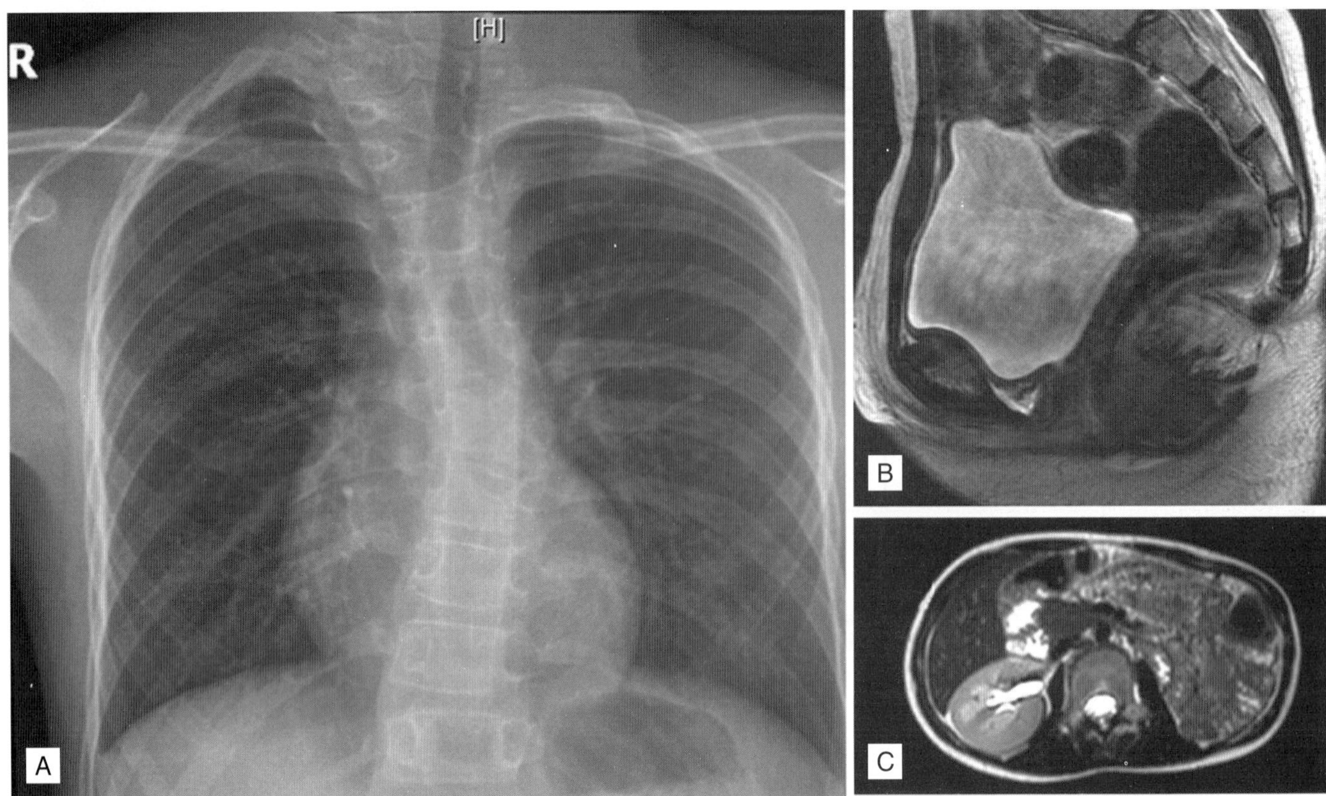

Figure 85.22 MURCS (Müllerian aplasia, renal agenesis, and cervicothoracic somite dysplasia) association. (A) Chest radiograph of a 12-year-old girl showing multilevel vertebral segmentation anomalies. (B) On MRI T2 high-resolution sagittal image, the uterus is absent and (C) axial T2 image shows empty left renal fossa.

- Abnormal medial course of the colon occupying the renal fossa ("loop to loop colon" sign) and a lying down (pancake) adrenal gland due to long slender shape of the ipsilateral adrenal gland due to empty renal fossa are observed in renal agenesis/ectopia [30]
- When the normal medial rotation of kidney does not occur during ascent, it results in a malrotated kidney with the pelvicalyceal system facing anteriorly or laterally (Figs. 85.23 and 85.24)

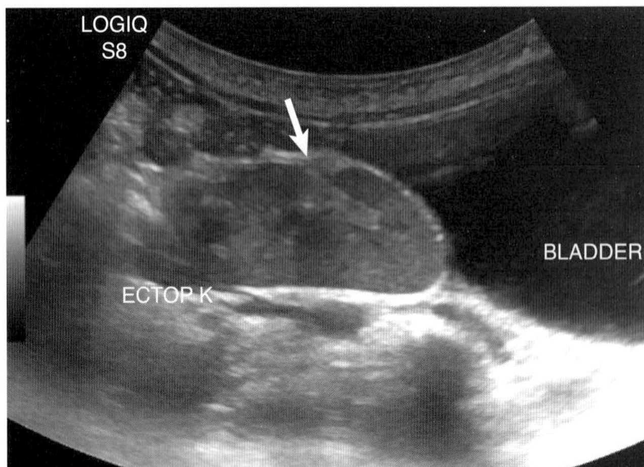

Figure 85.23 Ectopic kidney. Ultrasonography in a 4-year-old child shows an ectopic pelvic kidney and associated malrotation with anteriorly facing renal hilum (*arrow*).

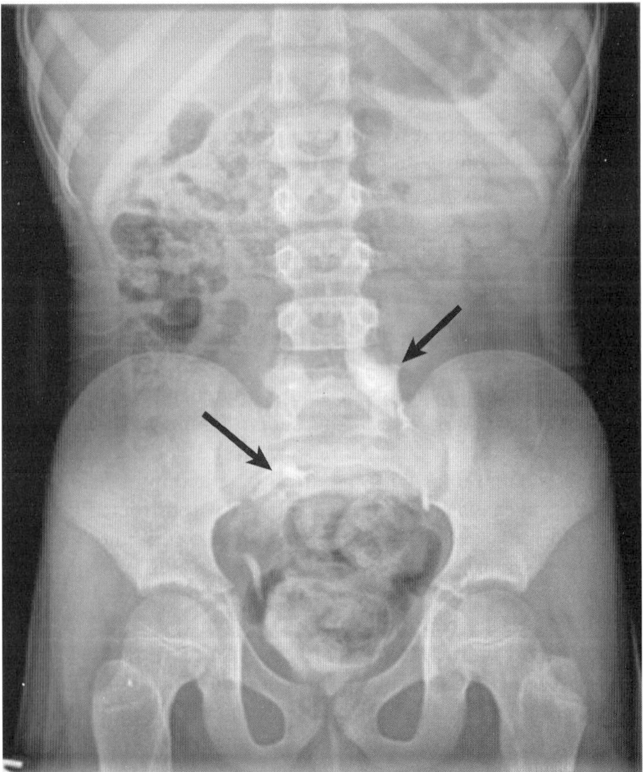

Figure 85.24 Bilateral pelvic kidneys with associated malrotation. IVU of an 11-year-old child, 7 minutes urogram showing bilateral pelvic kidneys (*arrows*) with associated malrotation.

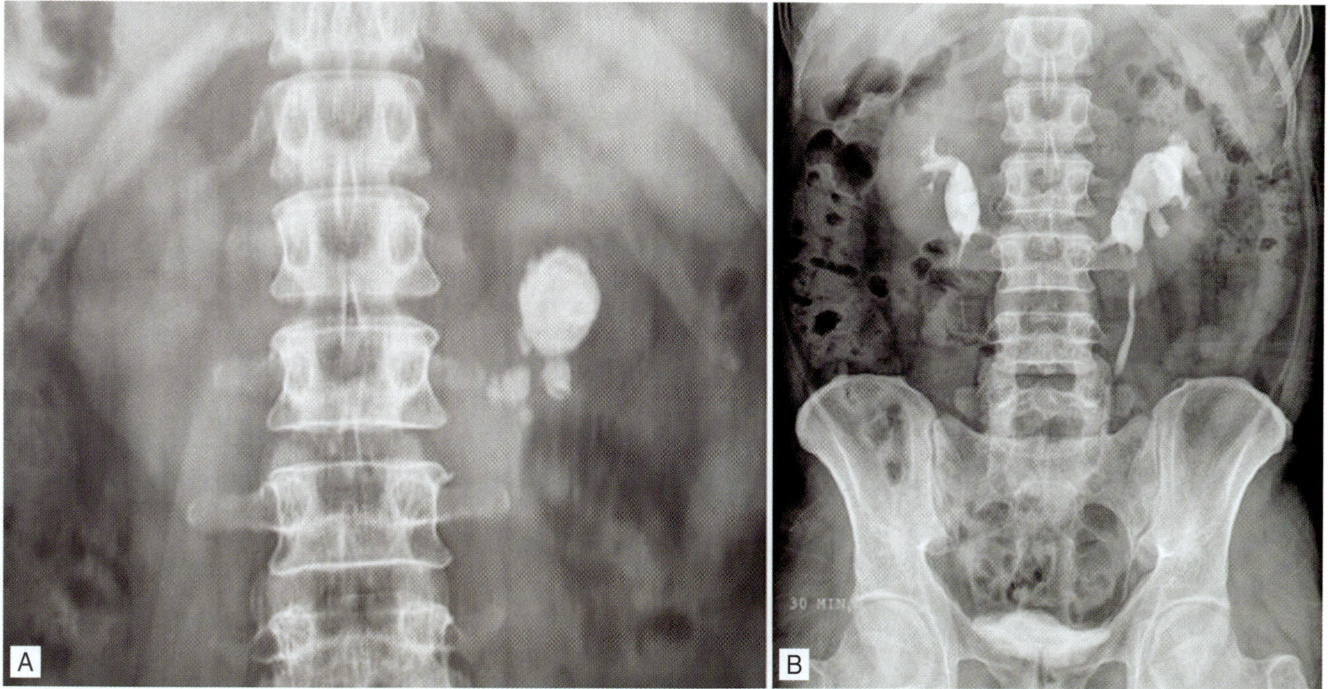

Figure 85.25 Horseshoe kidney. (A) IVU plain tomogram and (B) 20-minute urogram shows medially oriented lower pole of the kidneys and malrotated pelvicalyceal system bilaterally which is anteromedially oriented. Note the calculi in the *left side* moiety.

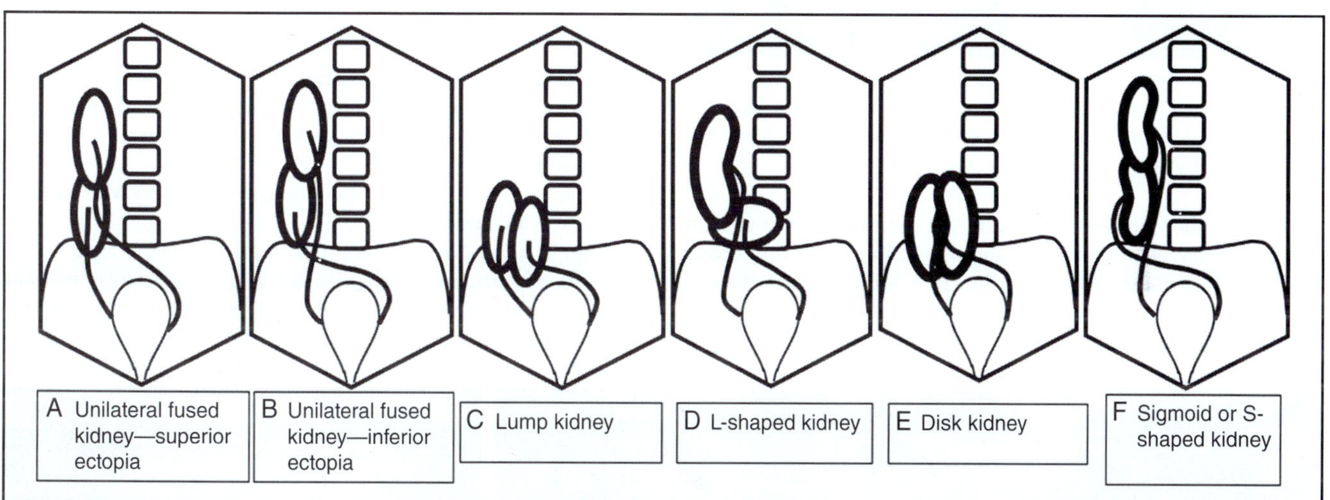

Figure 85.26 (A–F) Illustration of different types of fusion in crossed renal ectopia.

Abnormalities of Fusion

Horseshoe kidney is the commonest renal fusion anomaly with a quoted incidence of 0.25% in the general population [31]. The lower poles are medially aligned and fused in the midline, by a bridge of tissue called isthmus which can be parenchymal or fibrous. The isthmus lies mostly anterior to the aorta and IVC at the level of, and inferior to, inferior mesenteric artery (IMA). IMA prevents the further ascent of the fused kidneys. *They are usually asymptomatic but there is an increased incidence of PUJ obstruction, VUR, ureteric duplication, and Wilm's tumor reported* [32]. The metanephric blastema fuses together very early in the development before rotation begins and hence, an associated malrotation is seen in almost every case. On IVU, the lower calyces of both moieties come close together in the midline as if they are shaking hands with each other ("handholding calyces") (Fig. 85.25).

Crossed ectopia could be fused (majority, ~85%) or unfused (~10%). Very rarely, a solitary crossed ectopia and bilateral crossed ectopia can occur [33]. In crossed ectopia, the ureter crosses over to the normal side with normal insertion into the bladder. Various types of fusion can occur in crossed ectopic kidneys with varying degrees of rotational abnormalities in the ectopic and normal positioned kidney (Figs. 85.26 and 85.27). When normal rotation of both kidneys has happened, the fused kidneys will have renal pelvis facing in opposite direction and the ureters cross one over the other giving rise to a S shaped/sigmoid kidney. When parenchymal fusion occurs along the medial

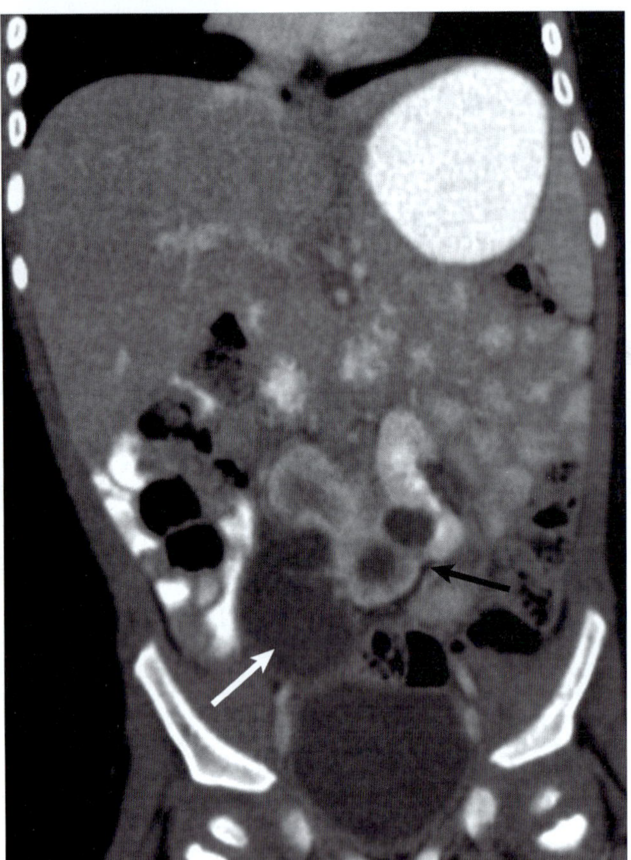

Figure 85.27 Crossed ectopia. Contrast enhanced CT coronal sections of a 3-year-old male child showing right crossed ectopia with "L" type fusion (*black arrow*). Associated right PUJ obstruction noted with dilated renal pelvis (*white arrow*).

border of the kidneys, it results in pancake/ring/doughnut shaped kidney. When there is extensive fusion along the medial border it forms a disc/shield shape. In a lump kidney, there is substantial fusion between the two kidneys, not necessarily along the medial border [34].

Congenital Anomalies of the Pelvicalyceal System and Ureter

Megacalicosis/Polycalicosis

Dilatation of calyces in the absence of obstruction with a normal caliber renal pelvis and ureter constitute magacalyces. The calyces have a faceted appearance with absent papillary impression. It can be unilateral or bilateral (Fig. 85.28). Though exact pathogenesis is not clear, underdevelopment of renal medullary pyramids has been suggested as a possible cause for this morphologic appearance of calyces. Often there is also increased number of calyces and calyces have a polygonal appearance when it is called mega-polycalycosis. The number of calyces increases to 20–25, where as normal kidney has 10–14 calyces. The interlobar arteries are not displaced/stretched in contrast to hydronephrosis, and the renal cortical thickness is maintained. Function of the kidney is preserved in megapolycalycosis but there is an increased risk of infection and stone formation due to stasis [35,36]. Megacalycosis can sometimes coexist with primary megaureter which is important to recognize and avoid interpreting the calyceal dilatation as due to obstructing primary megaureter. The key would be to assess the renal pelvis morphology, which would be normal in morphology and caliber in congenital primary megaureter whereas it will be dilated in obstruction (Fig. 85.29). If in doubt, renal scintigraphy can be done to assess the ureteric drainage to quantify the degree of obstruction before operative decision is made [36].

Pyelocalyceal Diverticulum

Calyceal diverticulum is a congenital outpouching from the renal collecting system lined by transitional epithelium. Stone formation is the most common complication reported in 9.5–50% of patients [37,38].

- Type 1 pyelocalyceal diverticulum communicates with a minor calyx or infundibulum
- Type 2 communicates with renal pelvis or major calyx

Mean size is around 10 mm, though larger diverticulae measuring a few centimeters can be seen. On USG, an anechoic cyst will be seen indistinguishable from other cortical cysts, unless a

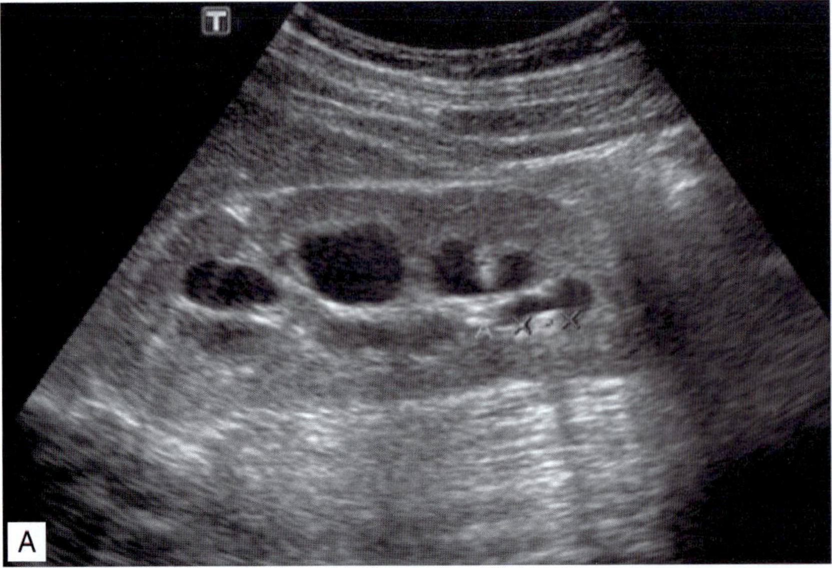

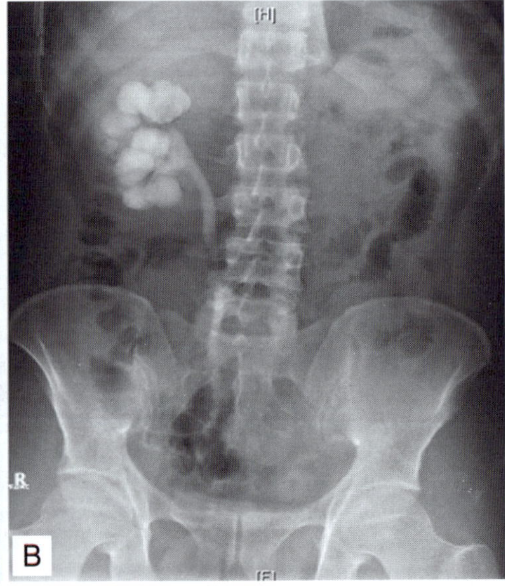

Figure 85.28 Congenital megacalycosis. (A) Ultrasonogram and (B) IVU 20 minute urogram showing dilated polygonal shaped calyces with normal renal pelvis, ureter and maintained cortical thickness in the right kidney. Stasis calculus is demonstrated in the lower pole calyx (*calipers* in A).

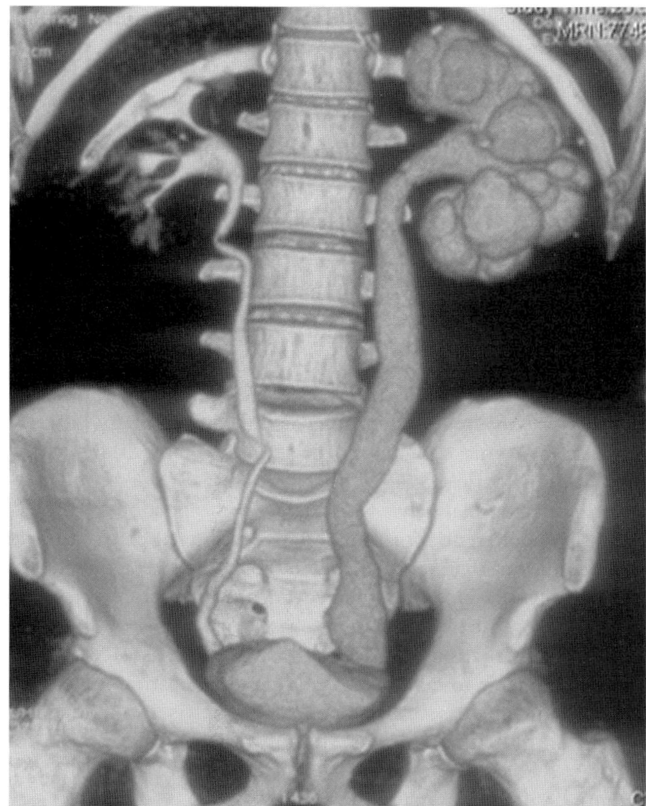

Figure 85.29 Left megapolycalycosis and left megaureter. Three-dimensional reconstructed CT image showing increased number of calyces which are enlarged and polygonal shaped, normal caliber renal pelvis and tapered narrowing of the juxtavesical segment of ureter.

mobile calculus is demonstrated within. On IVU, the outpouching from the pelvicalyceal system will show gradual filling-in of contrast. The same finding can be observed in CT urography (Fig. 85.30). Intervention and ablation is required if complicated with infection/calculi.

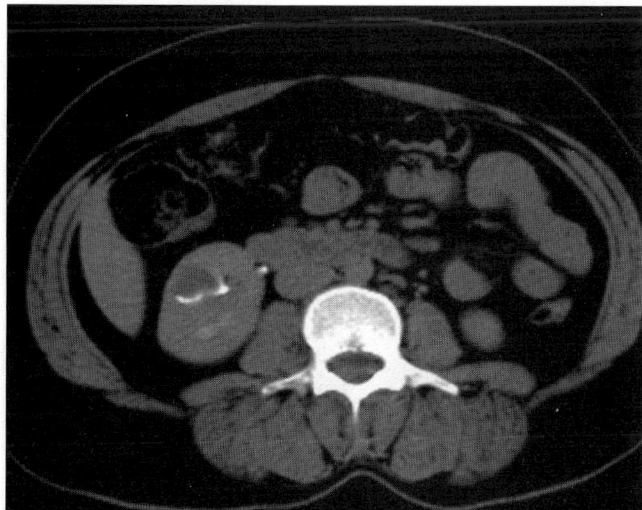

Figure 85.30 Type 1 pyelocalyceal diverticulum. CT axial section, urographic phase shows a cystic lesion in the interpole in close relation to a calyx with contrast extending from the calyx to the cyst in this excretory phase film.

Infundibular and Infundibulopelvic Stenosis

This is an extremely rare anomaly where there is congenital narrowing of the infundibulum with resultant hydrocalycosis. Associated stenosis of pelvis can occur resulting in infundibulopelvic stenosis [39]. Infundibular narrowing can be due to intrinsic cause or extrinsic cause like an extrinsic vascular compression. Congenital intrinsic infundibulopelvic stenosis needs to be differentiated from intrinsic stenosis due to acquired causes like infection, neoplasm or trauma. It can be unilateral or bilateral. It is considered a milder form of disease in the spectrum of obstructive renal dysplasias, the most severe form being infundibulopelvic atresia causing multicystic dysplastic kidney (MCDK) [40].

Ureteropelvic Duplication Anomalies

Pathophysiology and Clinical Presentation

Duplication of the collecting system is considered as one of the commonest developmental anomalies of the kidney. Reported prevalence of duplex kidneys ranges from 0.3% to 6% [41]. Varying degrees of duplication can occur, ranging from a bifid pelvis to ureters joining at any level along its course and complete duplication of ureters. Complete duplication occurs when two separate ureteric buds arise from the mesonephric duct. In complete duplication, the upper pole moiety ureter inserts medially and at a lower level in the urinary bladder compared to the lower pole moiety ureter. This upper moiety ureter could also have an ectopic insertion and can sometimes be associated with a ureterocele, causing obstruction of the upper pole moiety. The lower pole moiety inserts at a higher and lateral position in the bladder making it prone for VUR. This pattern of ureteric insertion in complete duplication of ureters is called the *Weigert Meyer rule* (Fig. 85.31).

Duplex kidney could be an incidental finding in many patients. However, some patients present with complications like VUR or

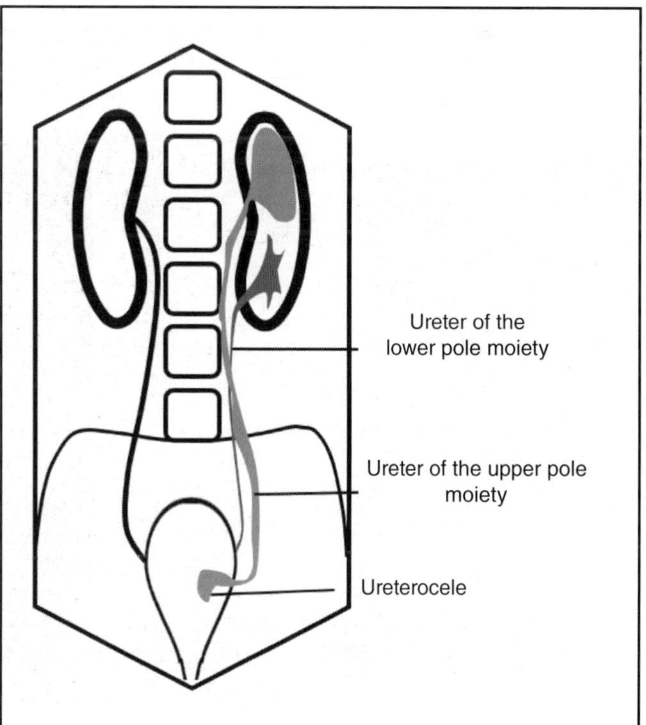

Figure 85.31 Illustration of Weigert Meyer rule in complete duplication.

obstruction. Ectopic ureteric insertion presents with clinical features related to urinary tract infection, obstruction or dribbling of urine depending on the site of ectopic insertion. Obstruction can be due to various reasons including a ureterocoele or associated UPJ in duplex kidneys. Rarely ureterocele can prolapse into the posterior urethra causing bladder outlet obstruction symptoms. Imaging helps to identify the cause of obstruction, demonstrate VUR if present and delineate the course and site of ectopic ureters in a complicated duplex system [42].

Imaging Features

- USG can diagnose a duplex collecting system when there is an enlarged kidney with two distinct collecting systems separated by a bridge of normal renal parenchyma. Hydroureteronephrosis with associated polar parenchymal scars and patulous VUJ suggests VUR
- "Faceless kidney" sign is a CT sign described in duplex kidney. On axial images, a section through the intervening parenchyma between the two collecting systems do not show the normal sinus signature. Since the normal face of the kidney is lacking, it has been termed the "faceless" kidney (Fig. 85.32)
- An obstructed grossly hydronephrotic upper moiety can cause mass effect on the lower pole moiety with a characteristic "drooping lilly" appearance of lower moiety pelvicalyceal system on IVP (Fig. 85.33)
- MRU is the technique of choice to clearly delineate the urinary tract anatomy, course of the ectopic ureter and site of ectopic insertion, especially when there is a poorly functioning moiety [42]
- Isotope studies/dynamic MRU help to assess the function of the two moieties
- Traditional imaging methods which use ionizing radiation like IVU and CT are largely being replaced by MRU in the evaluation of complicated duplex systems. Scintigraphy helps to assess drainage and split renal function in an obstructed system. Though dynamic MRI can also be used for this assessment, its performance in comparison to scintigraphy needs to be evaluated prospectively [43]

UPJ Obstruction

UPJ obstruction is defined as an anatomical or functional obstruction to the flow of urine from renal pelvis into the ureter at the pelviureteric junction. The exact etiology of congenital UPJ obstruction is not clear. An intrinsic mural abnormality is considered more likely than other causes like valves. Secondary UPJ obstruction is a result of strictures due to various causes and tumor. Occasionally, crossing vessels have been implicated in the pathogenesis of UPJ obstruction, and it is important to identify then preoperatively if present to avoid failed pyeloplasty [44].

Both anatomic and functional studies are important in the evaluation of patients with UPJ obstruction. USG can demonstrate a dilated renal pelvis which is out of proportion to calyceal dilatation. Differentiation from a large extrarenal pelvis requires demonstration of functional obstruction. On IVU, long standing UPJ obstruction and gross hydronephrosis produces negative pyelogram on the nephrographic phase (Fig. 85.34). In intermittent UPJ obstruction and doubtful cases, Lasix assisted urography is invaluable to demonstrate a functional obstruction, where hold up and increase in diameter of the pelvis can be demonstrated on diuretic stress after administration of injection Furosemide. Radioisotope studies can quantitatively assess the differential renal function.

Ureterocele

Ureterocele refers to the cystic dilatation of terminal ureter in the intravesical intramural segment. They can be either orthotopic or ectopic, the latter occurring at an ectopic site of insertion of ureter. Failure of resorption and canalization of an embryonic membrane (Chwalla's membrane) that covers the ureteric orifice in the

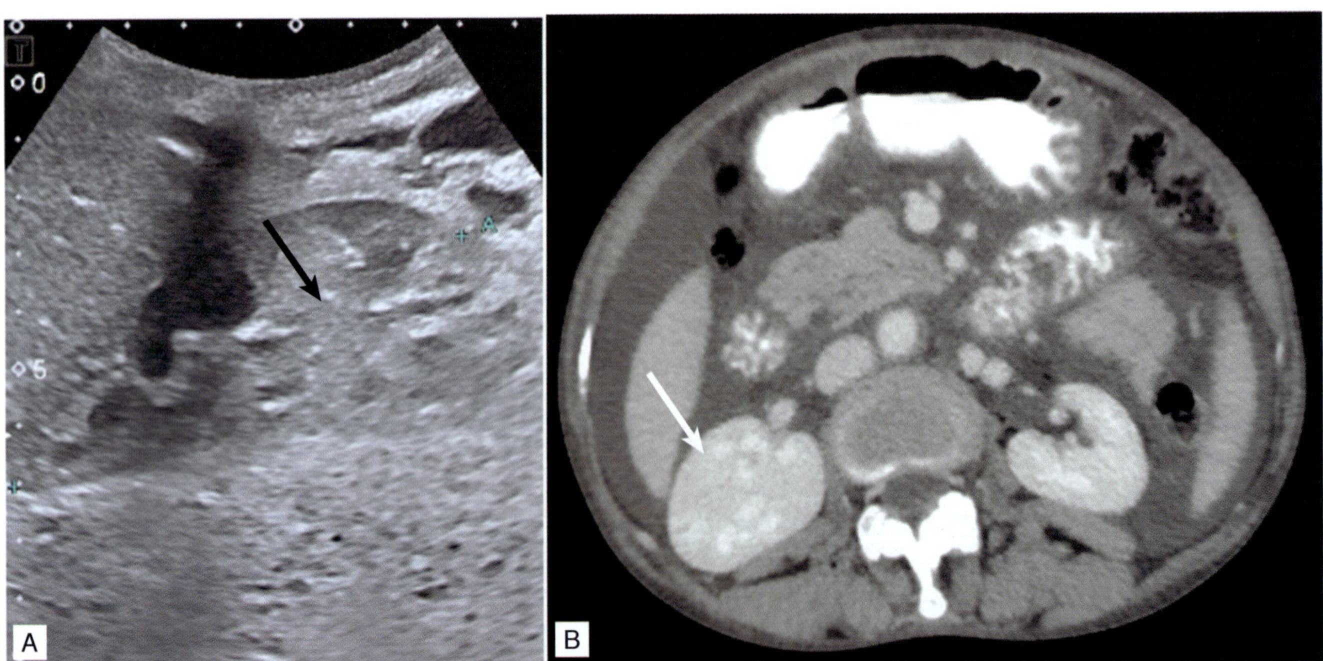

Figure 85.32 (A) Ultrasonogram of duplex kidney showing a bridge of normal renal parenchyma separating the central renal sinus echo (*black arrow*). (B) Contrast enhanced CT axial section of the patient demonstrating the "faceless" kidney sign (*white arrow*), where there is absence of the normal sinus signature in this section which passes through the intervening parenchyma between the two collecting systems.

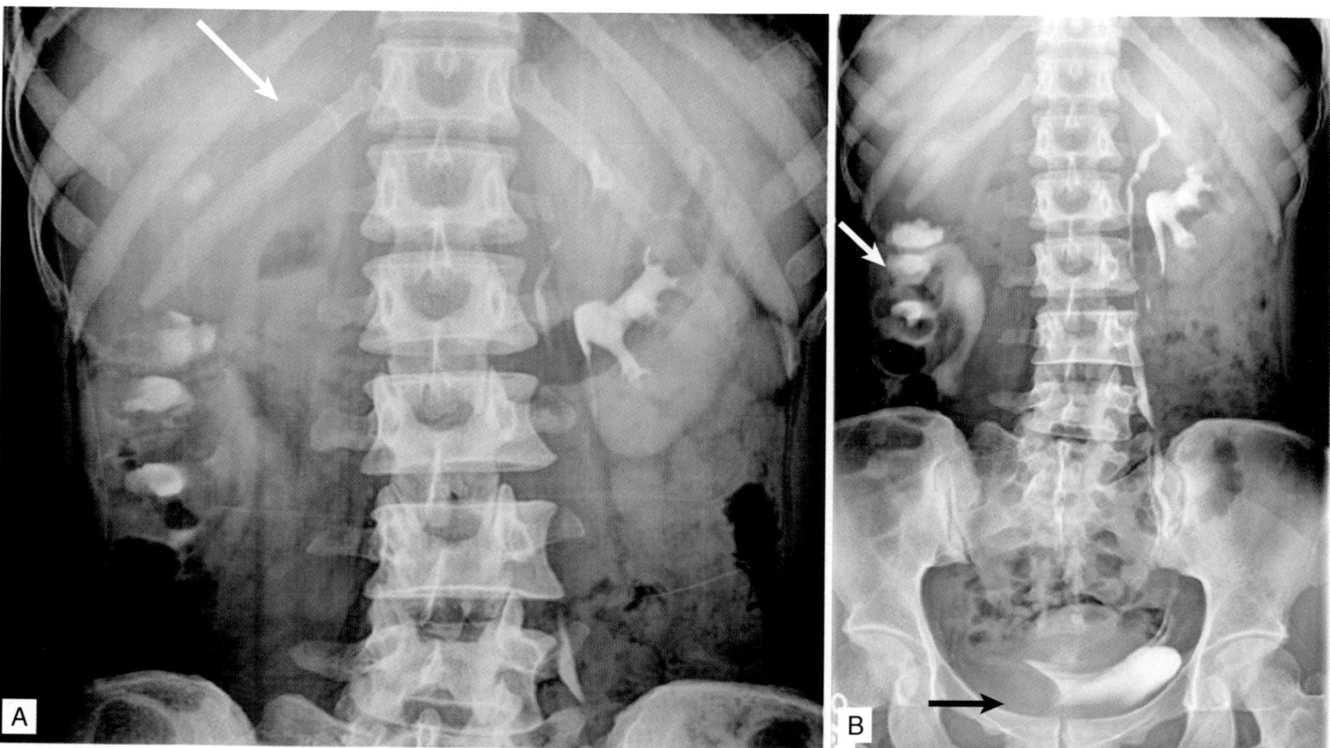

Figure 85.33 IVU study, 5 minute pyelogram image (A) shows bilateral duplex collecting system with poorly functioning hydronephrotic right upper pole moiety seen as a rim nephrogram (*white arrow*). Right upper moiety obstruction is due to an obstructing ureterocele seen as well-defined oval filling defect projecting into the bladder on the 20 minute urogram, *black arrow* in (B). Mass effect on the right lower moiety by the hydronephrotic right upper moiety producing the characteristic "drooping lilly" appearance, *white arrow* in (B).

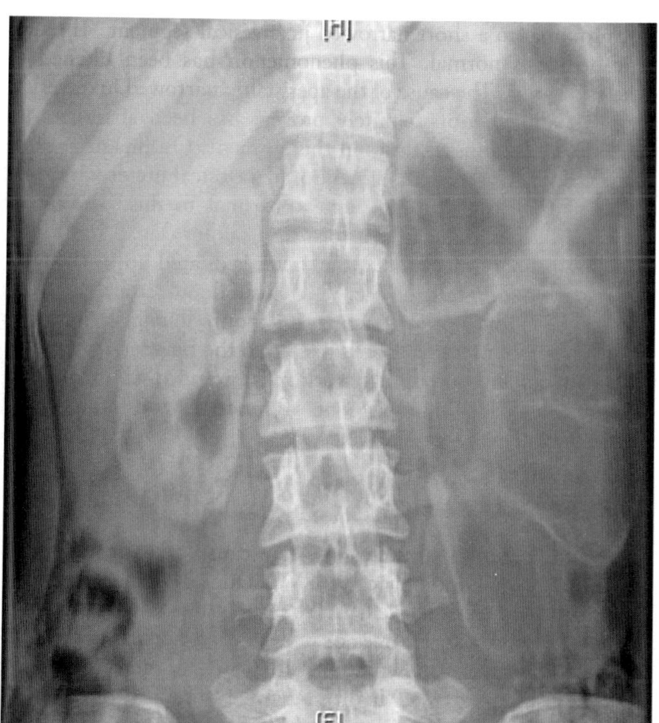

Figure 85.34 Negative pyelogram. IVU nephrotomogram image showing "rim nephrogram" also called "negative pyelogram" in a grossly hydronephrotic enlarged left kidney with thinning of renal parenchyma due to UPJ obstruction. A rim of enhancement is seen outlining the lucency produced by the dilated pelvicalyceal system.

fetus with obstruction at VUJ and ballooning of the segment just proximal to it has been postulated as one of the causes of ureterocele [45].

On ultrasound, cystic dilatation of the terminal ureter can be demonstrated in continuity with the dilated proximal ureter. Scanning should be done with distended bladder and filling up and collapse of the ureterocele with urine can be demonstrated during a ureteric jet. On MCU, the ureterocele is seen as a filling defect in a contrast filled bladder. On IVU, contrast filled rounded or oval density is seen within the bladder with a surrounding radiolucent halo representing the wall of ureterocele forming the classic "cobra head"/"onion bulb" appearance (Fig. 85.35). If it is a poorly functioning kidney or moiety, a rounded or oval filling defect will be seen in a contrast filled bladder [45,46].

Primary Megaureter

Megaureter is a general term used to denote a dilated ureter, with a caliber of more than or equal to 7 mm in children. This may or may not be associated with upper tract dilatation. Primary megaureter refers to ureteric dilatation due to congenital abnormalities in the vesicoureteric junction or the juxtavesical segment of the ureter. It can be of three types:

- Obstructed
- Refluxing
- Unobstructed and nonrefluxing

Ureteric dilatation due to other pathologies involving bladder, urethra, etc. is classified as secondary megaureter and can be called hydroureter.

spondyloepiphyseal dysplasia congenita (see below). Understanding the *sequence of ossification centers* at the elbow is critical to interpreting trauma radiographs, particularly in recognizing the internal epicondyle's avulsive injuries. Epiphyses and apophyses do not always develop in a uniform manner, and may appear fragmented during the process of ossification, for instance as often seen at the calcaneus. Use of a reference text of normal variants is invaluable for differentiation of normal development from pathology—such as fracture, erosions, or AVN [1]. Formal *evaluation of ossification maturity* is the basis of bone age assessment (see later).

Normal Pediatric Bone Marrow

Pediatric bone marrow *converts progressively* from largely *red marrow at birth* to the *adult yellow marrow* pattern. Red marrow contains approximately 40% fat and 60% hemopoietic cells, compared with 80% fat in yellow marrow—largely accounting for its different signal characteristics on MRI [5]. Bone marrow signal changes that may be considered pathological in adults can be seen normally in asymptomatic children. An understanding of the normal pattern of changes is required to be able to identify pathologic marrow changes in children.

Key Facts

- Neonates—essentially *all marrow* is hemopoietic *red marrow*
- *Infancy—conversion* from red to yellow marrow begins in the *appendicular skeleton*
  - By one year of age—the marrow of the hands and feet is predominantly yellow
- As *epiphyses* appear, they convert to yellow marrow within just a few months
- The conversion from red to yellow marrow continues progressively in an appendicular to axial direction until early adulthood [5]
- *In the spine,* the vertebral bodies should not be lower T1 signal than the disks after 5 years of age [6], and normally before (Fig. 86.5)
- *Patchy marrow signal* on T2/STIR MRI sequences is *very common in children* and adolescents and often a nonspecific finding [7]

Imaging Techniques: Magnetic resonance imaging (MRI) is the most common imaging technique for the assessment of marrow changes.

Given the reduced fat composition of red versus yellow marrow, there will be less signal loss on fat-suppressed sequences and out-of-phase imaging in areas containing red marrow.

T1 is the most sensitive sequence for detecting pathological marrow infiltration, with STIR sequences helpful for detecting edema—allowing for the normal patchy STIR signal in normal children.

Upper Limb Disorders

Reduction Defects: An Overview

Reduction defects are congenital anomalies reflecting *disordered early limb development*, typically resulting in failure of formation of skeletal elements. Classification of reduction defects is given in Table 86.2 and illustrated in Fig. 86.6 [8].

Longitudinal Deficiencies of the Hand and Forearm

These disorders feature hypoplasia of the radial or ulnar aspects of the upper limbs including the hands.

Radial Longitudinal Deficiencies

Radial longitudinal defects are relatively common and involve hypoplasia or absence of the radius ± thumb. With more severe radial hypoplasia, the wrist is unstable and subluxes radially, termed a *"Radial Club Hand"* (Fig. 86.8).

Key Facts

- Thumb is usually hypoplastic or absent
- 30–50% cases are bilateral
- Radial deficiencies of the upper limb have a number of syndromic associations
  - *VACTERL* association (vertebral anomalies, anal atresia, cardiac abnormalities, tracheo-esophageal fistula, renal agenesis, limb defects)
  - *Thrombocytopenia Absent Radius* syndrome (TAR): an autosomal recessive disorder resulting from mutations in

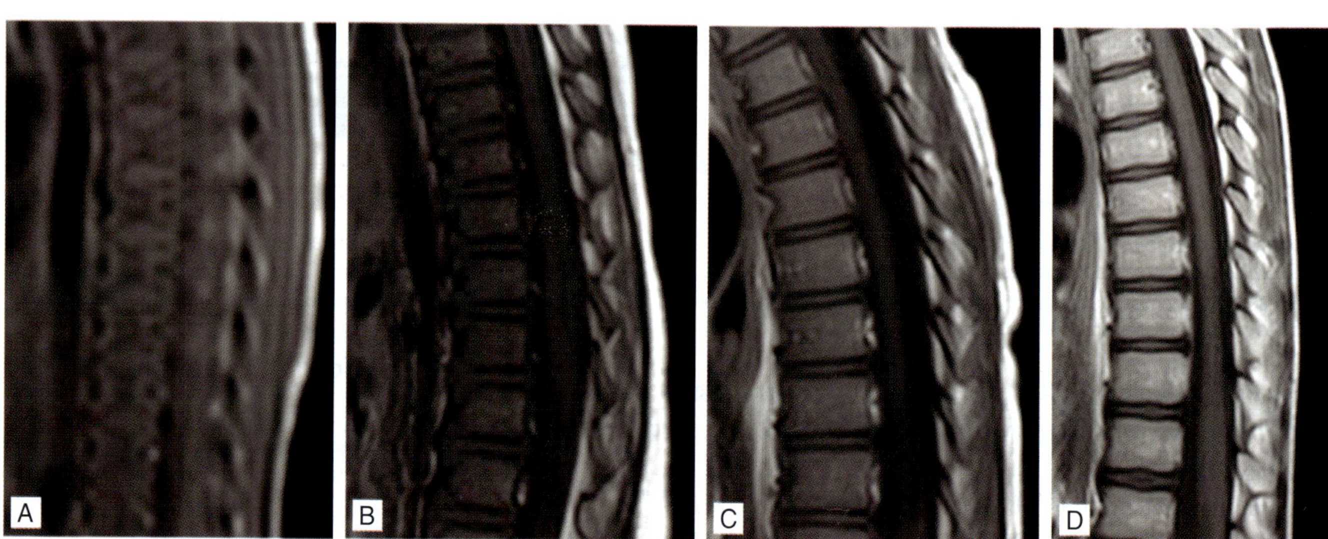

Figure 86.5 The progression of change in normal vertebral marrow signal on T1 sequences. (A) At 1 month, the discs are lower signal than the adjacent vertebral bodies due to their high red marrow content. (B) At 1 year of age, the vertebral bodies and discs are similar signal. (C) At 3 years, the vertebral bodies are becoming higher signal than the discs, as the proportion of fatty yellow marrow increases. (D) By 5 years of age, the vertebral bodies should be reliably higher signal than the discs.

TABLE 86.2 General Classification of Limb Reduction Defects

Type	Definition	Examples
Terminal transverse defects	Absence of distal structures of limb with largely preserved proximal structures	■ Amelia: absent whole limb ■ Hemimelia: absent forearm and hand/foreleg and foot ■ Acheira: absent hand ■ Apodia: absent foot ■ Adactyly: absent digits
Proximal intercalary defect	Absence or severe hypoplasia of proximal part of limb, distal structures preserved	■ Absent humerus ± absent forearm (Fig. 86.7) ■ Absent femur ± foreleg ■ Absence of proximal and middle segments together is sometimes termed "phocomelia"
Longitudinal defect	Absence or severe hypoplasia of lateral part of limb	■ Preaxial (radial or tibia) ■ Postaxial (ulnar or fibular)
Split hand-foot	Absence of central digits	■ Cleft hand/foot ■ Monodactyly (central deficiency and absent thumb/toe)

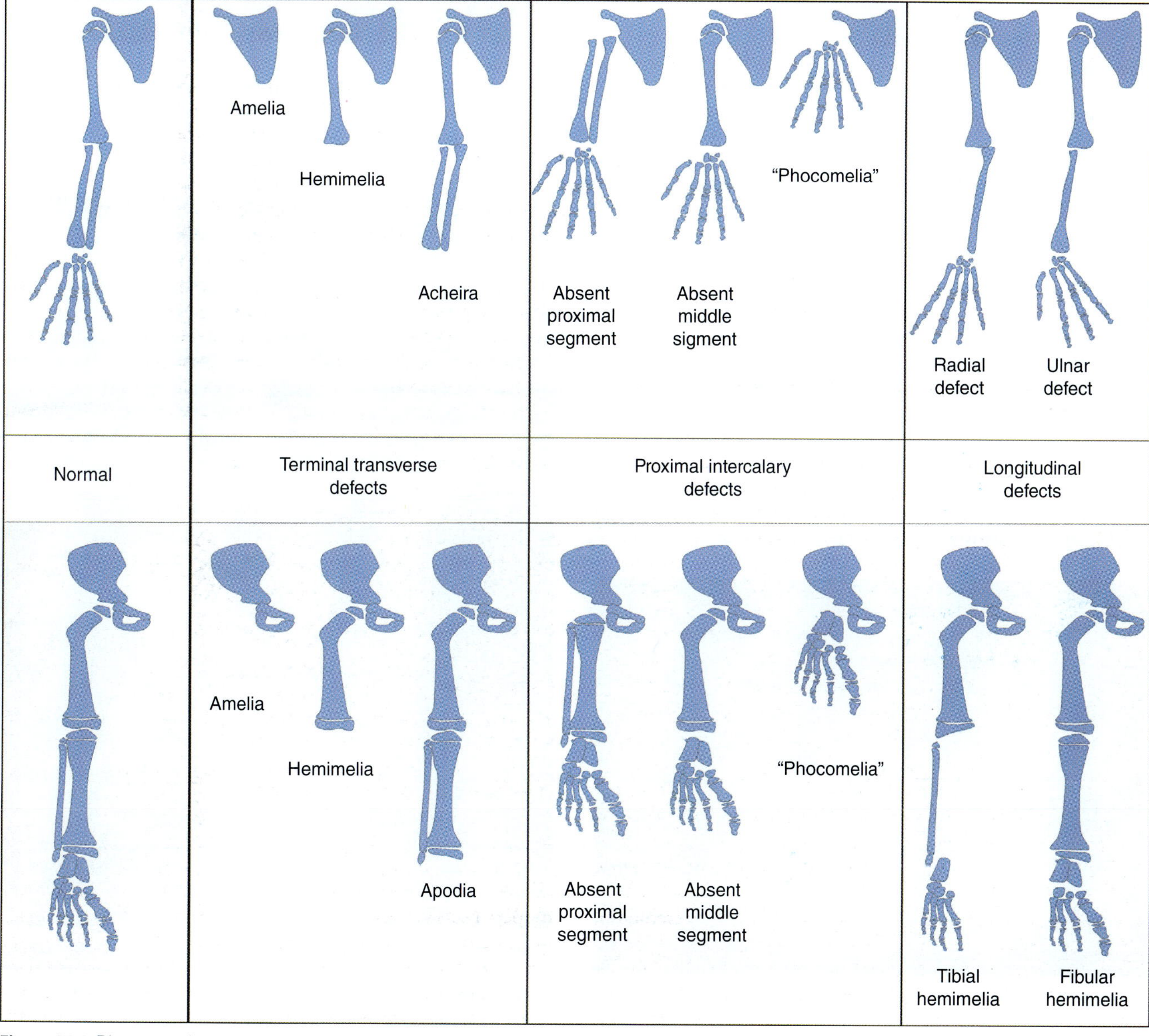

Figure 86.6 Diagrammatic overview of classification of limb reduction defects.

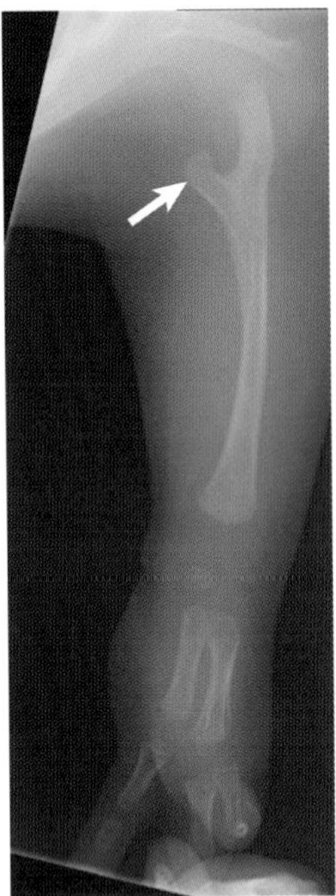

Figure 86.7 Proximal intercalary defect. Left upper limb radiograph in 2-year-old male with congenital malformation. The humerus is absent. There is a single forearm bone which is proximally bifid (*arrow*). Note 3 ray hand.

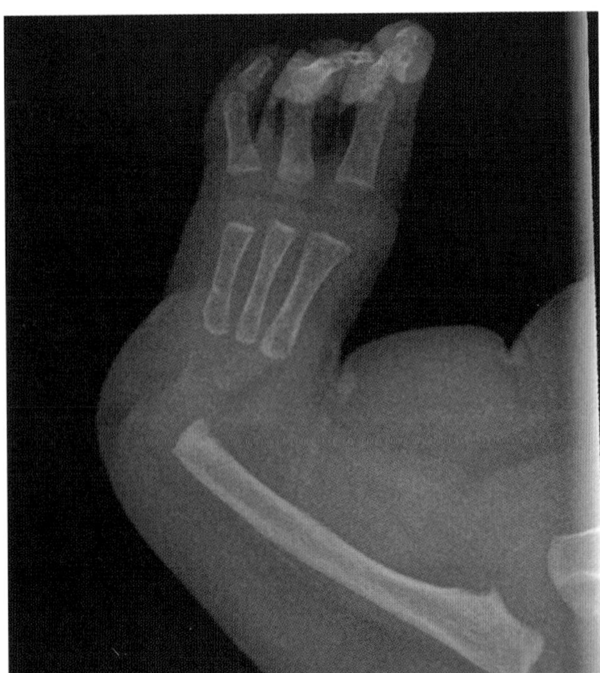

Figure 86.8 Radial club hand. Radiograph of right forearm in 20-week-old male with isolated right upper limb deformity. The radius is absent. The thumb is absent and there is three-ray oligodactyly.

RBM8A; the thumb is almost always present in TAR (Fig. 86.9)

- *Fanconi anemia*; a group of mostly autosomal recessive conditions resulting in impaired DNA repair and aplastic anemia. Thumb may be present or absent. Affected individuals are thought to be highly *sensitive to radiation*
- *Holt-Oram* syndrome: in this autosomal dominant disorder due to mutations in TBX5, hand anomalies are associated with cardiac (usually ventricular septal) defects. The classical manifestation is a thumb which lies in the same plane as the fingers, and which may be triphalangeal; a *"finger-like" thumb* (Fig. 86.10). Alternatively, thumb and/or radial hypoplasia may be present, and sometimes carpal synostosis

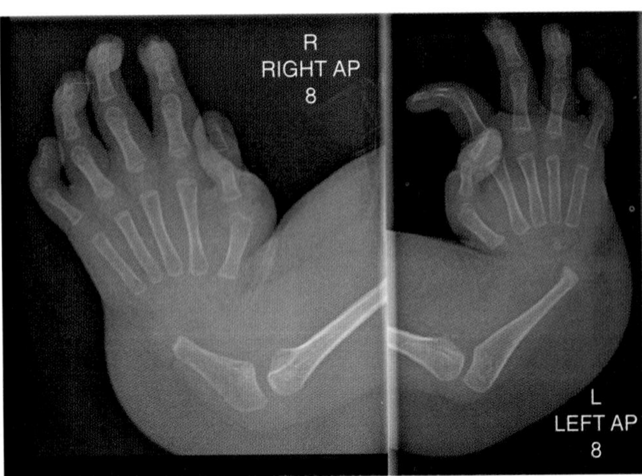

Figure 86.9 TAR syndrome. Radiograph of right forearm in 20-week-old male with isolated right upper limb deformity. The radius is absent. The thumb is present and there is three-ray oligodactyly.

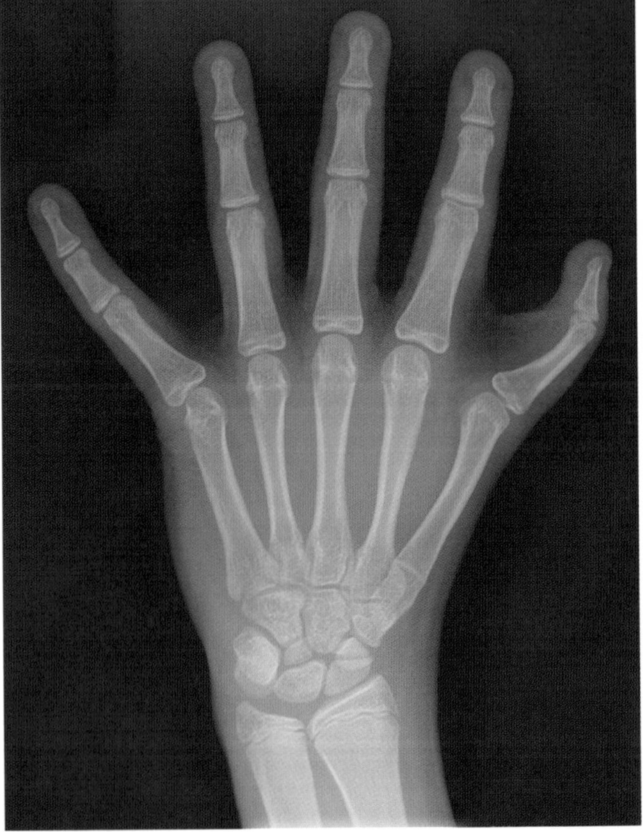

Figure 86.10 Holt-Oram syndrome. Hand radiograph in 14-year-old male with deletion of the TBX5 gene. The thumb lies in the same plane as the fingers giving it a finger-like appearance. In this case, the thumb is biphalangeal, but a triphalangeal thumb may also occur in this setting.

Imaging Techniques

- Plain radiographs of forearm, with a separate AP view of the hand for initial evaluation
- Delineation of tendon structures via ultrasound (USG) or MRI can aid the reconstructive surgeon in the specialist setting

Imaging Findings

- Radial hypoplasia usually results in distal shortening of the radius and radial subluxation of the wrist
- Thumb hypoplasia ranges from complete absence of the thumb, through a rudimentary thumb loosely attached to the hand, to a small but normally formed digit

Treatment: A severely hypoplastic thumb is treated with amputation, usually followed by *pollicisation of the index finger* to restore pincer grip. Milder thumb hypoplasia may require less drastic surgical interventions such as metacarpophalangeal (MCP) joint stabilization.

A radial club hand with poor function is treated by centralization and stabilization of the carpus, if necessary supported by tendon modifications and ulnar osteotomies [9].

Ulnar Longitudinal Deficiencies

In these disorders a hypoplastic or absent ulna is usually associated with absent 5th ± 4th fingers (Fig. 86.11).

Key Facts

- These are 3–4 times *rarer than radial deficiencies*
- More commonly isolated rather than syndromic when compared with radial deficiencies
- Exceptions include:
  - *Ulnar-mammary syndrome* due to mutations in or deletions of TBX3
  - *Femur-fibula-ulna syndrome*, a sporadic disorder combining femoral deficiency with fibular and ulnar longitudinal deficiencies

Imaging Technique and Findings

- Imaging technique as per radial deficiencies
- Mild deformities involve the carpals and hand only
- In the most severe deformities, ulna is absent and there is proximal radio-humeral synostosis

Treatment: Many cases can be managed via nonoperative supportive interventions. Surgical options to improve wrist stability may result in loss of forearm rotation [10].

Symbrachydactyly

This term describes a range of *unilateral terminal transverse defects* of the hand with deficient finger formation.

Key Facts

- Etiology uncertain, probably reflects interruption of fetal blood supply to developing limb bud
- Usually isolated, but symbrachydactyly is the typical hand malformation seen in *Poland syndrome*(absent pectoral ± latissimus dorsi muscles with variable skeletal defects)

Imaging Technique and Findings

- Plain radiographs are sufficient in most cases. Tendon imaging may be used in a specialist setting
- Range from short but structurally normal fingers (± syndactyly) to "peromelia," absent fingers with rudimentary "nubbins" (Fig. 86.12)
- Rudimentary fingers may contain small elements of bone
- The thumb is typically the least severely affected and may be normal
- Syndactyly, usually soft tissues only, may also be present.

Treatment

As the condition is unilateral in almost all cases, most individuals function well. Nonoperative supporting measures are helpful. Establishing a pincer grip through webspace release and syndactyly division can help some. Toe-to-hand phalangeal transfers have been successful [11].

Amniotic Band Syndrome (ABS)

Amniotic band syndrome is a *disruption-deformation sequence* thought to result in most cases from early rupture of the amnion

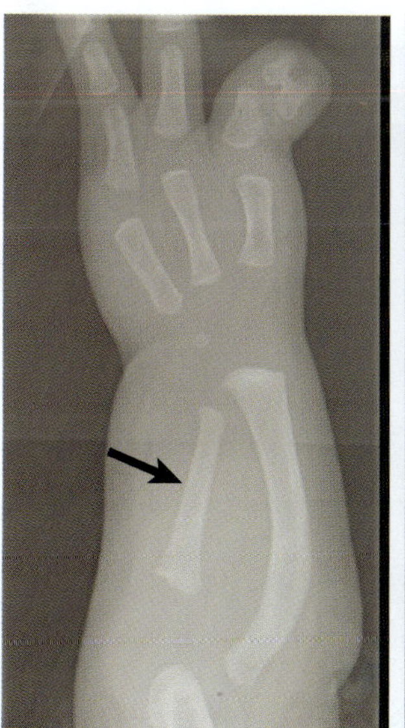
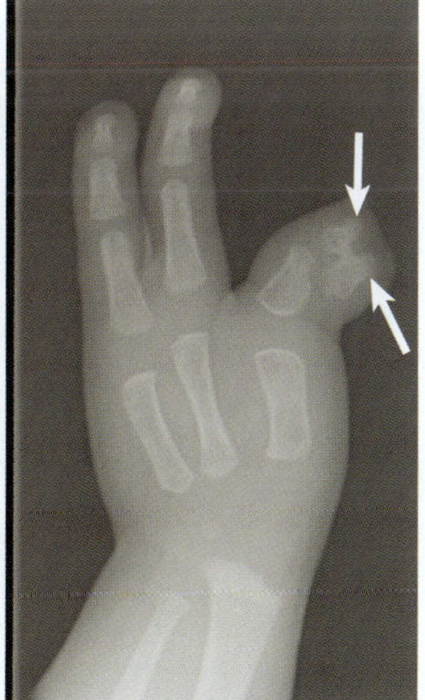

Figure 86.11 Ulnar longitudinal deficiency. Radiographs of forearm and hand in 15-month-old male with unilateral upper limb malformation. The ulna (*black arrow*) is short and slender. The radius is bowed. There is thumb duplication (*white arrows*) with syndactyly. The 4th and 5th rays are absent.

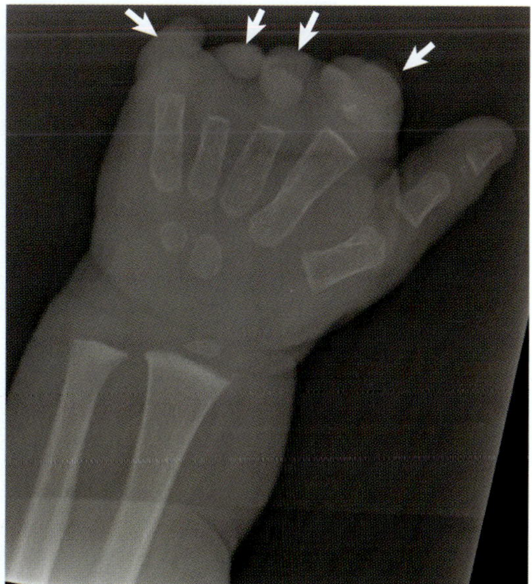

Figure 86.12 Symbrachydactyly. Radiographs of left hand in 15-month-old male. The fingers are absent with rudimentary nubbins (*arrows*) only ("Peromelia"). The thumb is present and only mildly hypoplastic.

leading to *fetal entrapment* by strands of amniotic tissue; the commonest manifestation is *amputation of digits.*

Key Facts

- Amputations may occur at any level, and typically are *bilateral but asymmetrical*, which helps distinguish from symbrachydactyly
- The thumb may be spared as it is protected by the palm of the hand
- *Constriction bands* in the limbs may be present with soft tissue swelling distal to the bands
- Nonmidline craniofacial defects and rarely spinal defects are occasionally present

Imaging Techniques

Plain radiographs are sufficient for most cases. MRI can be useful to evaluate soft tissues distal to a constriction band. MRI is also useful for craniofacial and spinal defects. Vascular imaging is sometimes needed in presence of vascular compromise.

Imaging Findings

Typical hand findings of bilateral, asymmetric amputations favoring the central digits and often sparing the thumb (Fig. 86.13).

Treatment

Surgical relief of contraction bands. Nonoperative and operative interventions to maximize hand function on a case-by-case basis.

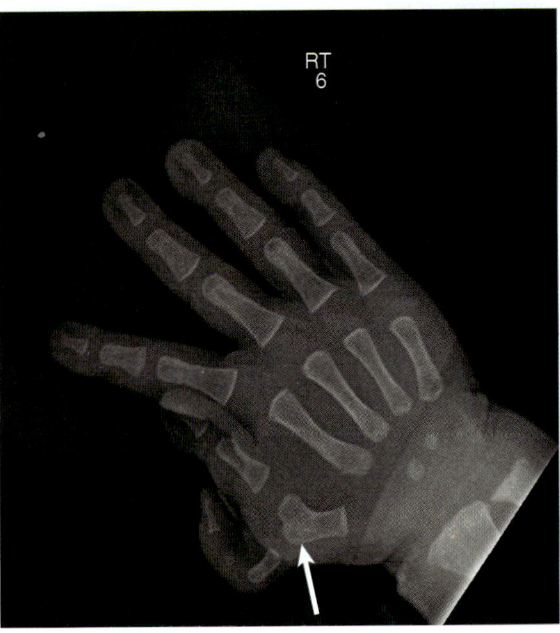

Figure 86.14 Preaxial (radial) polydactyly. Right hand radiograph in 12-week-old male. There is duplication of the thumb with a y-shaped 1st metatarsal (*arrow*). The accessory thumb is triphalangeal.

Polydactyly

Polydactyly refers to *extra digits* in the hands and/or feet.

Key Facts

- Extra digits along the borders of the hand/foot are termed *preaxial polydactyly* if on the radial/tibial side (Fig. 86.14) and *postaxial polydactyly* if on the ulnar/fibular side (Fig. 86.15)
- Extra digits within the borders of the hand and foot are termed *meso-axial or central polydactyly*
- Polydactyly is commonly isolated, but there is a wide range of *syndromic associations* including
  - Skeletal dysplasia, particularly the *ciliopathies* including *Bardet-Biedl* syndrome, *Ellis-Van-Creveld*, *Oro-Facial-Digital syndromes*
  - Some fetal toxicity syndromes including *diabetic embryopathy* (duplication of the hallux with tibia deficiency) and *fetal valproate syndrome*
  - *Smith-Lemli-Opitz syndrome*, a disorder of cholesterol biosynthesis with multiple manifestations including polydactyl and syndactyly of 2nd and 3rd toes
  - Aneuploidies, particularly *Trisomy 13*
  - Rarely as part of the *VACTERAL* association

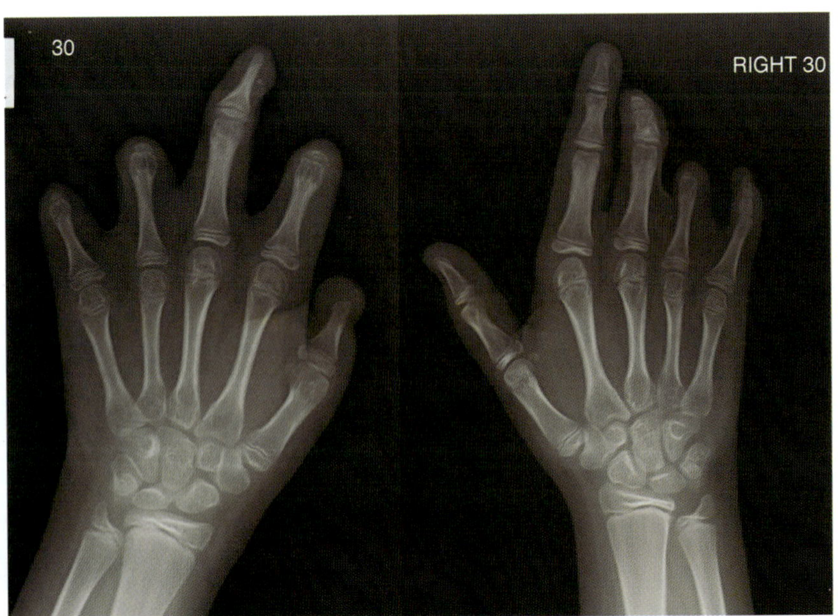

Figure 86.13 Amniotic band syndrome. Radiographs of both hands in 10-year-old female. There are amputations asymmetrically involving both hands. Right thumb and index finger are spared.

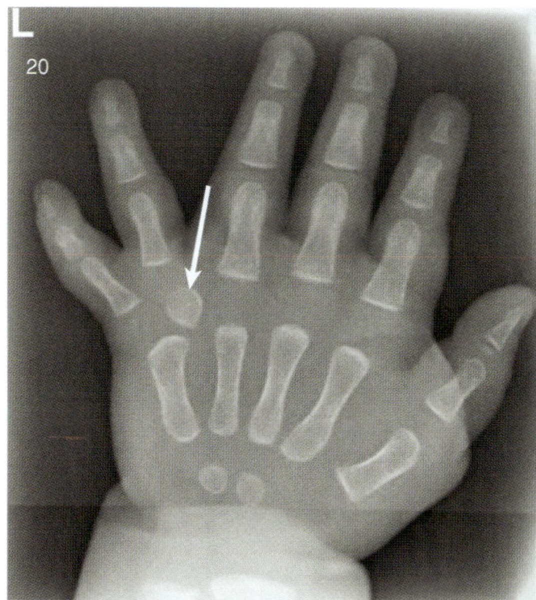

Figure 86.15 Postaxial (ulnar) polydactyly: left hand radiograph in 28-week-old female showing duplication of the little finger with a supernumerary phalanx (*arrow*) at the base of the 5th and 6th fingers.

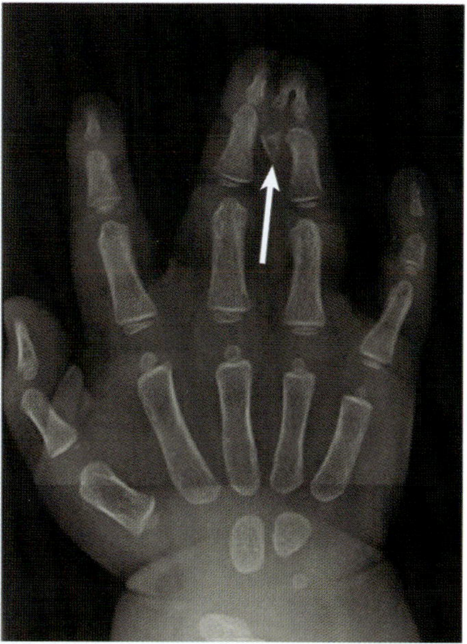

Figure 86.16 Synpolydactyly. Right hand radiograph in 14-month-old female. The middle and ring fingers are fused with accessory middle and distal phalanges (*arrow*) within the fused tissue. This pattern is associated with HOXD13 mutations.

Imaging Technique and Findings

- Radiographs are useful to define bony anatomy including syndactyly before surgery
- A skeletal survey is indicated if there is suspected underlying skeletal dysplasia
- Extra digits may be complete or involve part of a digit
- Bony syndactyly of accessory metacarpals or metatarsal is common

Syndactyly and Polysyndactyly

Syndactyly is abnormal connection between adjacent digits.

Key Facts

- Syndactyly is described as *complete* or *incomplete* based on the length of the connections, and simple (soft tissue only) or complex (soft tissue and bone)
- When associated with polydactyly the term *polysyndactyly* is used; *synpolydactyly* is a specific combination of 3–4 syndactyly in hands (Fig. 86.16) and 4–5 syndactyly in the feet with an extra digit buried in the syndactylous mass, and is usually due to *HOXD13* mutations
- Syndactyly may be isolated but again there are a number of syndromic associations, including:
  - Acrocephalosyndactylies, e.g., *Apert syndrome* (see skeletal dysplasia section)
  - Acrocephalopolysyndactylies, e.g., Carpenter syndrome
  - Greig syndrome
  - Most causes of polydactyly may feature syndactyly

Ectrodactyly

Ectrodactyly describes central deficiencies of the hand (or foot) with a soft tissue cleft.

Key Facts

- May be an isolated, often autosomal dominant trait
- Occasionally part of Ectrodactyly-ectrodermal dysplasia-clefting syndrome (Fig. 86.17)
- Hands are more commonly involved than feet

Imaging Technique and Findings

- Plain radiographs are normally sufficient
- There is variability in imaging appearance: central rays are usually absent, but abnormal bones with syndactyly or transverse orientation are sometimes present in cleft

Congenital Anomalies of Distal Radio-Ulnar Joint Alignment

Madelung Deformity

Premature fusion of the medial, volar aspect of the distal radial growth plate, resulting in *bowing of the radial shaft with a triangular shaped carpal deformity* (Fig. 86.18). Acquired injury to the growth plate, or physical distortion of normal distal radius and ulna growth can cause a similar "madelung-type" deformity.

Causes

- True Madelung deformity
  - Isolated (more common in females, typically presents in adolescence)
  - Leri-Weill dyschondrosteosis (see the Mesomelic dysplasia section)
  - Turner's syndrome
- Acquired Madelung-type deformity
  - Local injury—trauma, infection, vascular insufficiency
  - Deformation of growth—added bone within the distal radio-ulnar joint, e.g.,
    - Ollier's disease
    - Multiple hereditary osteochondromas (exostoses)

Imaging Findings

- Radial and dorsal bowing of the radius with dorsal distal ulnar subluxation
- Exaggerated medial inclination of the distal radial articular surface and positive ulnar variance

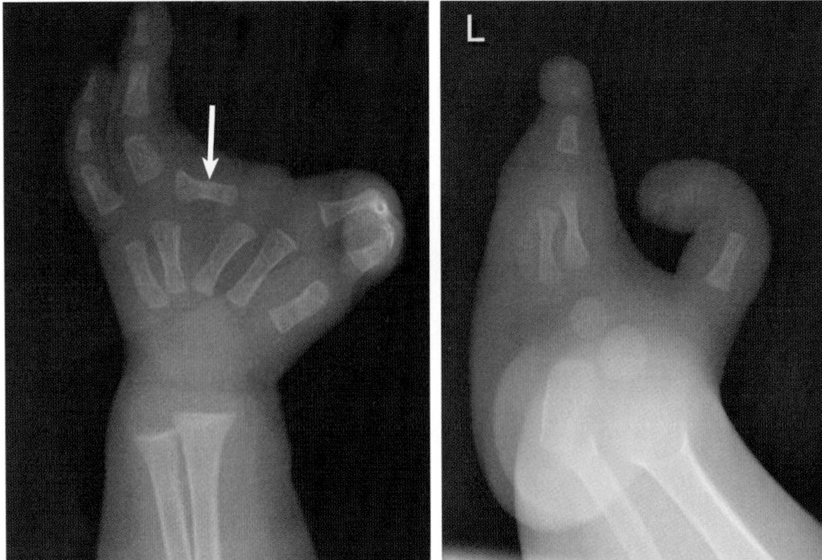

Figure 86.17 Ectrodactyly. Radiographs of left hand and foot in 30-week-old male with partial chromosome 7 deletion and ectrodactyly, ectodermal dysplasia, cleft lip/palate syndrome type 1. There is a large central cleft in the hand, with a transversely oriented tubular bone at the base of the cleft (*arrow*). The foot shows oligodactyly with a deep cleft between hallux and syndactylous fibular rays.

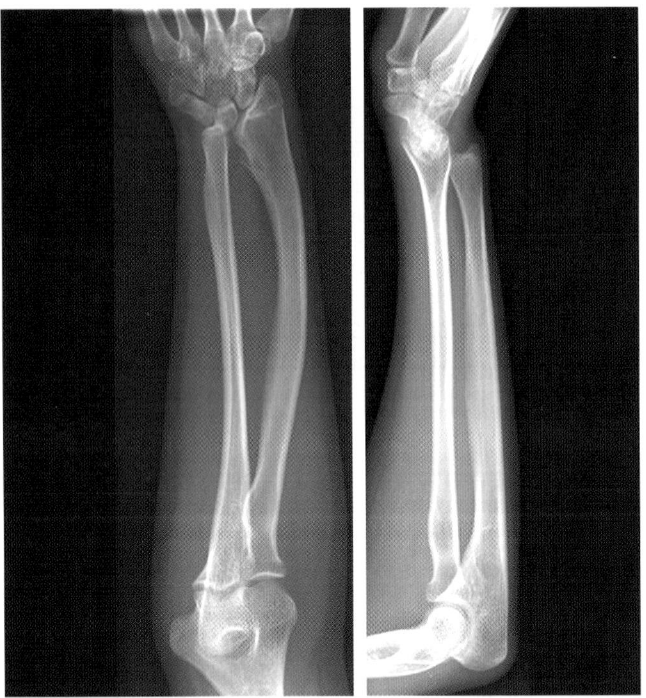

Figure 86.18 AP and lateral forearm radiographs of a 13-year-old girl with bilateral Madelung deformity and mild short stature, and a pathogenic mutation in the SHOX gene; in keeping with Leri-Weill.

- V-shaped subluxation of the proximal carpal row
- Small distal radial epiphysis medially
- Anomalous radiolunate ligament (Vickers ligament) in the "true" form [12]

Treatment: Indicated for *deformity, impaired function, or pain due to ulnocarpal impaction.* Conservative measures tend to be unsuccessful. Many surgical options are available, with variable success rates, including distal radial osteotomy or physiolysis, Vickers ligament release, and ulna shortening [13].

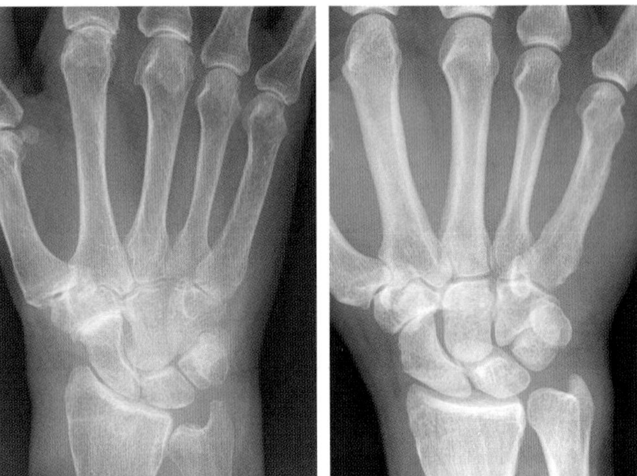

Figure 86.19 Negative (*left*) and positive (*right*) ulnar variance. Note, it is the position of the ulna articular surface that is assessed, not the ulnar styloid.

Ulnar Variance

Describes the relative positions of the articular surfaces of the ulna and radius at the wrist (Fig. 86.19). *It is independent of the length of the ulnar styloid process.* Measurements are derived from PA radiographs taken in a neutral forearm rotation, elbow flexed at 90 degrees and shoulder abducted to 90 degrees.

Positive Variance: When the distal ulna articular surface is >2.5 mm beyond the radius. It predisposes to *ulnar impaction syndrome and injury to the triangular fibrocartilage complex.*

Negative Variance: When the distal ulna appears short at the wrist, >2.5 mm proximal to the radial surface. It has been associated with *Kienbocks disease* (avascular necrosis of the lunate). A causative role for negative ulnar variance has not been proven, although surgical techniques equalizing the length of the forearm bones do provide symptomatic relief in some patients.

Congenital Dislocation of the Radial Head

The cardinal feature is nontraumatic dislocation at the radiocapitellar joint, i.e., *the longitudinal axis of the radius failing to bisect the capitellum.* Congenital dislocation of the radial head may be an isolated abnormality, or seen as part of a genetic syndrome. The main differential for a congenital dislocation of the radial head is an acquired, traumatic dislocation.

Distinguishing Features (Fig. 86.20)

- Small dome-shaped radial head
- Hypoplastic capitellum
- Prominent ulnar epicondyle
- Bowing of the ulna
- More commonly bilateral
- More commonly posterior dislocation

Note, if a traumatic dislocation occurs at birth and is detected late, secondary bony remodeling may have occurred and it may be indistinguishable from a true "congenital" deformity.

Associated syndromes include Ehlers-Danlos, Klinefelter, Nail-patella, Klippel-feil, and Apert.

Treatment: Often asymptomatic. If there is limitation of movement or pain, ulnar, and radial osteotomies combined with annular ligament reconstruction, or radial head excision may be considered.

Supracondylar Process

A *normal anatomic variant* present in approximately 1% of individuals. It is a bony spur projecting from the anteromedial surface of the distal humerus, approximately 5 cm above the elbow (Fig. 86.21). Considered to be a vestigial remnant, it is sometimes known as an "avian spur."

Key Facts

- Usually an asymptomatic, incidental finding
- May be associated with a fibrous band *(Struthers ligament)* extending from the supracondylar process to the medial epicondyle, which can cause median nerve or brachial artery compression [14]

Imaging: Whilst easily seen on an oblique view of the elbow, it may not be apparent on true AP and true lateral views.

Treatment: Surgical decompression for symptomatic cases associated with a Struthers ligament.

Carpal Coalition

Carpal coalition may occur in isolation, or as part of a syndrome. Isolated carpal coalitions are usually transverse, e.g., lunate-triquetrum and capitate-hamate (Fig. 86.22), and can be inherited [15]. In syndromes they may be longitudinal or more extensive [16]. Similar appearances may develop following acquired bony injury. Fusions may be described osseous, fibrous, or cartilaginous.

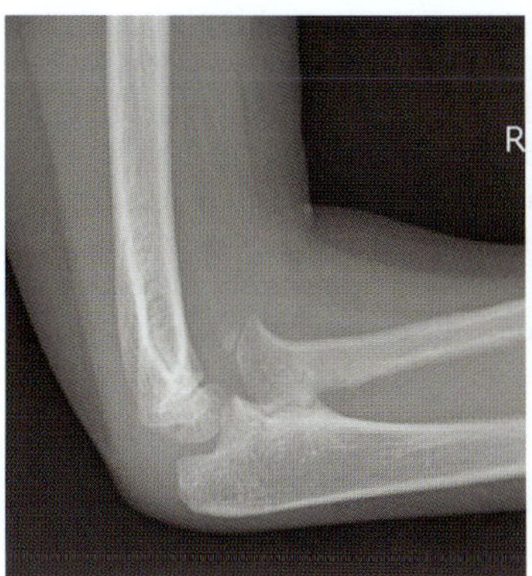

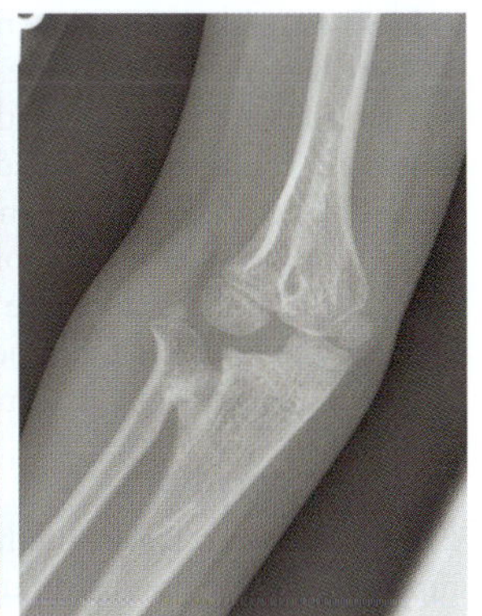

Figure 86.20 8-year-old boy with inability to pronate elbows. The right radial head is subluxed with a small, abnormally positioned epiphysis, widened metaphysis and partial bony synostosis between the proximal radius and ulna. The proximal ulna metaphysis also appears abnormally broad. The synostosis is in keeping with a "type 2" appearance—that is, just distal to the radial epiphysis and associated with congenital dislocation. This is associated with genetic causes including karyotype abnormalities (e.g., mosaic XXXY).

Key Facts

- Isolated
  - Inherited as an autosomal dominant Mendelian characteristic
  - Most common within the same carpal row, particularly lunate-triquetrum
  - More common in females (2:1)
  - Regional variation in prevalence. White Caucasian 0.1%, Afro-Caribbean 0.4–0.8% [15]
- Syndromic
  - Coalitions between the proximal and distal rows—particularly if bilateral, were classically thought more likely to indicate a syndromic association [16]. An increasing number of case reports in recent years though have described inter-row fusions in nonsyndromic patients
  - Consider Ellis-van Creveld, Holt-Oram, Turner's, Carpal-tarsal coalition, Oto-palatal-digital syndromes
- Acquired
  - Acquired fusion rather than a primary failure of segmentation
  - More likely to be incomplete
  - Consider history of prior trauma, infection or inflammatory arthropathy

Pelvis and Lower Limb

Hip Pain in Children

Hip pain in children is a relatively common presentation, with the likely cause highly dependent on patient age. In preverbal children, specific localization of pain is difficult, and hip pathologies may present as a nonspecific limp, or reluctance to use the limb. Reference to the ACR appropriateness criteria for work-up of a limping child under the age of 5 is suggested [17]. Differentials based on age are considered in Table 86.3. The individual pathologies are considered in more detail in the following sections.

Developmental Dysplasia of the Hip

This is a very important condition for the radiologist because success in its treatment depends upon *early recognition.* The incidence

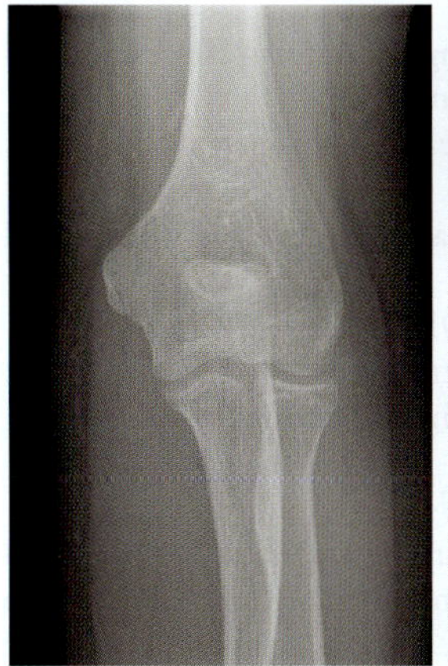

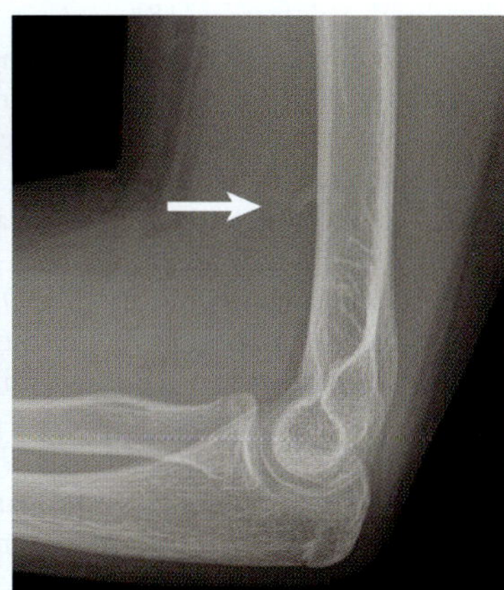

Figure 86.21 A 13-year-old boy with restriction of elbow movement. The supracondylar spur is not apparent on the AP projection, but well seen on the lateral view in this case (*arrow*).

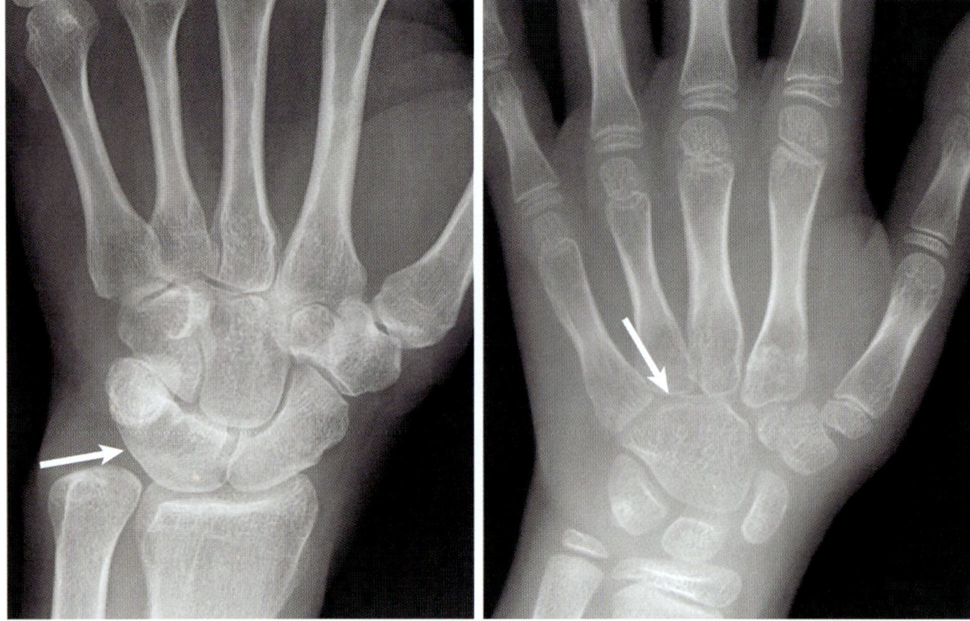

Figure 86.22 Incidental luno-triquetral coalition (*arrow*) presenting in a young adult (*left*) and more extensive capito-hamate coalition (*arrow*) seen in a 10-year-old during a skeletal survey for suspected dysplasia (*right*).

TABLE 86.3 Differential Diagnosis of Hip Pain/Limp in Children

Age	<4 Years of Age	4–8 Years	>8 Years of Age
Common causes	Transient synovitis Septic joint/osteomyelitis Referred pain Trauma (including NAI)	Transient synovitis Perthes Septic joint/osteomyelitis	Slipped upper femoral epiphysis Septic joint/osteomyelitis Trauma (including overuse, e.g., avulsion fractures)
Also consider	Developmental dysplasia of the hipJuvenile idiopathic arthritisTumors ▪ Leukemia ▪ Metastases (e.g., neuroblastoma) Langerhan's cell histiocystosis (pelvis more common <5 years old)	Tumors ▪ Leukemia ▪ Ewings Juvenile idiopathic arthritis	Tumors ▪ Osteoid Osteoma ▪ Leukemia ▪ Ewings ▪ Osteosarcoma Juvenile idiopathic arthritis

of hip instability at birth is 5–10/1000, and of frank dislocation 1–1.5/1000. It is more common in girls. Screening USG should be undertaken for babies with abnormal hip examination and for those with risk factors [18].

Abnormal Physical Examination Findings Warranting Hip Ultrasound

- Positive Barlow and Ortolani maneuvers
- Asymmetric thigh or buttock creases, asymmetric leg length, or restricted abduction

Risk Factors Warranting Hip Ultrasound, Even With Normal Physical Examination Findings

- First degree family history of DDH
- Breech presentation in the third trimester
- History of incorrect tight lower limb swaddling

Imaging Techniques and Findings

Ultrasound: Ultrasound is the primary investigation for suspected developmental dysplasia of the hip in children from 6 weeks to 6 months of age. Before 6 weeks of age, there is a higher rate of "false positive" immature hips which normalize without intervention.

There are two key techniques, the Graf static technique, and Harcke dynamic method. A combination of the two techniques was recommended as the standard in the ACR 1999 consensus guidelines, with a two-view minimum standard [19].

For the Graf method, the image is obtained with the child on his/her side with the hip slightly flexed, the transducer parallel to the ilium and the image obtained in the coronal plane. The measurement of Graf angles may be made in the assessment of hip dysplasia to determine the degree of dysplasia and plan management (Figs. 86.23 and 86.24). The standard view—with a linear probe, includes the horizontal iliac bone, the cartilaginous labrum, triradiate cartilage, cartilaginous femoral head and proximal femur [20].

Graf Classification

For the dynamic Harke method, a similar lateral approach is also most commonly used, although the child may be lying in a lateral decubitus or supine position. The four basic lateral views are in the coronal plane in neutral (15–20 degrees of hip flexion) and flexion (hip at 90 degrees), and in the transverse plane in neutral and flexion. The hip is imaged with and without stress, using a technique akin to the Barlow and Ortolani maneuvers. At a minimum, there should be two orthogonal views, one with the hip under stress.

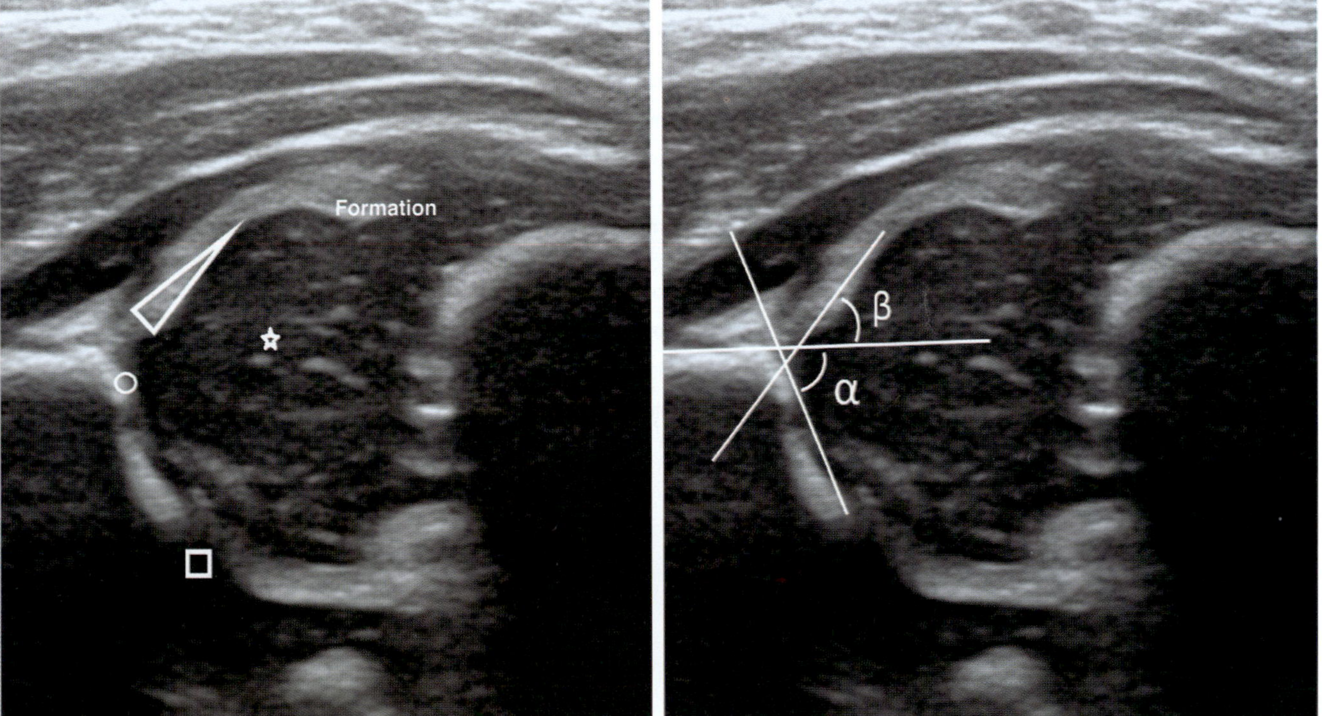

Figure 86.23 Essential landmarks for measurement of Graf angles are demonstrated on the left: the *triangle* denoting the echogenic cartilaginous labrum, the *circle* the point of transition from concave acetabulum to convex ilium, and the *square* the triradiate cartilage. On the right: these landmarks are used for calculation of alpha and beta angle measurements. *Asterisk* indicates femoral head.

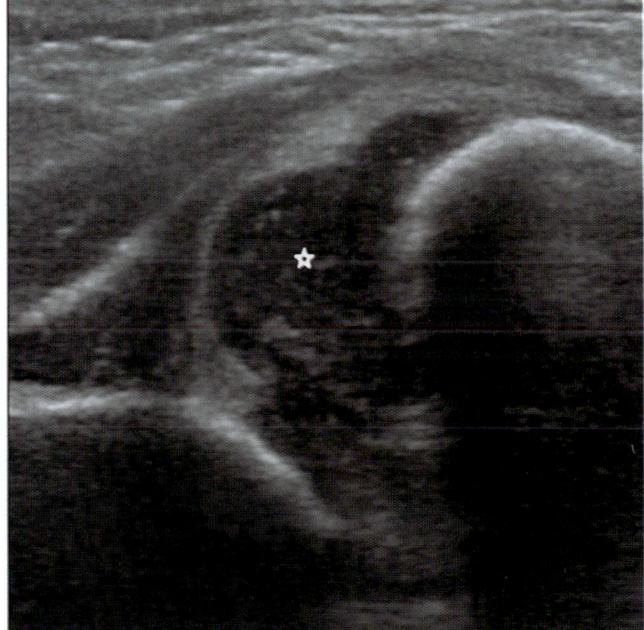

Figure 86.24 2-week-old female born breech, with a positive Ortolani test on the left hip. The bony acetabular margin is flattened and bony roof poor, with the hip eccentrically located. The alpha angle is 40 degrees. The cartilaginous labrum is displaced upwards (Graf III), although on the point of slipping between the femoral head and lateral acetabular margin the labrum appears normal (Graf IV). *Asterisk* indicates femoral head.

Ultrasound Reporting Checklist

- Clinical indication
- Presence of dislocation/subluxation, including stability of the hip
- Femoral head coverage
- Bony ossific rim morphology
- Cartilaginous labrum morphology
- Alpha and beta angles
- Femoral head ossification
- Conclusion, including Graf classification (Table 86.4)

Plain Film

Is the preferred technique for investigation once the child is over 6 months, but may be useful from 4 months, due to progression of femoral head ossification. Features indicating DDH (Fig. 86.25):

- Ossification of the femoral ossific nucleus may be delayed on the dysplastic side
- The femoral head is displaced upwards and outwards
- The acetabulum is shallow, with an acetabular angle greater than 30 degrees;
  This is the angle subtended by a line drawn through the centers of both Y-cartilages (Hilgenreiner's line) and a line parallel to the acetabular roof

MRI/CT

May be helpful in select cases, for instance for confirming successful reduction of the femoral head postoperatively. Cartilage sensitive MRI sequences facilitate identification of the nonossified femoral head. The two available forms are Double Echo Steady State (DESS, Siemens) and Multi-Echo iN Steady-state Acquisition (MENSA, GE). These are gradient echo sequences with a prolonged unbalanced readout gradient which generate combined free-induction-decay and echo-type signals.

Treatment

For Graf 2a hips, follow-up is undertaken until 3 months of age or hip normalization. For Graf 2b hips and above, splinting with a Pavlik harness is the first-line for treatment and is normally applied for 4–6 weeks. Surgical options are available for cases where the hips are found to be irreducible, or the Pavlik harness

TABLE 86.4 Graf Classification for Developmental Dysplasia of the Hip

Graf	Description	Bony Roof	Ossific Rim	Labrum	Alpha Angle	Beta Angle
1	Mature	Good	Sharp	Long and narrow, covers femoral head	>60	NA
2a	Immature (<3 months old)	Deficient	Rounded	Covers femoral head	50–59	NA
2b	Delayed development (>3 months old)	Deficient	Rounded	Covers femoral head	50–59	NA
2c	Stable or unstable	Deficient	Rounded/flat	Covers femoral head	43–49	<77
2d	Decentering	Severely deficient	Rounded/flat	Compressed	43–49	>77
3	Dislocated	Poor	Flat	Displaced upwards and abnormal echogenicity	<43	NA
4	Dislocated	Poor	Flat	Interposed	<43	NA

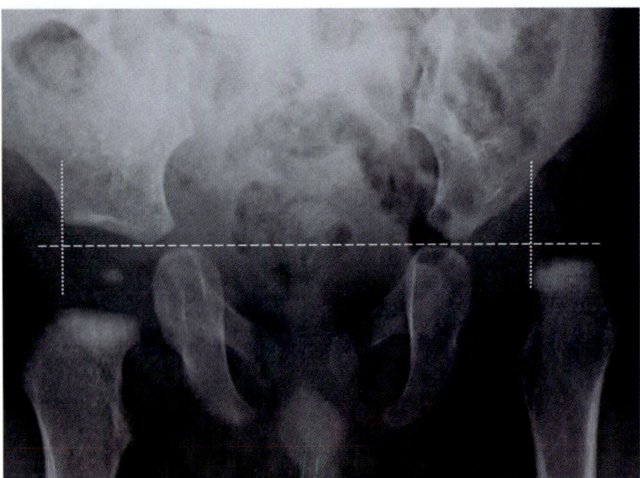

Figure 86.25 A late presentation of DDH in an 8-month-old boy. The left hip is laterally and superiorly subluxed. There is relatively delayed ossification of the left upper femoral epiphysis. The right hip is normal. Lines and angles for assessment of DDH on a well-centered plain film are shown: Hilgenreiner line (*dashed*)—a horizontal line between triradiate cartilages. Perkin line (*dotted*)—drawn perpendicular to the Hilgenreiner line, contacting the lateral aspect of the acetabulum. The femoral head (or metaphysis if unossified) should be in the inner lower quadrant. The acetabular angle is measured between the Hilgenreiner line and the roof of the acetabulum, it should be less than 30 degrees.

has failed. These range from closed reduction and spica for children under 18 months of age, to open reduction and femoral osteotomy—generally reserved for children over 2 years of age.

Perthes Disease/Avascular Necrosis of the Hip

Perthes disease is an idiopathic avascular necrosis of the femoral head. It is more common in boys. Typical age range from 5 to 8 years (although may range from 3 years to 12 years). Most commonly unilateral, but if bilateral typically asymmetric. If symmetry is present, *hypothyroidism* or *multiple epiphyseal dysplasia* should be excluded. There is no increased familial incidence, but parents of affected children are often elderly. Many of the affected children have a below-average birth weight and, at presentation, show skeletal growth retardation in the hands. This is especially seen in boys. There is an increased incidence of associated congenital anomalies, including congenital heart disease, pyloric stenosis, hernia, renal anomalies, and undescended testes.

Following ischemia, the ossific nucleus of the epiphysis necroses, causing growth arrest. The overlying cartilage, which is supplied by synovial fluid, survives and thickens especially in the nonweight-bearing regions, medially, and laterally. Dense, necrotic bone resorbs and is slowly replaced by vital bone. The predisease shape of the necrotic nucleus does not return to normal and the nucleus ends up flat in whole or in part.

Stages of the Disease

These occur within each group. There is an *initial* phase of onset, with widening of the joint space and increased density of all or part of the ossific nucleus, which is followed by collapse of part or all of the nucleus, according to group. *Repair* removes the fragmented, crushed necrotic bone. *Healing* shows as an increase in size and re-ossification. *Remodeling* then occurs and is aided when the femoral head is completely contained within the acetabulum. Uncovering of the lateral margin of the femoral head has a bad prognosis.

The metaphyseal lesion leads to an abnormal femoral neck. The most severely involved cases have a broad, short neck, i.e., the neck length/width ratio is lower than normal.

Imaging Findings

- Radiographs (Fig. 86.26)
  - *Lateral displacement of the femoral head.* Early on, and in the irritable hip syndrome, displacement of the femoral head (Waldenström's sign) is seen, possibly due to effusion or to thickening of the ligamentum teres. Later, the superior part of the joint may also be widened
  - Subchondral lucencies/fracturing. This sign is seen early in the disease but is transient. It is best seen in the "frog" lateral view
  - *Reduction in size of the ossific nucleus of the epiphysis.* This is found in some 50% of cases and is due to growth retardation. The medial joint space then seems wider
  - *Increase in density of the femoral ossific nucleus.* This is due to trabecular compression, dystrophic calcification in debris and creeping substitution repair, with laying down of new bone on the pre-existing trabeculation
  - As disease progresses, coxa magna may result
- MRI
  - May show marrow edema in early cases
  - MRI changes are seen in bone and cartilaginous structures of the femoral head and acetabulum. The ossific nucleus flattens and the normal bright signal related to marrow fat diminishes following loss of the normal circulation. The signal seen from this region varies with the stage of disease

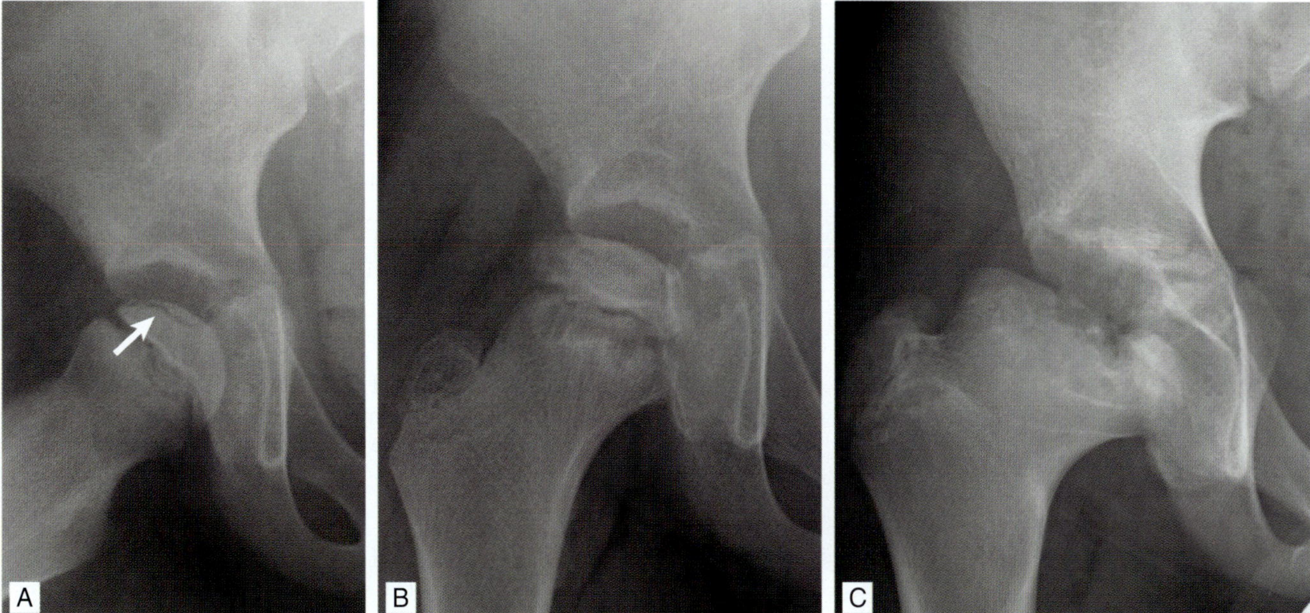

Figure 86.26 Boy with limp. (A) at 8 years, (B) 8.5 years, and (C) 12 years of age. The natural history of Perthes disease is shown, with initial subchondral lucencies (*arrow*) progressing to flattening, sclerosis and fragmentation, and later development of a coxa magna with secondary acetabular irregularity.

and healing, and may range from low early on in the disease to a mixture of high and low when revascularization occurs or if cysts are present. The bone deformity is visualized. Metaphyseal irregularity is seen and an abnormal relationship of the entire head to the acetabulum shown. Dynamic contrast-enhanced MRI may demonstrate reduced perfusion
- MRI also shows thickening of the nonossified cartilage of the femoral head, especially laterally, and of the acetabulum, especially the labrum. The degree of acetabular covering of the developing femoral head, as well as articular congruity is well seen in MRI

Differential Diagnosis

- Secondary avascular necrosis—underlying predisposing factors need to be sought (Fig. 86.27)
- Meyer's dysplasia—irregular, variant ossification of the femoral heads which should be asymptomatic, normally symmetric, and expected to normalize by approximately 5 years of age
- Skeletal dysplasia
  - Multiple epiphyseal dysplasia—other epiphyses will be affected
  - Mucopolysaccharidosis, particularly Morquio—will show other clinical and radiographic features (described later)

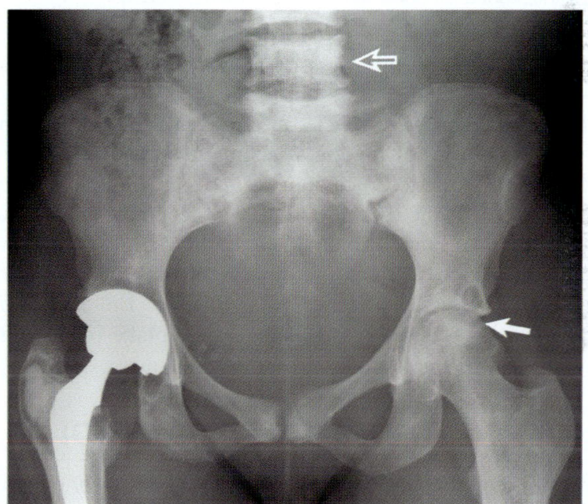

Figure 86.27 17-year-old with avascular necrosis of the left hip. There is left femoral head subchondral sclerosis and lucency (*block arrow*), and fragmentation of the articular surface. There are secondary degenerative changes in the left acetabulum. There has already been a right total hip replacement due to prior right hip avascular necrosis, and there is patchy bony sclerosis and "cod-fish" vertebral shape (*open arrow*) in keeping with underlying sickle cell disease.

Slipped Upper Femoral Epiphysis (SUFE)

SUFE is an idiopathic Salter-Harris type 1 fracture across the proximal femoral growth plate. It is bilateral in a third of cases. More common in boys, obese children, and typically between 12 and 15 years of age. Treatment involves fixation of the femoral head in situ (without relocation). Avascular necrosis of the femoral epiphysis is a potential complication. Deformity resulting from remodeling of the femoral head can cause a cam-type femoroacetabular impingement and early osteoarthritis.

This topic is covered in more detail in the Skeletal trauma (pediatric) chapter along with the Salter-Harris classification.

Imaging findings (Fig. 86.28)

- Sensitivity on radiographs is much increased in the frog-leg lateral position
- On an AP radiograph, features may be subtle, including widening of the physis, abnormal line of Klein, and reduced overlap of the medial aspect of the metaphysis with the posterior acetabulum
- Preoperative dynamic contrast-enhanced MRI can demonstrate altered perfusion within the slipped epiphysis, with subtraction images aiding identification of focal or global devascularization. This can aid prognostication and parental counseling regarding the risk of postoperative avascular necrosis

Distal Femoral Metaphyseal Irregularity

Also known as a cortical desmoid or an avulsive cortical irregularity, these are classic "do not touch" abnormalities which are

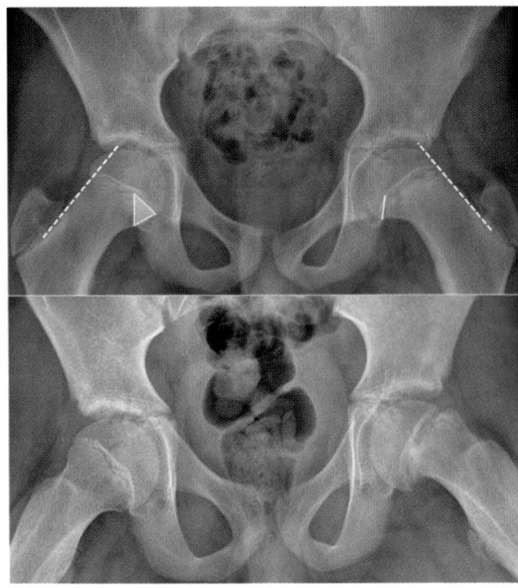

Figure 86.28 13-year-old boy presenting with left hip pain. AP view demonstrates the line of Klein—drawn along the lateral margin of the femoral neck—failing to intersect with the femoral head on the *left side*. The metaphyseal overlap sign is also seen—with the normal small triangle of overlap between the posterior acetabular margin and the medial aspect of the proximal femoral metaphysis absent on the *left side*. The frog-leg lateral projection demonstrates the slipped left upper femoral epiphysis more easily.

benign and self-limiting. They are seen most often in boys aged 10–15 years, as incidental findings.

These focal cortical lucencies in the distal femoral metaphysis are seen at the site of tendon attachments—predominantly the medial head of the gastrocnemius muscle on the posteromedial surface, although the lateral head of gastrocnemius and adductor magnus insertions may also be affected. On MRI, they are low T1 signal, and high T2 signal—although there may be a rim of peripheral low signal sclerosis (Fig. 86.29). The lesions may enhance with gadolinium, and may show uptake on bone scan due to associated inflammation/trauma.

Proximal Focal Femoral Deficiency (PFFD)

PFFD is a *congenital defect of upper femoral development* ranging in severity from mild femoral shortening with coxa vara to complete absence of the proximal third of the femur and no hip joint [21].

Key Facts

- Rare entity, affecting approximately 1:50,000
- Bilateral in~15%, usually asymmetrical
- May be associated fibular deficiency (see below)
- Associated sporadic syndromes: *femur-fibula-ulna complex, femoral hypoplasia-unusual facies syndrome*
- Rarely part of WNT1A associated genetic disorder (*Al-Awaadi-Raas-Rothschild syndrome*)

Imaging Techniques

Plain radiographs of pelvis and affected femur. AP radiographs of remaining lower limb bones (a leg length radiograph if able to stand). MRI is useful in preoperative planning. CT is useful for peri and postoperative trouble-shooting.

Imaging Findings

The **Paley classification** is commonly used to describe the clinical and imaging findings in PFFD (Table 86.5 and Fig. 86.30).

Treatment

Requires specialist orthopedic management. Depending on imaging findings, reconstruction may be attempted. Successful treatment addresses the deformity and establishes bony continuity of the upper femur, and corrects acetabular dysplasia. Lengthening may be performed later. The surgical results are monitored by radiographs (typically standing "leg lengths" views), supplemented by cross sectional imaging. Alternatively, a prosthetic may be used to restore limb length and function (with or without amputation).

Fibular Deficiency

A *longitudinal deficiency* of the lower limb with hypoplasia of the fibular side elements; sometimes termed fibular hemimelia or postaxial hypoplasia of the lower limb.

Key Facts

- Typically isolated
- Commonest congenital long bone deficiency
- Sometimes associated with short femur or proximal focal femoral deficiency, occasionally short ulna (femur-fibula-ulna syndrome)

Imaging Technique

Plain radiographs including standing leg lengths films to guide surgical treatment. MRI is sometimes helpful to assess knee ligaments.

Imaging Findings

- Fibula is either partially present (type I) or absent (type II)
- Disorder does not just affect the fibula: other components (Fig. 86.31), variably present, include:
  - Tibial shortening (milder than fibular shortening) ± anteromedial bowing
  - *Hypoplasia of the lateral femoral* condyle leading to genu valgum
  - Deficiency of the *cruciate ligaments* leading to undeveloped tibial spines and knee instability
  - *Ball-and-socket ankle joint* (rounded talar dome with concave tibial plafond) leading to ankle instability
  - *Tarsal coalition*
  - Absent lateral rays of the foot

Treatment

Nonoperative treatments include shoe raises and bracing. Contralateral epiphysiodesis to reduce limb length discrepancies in mild cases. Limb lengthening procedures for more severe cases. Most severe cases with nonfunctional foot best treated with amputation and prosthesis.

Tibial Dysplasia

Longitudinal deficiency of the tibial side of the lower limb.

Key Facts

- Rarer than fibular deficiency
- May be inherited as autosomal dominant trait

Imaging Techniques

Plain radiographs, with standing leg lengths films when possible.

Imaging Findings

Different patterns of tibial dysplasia are described by the *Jones classification* (Table 86.6 and Fig. 86.32) [22].

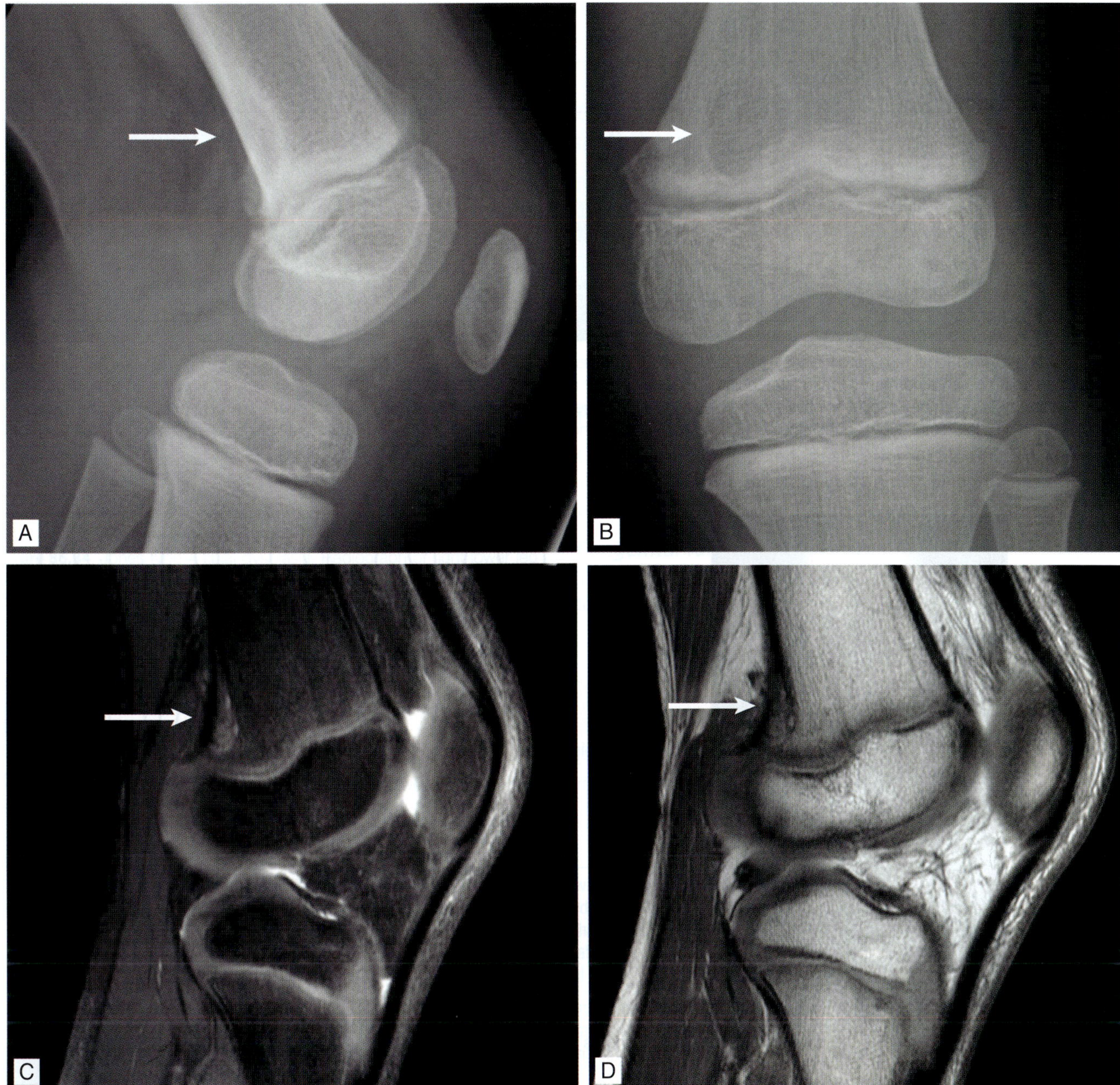

Figure 86.29 A distal femoral cortical irregularity at the site of insertion of the medial head of gastrocnemius. (A) On the lateral radiograph, the irregularity appears as a saucer-shaped lucency along the cortical surface (*arrow*). (B) The lucency can be seen en-face on the AP radiograph (*arrow*). (C) This corresponds with high signal along the cortex (*arrow*) on the proton density fat-saturated MRI image, (D) with a thin sclerotic rim (*arrow*) seen around its margin also on the nonsaturated proton density sequence.

TABLE 86.5 The Paley Classification of Proximal Focal Femoral Deficiency

Paley Type	1	2	3
Essence	Intact short femur	Pseudoarthrosis between proximal femur and femoral head	Major deficiency
Imaging appearance	Short but normally shaped femur (may show varus bowing), may have severe coxa vara, femoral head present.	Blunt proximal end of femur, femoral head may be present or fused to pelvis. Acetabulum present.	Sharp proximal end of femur, deficient femoral head (may be fused to pelvis), poorly formed acetabulum
Treatment	Limb lengthening ± hip reconstruction	Hip reconstruction and limb lengthening	1. Hip reconstruction 2. Transfer of knee to hip if reconstruction not possible 3. Amputation and prosthesis in worst cases

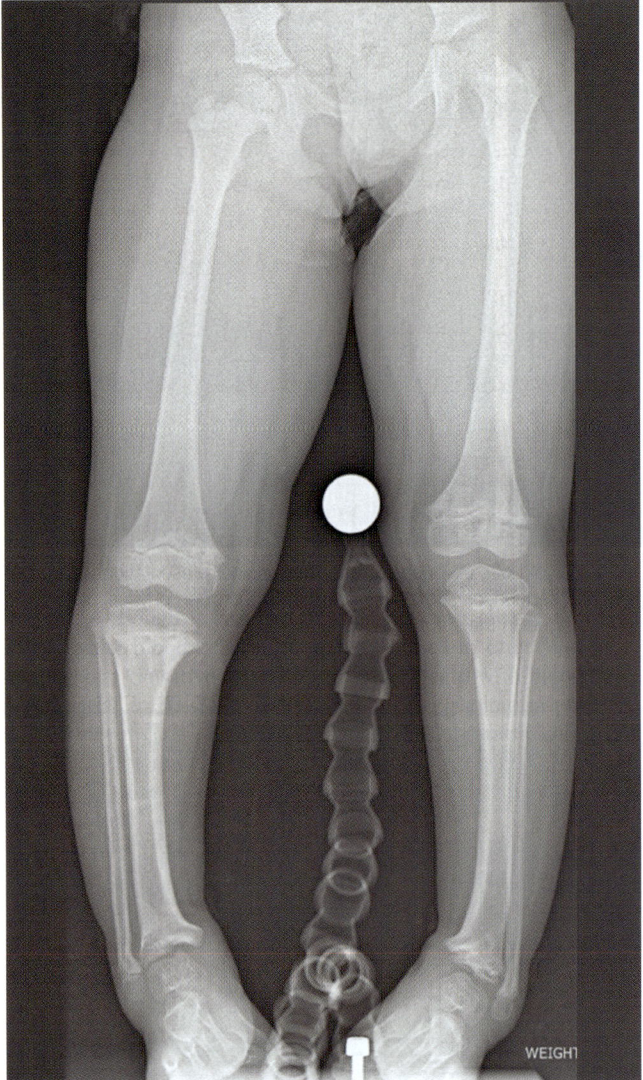

Figure 86.55 The late sequelae of disseminated meningococcus infection in the neonatal period, with asymmetric involvement at multiple joints.

- Transient synovitis is expected to self-resolve with supportive measures only

Table 86.11 provides a checklist for reporting pediatric bone infection.

TABLE 86.11 Reporting Checklist for Pediatric Bone Infection

Reporting Checklist for Pediatric Bone Infection
Is infection present?
Location of infection, multifocality
Presence of drainable collections
Associated complications—thrombophlebitis, soft tissue (pyo)myositis, fracture, chronic infection
Poor prognostic signs—marrow ischemia, large subperiosteal abscess
Recommendations on further investigations—imaging and laboratory tests

Periosteal Reaction in Children

The differential diagnosis of periosteal reaction in children can be narrowed by first considering the localization of the periosteal reaction, and the age of the child.

Localization

- Focal/unilateral: localized processes such as infection (Fig. 86.56), trauma and tumor need to be considered first
- Diffuse/bilateral: more likely due to a systemic process, although prenatal and neonatal infection are more likely to be disseminated. Metastases may also be multifocal

Age

- Under 6 months of age:
  - Physiological periosteal reaction—normal variant, typically 1–5 months of age, bilateral symmetrical, <2 mm thick along diaphysis of long bones (Fig. 86.57)
  - Infantile cortical hyperostosis (Caffey's disease, see skeletal dysplasia section) —soft tissue swelling and laminated

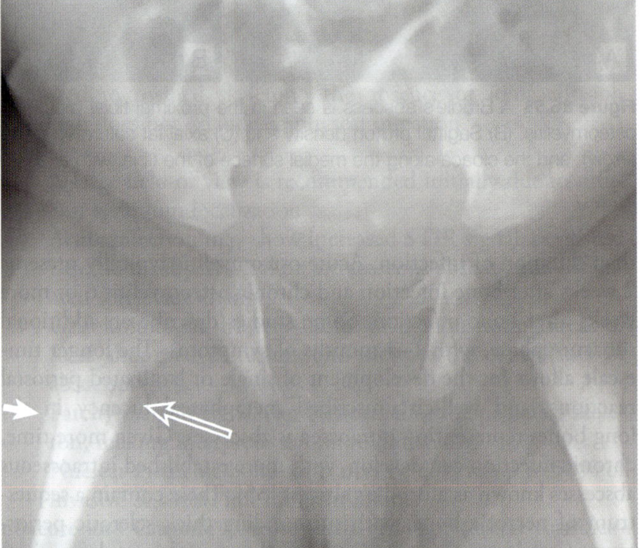

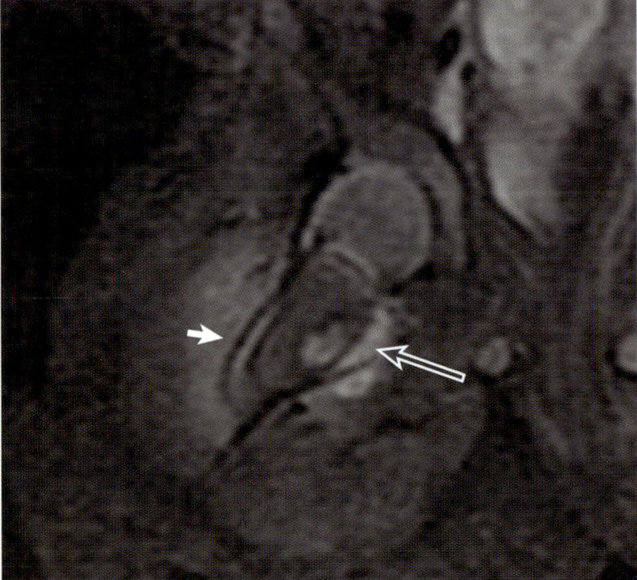

Figure 86.56 3-week-old baby with right hip and leg retracted with no active movement, due to osteomyelitis. Pathological periosteal reaction is demonstrated along the right proximal femur (*solid arrows*), with a subtle lucency in the medial aspect of the proximal femoral metaphysis due to an intraosseous abscess (*open arrows*), shown on radiograph and MRI. There is no joint effusion nor involvement of the epiphysis.

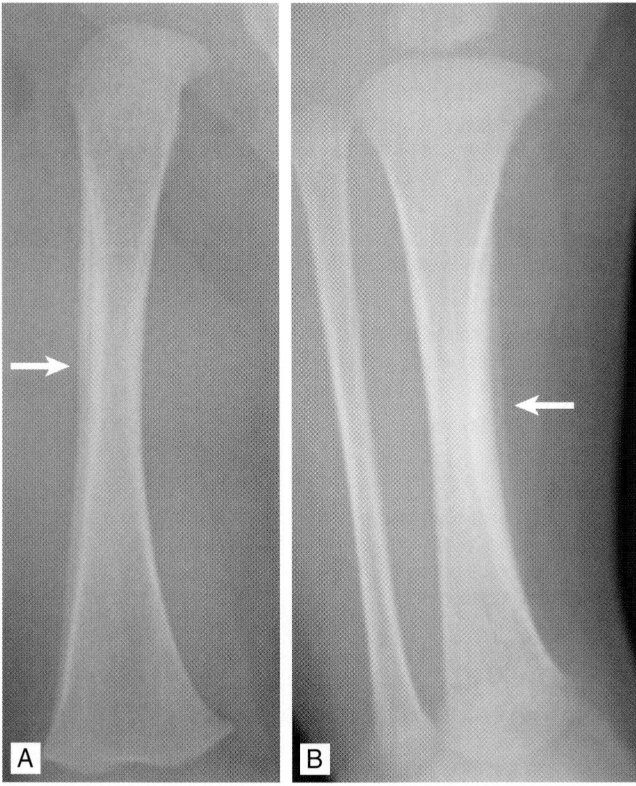

Figure 86.57 Physiological periosteal (*arrows*) reaction is demonstrated in the femur (A) and (B). It affects just the diaphysis, and is <2 mm thick.

periosteal reaction, typically of mandible, scapula, clavicle, ulna, and occasionally ribs
- ◦ Prostaglandin treatment—resolves after end of treatment
- Over 6 months of age:
  - ◦ Hypertrophic osteoarthropathy
  - ◦ Arthritides, most commonly Juvenile idiopathic arthritis (JIA)
  - ◦ Metabolic and nutritional, including hypervitaminosis A/D, scurvy, hyperparathyroidism

Osteochondroses

The osteochondroses are a heterogeneous group of conditions characterized by abnormal endochondral growth and ossification affecting epiphyses and epiphyseal equivalents. They are linked by similar radiographic appearances of flattening, sclerosis, and fragmentation within the developing growth centers. The etiology of the conditions is not well understood, but the fundamental radiographic changes are generally attributed to aseptic ischemic necrosis, with revascularisation and repair seen over time in some cases. Predisposing factors may include trauma, overuse, and genetic factors—however, many cases are idiopathic. The range of osteochondroses is summarized in Table 86.12.

Rheumatological Disorders

Juvenile Idiopathic Arthritis (JIA)

JIA encompasses a range of *chronic arthritides of childhood* onset, characterized by inflammation primarily involving synovial membranes.

Key Facts

- *Commonest rheumatological disorder* of childhood
- JIA is currently divided into *seven subtypes* (see Table 86.13)

Imaging Techniques and Findings [39,40]: *Plain radiographs* are typically *normal in early JIA*, but may be useful in *excluding various differential diagnoses*, e.g., Perthes disease, skeletal dysplasia, trauma. Erosive changes may be present in established disease.

Ultrasound is useful in confirming clinical diagnosis of *synovitis*, and in complex joints such as the ankle and wrist in particular is useful for *distinguishing between tenosynovitis and arthritis*.

MRI is valuable in demonstration of *axial skeletal involvement,* particularly in the cervical spine, and for sacroiliitis or enthesitis in the pelvis in suspected enthesitis-related arthritis (Fig. 86.58), and in evaluation of *Temporo-Mandibular Joint involvement*, which is common. MRI of the appendicular skeleton may allow evaluation for some alternative diagnoses, e.g., pigmented villonodular synovitis, intra-articular vascular anomalies. Bone marrow edema is a less useful sign in children than in adults as areas of apparent bone marrow edema are a common incidental finding in healthy children. Similarly, normal developmental pits and subchondral bone irregularity can be mistaken for erosions.

Management: Children with a small number of joints involved may initially be treated with *localized joint injections*, which may be image guided. Involvement of 5 or more joints is an indication for *systemic treatment* with a range of disease-modifying drugs.

Juvenile Dermatomyositis (JDM)

JDM is a rare autoimmune connective tissue characterized by *muscle weakness, elevated serum muscle enzymes* and a characteristic *skin rash*.

Key Facts

- *Typical rash* consists of Gottron's papules of extensor surfaces and heliotropic rash of the eyelids
- Affects girls more than boys, typical onset 5–10 years
- Muscle biopsy usually still performed to establish diagnosis, but not always necessary if clinical and MRI findings typical
- In some cases JDM may overlap with other connective tissue disorders, particularly scleroderma

Imaging Techniques and Findings: MRI of gluteal and thigh muscles, with *STIR sequences* most useful. MRI shows *muscle edema* (Fig. 86.59), which may also involve adjacent fascia and subcutaneous tissues. MRI can also demonstrate muscle wasting and calcinosis in late disease. MRI is more sensitive than muscle enzyme testing [41].

Plain radiographs and USG can be used to demonstrate areas of calcinosis in late disease.

Chronic Nonbacterial Osteomyelitis/Chronic Recurrent Multifocal Osteomyelitis

Chronic nonbacterial osteomyelitis is an *autoinflammatory disorder* characterized by sterile bone lesions. The term chronic recurrent multifocal osteomyelitis (*CRMO*) is widely used in pediatric medicine; the condition described in adults as *SAPHO* (synovitis, acnes, pustulosis, hyperostosis, and osteitis) is likely the same disorder, with broadly similar manifestations [42].

Key Facts

- Rare in first 5 years of life, typically presents in second decade
- Slight female predominance
- Typically present with pain and signs of inflammation
- Skin disease (typically acne) present in ~40% of children
- ~40% of cases are monostotic, median number of sites is 3
- *Clavicle* commonest site of monostotic and polyostotic disease
- Other commonly involved sites include tibiae, femora, vertebrae, foot bones and mandible

TABLE 86.12 The Osteochondroses

Name	Affected Bone	Features
Scheuermann	Vertebral ring apophysis	12–17 years, slight male preponderance, 75% thoracic spine. At least 3 adjacent vertebrae wedged >5 degrees, with thoracic (>40 degree) or thoracolumbar (>30) kyphosis.
Panner	Capitellum	Children 5–10 years History of throwing Resolves with rest and anti-inflammatories
Kienbock	Lunate	20–40 years adults. Repetitive microtrauma, e.g., manual labor Association with negative ulnar variant
Legg-Calve-Perthes (Perthes)	Femoral head	Classically boys 4–8 years. Mostly unilateral. If bilateral, asymmetric. Can result in deformity. (see hip section)
Sinding-Larson-Johansson	Inferior pole of patella	Adolescents 10–14 years, particularly jumping/kicking. Point swelling and focal tenderness. Soft tissue changes seen first on ultrasound/MRI. Resolves with supportive management,
Osgood-Schlatter	Tibial tubercle	Adolescents 10–14 years, particularly jumping/kicking. Bilateral in 25–50%. Point swelling and focal tenderness. Radiographic changes overlap with normal variation. Soft tissues changes on ultrasound/MRI can confirm. Most cases resolve with supportive management.
Blount	Medial compartment of knee	Bimodal distribution—infantile and adolescent forms. Medial tibial fragmentation, medial meniscal hypertrophy (see leg bowing section)
Sever	Calcaneal apophysis	Radiographic changes overlap with normal variation. MRI—bone and soft tissue edema, tendon thickening.
Kohler	Navicular	Radiographic changes overlap with normal variation—however, tends to be painful and in older children
Freiberg	Head of 2nd/3rd metatarsal	Especially adolescent females, repetitive trauma. Can predispose to early OA.

TABLE 86.13 Classification of JIA Subtypes

Category	Features	Frequency	Age of Onset
Systemic arthritis	Arthritis with or preceded by fever, with other systemic features, e.g., rash, lymphadenopathy, hepatosplenomegaly, serositis	5–15%	Any
Oligoarthritis	Arthritis affecting 1–4 joints during first 6 months of illness.	30–60%	Early childhood
Rheumatoid factor positive polyarthritis	Arthritis involving 5 or more joints in first 6 months, positive rheumatoid factor	3–7%	Late childhood/adolescence
Rheumatoid factor negative polyarthritis	Arthritis involving 5 or more joints in first 6 months, negative rheumatoid factor	10–25%	Bimodal, pre and post 6 years
Enthesitis-related arthritis	Arthritis or enthesitis and 2 of: sacro-iliac involvement, HLA B27 antigen, male aged over 6, anterior uveitis (in child or first degree relative), ankylosing spondylitis, inflammatory bowel disease, Reiter's syndrome	5–10%	Late childhood/adolescence
Psoriatic arthritis	Arthritis and psoriasis and 2 of: dactylitis, nail pitting, onycholysis, family history of psoriasis	3–10%	Bimodal, pre/post 6 years
Undifferentiated arthritis	Arthritis not fulfilling other criteria	10–20%	

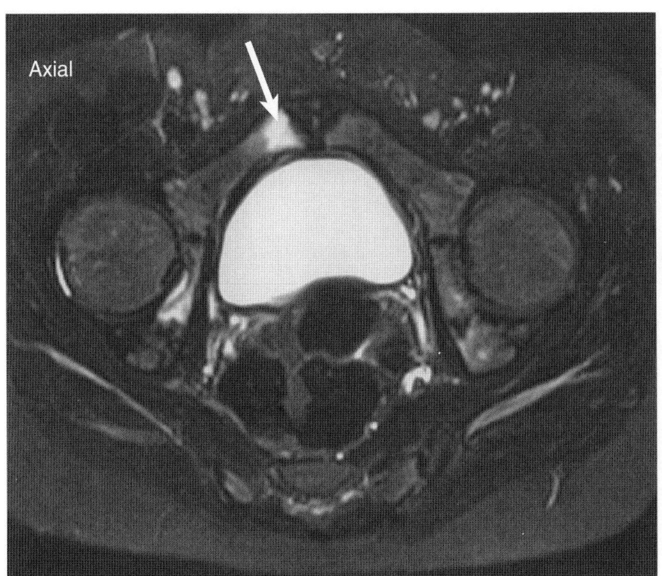

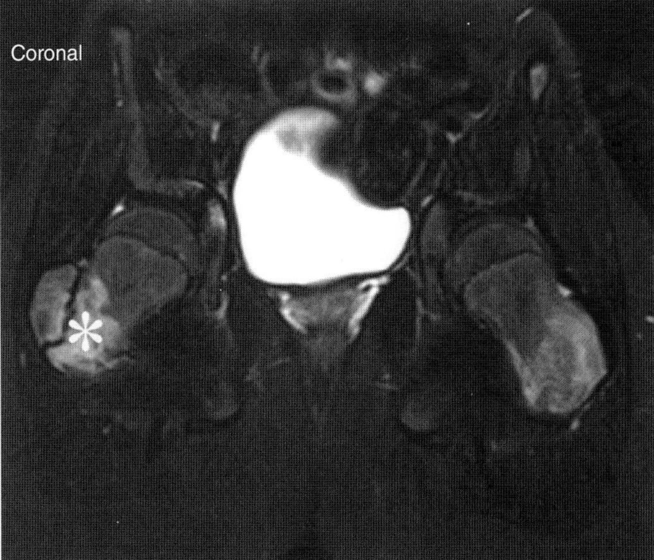

Figure 86.58 Enthesitis-related arthritis. Axial and coronal STIR MRI sequences in 13-year-old male with HLA-B27 antigen. There is inflammatory signal change in the right pubic body (*white arrow*) and in the femoral necks adjacent to both greater trochanters. Minor SI joint inflammation was also shown.

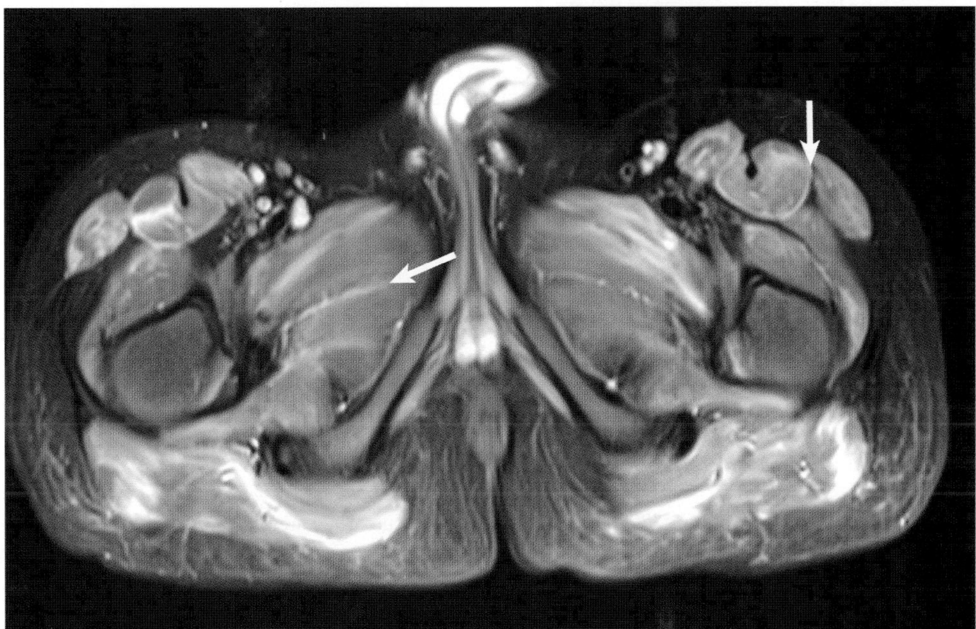

Figure 86.59 Juvenile dermatomyositis. Axial STIR MRI of pelvis in 6-year-old male with skin rash and muscle weakness. There is widespread inflammatory signal change within the pelvic musculature, most pronounced in the gluteal muscles; some edema of the deep intermuscular fascia is also shown (*arrows*).

- *Synovitis in adjacent joints* is common (approximately 50%); sacro-ileitis/spondyloarthropathy/enthesitis-related arthritis also appear to be associated in a minority of cases

Imaging Techniques: Plain radiographs are typically performed in first instance. Further evaluation with MRI useful in most cases. Screening for additional lesions via *whole body MRI or bone scintigraphy* can be very helpful, as multifocal involvement at typical sites is strongly supportive of the diagnosis.

Imaging Findings: Early appearances may be similar to infectious osteomyelitis with metaphyseal predominance, osteolytic changes on radiographs, inflammatory signal changes on MRI and periosteal reaction. Hyperostosis may develop over time (Fig. 86.60).

Management: CRMO may be considered a *diagnosis of exclusion*. A provisional diagnosis of CRMO may be applied for polyostotic disease in typical sites, especially in the presence of suggestive skin lesions. Other clinical settings, particularly *monostotic* disease usually require *tissue diagnosis* to exclude infection or neoplasia. Many patients will receive antibiotics at first presentation owing to overlap with infectious osteomyelitis. Symptomatic treatment with NSAIDS is helpful. Systemic treatment with steroids, rheumatological disease-modifying drugs and bisphosphonates have been successfully employed. The disease shows a benign course with complete symptomatic remission in approximately 2/3 of affected children, usually over 1–4 years.

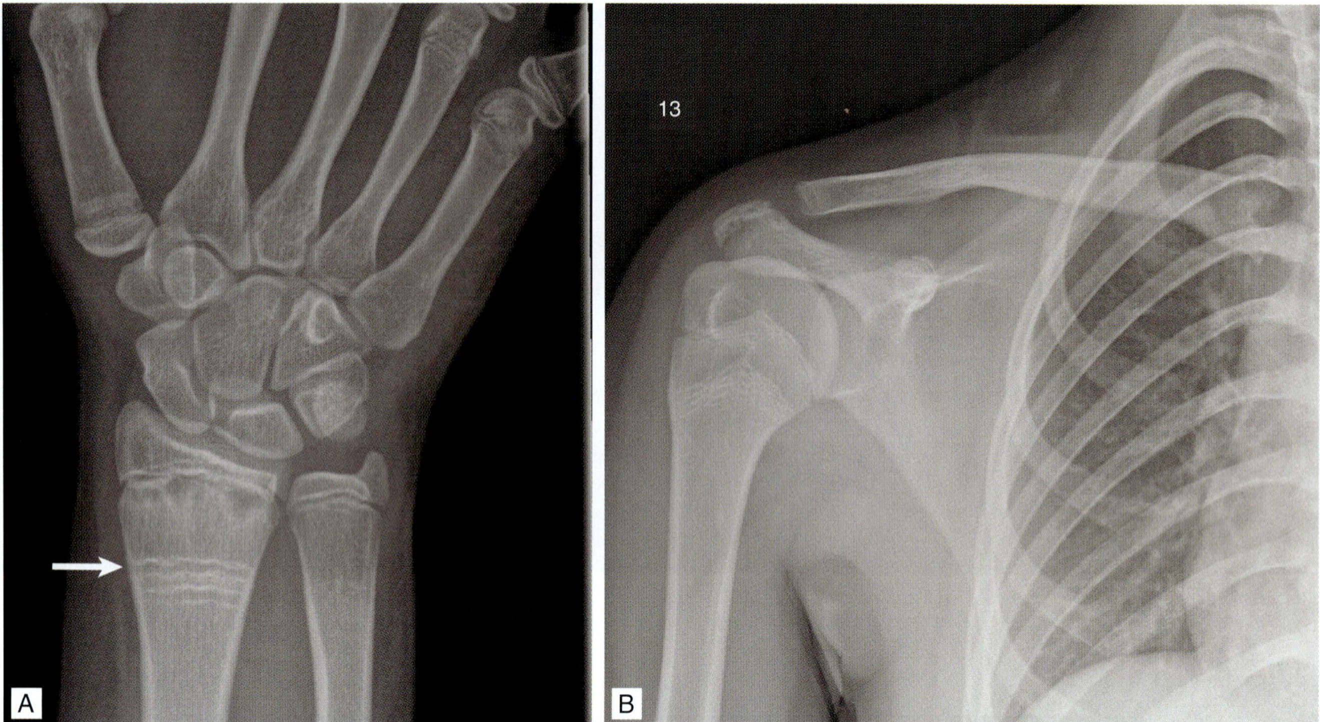

Figure 86.60 Chronic recurrent multifocal osteomyelitis. (A) Radiographs of right wrist and (B) shoulder in 13-year-old female with long history of recurrent bone pain. There is irregular osteolysis of the distal radial metaphysis reflecting recent inflammation. Transverse bands in the more proximal metaphysis (*arrow*) reflect prior treatment with intravenous bisphosphonates. The right clavicle shows expansion and hyperostosis in its medial two-thirds, reflecting chronic inflammation.

Langerhans Cell Histiocytosis (LCH)

LCH is a disorder of cells of the mononuclear phagocyte system with both *neoplastic and immunodysregulatory* components which may involve multiple organ systems including bone, skin, reticulo-endothelial system, liver, lungs, and brain (particularly hypothalamic-pituitary axis) [43].

Key Facts

- Slightly commoner in females
- 80% of childhood cases feature skeletal lesions
- Classified as
  - Single System Single Site (SS-s); 65% of cases, 80% skeletal
  - Single system multi-site (SS-m)
  - Multisystem type (MS)
- MS form commoner in younger children and has worst prognosis

Imaging Technique: Radiographs of index lesion. Skeletal survey (including bilateral limbs, but hands and feet not needed). Ultrasound first line for abdominal involvement and lymph nodes.

Imaging Findings (Fig. 86.61): LCH can involve any bone; 50% of lesions involve the *axial skeleton*. At presentation lesions are lytic, and may have an aggressive appearance. With healing they become better defined.

- Cranial vault lesions produce a lytic lesion that involves the outer table more than the inner table, producing a *"beveled" edge*. There is no marginal sclerosis at presentation, this may appear with healing
- Skull base lesions may be subtle on radiography
- Vertebral body lesions lead to severe vertebral body collapse (*"vertebra plana"*)
- Femoral and humeri are commonest long bone sites

Management: SS-s disease may be managed conservatively (depending on site) and has a good prognosis. SS-m and MS disease is usually treated systemically with chemotherapeutic agents, e.g., Vinblastine and prednisolone, with more intensive chemotherapy offered to nonresponders. Bone marrow transplantation has been performed for some intransigent cases [44].

Generalized Skeletal Disorders: Genomic and Chromosomal

Overview of Genetic Disorders of the Skeleton

Skeletal dysplasias are genetic disorders with major involvement of skeletal tissue. They are both *rare* and extremely *heterogeneous*; the commonest disorders affect only approximately 1:20,000 people, and *over 450 distinct disorders* are recognized. The genetic basis for the great majority of these entities has now been established, and genetic testing is routinely available to confirm diagnosis for most disorders. Nonetheless, radiologists with skeletal dysplasia expertise continue to play a *pivotal role* in establishing a diagnosis by precise definition of the *skeletal phenotype*, to allow correct ordering of genetic tests and interpretation of their sometimes ambiguous or uncertain results.

Skeletal dysplasias typically present with *disproportionate short stature*, which may manifest as early as 20-weeks' gestation or as late as early adolescence. Other clinical pointers to a skeletal dysplasia include facial dysmorphism or a pedigree suggesting a genetic disorder.

Early referral of a child with suspected skeletal dysplasia to a *clinical geneticist* with an interest in these disorders is the most important step. In most cases, a *radiographic skeletal survey* will be indicated (see below); this should be interpreted by an appropriately qualified individual, typically a pediatric radiologist with musculoskeletal interest. Having established a phenotype and a differential diagnosis, genetic testing will usually be performed. For commoner disorders with a clear phenotype such as *achondroplasia* this may be testing for a single gene.

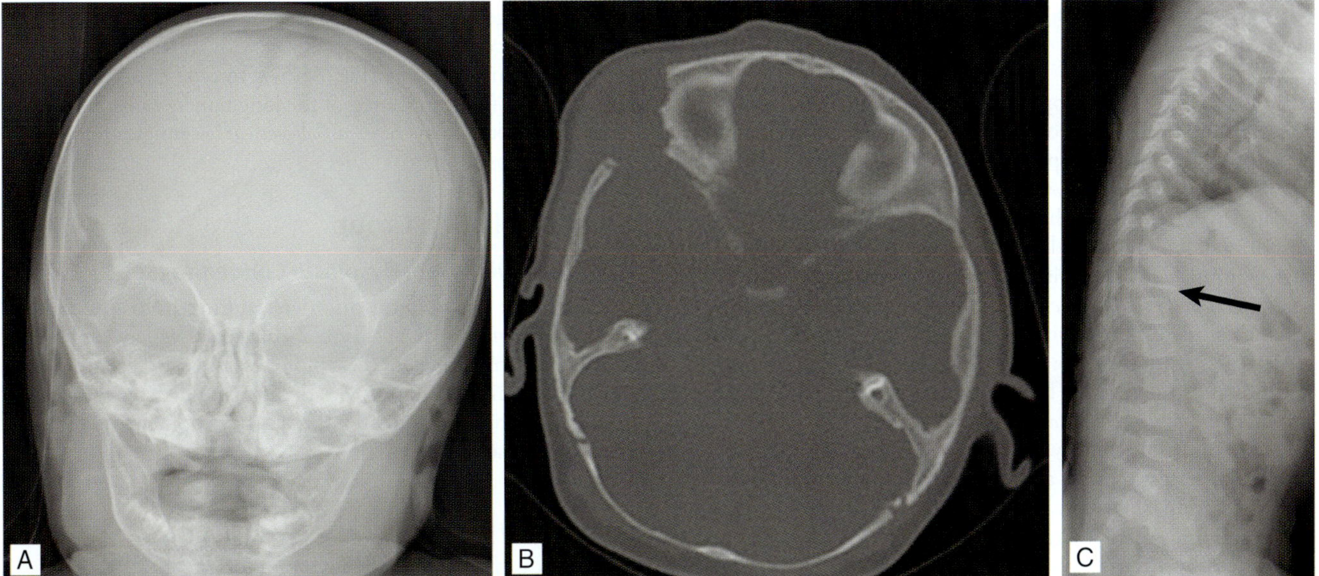

Figure 86.61 Langerhans cell histiocytosis. (A) Radiograph and (B) axial CT of skull in 30-month-old female presenting with a right supraorbital mass. There is purely lytic destruction of the right lateral supraorbital margin. Lateral spinal radiograph (C) from skeletal survey in same child shows a dense, flat vertebral body at T12 (*arrow*), "vertebra plana." A left femoral lytic lesion was also shown.

In most cases, a wider testing strategy using *next generation genetic sequencing* is undertaken; this may take the form of: testing for a *small panel* of genes; testing for all genes known to cause skeletal dysplasia; testing for all genes known to cause human disease (*clinical exome*); testing for all genes (*whole exome sequencing*); or testing the whole genome (*whole genome sequencing*).

The results of these genetic tests may give a clear confirmation of diagnosis, but in many cases, the testing reveals multiple gene variants which may or may not be pathogenic; at this point, a further review of the phenotype can help to establish which if any are the cause of the disease.

Imaging Investigations

Unlike in nonaccidental injury, where the entire skeleton must be imaged, radiographs for dysplasia diagnosis are more select.

Recommended radiographs of:

- Axial skeleton: skull (two views, to include the mandible), whole spine (AP and lateral), chest, pelvis
- Limbs: unless the disorder is asymmetric, only one side needs to be imaged—whole upper limb and lower limb, and hand (preferably the nondominant side for bone age). There is much natural variability in foot development, and foot radiographs often are noncontributory, but can be important for some conditions

Terminology

The terminology in skeletal dysplasias can be confusing, particularly as there is inconsistent, largely historical naming of some conditions. Table 86.14 provides definitions for some of the more commonly used terms; some of these terms may be combined, e.g., "acromesomelic" means shortening of distal and middle limb segments:

TABLE 86.14 Commonly Used Terms in Skeletal Dysplasia Diagnosis

Term	Definition	Example/Notes
Dysplasia	Developmental disorder of chondro-osseous tissue—bones and joints	Spondyloepiphyseal dysplasia (due to collagen 2 gene defect)
Dysostosis	Inherited congenital malformation of single (multiple) skeletal elements Typically reflects mutation in genes determining early skeletal patterning (normally <6 weeks)	Holt-Oram or Isolated polydactyly Note—there is much inconsistency around the use of this term: dysostosis multiplex (which has an evolving skeletal phenotype) is technically a dysplasia.
Disruption	Malformation of bone secondary to nongenetic causes Normally due to one hit	E.g., due to warfarin/diabetes/amniotic bands
Spondylo-	Of the spine	Spondyloepiphyseal dysplasia—involves spine and epiphyses
Chondro-	Of cartilage	Chondrodysplasia
Acro-	Distal segment	Acrodysostosis—shortening in the hands
Meso-	Middle segment	Mesomelia—shortening of forearms/tibia/fibula
Rhizo-	Proximal segment	Rhizomelia—shortening of humerus/femur

Classification of Skeletal Dysplasias: the Nosology

Although a variety of approaches to the classification of this complex and highly heterogeneous group of disorders have been attempted, the most comprehensive and up to date is the *Nosology of the International Skeletal Dysplasia Society*, most recently updated in 2019 [45]. The nosology assigns *461 distinct disorders* (425 of which have a known genetic basis) to *42 groups*. The first 9 groups consist of disorders due to mutations in *particular genes or related groups of genes*; e.g., group 1 is the FGFR3 group (including achondroplasia), whilst group 9 is the skeletal ciliopathies (mutations in genes involved in immotile cilia formation and function). The remaining groups are based on shared *radiological, clinical or pathogenetic features*, e.g., group 10 is the multiple epiphyseal dysplasia, group 25 is the osteogenesis imperfecta group and group 27 is the lysosomal storage disorder group. A review of the nosology will give readers an appreciation of the wide range of disorders that may present for assessment by a radiologist. We summarize a select few of these disorders below; a more comprehensive review is available elsewhere [46].

FGFR3 Group

Achondroplasia

Achondroplasia is the most common short limb dwarfism, and the prototypical dysplasia in the FGFR3 group. A gain of function mutation in the fibroblast growth factor receptor 3 gene results in disordered chondrocyte differentiation in the growth plate and deficient growth of bones formed by enchondral ossification.

Key Facts

- The disorder is autosomal dominant, although most cases are due to de novo mutations. Homozygosity for the gene is lethal
- It is difficult to detect antenatally until the third trimester with many cases presenting at birth
- Clinically, there is disproportionate short limb dwarfism with disproportionately large head, kyphosis at the thoracolumbar junction in infancy and a trident hand configuration
- Muscular hypotonia and foramen magnum stenosis, leading to obstructive sleep apnea and cervico-medullary compression, are major causes of morbidity
- Whilst there are a number of promising treatments in development, currently standard management is targeted to specific complications

Imaging Findings

- Short long bones, with oval radiolucency in the proximal femora and humerus in infancy, and apparent broadening of bones in children and adults (Fig. 86.62)
- Decreasing interpedicular distance inferiorly in the lumbar spine on an AP view. Short pedicles with canal stenosis and posterior vertebral scalloping
- Large calvarium, with small skull base and foramen magnum (Fig. 86.63)
- Squaring of the iliac bones, horizontal trident acetabulum, "champagne glass" pelvic inlet

Thanatophoric Dysplasia

The most common lethal skeletal dysplasia. Most cases are sporadic and recurrence is extremely rare.

The changes are more severe than in achondroplasia, and can be detected from earlier in gestation, with wafer-thin platyspondyly and a narrow thorax (Fig. 86.64). In type 1 is typically bowing in addition to shortening of the long bones, whilst in the rarer type 2 the skull may have a "cloverleaf" configuration due to craniosynsotosis.

Type 2 Collagen Group

Spondyloepiphyseal Dysplasia Congenita (SEDC)

SEDC is the prototypical disorder resulting from mutations in *type 2 collagen* (COL2A1). Type 2 collagen is widely expressed in cartilage, particularly in the epiphyses and cartilage models of vertebral bodies. Mutations result in malfolded type 2 collagen molecules, and subsequent impaired development of the spine and epiphyseal dysplasia.

Key Facts

- *Autosomal dominant* disorder
- Most cases are due to de novo mutations
- May manifest as short limbs on antenatal scan at 20 weeks
- Evident at birth
- Key clinical features of *short trunk*, short limbs, *relatively normal hands and feet*
- Facial phenotype varies from near normal to mid-facial hypoplasia, micrognathia, and Pierre-Robin sequence
- May develop hypermetropia. At risk of retinal detachment

Imaging Techniques: *Skeletal survey* once diagnosis suspected (usually in first few weeks of life).

Flexion and extension lateral view of cervical spine if there are neurological concerns.

MRI of craniocervical junction for those with suspected cervical instability.

Key Imaging Findings (Fig. 86.65)

- *Immature vertebral body ossification*
  - Vertebral body heights similar to pedicles
  - Wide disc spaces
  - Vertebral body sizes reduce from L1 to L5 ("anisospondyly" or "meionospondyly")
- *Delayed appearance of epiphyses* and epiphyseal equivalents
  - Absent or small pubic bones at birth
  - Absent knee epiphyses at birth
- Rounded pelvic bones
- Abrupt horizontal cut-off of upper femora
- Rhizomelic limb shortening
- Relative *normal appearance of hands* and feet
- Relatively large appearing skull (may show mid-facial hypoplasia and micrognathia)

Management

- Surgical cervical stabilization required in some
- Adults develop precocious osteoarthritis and may require early joint replacement
- Regular ophthalmological assessment

Sulfation Disorders

This group of conditions are due to mutations in the "diastrophic dysplasia sulfate transporter" (DTDST) gene. The transporter is highly concentrated in chondrocytes, where it functions to move most of the cell's sulfate—critical for sulfation of proteoglycans and normal cartilage development. As with other groups there is a spectrum of severity; from the severe achondrogenesis to the milder recessive multiple epiphyseal dysplasia.

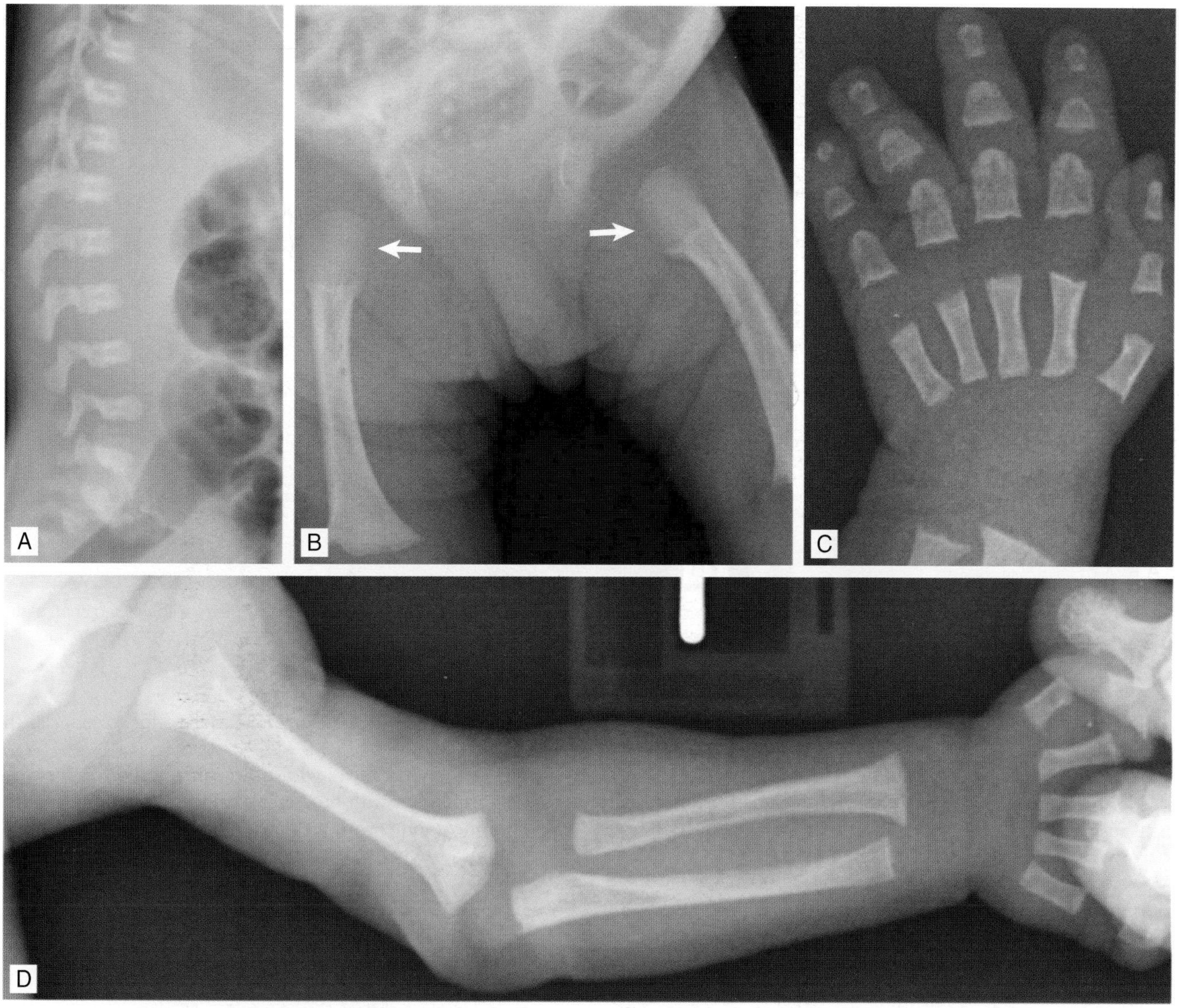

Figure 86.62 Neonate with achondroplasia. There were short long bones and frontal bossing on prenatal ultrasound. (A) There are bullet-shaped vertebral bodies and (B) phalanges, (C) oval-shaped lucency (*arrows*) of the proximal femurs, sloped proximal humerus metaphysis (D) and short long bones. The trident acetabulum is part obscured by overlying bowel. The nonwidening of interpedicular distance in the lumbar spine is seen later in infancy.

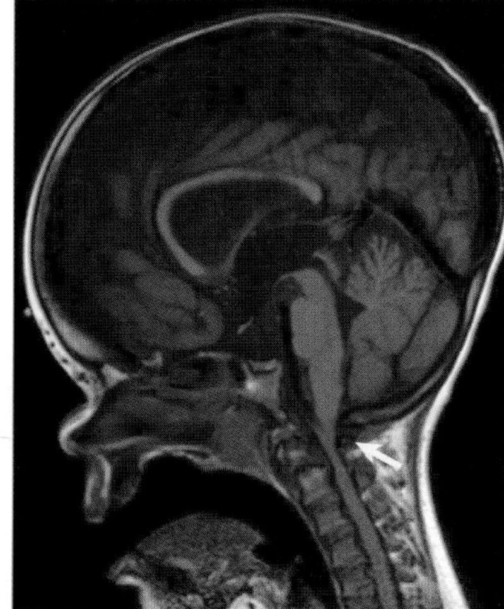

Figure 86.63 MRI of the cervical spine in the same child at the age of 5, demonstrating frontal bossing, and foramen magnum stenosis with compression of the cervical cord (*arrow*)—a major cause of morbidity in achondroplasia.

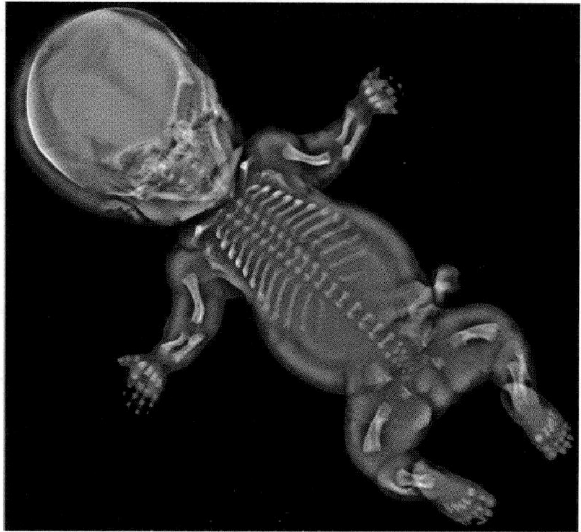

Figure 86.64 There is wafer-thin platyspondyly, shortening of long bones with disproportionate short limbs and bowing of humeri and femurs, a narrow thorax with short ribs, short metacarpals and phalanges, small square iliacs with broad acetabulae, and hypoplastic ilia. Relatively macrocephaly. The overall appearances are those of type 1 thanatophoric dysplasia.

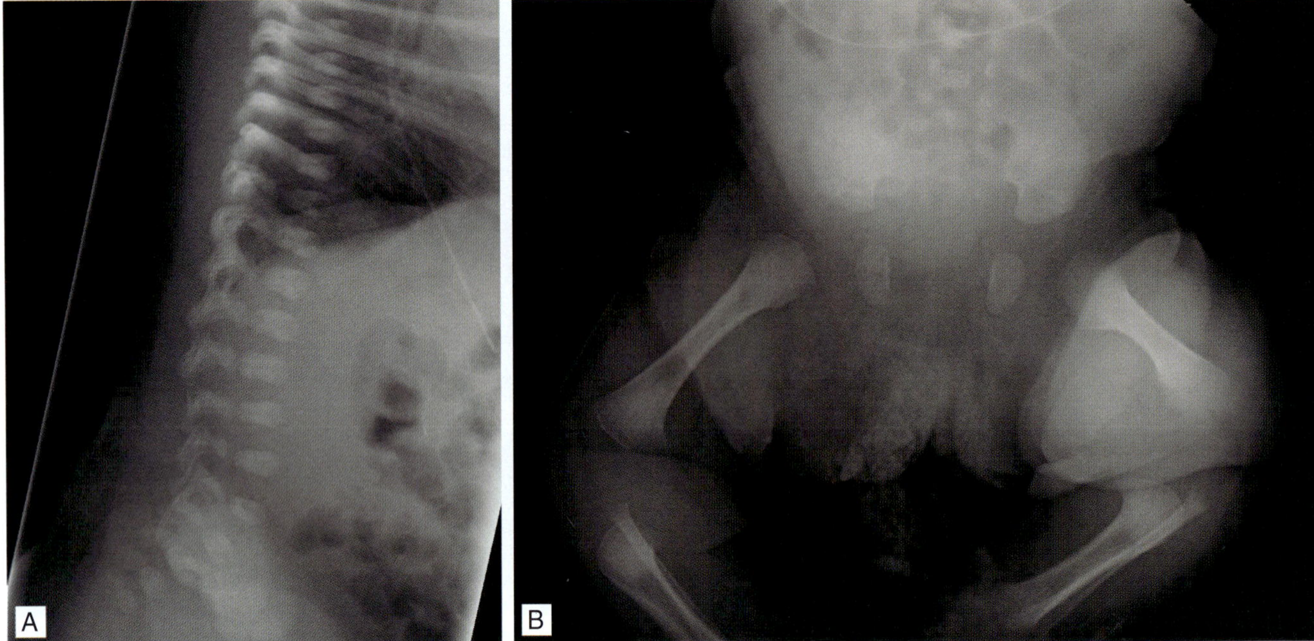

Figure 86.65 Spondyloepiphyseal dysplasia congenita. (A) Radiographs spine and (B) pelvis in 5-day-old female born at term with marked short stature. The vertebral bodies are small and "pear-shaped," and become progressively smaller from L1 to L5. The pubic bones and knee epiphyses are unossified, indicating ossification delay. A rounded appearance to the iliac bones and a "sawn-off" appearance of the upper femora is also shown.

Diastrophic Dysplasia

Key Facts

- Autosomal recessive
- Normally presents at birth although can be detected prenatally if suspected
- Very wide phenotypic variability
- Accordingly variable prognosis: increased perinatal and infant mortality, however normal life expectancy after infancy in the absence of significant spinal complications
- Small stature with short extremities, joint contractures, treatment resistant clubfeet, "hitch-hiker" thumb, "cauliflower" ears, progressive kyphoscoliosis after infancy

Imaging Findings (Fig. 86.66)

- Short, deformed tubular bones in hands and feet with metaphyseal widening
- Flat broad epiphyses—often seen best in the metacarpals ("melting snow")
- Oval shaped first metacarpal, proximally placed, adducted/dislocated thumb
- Delayed proximal femoral epiphysis appearance, broad club-like femur
- Progressive kyphoscoliosis, particularly cervical kyphosis

TRPV4 Group

The Transient Receptor Potential, Vanilloid group 4 (TRPV4) gene encodes the protein for a calcium permeable nonselective cation channel. This is required for normal calcium influx.

Metatropic Dysplasia

Metatropic dysplasia is at the severe end of the TRPV4 spectrum; Kozlowski type spondylometaphyseal dysplasia and autosomal dominant brachyolmia are examples of milder TRPV4-related conditions.

Key Facts

- Autosomal dominant, but with germline mosaicism
- There may be increased infant mortality due to reduced thoracic volume
- The phenotype evolves with time; initially short limbs with a long trunk, but with progressive truncal shortening
- Prominent joints with restricted mobility
- Odontoid hypoplasia can cause hypermobility of the cervical spine and medullary stenosis, often requiring operative stabilization
- There may be a tail-like appendage over the sacrum

Imaging Findings

- Marked dumb-bell shape to the long bones with shortening and metaphyseal flare (Fig. 86.67)
- Small dysplastic epiphyses
- Platyspondyly with broad flat vertebral bodies, irregular endplates, and "overfaced" pedicles (borders of vertebral borders lie lateral to lateral border of pedicles). Kyphoscoliosis may develop with time
- Irregular talus, calcaneus. Hypoplastic upper cervical spine. Early hyoid/cricoid cartilage calcification

Skeletal Ciliopathies

Short-rib Thoracic Dysplasia

Short-rib thoracic dysplasia, previously called as Asphyxiating thoracic dysplasia is characterized by *shortening of the ribs* causing respiratory embarrassment ranging from perinatal lethality to cosmetic deformity only. Also known as *Jeune's syndrome.*

Key Facts

- Prototypical *skeletal "ciliopathy."* Ciliopathies are a broad group of disorders involving mutations in genes involved in formation and function of cilia. Motile cilia are involved in fluid transport at mucosal brush borders. Immotile cilia have complex functions relating to intercellular signaling
- Shows *autosomal recessive* inheritance pattern
- Large number of different ciliopathy genes can produce this phenotype

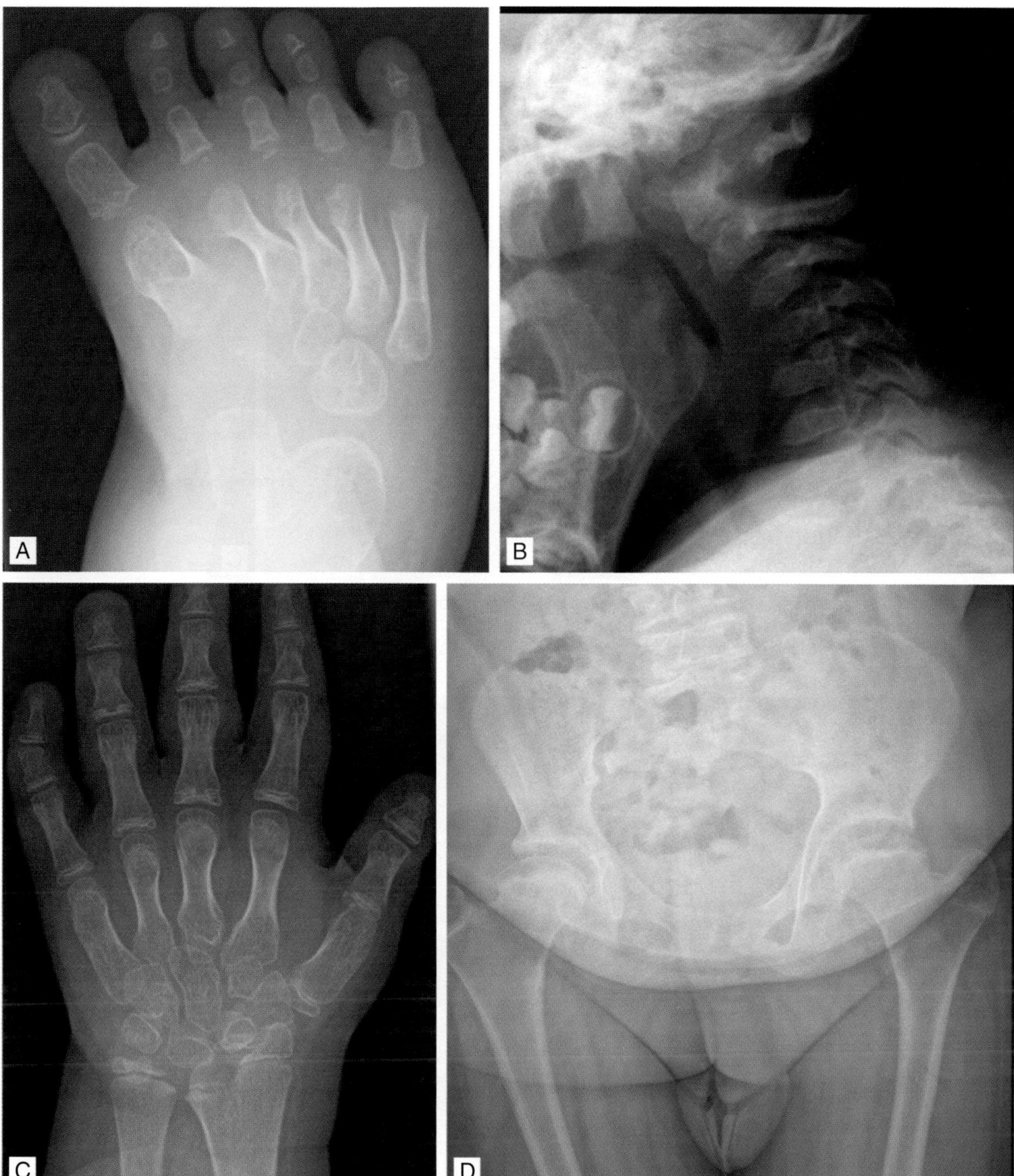

Figure 86.66 Diastrophic dysplasia. (A) Radiograph of left foot in 2-year-old male with diastrophic dysplasia. There is a club foot with a wide "sandal-gap" (1st interphalangeal space). (B) Radiograph of c-spine in same child at aged 2. The c4 vertebral body is hypoplastic and there is associated hyperkyphosis. (C) Radiograph of left hand in same child at age 9; there is brachydactyly. The metacarpal epiphyses show characteristic flattening, said to resemble "snow melting on a cabin roof." (D) Pelvic radiograph in same child aged 12 shows epiphyseal dysplasia with flattening of the femoral capital epiphyses.

- *Renal involvement* common, typically showing cortical cysts; may develop renal failure
- *Retinitis pigmentosa* develops in some

Imaging Technique: *Skeletal survey* to establish diagnosis. Abdominal ultrasound for demonstration of renal disease. Thoracic CT can be used to demonstrate impact of rib shortening on lungs.

Imaging Findings (Fig. 86.68)

- *Ribs globally shortened. "Trefoil-shaped"* axial cross section of chest wall on CT
- *Trident acetabulum* in infancy, resembling that seen in infants with achondroplasia
- Limb shortening typically showing *progressive distal-ward shortening* (hands and feet shorter than mesomelic segments, which are shorter than rhizomelic segments)
- Short tubular bones in hands may show *cone-shaped epiphyses*
- Polydactyly in 5–15%
- *Normal spine* helps distinguish from achondroplasia, along with lack of typical facial features

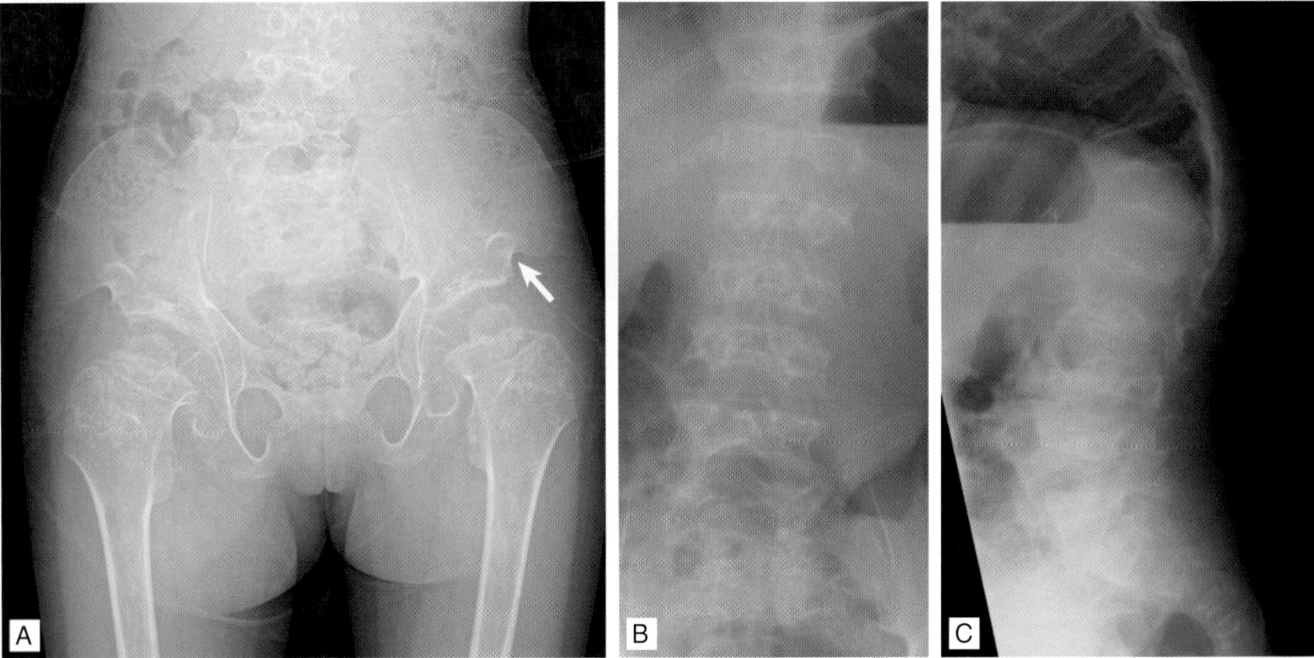

Figure 86.67 9 year old female with confirmed metatropic dysplasia. (A) Pelvic radiograph shows marked flaring of the iliac bones with supra-acetabular constriction (*arrow*). There is also marked flaring of the upper femoral metaphyses. (B) AP and (C) lateral views of the lumbar spine show marked platyspondyly and characteristic "overfacing" of the lumbar pedicles: the vertebral body margins extend lateral to the lateral borders of the pedicles on the frontal view.

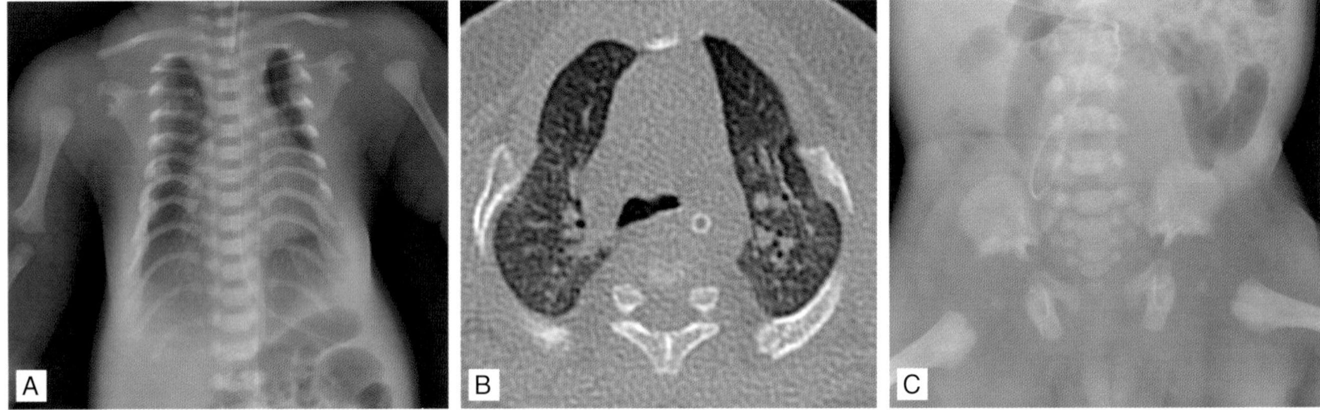

Figure 86.68 Short-rib thoracic dysplasia (A) Neonatal radiograph and (B) CT at aged 14 weeks of chest in female with respiratory insufficiency and narrow chest. The ribs are markedly short, producing a "trefoil" or "clover-leaf" shape to the chest in axial section. Neonatal pelvic radiograph (C) in same child shows a "trident" acetabulum, similar to that seen in achondroplasia; the spinal and upper femoral features of achondroplasia are not present.

Prognosis and Management: *Severe thoracic involvement* leads to *respiratory failure* and early death. Supportive treatment with oxygen, pressure-support and in some cases tracheostomy. *Surgical expansion of the chest wall* is performed in some centers and may improve outcome, but usually does not lead to elimination of ventilatory support. Milder chest deformity may improve over childhood. Milder cases may require renal replacement therapy or ophthalmological involvement later in life.

Chondroectodermal Dysplasia (Ellis-Van Creveld)

This ciliopathy is due to mutations in the EVC or EVC2 genes, which encode cilia-related proteins. Although there is some overlap in the radiographic appearance with Short-rib thoracic dysplasia—with short ribs, progressive distal-ward shortening of limbs, cone-epiphyses and polydactyly (Fig. 86.69)—the ectodermal changes help differentiate the conditions.

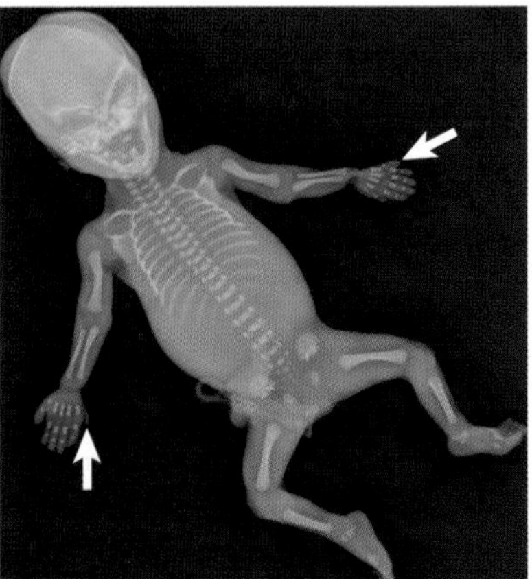

Figure 86.69 A fetus with Ellis-van Creveld. Note particularly the six-digit postaxial polydactyly (*arrows*), narrow thorax and trident acetabulae.

Key Facts

- Autosomal recessive inheritance with variable expression
- Up to 60% have a cardiac defect, and there is often pulmonary hypoplasia in infancy; complications of both of which largely account for the elevated infant mortality
- Variable dental abnormalities: neonatal teeth, small teeth, enamel hypoplasia, serrated incisal margins
- Short upper lip with multiple frenula
- Hypoplastic nails
- In the absence of cardiopulmonary complications, life expectancy is normal with dental intervention and corrective surgery as needed

Imaging Findings

- Progressive distal-ward shortening of limbs (hand shorter than forearm, shorter than humerus) resulting in predominant acromesomelic limb shortening
- Postaxial or axial hexadactyly (six digits, constant finding)
- Abnormal hands, with fusion or overlapping of the capitate and hamate and cone-epiphyses
- Slanting proximal tibial metaphyses and asymmetric, medially skewed proximal tibial epiphysis

Multiple Epiphyseal Dysplasia and Pseudoachondroplasia Group

Multiple Epiphyseal Dysplasia (MED)

In epiphyseal dysplasias, the epiphyses are small, and generally late to appear. Multiple epiphyseal dysplasia has both recessive and autosomal dominant forms, with multiple different genetic mutations resulting in distinct phenotypes. Nonetheless, similar localization of the pathology to epiphyses means joint pain and limitation is a common feature. Height is not necessarily reduced. It is important to consider hypothyroidism as a differential for multiple delayed epiphyses.

Key Facts

- Most MED is autosomal dominant
  - COMP mutations are most common, but COL9A1-3, and MATN3 mutations are also causative
  - In addition to the epiphyseal irregularity, there is also variable flattening and irregularity of vertebral bodies in the thoracic spine. The carpal bones may be irregular in outline (Fig. 86.70)
  - The hands are relatively spared
  - Secondary degenerative arthritis can be severe, with some patients unable to stand or walk by age 50 without treatment
- The recessive form of MED (25%) is due to a mutation in the DTDST gene and is classified as a sulfation disorder (above)
  - Flattened "snow melting" epiphyses in the hand, and double-layered patellae are two of the more distinctive features (Fig. 86.71)
  - Whilst the joint pain tends to be milder, clubfeet can be difficult to treat

Pseudoachondroplasia

Is due to a mutation in the COMP gene, and hence has some phenotypic overlap with one of the autosomal dominant forms of

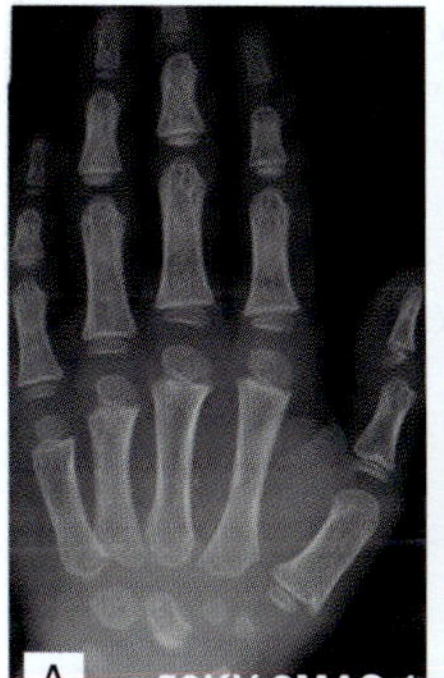

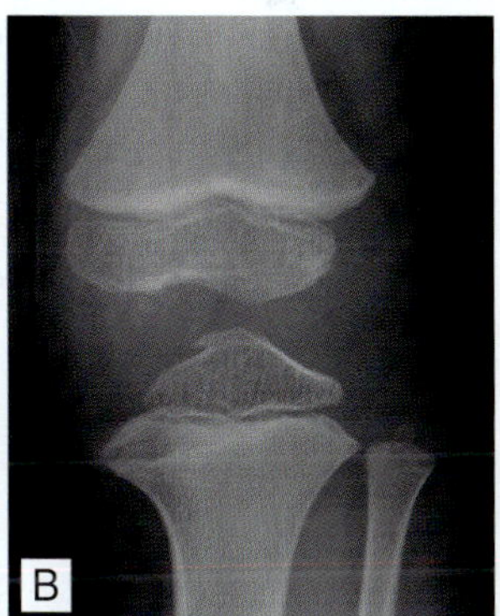

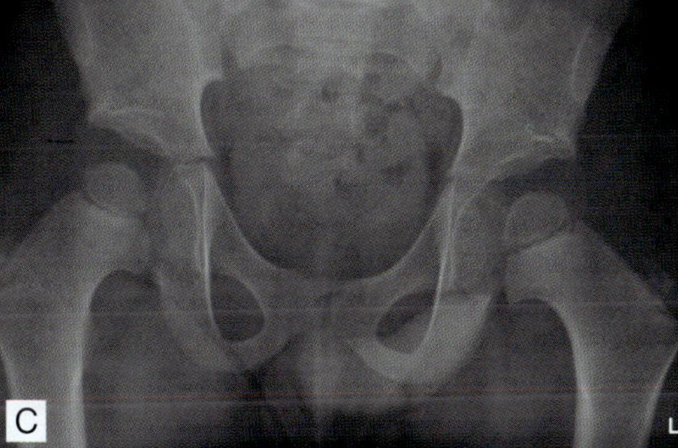

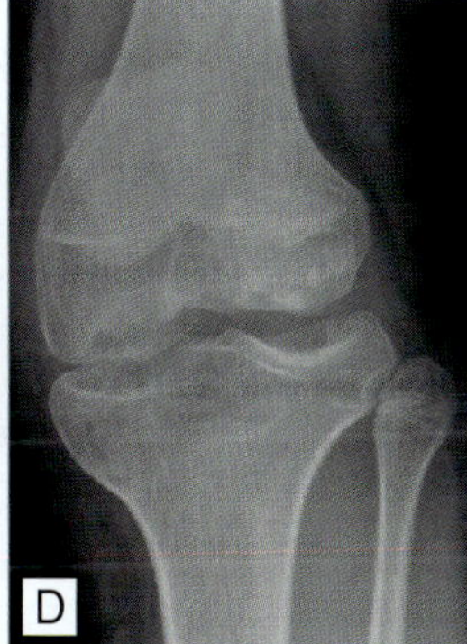

Figure 86.70 8-year-old boy presenting with joint pains. (A) Initial images at presentation show irregular carpal bones, and relatively small epiphyses. (B) The knees are more affected than the (C) hips. (D) By age 15, there is severe early onset arthritis, worst at the knees. The underlying diagnosis of autosomal dominant multiple epiphyseal dysplasia was genetically confirmed.

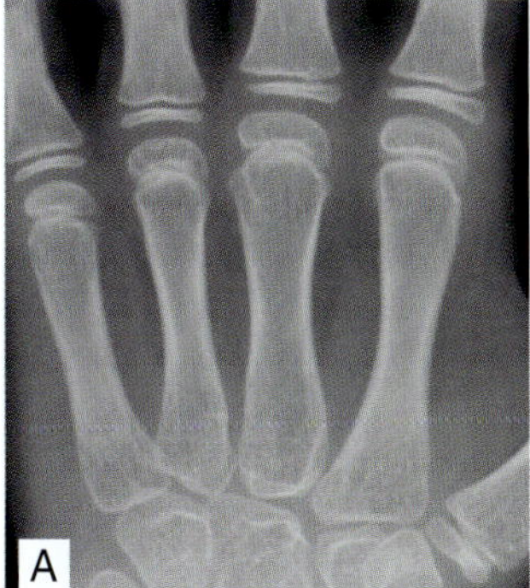

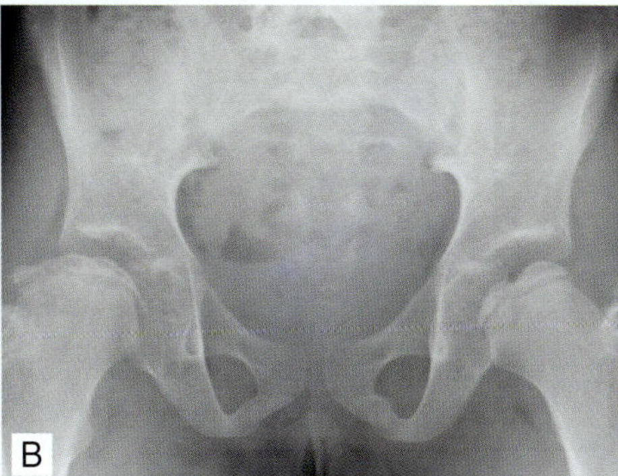

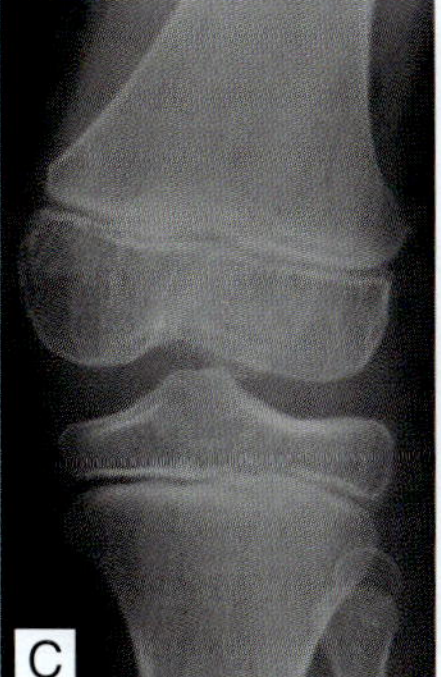

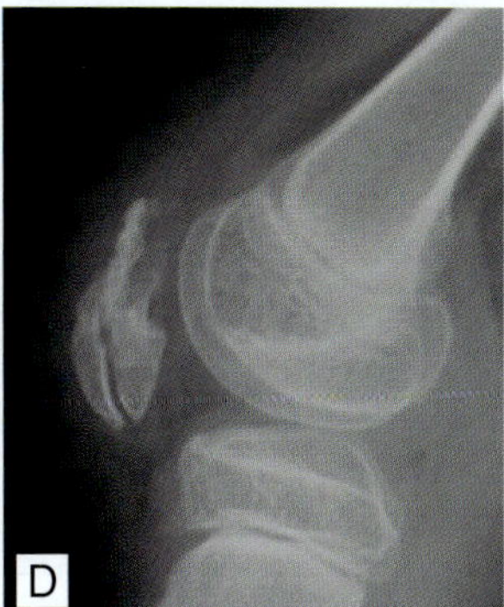

Figure 86.71 Radiographs of hand (A), pelvis (B), and AP left knee (C) and lateral left knee (D) in a 6-year-old boy. There is abnormal shaping and fragmentation of the epiphyses. Features suggesting that the multiple epiphyseal dysplasia in this case is recessive, due to a mutation in the DTDST gene, include the characteristic "snow-melting on roof" appearance of the metacarpal epiphyses (A), and the double-layered patella (D).

MED (above) but is at the more severe end of the spectrum. The COMP protein is normally found in extracellular matrix around chondrocytes, tendon, and ligament. The mutation causes toxic intracellular accumulation of malfolded COMP ("endoplasmicreticulum stress"), resulting in inflammation and oxidative stress within epiphyseal and growth plate cartilage. The chondrocyte arrangement in the growth plate becomes disordered, with acellular gaps between clusters of chondrocytes and reduced chondrocytes moving into the proliferative and hypertrophic zones needed for longitudinal growth.

Key Facts

- Autosomal dominant, with geminal mosaicism. 70% of cases are de novo mutations
- Manifests normally after infancy or later, with waddling gait and growth retardation
- Limbs are disproportionately short but the head and face normal
- There is joint hypermobility other than at the elbows, and knee deformities (windswept, genu valgum/varum) are common. Kypho/scoliosis develops in ~50%
- Cervical instability is seen in a minority, with risk of neurological impingement needing surgery

Imaging Findings

- Small, irregular epiphyses progressing to dysplastic joints
- Short tubular bones with wide, strikingly irregular metaphyses (Fig. 86.72)
- The carpal bones are small and deformed
- Moderate flattening of vertebral bodies with a biconvex shape and anterior "tonguing"

Metaphyseal Dysplasias

In metaphyseal dysplasias, there is generally irregularity of metaphyseal margins with large epiphyses. As a generalization, because the epiphyses and hence the joint surfaces are relatively preserved, although linear growth is impaired there are fewer arthritic complications compared to epiphyseal dysplasias.

Schmid, cartilage hair hypoplasia (McKusick), Schwachman-Diamond, and Jansen type are included in this heterogenous group.

Cartilage Hair Hypoplasia: An *autosomal recessive multisystem disorder* manifesting immune deficiency, sparse hair and a skeletal dysplasia of variable severity.

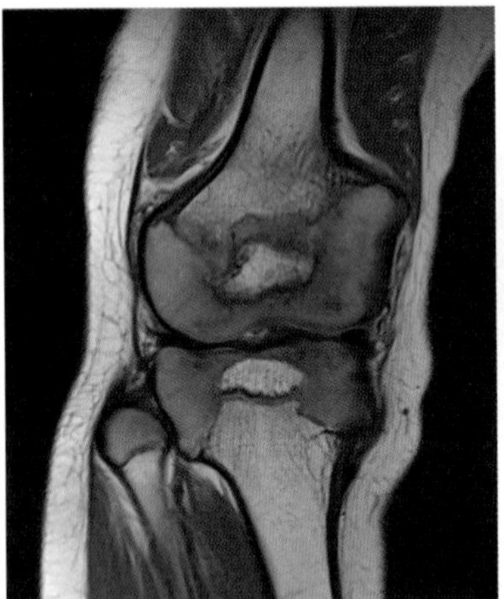
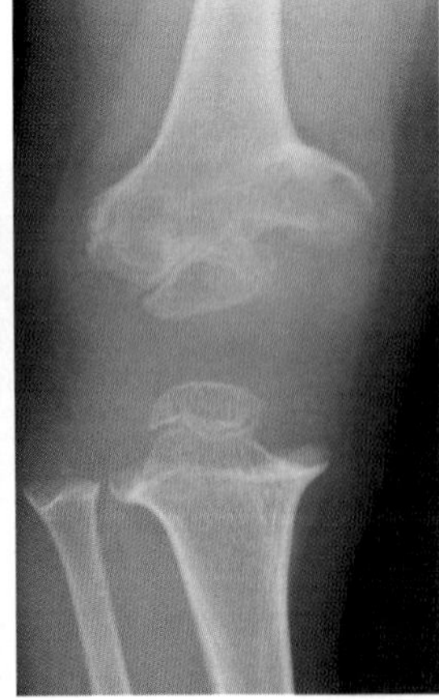

Figure 86.72 The striking cartilaginous hypertrophy of pseudoachondroplasia in a 6-year-old boy, demonstrated at the right knee on proton density MRI sequence (*right*); the resultant distorted metaphyseal and epiphyseal modeling is seen on plain film (*left*).

Key Facts

- Results from mutations in *RMRP*, a gene encoding a mRNA that is *not translated*, but instead regulates ribosomal function
- Rare overall, but common in *North American Amish* (founder effect)
- Results in abnormal function of various cell lines including t-lymphocytes, chondrocytes, and cells in hair follicles
- Immune deficit varies from severe combined immunodeficiency (SCID) necessitating bone marrow transplantation, to asymptomatic t-cell lymphopenia
- Skeletal involvement varies from extreme short stature to minimal involvement

Imaging Findings

- Neonatal severe presentation with short bowed femora, large round lower femoral epiphyses and brachydactyly
- Later presentation with stocky long bones, relatively long fibula, *brachydactyly with subtle coning of epiphyses* ('semilunar' epiphyses) (Fig. 86.73)
- Spine may show reduced progression of lumbar interpedicular distances (similar to achondroplasia)
- Pelvis usually normal

Management and Prognosis: Severe immune defects may require bone marrow transplantation.

Schmid Type Metaphyseal Dysplasia: An autosomal dominant skeletal disorder with short stature but relatively little functional impairment. It is important in radiology prospective as the metaphyseal changes early on can appear almost identical to rickets (Fig. 86.74). Bone density is however preserved.

Key Facts

- Due to a mutation in the COL10A1 gene resulting in endoplasmicreticulum stress in hypertrophic chondrocytes
- Typically presents around the second year of life
- Short stature, with disproportionate short limbs, bow legs and a waddling gait

Imaging Findings

- Cupping, fraying splaying of metaphyses, particularly in the lower limbs

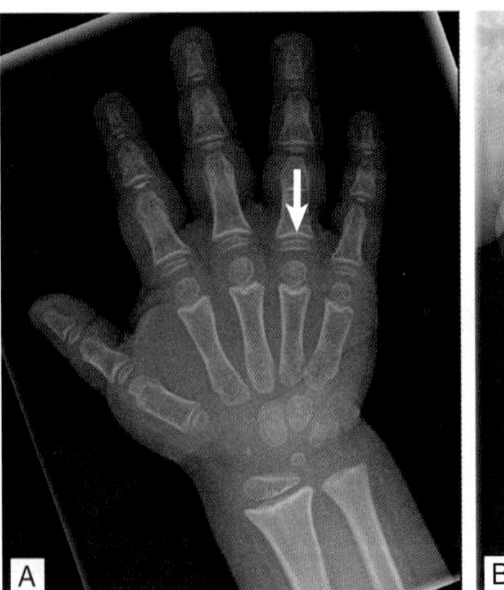

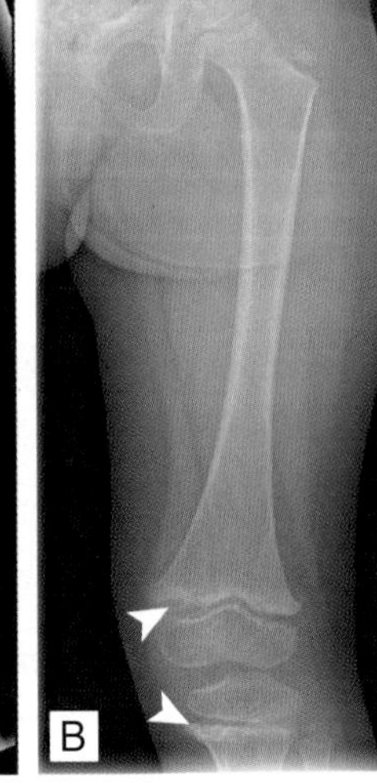

Figure 86.73 Cartilage hair hypoplasia. Radiographs of left hand (A) and left femur (B) from skeletal survey in 3-year-old female with short stature and family history of immunodeficiency. The hands are small with multiple areas of subtle coning of the metaphyses in the proximal phalanges (*arrow*) and 2nd to 5th metacarpals. There is irregular metaphyseal ossification in the lower femur and upper tibia (*arrowheads*).

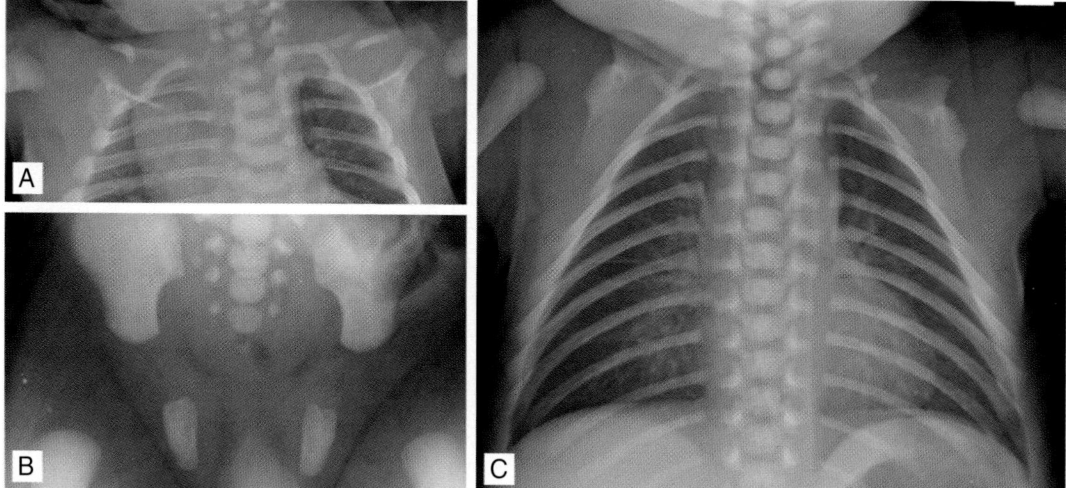

Figure 86.96 A 2-month-old baby presented with a palpable clavicular defect. (A) On plain film, there are bilateral mid-clavicular defects, and (B) there is absence of pubic bone ossification (normally expected by 22–24 weeks gestation) in keeping with cleidocranial dysplasia. There is some variability in phenotype, clavicular changes ranging from fairly mild defects seen in this case, to severe hypoplasia with a (C) "bell-shaped" chest.

- There may be shortening and deformity of the affected bones.
- Unlike other hemangiomas, the spindle-cell hemangiomas of Maffucci syndrome show phlebolith formation

Cleidocranial Dysplasia

This disorder results from dominant mutations in RUNX2, an important determinant of osteoblast differentiation, resulting in defective ossification of membranous bone.

Key Facts

- Normally manifests at birth, although can be detected in the second trimester
- Clavicular hypoplasia to varying degrees, narrow chest, small scapula
- Deciduous teeth can persist, and there can be impaction of supernumerary adult teeth
- Narrow pelvis and hypoplastic distal phalanges are less commonly seen

Imaging Findings

- Delayed ossification of the skull, delayed closure of sutures, median cleft in the occipital bone, Wormian bones, small maxilla
- Hypoplasia of the clavicles (more commonly middle/lateral), hypoplastic scapulae (Fig. 86.96)
- Delayed ossification and underdevelopment of the pubic bones and inferior ischium
- Pseudoepiphyses of the metacarpal and metatarsal bones, dysplastic little finger middle phalanx, hypoplastic distal phalangeal tufts, delayed carpal bone ossification

Craniosynostosis

Aperts Dyndrome: Aperts syndrome is the commonest of the *acrocephalosyndactylies*; it comprises brachycephaly due to *bicoronal craniosynostosis* with *central distal syndactyly* of the hands leading to a characteristic *"mitten-hand" deformity*.

Key Facts

- *Autosomal dominant* disorder (frequently due to a new mutation) resulting from mutations in *FGFR2*
- Associated with advanced paternal age
- Developmental delay present in some children
- *Pfeiffer syndrome* is a similar disorder with milder hand features but often more severe cranial dysmorphism

Imaging Techniques: Skeletal survey usually not needed as it is a clear clinical diagnosis. Radiographs of hands and feet to define bony anatomy before surgery. Volumetric cranial CT to plan craniosynostosis repair.

Imaging Findings (Fig. 86.97)

- Brachycephaly with bilateral coronal craniosynostosis and resulting *harlequin eye deformity*
- Maxillary hypoplasia
- *Bony syndactyly* of the central distal phalanges in the hands; short radially deviated distal phalanx of thumb; carpal synostosis in some
- *Cutaneous syndactyly* of central toes; broad hallux in varus; metatarsal bony syndactyly in variable patterns
- Glenoid hypoplasia and shoulder instability, occasional elbow anomalies
- Cervical spine segmentation anomalies, typically C-6 block vertebra

Management: Plastic surgical intervention restores some hand function. Cranial vault expansion to improve cosmesis and in some causes manage raised intracranial pressure.

Vertebral Dysostoses

Spondylocostal Dysostoses and Spondylothoracic Dysplasia

Key Facts

- There are autosomal recessive and dominant forms. Multiple gene mutations have been associated, although most affect the Notch signaling pathway
- Due to the genetic heterogeneity, there is broad phenotypic variability
- Scoliosis and/or kyphosis is congenital– there may be secondary respiratory impairment
- Associated cardiac and genitourinary malformations

Imaging Findings

- Normally greater than 10 contiguous vertebral segmentation defects (Fig. 86.98)
- Alternating left and right hemivertebrae produce the "pebble beach sign"
- The degree of scoliosis depends on the pattern of segmentation defects
- There may be associated rib anomalies—aplasia or fusion, and in some cases ribs may converge posteriorly ("crab chest").

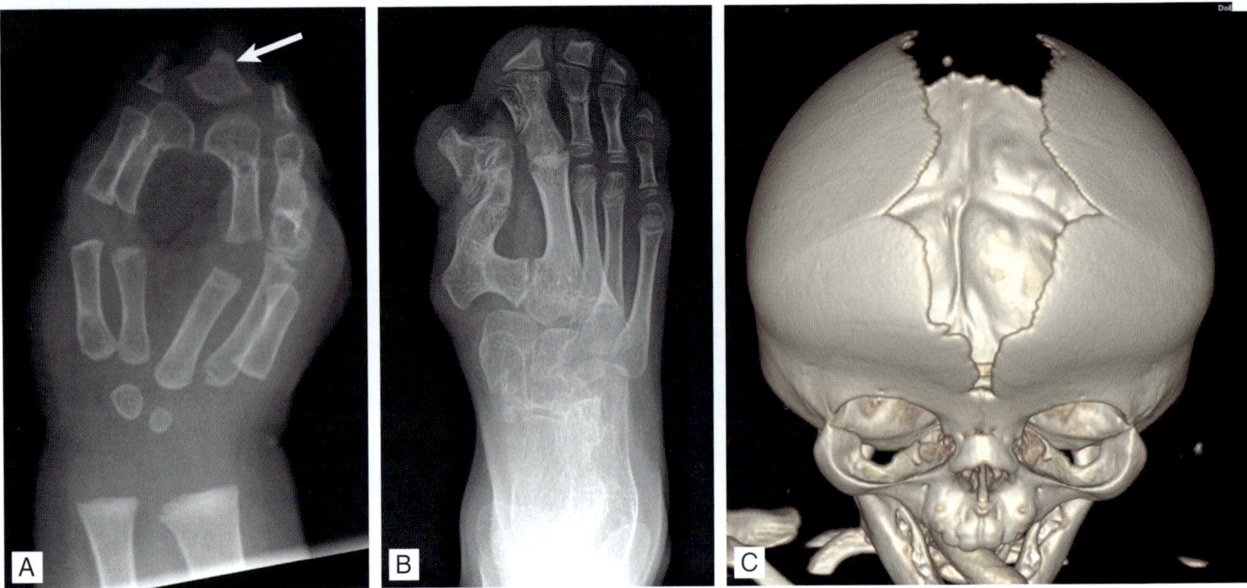

Figure 86.97 Apert syndrome. (A) Left hand radiograph in 36-week-old female showing "mitten-hand" deformity with central distal bony syndactyly (*arrow*). (B) Left foot radiograph in same child aged 6 years showing short broad hallux in varus, and soft tissue syndactyly of toes 2–5. (C) Volume rendered image from craniofacial CT in same child at aged 1 year showing bicoronal craniosynostosis.

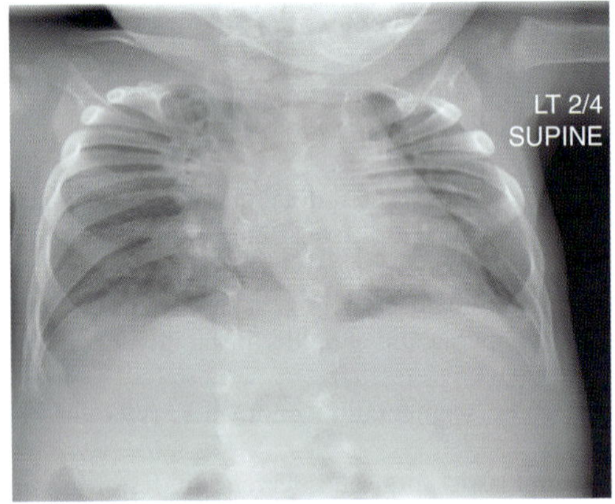

Figure 86.98 Spondylocostal dysostosis. Chest radiograph in 1-year-old female with short trunk. There are contiguous segmentation anomalies of the entire thoracic and lumbar spine, with posterior rib convergence producing the "crab-chest" appearance.

Respiratory complications are more common in these cases (previously termed "Jarcho-Levin syndrome")

Patellar Dysostoses

Nail-Patella Syndrome

Key Facts

- Autosomal dominant, normally presenting in late childhood
- Hypoplastic or absent patella, palpable posterior iliac horns, hypoplastic nails
- Restricted elbow and knee movements
- Nephropathy in approximately 25% in adulthood, which is the major cause of morbidity

Imaging Findings (Fig. 86.99)

- Hypoplastic or absent patella. Hypoplastic lateral femoral condyle
- Posterior iliac horns
- Hypoplastic radial head and capitellum—occasional radiocapitellar dislocation

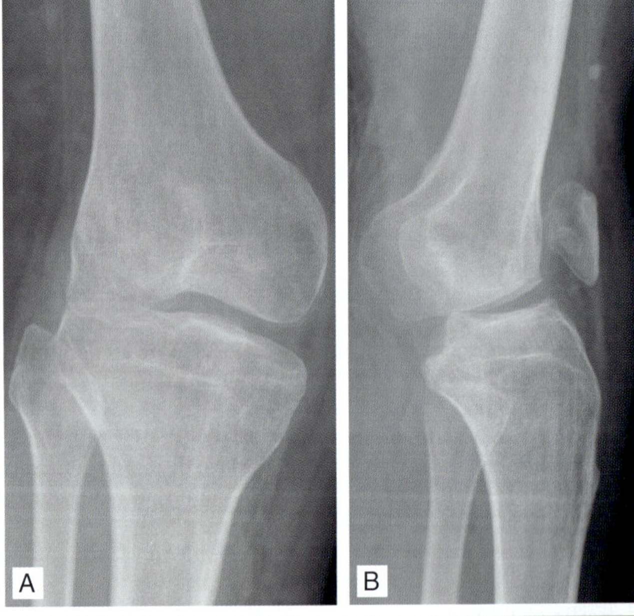

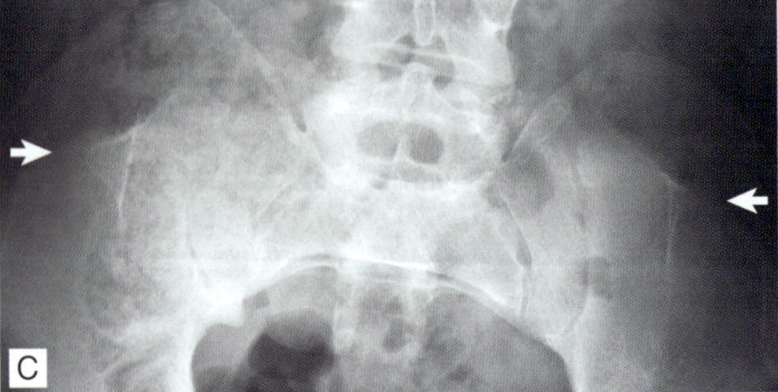

Figure 86.99 In nail-patella syndrome, there may be joint instability with recurrent dislocations, in addition to patella hypoplasia (A, B). Bilateral iliac horns (*arrows*) may be present (C).

TABLE 86.16 Skeletal Findings in Commoner Chromosomal Aneuploidies

Disorder	Karyotype	Skeletal Findings
Down syndrome (Fig. 86.100)	Trisomy 21	Accessory manubrial ossification centers (80%) 11 rib pairs (33%) "Bell-shaped" chest (80%) Alanto-axial instability (usually mild) Flared iliac wings Joint laxity, less frequently DDH
Turner syndrome (Fig. 86.101)	45 × 0	Shot 4th and 5th metacarpals Madelung deformity Skeletal features largely reflect haploinsufficiency for the SHOX gene
Edwards syndrome	Trisomy 18	Radial longitudinal deficiencies Overlapping 2nd and 3rd fingers Micrognathia
Patau syndrome	Trisomy 13	Postaxial polydactyly Overlapping digits Rocker-bottom feet Micrognathia

Skeletal Findings in Aneuploidies

Disorders involving abnormal numbers of chromosomes are termed aneuploidies, and may have wide ranging manifestations, reflecting abnormal imprinting or haploinsufficiency of large numbers of genes.

Skeletal findings in some of the commoner disorders are summarized in Table 86.16.

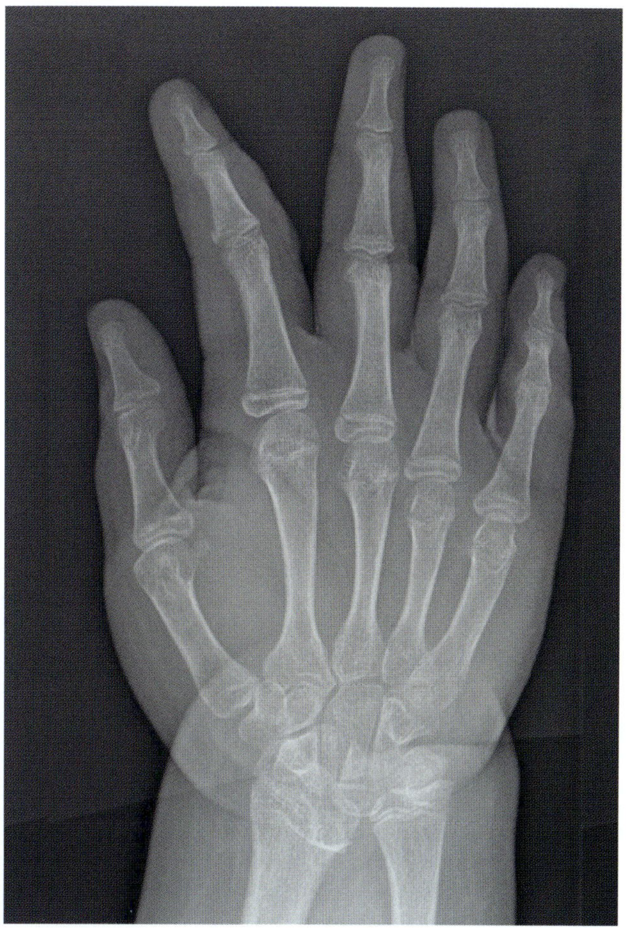

Figure 86.101 Turner syndrome; left hand radiograph in 14-year-old female with 45 × 0 karyotype. There is a Madelung deformity of the wrist. The 4th metacarpal is slightly short.

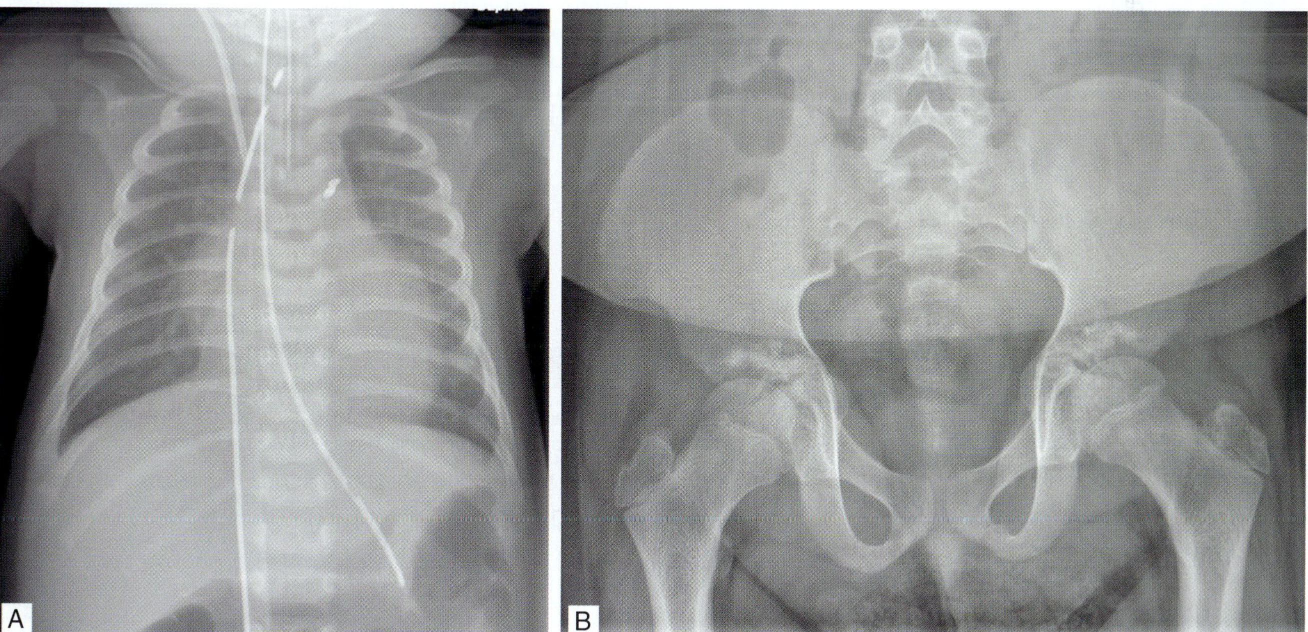

Figure 86.100 Skeletal features in trisomy 21. (A) chest radiograph in 4-week-old female with trisomy 21 post pulmonary artery band procedure for AVSD; there are 11 rib pairs, and the upper ribs are slightly short, producing a slightly "bell-shaped" chest. (B) Pelvic radiograph in 11-year-old male with trisomy 21 and acute leukemia. The iliac bones are markedly flared.

Generalized Skeletal Disorders: Metabolic

Rickets

A disorder of the growth plate, which has been considered synonymous with vitamin D deficiency, it includes a spectrum of conditions that result in prolonged low serum phosphate with or without hyperparathyroidism.

Key Facts

- *In vitamin D deficiency,*
  - The reduced gut absorption of calcium leads to hypocalcemia
  - This in turn leads to *secondary hyperparathyroidism*, which causes increased phosphate excretion in the urine and subsequent *hypophosphatemia*
  - Hypophosphatemia leads to *failure of apoptosis of mature hypertrophic chondrocytes* in the growth plate; these then accumulate, causing widening of the growth plate, and fraying and splaying of the metaphysis. This effect is potentiated by a direct action of elevated parathyroid hormone (PTH) on chondrocytes
  - Reduced availability of calcium and phosphate leads to diminished mineralization of osteoid during bone turnover, resulting in soft bones which bend *(osteomalacia)*, and sometimes *Looser zones* (pseudofractures, unmineralized seams of osteoid)
  - Prolonged hyperparathyroidism directly leads to loss of bone mass *(osteopenia)* and bone fragility
  - Thus, vitamin D deficient bone disease in children presents as a triad of rickets, osteomalacia, and hyperparathyroidism
- Causes of rickets are described in Table 86.17

Imaging Techniques

Radiographs of one wrist and knee are usually sufficient. Children with x-linked hypophosphatemic rickets require regular renal ultrasound for nephrocalcinosis. Leg length views for bowing deformities are helpful.

Imaging Findings (Fig. 86.102) [48]

- *Widening of the growth plate with splaying (widening) and fraying (irregular, patchy ossification) of the metaphyses*, most pronounced at sites of rapid growth (e.g., distal ulna); at the costochondral junctions, this produces the "rachitic rosary." These changes are often milder in FGF23 dependent rickets
- *Bowing of long bones due to osteomalacia*, femoral varus bowing and anterolateral bowing of tibiae are typical, and feature in all forms of rickets (Fig. 86.35B)
- Features of *hyperparathyroidism* (osteopenia, intracortical and subperiosteal bone resorption, brown tumors, salt and pepper skull) in PTH dependent forms of rickets, less pronounced or absent in FGF23 dependent ("phosphopenic") forms
- *Fractures* common in PTH dependent forms of rickets. Rarer in infants before mobility, although may occur in severe disease. Fractures unusual in FGF23 dependent forms, although Looser zones may occur

Management

Diagnosis is confirmed by biochemical evaluation, including serum calcium, phosphate, alkaline phosphatase (ALP), PTH and 25-OH Vitamin D levels. These determine subsequent consideration of differential diagnoses.

- If serum calcium and phosphate are low, but vitamin D levels are normal, testing for genetic forms of rickets are indicated; this includes measurement of renal tubular reabsorption of phosphate (for hypophosphatemic rickets), 1,25-OH Vitamin D levels (for 1-alpha hydroxylase deficiency) as well as genetic sequencing
- If the alkaline phosphatase level is low (usually elevated in rickets), hypophosphatasia must be considered
- If sercum calcium, phosphate, and PTH levels are normal, a metaphyseal chondrodysplasia should be considered (e.g., metaphyseal chondrodysplasia type Schmid; note that Jansen metaphyseal chondrodysplasia may present with low serum calcium and phosphate)

Treatment of vitamin D deficient rickets is with vitamin d supplementation. Restoration of normal serum biochemistry is rapid (within days). The earliest sign of healing rickets radiographically is the re-appearance of the "metaphyseal white line" at the zone of provisional calcification, and is apparent within days of restoration of normal biochemistry. Dense metaphyseal bands may subsequently develop. Bowing deformities may take months to remodel.

TABLE 86.17 Causes of Rickets

Category	Disorder
PTH dependent ("calcipenic") rickets Increased PTH activity leads to rickets through decreased renal reabsorption of phosphate. PTH also amplifies the effect of hypophosphatemia on the growth plate.	Vitamin D deficiency
	Dietary calcium deficiency. Commonest cause of rickets in some African countries. May compound vitamin D deficiency.
	1-alpha hydroxylase deficiency (autosomal recessive disorder) 1-alpha hydroxylase creates the active form of vitamin D, 1,25-OH Vitamin D
	Vitamin D receptor deficiency (autosomal recessive genetic disorder). Associated alopecia in most cases.
FGF23 dependent ("phosphopenic") FGF23 is a bone derived hormone which downregulates expression of renal phosphate transporters and inhibits 1-alpha hydroxylase. Excess FGF23 secretion leads to hyperphosphaturia and low serum phosphate. Hyperparathyroidism is usually mild or absent.	X-linked hypophosphatemic rickets (X-linked dominant disorder)
	Paraneoplastic rickets (associated with neoplasms of mesenchymal origin, includes linear sebaceous naevus syndrome)
Other	Renal tubular disorders (e.g., Fanconi syndrome) due to renal phosphate wasting

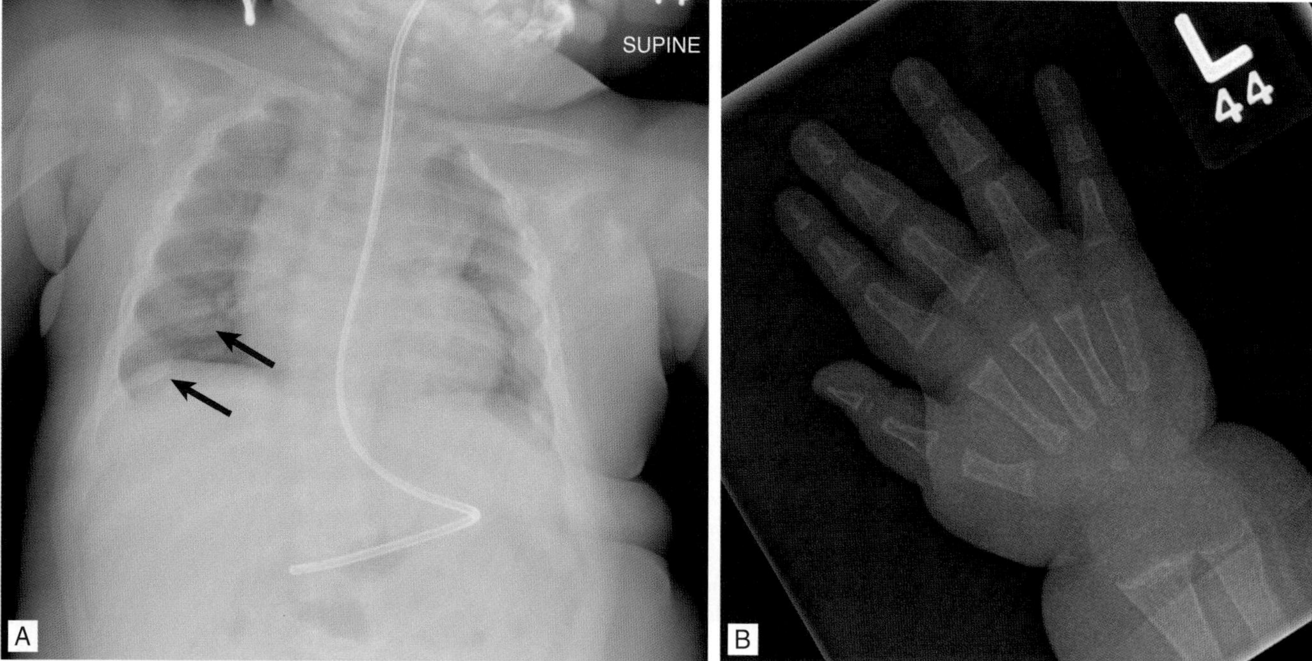

Figure 86.102 Nutritional rickets; 20-month-old male with vitamin d deficiency, hypophosphatemia, and hyperparathyroidism. (A) Chest radiograph shows that the anterior ribs are expanded ("rachitic rosary," *arrows*). (B) In the wrist there is splaying and fraying of the distal radial and ulnar metaphyses. There is marked osteopenia.

Metabolic Bone Disease of Prematurity (Osteopenia of Prematurity)

The active trans-placental transport of calcium and phosphorus occurs mostly in the third trimester, peaking between weeks 32–36 of gestation. Premature infants miss out on this crucial stage of mineralization. The time of presentation is typically 6–12 weeks after birth [49].

Risk Factors

- Placental insufficiency
- Very low (<1500 g) or extremely low (<1000 g) birth weight—20–50% babies
- Prolonged TPN (>4 weeks)
- Exclusive breastfeeding in preterm babies
- Neonatal complications such as necrotizing enterocolitis/chronic lung disease of prematurity/hyperbilirubinemia
- Diuretic/steroid use
- Immobility, e.g., sedation/paralysis

Clinical Features

- Enlargement of cranial sutures, frontal bossing
- Fractures, rickets
- Postnatal growth failure
- Typical biochemical profile: high alkaline phosphatase (>1000 IU/L), low serum phosphate (<1.8 mmol/L). Serum calcium levels may be normal, or conversely high due to low serum phosphate stimulating 1-alpha hydroxylase, which increases gut calcium absorption [49]

Imaging Findings

- Radiographs are the mainstay for diagnosis. DEXA and quantitative ultrasound may be used in a research setting
- The presentation varies widely from mild osteopenia, to frank rickets with multiple fractures (Fig. 86.103)

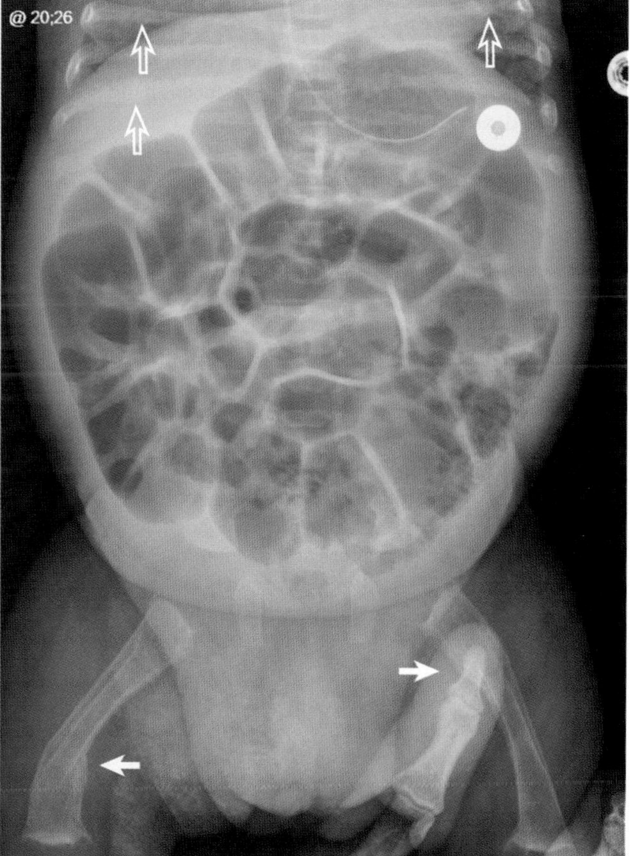

Figure 86.103 Bilateral healing femoral fractures (*solid arrows*) and healing rib fractures (*open arrows*) in an ex-24-week gestation premature infant. There is diffuse bony osteopenia, with splaying, fraying, and cupping of the metaphyses. In the correct clinical context, the appearances are in keeping with severe metabolic bone disease of prematurity.

- Most common fractures are of the long bones and ribs; metaphyseal and skull fractures not expected
- Nephrocalcinosis may be seen due to the secondary hypercalcaemia resulting from low serum phosphate
- A scoring system proposed by Koo suggests [50]
    - Grade 1: osteopenia
    - Grade 2: osteopenia with rachitic changes
    - Grade 3: osteopenia with rachitic changes and fractures
- Fractures may however occur in the absence of rachitic changes
- Biochemical and radiological changes can take 6–12 weeks to recover post treatment

Scurvy

Multisystem illness resulting from *vitamin C deficiency.*

Key Facts

- Vitamin C is required for *hydroxylation of proline residues* during *post-translational modification* of various *collagen* molecules
- Vitamin C deficiency leads to *impaired collagen synthesis*, particularly affecting bone, leading to *osteopenia*, and blood vessels, leading to a *bleeding tendency*

Imaging Techniques

Scurvy is often unsuspected, so may present incidentally. Radiographs of long bones are most helpful. MRI can also demonstrate the features.

Imaging Findings (Fig. 86.104)

- *Demineralization* most pronounced in submetaphyseal regions ("Trummerfield zone"), a metaphyseal lucent band adjacent to relative dense metaphyseal margin, the "Frankel line") and epiphyses ("Wimberger ring sign," relatively dense appearing epiphyseal margins)
- *Bone fragility*, including tendency to metaphyseal corner fractures ("Pelken spurs")
- *Periosteal reactions* reflecting subperiosteal hemorrhage
- Hemarthrosis

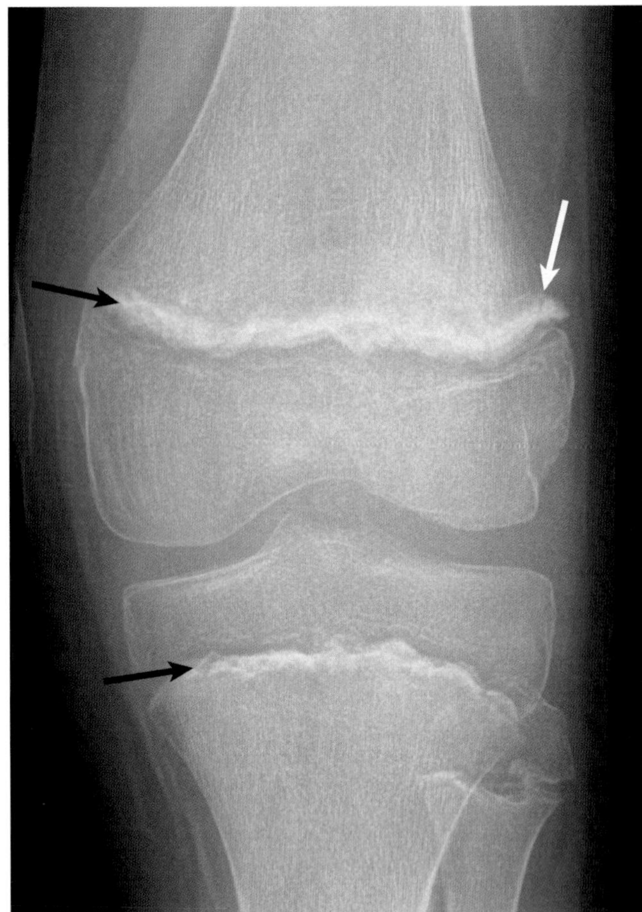

Figure 86.104 Scurvy; 9-year-old female with severe dietary issues and gingival swelling, shown to be severely vitamin C deficient. There is osteopenia. The metaphyses are irregular but the zone of provisional calcification is dense ("Frankel line," *black arrows*). There is a fracture of the lateral metaphyseal margin ("Pelken spur," *white arrow*).

Other Metabolic Bone Diseases in Childhood

Hyperparathyroidism

Secondary hyperparathyroidism is a key component of bone disease related to vitamin D deficiency (see above). Primary hyperparathyroidism (e.g., due to parathyroid adenoma) can produce similar radiological features to vitamin D deficiency, including rickets, as well as the typical features of subperiosteal bone resorption, lytic skull lesions and brown tumors (Fig. 86.105). Slipped epiphyses are common in children with hyperparathyroidism, and may occur at unusual sites, such as the proximal humerus.

Renal Osteodystrophy

Renal osteodystrophy is a complex disorder seen in patients with chronic renal failure. It predominantly results from loss of renal 1-alpha hydroxylase, the main site of vitamin D activation. This leads to impaired calcium absorption and subsequently secondary (and tertiary) hyperparathyroidism. Due to reduced glomerular filtration, in most cases, serum phosphate is elevated (unlike in vitamin D deficiency) and so rickets is not typically present (but may be in polyuric forms of renal failure with tubular dysfunction); osteomalacia may still be present owing to low serum calcium. Early disease may manifest typical features of hyperparathyroidism

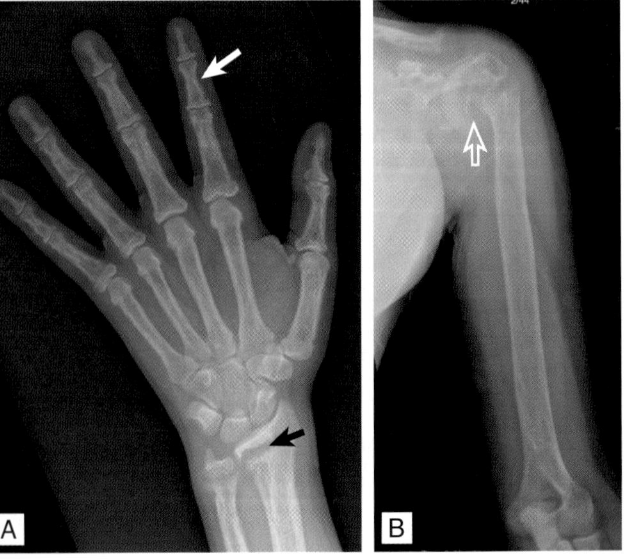

Figure 86.105 (A) Radiographs of right hand and (B) left humerus in 14-year-old female with hyperparathyroidism due to parathyroid adenoma. The typical subperiosteal bone resorption along the radial aspect of the middle phalanges is shown (*white arrow*). There is also rachitic widening of the distal radial growth plate (*black arrow*). There is a slipped upper humeral epiphysis (*white open arrow*).

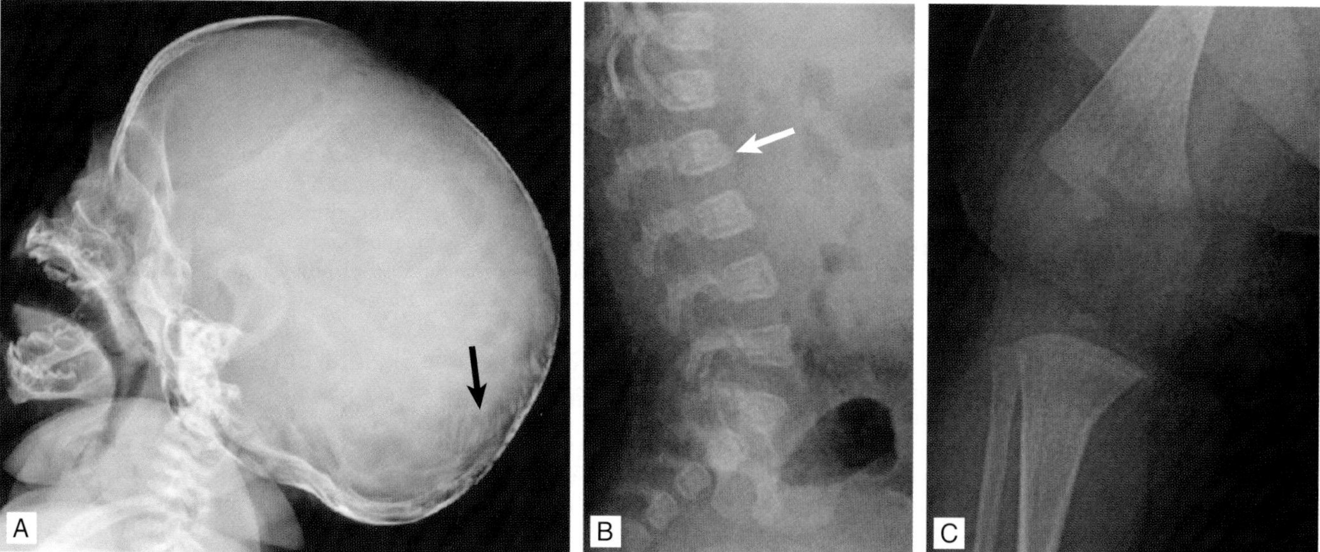

Figure 86.106 (A) Radiographs of skull, (B) lumbar spine and (C) right knee in 22-week-old male with failure to thrive. There are numerous small Wormian bones in the lambdoid sutures (*black arrow*). There is subtle platyspondyly. Inferior hook formation at L2 (*white arrow*) likely reflects hypotonia and prior gibbous deformity. The knee epiphyses show markedly delayed ossification. Subsequent testing confirmed pituitary dysfunction including severe central hypothyroidism.

(see above), but in many cases, chronicity leads to progressive parathyroid hormone resistance, which can produce paradoxical osteosclerosis, typically in vertebral body endplates.

Hypothyroidism

Thanks to neonatal heel-prick blood screening, skeletal manifestations of hypothyroidism are rarely seen in children today. Central hypothyroidism (due to deficient TSH production, often as part of generalized pituitary dysfunction) is not detected by neonatal testing, and occasionally can produce typical skeletal manifestations including platyspondyly, delayed bone age and multiple Wormian bone formation (Fig. 86.106). Hypothyroidism must always be excluded in children with unexplained Wormian bones or bone age delay.

Hypervitaminosis A

Excess vitamin A activity most typically occurs in children receiving 13-cis retinoic acid treatment, e.g., for neuroblastoma or some skin conditions. It may manifest radiologically as diffuse periosteal new bone formation, and occasionally with soft tissue calcification. A similar appearance can be seen in children receiving prolonged systemic prostaglandin therapy, e.g., for maintaining ductal patency in certain forms of congenital heart disease (Fig. 86.107).

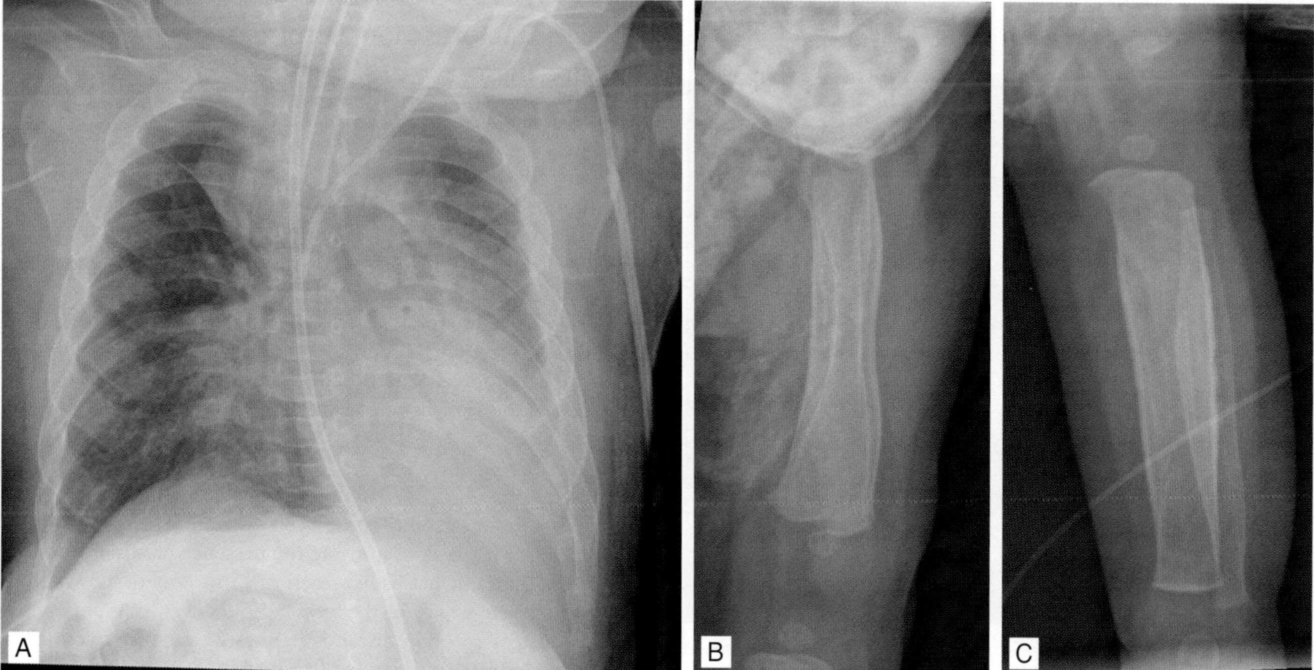

Figure 86.107 Radiographs of chest (A), left femur (B) and left tibia/fibula (C) in 18-week-old male with severe Tetralogy of Fallot on long standing prostaglandin infusions. The ribs are markedly broadened. There is abundant periosteal new bone formation in the femur, tibia, and fibula. (Courtesy: Dr Karl Johnson.)

Lead Poisoning

Lead poisoning still occurs in developing countries, and accounts for more than half a million deaths per annum; it may also occur in children who swallow foreign bodies. As well as causing neurological injury, lead also poisons osteoclasts. This leads to the appearance of dense metaphyseal new bone formation, producing characteristic dense metaphyseal bands.

Skeletal Findings in Haemoglobinopathies

Haemoglobinpathies such as sickle cell disease and thalassemia typically result in expansion of the medullary spaces of the skeleton. This can result in thinning of cortical bone and occasionally osteopenia and fractures. In the skull, the diploic space is widened, and in chronic, severe disorders, this may lead to the classical "hair-on-end" appearance; this is rare with modern treatment.

Sickle cell disease in addition is complicated by vaso-occlusive events, which can lead to bone infarction. This may manifest as medullary infracts or AVN of proximal humeral and femoral epiphyses. Vertebral end-plate infarcts classically manifest as "h-shaped" vertebrae due to end-plate depression (Fig. 86.108).

Nonaccidental Injury

Nonaccidental trauma (also known as suspected physical abuse, or inflicted injury) is sadly a significant cause of death and morbidity in young children. It accounted for approximately 30% of trauma deaths in children under 5 years, and over 40% of trauma deaths in children under 1 year of age in the United States from 2007 to 2014 [51].

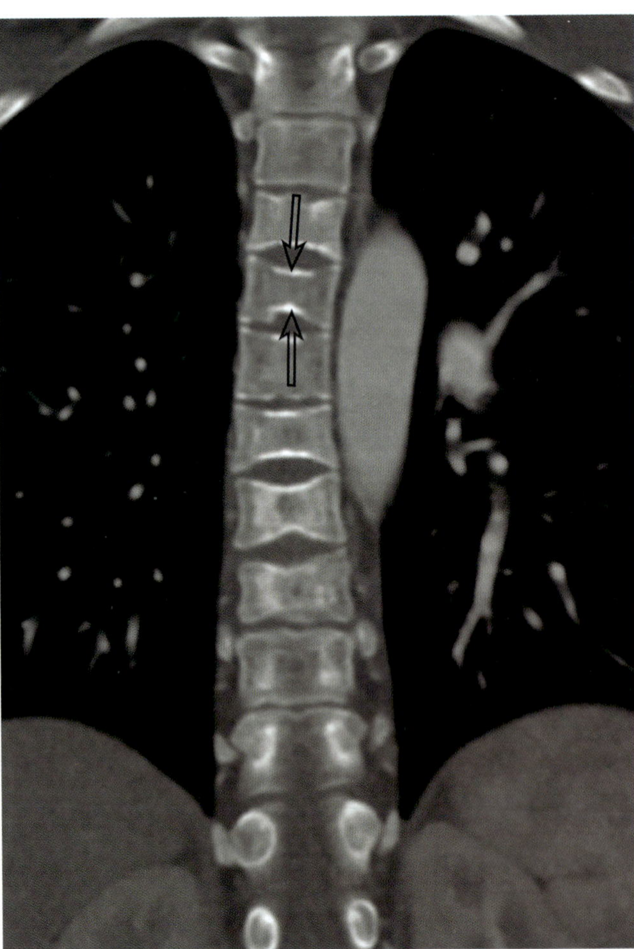

Figure 86.108 Coronally reformatted thoracic CT in 18-year-old female with known sickle cell anemia. Multiple typical vertebral end-plate depressions are shown (*arrows*).

Context and clinical history are key in the assessment of injuries; for instance, a femoral fracture in an active 6-year-old would raise much less concern than in a preambulant 1-year-old. Close discussion with the referring clinicians is essential. Whilst traumatic brain injury is the most common presentation, fractures are seen in approximately 30% of physical abuse cases, and a radiographic skeletal survey forms a crucial part of the work-up.

The Radiographic Skeletal Survey for Suspected Physical Abuse

Whilst in children over 2 years of age presenting with suspected physical abuse, targeted imaging of the area of suspected injury normally suffice. A full skeletal survey is recommended for children under the age of 24 months (Table 86.18). Each body region should be imaged with a separate exposure. A single "babygram" of the entire child provides inferior diagnostic image quality and is not advised.

A limited repeat radiographic skeletal survey for follow-up at 2 weeks—of the long bones, ribs, and any areas of suspicion on the first skeletal survey—increases the sensitivity for detecting fractures.

CT and MRI

CT head without intravenous contrast is the examination of choice for the emergent investigation of children with suspected abusive head trauma. MRI can be used in the nonemergent setting and can provide additional diagnostic information compared to CT head in up to 25% of children. In children under 2 years of age, a low threshold is recommended for performing head CT or MRI for screening for neurological injury, even in the absence of clinically apparent injury [52].

Suspected thoraco-abdominal visceral injury should be assessed with contrast-enhanced CT.

Specific Fractures More Suspicious of Inflicted Injury

- *Note, the most frequent presentation is with "common" fractures (e.g., femoral shaft) but with an inappropriate history (e.g., nonambulant child) (55)*
- Multiple fractures, fractures of different ages
- Posterior rib fractures
- Complex skull fractures (nonparietal, widened, branching, crossing suture lines, bilateral)
- Metaphyseal fractures ("corner" or "bucket handle," depending on the projection (Fig. 86.109). Due to considerable shearing or torsional force. Rare in older children
- Unusual locations: scapula, sternum spinous process

Dating of Fractures

Fracture dating is a complex medicolegal issue.

Important features to note are the presence or absence of soft tissue swelling and periosteal reaction [53]. Soft tissue swelling normally develops within the first 24 hours over long bone injuries. Periosteal reaction around diaphyseal and rib fractures is usually present around day 7–10 (rarely by day 4, always by day 14). Diaphyseal and rib fractures normally heal completely by

TABLE 86.18 Skeletal Survey for Suspected Physical Abuse in Children Under 2 Years of Age, Based on ACR Appropriateness Criteria [54]. Practice Varies in Other Countries

	Standard Imaging at Presentation	Supplementary Views as Needed
Appendicular skeleton	Humeri (AP) Forearms (AP) Hands (PA) Femurs (AP) Lower legs (AP) Feet (AP)	Lateral views of long bones AP and lateral selected joints
Axial skeleton	Thorax (AP, lateral, right, and left obliques; to include sternum, ribs, thoracic, and upper lumbar spine) Abdomen and Pelvis (AP) Cervical spine (lateral) Lumbosacral spine (lateral) Skull (frontal and lateral)	Townes view of skull
Other		Any other clinically abnormal or suspicious area

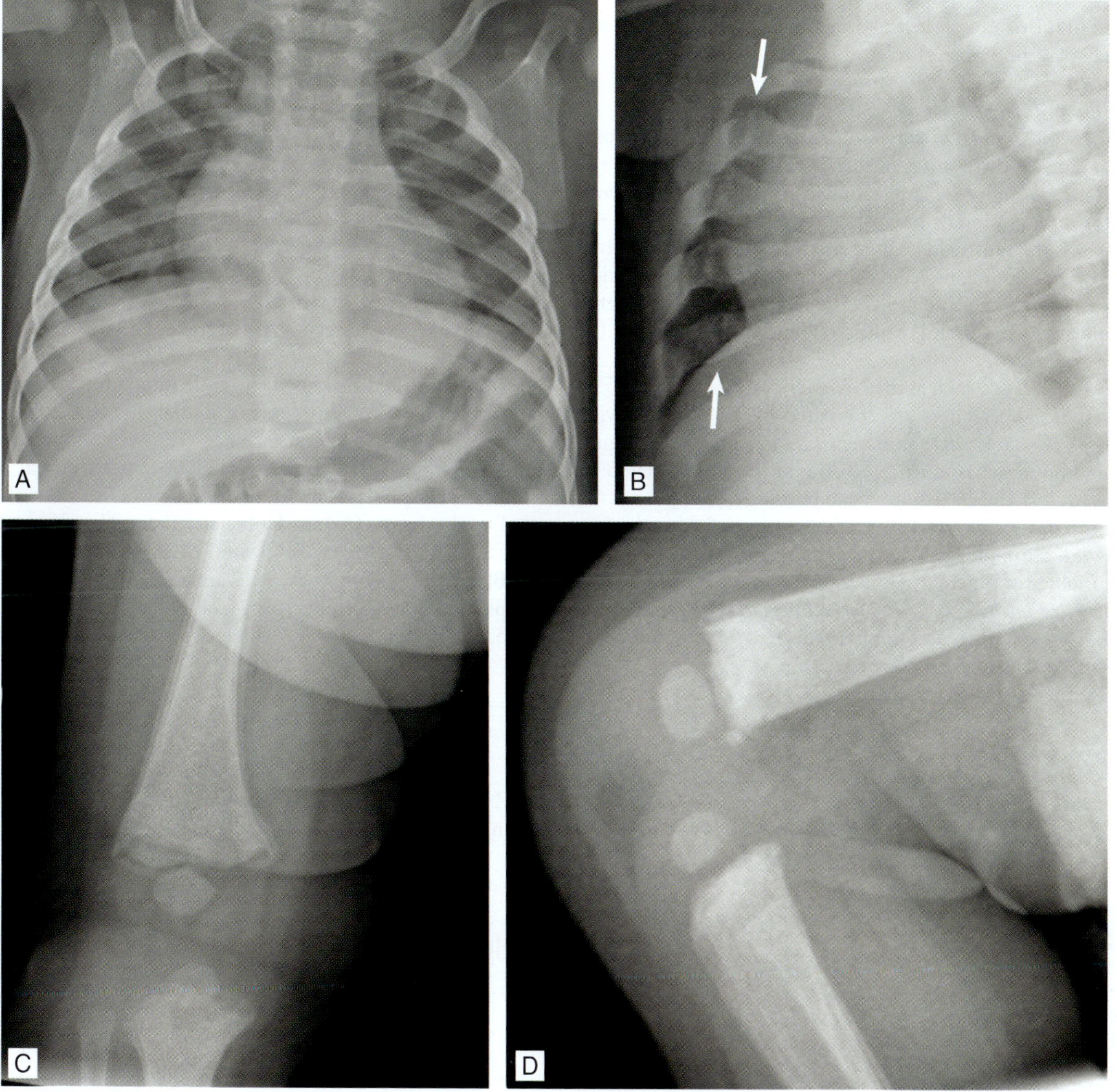

Figure 86.109 2-month-old boy, admitted with fracture of left femur and bruise, with inconsistent history, concerning for nonaccidental injury. Bilateral femoral metaphyseal fractures, seen with "bucket-handle" and "corner" fracture morphology on the AP (C) and lateral views (D) of the knee respectively. The row of right rib fractures (*between the arrows*) are much more conspicuous on the oblique rib views (B) than the AP chest radiograph (A).

3 months. Metaphyseal, costochondral, vertebral, and skull fractures are more difficult to date. More details of fracture dating is covered in chapter on pediatric skeletal trauma.

Differential Diagnosis

- Rickets
  - Note; in an infant with unexplained fractures, an isolated low vitamin D level with otherwise normal biochemistry, and the absence of other radiological markers of rickets, is thought inadequate to account for the fractures [54]
- Osteogenesis Imperfecta
- Metabolic bone disease of prematurity
- Birth injury (should have healed by 3 months of age)
- Normal metaphyseal variants
- Skeletal dysplasia—metaphyseal dysplasia (Menkes)

Bone Age Assessment in Children (Also See the Appendix of Bone Age Estimation)

Assessment of the degree of skeletal development ("bone age assessment") may play a number of roles in pediatrics, e.g.,

- Assessment of cause of *short stature*
- *Prediction* of *final adult height*
- Guidance for *timing of surgical interventions* (e.g., scoliosis repair, guided growth interventions in lower limbs)

An additional, *controversial* application is in attempting to *verify legal age* for immigration or forensic purposes.

The *hand* is the most widely used site for bone age assessment, typically the nondominant hand, although this is not essential. Although the wrist can also be assessed for bone development, carpal bone age is less useful. Multiple methods are available for evaluating bone age.

1) *Atlas based methods*, such as the *Greulich and Pyle* method [55]; radiographic appearances are compared by an observer with *gender-specific standards* for different ages in a printed or digital atlas, and bone age assigned according to the closest match
   - Pros: quick, cheap, requires little training
   - Cons: coarse scale (6–12 month gaps in scale), anchoring bias to chronological age, standards historical and not adjustable for different populations
2) *Scoring based methods*, e.g., *Tanner-Whitehouse* [56]; individual bones given a rating according to degrees of development, summarized scores give a bone age estimate
   - Pros: finer scale, less prone to bias
   - Cons: slower than atlas method, requires some training and experience
3) *Automated methods* standardized radiographs analyzed using AI-based algorithms [57,58]
   - Pros: fast, reproducible, continuous scale, no bias
   - Cons: expensive, may miss underlying bone disorders, e.g., dysplasia

The *hand* is a *less reliable* means of assessing bone age *under the age of 3* as most epiphyses are unossified. Although bone age assessment is less often required in this age group, methods using the *ossification of the ankle bones* have been described [59].

During the *adolescent* growth spurt, bone development can be very rapid, consequently specific *adolescent bone age systems* have been developed to provide a *finer scale* for this age group. Examples include the *Sauvegraine assessment of the elbow* (based on AP and lateral views) [60] and the *Risser staging of the iliac crest apophysis* (used in spinal surgery as can be assessed on AP spinal radiographs) [61].

Suggested Readings

- BY Chan, KG Gill, SL Rebsamen, JC Nguyen, MR imaging of pediatric bone marrow, Radiographics 36 (6) (2016 Oct) 1911–1930.
- NM Safdar, CK Rigsby, RS Iyer, AL Alazraki, SA Anupindi, DM Bardo, BP Brown, SS Chan, T Chandra, JR Dillman, SR Dorfman, ACR Appropriateness Criteria® acutely limping child up to age 5, J Am Coll Radiol 15 (11) (2018 Nov 1) S252–S262.
- J van Schuppen, MM van Doorn, RR van Rijn, Childhood osteomyelitis: imaging characteristics, Insights Imaging 3 (5) (2012 Oct 1) 519–533.
- R Hemke, N Herregods, JL Jaremko, G Åström, D Avenarius, F Becce F, et al., Imaging assessment of children presenting with suspected or known juvenile idiopathic arthritis: ESSR-ESPR points to consider, Eur Radiol 30 (10) (2020 May 12) 5237–5249.
- JW Spranger, PW Brill, C Hall, A Superti-Furga, S Unger, Bone Dysplasias: An Atlas of Genetic Disorders of Skeletal Development, Oxford University Press, New York, 2018.
- SL Wootton-Gorges, BP Soares, AL Alazraki, SA Anupindi, JP Blount, TN Booth, et al., ACR appropriateness criteria® suspected physical abuse—child, J Am Coll Radiol 14 (5) (2017 May 1) S338–S349.

87 Skeletal Trauma

SOPHIE WEST, SUJIT VAIDYA, DINA PEFANIS, ROY WHEELER

87.1 General Considerations

Introduction

Skeletal trauma is one of the most important aspects of orthopedic radiology, being by far the commonest problem presented to the musculoskeletal radiologist. Despite this fact however, trauma radiology continues to be a neglected aspect of this subspecialty. This may reflect an illogical approach to skeletal trauma historically, whereby fractures and dislocations were presented as a confusing list of unassociated injuries, often better known by eponyms. More recently, there has been a trend towards classifying fractures by the force of injury causing them. This allows a more logical and thoughtful approach, and enhances understanding of fracture patterns and associated injuries.

A fracture of a bone occurs when there is a break in the continuity of bone, which may be either complete or incomplete. When a loading force is applied to bone, it initially deforms elastically, and as the load is removed, the deformity of the bone is reversed and the bone returns to normal. As the loading force is increased, however, the elasticity of the bone is overcome, and a plastic "*fracture*" occurs, with the bone remaining deformed after cessation of the load. Finally, complete failure of the bone will occur, giving rise to a true fracture. Repetitive loading of a bone at "subfracture" levels may lead to the development of stress fracture (see below). Fractures are described in many different ways, as discussed below.

Terminology

The descriptive terms *open* or *closed* refer to whether the bone fragments communicate with the outside environment or not. If bone fragments penetrate the skin, the fracture is open, sometimes also referred to as a compound fracture (Fig. 87.1). If the fracture remains covered with intact skin, it is called closed. Although apparent on clinical inspection, various radiographic signs will suggest an open fracture (Box 87.1).

The nature of the fracture lines also describes the fracture. Generally, a single fracture line follows one of three major types: *transverse*, *oblique*, or *spiral*, although a combination of these may be present. In addition, if the injury produces more than one fracture line, the fracture is said to be *comminuted.*

Comminuted fractures will often produce a minor triangular fragment of bone, known as a "*butterfly*" fragment. A segmental fracture is one in which a segment of bone is isolated by fractures at each end. These are both illustrated in Fig. 87.2.

Fractures may also be termed *incomplete* or *complete*. Incomplete fractures occur most commonly in children, when bone resilience is greater, and are of three types. As mentioned above, plastic fractures occur when there is bending of the bone without cortical disruption, or acute angulation; *a "torus" or "buckle" fracture is the term applied to a fracture of the cortex on the compressive side of the bone* with an intact cortex on the tension side (Fig. 87.3). *Greenstick fracture is the converse of the torus fracture, occurring only on the tension side, with cortical disruption on the tension side and bending of the opposite cortex* (Fig. 87.4).

Fractures should also be evaluated for continuity and proximity of the fracture fragments. The term *apposition* refers to the position of the major fragments with respect to each other. *Fragments which are*

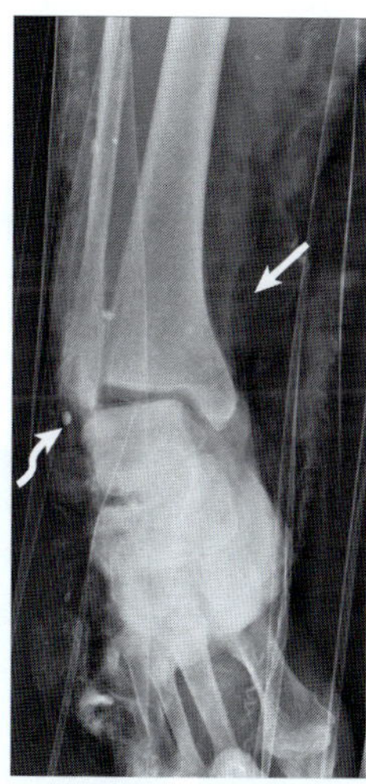

Figure 87.1 An open comminuted fracture dislocation of the ankle. Subcutaneous gas (*white arrow*), foreign material around the fracture site (*curved arrow*), absence of the distal fibula and the lateral midfoot and bone protrusion beyond normal skin margins all provide evidence of this being an open injury.

BOX 87.1 Radiographic Signs of Open Fracture

Obvious protrusion of bone fragments beyond the soft-tissue margins
Absence of portions of the bone
Gross soft-tissue disruption extending to the bone surface
Subcutaneous gas
Foreign material within the fracture

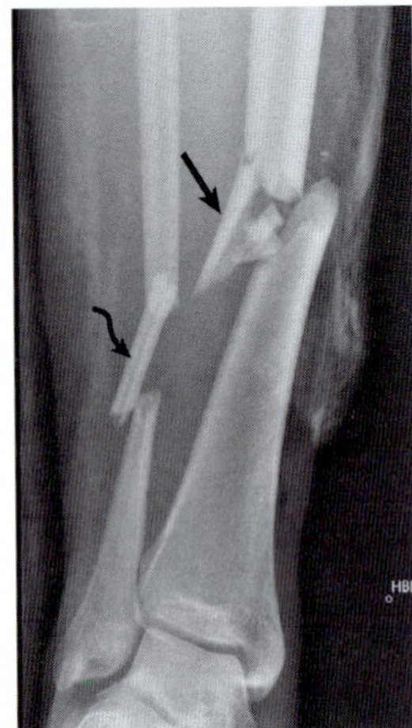

Figure 87.2 Comminuted fracture of the distal tibia with a "triangular" shaped butterfly fragment (*black arrow*) and a "segmental" fracture of the fibula (*curved arrow*). There is medial displacement but lateral angulation of the distal tibia.

not apposed are described as being distracted if the displacement is along the long axis of the bone, or displaced, away from the long axis. In such cases, the fracture should be described according to the direction of displacement of the distal fragment relative to the proximal bone.

Alignment refers to the relationship along the axis of major fragments. Abnormality of alignment may be described in two ways. The most logical description refers to the alignment of the distal fragment with respect to the proximal (Fig. 87.2). This has the additional advantage of following the same "rules" as apply to displacement. The alternative method, commonly used by orthopedic surgeons, is to describe the angulation as the direction of the apex of the angle at the fracture site.

Varus and *valgus angulation* are terms that are commonly used, particularly by orthopedic surgeons—they refer to the alignment of the distal fragment with respect to the midline of the body, *with varus indicating angulation of the distal fragment towards the midline and valgus the reverse.*

Impaction is the descriptive term for fractures in which the bone fragments are driven into each other.

Abnormality of rotation of the distal fragment is an important finding and should always be assessed. This requires visualization of both ends of the bone on the same radiograph, so that the orientation of the proximal and distal joints can be assessed. It is fundamental to have more than one view of a fracture to be able to assess it accurately.

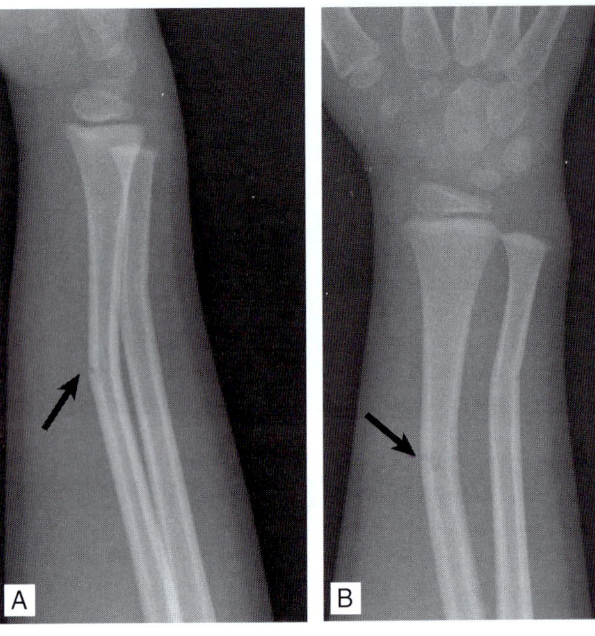

Figure 87.4 (A and B) Greenstick fracture of the radius (*arrows*) and ulna, there is a breach/break in the cortex on the volar side and bending of the opposite cortex.

Associated Soft-Tissue Abnormalities

Although the majority of fractures are readily identified, on occasion they may be difficult or impossible to see on initial radiographs, a classic example of this is a scaphoid fracture. Additional clues may be helpful in such cases. For example, fractures around a joint may provide evidence of a joint effusion or haemarthrosis, providing the joint capsule remains intact. This can be particularly useful at the elbow, where elevation of the fat pads, either anterior or posterior, although the latter is more specific, is good evidence of injury (Fig. 87.5) and at the elbow is often a sign of an occult radial head fracture.

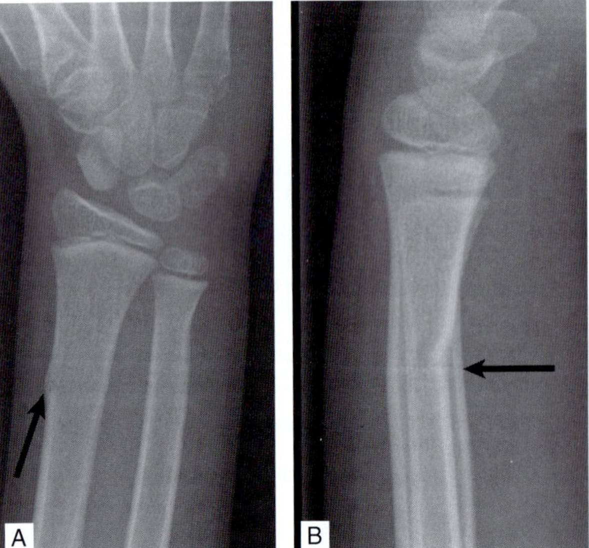

Figure 87.3 (A and B) Torus fracture of the distal radius (*arrows*). The cortex is buckled.

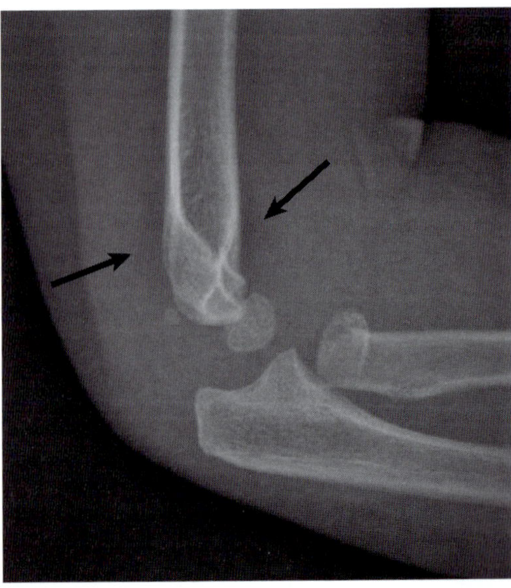

Figure 87.5 Lateral view of a pediatric elbow showing both anterior and posterior fat pad elevation (*arrows*) and a radial head fracture.

A fat–fluid level (lipohaemarthrosis) within a joint, most commonly seen in the knee with the radiograph made with a horizontal beam, is also firm presumptive evidence of an intra-articular fracture, the fat being derived from the bone marrow (Fig. 87.6).

Soft-tissue swelling in the retropharyngeal space has also been cited as being a reliable sign of cervical spine trauma when it is present, however the absence of swelling of the prevertebral soft tissues can still mean there is a significant bony or ligamentous injury in the cervical spine.

Fracture Healing

After a fracture has occurred, the process of healing begins. In the normal healing process, a hematoma initially forms between the bone ends, occasionally causing periosteal elevation. Granulation tissue then forms between the fracture fragments, with immature osteoid (callus) laid down on the bone surface acting as an early bridge. This first becomes calcified, but eventually woven bone is laid down, leading to firm bone union.

The early stages of bone formation are not visible radiographically, but in a healthy person, new bone formation is visible within 4–6 weeks, with the healing process complete in 4–6 months for a single fracture in a large tubular bone. Delay in union however may be evident by a delay in the appearance of new bone, and can occur from a variety of causes (see below).

Evaluation of Skeletal Trauma

The vast majority of injuries can be adequately visualized by *plain radiographs* and still remains the initial investigation of choice in the evaluation of an injury. However, while historically tomography and nuclear medicine studies were used to gain further information about an injury, in the modern radiology department CT and MRI are the mainstay of trauma evaluation. Modern multislice CT scanners, which utilize multi-planar reformats and 3D reconstructions can give far more accurate detail of fracture patterns, intra-articular involvement, and can detect occult fractures that are not always visible on plane film (Figs. 87.7–87.9). In addition, they can provide the operativing surgeon with valuable information allowing better planning of surgical approach and fixation planning.

Magnetic resonance imaging (MRI) can be helpful in detecting occult fractures, for example of the scaphoid or femoral neck,

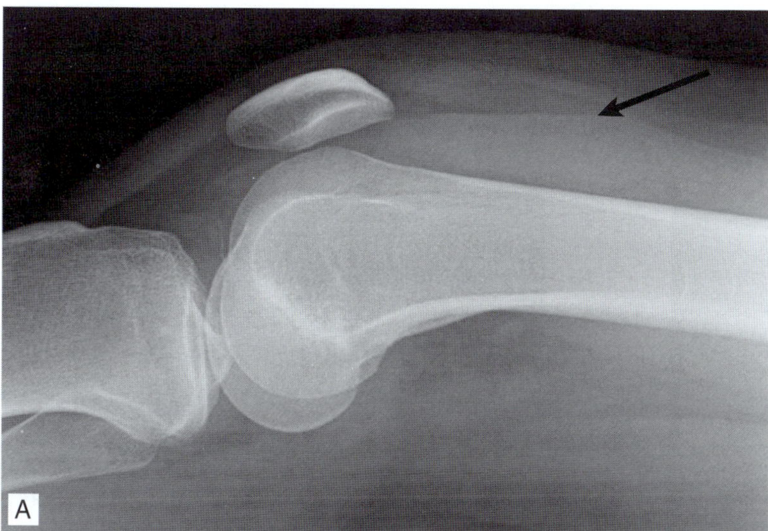

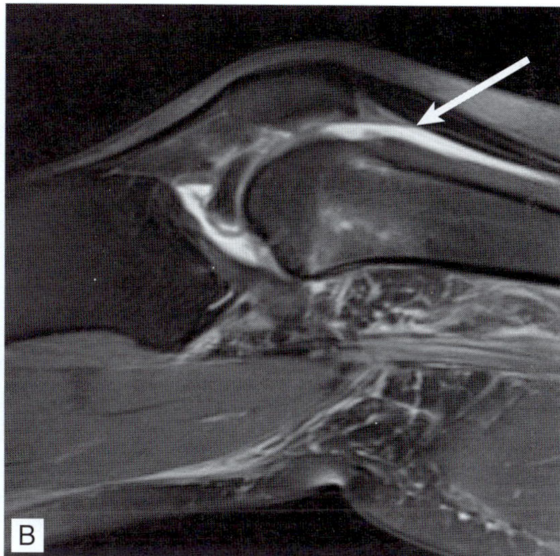

Figure 87.6 (A) Horizontal beam lateral of a knee showing a lipohaemarthrosis (*black arrow*). This indicates an intra-articular injury. (B) The lipohaemarthrosis on MRI PD Fat saturated sequence with the high signal fluid (*white arrow*) and the suppressed fat "floating" on top.

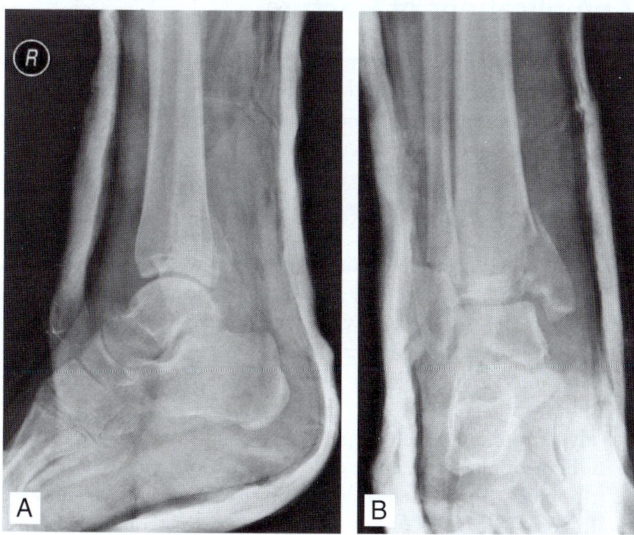

Figure 87.7 (A) Lateral view and (B) AP view plain film demonstrating a trimalleolar ankle fracture in cast.

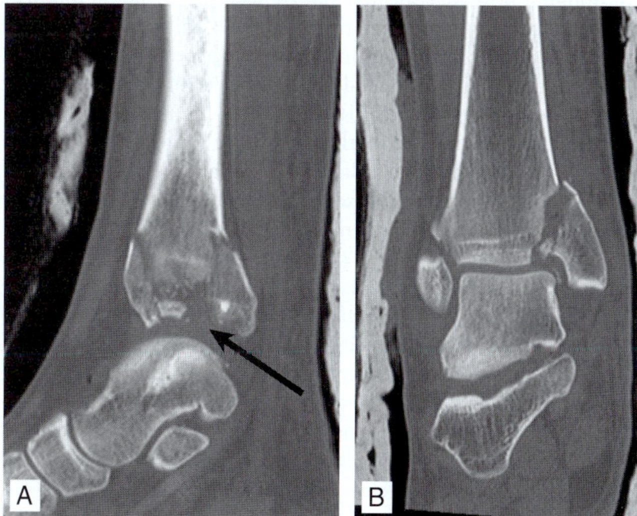

Figure 87.8 (A and B) CT scan with bony reconstructions demonstrates the extent of the intra-articular component (*black arrow*) of the fracture.

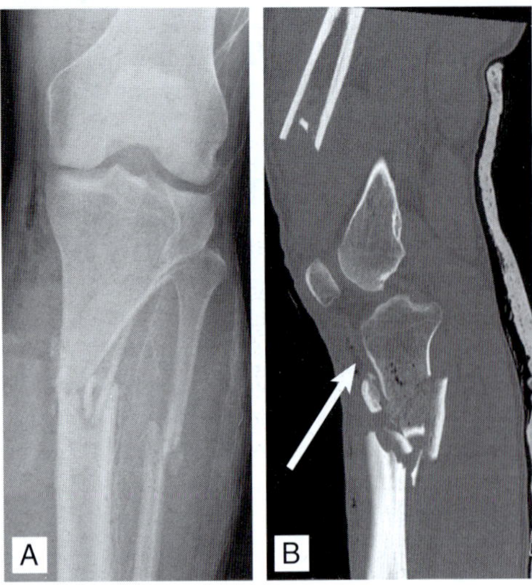

Figure 87.9 Plain film (A) and CT (B) of a proximal tibia fracture and distal femur fracture, again the extent of the injury is better appreciated on CT and gas in the soft tissues suggests an open injury (*white arrow*).

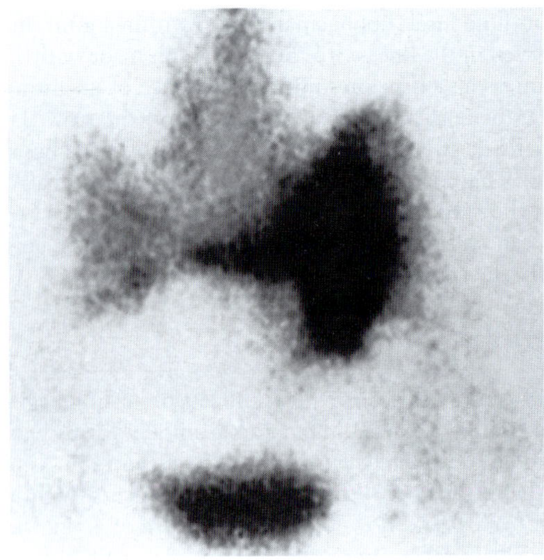

Figure 87.10 Stress fractures of the sacrum. This elderly patient underwent nuclear medicine bone scan for pain in the lower back. A characteristic pattern of increased tracer uptake indicates a stress fracture in the osteoporotic sacrum.

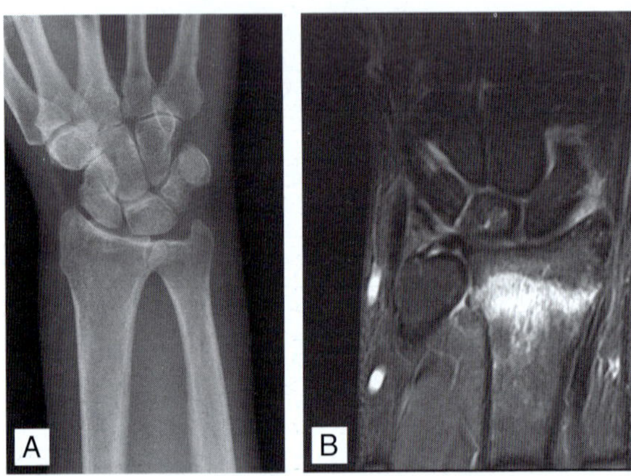

Figure 87.11 Plain film (A) of the wrist with no significant injury identifiable and (B) MRI on the same patient showing extensive marrow edema (bright white signal in the distal radius) and a fracture line in keeping with a distal radius fracture.

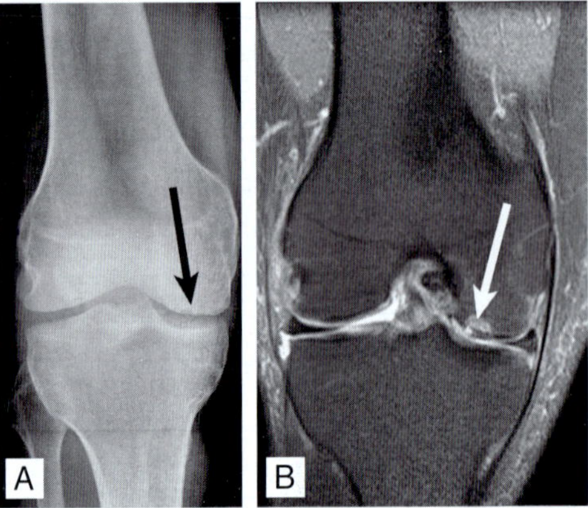

Figure 87.12 Radiograph (A) of the knee showing an osteochondral defect of the medial femoral condyle as evidenced by a semi-circular lucency along the joint line (*black arrow*) and the corresponding MRI (B) showing the defect as an area of bright signal (*white arrow*).

although a positive scan may not be seen for 24 hours following injury, especially in older patients. There is still a role for nuclear medicine in the identification of stress fractures of bone, particularly in the elderly with sacral stress fractures, often with a characteristic appearance (Fig. 87.10).

MRI has become the method of choice for evaluating injuries of and around the joints. It has the ability to detect not only injury to the surrounding soft tissues, but also it can identify occult injury to the bones themselves, such as "bone bruising" seen as bright signal on T2 fat suppressed and intermediate/low signal on T1 sequences (Fig. 87.11), osteochondral fractures (Fig. 87.12), and post-traumatic avascular necrosis (Fig. 87.13). Among its advantages are its ability to demonstrate soft-tissue detail, its capability of multiplanar imaging and its lack of ionizing radiation. These features are responsible for the rapidly increasing use of MRI in musculoskeletal radiology. Injuries to ligaments and tendons are readily identified by MRI (see relevant sections below), and muscle trauma can be appreciated (Figs. 87.14 and 87.15). This has greatly expanded the role of the radiologist in the traumatized patient.

Complications of Fracture

There are potential problems in all fractures. Although most uncomplicated fractures heal readily, in open fractures there is an increased potential for infection at the fracture site and careful scrutiny of the healing process is warranted.

Nonunion

Nonunion of a fracture is said to have occurred when there is no evidence of bony union after a period of 9 months from the original injury [1]. The reason why a fracture goes onto develop are usually multifactorial and are listed in Box 87.2.

Nonunion can be further categorized depending on the imaging findings [2]:

- Hypertrophic—which occurs despite abundant callous formation
- Oligotrophic—very little callous formation
- Atrophic—no callous formation, bony resorption at the fracture sites
- Infected—features of osteomyelitis and soft tissue infection
- Synovial pseudarthrosis

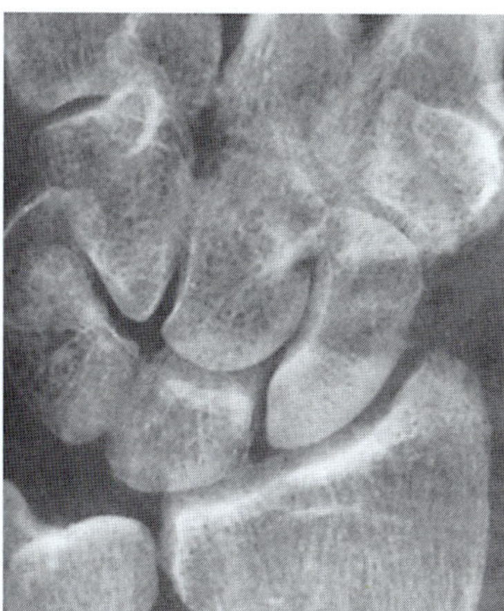

Figure 87.13 Post-traumatic avascular necrosis of the proximal pole of the scaphoid. Although the fracture of the waist of the scaphoid has "healed," avascular necrosis has occurred, with resulting sclerosis.

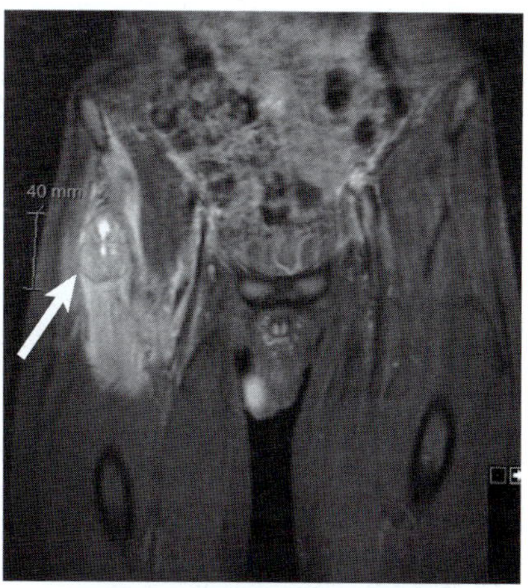

Figure 87.14 T1 TIRM coronal fat saturated sequence demonstrating a well-defined lesion (*arrow*) of mixed signal intensity in the region of the proximal rectus femoris muscle. The mixed signal pattern is common, indicating the complexity of the hematoma and variations in hemoglobin, deoxyhemoglobin, methaemoglobin and haemosiderin levels. Note the extensive increased signal in the adjacent muscles in keeping with associated muscle edema.

The tibia has long been singled out as a bone liable to *delayed union* or *nonunion*. The reasons for this are obscure, but poor vascular supply and thin subcutaneous soft tissue coverage are likely to play a part. In practice, however, it would appear that the reason for the high incidence of cases of delayed or non-union may be due to the large number of "high-energy" injuries seen in the tibia, particularly from pedestrian "bumper" injuries, with a large amount of resulting necrosis of soft tissue and bone at and around the fracture site. For this reason, there is a very low threshold to surgically fix these fractures. Figs. 87.16 and 87.17 demonstrate non-union despite immobilization/fixation.

The scaphoid is another bone that is worth mentioning in regards to delayed and nonunion. Fractures particularly of the proximal pole are prone to develop delayed or nonunion due to the arterial blood supply to the proximal pole entering from the distal aspect of the scaphoid. If not recognized this can go on to cause significant pain and morbidity for the patient (Fig. 87.18). MRI has a valuable role in identifying these fractures which can appear occult on plain film.

Malunion is the term given to a fracture which heals in an unsatisfactory anatomical position, either with excessive over-lap of fragments, giving rise to shortening of the bone, or unsatisfactory angulation or displacement of the distal fragment (Fig. 87.19). There are several reasons a bone may go on to develop malunion, these include delayed presentation, poor immobilization, and complexity of the initial injury. Another common reason is the patient, where, although fixation to attain a better anatomical reduction could be achieved, due to factors, for example age, or the presence of comorbidities, this is not carried out.

BOX 87.2 Causes of Delayed or Nonunion

Mechanical

Poor apposition
Inadequate stabilization (closed or open)
Massive initial trauma

Nonmechanical

Age—decreased osteoblastic activity
Dietary—vitamin deficiency (C and D)
Pathological fracture (underlying abnormality)
Infection
Poor vascular supply
Idiopathic

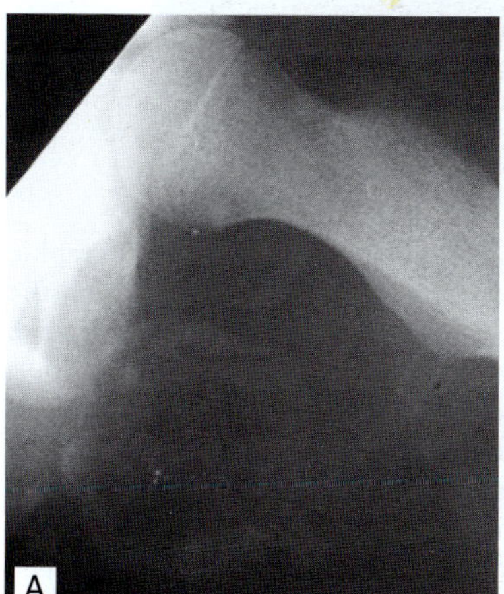

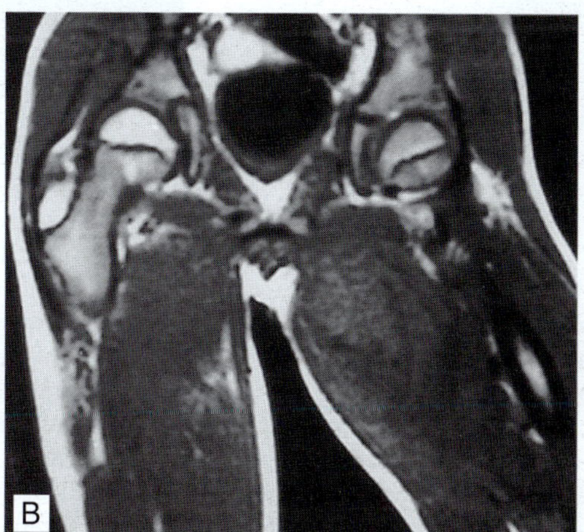

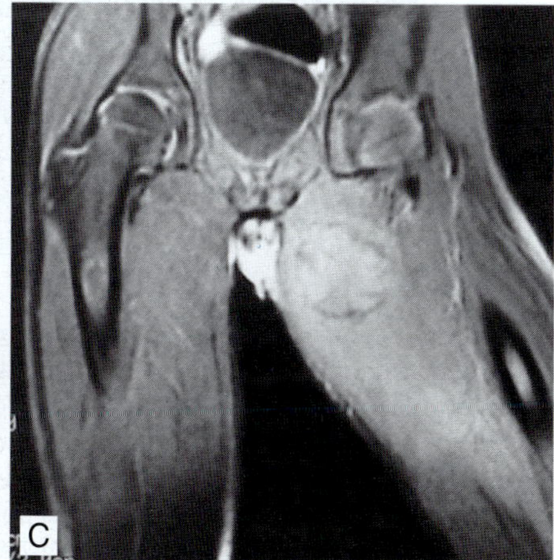

Figure 87.15 (A) A calcified "mass" in the thigh of this 16-year-old was worked to exclude tumor. (B) T1-weighted coronal MR images demonstrate a mass of low signal intensity, with surrounding low-signal-intensity edema, with increased signal intensity on T2-weighted images (image not shown). (C) There is also a well-defined, low-signal-intensity "ring" of calcification. Their appearances are characteristic of post-traumatic myositis ossificans.

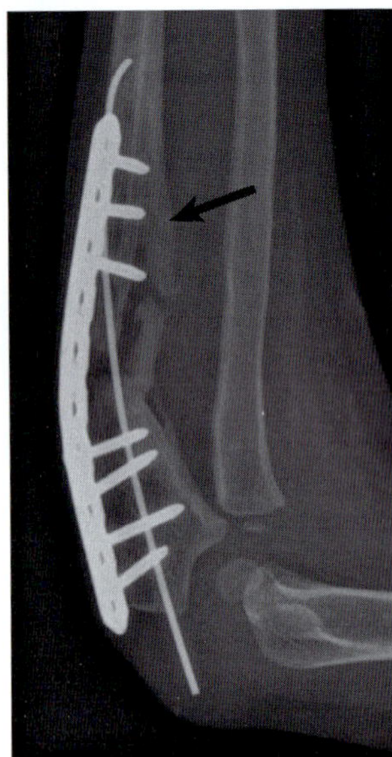

Figure 87.16 Nonunion of a proximal ulnar fracture in a child despite undergoing surgical fixation. While there is callous formation (*black arrow*) there is no evidence of union of the two ends of the fracture site with a large gap visible.

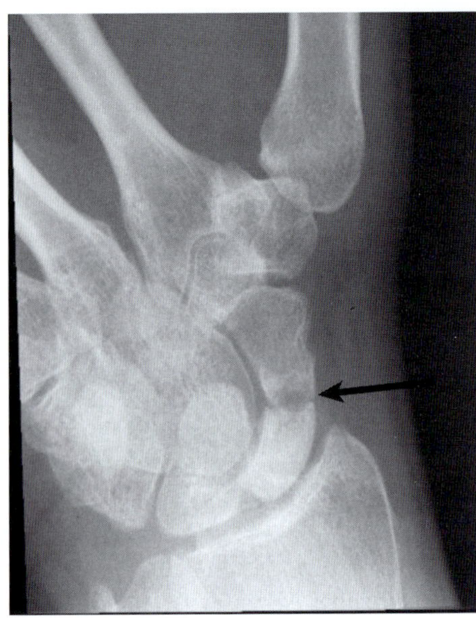

Figure 87.18 Nonunion of a scaphoid waist fracture, sclerosis can be seen at the two ends of the fracture site and a visible gap between the two ends (*black arrow*).

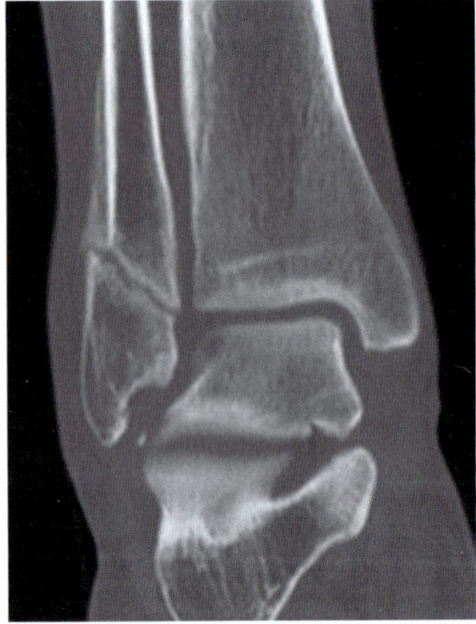

Figure 87.17 Nonunion of a distal fibula fracture seen on coronal bony reformats on CT. There is a persistent gap between the two fracture ends with evidence of sclerosis of the ends of the fracture sites.

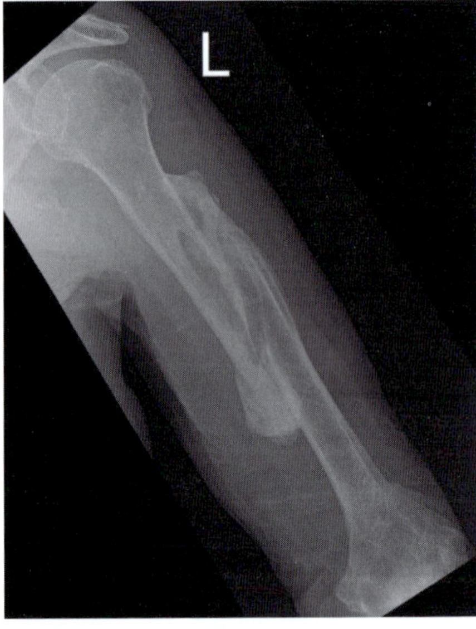

Figure 87.19 Malunion of a spiral fracture of the humerus. The bones have healed with shortening and overlap of the bony fragments.

Special Types of Trauma

Stress (Fatigue) Fractures

These fractures result from chronic repetitive forces which by themselves are insufficient to cause fracture, but over the course of time lead to the classical changes of a stress fracture. They occur in many bones, and usually at characteristic sites, often as the result of athletic activity: for example the "march" fracture of the second and third metatarsal head, the stress fracture of the mid and distal tibia and fibula in long-distance runners and ballet dancers, and fractures of the proximal fibula in paratroopers. The common sites are listed in Box 87.3.

The earliest diagnosis can be made by nuclear medicine scanning or MRI. A nuclear medicine bone scan will show increased activity before radiographic signs appear. When radiographic signs appear, they may take several forms, depending upon the stage of healing or the chronicity of the stress. A hair-like lucency may be seen traversing the bone. New bone formation around the fracture may be the only radiographic sign, or may accompany the cortical fracture (Fig. 87.20). MRI may also be useful in making the diagnosis before any changes are seen radiographically. If the patient continues the activity, a form of chronic fracture will occur, with abundant sclerotic periosteal new bone and a persistent lucent fracture line, with surrounding sclerosis (Fig. 87.21).

A type of stress fracture is said to account for the pars interarticularis defects seen in spondylolisthesis (Fig. 87.22), whereby

BOX 87.3 Common Sites of Stress Fracture

Tibial shaft
Metatarsals—shafts of 2-4th, base of 5th
Superolateral femoral neck
Pars inter-articularis of the lumbar spine
Calcaneus
Pubic rami
Sacrum
Ribs
Lateral malleolus
Navicular

the continuance of the stress leads to a complete fracture, followed by non-union. Alternatively, a congenital hypoplasia of the articular processes, or degenerative change within the posterior joints, may be the underlying cause. The defect in the pars is known as *spondylolysis*. When anterior displacement of the superior vertebral body on its neighbor is seen *spondylolisthesis* is said to have occurred. Mild degrees of spondylolisthesis can occur when there is loss of articular cartilage at the posterior intervertebral joints as in degenerative disease. More severe spondylolisthesis results from pars interarticularis defects, and is graded according to severity:

- Grade I up to 25% displacement of the vertebral body
- Grade II up to 50%
- Grade III up to 75%
- Grade IV 100% displacement

Avulsion Fractures

These occur from avulsion of bone fragments at the site of ligamentous or tendinous attachments throughout the skeleton. Of note are abnormalities which have previously been classified as osteochondritis, but which represent avulsion fractures from chronic or repeated trauma. This includes *Osgood–Schlatter disease* (Fig. 87.23) and *Sindig–Larsen disease* (Fig. 87.24) of the tibial tubercle and inferior patella respectively.

The diagnosis of Osgood–Schlatter disease is made clinically, although it can be suggested radiographically when there is clear elevation of fragments of the tibial tubercle separated from the underlying bone (Fig. 87.23). Apparent fragmentation alone without displacement does not constitute Osgood–Schlatter disease, and merely represents multiple unfused ossification centers.

Common avulsion injuries at the origin of muscle tendon insertions are seen at the inferior border of the ischium (hamstrings) (Fig. 87.25), anterior inferior iliac crest (rectus femoris; Fig. 87.26) and lesser trochanter (iliopsoas) (Table 87.1).

Pathological Fractures

Pathological fractures occur through bone that has been weakened by an underlying disease. This does not necessarily mean an underlying malignancy, although the term "pathological fracture" tends to suggest it. Pathological fractures occur through bone that is weakened by such conditions as osteoporosis or osteomalacia, bone tumors, whether benign (Fig. 87.27) or malignant (Fig. 87.28), or even tumor-like lesions of bone. In elderly patients, underlying malignancy should be considered, especially if the fracture occurs in a site other than those usually seen in osteoporosis such as the femoral neck, or in cases in which the severity of the injury is inappropriate to the fracture created.

Post-Traumatic Avascular Necrosis

This occurs from a traumatic severance of the blood supply to the bone or a fragment thereof. There are several bones in the body in which this is likely to happen in areas when the blood supply is easily compromised. Femoral neck fractures may interrupt the vascular supply to the femoral head, as can posterior dislocation of the femoral head, with or without overt fractures of the head or acetabulum. In fractures of the wrist involving the scaphoid, the proximal pole is at risk as the vascular supply enters the bone more distally (Fig. 87.18). Similarly, talar waist fractures threaten the proximal fragment. Post-traumatic avascular necrosis may occur in

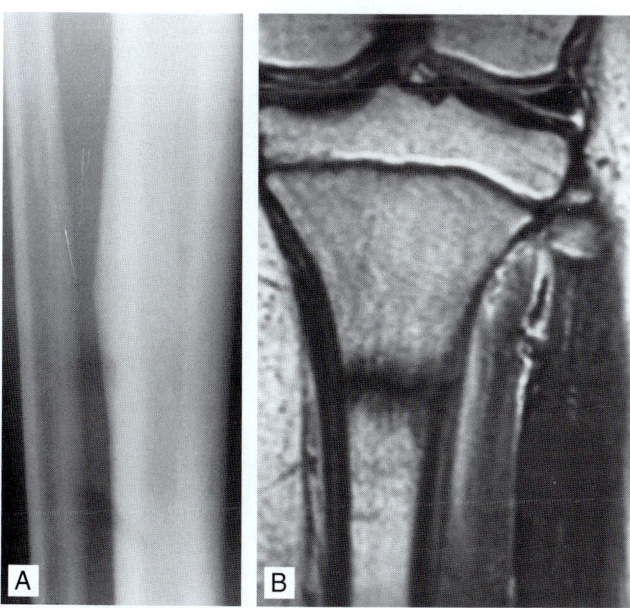

Figure 87.20 Stress fracture. (A) An area of increased sclerosis, with some dense periosteal new bone in the mid tibia. (B) MRI may be helpful in early diagnosis before the plain radiographic signs.

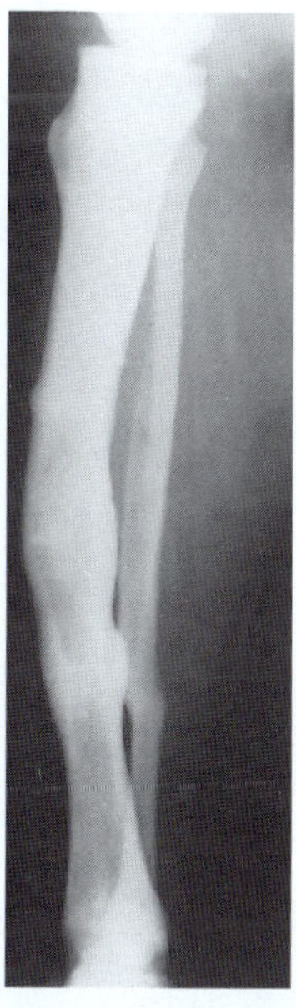

Figure 87.21 Multiple stress fractures are seen, some with obvious horizontal lucencies running perpendicular to the bone cortex. The patient was a jogger who refused to give up jogging despite the pain!

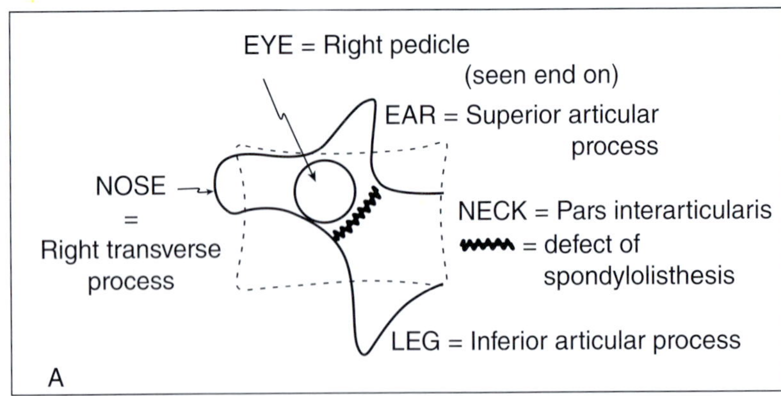

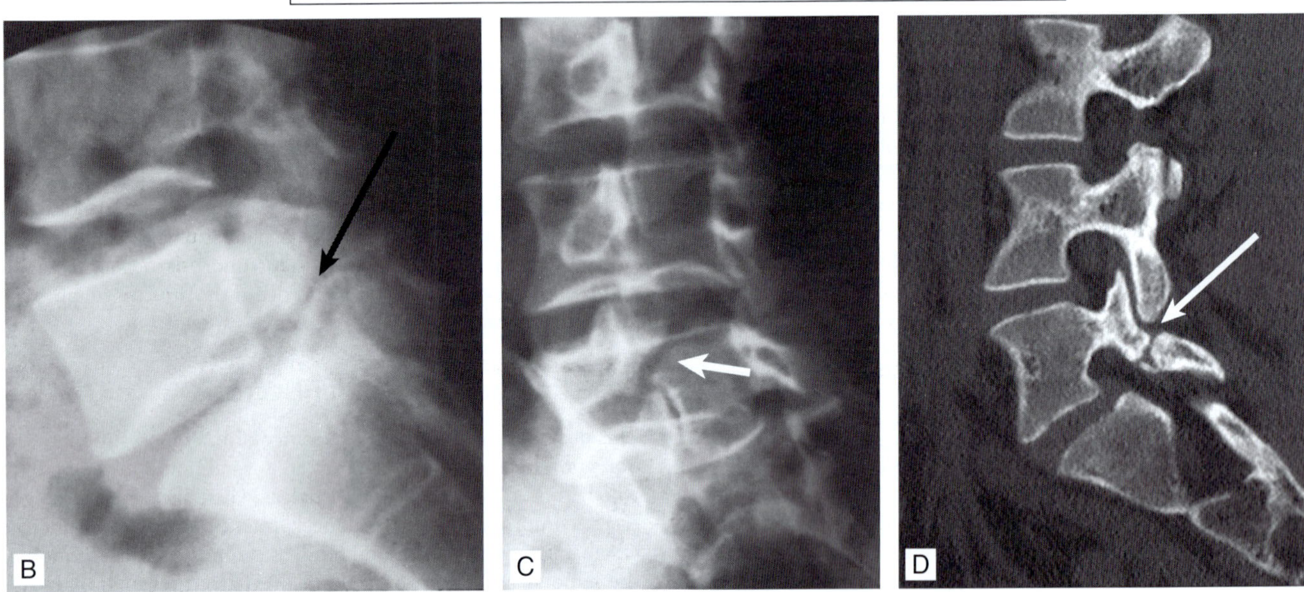

Figure 87.22 (A) Diagrammatic representation of an oblique view of a lumbar vertebra, presenting the "scotty dog" appearance. (B and C) X-ray and (D) CT scan demonstrating the pars interarticularis defect (*white arrow*) and associated anterior spondylolithesis of the L5 on S1 vertebral body.

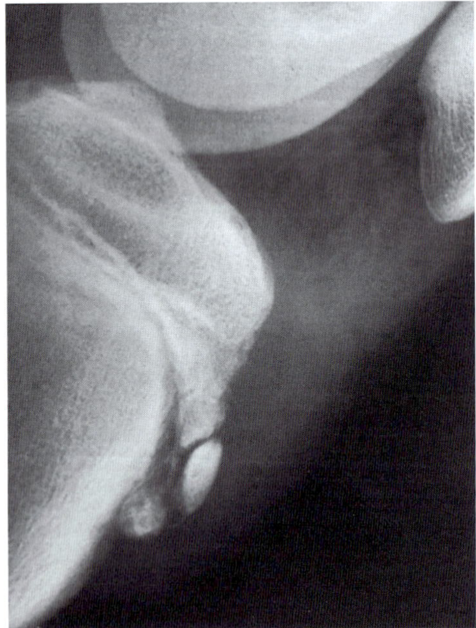

Figure 87.23 Osgood–Schlatter disease. Fragmentation may be seen and a portion of the tibial tubercle ossification center is elevated.

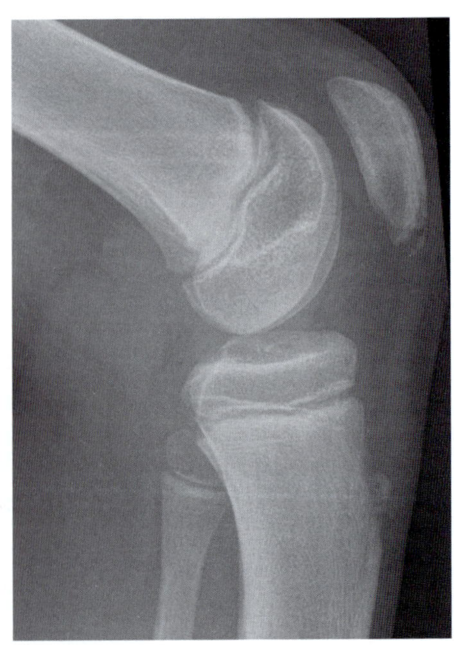

Figure 87.24 Sinding–Larson syndrome. Fragmentation at the distal pole of the patella is seen.

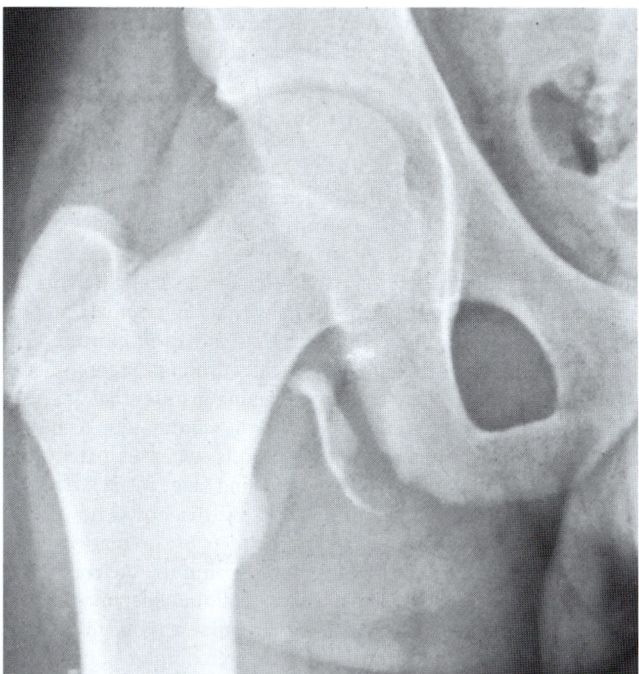

Figure 87.25 Note an avulsion of the inferior border of the ischium at the site of insertion of the hamstrings.

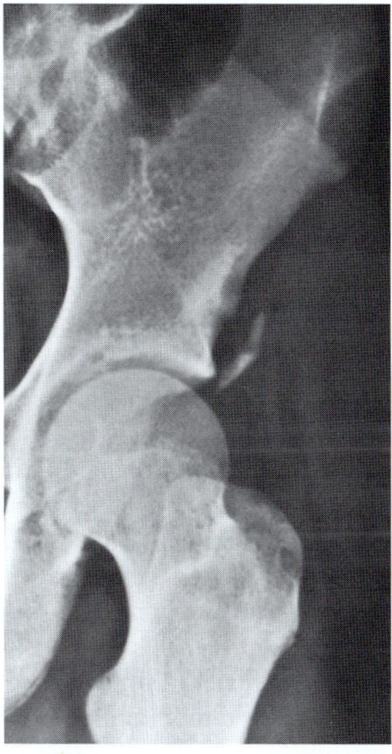

Figure 87.26 Avulsion fracture of the anterior inferior iliac crest: this is the origin of the rectus femoris muscle.

part of a bone as described above, but may also involve the growing epiphysis such as the head of the second or third metatarsal (*Frieberg's disease*) or even the whole of a small bone, for example lunate (*Kienbock's disease*) (Fig. 87.29). Frequently there is no clear history of predisposing fracture. However, there is evidence that even conditions such as *Perthes' disease* may result from trauma, and a traumatic effusion, which may also be responsible for the widening of the joint space that may be seen in the condition. This radiographic abnormality may be seen in the "*irritable hip syndrome*" of children, which may progress to frank necrosis of the femoral head. This has been attributed to interruption of the vascular flow, possibly on the venous side, by the formation of granulation tissue. A similar scenario has been suggested for septic arthritis (pus within the joint) and hemophilia (blood within the joint).

TABLE 87.1 Sites of Avulsion Fractures With Muscle Origin

Site of Avulsion Fracture	Muscle Origin
Anterior superior iliac crest	Sartorius
Anterior inferior iliac crest	Rectus femoris
Ischial tuberosity	Hamstrings
Greater trochanter	Gluteals
Lesser trochanter	Iliopsoas
Posterior calcaneus	Achilles tendon
Olecranon process	Triceps
Superior patella	Quadriceps
Inferior patella (Sinding–Larsen)	Patella ligament
Tibial tuberosity (Osgood–Schlatter)	Patella ligament

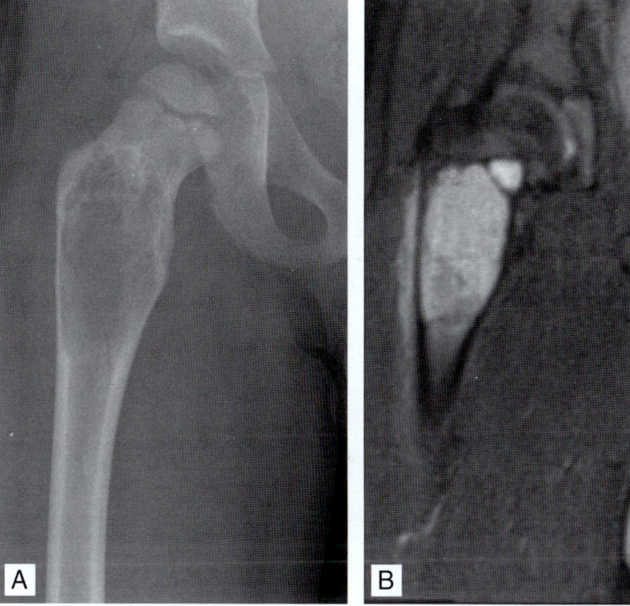

Figure 87.27 Plain film (A) and T1 TIRM coronal MRI (B) showing a bone cyst in the right proximal femur with a spiral fracture line passing through it, and visualization of the cyst on MRI, with edema in the adjacent muscle in keeping with a cortical breach.

In avascular necrosis, the necrotic bone usually becomes denser than the surrounding bone (Fig. 87.18), which in turn may become more osteopenic due to disuse. Studies on the femoral heads removed following fracture in the process of hip prosthesis implantation show that this is due to revascularization, when a thin layer of calcifying osteoid is laid down on the necrotic trabecula. This feature may occur anytime from 2 months to 2 years following injury. Eventually collapse and fragmentation are likely to occur. MRI scan may be useful in the diagnosis.

Drillers' Disease (Vibration Syndrome)

Drillers' disease is seen in workers using vibrating machinery, usually after five or more years of use. Degenerative cysts are found in the bones of the wrist, and occasionally the hand (Fig. 87.30). They

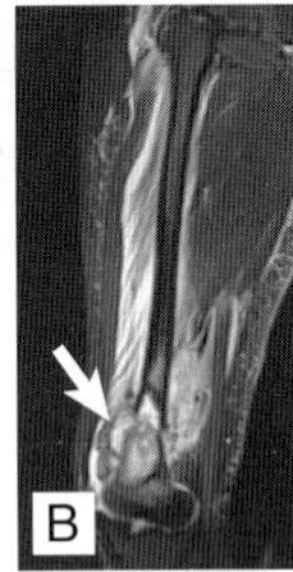

Figure 87.28 (A) plain radiograph of a horizontal beam lateral of a knee showing a pathological fracture through the distal femur. Note how the bone has a permeative appearance with multiple lucencies. The injury had occurred with minimal trauma. (B) The associated MRI reveals a tumor (osteosarcoma) of mixed signal intensity extending outside the bony margins into the surrounding soft tissues (*white arrow*) of the distal femur with a pathological fracture.

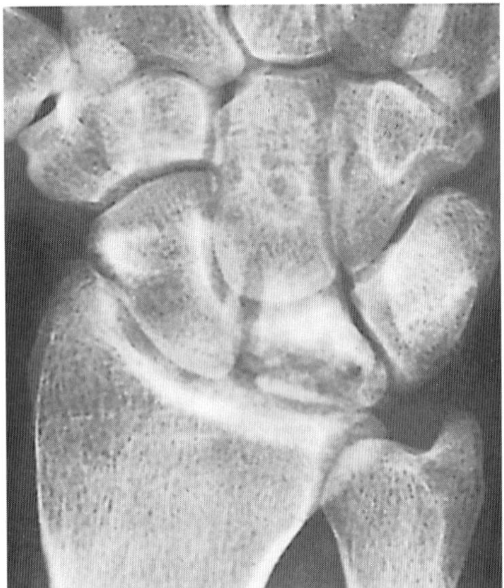

Figure 87.29 Kienbock's disease: in fact, a form of traumatic avascular necrosis of the lunate.

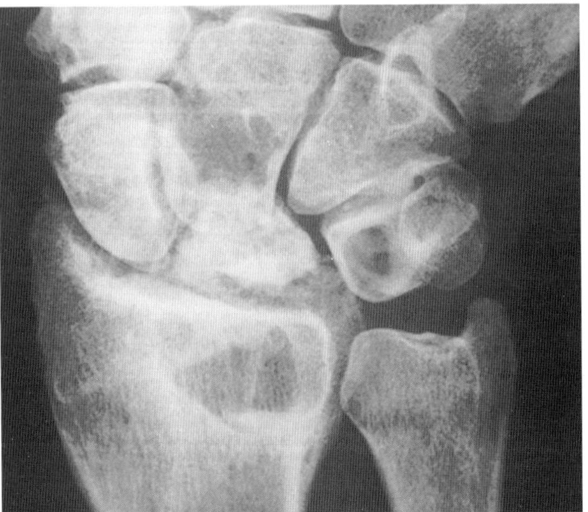

Figure 87.30 Vibration syndrome. Fragmentation and flattening of the lunate due to avascular necrosis is typical of Kienbock's disease, accompanied by extensive cystic changes in the surrounding bones. These abnormalities occurred in a worker using compressed-air drills, who had been exposed to this repeated trauma for many years. (Courtesy: Dr D.J. Stoker and Institute of Orthopaedics.)

are however indistinguishable from the cysts also seen that result from heavy manual labor, and the exact etiology is uncertain.

Complex Regional Pain Syndrome

This is also known as Sudeck's atrophy and is a rare clinical entity, which affects the extremities, where patients present with symptoms lasting longer than 6 months in duration and have a spectrum of symptoms which can include edema, changes in skin blood flow, abnormal motor activity, hyperalgesia or allodynia [3]. It usually affects people aged 50–70 with a slight female preponderance [4] and the clinical picture is usually disproportionate to the initial injury or precipitating event. Although predominantly a clinical diagnosis there are some imaging features that are pertinent to be aware of. Radiography is the commonest technique and the main features are of osteoporosis, which is patchy, and often periarticular and soft tissue swelling (Fig. 87.31). The role of MRI is mainly in excluding alternative diagnoses, however in these patients abnormal signal can be seen in the marrow, skin, joints, and bone and in the early phase within the skeletal muscle [5], however these are nonspecific. Radionuclide imaging can show increased blood flow and periarticular activity in all three phases in the affected limb [6]. These are complex patients that require management in a multi-disciplinary setting.

Transient Osteoporosis

This is a rare condition which usually affects the hip. Although this may represent a type of Sudeck's atrophy, a history of trauma is rare. Massive subarticular osteoporosis occurs, but this is self-limiting, however, with spontaneous resolution within 4–10 months.

Myositis Ossificans (Post-Traumatic)

This usually occurs without overt underlying bone injury. The exact etiology is uncertain, but it may be due to ossification of a hematoma or reactive periosteal elements which have been displaced into the soft tissues. The thigh is the commonest site. Interestingly, patients who have sustained a significant intracranial injury at the time of the axial injury have an increased risk of developing this. Hazy density in the soft tissues gives way to frank new bone formation, which may extend to the bone surface (Figs. 87.15 and 87.32). This may cause difficulty in distinguishing the lesion from parosteal osteosarcoma. Furthermore, unless adequate biopsy material is obtained, including the central and peripheral components of the lesion, histological differentiation may also be difficult. This is covered in more detail in Chapters 63 and 64 on bone tumor mimics and soft tissue tumors.

MRI has been shown to be a useful tool in the diagnosis of post-traumatic myositis ossificans, due to its ability to define the characteristic soft-tissue abnormality (Fig. 87.15), which also may be seen before the changes are evident radiographically. A similar type of calcification or ossification may occur around joints following dislocation, and in cases of severe closed head injury (Fig. 87.33). Ligamentous avulsions or chronic ligamentous trauma may also result in calcification, such as calcification of the medical collateral ligament of the knee in cases of chronic subclinical trauma (Fig. 87.34)—Pellegrini–Stieda lesion.

Compartment Syndrome

Rarely, trauma to a limb will give rise to a potentially devastating situation whereby the tissue pressure within a closed "compartment" causes progressive ischemia and ultimately necrosis. The

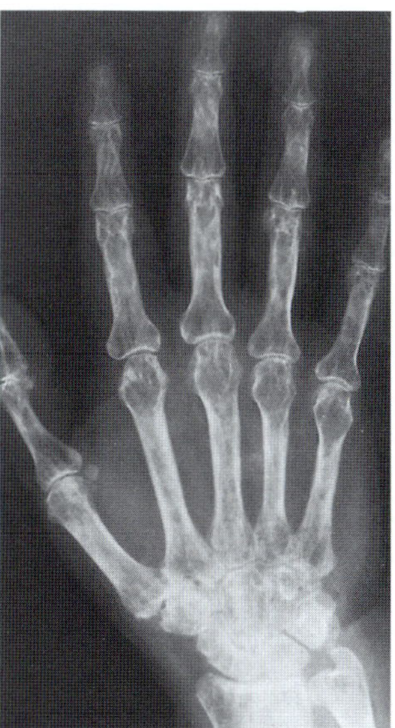

Figure 87.31 Sudeck's atrophy: there was minor trauma to the forearm some weeks earlier. Note gross osteoporosis of the bones of the hand, wrist and forearm, most marked at the bone ends, but also causing cortical "thinning" and resorption.

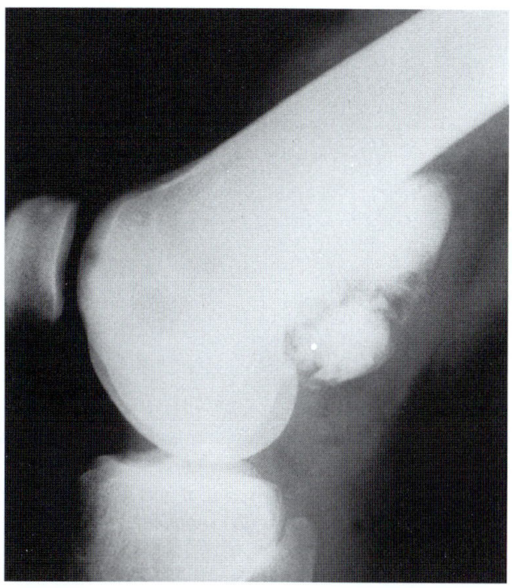

Figure 87.32 Post-traumatic myositis ossificans. A well-defined bone density arises from the cortex of the distal femur and extends into the soft tissues. There was a history of blunt trauma, but even so, this lesion needs to be differentiated from parosteal osteosarcoma.

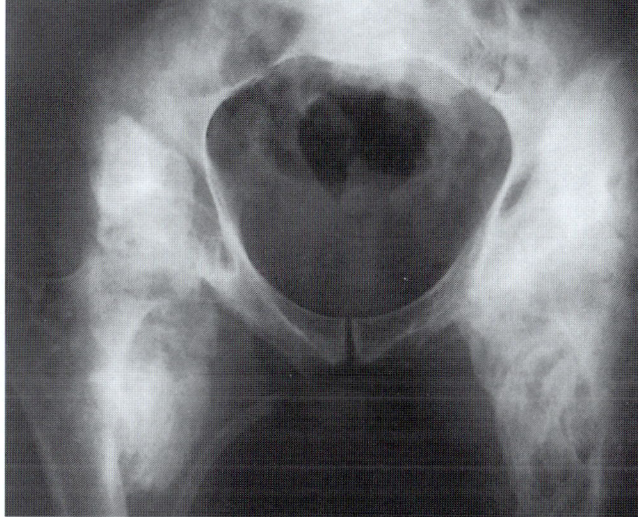

Figure 87.33 Myositis ossificans associated with paraplegia. Very extensive soft-tissue ossification is visible around both hip joints. (Courtesy: Dr D.J. Stoker and Institute of Orthopaedics.)

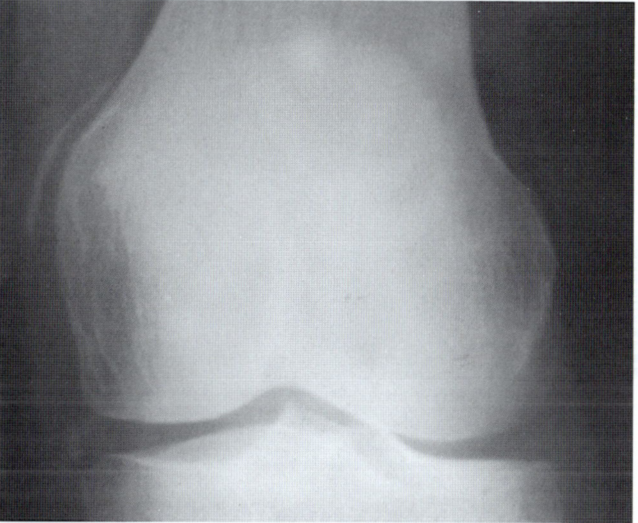

Figure 87.34 Pellegrini–Stieda lesion. Post-traumatic calcification is shown in relation to the medial femoral condyle following a tear of the medial collateral ligament. (Courtesy: Dr D.J. Stoker and Institute of Orthopaedics.)

compartments of the limbs consist of areas surrounded by rigid osseous and fascial planes. Tissue edema or hemorrhage may be the initiating factor and result from direct trauma and/or vascular interruption. The result of edema within a closed compartment is to raise the tissue pressure, thereby further decreasing vascular perfusion. Prompt fasciotomy is required. Volkmann's ischemia and contracture of the forearm, following fracture of the elbow, is probably a form of the compartment syndrome. Today the syndrome is most commonly seen in the leg as the result of road traffic accidents. It is a clinical diagnosis and there is little role for imaging.

Arterial Injury

Vascular trauma generally occurs as the result of penetrating injury, although it may be caused by sharp bone fragments from a fracture, either at the time of injury or during manipulation. The popliteal artery is commonly injured from fractures or dislocations around the knee. Brachial artery injury may also result from supracondylar fractures of the humerus or elbow dislocations, particularly in children. Branches of the internal iliac artery, especially the superior gluteal, pudendal and vesical, are at risk in pelvic ring fractures (see below), and are responsible for the massive blood loss and associated high mortality rates (Fig. 87.35).

Historically, vascular injury was evaluated almost exclusively by angiography. However, with the modern use of CT, the advent of trauma centers and the extensive progress that has occurred in recent years regarding early care of the polytrauma patient CT can provide high-quality angiographic images far more rapidly, and more effectively than angiography (Fig. 87.36). Advantages of CT over angiography are the fact the patient does not have to be sent to the angiographic suite and that the images are obtained in a

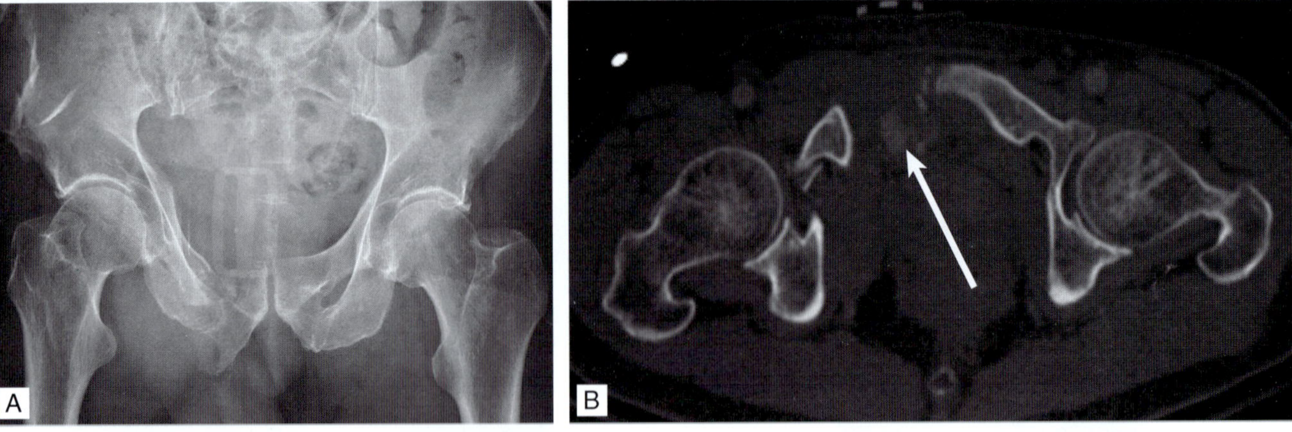

Figure 87.35 (A) Complex pelvic fracture involving the right sacro-iliac joint, ilac blade, acetabulum, and inferior and superior pubic rami. The patient had sustained the injury after falling from a roof and was haemodynamically unstable. (B) Corresponding axial CT scan showing the fractures and active extravasation of contrast (*white arrow*) in keeping with significant associated vascular injury.

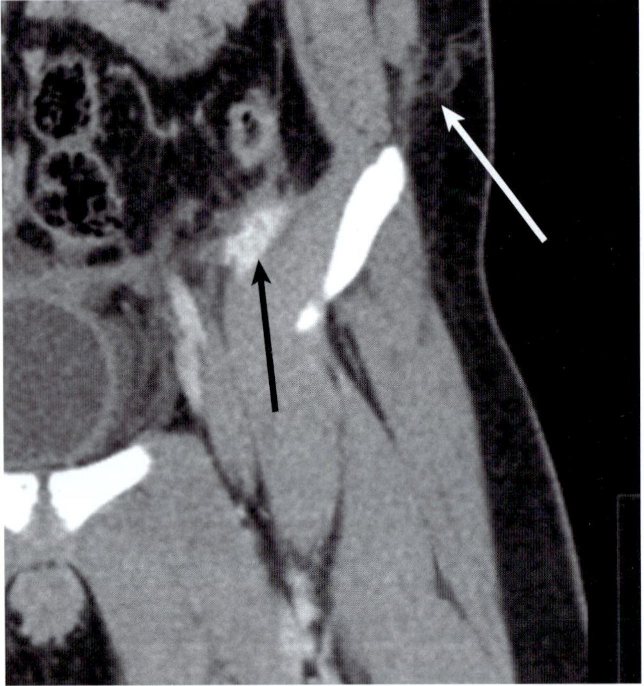

Figure 87.36 A further CT angiographic image demonstrating active extravasation of contrast (*black arrow*) and thus active hemorrhage in the iliacus muscle following a stab wound to the left side. The tract of the knife can be seen in the subcutaneous tissues (*white arrow*).

matter of seconds, with an intravenous injection rather than arterial catheterization. Also, with a variety of postprocessing capabilities, 3D or multiplanar representations can be obtained easily and rapidly. The main role of direct angiography in trauma is in the hands of the interventional radiologist where following CT, focused diagnosis and the capability to intervene and stop the bleeding is carried out. This can save the patient the need for a trauma laparotomy and the associated complications that can occur.

Joint Injuries

Dislocations occur when there is a complete loss of normal articular contact between the bones comprising the joint (Fig. 87.37). Subluxation refers to a partial loss of articular contact. Diastasis

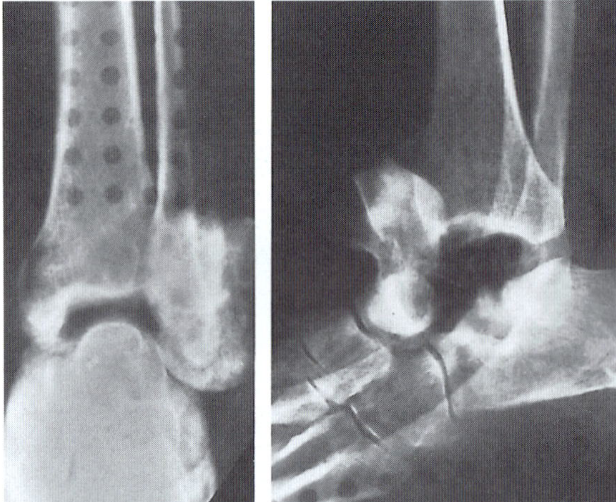

Figure 87.37 Complete dislocation of the talus.

refers to separation of fibrous joints, for example symphysis pubis, sacroiliac joint (Fig. 87.38).

Joint injuries may be difficult to diagnose radiographically, as they frequently comprise ligamentous injury without obvious bone involvement. In addition, subtle avulsion fractures adjacent to joints may be the only indicator of gross ligamentous injuries. These are most commonly encountered around the ankle, where avulsions of the medial and lateral malleoli indicate collateral ligament disruption. Other important areas are the base of the proximal phalanx of the thumb (Fig. 87.39) and corner avulsions of the tibial plateau. Plain radiographic signs of injury such as effusion or haemarthrosis may be helpful. Stress views of the involved joint have been advocated, but this may require the patient to be sedated, as they may be extremely painful to obtain.

Assessment of Joints

Arthrography has traditionally been used to assess joint abnormalities (Fig. 87.40). USG has also been used, particularly to assess the shoulder joint for injuries to the rotator cuff (see below), and CT is also useful in the shoulder, especially when combined with arthrography, when injuries of the glenoid labrum may be seen.

Most recently, however, MRI has made immense progress with its ability to define the soft tissues, ligaments, and tendons.

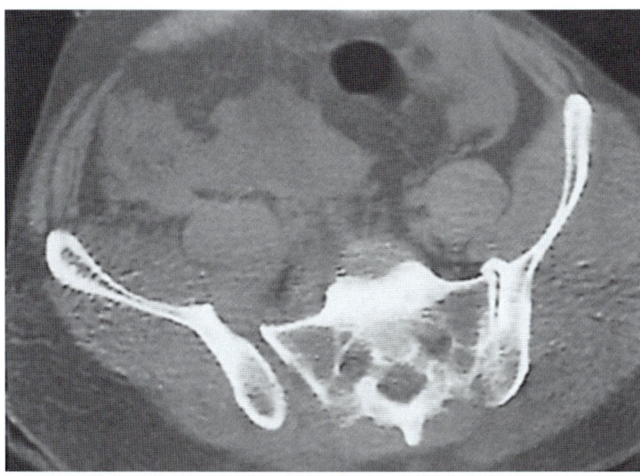

Figure 87.38 CT image demonstrates complete diastasis of the right sacroiliac joint.

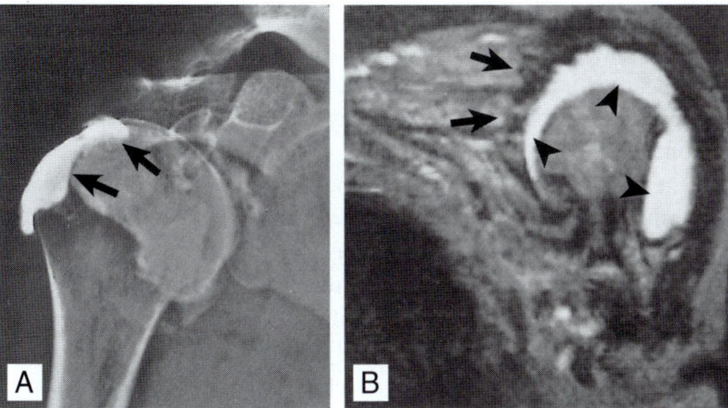

Figure 87.40 Rotator cuff tear. (A) Arthrography is performed by injecting contrast medium, with or without air, into the shoulder joint. Leakage of contrast into the subdeltoid bursa (*arrows*) indicates a rupture of the rotator cuff which normally separates the bursa from the joint. (B) MRI demonstrates a large joint effusion, shown as high signal on this FLASH image. The effusion, which shows markedly increased signal intensity on this sequence, has tracked into the subdeltoid bursa (*arrowheads*), indicating rotator cuff rupture. In this case the subscapularis is seen to be retracted, with an irregular lateral margin (*large arrows*) suggesting tear.

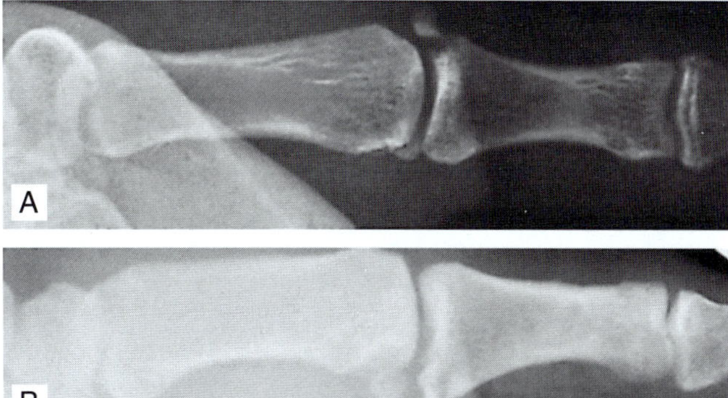

Figure 87.39 Avulsion fractures of the proximal phalanx of the thumb. (A) Fracture at the site of attachment of the radial collateral ligament. (B) Fracture at the site of the attachment of the ulnar collateral ligament. In practice, the adductor of the thumb inserts in the same area, and may also be avulsed.

Although originally finding favor for its ability to diagnose meniscal tears in the knee (Fig. 87.41), it can be useful for a variety of soft-tissue abnormalities around the knee (Fig. 87.42), shoulder, ankle and wrist, where ligamentous and tendinous abnormalities may be demonstrated.

Other Forms of Trauma

Trauma may occur from a variety of other causes, including *ionizing radiation, frostbite* and rarely *electrical burns,* and *dysbaric osteonecrosis* (*Caisson's disease*).

Frostbite may give rise to acro-osteolysis (Fig. 87.43), and in children, premature epiphyseal closure and growth arrest.

Osteonecrosis, also known as avascular necrosis, is characterized by a stereotypical pattern of cell death and a complex repair process of bone resorption and formation. Decreased blood flow occurs through three mechanisms: vascular interruption (usually traumatic), intravascular occlusion from thrombi or embolic fat, or intraosseous extravascular compression from lipocyte hypertrophy or Gaucher cells [7].

Bone changes include areas of irregular bone density, usually in the long bones, and due to medullary infarction, and subarticular

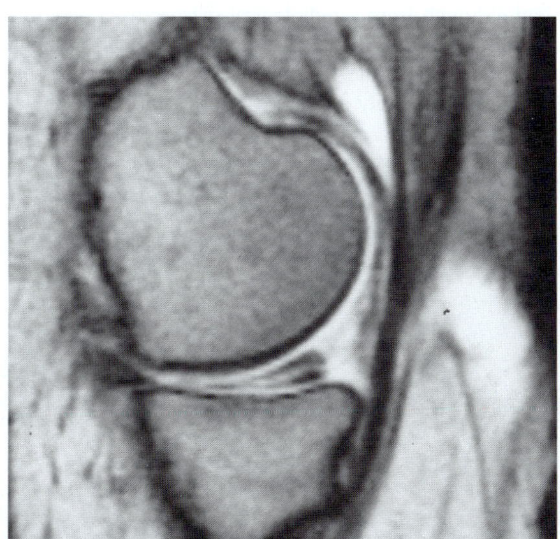

Figure 87.41 Tear of the posterior horn tear of medial meniscus. MRI image (T_2-weighted) demonstrates a linear area of higher signal extending to the articular surface.

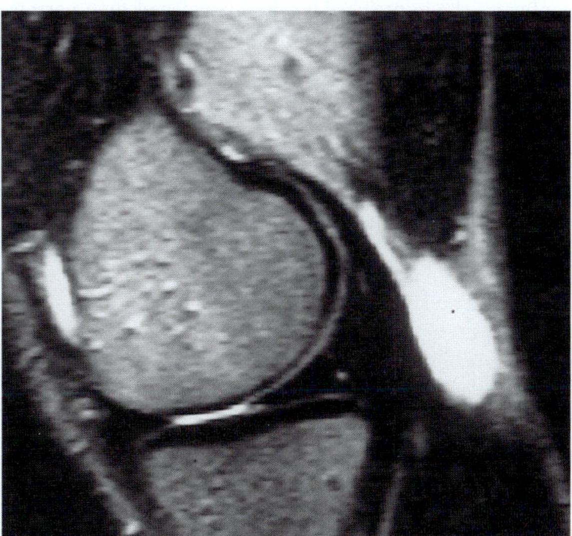

Figure 87.42 Baker's cyst. T_2-weighted sagittal image of the knee demonstrates a well-defined high-signal-intensity lesion posterior to the knee joint.

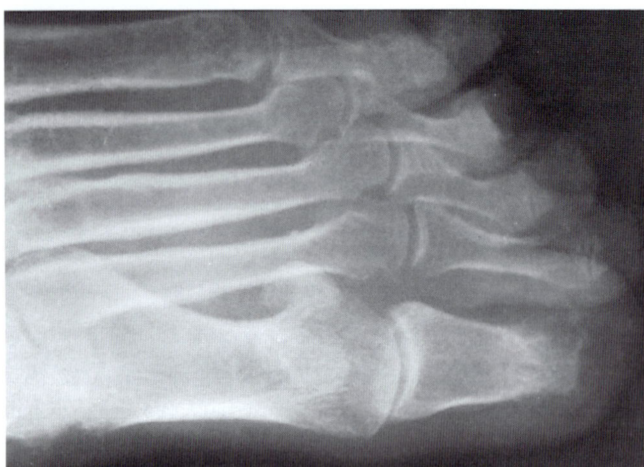

Figure 87.43 Frostbite. Note acro-osteolysis of the toes, with almost complete resorption of the distal phalanges.

infarctions, particularly in the humeral and femoral heads (Fig. 87.44). A similar pattern of subarticular bone infarction is seen in a variety of other conditions (Box 87.4). The changes of avascular necrosis are visible on nuclear medicine bone scan and MRI long before they can be seen radiographically.

Chronic Trauma to the Joints (Neuropathic Arthropathy)

Repeated trauma to the joints in the absence of normal pain and proprioceptive sensation will give rise to a severe destruction arthropathy, first described by Charcot (Figs. 87.45 and 87.46). Although seen originally in cases of neurosyphilis, there is a variety of causes (Box 87.5). Diabetes Mellitus is by far the commonest cause encountered today.

There are two patterns of Charcot joint -atrophic and hypertrophic. *Atrophic* form is most common and has an acute progression. It is characterized by resorption of the ends of the affected bone and joint destruction. It mainly occurs in non-weight bearing joints of the upper limb. *Hypertrophic* form has slow progression. It is characterized by joint destruction with periarticular debris or bone fragmentation and presence of osteosclerosis and osteophytes. The joint space is initially widened then narrowed.

Most joints show evidence of *disorganization*, increased bone *density*, *debris* within the joint capsule and bone *destruction*, giving rise to *deformity*—the so-called "5Ds."

BOX 87.4 Causes of Subarticular Bone Infarction—Avascular Necrosis

Sickle cell disease
Steroids
Trauma
Chronic alcoholism
Radiation
Rheumatoid arthritis
Amyloid arthropathy
Gaucher's disease
Pancreatitis
Caisson disease

Osteochondritis Dissecans (Osteochondral Fractures)

Osteochondritis dissecans is really a misnomer, as the lesions clinically referred to as osteochondritis are usually the result of trauma, and indicate an osteochondral or chondral fracture occurring at an articular surface. After injury the detached portion of the bone may remain in situ, may be mildly displaced or may become loose within the joint (Fig. 87.47)

The most common site of osteochondritis dissecans is the distal femur. The medial condyle is involved in 85% of cases with the lesion classically on the lateral aspect of the medial femoral condyle (Fig. 87.12). Other sites of osteochondritis dissecans include the posterior patella and talar dome (Fig. 87.48).

Other forms of osteochondral fractures occur, with direct trauma to the articular surface, as seen in the Hill–Sachs deformity of the humeral head, from anterior dislocations, and the anterior femoral head defect following posterior dislocation of the hip.

Fractures in the Thoracic and Lumbar Spine

Please see chapter on Neurological Trauma for information regarding cervical spine trauma.

Spinal fractures can occur in a wide variety of trauma, ranging from the simple fall from standing in the patient with osteoporosis to those with a significant mechanism of injury in the setting of polytrauma. There are several classification systems that are currently used and although from a radiological perspective a description of the injury is the most valuable tool, having an understanding of the biomechanics of how the fracture occurs and these classification systems can help identify associated injuries and guide the clinical

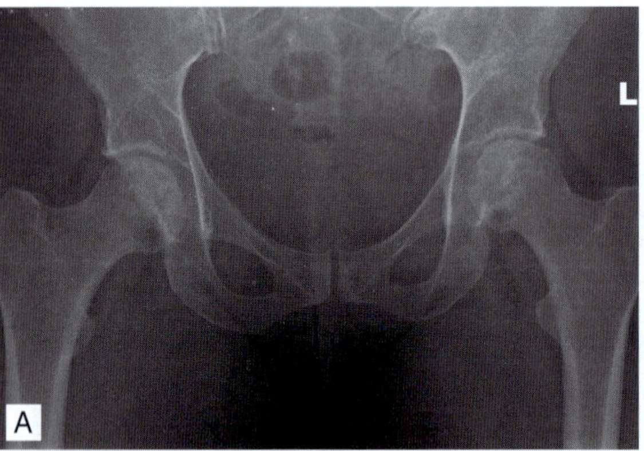

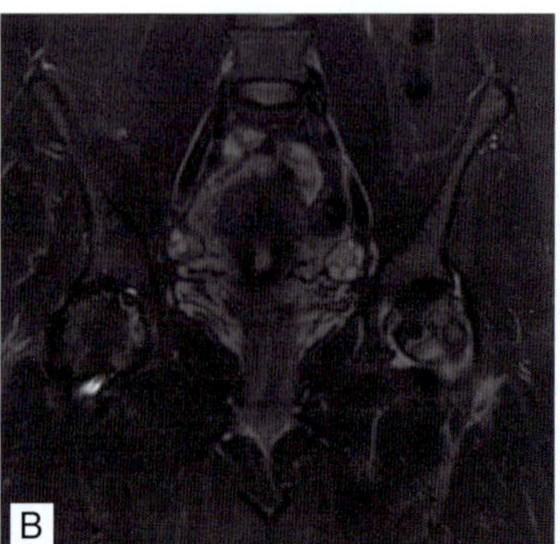

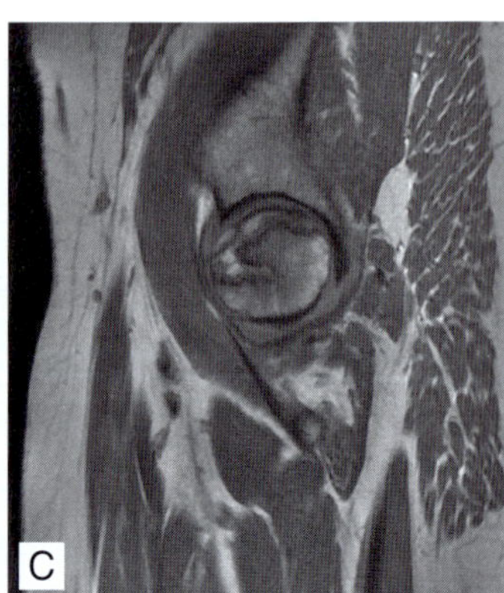

Figure 87.44 (A, B, and C) Avascular necrosis of the hips. Note mixed sclerosis and lucency in the femoral heads with collapse of the weightbearing surface, more marked on the left. The corresponding T1 saggital and PD SPAIR coronal fat saturated images demonstrate the serpiginous lines demarcating the avascular bone and the collapse of the femoral heads.

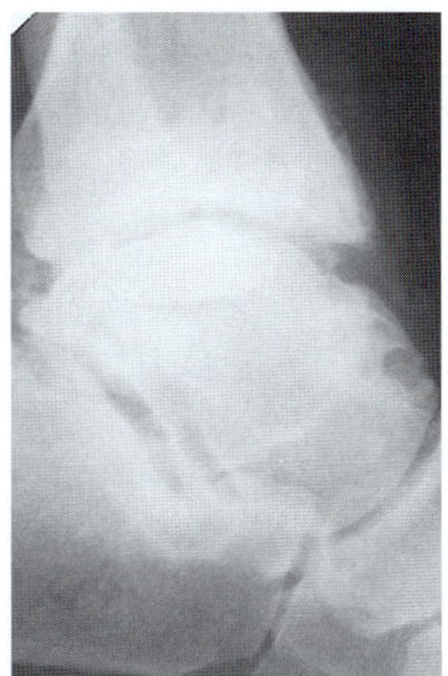

Figure 87.45 Early Charcot joint, diabetic patient. Note irregularity of the talar dome, with increased density seen around the ankle joint.

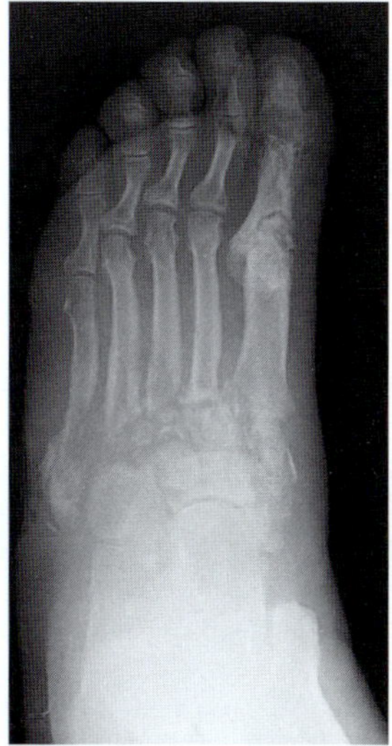

Figure 87.46 Charcot arthropathy of the foot, showing disorganization, increased bone density, debris within the joint capsule and bone destruction, giving rise to deformity.

teams. These include the AO thoracolumbar spine classification system [8], the thoracolumbar injury classification and severity score injury [9], and the Denis three column injury model [10].

There are common patterns of fractures seen in the thoracolumbar spine that are important to be aware of. If a patient has a suspected spinal fracture, or a confirmed fracture but only part of the spine has been imaged then CT imaging of the whole spine should be carried out with multi planar reformats [11]. If there is any concern about the force of a fracture going through the spinal canal or any obvious malalignment or encroachment of bony fragments in to the spinal canal, or any neurological defect the MRI of the whole spine should be carried out (Fig. 87.49). Neurosurgical teams should be involved early on in the management and diagnosis of these injuries.

Compression fractures: these can occur in younger patients with a significant history of trauma but are more common in the osteoporotic population with low velocity injuries. The common patterns are central compression and anterior compression fractures and can be a significant cause of pain and morbidity if not recognized (Fig. 87.50). The Genant classification can be used to assess the severity of the fracture pattern [12]

- **Grade 0:** normal
- **Grade 1:** mild fracture, <25% loss of height
- **Grade 2:** moderate fracture, 25% to 40% loss of height
- **Grade 3:** severe fracture, >40% loss of height

Burst fractures: these usually occur secondary to an axial loading force which goes through the spine and are more commonly seen in a fall or jump from height and landing on the feet or in motor vehicle collisions and while there is some overlap in the imaging appearances with compression fractures, due to the higher mechanism of injury the fracture always involves the posterior aspect of the vertebral body and often extends into the posterior elements and there is protrusion of fragments into the spinal canal [13] with the associated higher risk of neurological injury. These are usually unstable injuries.

BOX 87.5 Causes of Charcot Joints

Diabetes (Figs. 87.48 and 87.49)
Neurosyphilis
Syringomyelia
Spina bifida
Leprosy
Congenital indifference to pain

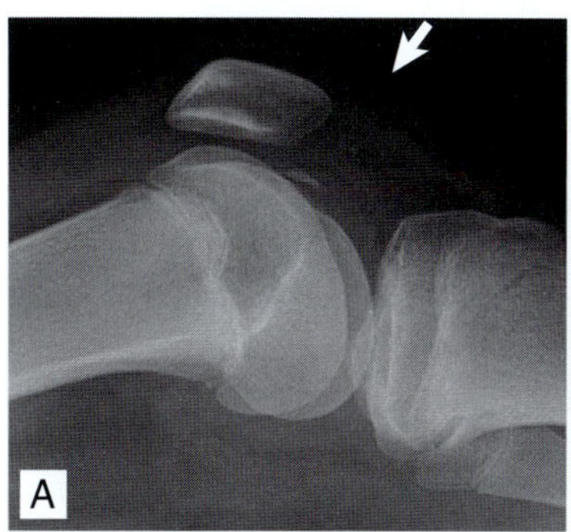

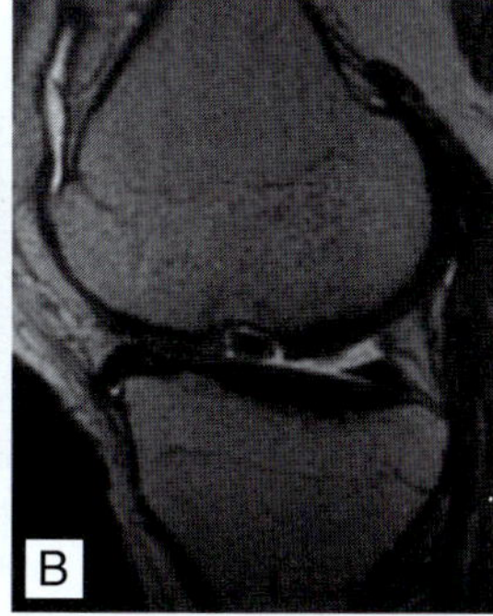

Figure 87.47 (A) Lateral x-ray of the knee showing a loose body within the anterior aspect from an osteochondral defect. (B) A saggital PD MRI demonstrating an established osteochondral defect still in situ in the fracture site.

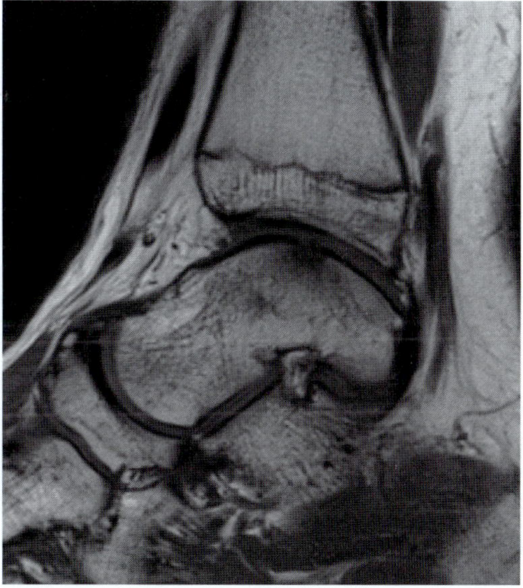

Figure 87.48 Saggital PD MRI of the ankle showing an osteochondral defect of the talar dome.

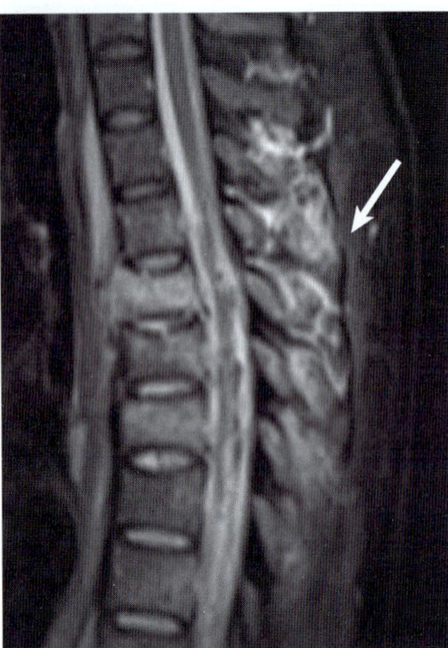

Figure 87.49 MRI of the mid thoracic spine in a patient with multiple spinal fractures. This is seen by increased signal in the vertebral bodies on this STIR sequence with associated loss of vertebral body height. There is significant increased signal in the interspinous ligaments and disruption of the supraspinous ligament (*white arrow*) illustrating how MRI can give far more information about the extent of a spinal fracture.

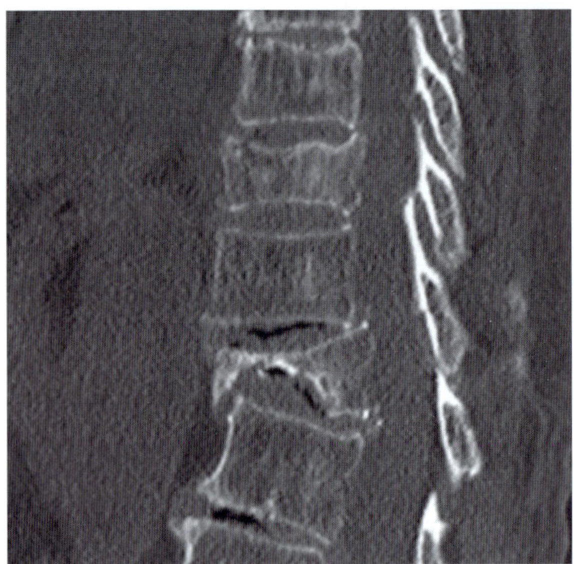

Figure 87.50 Osteoporotic fractures in the thoracolumbar spine—there is loss of the whole vertebral body height of T12 and a severe anterior wedge compression fracture of L2 with a degree of kyphosis secondary to this.

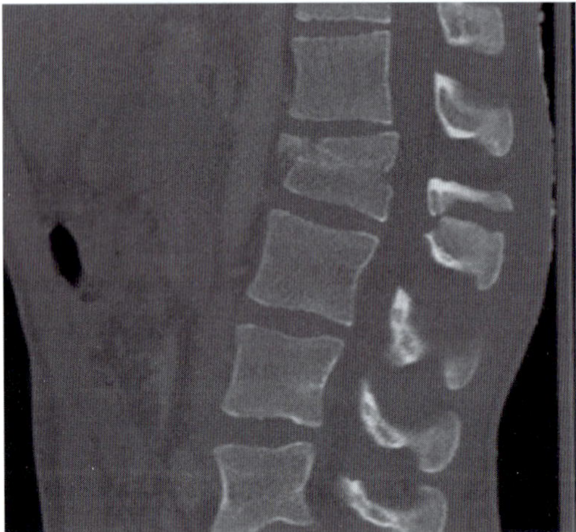

Figure 87.51 Chance fracture on saggital CT. Note the transverse fracture through the vertebral body that extends in a transverse pattern through the spinous process and the associated flexion/compression component by loss of the anterior vertebral body height.

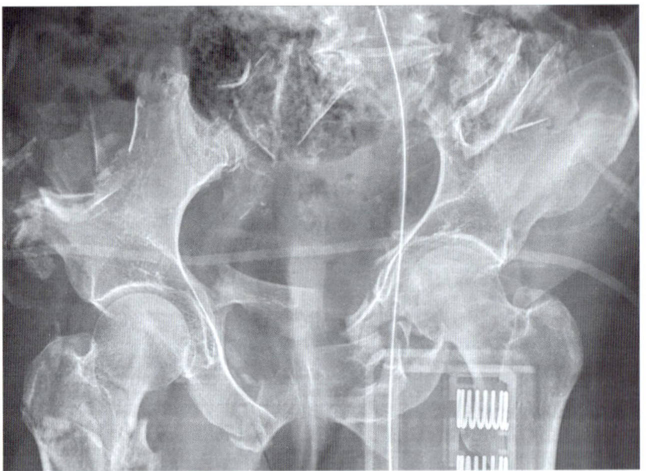

Figure 87.52 Spinopelvic dissociation—the L5/S1 vertebrae are completely dislocated from the pelvis, which is extensively fractured.

Chance fracture: this is a type of flexion and distraction injury that commonly occurs in restrained passengers in motor vehicle collisions secondary to the "lap" part of the seatbelt. It is a highly unstable injury that involves the vertebral body and the posterior elements [14] and due to the force created between the seatbelt and the more rigid thoracolumbar spine has a high incidence of associated abdominal injuries (Fig. 87.51).

Transverse process fractures: these can be as part of a more complex spinal injury or in isolation, however are important to recognize, as they are a source of pain for the patient.

Complex high-energy fractures/dislocations: these are unstable with high risk of associated ligamentous disruption and of associated spinal cord injury. The fracture patterns can be complex, involve the vertebral bodies and posterior elements, can have "perched" facet joints where there is a dislocation of the facet joints and mal-alignment of the vertebral column. Spino-pelvic dissociation is where the injury involves a fracture dislocation through the L5/S1 level in combination with a pelvic fracture leading to complete "dissociation" of the spine from the pelvis (Fig. 87.52).

87.2 Skeletal Trauma: Pediatrics

Dina Pefanis, Roy Wheeler

Approximately one-third of people sustain a fracture of a bone during their childhood [15]. The fracture patterns and causes differ in children when compared to adults, and the growing bones predispose to certain fracture patterns not seen in adults. The most common fracture location is the distal radius, and the most common cause of a childhood fracture is a fall [15,16].

Childhood fractures are often incomplete (torus or greenstick fractures) (Fig. 87.53), and plastic fractures, without cortical disruption, may occur. When describing a fracture, the terms buckle and torus may be used synonymously despite slight differences in the descriptive terms. Torus is derived from the Latin meaning swelling or round molding and has come to mean a ring-like bulge. Often the alternative radiographic projection will demonstrate a buckle fracture, indicating that the ring does not circumnavigate the bone. Greenstick fractures are a distinct fracture type with a break in one side of the cortex only (Fig. 87.54) and should not be confused with torus or buckle fractures.

Salter-Harris Fractures

Fractures involving the physis are common due to the relative weakness of the cartilage. Of all childhood fractures, nearly one fifth involve the physis [17]. The Salter-Harris classification is most commonly used (Figs. 87.55 and 87.56) to classify these fractures. Damage to the physis may cause partial or even complete growth arrest. However, despite its widespread use, the Salter-Harris classification is not, on its own, prognostic [18,19].

Fractures at the Elbow

The ossification centers at the elbow provide diagnostic clues based on the order in which they appear. *The mnemonic CRITOL indicates the order of ossification to be Capitellum, Radial head, Internal epicondyle, Trochlear, Olecranon, and Lateral epicondyle* (Fig. 87.57). The age at which ossification occurs is variable with ossification occurring earlier in girls [20–22]. However, the order ossification is more constant, and although there may be differences in the order of ossification [22,23], importantly, *the internal epicondyle always ossifies before the trochlear*. A displaced internal epicondyle ossification center may mimic a trochlear ossification center, and diagnosis should be made using the absence of the normal order of ossification, that is *apparent absent internal ossification center indicates displacement, if a trochlear ossification center is present* (Fig. 87.58).

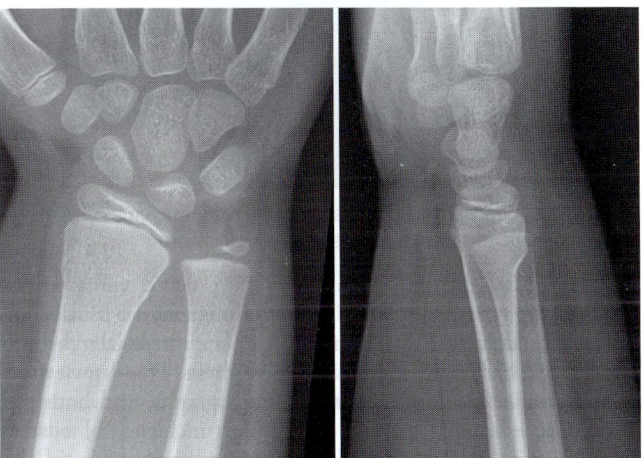

Figure 87.53 Torus fracture of the wrist. The cortex is buckled on the dorsal surface. The volar surface is intact.

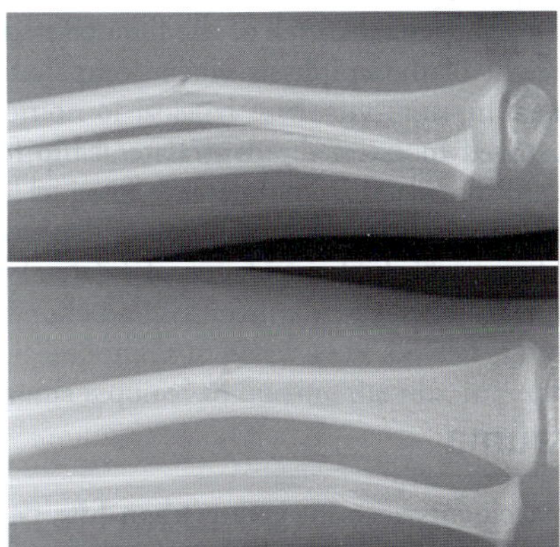

Figure 87.54 Greenstick fracture of the radius and buckle fracture of the ulna.

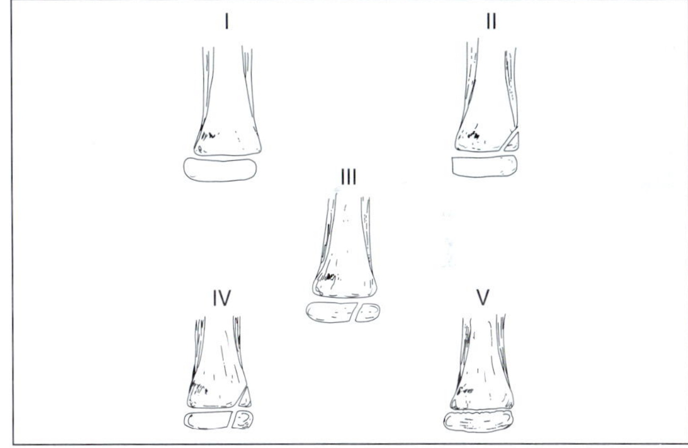

Figure 87.55 Salter-Harris classification. I, Injury through the physis only. II, Fracture through the physis and metaphysis. III, Fracture through the physis and epiphysis. IV, Fracture through the physis, metaphysis and epiphysis. V, Crush fracture of the physis.

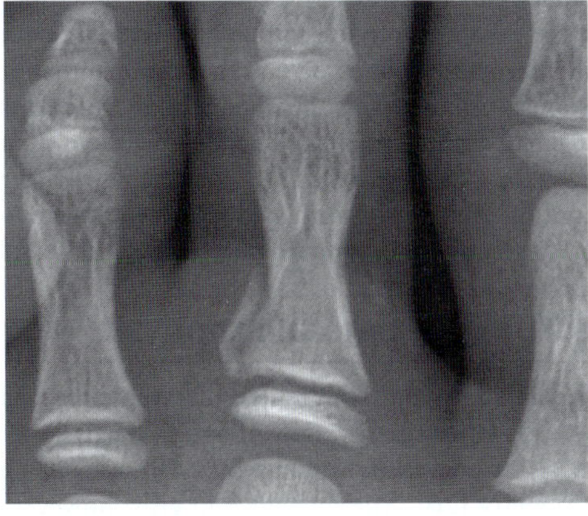

Figure 87.56 A Salter-Harris II fracture, the most common.

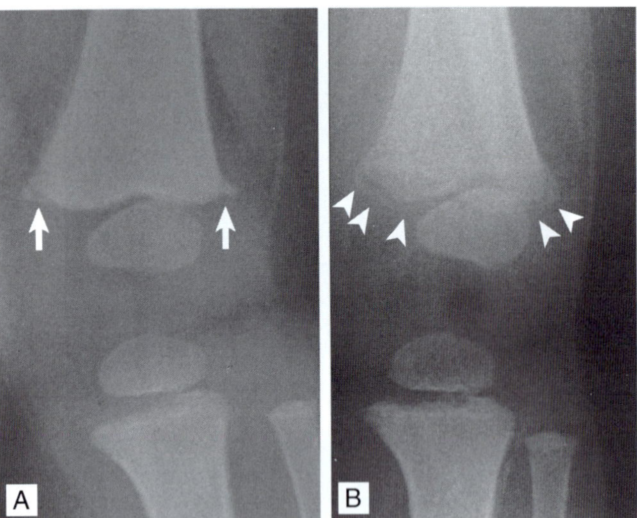

Figure 87.64 Classic metaphyseal lesions. (A) Radiograph demonstrating classic metaphyseal lesions appearing as corner fractures (*arrows*). (B) Radiograph of the same patient performed hours later. The slight difference in projection reveals a bucket handle fracture (*arrowheads*). Note the additional proximal tibial injury.

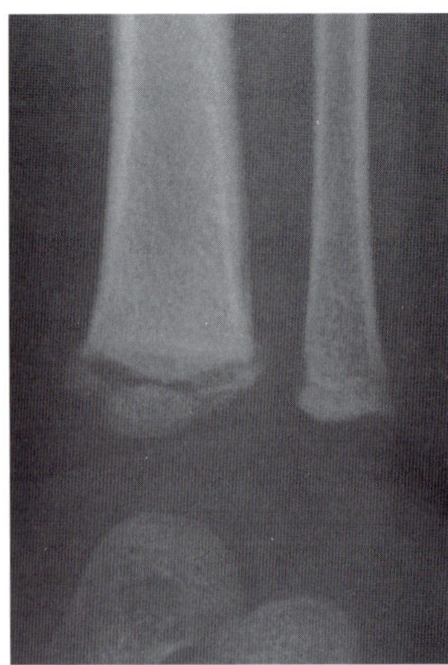

Figure 87.65 A distal tibial classic metaphyseal lesion appearing as a bucket handle fracture.

Classic Metaphyseal Lesions

Classic metaphyseal lesions (CML) or corner fractures are highly specific for physical abuse in young children [41]. These are thought to be caused by traction and torsion of the limb, although various maneuvers have been demonstrated to potentially cause the fractures [42]. The fracture occurs through the most immature portion of the metaphysis, separating a small fragment [43] which may appear as a corner fracture or a bucket handle fracture (Figs. 87.64–87.65).

Classic metaphyseal lesions often do not heal with periosteal reaction [44–46], may heal rapidly [47], and dating of these fractures is unreliable. There are instances of these being present in older children and in certain circumstances outside the context of physical abuse [48–53], particularly following caesarean section, but it should be noted that the incidence of long bone fracture during caesarean section is rare and the mechanism of injury is not incompatible with such a fracture. Outside rare cases with a clear history, classic metaphyseal lesions remain specific for abuse and should prompt a full skeletal survey [41,54].

Long Bone Fractures in Non-Ambulant Infants

In patients greater than 18 months of age, both femoral and humeral fractures are more likely to be accidental, but in those less than 18 months of age, the fractures are more likely to be caused by abuse [55,56]. Also, in the less than 18 months group, proximal humeral fractures are more likely to be secondary to abuse when compared to distal humeral fractures [57]. In older patients, the probability of abuse is increased with increasing numbers of risk factors such as other physical evidence of abuse and evidence of prior injuries [58].

Spiral Fractures

These may be specific for physical abuse in non-ambulant children since a rotational force is required. However, by the time the child is ambulant, a toddler's fracture is classically caused by twisting on a fixed foot, and this gives rise to a spiral fracture, which, in this case, is not suspicious for physical abuse. These are undisplaced and may often be faintly seen on only one projection (Fig 87.66), or the initial radiographs may be normal [59], so clinical suspicion and follow up imaging play a large role in the diagnosis. Most commonly, the fracture is in the middle or distal third of the tibia [59].

Rib Fractures

Due to the pliable nature of pediatric ribs, rib fractures are relatively uncommon when compared to adults, although major trauma commonly causes rib fractures and most are associated with other injuries [34]. *However, in the absence of major trauma and in children younger than one year of age, physical abuse should be suspected* [56,60]. Posterior rib fractures are thought to be caused by a grip with fingers behind the chest and thumbs anteriorly, such as the grip that may be used to shake a baby (Fig. 87.67).

Radiography has a sensitivity of 13.5% for the diagnosis of rib fractures, although CT demonstrates a sensitivity of 45%, it is marginally less specific (97.5% vs 97%) [61]. Both follow-up and oblique radiographs improve the sensitivity, and these should be performed if rib fractures are suspected and are diagnostically important [62–64].

It has been hypothesized that cardiopulmonary resuscitation using a two-thumb, hand encircling technique may cause rib fractures, however, data are not conclusive and may be complicated by birth trauma and metabolic bone disorders [65–67]. Studies before guidance suggesting a two thumb resuscitation method demonstrated that rib fractures were rare and not posterior in their location [68–70].

Fracture Age

Assessing the age of fractures is difficult and not exact [71], but often an estimate may be provided based on the appearance of subperiosteal new bone formation, callus formation, and remodeling. *In children without an underlying bone disorder such as osteogenesis imperfecta, subperiosteal new bone formation is first seen from*

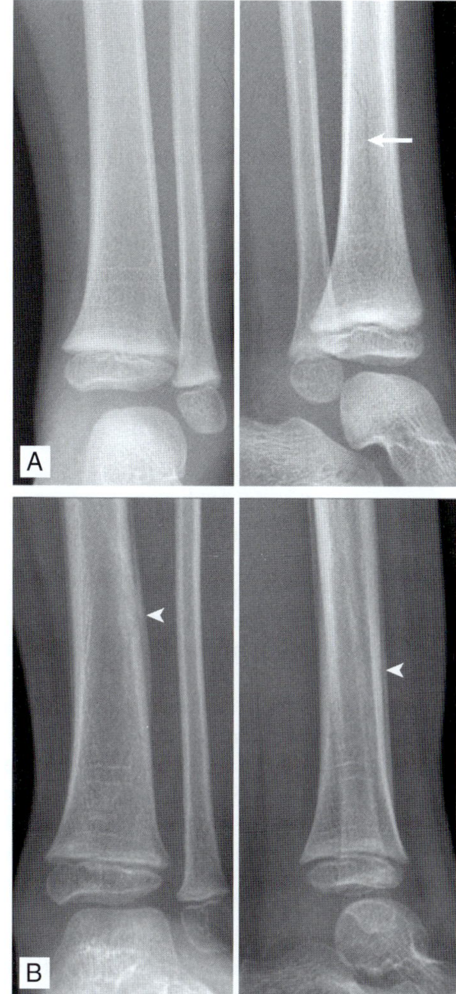

Figure 87.66 A Toddler's fracture. (A) Initial radiographs reveal a subtle linear fracture line (enhanced) on only one view (*arrow*). (B) Follow up radiographs reveal periosteal reaction (*arrowheads*).

4 days postinjury [72] to 23 days postinjury [73] and may last until 96 days. The mean fracture age at first demonstration of subperiosteal new bone formation is between ten and fifteen days [45,72–75]. Given this, any fracture with no evidence of healing, including subperiosteal new bone formation, is likely to be acute and less than 2 weeks old, more certainly less than 23 days old. More importantly, *a fracture demonstrating subperiosteal new bone formation will have occurred greater than 4 days previously* [45,72] and would be inconsistent with a history of a fracture occurring on the day of presentation.

Callus may be divided into soft and hard callus, but the definition of each is difficult—for the purposes of dating a fracture, it may be easier to refer to the first visualization of callus of any kind. *Consistent with the other stages of bone healing, callus formation is variable [72–74,76,77], but the earliest report of visualization is 7 days after injury [78]. Remodeling is the final stage, and it is first seen at 4 weeks post-injury* [76]. It should be noted that mean age at demonstration of mature callus can be as long as fifty-five days in immobilized femoral fractures [74] and it is possible that fracture evidence remains for a longer period in initially undetected fractures of other bones.

Mimics of Physical Abuse

Physiological Periosteal Reaction

Physiological periosteal reaction may be seen affecting the long bones of children aged 1–6 months [79], although the upper age limit has not been reliably studied. It is confined to the diaphysis and meta-diaphyseal region and does not extend to the end of the metaphysis. It is usually bilateral and symmetrical (Fig. 87.68), but not always so.

Osteogenesis Imperfecta

Osteogenesis imperfecta (Fig. 87.69) is a genetic disorder inherited in both autosomal dominant and autosomal recessive forms. There are 16 variants with varying features and degrees of severity

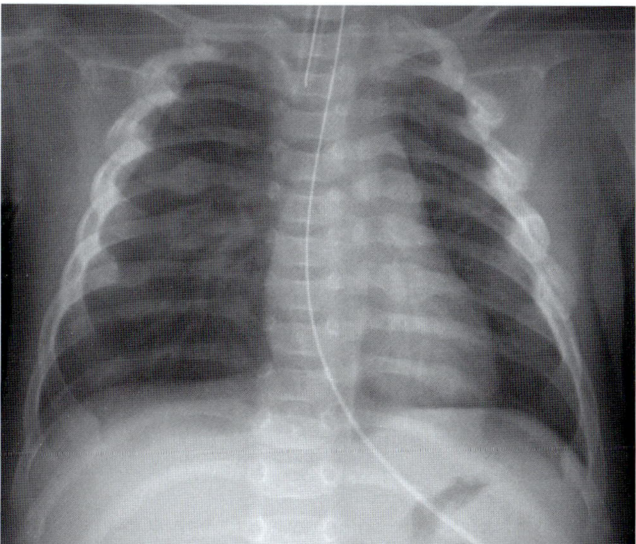
Figure 87.67 Rib fractures. There are multiple healing rib fractures, including posterior rib fractures, in a patient who suffered witnessed physical abuse.

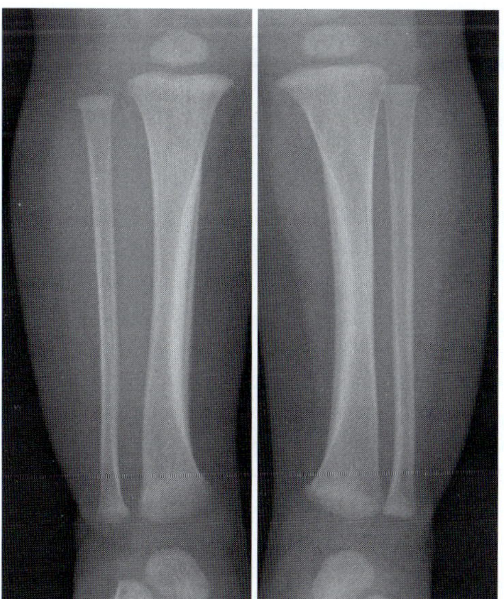
Figure 87.68 Physiological periosteal reaction. Note the bilateral, symmetrical appearance affecting the medial tibia. There is no extension to the end of the metaphysis.

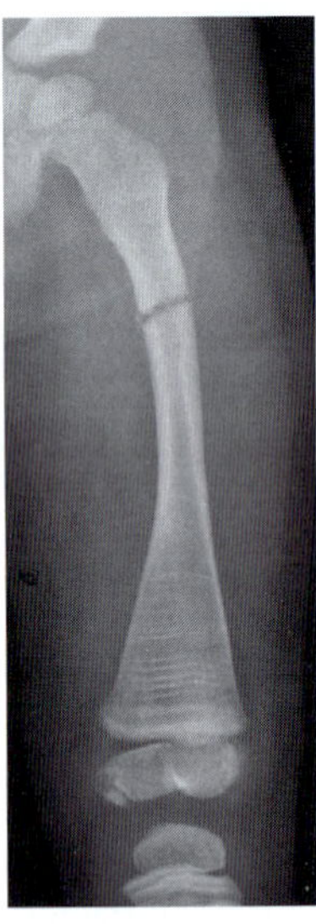

Figure 87.69 Osteogenesis imperfecta. Note the growth arrest lines and Erlenmeyer flask deformity of the distal femur.

ranging from mild to lethal. Multiple genes are responsible, and mutations usually result in defective collagen synthesis and bone fragility. The most common types of osteogenesis imperfecta are the autosomal dominant types I to IV, with defects in the COL1A1 and COL1A2 genes. The forms most likely to present a diagnostic problem are those not picked up before birth and those that are less severe.

- Type I osteogenesis imperfecta is mild, and the child may suffer from fractures sustained as a result of low-force trauma. A clinical clue may be a blue tint to the sclera
- Type II osteogenesis imperfecta demonstrates severe deformity and results in death within the first year of life
- Type III osteogenesis imperfecta presents with fractures at or before birth. The sclera have a blue tint, and there may be an abnormal number of Wormian bones –6% of children have five or more Wormian bones [80], but typically a cut-off of ten Wormian bones is used [81]
- Type IV osteogenesis imperfecta is more moderate in its severity and does not demonstrate a blue tint to the sclera. However, there may also be an abnormal pattern of Wormian bones

Osteopaenia is a feature, but *the diagnosis of osteopaenia based on radiographs is not accurate.* It is neither sensitive, nor is it specific [82,83]. *Unless there are clear signs of metabolic bone disease or connective tissue disease such as osteogenesis imperfecta, the radiograph cannot be used to estimate bone fracture risk* [84].

Birth Injuries

The most common birth-related fracture is a fracture of the clavicle. This occurs in approximately 2.9% of births [85] and is associated with increased birth weight and vacuum delivery [86–88]. Caesarian section does not eliminate the risk [87]. Many are not detected at the time of discharge [85,86]. Although fractures of the clavicle have been shown to undergo a well-described progressive healing process [89], dating the injury remains difficult, and the principles described earlier should be applied.

Birth related long bone fractures are much less common than clavicular fractures and are considered relatively rare [90]. Of these, femoral and humeral fractures are the most common with the most consistent risk factor being breech presentation. Also, it should be noted that whilst caesarean section is associated with a reduced incidence of birth trauma, including clavicular fracture [91], when compared to vaginal delivery, long bone fractures are more frequent [90,92].

Reports of rib fractures following birth trauma are present [60,93,94], and the fractures may be posterior in their location, but rib fractures during birth are either very rare or not picked up [60,95].

87.3 Skeletal Trauma: Upper Limb and Lower Limb

Dina Pefanis, Roy Wheeler

Upper Limb Fractures: the Shoulder and Upper Arm

Clavicle

The clavicle is a commonly fractured bone, with a bimodal distribution in young males due to high-energy trauma and in the elderly due to low-energy falls [96]. Plain films usually suffice for radiological assessment, with frontal and cephalic tilt views. Fractures are classified with respect to location; medial, middle, or lateral third [97]. Approximately 80% of clavicle fractures involve the midshaft [98] (Fig. 87.70). The degree of comminution, displacement, and shortening help determine operative management.

Sternoclavicular joint dislocation is easily overlooked on frontal radiographs and usually present in the context of a severely injured patient (Fig. 87.71). Therefore, if suspected, a CT chest with contrast should be performed to allow assessment for concomitant thoracic injuries. Most dislocations are anterior, but the rarer posterior dislocation is associated with more life-threatening injuries to the chest and mediastinal structures [99].

Acromioclavicular Joint

The acromioclavicular joint is stabilized statically by the acromioclavicular and coracoclavicular ligaments, and dynamically by the deltoid and trapezius muscles.

The usual mechanism of injury is direct impact onto the shoulder, which causes a medial compressive force stressing the ligaments sequentially.

Radiographically, increased acromioclavicular and coracoclavicular distance implies disruption of the respective ligaments and

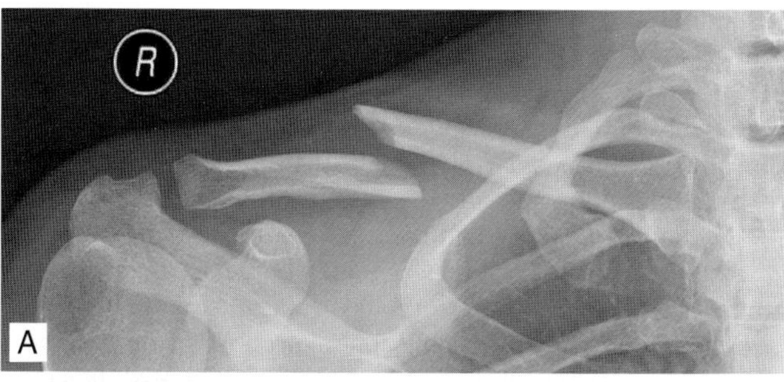

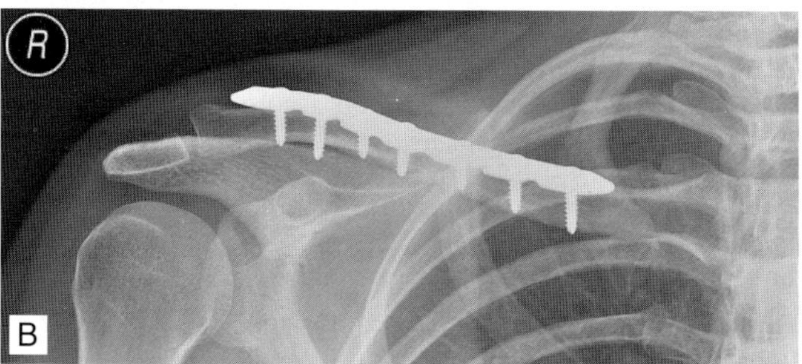

Figure 87.70 Frontal radiograph demonstrates a completely displaced fracture of the mid-clavicle (A) that was subsequently managed surgically with plate and screw fixation (B).

dislocation (Fig. 87.72). Another sign, and possibly the only sign of low-grade injury, is localized soft tissue swelling.

An acromioclavicular joint width of more than 7 mm in men and 6 mm in women is abnormal. The coracoclavicular interval normally measures 11–13 mm but varies according to projection. Imaging the contralateral side for comparison may help distinguish subtle low-grade injuries from normal variation.

The Rockwood classification system is commonly used by orthopedic surgeons to determine conservative versus operative management (Table 87.2). The grading of this classification system is based on the degree of involvement of the static and dynamic joint stabilizers as inferred by the direction and degree of clavicular displacement. Typically grade1 and 2 injuries are managed conservatively, and grade 4 and 5 injuries operatively. Controversy exists regarding the management of grade 3 injuries [100].

Scapula

Fractures of the scapula are relatively rare, comprising only 1% of all fractures. They usually result from high-energy trauma so are associated with other serious injuries in 80–95% of cases (e.g., haemopneumothorax, pulmonary, and spinal injuries) which should be actively evaluated for on a dedicated trauma CT and urgently communicated [101]. CT is therefore the preferred diagnostic tool rather than radiographs, and it also provides superior sensitivity and fracture characterization including 3D reformats. Initially the life-threatening injuries are prioritized for treatment, so the scapular fractures per se are not the primary concern and can be missed (Fig. 87.73).

Fractures are classified according to anatomical location and are grouped into fractures of the glenoid (intra-articular), extra-articular scapular neck, coracoid process, acromion process, and scapular body. The most common site of fracture (approximately 50%) is the scapular body [98].

More than 90% of scapula fractures are non- or minimally displaced so are managed conservatively. Management in principle depends on anatomic location, degree of displacement, and angulation. Fractures of the glenoid neck or articulating surface are more likely to require surgery [98].

With scapular neck fractures, look for concomitant acromioclavicular joint separation or clavicle fracture as this implies an unstable superior shoulder suspensory complex or *"floating shoulder"* which would require surgical repair [102] (Fig. 87.74). This ensues from high-energy mechanisms of injury and associated with neurovascular injury to the upper limb.

Glenohumeral Dislocation

The glenohumeral joint is the most commonly dislocated large joint, owing to its large range of motion and inherent instability. Most dislocations are anterior (85–98%), with far less common posterior (2–5%) and inferior (0.5%) dislocations [98].

The usual mechanism of injury is fall onto the outstretched hand. Seizures and electrocution are associated with posterior and bilateral dislocations. Risk factors for recurrent dislocations include young adult/adolescent males participating in contact sports, hyperlaxity, and severity of the initial trauma.

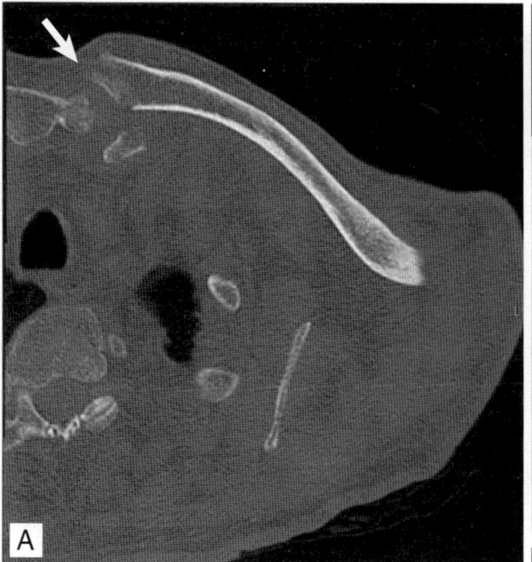

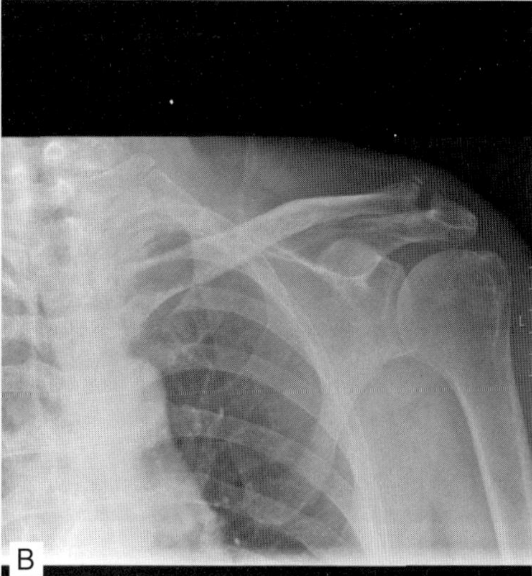

Figure 87.71 (A) Axial CT of a fracture-dislocation of the left sternoclavicular joint with medial clavicle fracture (*arrow*). (B) The left shoulder frontal radiograph where this abnormality is not discernible that warranted the CT due to the high clinical suspicion.

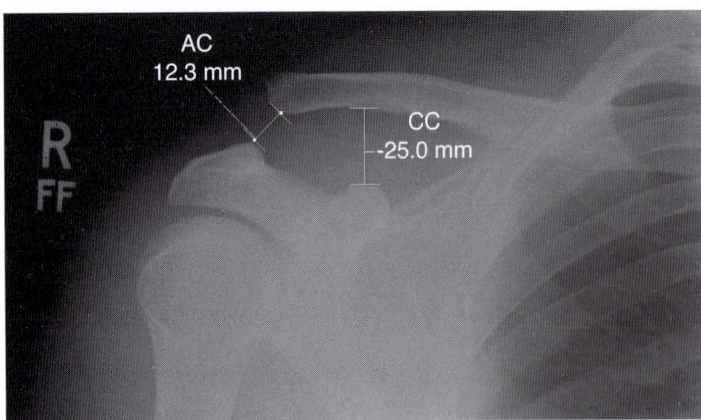

Figure 87.72 Frontal radiograph demonstrating a right acromioclavicular joint dislocation with superior displacement of the distal clavicle in relation to the acromion and abnormal widening of the acromioclavicular (AC) and coracoclavicular (CC) intervals. This is a Rockwood grade 3 injury.

The main diagnostic tool in the acute setting are radiographs, with a combination of anteroposterior and scapular Y or axillary views. Anterior dislocations are relatively straightforward to diagnose, but posterior dislocations can be more challenging. The role of initial imaging is to also detect any impediments to reduction and injuries predisposing to recurrent instability [102].

CT better characterizes the degree of glenoid and humeral head deficiency that corresponds to the risk of recurrent dislocation and guides operative planning. MRI (including MR arthrography) is useful for assessing the related labroligamentous injuries such as Bankart variants and the rotator cuff.

In an **anterior** dislocation (Fig. 87.75), the posterosuperolateral aspect of the humeral head impacts on the anteroinferior glenoid giving the characteristic imaging appearances. A *Hill Sachs lesion* is an impaction fracture at the posterolateral humeral head. It is present in approximately 80% of first presentations and up to 100% of recurrent dislocations [103]. A large Hill-Sachs lesion may engage the anterior glenoid rim even within a normal range of motion requiring surgical management. On radiographs, it appears as a defect in the posterolateral humeral head. Smaller defects are better detected on CT or MRI (Fig. 87.76). This should not be confused with the normal physiological depression.

A *Bankart lesion* is defined as detachment of the anteroinferior labrum from the glenoid and is diagnosed on MRI (see Figs. 87.77 and 87.78).

Less commonly, there is a fracture of anteroinferior glenoid termed a *Bony Bankart* (Fig. 87.79). CT including 3D

TABLE 87.2 Description of the Rockwood Classification System

Injury Grade	AC Ligaments	CC Ligaments	Trapezius and Deltoid Clavicular Attachments	Clavicle Displacement*	AC Distance on X-Ray	CC Distance on X-Ray
I	Sprain	Intact	Intact	None	Normal	Normal
II	Ruptured	Sprain	Minimally detached	50% superior	Widened	Slightly increased <25%
III	Ruptured	Ruptured	Detached	100% superior	Widened	Increased 25–100%
IV	Ruptured	Ruptured	Detached	Posteriorly	Can be normal	Can be normal
V	Ruptured	Ruptured	Detached	>100% superior	Widened	Increased 100–300%
VI	Ruptured	Ruptured (subcoracoid type only)	Detached	Inferior†	–	Decreased

AC, acromioclavicular; *CC*, coracoclavicular.
Adapted from: F Alyas, M Curtis, C Speed, A Saifuddin, D Connell, MR Imaging appearances of acromioclavicular joint dislocation, RadioGraphics, 28 (2) (2008) 463–479.
*Relative to the inferior border of the acromion.
†Below the acromion or subcoracoid.

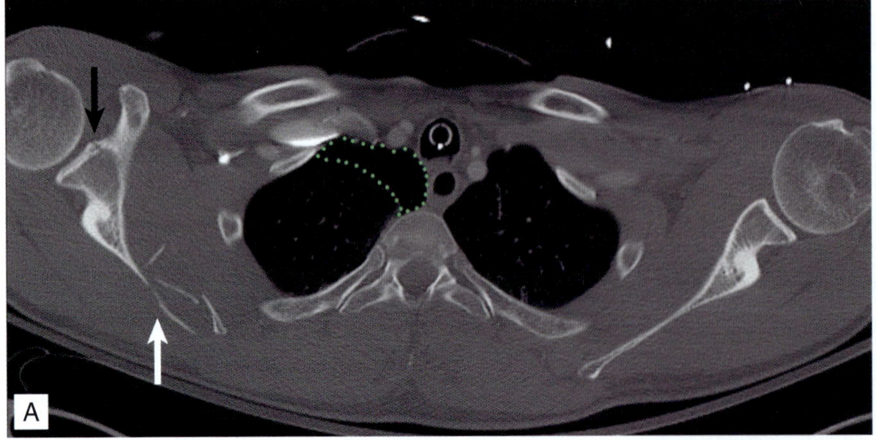

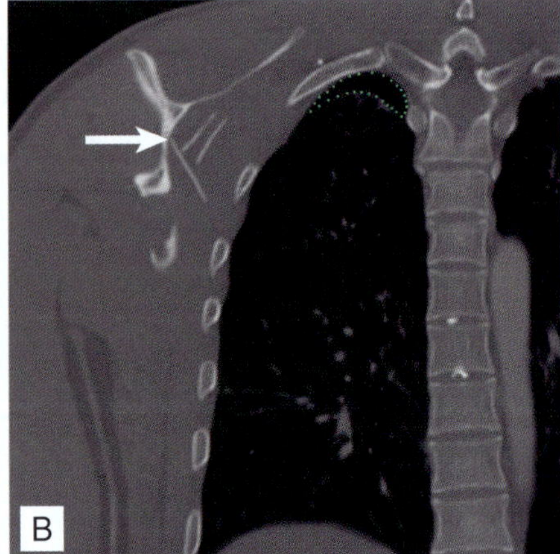

Figure 87.73 (A) Axial and (B) coronal CT slices of the chest, part of a contrast-enhanced whole body trauma CT scan. There is a comminuted right scapula blade fracture (*white arrows*) with extension into the glenoid fossa (*black arrow*). This is a high-energy trauma with more severe associated injuries—note the patient is intubated, and there is a right pnemothorax (*green dotted outline*). This patient also sustained severe traumatic brain, spinal and intra-abdominal injuries seen elsewhere on the CT.

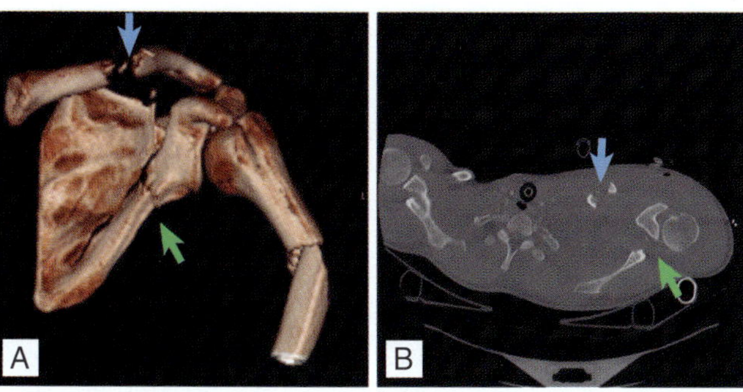

Figure 87.74 CT of a patient who sustained a high-energy motorcycle versus car accident. (A) 3D bony reconstruction and (B) axial CT slice bone windows demonstrate a displaced comminuted mid-clavicle fracture (*blue arrow*) and displaced scapular neck and body fractures (*green arrow*) constituting a floating shoulder or unstable superior shoulder suspensory complex. The patient had associated left subclavian artery and brachial plexus injuries. Notice also the displaced left humeral shaft and left first rib fractures as well as the fact the patient is intubated.

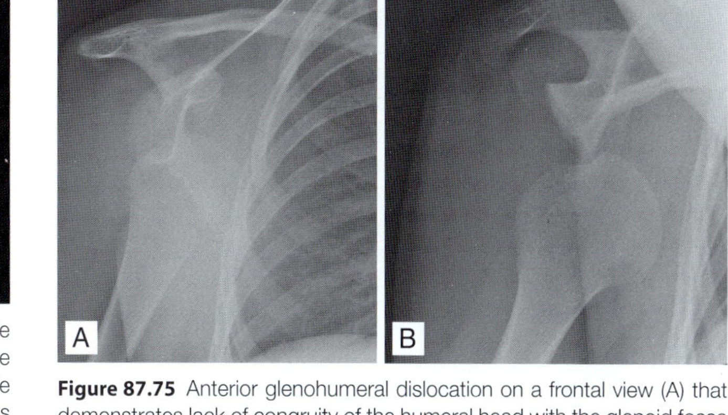

Figure 87.75 Anterior glenohumeral dislocation on a frontal view (A) that demonstrates lack of congruity of the humeral head with the glenoid fossa outline, and the humeral head is located inferior to the coracoid process. On the modified axial view (B) the humeral head is seen anterior to the glenoid fossa in the direction of the coracoid process. An indentation present at the superolateral humeral head where it engages the glenoid represents a subtle Hill-Sachs lesion.

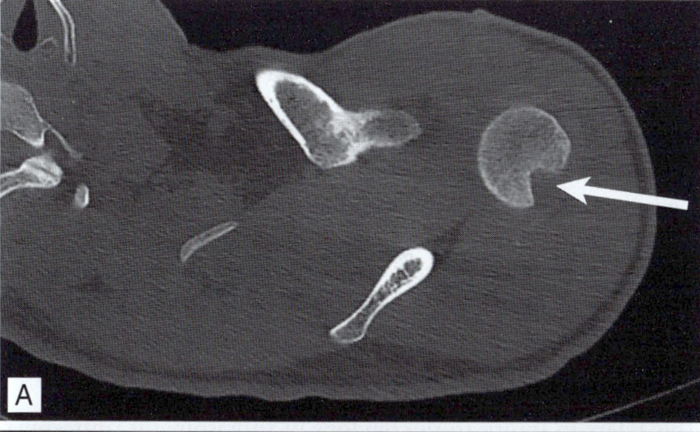

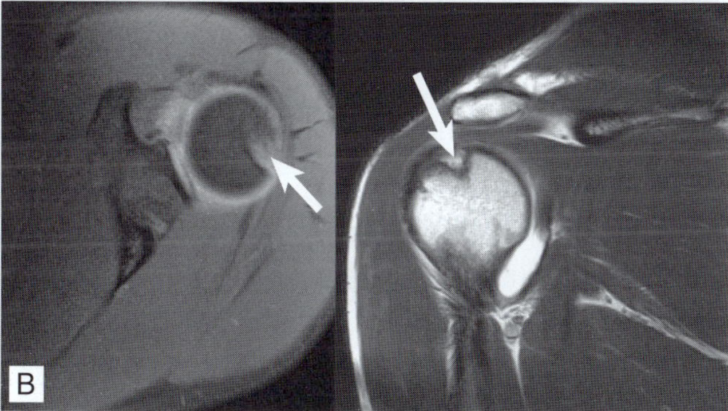

Figure 87.76 (A) Axial CT demonstrates a Hill-Sachs defect (*arrow*) in the posterolateral humeral head. Note that this defect is present at the most superior aspect of the humeral head above the level of the coracoid, in contradistinction to a normal physiologic groove that is more inferior. (B) MR arthrogram shoulder A axial T1 fat saturated (left) and coronal T1 view (right) also demonstrating the Hill-Sachs lesion (*arrowed*).

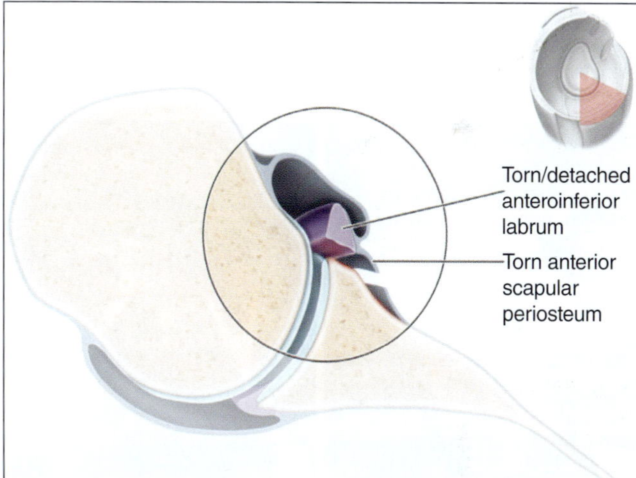

Figure 87.77 Schematic of a Bankart lesion. (Reproduced from: T Pope, HL Bloem, J Beltran, WB Morrison, DJ Wilson, Chapter 9: Glenohumeral Instability, in: Musculoskeletal Imaging, second ed., Elsevier. p. 120, ISBN: 978-1-4557-0813-0.)

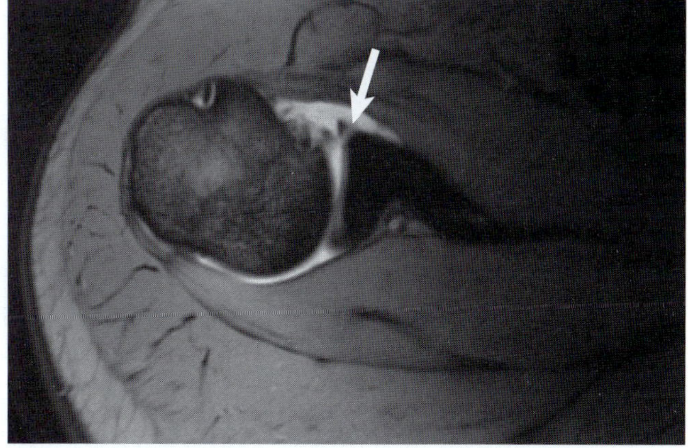

Figure 87.78 MR shoulder arthrogram axial fat-saturated sequence demonstrates a Bankart lesion (*arrow*); a tear in the anteroinferior labrum.

reconstructions can better depict the degree of bone loss (Fig. 87.80); more significant amounts of bone loss (usually above 15–25%) are associated with higher risk of re-dislocation and may necessitate surgical bone grafting.

Posterior glenohumeral dislocation can be challenging to diagnose on radiographs so should be carefully scrutinized (Fig. 87.81). They result classically from seizures or electric shocks.

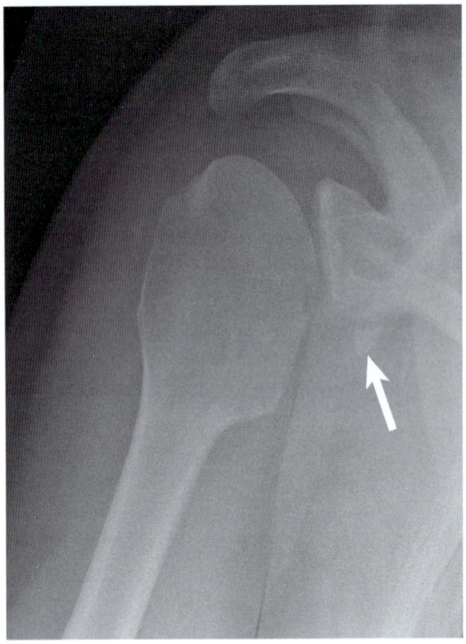

Figure 87.79 Postreduction frontal radiograph demonstrates a bony fragment (*arrow*) inferomedial to the glenoid in keeping with a bony Bankart.

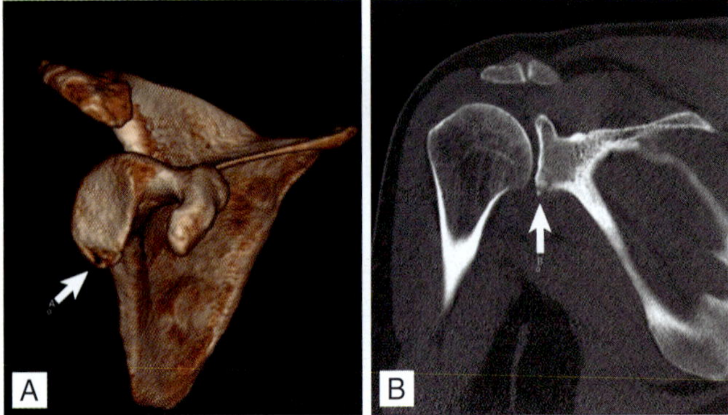

Figure 87.80 (A) CT 3D bony reconstruction and (B) coronal CT shoulder demonstrating a subtle bony Bankart fracture that is not discernible on radiographs. There is <25% of the glenoid surface area affected, easily quantified on CT. Note if the bony defect is greater than 20–25% of the articular surface area it is deemed unstable and a surgical soft tissue stabilization alone would result in an unacceptable failure rate.

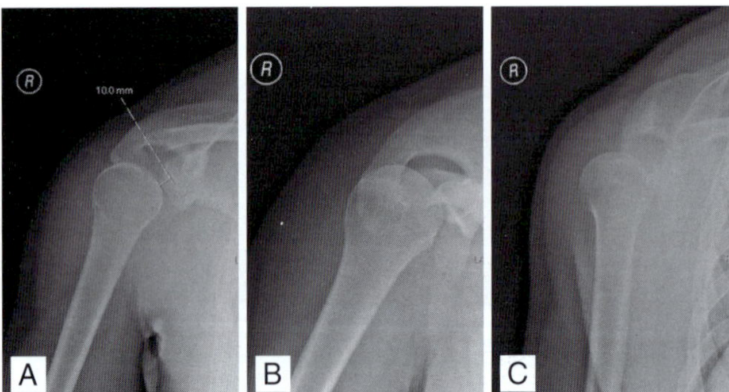

Figure 87.81 Radiographs of the right shoulder demonstrating a posterior glenohumeral dislocation. (A) Frontal view demonstrates the humeral head in an internally rotated position giving the classic "lightbulb" appearance. There is also lack of parallelism with the glenoid fossa and abnormal joint space widening >6 mm or "rim sign". (B) Axial and (C) scapular Y-views show the posterior position of the humeral head in relation to the glenoid fossa.

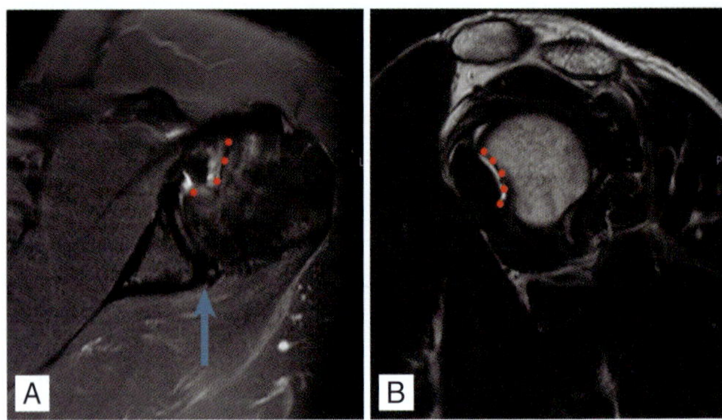

Figure 87.82 MRI scan following posterior glenohumeral dislocation (A) Axial T2 fat-saturated and (B) sagittal T2 images demonstrate a reverse Hill-Sachs lesion (*red dotted line*) that is the characteristic compression fracture of the anteromedial humeral head. There is associated mild bone marrow edema signal (A) signifying a subacute injury. The anterior humeral head had impacted on the posterior glenoid resulting in the corresponding posterior labral tear (*blue arrow*); a reverse Bankart lesion.

Posterior dislocation results in the reverse pattern of bony and labral injury to an anterior dislocation; *reverse* Hill-Sachs and *reverse* Bankart lesions (Fig. 87.82).

Inferior glenohumeral dislocation (or luxation erectae) is exceedingly uncommon and results from impact on a hyperabducted arm (Fig. 87.83). The humeral head impinges upon the acromion, which in turn acts as a fulcrum and causes an inferior displacement of the humeral head with the arm "locked" in abduction.

Rotator Cuff Injury

This refers to injury to the tendons of supraspinatus, infraspinatus, subscapularis, and teres minor. This can be acute traumatic or chronic, likely coexisting with tendinosis particularly in older patients. Rupture can be partial or full thickness. Diagnosis is with USG or ideally MRI. A complete supraspinatus tear can

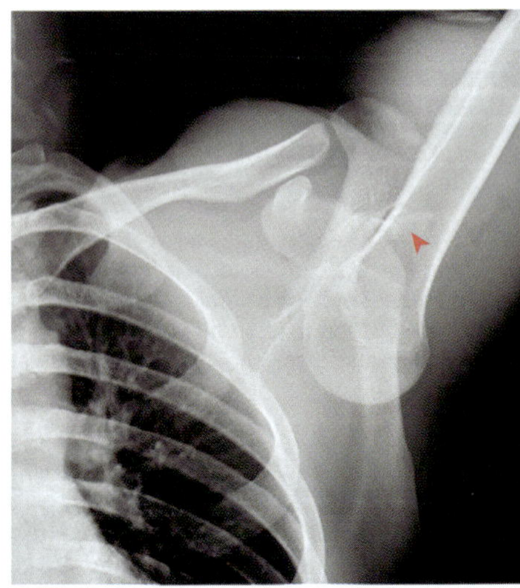

Figure 87.83 Frontal shoulder radiograph shows fixed hyperabduction of the left arm, and the humeral head projected medial and inferior to the glenoid. A few bony fragments (*red arrowhead*) are projected just lateral to the glenoid that on subsequent CT were shown to arise from the greater tuberosity of the humerus.

however be suspected on a radiograph where there is a reduced acromiohumeral distance <6 mm (Fig. 87.84).

Proximal Humerus

Fractures of the proximal humerus are common accounting for approximately 5.7% of all extremity fractures [104]. It characteristically affects older osteopenic females who fall onto an outstretched hand. The commonest site is the surgical neck, that is likely to be impacted and the fracture may extend into the adjacent tuberosities (Fig. 87.85).

CT is the technique of choice for assessing complex and comminuted fractures, as it can better characterize the number of fragments and degree of displacement. The Neer classification is widely adopted by orthopedic surgeons to aid management (Table 87.3) [102]. A fracture part is defined as displaced if there is at least 1 cm of displacementor or 45 degrees of angulation.

Most fractures (85%) are one-part fractures that are usually treated non-operatively. Two-part fractures may require surgical repair, and three- and four-part fractures may require surgical repair or shoulder arthroplasty [102].

Displaced fractures of the anatomic neck predispose the patient to humeral head osteonecrosis, as this is the site of capsular insertion and blood supply to the humeral head.

Greater tuberosity fractures are at the site of rotator cuff tendon insertion so imply a bony avu[illegible]njury. They can be difficult to identify on radiographs, so MRI is useful in detecting these injuries.

Humeral shaft fractures usually result from direct trauma, and mostly located in the mid-shaft (Fig. 87.86). The direction and degree of fracture displacement depends on the fracture location in relation to muscular attachment and pull. Distal third and spiral groove fractures are associated with radial nerve damage.

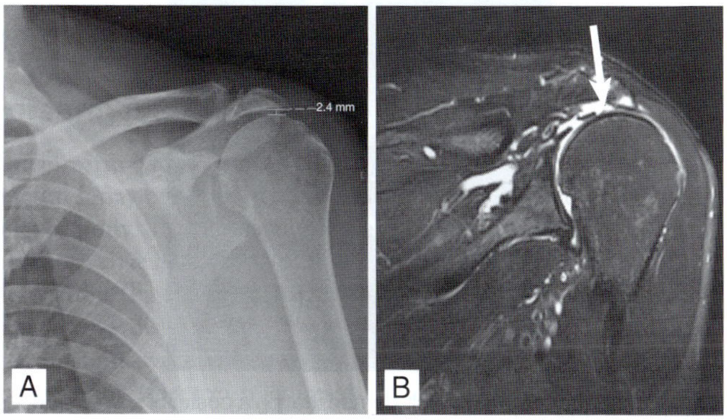

Figure 87.84 (A) Frontal radiograph of the left shoulder show a reduced acromiohumeral interval and (B) coronal T2 fat-saturated MRI of the same patient demonstrates a complete tear of the supraspinatus tendon with a fluid-filled gap (*arrow*).

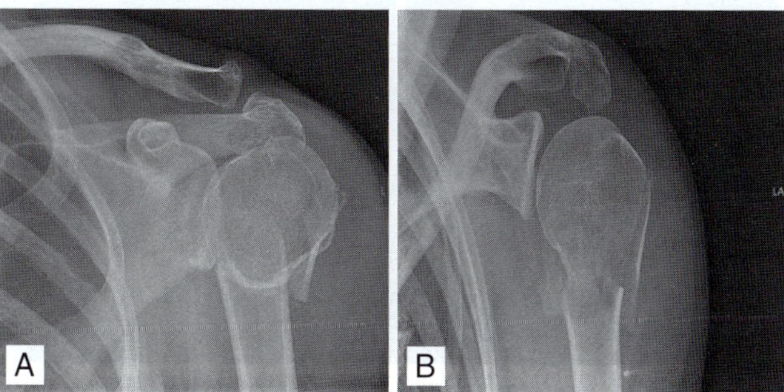

Figure 87.85 (A) Frontal and (B) axial radiographs of the left shoulder demonstrating a comminuted and significantly impacted fracture involving the surgical neck (Neer 2-part fracture). The greater tuberosity is also fractured but not significantly displaced (<1 cm) that was more accurately assessed on the patient's subsequent CT.

The Elbow

Distal Humerus Fracture

The usual mechanism of injury in adults is axial loading of the humerus, with varying degrees of elbow flexion determining the fracture pattern [105]. The distal humerus has medial and lateral structural columns that provide load-bearing stability to the arm. The number of columns and articular surface involvement, as well as degree of comminution determine management and should be described. Most fractures are intra-articular.

Radial Head Fracture

Radial head and neck fractures are the commonest type of elbow fracture in adults, and the usual mechanism is a fall onto the outstretched hand. Undisplaced fractures may not be discernible

TABLE 87.3 Neer Classification of Proximal Humerus Fractures

1-part	No fracture fragment meets criteria for displacement
2-part	One displaced fracture segment relative to the other 3 segments
3-part	Two displaced fracture segments relative to the other 2 segments
4-part	All four segments are displaced

The possible contributory fracture segments are the (1) articular head (2) surgical neck (3) greater tuberosity, and (4) lesser tuberosity.

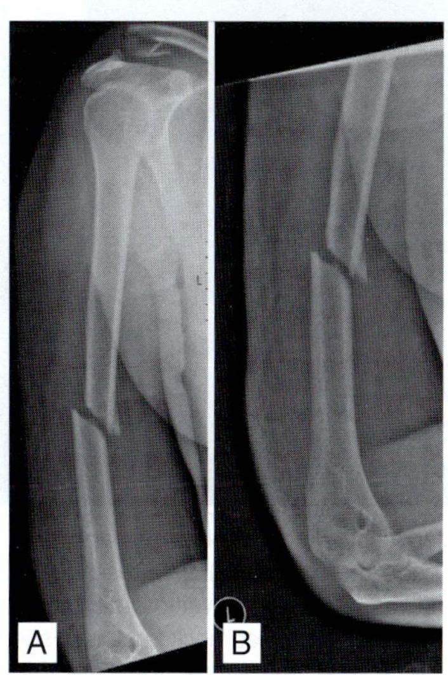

Figure 87.86 (A) Frontal and (B) lateral radiographs of the humerus demonstrate a mildly comminuted transverse fracture of the humeral shaft.

TABLE 87.5 Assessment of Carpal Alignment

Radiograph positioning	Is there a true posteroanterior and lateral view?
Joint spaces	Parallelism and symmetry
Carpal arc alignment	Disruption indicates ligamentous injury or fracture
Carpal bone shape	Lunate and scaphoid
Carpal axis	Normal, DISI or VISI deformity

Adapted from: Radiology Assistant. https://radiologyassistant.nl/musculoskeletal/wrist/carpal-instability.

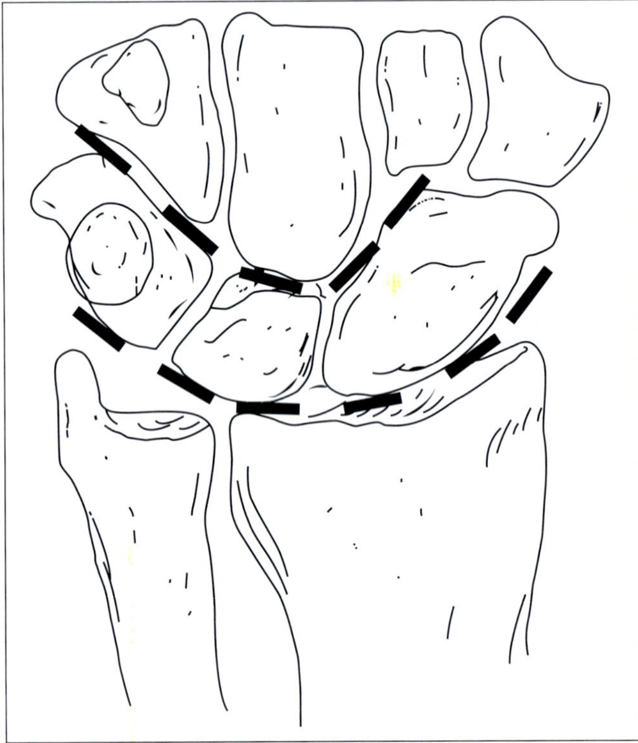

Figure 87.102 Schematic of the carpal arcs. The proximal and distal carpal lines define the normal carpal relationship on the PA radiograph.

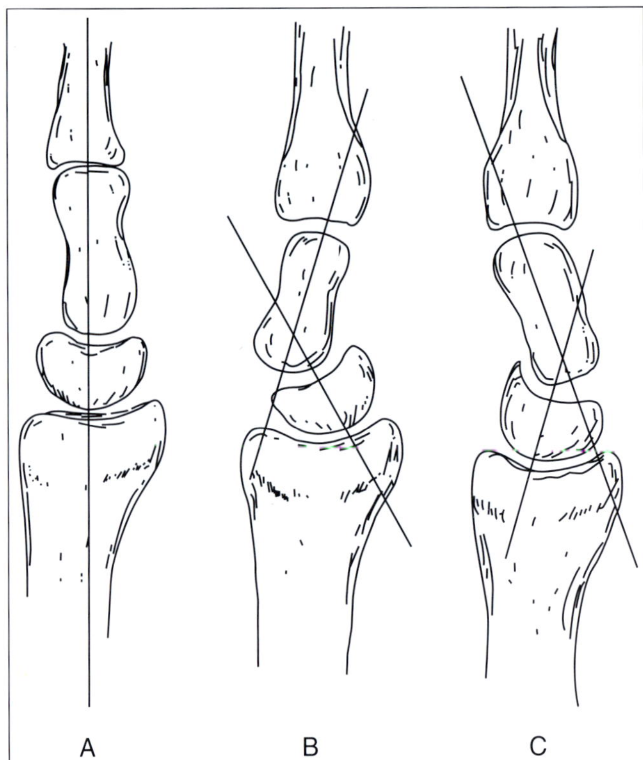

Figure 87.103 (A) Normal alignment of the wrist allows a continuous line to be drawn through the radius, lunate and capitate. (B) Abnormal alignment: palmar flexion instability (volar intercalary segment carpal instability: VISI). The lunate is rotated towards the palmar surface of the wrist, with the capitate rotated towards the dorsal surface. (C) Dorsiflexion instability (dorsal intercalary segment carpal instability: DISI)—the converse of B.

Perilunate injuries may occur with or without a fracture. A purely ligamentous injury is termed a "lesser arc" injury. More commonly a "greater arc" injury occurs, that involves a perilunate dislocation with a fracture of one or more of the bones around the lunate (scaphoid, trapezium, capitate, hamate, or triquetrum).

- *Stage I* represents tearing of the scapholunate ligaments with rotary subluxation of the scaphoid and *scapholunate dissociation*. This is identified by widening of the scapholunate joint >3 mm (Terry Thomas sign) and a scapholunate angle >100°. This is the commonest type of perilunate injury (Fig. 87.106)
- *Stage II* injuries involve disruption of the capitolunate joint causing *perilunate dislocation.* This is recognized on the lateral radiograph as dorsal dislocation of the capitate in relation to the lunate, while the lunate retains normal articulation with the radius (Fig. 87.107) [110]
- *Stage III* injury is additional disruption of the lunotriquetral joint and further midcarpal instability
- *Stage IV* represents the rarest and most severe injury with *lunate dislocation*, due to final failure of the dorsal radiocarpal ligament. The normal anatomy of the proximal carpal row is lost, and the lunate is usually seen to abnormally overlap the capitate, hamate and triquetrum on the PA view, also taking on a triangular, rather than a rectangular shape. On the lateral view, the lunate is volarly dislocated and rotated with respect to the distal radius. The capitate maintains its alignment with the distal radius. This is known as the "spilled teacup" sign (Fig. 87.108)

CT with the capability of multiplanar/3D and volumetric reformats can help delineate these complex injuries and subtle fractures.

Hand Fractures

Hand injuries are common and usually present minimal diagnostic difficulty. A few of the more challenging types are discussed below.

A *Bennett's fracture* is a 2-part fracture-dislocation of the base of the first metacarpal with involvement of the articular surface, usually associated with "dislocation" of the major fragment (Fig. 87.109).

In contrast a *Rolando fracture* is a comminuted intra-articular fracture of the thumb metacarpal base (Fig. 87.110), which is more unstable and difficult to reduce.

Another significant thumb injury is *"skier's thumb"* (or gamekeeper's thumb) that is avulsion of the ulnar collateral ligament (UCL) at the first metacarpophalangeal joint. This usually results

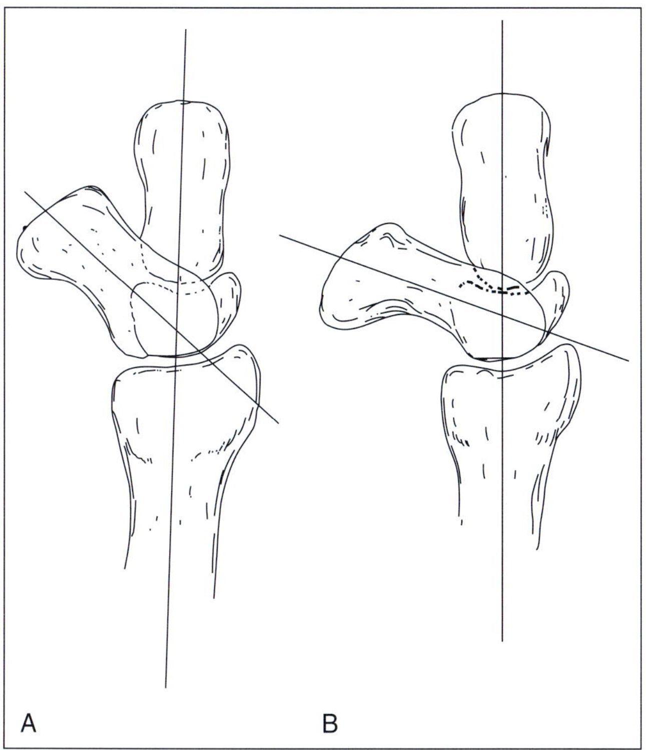

Figure 87.104 (A) In the normal wrist, the scaphoid long axis at approximately 45° (30–60°). (B) Rotatory subluxation: the long axis of the scaphoid is tilted in a volar direction.

TABLE 87.6 Stages of Perilunate Dislocation

I	Scapholunate dissociation
II	Capitolunate dislocation
III	Lunotriquetral dislocation
IV	Lunate dislocation

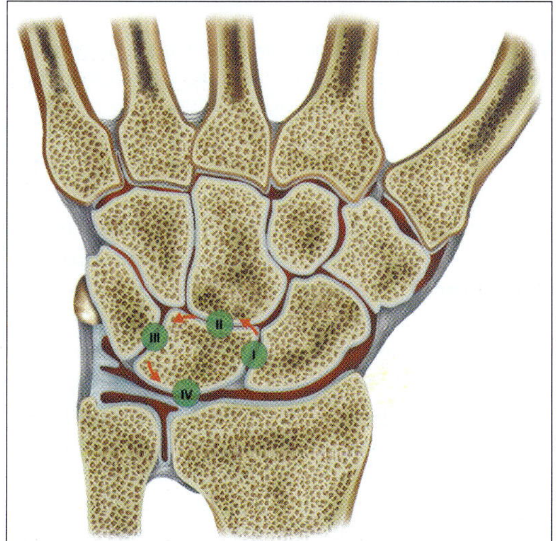

Figure 87.105 Schematic of the four stages perilunate dislocation. (Reproduced from: T Pope, HL Bloem, J Beltran, WB Morrison, DJ Wilson, Chapter 14: Acute Osseous Injury to the Wrist, in: Musculoskeletal Imaging, second ed., Elsevier, p. 187, ISBN: 978-1-4557-0813-0.)

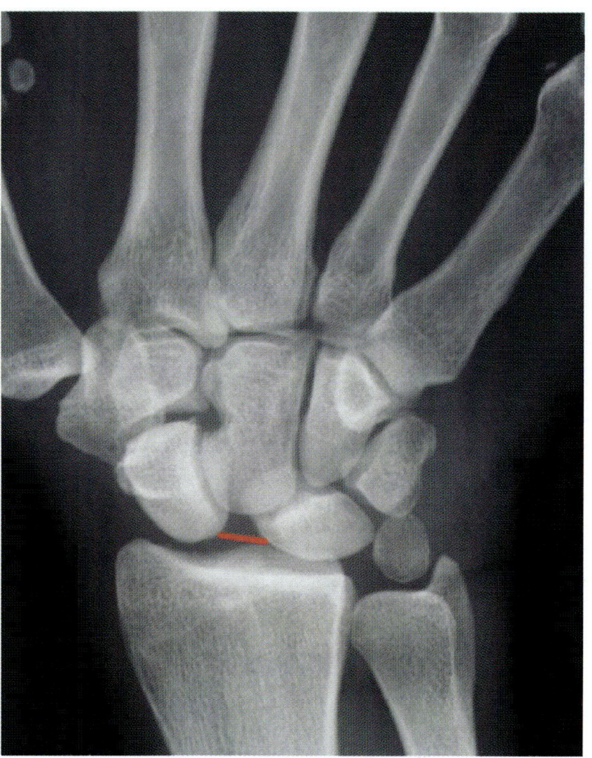

Figure 87.106 Frontal wrist radiograph demonstrates abnormal widening of the scapholunate interval implying scapholunate dissociation. This is also known as the Terry Thomas or Madonna sign.

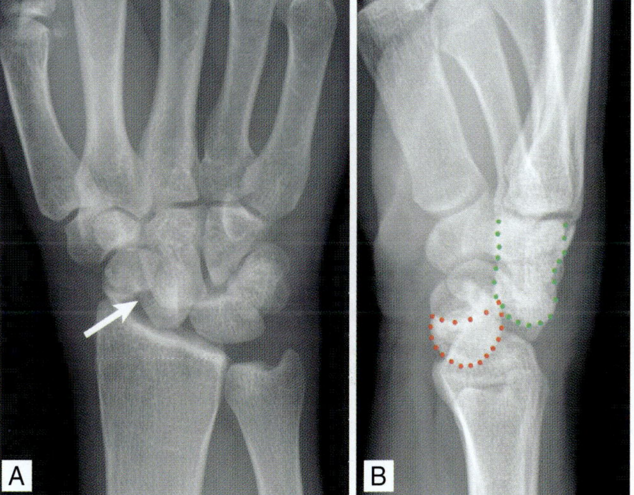

Figure 87.107 Perilunate dislocation (transscaphoid). (A) Frontal radiograph demonstrates a displaced scaphoid waist fracture (*arrow*) and an abnormal triangular shape of the lunate with disruption of the carpal arcs as the capitate and lunate/scaphoid overlap. (B) Lateral view shows dorsal subluxation of the capitate (*green dots*) in relation to the lunate (*red dots*).

from forceful abduction and hyperextension of this joint and involves avulsion of the proximal phalanx insertion of the ligament. Bony avulsion occurs in approximately 50% [111] (Fig. 87.111). If no bony fragment is evident on the radiograph but clinically there is valgus instability, further investigation with USG or ideally MRI is indicated. MRI is also useful to exclude a *Stener lesion* (Fig. 87.112); a complication of the injury when the torn UCL is retracted superficial to the adductor aponeurosis that acts as a block to healing and necessitates surgery. Surgery is also

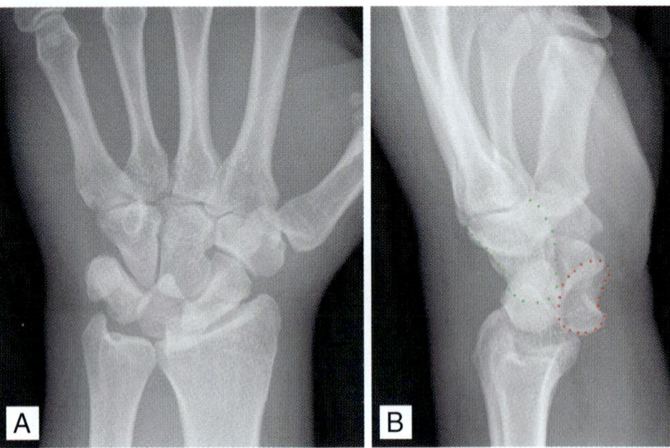

Figure 87.108 Lunate dislocation. (A) Frontal radiograph demonstrates an abnormal triangular shape of the lunate with disruption of the carpal arcs. (B) Lateral view shows the lunate (red dots) is volarly dislocated and tilted with respect to the distal radius. The capitate (green dots) remains aligned with the radius. The abnormal appearance of the lunate is likened to a "spilled teacup."

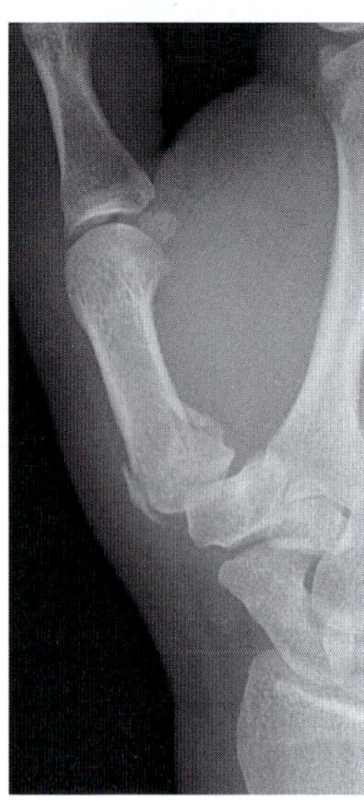

Figure 87.110 Oblique radiograph of the thumb showing a Rolando fracture.

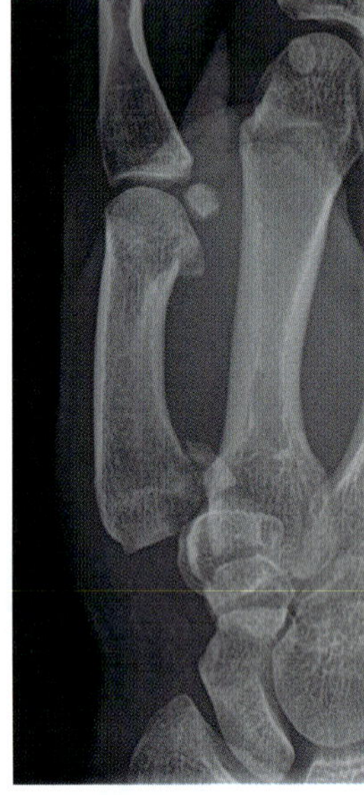

Figure 87.109 Lateral thumb radiograph demonstrate a Bennett's fracture; a base of thumb metacarpal avulsion fracture (volar fragment) that remains articulated with the trapezium due to the intact attachment of the anterior oblique ligament. The remaining thumb metacarpal base is subluxed dorsally.

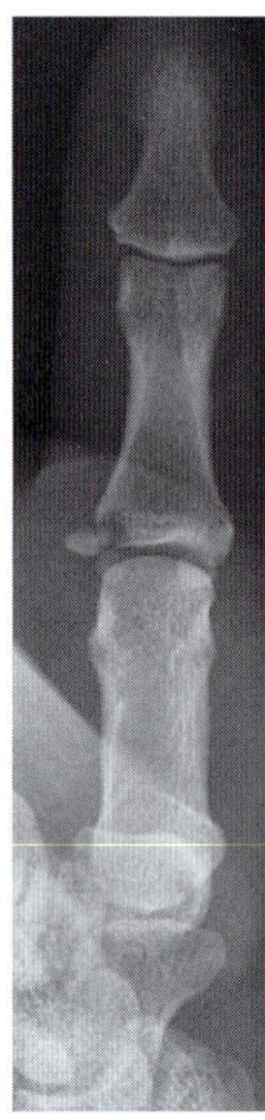

Figure 87.111 Frontal radiograph showing a fracture of the ulnar aspect of the thumb proximal phalanx at the metacarpophalangeal joint in keeping with bony avulsion of the distal UCL insertion.

indicated for significantly displaced bony fragments or fracture involving >20% of the articular surface.

A *"Boxer's fracture"* is the commonest fracture of the metacarpal bones, usually due to punching an object with a clenched fist that causes axial compression along the length of the bone. This is classically a transverse fracture of the fifth (or fourth) metacarpal neck with volar angulation and shortening (Fig. 87.113).

The Lower Limb

Fractures of the Hip

Fractures involving the femoral head, femoral neck and the trochanters are commonly known as hip fractures. These fractures are frequently seen in the elderly population secondary to a fall and co-existing low bone mineral density. They are associated with significantly increased morbidity and mortality if not appropriately treated [112]. In the elderly underlying pathology such as metastasis should always be excluded especially in the context of little force. Non-displaced hip fractures can be challenging to identify with plain film, especially in the osteoporotic patient. A faint ill-defined linear density across the femoral neck, interruption of trabecular lines, and subtle cortical disruptions may be the only radiological signs. If there is doubt about the presence of a hip fracture, the gold standard for fracture identification is MRI as CT is not as sensitive, especially in patients with osteopenia. Images will demonstrate a linear band of low signal T1 with associated high T2/STIR signal signifying a fracture line (Fig. 87.114). There may also be a subperiosteal fluid, hematoma and soft tissue edema.

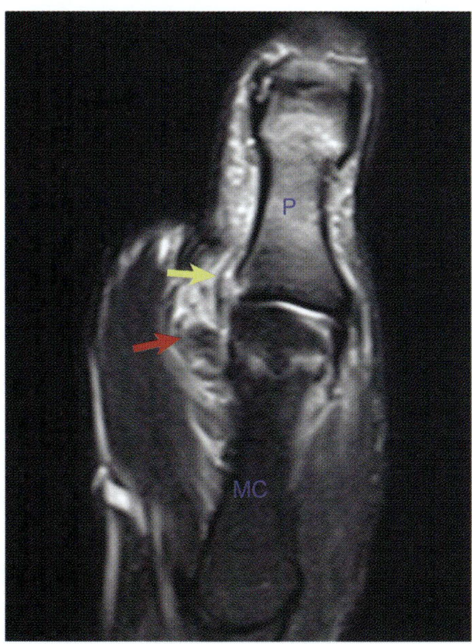

Figure 87.112 Coronal T2 fat-saturated sequence of the thumb shows complete avulsion and retraction of the distal attachment of the UCL (*red arrow*). This is now located superficial to the adductor aponeurosis (*yellow arrow*) giving a "yo-yo on a string" appearance. Proximal phalanx (P) and metacarpal (MC) of the thumb are labeled.

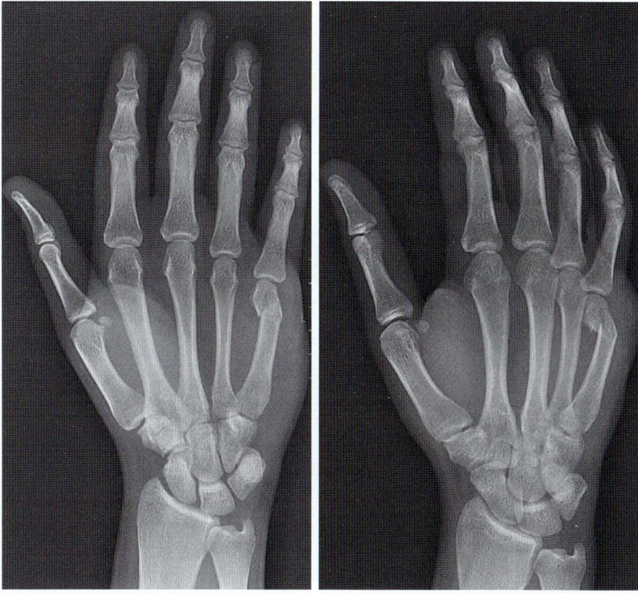

Figure 87.113 Frontal and oblique radiographs of the hand demonstrate a boxer's fracture of the little finger metacarpal neck, with volar angulation and shortening.

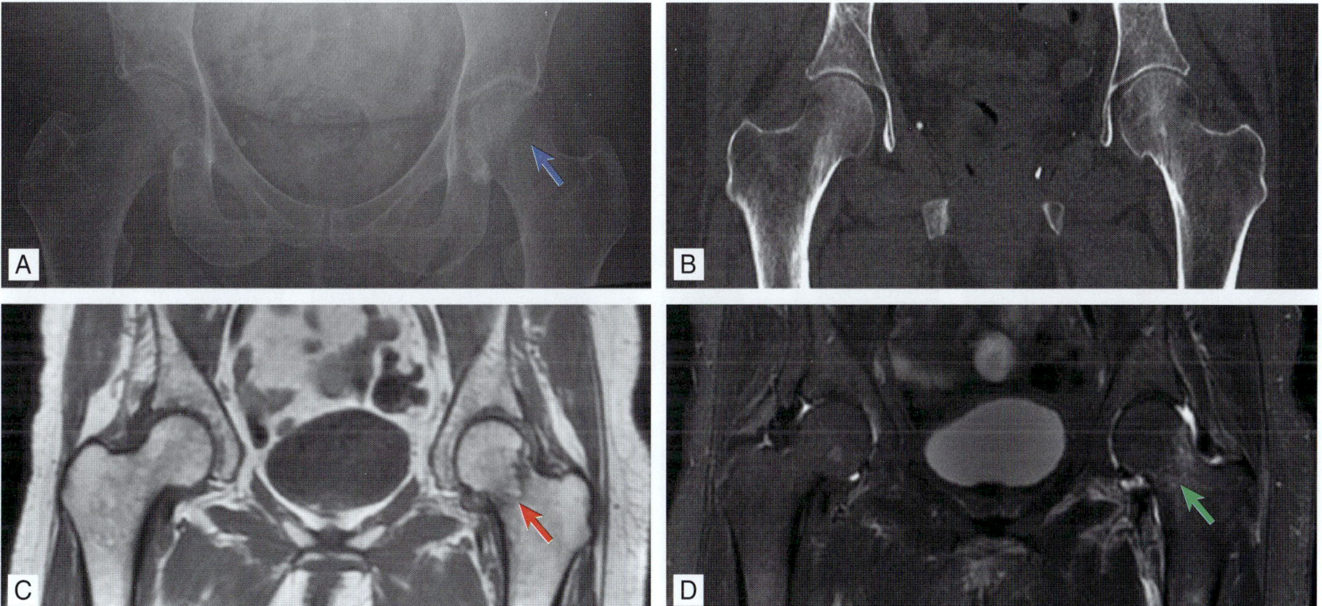

Figure 87.114 Fracture of the neck of femur. (A) Pelvic radiograph demonstrating a faint lucent line through the subcapital neck of the left femur (*blue arrow*). It would be easy to overlook this finding as there is no obvious cortical disruption. The CT (B) does not demonstrate a clear fracture. Noticeable linear signal abnormalities through the neck of femur represents a fracture on the MRI images (C) T1 weighted (*red arrow*) and (D) T2 weighted (*green arrow*).

It is important to diagnose and differentiate between intracapsular and extracapsular fractures. Intracapsular fractures are those from the femoral head to the basocervical region of the femoral neck, which is just proximal to the trochanters. Extracapsular fractures are either intertrochanteric (between the greater and lesser trochanter) or subtrochanteric (Figs. 87.115 and 87.116). The majority of the femoral head's blood supply is from extracapsular medial and lateral circumflex femoral artery branches. A small artery in the ligamentum teres (foveal artery) is not sufficient in isolation to perfuse the femoral head in adults. Any intracapsular neck of femur fractures risk compromising the blood supply to the femoral head with consequent avascular necrosis. Treatment of such fractures usually requires replacement of the femoral head with a metal polymer (Fig. 87.117).

Femoral stress fractures arise due to either repeated abnormal mechanical strain onto normal bone (fatigue fractures) or due to normal stresses transmitted to bone of abnormal density (insufficiency fractures). Fatigue fractures most commonly involve the medial cortex of the proximal third of the femur whereas

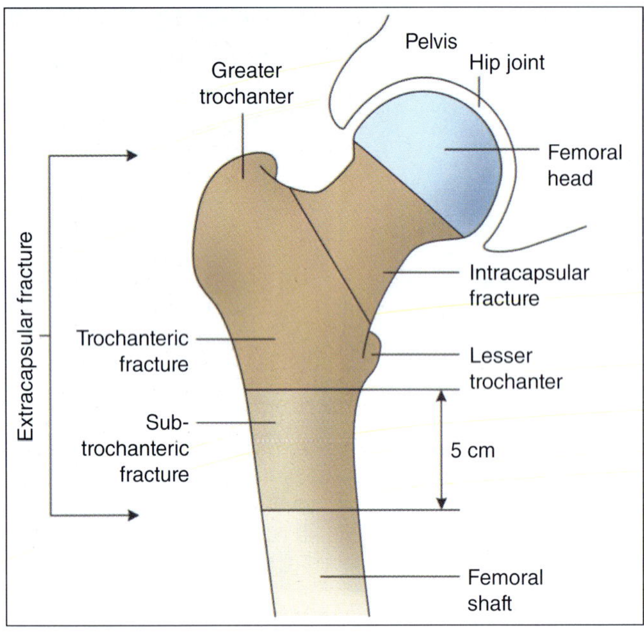

Figure 87.115 Image of the proximal femur and hip with annotations of the intracapsular and extracapsular fracture areas.

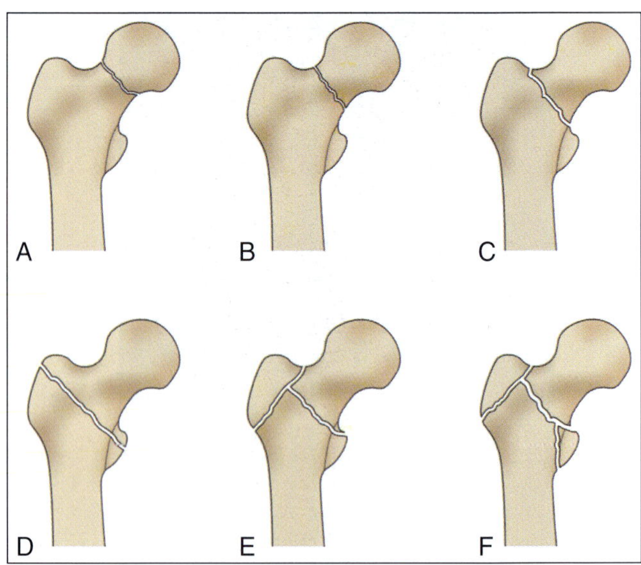

Figure 87.116 Intracapsular neck of femur fractures are subcapital (A), transcervical (B), or basicervical (C). Extracapsular neck of femur fractures include intertrochanteric fractures which can be two-part (D) or comminuted (E and F).

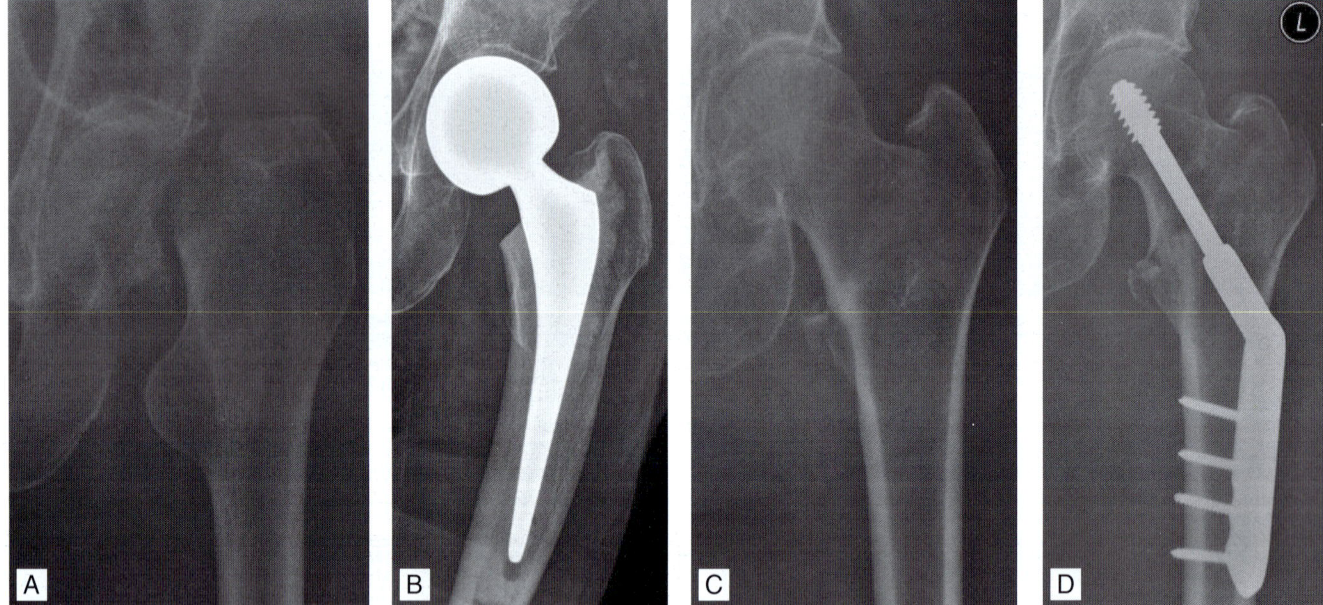

Figure 87.117 Preoperative and postoperative radiographs of neck of femur fractures. (A) Displaced intracapsular neck of femur fracture which likely result in avascular necrosis of the femoral head. (B) Patients with such injuries generally require a complete femoral head prosthesis. (C) An extracapsular, neck of femur. fractures generally have a preserved blood supply to the femoral head. (D) Such fractures can be treated with a dynamic hip screw.

insufficiency fractures involve the lateral cortex of the femur distal to the greater trochanter (Fig 87.118). If a stress fracture is identified on one side the patient is at risk of developing a further stress fracture in the contralateral limb [113].

Subtrochanteric fractures account for 25% of proximal femoral fractures with a bimodal distribution. They are seen in young male adults following high velocity trauma such as road traffic accident and also in elderly female patients whom take bisphosphonate medication for osteoporosis [114,115] (Fig 87.119). Such fractures are uncommon in other circumstances and should be treated with caution as patients may have an underlying bone pathology.

Femoral shaft fractures are uncommon injuries and when seen are in the context of significant trauma. If no significant trauma is identified an underlying bone pathology should be suspected.

Distal femoral fractures are rare, accounting for 3–6% [116] of femoral fractures with a bimodal distribution as with subtrochanteric fractures. They are frequently comminuted and intra-articular, involving the femoral condyles and metaphysis (Fig. 87.120). They

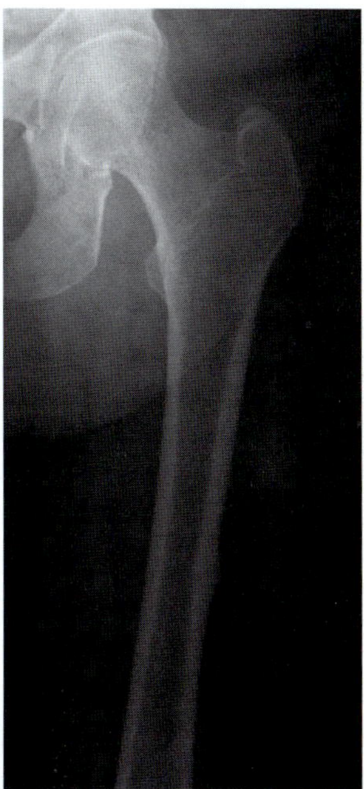

Figure 87.118 Femoral insufficiency fracture. There is thickening and beaking of the lateral cortex of the femoral shaft consistent with an insufficiency type of stress fracture. A fatigue fracture will have similar appearances but involve the medial cortex.

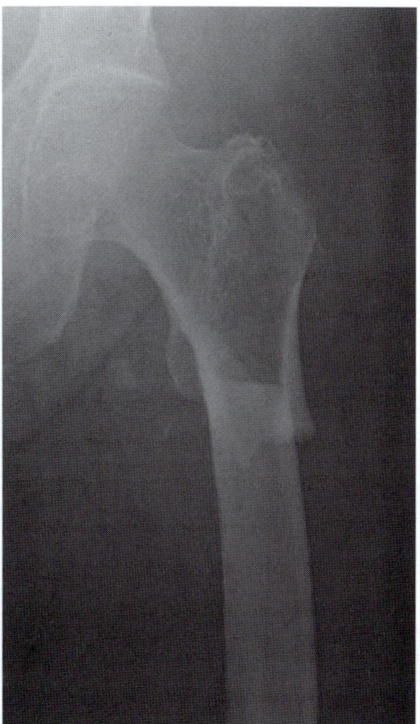

Figure 87.119 A transverse fracture through an area of lateral cortical thickening involving the subtrochanteric region of the femur. This is an atypical subtrochanteric femoral stress fracture due to abnormal bone mineral density. These types of fractures are often seen in patients taking bisphosphonate medication.

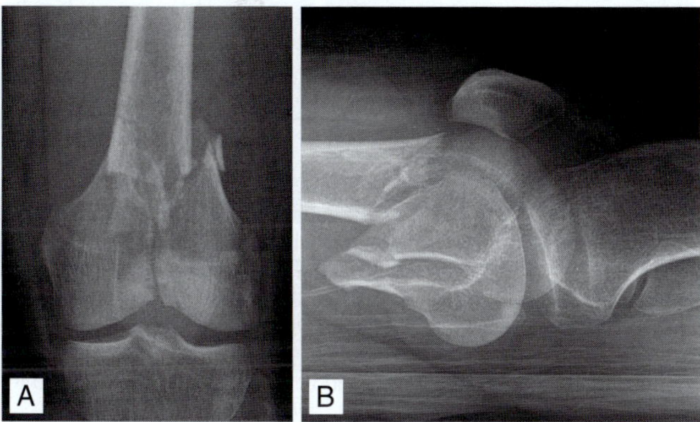

Figure 87.120 Supracondylar fracture of the femur with comminution and extension to the articular surface.

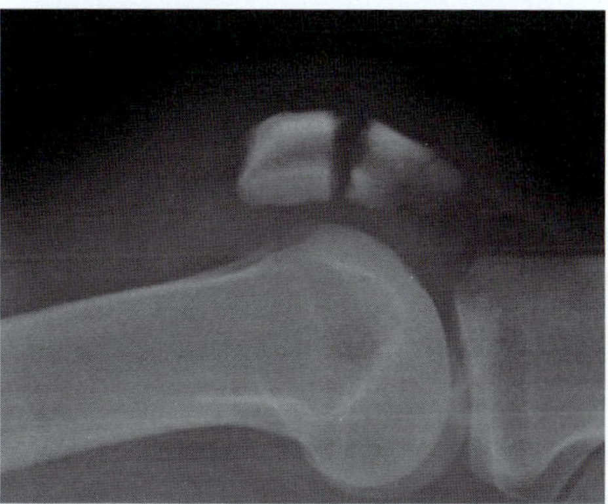

Figure 87.121 Patella fracture. Lateral knee radiograph demonstrating a comminuted and displaced transverse fracture through the body of the patella. There is also a joint effusion and prepatellar soft tissue swelling evident.

are frequently seen in the context of high-energy trauma or in the elderly as a result of a fall [117].

Fractures of the Knee

Fractures around the knee include femoral fractures (see above), patellar fractures, and tibial plateau fractures.

Patellar fractures can sometimes be challenging to diagnose in the absence of a clear history of direct trauma to the knee joint and are sometimes missed on AP knee radiographs and a lateral radiograph is important to have to hand in such queries (Fig. 87.121). It is important to differentiate acute fractures from that of normal variants such as bipartite or tripartite patella. Unlike a fracture these normal variants are well corticated. They occur in roughly 2% of the population and involve the superolateral patella in 80%, lateral patella margin in 15% and patella tip in 5% [118]. The absence of any prepatella soft tissue swelling or joint effusion on a lateral radiograph should raise suspicion for the presence of a bipartite patella. Patella dislocations are obvious clinically, however, many patients present post reduction with no evidence of trauma radiologically. MRI can be used to identify the pattern of soft tissue injury that is characteristic of a patella dislocation in such instances or to identify alternative pathology (Figs. 87.122 and 87.123).

Tibial plateau fractures are synonymous with the presence of a fat–fluid level within the suprapatellar bursa on a lateralradiograph (Fig. 87.124). The extent of injury is often not possible to identify with plain film and it is common to perform a CT to identify the extent of the fracture and also to identify, the presence of any depressed fragments (Figs. 87.125 and 87.126). Such fractures may be missed in osteopenic bones and subtle signs like a small articular step or the margin of the lateral tibial plateau overhanging the outer edge of the femoral condyle are important to identify. The Schatzker classification system for tibial plateau fractures is widely used by orthopaedic surgeons and subdivides

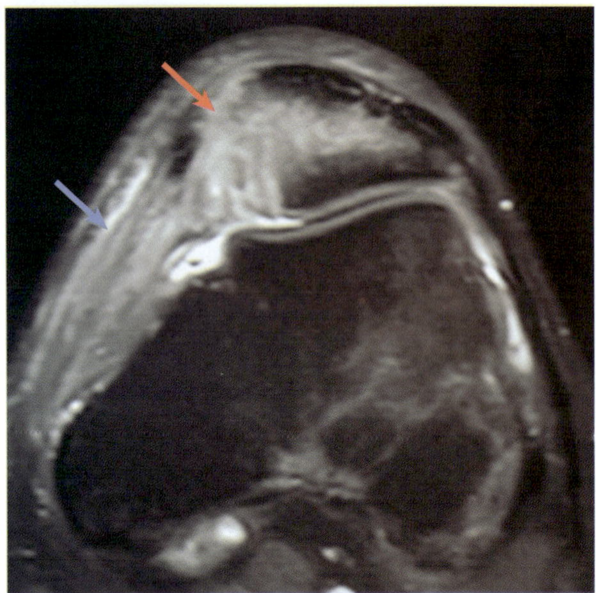

Figure 87.122 MRI following a recent patella dislocation. The medial retinaculum should be a thin dark band but it is indistinct as it is torn and edematous (*blue arrow*). There is extensive patella bone marrow edema along with a fracture involving the medial patella facet (*red arrow*). There is contralateral femoral condyle marrow edema secondary to patella impaction.

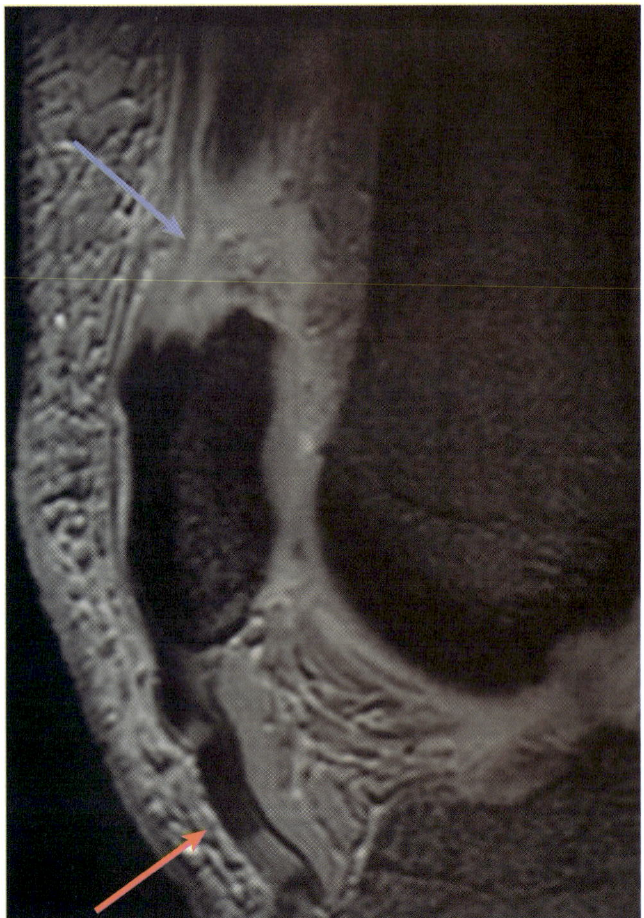

Figure 87.123 Quadriceps rupture. The normally low signal band of the quadriceps tendon insertion on the patella has been filled with high signal fluid (*blue arrow*). The tendon fibers of the quadriceps have retracted. The patella tendon is no longer under tension and slack in appearance (*red arrow*).

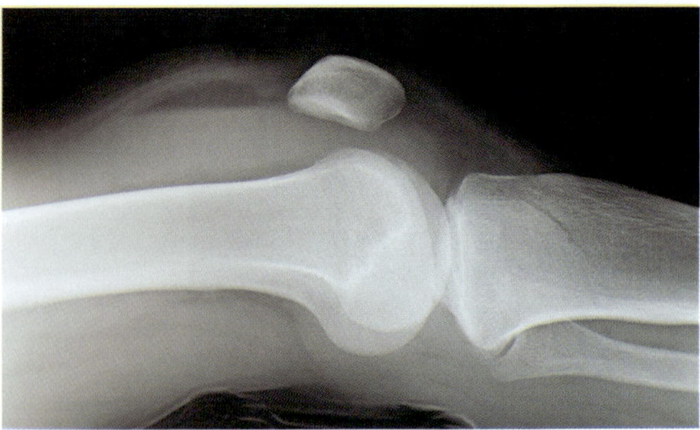

Figure 87.124 A fluid level within the supra-patella bursa seen on this lateral radiograph is due to the presence of both fat and haematoma. This is known as lipohaemarthrosis and is synonymous with an intracapsular fracture of the knee. If not seen on plain radiograph, a CT is indicated.

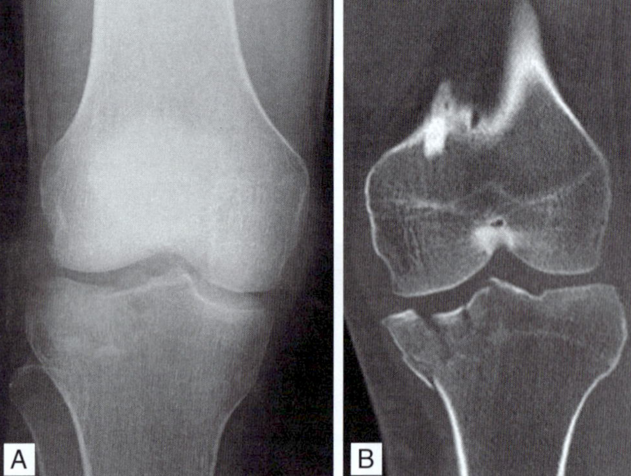

Figure 87.125 A fracture to the lateral tibial plateau. (A) Forced knee abduction results in the lateral femoral condyle impacting the lateral tibial plateau resulting in the plateau becoming depressed. (B) CT demonstrates the fracture in greater detail and that the fractures extends to the tibial metaphysis laterally and the tibial spine medially.

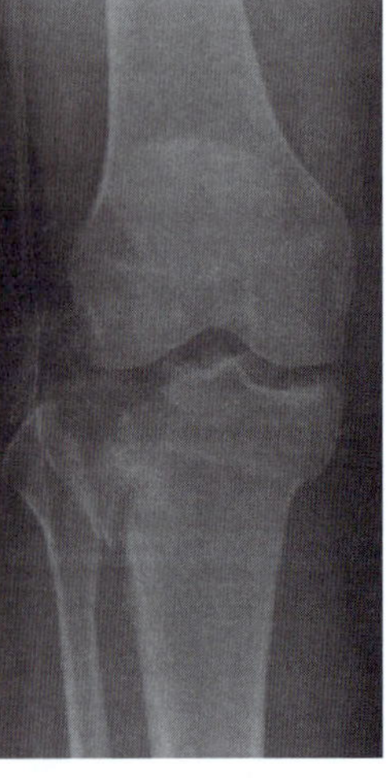

Figure 87.126 A severe fracture of the tibial plateau. The lateral plateau is depressed, comminuted and has been displaced laterally. There is also a transverse metaphyseal fracture.

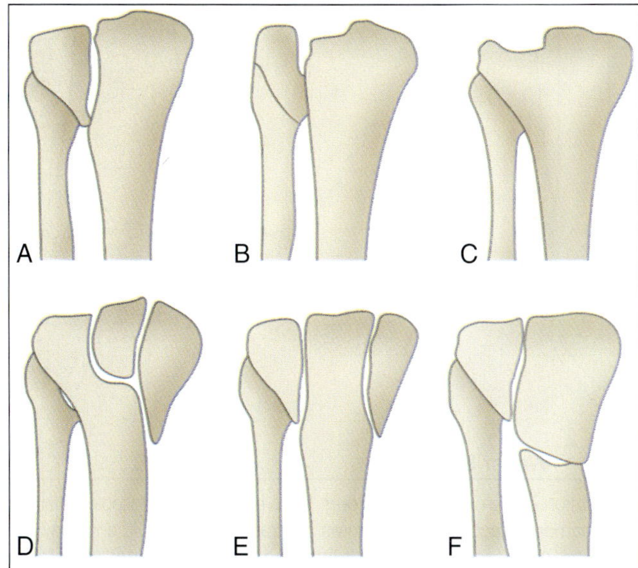

Figure 87.127 The six subtypes of tibial plateau fractures as described in the Schatzker classification. (A) Type I—Split fracture of the lateral tibial plateau. (B) Type II—Split depression fracture of the lateral tibial plateau. (C) Type III Central depression of the lateral tibial plateau. (D) Type IV—Split fracture involving the medial tibial plateau. (E) Type V—Bicondylar tibial plateau fracture. (F) Type VI—Dissociation between diaphysis and metaphysis.

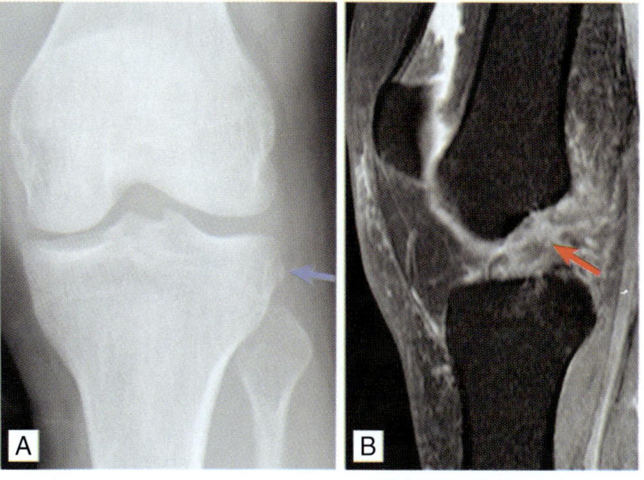

Figure 87.128 Segond fracture with associated soft tissue injury. (A) A small bone avulsion (*blue arrow*) representing the "lateral capsular sign" on a frontal knee radiograph, also known as a Segond fracture. These fractures are associated with significant soft tissue knee injuries, commonly involving the anterior cruciate ligament and medial meniscus. (B) In this instance the MRI demonstrates that the anterior cruciate ligament is torn (*red arrow*) as the ACL fibers have been replaced by heterogeneous high signal intensity edema and hematoma.

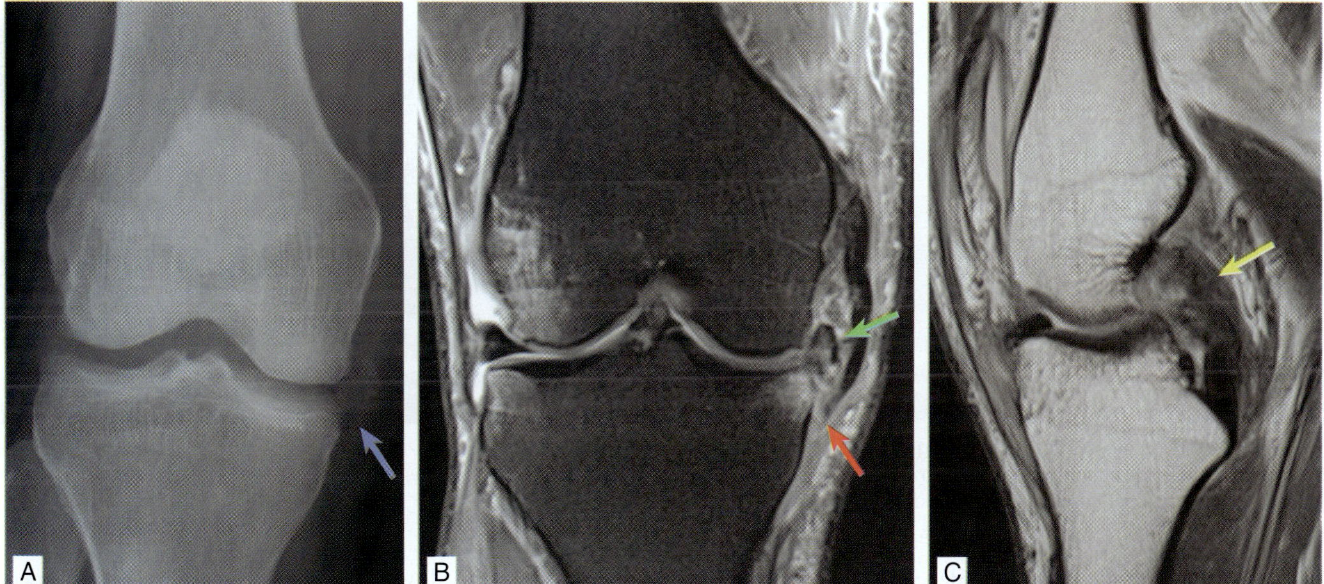

Figure 87.129 Reverse Segond fracture with associated soft tissue injuries. (A) There is an avulsion fracture involving the medial tibial plateau (*blue arrow*). This type of fracture occurs following valgus stress and external rotation of the knee. (B and C) MRIs demonstrating the associated soft tissue injuries. There is an avulsion of the deep fibers of the medial collateral ligament (*red arrow*). The normally black band is replaced by high signal intensity at the tibial insertion. The medial meniscus is torn and extruded with intrasubstance abnormal high signal extending through the body of the meniscus (*green arrow*). The posterior cruciate ligament is also torn as the normally well-defined low signal ligament has been replaced by amorphous mixed signal intensity haematoma (*yellow arrow*).

tibial plateau fractures into six categories based on CT or MRI appearances [119] (Fig. 87.127). The classification system helps to predict the degree of articular surface damage, soft tissue injury, timing of surgery and operative approach. The use of MRI is frequently employed should ligamentous or meniscal injury be queried. Certain fractures such as the Segond (Fig. 87.128) and reverse Segond (Fig. 87.129) fractures are associated with significant ligamentous injury and knee instability.

Fractures of the shaft of the tibia are usually oblique or spiral, although transverse fractures also occur. There is invariably an associated fracture of the fibula, again indicating the association of double injuries with bony "ring" structures. Complications of

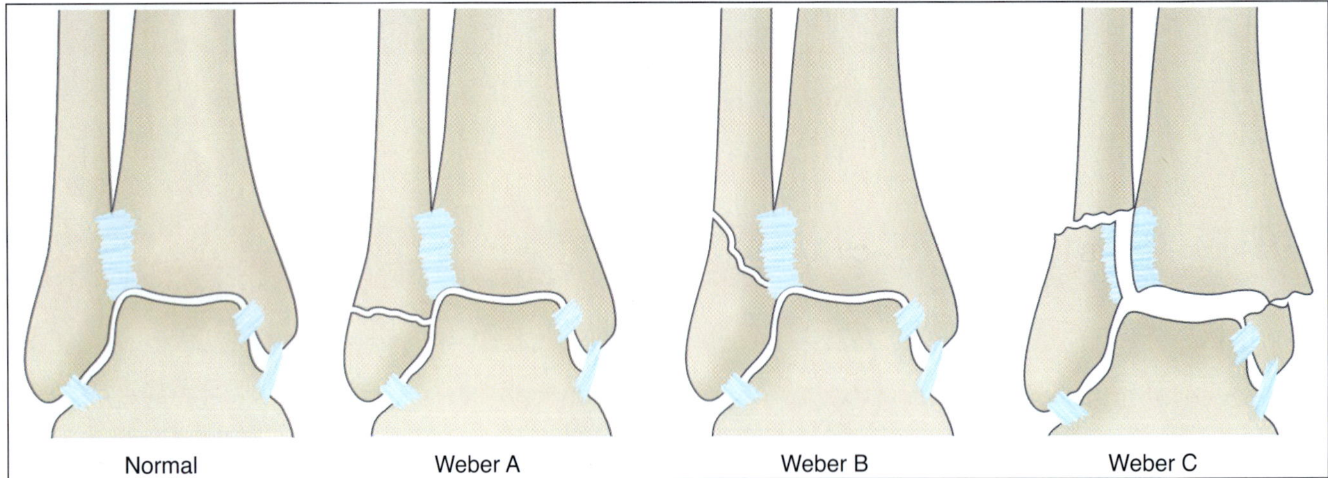

Figure 87.130 The three patterns of ankle fracture according to the Weber classification system. Type A fractures involve the lateral malleolus distal to the syndesmosis. The medial malleolus is frequently also fractured with the deltoid ligament intact. Type B fractures are trans-syndesmotic and may also have a synchronous medial malleolus fracture or deltoid ligament injury. Type C fractures occur above the level of the syndesmosis. The medial malleolus and deltoid ligament are frequently also injured. If the medial malleolus is injured or the medial clear space widened but no lateral malleolus injury is identified, the proximal fibula should be imaged to exclude a high fibula injury (Maisonneuve fracture).

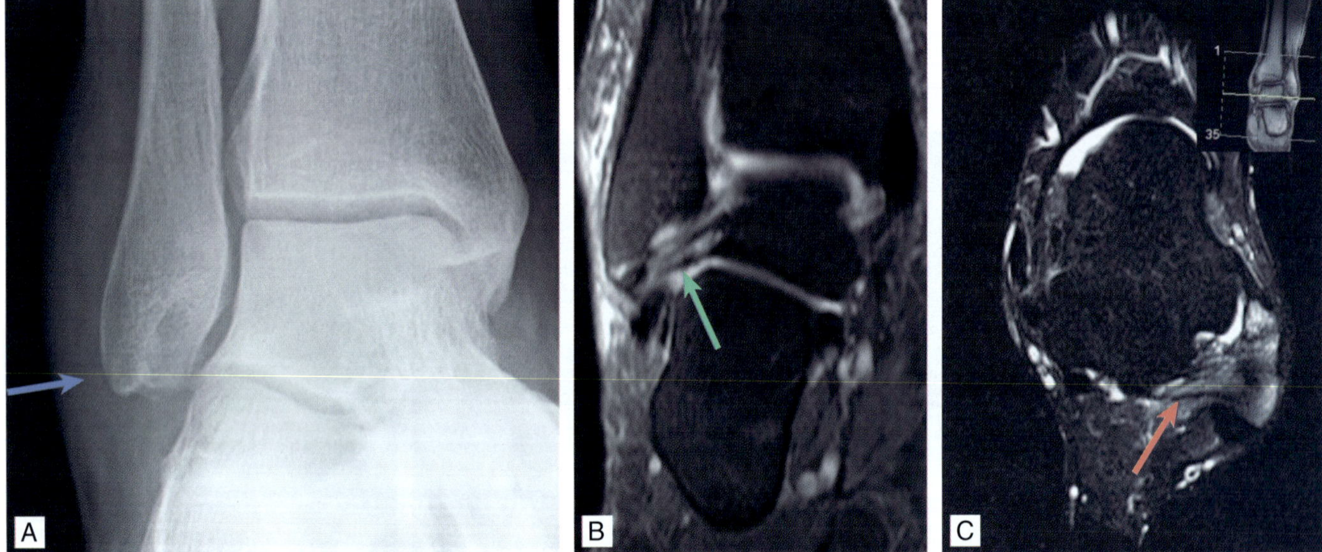

Figure 87.131 (A) There is soft tissue swelling adjacent to the medial malleolus along with a small avulsion fracture to the fibula tip (*blue arrow*). (B) The MRI demonstrates the fracture with linear high signal of the fibula tip. The talofibular ligament (*green arrow*) is strained. (C) Axial MRI showing the posterior calcaneofibular ligament (*red arrow*) is strained.

tibial fractures include a high incidence of open injuries and delayed union, usually the result of high-energy impact forces.

Fractures of the Ankle and Foot

The ankle is the most frequently injured joint and fractures are often seen in the context of sporting trauma or axial loading onto a rotated joint. Classification systems play an important role in piecing together the constellation of both bone and ligamentous injury and thus the degree of ankle stability. The Weber classification system focuses on the integrity of the tibiofibular syndesmosis with fractures being classified as

- type A (infrasyndesmotic),
- type B (transsyndesmotic), and
- type C (suprasyndesmotic) [120,121] (Fig. 87.130).

These fractures are identical to those described by Lauge-Hansen, which concentrates, on the mechanism of trauma in terms of directional force on the ankle joint, those being supination-adduction, supination-external rotation, and pronation-external rotation. On plain film, the medial and lateral clear spaces are crucial review areas as their widening can indicate ankle ligamentous injury. CT can be used to evaluate for the fracture morphology, intra-articular involvement, the presence of any osteochondral defects or intra-articular lose bodies or for the presence of occult talar fractures if suspected however not evident on plain film. MRI is generally reserved for evaluating the pattern of ligamentous and tendinous injury (Figs. 87.131 and 87.132).

Maisonneuve fractures occur due to forced pronation and external rotation resulting in a combined proximal fibula fracture and unstable ankle injury (Fig. 87.133). This is evident from widening

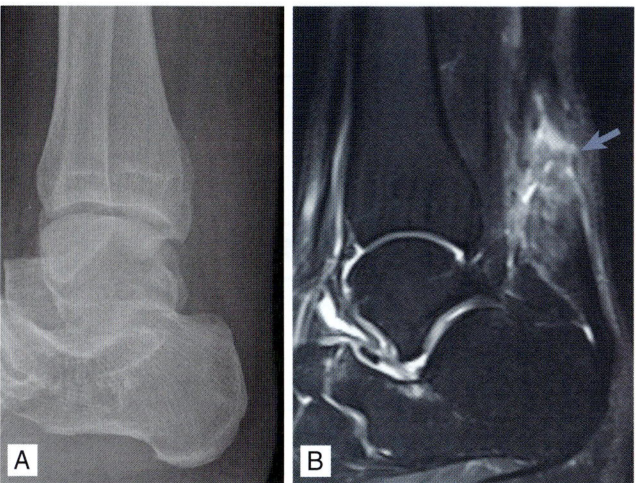

Figure 87.132 Achilles rupture. (A) Swelling and edema involving the posterior soft tissues of the ankle with an indistinct dorsal fat pad (Kager's triangle). (B) The MRI demonstrates a full thickness Achilles tendon tear (*blue arrow*). There is gross swelling, edema, and retraction of the tendon proximal to its insertion along with inflammation of the surrounding soft tissues.

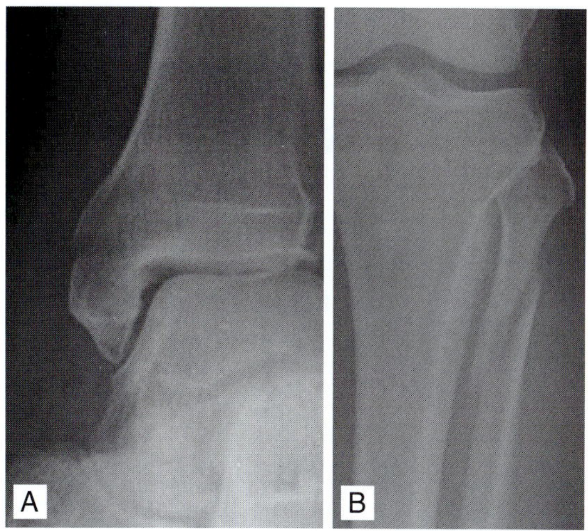

Figure 87.133 Maisonneuve fracture. Forced pronation and external rotation of the ankle has resulted in a fracture to the lateral malleolus (A) and a proximal spiral fibula fracture (B).

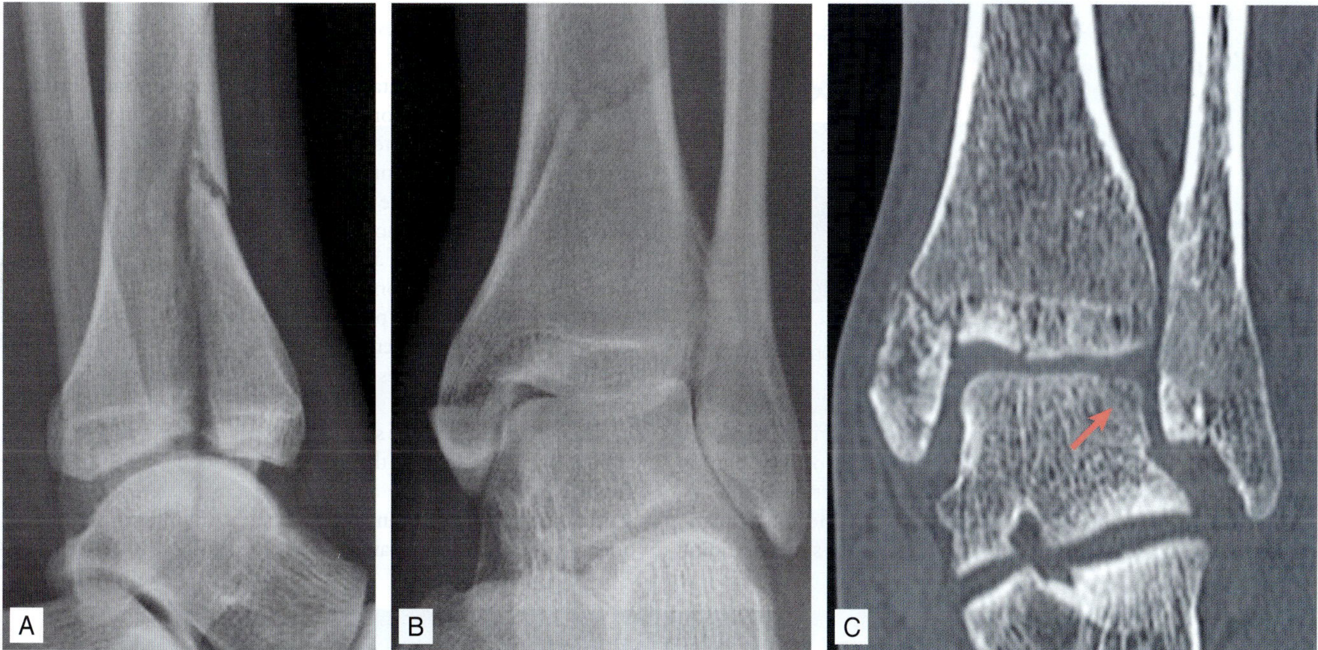

Figure 87.134 Pilon fracture. (A and B) Significant axial loading onto the ankle resulting in the distal tibia to be driven into the talus. The distal tibia fracture extends into the metaphysis. The joint space is narrowed. (C) CT demonstrating the medial malleolus fracture in more detail along with a small talar dome fracture (*red arrow*).

of the medial and lateral clear space with or without the presence of medial malleolus fracture. If suspected a radiograph to visualise the more proximal fibula is indicated. There is often significant concomitant ligamentous injury involving the deltoid ligament and distal tibiofibular syndesmosis.

Pilon fractures involve high energy axial loading onto ankle joint which drives the talus into the tibial articular surface (tibial plafond). This results in an impacted and comminuted distal tibial fracture extending to the metaphysis (Fig. 87.134). 75% of Pilon fractures are associated with distal fibula fractures [122]. Commonly the fracture is in three parts with intact ankle ligaments. These comprise of a medial malleolar fragment with intact deltoid ligament, a posterolateral fragment with intact posterior inferior tibiofibular ligament and an anterolateral fragment with an intact anterior inferior tibiofibular ligament [123].

Tarsal bone fractures are uncommon and account for 2% of all fractures with Calcaneal fractures accounting for 50–60% of these [124]. Calcaneal fractures are a frequent finding in falls from a height, and may be associated with fractures of the thoracolumbar spine. The talus acts as a wedge driving down into the calcaneal body causing depression and widening. Calcaneal fractures can be difficult to appreciate on plain radiograph, flattening of Bohler's angle may be a helpful sign (Fig. 87.135). CT is particularly useful in the evaluation of calcaneal fractures and in particular to assess

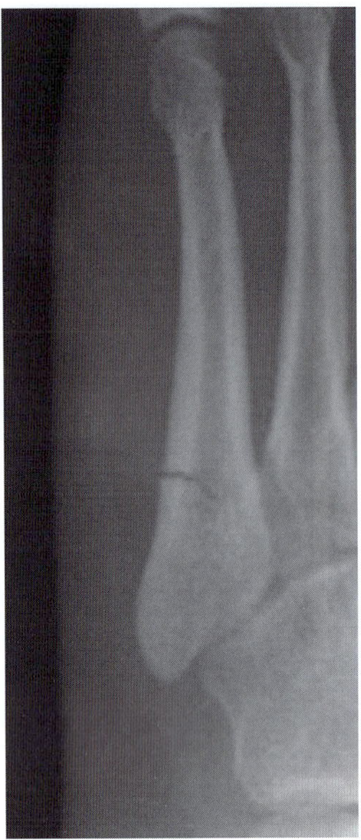

Figure 87.141 Jones's fracture. A transversely orientated fracture of the proximal 5th metatarsal diaphysis.

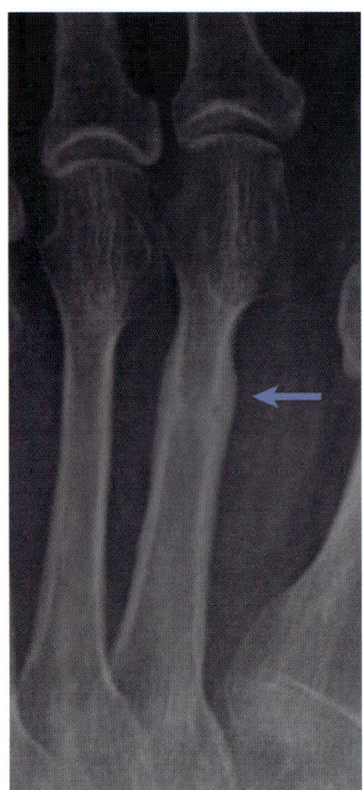

Figure 87.142 Stress fracture. The 2nd metatarsal diaphysis is a common site for stress fractures in the foot. These fractures are often subtle on the initial radiograph but are more evident on subsequent films when a sclerotic fracture line and periosteal thickening are apparent (*blue arrow*).

scan being the earliest signs. MRI will be able to demonstrate the presence of bone marrow edema and subperiosteal fluid if the radiograph is normal. Follow up radiographs will demonstrate diaphyseal periosteal reaction and sclerosis confirming the presence of a stress fracture (Fig. 87.142).

Suggested Readings

- TH Berquist, MRI of the Musculoskeletal System, third ed., Lippincott–Raven, Philadelphia, 1996.
- K Bohndort, Injuries at the articulating surface of bone, Eur J Radiol 22 (1996) 22–29.
- RB Greaney, FH Gerber, RI Laughlin, et al., Distribution and natural history of stress fractures in US marine recruits, Radiology 146 (1983) 339–346.
- JS Fisher, JJ Kazam, D Fufa, RJ Bartolotta, Radiologic evaluation of fracture healing, Skeletal Radiol 48 (2019) 349–361.
- JM Kazley, S Banerjee, MM Abousayed, AJ Rosenbaum, Classifications in brief: garden classification of femoral neck fractures, Clin Orthop Relat Res 476 (2) (2018 Feb) 441–445.
- RA Marshall, J Mandell, MJ Weaver, M Ferrone, A Sodickson, Imaging features and management of stress, atypical, and pathologic fractures, Radiographics 38 (7) (2018 Nov), doi:10.1148/rg.2018180073.
- KE Halliday, NJ Broderick, JM Somers, R Hawkes, Dating fractures in infants, Clin Radiol 66 (11) (2011 Nov) 1049–1054.
- F Canavese, A Samba, M Rousset, Pathological fractures in children: diagnosis and treatment options, Orthop Traumatol Surg Res 102 (1, Suppl.) (2016 Feb) S149–S159.
- M Paddock, A Sprigg, AC Offiah, Imaging and reporting considerations for suspected physical abuse (non-accidental injury) in infants and young children. Part 1: initial considerations and appendicular skeleton, Clin Radiol 72 (3) (2017 Mar) 179–188.
- A Fassier, P Gaucherand, R Kohler, Fractures in children younger than 18 months, Orthop Traumatol Surg Res 99 (1, Suppl.) (2013 Feb) S160–S170.
- M Paddock, A Sprigg, AC Offiah, Imaging and reporting considerations for suspected physical abuse (non-accidental injury) in infants and young children. Part 2: axial skeleton and differential diagnoses, Clin Radiol 72 (3) (2017 Mar) 189–201.
- R Moverley, N Little, A Gulihar, B Singh, Current concepts in the management of clavicle fractures, J Clin Orthop Trauma, 11 (2020) S25–S30.
- SE Sheehan, G Gaviola, A Sacks, R Gordon, LL Shi, SE Smith, Traumatic shoulder injuries: a force mechanism analysis of complex injuries to the shoulder girdle and proximal humerus, Am J Roentgenol 201 (3) (2013 Sep) W409–W424.
- AM Ropp, DL Davis, Scapular fractures: what radiologists need to know, Am J Roentgenol 205 (3) (2015 Sep) 491–501.
- SE Sheehan, GS Dyer, AD Sodickson, KI Patel, B Khurana, Traumatic elbow injuries: what the orthopedic surgeon wants to know, Radiographics 33 (3) (2013 May) 869–888.

- T Pope, H Bloem, J Beltran, W WD Morrison, Acute osseous injury to the wrist, in: Musculoskeletal imaging, second ed., Elsevier Saunders, Philadelphia, PA, 2014, p. 185.
- LR Scalcione, LH Gimber, AM Ho, SS Johnston, JE Sheppard, MS Taljanovic, Spectrum of carpal dislocations and fracture-dislocations: imaging and management, Am J Roentgenol (2014) 541–550.
- SE Sheehan, JY Shyu, MJ Weaver, AD Sodickson, B Khurana, Proximal femoral fractures: what the orthopedic surgeon wants to know, Radiographics 35 (5) (2015 Sep) 1563–1584.
- BK Markhardt, JM Gross, JUV Monu, Schatzker classification of tibial plateau fractures: use of CT and MR imaging improves assessment, Radiographics 29 (2) (2009 Mar) 585–597.
- NG Lasanianos, NK Kanakaris, Ankle fractures, in: Trauma and Orthopaedic Classifications: A Comprehensive Overview, Springer-Verlag, London, 2015, pp. 367–370.

88

Neuro, Head, and Neck Trauma

CURTIS OFFIAH, MERVYN CHONG

Introduction

Trauma to the head and neck region is a frequent cause of emergency department (ED) attendance with over 2.5 million ED visits for head trauma in the United States in 2014 [1]. The spectrum of potential injuries in this region is vast including osseous, soft tissue, and vascular injury. Imaging plays a major role in the diagnosis of these injuries and knowledge of imaging strategies, typical patterns of injury, radiological findings, and associated complications are vital for the reporting radiologist.

Multidetector computed tomography (MDCT) is the primary technique in imaging of acute neuro/head and neck trauma with scanning protocols depending on the traumatic mechanism and briefly described below.

For intracranial injury and skull fractures, noncontrast head CT with thin axial slices and multiplanar reformats are standard. For suspected facial bone fractures noncontrast facial CT is first-line (with or without the inclusion of intracranial imaging). Noncontrast CT cervical spine is performed for suspected cervical spine trauma.

The indications for CT head examination for head and cervical spine injury in adults in the UK are generally taken from guidance by the National Institute for Health and Clinical Excellence (NICE) [2]. The American College of Radiology (ACR) appropriateness criteria cite the Nexus Criteria and Canadian Cervical Spine rule in their guidance for cervical spine imaging [3]. The ACR appropriateness criteria for imaging in head trauma refer to the use of a validated clinical decision rule as a criterion for imaging, of which the most well-known is the New Orleans Criteria and Canadian CT Head Rule [4].

CT angiography (CTA) of the neck with or without extension to the vertex is utilized in penetrating neck trauma to assess for vascular injury. CTA is also used in screening for blunt cerebrovascular injury (BCVI). MR angiogram occasionally may be used instead of CT angiogram but may be challenging in intubated and ventilated patients outside major trauma units where specialized adapted magnetic resonance imaging (MRI)-compatible anaesthetic equipment may not be available.

Brain MRI is particularly useful as a second-line investigation in neurotrauma where there is a concern for traumatic axonal injury (TAI) and in assisting prognostication. Haem-sensitive sequences such as gradient echo and susceptibility-weighted imaging (SWI) are especially beneficial in demonstrating the hemosiderin staining associated with hemorrhagic TAI, the extent and severity of which is generally under-represented on CT.

The use of more specialized MR techniques such as cisternography may be performed in the assessment for cerebrospinal fluid (CSF) leak, a frequent concern in fracture of the skull base.

MRI is the imaging technique of choice for assessment of the soft tissues in spinal trauma, demonstrating ligamentous and spinal cord injury, and intraspinal hematoma. MRI is also beneficial in discerning marrow edema of a recent vertebral fracture.

Intracranial Trauma

Introduction

Intracranial trauma encompasses a number of injury patterns that can be considered as intra-axial or extra-axial injuries. Secondary injuries may also occur including brain herniation, infarction, and hydrocephalus. Intracranial vascular injury represents another important area of consideration.

Imaging Approach

Nonenhanced head CT remains the imaging technique of the first choice in suspected traumatic brain injury, and early follow-up due to its speed, accessibility, higher sensitivity for fracture (allowing earlier identification of fracture complications), and no limitation in terms of screening for MRI contraindications such as metallic foreign body [5].

It is generally advised that CT protocols utilize MDCT with axial views acquired from the vertex to the foramen magnum. Liberal use of multiplanar reformats of bone algorithms as well as volume-rendered reconstructions are recommended in the evaluation of pediatric trauma, particularly in the setting of suspected abusive head trauma. When imaging of the facial bones is required the CT acquisition is extended to include the facial bones and/or mandible as required. Facial bone reformats are configured in coronal and sagittal plane in thin-section (1 mm) aligned to the hard palate, with a bone algorithm applied. Multiplanar facial soft tissue reformats are also performed.

Injury Type and Findings

Extradural Hematoma (EDH)

These hematomas arise within the extradural space, between the superficial layer of the dura mater, and the inner table of the skull (Figs. 88.1 and 88.2). *They may be arterial or venous in origin, classically have a biconvex or "lentiform" contour and are of high density (representing acute clot). A "swirl sign"* (Fig. 88.1) *is described where there is low density mixed within the hematoma and is suggestive of active hemorrhage* [6]. The mass effect from the hematoma typically displaces the lateral ventricles to the

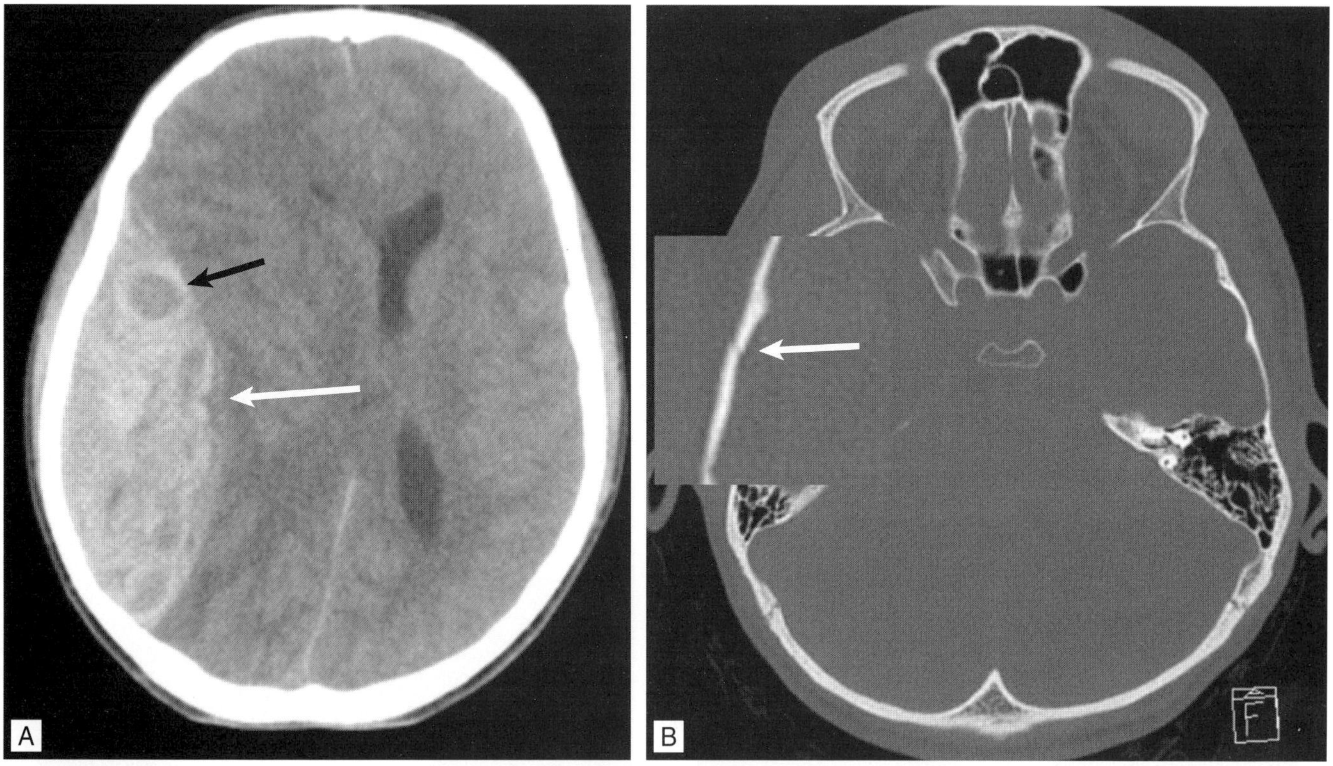

Figure 88.1 20-year-old male who suffered an alleged punch to the face and resultant accelerated fall striking head on the ground. (A) CT scan demonstrates a large right acute extradural hematoma (*white arrow*). Note the areas of unclotted blood within the extradural hematoma (*black arrow*) consistent with active bleeding—the so-called "swirl sign"; there is severe mass effect with midline shift and subfalcine herniation to the left. (B) The bone reconstructions demonstrate a fracture (*magnified and highlighted with white arrow*) which extended through a right middle meningeal artery branch vascular channel in the squamous temporal bone.

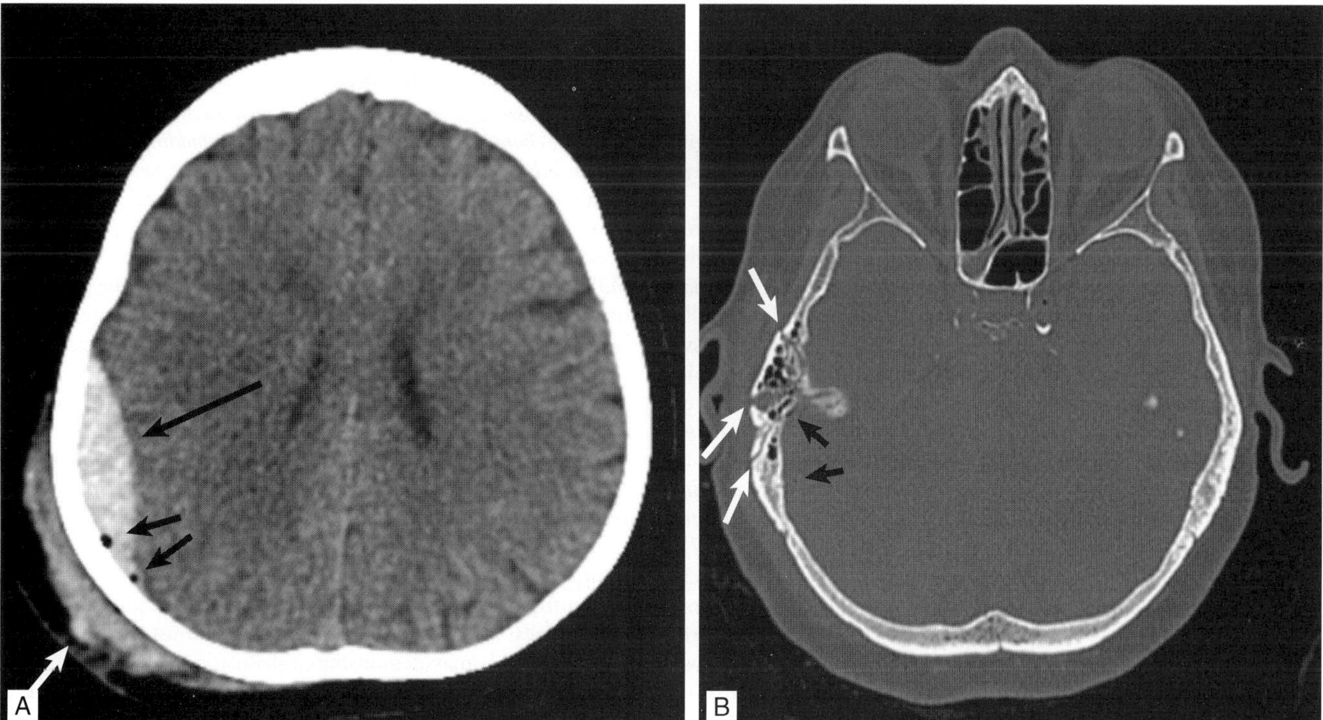

Figure 88.2 56-year-old male who fell from standing sustaining head injury. (A) CT scan demonstrating right parietal acute extradural hematoma (*long black arrow*) with some locules of gas within the hematoma (*short black arrows*) related to underlying skull base fracture extension. Associated scalp soft tissue hematoma evident (*white arrow*). (B) Associated comminuted fractures through the right lateral skull base (*white arrows*) and secondary pneumocephalus (*short black arrows*).

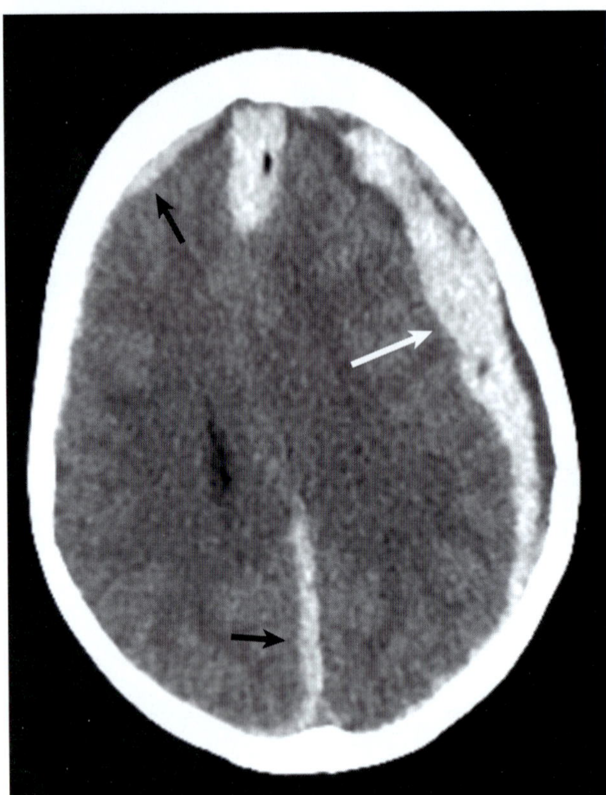

Figure 88.3 73-year-old female with bilateral acute subdural hematomas related to the left (*white arrow*) and right (*black arrows*) cerebral hemispheres, larger on the left demonstrated on CT scan. The left subdural hematoma (*white arrow*) exhibits some mixed density with features suggestive of acute hemorrhage into pre-existing older chronic sudural hematoma but similar appearances can be seen with underlying coagulopathy.

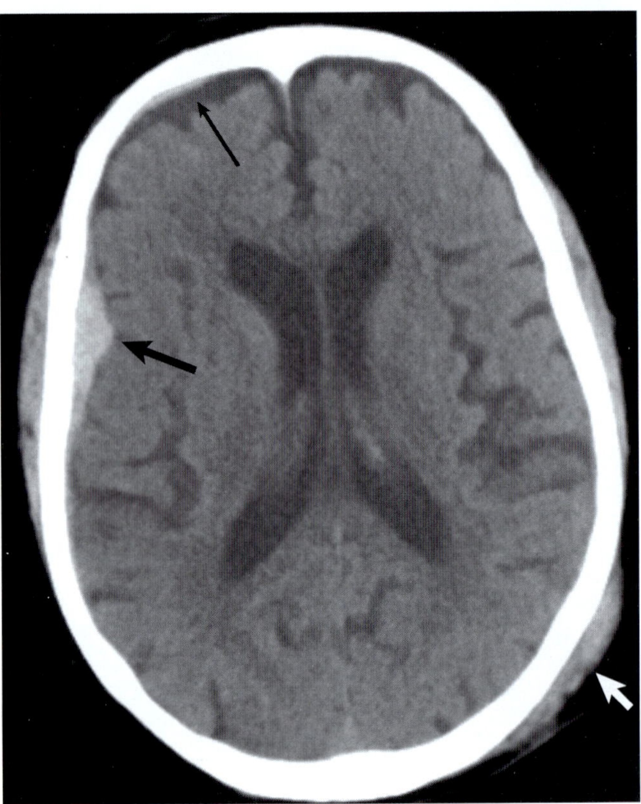

Figure 88.4 83-year-old male who sustained a fall striking the *left side* of the head (*short arrow*) resulting in contrecoup right cerebral hemispheric convexity subdural hematoma (*black arrows*) demonstrated on CT scan—note that acute subdural hematoma may not always exhibit the crescentic morphology in their entirety (*thick black arrow*).

contralateral side, there is frequently swelling of the ipsilateral cerebral hemisphere.

A pterional extradural hematoma is generally of arterial origin and is caused by injury to the middle meningeal artery by overlying skull fracture (Fig. 88.1B).

Venous extradural hematomas may also be seen in fractures that cross a dural venous sinus. Injury to the superior sagittal sinus or sphenoparietal sinus may result in a venous extradural hematoma at the vertex or an anterior temporal pole (anterior middle cranial fossa) extradural hematoma, respectively. Posterior fossa venous EDH may occur with injury to the transverse or sigmoid sinuses or the jugular bulb and is associated with a risk of brainstem and fourth ventricle compression and obstructive hydrocephalus.

An identifying feature of EDH is that they do not cross cranial sutures. This is due to the superficial dura being strongly adherent to the inner table of the calvarium at the suture sites [7]. The rare exception to this rule is where the suture itself is involved by a fracture [5]. Extradural hematomas do, however, cross the midline, e.g. when they are overlying the falx cerebri/interhemispheric fissure and superior sagittal sinus (in contrast to subdural hematomas, as later described).

The treatment of EDH is with surgical evacuation. In occasional cases, smaller EDHs may potentially be treated with middle meningeal arterial embolization [8]. Anterior temporal EDH specifically, however, has a benign course and does not generally require surgery [9].

Subdural Hematoma (SDH)

Subdural hematomas arise between the dura and arachnoid mater. *These are characteristically crescentic in shape, moulding to the contour of the underlying cerebral convexity* (Fig. 88.3). The vessel of origin is usually a bridging cortical vein as it crosses the dura. There is often associated swelling of the underlying brain parenchyma. *In contrast to extradural hematomata, subdural hematomas do cross suture lines.* SDHs, however, do not cross dural reflections, such as the falx cerebri or the tentorium [7]. Caution is advised as not all acute subdural hematomas exhibit the classical crescentic morphology (Fig. 88.4).

As SDHs mature from acute to chronic, they change in density due to maturation of blood products from hyper- to hypo-dense (Fig. 88.3). *While "acute-on-chronic" SDH may result in mixed attenuation characteristics (often from rehemorrhage from internal membranes of granulation tissue), low-density contents can be seen in the hyperacute phase before clot formation, in severe anaemia, in pre-existing coagulopathic states, or in CSF-blood admixture where there is an associated tear in the arachnoid mater.* A more useful feature in identifying chronicity of a SDH is the identification of internal membranes, which tend to enhance if IV contrast is administered. Chronic SDHs may demonstrate calcification [5].

SDH that requires surgery is treated with evacuation by burr hole drainage or craniotomy.

Subdural Hygroma

These are collections of CSF within the subdural space that occur as the result of a tear in the arachnoid mater (Fig. 88.5).

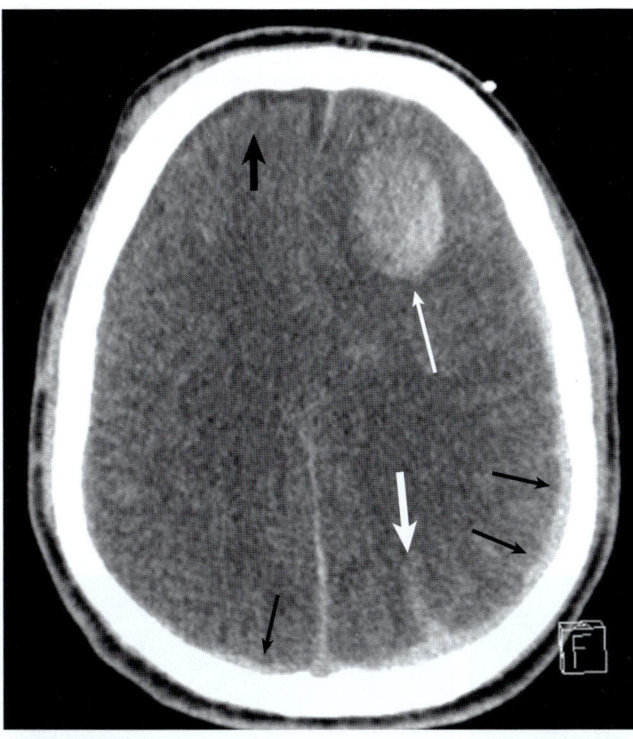

Figure 88.5 28-year-old male hit by a train. CT scan was performed 24 hours later demonstrating bilateral acute subdural hematomas (*long thin black arrows*) but evolving shallow hygromatous component is evident over the right frontal lobe convexity (*short thick black arrow*). Note progressive left frontal hematoma (*long thin white arrow*) and areas of left parietal acute traumatic subarachnoid hemorrhage (*thick white arrow*).

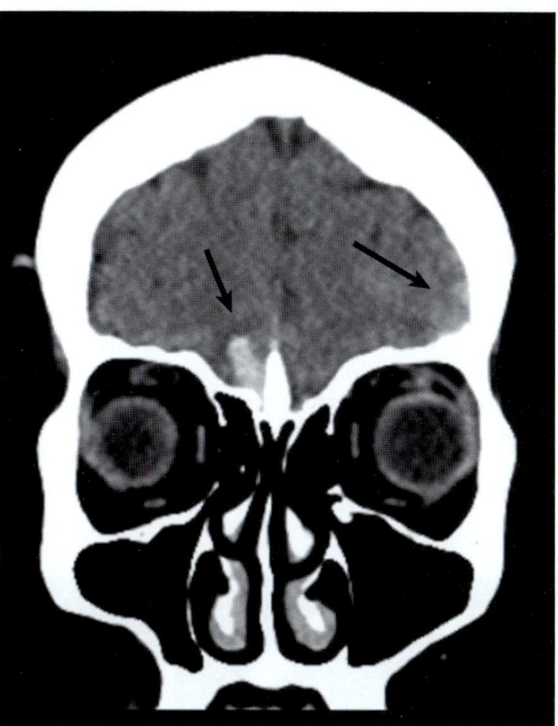

Figure 88.6 56-year-old female fell and struck the back of the head resulting in contrecoup left subfrontal and right frontal brain parenchymal hemorrhagic contusions (*black arrows*) demonstrated on CT scan.

As with all subdural collections, these cause displacement of the vessels within the subarachnoid space, which allows distinction of these from a prominent subarachnoid space. Subdural hygromas may arise within the first 24 hours of trauma, although their mean time of onset is more delayed at 9 days post injury [10].

A chronic subdural hematoma may have a similar appearance as both this and a hygroma will be of CSF density. A potential distinguishing feature is the absence of internal membranes of granulation tissue within the subdural hygroma but more typically, distinction is possible because of the temporal association with recent significant head injury. Definite differentiation is not always possible and indeed a CSF–blood admixture mix of hygroma and hematoma may be present [5,11].

Traumatic Subarachnoid Hemorrhage

This is hemorrhage occurring within the subarachnoid space between the arachnoid and pia mater. In traumatic subarachnoid hemorrhage (SAH), this generally occurs at the coup or contrecoup site relative to the head impact, is of a small volume, and is sulcal in location (Fig. 88.5).

When seen as an isolated finding, traumatic SAH is associated with a lower likelihood of clinical deterioration than when hemorrhage in another compartment is also present [12]. *Midline traumatic SAH within the perimesencephalic cisterns and interhemispheric fissure on initial head CT has been shown to be associated with an increased incidence of TAI on follow-up imaging* [13]. Traumatic SAH within the interpeduncular and perimesencephalic cisterns increases the possibility of associated brainstem injury [13].

Vasospasm may occur as a delayed complication in traumatic SAH but this is much less frequently seen than in aneurysmal SAH [14]. While uncommon, aneurysmal SAH can be present in a patient presenting with traumatic injury and this should be considered, particularly where there is isolated SAH within the basal cisterns [5].

Intraventricular Hemorrhage

Traumatic intraventricular hemorrhage may be a primary finding from a ruptured subependymal vein or secondary extension from either intraparenchymal hematoma or redistributed SAH [5]. Intraventricular hemorrhage within the occipital horns may be of small volume and may be overlooked. The presence of IVH on initial CT head imaging has been shown to correlate with an increased risk of TAI [15].

Parenchymal Contusion

Parenchymal contusions may be hemorrhagic or nonhemorrhagic. Hemorrhagic contusions appear as focal intracerebral hemorrhages, often with surrounding edema, while nonhemorrhagic contusions are typically of low density and may appear similar to isolated focal cerebral edema. Contusions typically occur at coup and contrecoup sites. The most common locations are at the inferior frontal and (Fig. 88.6) anterior–inferior temporal lobes due to the impact of the parenchyma against the inner table [5]. Hemorrhagic areas may not be identifiable on CT in the very acute stage. MRI has been found to be more sensitive than CT in identifying contusions, especially smaller and nonhemorrhagic contusions [5,16].

While an initial increase in the size of contusions in the first 48 hours postinjury is frequently present and not unexpected (referred to as "blossoming"), [17] *interval evolution of unidentified contusions and/or a doubling in contusion volume on follow-up imaging have been found to be associated with worsened clinical outcomes* [18].

Traumatic Axonal Injury (TAI)

TAI occurs as a result of tractional or shearing forces on axons. The most susceptible regions of the brain are the white matter tracts and areas of abrupt change in neuroparenchymal density such as the gray–white matter junction.

The terms TAI and diffuse axonal injury (DAI) are frequently used interchangeably although DAI is better reserved for multifocal injuries where there are greater than 3 lesions, and TAI for those cases with 3 or fewer lesions [5,19,20].

TAI can be hemorrhagic or nonhemorrhagic. Most commonly they appear as punctate foci of hemorrhage at characteristic locations such as the gray–white matter junction (particularly the frontal lobe), corpus callosum (with predilection for the splenium) (Fig. 88.7A–E), internal capsules, dorsal midbrain and pons.

MRI is more sensitive than CT for both hemorrhagic and nonhemorrhagic lesions. Hemorrhagic lesions on MRI are best demonstrated using blood-sensitive sequences such as SWI and T2* (GRE) imaging (Fig. 88.7B and E). Restricted diffusion may be present in acute DAI lesions (Fig. 88.7C and D).

TAI is graded from 1 to 3 with a higher grade indicating greater injury severity and has potential prognostic implications. *Grades 1–3, respectively, refer to involvement of the subcortical white matter, deep brain parenchyma, typically corpus callosum, and brainstem* [21].

TAI is associated with a much greater morbidity and mortality than other intracranial injuries. Management is with close monitoring of intracranial pressure and potential craniectomy to avoid herniation [5].

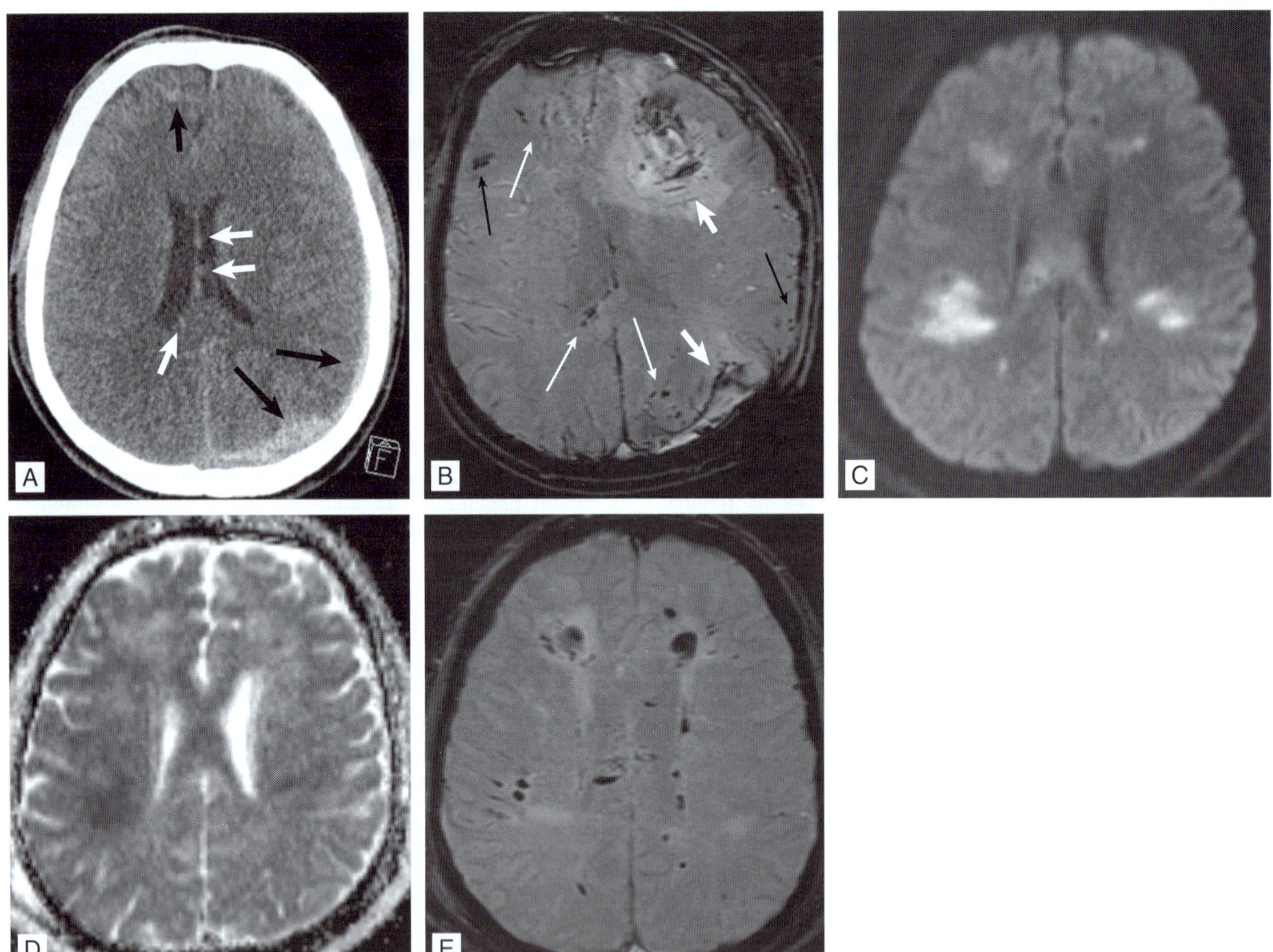

Figure 88.7 28-year-old male who jumped in front of a train. (A) Acute left subdural hemorrhage (*long black arrows*), right frontal traumatic subarachnoid hemorrhage (*short black arrow*) and grade 2 traumatic axonal injury in the splenium of the corpus callosum and septum pellucidum (*white arrows*). (B) Axial susceptibility-weighted image performed several days after neurosurgical left decompressive craniectomy demonstrates grade 1 and grade 2 traumatic axonal injury (*long thin white arrows*), as well as blossomed left frontal lobe traumatic intraparenchyma hematoma (*short thin white arrow*) with surrounding edema and areas of parenchymal hemorrhagic contusions (*long thin black arrows*).
31-year-old male driver of a car that collided with a stationary vehicle at high speed. (C) Axial echo-planar b1000 diffusion-weighted image demonstrates grade 2 multifocal traumatic axonal injury—high signal lesions consistent with restricted diffusion typical of early traumatic axonal injury MRI appearances and confirmed on ADC image (D). (E) Susceptibility-weighted imaging of the same patient—multiple hypointense foci, again, in keeping with grade 1 and grade 2 hemorrhagic traumatic axonal injury.

Diffuse Brain Swelling

Diffuse swelling of the brain parenchyma may occur post-trauma and is thought to be due to dysfunction of cerebral autoregulation and/or disruption of the blood–brain barrier [22].

Vascular Injury

Multiple vascular injuries can occur as a result of head trauma. These include arterial dissections particularly in skull base fracture, pseudoaneurysm (most commonly of the vertebral artery followed by the anterior cerebral artery), active hemorrhage, arterial occlusion, traumatic carotid-cavernous fistula, traumatic dural arteriovenous fistula, and venous thrombosis (particularly where a fracture crosses a dural venous sinus) [5,23,24].

Cervical spine fractures are the subgroup of nonvascular injuries found to have the greatest association with BCVI [25–27]. Vascular injuries are discussed in more depth in a dedicated section "*Blunt Cerebrovascular Injury.*"

Secondary Brain Injury

Herniation from a primary brain injury can lead to secondary complications including cerebrovascular infarction, hydrocephalus, and secondary hemorrhage [5,28–30].

- Subfalcine herniation (Fig. 88.8) can cause compression of the anterior cerebral artery against the falx cerebri leading to anterior cerebral artery territory infarction and may cause lateral ventricular dilatation/entrapment through occlusion of one of the foramina of Monro
- Downward transtentorial herniation (Fig. 88.9A) can cause posterior cerebral artery compression and posterior cerebral artery territory infarction (Fig. 88.9B and C), as well as compressive third nerve palsy with ipsilateral pupillary dilatation (the "blown" pupil). More severe and bilateral downward transtentorial herniation can compress small perforating arteries leading to hypothalamic and basal ganglia infarction
- Severe cerebellar tonsillar herniation may result in posterior inferior cerebellar artery compression and infarction and can also obstruct the fourth ventricular apertures and secondary hydrocephalus
- Ascending transtentorial herniation can cause effacement of the quadrigeminal cistern, compression of the midbrain, and hydrocephalus from obstruction of the Sylvian aqueduct
- Duret hemorrhages (Fig. 88.9A) are secondary midbrain hemorrhages due to severe downward transtentorial herniation

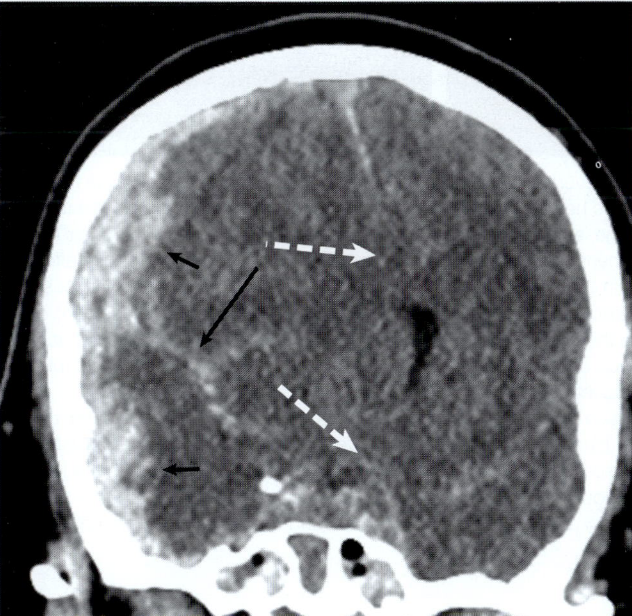

Figure 88.8 60-year-old male who fell from ladder (and was on antiplatelet therapy). The large volume acute right cerebral hemispheric subdural hematoma (*short thin black arrows*) is causing severe midline shift with subfalcine herniation (*broken white arrow*) and right descending transtentorial herniation (again, the direction of which is indicated by the *broken white arrow*). Note displacement and compressive effect on the third ventricle. Traumatic subarachnoid hemorrhage is also evident (*long thin black arrow*).

Penetrating Craniocerebral Trauma

This is distinct from blunt cranial trauma. This may take the form of sharp force penetrating injury (e.g., from a knife or axe) or projectile penetrating injury, typically from a gunshot or blast injury (with associated in-driven secondary foreign bodies created by the later mechanism). Such penetrating craniocerebral trauma will require noncontrast CT head for imaging assessment and frequently additional CT angiography may be required in obtunded patients or where there is clear evidence of significant hemorrhagic vascular injury on the noncontrast CT head scan or evidence that the penetrating injury has transgressed more than one lobe or more than one hemisphere. Interrogation of the images on bone windows will greatly assist in identifying, e.g., bullet fragments or broken-off blade tips. In addition, the scanogram (scout) images of the CT scan can also be very useful in identifying bullet fragments and potential additional penetrating injuries that may be extracranial (Fig. 88.9D–F).

Key Points for Intracranial Trauma

- Intracranial hemorrhage can be categorized into extra-axial (extradural, subdural, subarachnoid, and intraventricular) and intra-axial
- The "swirl" sign is suggestive of active hemorrhage into an extradural hematoma
- Subdural hematomas of mixed density should not automatically be assumed to be acute-on-chronic
- Isolated SAH is less associated with clinical deterioration than when accompanied by another intracranial hemorrhage. Perimesencephalic SAH, however, is associated with a higher incidence of TAI and brainstem injury
- An increase in the size of parenchymal contusions within 48 hours of injury is not unexpected; however, newly identifiable contusions or doubling in contusion volume are associated with poorer clinical outcomes
- Secondary brain injury relating to mass effect should be assessed for including ACA and PCA territorial infarction relating to subfalcine and downward transtentorial herniation

Skull Including the Skull Base

Calvarial Fractures

The calvarium (or skull vault) comprises the frontal and occipital bones and the paired parietal and temporal bones. Calvarial fractures are seen in both blunt and penetrating trauma. Depression of skull

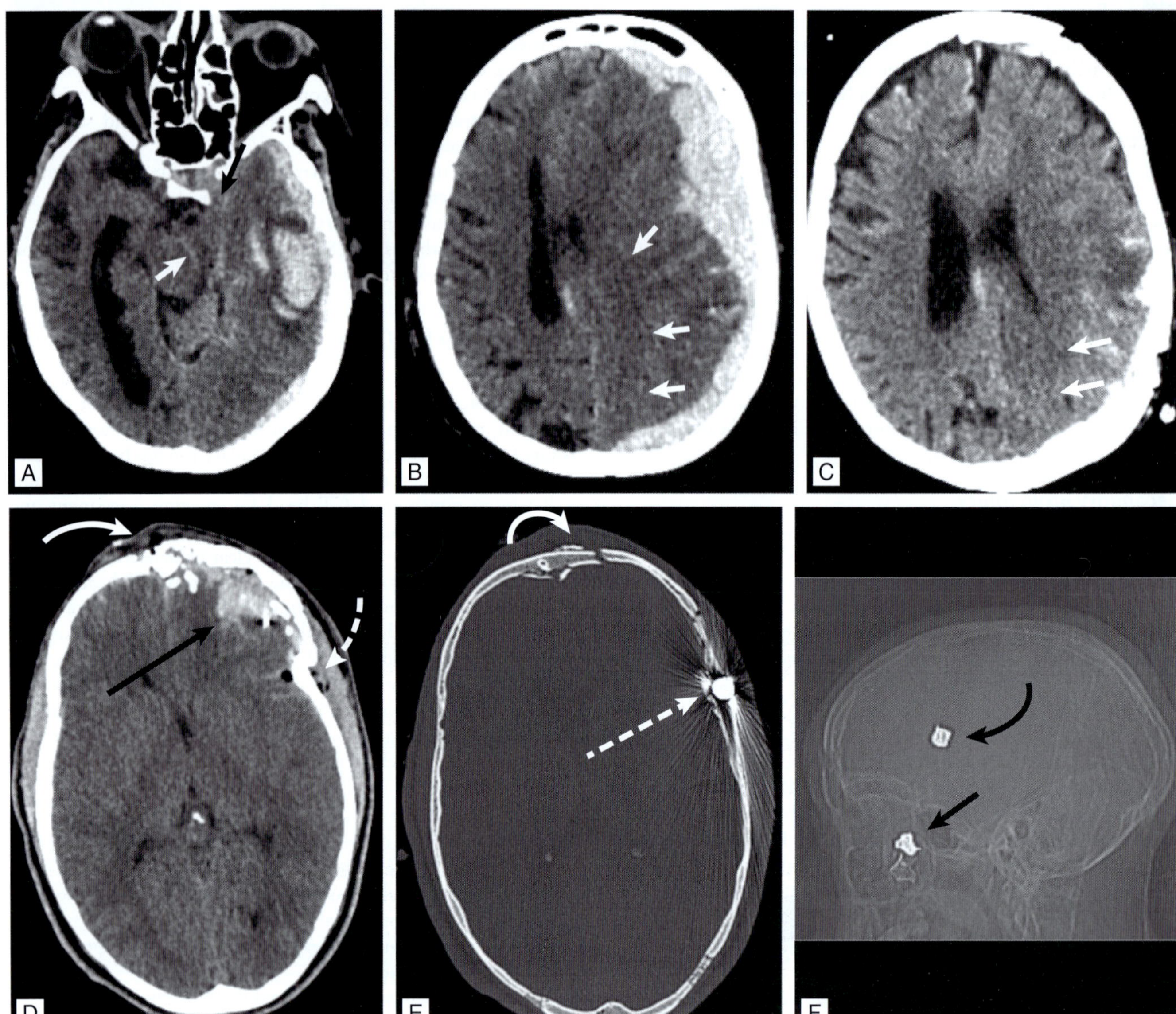

Figure 88.9 64-year-old male who sustained a fall admitted following discovery several hours after the fall. (A) CT scan demonstrates large traumatic left temporal lobe parenchymal hematoma with some evolving edema around the hematoma and traumatic left subdural hemorrhage and subarachnoid hemorrhage extending over the vermis. The mass effect associated with the left hemispheric traumatic hemorrhage is causing left uncal herniation (descending transtentorial herniation) (*thick black arrow*) resulting effacement of the left perimesencephalic cistern and compressive effect on the midbrain with some Duret hemorrhage within the *left side* of the midbrain (*small white arrow*). (B) CT scan demonstrates early left posterior cerebral artery ischemia with loss of gray–white matter differentiation (*white arrows*) resulting from herniation syndrome causing effacement of left perimesencephalic cistern and left posterior cerebral artery compromise. Note the large left acute subdural hemorrhage and traumatic subarachnoid hemorrhage. (C) Early postoperative CT scan following neurosurgical evacuation of the acute subdural hemorrhage with further interval establishing demarcation of the left posterior cerebral artery territory ischemic changes (*arrows*).
22-year-old male victim of gunshot injuries to the head. (D) CT scan on soft tissue brain algorithm demonstrates gunshot injury entry wound (*curved white arrow*) and hemorrhagic bullet wound track through the left frontal lobe (*black arrow*) with associated extra-axial as well as intra-axial hemorrhage and cranial exit wound (*curved broken white arrow*) in the left temple region. (E) CT scan on bone algorithm better demonstrates the location of the bullet (*broken straight arrow*) in relation to the penetrating bullet entry wound and associated skull fractures at entry site (*curved arrow*). (F) CT scanogram confirms the second penetrating bullet injury of the sinonasal-facial region extracranially with second deformed bullet evident (*straight arrow*) in addition to the other cranial bullet (*curved arrow*).

fractures increases the risk of meningeal tear and dural vessel injury. Fractures of the skull vault have been classified as linear, stellate, and depressed, with the majority being linear. On occasion, these can cause diagnostic uncertainty when they simulate or are simulated by normal vascular channels. In general, vascular grooves are less lucent and less sharply marginated, and are seen to branch and make curves rather than sharp angles.

Fractures traversing a dural venous sinus or the jugular bulb have been shown in approximately two-thirds of cases to be associated with underlying venous injury, either by compressive extra-axial hematoma, and/or thrombosis [31–34]. Sutures should be inspected for diastasis secondary to fracture extension.

Basic skull base anatomy is covered in the dedicated skull base chapter.

TABLE 88.1 Major Associated Complications of Skull Base Fractures [24]

- Anterior skull base (ASB)
  - Intraorbital injury
  - Sinonasal CSF leak/meningoencephalocele
  - CN I injury
  - Epistaxis from ethmoidal artery injury
- Central skull base (CSB)
  - Vascular injury—ICA occlusion, dissection, pseudoaneurysm, aneurysm, carotid-cavernous fistula
  - CN II–VI injury
- Temporal bone/Lateral skull base (LSB)
  - ICA injury
  - CN VII–VIII injury
  - Mastoid CSF leak/meningoencephalocele
- Posterior skull base (PSB)
  - Venous injury
  - Vertebrobasilar injury
  - CN IX–XII injury
  - Craniocervical junction and C spine injury

CN, Cranial Nerve.

Introduction to Skull Base Trauma

The skull base is fractured in up to 16% of nonpenetrating head injuries [24,35]. This typically occurs in high-velocity trauma such as motor vehicle accidents. Significant complications associated with skull base fractures are listed in Table 88.1 [24]. The radiologist needs to be able to recognize and report these injuries as their presence is a key factor in decision making regarding skull base fracture management.

Anterior Skull Base (ASB) Fractures

Anterior skull base fractures are most commonly due to blunt direct trauma to the frontal region.

The osseous structures at specific risk are the frontal sinus, cribriform plate, fovea ethmoidalis (Fig. 88.10A), lesser wing of sphenoid, and planum sphenoidale.

The complications most associated with anterior skull base fractures are intraorbital injuries, sinonasal CSF leak, meningoencephalocele (Fig. 88.10A–C), and olfactory nerve injury. Severe epistaxis is also a potential complication due to injury to the anterior or posterior ethmoid arteries within their foramina in the lateral margins of the ethmoid bone [24].

Olfactory Nerve Injury

Fracture of the cribriform plate may involve the olfactory grooves within, leading to olfactory nerve injury and anosmia. This is reported in up to 7% of anterior skull base fractures. Approximately 10% of cases spontaneously recover function in the long term [36].

CSF Leak

Traumatic CSF leak has been reported in 10–30% of skull base fractures [24,37,38]. This occurs due to skull base fracture with an associated tear of the underlying dura causing CSF from the subarachnoid space to enter the nasal cavity via the paranasal sinuses. The fluid is usually clear, colorless, and contains glucose. The presentation may be delayed by initial edema and hemorrhage or may occur late due to chronic, progressive, dural breach by fracture fragments [24,39]. The most concerning complication in CSF leak is an increased risk of meningitis from intracranial communication with the sinonasal flora.

Most CSF leaks resolve spontaneously with conservative bed rest, head elevation, and stool softeners. Some may require lumbar or external ventricular drainage, and persistent leaks are an

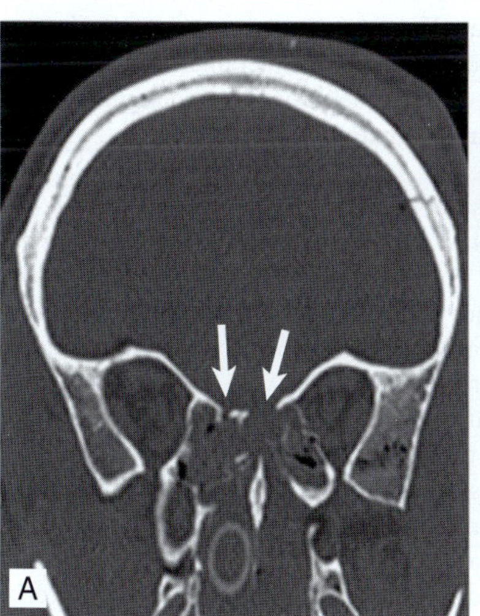

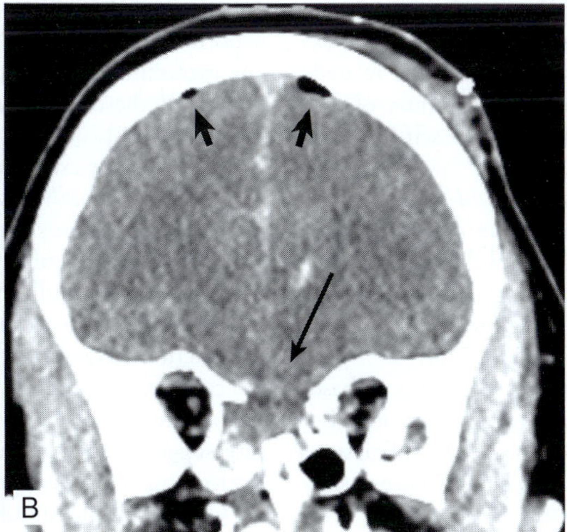

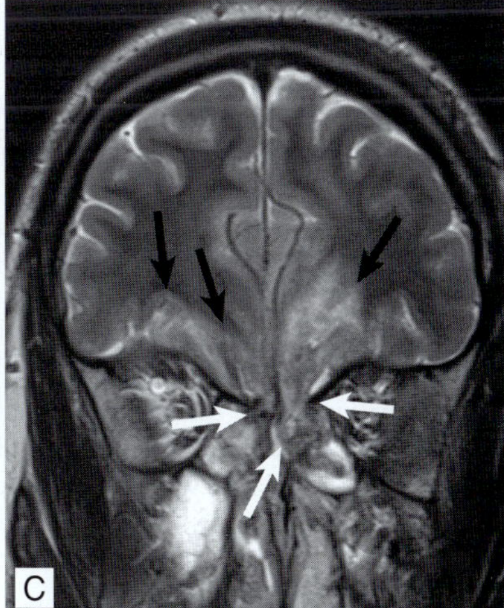

Figure 88.10 31-year-old male driver in high-speed motor vehicle collision—car versus tree. (A) Coronal CT scan image on bone windows shows severe anterior skull base fracture disruption and traumatic dehiscence (*white arrows*). (B) Coronal CT scan image demonstrates associated severe frontal/subfrontal brain parenchymal injury associated with the anterior skull base traumatic disruption and associated traumatic cephalocoele (*long thin black arrow*). Secondary extra-axial pneumocephalus is present (*short black arrows*). (C) subsequent early MRI brain scan—coronal T2-weighted image demonstrates the extent of traumatic cephalocoele of traumatized subfrontal brain parenchyma (*white arrows*) present bilaterally but more marked on the left; the patient had developed CSF leak by this time also. The abnormal subfrontal brain parenchymal signal changes consistent with traumatic damage are also evident (*black arrows*).

indication for surgery [24,40]. Radiological features correlating with a persistent leak likely to require surgical repair include defect size >1.5 cm, severe fracture comminution, and meningoencephalocele [24,41].

Frontal Sinus

Frontal bone fractures from a direct anterior impact frequently involve the anterior table of the frontal sinus and may extend further to the posterior table. Fracture of the posterior table with an underlying dural tear is associated with a risk of CSF leak and meningitis [24].

When there is fracture of the floor of the frontal sinus the frontal sinus outflow tract/frontal recess should be carefully interrogated for injury. Complications of outflow tract injury include frontal sinus mucocele, osteomyelitis, and intracranial infection including brain abscess [42,43].

Outflow tract injury is also important in determining surgical management. Fractures of the anterior table of the frontal sinus can be repaired with plates and screws if the outflow tract is preserved. In severe injury to the drainage pathway, frontal sinus cranialization is performed and the outflow tract is removed. In frontal sinus cranialization, the sinus mucosa is removed, preventing the development of mucocele and mucopyocele [43–45].

Central Skull Base (CSB) Fractures

Fractures of the central skull base are frequently posterior extensions of anterior skull base fractures, or transverse fractures from lateral high-impact trauma to the temporal, parietal, zygomatic, and/or lateral frontal bones [24].

Complications

Intracranial: Since CSB fractures are often due to high-velocity injuries intracranial hemorrhage (especially temporal lobe contusions) and TAI is a common association [24].

Vascular: Fractures of the clivus, orbital apex, petrous ridge, occiput, and occipital condyles are the skull base injuries most commonly associated with BCVI [46].

Anterior Middle Cranial Fossa Epidural Hematoma: The anterior middle cranial fossa extradural hematoma (also referred to as "benign venous epidural hematoma") is a specific finding related to fracture of the greater wing of sphenoid, due to injury of the sphenoparietal venous sinus, and generally follows a self-limiting course [9].

Carotid-Cavernous Fistula: *Post-traumatic carotid-cavernous fistula is a rare but important vascular complication of central skull base trauma.* Clinical presentation is with exophthalmos, orbital bruit, chemosis, visual loss, and ophthalmoplegia. There is a risk of blindness, stroke, and death, re-emphasising the importance of CTA in patients with central skull base fractures [24,47].

Cranial Nerve and Sympathetic Chain Injury: Central skull base fractures are associated with cranial nerve injury which may be acute from laceration, or delayed from traction or edema. Fracture involvement of a relevant skull base foramen should raise suspicion for cranial nerve injury [24].

Orbital apex fractures may cause optic (II) nerve injury through entrapment or compressive hematoma [24,48].

Injury to the cavernous sinus can affect cranial nerves III, IV, V1, V2, and/or VI which traverse within the sinus and its lateral wall.

An incomplete Horner syndrome (ptosis and meiosis) can arise from injury to the postganglionic sympathetic chain near the ICA, in fractures of the carotid canal or near Meckel's cave. This syndrome can also occur if damage occurs to the sympathetic chain within the neck adjacent to the carotid space from cervical carotid artery dissection [24].

CSF Leak: CSF leak is less common in central than in anterior skull base fractures. This is more frequently seen in transversely oriented fractures [49].

Clival Involvement: Fracture involvement of the clivus is relatively uncommon, however, is associated with high mortality, (reportedly 24–80%) related to its proximity to the brainstem and risk of significant neurological and vascular injury [50].

Transverse clival fractures are more commonly associated with cranial nerve and internal carotid artery injuries. Longitudinal clival fractures are usually associated with vertebrobasilar arterial injury, brainstem ischemia, and injury to the craniocervical junction. A traumatic VI nerve palsy may occur in clival fractures due to involvement of the Dorello canal, located at the posteromedial part of the petrous apex [24].

Posterior Skull Base (PSB) Fractures

Posterior skull base fractures arise most commonly from posterior or posterolateral impact to the occiput and can involve the posterior clivus (basiocciput) [24].

Occipital condyle fractures occur although are relatively uncommon. The most widely used classification system (Anderson and Montesano), divides these into three types dependent on imaging appearance on imaging and probable mechanism of injury [24,51].

- Type 1 is condylar impaction with comminution due to an axial load
- Type 2 is a posterior skull base fracture extending in linear fashion into the condyle
- Type 3 is an avulsion fracture at the attachment site of the alar ligament

Complications

Intracranial and Vascular: Posterior skull base fractures have a reported high incidence of associated intracranial injury, including extradural, subdural, and cerebellar intraparenchymal hematoma. Of these, extradural hematomas occur with the greatest frequency [24].

Posterior fossa extradural hematomas are generally venous in origin. These can rapidly expand and cause sudden neurological deterioration due to compression of the fourth ventricle and/or brainstem. They are the result of injury to the transverse or sigmoid venous sinus or jugular bulb. Surgical decompression is indicated for large hematomas with mass effect [52].

Fractures extending into the jugular foramen or venous sinuses or can lead to venous thrombosis [53]. On noncontrast CT examination, the venous sinuses should be reviewed for hyperdensity suggestive of clot, and there should be a low threshold for performing a CT venogram [24].

Consideration should be given to vertebrobasilar arterial injury when there is fracture of the clivus at the basiocciput and the occipital condyles. CT angiography and an MRI of the C spine should be performed [24,54].

Cranial Nerve: The lower cranial nerves IX–XII are at risk of injury in fractures of the posterior skull base. Hypoglossal nerve palsy can also occur as a result of internal carotid artery traumatic dissection injury below the skull base.

Key Points for Skull Base Trauma
- A knowledge of skull base anatomy is vital to understand the structures involved in fractures and potential complications
- Anterior skull base fractures carry a potential risk of CSF leak and meningitis
- Frontal sinus fractures involving the posterior table may require frontal sinus cranialization to prevent mucocoele and mucopyocoele
- There is a particularly high risk of BCVI and carotid-cavernous fistula in central skull base fractures and CT angiography should be performed
- Posterior skull base fractures may be associated with extradural hematomata and compression of the fourth ventricle and brainstem

Temporal Bone Trauma

Introduction

Temporal bone injury is reported in 3–22% of patients with skull fracture. The most common mechanisms include motor vehicle accident, physical assault, and fall [55,56].

The identification of temporal bone trauma and complications is usually made on the unenhanced (noncontrast) CT undertaken for evaluation of general head trauma using a slice thickness of less than 1 mm.

The primary sign of temporal bone fracture is the presence of a fracture line. Secondary signs that should raise suspicion include:
- *Opacification of the external auditory canal, mastoid air cells, and middle ear cavity*
- *Air within the intracranial compartment adjacent to the temporal bone, within the labyrinth and the temporomandibular joint*

Temporal Bone Fracture Classification

Temporal bone fractures have traditionally been classified as transverse, longitudinal, or mixed with respect to the long axis of the petrous temporal bone.
- Longitudinal fractures are more common at 50–80% with transverse fracture comprising 10–20%
- Transverse fractures are more commonly associated with facial nerve injury near the internal auditory meatus or at the labyrinthine segment
- Longitudinal fractures are less commonly associated with facial nerve injury, and if nerve injury is present this is often at the geniculate ganglion [55–57]

In more modern practice, violation of the otic capsule has been shown to be of greater clinical relevance than *fracture orientation, with better prediction of the complications of sensorineural hearing loss, intracranial, vascular, and facial nerve injury* [58–61]. It is recommended that reports include the direction and location of the fracture, and whether or not the otic capsule is involved [55].

Complications

Hearing Loss (CHL and SNHL) and Vertigo

Hearing loss: Hearing loss is the most frequent complication of temporal bone trauma and may be conductive, sensorineural, or mixed [55,61].

Causes of traumatic conductive hearing loss (CHL) include perforation of the tympanic membrane (TM), hemotympanum, and ossicular disruption. If persistent for more than 6 weeks, an ossicular chain injury should be suspected [55,62,63].

Sensorineural hearing loss (SNHL) is due to involvement of the otic capsule or cochlear nerve. Traumatic SNHL may be due to fractures violating the labyrinth or the cochlear nerve within the internal auditory canal (IAC) or intralabyrinth hemorrhage (with or without fracture).

Presence of pneumolabyrinth is an important secondary sign of otic capsule-violation (Fig. 88.11A and B) which should be considered to indicate a fracture in the absence of an identifiable line on imaging. Labyrinthitis ossificans is a longer-term complication which may be identifiable on CT (labyrinthine calcification) and MR imaging (loss of normal labyrinthine signal).

Vertigo: Vertigo may occur due to fracture of the vestibule, semicircular canals, vestibular aqueduct or vestibular nerve, from labyrinthine concussion, nerve root entry zone shearing injury, brainstem injury, perilymphatic fistulae and disruption of otoliths. Vertigo generally self resolves at 6–12 months post-trauma in the majority [64].

Axial CT is most useful for evaluation of the labyrinth and fracture of the vestibular structures. Stenvers and Poschl reconstructions (parallel and perpendicular to the long axis of the petrous bone) can help as the posterior and superior semicircular canals are viewed in profile.

Ossicular Injury

Ossicular injuries (Fig. 88.12A and B) include ossicular joint dislocation and ossicular fracture. Ossicular injuries are more

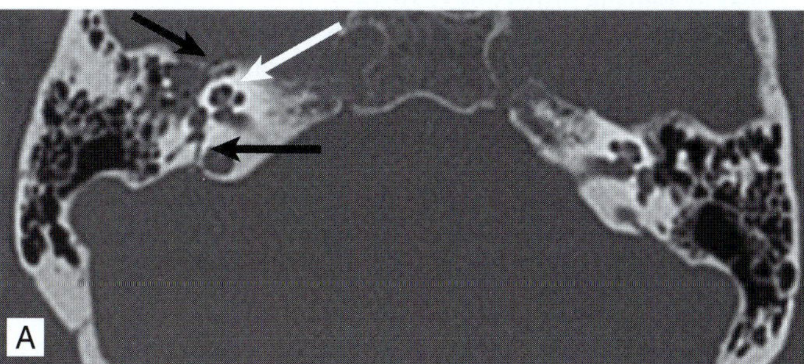

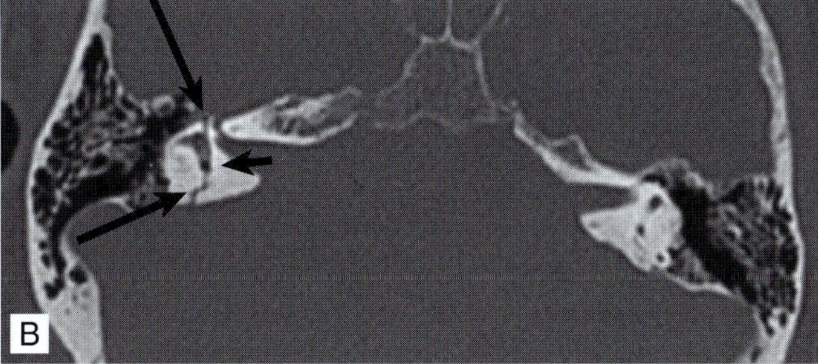

Figure 88.11 82-year-old female pedestrian struck by car. (A) CT scan demonstrates right otic-involving transverse petrous temporal bone fracture extending through the posterior semicircular canal and vestibule (*black arrows*). Note the hemotympanum. Also, note right cochlea pneumolabyrinth—small locules of gas in the right cochlear labyrinth secondary to the otic-involving fracture (*white arrow*). (B) CT scan demonstrates fracture extension through the right lateral semicircular canal and toward the labyrinthine segment of the right facial nerve and geniculate ganglion (*long black arrows*); pneumolabyrinth is present (*short black arrow*).

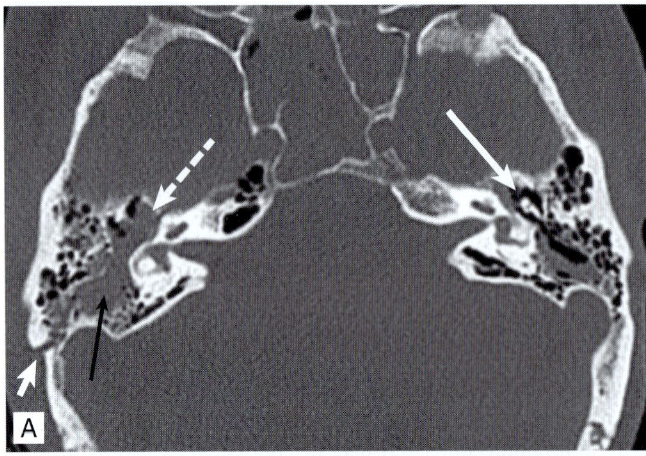

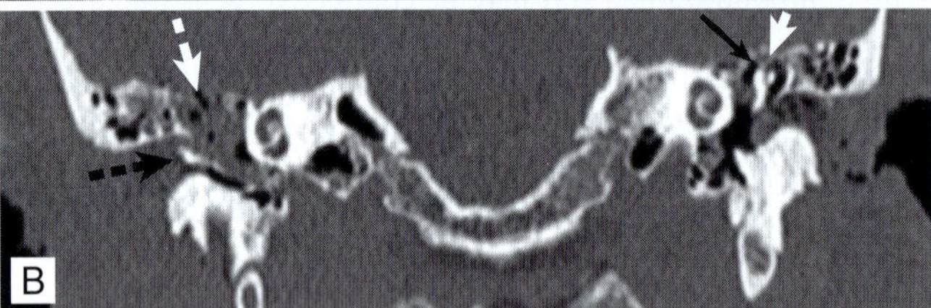

Figure 88.12 72-year-old male pedestrian struck by cyclist. (A) CT scan demonstrates mixed right temporal bone fracture with compete loss of right ossicular integrity—the right incus and malleus are completely absent from normal location (*broken white arrow*)—compare with normal *left side* (*long thick white arrow*). There is hemotympanum (and middle ear cavity perilymph) (*long thin black arrow*). One of the right petrous temporal bone fracture lines is demonstrated (*short white arrow*). (B) coronal CT image—the normal left incudo-mallear articulation is evident (*short white arrow*) compared with absence of the incus and malleus from their normal location on the right (*broken white arrow*). The right malleus is dislocated, and inferiorly and laterally displaced into the medial bony right external auditory canal and contiguous lateral aspect of the inferior mesotympanum (*broken black arrow*) compared with the normal location of the left malleus (*long thin solid black arrow*). The stapes were also dislocated from the oval window (not shown) resulting in a perilymph fistula.

common in longitudinal fractures than in transverse, and dislocations are more common than fractures.

Ossicular Dislocation: *The incudostapedial joint is reported to be the most common site of ossicular dislocation* [65].

The next most common dislocation is of the incudomalleolar joint (shown as separation of the "ice cream" (head of malleus) and "ice cream cone" (body and short process of incus).

Complete incus dislocation is present when there is both incudostapedial and incudomalleolar joint dislocation [64].

Dislocation of the stapedial footplate is rare and may be associated with perilymphatic fistula (PLF) formation at the oval window [65].

Ossicular Fractures: *The most frequently fractured ossicle is the incus (especially at the long process),* followed by the crura of the stapes. The malleus is the least frequently fractured ossicle [66].

Treatment: TM perforation, hemotympanum, and minor ossicle subluxation often spontaneously resolve and are treated conservatively. If CHL persists beyond 6 months surgical repair of the ossicular chain may be indicated [55,67].

Perilymphatic Fistula

PLF occurs due to formation of an abnormal communication between the perilymph and middle ear cavity (Fig. 88.12A and B). Post-traumatic PLF may occur with injury to the oval or round window [68].

Symptoms of persistent vertigo and intermittent SNHL and/or CHL begin within 24–72 hours postinjury. PLF should be considered with fractures through the stapes footplate or round window on CT. Secondary signs in absence of a temporal bone fracture include pneumolabyrinth and unexplained dependent fluid in the middle ear [55,69].

CSF Leak

Temporal bone fractures with underlying dural injury are associated with risk of CSF leak and meningitis, particularly if involvement of the tegmen tympani, tegmen mastoideum, or posterior petrous ridge. This can present as otorrhea via the TM or rhinorrhea via eustachian tube drainage (where the TM is intact). CSF leak is more commonly seen in otic capsule-violating fractures than in those where the capsule is spared [55,58,59].

Imaging Findings: Coronal and sagittal reconstructions are best for CT assessment of the tegmen. Reports should include location and size of any defect, orientation of displaced fragments through the defect, and presence of an encephalocele.

Factors increasing the risk of persistent CSF leak include widely spaced fracture defect and a bony spicule oriented perpendicularly to the dura.

MRI of the temporal bone with high-resolution T2WI and postcontrast T1WI of the temporal bone can be performed to look for the location and size of any encephalocele, and demonstrate dural enhancement as secondary signs of dural tear, CSF leak, and focal meningitis [55,70].

Treatment: Most post-traumatic CSF leaks self-resolve within 7 days with conservative management. If persistent CSF leak beyond day 10 surgical closure may be performed [70].

Facial Nerve Injury and Canal Fractures

Due to its long course through the temporal bone, the facial nerve is at risk of injury at multiple points. Identifiable injury is considered relatively uncommon [55,70–72].

Facial nerve palsy is more commonly associated with otic capsule-violating fractures. Otic capsule-sparing fractures are, however, the more frequent subtype and so the majority of cases are seen in this subgroup [70]. Fractures of the canal are also more common in transverse fractures than longitudinal fractures [73].

The most common sites of injury are the distal labyrinthine segment, at the geniculate ganglion, and the intracanalicular (IAC) segment (Fig. 88.13) [64].

Compression of the nerve by a fracture fragment may be visible and is important to identify as it is likely to be treatable by early surgical management. High-resolution MRI can demonstrate perineural hematoma, and abnormal enhancement may be seen in scarring or fibrosis [55,74].

Treatment: Optimal management is a controversial topic. Delayed onset palsy has relatively good prognosis without surgery. Surgery may be utilized in complete, immediate paralysis, or cases of progressive loss of function. Aims of surgery are to evaluate and decompress the facial nerve, and may involve nerve rerouting, re-anastomosis, or sural nerve graft [55].

Vascular Injury

A previous series found that 24% of skull base fractures show carotid canal involvement and 11% of fractures were positive for vascular injury [75] and a fracture extending through the carotid canal requires CT angiography to assess for vascular injury [55].

There is a risk of venous injury and CT venogram should be performed in fractures involving the jugular foramen or traversing the sinuses [55].

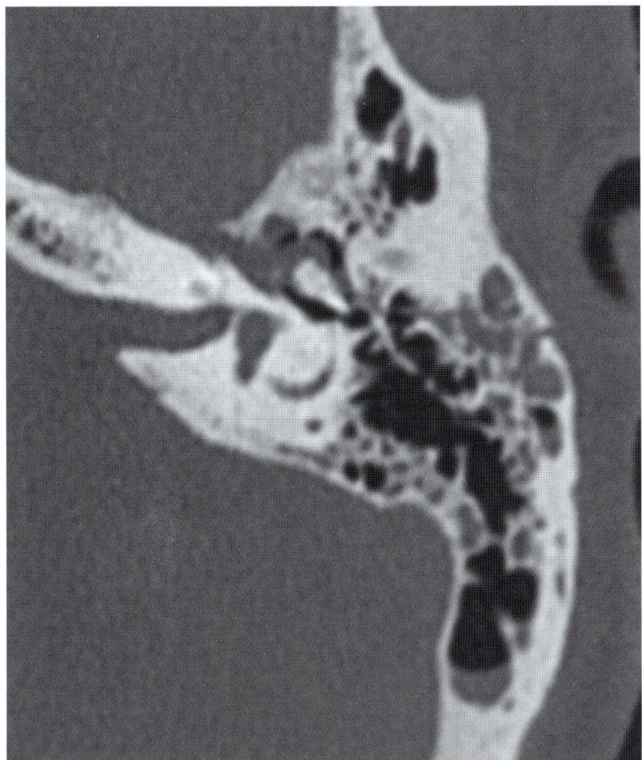

Figure 88.13 Temporal bone fracture. 56-year-old male cyclist postmotor vehicle collision. Axial CT of the left temporal bone demonstrates a complex/mixed temporal bone fracture with extension into the left geniculate ganglion.

Key Points for Temporal Bone Trauma

- Air within the intracranial compartment near the temporal bone, and within the labyrinth should raise suspicion for occult temporal bone fracture in the absence of a visualized fracture line
- Facial nerve injury is more common in transverse temporal bone fractures than longitudinal. Otic capsule-violation are a better predictor of complications than fracture orientation. It is suggested that fracture location, orientation, and otic capsule status are reported
- The incus is the most commonly fracture ossicle, and the incudo-stapedial joint is the most common site of dislocation
- Fractures of the tegmen tympani, tegmen mastoideum, and posterior petrous ridge place the patient at risk of CSF leak and meningitis
- Fractures of the carotid canal warrant intracranial CT angiography to assess for internal carotid artery injury

Facial Trauma—Midface, Orbits, Nasoseptal, and Mandible

Introduction

Facial fractures can be complex, traversing multiple bones and foramina, potentially daunting for the reporting radiologist. There are, however, several key fracture configurations that commonly occur and have specific clinical and surgical relevance. Knowledge of these can act as a basis for reporting more complex fractures and make the process more straightforward.

Midface Fractures

Zygomatico–Maxillary Complex (ZMC) Fractures

Zygomatico–Maxillary complex or tetrapod fractures are the second most common category of midface fracture (Fig. 88.14) [76]. These were previously incorrectly referred to as "tripod" fractures given the visualization of only three of the four key components on plain radiograph [77].

The four core sites are as follows:

- Lateral orbital rim
- Inferior orbital rim
- Zygomatic arch
- Zygomaticomaxillary buttress (the lateral vertical facial buttress, extending from the alveolar process of the maxilla inferiorly through the body and zygomatic process of maxilla, the zygoma, and lateral orbital wall to the frontozygomatic suture)

Given that part of the lateral orbital wall and floor arise from the zygomatic bone, orbital volume may be increased or decreased as a result of displacement and/or rotation of the ZMC fragment, with the risk of facial asymmetry and enophthalmos [43,78]. Depression of the zygomatic arch can lead to restriction in mouth opening due to compression of the masticatory muscles or impingement of the mandibular coronoid [77,79].

Grading systems such as the Zingg classification have been suggested which increase in severity from incomplete ZMC fractures not involving all four limbs (A), to classic tetrapod (B) through to severe comminution (C). CT fracture grade and surgical findings of fracture instability have been found to correlate [43,80].

Le Fort Fractures

Le Fort fractures are craniofacial dissociation injuries. The classically described core component in these is fracture of the pterygoid plates, which form the posterior maxillary buttress and interface between the skull base (sphenoid) and midface [77].

René Le Fort described the classification following cadaveric experiments demonstrating commonly occurring fracture patterns after blunt facial trauma [81]. While many facial fractures do not

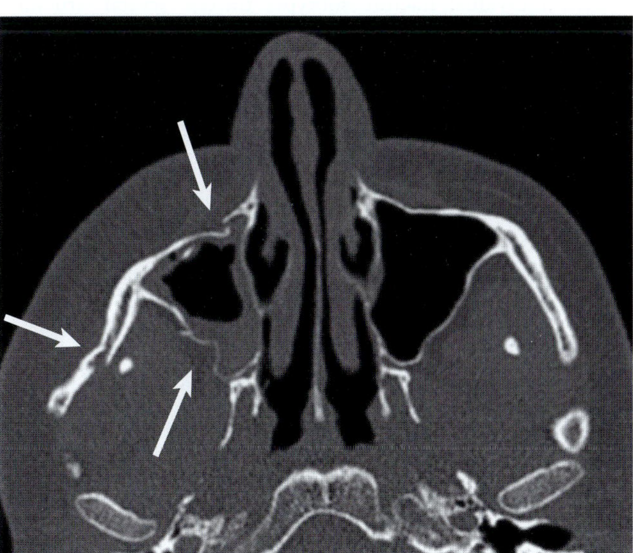

Figure 88.14 36-year-old male victim of alleged assault. CT scan demonstrates right zygomatico–maxillary complex fracture (fractures of the complex annotated with *white arrows*).

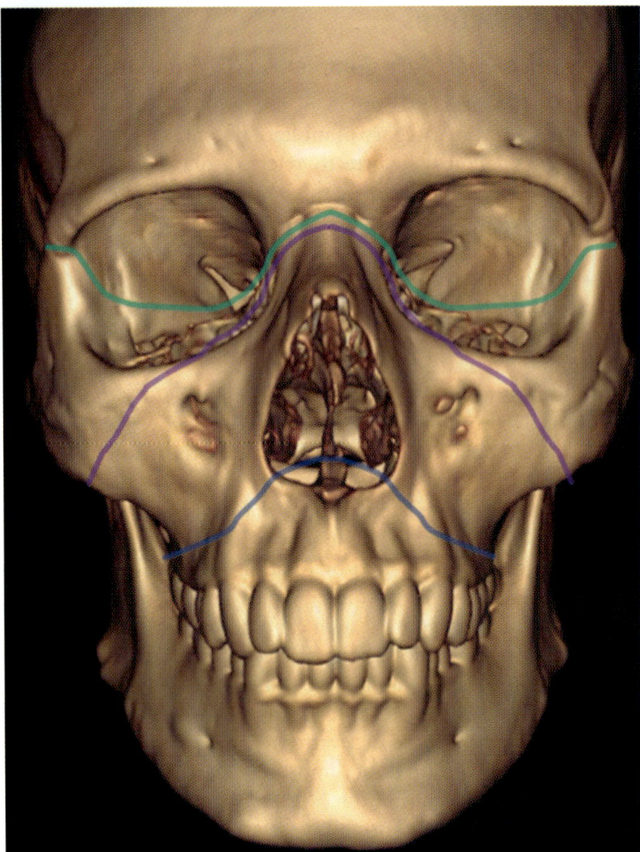

Figure 88.15 Le Fort classification. Frontal volume-rendered reconstructions of a normal CT of the facial bones demonstrating the Le Fort Fracture Classification. The morphology of each fracture type is demonstrated (I = Blue, II = Purple, III = Green). Le Fort type I injuries involve the nasal pyriform aperture, type II injuries involve the inferior orbital rim, and type III injuries involve the lateral orbital wall and zygomatic arch.

fit simply into the Le Fort classification, it remains useful as a common descriptive language between radiologists, emergency physicians, and maxillofacial surgeons [43,82].

The individual fracture subtypes traverse several structures, however, use of a single key component can help simplify recognition of the distinction between Le Fort I–III injuries (Figs. 88.15 and 16A) [77,83].

- Le Fort I—Floating Palate—Lateral and medial walls of maxillary sinus with posterior extension to the piriform aperture. *Single key component: nasal piriform aperture (the anterior bony nasal opening formed superiorly by the nasal bone and laterally and inferiorly by the maxilla).*
- Le Fort II—Floating Maxilla—Pyramidal fractures involving the frontonasal suture, inferior orbital rim/floor, and maxillary sinuses. *Single key component: inferior orbital rim.*
- Le Fort III—Floating Face—Frontonasal suture to frontozygomatic suture and zygomatic arch. Often a combination of ZMC and naso-orbito-ethmoidal (NOE) fracture. *Single key component: zygomatic arch.*

Combinations of the Le Fort subtypes can be present on the same side of the face.

Le Fort II and III represent severe injuries and a CT angiogram of the neck to vertex is advised to screen for blunt vascular injury.

Nasoseptal Fractures

The nasal bones are the most commonly fractured facial bones (Fig. 88.17) [76].

Anatomically the bony nasal structure consists of the two nasal bones, frontal bone and frontal processes of the maxilla.

Correction of deformity is aimed at restoring a normal nasal pathway and avoiding turbulent flow which can be a risk factor for sinusitis [77,84].

Sinusitis may occur as a complication of fracture fragment displacement into the maxillary sinus.

Naso-Orbito-Ethmoid Fracture (NOE)

Extension of proximal nasal bone fractures to the frontal bone, cribriform plate, midface, and orbit gives rise to an NOE-type fracture. Intracranial and orbital injuries are more frequently associated NOE fractures and intracranial imaging is usually warranted (Fig. 88.16B). NOE fractures usually occur in combination with other facial fractures [85].

The major feature of NOE fracture is that a central NOE fracture fragment is separated along at least four of five fracture lines. These are referred to as "cardinal tracts" and are as follows:

- Lateral nose and piriform aperture
- Nasomaxillary buttress

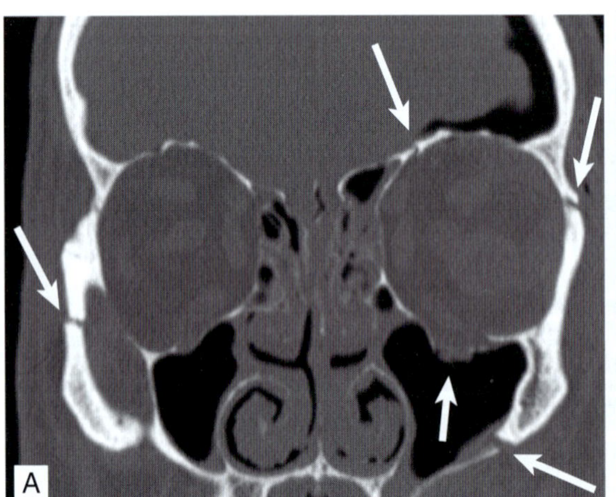

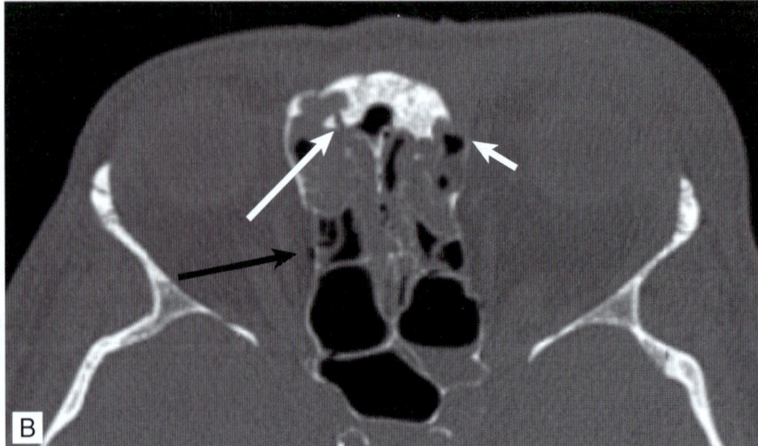

Figure 88.16 59-year-old male who fell on face due to collapse. (A) CT scan showed mixed left and right hemi-Le Fort I, II, and III fractures and left orbital floor fracture—some of the typical fracture line sites of Le Fort fractures are shown (*white arrows*) but not all. (B) CT scan of the same patient also demonstrates some fracture changes related to left naso-orbito-ethmoidal complex fracture (*short white arrow*) and right fronto-nasal duct fracture (*long white arrows*). Right orbital emphysema (*black arrow*) is shown associated with right medial orbital wall fractures.

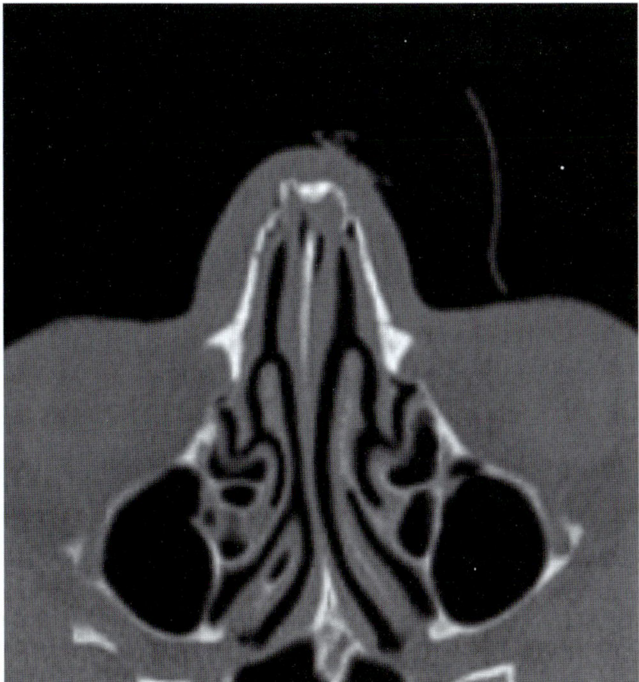

Figure 88.17 Nasal fractures. 35-year-old female following a fall onto face. Axial CT of the facial bones demonstrates displaced fractures of the nasal bones bilaterally with associated external subdermal nasal soft tissue swelling and injury and fracture of the bony nasal septum (not shown) and associated septal mucosal and submucosal gas secondary to intranasal septal mucosal laceration.

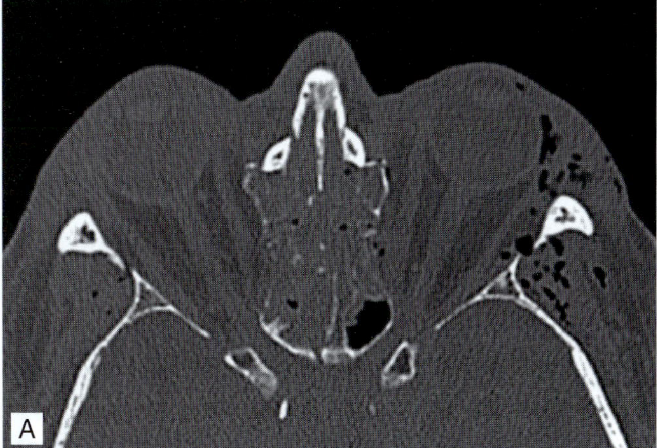

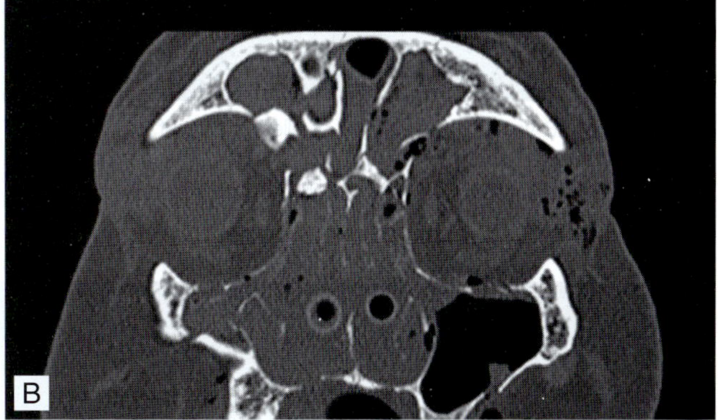

Figure 88.18 NOE fracture. 65-year-old male following a fall from height. Axial (A) and coronal (B) CT of the facial bones demonstrates severe complex bilateral facial fractures including a bilateral naso-orbito-ethmoid fracture. There is comminution and displacement at the medial NOE fracture component bilaterally. There are also fractures involving the orbital walls, anterior skull base, maxillary sinuses and hard palate.

- Inferior orbital rim/floor
- Medial orbital wall
- Frontomaxillary suture

The central NOE fragment is the insertion site for the medial canthal tendon, the stability of which is a key factor in operative decision-making. Although the tendon itself is not visible on CT, severe comminution of the medial orbital wall is a useful imaging sign suggesting compromised stability (Fig. 88.18).

Other complications associated with NOE fractures are impairment of lacrimal and mucociliary drainage through injury to the nasolacrimal duct, frontonasal duct (frontal recess), and frontal sinuses. The involvement of these influences surgical management and they should be reported [43].

Orbital Fractures

Blow-Out Fracture

The term "blow-out" fracture is used where there is enlargement of orbital volume due to fracture of the medial orbital wall and/or floor with outward fracture displacement. The medial orbital wall and floor are relatively weaker than the lateral wall and roof and are hence more commonly fractured in primary orbital fractures. The orbital rim itself is usually spared.

Primary orbital fractures are associated with higher risk of globe and optic nerve injury than the orbital extension of other local facial fractures. Other risks include enophthalmos from the increased orbital volume, and herniation of soft tissues through fracture defects (Fig. 88.19A and B). Diplopia may occur due to fat and/or muscular herniation and entrapment, and smaller fracture size is a useful predictor (soft tissue entrapment is more commonly associated with small and medium-size orbital floor fractures rather than large defects [86]). *Of note, the extra-ocular muscles do not specifically need to be incarcerated for there to be clinical entrapment. The sheaths of these muscles are connected to fibrous septae within the orbital fat and therefore herniation of any soft tissue should be flagged in the report* (Fig. 88.19B).

Blow-In Fracture

Blow-in fractures where there is orbital volume reduction from fracture fragments prolapsing into the orbit are less common [77].

Orbital Roof Fractures

Orbital roof fractures frequently are part of more extensive anterior skull base fractures and may be associated with the risk of intracranial injury, CSF leak, and/or traumatic meningoencephalocele as well as intraorbital subperiosteal hematoma related to the orbital roof (Fig. 88.20). These are discussed further in the intracranial and skull base trauma sections [77].

Orbital Soft Tissue Injuries

Soft tissue injuries identified on CT include optic nerve injury, anterior chamber hemorrhage, corneal laceration (with anterior iris prolapse), lens dislocation, globe rupture/open globe injury (Fig. 88.21), retinal detachment (Fig. 88.22), and intraorbital foreign body [87].

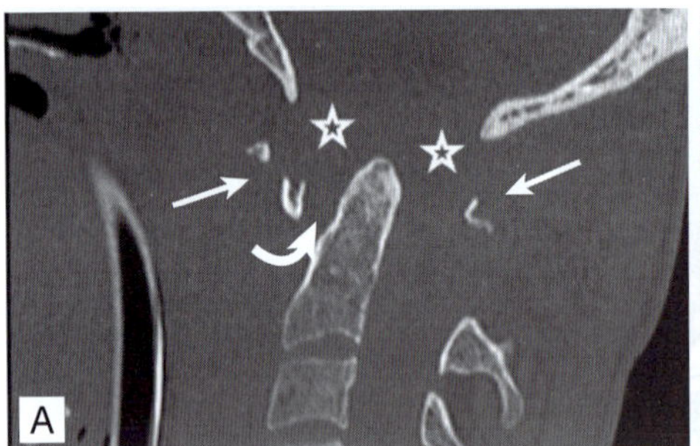

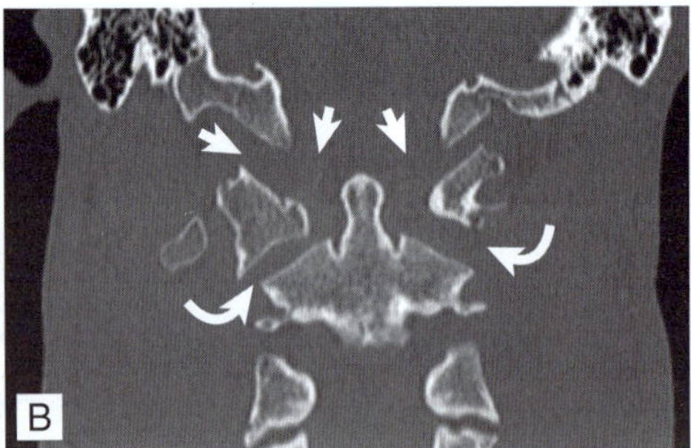

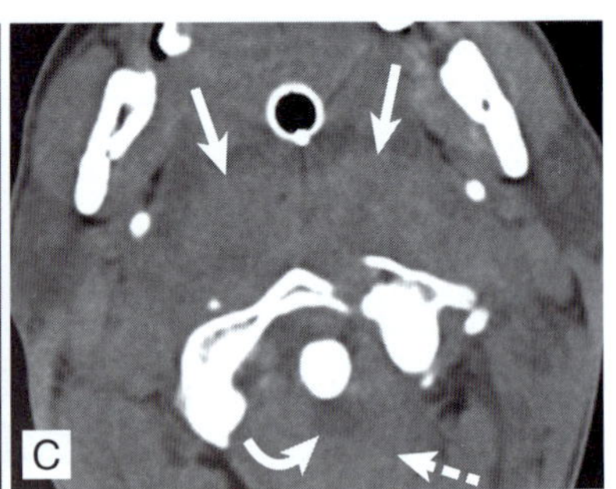

Figure 88.26 31-year-old male cyclist in collision with car. (A) Sagittal CT reconstruction on bone algorithm demonstrates severe atlanto-axial fracture-dissociation mechanism with fracture and distraction-subluxation evident. Note the abnormally widened relationship (*white stars*) between basion/opisthion and the C1 vertebral fracture elements (*long thin arrow*) and the C2 odontoid process (peg) and the abnormally widened atlanto-dental interval (*curved white arrow*). (B) Coronal CT reconstruction on bone algorithm demonstrated the atlanto-occipital distraction (*short arrows*) and fracture injury as well as atlanto-axial fracture-subluxation (*curved arrows*). (C) Axial CT reconstruction on soft tissue windows demonstrates large volume prevertebral hematoma (*straight solid arrows*), the presence of posterior atlanto-occipital hematoma (*broken white arrow*) associated with the craniocervical junction fracture-distraction injury and the relationship to the spinal cord (*curved white arrow*).

the axis or subaxial cervical spine [91,96]. The associated other C-spine fractures and integrity of the transverse ligament are the main factors in determining a need for surgery [89,91].

Atlas fractures are divided into five subtypes by the modified Jefferson classification. The most common patterns are type I and type III. Type II is rare.

- Type I fracture involves only the posterior arch
- Type II fracture involves only the anterior arch
- Type III is the classical *Jefferson burst fracture* with bilateral posterior arch fractures with unilateral or bilateral anterior arch fracture
- Type IV is fracture of the lateral mass
- Type V is a transverse fracture of the anterior arch [91,95,97]

Atlas fractures are predominantly a result of axial loading injuries [23,98]. Transverse ligament injury is a common association. An atlanto-dens interval of >3 mm in adults and >5 mm in children is highly suggestive of transverse ligament disruption and MRI assessment should be performed.

"Pseudospread" of the atlas is a normal variant on plain radiograph most commonly seen in children under 7 years of age and is due to the ossified lateral masses of the atlas being projected beyond the ossified articular surface of the axis [91,99].

Axis (C2) Fractures: Injuries to the axis comprise 17–20% of C-spine fractures [89,100]. The three main injury patterns are fractures of the odontoid, axis body, and hangman fracture [91,101].

Odontoid Fracture: This is the most common axis fracture. These are more common in elderly patients which may be due to a greater proportion of force being transmitted to the dens in the spondylotic spine.

Fractures of the dens are classified as types I–III by Anderson and D'Alonzo [102].

- Type I fractures through the upper part of the dens, are the least common. Nonoperative management with collar or halo immobilization leads to a fusion rate near 100%
- Type II fractures at the junction of the dens and the body of the axis are the most common. They are more susceptible to nonunion (probably due to a relatively poor blood supply at the dens-body junction) and may need surgical fusion

A subtype of Type II fracture is the IIa where "chip" fragments are present at the anterior and posterior aspect of the base of the dens

TABLE 88.2 Normal Measurements on CT at the Craniocervical Junction [89]

Interval	Plain Radiograph Cut-off Value	CT Cut-off Value	Ligaments Involved
Basion-Dens interval	12 mm	8.5–9.5 mm	Alar ligaments Tectorial membrane
Atlantodental interval	3 mm (men), 2.5 mm (women)	2 mm	Atlanto-occipital joint capsules Alar ligaments Tectorial membrane
Atlanto-occipital interval		4 mm (summed) or 2.5 mm (single atlanto-occipital interval)	Atlanto-occipital joint capsules Alar ligaments Tectorial membrane
Atlantoaxial interval		2.6–4.0 mm (midsagittal) 1.2 mm (lateral margins) 1 mm (posterior and anterior margins)	C1-C2 joint capsules Alar ligaments Tectorial membrane
Powers ratio*	Abnormal if >1.0	Abnormal if >1.0 (Anterior atlanto-occipital distraction)	Transverse ligament Atlanto-occipital joint capsules Tectorial membrane Alar ligament

*Powers Ratio: the distance measured from the tip of the basion to the posterior arch of C1 divided by the distance from the opisthion to the anterior arch of C1.

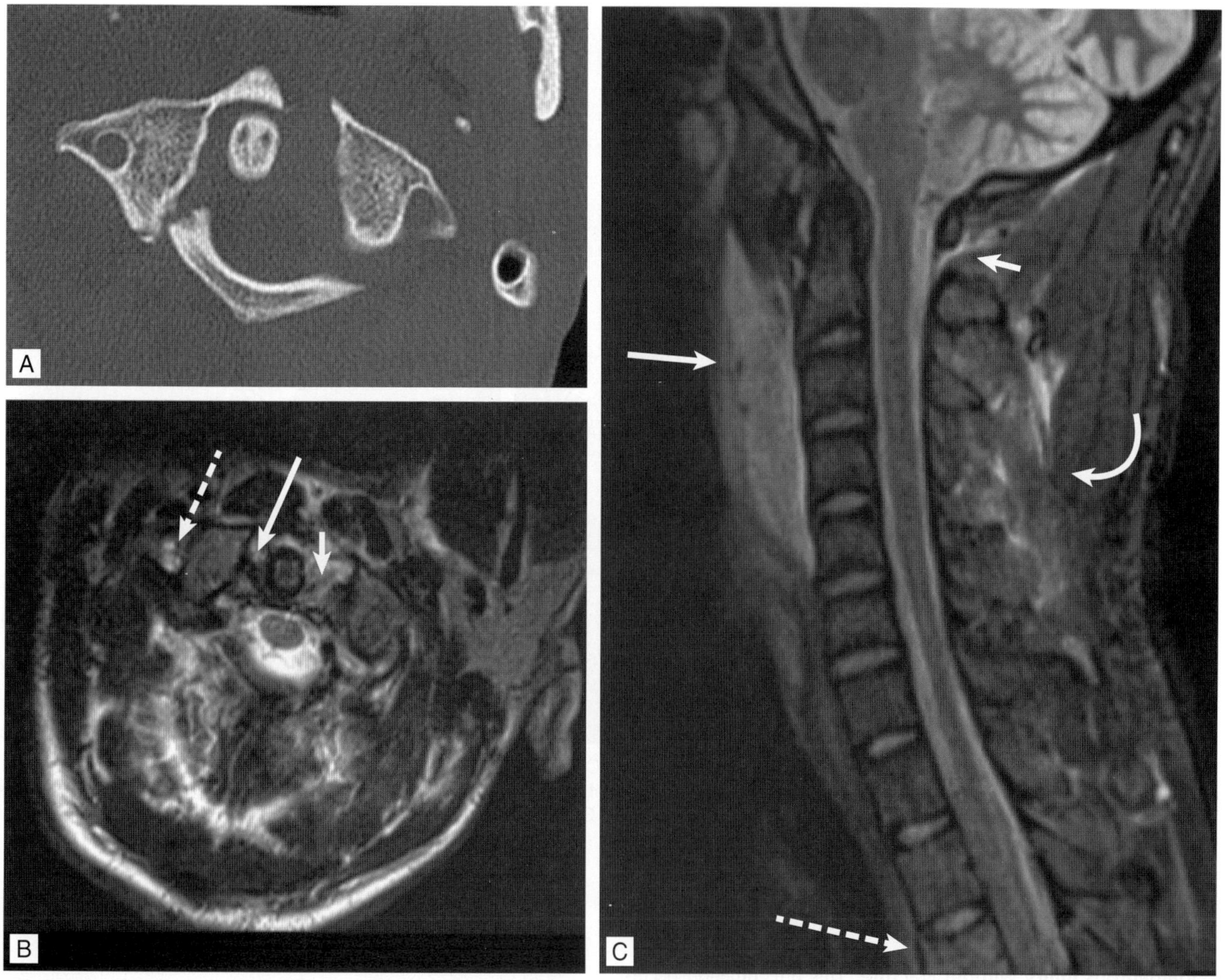

Figure 88.27 28-year-old male who fell from a height. (A) CT scan demonstrates Jefferson-type fracture of the atlas (C1 vertebra). Widened left lateral atlanto-dental interval in keeping with associated transverse ligament disruption. (B) Axial T2-weighted MR image through craniocervical junction of the same patient—the *left side* of the transverse atlantal ligament disruption is demonstrated (*short white arrow*)—compare with the intact *right side* of the ligament (*long white solid arrow*). Associated traumatic vascular dissection injury of the right vertebral artery is evident with loss of normal flow void at the level of the C1 lateral mass (*long white broken arrow*). (C) Sagittal STIR sequence demonstrates large prevertebral soft tissue hematoma (*long solid white arrow*), posterior atlanto-axial membrane injury (*short white arrow*), subaxial posterior ligamentous complex injury (*curved white arrow*) and abnormal marrow edema in keeping with compression injury of the T3 vertebral body on edge of the image (*long broken white arrow*).

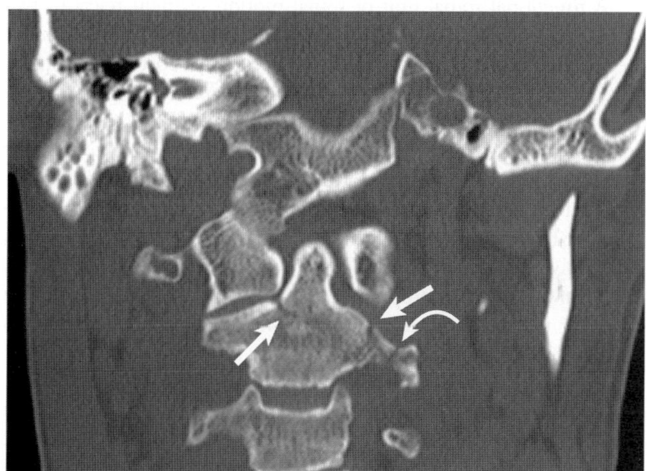

Figure 88.28 48-year-old male pedestrian struck by a car. Type 3 fracture of the C2 odontoid process (peg) is demonstrated (*straight white arrows*). There is also a fracture of the left lateral mass of the C2 vertebra (*curved white arrow*).

which lead to nonunion, and may require earlier surgical stabilization and fusion [91,103].

- Type III (Fig. 88.28) is the next most common and extend through the C2 body into its cancellous part. These are potentially unstable although there is healing with immobilization in 88% of cases

Hangman Fracture: These are bilateral pars interarticularis fractures of the axis although any part of the axis ring can be involved including lamina, pedicle, or posterior axis body (Fig. 88.29) [89,101]. They comprise 22% of axis fractures and 4% of all cervical fractures [89,104]. The fracture configuration was first described in 1913 in association with judicial hanging, however the "Hangman" name was only given to them in 1965, by which point it referred to the fractures mostly seen post-MVC due to severe, sudden deceleration injury, or after a fall [89,105,106]. If the patient has survived, spinal cord and nerve root injury are reported to be low due to the relative wide calibre of the canal at this level. The majority are treated with immobilization. The most severe distractive flexion injuries with bilateral facet dislocation require surgical stabilization [89,91].

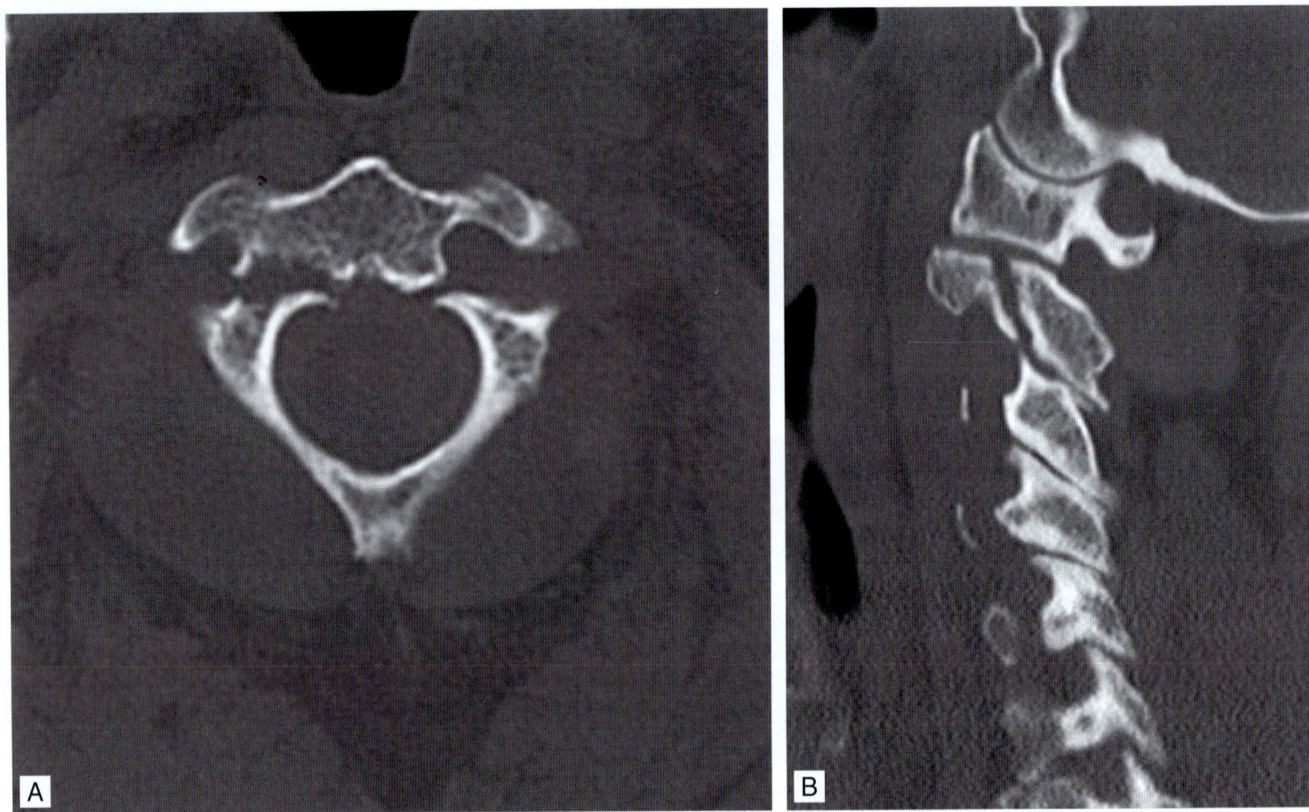

Figure 88.29 Hangman fracture. 62-year-old male found on floor. Axial (A) CT images of the cervical spine demonstrate bilateral fractures of the pars interarticularis of C2 with involvement of the foramina transversaria and risk of traumatic vertebral artery injury. Parasagittal image (B) of the same patient demonstrates the appearance of the right C2 pars fracture (contralateral left C2 pars fracture not shown).

Axis Body Fracture: These have a variety of configurations and can include burst injury. They are frequently stable and treated nonsurgically [89].

Ligamentous Injury Without Fracture: This phenomenon occurs in both children and adults and may have long-term sequelae if not identified acutely. Traumatic alar ligament injuries usually occur near the condylar insertion with potential compression or dissection of the vertebral artery and spinal accessory nerve injury [107]. In the absence of a fracture, MRI evidence of injury to the less clinically significant ligaments such as the apical ligaments or effusion associated with the supra-odontoid space may be indicators of associated strain injury of the more important stabilizing ligaments [91].

Traumatic Atlanto-Axial Rotatory Subluxation (AARS) and Fixation: This is more commonly seen in children and relatively rare in adults [89,91].

Two-thirds of normal rotation of the cervical spine occurs at the atlanto-axial joint. The normal range of rotation at the atlantoaxial joint in adults can be as high as 52° to one side [89,108].

Spasmodic torticollis arising from the sternocleidomastoid contraction should be distinguished clinically from AARS—in torticollis, it is the sternocleidomastoid muscle contralateral to the rotation which is in spasm. In AARS, it is the ipsilateral, lengthened sternocleidomastoid muscle which is in spasm attempting to correct the deformity [91,109].

Subaxial Cervical Spine

Subaxial cervical spine fractures generally occur in predictable configurations [110]. A mechanistic approach can be useful in conceptualizing injuries to the subaxial cervical spine. An awareness of these mechanisms and injury patterns allows for a comprehensive assessment of the cervical spine on CT and in particular helps to identify subtle but important abnormalities which might be missed [110,111].

Relevant Anatomy

The subaxial cervical spine encompasses the C3–C7 vertebrae and their associated discoligamentous structures. The discoligamentous complex (DLC) comprises the intervertebral discs and spinal ligaments including the anterior longitudinal ligament (ALL), PLL, facet joint capsule, ligamentum flava, interspinous and supraspinous ligaments [110].

A functional spinal unit or spinal motion segment refers to two adjacent vertebrae connected by the DLC. From a biomechanical perspective, this can be divided into anterior and posterior columns.

- *The anterior column is anterior to and inclusive of the PLL, comprising the vertebral body, intervertebral disc, ALL, and PLL*
- The posterior column is posterior to the PLL and consists of the neural arch and the posterior ligamentous complex (PLC)

The vertebral bodies and intervertebral discs transmit the compressive loads on the spine while the ligaments bear the rotational, distractive, and shear forces [110].

General Concepts: Compressive traumatic forces generally result in burst or wedge fractures. Distractive force results in ligamentous disruption or dislocation. Rotation-shear forces result in combined osseous and ligamentous fracture–dislocation injuries [110].

The following checklist has been suggested as a framework for CT evaluation of the cervical spine (Table 88.3) [110]. On the midsagittal image, bony alignment should be assessed using the anterior and posterior vertebral lines (Fig. 88.30). The posterior vertebral line is considered to be the most reliable and accurate indicator of antero–posterior alignment [110].

TABLE 88.3 Checklist for Assessment of the Subaxial Cervical Spine [110]

Bone	Vertebral Body	Neural Arch
	▪ Height loss ▪ Wedging ▪ Cortical step ▪ Fracture ○ Comminution ○ Involvement of posterior cortex of vertebral body ○ Retropulsion of fragments	▪ Intact or fracture ▪ Comminution ▪ Orientation of fracture ▪ Vertical vs horizontal ▪ Unilateral vs bilateral
Joints	Intervertebral Disc	Facet Joint
	Focal anterior or posterior widening or asymmetry in coronal plane	▪ Diastasis, subluxation, dislocation ▪ Focal anterior vs posterior widening ▪ Unilateral vs bilateral ▪ Associated articular process fracture
Ligaments	ALL/PLL	PLC
	▪ Preservation inferred from the alignment of anterior posterior vertebral lines ▪ Abnormal: ○ Anterior vs posterior translation ○ Triangular avulsion at the corners of vertebral end plates	▪ Preservation inferred from the normal alignment, interspinous distance and facet joint morphology ▪ Abnormal: ○ Anterolisthesis ○ Focal kyphosis ○ Interspinous widening ○ Facet joint abnormality
Curvature	▪ Normal, smooth lordosis or any abnormal focal kyphosis	–
Alignment	▪ Anterior/posterior vertebral lines assessed on sagittal plane	▪ Spinolaminar and interspinous lines on sagittal plane ▪ Interspinous and articular pillar lines in coronal plane
Measurement	–	▪ Interpedicular, interspinous, and interlaminar distances ▪ A difference of more than 2 mm between adjacent segments is considered abnormal, although usage of measurements may be limited by interobserver variability

Facet joints are best evaluated on parasagittal images and can also be assessed on axial images where they have a "hamburger bun" appearance when normally aligned. Normal facet joint space should be less than 2 mm.

Fractures and Key Injury Patterns

Hyperflexion Injury

Compressive Hyperflexion: The compressive force is to the anterosuperior margin of the vertebral body. With increasing force the injuries progress from anterior vertebral body wedging, to development of a vertically oriented fracture line forming a triangular or quadrangular anterior "teardrop" fragment. With further increase in force the posterior disc, PLL, and PLC may fail leading to a highly unstable injury (the flexion teardrop fracture) [110].

The CT features of the flexion teardrop fracture include:

- Oblique fracture in coronal plane from anterior aspect of superior end plate to inferior end plate, separating a small anterior fragment from the remainder of the vertebral body
- Posterior subluxation of the remaining injured vertebral body on the vertebra below
- Signs of PLC injury [110]

Vertical Compression/Axial Loading: Energy is absorbed by the vertebral bodies and intervertebral discs with a resultant "burst" (horizontal spread) of fragments. Fragments may be retropulsed into the spinal canal. The loss of vertebral body height is generally symmetrical with minimal kyphosis.

A minor vertical compression leads to central cupping of end plates or sagittal/coronal split fracture. A greater force may lead to the typical burst fracture where there is vertebral body height loss and comminution, centrifugal dispersal of fragments, and a fracture line extending to posterior cortex with a retropulsed fragment [110].

Distractive Hyperflexion: In these injuries the center of rotation is considered to be anterior to the vertebral body with the neck in flexion, leading to primary failure of the posterior elements [110,112]. Ligamentous disruption progresses from posterior to anterior, in sequence from the supraspinous ligament to the interspinous ligament, facet capsules, and ligamentum flavum. If there is an even greater force of injury there may be failure of anterior column ligaments.

CT features include the following:

- Interspinous widening
- Interlaminar widening
- Facet joint subluxation or dislocation
- Widened posterior disc space
- Focal kyphosis
- Anterior subluxation of vertebral bodies [113]

Bilateral facet dislocation is the most severe injury of the flexion-distraction spectrum and there is usually a severe associated

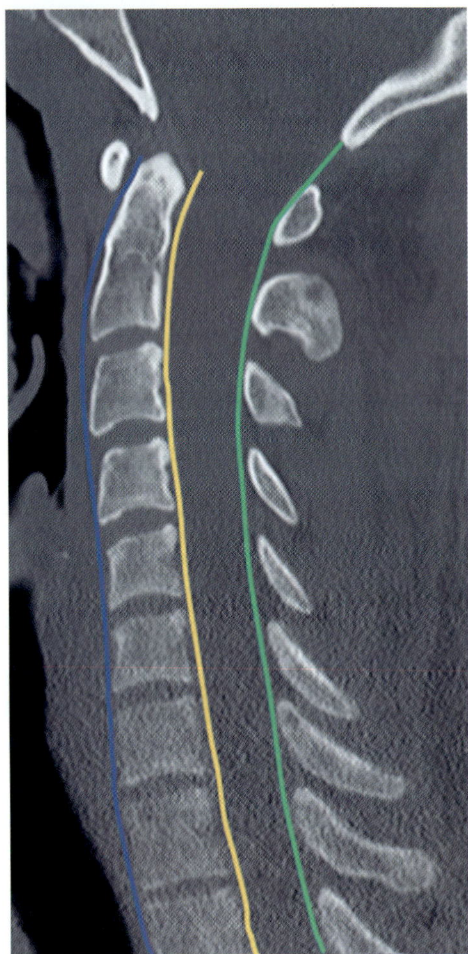

Figure 88.30 Mid-sagittal normal cervical spine CT image demonstrating normal alignment. The anterior spinal line (*blue*), posterior spinal line (*yellow*), and spinolaminar line (*green*) are illustrated. These are useful lines of reference in the identification of anterior or posterior translational and distraction injuries.

neurological injury (Fig. 88.31) [114]. PLL disruption is also frequently seen in association, as is traumatic disc herniation with disruption of the posterior annulus. Disc herniation should be confirmed at MRI before stabilization of the facet dislocation. Fracture of the posteroinferior cortex of the vertebral body is often seen. Unilateral facet joint dislocation may occur when the center of rotation is off-midline and is also a highly unstable injury.

Sagittal plane is best for identifying facet joint dislocations [110]. Normal facet joints show >50% overlap of the articular surfaces. *Subluxation of the facet joints is present where there is <50% overlap of articular surfaces, or diastasis of >2 mm* [113]. When the inferior articular process of the cranial vertebra is sat on the tip of the superior articular process of the caudal vertebra this is referred to as a "perched" facet. Further anterior displacement of the inferior articular process of the cranial vertebra constitutes a "locked" or "jumped" facet (Fig. 88.31A and B). Axial images may demonstrate the "reverse hamburger bun" sign [110].

Hyperextension Injury

Hyperextension Compression: In these injuries, the spinal motion segment is extended and there is compression to the posterior column at the neural arch, including fracture of the lateral mass, laminae, or pars interarticularis. If there is bilateral pedicle or lateral mass fracture traumatic anterior spondylolisthesis may occur. The spinolaminar line may still be intact at the level of the anterolisthesis [110].

Hyperextension Rotation: There is resultant asymmetric, hyperextension compression injury of the posterior column with asymmetric or unilateral fractures of the articular pillars or processes. If there is concomitant fracture of the ipsilateral pedicle and lamina there can be traumatic isolation of the cervical articular pillar with potential rotational instability of the facet above and below [110].

Hyperextension Distraction: In these injuries, the center of rotation is posterior to the vertebral column with the neck in extension. The result is tensile failure of the anterior column. These are mainly ligamentous disruptions progressing from anterior to posterior, starting with ALL. These are common in patients with degenerative or ankylosed spine, including ankylosing spondylitis and diffuse idiopathic skeletal hyperostosis, including with low energy mechanisms [110,115].

On CT, the abnormality may be subtle due to the predominantly ligamentous nature of the injury. Prevertebral soft tissue thickening may be the only apparent feature on CT [110]. Anterior disc space widening is the hallmark feature and is due to rupture of the ALL and anterior annulus [116]. An avulsion of the anterior body may also occur through an intact ALL (the extension teardrop fracture) or there may be fracture of an anterior osteophyte or syndesmophyte.

As the hyperextension force increases, there may be a hyperextension-dislocation injury where there is transient posterior dislocation of the cranial vertebra over the caudal vertebra with disruption of the ALL, anterior annulus, disc, posterior annulus, and PLL. This is frequently associated with a major neurological injury, most commonly a central cord syndrome. A high index of suspicion is required, e.g., in patients with lower facial trauma and clinical central cord syndrome [110]. There may again be widening of the anterior disc space and diffuse prevertebral soft tissue swelling.

Less commonly seen features on CT include disc vacuum phenomenon, and avulsion of the anteroinferior margin of the involved vertebra. Horizontal fracture through the vertebral body or purely through the fused disc space may occur in the ankylosed spine. MRI is indicated to assess discoligamentous injury and spinal cord compression/injury and should be performed particularly in the elderly or ankylosed spine with minor trauma if there is a neurological deficit.

Rotation Injury: The most commonly utilized sign is malalignment of the spinous process in the coronal plane. On CT, one of the most accurate indicators is asymmetry of the uncinate processes [110,117].

Other useful CT indicators include asymmetric disc space with a rotated vertebral body (in coronal plane) and rotation of fracture fragments.

Thoracolumbar Spinal Trauma

Introduction

The concepts of thoracolumbar spinal trauma demonstrate some overlap with the cervical spine although the injury configurations vary relating to inherent differences in biomechanics of the injuries sustained (Fig. 88.32).

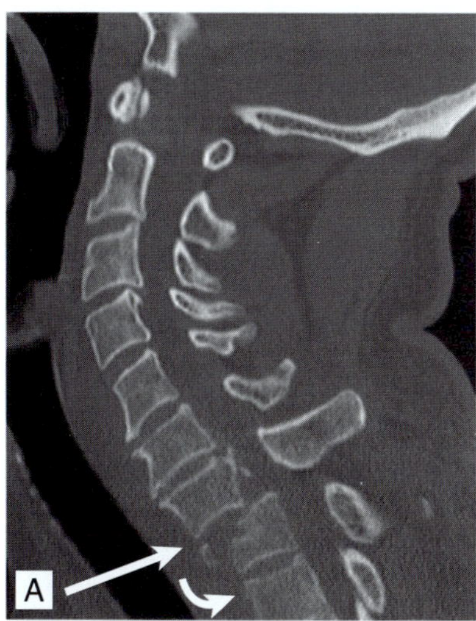

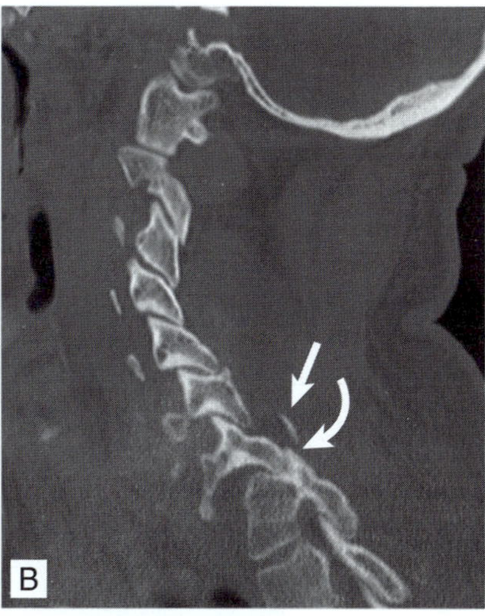

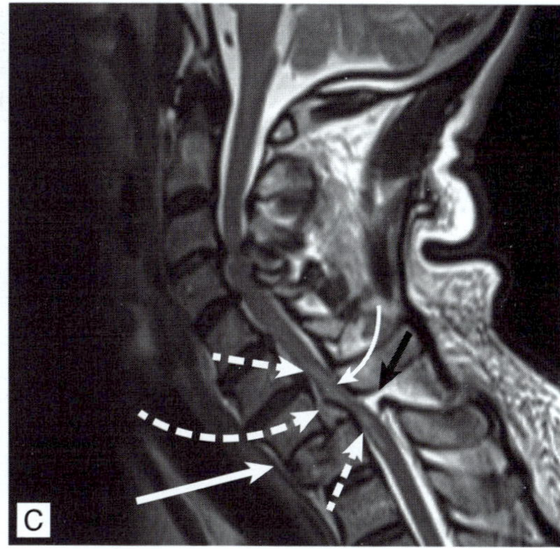

Figure 88.31 56-year-old male suffered fall from significant height. (A) Sagittal CT reconstruction on bone algorithm demonstrates C7-T1 fracture subluxation (*straight arrow*) associated with bilateral facet dislocation ("jumped facets") (not shown). Compression fracture of the T2 superior endplate is also evident (*curved arrow*). (B) Sagittal CT reconstruction on bone algorithm demonstrates "jumped" right C7-T1 facet joint dislocation (*curved arrow*) and associated fracture fragment from the right C7 inferior articular facet (*straight arrow*). Left C7-T1 "jumped" facet was also present (not shown). (C) Sagittal T2-weighted MRI sequence demonstrates the C7-T1 fracture-subluxation (*thick solid white arrow*) associated with the bilateral facet dislocation at the same level (not shown) and the disrupted ligamentum flavum (*black arrow*) at the C7-T1 level and the compressive effect caused by the subluxation and associated subligamentous epidural hematoma (*broken thin curved white arrow*) stripping the posterior longitudinal ligament at the C7-T1 level. Compressive cord signal is present (venous edema) (*broken straight white arrows*) and there is a small petechial hemorrhagic focus within the affected cord parenchyma (*thin curved solid white arrow*).

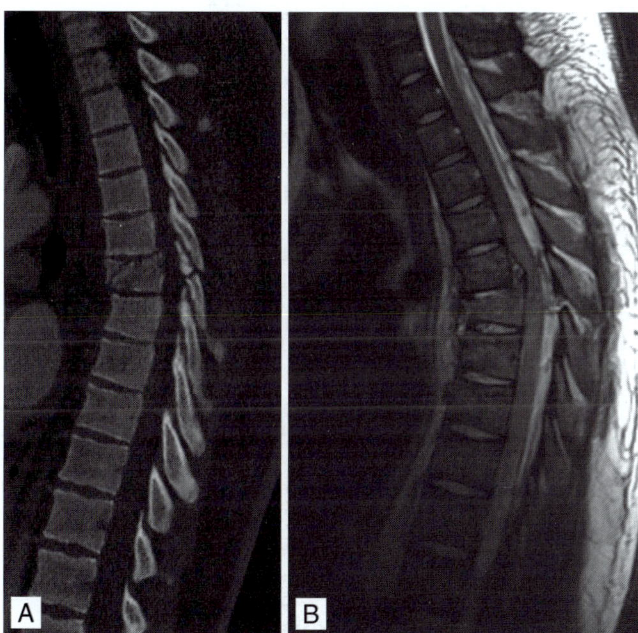

Figure 88.32 Thoracic spinal ligamentous injury. 25-year-old male post-fall from height. Sagittal CT (A) demonstrates a three-column fracture involving the T6 vertebra with evidence of flexion-axial loading injury. Subsequent sagittal T2W MRI (B) shows worsening alignment with anterior translation of T5 and T6 and ligamentous disruption including both the posterior longitudinal ligament and ligamentum flavum of the posterior ligamentous complex. There is indentation of the ventral spinal cord by fracture disruption and localized subligamentous epidural hematoma beneath the posterior longitudinal ligament; there is intramedullary spinal cord signal abnormality consistent with cord contusion.

Multiple injury classification systems have been proposed with the most commonly used being the Denis three-column classification in which the vertebral column is divided into anterior, middle, and posterior columns whereby *any involvement of the middle column suggests an unstable injury*.

- The anterior column includes the ALL, anterior annulus, and anterior two-thirds of the vertebral body
- The middle column includes the posterior one-third of the vertebral body, the posterior annulus, and PLL
- The posterior column includes the posterior elements (pedicles, facets, laminae, and spinous process) and the PLC (ligamentum flavum, interspinous ligament, supraspinous ligament, and facet joint capsules) [111]

Other more recent classifications have been proposed such as the thoracolumbar injury classification and severity score (TLICS), which generates a score based on fracture morphology, ligamentous injury, and neurological involvement to help guide conservative or surgical management [118].

Thoracolumbar Injuries by TLICS Classification

The TLICS system classifies injury morphology into compression, translation, and distraction injuries (Tables 88.4 and 88.5).

Compression fractures are demonstrated as a visible loss of vertebral body height or disruption of the endplate. Less severe injuries may involve only the anterior part of the vertebral body. With increasing force, a burst fracture may occur where the posterior vertebral body is involved and there is retropulsion into the spinal canal [118,119].

Translational injuries appear as horizontal displacement or rotation of two vertebral bodies with respect to one another. They are characterized by spinous process rotation, unilateral, or bilateral facet fracture-dislocation, and vertebral body subluxation [118,119].

Distraction injuries appear as dissociation in the vertical axis. The disruption may involve both anterior and posterior ligaments and the vertebrae. A chance-type fracture falls into this category. The *chance fracture* (Fig. 88.33) was initially described as a specific injury caused by forceful forward flexion,

TABLE 88.4 Thoracolumbar Injury Classification and Severity Score Classification System [118]

Injury Category	Point Value
Morphology	
Compression	1
Burst	2
Translation or rotation	3
Distraction	4
PLC status	
Intact	0
Injury suspected or indeterminate	2
Injured	3
Neurological status	
Intact	0
Nerve root involvement	2
Spinal cord or conus medullaris injury	
– Incomplete	3
– Complete	2
Cauda equina syndrome	3

TABLE 88.5 Total Thoracolumbar Injury Classification and Severity Score and Treatment Recommendation [118]

TLICS Score	Treatment Recommendation
0–3	Nonsurgical
4	Nonsurgical or surgical
≥5	Surgical

TLICS, thoracolumbar injury classification and severity score.

typically sustained by a passenger in a motor vehicle collision (MVC) wearing a lap-seatbelt [119,120]. There is an anterior vertebral body compression fracture with a transverse fracture line extending through the posterior vertebral body into the posterior elements, coupled with posterior element distraction [118,119].

Disruption of the PLC is inferred on radiograph or CT as widening of the interspinous space, avulsion of the superior, or inferior aspects of contiguous spinous process, facet joint widening, "empty" facet joints, perched or dislocated facet joints, and vertebral body translation or rotation [111,118].

There can be various forms of neurological injury including nerve root injury, complete spinal cord injury, incomplete cord injury, or cauda equina syndrome. The role of imaging is to detect the presence of cord or nerve root injury and cord or cauda equina compression on MRI [111,118].

MRI Assessment of the Soft Tissues in Spinal Trauma

At the authors' institution, if there has been spinal trauma significant enough to warrant spinal MRI imaging, MRI of the whole spine is generally performed.

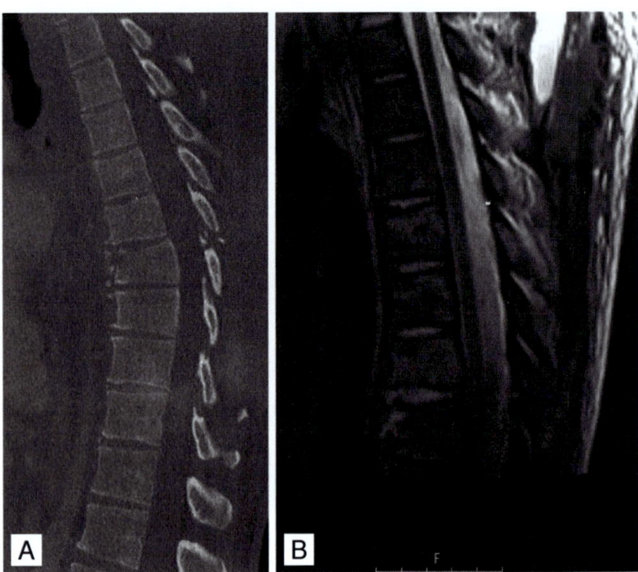

Figure 88.33 Chance fracture. 39-year-old motorcyclist postcollision with lamppost. Sagittal CT of the thoracic spine shows a chance fracture extending through the T7/T8 level (A) with characteristic three-column involvement. Subsequent sagittal T2W MRI (B) demonstrates disruption of the T7/T8 intervertebral disc and the posterior ligamentous complex in addition to marrow edema in adjacent vertebral levels secondary to axial loading/compression mechanism of injury.

Ligamentous Injury

The majority of the spinal ligaments appear on MRI as low signal intensity bands on all sequences, with the main exception being the interspinous ligament which is normally of striated low and high-signal on T1W images (due to interspersed fat) [121,122].

A ligamentous tear may be partial or complete. Partial tears are indicated by a high signal area on short TI inversion recovery (STIR) sequences due to edema and hemorrhage combined with some intact, preserved fibers. Complete tears show the absence of intact fibers with associated edema and hemorrhage [121,123].

Other types of injury include an intact ligament being stripped off the bone and combined bony-ligamentous injury [121].

Injuries to the facet joint capsules are shown as widening of the joint and increased fluid signal within the joint space [121,124].

It should be stressed that the ligaments are components of the spinal columns. The PLC forms a core component of the TLICS assessment and from the perspective of the Denis classification, ligamentous injury can upstage a single column bony injury to a two-column injury [121,123].

Acute Traumatic Disc Herniation

Traumatic disc herniation is most frequently associated with vertebral fracture-dislocation and hyperextension injury due to injury to the annulus fibrosus and herniation of the nucleus pulposus. There may be disc injury (hematoma) without herniation which appears as asymmetric widening/narrowing of the disc and abnormal signal from edema. There may be compression of the spinal cord by the disc herniation [121,125].

Extramedullary Hemorrhage

The most common traumatic extramedullary collection is the epidural hematoma. In the acute phase, epidural hematomatas are isointense to mildly hyperintense on T1W and hyperintense on T2W imaging. Imaging should be extended to capture the full craniocaudal extent of the hematoma. Hemorrhage may also occur within the subdural and subarachnoid spaces.

Spinal Cord Injury

Spinal cord injury can be hemorrhagic or nonhemorrhagic, both of which may be demonstrated on MRI.

Sagittal and axial T2W (Fig. 88.31C) and T2*W (GRE) images are considered to be the most useful with hyperintense intramedullary T2 signal suggestive of cord edema and hypointense signal representing hemorrhage (best shown on GRE images) [121,126]. There may be expansion of the cord due to edema.

Clinical neurological status at presentation is the best predictor of long-term function; however, cord hemorrhage on MRI is particularly important as it is associated with poorer prognosis. Other findings reported to be of prognostic value are the extent of cord hematoma and edema, and spinal cord compression by extra-medullary hematoma [121,127].

Key Points for Spinal Trauma

- Be familiar with the normal alignment and intervals at the craniocervical junction as injury may be subtle and consequences severe
- If a cervical spine fracture is present the remainder of the spinal axis should be imaged. Further injuries are present in 10–15%
- The transverse atlantal ligament is the primary stabilizer of the craniocervical junction
- Ligamentous injury may occur without fracture. Mild mal-alignment on CT may be the only feature
- The TLICS Classification utilizes morphology, status of the PLC and neurological status to help determine stability and the need for surgical treatment of thoracolumbar vertebral injury
- MRI is the optimum imaging technique for evaluating the spinal soft tissues including the ligaments and cord, and for compressive intraspinal hematoma

Blunt Cerebrovascular Injury (BCVI)

Introduction

BCVI refers to nonpenetrating traumatic injury to the cervicocranial carotid and vertebral arteries. While these are relatively rare injuries, they are associated with a high morbidity and mortality risk from stroke and death if untreated [23,128,129].

The prevalence of BCVI is thought to be 1.0–1.6% in all trauma cases although as the majority of injuries are clinically silent at initial imaging true prevalence is difficult to delineate [23,130].

Mechanisms and Pathophysiology of Injury

High-speed MVCs are responsible for more than 50% of BCVI although lower impact mechanisms are also frequently implicated [23]. When BCVI occurs with relatively minor trauma consideration should be given to the possibility of an underlying connective tissue disorder such as Marfan or Ehlers–Danlos syndrome.

The type of trauma to the vessel may be a stretching, twisting, or compression injury. The traumatic force results in an intimal arterial injury with intraluminal blood then dissect through the intimal defect. Distal propagation of the dissection can cause flow-limiting stenosis or occlusion. The intimal injury creates a locally prothrombotic environment with the risk of distal embolization and vessel occlusion [23,131–134].

Traumatic pseudoaneurysms are focal outpouchings at a defect in the vessel wall. This may be contained by the adventitia or the surrounding extravascular soft tissues and the sac may compress the source vessel causing stenosis or occlusion. There is also a risk of thrombus within the sac and distal embolization of clot.

The most severe subtype of BCVI is arterial transection, in which there is arterial hemorrhage into the adjacent cervical and/or facial soft tissues and massive stroke or exsanguination may occur without emergent treatment. Following transection, traumatic arteriovenous fistula may occur although these are not commonly seen as patients tend not to survive to undergo imaging.

Carotico-cavernous fistula may occur in traumatic skull base fracture or rupture of cavernous ICA injury and has been discussed in the skull base section.

BCVI also encompasses venous injury, for example, laceration of a vein by bony fragments or external compression. Venous mural injuries include pseudoaneurysm and transection and are more common after penetrating injury than blunt trauma. Extradural hematomas may also lead to compression of venous sinuses and subsequent dural venous sinus thrombosis.

Screening for BCVI

Screening for BCVI in modern practice is primarily performed with CT angiogram from the aortic arch to the vertex with reported sensitivity of 66–98% and specificity of 92–100% [135–139].

Numerous screening criteria have been proposed including by the Eastern Association for Surgery of Trauma and Western Trauma Association/Modified Denver Criteria. The summarized list of imaging risk factors is included in Table 88.6 [23,134].

Of note, as a group of nonvascular injuries, cervical spine fractures have the strongest association with BCVI. Of these, injuries of the upper cervical spine, ligamentous disruption, and traumatic subluxation/dislocation show the greatest associated risk [23]. High-grade facial fractures also carry significant risk of BCVI (Fig. 88.34A–C).

TABLE 88.6 Screening Criteria for Blunt Cerebrovascular Injury [23]

Screening for BCVI: [23]

- Imaging risk factors
  - Ischemic stroke on imaging
  - Specific high energy mechanism injuries indicated by:
    - Le Fort II or III fracture
    - Skull base fracture with carotid canal involvement
    - Diffuse axonal injury with GCS ≤ 8
  - Cervical spine fracture or subluxation—depends on criteria source
    - Vertebral body fracture
    - Transverse foramen fracture
    - Subluxation or ligamentous injury at any level
    - Any fracture from C1 to C3
  - Near-hanging with anoxia
  - Clothesline-type injury or seat belt abrasion with swelling/pain and/or altered mental status
  - Mandible fracture
  - Complex skull fracture
  - Scalp degloving
  - Thoracic vascular injury
  - Thoracic injury

MRI (including MR angiography) is not generally utilized for BCVI screening.

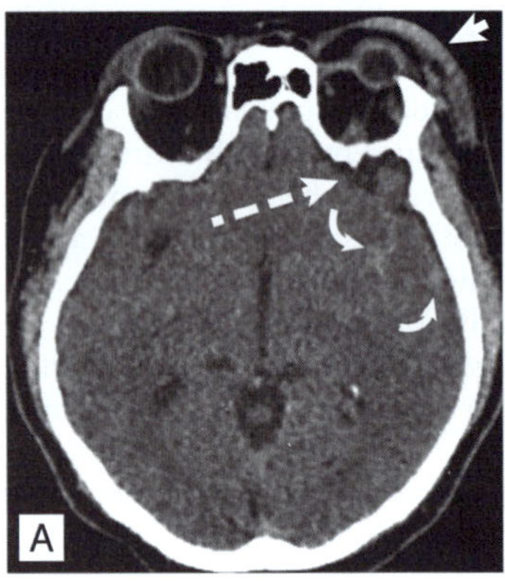

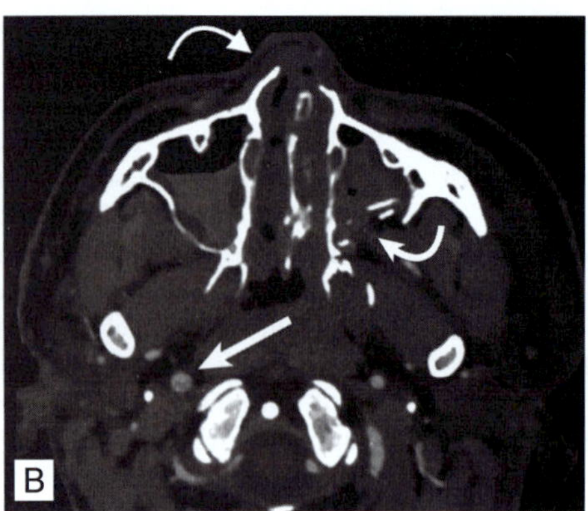

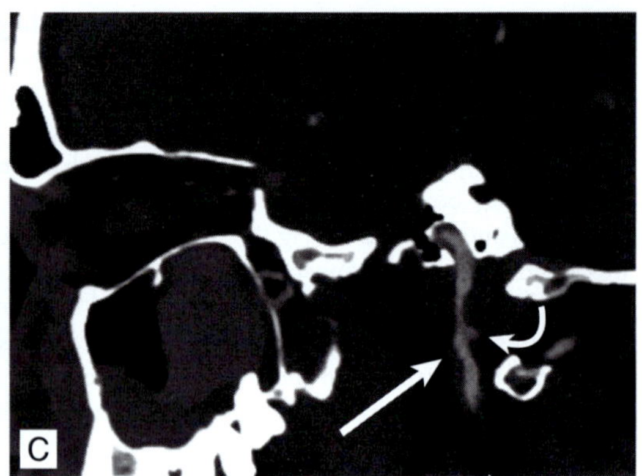

Figure 88.34 50-year-old male fell from an electric scooter at speed sustaining craniofacial injury including severe facial fractures. (A) CT scan demonstrates traumatic subarachnoid hemorrhage (*curved white arrow*) and shallow subdural hygroma (*broken white arrow*) and associated left periorbital soft tissue hematoma (*short white arrow*). (B) Axial CT angiogram image demonstrates traumatic vascular dissection injury of the right internal carotid artery just below the skull base at the craniocervical junction level with intimal flap and subintimal hematoma and localized dilatation of the vessel (*compare to the normal left side*). (C) Sagittal oblique reconstructed CT angiogram image demonstrates the longitudinal morphology of the traumatic dissection injury of the right internal carotid artery and its relationship to the skull base—note irregularity and narrowing (*straight arrow*) in keeping with subintimal hematoma and mural hematoma related to the vessel wall and small subadventitial pseudoaneurysm (*curved arrow*).

CT venography is the examination of choice where there is suspicion of venous injury. There are no official WTA or EAST recommendations; however, any fracture extension to the dural venous sinuses and/or jugular bulb should raise concern for venous injury.

Appearances on Imaging

- Intramural hematoma (IMH) is seen as long segments of mural thickening and may be eccentric or circumferential. IMH in the subacute phase on MRI is hyperintense on fat-saturated T1WI (and PDw images). In the acute phase (1–3 days) and chronic (>14 days), IMH tends to be T1-isointense
- Dissection at cross-sectional imaging shows a linear filling defect within the vessel lumen. A "double lumen" sign with contrast opacification of the false and true lumens is pathognomonic however this may not be seen. On MRI, the false lumen is hyperintense on fat-saturated T1WI
- Pseudoaneurysms are seen as a focal outpouching through an expansion in the vessel wall (Fig. 88.34B and C)
- Arterial occlusion in the cervical carotid artery is often seen as a tapering before total occlusion, whereas vertebral occlusion more commonly shows an abrupt cutoff
- Transection at CTA and DSA shows as an irregular extravasation of contrast surrounding the source vessel. On delayed images, the contrast will disperse
- AVF can be subtle on CTA. Early venous filling in arterial phase (i.e., arterio-venous shunting) and dilatation of draining veins are the major features (Fig. 88.35). These are more clearly shown on DSA (Fig. 88.35D). *Features of caroticocavernous fistula include proptosis, superior ophthalmic vein enlargement, orbital edema, and asymmetric early cavernous sinus opacification in the arterial phase*
- Hyperdensity within a dural venous sinus on noncontrast CT raises suspicion for thrombus and warrants a CT venogram to confirm or exclude a filling defect. Gyral enhancement and prominent intramedullary veins may also be seen due to venous backflow

Pitfalls

Atherosclerosis, carotid fibromuscular dysplasia, vasospasm, and vasculitis may mimic BCVI.

Vasospasm in particular is common after severe trauma and transient vasospasm may mimic low-grade BCVI. Vasospasm typically resolves over several hours, while BCVI will have a longer duration or persist [23].

Normal vascular variants such as coiled ICAs can mask or mimic small pseudoaneurysms. Congenital hypoplasia may mimic luminal stenosis or occlusion. The vertebral arteries are more commonly hypoplastic than the ICAs, and this is typically uniform throughout the length of the vessel. The skull base, the carotid canal, and at the tortuous V3 segment of the vertebral arteries are locations at which vascular injuries have been found to be more easily overlooked [135,139].

Treatment

Treatment of BCVI is with antithrombotic (antiplatelet or anticoagulant) therapy. Low-grade injuries are treated medically unless there is contraindication. Higher grade injury with definite signs of active bleeding or haemodynamic compromise generally warrant surgical or endovascular treatment. Pseudoaneurysms rarely resolve without intervention and early intervention should be considered when lesions are symptomatic or if they grow to a diameter of 1.0–1.5 cm.

Follow-up imaging with CTA is frequently used to help determine duration of antithrombotic therapy. A repeat CTA at 7–10 days is advised to assess for progression or resolution of injury [141].

Key Points for BCVI

- Be aware of the screening criteria for BCVI. If any of these are met CT angiography of the neck and/or intracranial vessels should be performed
- BCVI encompasses arterial and venous injury. The spectrum of arterial injury includes dissection, intramural hematoma, pseudoaneurysm, complete occlusion, transection, and AV fistula
- Features of traumatic caroticocavernous fistula include cavernous sinus expansion, asymmetric early venous enhancement in the arterial phase, enlargement of the superior ophthalmic vein and proptosis
- Vasospasm is common after trauma and may mimic BCVI

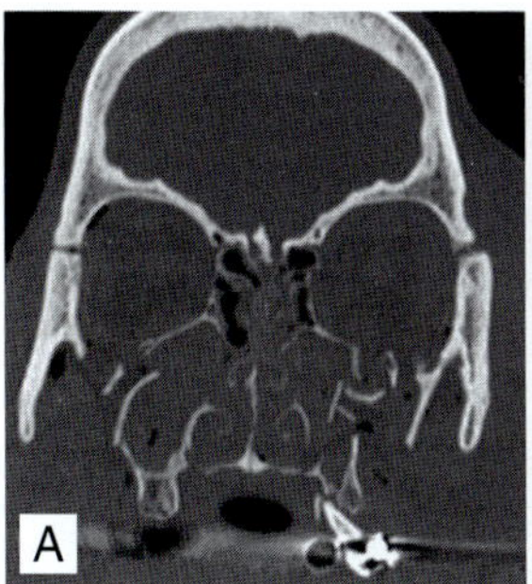

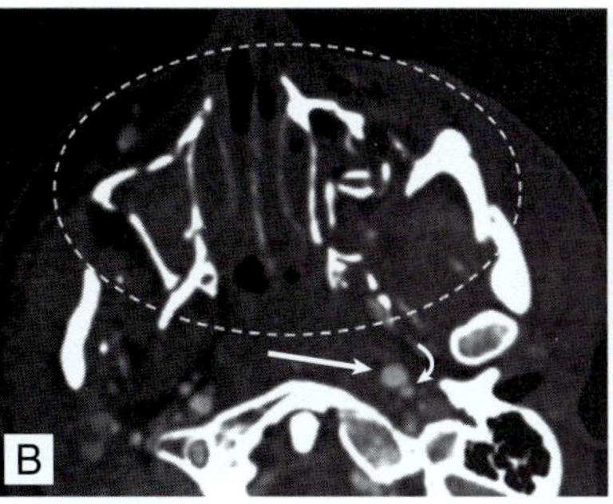

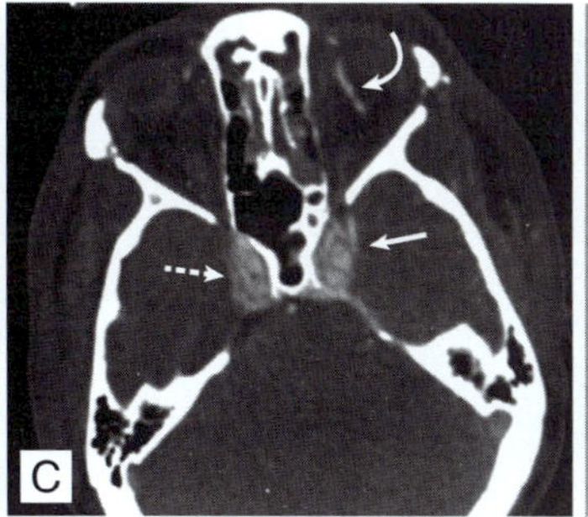

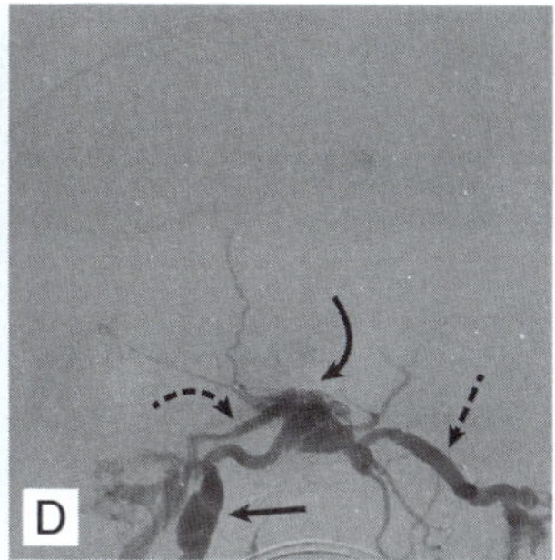

Figure 88.35 39-year-old female pedestrian struck by a car suffered severe mixed Le Fort I, II, and III facial fractures. (A) Coronal CT reconstruction on bone algorithms demonstrates severe mixed Le Fort I, II, and III facial fractures bilaterally. (B) Axial CT angiogram image demonstrates traumatic dissection injury of the left internal carotid artery (*straight arrow*) just below the skull base with associated subadventitial pseudoaneurysm (*curved arrow*). Severe midfacial fractures are demonstrated (oval). (C) Axial CT angiogram image more cranially of the same patient also demonstrates traumatic direct left carotico-cavernous fistula (*straight arrow*) with arteriovenous shunting also evident in the contralateral right cavernous sinus (*broken arrow*) and early mild arteriovenous shunting into the left superior ophthalmic vein (*curved arrow*) at this time. (D) Lateral digital subtraction catheter angiogram performed a few days later (early phase left internal artery injection run) demonstrates traumatic direct left carotico-cavernous fistula (*curved solid black arrow*) with arterial phase shunting into the left superior ophthalmic vein (*broken straight black arrow*) and also into the inferior petrosal sinus (*broken curved black arrow*). Note other sites of right internal carotid artery traumatic dissection injury just below the skull base (*straight solid black arrow*) (also demonstrated on CT in (B)).

Penetrating Neck Trauma

Introduction

Penetrating neck trauma may be due to projectile mechanisms (including gun and blast injury) or nonprojectile sharp force mechanisms (e.g., knife and other sharp implements).

In modern practice MDCT with CT angiography is the standard mode of primary investigation, superseding surgical exploration. CTA allows identification of the wound track and assessment of vascular injury, the upper aerodigestive tract and the cervical spine (Fig. 88.36).

When describing the site of penetrating neck trauma, three anatomical zones are traditionally described.

- Zone 1 extends from sternal notch and clavicles to cricoid cartilage
- Zone 2 from cricoid to mandibular angle
- Zone 3 from mandibular angle to the skull base

These were originally used to help decide which patients would undergo surgical exploration or initial conservative management in the pre-CTA era; however, it remains useful as a common descriptive language between surgeon and radiologist. It should be noted, however, that injuries frequently traverse multiple zones [141].

Immediate surgical intervention without imaging remains indicated in patients with expanding hematoma, severe external hemorrhage, hypovolaemic shock, airway compromise, and massive subcutaneous emphysema [141–145].

Extracranial Vascular Trauma

Extracranial vessel injury is the most common subset of penetrating neck trauma. Arterial injury comprises 15–25%, with 80% of these involving the carotid and up to 43% involving the vertebral arteries [141,142,146].

The associated morbidity and mortality are mainly duc to stroke and exsanguination. Vascular injury secondary to penetrating neck trauma is well demonstrated on multidetector CT angiography (MDCTA). Injury subtypes include pseudoaneurysm formation, arteriovenous fistula, vessel transection, intimal injury and flap formation, dissection, active hemorrhage, and partial or complete occlusion of the carotid or vertebral arteries.

Venous injury may also occur secondary to penetrating trauma and may be missed on physical examination and can be life-threatening because of potential for exsanguination. Early venous opacification on CTA imaging may assist in assessing for venous irregularities or filling defects suggesting the need for a dedicated CT venogram particularly with craniocerebral penetrating trauma [147].

Careful assessment for the presence of any metallic foreign body is crucial as patients may require MR imaging particularly with injury to the cervical spine or craniocervical junction [141].

Catheter angiography has a role in confirmation and interventional management of injuries identified on CTA [141].

Upper Aerodigestive Tract

Oesophageal and Pharyngeal Injury

Penetrating injury to the cervical oesophagus injury is uncommon but identification and a high index of suspicion are crucial in view of the significant risks of mediastinitis, sepsis and death, especially if diagnosis is delayed [141,148].

Water-soluble contrast swallow is reported to be less sensitive for detecting hypopharyngeal injury than oesophageal and for these, flexible nasendoscopy is recommended [141,149]. In penetrating pharyngeal injury, the potential for airway compromise must also be considered [147,150].

Laryngotracheal Injury

Laryngotracheal trauma is relatively uncommon; however, it carries a risk of life-threatening airway compromise and a high index of suspicion is also required [141,151].

Extensive subcutaneous emphysema on CT, disproportionate for the local penetrating injury should raise the suspicion for traumatic disruption of the larynx or trachea.

Facial Injury

Penetrating injury to the face is frequently associated with concomitant intracranial injuries and carries a risk of significant morbidity and mortality. Imaging is normally performed with noncontrast CT head and facial bones although if there is suspected vascular injury MDCTA is indicated. In high energy

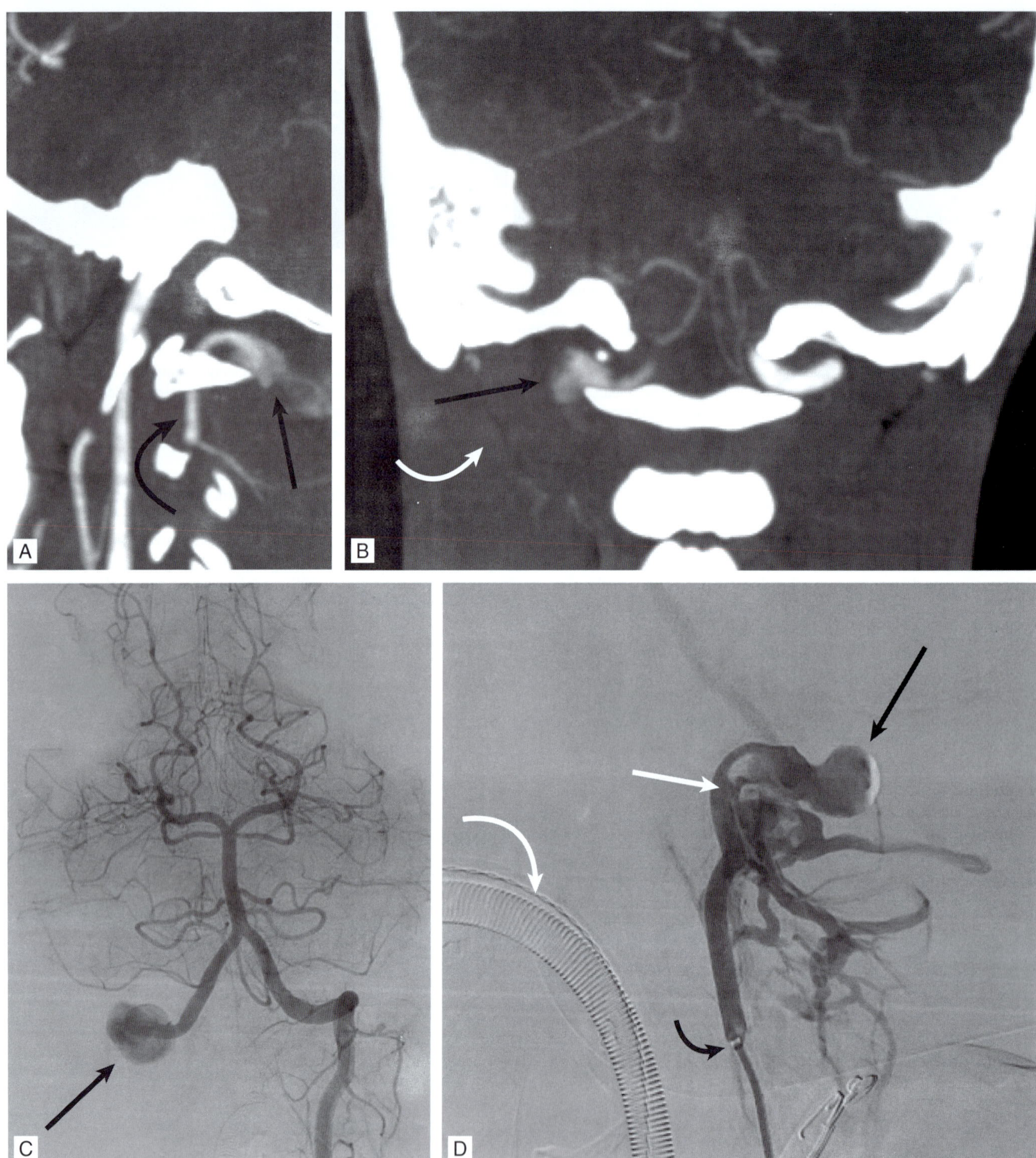

Figure 88.36 19-year-old male stabbed to the right suboccipital region. (A) Sagittal oblique MIP CT angiographic image demonstrates stab wound injury to the right vertebral artery (*curved arrow*) in its V3 segment with subadventitial pseudoaneurysm formation. (B) Coronal MIP CT angiographic image demonstrates right vertebral artery pseudoaneurysm associated with stab injury. Note right suboccipital soft tissue hematoma and loss of perivertebral deep cervical fascia planes (*curved white arrow*) associated with the stab wound track (compare to contralateral side). (C) Frontal digital subtraction catheter angiogram performed a few days later (selective left vertebral artery injection run) demonstrates subadventitial pseudoaneurysm of the right vertebral artery in its V3 segment (*arrow*). (D) Lateral digital subtraction catheter angiogram performed a few days later (early phase selective right vertebral artery injection run) demonstrates subadvential pseudoaneurysm (*black arrow*) of the V3 segment of the right vertebral artery and an associated traumatic arterio-venous fistula (*long white arrow*) proximal to the pseudoaneurysm shunting into adjacent veins. Note the catheter tip (*curved black arrow*) and the endo-tracheal tube (*curved white arrow*).

projectile injuries, fractured fragments of bone and teeth may act as "secondary projectiles" causing further damage [147]. As with pharyngeal and laryngotracheal injury, projectiles entering the oral cavity are at risk of migration and aspiration [141,147,152]. *Wooden foreign bodies merit special mention as their density may grossly approximate gas and hence be incorrectly dismissed. The appearance of a geometric focus of "gas" should raise suspicion for a wooden foreign body* [141].

Spinal Injury

The cervical spine should be carefully interrogated in penetrating neck trauma as both high energy projectile and low energy non-projectile instruments can cause vertebral fracture and there is a risk of dural breach and spinal cord injury. *Reports should include the presence of foreign body and features of dural breach, including intracanalicular gas, bone, or foreign body* [151,153].

Key Points for Penetrating Neck Trauma

- CT angiography is the standard imaging technique for the assessment of penetrating neck trauma
- Immediate surgical intervention is indicated in airway compromise and severe external hemorrhage
- Venous injury should be considered in addition to arterial injury
- Carefully assess for metallic foreign bodies as spinal MRI imaging may be required
- A high index of suspicion is required for oesophageal and pharyngeal injury as there is a high associated mortality risk if diagnosis is delayed
- Wooden foreign bodies may be misdiagnosed as "gas" within the craniofacial soft tissues on CT
- Gas within the spinal canal is highly suspicious for a dural breach and risk of spinal cord injury

Suggested Readings

- AD Schweitzer, SN Niogi, CJ Whitlow, AJ Tsiouris, Traumatic brain injury: imaging patterns and complications, Radiographics 39 (6) (2019 Oct) 1571–1595.
- AM Rutman, JE Vranic, M Mossa-Basha, Imaging and management of blunt cerebrovascular injury, Radiographics 38 (2) (2018 Mar) 542–563.
- C Offiah, S Twigg, Imaging assessment of penetrating craniocerebral and spinal trauma, Clin Radiol 64 (12) (2009 Dec) 1146–1157.
- CE Offiah, E Day, The craniocervical junction: embryology, anatomy, biomechanics and imaging in blunt trauma, Insights Imaging 8 (1) (2017 Feb 4) 29–47.
- C Offiah, E Hall, Imaging assessment of penetrating injury of the neck and face, Insights Imaging 3 (5) (2012 Oct 4) 419–431.
- KL Baugnon, PA Hudgins, Skull base fractures and their complications, Neuroimaging Clin N Am 24 (3) (2014 Aug) 439–465, vii–viii.
- TA Kennedy, GD Avey, LR Gentry, Imaging of temporal bone trauma, Neuroimaging Clin N Am 24 (3) (2014 Aug) 467–486, viii.
- YY Kurihara, A Fujikawa, N Tachizawa, M Takaya, H Ikeda, J Starkey, Temporal bone trauma: typical CT and MRI appearances and important points for evaluation, Radiographics 40 (4) (2020 Jul) 1148–1162.
- A Uzelac, AD Gean, Orbital and facial fractures, Neuroimaging Clin N Am 24 (3) (2014 Aug) 407–424, vii.
- D Dreizin, AJ Nam, SC Diaconu, MP Bernstein, UK Bodanapally, F Munera, Multidetector CT of midfacial fractures: classification systems, principles of reduction, and common complications, Radiographics 38 (1) (2018 Jan) 248–274.
- Y Kumar, D Hayashi, Role of magnetic resonance imaging in acute spinal trauma: a pictorial review, BMC Musculoskelet Disord 17 (2016 Dec 22) 310.

89

Trauma of the Torso

SUSAN CROSS

Introduction

Trauma is a significant public health problem and remains a leading cause of death and disability worldwide [1]. It is one the commonest causes of death under the age of 40. As such, the impact of fatal and nonfatal injuries on healthcare systems and costs due to loss of work force is huge [2,3]. Nearly one-quarter of global deaths attributable to trauma per year are as a result of road traffic accidents, approximately one-third are as a result of violence (including suicide and homicide) with the remainder of the main causes secondary to falls, drowning, burns, and poisoning [4].

The classic concept of trimodal distribution of trauma deaths was first described over 20 years ago and played an important role in the development of regionalized trauma networks [5]. Despite the advancements in trauma networks, prehospital care, and injury prevention, the first and highest peak of deaths, occurring immediately or within 60 minutes of injury, remains fairly stable at 50–60%. This reflects the devastating nature of injuries to the central nervous and cardiovascular systems [6]. The second peak is the early phase, widely defined as deaths within 24 hours of arrival at a trauma center (excluding immediate deaths) and accounting for 25–30% of all trauma deaths. The cause of death in this group is due to hemorrhage, most commonly from injuries to the liver, heart, or major blood vessels and neurological injury. The late phase which includes deaths occurring days to weeks after the injury is largely attributable to infection and multiorgan failure and accounts for approximately 10% of all deaths. A number of studies have shown the number of deaths in this late phase to have declined dramatically over time [7,8].

Imaging of the chest, abdomen, and pelvis plays a crucial role in the management of the severely injured patient, helping to identify bleeding and infection in the early and late phases, respectively.

The aims of this chapter are as follows:

- To understand how best to image the severely injured patient on arrival in the resuscitation room and beyond
- To recognize immediately and potentially life-threatening injuries on x-ray, ultrasonography (USG) in the form of fast and multidetector CT (MDCT)
- To identify intrathoracic and intraabdominal injuries that are significant to the trauma surgeons and interventional radiologists, with pearls and pitfalls where appropriate
- To understand the clinical impact of the American Association of Surgery for Trauma (AAST) grading of intra-abdominal solid organ injuries, upon management of the severely injured patient
- To understand the importance of how the mechanism of injury matters, particular in bowel and mesenteric injury
- To apply what we have covered in the course of the chapter to important clinical scenarios

While evaluation of the neuro spinal axis is outside the scope of this chapter, it is important to appreciate that the presence of acute severe intracranial injury and/or unstable spinal pathology in the multiply injured patient will contribute to decision-making pathway for the trauma team. Therefore, reference will be made to this where appropriate.

Imaging of the Severely Injured Patient

When a severely injured patient arrives in the resuscitation room, there are a number of pathways available to them. Their injuries may, e.g., necessitate a trauma laparotomy, urgent neurosurgical review, interventional radiology procedure, orthopaedic intervention, observation and treatment in intensive therapy or high dependency units (ITU/HDU) or the trauma ward; or a combination of these. It may even be, that after a period of observation in the emergency department, the patient is discharged. Instrumental to where the patient goes next will be the hemodynamic status of the patient and the imaging findings.

The primary imaging survey consists of a portable anteroposterior (AP) chest radiograph (CXR), AP pelvic radiograph, and USG in the form of focussed assessment with sonography in trauma (FAST). *These should be incorporated as an adjunct, into the clinical primary survey, but should not impede definitive investigation (in the form of CT) or definitive treatment* [9]. *They are of particular value in the hemodynamically unstable patient, where they can help to identify the source of bleeding, particularly if the patient is too unstable to proceed to definitive imaging with CT* [10]. For example, in a hemodynamically unstable blunt polytrauma patient with a normal pelvic and chest radiograph but a positive FAST scan, the source of bleeding is most likely to be from the abdominal cavity.

The chest radiograph is useful to screen for immediately life-threatening injuries, e.g., tension pneumothorax (Fig. 89.1) and large hemothorax (Fig. 89.2). It can also evaluate endotracheal tube placement if there has been emergent intubation prehospital (Fig. 89.3). It should be noted that evaluation for potentially life-threatening mediastinal hematoma from major vessel injury on the supine chest radiograph is challenging. The finding of mediastinal widening on a supine chest radiograph is nonspecific for traumatic injuries, especially for aortic injuries [11]. More discriminating findings include loss of the aortopulmonary contour, abnormality of the aortic arch, and presence of a left apical cap (Figs. 89.3 and 89.4). In up to 7% of cases of traumatic aortic injury (TAI), the chest radiograph may be normal [12]. *In reality, those patients with rapid deceleration mechanism of injury and high clinical suspicion of TAI should undergo further evaluation with MDCT to confirm or refute this diagnosis, irrespective of the chest radiograph findings* [13].

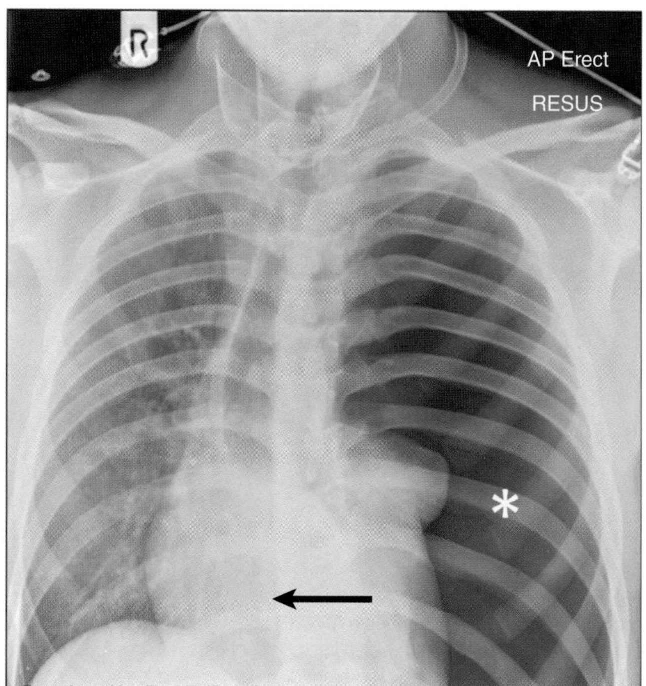

Figure 89.1 Penetrating trauma. Stab wound to left posterior chest wall. AP erect CXR taken in emergency department demonstrates complete paucity of vascular lung markings on the left (*asterisk*) with complete collapse of left lung. There is mediastinal shift away from this (*black arrow*), consistent with a left-sided tension pneumothorax. This requires urgent decompression.

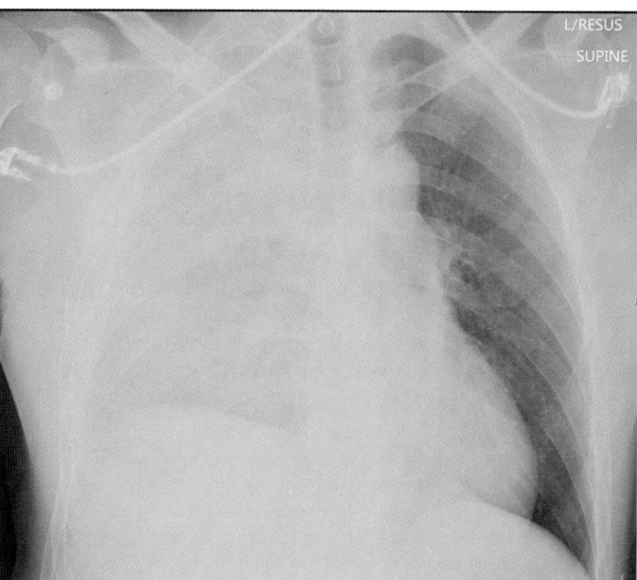

Figure 89.2 Blunt trauma. Crush injury between lorry and wall. Hemodynamically unstable. Supine AP chest radiograph taken as part of primary survey. This demonstrates complete increased opacification of the right hemithorax due to blood layering posteriorly along the pleural space while patient is in the supine position. Vascular markings still evident in the right lung (compare with Fig. 89.1). There is mediastinal shift away from the opacification. Chest radiograph findings are consistent with a large right hemothorax. This is a potential source of the patient's hemodynamic compromise.

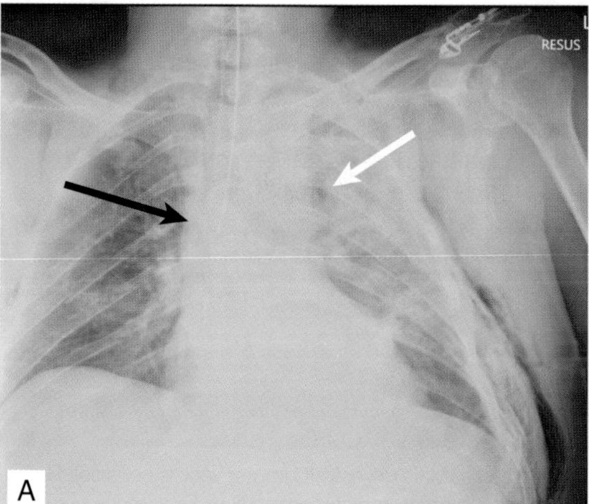

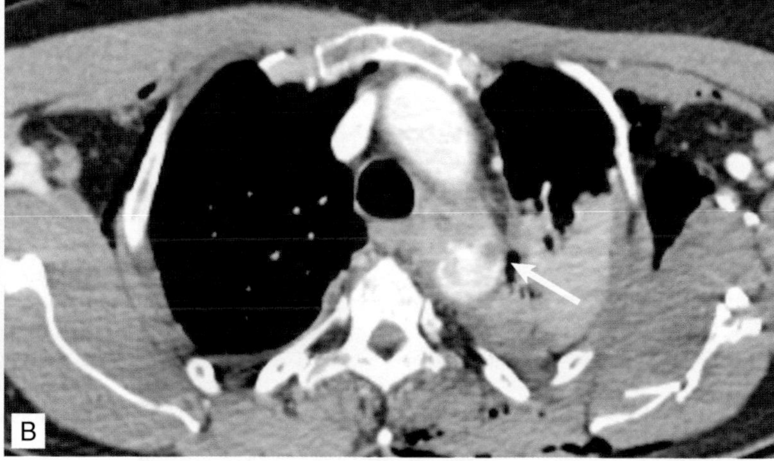

Figure 89.3 Blunt trauma. Cyclist versus taxi. Hemodynamically stable. Intubated at the scene. (A) Supine AP radiograph confirms endotracheal tube (ETT) is too low, the distal tip of which lies within the right main bronchus (*black arrow*). Note the loss of the normal aortic arch and loss of normal aortopulmonary contour (*white block arrow*) together with multiple left-sided rib fractures and extensive surgical emphysema within the soft tissues of the chest bilaterally (L>R). (B) Acute traumatic aortic injury was confirmed on subsequent CT, evidenced by intraluminal thrombus at the origin of the descending aorta (*white block arrow*) with periaortic hematoma with loss of the fat plane around the aorta. This was confirmed as aortic transection at the aortic isthmus and was treated successfully with thoracic endovascular aortic repair (TEVAR).

Mortality in patients with pelvic fractures with hemodynamically instability has been shown to range from 20% to 50% [14–16]. If a blunt polytrauma patient is hemodynamically stable and is proceeding directly to CT for definitive imaging, then a pelvic radiograph will offer little, if any, incremental help in decision making around the next best step in their management [10]. However, a pelvic radiograph confirming unstable pelvic fractures, in a hemodynamically unstable patient, is useful, particularly if they are not able to proceed to MDCT (Fig. 89.5). It will also confirm the adequate placement of the potentially lifesaving pelvic binder [17] (Figs. 89.5 and 89.6). *All polytrauma patients also require a postbinder pelvic x-ray after resuscitation even in the presence of a "negative" CT because a well-applied pelvic binder can mask a catastrophic pelvic ring injury* (Fig. 89.7).

Bedside USG in the form of a FAST scan can be useful in the early resuscitative phase, particularly when it is positive in the

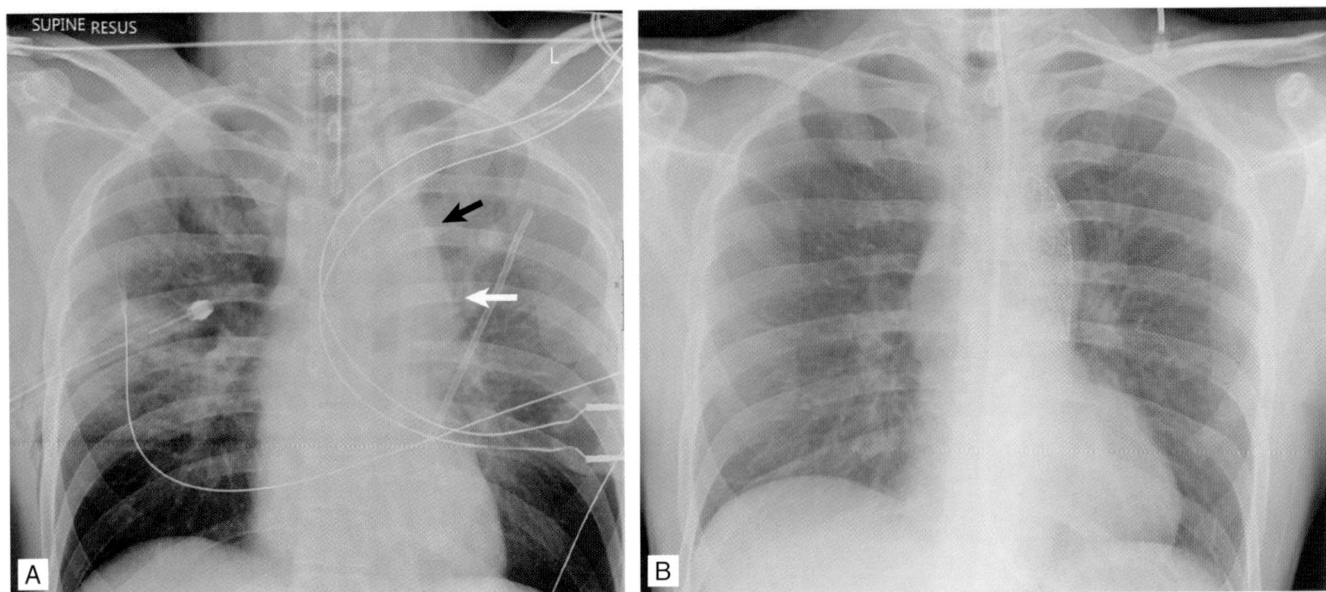

Figure 89.4 Blunt trauma Motorcyclist versus car. Hemodynamically stable in emergency department. (A) Supine AP CXR taken as part of primary survey. ETT in situ appropriately sited. Artefact from tubes and leads extraneous to patient can be distracting. Right-sided intercostal chest drain in situ. Ill-defined air space opacifications in right mid zone in keeping with lung contusions. Note the abnormal contour of aortic arch (*black arrow*) and loss of the aorto-pulmonary contour (*white arrow*). Subsequent CT confirmed aortic transection with large pseudoaneurysm at the aortic isthmus. (B) Erect AP CXR in the same patient at day 13 post-thoracic endovascular aortic repair TEVAR, for comparison. Nasogastric tube in situ. Note the TEVAR stent in situ and now normal aortic arch and aortopulmonary contours.

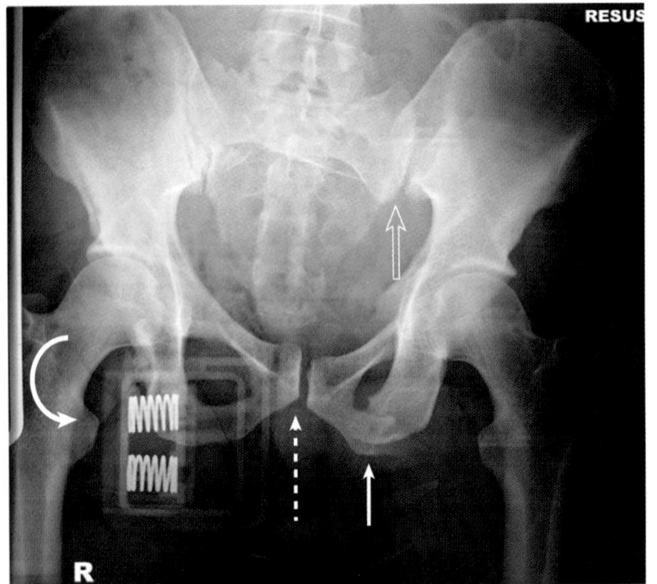

Figure 89.5 Blunt trauma. Pedestrian versus truck. Hemodynamically unstable in emergency department. AP pelvic radiograph demonstrates widening of the left sacroiliac joint (*block arrow*), malalignment of the pubic symphysis (*dashed arrow*), displaced fractures of the left superior and inferior pubic rami (*white arrow*). This unstable fracture pattern is susceptible to significant blood loss. The pelvic binder (*curved arrow*) is an immediate measure to compress the fractured pelvis in an effort to stop the bleeding. It should be positioned at the level of the greater trochanters, as in this case.

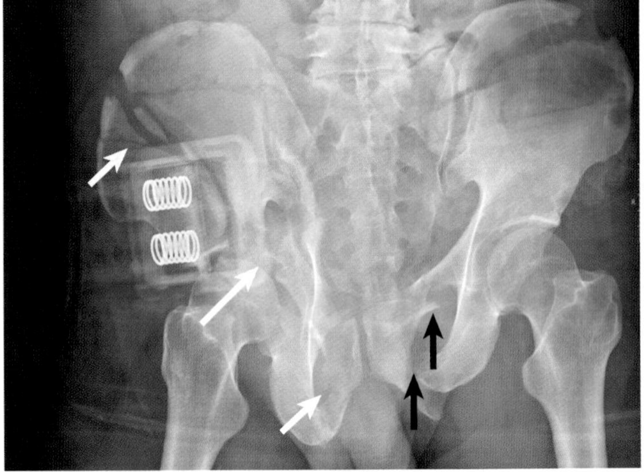

Figure 89.6 Blunt trauma. Male driver MVC (motor vehicle collision). Hemodynamically unstable. AP pelvic radiograph demonstrates complex pelvic fracture pattern resulting in combined lateral compression and vertical shear combined type injury with marked comminution of the right acetabulum extending into the right iliac blade and right pubic rami (*white arrows*) and disruption to left sacroiliac joint extending into the left iliac blade with displaced fractures of left superior and inferior pubic rami (*black arrows*). This unstable fracture pattern is susceptible to significant blood loss. Note the pelvic binder is a little high and needs repositioning ideally at the level of the greater trochanters if possible. The patient was hemodynamically unstable and proceeded directly to the theatre for damage control surgery (DCS) and pelvic packing. WBCT was performed post-DCS surgery for complete injury assessment. *WBCT*, whole body CT.

hemodynamically unstable patient. Typically, the FAST scan involves evaluation of the hepatorenal fossa, splenorenal fossa, and pelvis to assess for free intraperitoneal fluid (blood), and the xyphoid view to assess for hemopericardium (Fig. 89.8). It can also be extended to assess for pneumothorax and hemothorax [18]. *It is important to recognize that the FAST scan may not detect clinically significant bleeding within the abdomen, e.g., within the retroperitoneal cavity or within solid or hollow viscus organs* [19] (Fig. 89.9). Surgical emphysema and body habitus may also limit interpretation. Therefore a negative FAST scan, in the

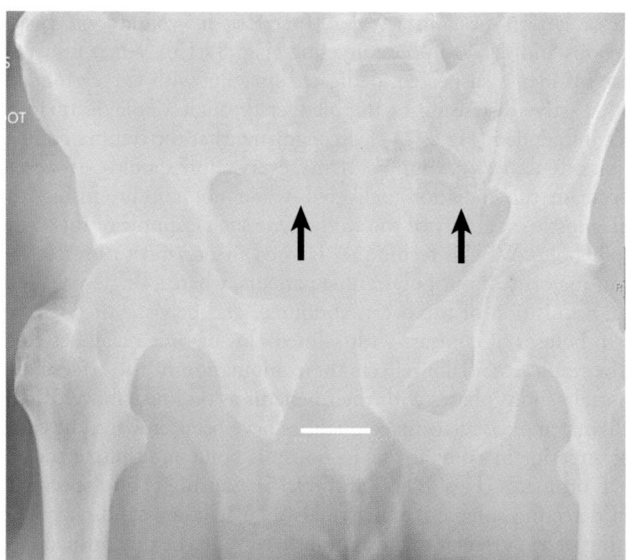

Figure 89.7 Blunt trauma. Pedestrian versus car. Hemodynamically unstable in emergency department. AP pelvic radiograph out of pelvic binder demonstrates an open book pelvic injury resulting from AP compression type injury with pubic symphysis diastasis (*white line*) and fractures of the sacral ala (*black arrows*). This fracture pattern is susceptible to significant blood loss.

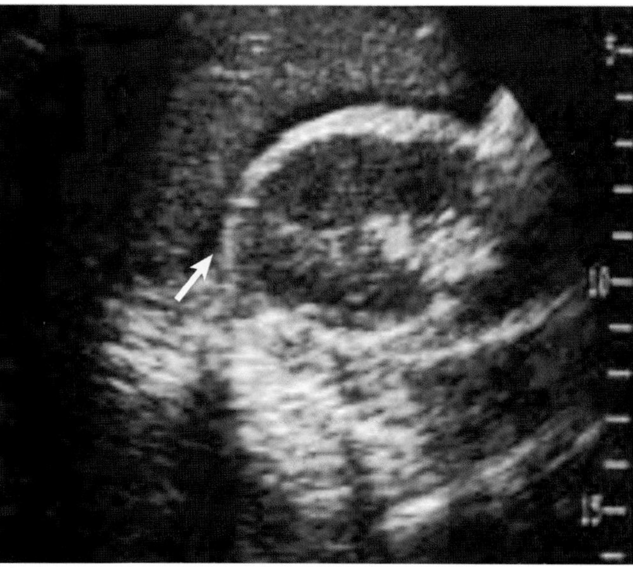

Figure 89.8 Blunt trauma. Selected USG image (scanning in right upper quadrant) confirming anechoic free fluid in hepatorenal fossa (*white arrow*). FAST positive scan.

trauma patient with a significant mechanism of injury, must be confirmed by either CT or in the case of limited resources, e.g., the mass casualty scenario, by follow-up FAST scan and observation [20].

Multidetector CT is now well established as the definitive imaging investigation in the polytrauma patient and its diagnostic accuracy for detecting clinically significant intrathoracic and intraabdominal injuries has been well documented [21–23]. *Whole body CT (WBCT) (vertex to pubic symphysis) can provide a rapid and comprehensive overview of injuries and help to direct the order and way in which these injuries should be treated.* There are a number of WBCT protocols that are in use, all of which involve the use of intravenous contrast to evaluate the torso [10,24,25]. Acquiring imaging in the portal venous phase maximizes the detection of intraabdominal solid organ injuries (Figs. 89.10 and 89.11). Arterial phase imaging enables the detection and characterization of solid organ vascular lesions such as pseudoaneurysms and arteriovenous fistulas, which are often not apparent in the portal venous phase [26,27]. In the context of multiple pelvic fractures, it can also facilitate the characterization of active extravasation as being arterial in origin, rather than osseous or venous [28]. This can provide a "roadmap" for the interventional radiologist if angioembolization is appropriate. Selective acquirement of delayed phase imaging will help further characterize injuries of the urinary tract, which is discussed in detail later in the chapter (Fig. 89.12). Active bleeding manifests as amorphous

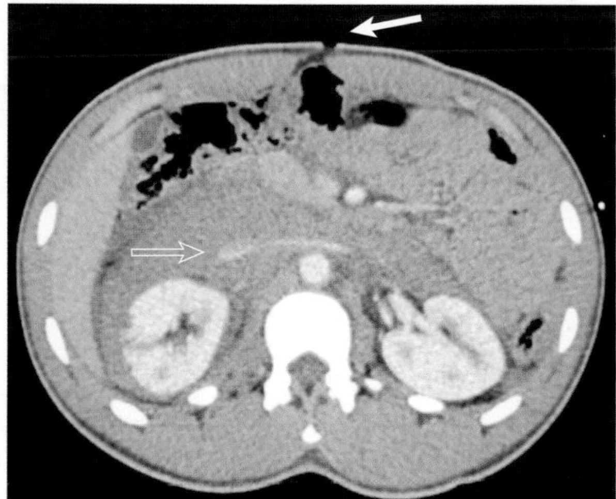

Figure 89.9 Penetrating trauma. Isolated stab wound to epigastric region. FAST scan negative. Patient tachycardic but normal blood pressure. Skin defect from isolated penetrating stab wound to epigastric region (*white arrow*). Large retroperitoneal hematoma (*block arrow*). Trauma laparotomy confirmed IVC injury with through and through injury to the SMV. *SMV*, superior mesenteric vein.

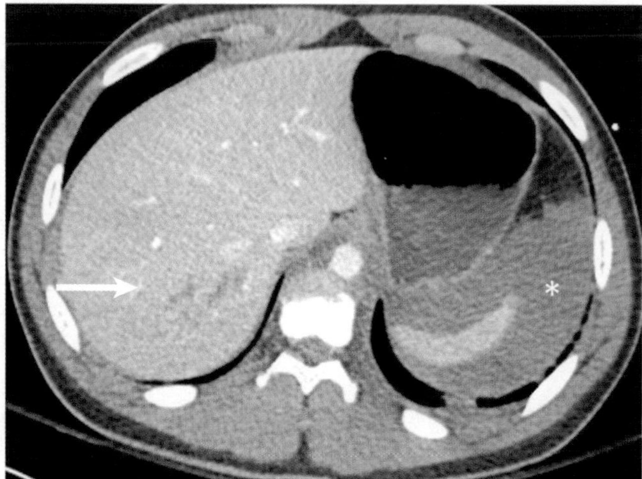

Figure 89.10 Blunt trauma. Cyclist versus car. Axial CT image in portal venous phase demonstrates homogeneous enhancement of the liver with clear delineation of a linear low attenuation liver laceration, AAST Grade II liver injury, which does not breach the liver capsule (*white arrow*). The large volume of hemoperitoneum seen in this image in the left upper quadrant (*asterisk*) was secondary to bowel injury confirmed at laparotomy.

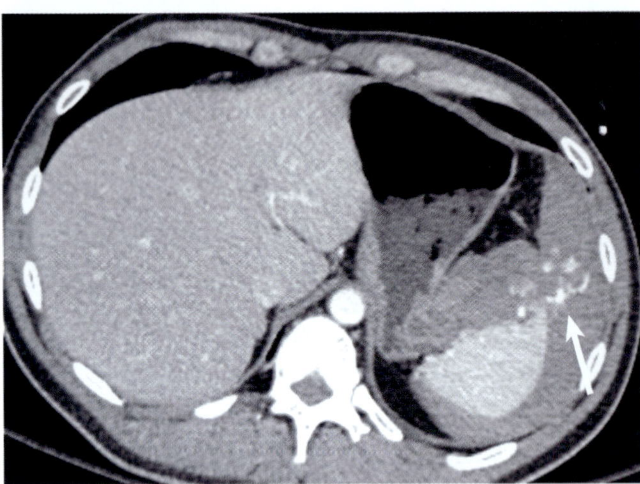

Figure 89.11 Blunt trauma. Motorcyclist versus car. Hemodynamically stable axial CT image acquired with single-pass split bolus technique. Note the homogenous enhancement of the liver and the spleen. There is active extravasation from splenic injury into the peritoneal cavity (*white arrow*) with hemoperitoneum. AAST grade V splenic injury. This was an isolated high-grade splenic injury and the patient remained hemodynamically stable. Decision made to proceed with nonoperative management (NOM) with adjunctive successful angioembolization.

extravasation of contrast that increases in volume on portal venous and delayed phase imaging (Fig. 89.13). When injury to the bladder is suspected, dedicated imaging with CT cystogram, with active distension of the bladder through a Foley catheter is recommended (Fig. 89.14). Recognizing that the trauma population often involves young patients, every effort should be made to decrease the radiation delivered while not compromising the diagnostic capability of the study. One such example of this is the split bolus WBCT technique, favored in our institution for the vast majority of our polytrauma patients, where a single-pass helical acquisition of the chest, abdomen, and pelvis is preceded by two boluses of contrast with saline bolus or time delay between. The result essentially reflects the combination of the arterial and portal venous phases with their benefits as outlined above. Parenchymal and vascular image qualities have been shown to be equal or superior in comparison to nonsplit bolus multiphase trauma CT protocols (Figs. 89.13 and 89.15). Sensitivity and specificity in detecting splenic parenchymal vascular lesions and characterizing pelvic vascular extravasation have yet to be determined [29] (Figs. 89.15 and 89.70).

There have been a number of studies and systematic reviews which have assessed the benefits and risks of immediate WBCT scan compared with selective CT in major trauma patients [30–36]. All of these have agreed that there is a time benefit to

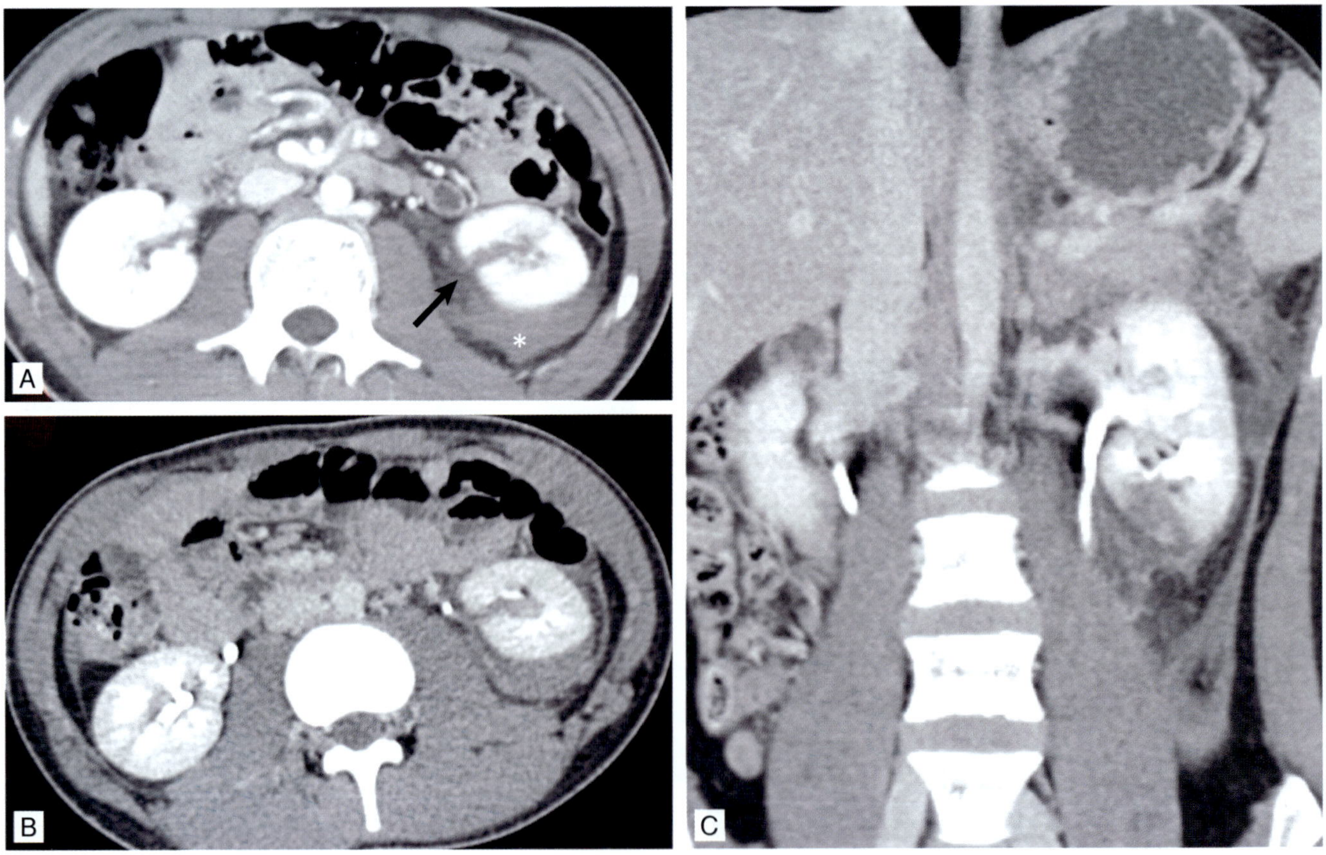

Figure 89.12 Blunt trauma. Fall from horse. Hemodynamically stable. Axial CT (soft tissue windows) acquired with split bolus protocol and demonstrates focal linear laceration in lower pole of the left kidney (*black arrow*) with perirenal hematoma (*asterisk*). This is at least an AAST grade III injury. We need to decide whether it involves the pelvicalyceal system which would upgrade the injury and potentially alter management. (B and C) The patient was hemodynamically stable and decision was made to perform a delayed phase scan (at 5 minutes) to allow further assessment of the left pelvicalyceal (PC) system and proximal ureter. Selected axial and coronal reformats confirm no urine leak from the PC system or left ureter during this phase, therefore this injury remains classified as AAST grade III.

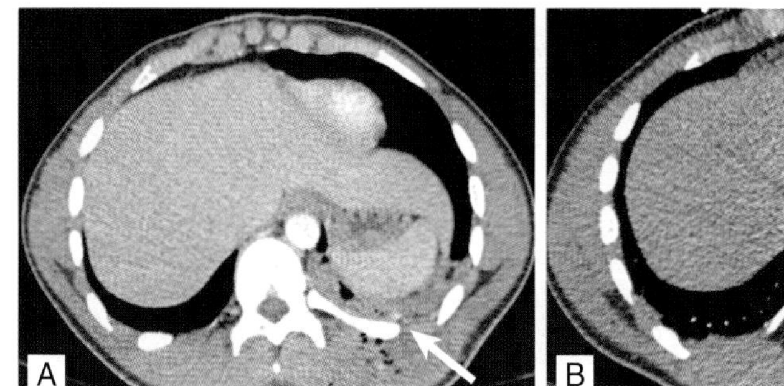

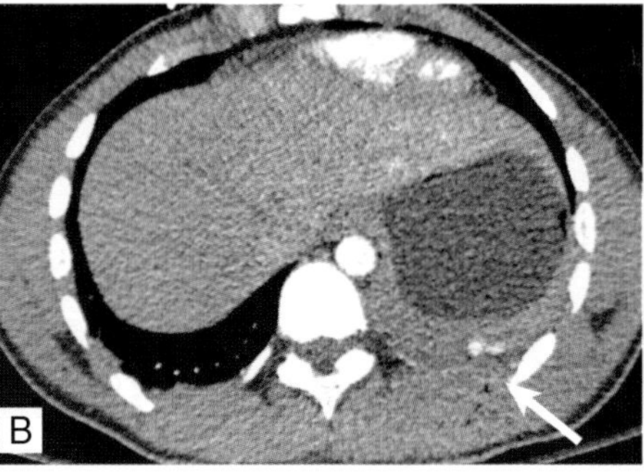

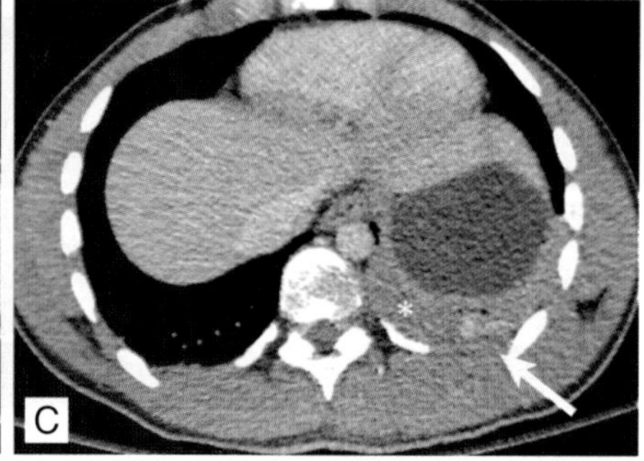

Figure 89.13 Penetrating trauma. Stab wound to lower left posterior chest. Hemodynamically stable in emergency department. Axial CT image (acquired with split bolus protocol) shows surgical emphysema and hematoma in superficial soft tissues of the left chest wall. There is a shallow hemothorax with small focus of active extravasation related to an intercostal vessel (*white arrow*). Large bore chest drain was inserted was inserted with drainage of approximately 400 mL of blood. (B and C) Patient initially stabilized but then further increase in volume of blood from the left chest drain with drop in systolic blood pressure 5 hours after admission. Repeat dual-phase CT was performed. Arterial phase (B) shows focal of active extravasation has increased in size (*white arrow*) from the previously noted CT with increase in size of hemothorax (*asterisk*). Delayed phase at 90 seconds. (C) shows increased amorphous pooling of contrast at this site consistent with active bleeding. Patient proceeded to interventional radiology for coil angioembolization of the ninth intercostal artery.

WBCT scanning; however, while WBCT has been shown to be a predictor of survival in a number of these studies, a consensus has not been reached on overall survival benefit. However, diagnostic accuracy of MDCT together with rapid scan time has meant that many trauma centers incorporate WBCT scanning (vertex to pubic symphysis) into the trauma survey either as a supplement or replacement to conventional imaging in the severely injured patient. It should be noted that as far as possible CT evaluation of the torso should be performed with the arms up, unless prevented from doing so due to fracture or injury. This provides the best quality evaluation of the solid organs by reducing streak artifact from the arms (Fig. 89.16) and also reduces radiation dose by up to 45%, when compared with arms down by sides [37]. Oral contrast is not routinely administered in the emergency setting of blunt abdominal trauma.

There will always be a number of hemodynamically unstable severely injured patients who require immediate life-saving surgery. *The decision to proceed to CT with a hemodynamically unstable patient is at the trauma team leaders discretion and should only be performed where there is a well-organized trauma team and appropriate structural requirements to facilitate this safely* [38]. *Often these patients will proceed to WBCT after immediate life-saving surgery to ensure complete evaluation of the retroperitoneum, mediastinum and neurospinal axis; to further characterize solid organ injuries; to assess for vascular injuries that may require angioembolization or to assess for source of ongoing hemodynamic instability* (Figs. 89.17 and 89.18). This is particularly helpful in patients post damage control surgery (DCS) for high velocity penetrating trauma (Fig. 89.19). Of note, it is worth performing a noncontrast CT scan of the abdomen and pelvis in patients who are having WBCT post

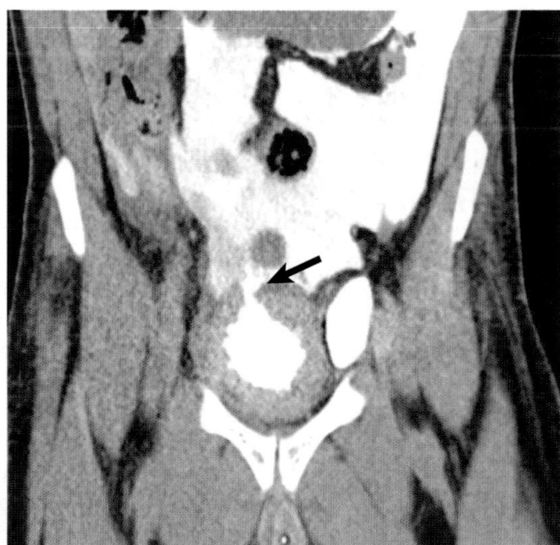

Figure 89.14 Restrained driver. Hemodynamically stable but FAST positive. Coronal reformat from CT cystogram demonstrates focal defect in the dome of the bladder (*black arrow*) with free intraperitoneal spill of water-soluble contrast. This confirms intraperitoneal bladder rupture which necessitates laparotomy repair (Type). The initial FAST scan was positive due to the free intraperitoneal spill of urine (an important learning point that free fluid in a FAST scan, although most likely, is not always blood).

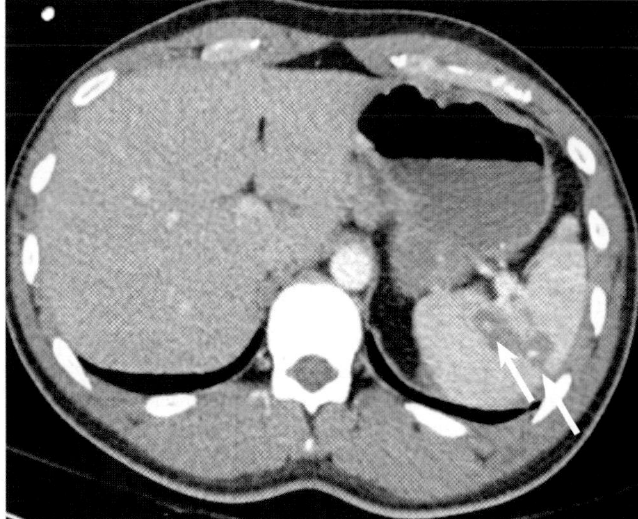

Figure 89.15 Pedestrian versus car. Hemodynamically stable in emergency department. Axial CT image acquired using split bolus protocol with splenic laceration with intralesional focal of vascular injury (*white arrows*). Small volume of perisplenic hematoma but not active extravasation outside the splenic capsule into the peritoneum. AAST grade IV splenic injury. Patient proceeded to interventional radiology. Discrete pseudoaneurysm not identified on the diagnostic angiogram and patient proceeded to proximal splenic angioembolization with coils.

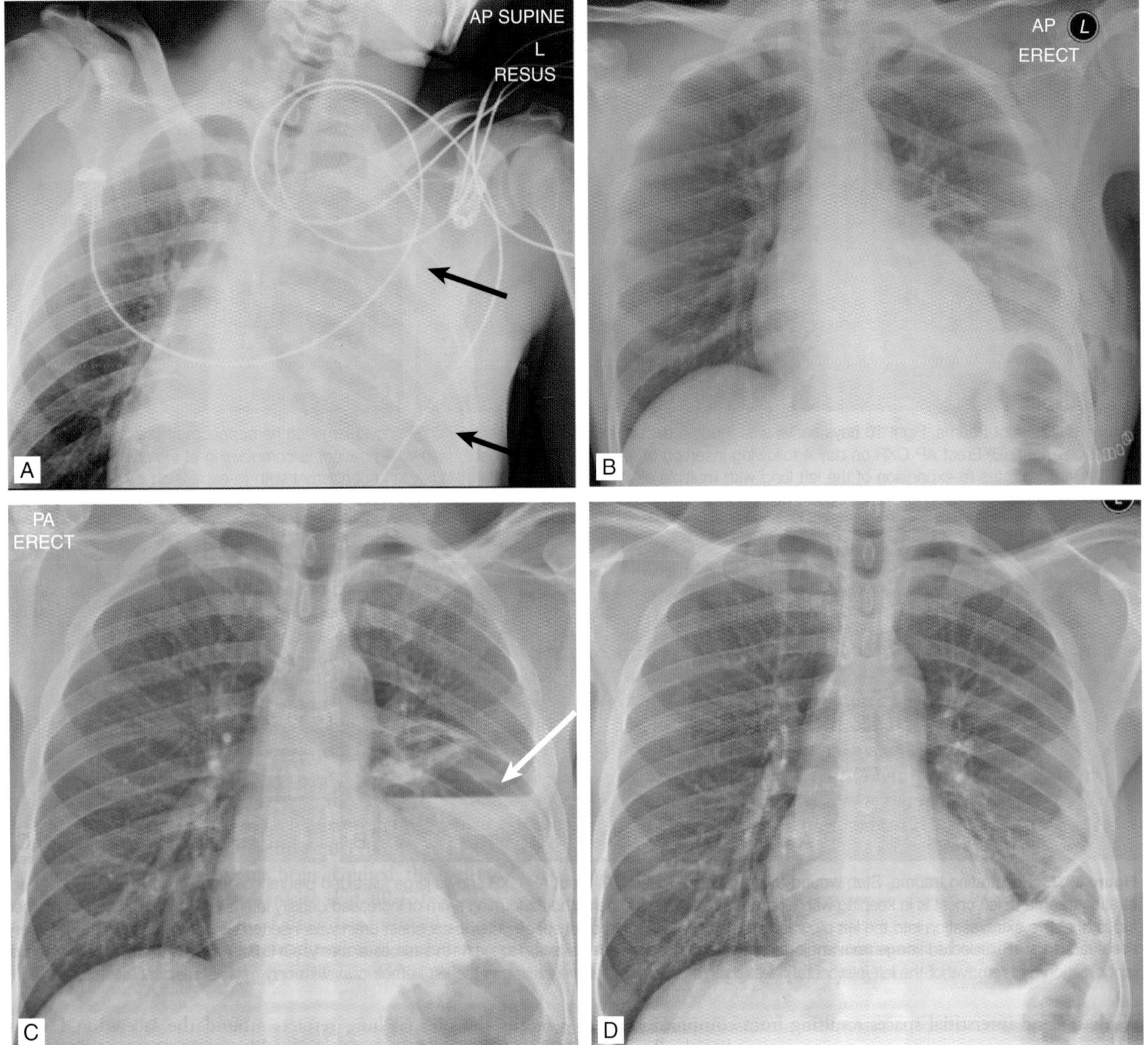

Figure 89.24 Penetrating trauma. Stab wounds to left chest. (A) Supine AP CXR on admission in resus bay demonstrates increased opacification of the left hemithorax, with rim of increased density at the lateral surface and apex (*black arrows*) all consistent with a large left-sided hemothorax. (B) AP erect CXR at day 6 following removal of large-bore chest drain confirms resolution of the large left hemothorax with residual consolidation and atelectasis in left lower lobe and minor surgical emphysema in soft tissues of the left chest wall. USG at this time confirmed minimal residual pleural collection. (C) PA erect CXR at day 14. Patient represents with pyrexia and worsening shortness of breath. CXR confirms left hydropneumothorax with air–fluid level (*white arrow*). Patient underwent VATs decortication for treatment of large left-sided empyema. (D) AP erect CXR post VATS decortication 4 weeks following injury. There is residual atelectasis and blunting of left costophrenic angle. Patient is now apyrexial with no other respiratory symptoms.

They can occur anywhere along the aorta but the majority are at the isthmus (85–90%), followed by distal thoracic aorta (5%), abdominal aorta (5%), and aortic root (1%) in order of descending frequency, most often at sites of relative aortic fixation. Abdominal aortic injury can be associated with lower thoracic and lumbar vertebral body fractures (Fig. 89.64)

- Chest radiograph findings of TAI are sensitive but not specific and described earlier in the chapter. The imaging technique of choice for suspected TAI is MDCT and if the initial MDCT is equivocal then repeat cardiac gated CT is recommended [45,46]
- Direct signs of aortic injury on MDCT include pseudoaneurysm formation, periaortic hematoma with loss of fat plane around the aorta, abnormal aortic contour, intimal flab and thrombus, active extravasation, and aortic pseudocoarctation (narrowing of the distal thoracic aorta due to hemorrhage) [12] (Figs. 89.3, 89.29, 89.30, and 89.32)
- Mediastinal hematoma with preservation of the fat plane around the thoracic aorta will not be from TAI and should prompt further evaluation of the mediastinal structures, in particular the aortic branch vessels (Fig. 89.31). *Periarterial hematoma in the superior mediastinum is an important indirect sign of possible brachiocephalic or subclavian injury*
- Multiplanar and volumetric reformats (particularly the sagittal oblique plane) are invaluable to confirm axial findings, characterize the TAI, and determine optimum treatment, particularly as the treatment of choice is more often endovascular stent graft repair [13,46] (Fig. 89.30)

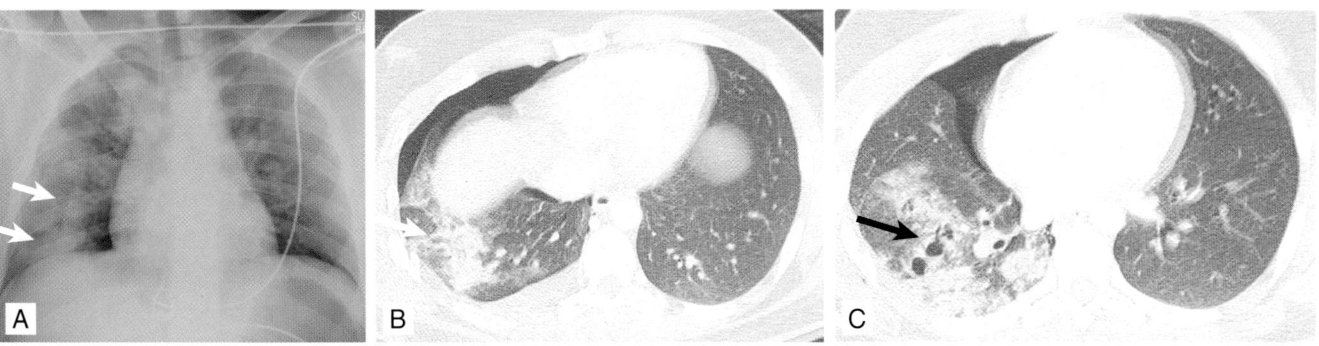

Figure 89.25 Blunt trauma. Pedestrian versus car. Supine CXR demonstrates multiple air space opacities in right hemithorax (*white arrows*). (B and C) Corresponding axial CT imaging on lung windows characterizes these much better as lung contusions (*white arrow*) and lung lacerations (*black arrows*) respectively. Note also the right hemopneumothorax is much better delineated on the subsequent CT. Multiple right-sided rib fractures are seen on the CXR primarily because a number of them (6th–8th ribs) are displaced. Characterization of rib fractures (including site, number, degree of displacement) should be performed on CT.

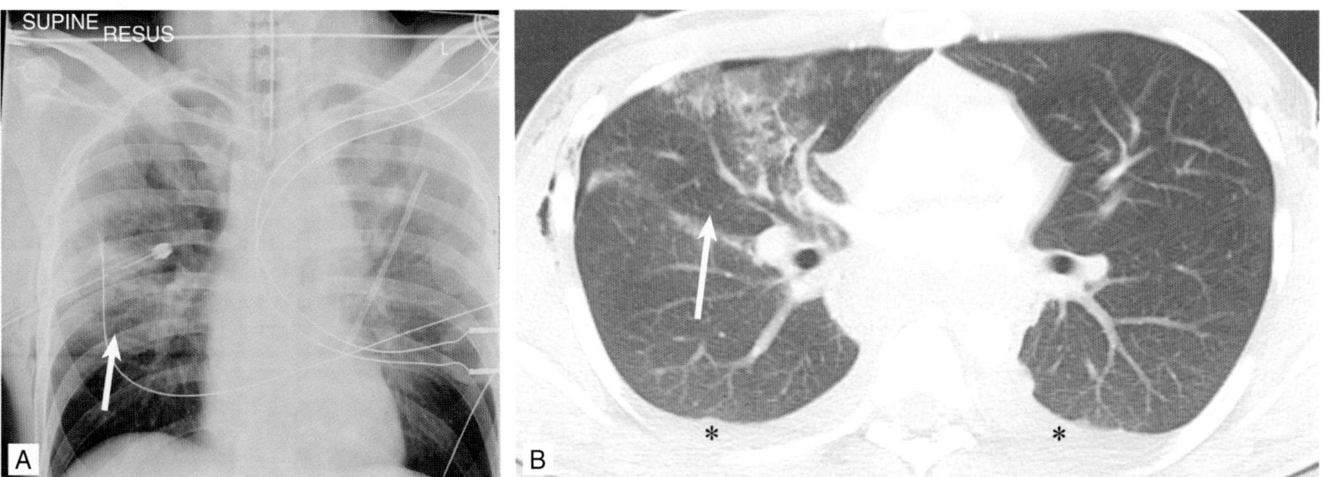

Figure 89.26 Blunt trauma. Motorcyclist versus car. (A) Supine CXR confirms appropriate siting of ETT (at level of medial clavicles). Right intercostal drain in situ. Ill-defined air space opacifications in right upper and mid zones (*white arrows*), confirmed on subsequent CT as lung contusions. (B) Axial CT image (lung windows) demonstrates ill-defined ground glass change on the right consistent with lung contusion (*white arrow*). Note also shallow bilateral hemothoraces (*asterisk*) and surgical emphysema in right chest wall from recent at scene thoracostomy and subsequent chest drain insertion (not shown).

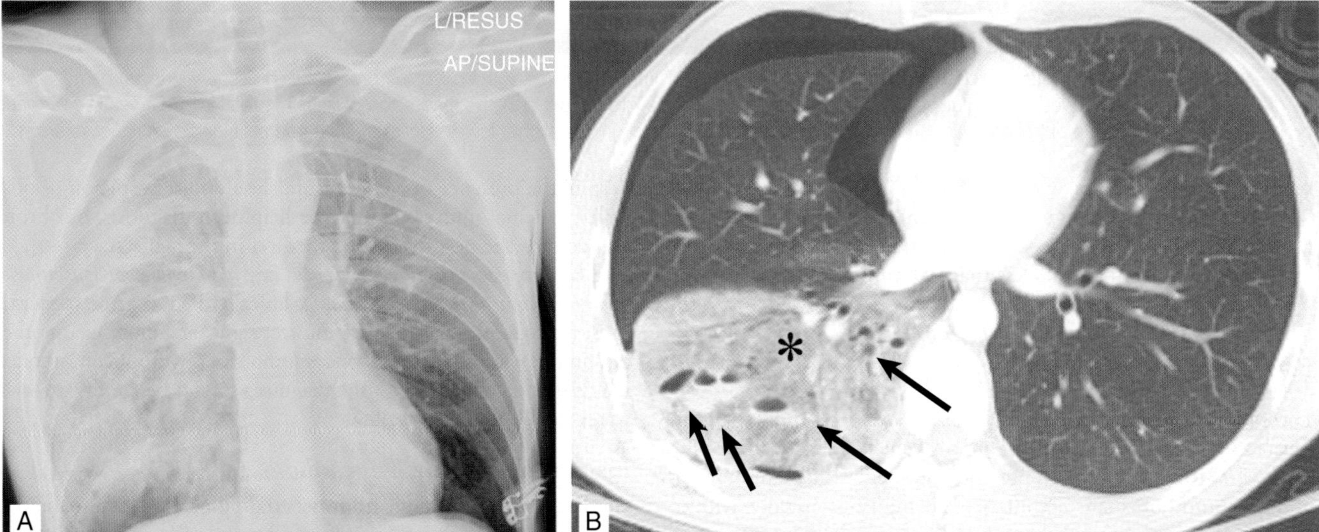

Figure 89.27 Blunt trauma pedestrian versus car. (A) Supine CXR demonstrates multiple displaced right sided rib fractures with diffuse increased opacification throughout right hemithorax consistent with hemothorax layering posteriorly along the pleural space. Further ill-defined nodular air space opacities in the right mid and lower zones are better characterized on the subsequent CT. (B) Axial CT image (lung windows), confirms right-sided hemopneumothorax. The ill-defined air space opacites seen on the x-ray are a combinaton of lung contusion (*asterisk*) and partially blood-filled lung lacerations (*black arrows*).

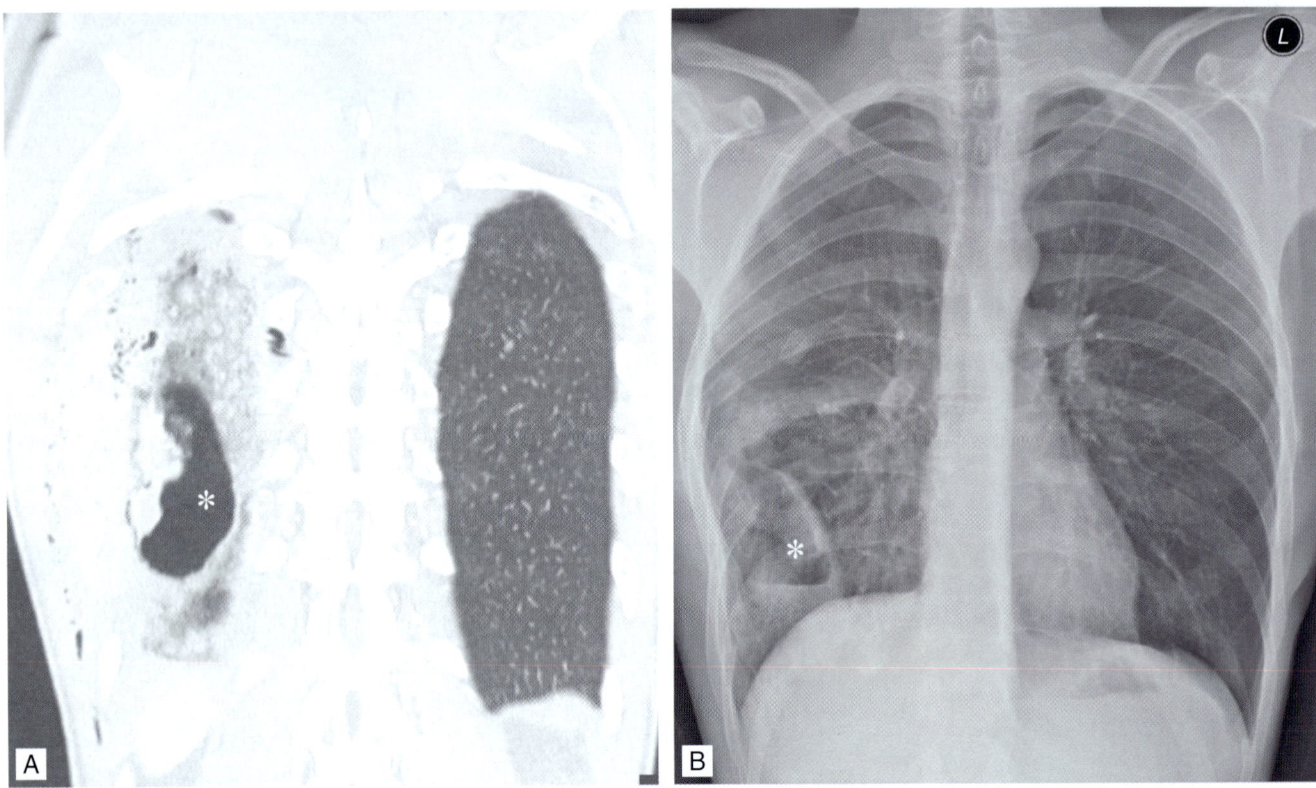

Figure 89.28 Blunt trauma pedestrian versus car. (A) Coronal CT reformat, lung windows, on admission, confirms large traumatic lung laceration on the right (*asterisk*). (B) CXR day 10—the large right lung laceration persists with air-fluid level within it (*asterisk*). Multiple right-sided rib fractures persist. Lung lacerations can persist for weeks to months, therefore it is important to correlate any CXR findings with previous imaging and history.

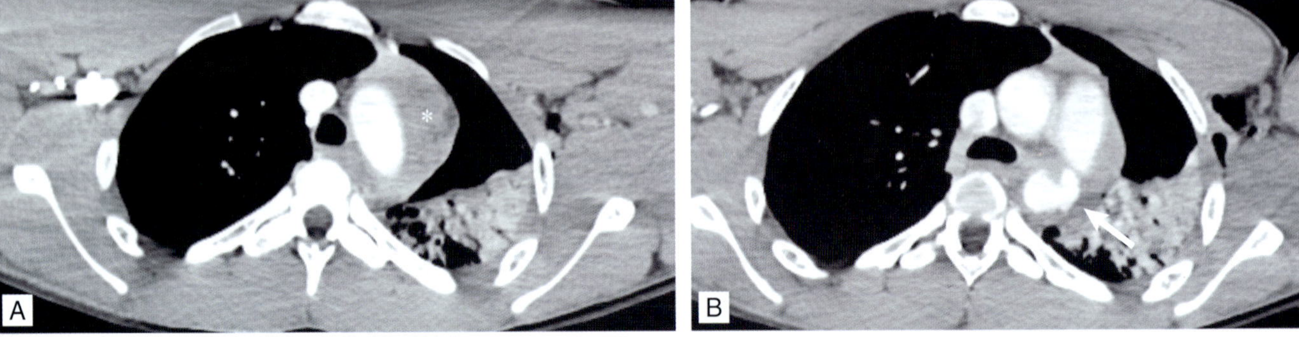

Figure 89.29 Blunt trauma motor vehicle collision at 70 mph. (A) Axial CT image acquired with split bolus protocol (soft tissue windows) demonstrates mediastinal hematoma with loss of the fat plane around the aorta (*asterisk*). This should alert the reader to potential mediastinal great vessel injury and prompt careful interrogation of the aorta and the major arch vessels. (B) Axial CT image slightly lower confirms acute traumatic aortic injury (*white arrow*).

- Treatment is usually within 24 hours of diagnosis but one must take into account other significant comorbid injuries that may necessitate more urgent treatment. Minimal aortic injures, described as intimal tears less than 10 mm in length, typically follow a nonoperative course and can be followed up with CTA until resolution [45] (Fig. 89.32)

Tracheobronchial and Esophagus Injuries

Laceration or rupture of a major airway is an uncommon result of severe chest trauma, usually in a motor vehicle collision. Fracture of the first three ribs is often present, and mediastinal emphysema and pneumothorax are common. The injury is usually within 2.5 cm of the carina with bronchial laceration being more common than tracheal laceration. If the bronchial sheath is preserved there may be no immediate signs or symptoms, but tracheostenosis or bronchiectasis may occur later. Peristent pneumothorax despite the presence of a chest drain should raise suspicion of possible bronchial injury. CT may be helpful in diagnosis, but bronchoscopy is the best diagnostic method in the acute stage [44].

Blunt esophagus rupture is extremely rare with most esophagus injuries occurring from penetrating trauma. Clinically there is acute mediastinitis; radiographically there are indirect signs including pneumomediastinum, with or without a pneumothorax or hydropneumothorax, which is usually left-sided. The diagnosis should be confirmed by a water-soluble contrast swallow.

Injuries to Heart and Pericardium

Cardiac injury may result from penetrating or blunt trauma and is rare accounting for less than 10% of all trauma admissions. Penetrating injuries are usually rapidly fatal (mortality of approximately 80% in gunshot wounds and 60% in stab wounds) but may cause tamponade, ventricular aneurysm, or septal defects. Survival is directly

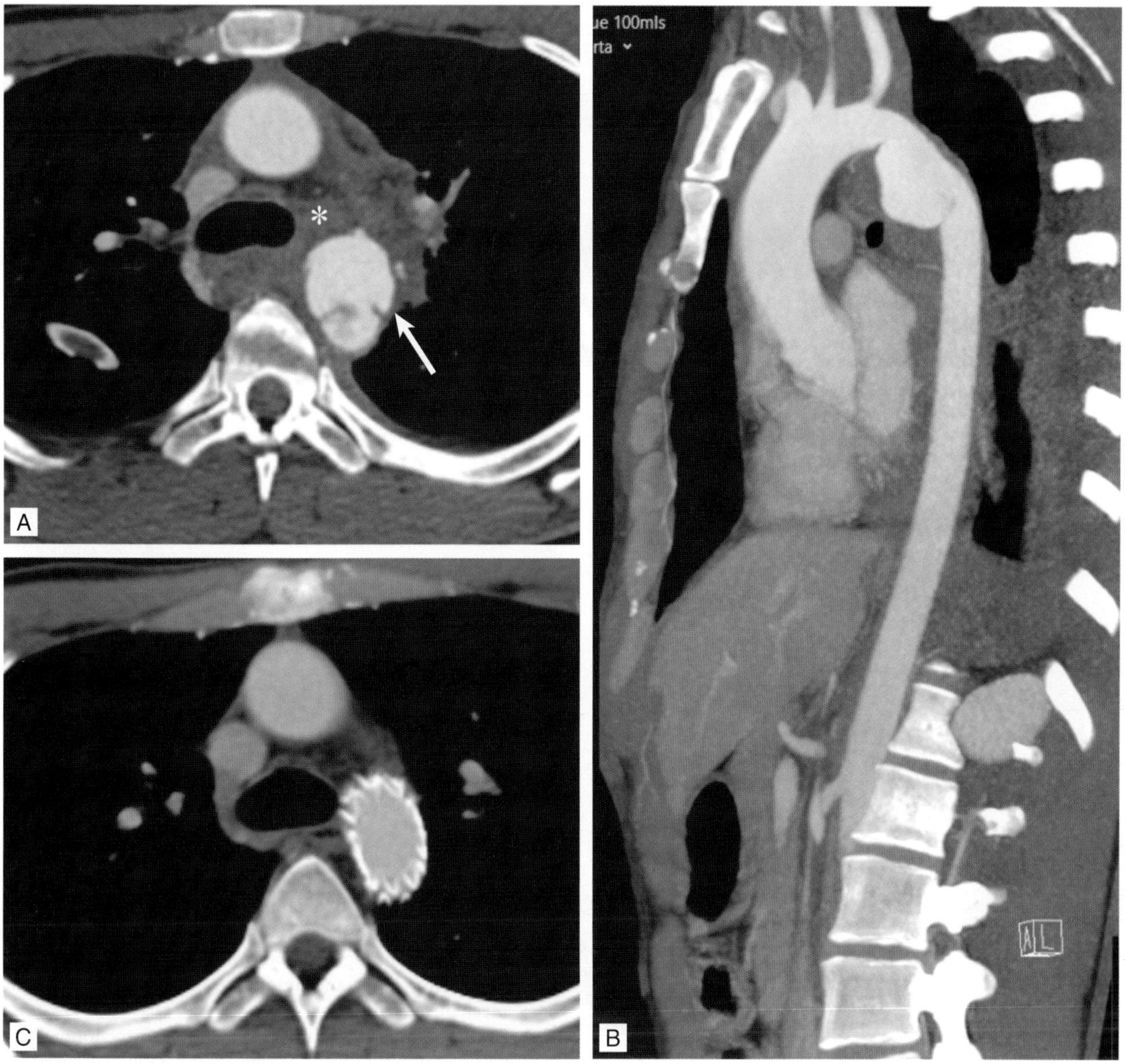

Figure 89.30 Blunt trauma. Motorcyclist versus car. (A) Axial postcontrast CT acquired using split bolus protocol demonstrates focal traumatic pseudoaneurysm formation at the aortic isthmus consistent with acute TAI (*white arrow*). Note the periaortic hematoma with loss of fat plane at the aorta (*asterisk*). (B) Oblique sagittal reformat is useful to delineate the aortic injury further in this region and can help in preoperative planning as distance of the injury from the left subclavian artery is important. (C) Axial image from dedicated CTA of the thoracic aorta 3 months after injury at a similar level confirms resolution of the periaortic hematoma and no endoleak from the thoracic aortic stent.

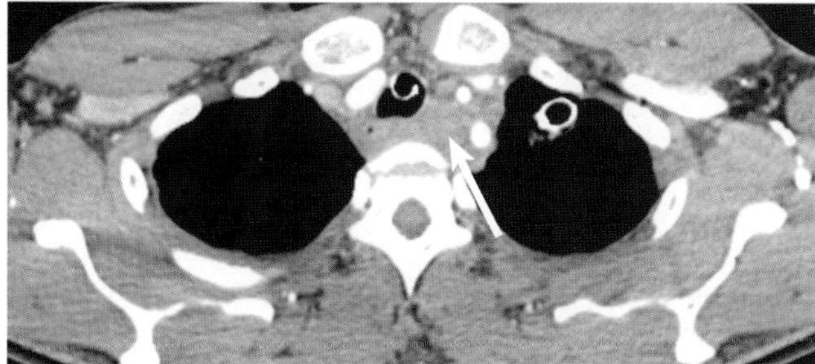

Figure 89.31 Blunt trauma. Motorcyclist versus car. ETT and left-sided intercostal drain in situ. Acute mediastinal hematoma surrounding the left subclavian artery (*white arrow*). Close interrogation of the aortic arch branch vessels should be performed to ensure no direct signs of vessel injury. Interrogation of the thoracic spine at this level is also warranted. *ETT*, endotracheal tube.

related to initial hemodynamic status [47]. Blunt trauma may cause myocardial contusion and infarction and may be associated with transient or more permanent rhythm disturbance. *There is no single test to rule blunt cardiac injury in or out but a combination of normal ECG and normal cardiac enzymes has a negative predictive value of 98% for significant blunt cardiac injury* [48]. CT has low sensitivity in detecting cardiac injuries but imaging findings include hemo- or pneumo-pericardium, intramural hematoma, and cardiac herniation if pericardial tear (Figs. 89.33 and 89.34). Coronal multiplanar reformats are helpful to identify shallow hemopericardium.

Injuries to Thoracic Cage

Rib Fractures

- Rib fractures are the commonest skeletal injury in blunt chest trauma. The chest radiograph has limited sensitivity

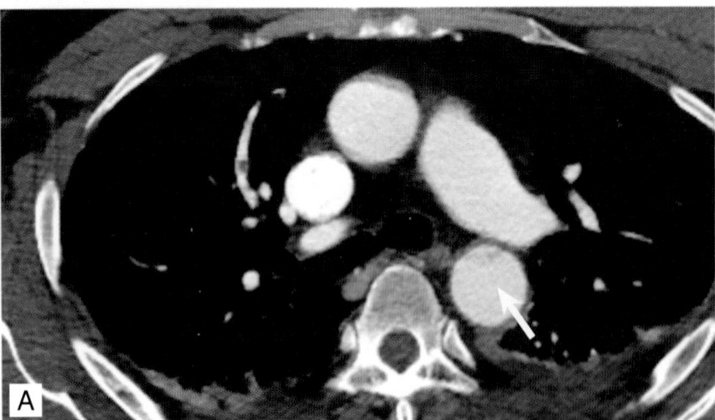
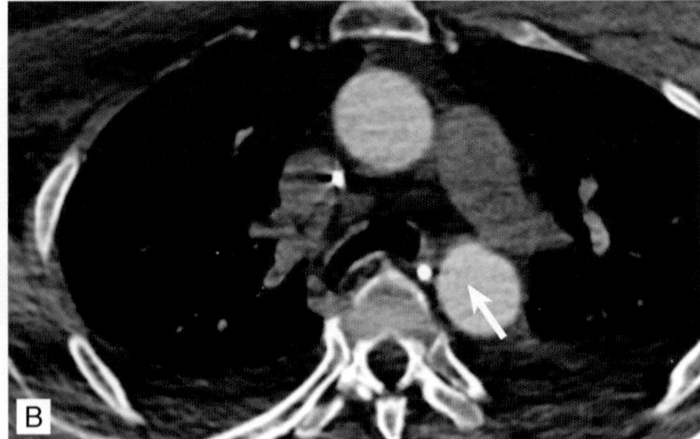

Figure 89.32 Blunt trauma. Pedestrian versus car. (A) Axial CT acquired using split bolus technique confirms focal intimal flap at aortic isthmus consistent with grade 1 acute TAI or minimal aortic injury (*white arrow*). Decision made to follow up with dedicated CTA at 48 hours. (B) Axial CT image (arterial phase) at 48 hours demonstrates almost complete resolution of the intimal flap tear. Repeat CTA at day 7 was normal.

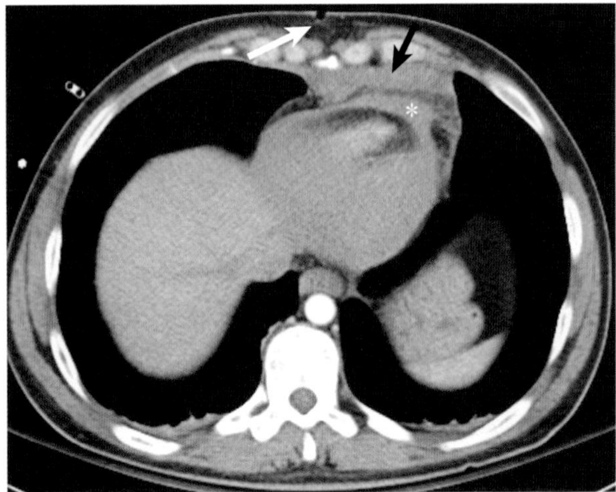

Figure 89.33 Penetrating trauma. Self-inflicted stab wounds to praecordial region. Axial CT image following IV contrast demonstrates focal skin defect anteriorly in the midline (*white arrow*). There is retrosternal hematoma (*black arrow*) and high attenuation fluid within the pericardium in keeping with hemopericardium (*asterisk*).

for the detection of rib fractures but can delineate complications from them including significant pneumo- and hemo-thorax (Fig. 89.2). CT is excellent at not only identifying number and location of rib fractures but importantly any associated thoracic injuries. Multiplanar reformats are useful to aid fracture detection, especially if they are undisplaced

- Fractures of the first three ribs are indicative of high-velocity injury and should prompt careful evaluation of the mediastinal great vessels, in particular the subclavian arteries, while fractures of the lower three ribs may be associated with hepatic, splenic or renal injury [49] (Fig. 89.35)
- Overall morbidity and mortality increases with the increasing number of fractures, particularly so in the elderly population, therefore early identification and aggressive pain control measures including regional analgesia with percutaneous catheter infusion are crucial [50]
- Another complication of rib fractures includes a flail segment. Flail chest occurs when there are three or more contiguous ribs with fractures in two or more places. It is usually apparent clinically, the affected part of the chest wall being paradoxically sucked in during inspiration, possibly compromising the underlying lung, and leading to increased requirement for mechanical ventilation
- At this point, it is important to mention costochondral fractures which commonly occur in high energy trauma, often occur with multiple consecutive rib fractures and also contribute to chest wall instability [51]. These can be more subtle and careful interrogation of the entire rib from costovertebral to costochondral junction with the aid of multiplanar reformats is important

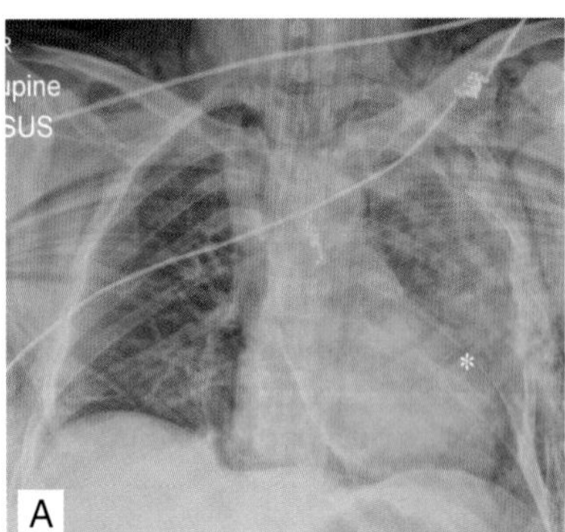
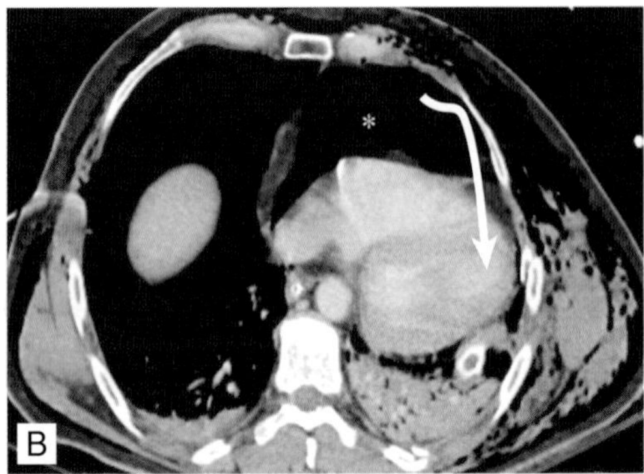
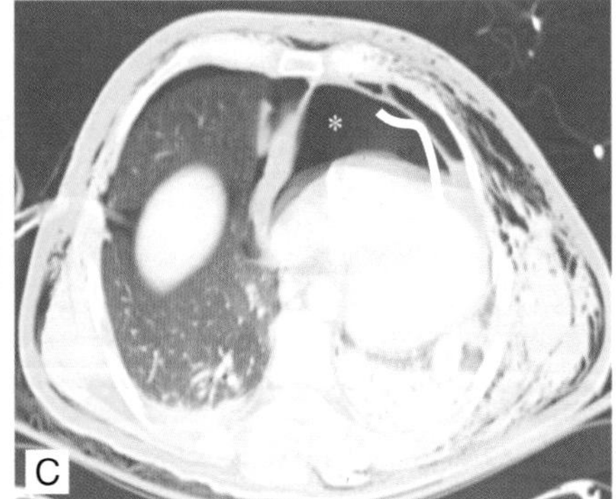

Figure 89.34 Blunt trauma. MVC (motor vehicle collision) left-sided impact. (A) Supine AP CXR demonstrates extensive surgical emphysema outlining the pectoral musculature and soft tissues of the chest wall bilaterally. There are multiple displaced left-sided rib fractures. In addition, there is evidence of pneumopericardium (*asterisk*). (B and C) Axial CT (soft tissue and lung windows) demonstrates pneumopericardium (*asterisk*). There is also posterior displacement of the heart with clockwise rotation of the left ventricle apex all consistent with traumatic pericardial rupture (*arrow*).

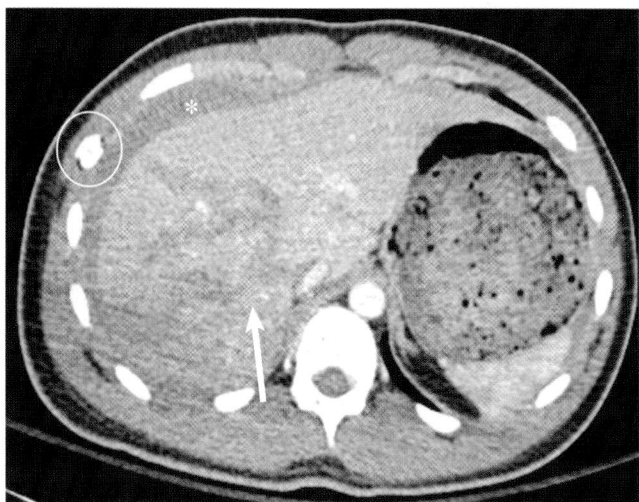

Figure 89.35 Blunt trauma. Fall from height onto wall. Axial CT image following IV contrast demonstrates branching central liver lacerations (bear claw appearance) which extend to the liver capsule posteriorly (*white arrow*). There is associated hemoperitoneum (*asterisk*). No active extravasation either within the liver parenchyma or into the peritoneal cavity. AAST Grade IV liver injury. Associated right rib fracture (*circle*).

- Surgical fixation of flail chest injuries has been shown to reduce pulmonary complications, ITU stays and mortality in *selected* patients [52] (Fig. 89.36). At our institution, there is multidisciplinary team discussion of each case to aid decision making around conservative or surgical management of these patients. *Regardless of whether the multiple rib fractures constitute "flail chest," the importance of early good regional anaesthesia cannot be emphasized enough in these patients*

Sternal Fractures

Sternal fractures are most often as a result of direct impact to the chest or deceleration injuries, typically occurring at the body or manubrium. They are most commonly detected using MDCT and sagittal reformats are particularly helpful in detecting the minimally displaced fractures (Fig. 89.37). They may be associated with retrosternal hematoma and if present should prompt careful interrogation of the heart, mediastinal structures and thoracic spine, particularly when as a result of a fall from a height greater than 20 feet [22,48].

Clavicle Fractures

Fractures of the clavicle may be associated with injury to the subclavian vessels or brachial plexus (scapulothoracic dissociation or floating shoulder) and posterior dislocation of the clavicle at the sternoclavicular joint may cause injury to the trachea, oesophagus, great vessels, or nerves of the superior mediastinum.

Scapula Fractures

Fractures of the scapula are rare and usually as a result of high energy trauma, e.g., fall from height or motor vehicle collisions. Their presence should again prompt careful interrogation for other thoracic injuries, including integrity of the shoulder girdle and adjacent neurovascular bundle. Management is typically conservative unless there is significant displacement.

Injuries to the Diaphragm

- Laceration of the diaphragm may result from penetrating or nonpenetrating trauma to the chest or abdomen. Ruptures of the left hemidiaphragm are encountered more frequently in clinical practice than ruptures on the right, possibly because of the protective effect of the liver. The typical plain film appearance is of obscuration of the affected hemidiaphragm and increased shadowing in the ipsilateral hemithorax due to herniation of stomach, omentum, bowel, or solid viscera (Fig. 89.38), although such herniation may be delayed
- A number of direct and indirect CT signs have been described (Figs. 89.39–89.45). In cases of isolated penetrating trauma,

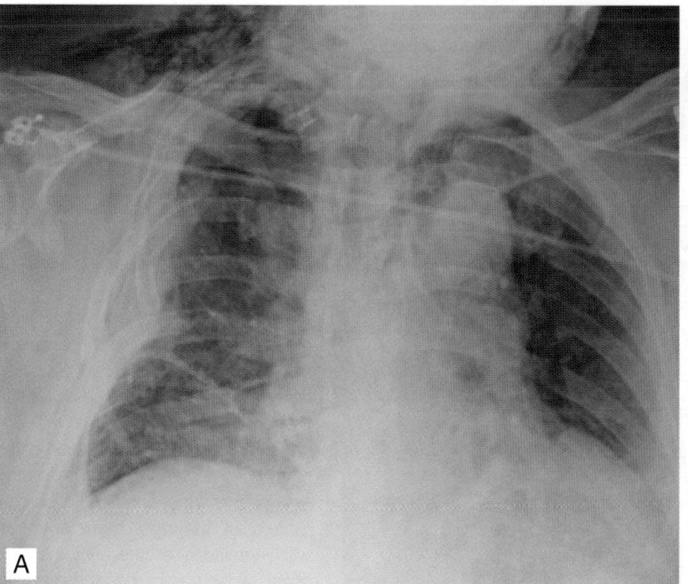

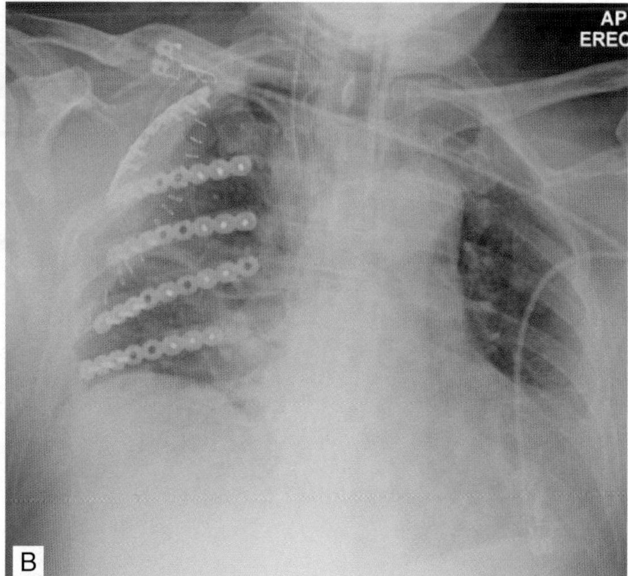

Figure 89.36 Blunt trauma. Elderly patient fall from standing onto the right side. (A) Semierect AP CXR demonstrates multiple displaced right sided rib fractures with radiological flail segment confirmed on CT. Large bore intercostal drain was placed for the associated pneumothorax. However, despite early and aggressive pain control measures, the patient developed increased respiratory distress. Decision was made to proceed to right-sided surgical fixation on day 4 following the injury with excellent clinical response. (B) CXR following right-sided rib plate fixation.

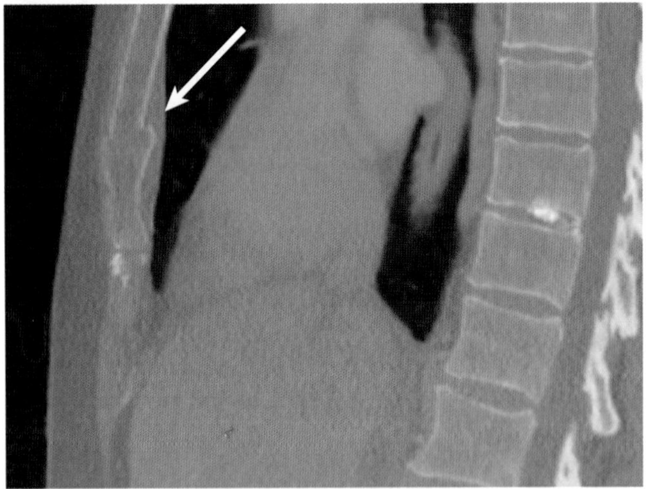

Figure 89.37 Blunt trauma. Fall from height. Sagittal reformat on bone windows demonstrates minimally displaced fracture through body of sternum. Sternal fractures can be easily overlooked on axial CT imaging and the coronal and in particular sagittal reformats should be reviewed to ensure no injury. Sternal fractures resulting from significant mechanism of blunt trauma should prompt careful review of the heart, mediastinal great vessels, and the spine to ensure no associated injury.

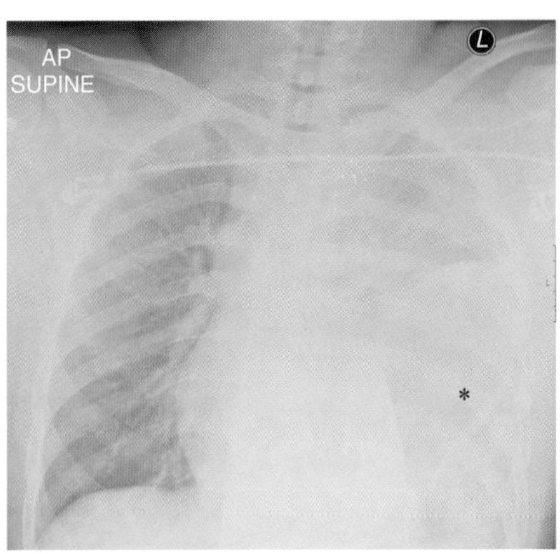

Figure 89.38 Blunt trauma. Restrained driver MVC. AP supine CXR, taken as part of the primary survey, demonstrates loss of left hemidiaphragm with abnormal gas-filled structure in the left hemithorax due to herniation of bowel into left chest (*asterisk*).

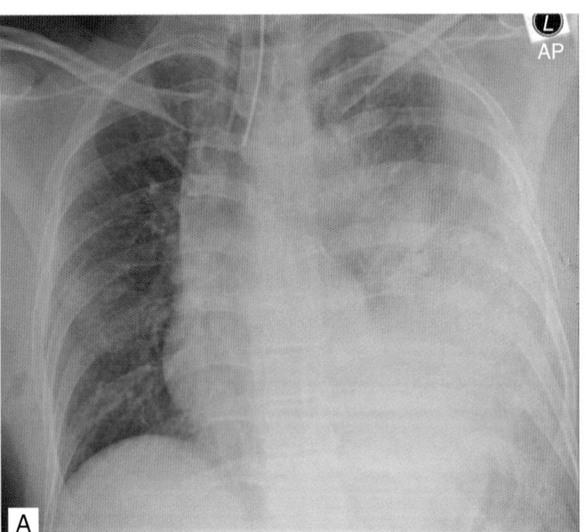

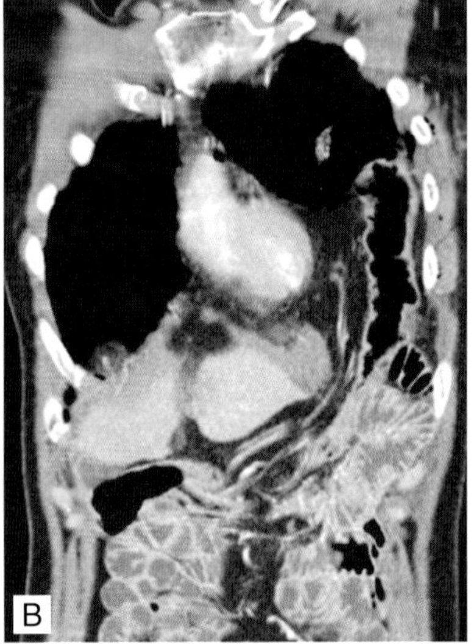

Figure 89.39 Blunt trauma. Passenger high-speed MVC. Hemodynamically stable. (A) AP supine CXR taken as part of the primary survey. ETT in situ appropriately sited. There is tracheal deviation to the right and increased shadowing in the lower left hemithorax with complete loss of the left hemidiaphragm. (B) Coronal CT reformat confirms left hemidiaphragm rupture with herniation of splenic flexure and small bowel loops into the left chest. (Indirect sign of diaphragm injury). Patient proceeded to theatre for laparotomy. *ETT*, endotracheal tube.

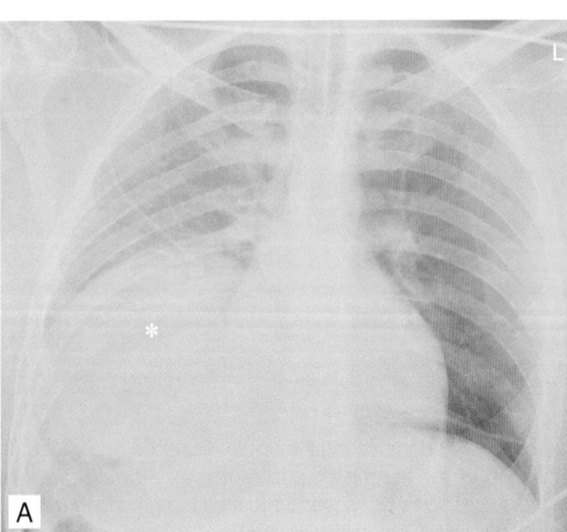

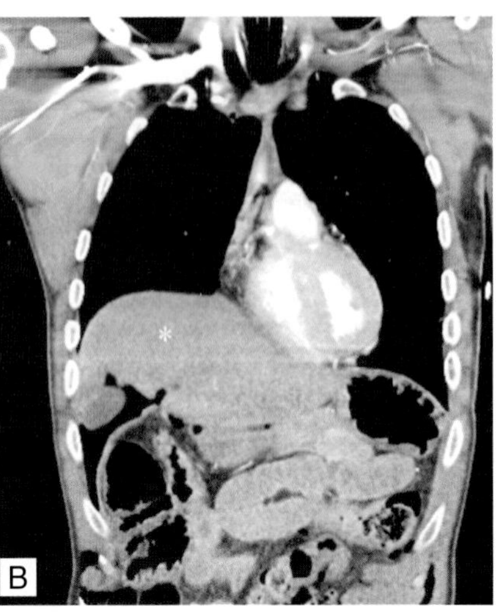

Figure 89.40 Blunt trauma. Patient crushed between wall and car. Supine AP CXR. ETT in situ appropriately sited. Homogeneous increased opacification of right lower zone with the appearance of marked elevation of the right hemidiaphragm. Coronal reformat of the subsequent CT confirms rupture of the right hemidiaphragm with herniation of the liver into the chest (which explains the appearances seen on the CXR) (*asterisk*). Intrathoracic herniation of viscera is an indirect sign of diaphragmatic injury. *ETT*, endotracheal tube.

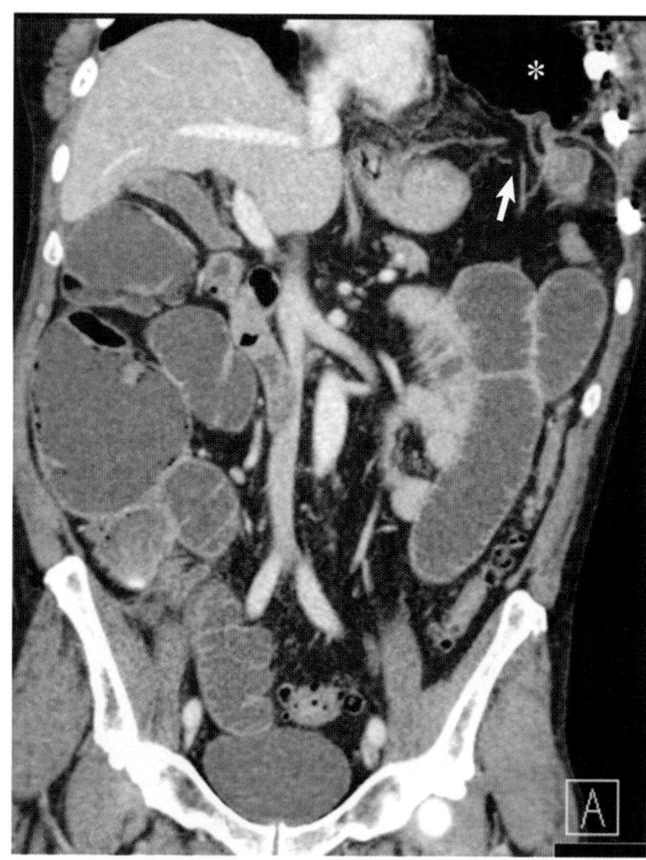

Figure 89.41 Blunt trauma 12 months previously. Patient who had been involved in a MVC 12 months previously. At initial injury patient had sustained a number of rib fractures. The patient represented with clinical evidence of bowel obstruction. Coronal CT reformat demonstrates defect in left hemidiaphragm (*white arrow*) with herniation of splenic flexure (*asterisk*) through the defect into the chest with associated bowel obstruction.

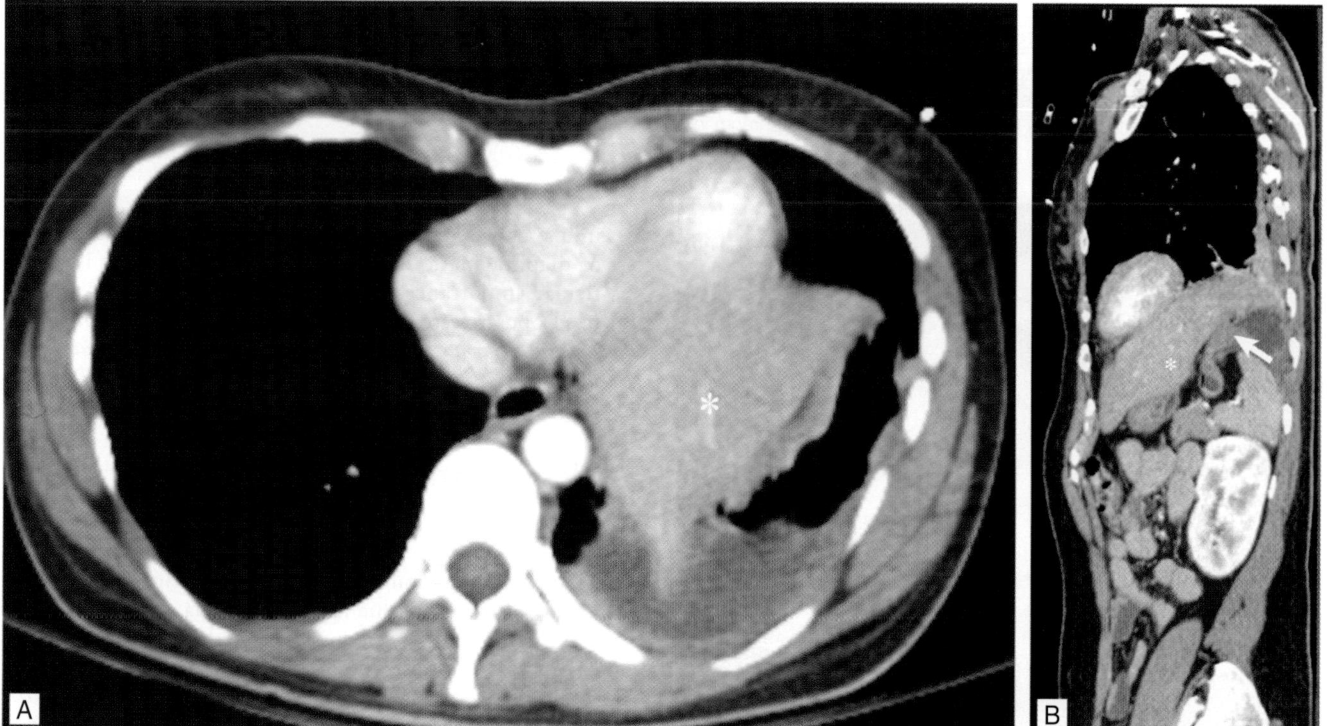

Figure 89.42 Blunt trauma. Pedestrian versus van. Axial and coronal images demonstrate intrathoracic herniation of left lobe of liver (*asterisk*) and part of the stomach (*white arrow*) through defect in the left hemidiaphragm (an indirect sign of diaphragm injury). This case illustrates the importance of evaluation of the multiplanar reformats to fully interrogate the diaphragm.

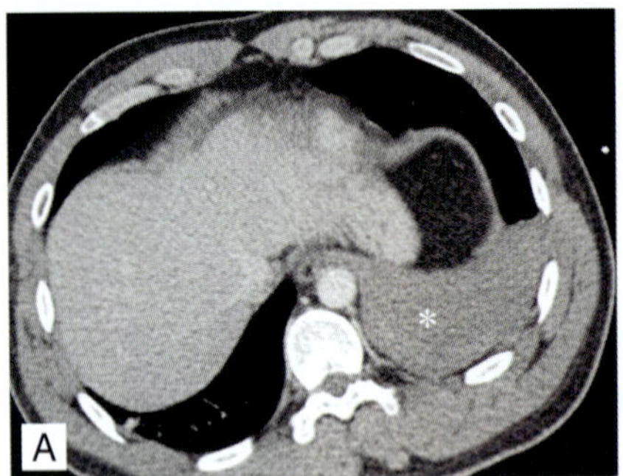
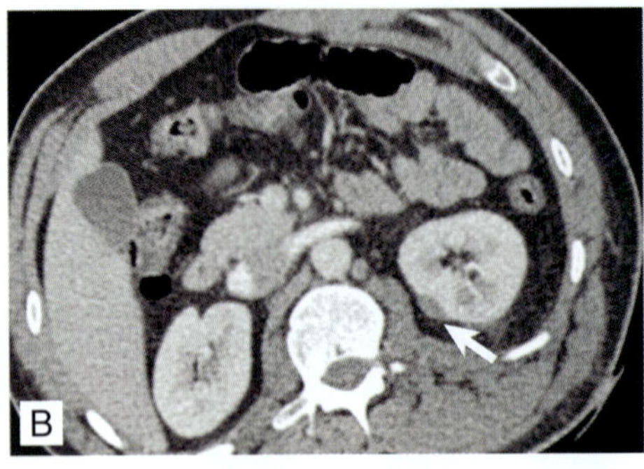
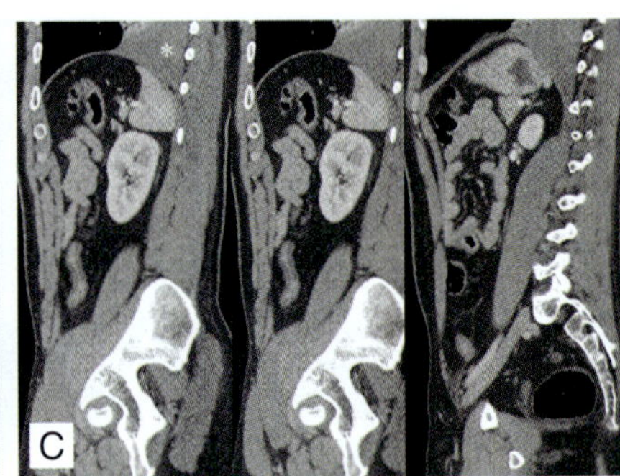

Figure 89.43 Penetrating trauma. Single stab wound to left flank. (A and B) Selected axial CT imaging acquired using split bolus protocol demonstrates moderate left hemothorax (*asterisk*) and AAST grade I renal injury (*white arrow*). (C) These contiguous injuries above and below the diaphragm in the context of isolated penetrating trauma to left flank should raise index of suspicion of diaphragmatic injury and prompt careful evaluation of multiplanar reformats (MPRs) (Indirect sign of diaghragmatic injury). Note in this case the sagittal reformats did not reveal the diaphragmatic injury but decision made to proceed to laparotomy to evaluate further given the indirect sign on CT. A 10 cm tear of the left hemidiaphragm was confirmed at laparotomy and repaired.

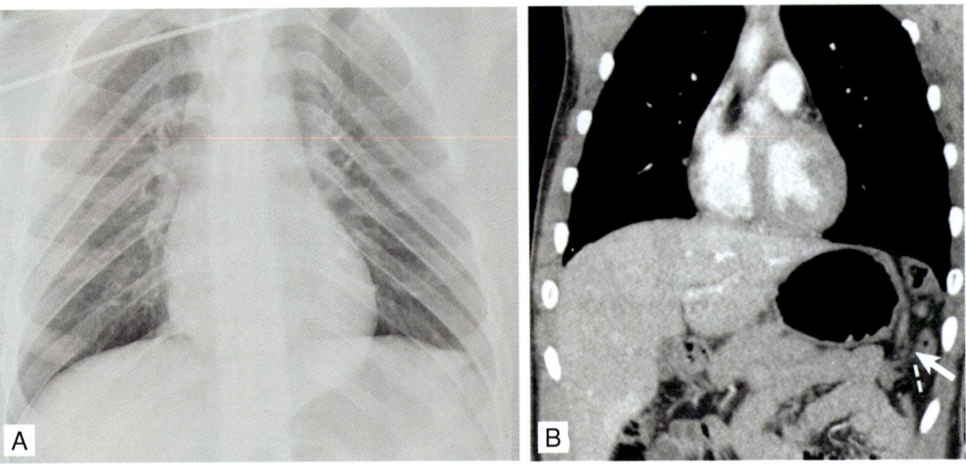

Figure 89.44 Penetrating trauma. Stab wound to left upper quadrant. Hemodynamically stable. (A) Supine CXR, taken as part of primary survey, is essentially normal. In particular the left hemi diaphragm appears intact. (B) Coronal CT reformat confirms focal discontinuity (*dashed line*) of the left hemidiaphragm with dangling diaphragm sign (*white arrow*), both direct signs of diaphragm injury. Note the herniation of omentum and bowel through the defect laterally but not above the medial hemidiaphragm which gives the seemingly normal appearance of the left hemidiaphragm on the initial CXR. Patient proceeded to laparotomy for repair of the left hemidiaphragm injury.

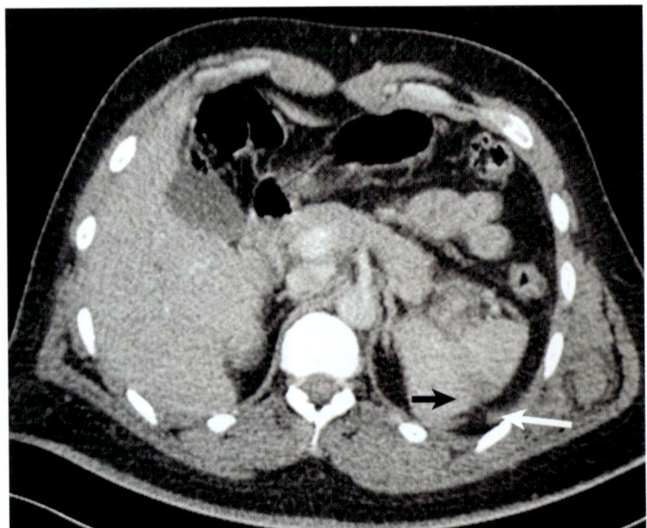

Figure 89.45 Penetrating trauma. Stab wound to left flank. Focal discontinuity of left hemi diaphragm (*white arrow*)—a direct sign of diaphragmatic injury Note also the AAST grade II splenic injury adjacent to this (*short black arrow*).

injury above and below the diaphragm is an indirect sign of diaphragmatic injury [53] (Fig. 89.43). This is of particular importance on the left as these injuries typically need operative repair (Fig. 89.41). *A review of coronal and sagittal reformats on MDCT is essential as more subtle diaphragmatic injuries may not be obvious on the axial imaging* (Fig. 89.42)

Abdominal Trauma

Introduction

Most traumatic abdominal injuries presenting to the emergency department are due to blunt trauma, the majority as a result of road traffic accidents, followed by falls, assault and sports related injuries. The most common cause of penetrating abdominal trauma is a stab wound or gunshot [24]. *Initial management of traumatic abdominal injuries will depend on hemodynamic stability and whether there are definitive indications for trauma laparotomy identified either clinically or, more often, on MDCT (e.g., bowel or intraperitoneal bladder injury)*

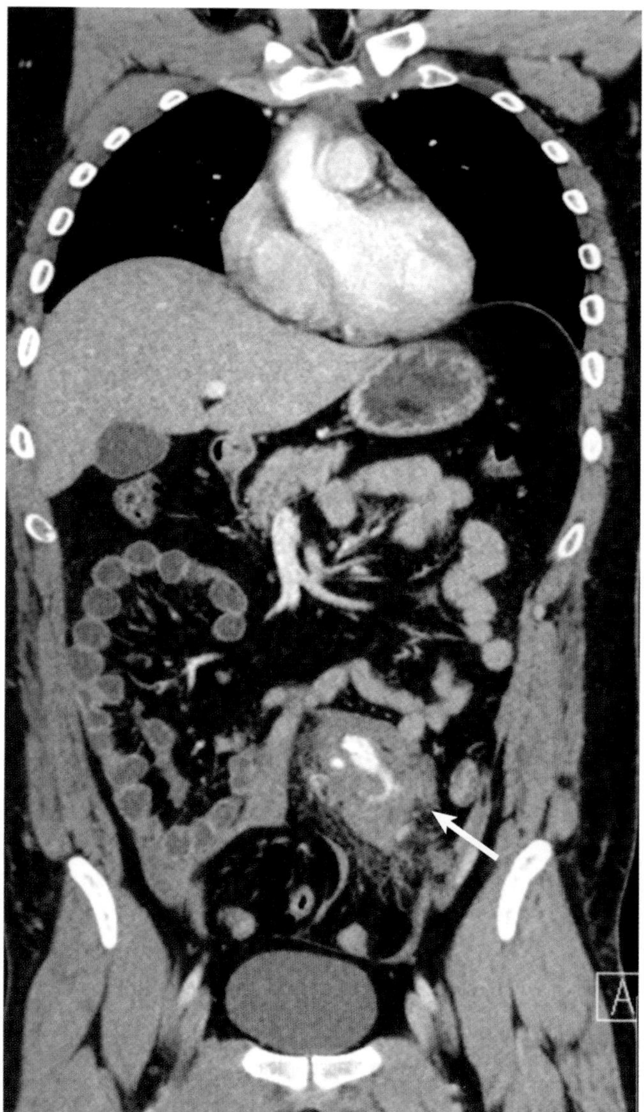

Figure 89.46 Blunt trauma. Restrained driver MVC. Hemodynamically labile. Initial responder to resuscitation. Coronal CT reformat acquired with split bolus protocol demonstrates mesenteric hemorrhage with focus of active extravasation (*white arrow*). Patient was peritonitic and proceeded directly to laparotomy. Large mesenteric tear was repaired.

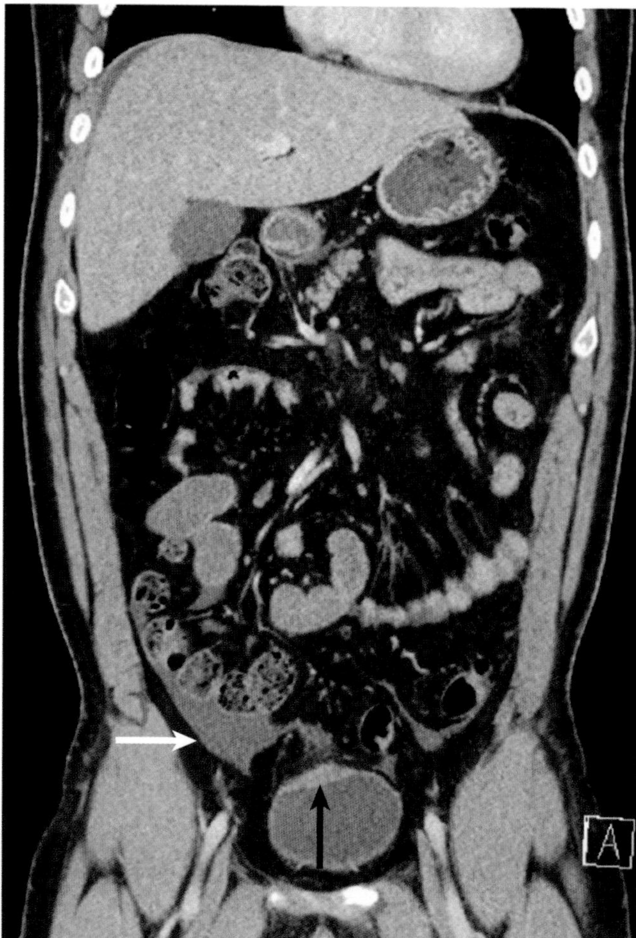

Figure 89.47 Blunt trauma. Pedestrian versus car. Hemodynamically stable. Complaining of abdominal pain. Coronal CT reformat acquired with split bolus protocol demonstrates free fluid within the right lower quadrant (*white arrow*). There is no solid organ or bowel injury identified on CT to account for this. However, there is focal bladder wall thickening at dome of bladder (*black arrow*). A dedicated CT cystogram was not performed as patient was clinically peritonitic and the index of suspicion for intraperitoneal bladder rupture was high based on these CT findings. Patient was taken to theatre for intraperitoneal bladder repair.

(Figs. 89.46–89.48). In the hemodynamically stable blunt trauma patient, management of solid organ injury has evolved to that of primarily nonoperative management (NOM) with increasing reliance on MDCT for diagnosis and classification of injuries [54]. The most widely accepted grading system for blunt splenic, hepatic and renal injuries is the revised organ injury scale (OIS) of the AAST. Its initial purpose was to provide anatomic description of injury (based on surgical findings) rather than guide clinical pathways [55]. The 1994-AAST revision did not include active contrast extravasation or intraparenchymal vascular injuries, both of which have been shown to be a major factor in failure of NOM of solid organ injuries (Figs. 89.11 and 89.15). A novel CT-based grading system for splenic injury was proposed in 2007 by Marmery et al., which proved to better predict the need for splenic artery embolization (SAE) or operative management (OM) [56]. *In 2018, AAST published an OIS update, incorporating CT diagnosed vascular injury and active bleeding into the liver, spleen, and kidney injury grading.* This has since been validated in a study by Morell-Hofert et al. in 2020 which showed that the revised 2018 version was superior to the 1994-AAST classification in terms of correlation with primary or secondary OM in blunt splenic and hepatic trauma [57]. As such, timely and accurate CT interpretation of solid organ injuries is crucial to aid management decisions and will be described in the following subsections.

There is no consensus on follow up imaging after NOM of solid organ injury. As such decisions around whether to repeat CT is often guided by the patient's clinical status or deterioration in blood tests [58] (Figs. 89.51 and 89.54). Routine postdischarge scans are often felt unnecessary [59].

Injury to the Spleen

The spleen is the most commonly injured organ in blunt abdominal trauma, accounting for up to 40% of all solid organ injuries.

- Hemobilia, due to the communication of the vascular tree with the biliary tree, also usually presents in a delayed fashion with pain, jaundice, and gastrointestinal bleeding. CT may demonstrate the presence of high-attenuation blood in a dilated biliary tree. The use of interventional assessment and selective embolization has reduced the morbidity and mortality of operative intervention

Management of Hepatic Injuries

NOM of blunt hepatic injuries is the treatment of choice in hemodynamically stable patients, irrespective of injury grade or patient age [67]. Angioembolization should be considered as an adjunct to this in the hemodynamically stable patient where there is clinical evidence of ongoing bleeding; imaging evidence of arterial bleeding; or suspicion of the ongoing arterial source of bleeding despite operative intervention [64] (Figs. 89.18 and 89.53). *Explorative laparotomy should be considered for those patients that are hemodynamically unstable, regardless of grade of liver injury* (Fig. 89.18). There may also be other injuries present that necessitate laparotomy regardless of hemodynamic status or grade of injury (Fig. 89.10).

The patient must be appropriately resuscitated and in an environment that permits constant physiological monitoring and ready access to surgery should there be clinical deterioration. *The role of CT, therefore, is to identify and characterize the liver injuries, determine the quantity of hemoperitoneum, and exclude the presence of other organ involvement.* It is advisable to use the AAST OIS grading scale when reporting CT findings of liver trauma and where possible describe proximity of the injury to hepatic veins and porta hepatis which increase the risk of NOM failure and biliary injury, respectively [68]. The AAST OIS 2018 update now incorporates CT findings and importantly, as with the spleen, vascular injury is now included in the higher grades, which may help to further guide clinical pathways [55,57] (Table 89.2). *A difference between the liver and splenic new AAST injury grading is that intraparenchymal bleeding of the liver is Grade III, whereas intraparenchymal bleeding within the spleen is Grade IV.* Grade IV liver injury now includes active bleed beyond the parenchyma (Fig. 89.53). The presence of active contrast extravasation or pooling, or of traumatic vascular malformations, are warnings that conservative management alone may fail and should at least prompt either angiographic assessment or follow up imaging to assess for post-traumatic pseudoaneurysm, biloma formation or hemobilia (Fig. 89.54).

Complications and Injury Resolution

- Following hepatic trauma, delayed complications occur in a fifth of patients overall, although these are more common in surgically treated patients. The main liver complications are delayed hemorrhage and infective collections. Involvement of

TABLE 89.2 Liver Injury Scale—2018 Revision

AAST Grade	AIS Severity	Imaging Criteria (CT Findings)	Operative Criteria	Pathologic Criteria
I	2	▪ Subcapsular hematoma <10% surface area ▪ Parenchymal lacration <1 cm in depth	▪ Subcapsular hematoma <10% surface area ▪ Parenchymal laceration <1 cm in depth Capsular tear	▪ Subcapsular hematoma <10% surface area ▪ Parenchymal laceration <1 cm capsular tear
II	2	▪ Subcapsular hematoma 10–50% surface area; intraparenchymal hematoma <10 cm in diameter ▪ Laceration 1–3 cm in depth and ≤10 cm length	▪ Subcapsular hematoma 10–50% surface area; parenchymal hematoma <10 cm in diameter ▪ Laceration 1–3 cm in depth and ≤10 cm length	▪ Subcapsular hematoma 10–50% surface areal intraparechymal hematoma <10 cm in diameter ▪ Laceration 1–3 cm depth and ≤10 cm length
III	3	▪ Subcapsular hematoma >50% surface area; ruptured subcapsular or parenchymal homatoma ▪ Intraparenchymal hematoma >10cm ▪ Laceration >3 cm depth ▪ Any injury in the presence of a liver vascular injury or active bleeding ocetained within liver parenchyma	▪ Subcapsular hematoma >50% surface area or expending; ruptured subcapsular or parenchymal hematoma ▪ Intraparenchymal hematoma >10 cm ▪ Laceration >3 cm in depth	▪ Subcapsular hematoma >50%-surface area; ruptured subcapsular or intraparenchymal hematoma ▪ Intraparenchymal hematoma >10 cm ▪ Laceration >3 cm in depth
IV	4	▪ Parenchymal disruption involving 25–75% of a hepatic lobe ▪ Active bleeding extending beyond the liver parenchyma into the peritoneum	▪ Parenchymal disruption involving 25–75% of a hepatic lobe	▪ Parenchymal disruption involving 25–75% of a hepatic lobe
V	5	▪ Parenchymal disruption >75% of hepatic lobe ▪ Juxtahepatic venous injury to include retrohepatic vena cava and control major hepatic veins	▪ Parenchymal disruption >75% of hepatic lobe ▪ Juxtahepatic venous injury to include retrohepatic vena cava and central major hepatic veins	▪ Parenchymal disruption >75% of hepatic lobe ▪ Juxtahepatic venous injury to include retrohepatic vena cava and central major hepatic veins

Vascular injury is defined as a pseudoancurysm or arterioveocus fistula and appears as a focal collection of contrast that decrease in attenuation with delayed imaging. Active bleeding from a vascular injury presents as extra-vascular contrast, focal or diffuse, that increase in size or attenuation in delayed phase. Vascular thrombosis can lead to organ infarction.
Grade based on highest grade assessment made on imaging, at operation or on pathologic specimen.
More than one grade of liver injury may be present and should be classified by the higher grade of injury.
Advance one grade for multiple injuries up to a grade III.

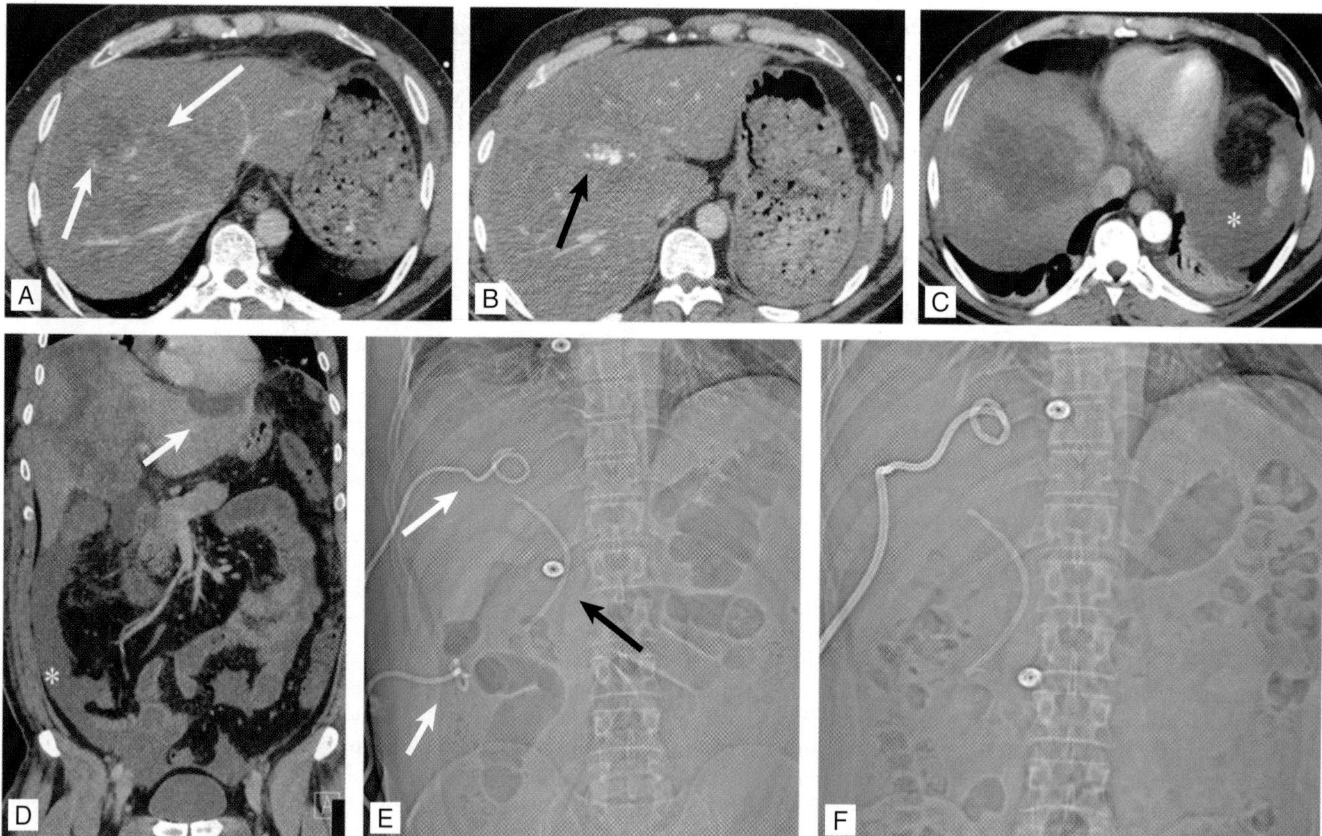

Figure 89.54 Blunt trauma. Crush injury between van and wall. Hemodynamically stable. (A and B) Selected axial CT images demonstrate multiple ill-defined low attenuation lacerations and hematoma within the substance of the liver (*white arrows*) with focal intraparenchymal contrast extravasation (*black arrow*). AAST grade III injury. Given it is isolated high-grade liver injury and patient remained hemodynamically stable, patient proceeded to nonoperative management (NOM). (C and D) Day 5 inflammatory markers rising. Repeat dual-phase CT performed. No intraparenchymal vascular injury on arterial phase. Portovenous phase scan shows evolution of the central liver injury with development of subcapsular biloma (*white arrow*) and free bile leak into the peritoneum (*asterisk*). Interval increase in low attenuation fluid within the abdomen and pelvis following high-grade liver injury should raise suspicion for intraperitoneal bile leak. (E and F) Selected scout images from CT scans performed at day 13 and day 46, respectively, demonstrate how protracted the course of these injuries can be. There have been interval percutaneous drainages (*white arrows*) and placement of a biliary stent endoscopically (*black arrow*) to encourage resolution of bile leak.

the biliary system may result in bilomas, hemobilia, bile peritonitis, and delayed strictures of the extrahepatic biliary tree

- Unless there are clinical signs or parameters suggesting such complications, there is little value in the routine follow-up of hepatic injuries to monitor resolution. Serial CT following injury to the liver demonstrates that, unless there is persistent hemorrhage, there should be significant reduction of hemoperitoneum within 3–7 days
- Intraparenchymal lacerations or hematomas initially expand and become more sharply defined as the damaged peripheral parenchyma is resorbed. The attenuation of the focal abnormality often falls owing to clot lysis and water osmosis. The time course of resolution of injuries over weeks or months often exceeds that of comparable splenic injuries, due to the inhibitory effect of stasis of bile products at the injury margins (Fig. 89.54)
- Injuries may heal completely or result in small cysts or serous collections. Focal intraparenchymal collections developing following hepatic trauma may relate to resolving hematomas, abscesses, or contained bile leaks termed bilomas. Distinguishing one from the other can be difficult, relying largely on the clinical context but often ultimately on diagnostic aspiration
- Infective abscesses may develop thick enhancing walls and on occasion contain gas bubbles. The latter finding has, however, been described in sterile resolving lacerations. Extension of the infection may result in subcapsular empyemas, which may demonstrate enhancement along their margin
- Bilomas tend to occur following deep injuries to the central periportal biliary tree. They usually present weeks to months after injury as simple thin-walled cysts with low-attenuation contents. Occasionally, however, septations may develop due to secondary infection or hemorrhage. Their communication with the biliary tree can be confirmed by hepatobiliary scintigraphy. MRI may help distinguish bilomas from hematomas if required [65]
- Biliary peritoneal leaks may result in biliary peritonitis following secondary infection. The suspicion of such a leak may be raised by the peristence or increase of low attenuation of the peritoneal fluid (0–20 HU compared with >50 HU in hemoperitoneum) after recent trauma, although this is usually confirmed by diagnostic aspiration (Fig. 89.54). *A high degree of suspicion by the radiologist, from the index CT findings together with follow up imaging in the days and weeks following the trauma, is integral to diagnosing bile leaks as the signs and symptoms of this delayed complication can be vague and nonspecific*
- Trauma patients with liver injury and free intraperitoneal bile leak have been shown to have prolonged hospital stays and

increased requirements for therapeutic procedures [69]. A multitechnique approach to management of post-traumatic bile leaks is often required with percutaneous drainage or endoscopic-surgical intervention often the treatments of choice (Fig. 89.54)

Injury to the Kidneys and Ureters

Renal trauma accounts for 8–10% of all abdominal trauma. The vast majority are due to blunt trauma from motor vehicle collisions, assaults, or fall from height. The remainder is largely attributable to stabbings, gunshot, and iatrogenic procedures. Certain anatomical variants predispose to renal injury. These include horseshoe, cross-fused, and pelvic or transplanted kidneys. This susceptibility is due to their relatively anterior location and the potential for compression against the spine. The presence of congenital or acquired cystic disease, hydronephrosis, and solid vascular lesions (e.g., angiomyolipomas, renal cell carcinomas) also predisposes to injury.

Imaging Features

- Contrast-enhanced MDCT is the imaging technique of choice for renal trauma and other associated injuries. Although it has become clear that CT is an excellent tool for the detection and characterization of renal injuries, more debate has centered on the indications for imaging in suspected renal trauma. In adults with blunt trauma the presence of gross hematuria or the combination of microscopic hematuria and shock (<90 mmHg systolic) are indications for imaging to exclude renal injury and other associated intra-abdominal injuries. 25% of patients with gross hematuria will have significant renal injuries. In a meta-analysis of 2873 patients with blunt trauma, microscopic hematuria and no shock, only 10 significant injuries were identified. Of these, only one did not have other associated injuries that would have necessitated abdominal imaging or surgery that would have identified the renal injury. Thus, the restriction of imaging to those patients with microscopic hematuria and shock is justified, with a failed detection rate of only 0.03%. While it has been stated that renal pedicle abruption can rarely occur without hematuria, a review of the literature reveals all such injuries have been associated with other significant injuries that necessitated imaging
- Unlike blunt trauma, the indications for renal imaging in penetrative trauma are based solely on the site of injury and are irrespective of the presence of hematuria. This approach is justified because the rate of significant renal injuries can be as high as 67% in penetrating trauma, as opposed to 4% in blunt trauma. Moreover, penetrating injuries are more likely to result in renal loss. In a large series of proven, stab injuries to the kidney 9% had no hematuria. Other studies have demonstrated no relationship between the degree of hematuria and the severity of renal injury
- *Normality of renal appearances on CT effectively excludes any significant renal injury.* Portal venous phase imaging delineates renal lacerations (linear disruptions that may extend into the medulla), renal contusions (ill-defined globular areas of low attenuation), subcapsular hematomas (crescentic fluid collections confined by renal capsule that distort the underlying renal parenchyma) and perinephric hematomas (acute high attenuation perinephric fluid with ill-defined margins usually bounded by Gerota's fascia) [70,71] (Fig. 89.55)
- Later phase excretory images (5–10 min) should be used when there is significant fluid around the renal pelvis or renal lacerations that appear to extend to the medulla to assess for urine leak from collecting system injury [72] (Figs. 89.12 and 89.56). Delayed phase imaging may also be useful in distinguishing between active bleeding and pseudoaneurysms. However, if the patient is hemodynamically unstable then this phase can be performed at a later time
- More severe renal injuries are well delineated by CT and this has resulted in a reduction of exploratory staging surgery. Fractured and shattered kidneys are accurately defined, as well as the extent of the devascularized fragments. CT may often determine the presence of pedicular injuries, reducing the need for angiography. This results in expedited surgery, increasing the success rate of revascularization
- Renal arterial injury is characterized by absent renal perfusion or a rim nephrogram, abrupt cut-off of the renal artery with periarterial hematoma and retrograde filling of the renal vein. Renal vein injuries are often underdetected and are suggested when the kidney is enlarged with an, often thick, rim nephrogram. An expanded renal vein with thrombus is diagnostic
- Ureteropelvic junction disruptions are characterized by medial perirenal collections, good renal excretion, an intact calyceal system and focal extravasation (Fig. 89.56)
- The AAST renal injury scale has also been updated in 2018 to include vascular injuries and renal collecting system injuries [55] (Table 89.3). *It is worth recognizing that Grade IV encompasses a heterogenous group of injuries. For example, segemental vascular injuries are included in this subgroup but are known to be lower risk and tend to be managed conservatively (Fig. 89.59). Also, all collecting system injuries are classified as Grade IV, however, ureteropelvic junction and renal pelvis injuries carry higher risk than lateral pelvicalyceal injuries* (Fig. 89.56)

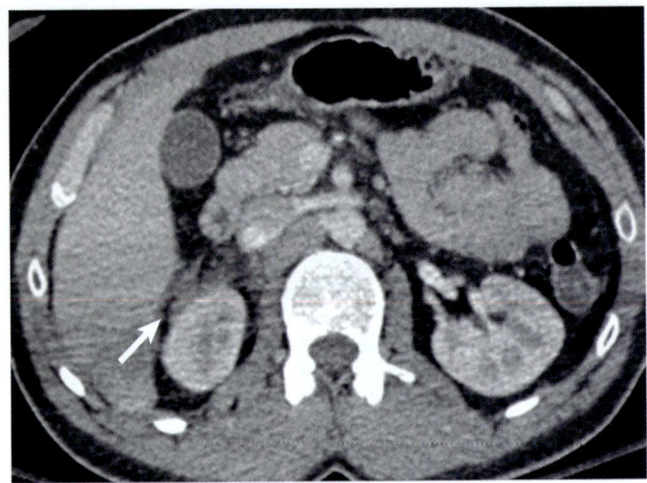

Figure 89.55 Blunt trauma. Fall from height. Hemodynamically stable. Axial CT image following IV contrast administration demonstrates small volume of perirenal hematoma anteriorly at the right kidney confined within the perirenal fascia (*white arrow*). AAST grade II renal injury. This was managed nonoperatively.

Management

Consensus has been established that providing the patient is hemodynamically stable and there are no associated injuries requiring treatment, grade I–II injuries can be successfully treated nonoperatively (Fig. 89.55). These injuries are considered minor and constitute the vast majority of renal injuries (75–98%). AAST Grades III–V renal injuries should be promptly recognized and communicated to the

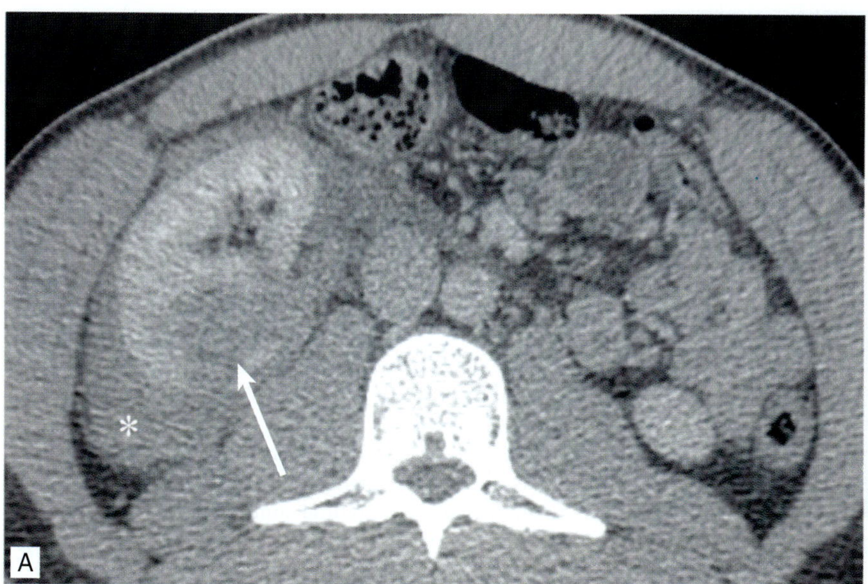

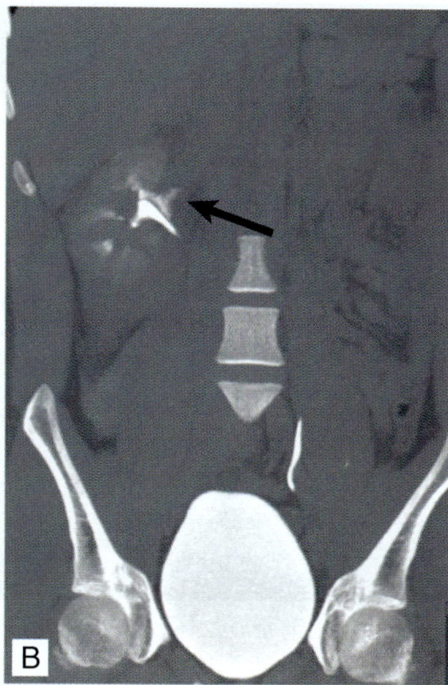

Figure 89.56 Blunt trauma. Pedestrian versus car. Hemodynamically stable. (A) Axial CT image following IV contrast administration demonstrates focal intraparenchymal contusion and laceration extending to renal capsule medially (*white arrow*) with perirenal hematoma (*asterisk*). (B) Delayed phase scan performed at 10 minutes as patient remained hemodynamically stable. Coronal reformat on bone windows delineates leak of contrast from renal pelvis (*black arrow*) upgrading this to AAST grade IV injury. This was treated with ureteric stent insertion.

TABLE 89.3 Kidney Injury Scale—2018 Revision

AAST Grade	AIS Severity	Imaging Criteria (CT Findings)	Operative Goals	Pathologic Criteria
I	2	▪ Subcapsular hematoma and/or parenchymal contusion without laceration	▪ Nonexpanding subcapsular hematoma ▪ Parenchymal contusion without laceration	▪ Subcapsular hematoma or parenchymal contusion without parenchymal laceratice
II	2	▪ Perirenal hematoma confined to Gerota fascia ▪ Renal parenchymal laceration ≤cm depth without urinary extravasation	▪ Nonexpanding peri-renal hematoma confined to Gerota fascia ▪ Renal parenchymal laceration ≤1cm depth without urinary extravasation	▪ Perirenal hematoma confined to Gerota fascia ▪ Renal parenchymal laceration ≤1 cm depth without urinary extravasation
III	3	▪ Renal parenchymal laceration >1 cm depth without collecting system rupture or urinary extravasation ▪ Any injury in the presence of a kidney vascular injury or active bleeding coetained within Gerota fascia	▪ Renal parenchymal laceration >1 cm depth without collection system rupture or urinary extravasation	▪ Renal parenchymal laceration >1 cm depth without collecting system rupture or urinary extravasation
IV	4	▪ Parenchymal laceration extending into urinary collecting system with urinary extravasation ▪ Renal pelvis laceration and/or complete ureteropelvic disruption ▪ Segmental renal vein or artery injury ▪ Active bleeding beyond Gerota fascia into the retroperitoneum or peritoneum ▪ Segmental or complete kidney infarction(s) due to vessel thrombosis without active bleeding	▪ Parenchymal laceration extending into urinary collection system with urinary extravasation ▪ Renal pelvis laceration and/or complete ureteropelvic disruption ▪ Segmental renal vein or artery injury ▪ Segemental or complete kidney infarction(s) due to vassel thrombosis without active bleeding	▪ Parenchymal laceration extending into urinary collection system ▪ Renal pelvis laceration and/or complete uretropelvic disruption ▪ Segmental renal vein or artery injury ▪ Segmental or complete kidney infarction(s) due to vessel thrombosis without active bleeding
V	5	▪ Main renal artery or vein laceration or avulsion of hilum ▪ Devascularized kidney with active bleeding ▪ Shuttered kidney with loss of identifiable parenchymal renal aratomy	▪ Main renal artery or vein laceration or avulsion of hilum ▪ Devascularized kidney with active bleeding ▪ Shuttered kidney with loss of identifiable parenchymal renal anatomy	▪ Main renal artery or vein laceration or avulsion of hilum ▪ Devascularized kidney ▪ Shuttered kidney with loss of identifiable parenchymal renal anatomy

Vascular injury is defined as a pseudoaneurysm or arteriovenous fistula and appears as a focal collection of contrast that decreases in attenuation with delayed imaging. Active bleeding from a vascular injury presents as extra-vascular contrast, focal or diffuse, that increases in size or attenuation in delayed phase. Vascular thrombosis can lead to organ infraction.
Grade based on highest grade assessment made on imaging, at operation or on pathologic specimen.
More than one grade of kidney injury may be present and should be classified by the higher grade of injury.
Advance one grade for bilateral injuries up to Grade III.

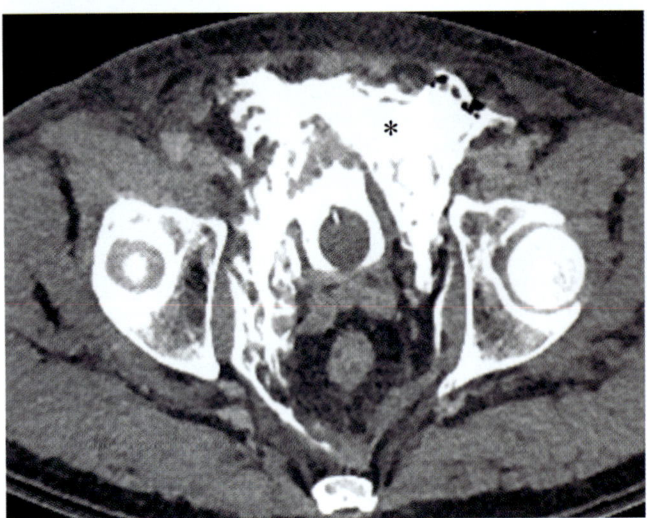

Figure 89.57 Blunt trauma. Male fall from height. Axial image from CT cystogram confirms contrast extravasation from catheterized bladder into space of retzius (*asterisk*) and along the pelvic sidewalls, consistent with extraperitoneal bladder rupture. No intraperitoneal spill of contrast. Although in this case, the nature of the bladder injury is obvious, the CT cystogram should be carefully evaluated in all 3 planes to assess for more subtle bladder injuries. The timing of the CT cystogram is dependent on hemodynamic status particularly if there is an unstable pelvic fracture pattern. The more pressing issue of achieving hemostasis should be the first priority. Delineating the nature of the suspected bladder injury is important but can be delayed until the patient is stabilized.

Trauma surgeon because they may require angioembolization, endourologic or surgical treatment depending on the nature of the injury that has placed it in this higher grade of injury [70,73] (Fig. 89.56). Devitalized segments were once considered an absolute contraindication to NOM; however, if there are no associated bowel or pancreatic injuries, these have been demonstrated to be treated with similar success nonoperatively. Complete ureteropelvic disruptions are an indication for surgery, although partial tears can be treated by antegrade stenting. Renal pedicle injuries have the worst overall prognosis, with poor operative revascularization rates; however, endovascular stenting may prove a viable alternative. *The indications for angiography in renal tract injuries remain predominantly the investigation of delayed or protracted bleeding and the treatment of CT-detected traumatic vascular malformations.* Angiography and selective embolization have increased success rates of NOM of higher-grade injuries, with hemostasis successfully achieved in approximately 90%. Angiographic techniques result in a greater preservation of renal parenchyma and are, therefore, the first line of treatment in transplant kidneys.

Injury to the Bladder

- Bladder injury may be the result of blunt or penetrative injuries. The propensity to injury depends largely on the degree of bladder distension at the time of injury. Hematuria is almost invariably present in bladder injuries and is usually gross in nature. Injuries may be classified as contusions or lacerations that may result in rupture
- Intraperitoneal ruptures are usually the result of blunt trauma to a distended bladder (Fig. 89.14). By contrast, extraperitoneal ruptures are associated with pelvic fractures in over 95% of cases (Fig. 89.57). Although traditionally these are believed to be due to direct bony penetration, many injuries probably also occur due to shearing injuries of the bladder base. Isolated extraperitoneal injuries are more common (50–85%) than isolated intraperitoneal ruptures (15–45%) or combined injuries (0–12%)
- Conventional CT with intravenous contrast may detect contusions of the bladder wall appearing as wall thickening or hyperdense intravesical hematoma (Fig. 89.47). However, CT is poor at depicting bladder lacerations, due to inadequate distension and the absence of intravesical contrast at the time of pelvic scanning. Delayed scanning at 5 minutes is still insensitive due to inadequate vesical distension
- Cystogram can be performed in those trauma patients who proceed for angiography and angioembolization. However, *CT cystography is the technique of choice to delineate bladder injury and indicated in hemodynamically stable patients with frank hematuria and pelvic fractures* (Fig. 89.57) Gross hematuria without pelvic fractures and microscopic hematuria with pelvic fractures are relative indications if there is clinical suspicion for bladder injury [74]
- Foley catheter placement should only be performed after clinical confirmation of urethral continuity. The bladder is drained and approximately 350 mL of dilute (3–5%) water-soluble iodinated contrast is instilled by gravity drip infusion. This is followed by axial scanning from iliac crests to lesser trochanters of femurs with coronal and sagittal reformats. It is vital to interrogate the urinary bladder in three planes and to adjust the window width and level settings to ensure complete and accurate diagnosis [75]
- Classification schemes for bladder injury include the AAST classification and the image-based classification which helps to stratify patients in terms of subsequent management. In this, radiology-based classification system there are five types of injury of which Type II (intraperitoneal rupture) and Type V (combined intra- and extra-peritoneal rupture) require surgical repair (Table 89.4) [75,76]

Injury to Pancreas

Injury to the pancreas is relatively uncommon, occurring in less than 2% of blunt abdominal trauma [77]. Such injuries are often the result of compression of the neck and body of pancreas against the spinal column by steering wheels and seat belts in adults and bicycle handlebars in children [78]. These mechanisms of injury result in associated with injuries to the duodenum, spleen, kidneys, or

TABLE 89.4 Imaging-Based Classification of Urinary Bladder Injury Following CT Cystogram

TYPE II AND TYPE V REQUIRE OPERATIVE REPAIR

Type of Bladder Injury	Pathology
Type I UB (urinary bladder) injury	Urinary bladder contusion
Type II UB injury	Intraperitoneal urinary bladder rupture
Type III UB injury	Interstitial urinary bladder injury (contrast extension into bladder wall but no extension into extra or intraperitoneal spaces)
Type IV UB injury	Extraperitoneal urinary bladder rupture (simple IVa contrast confined to prevesical space; complex IVb contrast may dissect into variety of fascial planes and spaces)
Type V UB injury	Combined intra and extraperitoneal urinary bladder rupture

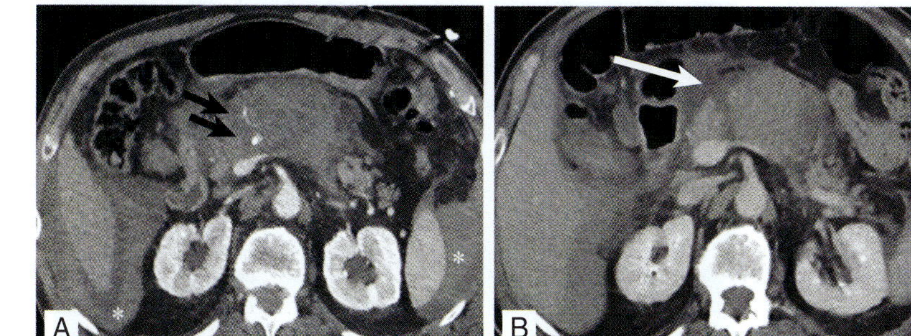

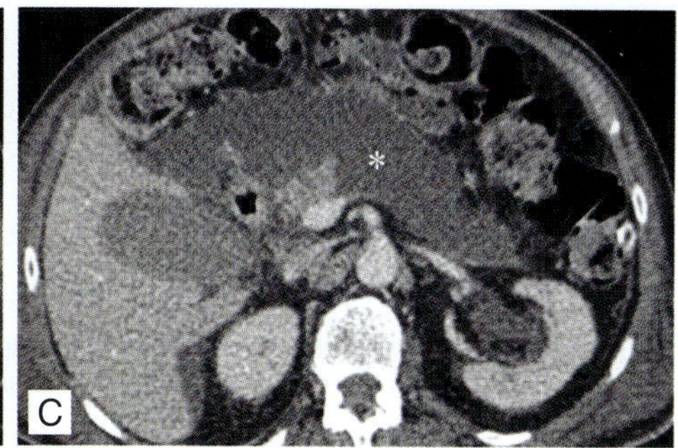

Figure 89.58 Blunt trauma. Fall from standing onto a low wall. Hemodynamically labile responding to fluids. (A) Axial image from CT acquired using split bolus protocol demonstrates extensive hematoma within and around the head and body of pancreas with foci of active extravasation (*black arrows*) (direct sign of pancreatic injury). Note also the extensive perihepatic and peri splenic hemoperitoneum (*asterisk*). Patient proceeded to interventional radiology for diagnostic angiogram but no active bleeding was identified and patient's hemodynamic status stabilized. (B) Follow-up dual-phase CT performed 48 hours later to further characterize the pancreatic injury. Note the full thickness laceration (a direct sign) through the proximal body of the pancreas (*white arrow*) with reduction in volume of hemoperitoneum. The full-thickness laceration was not appreciated on the index scan due to the extensive acute hematoma. Note that the laceration is to the left of the SMV making it within the distal pancreas anatomically. This observation is important as it has implications on the nature of the surgery required. Distal pancreatectomy with splenectomy was performed. (C) CT scan performed at 3 weeks following distal pancreatectomy and splenectomy due to increasing inflammatory markers. Postoperative low attenuation collection in surgical bed (*asterisk*) from stump leak which was drained percutaneously by interventional radiology. *SMV*, superior mesenteric vein.

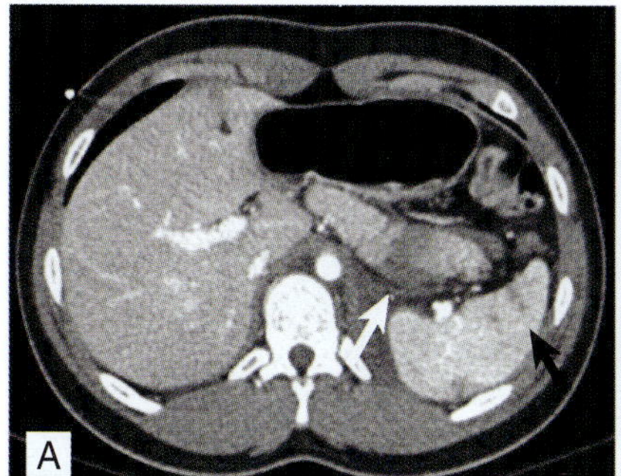

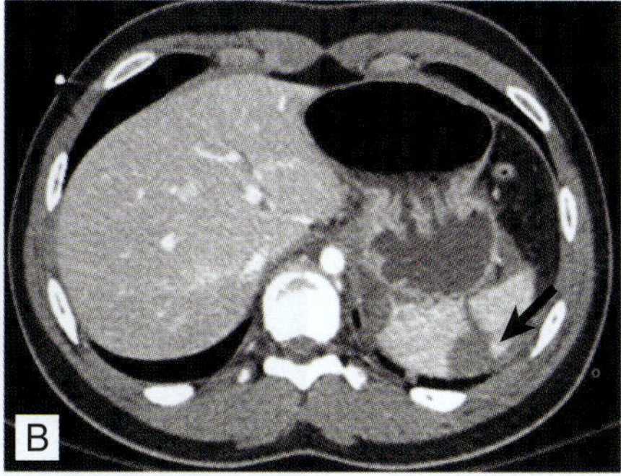

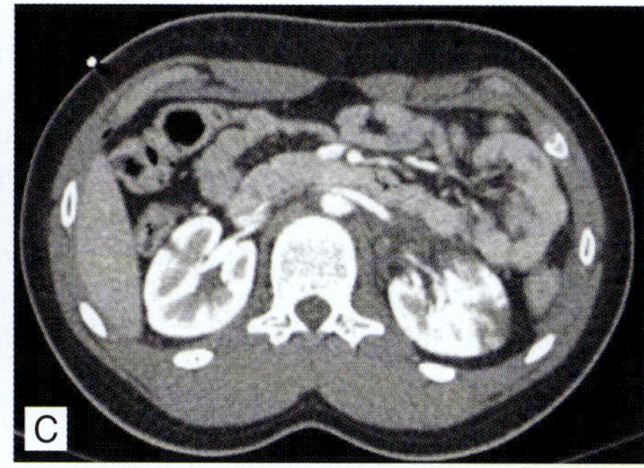

Figure 89.59 Blunt trauma. Person versus train. (A) Axial CT demonstrates linear low attenuation laceration through the distal body of pancreas (direct sign of pancreatic injury) (*white arrow*). There is also peripancreatic hematoma with loss of fat plane around the distal pancreas (indirect sign of pancreatic injury). Blunt pancreatic injury is rare and is rarely an isolated injury. (B) Note the lacerations within the spleen (AAST grade III) (*black arrows*). (C) There are multiple segmental infarcts within the left kidney with hematoma at the left renal pedicle but patent main renal vessels (AAST grade IV) and focal laceration in the right kidney (AAST grade 1).

lumbar spine in over 90% of cases. It is these associated injuries that are largely responsible for the increased mortality levels of 10–25% in combined injuries, compared with 3–10% for isolated injuries.

Imaging Features

- Pancreatic injuries can be subtle or overlooked on initial CT appraisal, particularly when there is extensive multiorgan trauma. Up to 40% of pancreatic injuries may not be visible on CT obtained within 12 hours of trauma and initial clinical and biochemical parameters are often nonspecific and unreliable [77]
- Direct CT findings include pancreatic swelling or enlargement, laceration, transection, or inhomogenous enhancement (Fig. 89.58). Indirect CT findings include thickening of the anterior pararenal fascia; induration of the peripancreatic fat; extra or intraperitoneal fluid; fluid in the lesser sac; peripancreatic fluid between the splenic vein and pancreas; associated left upper quadrant, hepatobiliary or duodenal injuries (Fig. 89.59)
- If there is delay in diagnosis, pancreatic injuries often become more apparent owing to the development of localized edema and autodigestion due to pancreatic enzyme leakage. Additional imaging is often required as the injury evolves or to further evaluate for duct integrity in the form of follow up dual-phase CT or MRCP, respectively [77,79] (Fig. 89.58)
- For equivocal findings about duct integrity on MRCP, ERCP is recommended. Although this is an invasive test, it also has the advantage of facilitating intervention, by means of stent placement, in otherwise well and stable patients

Classification and Management of Pancreatic Injuries

Pancreatic injuries may be graded using the AAST OIS scale (Table 89.5) [80]. The 2018 update does not include vascular injuries; however, it is still important to report these as it has impact on management (Fig. 89.58).

Key points to appreciate and comment on:

- The proximal pancreas is defined as to the (patients) right of the superior mesenteric vein (SMV). This is important as it alters the surgical approach, if warranted
- Integrity of the main pancreatic duct. This is important as ductal injury significantly increases morbidity and mortality due to development of pancreatic pseudocysts, fistulas and abscesses
- All high-grade injuries infer pancreatic duct injury
- Advance up to grade III for multiple low-grade injuries

Management depends on grade/severity of injury; location of injury; other concomitant abdominal injuries and time elapsed after injury. If the main pancreatic duct is involved, then surgery is preferred. Interventional radiology has a significant role

TABLE 89.5 Pancreas CT Grading

CT Grading	Blunt Pancreatic Injury*
Grade 1	Minor contusion without duct injury
Grade 2	Major contusion without duct injury or tissue loss
Grade 3	Distal transection or parenchymal injury with duct injury
Grade 4	Proximal transection (to the right of the superior mesenteric vein) or parenchymal injury involving the ampulla
Grade 5	Massive disruption to the pancreatic head

*Grade based on most accurate assessment of radiology, surgery, or autopsy. Advance one grade for multiple injuries.

supporting treatment of complications of traumatic pancreatitis and drainage of postoperative collections (Fig. 89.58).

Injury to Bowel and Mesentery

Bowel and mesenteric injuries occur in approximately 5% of blunt abdominal trauma cases and are, therefore, relatively unusual injuries. These injuries often demonstrate subtle or minimal signs on CT imaging and can hence cause interpretative problems [80]. Even when the diagnosis is suspected, several of the described signs of injury have a low diagnostic specificity. *Detection of these injuries is of importance as, in contradistinction to the trend to NOM of solid intra-abdominal organ injuries, the optimal treatment for bowel and mesenteric injuries remains early surgical repair. A delay in diagnosis, and hence treatment, increases morbidity and mortality* [81].

Deceleration injuries tend to cause shearing forces at the points of fixation of the bowel, such as the retroperitoneal duodenum, the ligament of Treitz, the ileocaecal valve, and any incidental hernias. These forces may precipitate mesenteric tears or bowel wall injuries. Compressive forces tend to cause an increase in intraluminal bowel pressure resulting in direct rupture. Penetrating injuries tend to the affect the colon more due to its relative size and fixation. Blunt trauma injury to the colon is rare.

While seatbelts have undoubtedly reduced mortality in car accidents mainly due to a reduction in catastrophic brain injury, their introduction has led to a significant increase in intra-abdominal injuries, with a two- to three-fold increase in intestinal perforations and mesenteric devascularization [80] (Fig. 89.66). The association between abdominal ecchymosis (the "seatbelt" sign) and bowel and mesenteric injury has been well documented (Fig. 89.60). Interruption in mesenteric blood supply can result in bowel ischemia and infarction hours of days later. A similar association is reported between acute lumbar hernias and BMI, likely due to the increased intra-abdominal pressure elicited by rapid deceleration causing herniation of abdominal contents through sites of anatomical weakness in the superior and inferior lumbar triangles [83,84] (Fig. 89.61).

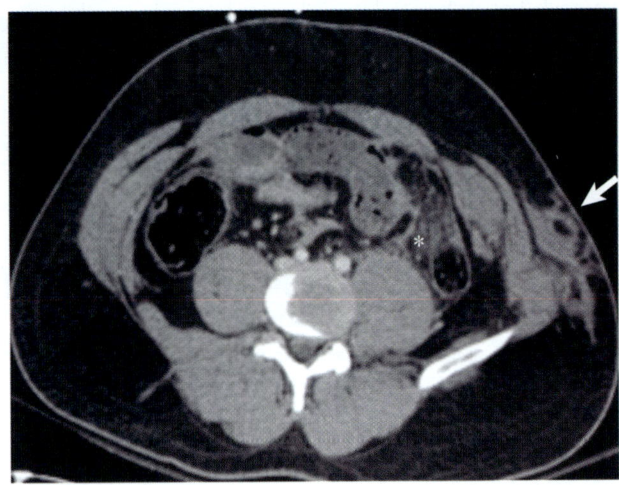

Figure 89.60 Blunt trauma. Restrained driver high-speed MVC. Axial CT image with IV contrast demonstrates characteristic seatbelt injury overlying the left iliac blade (*white arrow*). Mesenteric stranding is seen around the distal descending colon (*asterisk*). No direct signs of free intraperitoneal air or focal bowel wall discontinuity. Avulsed devascularized descending colon at laparotomy requiring stapled resection.

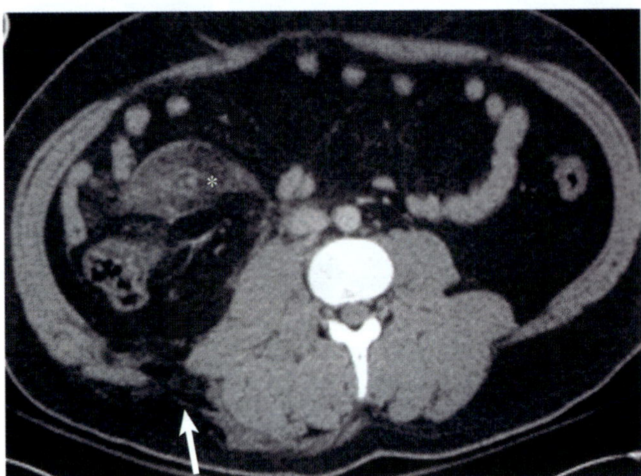

Figure 89.61 Blunt trauma. Restrained driver high speed MVC. Hemodynamically stable. Axial CT image, acquired with split bolus protocol, demonstrates acute right-sided traumatic lumbar hernia (*white arrow*) with focal stranding and hematoma in the terminal ileal mesentery (*asterisk*). No free intraperitoneal air on CT. Mesenteric root tear confirmed at laparotomy.

Imaging Features

- There are a number of signs on CT that help to diagnose bowel and mesenteric injury. The most specific signs for bowel injury in blunt abdominal trauma include focal bowel wall discontinuity (100%) and extraluminal air (95%) (Figs. 89.48 and 89.62). Detection of pneumoperitoneum is facilitated by the use of lung window settings but it may be present in fewer than 50% of cases at presentation
- Isolated free intraperitoneal air may be due to pneumothorax, chest tube placement, or diaphragmatic injury [85]. However, when free air is present in combination with other findings such as free intraperitoneal fluid or the seatbelt sign, it is highly predictive of bowel injury (Fig. 89.62). The location of extraluminal air can also help to localize the bowel injury, particularly in the setting of duodenal injury (Fig. 89.62). Oral contrast is not routinely administered in the emergency setting of blunt abdominal trauma therefore the other highly specific sign of oral contrast extravasation is rarely seen in this setting [86]
- The presence of hyperattenuating peritoneal fluid, particularly in the absence of an identifiable solid organ injury should also cause suspicion, except in the case of small amounts of low attenuation free fluid in the pelvis of women of reproductive age, which may be normal (Fig. 89.63)
- Other signs of bowel injury include focal bowel thickening due to intramural hematoma (commonest in the second part of the

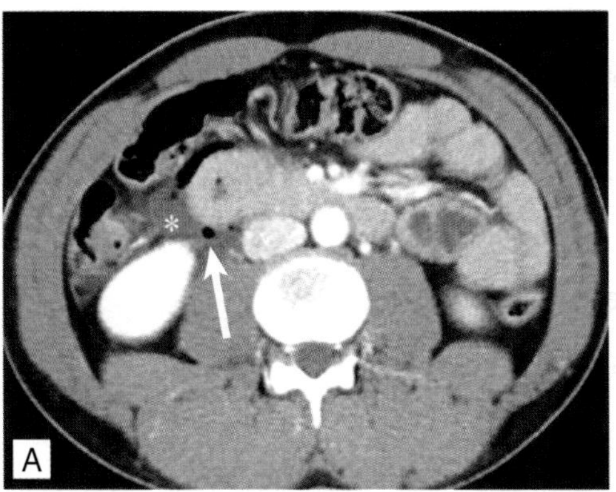

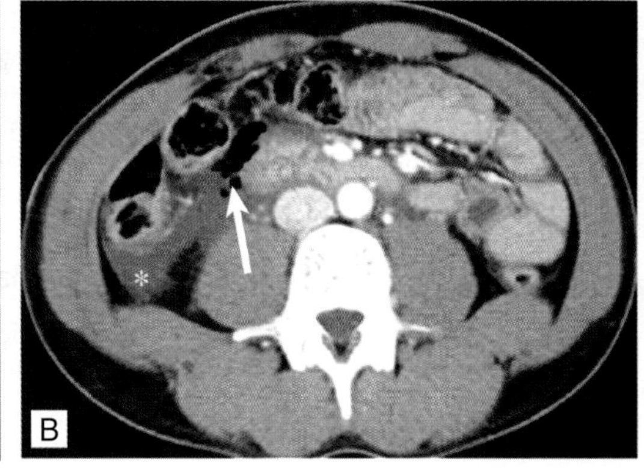

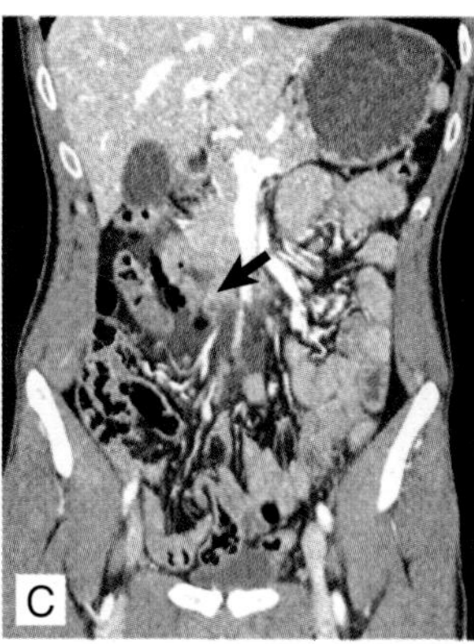

Figure 89.62 Blunt trauma. Restrained driver high speed MVC. Hemodynamically stable. (A and B) Axial CT images, acquired with split bolus protocol, demonstrate extraluminal free gas (*white arrows*) and fluid adjacent to duodenum (*white asterisk*) which is edematous with abnormal enhancement. Further fluid is present in right paracolic gutter (*white asterisk*). (C) Coronal CT reformat confirms focal bowel wall discontinuity at the third part of duodenum (*black arrow*). Duodenal rupture confirmed and repaired at laparotomy.

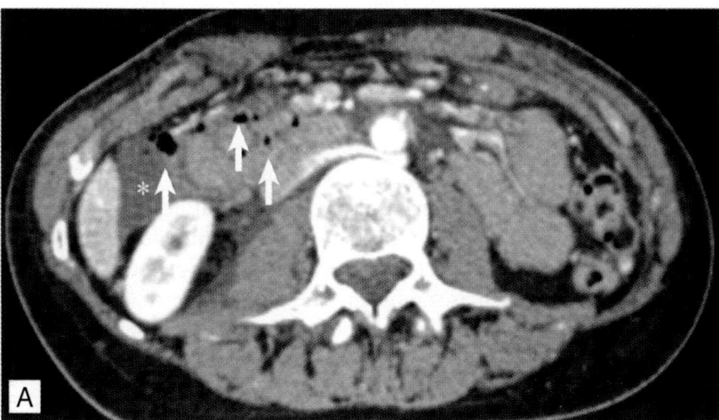

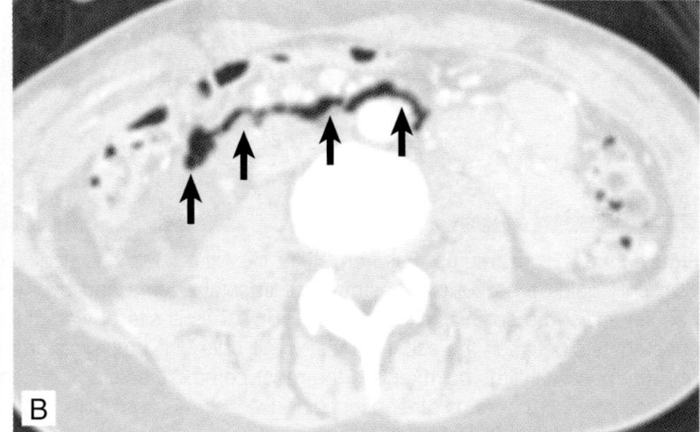

Figure 89.63 Blunt trauma. Restrained passenger MVC. Hemodynamically stable. Axial CT ((A) soft tissue and (B) lung windows) demonstrates multiple foci of extraluminal air within the abdomen which is within the retroperitoneum (*arrows*). There is associated retroperitoneal free fluid (*asterisk*). This is closely related to the second part of the duodenum which is markedly edematous and CT features are consistent with duodenal perforation. The retroperitoneal extension of fluid and air is explained by the retroperitoneal position of the second part of the duodenum. Of note this patient exhibited vague abdominal signs and was not overtly peritonitic because the pathology was centered on the retroperitoneal space.

duodenum) (Fig. 89.62) and abnormal bowel wall enhancement (Fig. 89.64). However, the low specificity for significant bowel injury in these signs in isolation does not justify immediate surgical intervention (Fig. 89.64). The presence of diffuse bowel wall thickening and intense enhancement without peritoneal fluid may simply be part of the hypoperfusion–reperfusion complex, commonly known as "shock bowel" and does not necessarily imply bowel rupture

- Mesenteric injuries may occur in isolation or in combination with bowel perforation. The presence of active vascular contrast extravasation with a large hematoma reflects a patient at high risk for subsequent bowel ischemia and rupture and is an indication for surgery (Fig. 89.46). However, lesser degrees of hematoma or "misting" of the mesentery do not necessarily indicate a need for surgery and may require follow-up examinations coupled with clinical observation (Figs. 89.65 and 89.67)

Management

There is no debate that patients who have sustained blunt or penetrating abdominal trauma, with peritonitis, evisceration or hemodynamic instability should undergo exploratory laparotomy. *However, challenges remain in selective NOM of hemodynamically stable nonperitonitic patients with penetrating torso trauma, particularly in low energy penetrating trauma such as stabbings.* A triple contrast CT protocol using intravenous, oral, and rectal contrast has been advocated for assessment of these patients, the rationale being that adding enteric contrast allows assessment for extravasation or leakage from bowel, a highly specific sign for bowel perforation [87]. However, although one prospective study of triple contrast CT for detection of bowel injury with surgical correlation showed 100% specificity when extravasation was present on CT, sensitivity of this sign was only 29%. More sensitive signs included direct extension of wound tract to bowel and focal bowel wall thickening. Other signs included mesenteric vascular extravasation, mesenteric fat stranding and interloop fluid [88] (Figs. 89.65–89.67) Interestingly, a recent international survey suggested that enteric contrast is used in a minority of centers for penetrating trauma, thought to be driven by perceived lack of benefit and delays in patient care [89]. A recent systematic review in 2018 evaluated the accuracy of CT for diagnosis of intraabdominal injuries requiring therapeutic laparotomy in stable, nonperitonitic pts with anterior abdominal stab wounds. It showed a high prevalence (8.7%, 95% CI 6.1–12.2%) of injuries requiring laparotomy in patients with a negative CT scan. Almost half (47%, 95% CI 30–64%) of those injuries involved the small bowel [90]. This finding has to be carefully balanced with the risks

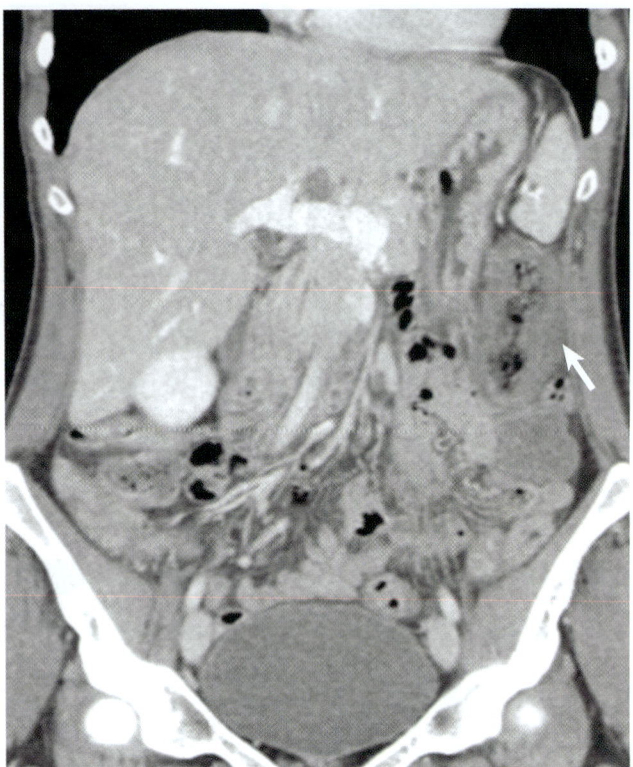

Figure 89.64 Blunt trauma. Fall from 4 m. (A) Axial CT image acquired with split bolus protocol demonstrates segmental edema and hypoenhancement of the splenic flexure (*white arrow*). This is site of watershed anastomosis between the ascending left colic artery and marginal artery of drummond (Griffiths point) and is the most common location for ischemic colitis. There were no other direct or indirect signs of bowel injury and no clinical peritonism. Patient was non operatively managed with serial observations and follow up CT confirmed resolution of presumed transient ischemia. Patient was discharged after 48 hours.

associated with nontherapeutic laparotomy. The importance of good clinical-radiological corroboration cannot be underestimated in this cohort of patients. Serial clinical observations, for developing peritonism, in selectively nonoperatively managed cohort of penetrating trauma, with follow up targeted diagnostic studies where necessary, remains a safe approach (Figs. 89.65 and 89.66).

Injury to Major Blood Vessels

- Blunt injuries to the inferior vena cava and the aorta are unusual except at the junction of the hepatic veins with the IVC. At this

Key Points: Pearls to Remember

- Mechanism of injury matters! Interrogate bowel and mesentery closely, particularly if the patient has been restrained occupant of high-speed MVC
- If mechanism of blunt trauma is severe, look for other markers of significant injury including seat belt sign, traumatic lumbar and abdominal wall hernias and traumatic abdominal aortic injury, which can be overlooked in the context of the multiply injured patient, but will help raise index of suspicion for potential bowel injury
- Have a high index of suspicion for bowel injury if bowel wall thickening and free intraperitoneal blood in absence of high-grade solid organ injury
- Challenges remain in selective NOM of hemodynamically stable nonperitonitic patients with penetrating torso trauma, particularly in low energy penetrating trauma such as stabbings. The importance of good clinical-radiological corroboration cannot be underestimated in this cohort of patients. A period of observation, for developing peritonism, in selectively nonoperatively managed cohort of penetrating torso trauma, with follow up targeted diagnostic studies where necessary, remains a safe approach

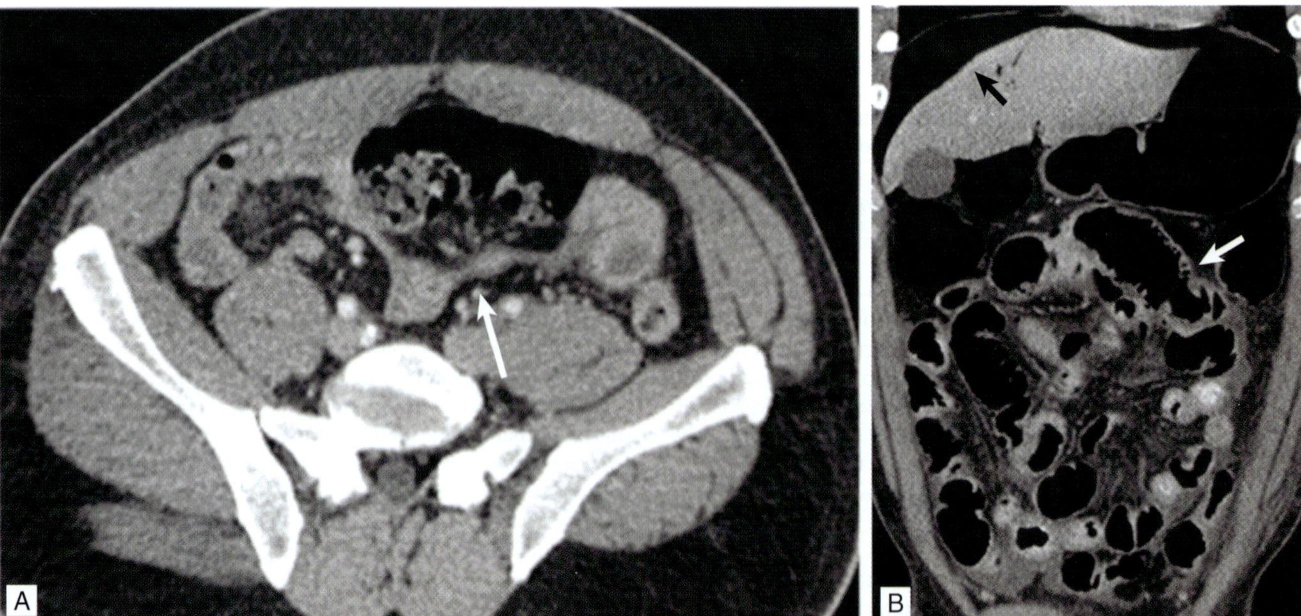

Figure 89.65 Blunt trauma. Restrained driver high speed MVC. (A) Axial CT image following IV contrast demonstrates subtle small volume of interloop fluid (*white arrow*). There was no solid organ injury and patient was intubated for concomitant head injury making clinical assessment for peritonism difficult. (B) Axial CT image with IV contrast 48 hours later on background of rising inflammatory markers and increased abdominal distension. Widespread free intraperitoneal air (*black arrow*) with poorly enhancing distended jejunum (*white arrow*). Ischemia and necrosis of jejunum and proximal ilium at laparotomy requiring resection.

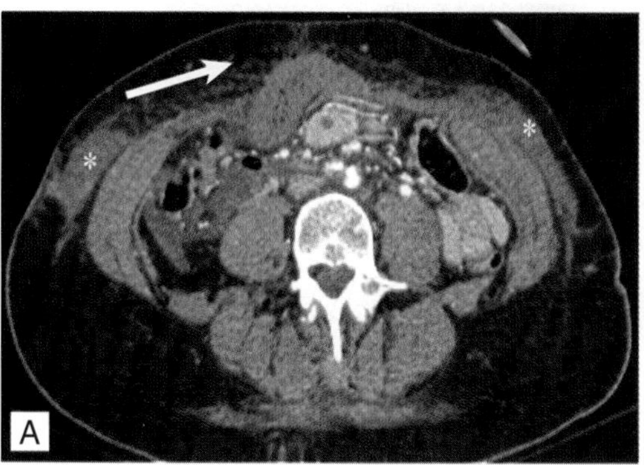
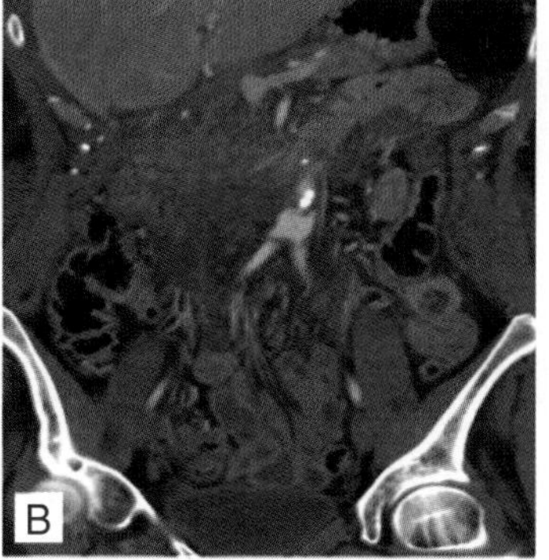
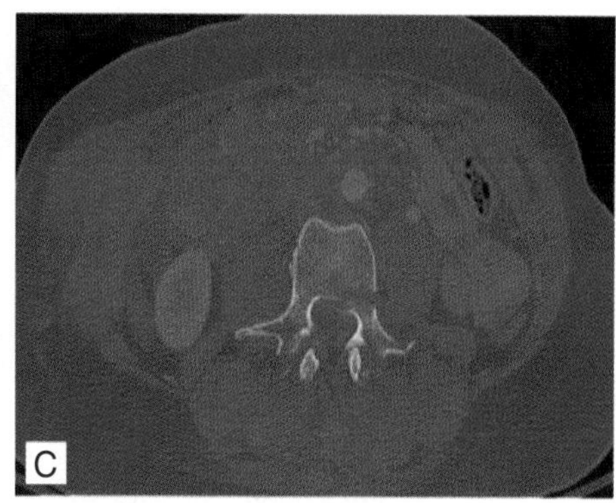

Figure 89.66 Blunt trauma. Restrained passenger in high-speed MVC. (A) Axial CT image acquired using split bolus CT protocol demonstrates acute traumatic abdominal wall herniation of devascularized bowel into the subcutaneous tissues anteriorly (*white arrow*). Note the radiological seat belt sign over the right and left sides of the abdomen (*asterisk*). Note also direct signs of distal aortic injury of focal narrowing of the vessel with intraluminal thrombus. (B) Coronal reformat confirms the axial CT findings of acute traumatic aortic injury in infrarenal aorta with intimal flap tear (direct sign of vascular injury) best appreciated on coronal reformat. Small bowel resection performed at laparotomy for devascularized segment. Patient proceeded to Interventional Radiology for endovascular stenting of the distal TAI. (C) Acute unstable chance type fracture also present at L3 which required ORIF after laparotomy and endovascular intervention. This case illustrates the importance of multidisciplinary approach to the acute severely injured polytrauma patient.

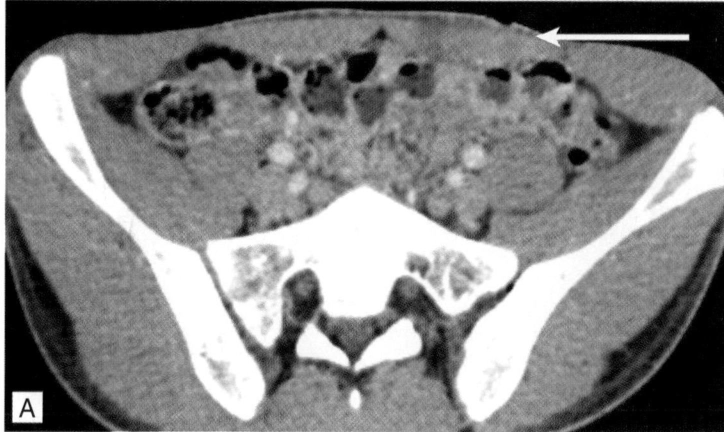
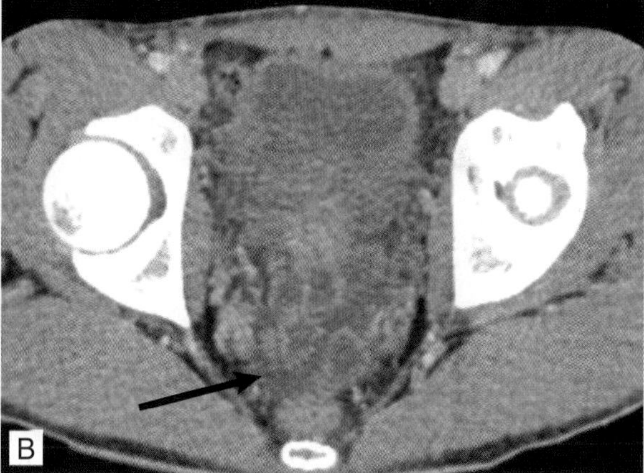

Figure 89.67 Penetrating trauma. Stab wound to left lower quadrant. (A) Axial CT image (with IV contrast) demonstrates skin defect in left lower quadrant (*white arrow*). Paucity of intraabdominalfat makes interpretation challenging. (B) Axial CT image more inferiorly demonstrates small volume of free intraperitoneal fluid in pelvis only (*black arrow*). Abdomen was soft and non peritonitic. Patient remained hemodynamically stable. Appreciating that routine laparotomy in hemodynamically stable patients may result in a 35 to 53% rate of non therapeutic laparotomies, decision made to proceed with serial observations. Patient remained well and was discharged 24 hrs later.

point, hepatic lacerations may extend directly into the IVC, which is relatively fixated by its opening into the diaphragm

- Injuries to the retroperitoneal infrarenal course of these vessels in the abdomen are unusual, and even less frequently imaged, as these patients are usually very hemodynamically unstable and have significant associated injuries. Injuries due to penetrating causes are relatively more common (Fig. 89.68) but still very rare unless they are due to gunshot wounds [91]. The mortality of patients surviving initial transfer to hospital with major caval or aortic injuries is very high and even for isolated injuries has been reported as 9% and 20% for caval and aortic injuries, respectively, and up to 75% for combined injuries
- Contrast-enhanced CT represents an excellent tool for the detection of these injuries. In caval injuries, the lumen of the IVC is often irregular or compressed by retroperitoneal hematoma and active vascular contrast extravasation may be observed. Injuries of the infrarenal IVC have a better prognosis than those of the retrohepatic IVC, due to the tamponading effect of the retroperitoneum (Fig. 89.9). These injuries may initially respond to fluid resuscitation and, therefore, delay presentation. A collapsed IVC, particularly in the absence of pericaval hemorrhage, should alert the careful observer to the possibility of extreme hypovolaemia [92]. This finding is useful in children and young adults, who can initially maintain their blood pressure despite significant volume loss
- Direct signs of vascular injury tend to be specific but less sensitive and include intimal tears, pseudoaneurysm, focal narrowing, intraluminal thrombus, discrete tear with active extravasation and arteriovenous malformation (Figs. 89.66, 89.69, and 89.72)
- Indirect signs tend to more sensitive but less specific including perivascular hematoma and variable degrees of end-organ hypoenhancement [93] (Figs. 89.31 and 89.68)
- In comparison with the thoracic aorta, injury of the abdominal aorta is rare and is well detected by CT. These injuries are usually infrarenal and are often associated with severe lower thoracic and lumbar vertebral body fractures (Fig. 89.66). The spectrum of CT findings in TAI and its management has been described earlier in the chapter
- *Mortality in patients with pelvic fractures with hemodynamic instability has been shown to range from 20% to 50%. Although the majority of bleeding in pelvic fractures is of venous or bony origin, up to 10% is arterial in origin, which although less common can cause more hemodynamic instability than venous bleeds* [64]. The vast majority of this arterial bleeding is from the

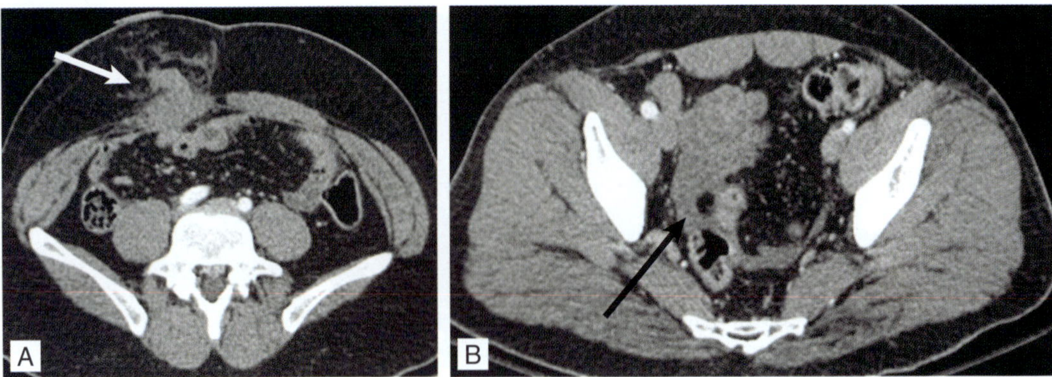

Figure 89.68 Penetrating trauma. Single stab wound to right paraumbilical region. Male patient. (A) Axial CT images demonstrate focal hematoma within deep subcutaneous tissues anteriorly down to the right rectus abdominus. (*white arrow*) (B) Small volume of high attenuation free fluid in pelvis. CT evidence of peritoneal breach. Patient remained alert, hemodynamically stable and abdomen was soft and not peritonitic. Decision made to serially observe. Peritonism developed 12 hrs later and patient taken for laparotomy. Through and through jejunal injury was repaired.

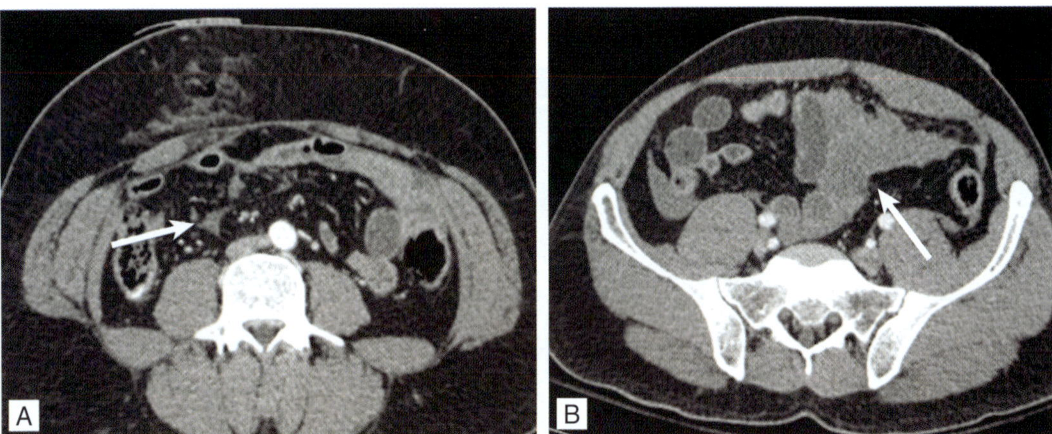

Figure 89.69 Penetrating trauma. (A) Axial CT image from patient with isolated stab wound to right lower quadrant demonstrates focal mesenteric hematoma (*white arrow*). Indirect sign of bowel or mesenteric injury in penetrating trauma. (B) Axial CT image from a different patient with isolated stab wound to left side of abdomen. Small volume of interloop fluid in pelvis (*white arrow*). Indirect sign of bowel or mesenteric injury in penetrating trauma.

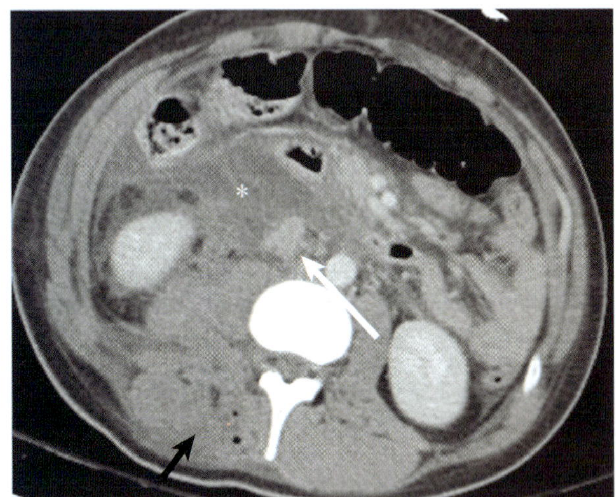

Figure 89.70 Penetrating trauma. Single stab wound to right paravertebral region. Initial responder to fluid resuscitation. Surgical emphysema and hematoma within the right paravertebral musculature (*black arrow*). Large volume of retroperitoneal hematoma (*asterisk*) with loss of fat plane around the IVC. The IVC has an irregular contour (*white arrow*). IVC injury confirmed at laparotomy.

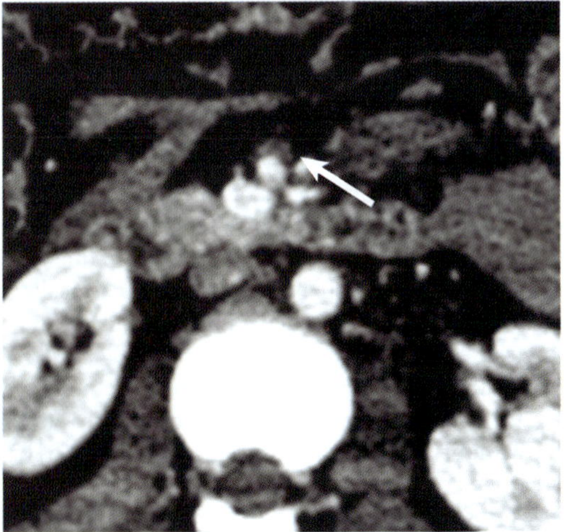

Figure 89.71 Blunt trauma. Motorcyclist versus bollard. Initial responder to fluid resuscitation. Axial CT image acquired with split bolus protocol. There is crescenteric low attenuation around the superior mesenteric artery (*white arrow*), a direct sign of vessel injury.

internal iliac arteries and their subdivisons, most commonly the superior gluteal and inferior pudendal arteries (Fig. 89.70 and 89.71). If hemodynamic status allows it, contrast-enhanced CT is a very useful noninvasive technique at detecting active bleeding sites or vascular abnormalities, with a sensitivity and specificity of approximately 85%. Associated pelvic injuries and hematomas are also simultaneously depicted

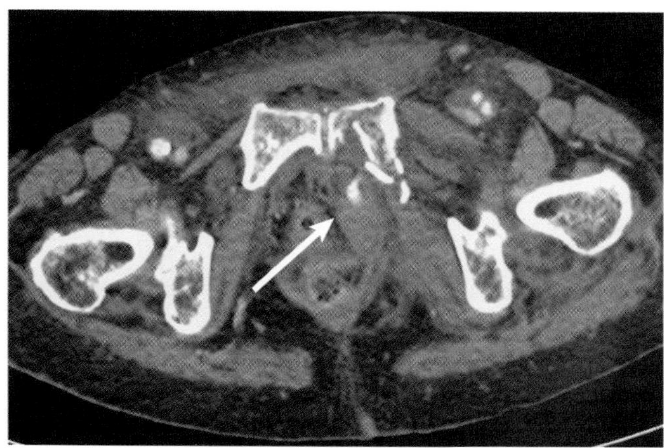

Figure 89.72 Blunt trauma. Pedestrian versus car. Axial CT image acquired using split bolus protocol demonstrating active extravasation posterior to the comminuted left pubic ramus fracture (*white arrow*).

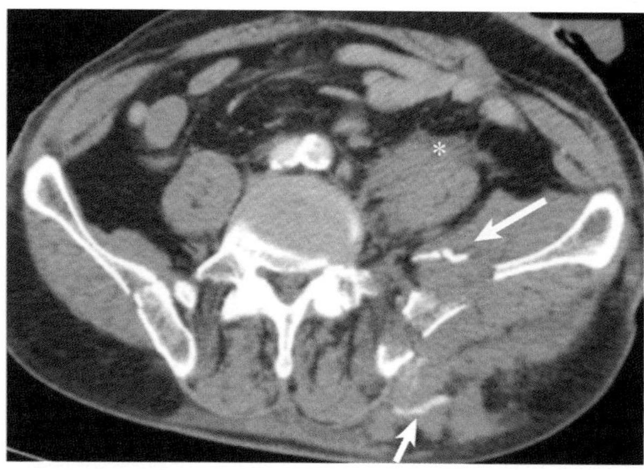

Figure 89.73 Blunt trauma. Male fall from height. Axial CT image demonstrating active extravasation anterior and posterior to the comminuted left iliac blade fracture (*white arrows*). Note hematoma tracking retroperitoneally along the left psoas and iliacus muscles (*asterisk*).

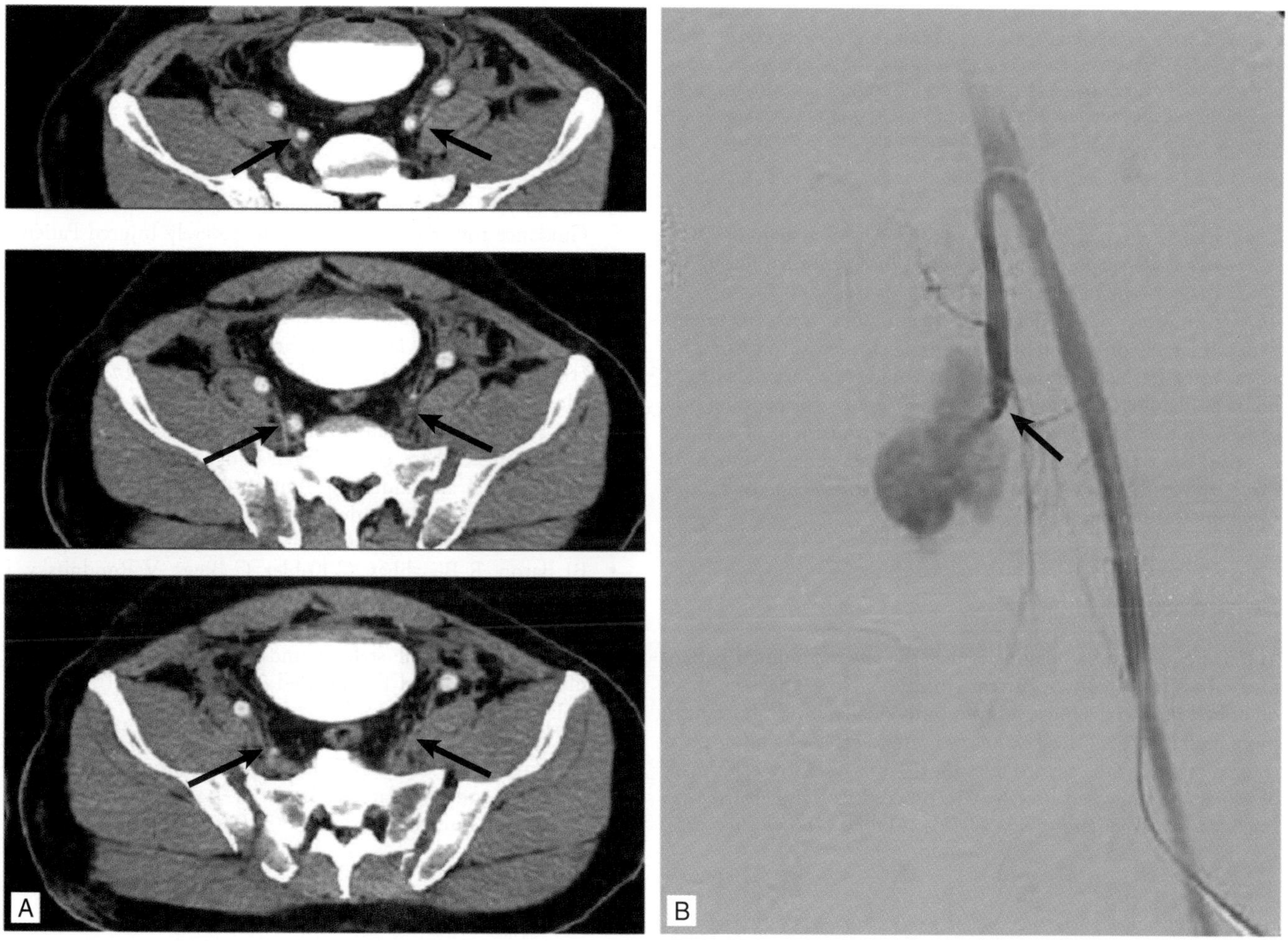

Figure 89.74 Blunt trauma. Male fell from height. (A) Selected axial CT images acquired in arterial phase demonstrate patent right internal iliac artery on the right throughout. Initial image shows patent left internal iliac artery then there is an abrupt termination of the vessel (direct sign of vessel injury). Note the displaced fracture though right iliac blade posteriorly extending into the right sacroiliac joint. Note also the abnormally widened left sacroiliac joint with pelvic sidewall hematoma bilaterally. Contrast within the bladder from CT imaging performed at initial receiving hospital. (B) Selected image from pelvic angiogram confirmed complete transection of the right internal iliac artery.

- Indications for pelvic angiography with possible angioembolization include:
  - Patient with pelvic ring fracture who is unstable despite pelvic binder and in whom intra thoracic or intraabdominal sources of bleeding have been excluded [64]
  - Presence of a vascular injury or active extravasation on CT in association with other signs of vascular injury on imaging such as large volume pelvic hematoma, pseudoaneurysm, vasospasm, or vascular "cut off" sign [64] (Figs. 89.72–89.74)

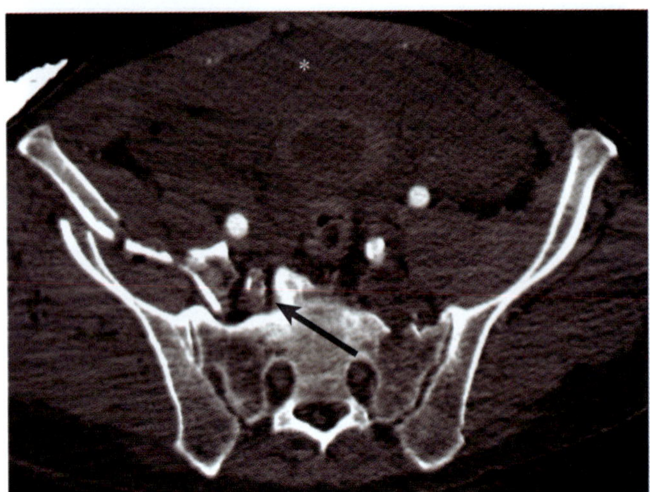

Figure 89.75 Blunt trauma. Pedestrian versus car. Hemodynamically unstable. Axial CT image (arterial phase). Markedly displaced fracture of the right iliac blade with intrusion of the fracture into the pelvis demonstrates complete occlusion of the right internal iliac artery (*black arrow*). A direct sign of vessel injury on CT. Compare with normal opacification of the left internal iliac artery. Note also the extensive hematoma around the bladder anteriorly (*asterisk*). Patient proceeded to dedicated CT cystogram to evaluate the bladder further after pelvic angio embolization and laparotomy for pelvic packing.

- When emergency pelvic packing is used as part of DCS, subsequent angioembolization in Interventional Radiology may also be necessary [94]

The utilization of angiographic techniques and treatments depends largely on the preplanning for such events. Angiographic suites must be in close proximity to emergency rooms, with 24 hours availability of staff. Although there are ever-expanding possibilities for endovascular stenting and the treatment of vascular injuries, the decision to use these techniques relies as much on these factors as on the local expertise and knowledge of trauma surgeons and radiologists.

Summary

The reality of trauma imaging is that the severely injured patient often has multiple concurrent injuries. Now that we have described how to diagnose injuries individually, it is important to piece it all together. The case below is an example of a blunt polytrauma patient with selected relevant CT images, a brief summary of salient findings and how best to proceed in terms of the next stage of management (Fig. 89.75) (Table 89.6). This case, although only one of multiple different scenarios, illustrates the importance of collaborative multidisciplinary approach to managing these patients.

TABLE 89.6 Summary of Salient Findings for the Blunt Polytrauma Patient in Fig. 89.75

Summary of Salient Findings	Management
Traumatic Aortic Injury	Alert Interventional Radiology (TEVAR)
Low grade splenic injury—AAST grade II	NOM (No active extravasation or vascular injury)
Low grade liver injury—AAST grade II	NOM (No active extravasation or vascular injury)
Bowel injury–specific sign of free intraperitoneal air in blunt trauma	Needs laparotomy
Head injury	Possible requirement for intracranial pressure (ICP) bolt but no immediate decompression required

Suggested Readings

- The Royal College of Radiologists, Standards of Practice and Guidance for Trauma Radiology in Severely Injured Patients, second ed., The Royal College of Radiologists, London, 2015.
- Expert Panel on Major Trauma Imaging, JY Shyu, B Khurana, JA Soto, WL Biffl, MA Camacho, et al., ACR appropriateness criteria® major blunt trauma, J Am Coll Radiol 17 (5S) (2020 May) S160–S174.
- RA Kozar, M Crandall, K Shanmuganathan, BL Zarzaur, M Coburn, C Cribari, et al., Organ injury scaling 2018 update: spleen, liver, and kidney, J Trauma Acute Care Surg 85 (6) (2018 Dec) 1119–1122. doi: 10.1097/TA.0000000000002058. Erratum in: J Trauma Acute Care Surg 87 (2) (2019 Aug) 512.
- BJ Baron, R Benabbas, C Kohler, C Biggs, V Roudnitsky, L Paladino, R Sinert, Accuracy of computed tomography in diagnosis of intra-abdominal injuries in stable patients with anterior abdominal stab wounds: a systematic review and meta-analysis, Acad Emerg Med 25 (7) (2018 Jul) 744–757. doi: 10.1111/acem.13380.
- S Chakraverty, K Flood, D Kessel, S McPherson, T Nicholson, CE Ray, et al., CIRSE guidelines: quality improvement guidelines for endovascular treatment of traumatic hemorrhage, Cardiovasc Intervent Radiol 35 (3) (2012 Jun) 472–482.

90

Acute Neurological Emergencies

ASHOK ADAMS

Introduction

The aim of this chapter is to review acute neurological emergencies and approach to imaging. Acute insults to the central nervous system can present in a variety of different ways and this chapter will present the most common clinical scenarios combined with imaging algorithms and differential diagnoses. Imaging of acute trauma and thromboembolic stroke are covered in other chapters and the primary focus of this chapter is on nontraumatic acute neurological emergencies.

Acute Onset Headache

Acute onset nontraumatic headaches represent approximately 2–4% of accident and emergency admissions and secondary causes of headaches are found in a small proportion [1]. This increases in the setting of sudden-onset acute headaches or thunderclap headache that peaks within 60 seconds. The presence of abnormal neurology increases the possibility of a secondary cause for the headache including the presence of Horner's syndrome, cranial nerve palsies, visual symptoms and visual aura, systemic symptoms as well as nausea and vomiting [2,3]. An underlying history of immunosuppression or neoplasia should also be sought [4]. Acute onset headache in the peripartum setting is dealt with separately in this chapter.

For the radiologist the spectrum of disease processes to consider are myriad and providing an accurate diagnosis or limited differential diagnosis is aided by the clinical information provided that also helps to guide subsequent imaging. An imaging algorithm is provided and, in our institution, a noncontrast computed tomography (CT) head is performed the first line given its accessibility and capability of identifying potential candidates for neurosurgical intervention. In the setting of acute onset headache, this can be supplemented by imaging of the vasculature and targeted at the arterial and/or venous system. If available, arterial or venous vascular imaging can be undertaken at the same time as routine brain CT or magnetic resonance imaging (MRI) of the intracranial compartment (Table 90.1).

- In the setting of a confirmed intracranial hemorrhage, imaging of the intracranial arterial and venous structures is undertaken
- If there is concern regarding thromboembolic disease, vascular dissection or vasculitis, imaging of the intra- as well as the extra-cranial vessels is performed

Intracranial Extra-axial Hemorrhage

Diffuse subarachnoid hemorrhage (SAH) is observed in the setting of trauma and in the nontrauma setting, this can occur secondary to aneurysmal rupture, arteriovenous malformation, or dural arteriovenous fistula [5]. Nontraumatic aneurysmal rupture in 85% of cases is most likely secondary to a saccular aneurysm rupture [6]. *The epicenter of the hemorrhage typically guides the source of the SAH and the most common sites include the anterior communicating artery, posterior communicating artery, middle cerebral artery bifurcation, and basilar artery.* Less frequently, the source of the SAH may be the internal carotid artery terminus, superior cerebellar artery, and posterior inferior cerebellar artery. The presence of SAH prompts further evaluation with an intracranial CT angiogram (CTA) to identify the source of hemorrhage and guide subsequent endovascular or surgical therapy if required (Fig. 90.1). It is also of benefit in assessing potential complicating

TABLE 90.1 Acute Onset Headache—Imaging Algorithm

1. Noncontrast CT head
   - Intracranial hemorrhage—parenchymal, subarachnoid, intraventricular, subdural, extradural
   - Cerebral edema and mass effect with trans compartmental shift (subfalcine, uncal, and transtentorial herniation)
   - Identify a potential space-occupying lesion
   - Sources of sepsis—sinuses, middle ear/mastoid, orbits, skull base
2. MR imaging
   - protocol including diffusion weighted imaging (DWI), gradient recall echo (GRE), or susceptibility weighted imaging (SWI), T2, FLAIR, and T1 weighted sequences
   - contrast-enhanced T1 weighted sequence and MRV and MRA as below
3. Angiographic studies
   - Arterial – CT arteriography (Intracranial and/or extracranial)
     – MR angiography (CE MRA, TOF MRA)
   - Venous – CT venography (45 seconds delay)
     – MR venography (two-dimensional time of flight MRV sensitive to flow perpendicular to plane, contrast-enhanced MRV)

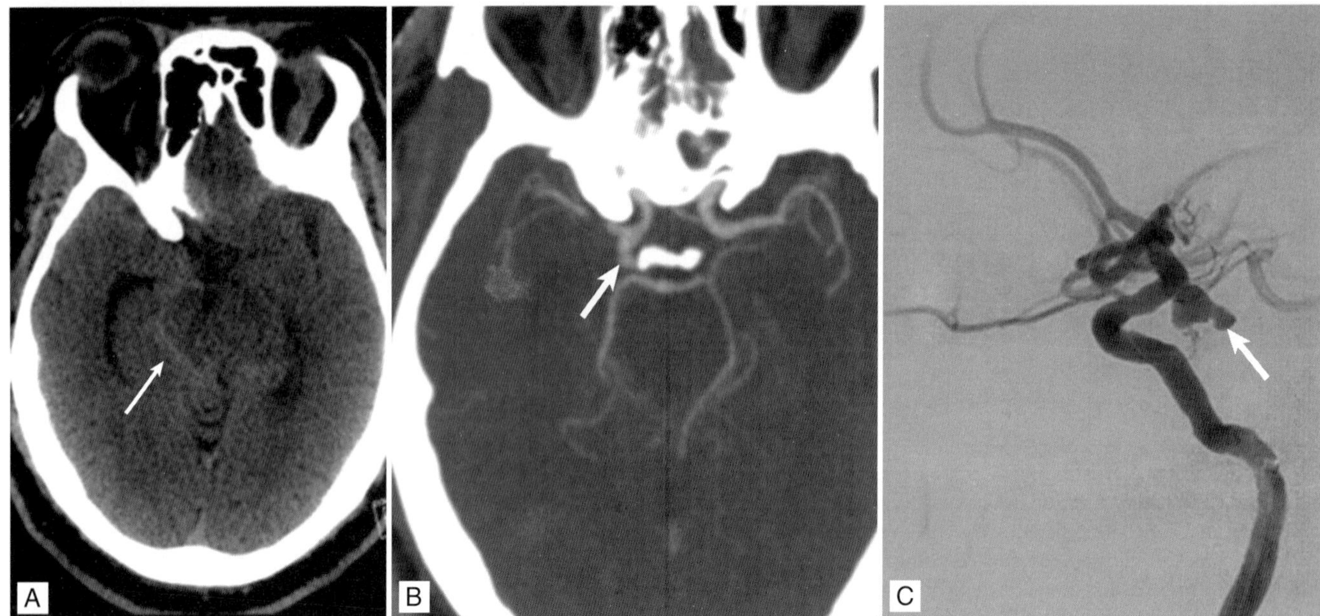

Figure 90.1 Axial noncontrast CT demonstrates acute subarachnoid hemorrhage in the right ambient cistern (*thin white arrow* in A). The CT angiogram (B) and digital subtraction angiogram (DSA) (C) confirmed a ruptured posterior communicating artery aneurysm (*thick white arrows*) that was successfully treated via an endovascular approach.

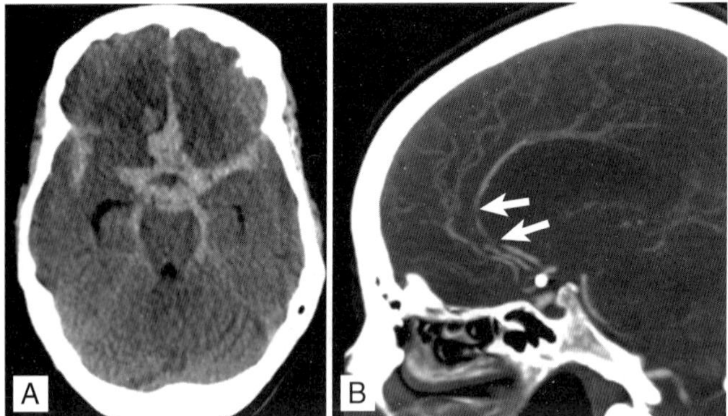

Figure 90.2 Axial CT head (A) confirms the presence of an extensive subarachnoid hemorrhage secondary to a ruptured anterior communicating artery aneurysm that was successfully treated via and endovascular approach (coil ball demonstrated on the CT angiogram). The CT angiogram (B) demonstrates multifocal irregularity affecting the anterior cerebral arteries (*white arrows*) compatible with vasospasm.

vasospasm (Fig. 90.2). Following CTA imaging this can be supplemented with MR imaging preferably with contrast-enhanced MRI and vessel wall imaging. Vessel wall imaging in particular is of benefit if an underlying vasculopathy is suspected and in patients with multiple intracranial aneurysms to guide targeted therapy [7,8].

In a patient with suspected or confirmed sepsis, the development of focal neurological signs or seizures should be viewed as concerning for infarction secondary to septic emboli. Infected mycotic aneurysms can affect the intracranial circulation and although rare, the intracranial compartment is the third most common site of involvement. There should also be a low threshold for vascular imaging, particularly in immunocompromised patients. Mycotic aneurysms more commonly affect the anterior circulation and are typically peripherally located and fusiform in morphology (Fig. 90.3). The evolution of the infective process affecting the vessel wall may lead to rupture of the wall may lead to pseudoaneurysm formation which can be lethal.

In a patient with confirmed SAH but in whom no aneurysmal source can be identified, the SAH may be secondary to perimesencephalic bleed that is typically venous in origin (Fig. 90.4). These patients have a low risk of rebleeding, vasospasm, and CSF flow impairment, and hydrocephalus with overall better outcomes [9]. The presence of blood anterior to the midbrain/pons, interpeduncular, and prepontine cisterns is characteristic and less likely to extend laterally into the sylvian fissures or demonstrate intraventricular extension. A retro clival hematoma is a rare entity that typically occurs in the post-traumatic setting in children but it can occur spontaneously and can be associated with intraventricular blood. As per a perimesencephalic bleed, the outcomes are favorable [10].

In the setting of a spontaneous convexity SAH, specific diagnoses to consider include reversible cerebral vasoconstriction syndrome (RCVS), cerebral venous sinus thrombosis (CVST), vasculitis, amyloid angiopathy, and underlying coagulopathy (Table 90.2). It may also reflect hemorrhagic transformation of parenchymal infarction [11].

Patients with CVST typically present with headache which is often the first symptom although the nature of the headache is variable. Focal deficits, seizures, altered consciousness, and papilledema can also occur. The venous thrombosis increases the venous pressure that can impair arterial perfusion that can then result in edema (both vasogenic and cytotoxic) and parenchymal hemorrhage that can be cortical with either subcortical or subarachnoid extension. On a noncontrast CT head, the venous thrombosis can be difficult to identify and the density of the sinus and measurement of the Hounsfield unit can add diagnostic confidence [12]. However, this should be interpreted with caution as it requires correlation with the patients hematocrit level [13,14]. The pattern of parenchymal involvement is dictated by the extent of involvement of the dural venous sinuses, superficial cortical veins and deep internal cerebral veins as well as the collateral drainage

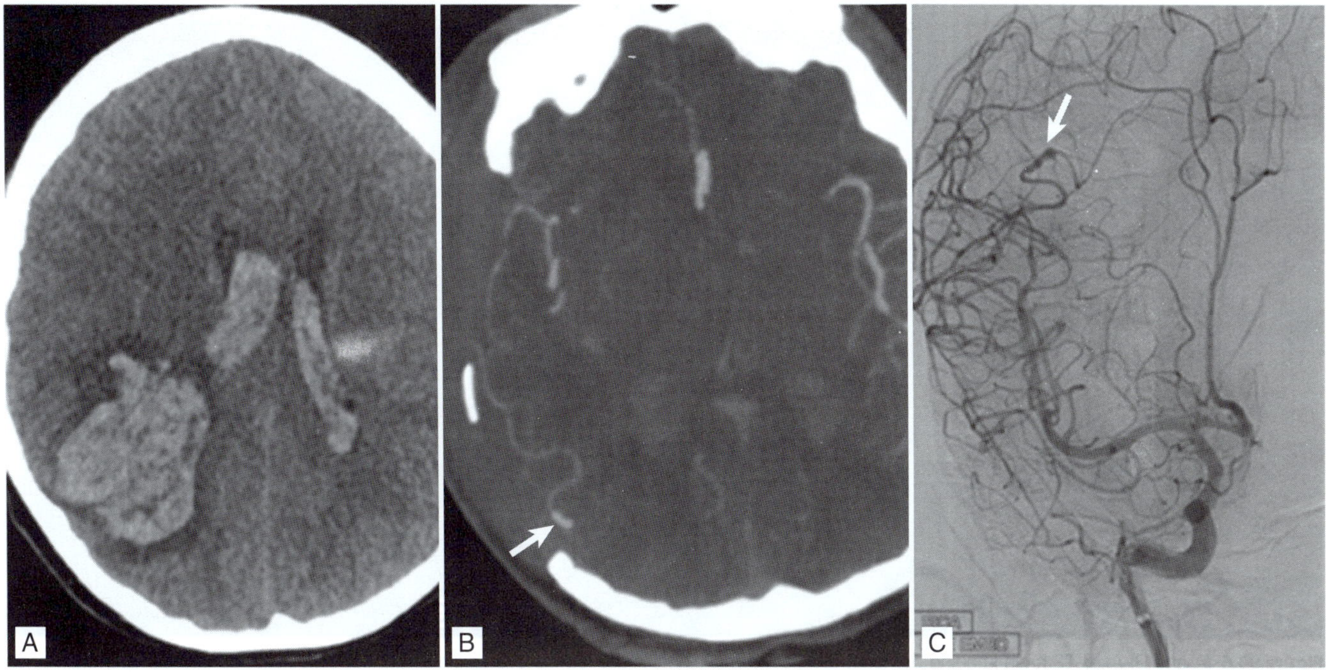

Figure 90.3 Axial CT head (A) performed in a patient with known infective bacterial endocarditis that presented with a drop in GCS. There is a large parenchymal hematoma with intraventricular extension. The CT angiogram (B) performed postdecompressive craniectomy and clot evacuation demonstrates a focal area of contrast suspicious for a fusiform mycotic aneurysm that was confirmed with a subsequent digital subtraction cerebral angiogram (C) to represent a mycotic aneurysm within a distal M4 segment of right posterior temporal artery (*white arrows*).

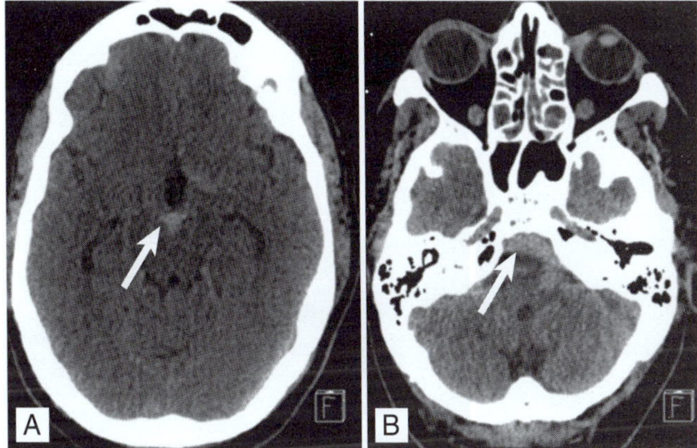

Figure 90.4 Axial noncontrast CT (A and B) demonstrating acute subarachnoid hemorrhage within the interpeduncular cistern and prepontine cistern (*white arrows*). There was a small volume of blood within the suprasellar cistern but no lateral extension into the sylvian fissure. The imaging features were suspicious for a perimesenencephalic hemorrhage, potentially venous in origin with subsequent negative CT angiogram and DSA (not shown). *DSA*, digital subtraction angiogram.

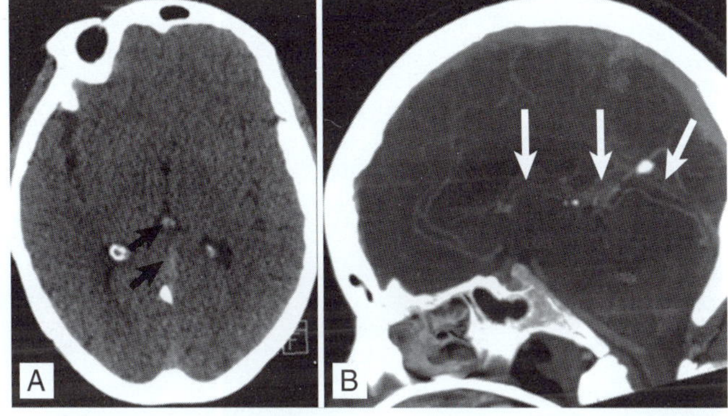

Figure 90.5 Axial CT (A) performed in a patient with sudden onset headache. There is abnormal hyperdensity along the pathway of the internal cerebral veins and vein of Galen suspicious for an internal cerebral vein thrombosis (*black arrows*). On the CT venogram (B), there were confirmed filling defects extending from the internal cerebral veins into the vein of Galen and straight sinus (*white arrows*).

TABLE 90.2 Differential Diagnosis Focal Convexity Subarachnoid Hemorrhage
Trauma
Cerebral venous sinus thrombosis
Vasculitis
Reversible cerebral vasoconstriction syndrome
Amyloid angiopathy
Coagulopathy

pathways (Fig. 90.5). MR imaging is a more sensitive test and can be combined with venographic imaging acquired as either a two-dimensional time of flight (TOF) MR venogram or contrast enhanced MR venogram [15] (Fig. 90.6). The appearance of the sinus thrombosis is dependent on the age of the thrombus and in the acute setting is isointense on T1 and hypointense on T2 thus can be overlooked. The brain parenchymal changes in terms of edema and hemorrhage are well depicted on the T2 weighted, FLAIR, and DW imaging sequences while the thrombus can be identified on either GRE or SWI sequences (Fig. 90.7).

Diagnosing vasculitis is challenging given the often nonspecific symptoms (e.g., fever, fatigue, night sweats, and weight loss) and

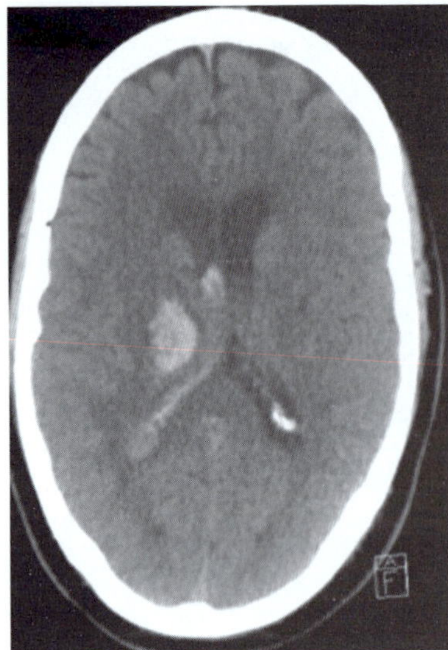

Figure 90.10 Axial CT performed in a patient with acute onset left-sided sensory symptoms confirming a right-sided thalamic hemorrhage with intraventricular extension in a patient with known poorly controlled hypertension.

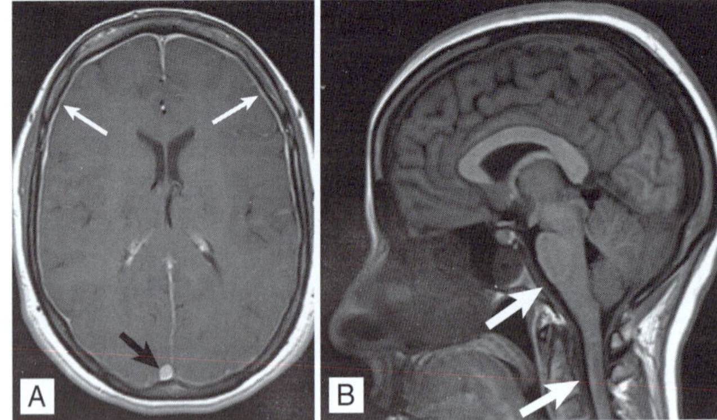

Figure 90.12 Axial T1 axial postcontrast imaging (A) in the same patient from Fig. 90.11 that demonstrates smooth and diffuse abnormal pachymeningeal enhancement (*thin white arrows*) with distension of the superior sagittal sinus that demonstrates a rounded morphology (*thick black arrow*). The sagittal T1 image (B) demonstrates distortion of the brainstem with reduction in the mamillopontine distance and there is an extra-axial retroclival collection that extends into the upper cervical spine (*thick white arrows*). The mamillopontine distance has been variably reported between 7 and 9 mm in normal individuals.

disease [18]. In the latter the parenchymal hematoma is located within the basal ganglia and cerebral white matter given the involvement of the small deep perforator vessels that are affected by arteriolosclerosis and lipohyalinosis (Fig. 90.10).

Cerebrospinal Fluid Space Abnormalities

Intracranial CSF hypotension should be considered in patients with new and persistent daily headaches that are positional in nature, worsened on standing with relief in the recumbent position [19].

- On a noncontrast CT the findings may be subtle and include the presence of subdural collections, distortion of the brainstem with "sagging" appearance, prominence of the dural venous sinuses, and prominence of the adenohypophysis (Fig. 90.11)
- Contrast enhanced MR imaging is the most sensitive test for identification of intracranial CSF hypotension with dural enhancement the most common imaging finding [20] (Fig. 90.12)
- Objective measures of brainstem distortion include mamillopontine distance (<5.5 mm) and pontomesencephalic angle (<50°) [21]
- Imaging of the whole spine included assessing for spinal extradural collections and for potential source of leak [22] (Fig. 90.13)

This may occur in patients with underlying connective tissue disorders, vascular abnormalities and intracranial hypotension can occur as a complication of spinal instrumentation or secondary to idiopathic intracranial hypertension (IIH).

IIH refers to a state of elevated intracranial pressure in the absence of a space-occupying lesion, hydrocephalus, or abnormal leptomeningeal process [23]. In patients with suspected IIH imaging should include CT or MR venography as transverse sinus stenosis is commonly identified in >90% patients [24] (Fig. 90.14). *Diagnostic criteria include papilledema, normal examination with*

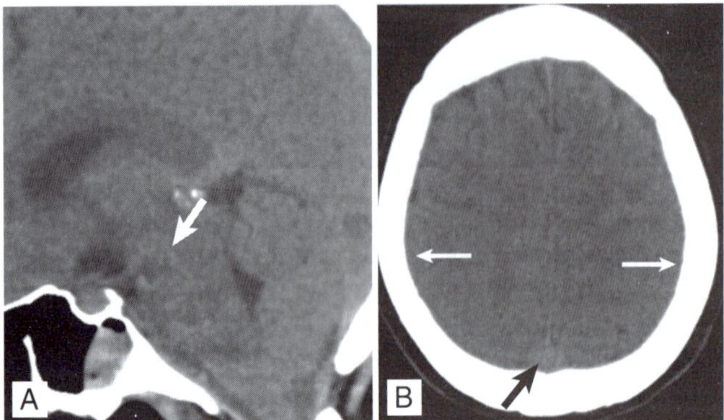

Figure 90.11 Sagittal (A) and Axial (B) CT images in a female patient presenting with postural headaches 2 weeks postpartum. The sagittal reformat demonstrates loss of the normal brainstem configuration with brainstem "sagging" (*thick white arrow*). There is a slight upper convex margin of the pituitary gland and the axial CT image demonstrates prominence of the superior sagittal sinus (*thick black arrow*) and the suspicious of bilateral subdural collections (*thin white arrows*).

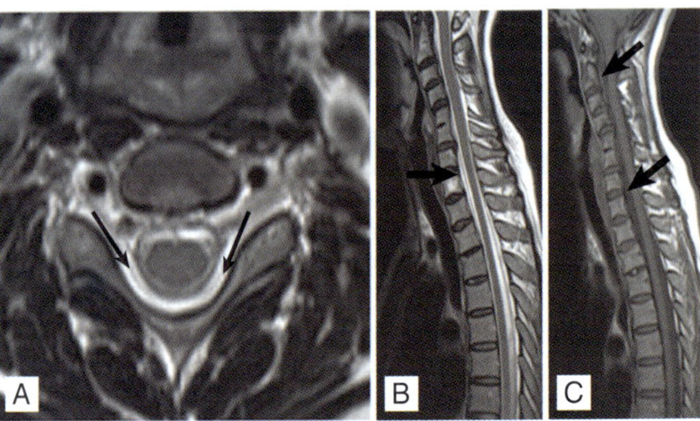

Figure 90.13 Axial T2 weighted imaging (A) at the level of C7/T1 in a patient with suspected CSF hypotension with extra-axial collections (*thin black arrows*) confirmed on the sagittal T2 (B) and T1 (C) weighted sequences (*thick black arrows*). The source for the leak was suspected to be due to the C6/7 degenerative change but was not confirmed on imaging however the patient responded well to therapy and a blood patch.

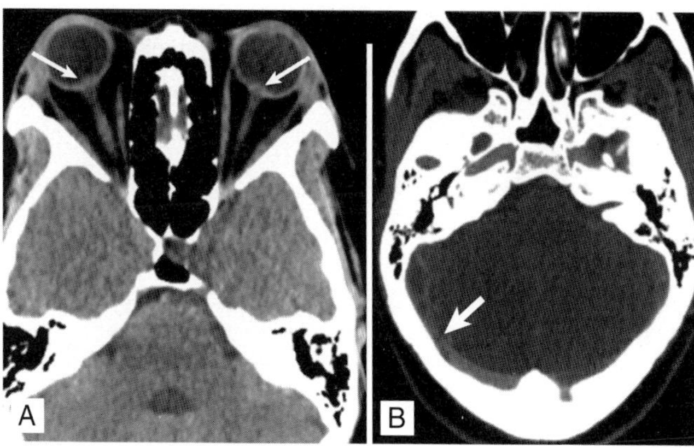

Figure 90.14 Axial noncontrast CT head (A) confirms the presence of bilateral optic nerve head protrusion correlating with bilateral papilledema (*thin white arrows*). The CT venogram (B) excluded a venous sinus thrombosis but it identified a transverse sinus stenosis (*thick white arrow*) in this patient with idiopathic intracranial hypertension.

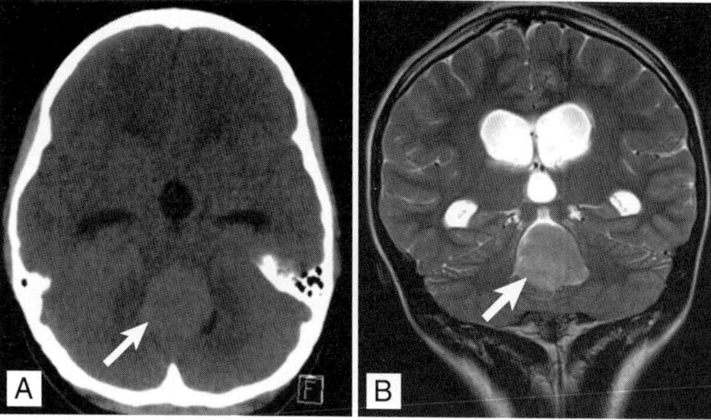

Figure 90.16 Axial noncontrast CT (A) in a 15-year-old female patient presenting with headaches, double vision, nausea, and vomiting. There is a hyperdense posterior fossa tumor (*white arrow*) with obstructive hydrocephalus. The coronal T2 weighted sequence (B) confirmed the presence of an intermediate T2 signal tumor (*thick white arrow*) that demonstrated marked cellularity on the DWI sequence with homogenous enhancement. This was confirmed to be a medulloblastoma.

the exception of abducens and facial nerve palsies, normal CSF with an elevated opening pressure of >250 mm in adults and >280 in children [25]. Other criteria demonstrable on imaging in addition to transverse sinus stenosis include an empty sella, globe flattening, and prominent subarachnoid spaces. Patients with IIH have a higher incidence of meningoceles and a potential complication of IIH also includes the development CSF hypotension secondary to a CSF leak [26] (Fig. 90.15).

Neoplastic Processes

A concern in the acute emergency setting in a patient with a new-onset headache is the exclusion of a neoplastic process [27]. Unfortunately, primary intrinsic gliomas, and other intracranial tumors as well as the secondary metastatic disease can all potentially present with headache (Fig. 90.16). In the setting of multiple foci of parenchymal hemorrhage, metastatic disease is a consideration, particularly in the setting of melanoma, renal, thyroid, cervical, and choriocarcinoma [28] (Fig. 90.17). Nonhemorrhagic lesions are often identified as areas of parenchymal edema on a noncontrast study that often prompts further evaluation with a contrast-enhanced CT or MRI. Complications of the lesion(s) include mass effect and trans-compartmental shift, hydrocephalus, and venous sinus thrombosis. Unique in this setting is the presence of a colloid cyst which, given its location, can result in obstruction of CSF flow [29]. The MR appearances and signal characteristics are dependent upon cyst composition and it can present with positional headaches (Fig. 90.18). Sudden death can occur from ball valve effect and obstruction of CSF outflow from the third ventricle [30].

Pituitary apoplexy (Fig. 90.19) can present with sudden onset headache that is typically retro-orbital in nature, accompanied by nausea and vomiting, visual symptoms, and ophthalmoplegia. It results from hemorrhagic infarction of a pituitary adenoma and can lead to SAH [31].

Infectious Processes

Intracranial sepsis can result from direct spread from sinugenic or otogenic sources or from hematogenous spread. Patients can present with headache with additional features including fever and systemic symptoms. This is covered in detail below in imaging the septic patient.

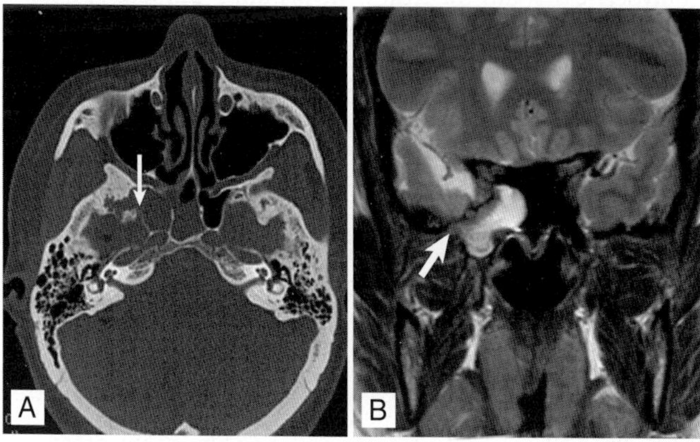

Figure 90.15 Axial CT (A) in a patient with idiopathic intracranial hypertension presenting with right-sided nasal discharge. There is opacification within the right sphenoid sinus with multiple arachnoid granulations and potential defect in the lateral wall of the right sphenoid (*thin white arrow*). The coronal T2 MRI (B) demonstrates a right sided meningoencephalocele (*thick white arrow*).

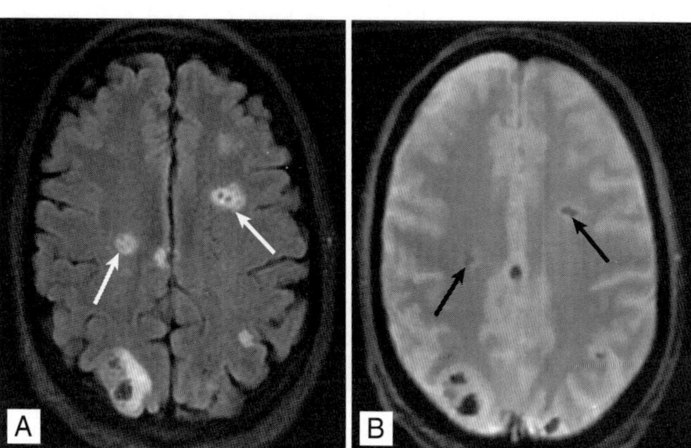

Figure 90.17 Axial FLAIR sequence (A) and an axial gradient recall echo sequence (B) in a patient with a known germ cell tumor. The imaging demonstrates multiple parenchymal lesions (*thin white arrows*) with evidence of susceptibility on the GRE (*thin black arrows*) consistent with hemorrhagic parenchymal metastases.

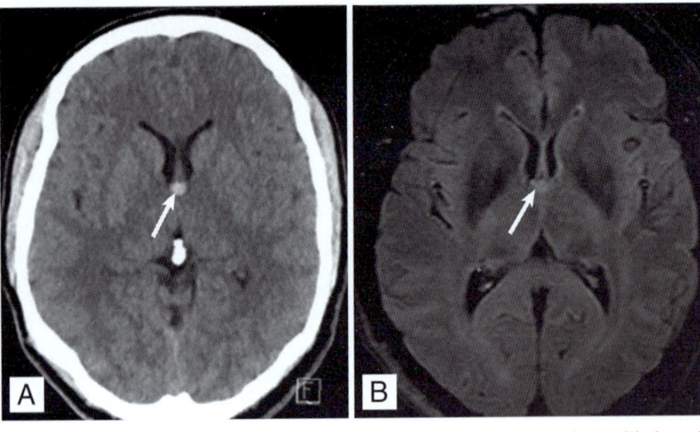

Figure 90.18 Axial CT head performed in a patient presenting with headache (A). There is a rounded hyperdense lesion in the third ventricle on the CT consistent with a colloid cyst (*thin white arrow*). On the axial FLAIR sequence (B), it returns high signal consistent with proteinaceous material.

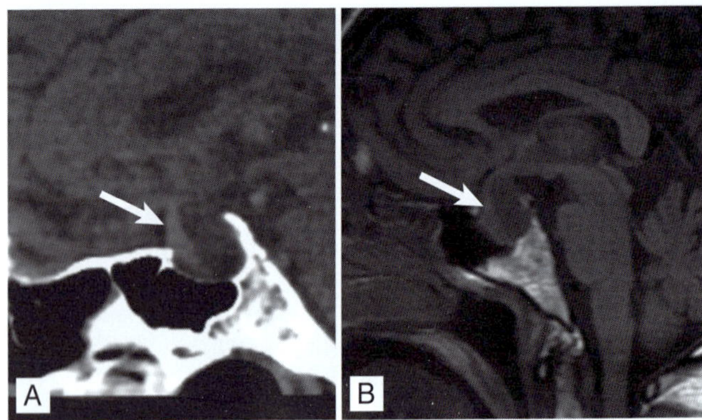

Figure 90.19 Sagittal CT (A) and T1 precontrast MR (B) images in a patient who presented with acute onset headache and opthalmoplegia. There is evidence of pituitary apoplexy and intralesional hemorrhage (*white arrows*) into a presumed pre-existing pituitary macroadenoma.

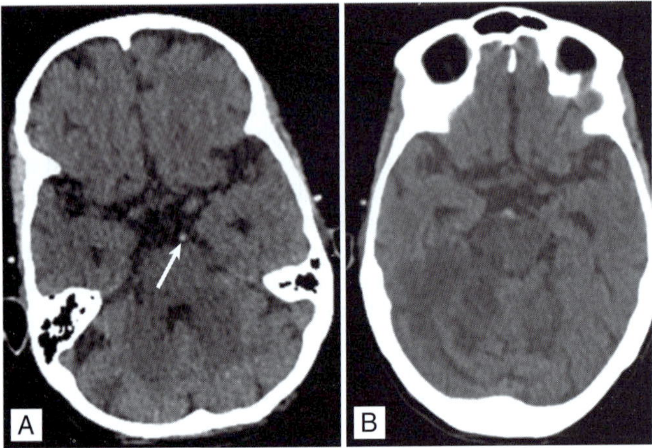

Figure 90.20 Axial CT performed in a patient who presented with a low GCS. There is hyperdensity within the basilar artery (*thin white arrow* in A) confirmed as a basilar artery thrombosis on CT angiographic imaging (not shown). The subsequent CT head (B) demonstrates persistent thrombus with extensive infarction affecting the brainstem, cerebellum, and right temporal lobe.

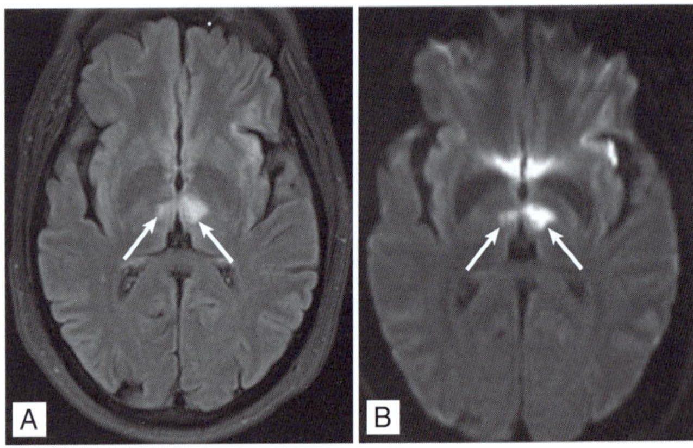

Figure 90.21 Axial FLAIR image (A) in a patient presenting with acute onset double vision and sensory symptoms with abnormal signal change in the ventromedial aspect of both thalami (*thin white arrows*) that was confirmed as areas of diffusion restriction on the DWI imaging (B) (*thin white arrows* on the b1000 image). The features were consistent with infarction within the artery of Percheron territory.

Comatose Patient

Imaging assessment in the patient with a reduced level of consciousness and low GCS presenting to the emergency department typically requires a combination of both CT and MR imaging [32]. Reduced consciousness and altered mental state may be secondary to disruption of the ascending reticular activating system (ARAS) that has an integral role in arousal state and consciousness. The ARAS has connections between the pons and dorsal midbrain with the cortex via the thalamus and hypothalamus [33]. In addition to disruption of this pathway other widespread cortical and global insults can result in reduced GCS and coma.

In the setting of acute trauma the mechanism of trauma is related to the severity of intracranial injuries and in the patient, with altered mental status this can be secondary to a number of factors including diffuse axonal injury, development of cerebral swelling, and edema and trans-compartmental shift that can be related to cerebral edema as well as other intra- and extra-axial hemorrhage [32].

In the nontrauma setting, it is imperative to exclude the possibility of a vertebral or basilar artery thrombosis that may result in brainstem ischemia and infarction as this is potentially reversible with institution of thrombolysis or mechanical thrombectomy to restore perfusion [34] (Fig. 90.20). This is identified as a hyperdensity within the vertebrobasilar circulation and this can be supplemented with CTA or MRA in equivocal cases and for treatment planning purposes. Areas of corresponding infarction within the vertebrobasilar territory aid in subsequent management decisions and potential reperfusion therapies. The presence of midbrain and bilateral thalamic infarcts should prompt consideration of infarction within the artery of percheron [35] (Fig. 90.21).

In patients with cardiorespiratory arrest or in cases with a suspected downtime the admission CT may be able to confirm the presence of a global hypoxic brain injury with

- global loss of gray–white matter differentiation,
- loss of clarity of the basal ganglia,
- cerebral swelling and generalized sulcal effacement,
- hyperdense cerebellum, and
- pseudo-SAH appearance (Fig. 90.22).

However, MR is more sensitive and provides more prognostic cases, especially in cases with suspected global hypoxic brain injury and no confirmatory findings on CT [36] (Fig. 90.23). Various patterns of cortical, ganglionic, white matter, and brainstem involvement can be observed [37]. Diffusion-weighted imaging represents the most sensitive imaging sequences with identification

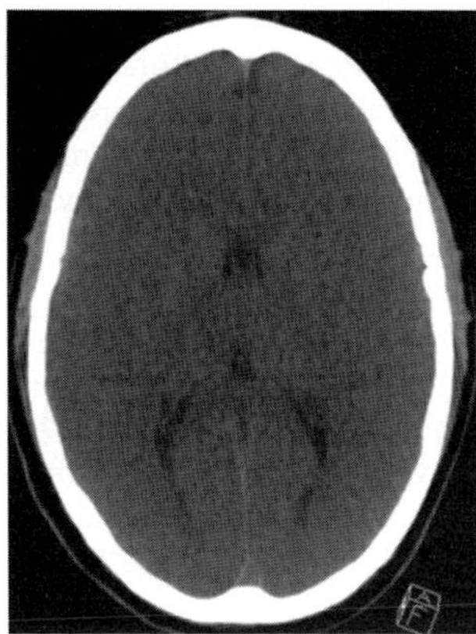

Figure 90.22 Axial CT head in a patient with an out-of-hospital cardiac arrest. There is cerebral swelling with loss of the gray and white matter differentiation and loss of clarity of the basal ganglia consistent with a hypoxic brain injury.

of diffusion restriction that may be difficult to appreciate on the conventional T2 and FLAIR imaging sequences (Fig. 90.24). The areas affected reflect areas of brain tissue that have high metabolic demand and thus are more susceptible to the effects of hypoxia.

A range of systemic abnormalities can induce a comatose state and this includes both metabolic disturbances and exposure to toxins. These can have both acute effects on the CNS while others can have chronic effects and thus the clinical presentation can be more subtle and insidious [38].

In this chapter, we will focus on metabolic disturbances and toxins that demonstrate immediate CNS toxicity and results in an acute presentation to the emergency department. Particular areas of the brain are particularly susceptible to toxic and metabolic insults that include the basal ganglia and cerebral white matter and typically this may occur in a symmetrical distribution. The differential diagnoses to consider in bilateral basal ganglia insults are listed in Table 90.3.

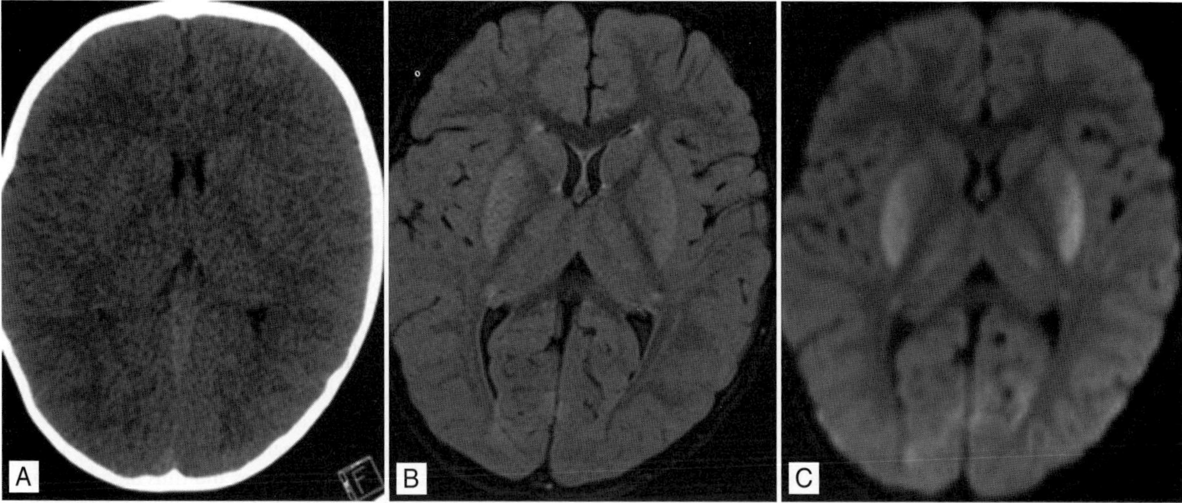

Figure 90.23 Axial CT (A) in a child who sustained neck trauma that was considered within normal limits but an MRI was performed given the mechanism of injury and clinical status. The axial FLAIR (B) and DWI imaging (C) (b1000 imaging shown) demonstrates abnormal signal change within the basal ganglia, internal capsules, occipital lobes, and hippocampi consistent with a hypoxic brain injury.

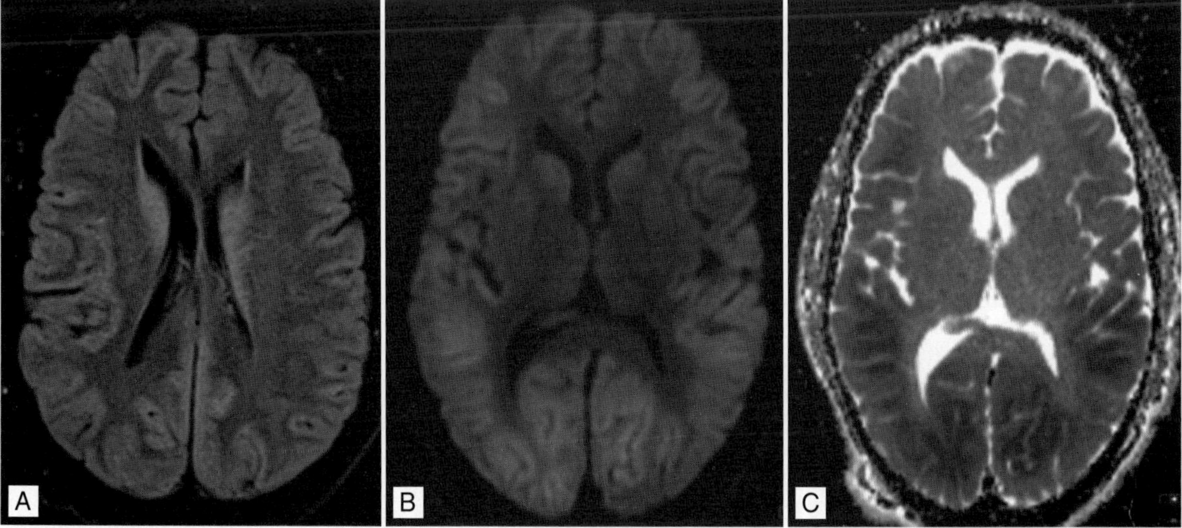

Figure 90.24 Axial FLAIR (A) and DWI (b1000 image (B) and ADC map (C)) in a patient who suffered a cardiac arrest following a road traffic accident. The FLAIR demonstrates subtle abnormal signal change within the caudate nuclei and affecting the cortex and subcortical white matter but this is accentuated and more readily appreciable on the b1000 imaging of the DWI sequences. This correlated with areas of low signal on the corresponding ADC map with features compatible with a global hypoxic brain injury.

TABLE 90.3 Bilateral Basal Ganglia Abnormalities

1. Vascular Internal cerebral vein thrombosis Artery of percheron infarct/basilar tip syndrome Global hypoxic/hypoperfusion ischemic injury
2. Toxic Carbon monoxide poisoning—globus pallidus necrosis Heroin—basal ganglia, cerebral white matter, and cerebellar involvement Methanol—visual disturbances, putaminal necrosis and white matter demyelination Cyanide poisoning—putaminal and globus pallidus involvement
3. Metabolic Glucose—Hyper glycaemia/Hypoglycaemia Hyperammonaemia/liver failure—globus pallidus changes Wernicke's encephalopathy Osmotic demyelination
4. Infective Viral aetiologies—flavivirus Postviral acute disseminated encephalomyelitis Immunocompromised—toxoplasmosis, cryptococcus
5. Inflammatory Neurobehcets disease
6. Neoplastic Lymphoma Glioblastoma multiforme

Alcohol (ethanol) is a commonly abused substance that is a potential neurotoxin that easily crosses the blood–brain barrier. It has a variety of acute and chronic effects on the CNS and it is a confounding factory in a significant proportion of emergency department admissions. Acute alcohol poisoning can result in cytotoxic edema affecting the cerebral white matter and thalami and can result in diffuse cerebral swelling [38]. Alcohol may result in Wernicke–Korsakoff syndrome in addition to other nonalcohol related causes of thiamine deficiency. The acute clinical presentation includes the triad of ocular dysfunction, ataxia, and altered mental status and the brain parenchymal areas commonly involved include the mamillary bodies, hypothalamus, medial thalamic nuclei, tectal plate, and periaqueductal gray (Fig. 90.25). These changes are difficult to discern on a noncontrast CT and MR imaging is more sensitive [39].

Osmotic demyelination syndrome (ODS) can result from acute electrolyte and osmolality disorders of which hyponatremia and rapid overcorrection are the most common. ODS typically affects the pons (pontine myelinolysis) however, extrapontine myelinolysis also commonly occurs affecting the thalami, basal ganglia, and cerebral white matter in particular [40]. MR imaging and diffusion weighted imaging is the most sensitive sequence in the setting of acute ODS demonstrating restricted diffusion in affected brain areas [39]. Development of hyperintense signal on T2 and FLAIR sequences with the corresponding hypointense signal on T1 weighted sequences develops in the first few days.

Acute hepatic encephalopathy results from hyperammonaemia that may be due to hepatic failure or other nonhepatic causes. Ammonia and its principal metabolite glutamine interfere mitochondrial metabolism and energy production and this accounts for the pattern of brain parenchymal involvement and magnetic resonance spectroscopy findings. Patients can present with nonspecific irritability, lethargy and vomiting that may progress to increasing drowsiness, seizures and subsequent coma.

- A noncontrast CT may demonstrate diffuse cerebral edema with cerebral sulcal effacement.
- On MR imaging there is abnormal T2 and FLAIR hyperintensity affecting the insula, cingulate gyri, and basal ganglia in particular although more diffuse cortical, thalamic, and white matter involvement may occur (Fig. 90.26). Restricted diffusion is typical and altered glutamate-glutamine peak at short echo times are seen on MRS [41].

The brain has significant demand for glucose being a metabolically active organ with no glycogen stores and thus blood glucose levels are tightly regulated. Disruption of glucose levels and either hypoglycaemia or hyperglycaemia has the potential to affect the CNS.

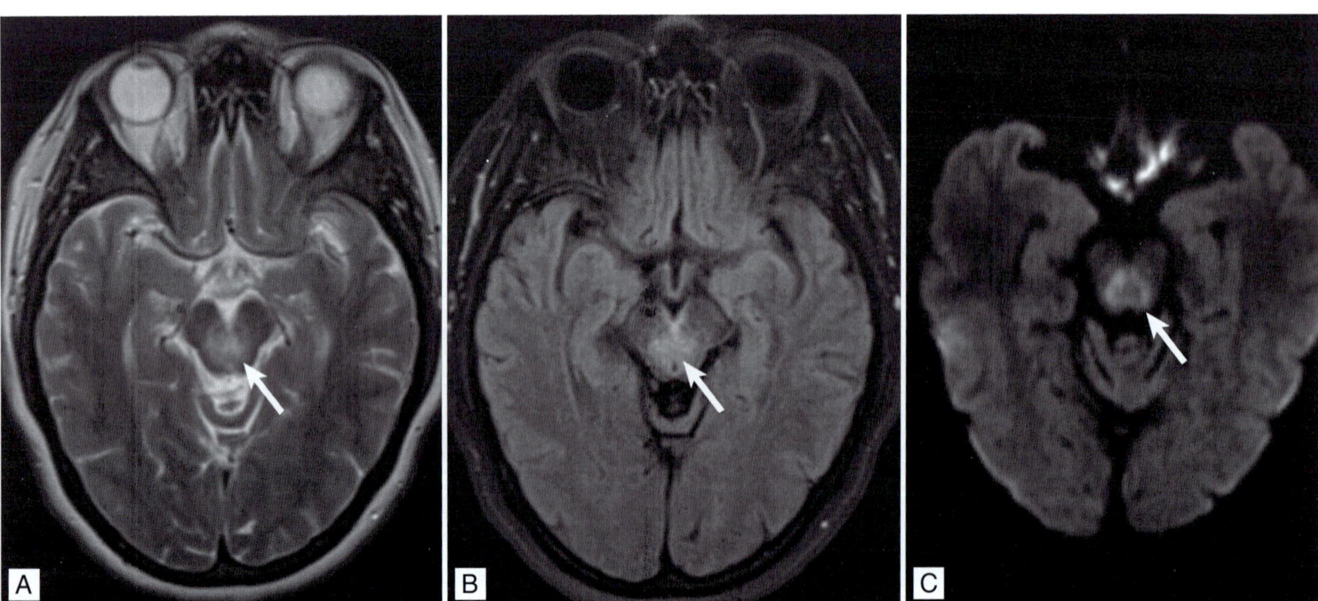

Figure 90.25 Axial T2 (A), FLAIR (B), and DWI (C) (b1000 image) in a patient with chronic alcoholism who presented with diplopia. There is abnormal signal change within the midbrain and periaqueductal gray consistent with Wernicke–Korsakoff syndrome. On the DWI the area of high signal on the b1000 image did not correlate with low signal on the ADC map and was not considered to represent diffusion restriction.

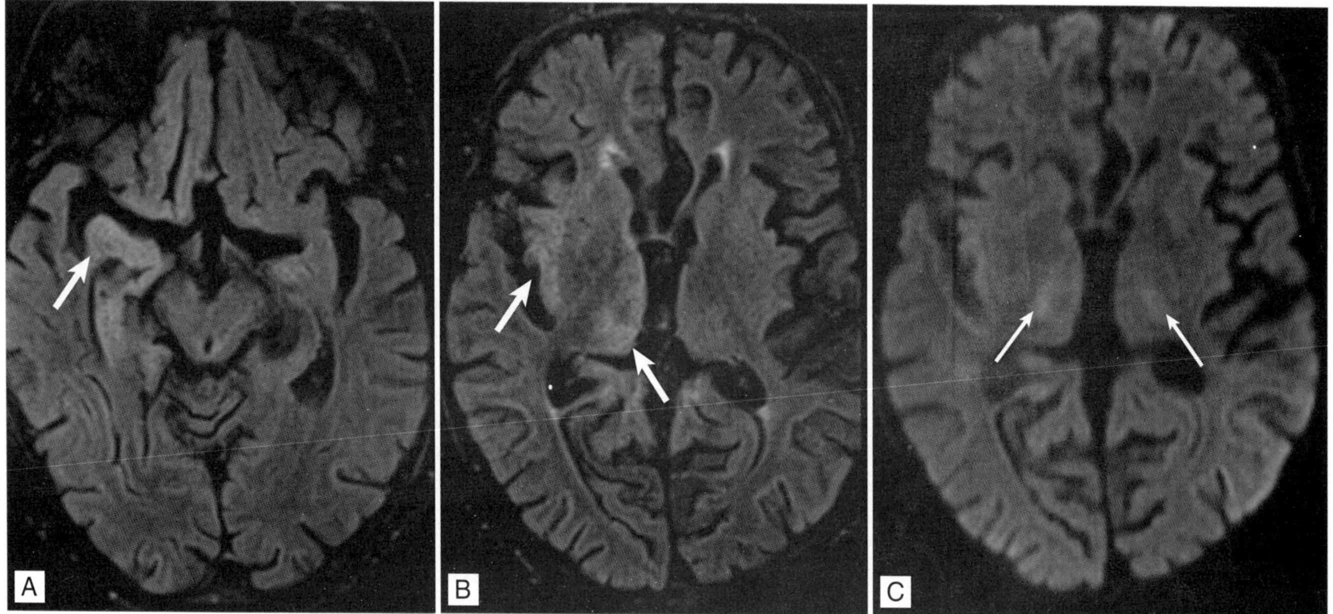

Figure 90.26 . Axial FLAIR imaging (A and B) in a hepatic encephalopathy with abnormal signal change noted in the right temporal lobe and right insula (with thalamic involvement (*white arrows*). The bithalamic involvement is accentuated on the DWI sequence (C) (*thin white arrows* on b1000 imaging).

Hypoglycaemic encephalopathy results from the direct effect of impaired intracellular metabolism and aerobic oxidation with further indirect effects resulting from the release of excitatory neurotransmitters. The pattern of brain parenchymal involvement includes cortical involvement with a predilection for the parieto-occipital lobes with subsequent cortical laminar necrosis [42]. The basal ganglia, hippocampi and amygdala can also be involved but areas not typically affected include the thalamus, brainstem and cerebellum.

- On an unenhanced CT head symmetrical hypodensities in the putamina and caudate nuclei can be present with sparing of the thalami. Cortical involvement can be identified as generalized cerebral swelling and sulcal effacement
- MR imaging demonstrates T2 and FLAIR signal hyperintensity in the affected parenchyma with the development of T1 shortening in areas of cortical laminar necrosis (Fig. 90.27)

The main differential to include would be hypoxic-ischemic encephalopathy given the requirements of oxygen and glucose for aerobic metabolism but HIE may involve the thalami and cerebellum.

In the acute emergency setting, *hyperglycaemia* may result in diabetic ketoacidosis or hyperglycaemic hyperosmolar state (HHS). Hyperglycaemia induced hemichorea and hemiballismus is less common and is evident on imaging as basal ganglia T1 shortening and signal hyperintensity with sparing of the thalamus [43]. These findings are typically unilateral but can be bilateral in nature (Fig. 90.28). The hyperglycaemic state results from reduced effects of insulin and impaired glucose utilization combined with accelerated glucose production. In diabetic ketoacidosis, this can be identified on imaging as areas of nonspecific vasogenic edema while clinically there is increased ketone production with resultant metabolic acidosis that also precipitates osmotic diuresis and loss of water, and electrolytes (Na+, K+). Correction of the metabolic disturbance can result in osmotic myelinolysis [40]. HHS results in hyperglycaemia with minimal ketone formation with

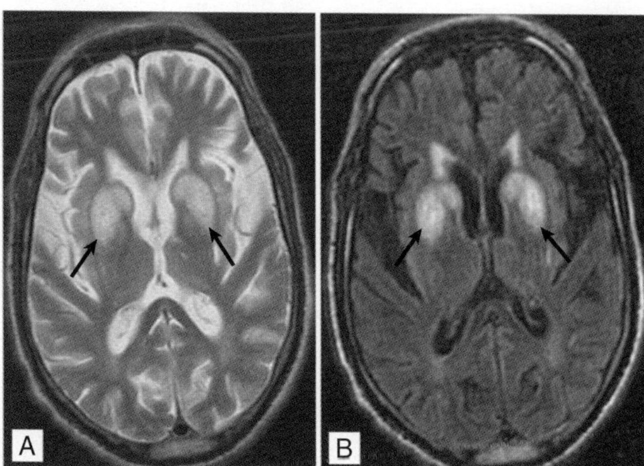

Figure 90.27 Axial T2 (A) and FLAIR (B) imaging in a patient presenting with low GCS secondary to hypoglycaemia. There was symmetrical abnormal signal change within the caudate nuclei and both putamina (*thin black arrows*).

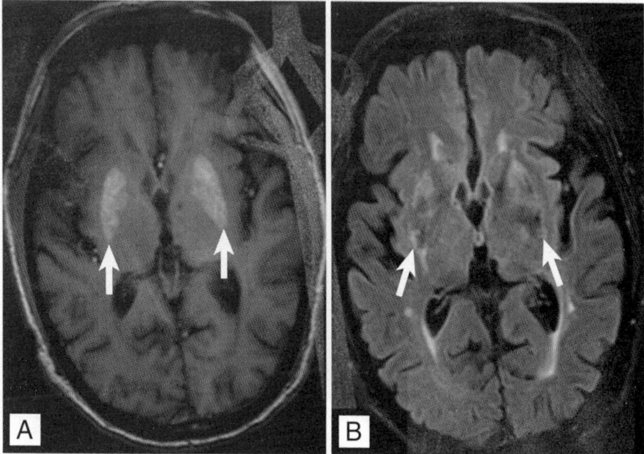

Figure 90.28 Axial T1 (A) and FLAIR (B) imaging in a patient with nonketotic hyperglycaemia presenting with generalized chorea. There was abnormal and symmetrical T1 hyperintensity affecting the putamina with heterogenous signal on the FLAIR (*white arrows*).

elevated glucose and bicarbonate levels. It typically results in white matter signal hypointensity within the parietal and occipital lobes, The affected cortical regions demonstrate T2/FLAIR signal hyperintensity with restricted diffusion [43].

The spectrum of potential toxins that affect the CNS is myriad and, in this chapter, we will focus on the most common presentations to the emergency department. This includes carbon monoxide (CO) poisoning, methanol intoxication, and illicit drug use including cocaine and heroin.

CO poisoning may occur due to accidental poisoning or in the setting of attempted suicide. It is a toxic, clear, and odorless gas formed from the incomplete combustion of hydrocarbons that combines with hemoglobin hence it impairs oxygen transportation. *The brain parenchymal areas involved include the globus pallida and cerebral white matter* [44].

- CT head imaging is typically normal although CO poisoning should be suspected if there are bilateral pallidal hypodensities
- On MR imaging the globus pallidus necrosis is observed as an area of T2/FLAIR signal hyperintensity and T1 signal hypointensity with peripheral T2 low signal and T1 shortening (Fig. 90.29)

The cerebral white matter involvement can be delayed and progresses from demyelination to necrosis. The main differential for the imaging appearances is that of HIE but in the setting of HIE other brain areas including the hippocampi and the other components of the basal ganglia while the white matter is less often affected.

Methanol poisoning can be deliberate or accidental. It is a strong CNS depressant and methanol is metabolized to formaldehyde and formic acid which can result in a metabolic acidosis. Clinical presentation includes visual disturbances and blindness, nonspecific GI symptoms of nausea, and vomiting with coma in severe cases. Changes are observed in the putamina and cerebral white matter. *Bilateral putaminal necrosis may hemorrhage with sparing of the globus pallida while cerebral white matter involvement has a predilection for the insula subcortical white matter* [44]. In addition to methanol, ethylene glycol poisoning should also be considered in the setting of putaminal necrosis.

Cocaine toxicity can result from both direct effects of the drug and its additives. It can be snorted, smoked, or injected but the effects are the same and it has a significant effect on the vasculature. It promotes platelet aggregation hence patients are at increased risk of thromboembolic strokes. Cocaine induces vasospasm and can result in systemic hypertensive crisis that also increases the risk of bleeding from existing aneurysms and vascular malformations. It also accounts for its association with posterior reversible encephalopathy syndrome (PRES) but cocaine use can also result in a vasculitis that also increases the risk of ischemia and infarction (Fig. 90.30).

Heroin is another toxin that can result in vasospasm and vasculopathy that results in ischemia that can also be secondary to emboli from impure additives. Heroin inhalation can produce a pattern of leukoencephalopathy affecting the hemispheric white matter, posterior limb of the internal capsule, cerebellar white matter brainstem [38] (Fig. 90.31).

Septic Patient

The radiologist plays a key role in imaging the patient with suspected intracranial sepsis in terms of potentially identifying the source of infection and the potential complications. If possible, it is important to establish whether the patient is immunocompetent or immunocompromised as this helps with refining potential differential diagnoses. In terms of imaging assessment, this can be broadly subdivided into extra-axial and intra-axial findings but there is frequent overlap with patients having abnormalities in multiple compartments. *The extra-axial findings to assess for include extradural collections, subdural collections, and leptomeningeal abnormalities while the intra-axial findings include identification of ring-enhancing lesions and specific assessment of the limbic and ganglionic structures.*

In our institution, primary assessment is undertaken with a noncontrast CT head supplemented with contrast-enhanced imaging prompted by identification of an intracranial abnormality on the initial CT or in the context of an immunocompromised patient or high index of suspicion of a meningoencephalitis. CT is of benefit in the acute setting to assess for potential

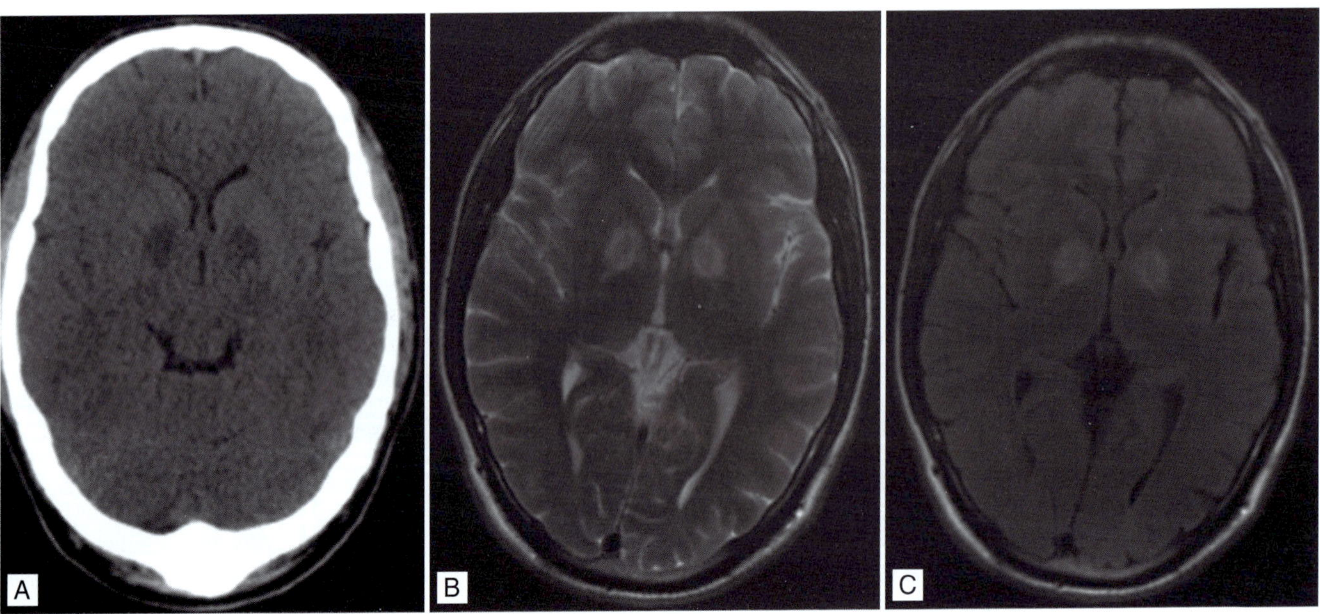

Figure 90.29 Axial CT (A) in a patient with suspected carbon monoxide poisoning who had a CT that confirmed low density within the globus pallida that correlated with abnormal signal hyperintensity on the axial T2 (B) and FLAIR (C) sequences.

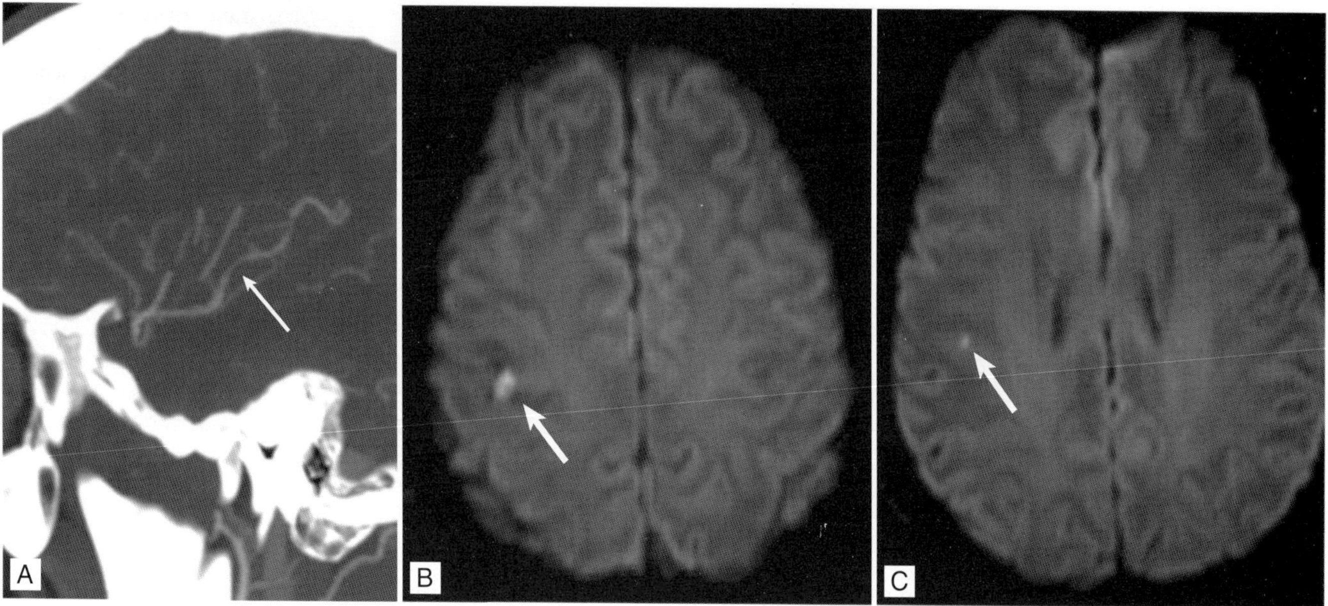

Figure 90.30 Sagittal CTA maximal intensity projection (A) that demonstrated irregularity within the right middle cerebral artery branches (*thin white arrow*). This was attributed to a cocaine induced vasculopathy with small foci of embolic infarction within the right MCA territory on the DWI sequences (*thick white arrows* in B and C).

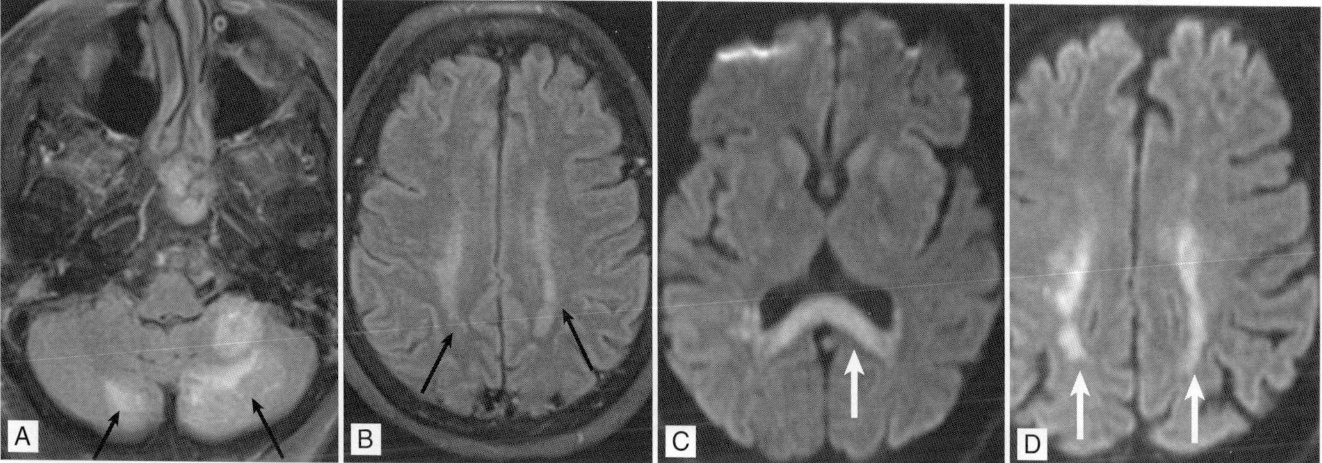

Figure 90.31 Axial FLAIR imaging (A and B) in a patient with opioid-induced toxicity with abnormal signal change within both cerebellar hemispheres with involvement of the supratentorial white matter with abnormal signal change within the centrum semiovale (*thin black arrows*). On the DWI sequences (C and D) this signal change demonstrated restricted diffusion within the splenium of the corpus callosum and centrum semiovale (*white arrows* on the b100 imaging of the DWI).

complications including hydrocephalus, assessment of mass effect, and trans-compartmental shift and intracranial hemorrhage. Contrast-enhanced imaging also enables assessment of both the arterial and venous structures depending on the timing of acquisition and provides an assessment of potential secondary vasculopathy and cerebral venous thrombosis.

In the majority of patients in whom there is a high index of suspicion of intracranial sepsis with normal initial CT findings, MR imaging is undertaken as it is inherently more sensitive. The routine imaging protocol includes a combination of T1 and T2 weighted sequences, a FLAIR sequence, diffusion weighted imaging, and T1 postcontrast imaging either as a volumetric postcontrast sequence to enable multiplanar reformats or a combination of both axial and coronal postcontrast sequences. In our institution, the use of MR spectroscopy is utilized in cases of diagnostic uncertainty and its potential role will also be discussed.

Identification of an extra-axial collection on a noncontrast CT head can be difficult, particularly in younger patients with preserved brain volume. However, extra-axial collection identification can be assisted by the administration of intravenous contrast.

- Extradural collections and empyema formation typically have a more benign course when compared to subdural empyemas [45]. There is dural enhancement and the collections can extend across midline although they are typically contained by sites of dural attachment to the inner table of the calvarium. Potential sources of infection to be assessed for include the sinonasal compartment, particularly the frontal sinuses, as well as the petromastoid air cells (Fig. 90.32). Extra-dural collections can also occur in the postoperative setting and following direct penetrating trauma. On MR imaging the extra-dural collections can demonstrate restricted diffusion with peripheral

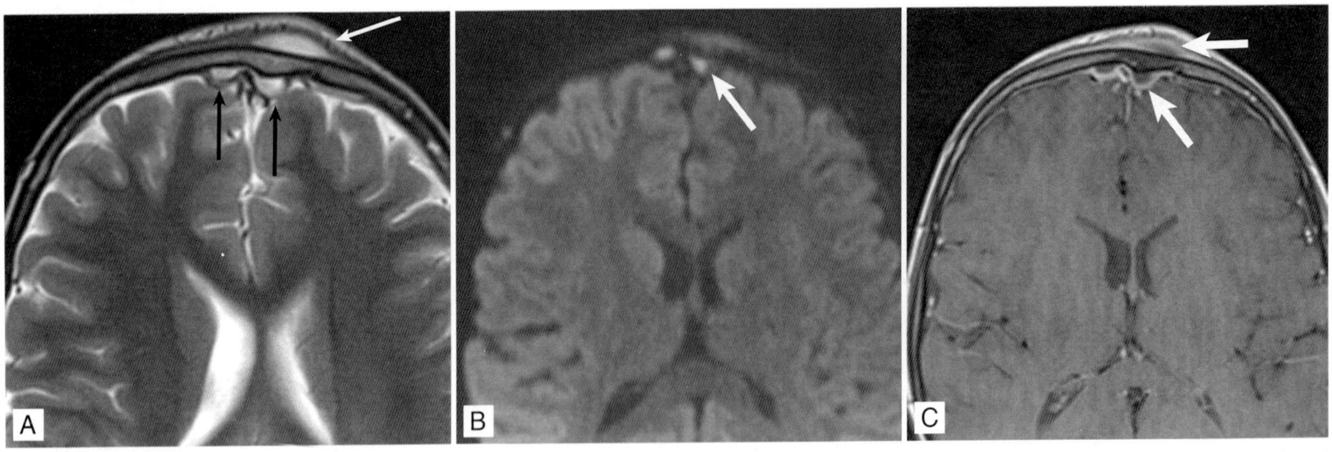

Figure 90.32 Axial T2 weighted sequence (A) in a patient with frontal sinusitis complicated by an extracalvarial subgaleal abscess (*thin white arrow*) and within the intracranial compartment a small extradural empyema (*thin black arrow*). The DWI (B) demonstrates pus with restricted diffusion within the extradural empyema with peripherally enhancing intra- and extra-cranial collections (*thick white arrows* in C).

enhancement of the collection on the postcontrast imaging but typically do not incite edema within the adjacent brain parenchyma

- The presence of a subdural collection in the setting of a septic patient typically indicates the presence of a subdural empyema and, as per extradural empyemas, the sinonasal compartment and petromastoid regions should be assessed for potential source of infection (Fig. 90.33). Subdural empyemas can extend over the cerebral convexities and result in local mass effect and can be associated with adjacent leptomeningeal and parenchymal changes. Patients can present with focal deficits and seizures and typically have less favorable outcomes when compared to extradural empyemas [46]. The subdural empyema demonstrates peripheral enhancement and restricted diffusion on the DWI sequences
- Involvement of the leptomeninges and associated leptomeningitis can be difficult to identify on CT imaging even with the administration of intravenous contrast. MR imaging is more sensitive in this regard and contrast-enhanced T1 weighted imaging demonstrates abnormal enhancement of the pia-arachnoid which can also identify on FLAIR imaging as sulcal hyperintensity [47]. The presence of pus in the subarachnoid spaces may also demonstrate linear foci of restricted diffusion (Fig. 90.34). There are newer imaging black blood imaging techniques that may improve imaging sensitivity of the vascular complications and vasculitis that can be associated with leptomeningitis and involvement of the perforating arterial vessels and vasculitis can also result in ischemia and infarction [48]. Meningitis can be secondary to bacterial, viral or fungal organisms and may be complicated by CVST, ventriculitis and basal meningitis that increases the risk of impaired CSF flow and hydrocephalus (Fig. 90.35)

The presence of intra-axial ring-enhancing lesions(s) has a differential that includes the presence of parenchymal abscesses in addition to metastatic deposits, tumefactive demyelination, hematoma, and parenchymal infarction [49]. The development of

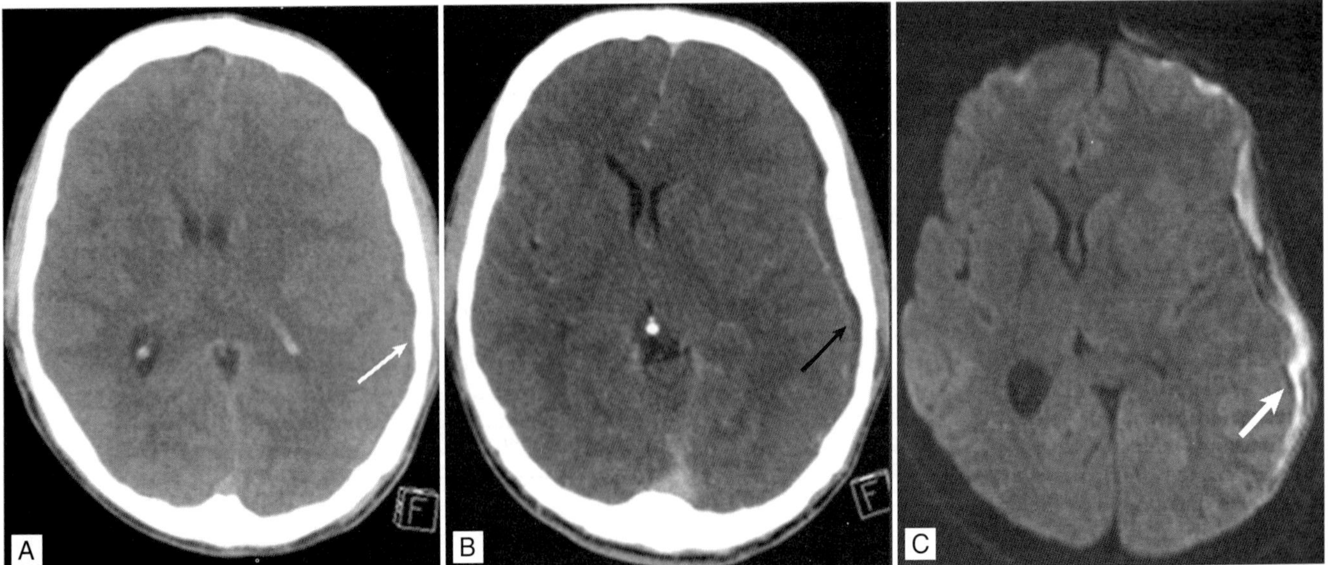

Figure 90.33 Axial noncontrast CT head (A) in a patient presenting with fever and headache. There is a low density subdural collection (*thin white arrow*) with peripheral enhancement (*thin black arrow* in B). This was a suspected subdural empyema secondary to sinusitis (not shown) and the collection demonstrated restricted diffusion on the DWI sequence (*thick white arrow* on b1000 image (C)).

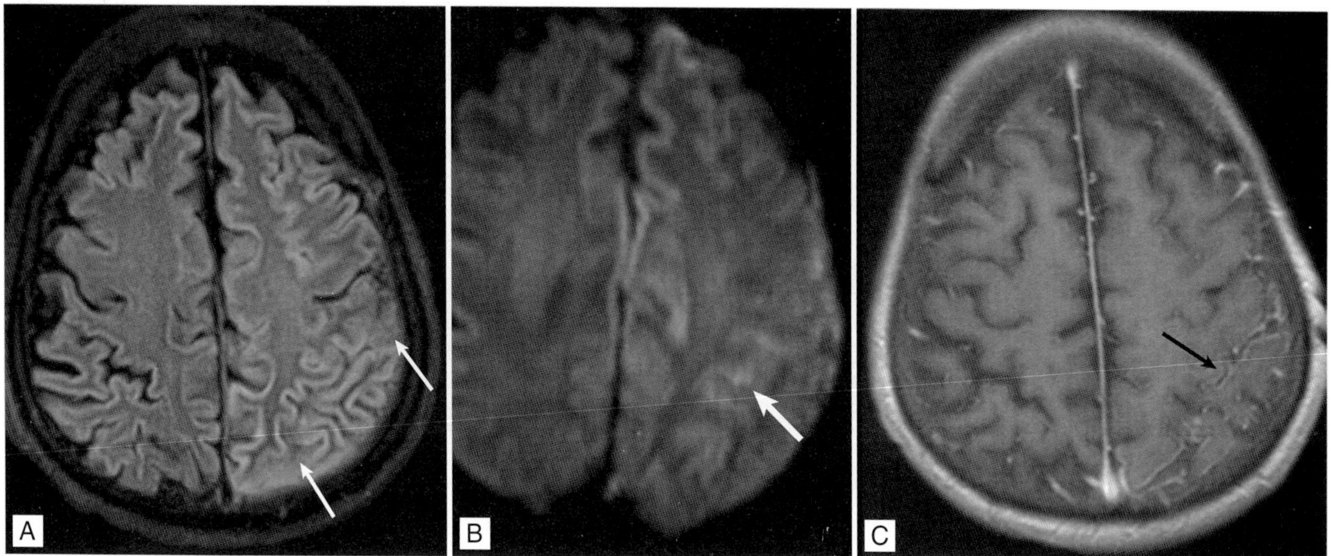

Figure 90.34 MR imaging performed in a patient with infectious meningitis. The axial FLAIR (A) demonstrates altered signal change within the CSF spaces particularly evident in the left parietal region (*thin white arrows*) that correlated with sulcal restricted diffusion (*thick white arrow* in B). There is pathological leptomeningeal enhancement (*thin black arrow* in C).

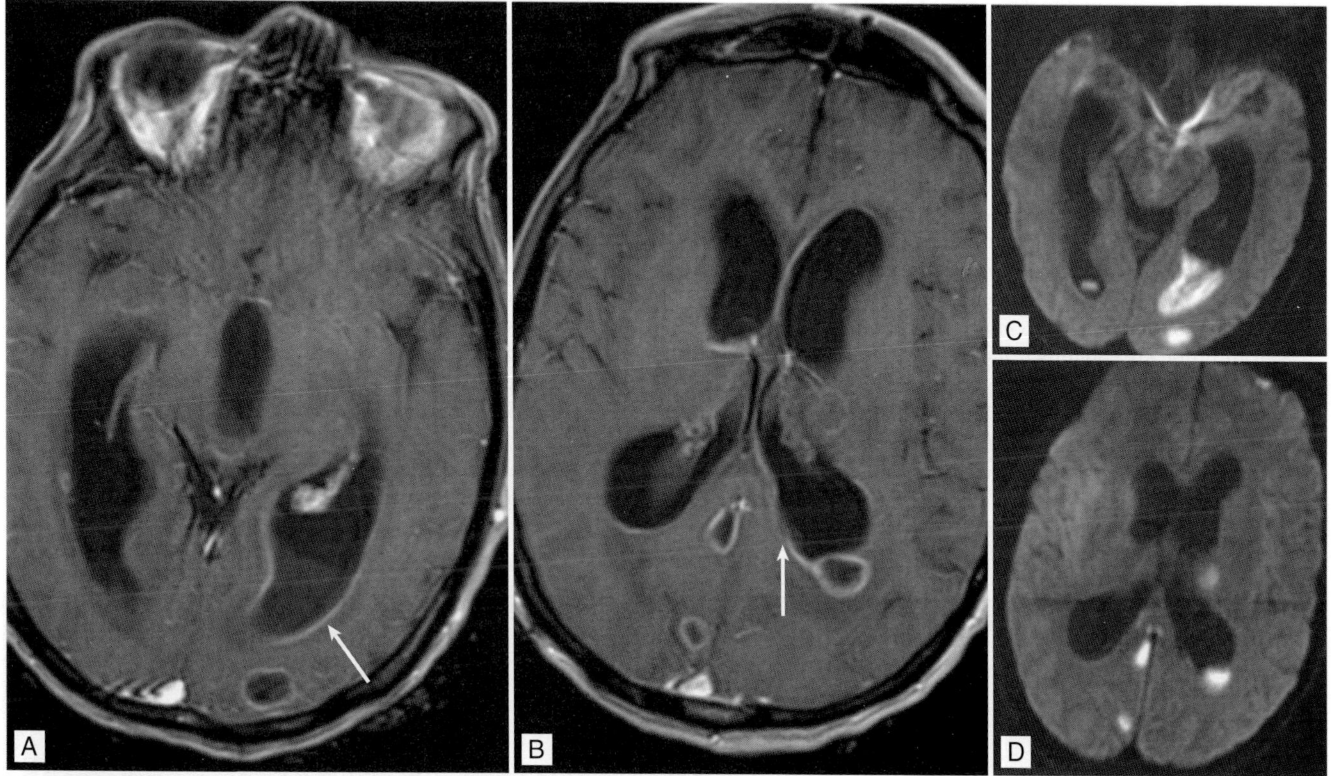

Figure 90.35 Axial T1 postcontrast images (A and B) in a patient with septic shock and low GCS. There are multiple ring-enhancing lesions with abnormal ependymal enhancement secondary to ventriculitis (*thin white arrows*) with complicating hydrocephalus. The pus within the ventricles and the parenchymal abscesses demonstrate restricted diffusion on the selected b1000 images from the DWI sequence (C and D).

parenchymal abscess evolves from early to late cerebritis followed by early abscess capsule formation and finally parenchymal abscess with capsule formation. *The enhancement pattern is typically smooth in nature as opposed to irregular enhancement that can be seen with neoplastic disease (Fig. 90.36). In addition, the enhancement is typically complete although it is typically thinner in relation to the ventricular side.* The abscess contains pus and given its internal viscosity will demonstrate internal restricted diffusion [50]. On T2 and GRE/SWI imaging, there is a peripheral low signal and the pattern of peripheral rim hypointensity can aid lesion characterization and diagnostic confidence [49]. MR spectroscopy within an abscess typically demonstrates elevated lactate (1.3 ppm), acetate (1.92 ppm) and succinate (2.4 ppm) peaks and presence of amino acids (valine and leucine) [51].

Patients presenting with suspected encephalitis can present with altered level of consciousness, fever, headache, focal deficits,

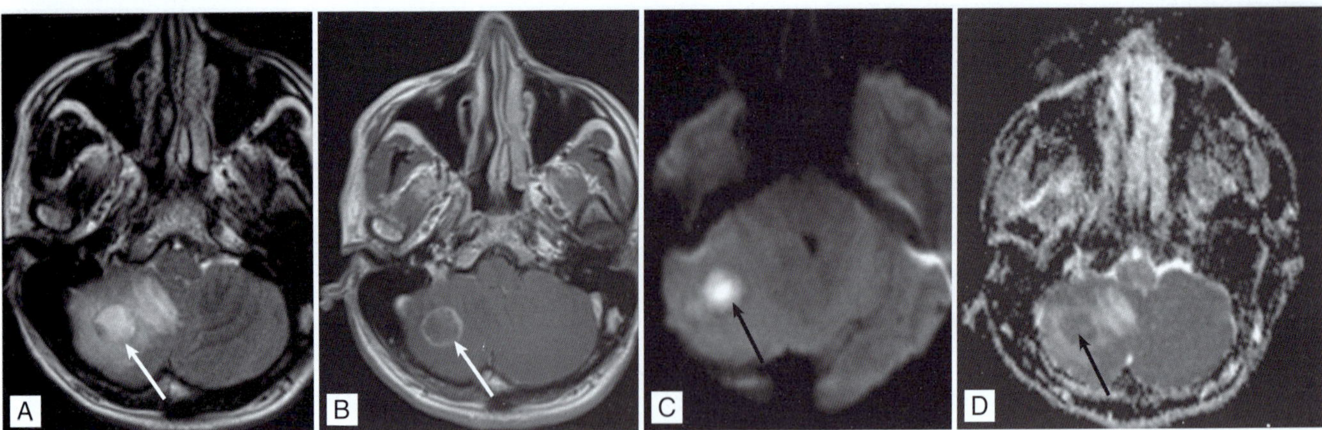

Figure 90.36 Axial T2 (A), postcontrast (B), DWI (C), and ADC (D) images demonstrates a rounded lesion within the right cerebellar hemisphere with surrounding signal change and peripheral enhancement (*thin white arrows*). This was associated with restricted diffusion (*thin black arrows*) and was confirmed to be a cerebellar abscess.

and seizures. Infectious encephalitis is most often due to Herpes Simplex virus (HSV-1 and HSV-2) [52]. *The pattern of intracranial involvement includes the mesial temporal lobe structures and it may be symmetrical or asymmetrical with potential for hemorrhage.* Other potential sites of involvement within the limbic system include the insula and inferior frontal lobes, cingulate gyri and thalamus while the ganglionic structures are typically spared [53] (Fig. 90.37). *Other viral aetiologies include Japanese encephalitis virus infection that typically affects the hippocampi with sparing of the rest of the temporal lobe* [54]. Other sites that can be affected include the thalami, basal ganglia, substantia nigra, pons and cortex. The parenchymal changes are best depicted on MR imaging as T2 and FLAIR signal hyperintensity with associated diffusion restriction. *West Nile virus demonstrates a different pattern of CNS involvement that includes the brainstem, thalami, cerebral white matter and anterior horns of the spinal cord* [55].

Autoimmune encephalitis is included in the differential based on imaging findings and includes both paraneoplastic and nonparaneoplastic aetiologies [56]. Paraneoplastic aetiologies are associated with antibodies that include anti-Hu and anti-CV2. The mesial temporal lobe structures, brainstem, and cerebellum can be affected including the striatum in the setting of anti-CV2 antibodies (Fig. 90.38). Nonparaneoplastic aetiologies include an association with NMDA receptor antibodies and the pattern of brain parenchymal involvement includes cortical T2 signal hyperintensity with variable enhancement and diffusion restriction.

The presence of basal ganglia abnormalities identified on CT and MR can be secondary to spectrum of aetiologies as described above, but in the setting of the acutely septic patient, there are specific infectious aetiologies that merit consideration. In this setting, knowledge of the patients' immune status is vital as both cryptococcosis and toxoplasmosis can affect the basal ganglia.

Cryptococcus neoformans is a ubiquitous fungus that can infect the CNS and result in either a meningitis, formation of focal lesions or cryptococcomas and result in gelatinous pseudocyst formation through involvement of the perivascular spaces that is typically noted in the basal ganglia, midbrain, dentate nuclei, and subcortical white matter [57]. While cryptococcus infections can occur in both immunocompetent and immunocompromised patients, it is typically encountered in patients with HIV infection with low CD4 counts (approximately 50–100 cells/μL).

- On unenhanced CT imaging the gelatinous pseudocyst formation affecting the basal ganglia demonstrates low density

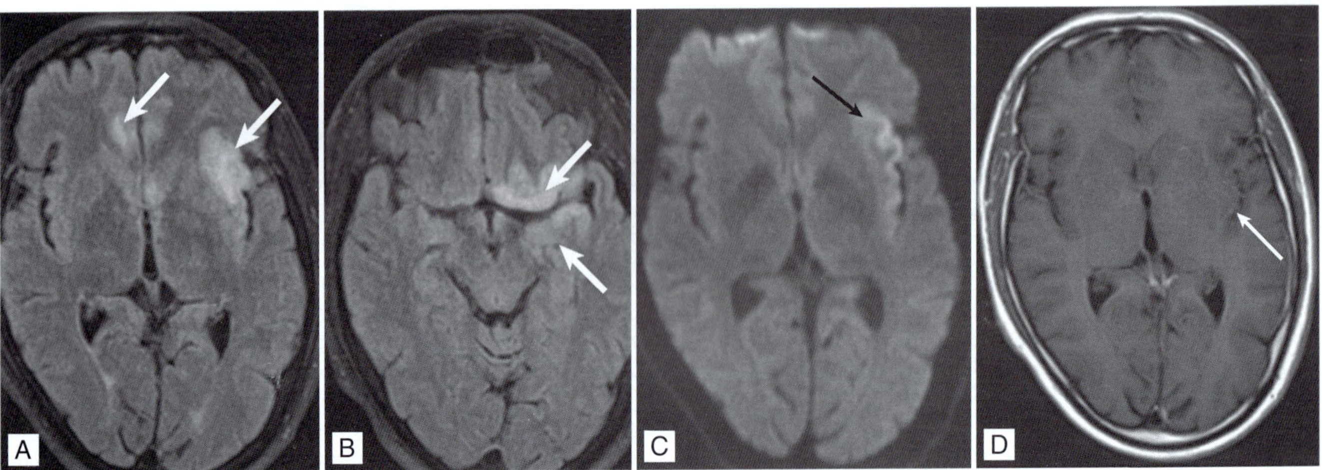

Figure 90.37 Axial FLAIR (A and B) imaging in a patient with Herpes simplex encephalitis with abnormal signal change involving the orbitofrontal brain parenchyma, left temporal lobe, left insula, and right cingulate gyrus. The cortical changes affecting the insula demonstrates restricted diffusion on the DWI sequence (*thin black arrow* in C) with the impression of faint leptomeningeal enhancement on the T1 postcontrast sequence (*thin white arrow* in D).

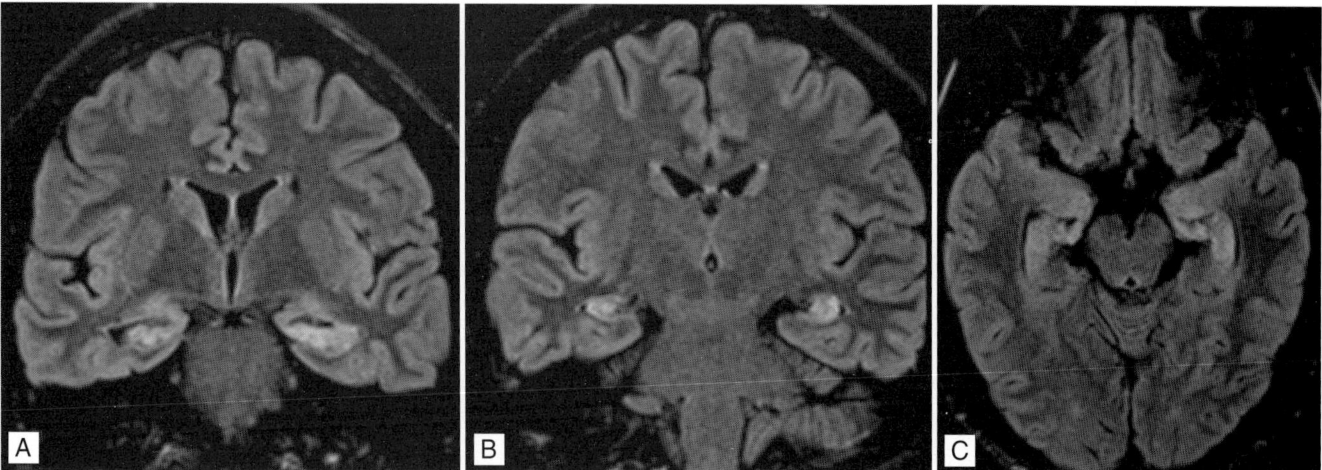

Figure 90.38 Combined coronal (A and B) and axial FLAIR (C) imaging in a patient with an autoimmune encephalitis with symmetrical abnormal signal change within both hippocampal formations and mesial temporal lobes.

- On MR imaging, this correlates with areas that are similar to CSF signal intensity, low on T1 with high signal on T2 that suppresses on FLAIR imaging (Fig. 90.39)

Toxoplasma gondii is a ubiquitous intracellular parasite that results in common opportunistic infection. In immunocompromised patients, it can result in an infective process that is typically multifocal with involvement of the basal ganglia, thalami, corticomedullary junction, and cerebellum (Fig. 90.40). *On CT, these are identified as hypodense lesions that me demonstrate nodular or ring enhancement while on MR imaging the lesions demonstrate alternating areas of high and low T2 signal change and may demonstrate an eccentric target sign* [58]. There is perilesional edema however, they demonstrate reduced relative cerebral blood volume that may help differentiate from other neoplastic entities, lymphoma being the most notable differential diagnosis to consider [59].

Aspergillus spp. can result in an angio-invasive fungal CNS infection that may occur secondary to inhaled fungal spores that invade the systemic circulation and as a consequence of hematogenous spread, infect the CNS. Alternatively, it can occur secondary to direct spread from the sinonasal compartment. Patients are typically immunocompromised and on CT imaging of the sinonasal compartment particularly attention to subtle bony changes and inflammatory fat stranding within the fat planes surrounding the sinuses is required given the aggressive angio-invasive nature of the fungal infection and high risk or morbidity and mortality if not identified and treated promptly [60] (Fig. 90.41). Within the intracranial compartment, the fungal infection can result in the formation of multiple abscesses while the angio-invasive nature of the infection can result in mycotic aneurysm formation and high risk of subsequent hemorrhage and ischemia/infarction.

Pseudomonas is a bacterium that is the main causative organism implicated in a necrotizing otitis externa that affects poorly controlled diabetic patients and the immunocompromised. Assessment of the tissues around the external auditory canal and upper deep fascial neck spaces in addition to the bony integrity of the

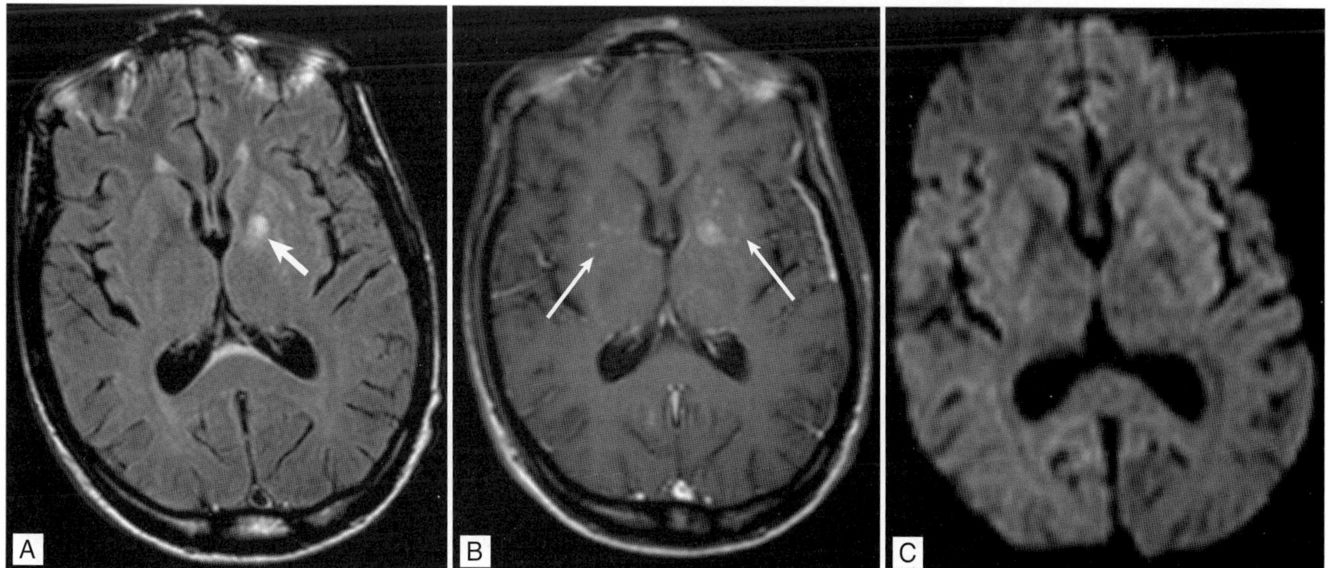

Figure 90.39 Axial FLAIR (A) imaging in a patient with cryptococcal meningitis demonstrating foci of signal hyperintensity within the basal ganglia (*thick white arrow*) with confirmed abnormal punctate enhancement bilaterally (*thin white arrows* in B). There was no associated abnormal restricted diffusion on the DWI sequence (C).

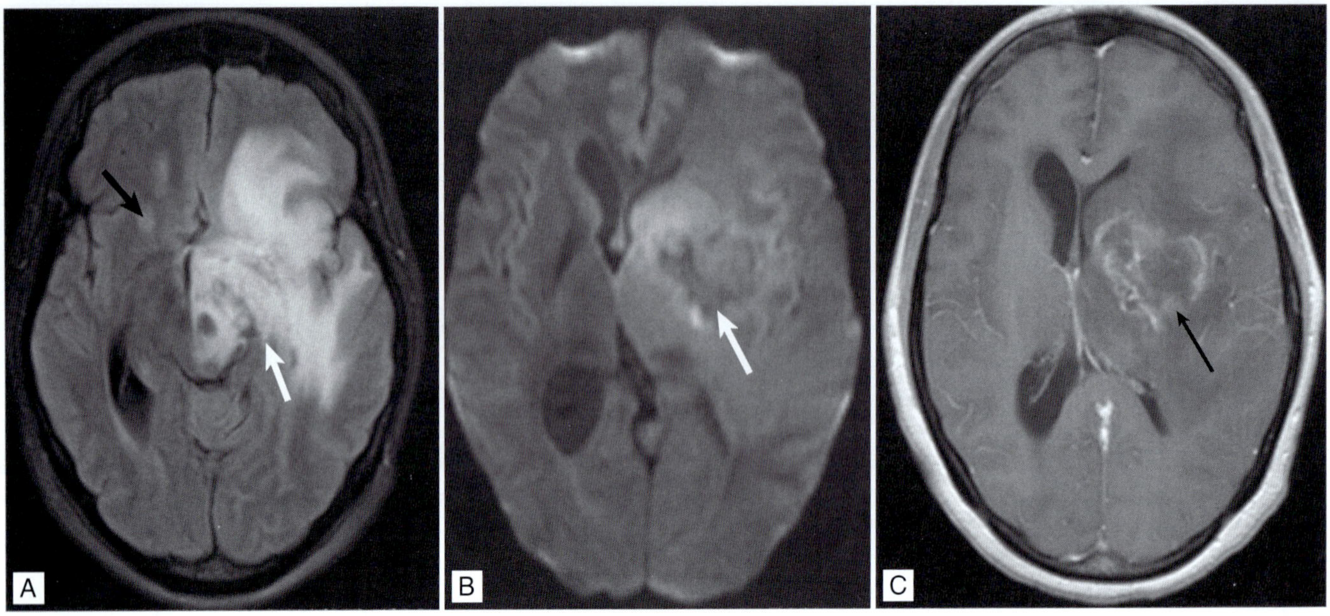

Figure 90.40 Axial FLAIR (A) sequence in a patient with new-onset right-sided weakness. There is an irregular lesion centered on the left basal ganglia with irregular peripheral enhancement and no significant internal restricted diffusion (*white arrows* in B (DWI) and C (postcontrast scan)). There is a small lesion in the right frontal lobe (*thin black arrow*) confirming multifocality. Initially suspected to represent a high-grade intra-axial neoplasm, the patient was confirmed to be immunocompromised and a stereotactic biopsy confirmed cerebral toxoplasmosis.

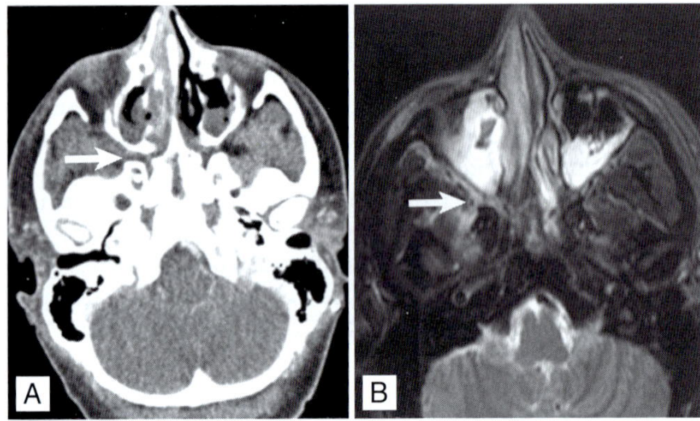

Figure 90.41 Axial CT head (A) in a patient with frontal headaches with a known hematological malignancy. There is mucosal thickening and inflammatory change within the paranasal sinuses but there is more concerning abnormal soft tissue and stranding within the right pterygopalatine fossa and retroantral soft tissues (*white arrow*) confirmed on the axial STIR sequence (B). The findings were compatible with an invasive fungal sinusitis that was confirmed following functional endoscopic sinus surgery.

external auditory canal is required to determine if there is an invasive fungal infection [61]. There is a risk of propagation to involve the posterior and central skull base with risk of potential vascular complications and intracranial extension (Fig. 90.42).

Neurocysticercosis caused by the parasitic pork tapeworm *Taenia solium* is endemic in certain parts of the world and is a common cause of seizures [62]. It can also present with headaches and depending on the pattern of CNS involvement can result in hydrocephalus. The imaging appearances of CNS involvement are dependent on the stage of the life cycle of the parasite.

- In the *vesicular stage* there is no host response and this appears as a small cyst and occasionally a scolex can be identified as an eccentric T1 hyperintense focus
- As the parasite dies this initiates a host response and this *colloid vesicular stage* is often the most symptomatic phase (Fig. 90.43). The cystic lesions demonstrate nodular or peripheral enhancement and the scolex can be increasingly difficult to identify. Given the immune response there is significant perilesional edema
- There is progression to the *granular nodular phase* where the cyst retracts and the edema improves
- the final *nodular calcified phase* is represented by calcified lesions with no significant surrounding edema

Mycobacterium tuberculosis remains a significant worldwide health problem associated with significant morbidity and mortality [63]. CNS infection with tuberculosis (Tb) typically has a nonspecific clinical presentation with fevers, weight loss, seizures, meningism, and focal deficits dependent upon the pattern of CNS involvement.

- Extra-axial involvement and Tb leptomeningitis can result in a florid basal meningitis that, given its location, can be complicated by hydrocephalus and arteritis affecting the basal perforator vessels that can result in areas of infarction (Fig. 90.44)
- A tuberculous pachymeningitis is a less common pattern of extra-axial involvement
- Intra-axial involvement is most commonly in the form of tuberculomas that differ from abscesses in the fact that the lesions are associated with a granulomatous inflammatory response and central caseous necrosis. On MR imaging, this is identified as lesions with central low T2 signal with no internal diffusion restriction and elevated lipid and lactate peaks on MR spectroscopy (Fig. 90.45)
- Tuberculous abscesses are rarer and typically occur in the immunocompromised. The MR signal characteristics are those of a typical abscess with an internal high T2 signal and diffusion restriction with a low T2 peripheral ring and surrounding edema
- Other patterns of CNS intra-axial involvement and cerebritis and tuberculous rhombencephalitis are less common

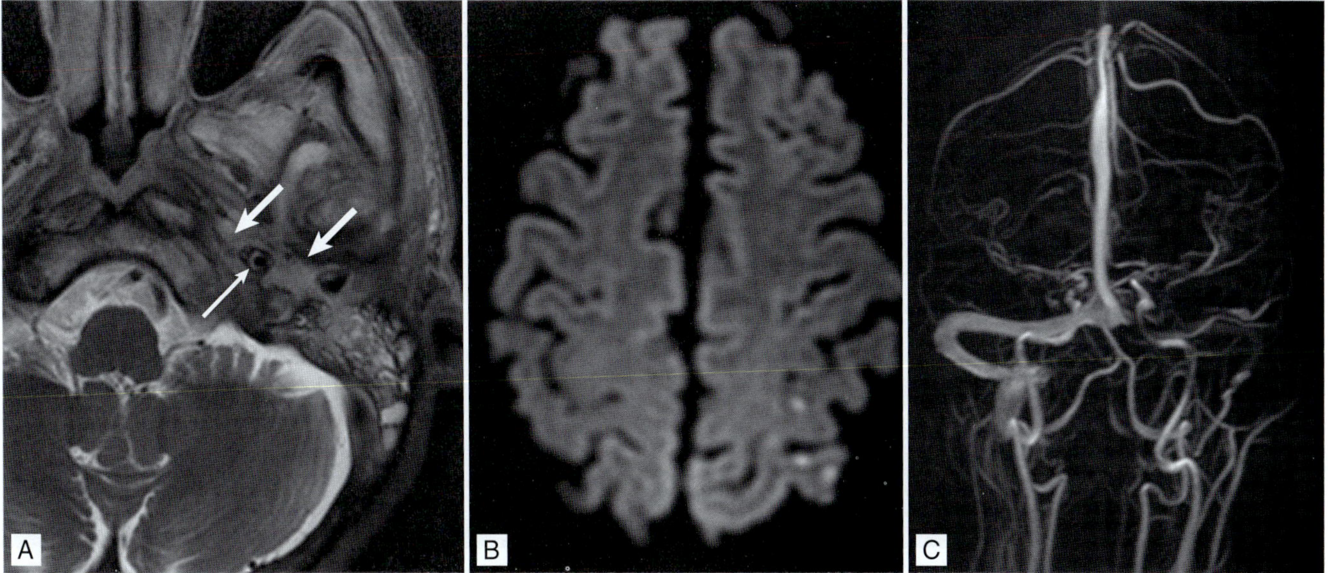

Figure 90.42 Axial T2 sequence (A) in a patient with a necrotizing otitis externa complicated by a skull base osteomyelitis with extension of inflammatory phlegmon to involve the upper deep neck spaces (*thick white arrows*) including the carotid space with an infectious arteritis (*thin white arrows*) that resulted in small embolic infarcts in the left MCA territory demonstrated on the DWI sequence (B). There was also a left-sided internal jugular vein thrombosis with loss of flow present on the MIP from the MR venogram (C).

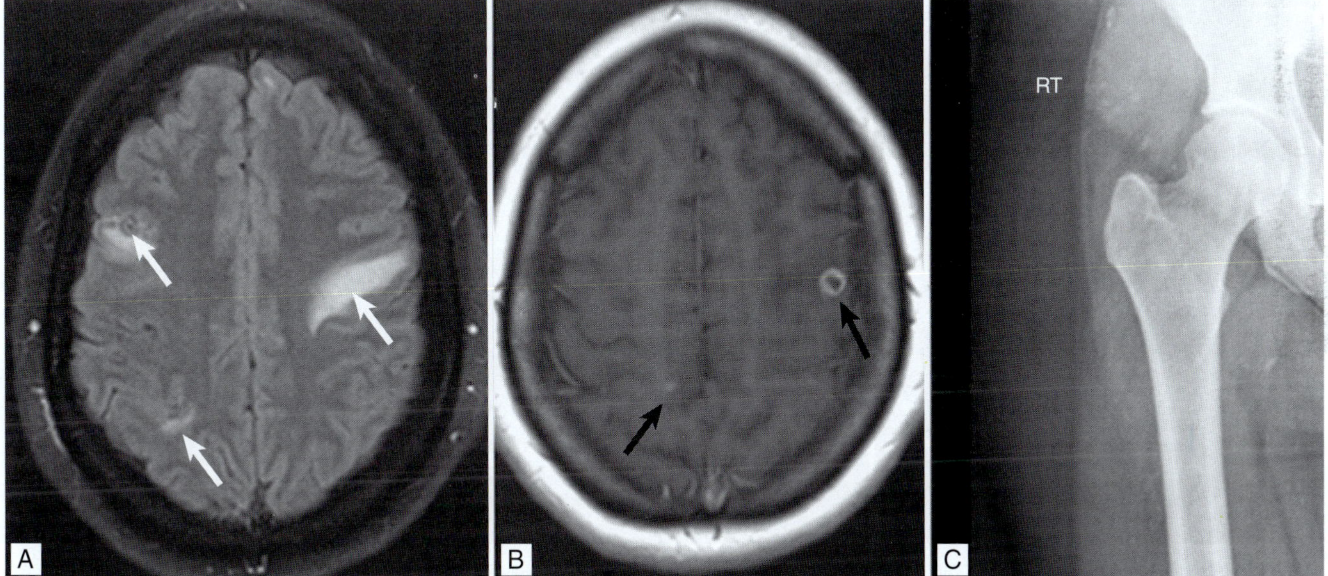

Figure 90.43 Axial FLAIR sequence (A) demonstrating multiple small lesions with surrounding edema (*white arrows*) and some of the lesions demonstrated a combination of punctate and ring enhancement (*black arrows* in B). There are soft tissue calcifications confirmed on the plain radiograph (C) in this patient with neurocysticercosis.

Neurological Emergencies in the Pregnant/Postpartum Patient

Acute neurological emergencies in pregnancy can result from exacerbations of pre-existing conditions as well as the development of a new neurological abnormality that is not unique to pregnancy [64]. This chapter will focus on those emergencies that are unique to or encountered with increasing frequency during pregnancy and in the postpartum period.

During pregnancy and the postpartum period there are a number of pathophysiological processes that can contribute to the spectrum of clinical presentations [65]. Elevated oestrogen levels result in the increased production of clotting factors and elevated risk of thromboembolic disease. Elevated progesterone levels are associated with increased venous distensibility and vascular leakage while elevated plasma and total blood volume can both contribute to elevated blood pressure.

Common symptoms and signs encountered in the pregnant patient include headache, visual symptoms, neurological deficits, and seizures with significant overlap in presentation between different neurological conditions discussed below.

In the emergency setting the imaging protocol typically includes a noncontrast CT head as first-line to assess for acute intracranial hemorrhage and parenchymal infarction and in the setting of seizure, to exclude a space occupying lesion. *A noncontrast CT head is*

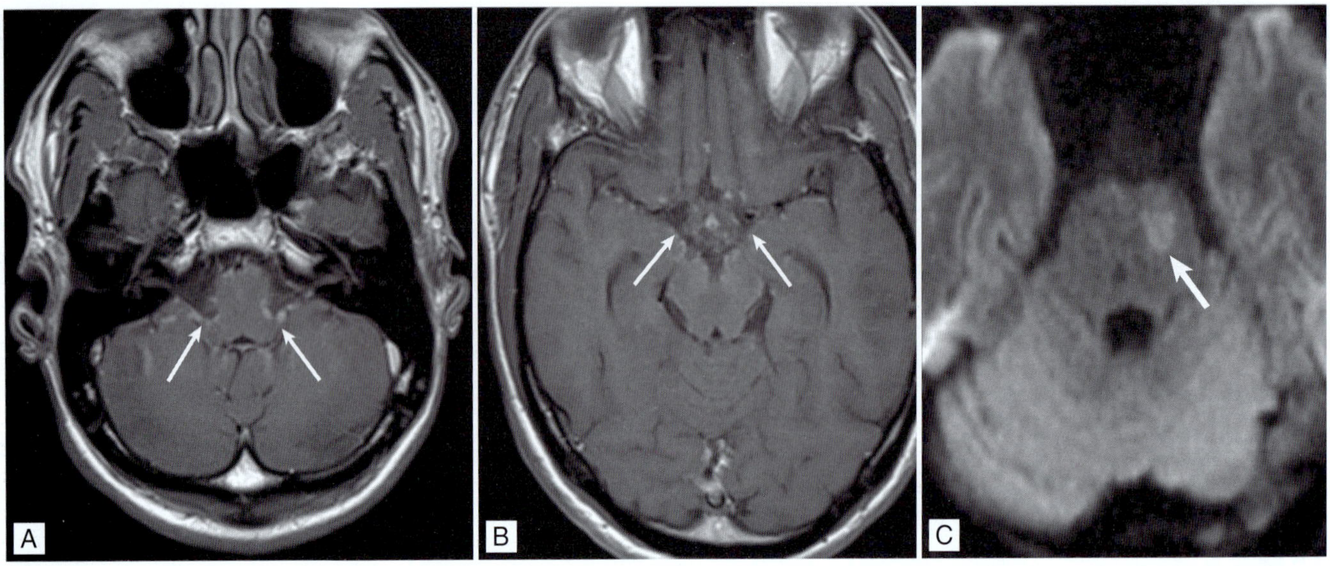

Figure 90.44 Axial T1 postcontrast imaging (A and B) in a patient with abnormal leptomeningeal enhancement and a confirmed basal meningitis due to Mycobacterium tuberculosis (*thin white arrows*). The patient had developed right sided symptoms due to a subacute left pontine infarct (*thick white arrow* in C).

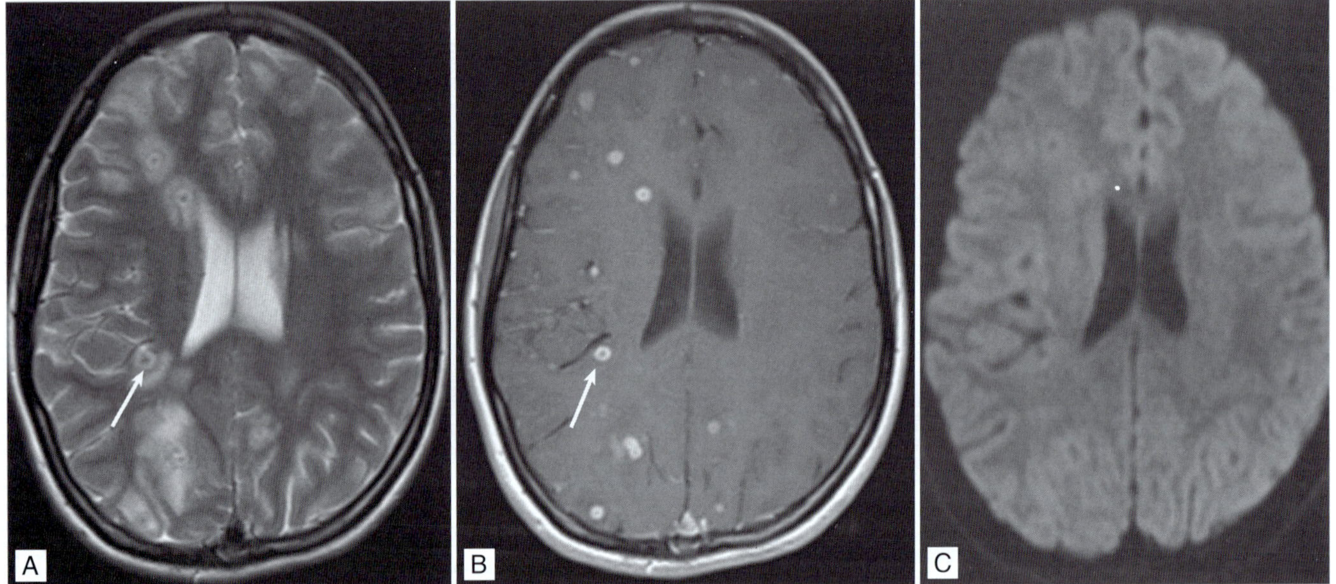

Figure 90.45 Axial T2 (A) and T1 postcontrast (B) imaging in a patient with multiple tuberculomata. The lesions demonstrate internal low T2 signal with surrounding high and low signal with peripheral enhancement (*thin white arrows*). The lesions do not demonstrate restricted diffusion (b1000 image from DWI sequence) (C).

a low dose procedure with minimal risk to foetus with benefits outweighing the risks in terms of excluding life-threatening diagnoses for the mother. In a proportion of patients with CVST, identification of hyperdense thrombus and complicating venous infarction or intracranial hemorrhage can establish the diagnosis on the initial noncontrast CT head. However, a normal CT head however does not exclude a number of clinical entities encountered during pregnancy and is supplemented by a CTA for suspected reversible cerebral vasoconstriction syndrome (RCVS) and aneurysmal SAH while CT venogram is performed if there is concern regarding a venous sinus thrombosis. If available, routine MRI brain with DWI supplemented by MR angiography, MR venography is preferable for exclusion of other entities such as PRES and hypertensive encephalopathy given its superior sensitivity.

Pre-eclampsia is graded on the basis of blood pressure and proteinuria progressing to eclampsia in the setting of a grand mal seizure [66]. In this setting, the presence of endothelial dysfunction, capillary leakage and vasogenic edema can result in PRES while vasoconstriction and the resultant elevated blood pressure can result in ischemia and cytotoxic edema that may progress to infarction.

RCVS encompasses a spectrum of disorders including call-Fleming syndrome [67]. The combination of oxidative stresses, endothelial dysfunction and increased sympathetic tone likely contribute to alterations in vascular tone and vasoconstriction thus RCVS may be the end point of a number of different pathological processes [68,69]. During pregnancy, the hormonal effect on the vasculature and alterations in BP, particularly during labor, can further increase in the risk of RCVS. There is a myriad of

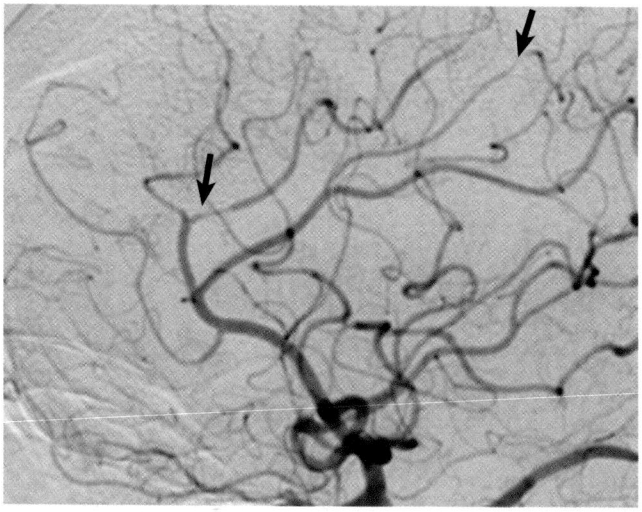

Figure 90.46 DSA lateral image from a right internal carotid artery injection in a patient with RCVS with focal areas of vascular irregularity and luminal narrowing (*black arrows*). Subsequent DSA imaging performed 3 months later was normal (not shown). *DSA*, digital subtraction angiogram.

potential triggers including vasoactive drugs, blood products, certain tumor types, and in the postpartum period [67]. Most commonly, the patient experiences a sudden onset thunderclap headache and other presentations include focal deficits/transient ischemic attacks, encephalopathy and seizures. It is typically a monophasic illness with no new symptoms after 4 weeks. The presence of nonaneurysmal, focal convexity SAH occurs earlier in the process with ischemia/infarction typically occurring as a later complication. On imaging, the noncontrast CT head can be normal but as stated, careful assessment for the presence of sulcal convexity SAH should be sought. CT or catheter angiographic imaging demonstrates the presence of segmental arterial vasoconstriction with identical appearances to vasospasm and primary angiitis that represent the main imaging differential diagnoses [69] (Fig. 90.46).

PRES is also considered in the spectrum of disorders associated with abnormalities of vascular tone and endothelial dysfunction. The clinical presentation is with similar symptomatology including headache, visual symptoms, encephalopathy, and seizures. Cerebral edema develops with involvement of the cortical and subcortical white matter with a predilection for the parietal and occipital lobes [70]. It can progress to ischemia and infarction and can be complicated by intracranial hemorrhage although in the majority of cases the vasogenic edema is reversible (Fig. 90.47).

CVST occurs with increased frequency in pregnancy and during the postpartum period as a consequence of the pathophysiological mechanisms outlined above. It is a potential cause of stroke in pregnancy that may also occur in the setting of other conditions including HELPP syndrome, thrombotic thrombocytopenic purpura. The association with vascular dissection in pregnancy is yet to be fully elucidated. *Other rarer entities to consider in patients with new focal neurological deficits include amniotic fluid embolism, air embolism and metastases secondary to a choriocarcinoma* [64].

In the postpartum period, the presence of nuchal/occipital/postural headaches that resolve on lying flat (worse on standing) raises the possibility of a *CSF leak* and *potential CSF hypotension*. The presence of a CSF leak can occur in the setting of spinal anaesthesia (typically 1–7 days postinstrumentation) but it can also occur spontaneously. Intracranial hypotension can be further complicated by the presence of SDH and CVST. The aim of imaging is to confirm the diagnosis, exclude complications and localize potential source of leak with the aim of guiding subsequent blood patch [22].

Visual symptoms in pregnancy may occur in the setting of PRES or ischemic stroke while during early pregnancy, hyperemesis gravidarum can result in thiamine deficiency and Wernicke's encephalopathy that may present with diplopia and eye movement disorders. The pituitary gland typically enlarges during pregnancy but pituitary apoplexy is rare. Bleeding or impaired blood supply can result in pituitary apoplexy while Sheehan's syndrome can result in hypopituitarism weeks/months after the postpartum bleed.

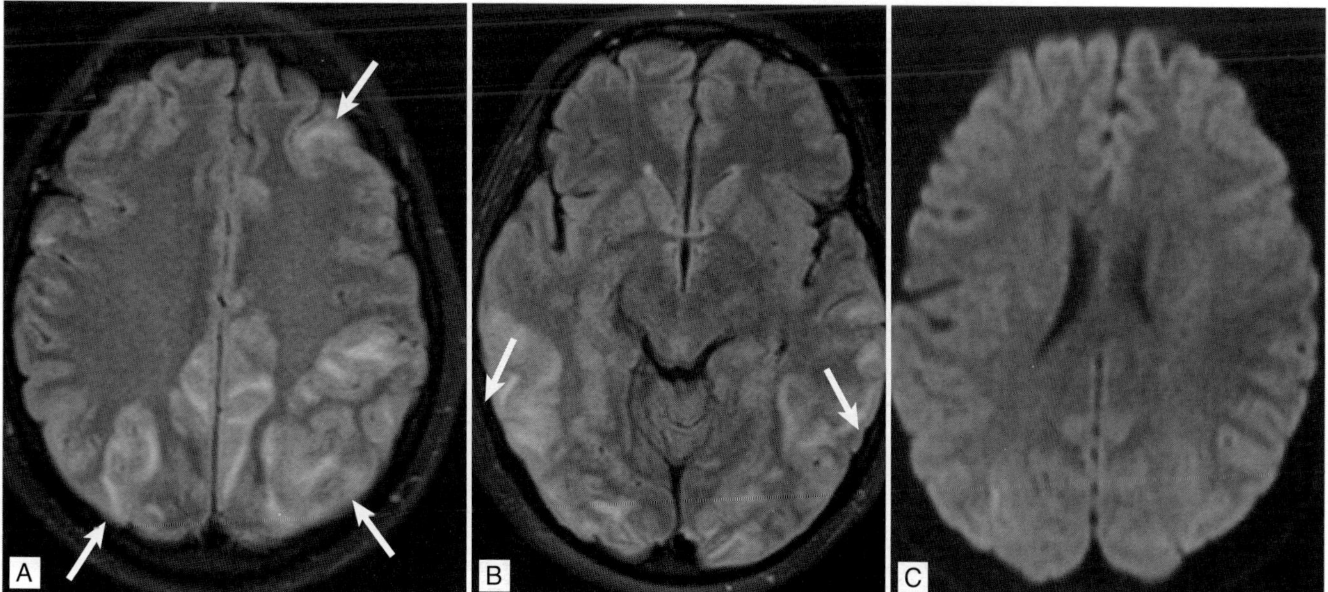

Figure 90.47 Axial FLAIR images (A and B) in a patient with hypertensive crisis and visual symptoms. There is abnormal cortical/subcortical signal change with a predilection for the parieto-occipital regions but with additional frontal and temporal lobe involvement (*white arrows*). This was due to PRES and there was no complicating infarction on the DWI sequence (C) (b1000 imaging shown).

Acute Onset Cranial Nerve Deficit(s)

In a patient presenting with an acute onset of cranial nerve palsy/palsies, the imaging protocol is guided by the pattern of cranial nerve involvement and suspicion of lesion localization. This requires the radiologist to have an understanding of the anatomy of the cranial nerves from nucleus to target organ (with the exception of the olfactory and optic nerves that have unique anatomy and do not have a CNS nucleus).

- Cranial nerves have an intra-axial component localized to the brainstem with respect to cranial nerves III-XII and supratentorial brain parenchymal component with cranial nerves I and II
- The intracranial but extra-axial component of the cranial nerves refers to their course from the CNS to the skull base neural foramina
- The extra-axial and extracranial course of the nerves relate to their pathway through the extracranial soft tissues and target end organs

While some of the cranial nerves have a purely motor (cranial nerves IV, VI, XI, XII) or sensory function (cranial nerves I, II, VIII), the rest of the cranial nerves have a combination of motor, sensory, and autonomic function.

Imaging in the acute setting typically involves a contrast-enhanced CT that does provide excellent bony detail of the skull base and neural foramina in addition to intracranial and extracranial soft tissue information that enables significant pathologies in the context of trauma and sepsis to be identified. However, in most clinical settings this will be followed by MR imaging and tailoring of the MR protocol is essential to depict the anatomical course of the cranial nerves and to highlight potential pathology. The use of T2 weighted imaging of the brain parenchyma enables identification of significant intra-axial pathology that is combined with DWI to assess for areas of potential infarction or inflammatory change. Imaging of the extra-axial and intracranial cisternal course of the cranial nerves can also be assessed on T2 weighted imaging that is best performed with a combination of axial and coronal sequences if a volumetric 3D imaging cannot be acquired. This is augmented by contrast-enhanced T1 weighted sequences and *pathological cranial nerve enhancement can sometimes be the only radiological abnormality identified* (Fig. 90.48). High resolution heavily T2 weighted sequences that accentuate the contrast between CSF and the cranial nerves (e.g., CISS, balanced FFE sequences, DRIVE, 3D-TSE) sequences aid assessment of small cranial nerve lesions and potential neurovascular conflicts. The extracranial course of the cranial nerves to be assessed should cover the soft tissues along the path of the nerve and target end organs. This is performed with axial T1, T2, and contrast-enhanced imaging and in our institution the T1 precontrast imaging is performed without contrast to assess the fat planes around the skull base and neural foramina and the marrow signal within the skull base itself. However other protocols that include DIXON sequences can provide both fat-suppressed and nonfat suppressed T1 weighted imaging [71].

In the presence of a single unilateral cranial nerve palsy imaging is targeted at the cranial nerve in question however in the presence of multiple cranial nerve palsies the pattern can guide and limit the differential diagnosis. With unilateral multiple cranial nerve palsies, there are specific sites where multiple cranial nerve palsies can be affected (Table 90.4) (Fig. 90.49). In the presence of multiple and bilateral cranial nerve palsies, this typically implies a more widespread systemic disorder and thus consideration of infectious, granulomatous, and neoplastic pathologies that will typically affect either the brainstem or cisternal courses of the nerves (Fig. 90.50).

TABLE 90.4 Multiple Cranial Nerve Neuropathies

1. Orbital apex/cavernous sinus syndromes Cranial nerves II, III, IV, Vi, VI may be affected Typically, inflammatory Tolosa-Hunt, IgG4 mediated diseases
2. Petrous apex/cavernous sinus syndrome Cranial nerves III, IV, Vi, VI may be affected Infective process propagating to petrous apex—Gradenigos syndrome
3. Jugular foramen syndromes Vernet syndrome affecting cranial nerves IX, X, XI Collet Sicard syndrome IX, X, XI, XII Skull base infections (central skull base osteomyelitis) or tumors including glomus lesions and nerve sheath tumors as well as posterior fossa meningiomas

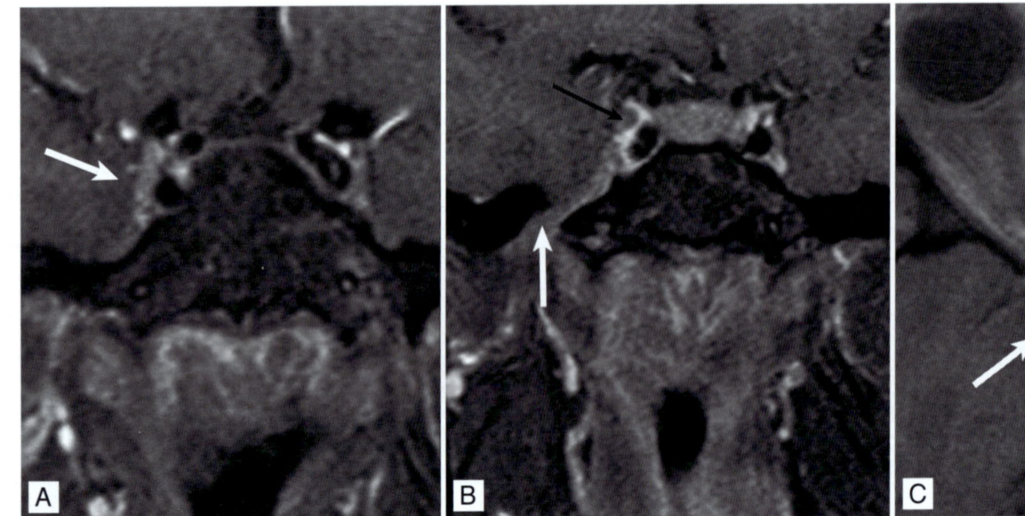

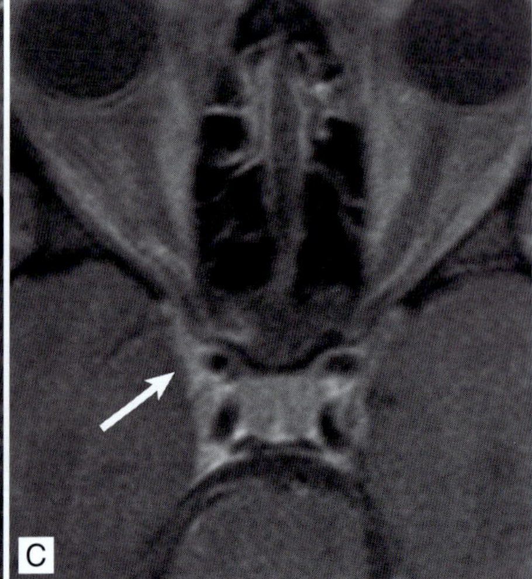

Figure 90.48 Coronal (A and B) and axial T1 (C) postcontrast imaging in a patient with right-sided retro-orbital pain with asymmetrical right cavernous sinus with asymmetrical thickening of the right oculomotor nerve (*thin black arrow*) and mandibular division of the right trigeminal nerve (*thick white arrow*). This was considered to represent a right-sided Tolosa Hunt syndrome and the patient responded to corticosteroid therapy with resolution of the abnormal imaging findings.

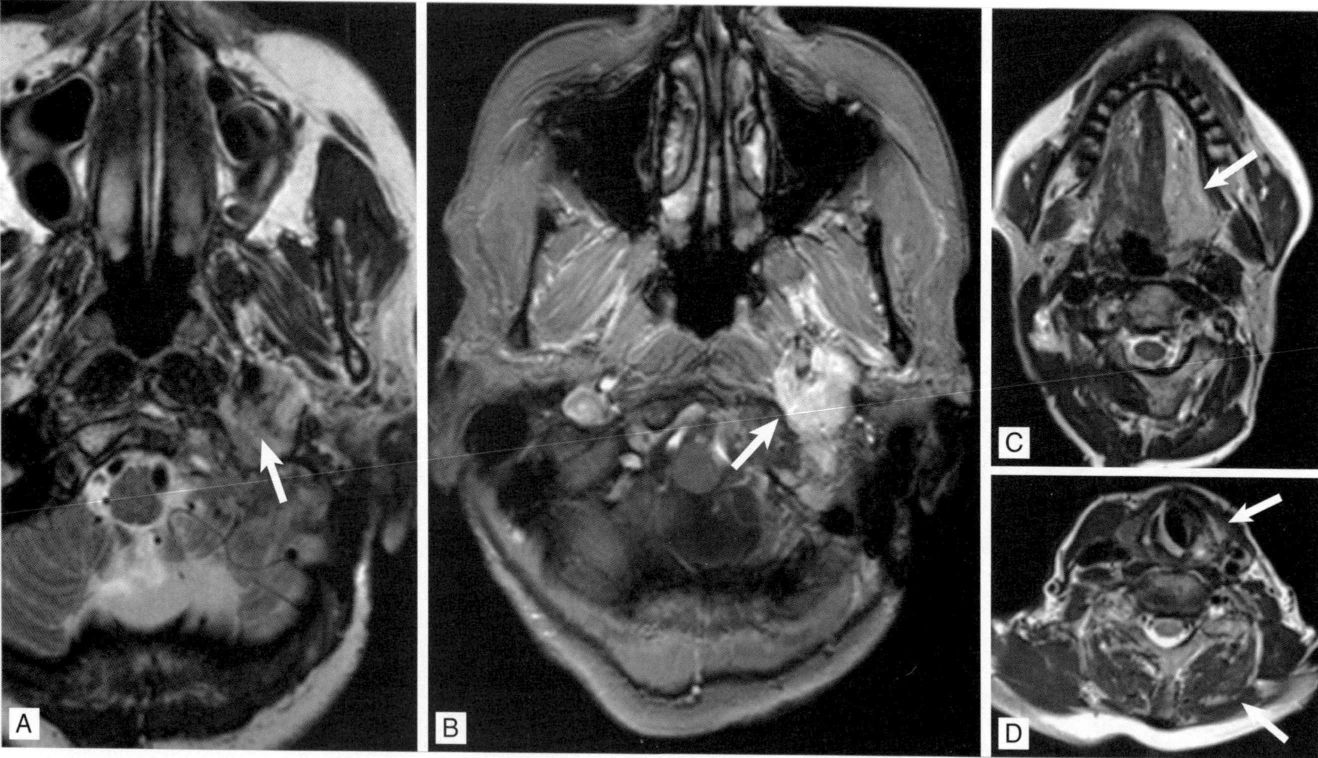

Figure 90.49 Axial T2 (A) and T1 postcontrast (B) imaging in this patient with a left jugular foramen syndrome secondary to a left-sided glomus jugulare tumor (*white arrows*). The soft tissue axial T2 sequences (C and D) confirmed the presence of a left-sided hypoglossal nerve palsy and tongue denervation and left accessory nerve palsy with sternocleidomastoid and trapezius muscle atrophy (*thick white arrows*). Additional left-sided vocal cord palsy and atrophy of the stylopharyngeus muscle secondary to vagus and glossopharyngeal nerve palsies respectively.

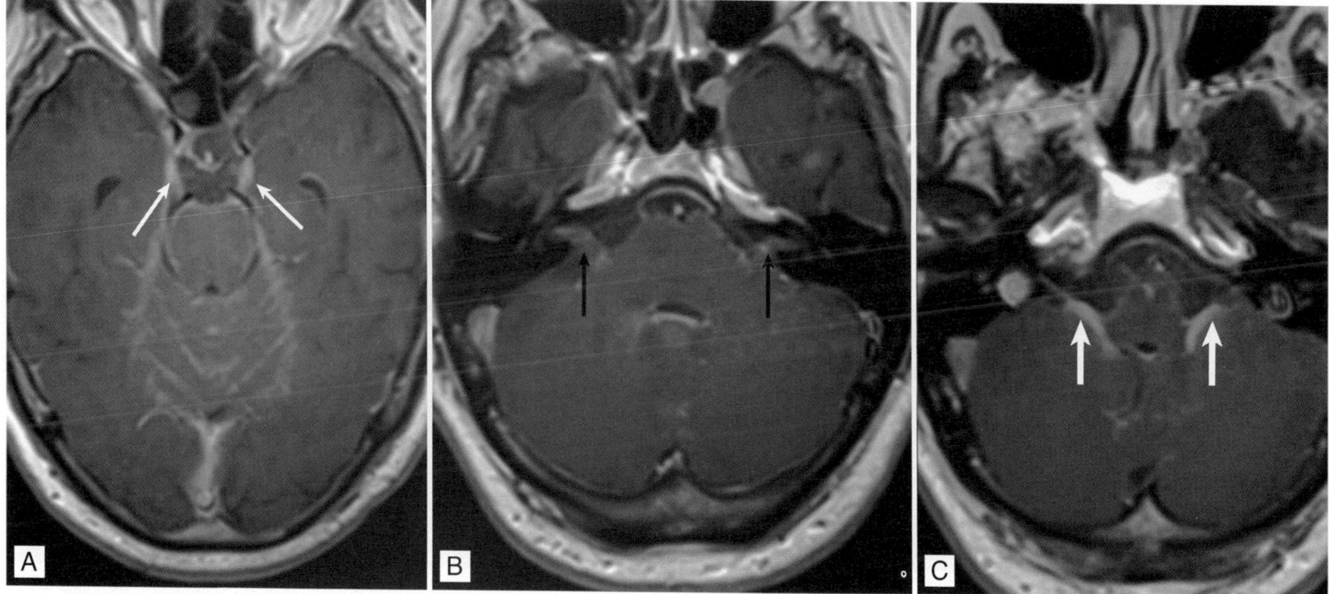

Figure 90.50 Axial T1 postcontrast imaging in a patient with carcinomatous meningitis with abnormal leptomeningeal enhancement that is well depicted in relation to the cerebellar folia. Symmetrical and bilateral abnormal cranial nerve enhancement is evident in relation to the oculomotor nerves (*thin white arrows* in A), facial/vestibulocochlear nerves (*thin black arrows* in B) and glossopharyngeal/vagal nerve complexes (*thick white arrows* in C).

Intra-axial pathologies that can present with acute cranial nerve palsies include acute stroke, infective, inflammatory, toxic, and neoplastic aetiologies [72]. Brainstem infarction results from thromboembolic disease affecting the basilar artery or its perforator branch vessels. With regards the extracranial course of the lower cranial nerves:

- The presence of an arterial dissection should be considered in any patient with an acute onset Horner's syndrome given the relationship of the sympathetic plexus to the internal carotid artery [3] (Fig. 90.51)
- In addition, an acute internal carotid artery dissection can result in an acute unilateral hypoglossal nerve palsy as the

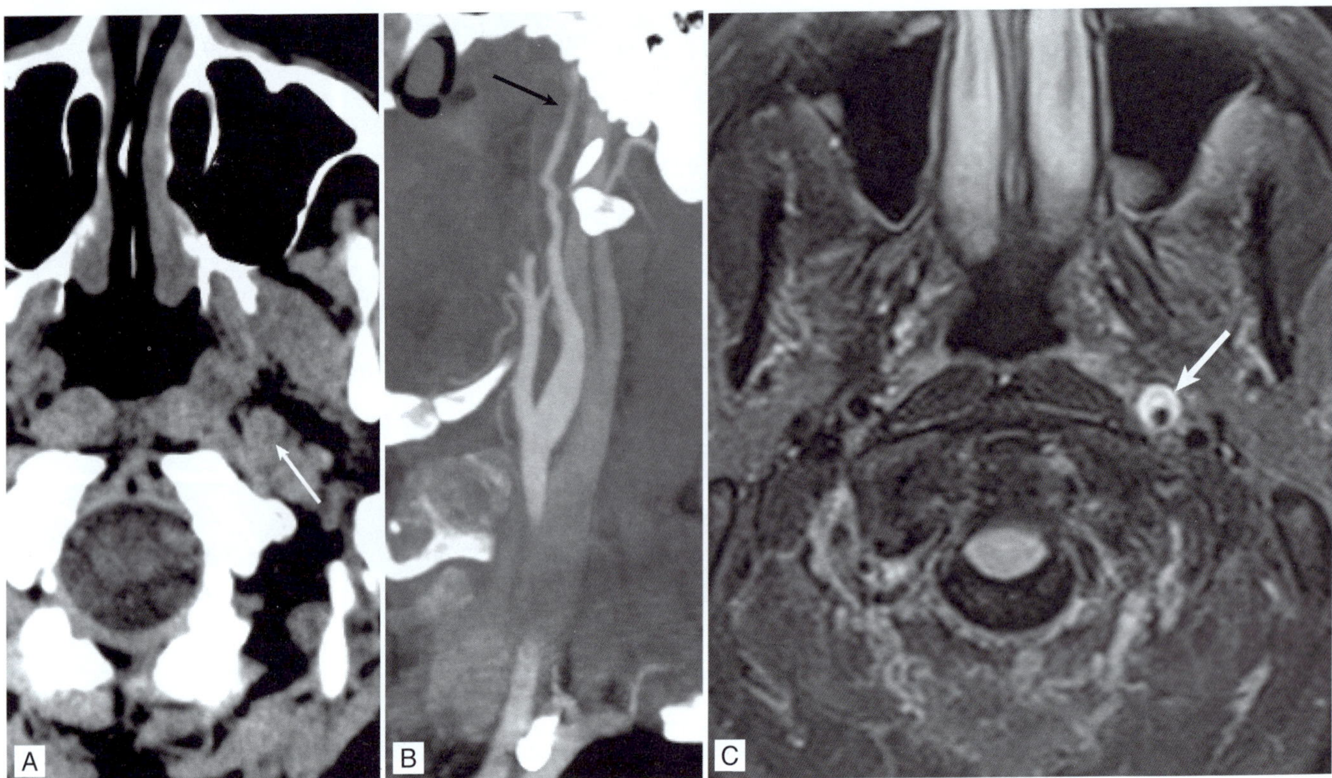

Figure 90.51 Axial CT head (A) in a patient with a left sided Horner's syndrome with an asymmetrical left internal carotid artery (*thin white arrow*). There is a confirmed left internal carotid artery dissection with luminal irregularity and tapering on the CTA (*thin black arrow* in B) with intramural hematoma evident on the axial FLAIR sequence (*thick white arrow* in C).

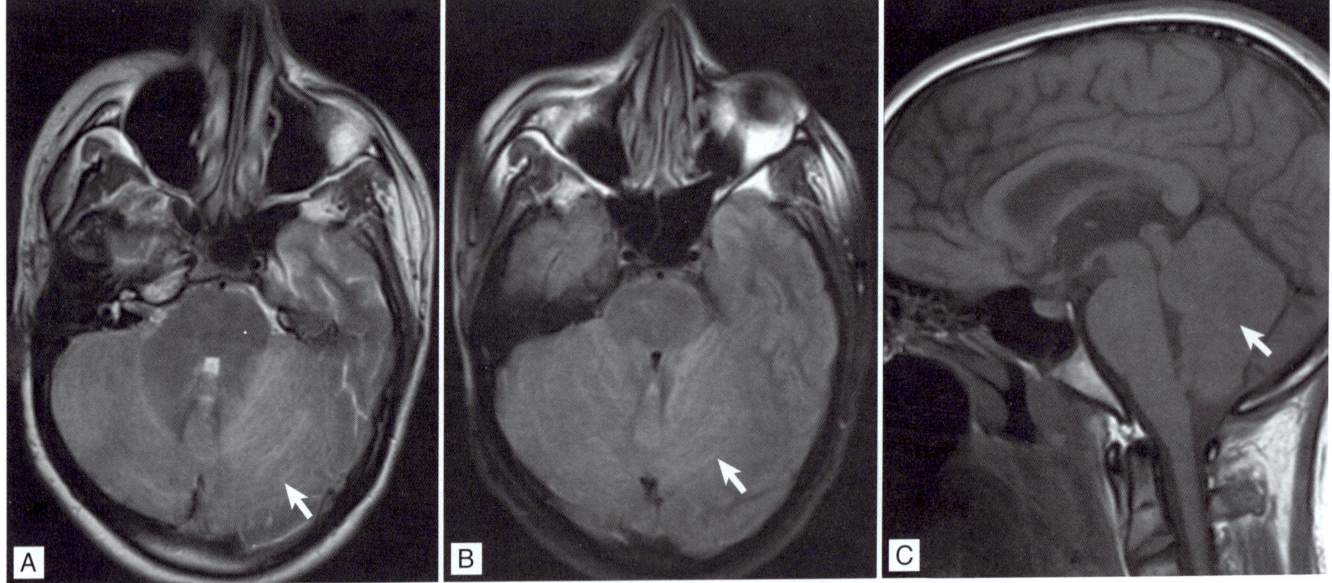

Figure 90.52 Axial T2 (A), FLAIR (B), and Sagittal T1 (C) sequences demonstrating abnormal hyperintense signal and swelling centered on the cerebellum (*white arrows*) secondary to a viral rhombencephalitis (adenovirus). There is distortion of the fourth ventricle with complicating hydrocephalus.

extracranial course of the XII nerve is intimately related to the carotid sheath and potential disruption of its vascular supply via the vasa vasorum can result in cranial nerve palsy [73]

- Another specific scenario to consider is the acute onset of an oculomotor nerve palsy particularly if there is involvement of the preganglionic parasympathetic fibers that are present along the superomedial surface of the nerve. This implies potential extrinsic compression on the pathway of the CN III and it is imperative that angiographic imaging is preformed to exclude an internal carotid artery or posterior communicating artery aneurysm [72]

An acute rhombencephalitis may be infectious in nature and typical organisms to consider include *Listeria monocytogenes* and viral entities (West Nile virus, Japanese encephalitis) [74]. These typically present with abnormal T2 signal change, potential mass effect/swelling and enhancement that may be parenchymal and/or leptomeningeal with potential DWI changes (Fig. 90.52). The differential for an infectious brainstem encephalitis would include

TABLE 90.5 Differential Diagnosis of Rhomboencephalitis

1. Infectious Viral [Enteroviruses, Herpes simplex virus (HSV-1, HSV-2), flaviviruses (West Nile virus, Japanese encephalitic virus) Bacterial (*Listeria monocytogenes, Mycobacterium tuberculosis*)
2. Inflammatory/autoimmune Neurobehcet's disease Systemic lupus erythematosus Multiple sclerosis, NMO spectrum disorders
3. Neoplastic/paraneoplastic Lymphoma High grade glioma Paraneoplastic syndromes (small cell lung cancer)

inflammatory aetiologies including neuro-behcets syndrome which is a multisystem, vascular inflammatory disorder [75] (Table 90.5). This is characterized by orogenital ulceration, uveitis, and skin lesions and typically sites of parenchymal involvement in the CNS include pons, midbrain and diencephalon with a higher risk of venous thrombosis (Fig. 90.53). Other acute brainstem inflammatory processes to consider include multiple sclerosis, neuromyelitis optica (NMO) spectrum disorders (assessment of anti-aquaporin 4 and anti-MOG antibodies). NMO in particular has a predilection for the area postrema and periaqueductal gray. Imaging of the entire neuraxis including brain, orbits and spinal cord can be undertaken to aid diagnosis. Osmotic myelinolysis or central pontine myelinolysis can occur as a result of rapid overcorrection of hyponatremia but it can also result from other insults [76]. While it typically affects the pons other extrapontine sites of involvement are also recognised [40].

Neoplastic infiltration of the brainstem typically presents with a more insidious onset of cranial nerve palsies however with more aggressive infiltrating tumors this progression can be more rapid. As per other aetiologies, this typically demonstrates abnormal T2 signal change with potential DWI changes and abnormal enhancement. With the associated mass effect this has the potential to obstruct the aqueduct of Sylvius and result in an obstructive hydrocephalus.

Cranial nerve involvement of the extra-axial course of the cranial nerves can result from a spectrum of infectious, inflammatory and neoplastic aetiologies.

- Specific infectious aetiologies to consider in the setting of a facial nerve palsy include Bell's palsy that is typically related to Herpes simplex virus
- Ramsay Hunt syndrome results from varicella zoster virus infection and results in sensorineural hearing and external ear vesicles in addition to the facial nerve palsy

Imaging is typically reserved for atypical cases of a facial nerve palsy where the suspected, viral neuritis fails to resolve or in the acute setting where the facial nerve palsy may result from an alternate infectious process. This latter is the case in diabetic and immunocompromised patients where the facial nerve palsy is involved from the direct spread of infection from a necrotizing otitis externa typically due to Pseudomonal infection [61]. As the infection can propagate into the posterior skull base other cranial nerve palsies may ensue including additional arterial and venous complications. In a persistent lower motor neuron palsy, the course of the facial nerve pathway from the pons to the muscles of facial expression including the parotid space is needed to exclude neoplastic processes such as a nerve sheath tumor or perineural spread of disease [77].

As stated in the setting of multiple bilateral cranial nerve palsies, the presence of abnormal leptomeningeal enhancement and cranial nerve enhancement should be sought. This would include infectious processes such as bacterial and tuberculous meningitis, vasculidites including ANCA mediated granulomatous polyangiitis, granulomatous processes such as sarcoidosis and carcinomatous meningitis and lymphoma. These can be difficult to distinguish on the basis of neuroimaging alone and requires correlation with other imaging modalities/body systems and CSF analysis.

Acute Spinal Cord Syndrome

In patients with an acute spinal cord syndrome, the suspected localization of the abnormality and targeted imaging is guided by the relevant motor, sensory and autonomic symptoms and signs. The technique of choice is MR imaging with a combination of sagittal T1, T2, STIR sequences with additional axial T1 and T2

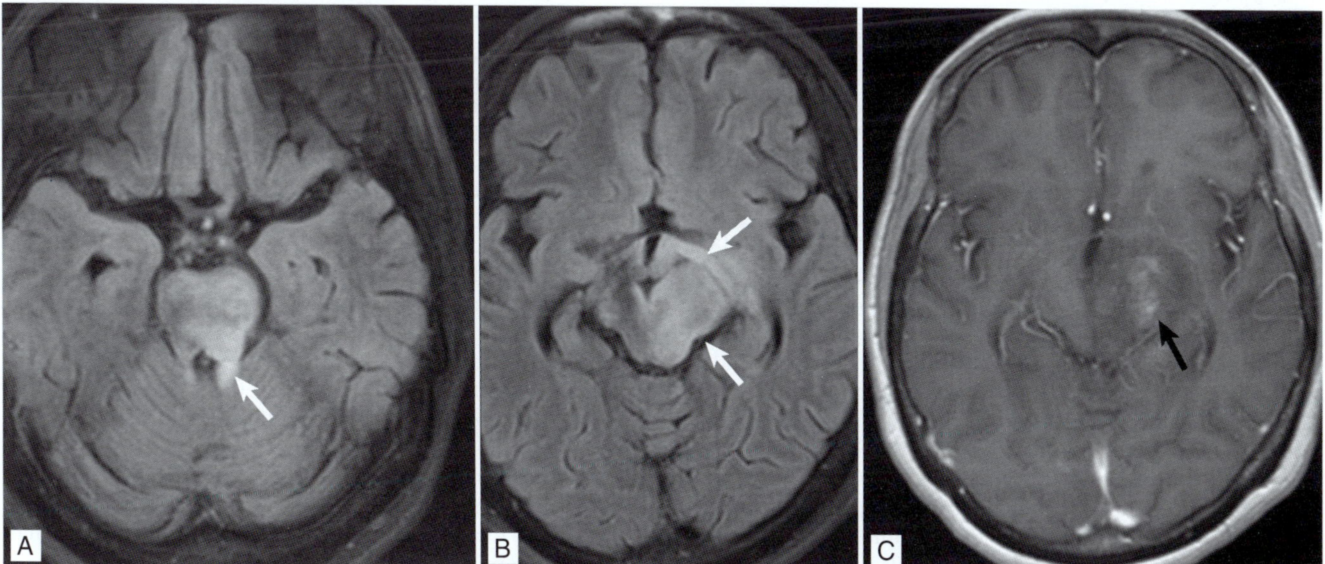

Figure 90.53 Axial FLAIR sequence (A and B) in a patient with neurobehcets syndrome with abnormal signal change within the brainstem extending into the superior cerebellar peduncle and into the left optic tract (*white arrows*). There is superior extension into the diencephalon with pathological enhancement (*black arrow* in C).

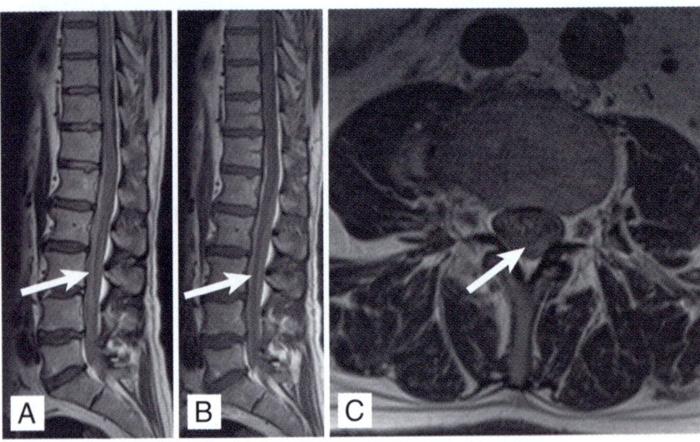

Figure 90.54 Sagittal T2 (A) and T1 (B) weighted sequences demonstrating extensive subarachnoid hemorrhage within the spinal canal (*white arrows*) confirmed on the axial imaging (C). The patient was on anticoagulant therapy.

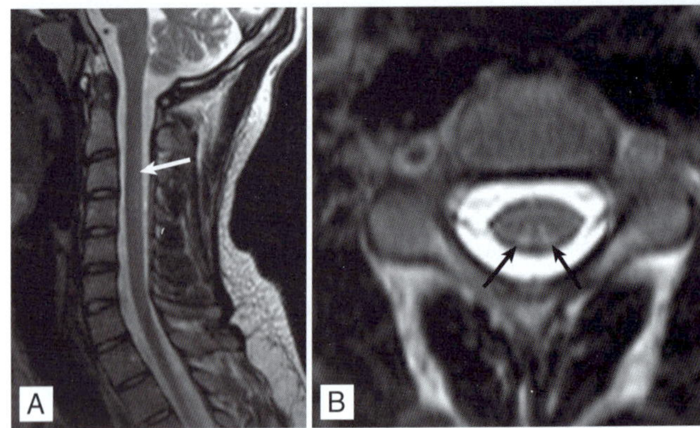

Figure 90.55 Sagittal T2 weighted sequence (A) in a 19-year-old patient who used recreational "popper"/nitrous oxide with the suspicion of cord signal change within the dorsal aspect of the cord (*thin white arrow*) that was confirmed on the axial T2 weighted imaging (B) (*thin black arrows*).

weighted sequences acquired in the areas of anatomical interest. Contrast-enhanced imaging is performed in the setting of suspected sepsis, inflammation, or neoplastic disease while high-resolution CISS sequences are utilized in specific scenarios including assessment of spinal cord herniation, CSF leaks and potential spinal vascular malformations and arteriovenous fistulae [78,79]. Acute spinal cord syndromes can be broadly subdivided into a complete cord and incomplete cord syndromes.

- In a *complete cord syndrome*, a whole cord segment is affected with resultant motor, sensory and autonomic signs below the level of the lesion. This can be secondary to trauma with transection of the cord, an extensive transverse myelitis or due to compression of the cord secondary to neoplastic infective processes and other rarer entities such as spontaneous intraspinal hemorrhage [80] (Fig. 90.54)
- *Incomplete cord syndromes* present with specific patterns of motor, sensory, and autonomic features depending on which part of the spinal cord is affected [81]. These patterns include dorsal cord syndromes, ventral cord syndromes, central cord syndromes, brown sequard syndrome, conus medullaris compression, and cauda equina compression

Dorsal cord syndromes present with disturbances of fine touch, proprioception and vibration sense with sensory ataxia, gait disturbances, and falls. With the increasing size of the lesion, this can extend to involve the autonomic pathways and corticospinal tracts. The differential diagnosis for abnormal signal change within the dorsal columns includes causes of subacute combined degeneration of the cord (SACD) including vitamin B12 deficiency, inflammatory (multiple sclerosis), infectious (tabes dorsalis, AIDS myelopathy), neurodegenerative processes (Freidreich's ataxia) while extrinsic compression and posterior cord infarcts are less common [82]. In the authors' institution, the incidence of SACD has increased secondary to abuse of nitrous oxide present in "poppers" that results in impairment of vitamin B12 metabolism [83] (Fig. 90.55).

A *ventral cord syndrome* presents with motor deficits secondary to disruption of the corticospinal tracts, autonomic disturbances, sensory disturbances secondary to disruption of the spinothalamic tracts. An insult to a hemicord will result in ipsilateral motor signs below the level of the cord while it will result in contralateral impairment of sensory symptoms (relating to pain and temperature sensation). The disruption of the spinothalamic tracts occurs a few segments below the level of the insult as the fibers ascend the cord before they decussate to the contralateral aspect of the cord before ascending to the thalamus. *Acute ischemia and infarction (typically arterial in origin) is the most common cause for a ventral cord syndrome but it can also occur secondary to trauma or disc degeneration* [84] (Fig. 90.56).

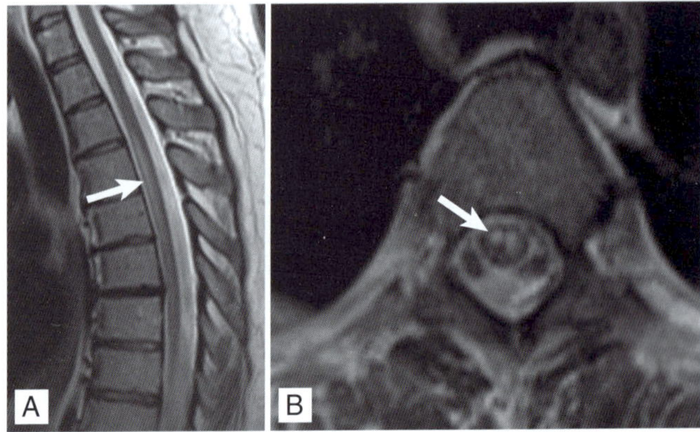

Figure 90.56 Sagittal T2 imaging (A) in a patient with a suspected spinal cord infarct that confirms abnormal signal change within the ventral aspect of the thoracic cord confirmed on the axial T2 sequence (*white arrows* in B).

A *central cord syndrome* initially results in a sensory disturbances in a cape distribution given decussating spinothalamic tracts in the ventral commissure. Given the somatotopic organization of the cord, this typically involves the upper extremities before the lower extremities. Lower motor neurons signs occur at the level of the insult with upper motor neuron signs present below the affected cord segment. This can occur secondary to injuries and lesions around the central canal. In elderly patients with existing degenerative changes, this can be secondary to hyperextension injuries while in younger patients, it typically occurs secondary to hyperflexion injuries. Syringohydromyelia can be primary/congenital in nature (e.g., basilar invagination, Arnold-Chiari malformations) or secondary to trauma and neoplastic processes. The most common neoplastic disorder to consider include ependymoma, astrocytoma, hemangioblastomas and metastases [85] (Fig. 90.57).

Brown sequard syndrome results from an insult to the hemicord that produces ipsilateral corticospinal and dorsal column deficits with contralateral spinothalamic tract disturbances [86]. It typically occurs secondary to blunt or penetrating trauma but can also be secondary to inflammatory processes, spinal cord herniation or disc herniation [78].

Conus medullaris compression and *cauda equina compression* have similar presentations, however, the compression of the conus medullaris also results in upper and lower motor neuron

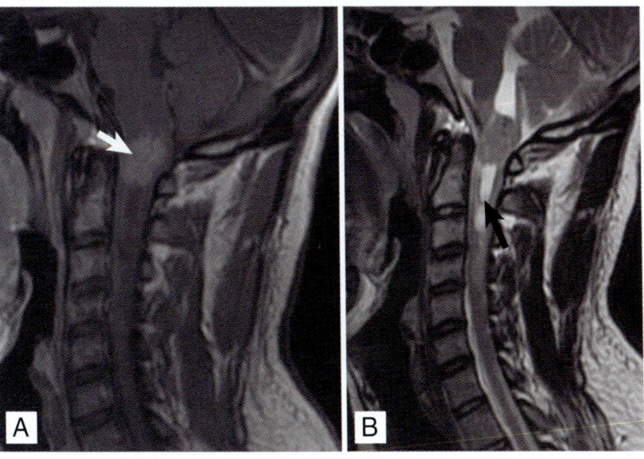

Figure 90.57 Sagittal T1 postcontrast (A) and T2 (B) imaging showed an enhancing intra-axial spinal cord tumor and confirmed astrocytoma at the cervicomedullary junction (*white arrow* in A) with a complicating cord syrinx (*black arrow* in B).

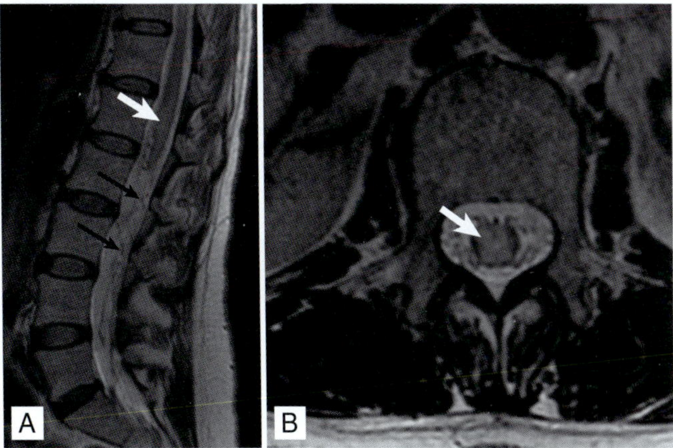

Figure 90.59 Sagittal T2 weighted imaging (A) demonstrating multiple serpiginous flow voids (*thin black arrows*) compatible with a spinal arteriovenous fistula complicated by edema within the distal cord and conus confirmed on the axial imaging (*white arrows* in B).

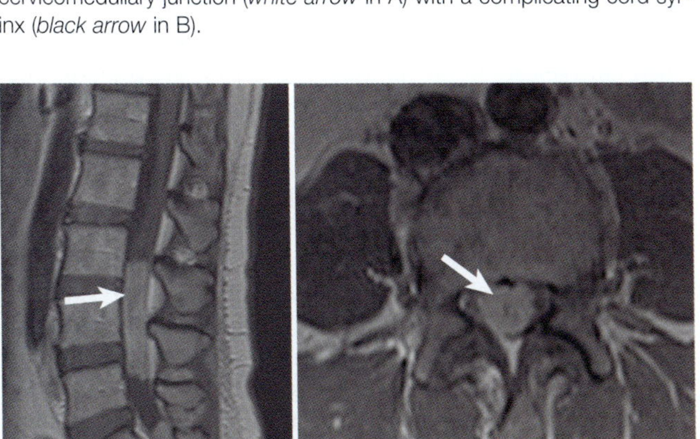

Figure 90.58 Sagittal (A) and axial (B) T1 postcontrast images demonstrating an enhancing intradural lesion affecting the cauda equina with a more inferior component within the inferior aspect of the thecal sac. The tumor was surgically resected and confirmed to represent a myxopapillary ependymoma.

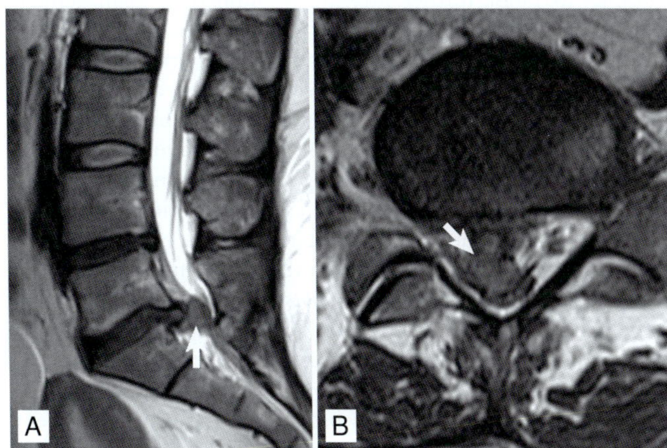

Figure 90.60 Sagittal (A) and axial (B) T2 weighted sequences in a patient with cauda equina syndrome secondary to a large L5/S1 disc extrusion (*white arrows*) that was compressing the thecal sac.

signs. The conus medullaris can be affected by disc herniations, trauma, tumors (e.g., myxopapillary ependymoma), infection, and vascular malformations (spinal dural AVM type I) (Fig. 90.58). The identification of a potential dural arteriovenous fistula is or paramount importance given the potential for curative endovascular or surgical intervention with a progressive course if left untreated that may result in irreversible damage to the spinal cord [87] (Fig. 90.59). Cauda equina syndrome results in a combination of lower motor neuron deficits, bladder and bowel disturbances and saddle anaesthesia. This is a neurosurgical emergency and commonly occurs secondary to disc herniation (Fig. 90.60) although it may also be secondary to trauma, neoplastic processes (leptomeningeal disease), arachnoiditis (type I–III) and Guillain–Barre syndrome.

Summary

In this chapter, we have provided a general overview of the most common acute neurological emergencies encountered in clinical practice by general radiologists and neuroradiologists. Relevant imaging algorithms have been provided for when these situations arise in clinical practice in addition to the important imaging manifestations to assess for in the emergency setting.

Suggested Readings

- A Micieli, W Kingston, An approach to identifying headache patients that require neuroimaging, Front Public Health 7 (2019) 52, doi:10.3389/fpubh.2019.00052.
- CA Potter, L Hsu, Emergent neuroimaging in the oncologic and immunosuppressed patient, Neuroimaging Clin N Am 28 (3) (2018) 397–417, doi:10.1016/j.nic.2018.03.004.
- SJ An, TJ Kim, B-W Yoon, Epidemiology, risk factors, and clinical features of intracerebral hemorrhage: an update, J Stroke 19 (1) (2017) 3–10, doi:10.5853/jos.2016.00864.
- C Torres, N Zakhari, S Symons, TB Nguyen, Imaging the unconscious "Found Down" patient in the emergency department, Neuroimaging Clin N Am 28 (3) (2018) 435–451, doi:10.1016/j.nic.2018.03.006.
- A Krainik, JW Casselman, Imaging evaluation of patients with cranial nerve disorders von Schulthess GK, in: J Hodler, RA Kubik- Huch (eds.), Diseases of the Brain, Head and Neck, Spine 2020–2023, Springer International Publishing, 2020, pp. 143–161, doi:10.1007/978-3-030-38490-6_12. IDKD Springer Series.

91

Acute Chest

REENA TANNA, JANAN JEYATHEESAN

Radiological Techniques

Chest Radiographs

Chest radiographs are by far the most common first-line investigation in the acute setting and provide many positive and negative findings to tailor further imaging or immediate management. Careful assessment of a technically good x-ray is key, and subsequently the production of a clear radiology report.

Currently, in most centers the x-ray source is a standard portable generator, and the image is captured on a computed radiography detector or a flat-panel digital detector, followed by immediate transfer to a picture archiving and communication system (PACS) [1]. The x-rays of intensive care ward patients need to be examined in the light of full clinical information because many of the pathological processes to which these patients are susceptible produce similar radiographic manifestations. Serial images need to be evaluated for general trends, as day-to-day changes may not be apparent, and special attention needs to be given to monitoring and life-support devices.

The injured patient is usually brought to the x-ray department, where, if possible, an erect posteroanterior (PA) x-ray should be taken. A high-kV technique is desirable to see mediastinal detail. If the patient is severely injured, it is necessary to make do with semi-erect or supine radiographs.

Computed Tomography

Computed tomography (CT) is the second most common modality when imaging the thorax. These scans vary significantly depending on the indication including the use of intravenous contrast, patient positioning, inspiration versus expiration, gated scanning, as well as newer techniques such as multispectral or dual-energy CT. The clinical indication and patient factors will dictate the exact protocol of the scan.

Ultrasonography (USG)

USG is an excellent method for examining the pleura, diaphragm, and subphrenic areas and has largely been replaced by the concomitant use of "Focussed Assessment with Sonography in Trauma" (FAST scanning) and chest x-rays (CXRs) [2].

Aortography, CT, and Trans-oesophageal USG

Aortography, *CT*, and *trans-oesophageal ultrasound* may be indicated when vascular injuries are suspected.

The best way to assess any scan of the chest is the same as with any form of imaging interpretation. A systematic approach, looking at all areas of the chest wall, pleura, lungs, and mediastinum, as well as any review areas identified by the reader (Fig. 91.1).

Nontraumatic Chest Emergencies

Chest emergencies in the nontraumatic setting are common presentations to the emergency department and make up a large proportion of the radiologist's workload. Common clinical presentations are chest pain, shortness of breath, cough, fever, and haemoptysis. It is important to be able to differentiate when certain diagnoses need urgent management to prevent significant morbidity or mortality.

The prevalence of *chronic lung disease* globally in 2017 was estimated to be 545 million people, with almost 4 million associated deaths [3]. Although these chronic conditions are not emergencies in themselves, it is the complications of these diseases that lead patients to attend hospital and where the role of imaging becomes important. Similarly, *cardiovascular disease* in the British population was recorded at nearly 272,000 in 2018 [4], and the number of deaths globally in 2016 reached an estimated 17.9 million [5]. These figures give an idea of the importance of detection of the primary condition, but more importantly, the associated morbidity

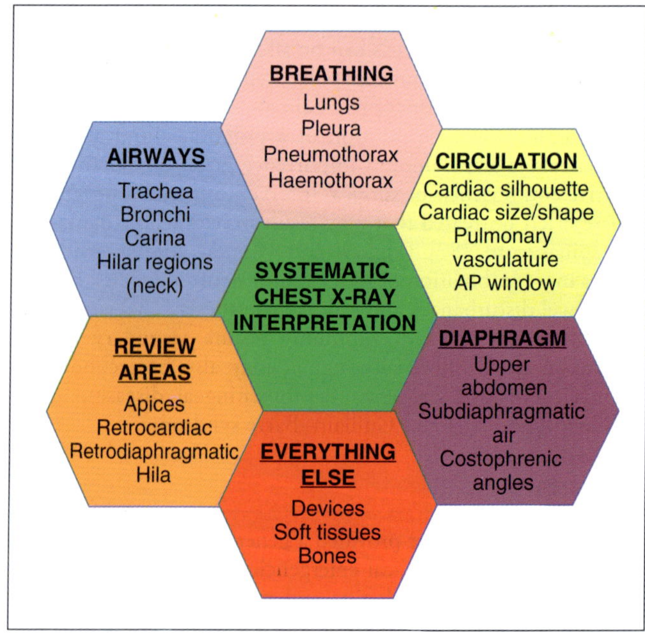

Figure 91.1 A systematic approach to assessing and reporting acute imaging of the chest, including all systems and review areas.

and mortality, some of which can be managed in a timely manner following appropriate image-guided diagnosis.

In most instances, a CXR will be enough to diagnose and direct management, however further imaging such as CT, nuclear medicine, or invasive angiography has a role in certain scenarios and is often adopted to gain more detail or a more definitive diagnosis.

Cough/Fever

One of the most common presentations in the acute setting is cough and fever. Although a simple *lower respiratory tract infection* accounts for many of these cases, there are certain differentials that must be considered following appropriate clinical history and examination, for example, atypical infections in the immunosuppressed patient.

Pneumonia

Airspace opacification or consolidation on a CXR is a classic finding in true *pneumonia*, and follow-up imaging 4–6 weeks following treatment is the usual advice given to ensure resolution. The appearance, distribution, and development of this consolidation can point the diagnostician toward a specific pathogen. For example, lobar consolidation with bulging fissures should automatically flag *Klebsiella* as a culprit (Fig. 91.2A and B). In the immunosuppressed patient, patchy perihilar ground-glass changes suggest *Pneumocystis pneumonia* [6].

High-resolution CT may be warranted in patients with unusual presentations or in those high-risk patients with clinical symptoms or refractory infections that do not have any x-ray changes. CT also demonstrates an array of findings dependent on the causative agent, but the most important use is to identify any complications of infections that might pose a risk to the patient's life.

Lung Abscess

Lung abscesses can be primary if they arise from the lung due to necrotizing pneumonias, immunodeficiency, or aspiration, or secondary from haematogenic spread or direct invasion from surrounding soft tissues, etc. They are an important entity to pick up on imaging as the mortality rate from untreated abscesses can reach up to 75% [7]. On x-ray, the classic appearance is of a rounded, thick-walled cavitating lesion, sometimes with an air-fluid level within. Contrast-enhanced CT should be adopted to clearly visualize the margins and any associated vascular or airway complications (Fig. 91.3). Features on CT are similar to radiographs, with thick-walled, discrete cavitating lesions containing fluid, with or without gas. There is often surrounding lung inflammation or atelectasis, and bronchovascular bundles can be seen tracing up to the wall, where they abruptly end. Management options include prolonged antibiotic therapy, and in some instances, surgical drainage [7].

Empyema

Empyema is infected pleural collections, usually developing as a complication of an existing pneumonia, or from any other means of introducing bacteria into the pleural space. This may be iatrogenic following thoracic surgery, from penetrating trauma, extension from a nonpleural infection such as the abdomen, or direct rupture from a lung abscess. Radiographs will demonstrate a pleural collection; however, USG or CT are better modalities to delineate an empyema from a simple effusion and to assess the size, complexity and any associated features that require urgent management [8].

Findings on USG include pleural thickening, septations, and loculated fluid (Fig. 91.4). The echogenicity of blood products will be more echogenic than pus, which will be more echogenic than simple fluid. Immediate drainage can be performed at the same time under direct visualization, which is the most common form of immediate management [9].

CT with contrast enhancement may show the "split pleura sign," where there is hyperenhancement of the parietal and visceral pleura (Fig. 91.5), separated by a fluid collection. Gas locules within the collection in the absence of previous instrumentation are indicative of an aerobic organism or may suggest fistulation with the small airways.

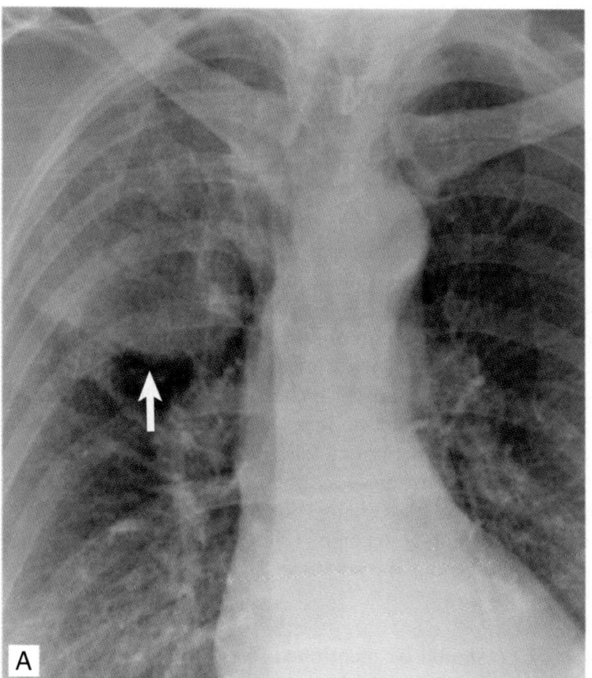

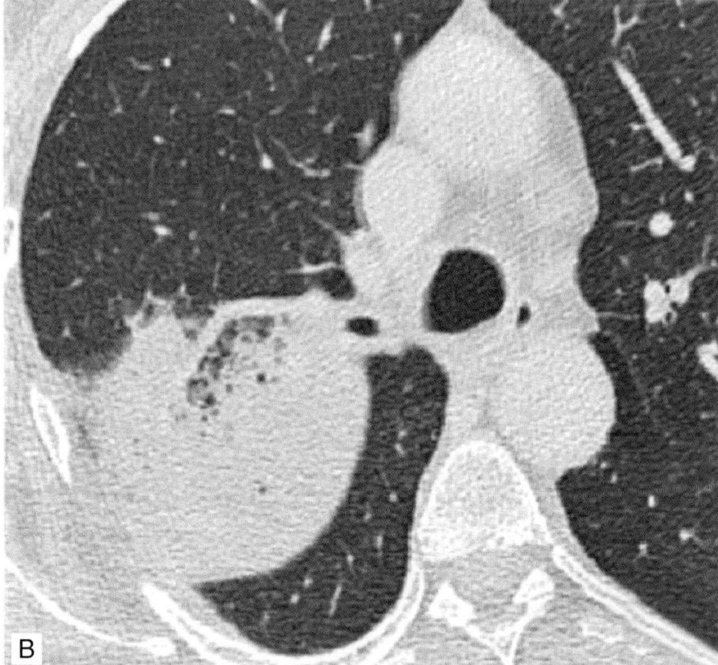

Figure 91.2 CXR (A) and CT (B). Consolidation with bulging of the adjacent fissure (*arrow*), a feature commonly seen in *Klebsiella* pneumonia.

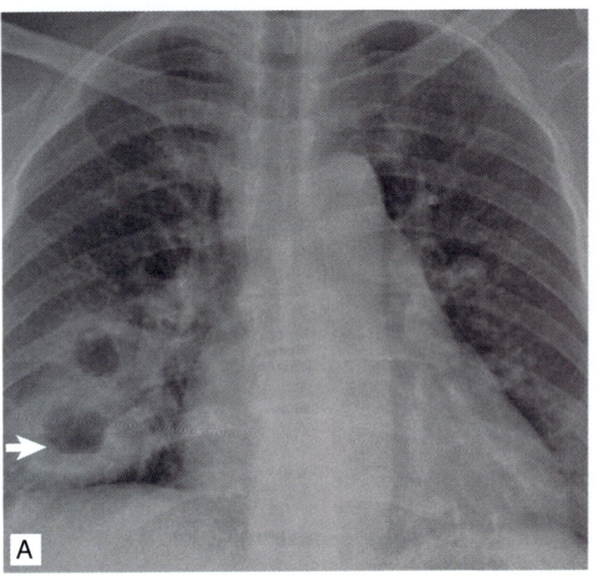

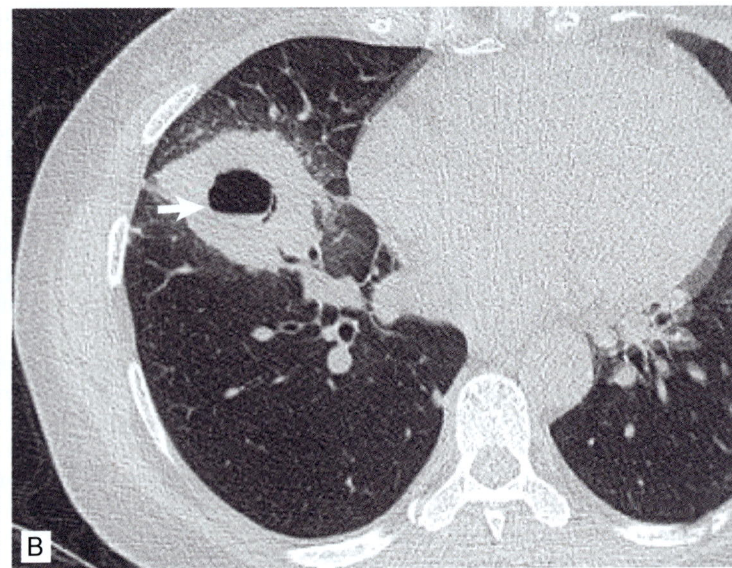

Figure 91.3 CXR (A) and axial CT (B). Lung abscess with irregular, thick-walled cavities, and surrounding ground-glass change. Air-fluid levels (*arrows*) are seen inferiorly on the CXR and dependently on the axial CT.

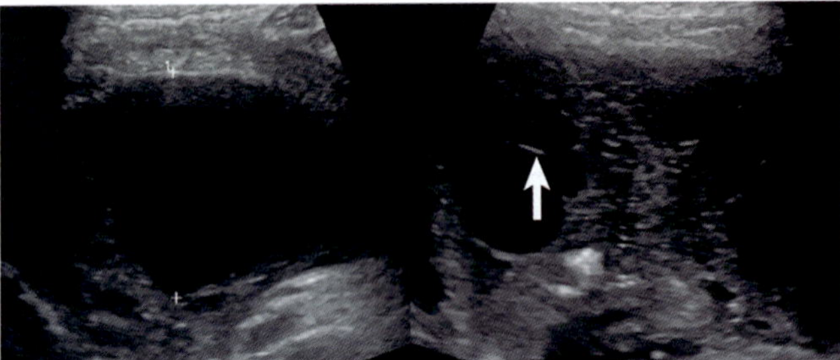

Figure 91.4 USG static images demonstrating a hypoechoic pleural fluid collection with a thickened pleura overlying the collection, and septations (*arrow*) in keeping with empyema.

TABLE 91.1 Imaging Differences to Distinguish Between Pleural Empyema and Pulmonary Abscess

Empyema	Lung Abscess
Smoother, thinner walls ("split pleura sign")	Thick, irregular walls
Abrupt interruption of bronchovascular bundles	Distortion and compression of bronchovascular bundles and lung parenchyma
Obtuse angle with pleura	Acute angle with pleura
Lentiform shape	Rounded shape, usually with an air-fluid level

Figure 91.5 Axial CT. Pleural collection with hyperenhancing pleura (*arrows*) known as the "split pleura sign," indicating empyema. Note the gas locules (*arrowhead*) within the fluid, another sign of an infected collection.

Septations are easily identified, as well as thoracic wall fat stranding or inflammatory change in the pulmonary tissue [9].

Empyema is sometimes difficult to differentiate from a lung abscess (Table 91.1), but certain imaging features can help to distinguish between the two [10].

Septic Emboli

Septic emboli occur when pathogen-laced thrombus fragments detach from an infective source in the body and travel via the bloodstream to the lungs, where they cause microinfarcts and abscesses. This is most commonly seen in intravenous drug users, diabetics, and in patients with infective endocarditis. Complications include lung abscesses, bronchopleural fistulas, pneumothoraces, or fatal sepsis. Small nodular opacification may be seen on CXRs, in a largely peripheral distribution. CT with contrast enhancement demonstrates peripheral, wedge-shaped areas of nodular, and ground-glass change or cavitation. CT can also demonstrate the "feeding vessel sign" (Fig. 91.6) which is an indication of haematogenous spread [11].

Pulmonary TB

Pulmonary TB should be mentioned in this section, as although the clinical presentation itself is not an "emergency," imaging plays a vital role in the detection and urgent referral to the

Figure 91.6 Axial CT bilateral, peripheral areas of consolidation, some showing internal cavitation (*arrow*) with a "feeding vessel sign" (*arrowhead*) in keeping with septic emboli.

appropriate infectious diseases teams to prevent spread. Currently, plain radiography is the only imaging modality in international guidelines for the diagnosis of TB (Fig. 91.7), alongside sputum microscopy for acid-fast bacilli. CT has a role, especially in refractory infections, radiographic occult disease, the assessment of complications and follow-up after management. Signs of active pulmonary TB on radiographs include multifocal, patchy consolidation with an upper lobe predilection with or without lymph node enlargement, miliary nodules, cavitating lesions, and occasional pleural effusions/empyema.

Coronavirus Disease (COVID-19)

Coronavirus disease (COVID-19) pneumonia was first presented in December 2019 and escalated within weeks to become a global pandemic. About 754 million cases and 6.83 million deaths of COVID-19 have been reported worldwide as of February 8th, 2023 [12]. There is ongoing research into this disease and whilst a lot is still unknown, it seems that COVID-19 will remain an especially important differential in patients with acute chest symptoms for the foreseeable future.

Radiographic features (Fig. 91.8) range from minor illness to more severe cases with complications including adult respiratory distress syndrome (ARDS) and lung fibrosis. Most cases in the acute setting demonstrate bilateral, peripheral, patchy airspace opacification, usually with a slight lower zone distribution [13].

CT is not routinely indicated for uncomplicated cases of COVID-19 as clinical history, radiographic signs, and *polymerase chain reaction* testing have adequate diagnostic value. However, the complication of COVID-19 pneumonia includes increased thromboembolic potential resulting in pulmonary emboli, significant respiratory compromise leading to ARDS, and long term effects of the infection and mechanical ventilatory support leading to fibrotic lung changes. These are all indications for CT evaluation and will have varying imaging findings [14]. CT findings in uncomplicated COVID-19 pneumonia are similar to those on CXR, with bilateral, patchy, peripheral ground-glass changes. Associated thoracic lymph node enlargement and pleural effusions are not commonly seen [15].

Shortness of Breath

Another common presentation in the acute setting is difficulty in breathing, dyspnoea, or shortness of breath. The most common causes are usually those that affect the main airways or lungs themselves, reducing or preventing adequate gas exchange.

Acute Exacerbations of Chronic Lung Disease

Acute exacerbations of chronic lung disease are a common cause of a sudden deterioration in respiratory function and presentation to the emergency department. Chronic conditions include asthma,

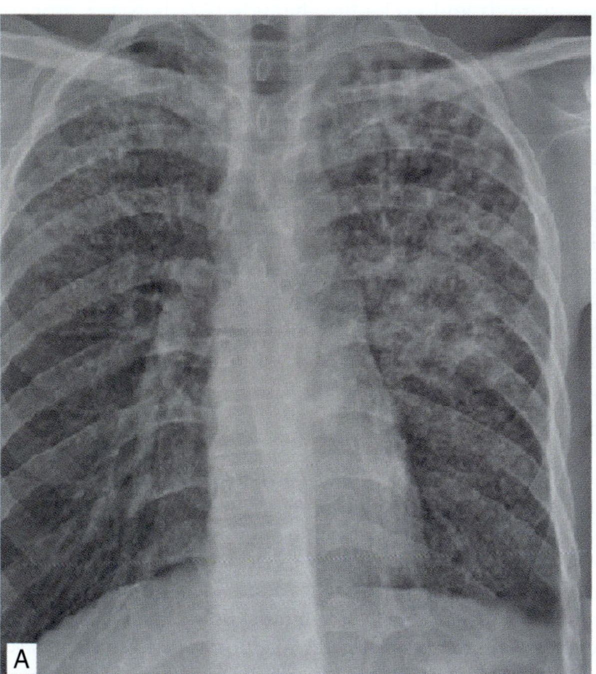

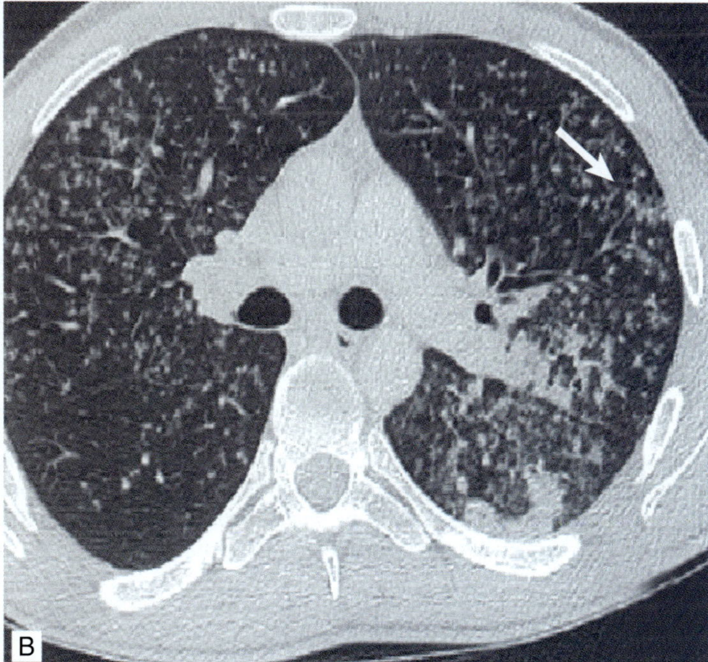

Figure 91.7 (A) CXR. Diffuse nodular (miliary) opacities predominantly affecting the upper lobes. (B) Axial CT shows peribronchial nodularity and "tree-in-bud" nodularity (*arrow*).

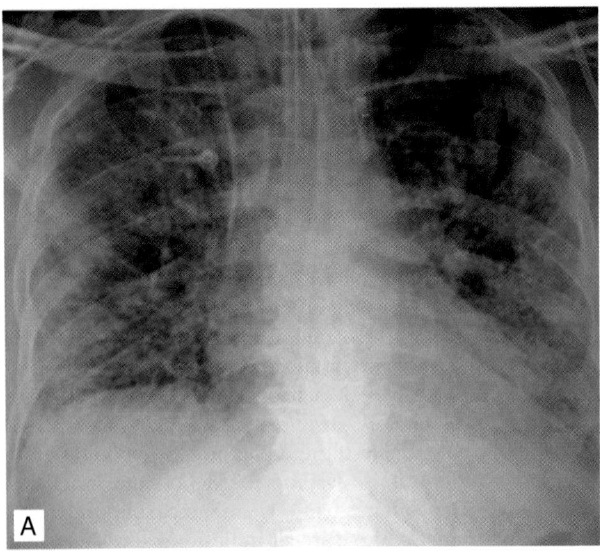

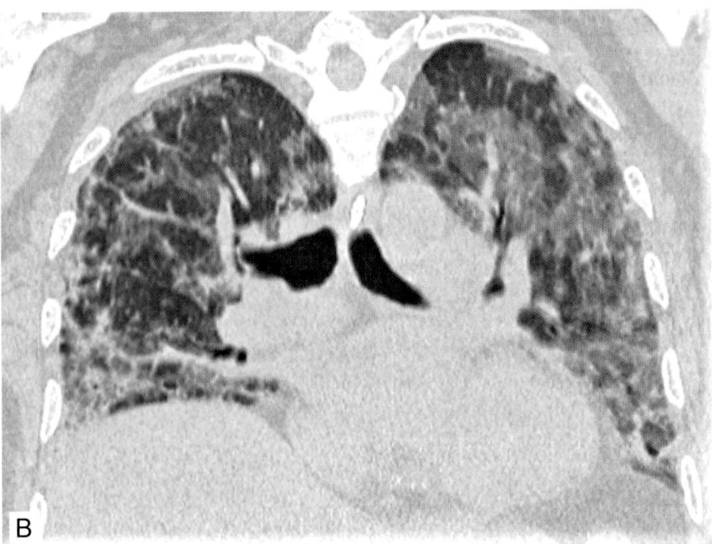

Figure 91.8 (A) CXR. Patchy bilateral, mainly peripheral ground-glass opacification seen in COVID-19 pneumonia. (B) CT correlate demonstrating patchy ground-glass changes in the absence of mediastinal lymph node enlargement, cardiomegaly, or pleural effusions.

chronic obstructive pulmonary disease (COPD) bronchiectasis, fibrotic lung disease, and cystic fibrosis (CF). Although an acute exacerbation is defined slightly differently in these entities, the overall result is the same: a reduction in respiratory function, possible progression of disease, reduced quality of life, and higher risk of disease-related mortality. It is important to identify these clinically; however, imaging can play a role in the diagnosis and monitoring of these cases [16].

Chest radiographs may show evidence of the underlying chronic condition, such as dilated airways in bronchiectasis or CF, or hyperexpanded lungs in COPD. Acute changes are varied depending on the cause of the exacerbation, but the most common findings include new infective/inflammatory consolidation, bronchial wall thickening, loss of lung volume, or areas of collapse (due to mucus plugging for example) or pleural effusions/edema (Fig. 91.9) [17]. CT is indicated in cases where radiographic findings are equivocal or where there is an unusual presentation, persisting symptoms despite appropriate treatment or when there is concern over associated complications, such as malignant transformation or abscess formation, etc.

Pulmonary Edema

Pulmonary edema can also present as acute shortness of breath and is usually cardiogenic in nature, however noncardiogenic pulmonary edema can be seen secondary to inhalation injuries, allergic reactions, acute renal dysfunction, and more severely in ARDS. It is the result of an increase in hydrostatic pressure, pushing fluid into the interstitium, and later into the alveoli [18].

Chest x-ray findings vary depending on the degree of edema but usually demonstrate increased vascular diameter bilaterally with upper lobe diversion, interstitial and interlobular septal thickening (Kerley B lines), and bilateral pleural effusions (Fig. 91.10). With worsening edema, there may be gravity-dependent ground glass changes and a *"batwing appearance"* representing centrally located alveolar edema [19].

Pleural Effusion

Pleural effusions are commonly associated with pulmonary edema; however, noncardiogenic causes are also common. There is usually at least 200 mL of fluid within the pleural space before a meniscus sign is seen on a PA radiograph, and 500 mL before the meniscus obscures the hemidiaphragm [20].

Acute Interstitial Pneumonitis

Acute interstitial pneumonitis is a rapidly progressing, noninfectious interstitial lung disease, the only acute process among the idiopathic interstitial pneumonias. It usually progresses over days or weeks in otherwise healthy individuals, causing nonspecific symptoms of myalgia, pyrexia, and malaise, with rapidly worsening respiratory function and dyspnoea [21]. There is diffuse alveolar damage which has almost identical imaging features to those in ARDS (discussed later). Management when the condition progresses to respiratory failure is usually supportive, with mechanical ventilation and the use of corticosteroids and cyclophosphamide [22] however prognosis is rather poor with more than 70% mortality rate at 3 months.

Lung Collapse

Anything that blocks the passage of air into the lungs can also lead to shortness of breath or difficulty in breathing. *Lung collapse* is seen when there is airway obstruction, either intraluminal such as an inhaled foreign body or mucous plugging, or from extrinsic compression such as a lung cancer. On plain radiographs, this will present as an opacity in differing positions dependending on which lobe of the lung is affected [23]. This is described in detail in the Chapter 17 on diseases of airways.

Chest Pain

The most common causes of chest pain in the acute setting are pulmonary emboli, myocardial infarction, and acute aortic syndrome (AAS). Various other, less common conditions present with chest pain, which in itself is a rather nonspecific symptom. It is important for referring physicians to have a good idea of the clinical picture and a list of differentials in order of likelihood and clinical urgency, to ensure the correct examination is performed. It is the role of the radiologist to help the physicians if there is any uncertainty, and to direct imaging appropriately to get the best results to help the patient.

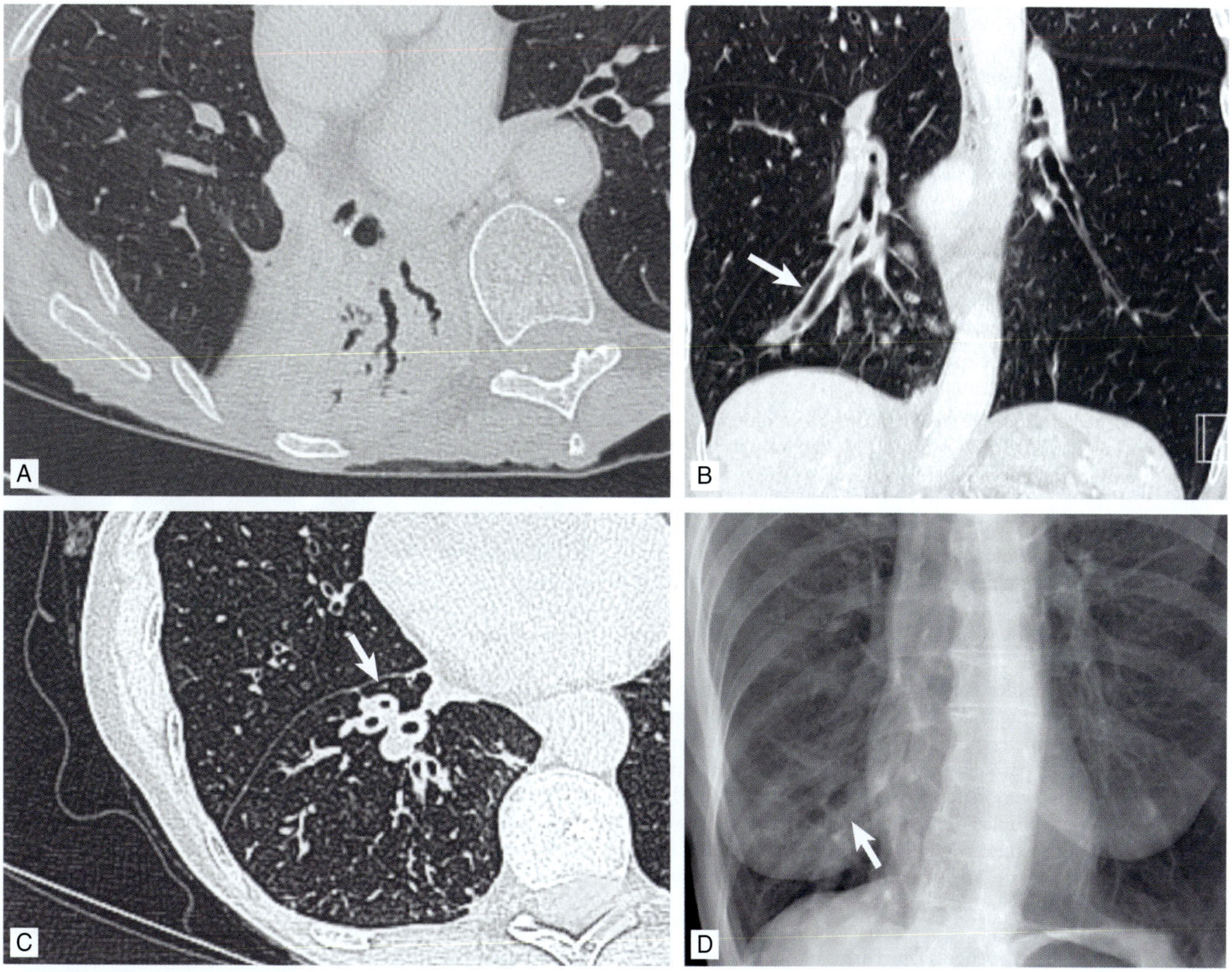

Figure 91.9 CT and CXR. Imaging features of bronchiectasis with dilatated, thickened airways (*arrows*) (B and C) and dense consolidation with air bronchograms (A) in acute infective exacerbation. CXR (D) shows "cystic" spaces (*arrow*) indicating dilated airways.

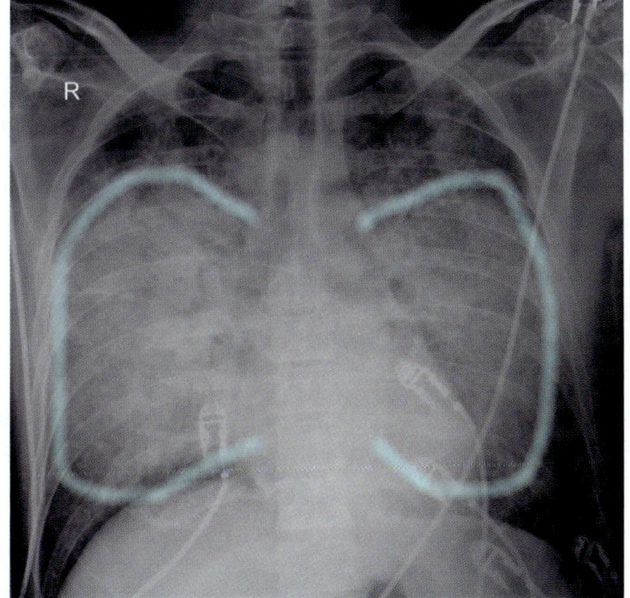

Figure 91.10 CXR. Classic radiographic "bat wing" appearance seen in pulmonary edema. (Image courtesy of Dr Zelena Aziz.)

Pulmonary Embolism

Pulmonary embolism (PE) occurs when thrombus, usually in the deep venous system of the limbs, is left untreated and fragments of thrombus break off, travel via the bloodstream to the right side of the heart and into the pulmonary circulation. These can then become lodged in the pulmonary arteries, depending on their size, causing ischaemia in the supplied lung [24]. Clinical presentation varies depending on the size and distribution of the emboli, from mild dyspnoea, tachycardia, and chest pain to more concerning haemoptysis or cardiac arrest. A chest radiograph is performed in the first instance, acting as an aid to identify any other cause for the patient's symptoms before following the algorithm in the investigation of PE's. Biochemical tests such as *D-dimer,* as well as a scoring system identifies the probability of there being a PE.

If the probability is high enough, and the radiograph has not highlighted any significant abnormalities, there are two main imaging pathways that can be taken [25]. A common investigation in those with high probability but clinical stability is a ventilation-perfusion scan (V/Q scan). Approximately 25% of patients with suspected PE having the diagnosis refuted by normal scintigraphy. PE's obstruct vessels, therefore causing a perfusion defect on a V/Q scan, however it should not affect the ventilation, unless

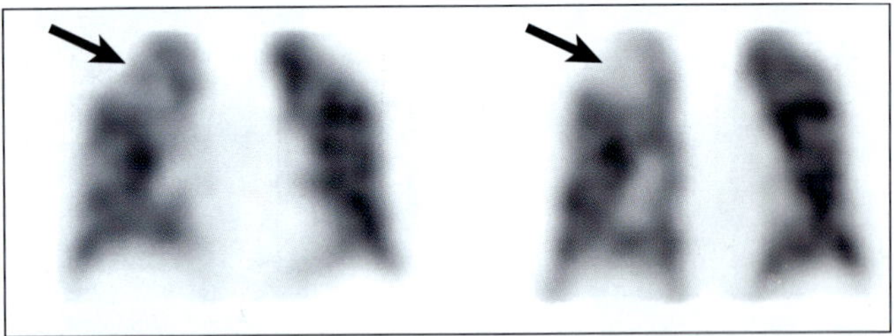

Figure 91.11 Single photon emission computed tomography (SPECT) perfusion scan. Perfusion defect in the right upper zone (*arrow*) with no CT correlate (not shown here), indicating a pulmonary embolus.

a lung infarct has occurred. This results in a ventilation-perfusion mismatch (Fig. 91.11).

The modified Prospective Investigation of Pulmonary Embolism Diagnosis II (PIOPED II) criteria are currently used to classify studies by probability (Table 91.2) [26].

An ideal test for PE would provide noninvasive direct visualization of thrombus within pulmonary arteries; *CT pulmonary angiography* (CTPA) comes close to fulfilling this description. The sensitivities and specificities for pulmonary emboli detection by CTPA at main, lobar, and segmental levels are almost always reported as greater than 90% [24,27]. Newer technologies such as *spectral* or *dual-energy CT* have led to improvements in image quality, requiring smaller volumes of intravenous contrast, and reduced beam hardening and streak artefact [28]. The CT signs of PE are now well defined, and the cardinal sign of an intraluminal filling defect, either partially or totally obstructive, remains the central diagnostic criterion for an embolus (Fig. 91.12). There may be features of complications such as interventricular bowing and reflux of contrast into the inferior vena cava, representing a degree of right heart strain. A dilated pulmonary trunk would suggest pulmonary hypertension, seen more commonly with chronic PE's. Finally, if there is any ischaemia in the lung, CT can demonstrate peripheral, wedge-shaped areas of opacification [29].

Myocardial Infarction

The clinical management of *acute myocardial infarction* is a complex matter, depending on the precise mode of presentation and the site and size of the infarct. The CXR is used as a guide to cardiac function and heart failure, but other imaging techniques are not routinely used in the first few days after

TABLE 91.2 Modified PIOPED II Classification

High Probability	Low Probability
▪ ≥2 large segmental perfusion defects ▪ 1 large segmental defect & ≥2 moderate segmental perfusion defects	▪ Multiple matching V/Q defects ▪ Corresponding V/Q defect and XR opacity in upper/middle zone OR large pleural effusion ▪ >3 small segmental perfusion defects
Intermediate Probability	**Very Low Probability**
▪ 1 moderate to <2 large segmental perfusion defects ▪ Corresponding V/Q defect and XR opacity in lower lung OR small pleural effusion ▪ Single moderately matched V/Q defect	▪ ≤3 small segmental perfusion defects **Normal** ▪ No perfusion defects and perfusion outlines normal lung contour

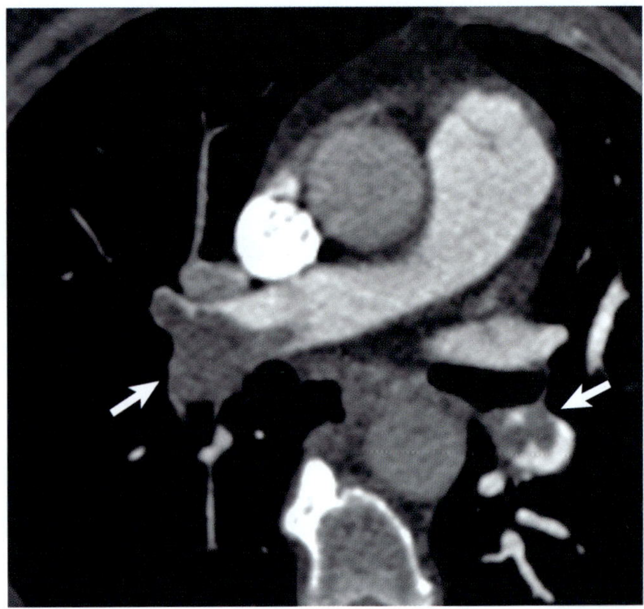

Figure 91.12 CTPA. Filling defects (*arrows*) in the right main pulmonary artery and left lower lobar pulmonary artery in keeping with extensive pulmonary emboli.

myocardial infarction unless there are haemodynamic complications.

The most common feature identified is the development of pulmonary edema, imaging findings of which have been discussed earlier. Serial radiographs may show pleural effusions which can develop if the left heart failure is prolonged. The presence of pulmonary edema indicates 1-year mortality of 44%. If there is no evidence of heart failure, this indicates a good prognosis with an 8% 1-year mortality.

If the serial radiographs taken over the first few days or weeks following myocardial infarction show progressive cardiac enlargement (Fig. 91.13A–C), this is an important adverse prognostic sign that should be further evaluated.

The *echocardiogram* will usually demonstrate the site, size, and severity of the infarct and will allow an assessment of overall left ventricular function.

Trans-oesophageal echocardigram is occasionally helpful in the acute phase but the potential imaging benefits must be seen in the context of the patient's clinical condition, and therefore this procedure should only be performed when there is a clear clinical management decision to be made.

The use of *Triple Rule Out CT* has been adopted in may centers around the world which has an indication in low to intermediate-risk patients, to assess for significant coronary artery disease, PE, and AAS. A modified CT coronary angiogram is performed, which images from just above the aortic arch to the top of the abdomen, using a split bolus of intravenous contrast, with ECG gating and the use of beta-blockers and GTN to optimize coronary image quality. TRO CT also has the advantage of being able to pick up any noncardiovascular causes for the patient's symptoms, for example, any pulmonary infections, pneumothoraces, etc.

Acute Pericarditis

Acute pericarditis occurs when there is inflammation of the pericardium, usually with an associated effusion and pericardial thickening. It is most commonly due to an infection, usually viral, bacterial, or tuberculous. Less commonly it can be associated with

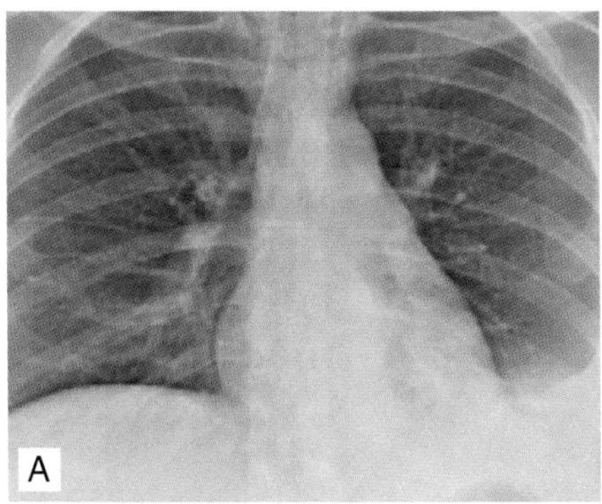

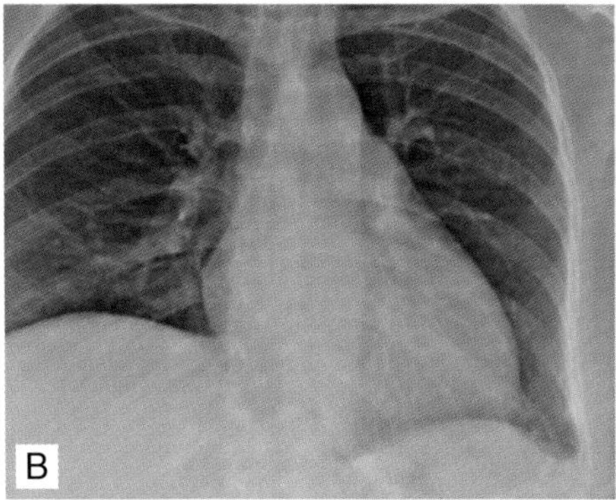

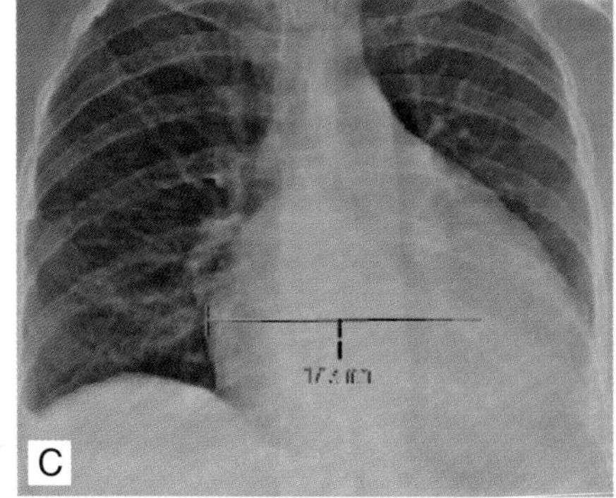

Figure 91.13 Sequential CXRs. Increase in the size of the cardiac silhouette on sequential radiographs (A–C) taken weeks apart. The cardiothoracic ratio (CTR) can be calculated on PA radiographs; however, there is an obvious increase in size indicating developing cardiomegaly.

inflammatory disorders such as scleroderma or rheumatoid arthritis, and following an MI, termed "Dressler's syndrome" [30].

Positional chest pain is the most common presentation, with many experiencing relief when sitting forwards. Chest radiographs have a role in excluding any other causes of chest pain or sepsis and may demonstrate changes to the cardiac contour if there is a significant enough pericardial effusion ("globular heart") (Fig. 91.14A). On CT, a purulent or loculated pericardial effusion may be seen, however, the presence of pericardial thickening is more specific (Fig. 91.14B). There may be hyperenhancement of the pericardium or areas of calcification in constrictive pericarditis [30].

MRI is extremely sensitive at detecting even small amounts of fluid within the pericardium and haemopericardium can be distinguished from conventional fluid (Fig. 91.14C). Often in constrictive pericarditis there is disproportionate dilatation of the atrium compared to the ventricles. If assessment of the valves excludes the diagnosis of regurgitation and imaging of the pericardium shows pathological thickening, then the diagnosis of constrictive pericarditis is likely.

Acute Aortic Syndrome

Acute aortic syndrome (AAS) is a spectrum of disorders affecting the aortic structure and integrity and is a medical emergency requiring prompt diagnosis and management. The unifying presentation is with sudden onset chest pain and usually a degree of haemodynamic instability. The main complication is aortic rupture, which is rapidly fatal, but this can be avoided with early recognition, accurate diagnosis, and appropriate, timely treatment. CT is the first-choice investigation in the acute setting, whereas MRI is usually reserved for any special circumstances, surveillance or further assessment, for example, haemodynamic assessment. Radiographs have a somewhat limited role, however nonspecific findings such as mediastinal widening may direct the clinical team to investigate further [31].

AAS encompasses the following: intramural haematoma, aortic dissection, penetrating ulcer, and unstable aortic aneurysm [32].

These conditions may all occur independently, or they may also occur together in any combination, to different degrees at different sites. Clinically, it is very difficult to differentiate these conditions, therefore imaging must be performed in a systematic way to enable a radiologist to assess each of these pathologies (Box 91.1).

CT is the preferred method of imaging for AAS in the acute setting, with sensitivity and specificity above 98% [33]. ECG-gated or flash scans should be carried out to prevent pulsation artefact, which can degrade image quality and produce false-positive signs of dissection, particularly around the aortic root. An unenhanced CT should be the first scan performed, to look for a high attenuation crescent shape in the aortic wall, indicative of an intramural haematoma (Fig. 91.15). Depending on their location and size, these may be treated conservatively, or with more aggressive measures such as endovascular repair (EVAR). This is because they can progress to dissection, rupture or aneurysm which all carry poorer prognoses [34].

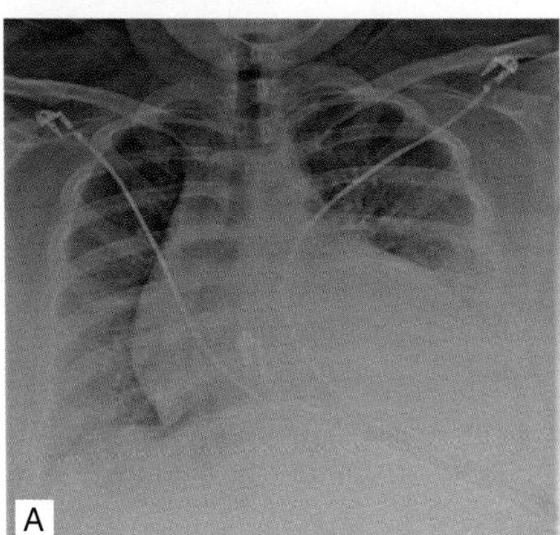

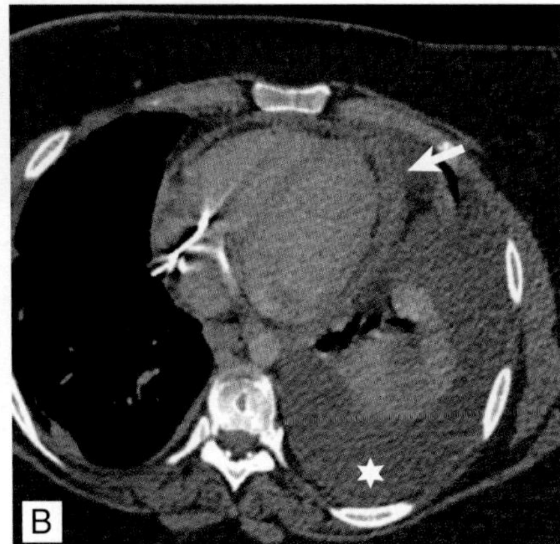

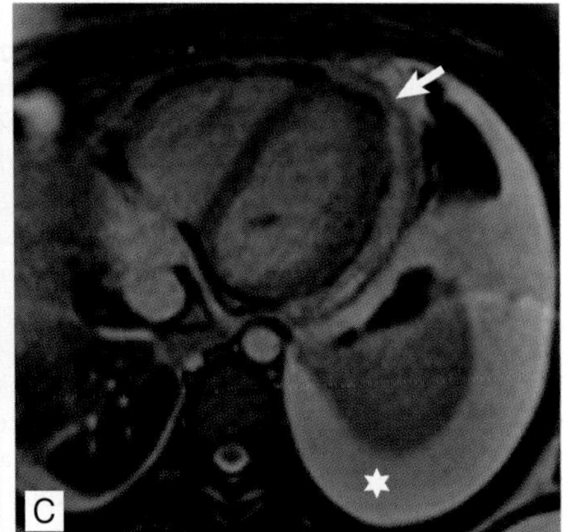

Figure 91.14 (A) CXR. Frontal radiograph demonstrates an enlarged cardiac contour in a patient with pericarditis. (B) Axial CT. Contrast-enhanced CT demonstrates a pericardial effusion with irregular thickening of the pericardium (*arrow*) in a patient with acute pericarditis. Incidental note made of a left pleural collection (*star*). (C) Axial T2 weighted MRI. High signal pleural (*star*) and pericardial effusions with a thickened pericardium (*arrow*) in a patient with acute pericarditis.

BOX 91.1 Acute Aortic Syndrome Imaging Peals

Unenhanced	High attenuation crescent indicates mural haematoma
Arterial phase	Dissection flap, true & false lumens indicate dissection
	Dilated aorta indicate aortic aneurysm
Delayed phase	End organ ischaemia

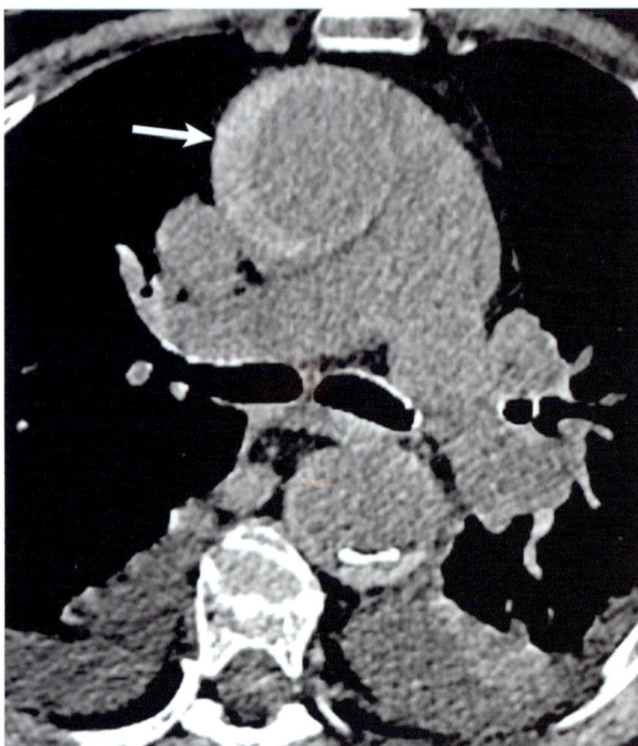

Figure 91.15 Axial CT. Unenhanced gated CT of the aorta demonstrates a high attenuation crescent along the lateral border of the ascending aorta (*arrow*) indicating an intramural haematoma as part of an acute aortic syndrome.

ECG-gated CT of the whole aorta with intravenous contrast in the angiographic phase is then performed to look at the aortic lumen size and integrity.

Aortic Dissection

Aortic dissection is a devastating disease that occurs as a result of degeneration of the thoracic aorta. Despite modern treatment, the mortality from this condition remains high, with death in 25% of patients with a dissection of the ascending aorta within the first 24 hours and a mortality of over 75% within the first month. Aortic dissection in younger patients usually occurs in high-risk groups such as patients with Marfan's syndrome, Ehlers–Danlos disease or in pregnancy.

The most common pattern of dissection involves the right anterior aspect of the ascending aorta and the posterior left lateral aspect of the descending aorta. Dissection in the descending aorta can extend down to the abdominal aorta and may then lead to dissection of the left renal artery with associated ischaemic change.

There are two major types of classification: De Bakey and Stanford, described in detail in the chapter "disorder of arteries" (Chapter 25).

CT signs of an intimal flap can be identified by demonstration of two lumens within the aorta originating from the point of the dissection tear (Fig. 91.16).

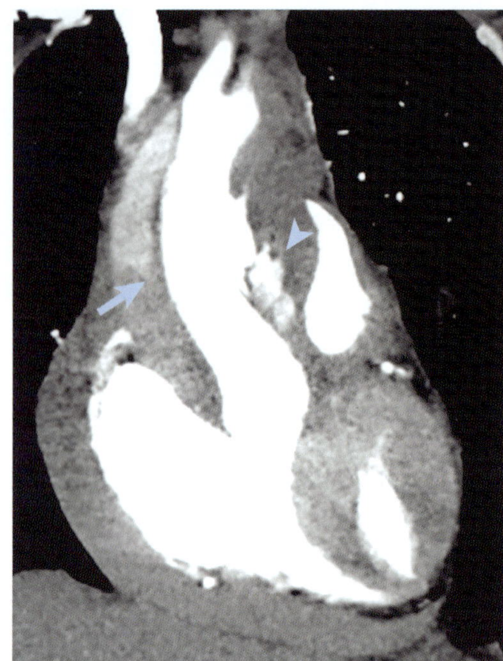

Figure 91.16 Coronal CT reformat. Ascending aortic dissection (*blue arrow*) with lower attenuation contrast filling the false lumen. Medially there is a blush of contrast (*blue arrowhead*) indicating aortic rupture and haemorrhage into the mediastinum and pericardial space.

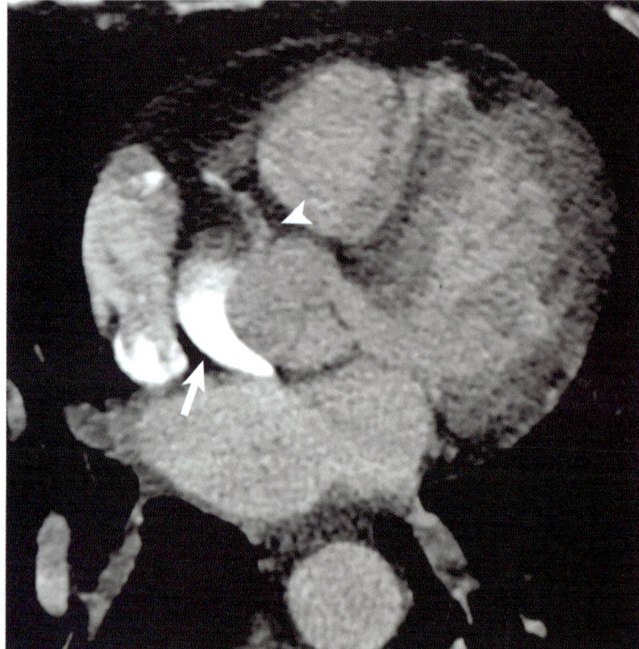

Figure 91.17 Axial CT. Images demonstrate a dissection flap involving the aortic root and extending to the aortic valve, with a crescent of high attenuation seen where the intravenous contrast enhances the false lumen (*arrow*) at the level of the right coronary artery origin (*arrowhead*).

Often a differential blood flow within the true and false lumens can be detected by the variable enhancement patterns following the intravenous contrast. Another important consideration is the need to determine whether the dissection extends into any of the great vessels arising from the aortic arch or the aortic valve (Fig. 91.17), which will be vital for the surgeons to know before any intervention.

Often in aortic dissection the CT will demonstrate periaortic haematoma caused by venous bleeding within the aortic wall. The technique may also demonstrate a pericardial effusion (haemopericardium), related to a tear extension into the aortic root. A dissection can extend into the aortic root leading to the development of aortic regurgitation, or into the origins of either coronary artery, leading to myocardial infarction.

It is important to be able to distinguish between the false and true lumens (Table 91.3) so that the surgeons or interventionalists can manage the correct one (Fig. 91.18). This can be challenging if there is a large dissection extending across the whole aorta, however there are several differentiating appearances that can help [35].

There are some pitfalls to be avoided in CT diagnosis of dissection.

- Linear artefacts across the aortic lumen can mimic an intimal flap.
- Leads or metallic lines on the patient's chest, or more commonly opacification of an adjacent venous structure such as the superior vena cava, can generate these artefacts.
- Occasionally periaortic structures can be interpreted as periaortic haematoma; a classic area that can give rise to confusion is the presence of fluid in the superior pericardial recess.
- Perhaps the most common misinterpretation is caused by tortuosity of the aorta, which can give rise to an apparent inward projection of the aortic wall (Box 91.2).

If further evaluation is required, or in those with contraindications to CT, MRI can be used for initial diagnosis, as well as for follow-up or surveillance (Fig. 91.19). Steady-state free procession MRI allows the possibility of diagnostic images with minimal scanning time in the acute setting. Contrast-enhanced MRI can also be adopted to visualize branching vessels, the presence of penetrating ulcers and any other luminal abnormality [36].

Transthoracic echocardiography is limited in the assessment of the aorta. Trans-oesophageal echocardiography, however, can give excellent detail of much of the aorta. Doppler studies will enhance diagnostic accuracy by showing flow in the true and false lumens as well as demonstrating the site of the tear in many cases.

TABLE 91.3 Imaging Features to Distinguish Between the True and False Lumen in Aortic Dissection

True Lumen	False Lumen
Smaller	Larger
Continuous with unaffected aorta	Discontinuous from unaffected aorta
Displaced medially	Lateral to or wrapped around the true lumen
Enhances more than false lumen	Slow flow—hypodense to true lumen
	"Cobweb sign" OR "beak sign"

BOX 91.2 Reporting a CTA

- Location of tear including the proximal and distal extents
- Aortic size (any evidence of aneurysm)
- Whether the major aortic branches arise from the false or true lumen
- Any associated complications, e.g., haemopericardium or rupture
- Signs of end-organ ischaemia or vascular occlusion

Penetrating Atherosclerotic Ulcers

Penetrating atherosclerotic ulcers can be seen on CTA as an outpouching of the aortic wall or into a thickened wall if it has not penetrated through all the intimal layers (Fig. 91.20). These can progress to IMH, dissection or rupture, and are often managed depending on size, progression and clinical symptoms [37].

The diagnosis of rupture depends on the identification of haematoma outside the aortic lumen but in close association with the course of the vessel (Fig. 91.21). The haematoma will not usually show contrast enhancement on CT examination unless there is severe bleeding. In some cases where the haematoma cannot be correlated with a bleeding site, the source of the haemorrhage may be periaotic veins or small arteries. There

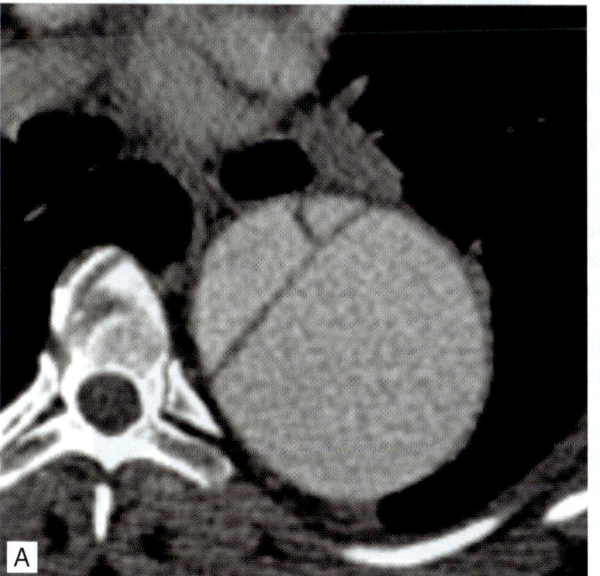

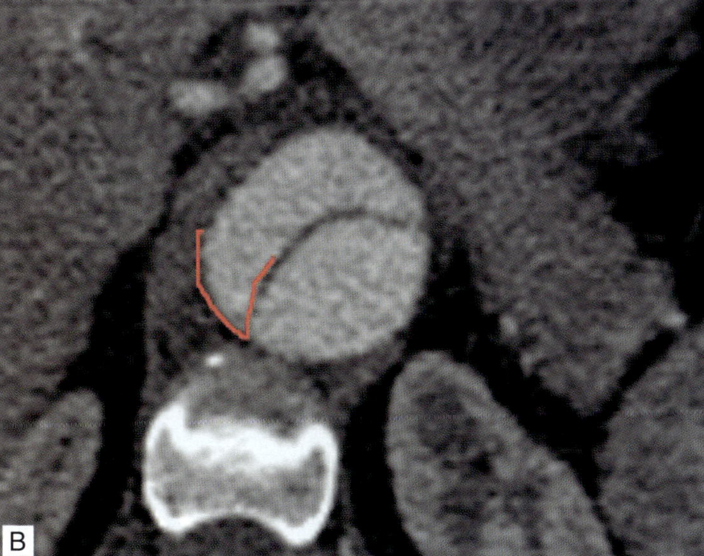

Figure 91.18 (A) Axial CT. Descending thoracic aorta dissection with "cobweb sign" representing strands of media crossing the false lumen. (B) "Beak sign" represents the acute angle formed by the false lumen in aortic dissection.

92

Acute Abdomen

ARMAN PARSAI, KHAWAJA SHAHABUDDIN, MAHRUKH QURESHI

The acute abdomen is the assigned diagnosis for acute or rapidly developing abdominal pain for which immediate (usually surgical) intervention/action is required until a specific diagnosis for the cause of the abdominal pain is found [1]. They account for 4–5% of accident and emergency (A&E) presentations [2]. Patients presenting to the A&E department will initially have a careful history taken by the attending physician as well as a meticulous physical examination. Based on these initial findings, the physician will consider imaging examinations to help establish the correct diagnosis. Causes of *"the acute abdomen"* can be broadly divided into "traumatic" and "nontraumatic." For the purposes of this chapter, we will only be discussing "nontraumatic" hepatopancreaticobiliary and gastrointestinal causes and their relevant imaging approach. More detailed descriptions are present in the individual chapters. Note that certain pathologies (e.g., pelvic or renal pathologies) are not covered in this chapter; these are covered in detail in other chapters elsewhere in the book.

The causes of *"the acute abdomen"* or acute abdominal pain as such range from the life-threatening to benign self-limiting disorders (Fig. 92.1). The patient will often present with vague abdominal symptoms and signs, making imaging crucial in diagnosis, risk stratification, and for guiding further management.

Conventional x-rays, ultrasonography (USG), and multidetector computed tomography (MDCT) are commonly used in the diagnostic work-up of patients with an acute abdomen.

Chest and Abdominal X-Rays (CXR and AXR)

An erect CXR has traditionally been used to exclude subphrenic air and hence a perforated viscus, and a supine abdominal x-ray to exclude bowel obstruction. However, the accuracy of these tests in investigating patients with acute abdominal pain may be as low as 53% [3]. Most patients will go on to have further detailed imaging in the form of an USG or more commonly a

ACUTE ABDOMEN: DIFFERENTIAL DIAGNOSIS BY ABDOMINO-PELVIC REGION

Cholecystitis Biliary colic Right lower lobe pneumonia Duodenal ulcer	Gastric ulcer	Gastric ulcer Pancreatitis Left lower lobe pneumonia
Right renal colic UTI Discitis	Pancreatitis Ruptured abdominal aortic aneurysm/dissection Appendicitis Discitis	Left renal colic UTI Ruptured abdominal aortic aneurysm/dissection Discitis
Appendicitis Mesenteric adenitis Ectopic pregnancy Ruptured ovarian cyst/hemorrhage Salpingitis/tubo-ovarian abscess Right colonic diverticulitis Epiploic appendagitis Ileocecal enteritis/typhlitis	Pelvic inflammatory disease Bladder calculus	Left colonic diverticulitis Ectopic pregnancy Ruptured ovarian cyst/hemorrhage Salpingitis/tubo-ovarian abscess Epiploic appendagitis

Figure 92.1 Acute abdomen: differential diagnosis by abdomino-pelvic region.

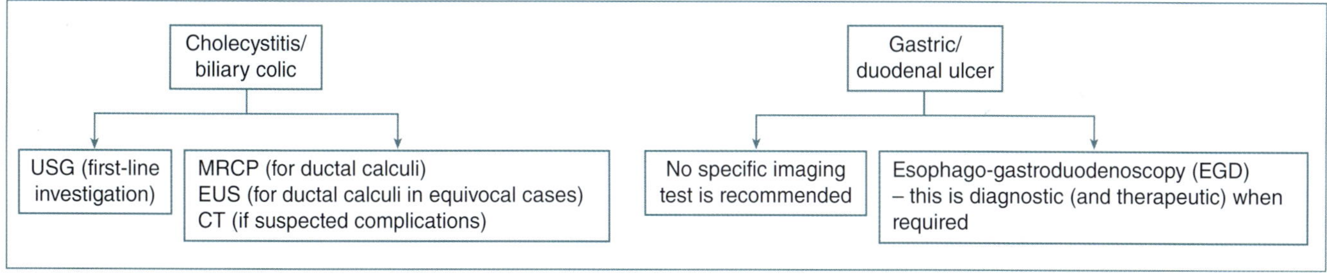

Figure 92.2 Imaging algorithm for the investigation of RUQ/epigastric pain.

contrast-enhanced CT (CECT) which has been found to be much more accurate. However, despite this lack of evidence, patients presenting to the emergency with acute abdominal pain will often have CXR and AXR as part of their work-up.

Ultrasonography

USG is used in the work-up of acute abdominal pain often when the patient is young and/or radiation exposure is an issue (e.g., pregnancy). It is often the first technique of choice when trying to establish or exclude a diagnosis of biliary colic/acute cholecystitis and acute appendicitis in a young patient. USG is also useful at investigating a point of maximal tenderness in the abdomen, hence often yielding the diagnosis versus clinical evaluation of that point of tenderness.

Multidetector Computed Tomography

The use of CECT in the evaluation of acute abdominal pain is now common practice and is regarded as the gold standard [4]. Although noncontrast CT may be an alternative [3], contrast administration improves accuracy. The exact CECT protocol used is decided by the reporting radiologist, but there is a consensus that portal venous phase imaging with an approximate delay of 70 seconds is recommended when imaging the abdomen for suspected GI/HPB causes of the abdominal pain [2,5].

Oral or rectal contrast medium (CM) is of little benefit when imaging patients with severe abdominal pain, as it delays the study, and the lack of contrast within the bowel loops does not appear to alter CT accuracy [6].

Magnetic Resonance Imaging (MRI)

Despite its lack of ionizing radiation and superior contrast resolution [7], MRI is not widely used in the acute abdominal setting due to the longer time taken. Patient co-operation and lack of motion are also difficult in acutely ill patients. Hence, the use of MRI in evaluating the acute abdomen is typically reserved for pregnant or pediatric patients where the radiation dose is an issue.

Hepatobiliary

There is a myriad of hepatobiliary causes for the acute abdomen ranging from acute cholecystitis to a hemorrhagic neoplasm. Imaging is key, as clinical examination and laboratory evaluation alone seldom reveals a specific diagnosis. CECT or USG are used in initial assessment, but the diagnosis may need further clarification with a nonurgent hepatobiliary MRI.

Gallbladder and Billiary System

Inflammation/Infection

Acute Cholecystitis

One of the most common causes of acute abdomen, 90% of cases are secondary to gallstones [8], the other 10% are due to severe illness or injury (acalculous cholecystitis), the latter having a worse prognosis. Approximately 40% of patients with acute cholecystitis develop complications, discussed ahead pictorially.

Imaging features

- USG is the technique of choice in initial assessment (Fig. 92.2) and allows assessment for the sonographic Murphy's sign, a reliable indicator of acute cholecystitis with a sensitivity of 92% [9]. USG and CT are less accurate for diagnosing acalculous cholecystitis compared with calculous cholecystitis.
- Gallbladder wall thickening in the presence of gallstones has a positive predictive value of 95% for the diagnosis of acute cholecystitis [9]. It is important to note that gallbladder wall thickening without tenderness may also be seen incidentally in conditions such as hypoalbuminemic states, hepatitis, and liver, renal, or heart failure, presumably due to raised portal or systemic venous pressures. The clinical picture will help differentiate. *Sonographic signs of acute cholecystitis include gallbladder wall thickening (>3 mm) or edema, gallbladder distension (>40 mm), and pericholecystic and perihepatic fluid* (Fig. 92.3).
- Acute cholecystitis on CT is associated with pericholecystic inflammatory fat stranding and fluid; hypo or hyperdense

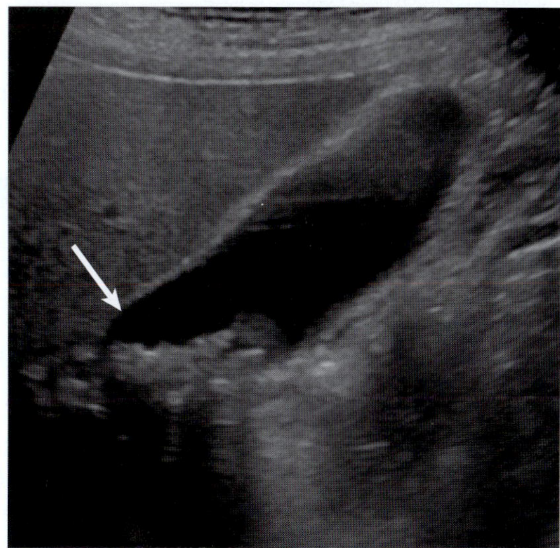

Figure 92.3 Dependent echogenic foci within the gallbladder lumen with posterior acoustic shadowing are typical USG appearances for gallstones.

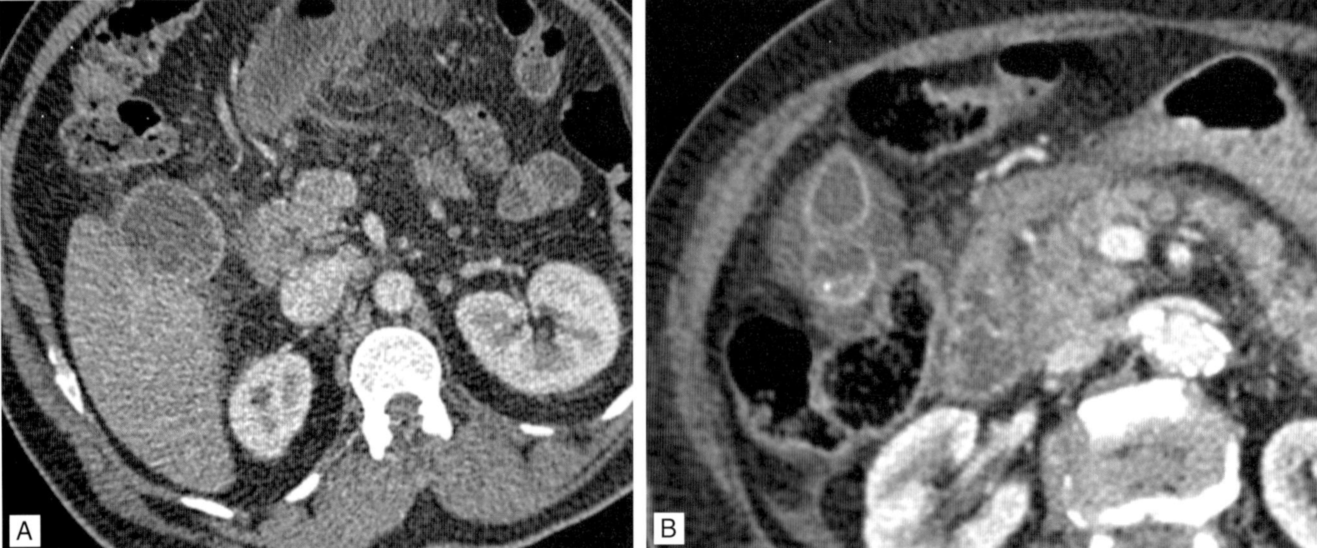

Figure 92.4 (A) Isodense gallstone in enhancing, thick-walled gallbladder with surrounding fat stranding in keeping with acute calculous cholecystitis. (B) Axial CT in another patient demonstrates hyperdense gallstones in the gallbladder with associated pericholecytsic fluid.

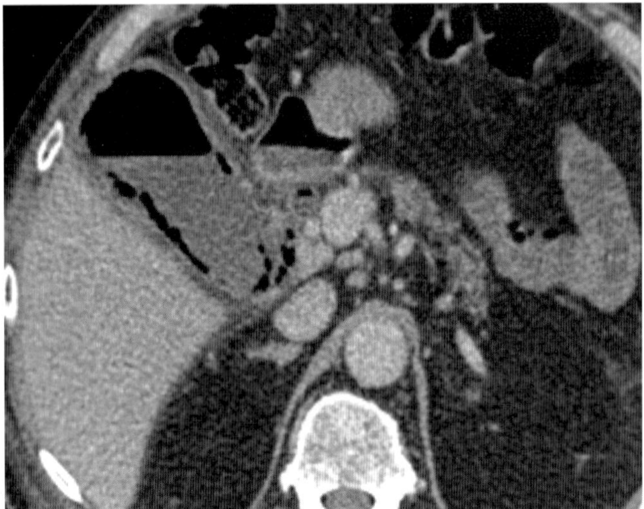

Figure 92.5 Intraluminal and intramural gas within inflamed gallbladder in keeping with emphysematous cholecystitis.

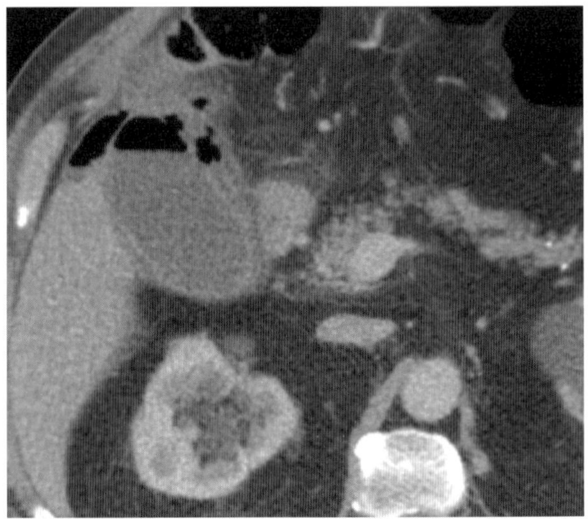

Figure 92.6 Gangrenous cholecystitis with wall which is poorly enhancing and has a perforation at its fundus.

gallstones and gallbladder fossa edema (Fig. 92.4). Complications of acute cholecystitis are better investigated with CT.

- Emphysematous cholecystitis is a serious complication typically diagnosed on CT by the presence of intraluminal or intramural gas, which could be mistaken for calculi on USG or MRI (Fig. 92.5). It is more commonly seen in diabetics and is usually associated with gas-forming organisms such as *Clostridium Welchi.*
- Gangrenous cholecystitis can occur in upto 39% of patients with acute calculous cholecystitis [10] and is associated with higher morbidity and mortality than uncomplicated cholecystitis. CECT findings of a poorly enhancing gallbladder wall, striated and reduced mural enhancement, and a pericholecystic abscess have been described with a specificity of approximately 90% in gangrenous cholecystitis [11]. Gangrenous cholecystitis can lead to perforation, usually at the fundus of the gallbladder [12] (Fig. 92.6).
- The three subtypes of gallbladder perforation include localized perforation, those that result in a cholecystoenteric fistula, and perforation with free intraperitoneal spillage and possibly loculated biloma formation. Despite the increased sensitivity of CT in detecting gallbladder perforation, a mural discontinuity is still only detected in 70% of cases [12].

Gallstone Ileus

This is diagnosed by the observation of *Rigler's triad, which comprises of pneumobilia, an ectopic gallstone, and bowel obstruction* (Fig. 92.7). CT is the technique of choice to demonstrate these signs as well as the cholecystoduodenal fistula and the level of small bowel obstruction. The culprit gallstone is usually larger than 2.5 cm. *Bouveret's syndrome* is a rare condition that results from the impaction of a discharged gallstone in the gastroduodenal junction, leading to gastric outlet obstruction.

Mirizzi Syndrome

This results from an impacted gallstone in the neck of the gallbladder or cystic duct causing extrinsic compression of the biliary tree and

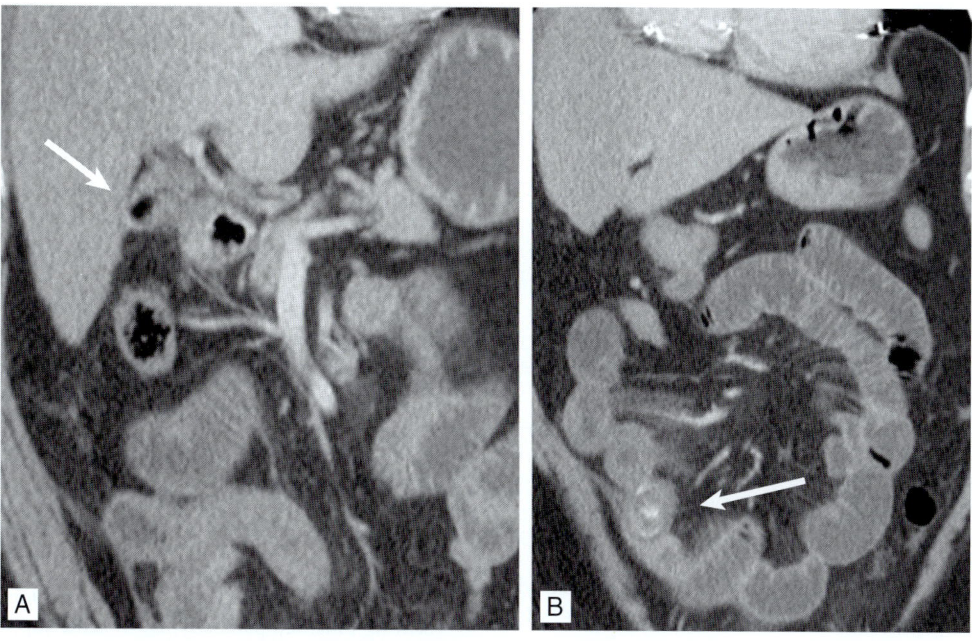

Figure 92.7 Intraluminal air within the gallbladder (*arrow* in A) in keeping with pneumobilia secondary to choleduodenal fistula as a result of the cholecystitis. Ectopic gallstone in distal ileum (*arrow* in B) causing proximal small bowel dilatation/obstruction.

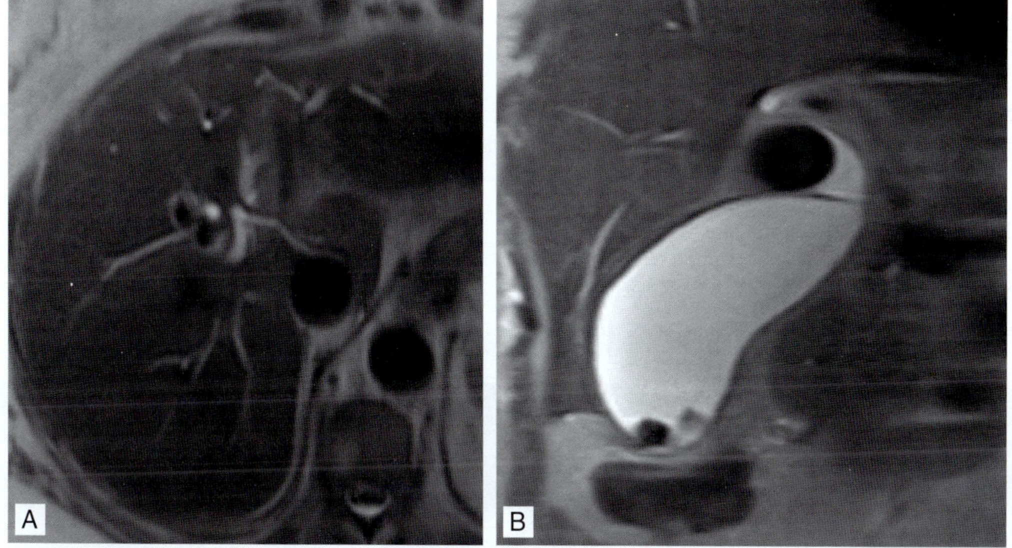

Figure 92.8 Axial T2w (A) and coronal T2w (B) sequences show a large gallstone in the gallbladder neck causing extrinsic compression of the CBD at the hilum and resultant mild upstream biliary dilatation.

resultant upstream intrahepatic biliary tree dilatation, in the context of a normal caliber CBD. These features are best demonstrated by magnetic resonance cholangiopancreatography (MRCP) (Fig. 92.8), although CECT can also be informative. A cholecystocholedochal fistula may form due to recurrent inflammation around the impacted gallstone in the cystic duct. Preoperative imaging can be extremely informative in this scenario as its presence and exact anatomy may warn the surgeon to perform an open cholecystectomy.

Biliary tree obstruction and ascending cholangitis:

- Biliary obstruction is highlighted by intrahepatic biliary dilatation with a transition point at the site of obstruction. The most common cause of biliary obstruction is choledocholithiasis; other etiologies include benign or malignant biliary strictures and parasitic disease (Table 92.1). Biliary obstruction and its

TABLE 92.1 Causes of Biliary Obstruction

Malignant Strictures	Benign Strictures
Cholangiocarcinoma	Primary sclerosing cholangitis
Carcinoma of the gallbladder	IgG4-related disease
Ampullary carcinoma	Mirizzi syndrome
Lymphoma	Recurrent pyogenic cholangitis
Intrabiliary metastasis	HIV cholangiopathy Sclerosing cholangitis induced by chemotherapy

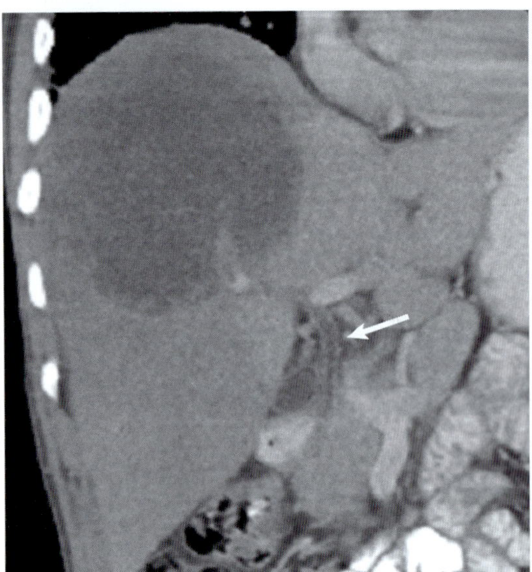

Figure 92.9 Cholangitis with cholangitic abscess formation. Note the enhancement along the CBD wall (*arrow*).

investigation is usually prompted by a clinically jaundiced patient with deranged cholestatic serum liver function tests.

- Initial assessment with a trans-abdominal USG can reliably detect biliary duct dilatation, where a cut off of 6 mm for a normal caliber common bile duct in a patient with no previous cholecystectomy can be used to evaluate biliary tree dilatation, as well as an intrahepatic bile duct caliber of 2 mm [13]. Trans-abdominal USG is however not as sensitive at detecting CBD stones [14]. CT is also good for demonstrating the biliary tree dilatation and the level of obstruction, but is poor at identifying choledocholithiasis (only 20% stones are high attenuation) [15]. MRCP is the investigation of choice when evaluating the biliary tree in obstructive jaundice.
- Biliary obstruction secondary to benign and malignant strictures does not necessarily occur acutely, but patients may present to the emergency department with obstructive jaundice and complicating cholangitis. Benign strictures are much less common than malignant ones, are often located at the hepatic hilum, and are usually iatrogenic or postoperative in etiology (e.g., postlaparoscopic cholecystectomy or postliver transplantation). Patients are usually asymptomatic but can occasionally present acutely. Biliary obstruction and subsequent stasis of bile within the biliary tree allows bacteremia to spread up from the duodenum [16] resulting in *ascending cholangitis*, which has a high mortality and usually requires urgent decompression, either percutaneously or endoscopically. Imaging allows the level of obstruction to be established and helps identify potential complications such as parenchymal abscess and portal vein thrombosis [17].
- Ascending cholangitis presents with an obstructed, dilated biliary tree along with smooth ductal wall thickening and enhancement (Fig. 92.9). Associated parenchymal inflammatory changes result in patchy and peribiliary parenchymal enhancement and wedge-shaped segments of hypoattenuation on CECT, representing inflamed parenchyma. In acute suppurative cholangitis, purulent dense material may be seen in the dilated biliary tree on CT [12] and will appear low signal relative to liver on T2-weighted MRI and intermediate on T1-weighted MRI [18]. Associated cholangitic abscesses may also be seen [19].

Liver

Acute Hepatitis

Acute hepatitis is usually secondary to a systemic infection by a viral agent. Probably the most important role of radiology in these patients is to rule out other diseases. At CT and MR imaging, findings in acute hepatitis are nonspecific and include hepatomegaly (Fig. 92.10) and periportal edema with heterogenous

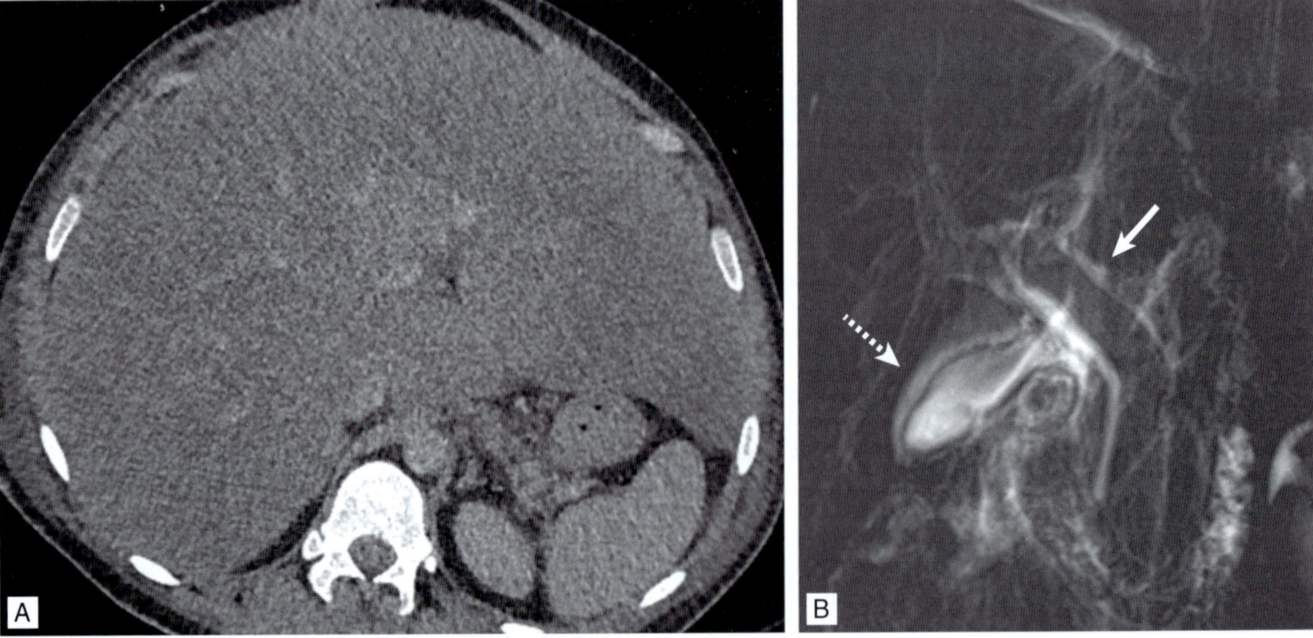

Figure 92.10 (A) Axial CT image demonstrates hepatomegaly in acute hepatitis secondary to hepatic steatosis. (B) Coronal MRCP projection of a different patient with hepatitis demonstrates periportal (*arrow*) and gall bladder wall edema (*dotted arrow*). *MRCP*, magnetic resonance cholangiopancreatography.

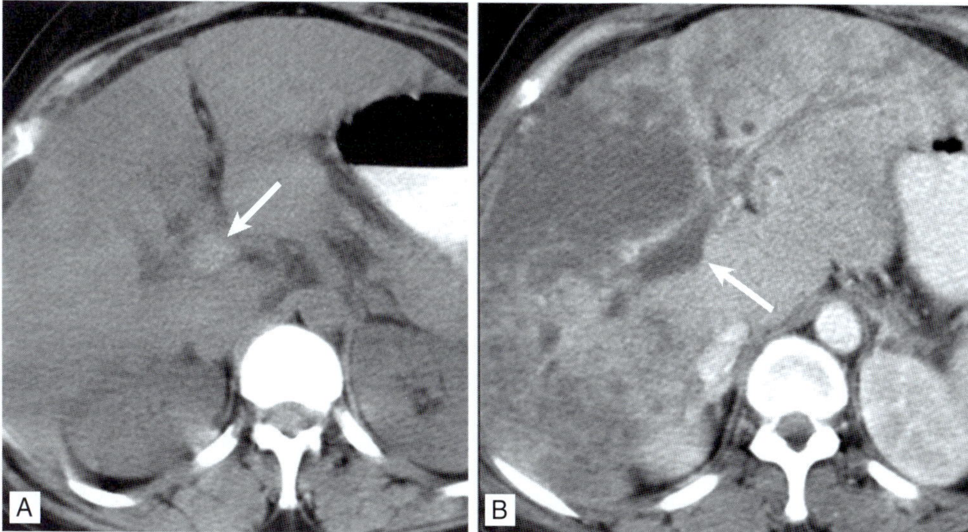

Figure 92.11 Noncontrast (A) and CECT (B) images demonstrate a hyperattenuating nonenhancing bland portal vein thrombus (*arrows*) with secondary perfusional abnormalities diffusely involving the liver.

TABLE 92.2 Imaging Features of Tumor Thrombus [18–20]

- US: Vascularity on color Doppler
- CT: Enhancement and expansion of portal vein on CECT
Enhancement and attenuation of thrombus similar to that of the tumor
- MRI: Similar SI to that of tumor
Restricted diffusion on DWI

enhancement of the liver parenchyma. Extra-hepatic findings include gallbladder wall edema and ascites.

Hepatic Vascular Disease

Portal vein thrombosis (PVT):

- PVT can be seen in many conditions including cirrhosis, abdominal tumors, and intra-abdominal inflammatory processes such as diverticulitis and appendicitis. PVT can be bland or tumoral (Table 92.2).
- Chronic PVT can result in the development of numerous periportal collateral vessels, which appear as a mass of veins in the porta hepatis. This is known as *cavernous transformation* and can occur 6–20 days after acute PVT [20]. These cavernomas and varices can cause secondary biliopathy due to the development of an ischemic stricture [21].
- PVT occurring secondary to infectious causes such as diverticulitis or appendicitis can present in a nonspecific manner clinically with fever, rigors, leukocytosis, and generalized abdominal pain. CECT becomes the investigation of choice to make the diagnosis. The imaging features include portal venous gas and low attenuation portal vein thrombus on the contrast-enhanced scan (Fig. 92.11). Occasionally acute thrombus can be seen as a hyper-attenuating density on a noncontrast CT. Secondary ancillary imaging findings may also include periportal edema and hepatic abscesses [22].
- Other causes of portal venous gas include bowel ischemia (most common) due to arterial or venous mesenteric thrombosis or intestinal obstruction [23]. Typically, peripheral branching air at CT helps differentiate portal venous gas from pneumobilia, which is typically more central.

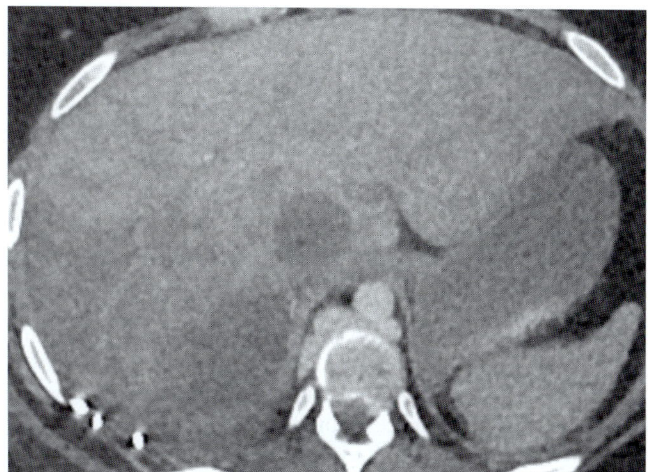

Figure 92.12 Thrombus in IVC and right hepatic vein (RHV) resulting in heterogenous enhancement of the liver.

Hepatic Vein Thrombosis and Budd–Chiari Syndrome

Budd–Chiari syndrome (BCS) results from hepatic venous outflow obstruction at the level of the hepatic veins or at the junction of the IVC and right atrium [24] (Fig. 92.12). BCS can be primary, with an endoluminal lesion such as a thrombus or web resulting in hepatic venous outflow obstruction, or secondary due to extrinsic compression by an adjacent mass.

Imaging features for BCS vary based on the extent and duration of the disease, but typically on Doppler USG there is absent, turbulent, or reversed flow in the hepatic veins, as well as hepatofugal flow in the portal vein [25]. CECT and CEMR are the investigations of choice in BCS [26]. In the arterial phase, differential contrast enhancement between the central and peripheral liver is usually seen, whereas in the portal venous phase there is washout in the central portion with increased peripheral hepatic parenchymal enhancement, known as the "flip-flop" pattern [27].

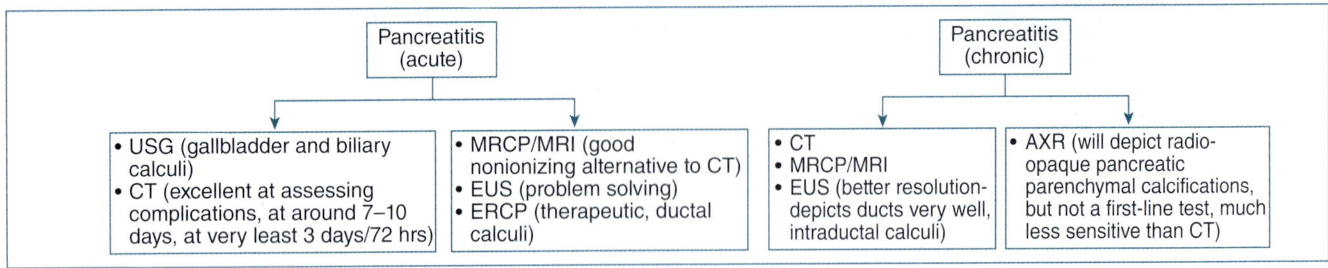

Figure 92.13 Imaging algorithm for pancreatitis according to RCR guidelines.

Pancreas

Acute Pancreatitis

Epidemiology

Acute pancreatitis is a condition that carries significant morbidity and mortality. It is the commonest pancreatic disease worldwide with no difference in incidence between genders [29]. The mortality rate ranges from 1 to 60 deaths per 100,000 people/year [29]. Alcohol-related pancreatitis is more prevalent in the Western world and Japan and has risen in parts of Asia.

Pathophysiology

A trigger such as gallstones or excess ethanol intake results in an insult to pancreatic acinar cells, resulting in the release of digestive enzymes and causing an inflammatory cytokine cascade, which can in severe cases cause a systemic inflammatory response syndrome [30].

Diagnostic Criteria: The revised Atlanta classification requires two or more conditions to be met for the diagnosis of acute pancreatitis:

- Abdominal pain
- Serum amylase or lipase level >3x upper limit of normal value
- Typical imaging findings [31].

Use of Imaging Modalities in Acute Pancreatitis: CECT is the imaging technique of choice for the assessment of acute pancreatitis and its complications (Fig. 92.13). A single portal venous phase is generally sufficient for this purpose, although supplementary arterial phase imaging can be helpful to assess for vascular complications. MRI is a good alternative (especially in cases of renal failure or contrast allergy) (Figs. 92.14 and 92.15). USG is an excellent technique for the detection of gallbladder calculi, besides being quick and inexpensive. The major drawback, however, is that the pancreas/peripancreatic tissues are often obscured by bowel gas [32].

Imaging can be performed at least 72 hours after the onset of symptoms, which allows time for complications to develop and any pancreatic necrosis to evolve. In the early phase of acute pancreatitis there can often be a mismatch between imaging findings and severity of disease, with a reduced sensitivity for the detection of necrotizing pancreatitis. However, imaging studies may be performed at an earlier stage in the disease to assess for an underlying treatable etiology such as calculi, or pancreatic malignancy [31]. If imaging is performed at least a week after the onset of symptoms, it allows more time for complications to develop and any pancreatic necrosis should be readily demonstrable.

Imaging is used in the later stages of the disease course for identification of complications, monitoring of existing collections, and guiding interventional procedures [32]. MRI can be very useful for the identification and follow-up of pancreatitis-related complications, for example, in distinguishing solid from liquid components or debris within collections, when this may be more difficult to ascertain on CT. This can then guide management, for example, drainage or surgery, and may ascertain the reason for the failure of drainage in an acute necrotic collection (ANC) or walled-off necrosis (WON) which has a high

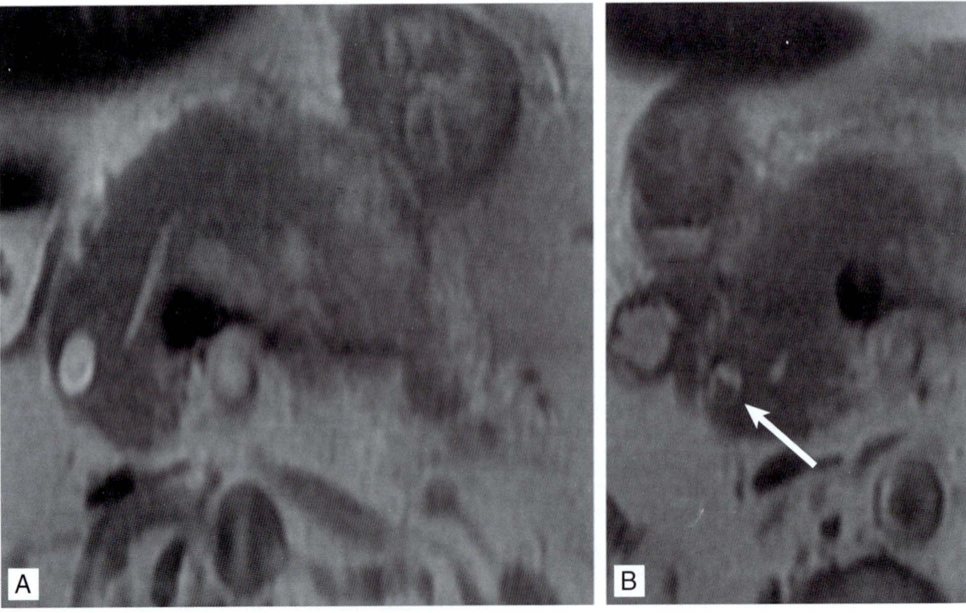

Figure 92.14 Acute gallstone pancreatitis. T2W coronal (A) and axial (B) demonstrate edematous body and tail of the pancreas with peripancreatic fluid and fat stranding. A calculus can be seen in the distal CBD (*arrow*).

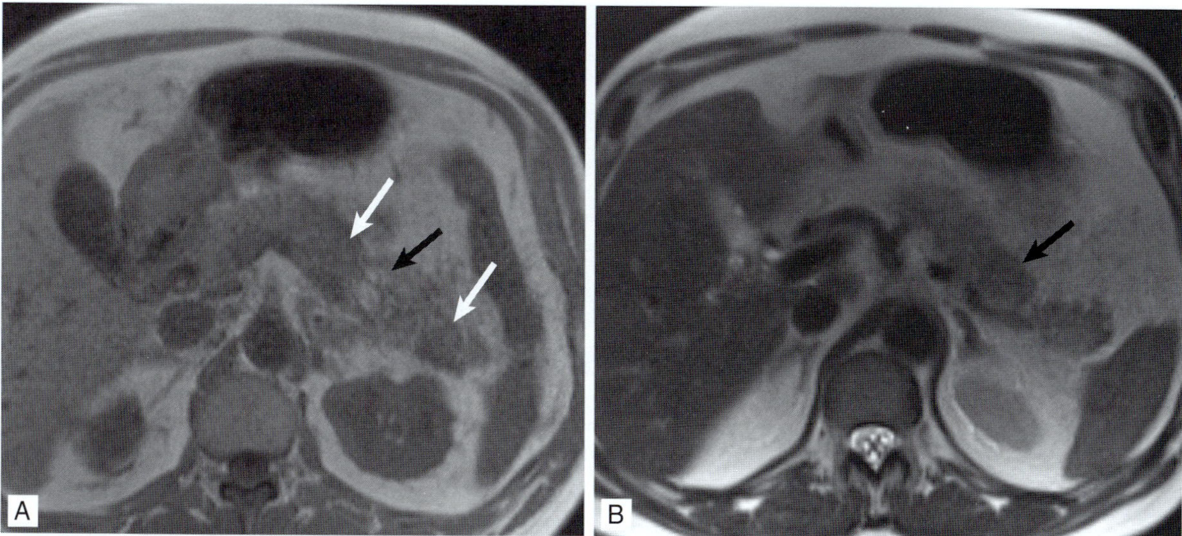

Figure 92.15 Acute hemorrhagic pancreatitis. Peripancreatic inflammatory stranding surrounding the body and tail of pancreas. The T1-weighted image (A) demonstrates low-signal changes (*white arrows*) demonstrating interstitial edema. Focal high-signal change is also visible within the gland (*black arrow*) in keeping with hemorrhagic change. Corresponding area is marked with an *arrow* on the T2-weighted sequence (B).

proportion of solid material. In this instance, the drain may require upsizing or necrosectomy may be opted for.

To apply the relevant nomenclature when reporting imaging studies using the Atlanta classification, it should be noted that the first day of onset of acute pancreatitis coincides with the first day the patient experiences pain and not when they first seek medical help.

Acute pancreatitis is split into early (<7 days) and late (>7 days) phases. Patients whose clinical course terminates within the early phase and who do not present with local complications or features of organ failure are classed as having mild acute pancreatitis with very low mortality rates. Patients with a clinical course lasting beyond 7 days with local complications and transient organ failure lasting <48 hours are classed as having moderately severe acute pancreatitis. Patients in the severe acute pancreatitis group will experience organ failure for >48 hours.

Imaging Characteristics of Acute Pancreatitis

- *Acute pancreatitis can be divided into two categories: interstitial edematous pancreatitis (IEP) and necrotizing pancreatitis* (Figs. 92.16 and 92.17). In IEP, the pancreatic parenchyma can enhance homogenously or show areas of reduced enhancement, due to interstitial edema. There is often enlargement of the gland and surrounding inflammatory change, small volume free fluid, and occasionally, peripancreatic fluid collections.

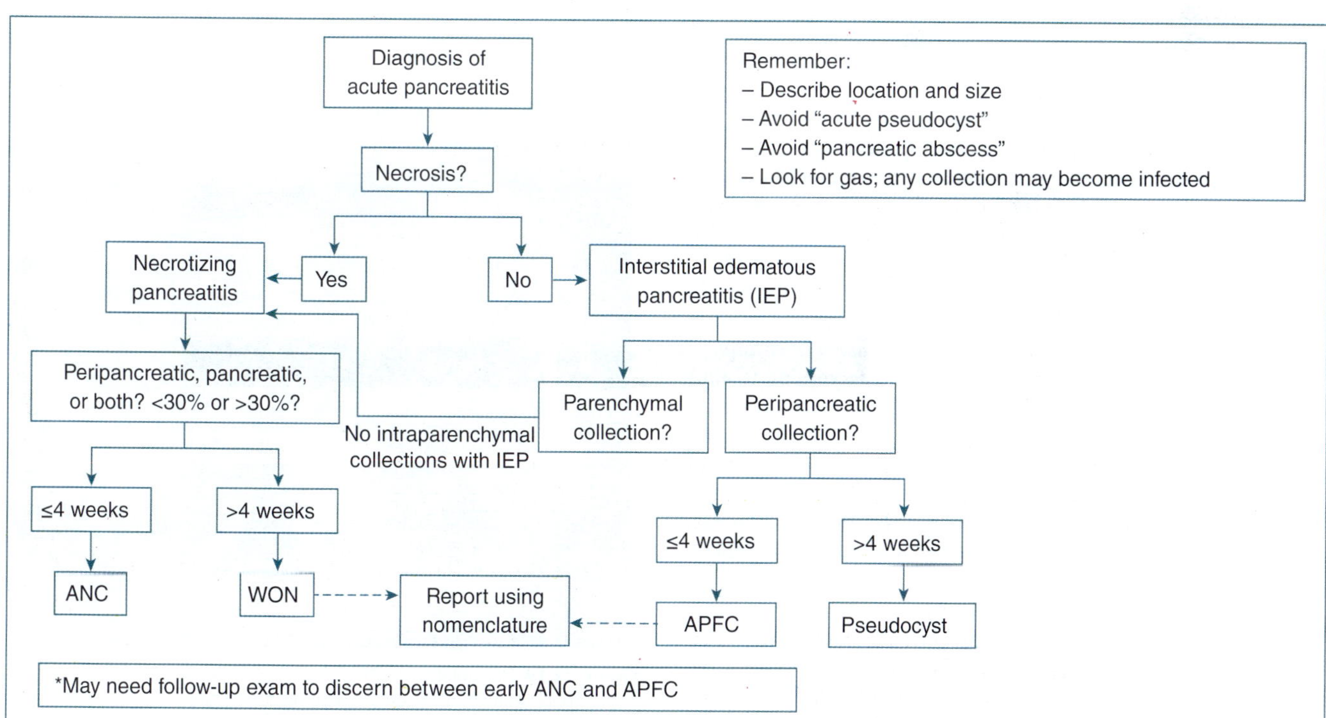

Figure 92.16 Decision tree for reporting according to the revised Atlanta classification. Taken from Radiographics: Revised Atlanta classification for Acute Pancreatitis: A Pictorial Essay (2019).

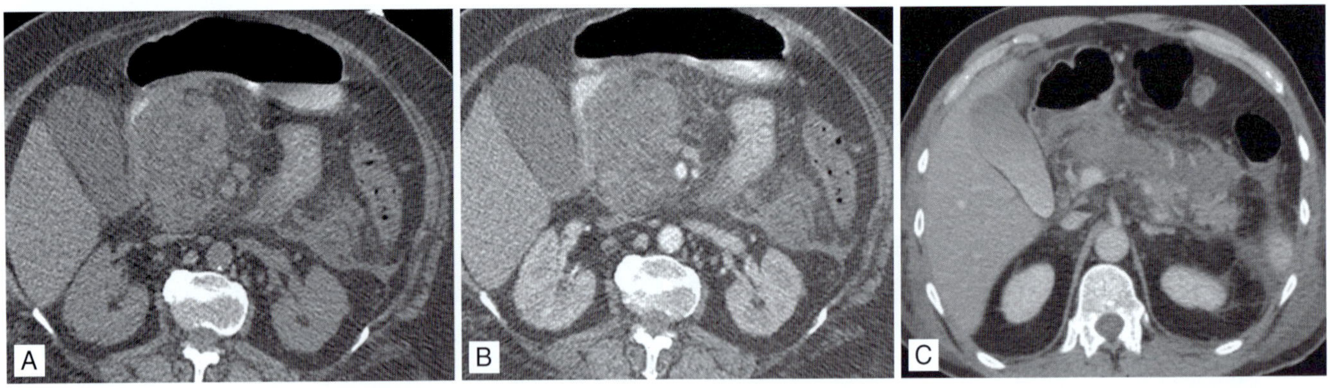

Figure 92.17 (A and B) Axial noncontrast and contrast CT images of acute peripancreatic fluid collection. Two weeks post onset of abdominal pain. Fluid attenuation collection adjacent to the pancreatic head and uncinate process with no discernible wall. (C) Acute necrotic collection. Two days after onset of abdominal pain. A large proportion of the pancreatic parenchyma is replaced by necrotic fluid and there is no discernible wall. There are intervening areas of intact parenchyma.

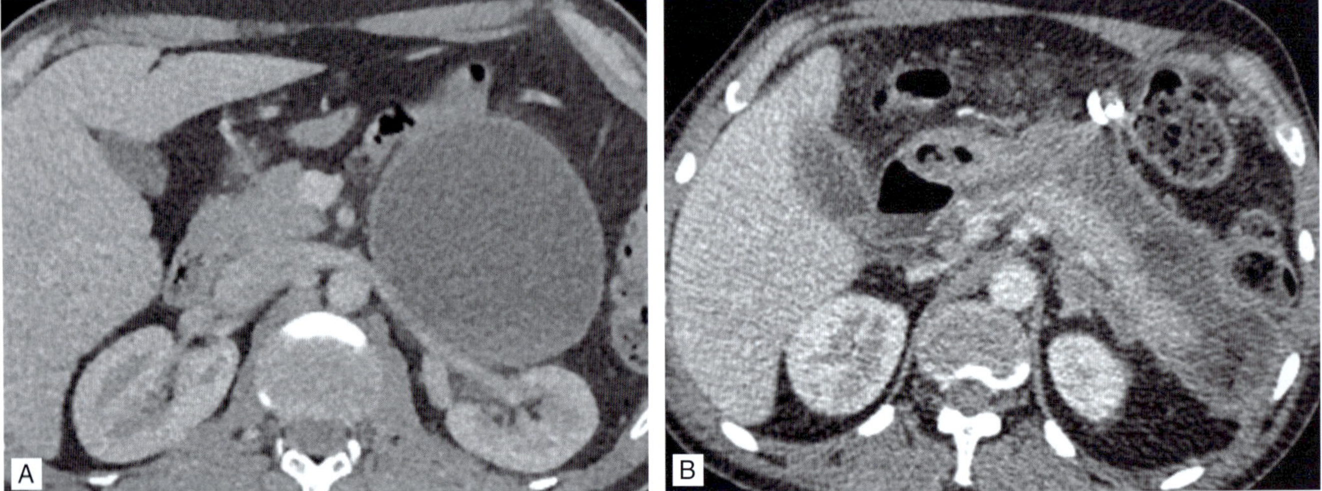

Figure 92.18 (A) Pseudocyst. Four weeks postonset of abdominal pain. Large peripancreatic fluid attenuation collection. There are no solid-appearing components or fat globules. (B) Walled-off necrosis. Study was performed 2 months after initial presentation. Areas of fat density can be seen interspersed amongst the peripancreatic fluid collections, which are well organized with enhancing walls.

Necrotizing pancreatitis makes up 5–10% of cases of acute pancreatitis and can be pancreatic only, peripancreatic only, or combined pancreatic and peripancreatic. It is important to note that not all pancreatitis-related collections are solely composed of fluid and may contain nonliquefied components such as fat. *The phrase "pancreatic abscess" has fallen out of favor and should no longer be used in reporting terminology. Similarly, "acute pseudocyst" should not be used as a general term to describe any pancreatitis-related collection, because not all are solely composed of fluid.*

- The Atlanta classification groups collections according to time scale (4 weeks being the cut-off) into acute peripancreatic fluid collections (APFC), ANC, pseudocyst, and WON (Fig. 92.18). Collections containing nonliquefied components, whether fat or soft tissue (even if in small quantities), are considered necrotic).
- *An uncommon complication of acute pancreatitis is disconnection of the main pancreatic duct,* due to ductal necrosis. The pancreatic segment upstream of the necrosis becomes isolated from the duodenum. A persistent end-fistula results, with continuous leakage of pancreatic secretions into peripancreatic tissues. *Recognition of this entity may avoid the need for unnecessary conservative drainage procedures which are unlikely to be effective.* The key sign of a disconnected duct is an intraparenchymal focus of necrosis or collection, with a viable segment of parenchyma upstream (Fig. 92.19). The upstream duct may or may

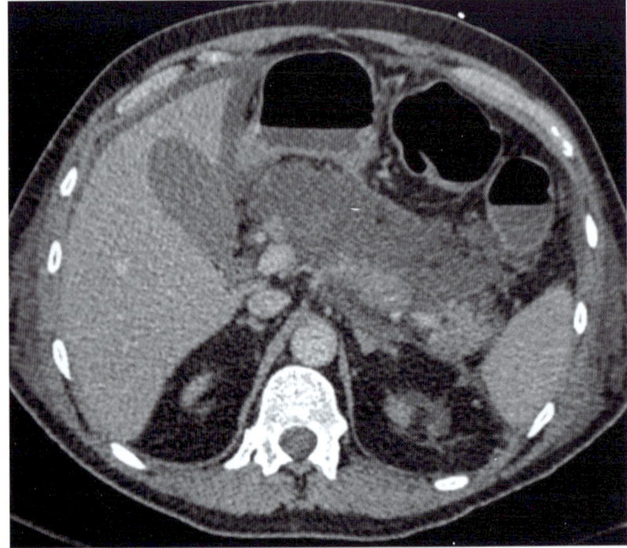

Figure 92.19 Developing WON. This patient is also at risk of a disconnected pancreatic duct. There are interdigitating areas of intact pancreatic parenchyma. Fat globules are also visible. The collection is beginning to organize with the development of an enhancing wall anteriorly, although this is incomplete toward the tail of pancreas.

not be dilated. A confident diagnosis of disconnected duct requires: (1) necrosis of ≥20 mm of pancreas, (2) viable upstream pancreatic tissue, (3) extravasation of contrast injected into the main pancreatic duct at ERCP [33].

- Pancreatitis-related collections can become infected. *On imaging, gas within a collection is the only definitive finding suggestive of this.* It is also important to exclude fistulous communication with a hollow viscus and any previous intervention (sampling or drainage) (Fig. 92.20). *The presence of wall enhancement implies that a collection has matured/organized and is seen in both pseudocysts and WON. Therefore, it is not a reliable marker of infection* [44]. Pseudoaneurysms are another important but potentially treatable complication of acute pancreatitis, usually seen in arteries adjacent to the pancreas such as the splenic artery, gastroduodenal artery, or its branches (Fig. 92.20). This is explained in more detail in the section on splenic artery pseudoaneurysm section.

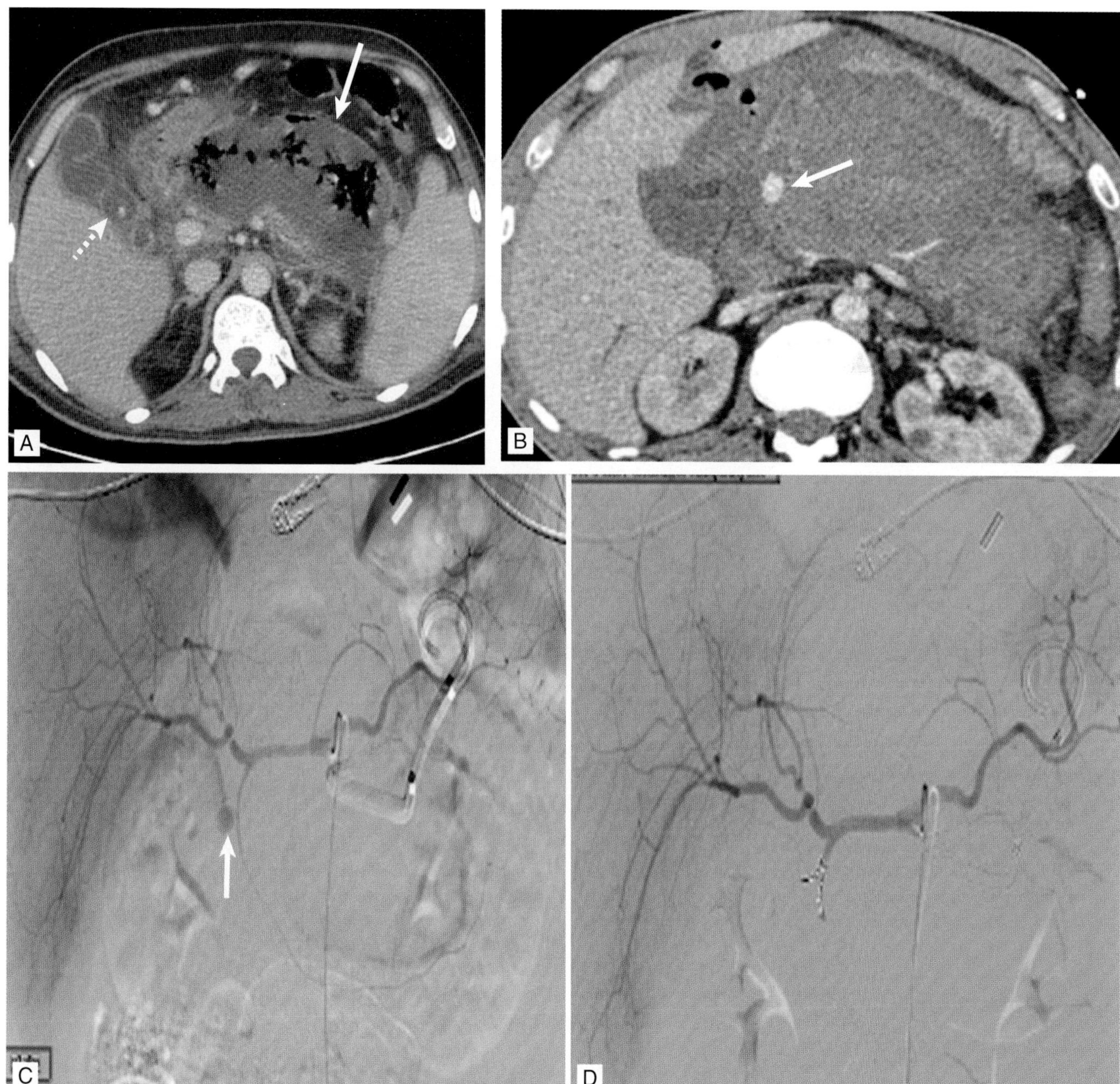

Figure 92.20 (A) Gas-containing pancreatic peripancreatic collection (*solid arrow*). Patient with acute pancreatitis presented with signs of sepsis, 2 weeks after start of symptoms. A calcified gall stone is also seen (*dotted arrow*). (B) Status day 8 of acute pancreatitis in another patient. Axial CECT image reveals hemorrhage into a pseudocyst. A pseudoaneurysm is visible (*arrow*) and there is dependent contrast material, indicating active bleeding. (C and D) Celiac axis digital subtraction angiogram. The bleeding point is identified in the superior pancreaticoduodenal artery (SPA), arising from the gastroduodenal artery (GDA) (*arrow*). The second image demonstrates coils placed across the GDA and SPA, achieving homeostasis.

Key Points: Acute Pancreatitis

- Day 1 of the presentation of acute pancreatitis corresponds to the first day the patient experiences pain.
- Imaging for acute pancreatitis should be performed a minimum of 3 days to over a week after the onset of symptoms, which increases the sensitivity of detection of complications (particularly pancreatic necrosis).
- The phrases "pancreatic abscess" and "acute pseudocyst" can be misleading and should be avoided.
- In the early phase ≤4 weeks, pancreatitis-related collections are classified as either APFC or ANC, according to absence/presence of nonliquid components. In the late phase > 4 weeks, pancreatitis-related collections are classified either as pseudocysts or WON, according to absence/presence of nonliquid components.
- Disconnected duct is an important, uncommon complication. Identification can obviate the need for ineffective conservative drainage measures.
- The presence of gas in a collection is the only reliable sign of infection. Other causes should be excluded before this diagnosis, e.g., fistula with a hollow viscus, prior intervention. Wall enhancement is seen in both pseudocyst and WON and is not a reliable indicator of infection.

What to Include in the Radiology Report

- Necrosis (present or absent)? Location
- % of gland involved
- Complications? Location(s)
- Evidence of disconnected duct?
- Fluid-containing collection? Or, nonliquefied component?
- Rim-enhancing/walled collection? Any gas?
- Subtype of pancreatitis? (IEP or necrotizing)
- Name type of collection(s) (according to Atlanta classification)
- Mention use of Atlanta classification

TABLE 92.3 Causes of Splenic Infarction

Inflow Disruption	Intrinsic Splenic Circulatory Disruption	Outflow Disruption
Splenic artery thrombus/embolus Vasculitides	Hemoglobinopathies, for example, sickle cell anemia Lymphoproliferative disorders Vasculitides Hypercoagulable states, for example, factor V Leiden mutation, malignancy	Splenic vein thrombosis Hypercoagulable states Pancreatitis Portal hypertension

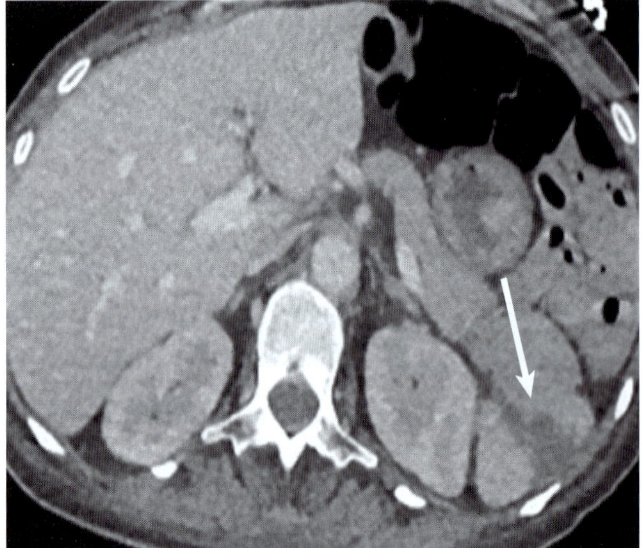

Figure 92.21 Splenic infarction (*arrow*).

Spleen

Albeit infrequent, it is important to recognize some key splenic emergencies, especially given that the spleen is a highly vascular organ and prone to severe hemorrhage. As with acute pancreatitis, CT is the primary technique for assessment of splenic emergencies, with USG used in follow-up to assess for evolution and is limited in primary assessment [34,35].

Splenic Infarction

Splenic infarction can arise as a result of an interruption to the inflow of blood to the spleen (arterial supply), congestion of the internal splenic circulation, or reduced venous outflow, resulting in indirect impedance to inflow via increased hydrostatic pressure (see Table 92.3) [36–38]. In the early stages of splenic ischemia, the affected area is edematous due to the inflammatory insult, giving rise to poorly demarcated areas of reduced attenuation/hypoechogenicity. With time, the edema evolves into well-defined wedge-shaped areas of lower hypoattenuation/hypoechogenicity (Fig. 92.21). Chronic changes include volume loss in the affected area and calcification [34,35].

Splenic Venous and Arterial Thrombosis

Splenic venous thrombosis is a fairly common sequela of pancreatic cancer, and less commonly pancreatitis [34]. Splenic artery thrombosis, on the other hand, is a relatively rare entity. *Complete arterial occlusion (Fig. 92.22) can result in infarction of the entire spleen, but preserved capsular enhancement, as the splenic capsule is supplied by the short gastric arteries* [39].

Splenic Artery Aneurysm

Most are detected incidentally and are asymptomatic, with a quoted prevalence ranging between 0.2% and 10.4%. The etiology is unclear but associated with hypertension, cirrhosis, portal hypertension, pregnancy, and liver transplant. The rate of rupture is reported at around 2–3% and patients will present with a combination of sudden left upper quadrant abdominal pain, hypovolemic shock and gastrointestinal hemorrhage. Most splenic artery aneurysms are small, often <3 cm, and usually

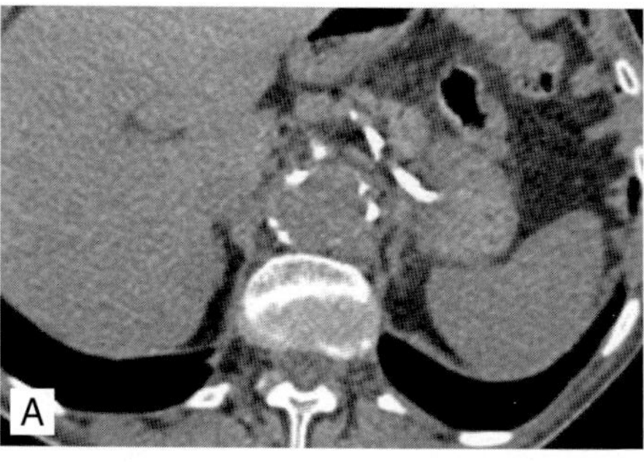

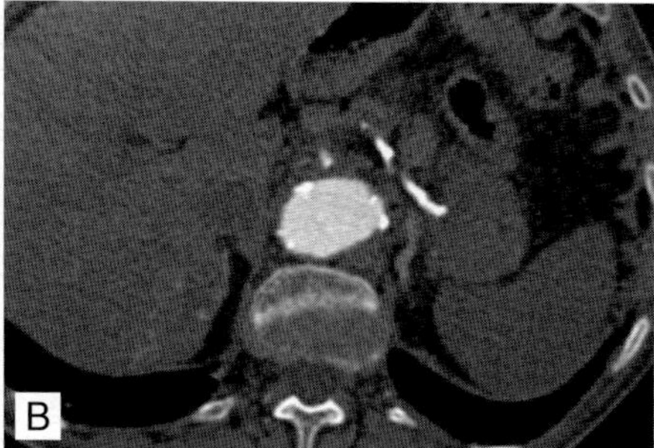

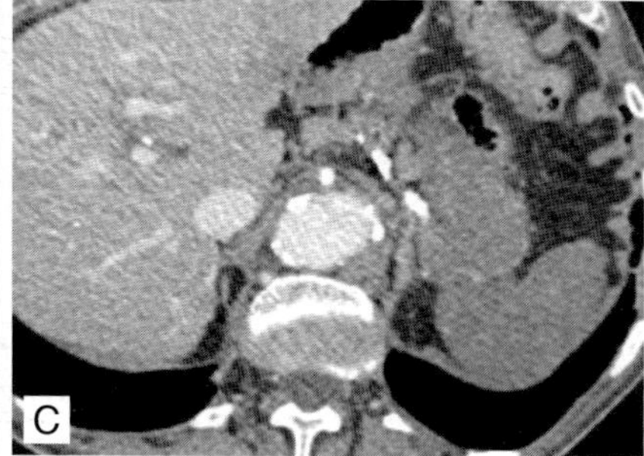

Figure 92.22 Splenic artery occlusion. Axial precontrast (A), arterial (B), and delayed (C) phase acquisitions. Precontrast phase image demonstrates heavy calcific atheromatous disease of the splenic artery. No splenic artery opacification is evident in the arterial phase, with absence of the typical "zebra" pattern of splenic parenchymal enhancement. The delayed phase image demonstrates lack of splenic enhancement, consistent with ischemic change.

located at the distal aspect of the artery. *Asymptomatic aneurysms ≥20 mm or asymptomatic high-risk groups* (portal hypertension, pregnancy, and liver transplant) *should be treated to avoid future risk of rupture* [40,41].

Aneurysms in the proximal and middle thirds of the splenic artery can be safely resected with splenic preservation. In the distal third, splenectomy ± distal pancreatectomy is the preferred option [42,43]. Endovascular treatment has reduced rates of success (75–85%) [43] compared with open surgery but avoids the associated perioperative complications [44] (Fig. 92.23).

Splenic Artery Pseudoaneurysm

Pseudoaneurysms of the splenic artery usually always present with symptoms, in contrast to splenic artery aneurysms [41]. The most frequent symptoms include abdominal pain, melena or hematochezia, pancreatic duct hemorrhage, and hematemesis [40]. The risk of rupture in pseudoaneurysm is much higher than in true aneurysm (up to 37% in one center) as it is invariably associated with coexisting disease, for example, pancreatitis or peptic ulcer and hence timely intervention is critical [41,45]. *The pathologic hallmark of a true aneurysm is that it contains all three layers of the arterial wall, whereas a pseudoaneurysm only contains the tunica media and intima, indicative of a mural breach* [41]. At rupture, high mortality rates of up to 90% are reported [45].

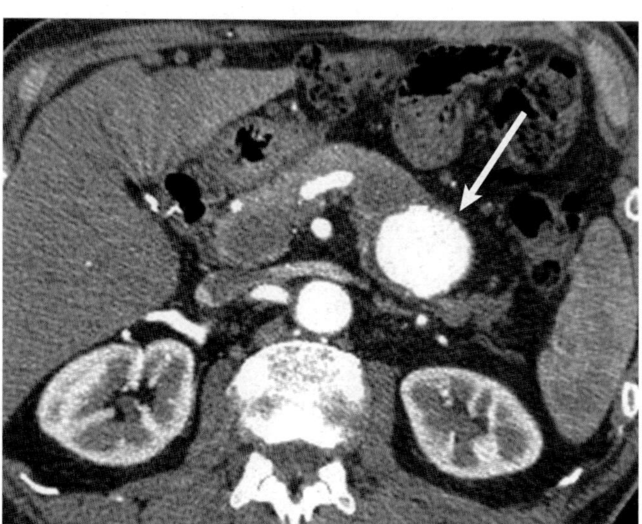

Figure 92.23 Splenic artery aneurysm. Axial arterial phase CT image demonstrates a 30 mm splenic artery aneurysm (*arrow*). The patient underwent successful coil embolization (not shown).

On CT imaging, pseudoaneurysms can be of higher attenuation than adjacent tissues on noncontrast imaging and enhance avidly postcontrast administration (Fig. 92.20). Adjacent hematoma and or thrombus may also be present. Splenic artery pseudoaneurysms have been found within peripancreatic pseudocysts as small foci of enhancement surrounded by low-attenuation fluid [46,47].

Splenic Sequestration

A rare consequence of sickle-cell anemia, acute splenic sequestration crisis (ASSC) occurs when large volumes of sickle-shaped cells become trapped in the splenic microcirculation. This, in turn, results in massive splenomegaly, reduction in circulating red blood cells, and anemia. The splenic enlargement results in mechanical stretching of the capsule causing discomfort and pain. If left untreated, the spleen can rupture which will result in severe hemorrhage and death. *Radiological features of this condition include splenic enlargement, patency of the splenic artery, and vein and peripheral parenchymal lesions,* which are hypoattenuating on CT (or reduced echogenicity on US) and hyperintense on T1/T2-weighted MRI sequences, postulated to be due to sub-acute hemorrhage [34,48]. Blood flow within the splenic vein is maintained due to retrograde flow from the portal vein [34].

Acute Splenic Infection/Abscess

The spleen can be a source of primary or secondary infection. Primary splenic infection with abscess formation is rare [49,50]. There is usually an underlying etiological factor such as infective bacterial endocarditis, intravenous drug abuse, alcohol abuse, trauma, hemoglobinopathies, hematological malignancy, and other immunocompromised states [39].

Pyogenic abscess usually presents as a single hypoattenuating or hypoechoic lesion on CT/USG, which may also demonstrate internal septations, a hyperenhancing rim, and gas. The presence of the latter two findings on imaging is specific for the diagnosis [34] (Fig. 92.24). *Streptococcus viridians* and *Klebsiella pneumoniae* are common pathogens implicated in pyogenic splenic abscess [50]. Multiple abscesses/microabscesses are more commonly observed in the setting of immunocompromised patients, often due to *Candida albicans* infection and less commonly with other pathogens such as *Mycobacterium tuberculosis, Pneumocystis jiroveci,* and *Histoplasma capsulatum*. An important mimic of splenic abscess, infarct, and laceration is lymphoma, which can present as single or multiple splenic lesions. High FDG PET-CT uptake can indicate the diagnosis [51].

Key Points: Non-Traumatic Acute Splenic Pathologies

- Complete arterial occlusion can result in infarction of the entire spleen, but preserved capsular enhancement, as the splenic capsule is supplied by the short gastric arteries.
- Splenic artery aneurysms are often detected incidentally. The risk of rupture is increased with portal hypertension, pregnancy, and liver transplant. Asymptomatic aneurysms ≥20 mm or asymptomatic high-risk groups should be treated to avoid the future risk of rupture. MPR/curved MPR can be useful in differentiating splenic artery aneurysms from hypervascular pancreatic neoplasms, for example, NET.
- Pseudoaneurysms of the splenic artery almost always present with symptoms, in contrast to splenic artery aneurysms. The risk of rupture is greater than for true aneurysm and prompt diagnosis and treatment is required to avoid serious morbidity/mortality. On imaging, pseudoaneurysms will follow the blood pool on the arterial and delayed phase imaging. Contrast this with active hemorrhage, where CM accumulates over time on imaging phases and is not focal/well-circumscribed.
- Specific features of pyogenic splenic abscess: a rim-enhancing parenchymal lesion and presence of gas within the lesion.
- Microabscesses are more common in immunocompromised patients.
- Radiological features of ASSC: splenic enlargement, patency of the splenic artery/vein, and peripheral parenchymal lesions.

What to Include in the Radiology Report: Acute Splenic Pathologies

Any parenchymal lesions?
- Solitary/Multiple
- Size?
- Position?
- Shape?

Preserved capsular enhancement?
Intralesional gas? Rim-enhancing lesion?
Patency of the splenic vasculature—any thrombus?

Gastrointestinal Tract

Gastric and Duodenal Ulcer

Peptic ulcers can penetrate deep to the serosa and lead to perforation. The known risk factors are infection by Helicobacter pylori, use of NSAIDS or corticosteriods, and Zollinger–Ellison disease, amongst others [52]. Duodenal ulcers are two to three times more frequent compared to gastric ulcers, with the duodenal bulb being the most common location. The most common location of gastric ulcers is the lesser curvature, posterior wall of the body or antrum.

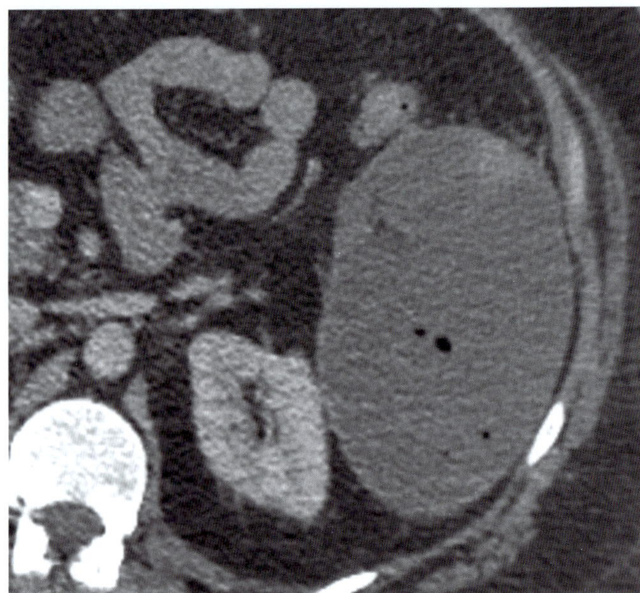

Figure 92.24 Infected splenic abscess, containing gas locules.

Clinically, the patient has epigastric pain not relieved by food or antacids.

Most often an MDCT scan with or without oral contrast is done when the patient presents with an acute abdomen [53]. A superficial ulcer is often not visualized, while deeper ulcers are usually seen as an outpouching of contrast in the gastric or duodenal wall. There is often associated wall thickening and luminal narrowing of the stomach or duodenum associated with submucosal edema and surrounding inflammatory fat stranding [54].

If the ulcer has eroded through the gastric or duodenal wall, free air can be detected in the peritoneal cavity or retroperitoneal fat (Fig. 92.25). The ulcer can also erode through a small artery leading to extravasation and pooling of contrast in the lumen of the stomach and duodenum with the patient vomiting large amounts of blood. An underlying carcinoma is associated with a small percentage of duodenal

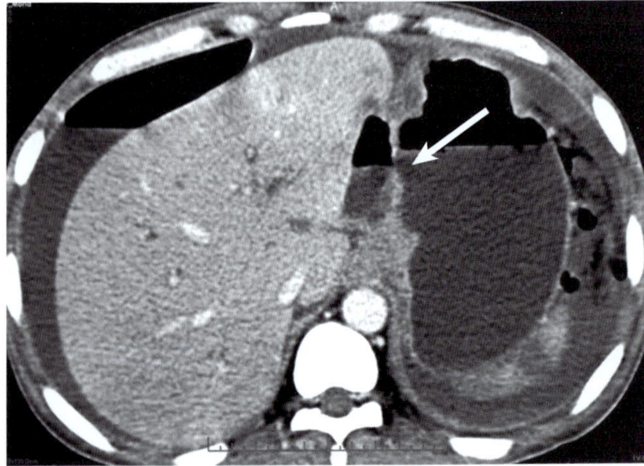

Figure 92.25 Axial CECT demonstrates a defect in the gastric wall (*arrow*) with fluid collection adjacent to it, consistent with a perforated ulcer, with pneumoperitoneum and ascites.

(<1%) and gastric (<5%) ulcers; enlarged lymphhodes or focal liver lesions should raise suspicion [55].

Appendicitis

Pathophysiology and Clinical Features

The appendix is a blind tube that arises from the cecal pole, consisting histologically of the same elements as rest of the gastrointestinal tract. The acute inflammation of the appendix is related to obstruction of its lumen. The physiopathology of this obstruction is related to an appendicolith/foreign body or hypertrophy of the lymphoid tissue (Peyer's patch) in the appendix. The build-up of secretions in the appendix leads to distension, inflammation, venous congestion with exudation, and finally necrosis and perforation [56]. When there are only local inflammatory changes in the appendix with no evidence of abscess or perforation, it is often designed as "simple appendicitis." However, when there is an associated inflammatory collection (abscess) or perforation, the term "complicated appendicitis" is often used [57].

Appendicitis is common, involving 7% of all individuals in the western world [58]. There is no age or gender preponderance. The most common symptoms are periumbilical pain radiating to the right lower quadrant. However, up to one-third of patients have atypical symptoms and the diagnosis is only made on imaging. Blood tests are highly variable and therefore not reliable.

Imaging Features

- The best imaging modalities are USG and CECT [59]. The sensitivity and specificity (95% each) of MDCT has been shown in multiple studies to be slightly better compared to USG (sensitivity 85%, specificity 90%) [60]. However, USG is usually the first technique for investigation due to the easy access and absence of radiation.
- Abdominal radiographs are usually not contributive in the acute setting, but can show a calcified appendicolith in 5–10% cases, air-fluid levels in the right lower quadrant ileal loops due to ileus, effacement of the right psoas margin or free intraperitoneal air when there is perforation [61].
- The best diagnostic sign for appendicitis is the size of the appendix. Studies have shown that a cut-off of >6 mm yields a sensitivity of 100% but a low specificity of 64%. However, when a cut-off of ≥7 mm is used, the sensitivity decreases to 94% but the specificity increased to 88% [59]. Therefore in current practice 6 mm is preferred as the cut-off to safely exclude disease.
- On grayscale USG, appendicitis is seen as a noncompressible tubular aperistaltic blind-ending structure at the tip of the cecum which is distended and measures ≥7 mm in diameter (Fig. 92.26). The appendix is usually located by finding the ascending colon and moving inferiorly to identify the cecum. The appendix usually lies just inferior to the cecal pole. The appendicolith can be visualized as an echogenic focus with posterior shadowing. The operator can trigger focal pain over the appendix by positioning and pressing the probe on the appendicitis (sonographic "McBurney" sign). Often, there is a small amount of hypoechoic fluid in the right lower quadrant. In complicated cases, an abscess or collection is usually seen. Color Doppler shows increased flow within the wall of the appendix [62].
- MDCT is usually performed when USG is inconclusive or when there is high suspicion of appendiceal perforation or in obese patients, both of which can decrease USG image quality (Fig. 92.27) [63]. The appendix is usually dilated and measures >7 mm, with abnormal enhancement of the appendiceal wall with mucosal hyperattenuation and submucosal mural edema and hypoenhancement. There is usually associated periappendiceal fat stranding and the dense appendicolith is often visualized. The cecum can be also thickened and there is also often focal dilatation and air/fluid levels in the terminal ileum.

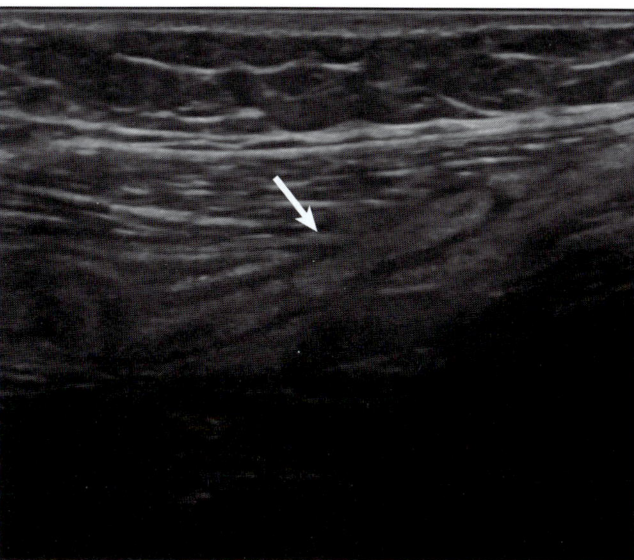

Figure 92.26 Appendicitis seen on USG. The appendix (*arrow*) is seen as a distended tubular structure (>7 mm) extending from the cecum. The echogenic lining represents the mucosa and the low echogenic band surrounding it is the muscular layer.

- In necrotic appendicitis, there is no enhancement of the appendix and in complicated, perforated appendicitis hypoattenuation of the mucosa and muscular layers can be seen with mural defects, often with a collection that lies close to the cecum or in the pelvic peritoneal recesses (recto-vesical or recto-uterine cul de sac). In cases of perforation, there may also be small air locules below the anterior abdominal wall and diaphragm.
- The differential diagnosis on clinical examination includes omental infarction (fat infarction of the omentum), which also presents with right lower quadrant pain and tenderness (without fever). This can be easily differentiated in radiology as it presents as a focal area of omental fat stranding, often with a hyperattenuating rim.
- The treatment of noncomplicated appendicitis usually involves antibiotics and early surgery. In complicated appendicitis, antibiotic therapy, radiological drainage of the abscesses/collections, and surgery are the treatment of choice [64].

Diverticulitis

Pathophysiology and Clinical Features

Diverticulitis is inflammation of colonic diverticula, which are acquired herniation of mucosa and submucosa through the muscular layers of the colon. The simple outpouching of diverticula through the colonic wall without inflammation is called diverticulosis. Diverticula are small saccular outpouchings of the colon and measure 0.5–1 cm. The pathophysiology of the diverticuli is related to increased pressure in the lumen of the colon with herniation of mucosa and submucosa at the site of vasa recta perforation of the colonic wall which are its weak points. The diverticuli are not composed of whole layers of the colonic wall and are therefore pseudodiverticuli rather than true diverticuli. Fecal impaction at the neck of the diverticulum causes inflammation of

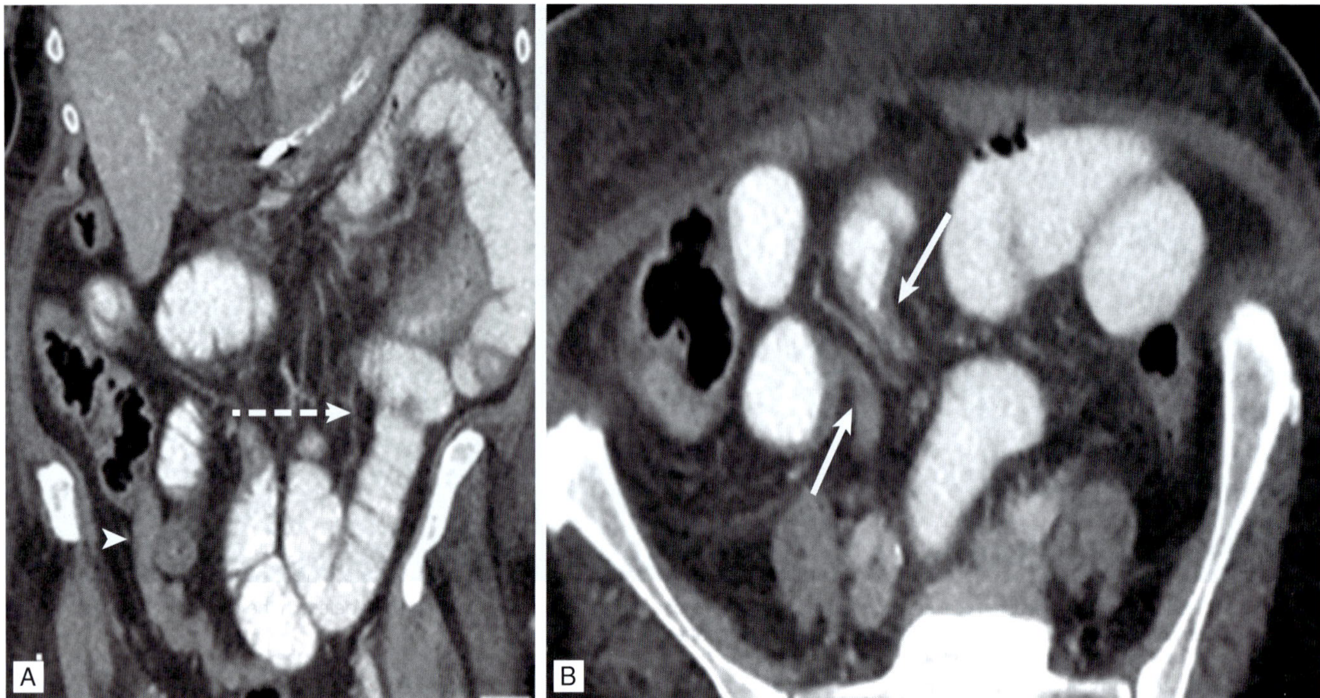

Figure 92.34 CECT in a middle-age man with acute abdominal obstruction. The coronal images (A) demonstrates complete collapse of the terminal ileum (*arrowhead*) and markedly distended proximal small bowel (*dashed arrow*). There are two focal areas of sudden narrowing ("transition points") seen on the axial image (B) in keeping with obstruction (*solid arrows*). On surgery, the obstruction was caused by a fibrous band crossing two segments of small bowel and causing obstruction (also called closed loop).

the colon leading to the volvulus which resemble beaks (called "beaking"). The twisting of the colon leads to twisting of the mesentery and accompanying vessels ("whirl sign"). If the colon remains twisted, it can lead to ischemia, infarction and perforation, which can be also assessed with MDCT [81].

Conclusion

Imaging plays a crucial role in the management of patients with nontraumatic acute abdominal pain. CECT remains the primary imaging technique and gives invaluable diagnostic information. USG may also serve as an initial diagnostic test, particularly for evaluation of the gallbladder or the abdomen as a whole in pediatric or pregnant patients, when the radiation from CECT is an issue. MRI is becoming used more frequently in select patient populations, but is not always suitable for the acutely unwell patient and has limited variable availability out of normal working hours.

Suggested Readings

- J Stoker, A Van Randen, W Laméris, MA Boermeester, Imaging patients with acute abdominal pain, Radiology 253 (2009) 31–46.
- NG Ditkofsky, A Singh, L Avery, RA Novelline, The role of emergency MRI in the setting of acute abdominal pain, Emerg Radiol 21 (2014) 615–624.
- RM Gore, The acute abdomen. Radiol Clin North Am 53 (6) (2015) 1093–1348.

93 Introduction to Interventional Radiology

ABHAY KUMAR KAPOOR, SANJAY BAIJAL

Before the era of interventional radiology (IR), treatments of various disease were compartmentalized mainly into medical and surgical protocols. A large number of patients used to be refused any treatment because they were poor candidates for administration of any kind of anesthesia, or the risks of surgery were deemed too high. This necessitated the need for development of innovative techniques for percutaneous procedures as well as endoscopic procedures. The whole thought process began to use imaging to direct targeted therapies for various organ systems, leading to development of the subspeciality of therapeutic IR. Innovations have been fairly rapid in IR, starting with a new idea, use of existing tools, or development of new ones to meet the challenge and finally gain acceptance in clinical practice. The new procedures are tested against preexisting standard of care treatments with regards to outcome, cost, and safety. There are many diseases that at one point of time were thought to be incurable or had to be dealt with a major surgery with associated morbidity that are now easily managed with a minimally invasive percutaneous approach using image guidance.

History

Initial angiograms were performed by surgeons through a direct cutdown [1]. Later, when radiologists started performing angiography, it was only for diagnostic purpose. This practice continued until the mid-1970s with progress to contrast studies in veins and lymphatics to perform presurgical vascular mapping [2].

The major breakthrough in IR dates back to 1953 when Swedish radiologist Sven Ivar Seldinger devised the technique for percutaneous replacement of needle by a catheter [3]. Before this, major complications were associated with vascular procedures because large-bore needles or trocars were used to gain vascular access [4]. With introduction of the Seldinger technique, catheterization became safer, and angiographic procedures were subsequently refined [2].

Charles T. Dotter popularized the use of catheters for various vascular procedures in 1963 and published his case describing dilation of atherosclerotic lesions in femoral artery with serial dilators using Seldinger's method [5]. During this period in the early 1960s, angiographic techniques were refined and used extensively to diagnose pathologies in all organ systems [6,7]. Use of preshaped catheters came into vogue in this period, allowing pharmacoangiography [8].

With the advent of preshaped catheters, endovascular treatment of gastrointestinal bleeding was started. Initially, this was done for bleeding esophageal varices by selective infusion of vasopressin in the superior mesenteric artery [9]. Following the success in treating varices, patients with arterial and capillary or mucosal bleeding were treated by selectively infusing vasoconstrictor in the supply vessel or with embolic materials [10].

In 1974, German-born physician-scientist Andreas Grüntzig used a balloon catheter to reopen a stenosed femoral artery [11]. Grüntzig and Charles T. Dotter were nominated for the Nobel Prize in Physiology or Medicine in 1978 for balloon angioplasty to treat patients with atherosclerotic vascular disease [11]. The next landmark in IR was with the invention of balloon-expandable vascular stent by Julio Palmaz in 1990.

Simultaneously during this period, selective coronary angiographies were also performed, and the technique of F. Mason Sones [12], who performed the first right coronary artery angiogram in 1958, began to be refined by radiologists [13]. However, because most radiologists were not keen on performing cardiac catheterization, the procedure was taken over by cardiologists [14].

Nonvascular interventions rapidly grew in the 1970s with procedures evolving in all organ systems. Percutaneous biliary drainage and nephrostomy were regularly used for various indications. The self-expanding metal stent for biliary use was devised by Cesare Gianturco in 1985 [15] and made a big impact on the treatment of patients with malignant biliary obstruction. The Hybrid Gianturco expandable stent was later devised by Sumit Roy and Sanjay S. Baijal in 1994 [16], and its use in the clinical setting of urethral stricture and Budd-Chiari syndrome was reported in 1995 and 1996, respectively [17,18]. Likewise, drainage of various abscesses percutaneously made a major impact on patient treatment [19,20].

Neurointerventions started in 1927 when the Portuguese physician and neurologist Egas Moniz at the University of Lisbon introduced cerebral angiography by direct puncture of the carotid artery [21]. However, the use of the modality remained limited to diagnostic angiographies until Luessenhop and Spence described endovascular embolization of cerebral arteriovenous malformation in 1960 [22]. Further progress happened in 1970 when Pierre Lasjuanias described the cerebral vascular microanatomy and Fedor Serbinenko developed a technique to treat patients with intracranial aneurysms and carotid cavernous sinus fistulas using detachable balloons [23] The 1980s saw the advent of endovascular stroke management as described by Zeumer and Theron [24,25]. Early 1990 saw the introduction of Gugliemi detachable coils, and by the end of the decade, endovascular coiling was a well-established option used to treat cerebral aneurysms [26]. In the 2000s, advanced techniques such as balloon-assisted coiling, stent-assisted coiling, flow diversion, and Onyx embolization made remarkable improvements in the outcomes of neurointerventions [27].

Significant technologic advances in the past two decades in the field of imaging equipment and medical hardware have led to a large increase in the diseases treated by IR. The newer procedures added to the list included transjugular intrahepatic portosystemic shunt (TIPS), uterine artery embolization, stent graft placement, ablative techniques to treat tumors and transarterial therapies (transarterial chemoembolization), transarterial radioembolization, and chemoinfusion to selectively treat primary and metastatic liver tumors [4].

Preprocedure Checklists

Before any needle-based procedure, it is very important to evaluate the patient's coagulation profile. Consensus guidelines regarding periprocedural management for percutaneous image-guided interventions published by the Society of Interventional Radiology (SIR) [28,29] clearly define the various requirements. These guidelines are endorsed by the Canadian Association for Interventional Radiology and the Cardiovascular and Interventional Radiological Society of Europe.

Systemic Disease Evaluation

1. **Chronic liver disease (CLD):** It is difficult to assess the hemostasis in patients with CLD because the prothrombin time (PT) and international normalized ratio (INR) and partial thromboplastin time evaluate any decrease in procoagulant factors without assessing the effect of concomitant decrease in natural anticoagulants because both are synthesized by the liver [28]. Similarly, although the platelet count is reduced because of multiple factors, the adhesive function of these platelets is actually enhanced [28].
2. **Chronic kidney disease (CKD):** Higher bleeding rates are associated with CKD because of abnormal platelet–endothelial interaction and anemia. Another important point to be considered is the bioavailability of many anticoagulant agents, including low-molecular-weight heparin (LMWH), fondaparinux, and direct oral anticoagulants, requiring prolonged stoppage time before any elective procedure.
3. **Cancer:** Because patients with cancer are at increased risk of venous and arterial thromboembolism, many of them receive some form of anticoagulation. It is very important to elicit this history and stop the medication before the procedure.

Preprocedure Tests

SIR guidelines have discussed the need for laboratory tests depending on the risk category of the procedure. Accordingly, procedures have been categorized into high risk or low risk for bleeding. *High-risk procedures have been defined as the ones having a greater than 1.5% rate of bleeding or the bleeding maybe occurring at sites where it will be difficult to diagnose or treat (e.g., lung parenchyma or within the abdomen)* [29]. Low-risk procedures are the ones expected to rarely bleed (rate of <1.5%), or bleeding occurs in areas where it is easy to diagnose and control. No preprocedural assessment has been recommended for patients with low bleeding risk. The requisites for patients with higher risk of bleeding are

1. hemoglobin,
2. platelet count,
3. PT or INR,
4. activated partial thromboplastin time (aPTT) or anti-Xa testing recommended for patients receiving unfractionated heparin,
5. thromboelastography (TEG) levels are recommended for patients with cirrhosis [30,31]. TEG is an assay that measures the global viscoelastic properties of whole-blood clot formation.

The categorization of various procedures into low- and high-risk categories as per SIR guidelines is reproduced in Table 93.1.

TABLE 93.1 Categorization of Procedures Associated With Bleeding Risk

Screening Coagulation Laboratory Test	Procedure
Low Bleeding Risk	
PT/INR: not routinely recommended except for patients with higher bleeding risk	Catheter exchanges (gastrostomy, biliary, nephrostomy, abscess)
Platelet count and hemoglobin: not routinely recommended	Diagnostic arteriography and arterial interventions: peripheral, sheath <6 Fr
Thresholds	Diagnostic venography
INR: correct to within range of ≤2.0–3.0	Dialysis access interventions
Platelets: transfuse if <20 × 10^9/L	Paracentesis
	Facet joint injections and medial branch nerve blocks (thoracic and lumbar spine)
	Nontunneled chest tube placement for pleural effusion
	Nontunneled venous access and removal (including PICC placement)
	Superficial abscess drainage or biopsy (palpable lesion, lymph node, soft tissue, breast, thyroid, superficial bone)
	Transjugular liver biopsy
High Bleeding Risk	
PT/INR: routinely recommended	Ablations
Platelet count and hemoglobin: routinely recommended	Arterial interventions: >7-Fr sheath
Thresholds	Biliary interventions
INR: correct to within range of ≤1.5–1.8	Deep abscess drainage
Platelets; transfuse if <50 × 10^9/L	Deep nonorgan biopsies (e.g., spine, soft tissue in intraabdominal, retroperitoneal, pelvic compartments)
	Solid organ biopsies
	Transjugular intrahepatic portosystemic shunt
	Percutaneous nephrostomy

INR, international normalized ratio; *PICC,* peripherally inserted central catheter; *PT,* prothrombin time.

Adapted from IJ Patel, S Rahim, JC Davidson, et al., Society of Interventional Radiology Consensus Guidelines for the Periprocedural Management of Thrombotic and Bleeding Risk in Patients Undergoing Percutaneous Image-Guided Interventions—Part II: Recommendations, J Vasc Interv Radiol 30 (2019) 1168–1184.

The interpretation of the laboratory parameters and the need for correction as per the SIR guidelines is as follows:

1. **Low bleeding risk**
   Platelet count >20 × 10^9/L
   INR ≤2.0 to 3.0
   INR needs correction to within 2.0 to 3.0 or less; platelet transfusion if platelet count is <20 × 10^9/L.
   For arterial access, the INR thresholds are <1.8 for femoral access and <2.2 for radial access.
2. **High bleeding risk**
   Platelet count >50 × 10^9/L
   INR <1.5

In CLD, American Association for the Study of Liver Diseases' position paper on liver biopsy concluded that no specific PT/INR or platelet count cutoff can be reliably predicted, and the decision to perform the procedure with abnormal laboratory parameters should be reached as per the results of local practice [32,42]. Fibrinogen level correction can be helpful in these cases.

Anesthesia-Related Prerequisites

Patients requiring sedation or anesthesia need to undergo a preanesthesia checkup for evaluation of their fitness for anesthesia. This is very important for any procedure that is expected to go on for a longer duration or where any complication is expected, such as lung biopsy in patients with emphysematous lungs. Sedation may be required for apprehensive patients and in children. Fasting instructions need to be given to the patient depending on the type of anesthesia and procedure. These instructions are very important to decrease the risk of dehydration and hypoglycemia. The instructions need to be modified for patients with diabetes in consultation with an endocrinologist. Mostly 4 to 6 hours of fasting is suffice for sedation or general anesthesia [33]. Clear fluids can be allowed up to 2 hours before the procedure. Infants can be allowed clear fluids up to 2 hours, breast milk up to 4 hours, and infant formula milk up to 6 hours before elective procedures. Nonhuman milk and a light meal can be allowed up to 6 hours before the procedure.

Prerequisites Related to Drugs for Chronic Ailments

It is important to take the history of any other medication the patient is taking. If the patient is taking antihypertensive or hypothyroid medication, these should be taken with a sip of water in the morning on the day of procedure. Modification of oral hypoglycemic agents or insulin for patients with diabetes is more complex and beyond the scope of this chapter. This needs to be done in consultation with an endocrinologist.

Prerequisites for Anticoagulation and Antiplatelet Medication

Patients who have undergone coronary stenting or have a history of acute coronary syndrome receive antiplatelet therapy. As per current guidelines, dual antiplatelet therapy (DAPT) for a minimum of 1 month is required for patients receiving bare-metal stents and 6 to 12 months for patients receiving drug-eluting stents [34,35]. The recommendation for patients with a history of acute coronary syndrome is 12 months of DAPT [36]. Patients who have nonvalvular atrial fibrillation taking long-term anticoagulation to reduce the risk of systemic embolization and stroke [37]. Similarly, patients with deep vein thrombosis (DVT) take anticoagulation medication.

Discontinuation of antiplatelet or anticoagulation medication in any of these patients can expose them to a high risk of stent occlusion, myocardial infarction, or thromboembolism. *Hence, these medications should be discontinued preferably in consultation with the clinician who has started these drugs, and the patient should be made aware of the possible risks.*

If the patient is on anticoagulation with LMWH or vitamin K antagonists, these need to be stopped as shown in Table 93.2.

Unfractionated heparin needs to be stopped for only 4 to 6 hours before the procedure, but LMWH needs to be stopped for 24 hours. The effects of heparin can be monitored with aPTT. Vitamin K antagonists need to be stopped for 3 to 5 days. Their effect is monitored by the INR.

Patients taking antiplatelet drugs need to stop these drugs for 5 days before the procedure. Patients taking dual antiplatelets can continue with Ecosprin until 24 hours before the procedure while discontinuing clopidogrel for 5 days. Bridging therapy with heparin may be considered for patients who are at high risk for thromboembolic events.

Most of the withheld drugs can be restarted after 6 to 8 hours because this is the approximate duration required for clot stabilization [38]. However, it is safer to restart after 24 hours unless there is urgency to restart.

Patient Preparation

Apart from the laboratory tests for coagulation profile as mentioned earlier, the following important points should be looked into before the procedure:

1. Renal function test: if contrast is going to be used.
2. Viral markers: required for adequate precautions for the staff and appropriate disposal of the contaminated material. HIV, hepatitis B surface antigen, and anti–hepatitis C virus are the commonly done viral markers.
3. Shave and prepare the part to be intervened (e.g., the groin for angiography).
4. All previous imaging should be available for review.
5. Bowel preparation: for procedures using a transrectal approach such as prostatic biopsy or transrectal ultrasound-guided drainage of pelvic collection. This is normally done with laxatives for 2 days before the procedure along with antibiotics, which are continued for 3 days after the procedure. Such procedures require overnight fasting.

Postprocedure Checklist

Every procedure has its own set of complications that need to be checked before discharging the patient. *The most common universal complications after a procedure are bleeding and infection.* These need to be excluded before discharge, and patients need to be counseled about their symptoms in case of delayed complications.

The duration of monitoring required post procedure is very variable depending on the procedure done. For low-risk procedures such as superficial fine-needle aspiration cytology or biopsy done on an outpatient basis, no monitoring maybe required. However, patients should be informed to seek medical advice if they experience an increasing intensity of pain or have palpitations (tachycardia), to exclude any hemorrhagic complication.

All high-risk procedures should preferably be done in day care or regular admission. Vital monitoring for at least 4 hours is essential. In cases of femoral arterial puncture in which a closure device has not been used, 6 hours of bed rest and vital

TABLE 93.2 Management Recommendations for Anticoagulant and Antiplatelet Agents

Medication	Low Risk for Bleeding	High Risk for Bleeding
Anticoagulants		
Unfractionated Heparin		
Withholding	Do not withhold	Withhold IV heparin for 4–6 hr before procedure; check aPTT or anti-Xa level; for BID or TID dosing of SC heparin, procedure may be performed 6 hr after last dose
Reinitiation	NA	6–8 hr
LMWH: Enoxaparin (Lovenox), Dalteparin (Fragmin)		
Withholding	Do not withhold	Enoxaparin: withhold one dose if prophylactic dose is used; withhold two doses or 24 hr before procedure if therapeutic dose is used; check anti-Xa level if renal function impaired; dalteparin: withhold one dose before procedure
Reinitiation	NA	12 hr
Warfarin (Coumadin) Withholding	Target INR, 3.0; consider bridging for high thrombosis risk cases	Withhold 5 days until target INR (1.8); consider bridging for high thrombosis risk cases; if STAT or emergent, use reversal agent
Reinitiation	NA or same-day reinitiation for bridged patients	Resume day after procedure; high thrombosis risk cases may benefit from bridging with LMWH and multidisciplinary management, especially if a reversal agent is used along with vitamin K
Antiplatelet Agents: NSAIDs		
Aspirin Withholding	Do not withhold	Withhold 3–5 days before procedure
Reinitiation	NA	Day after procedure
Clopidogrel (Plavix) Withholding	Do not withhold	Withhold for 5 days before procedure
Reinitiation	NA	6 hr after procedure if using 75-mg dose but should occur 24 hr after procedure if using a loading dose (300–600 mg)

aPTT, activated partial thromboplastin time; *BID*, twice a day; *INR*, international normalized ratio; *IV*, intravenous; *LMWH*, low molecular weight heparin; *NA*, not applicable; *SC*, subcutaneous; *TID*, three times a day.

Adapted from IJ Patel, S Rahim, JC Davidson, et al., Society of Interventional Radiology Consensus Guidelines for the Periprocedural Management of Thrombotic and Bleeding Risk in Patients Undergoing Percutaneous Image-Guided Interventions—Part II: Recommendations, J Vasc Interv Radiol 30 (2019) 1168–1184.

monitoring are mandatory. Advice to monitor the puncture site for any bleeding should be given. The peripheral pulse can be checked to look for patency of the punctured artery. Before discharge, ultrasonography (USG) of the groin may be done to rule out any hematoma.

Patients who have undergone biliary drainage should undergo USG the next day to look at any residual biliary dilation in addition to hemogram to evaluate for any biliary sepsis. Liver function testing (LFT) can be done 48 to 72 hours later to assess the reduction in serum bilirubin. After chemoembolization, patients need to undergo LFT to detect postembolization complications.

The discharge summary should mention about any antibiotics that are prescribed and the duration for which they need to be taken. Likewise, follow-up imaging and review should be recorded.

Overall Contraindications

It is the benefit versus complications that decide for or against any procedure. The general contraindications for elective procedures are as follows:

1. Uncorrectable coagulopathy
2. Ongoing sepsis before any stenting
3. Ascites when abdominal biopsy is required

Basics of Fine-Needle Aspiration Cytology or Biopsy

Tissue sampling has become one of the mainstays of patient management in the current era of evidence-based medicine. Advances in imaging with better resolution of USG and rapid computed tomography (CT) acquisition (Fig. 93.1) along with robotic guidance systems have made it possible to acquire sample from places that were earlier thought to be inaccessible. The first liver aspiration biopsy was done in 1883 by Ehrlich and Menghini, described as "one-second needle biopsy of the liver" in 1958 [39].

It is very important to decide whether FNAC or core biopsy is required. Various factors that help decide this are

1. location of the tumor,
2. type of tests required on the sample,
3. safety of procedure.

FNAC is the first line of approach for superficial lesions such as those of the thyroid and salivary glands [40]. However, if two FNACs are inconclusive to diagnose a thyroid lesion, core biopsy should be performed [41].

If multiple samples are needed for histopathology and to test for various infections, core biopsy using a coaxial technique is preferred. Similarly, if a suspected tumor needs to be evaluated

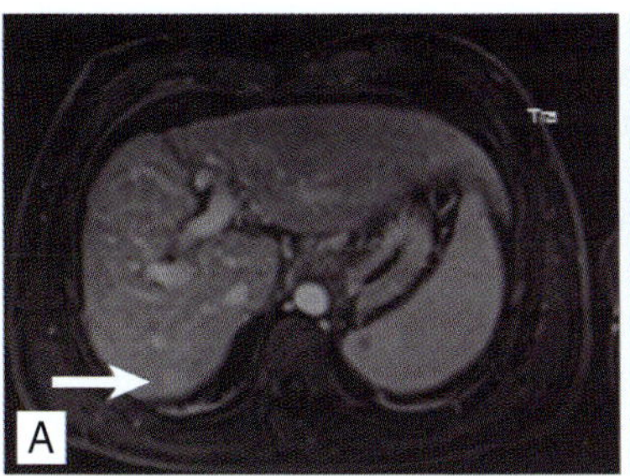
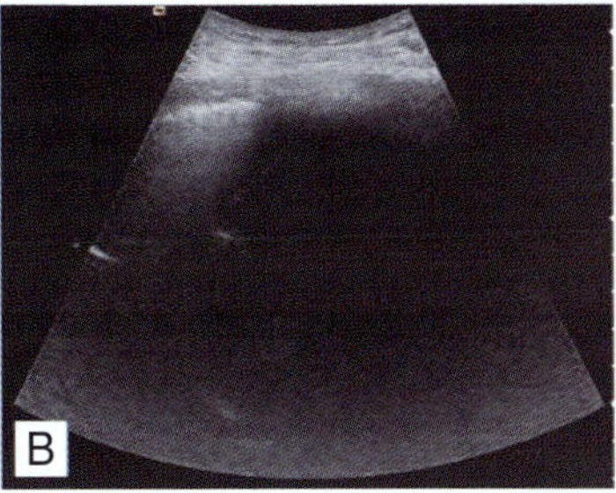
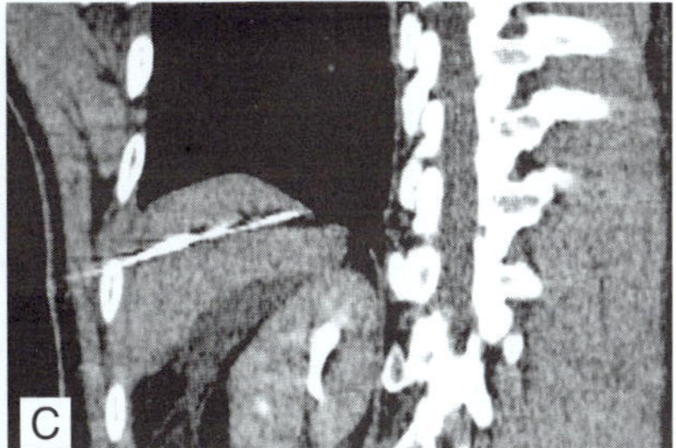
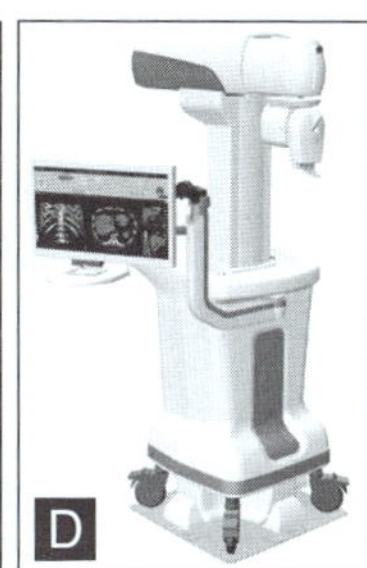

Figure 93.1 (A) Lesion (*white arrow*) in segment VII of the liver is seen in portal venous phase on magnetic resonance imaging. (B) Lesion not visualized on ultrasonography because of a pulmonary air shadow. (C) Reformat computed tomography image showing caudocranial placement of the needle with robotic guidance. (D) MAXIO® treatment plan–controlled robotic navigation system (Perfint Healthcare).

with immunohistochemistry (IHC) markers for starting the appropriate therapy, biopsy is preferred over FNAC.

FNAC is also the preferred mode of sampling of liver lesions in the presence of biliary dilation because biopsy in such cases can lead to biliary leak [42]. Biopsy can be done if histopathology is going to significantly alter the management, provided the patient has been counseled regarding the relatively higher risk of biliary leak compared with other patients whose ducts are not dilated. In such cases, plug biopsy should be performed using a coaxial system to plug the track with coils or Gelfoam. FNAC also plays a role when transpancreatic sampling has to be done.

Hardware

Most FNACs can be done using a 22-gauge needle, with the choice of length depending on the depth of the lesion. Superficial lesions can be sampled using hypodermic needles, and Chiba needles are used for deeper lesions (Fig. 93.2). However, if the sample in the first pass is hemorrhagic, one should use a 26-gauge needle for further samples to get better cellularity. A 20-cc syringe is attached to the hypodermic needle while advancing in the lesion. If a needle with a stylet is being used, it is removed when the needle is in the lesion, and a 20-cc syringe is then attached for aspiration.

A wide range of hardware is available for soft tissue biopsy. The common size in use along with their indications are listed in Table 93.3.

A **coaxial biopsy system** is preferred whenever multiple cores are required because this helps in acquisition of sample with only a single puncture of the desired organ capsule. This technique helps in reducing the complication rate of bleeding, which is mostly associated with multiple punctures. This also helps in reducing the complication rate of pneumothorax while sampling lung lesions because the pneumothorax rate is directly proportional to the number of punctures in the pleura. This is also the reason why a transfissural route is not preferred. The added advantage of a coaxial system in CT-guided cases is accurate documentation of the tissue sampled.

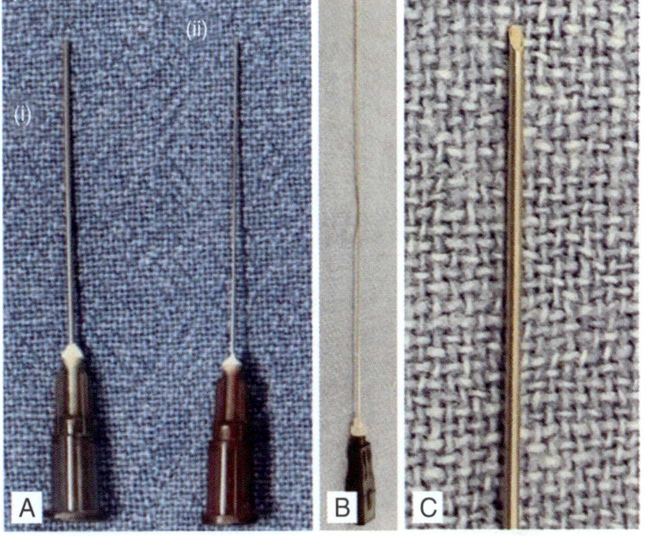

Figure 93.2 (A) 22-gauge (i) and 26-gauge (ii) needles. (B) A 22-gauge Chiba needle. (C) Short bevel of a 22-gauge Chiba needle.

The Tru-Cut biopsy needles are either automatic or semiautomatic (Fig. 93.3). *Whereas the automatic needles are mostly*

TABLE 93.3 Commonly Used Biopsy Needles

Gauge	Length (cm)	Type	Organ	Biopsy Type
18	10/16	Automatic	Liver	Non-target
18	10	Semiautomatic	Thyroid, parietal, cervical	Superficial lesions
18	16	Semiautomatic	Liver, lung, abdominal lymph nodes	Deep lesions
18	25	Automatic	Prostate, ovarian mass	TRUS, TVS sampling
16	10/16	Automatic	Kidney, omentum	Nontarget
14	10/16	Automatic	Breast	Hard lesions
13	10/15	Manual	Bone lesions	
11	10/15	Manual	Bone lesions	

TRUS, transrectal ultrasound guided scan; *TVS*, transvaginal scan.

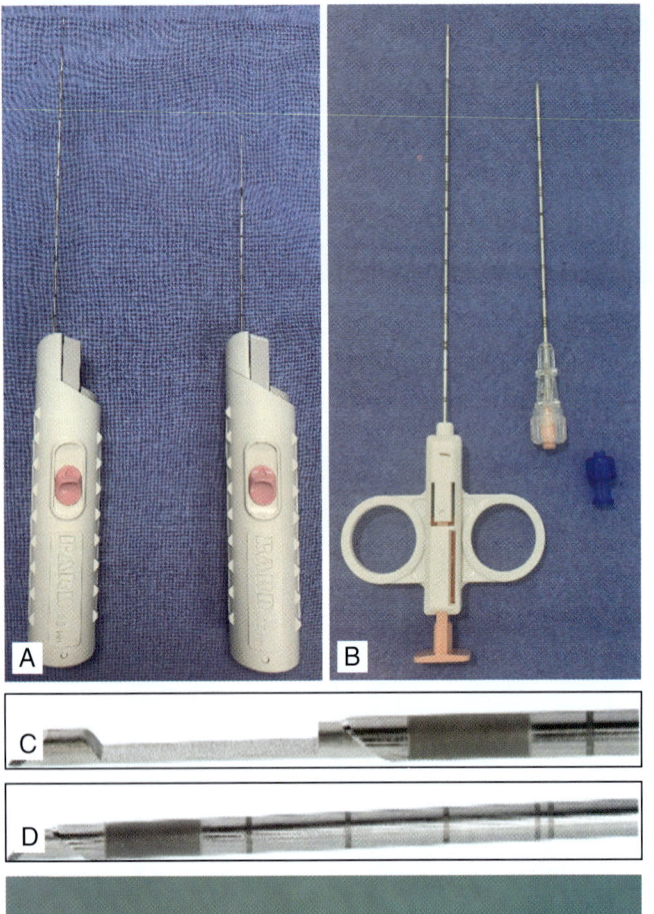

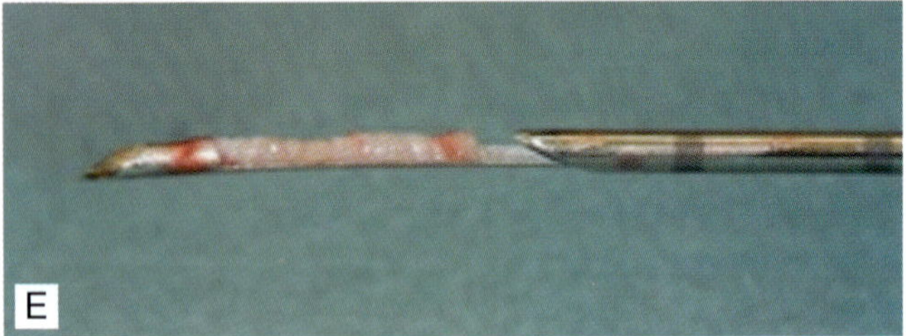

Figure 93.3 (A) 18-gauge 16-cm and 10-cm automated biopsy guns. (B) 18-gauge 16-cm semiautomatic biopsy gun. (C) Open sample notch of a biopsy gun. (D) Closed sample notch of a biopsy gun. (E) Open sample notch with tissue core post biopsy.

used for nontarget organ sampling, semiautomatic needles are mostly used with a coaxial biopsy system to sample any lesion in solid organs. The coaxial biopsy system gives the added option of plugging the biopsy track using coils, Gelfoam, or both (Fig. 93.4). A newer automatic biopsy gun takes a full core of the tissue compared with the semilunar core in the older guns (Fig. 93.5).

Organ-Specific Biopsy

Renal Biopsy

A 16-gauge needle is the preferred size for nontarget renal biopsy. Renal biopsy is taken from the lower pole in native kidneys because of better visualization and easy access, but the upper pole is preferred in transplant kidneys because this is more superficial in location, and there are lesser chances of injury to gut in this approach. It is important to take the sample from cortex and not transgress the medulla. Generally, the pathologists prefer more than 10 glomeruli within the sample for accurate reporting [43]. Most centers perform renal biopsy using automated biopsy guns with some studies showing no significant difference in the complication rate between automated versus coaxial needles [44]. Bleeding is the most common complication after percutaneous renal biopsy with a rate of 3.5% for gross hematuria and 0.9% requiring blood transfusion [45].

Most of the renal sampling requires two cores, one in formalin for histopathology and one in saline for immunofluorescence. The core in saline can also be used for electron microscopy. However, if electron microscopy is very important, as in cases of suspected Alport disease, immunotactoid disease, and minimal change nephropathy, an extra core should be taken, or a second core should be cut and half sent in glutaraldehyde [46].

Renal tumors are not often sampled. Most renal masses are diagnosed and characterized on imaging and subjected to appropriate treatment. The smaller renal masses up to 3 cm, which are treated percutaneously by radiofrequency ablation or cryoablation, can undergo percutaneous biopsy at the time of ablation to avoid needle-track seeding. If the patient has metastatic disease or is going to be treated with chemotherapy, biopsy may be taken using a coaxial biopsy system so that the track can be plugged because most of these tumors are very vascular, and there is a possibility of significant bleed after a biopsy. The needle-track seeding after renal biopsy is relatively uncommon and has been reported only 16 times until 2019 in an article by Renshaw et al [47]. This is more commonly seen in papillary renal carcinoma and if multiple punctures of the lesion have been made and with needle gauge of 20 gauge or larger [47].

Bone Biopsy

Bone biopsy is done either for bone marrow aspiration or to do sampling of any lesion suspicious for metastasis. Most of the primary bone tumors are not sampled because the diagnosis is made on imaging. However, if there is a diagnostic dilemma, sampling can be done. *It is important to discuss the surgical plan with the orthopedic surgeon before sampling because one should plan the needle entry site in an area that will get excised during surgery to prevent track seeding.*

Bone sampling is usually done using a 13-gauge needle. Use of a coaxial biopsy needle is preferred because there is a possibility of getting no tissue after the biopsy needle is removed. This can happen because unlike the soft tissue biopsy needles, bone biopsy needles do not have a tissue-cutting system (Fig. 93.6). The needle is preferably kept perpendicular to the bone, and the shortest path to the lesion is preferred. A longer path may be chosen to avoid transgression of the joint capsule.

Transvenous Sampling

Various situations such as deranged coagulation parameters or ascites preclude a patient from undergoing percutaneous sampling of liver as the risk of bleeding is high. These can be sampled using a transjugular approach. When deep cannulation of the right hepatic vein (RHV) is achieved, over a stiff guidewire, the angled metal cannula of the transjugular liver biopsy set (Fig. 93.7) is advanced into the RHV. The wire is then replaced with a 65-cm, 18- or 19-gauge, 20-mm biopsy needle, and using USG and fluoroscopy guidance, the needle is advanced into the liver parenchyma and a sample taken

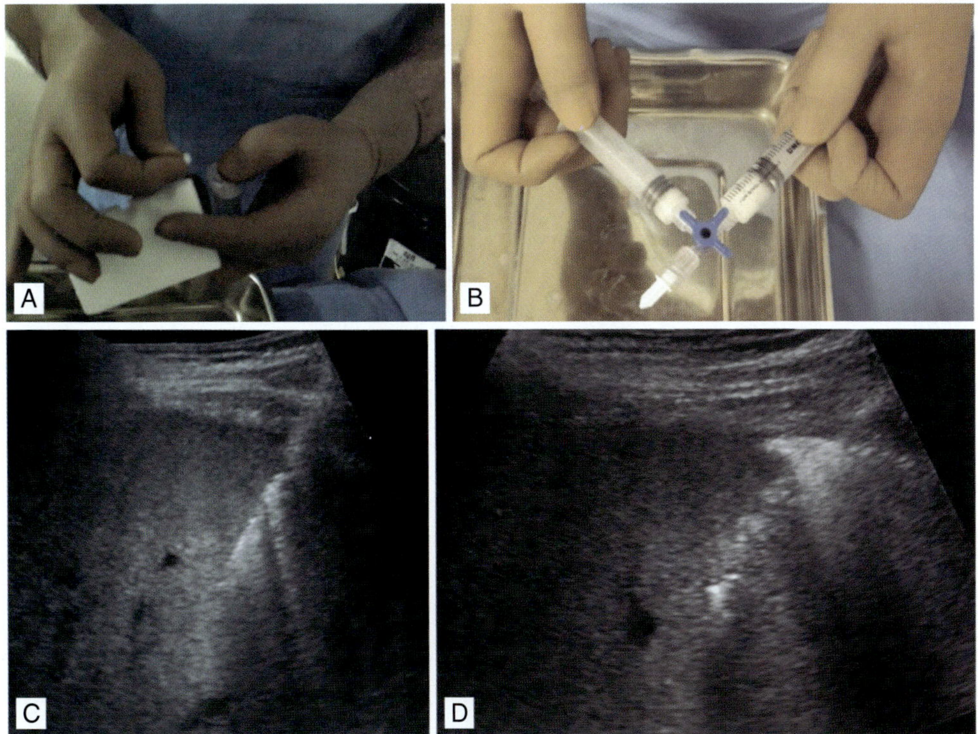

Figure 93.4 Plug liver biopsy. (A) Gelfoam pledgets being loaded in a 5-mL syringe. (B) Gelfoam pledgets being mixed with equal amount of normal saline. (C) Gelfoam mixture in the track of a biopsy needle. (D) Gelfoam mixture seen in the perihepatic region.

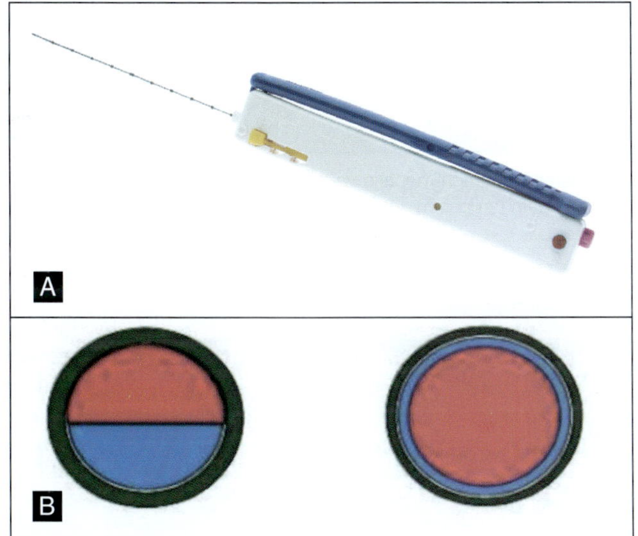

Figure 93.5 (A) BioPince full core biopsy needle by Argon Medical Devices. (B) Conventional side notch half core sample compared with a BioPince full core sample.

(Fig. 93.8). The advantage of using USG guidance is to prevent inadvertent capsular puncture or portal vein puncture. A similar procedure can be done for sampling the right kidney (Fig. 93.9). This may be required in cases of CKD in which the platelet function is deranged.

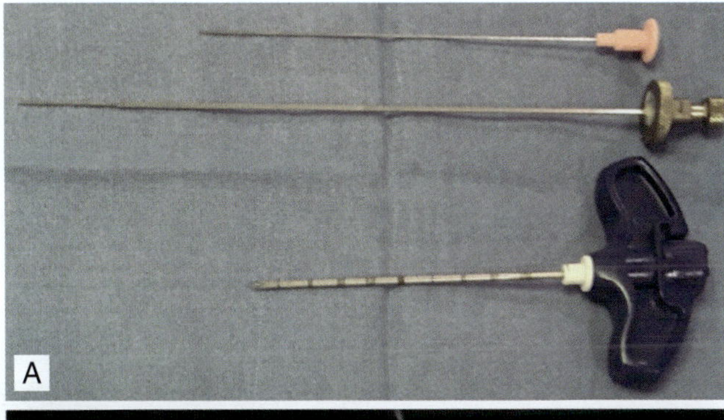

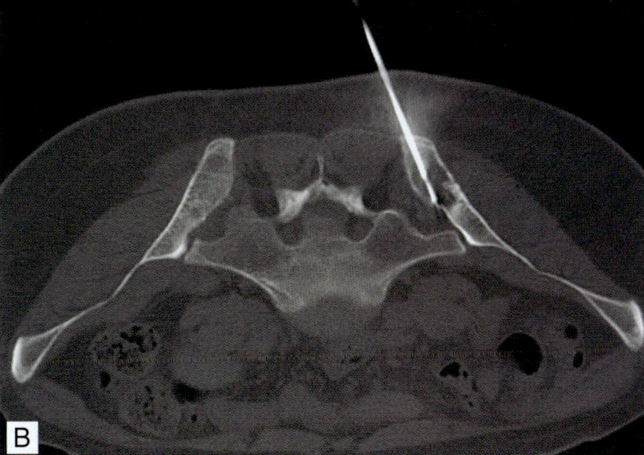

Figure 93.6 (A) 13-gauge coaxial bone biopsy needle. (B) Bone biopsy needle in the right iliac bone lesion.

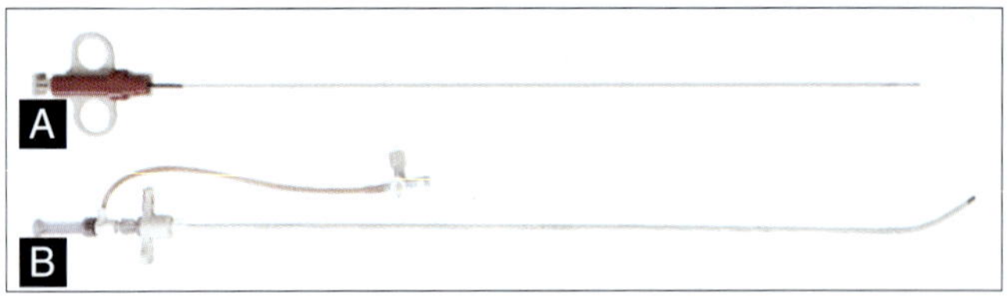

Figure 93.7 Transjugular liver biopsy kit (TLAB, Argon Medical Devices). (A) 19-gauge 60-cm biopsy needle. (B) 7-Fr 51-cm introducer sheath with a curved metal stiffener.

Intraductal Sampling

In cases of cholangiocarcinoma or carcinoma of the gallbladder, percutaneous sampling is not possible sometimes because of the central location of lesion or nonvisualization on USG. These patients usually have intrahepatic biliary radical dilation and require percutaneous transhepatic biliary drainage (PTBD) to be able to start chemotherapy after the bilirubin level comes to within normal limits. The PTBD track can be used to do intraductal punch biopsy (Fig. 93.10) or brush cytology (Fig. 93.11) from the site of occlusion. The same can be done during endoscopic retrograde cholangiopancreatography if PTBD is not being done.

Transrectal Biopsy

This is the common approach for doing prostatic biopsy but can also be used for sampling other pelvic lesions in women if the transvaginal approach cannot be used. An 18-gauge automated biopsy gun is used for sampling the prostate. Normally, 12 cores are taken from different areas. A transperineal approach can also

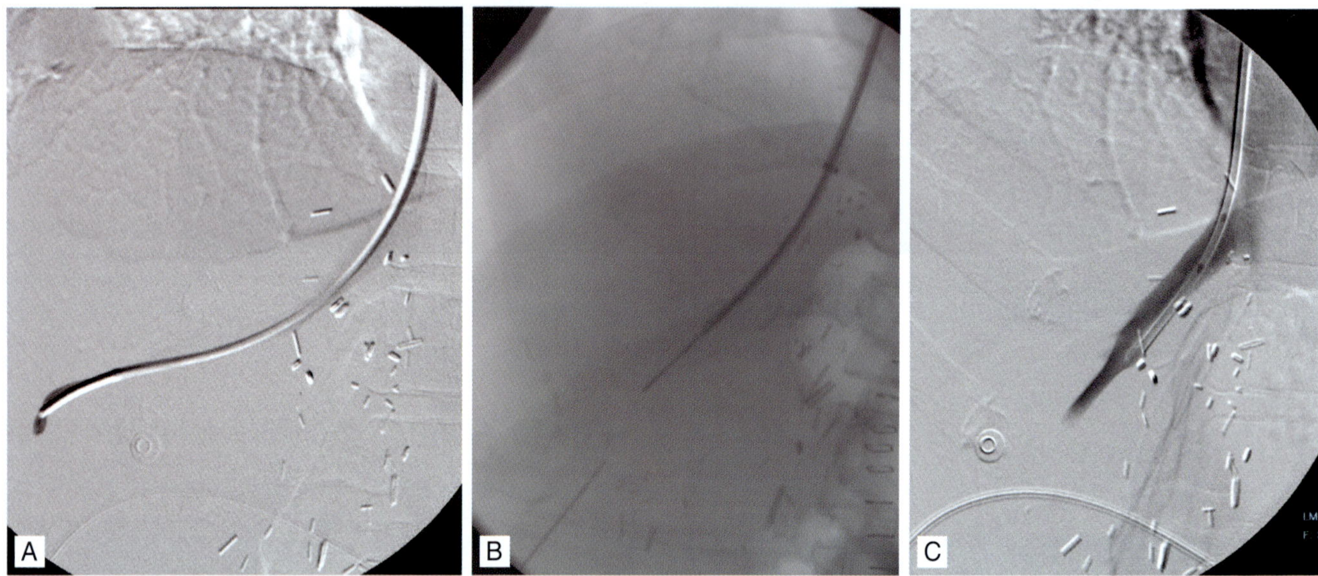

Figure 93.8 Transjugular liver biopsy. (A) 5-Fr multipurpose angiographic (MPA) catheter in the right hepatic vein. (B) Introducer sheath with exposed sample notch of biopsy needle. (C) Check venogram post biopsy from the introducer sheath to confirm no extravasation of contrast.

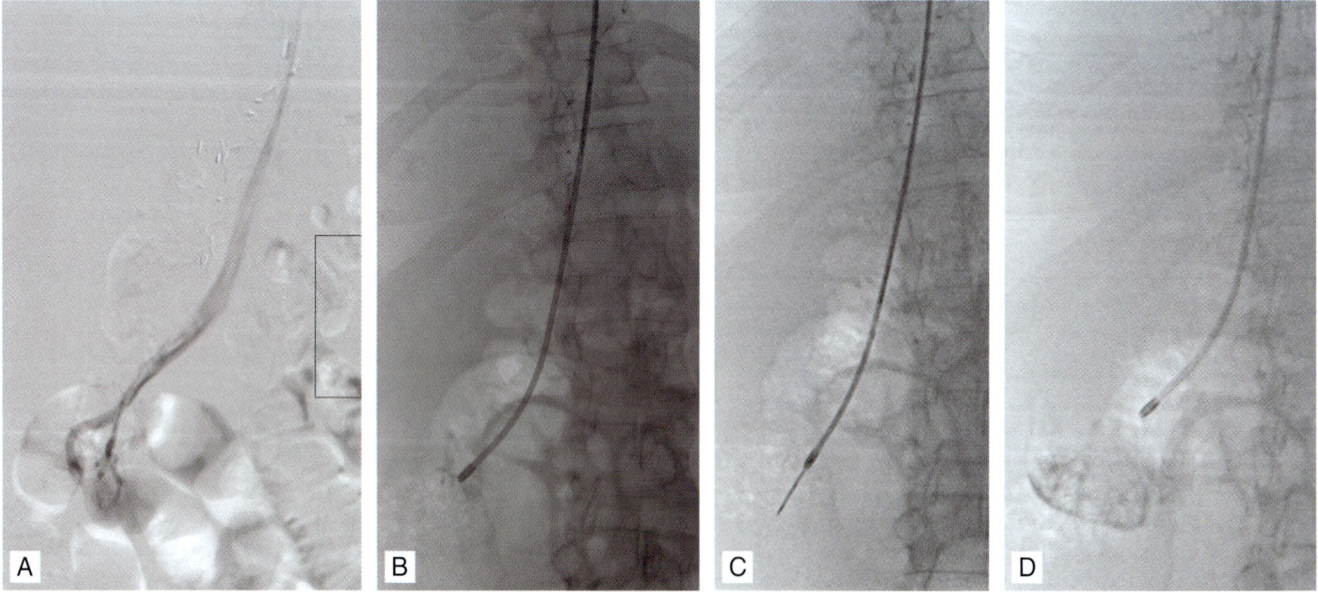

Figure 93.9 Transjugular kidney biopsy. (A) Venogram in the renal vein. (B) Introducer sheath in the renal vein. (C) Exposed sample notch of biopsy needle in renal parenchyma. (D) Check venogram showing small extravasation of contrast.

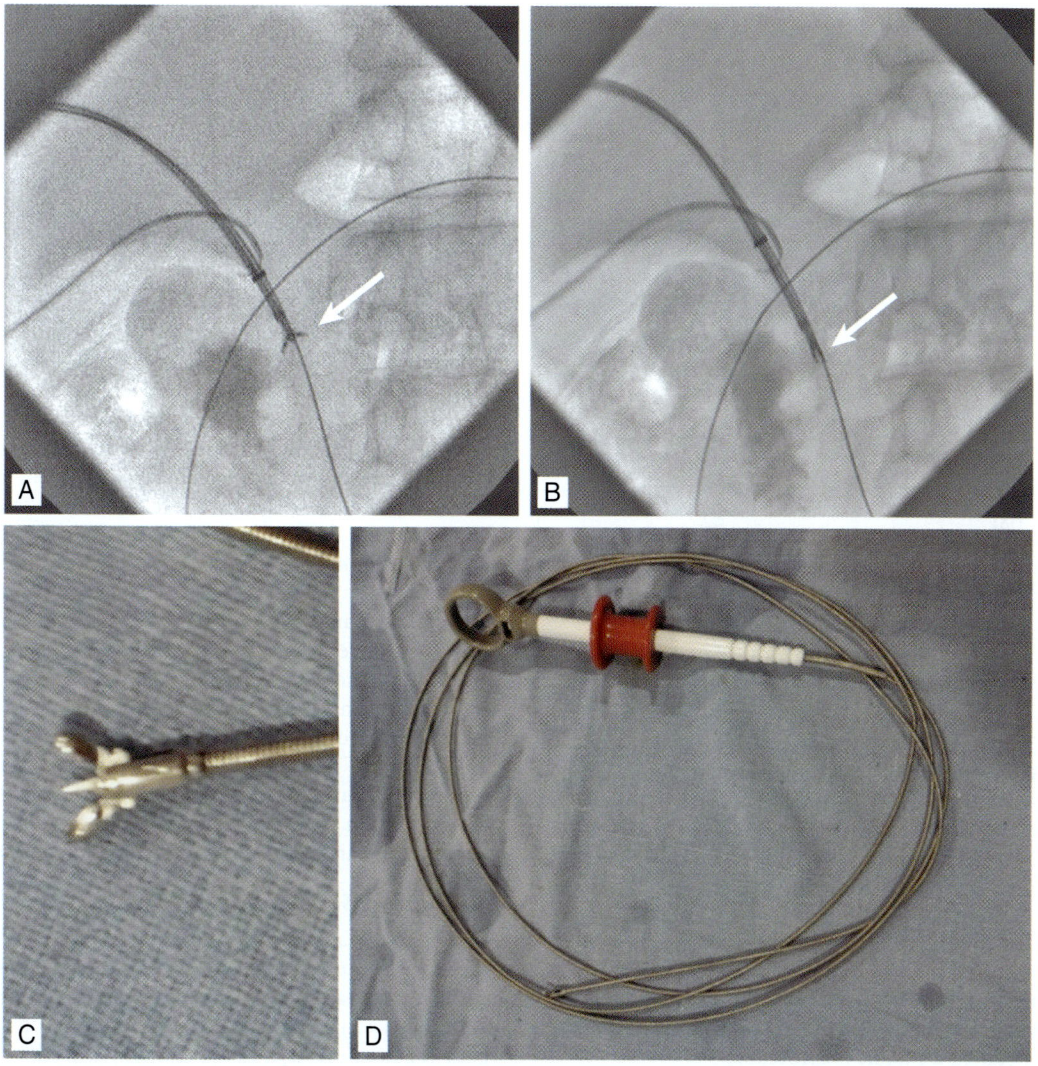

Figure 93.10 Intraductal punch biopsy. (A) Fluoroscopy image of open punch biopsy forceps (*white arrow*) at the site of biliary obstruction. (B) Fluoroscopy image of closed punch biopsy forceps (*white arrow*). (C) Picture of exposed punch biopsy forceps tip. (D) Punch biopsy forceps.

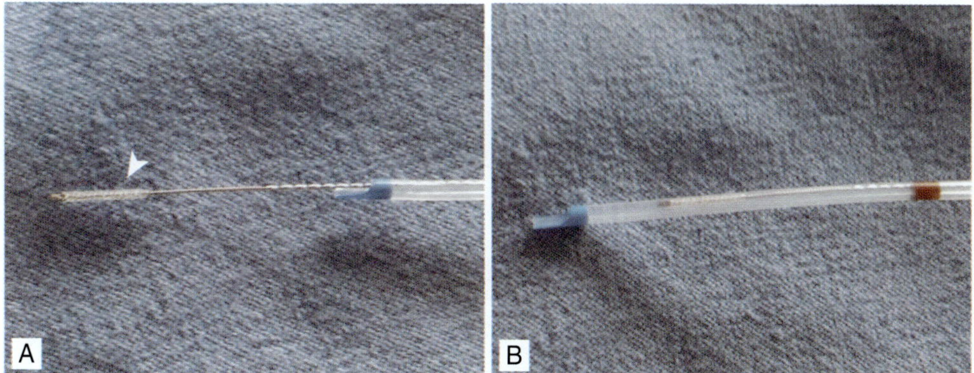

Figure 93.11 Intraductal brush cytology. (A) Exposed brush (*arrowhead*). (B) Brush withdrawn in the sheath.

be used for prostatic sampling if the patient is apprehensive of the transrectal approach. Bowel preparation is very essential for this and has been discussed under Preprocedural instructions.

In the initial years, the presence of prostatic nodule or evidence of metastatic disease was the indication for *prostatic biopsy*. With increasing use of prostate-specific antigen in adults older than the age of 50 years, sampling the prostate without any evidence of nodularity on digital rectal examination is common.

Previously, 6 core biopsies used to be taken, 3 on each side. Currently, it is standard to obtain 12 cores [48] (Fig. 93.12).

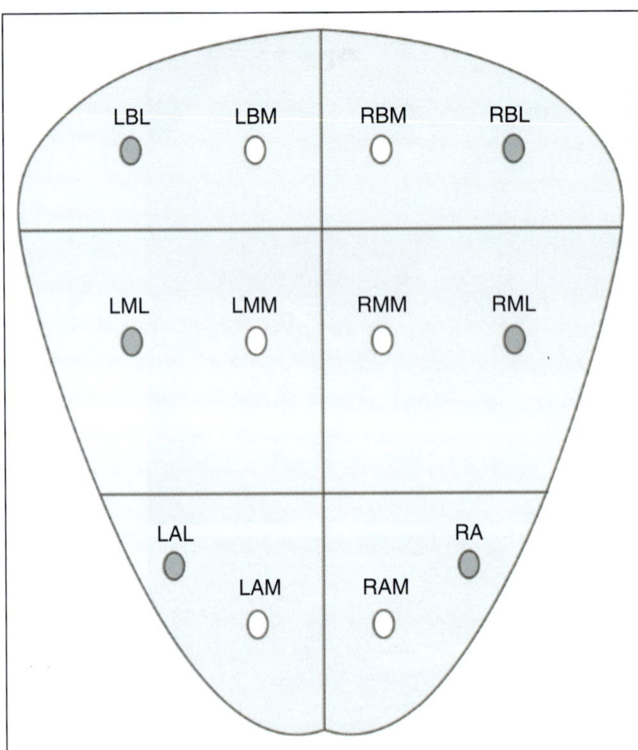

Figure 93.12 Schematic representation of nontarget prostatic biopsy. *LAL,* left apex lateral; *LAM,* left apex medial; *LBL,* left base lateral; *LBM,* left basal medial; *LML,* left mid lateral; *LMM,* left mid medial; *RAL,* right apex lateral; *RAM,* right apex medial; *RBL,* right base lateral; *RBM,* right basal medial; *RML,* right mid lateral; *RMM,* right mid medial.

Bowel preparation with laxatives 2 days before the procedure is done, failing which enema is given preprocedure. Patient is on oral antibiotic cover started 24 hours preprocedure.

The possibility of urethral injury needs to be kept in mind, and patients are followed up by observing the color of the first three samples of urine after the procedure. The reddish discolouration of urine should gradually diminish in prospective samples. Rectal bleeding is another known complication that may also require treatment.

Transvaginal Sampling

This route is used to sample pelvic masses whether they are primary lesions or metastatic or recurrent growths. Percutaneous sampling of ovarian masses is avoided because this can lead to peritoneal seeding of the tumor cells (Figs. 93.13 and 93.14).

Trans-Hollow Viscus

This is not a standard approach but can be used when sampling is important and no other approach route is available. This approach can be used to sample through the gallbladder for an intraluminal gallbladder neck mass. Coaxial biopsy system should be used, and after biopsy, the outer of the coaxial system should be used to completely empty out the gallbladder to prevent any bile leakage after the procedure (Fig. 93.15). It is preferred to go through the liver tissue into the fundus for such sampling because this approach provides compression on the site of entry after the needle is removed.

Similarly, sampling can be done through the urinary bladder. A Foley catheter should be kept in situ in the bladder before the procedure. After the biopsy has been done, the Foley catheter should be connected to bag to keep the bladder empty for 24 hours to avoid any urinary leak (Fig. 93.16).

Biopsy can be done through the stomach and small bowel using a 18-gauge needle but does not require postprocedure decompression. Sampling through the large gut is not done because this can lead to fecal contamination and peritonitis.

Mediastinal Sampling

The preferred approach for anterior mediastinal lesions is extrapleural. One needs to take precautions not to puncture the internal mammary artery because it often lies in the path. If required, a salinoma can be created to dissect through tissues to create a path for needle entry. This is done by injecting 5 to 10 mL of normal saline using a thin needle (22 gauge) between the vessel and intended path to create a space for the biopsy needle. A transsternal approach can also be used if this can avoid pleural

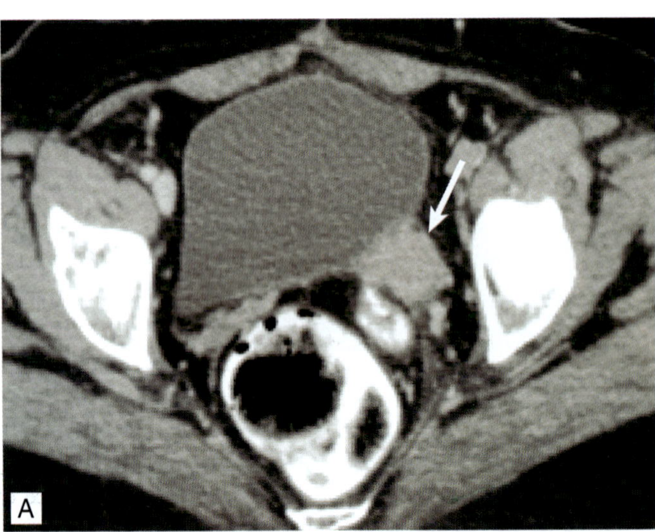

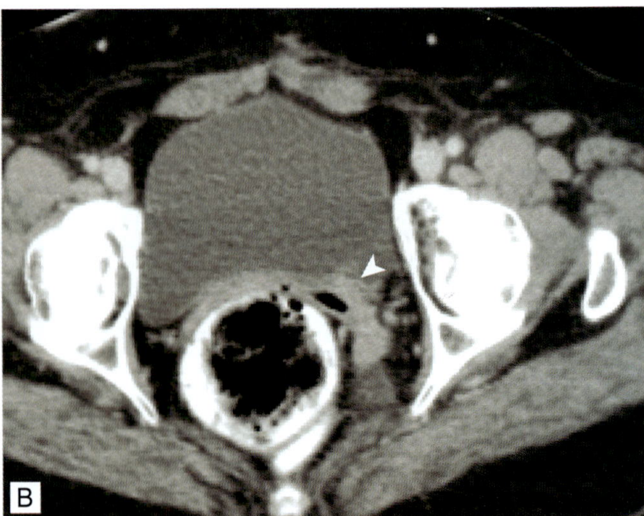

Figure 93.13 (A) Axial computed tomography sections of pelvis showing a perivesical nodule (*arrow*). (B) Nodule appreciated close to the left fornix (*arrowhead*).

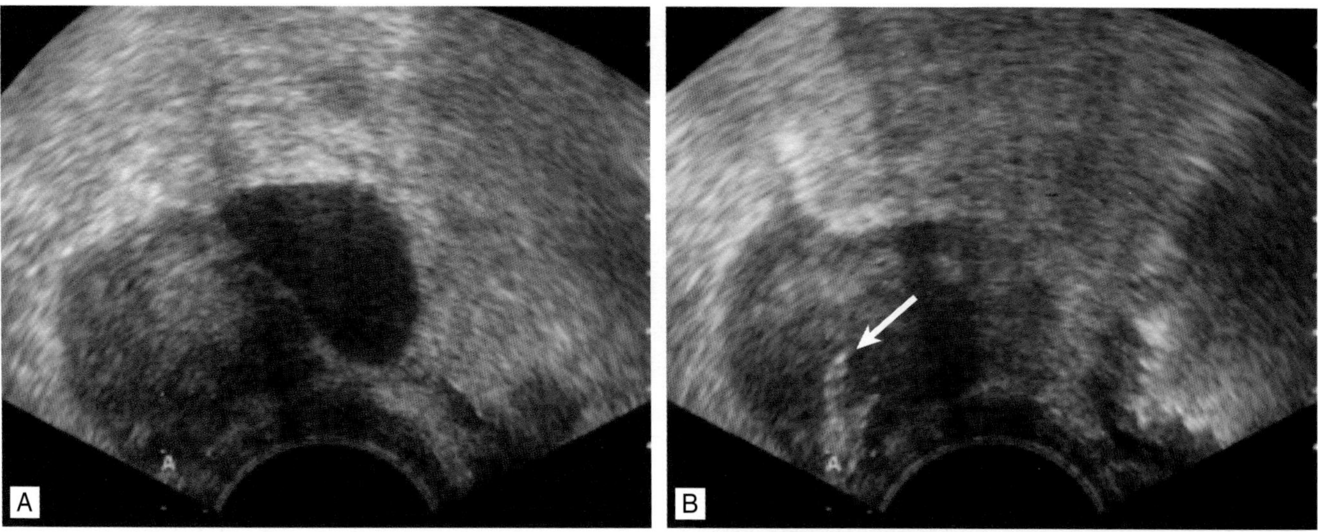

Figure 93.14 (A) Transvaginal ultrasound images showing the lesion (as seen in Fig. 93.13) from the left fornix. (B) A biopsy needle in the lesion (*arrow*).

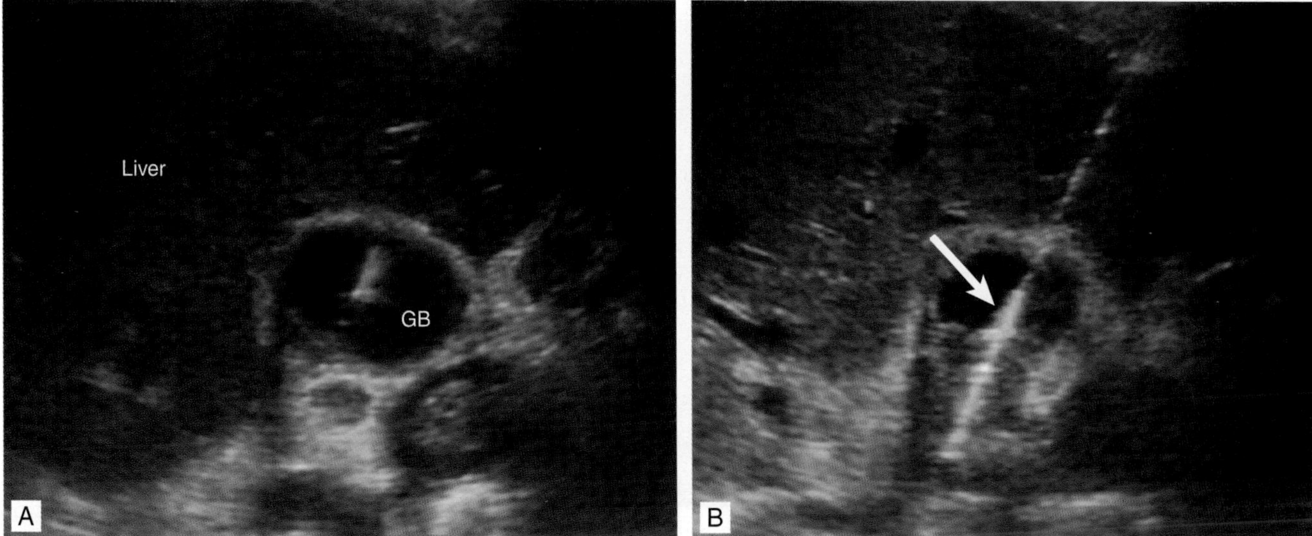

Figure 93.15 Per-abdomen ultrasound images show transhepatic needle in the gallbladder (GB) fundus (A) and the biopsy needle (*arrow*) in the GB neck mass (B).

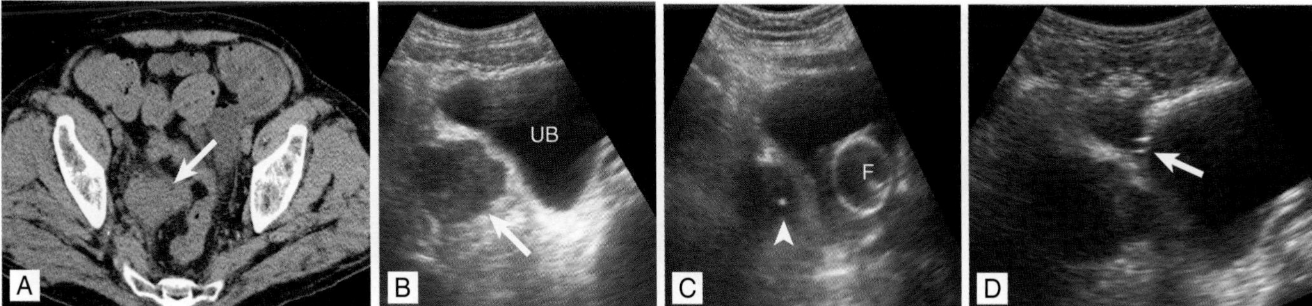

Figure 93.16 (A) Axial computed tomography image of the pelvis shows the pelvic lesion (*arrow*). (B) Per-abdomen ultrasound image shows the lesion (*arrow*) in relation to the urinary bladder (UB). (C) A Foley catheter (F) in the urinary bladder and needle tip (*arrowhead*) in the lesion. (D) The needle is seen reaching the lesion through a transvesical route (*arrow*).

puncture. In this case, a bone biopsy needle is used to go through sternum, and a soft tissue biopsy needle is advanced coaxially for final sampling from the mass (Fig. 93.17). While sampling paracardiac lesions, the needle tip should be kept away from the pericardium (Fig. 93.18).

Pulmonary Lesions

If there are any pleural-based lesions, they are easily sampled on USG guidance. For deeper lesions, CT guidance is required. Because pulmonary lesions move with respiration, it is very important to counsel the patient that the sampling needs to be

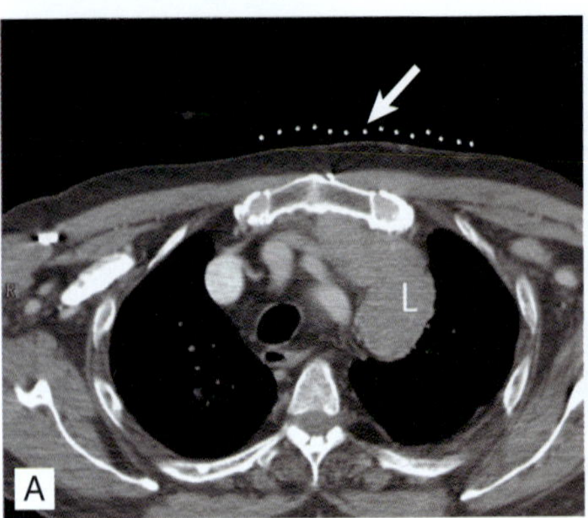

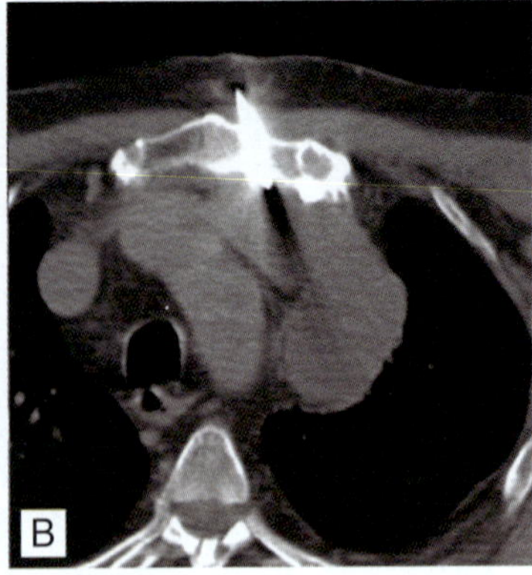

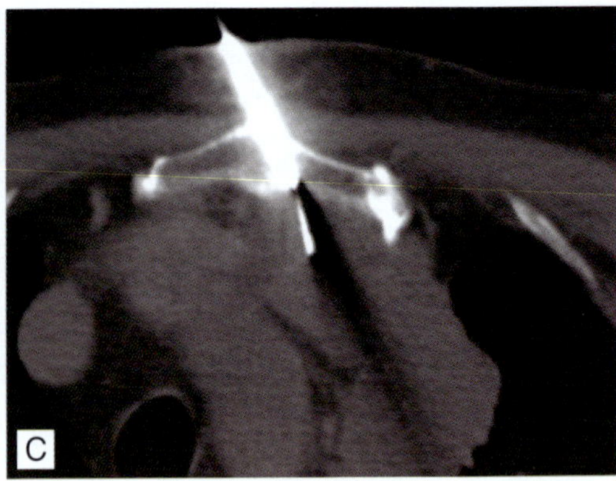

Figure 93.17 Case of myasthenia after thymectomy with a recurrent retrosternal lesion. (A) Axial computed tomography scan images show the lesion (L) and the planning grid (*arrow*). (B) Bone biopsy needle through the sternum. (C) Soft tissue biopsy needle through the bone biopsy needle in the lesion.

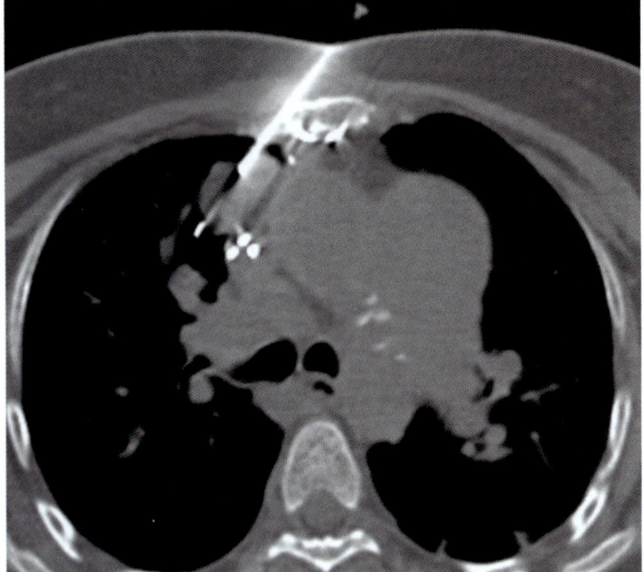

Figure 93.18 Parasternal approach with needle between sternum and internal mammary artery for para cardiac mass. Needle tip is not pointing towards the heart.

done in quiet, shallow respiration. Breath-holding can make it difficult to target the lesion and is best avoided. Planning of the needle path should be done using a path where fissures are not being traversed because this increases the risk of pneumothorax (Fig. 93.19).

The sample collection for pulmonary lesions is different from the rest of the tissues as IHC markers are mostly needed to classify tumors. Hence, multiple cores (three to four) should be taken in formalin, and an extra core of tissue is required in a special medium (phosphate buffered solution). The detailed evaluation required on the tissue and prevalence of different types of lung cancer as given in World Health Organization (WHO) classification of lung tumors [49] is given in Fig. 93.20.

Testicular Sampling

This is required mostly for diagnosis in cases of infertility with azoospermia on semen analysis or for testicular sperm extraction. Most of the testicular tumors are diagnosed on imaging and taken up for surgery without sampling. However, in cases in which the diagnosis is in doubt or to rule out carcinoma in-situ in patients presenting with microlithiasis with associated risk factors such as undescended testis, testicular atrophy, infertility,

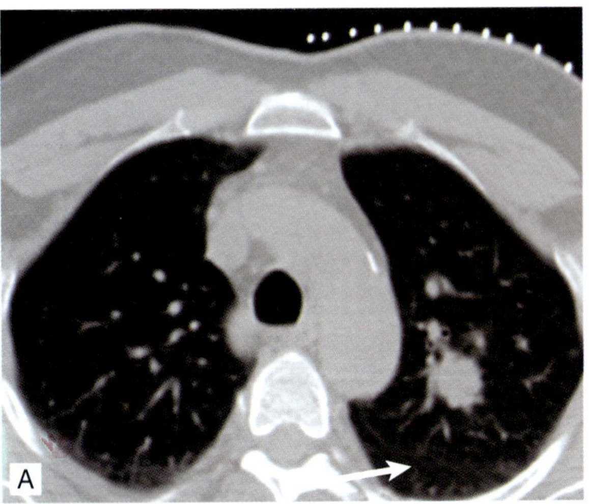

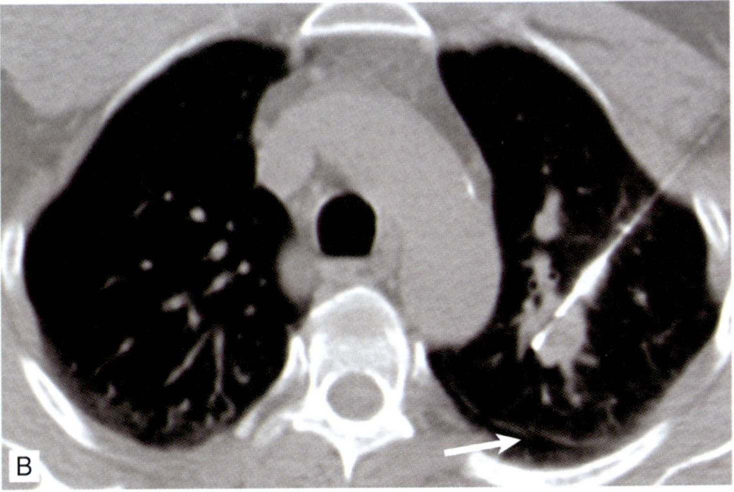

Figure 93.19 (A) Axial section computed tomography scan shows an oblique fissure (*arrow*) in the posterior approach to sample the left upper lobar mass. (B) Longer route using the anterior approach used to sample the lesion to avoid traversing the fissure (*arrow*).

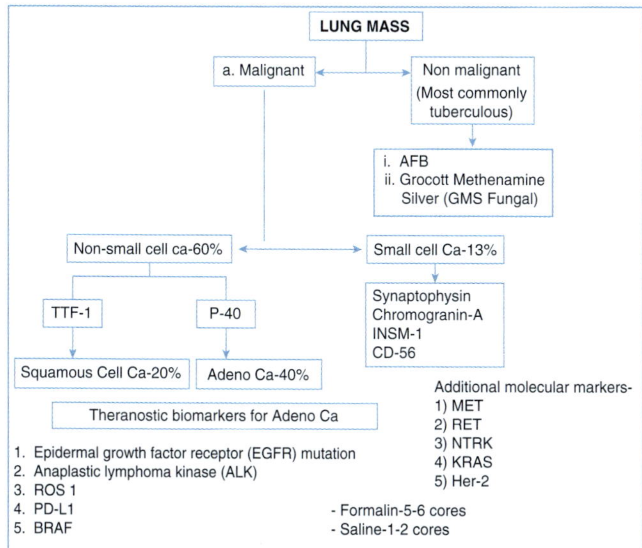

Figure 93.20 Chart evaluation of lung biopsy required as per WHO classification.

or a history of unilateral germ cell tumor, percutaneous sampling is required [50]. Testicular sampling can be done in the cover of testicular nerve block, which renders the procedure painless.

In cases of infertility, a 22-gauge needle is used, and the aspirate is used to either prepare slides for diagnostic purpose or the aspirate is used for testicular sperm aspiration. If the aspirate does not give a good yield of sperm, percutaneous biopsy with an 18-gauge coaxial biopsy needle is done for testicular sperm extraction.

Spleen Biopsy

The spleen can be affected in multiorgan disease and is considered for sampling if there is no other safer alternative site available. Splenic biopsy is often avoided because of the perceived higher risk of hemorrhage. In a metaanalysis by Mathew et al. [51], including four studies (639 patients) for diagnostic accuracy and nine studies (741 patients) for complication rate, it was concluded that pooled sensitivity was 87% and pooled specificity was 96.4%, but major complication rate with 18-gauge needles was 1.3%. These findings are just marginally higher than those encountered with biopsy from liver or kidney.

It is considered safer by the authors to use 18-gauge coaxial biopsy needle and plug the track with Gelfoam or glue. As in liver lesion sampling, the needle path to the lesion through normal tissue is preferred.

Adrenal Biopsy

With improvements in imaging, the need for adrenal sampling has decreased over the years. However, this may be required in the following situations:

a. Staging of known malignancy
b. Identifying an unknown primary malignancy
c. Differentiating benign from malignant adrenal mass when imaging is equivocal

Adrenal adenomas can be diagnosed with a sensitivity of 98% and specificity of 92% by CT. This accuracy can further increase with the use of magnetic resonance imaging [52]. Pheochromocytomas are characteristically arterially enhancing lesions and can be diagnosed with a sensitivity of 83% to 100% and a specificity of 95% to 100% by iodine-123-metaiodobenzylguanidine (^{123}I-MIBG) [52]. Urine and plasma metanephrines should be done to screen patients if pheochromocytoma is suspected. This is very important because the patient may go into hypertensive crisis due to catecholamine secretion precipitated by the biopsy. A pharmacologic blockage (adrenergic blockade) may be used before the procedure when there is high suspicion for pheochromocytoma. During the procedure, direct-acting vasodilators (nitroprusside) should be kept ready.

The larger adrenal lesions can be sampled using USG guidance; for the smaller lesions, CT guidance is required. A caudocranial angulation helps reach the lesion without transgressing the pleura or lung.

The left adrenal gland can be easily sampled using endoscopic ultrasound guidance with a transgastric approach, but right adrenal lesions need percutaneous sampling.

Pelvic Sampling

Pelvic masses originating from the uterus, ovaries, or fallopian tubes usually undergo debulking surgery as the first step followed by chemotherapy later on [53]. Image-guided biopsy does not figure in the protocol for staging of cervical cancer also. However, patients unfit for surgery or in those in the late stage of cancer may need tissue sampling before chemotherapy can be started. Biopsy is also essential in patients with preexisting cancer that can metastasize to ovary (e.g., breast, gastrointestinal tract, melanoma) [54].

If patients with pelvic malignancy have extrapelvic disease in the form of abdominal lymphadenopathy, omental caking, or pulmonary lesions that are suspicious for metastasis, these should be preferred for sampling. If there is no suspicion for extrapelvic disease, the transvaginal route should be preferred over the percutaneous route because there is a risk of peritoneal seeding of tumor cells in percutaneous sampling.

Endoscopic Sampling

For abdominal or mediastinal lesions that are difficult to access percutaneously, options of endoscopic USG or endobronchial ultrasound-guided sampling should be considered.

Basics of Aspiration

This is required in smaller collections or to decide whether drainage is required.

Indications for Diagnostic Aspirations

1. To rule out infection by fluid cell count and to decide on antibiotic by culture/sensitivity
2. To look for hemorrhage in collection
3. For malignant cytology
4. To confirm pancreatic duct leakage by doing fluid amylase level
5. To diagnose chyle leak from fluid triglyceride level

Most of the diagnostic tests can be done with a sample of 20 mL. However, for malignant cytology, an attempt should be to give at least 100 mL of fluid.

Diagnostic aspirations can be done using a 22-gauge needle. If a patient has a coagulation disorder, a 26-gauge needle is preferred, and for thick collections, an 18- or 16-gauge needle is preferred.

One should ensure the availability of the appropriate containers and media for securing the sample. A sterile container is required for aerobic and anaerobic culture of any purulent collection such as liver abscess. Specific blood culture bottles are used for culture of sterile fluids such as pleural effusion and ascites. If only a few drops of pus are aspirated, one should send the sample in sterile swabs.

Basics of Drainage Procedures

Percutaneous drainage of abdominal collections, empyema gallbladder, liver abscess, or pyonephrosis plays a major role in management of patients in sepsis. These patients remain unfit for surgical procedures because of severe sepsis. When sepsis has been controlled by percutaneous drainage, the patient can be taken up for final surgical management if required.

There is also a requirement for drainage procedures in postsurgical situations for residual or new loculated collections. The mortality rate for undrained collections can vary from 45 to 100% [55]. Common indications for therapeutic drainage are as follows:

1. Drainage of infected fluid (e.g., postoperative; pancreatitis; liver, renal, or splenic abscess)
2. Relief from respiratory distress (pleural drainage)
3. Relief from abdominal distension (ascitic drainage)
4. External drainage of urine in obstructed kidney or urinary bladder
5. Special procedures such as cholecystostomy for obstructed gallbladder or cecostomy to relieve large gut obstruction

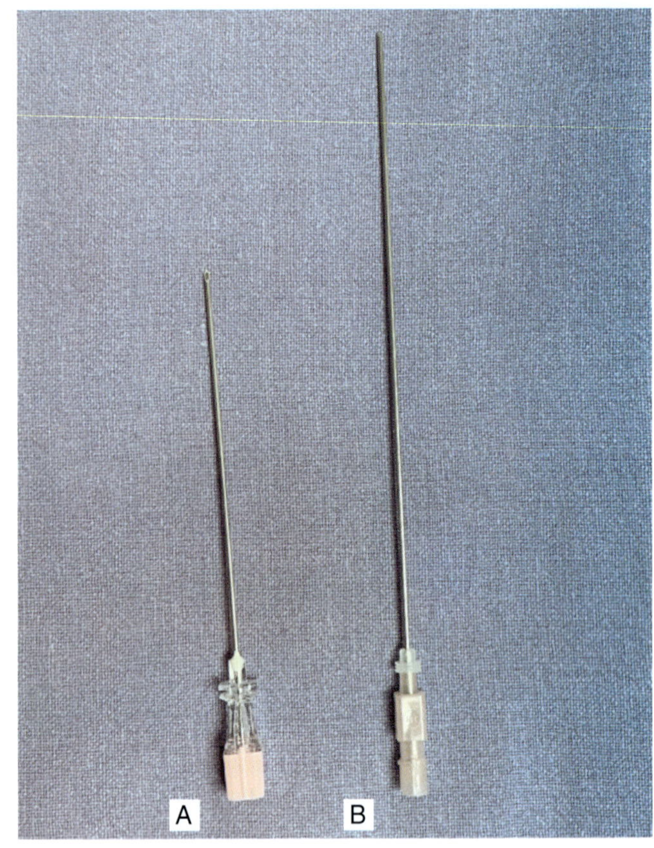

Figure 93.21 Chiba needles: 18 gauge, 9 cm (A). and 15 cm (B).

Hardware

Needles

Most of the drainage procedures require an 180-gauge Chiba needle (Fig. 93.21). Although most of the procedures can be done with a 9-cm needle, few deeper collections may require a 15-cm or longer needle. The longer needles are especially helpful for drainage of septated collections where the long needle can be maneuvered to break the septae. Some collections having narrow access are best drained using an access set (Fig. 93.22) containing a 22-gauge needle with an 0.018-inch guide wire over which a 4-Fr sheath with its stiffener can be sent into the collection for exchanging with a 0.03-inch Amplatz ultra-stiff guidewire.

Wires

Most of the collections are drained using an 80-cm, 035-inch Amplatz ultra-stiff guidewire, but deeper collections where a long track has to be dilated require a 145-cm, 0.035-inch Amplatz super-stiff guidewire is useful (Fig. 93.23).

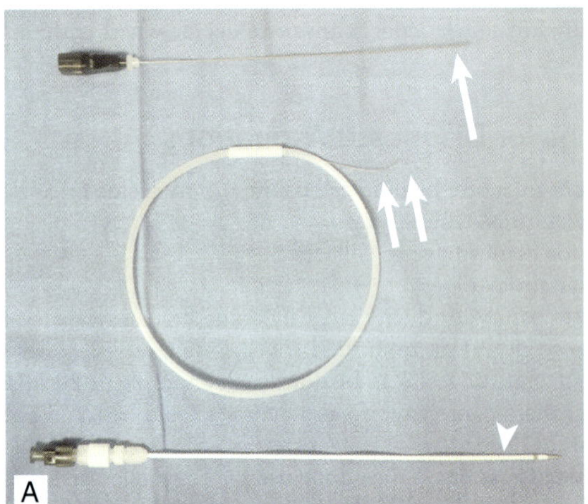

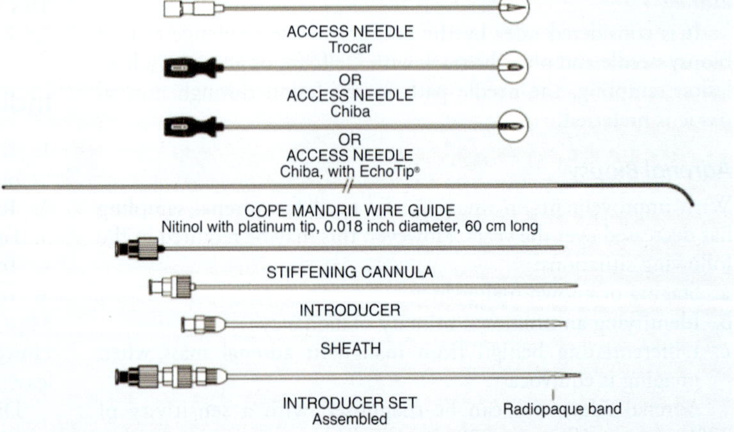

Figure 93.22 Neff percutaneous access set (Cook Medical). (A) A 22-gauge needle (*arrow*), 0.018-inch wire (*double arrow*), and 4-Fr assembled sheath (*arrowhead*). (B) Pictorial representation of a Neff set.

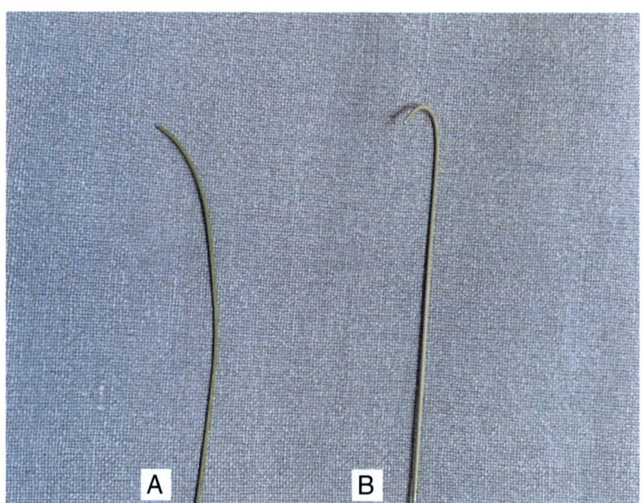

Figure 93.23 (A) Amplatz 0.035-inch, 80-cm ultrastiff wire. (B) Amplatz 0.035-inch, 145-cm super-stiff wire.

Dilators

Two types of dilators are available (Fig. 93.24):

1. **Fascial:** These have a short taper and are the commonly used dilators.
2. **Coons:** These have a long, smooth distal taper, making the transition over the wire easier. These are *not* suited for dilating small cavities as in cholecystostomy or nephrostomy.

Whenever a larger bore catheter is to be placed, serial progressive dilation makes it easier to dilate up to the desired size.

Catheters

These come in different shapes meant for draining different type of collections (Fig. 93.25). All catheters come in different sizes ranging from 5 to 32 Fr. The most common shapes are as follows:

1. **Pigtail catheter:** These are most commonly used for drainage of collections anywhere in the body (e.g., pleural, postoperative collections, abscess drainage).

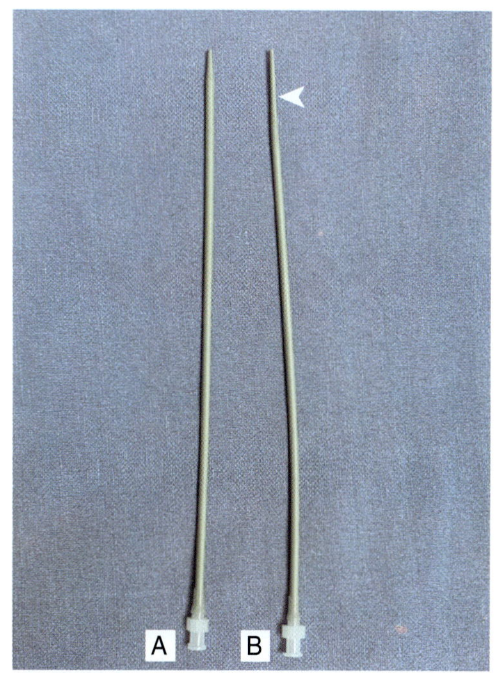

Figure 93.24 Dilators. (A) Twelve-Fr fascial. (B) Coons, showing the smooth distal taper (*arrowhead*).

2. **Malecot catheter:** These are most commonly used in places that cannot accommodate a larger size of the pigtail catheter (e.g., nephrostomy).
3. **Straight catheter:** These are most commonly used to drain thick collections (e.g., pancreatitis collection, empyema).

Drainage Bags

There is a wide array of drainage bags, but the most common ones in use are

1. **Urobag:** These are attached to the drainage catheter and come in different capacities ranging from 1 to 2 L.

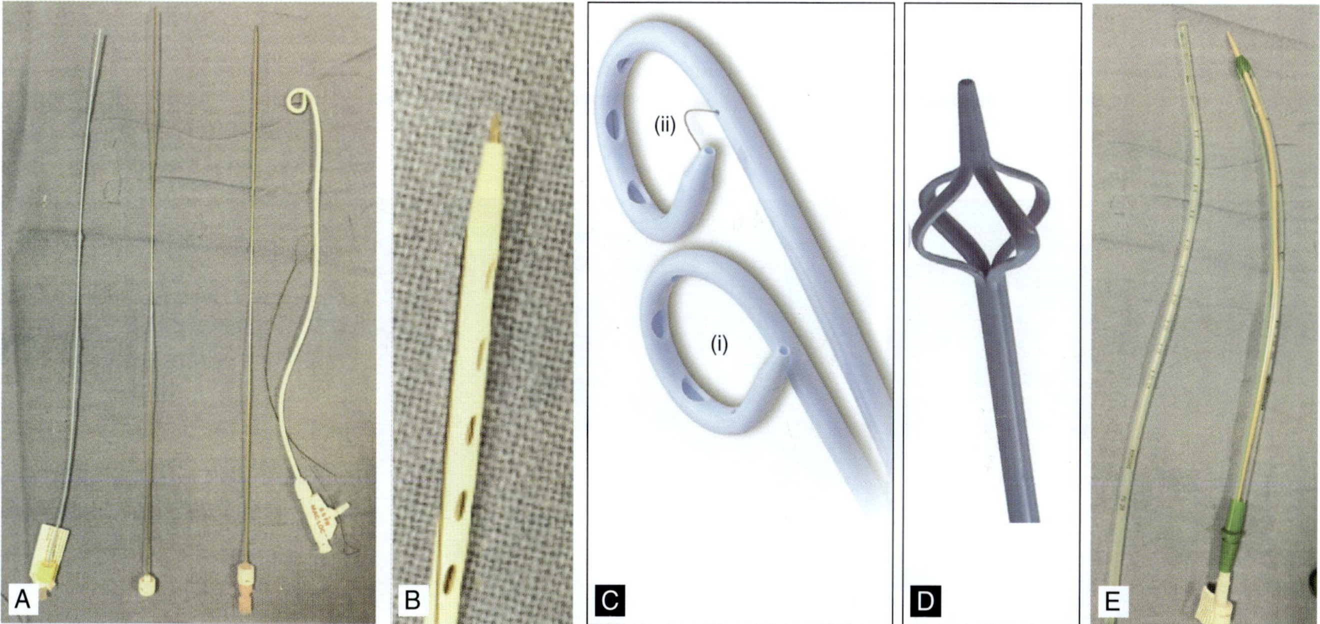

Figure 93.25 Catheters. (A) Pigtail catheter with a metal and soft stiffening cannula. (B) An assembled pigtail catheter with the trocar tip seen distally. (C) Nonlocking (i) and locking loop (ii) pigtail catheters. (D) Malecot catheter. (E) Straight catheter.

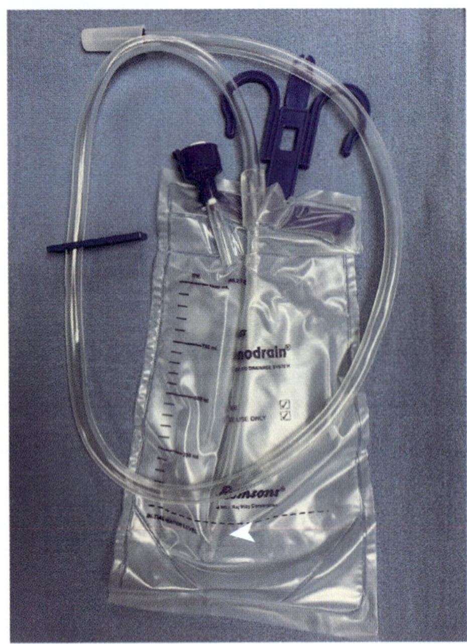

Figure 93.26 Water seal drainage bag with tubing reaching under the water seal (*arrowhead*).

2. **Water seal drainage bag**: These are used to drain pleural fluid and have a water seal mechanism to prevent any backflow of air into the pleural cavity (Fig. 93.26).
3. **Suction drainage bag:** These are most commonly used in surgical drains but can also be used for draining some thick collections.

Most of the drainage procedures are preferably done using the Seldinger technique, but the trocar technique is preferred for suprapubic cystostomy and superficial hydatid cysts.

Pleural Drainage

Anechoic large pleural collections can be drained using 10- or 12-Fr catheters. An intercostal approach is used for pleural collections. Care should be taken to avoid leaving the catheter in a subpulmonic location because it can get trapped and stop draining after a small amount of fluid is drained.

The septated pleural collections need a larger bore catheter from 16 to 32 Fr. The pleural drainage catheters need to be connected to a water seal drainage bag. The output of the catheter should be measured daily, and the pleural catheter can be removed when the output is less than 100 mL in the preceding 24 hours [56] and there is no residual pericatheter collection. *To avoid reexpansion pulmonary edema, it is not recommended to drain more than 1 to 1.5 L of fluid in a day because this can lower the pleural pressures alarmingly* [57].

Ascitic Drainage

Ascites can be drained using thin catheters with caliber of 5 F if there are no septations. The septated collections need larger bore catheters with multiple side holes to be able to achieve complete drainage. It is important to avoid injury to the inferior epigastric artery during ascitic drainage from either flank (Fig. 93.27).

Large-volume paracentesis in patients with cirrhosis should be done under cover of albumin infusion to prevent hypoalbuminemia and its associated complications.

Liver Abscess

Untreated hepatic abscess can be fatal because of complications such as development of sepsis or peritonitis from rupture into the peritoneal space. These can also cause respiratory distress by rupture into the pleural cavity. All abscesses with impending rupture (margins within 10 mm of the liver capsule) [58] should be treated with percutaneous needle-based aspiration or catheter-based drainage along with appropriate antibiotics (Fig. 93.28). Centrally located small abscesses may be treated with only antibiotics. Liver abscesses are preferably drained with an approach through normal parenchyma rather than direct puncture of the abscess cavity. Most of the abscesses heal early, but some catheters keep draining large amount of bile because of biliary communication within the abscess cavity. This can be managed by endoscopic papillotomy with or without plastic stent placement in the relevant bile duct for biliary diversion.

Cholecystostomy

Patients with acute cholecystitis (calculous or acalculous), empyema, or perforated gallbladder caused by impacted

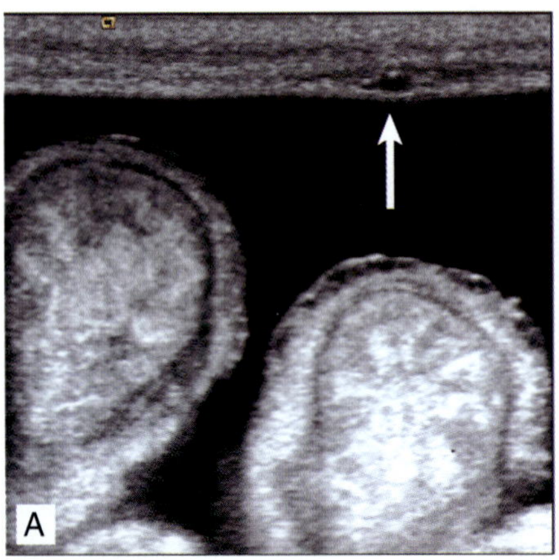

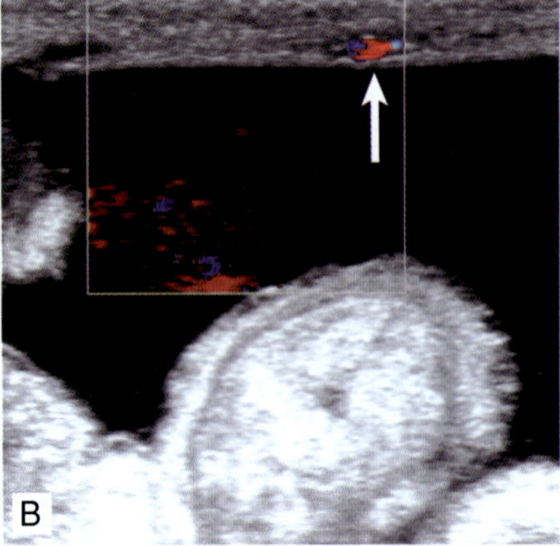

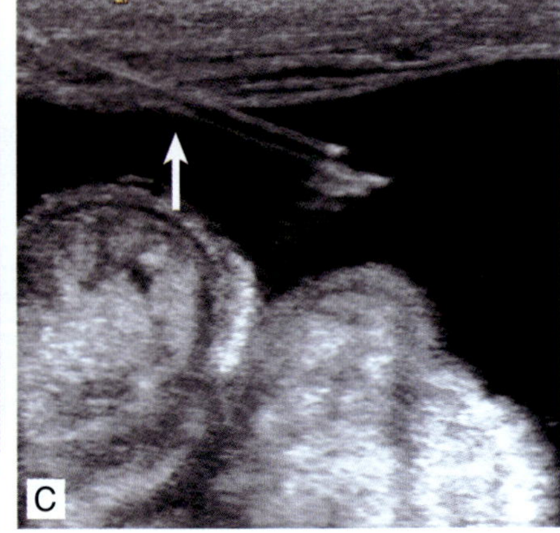

Figure 93.27 (A) Inferior epigastric artery (*arrow*) seen on a high-frequency ultrasound image (*grayscale*) during ascitic drainage. (B) Color flow seen in the inferior epigastric artery (*arrow*) on Doppler. (C) Ascitic drainage needle (*arrow*) seen away from the vessels.

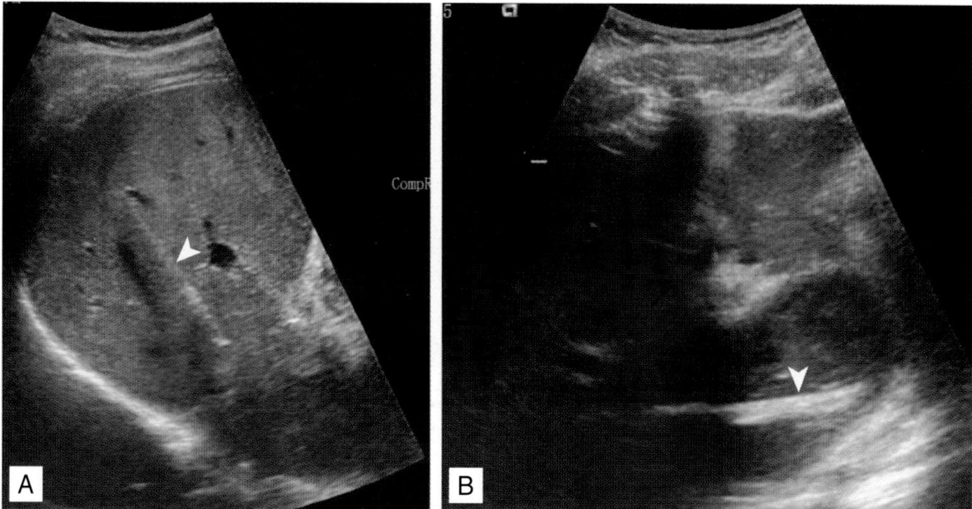

Figure 93.28 Percutaneous drainage of impending rupture caudate lobe abscess. (A) The needle (*arrowhead*) is seen advancing from the intercostal approach. (B) The catheter (*arrowhead*) is seen in the abscess with ultrasonography done from the epigastrium.

calculus or any other reason who are poor surgical candidates because of sepsis or comorbid conditions should be treated with percutaneous cholecystostomy (PC). After sepsis has been controlled and co-morbid conditions optimized, definitive surgery can be performed. The drainage catheter can be placed using a transhepatic or transperitoneal approach (Fig. 93.29). A transhepatic approach is preferred because of less risk of biliary leak, early track maturation, and better stability of the catheter [59]. It is important to counsel the patient that the catheter needs to remain in situ for at least 4 weeks until track matures unless surgery happens earlier [59]. PC may be the only treatment required for cases of acalculous cholecystitis [60]. After 4 weeks, the catheter can be removed either by giving a trial of capping for 24 hour or after doing cholecystogram

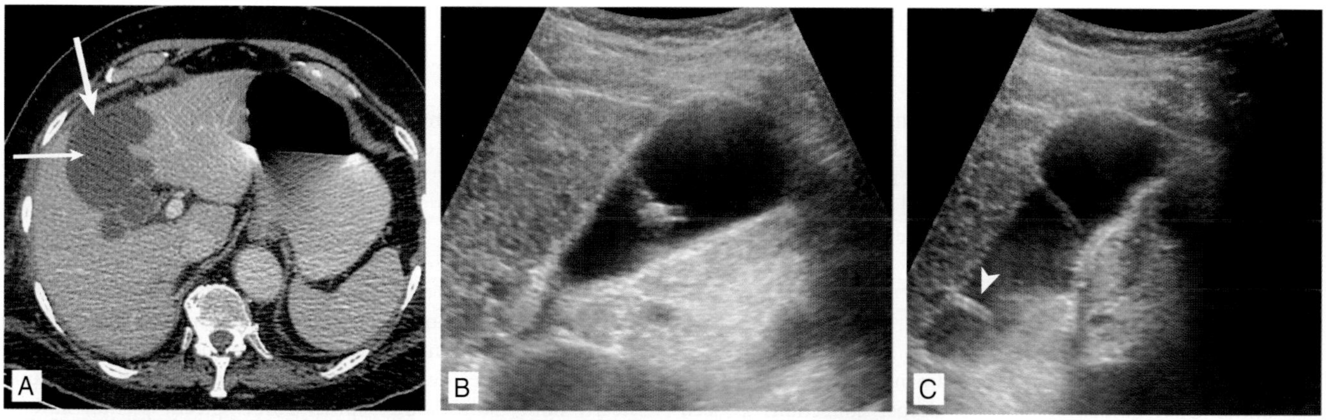

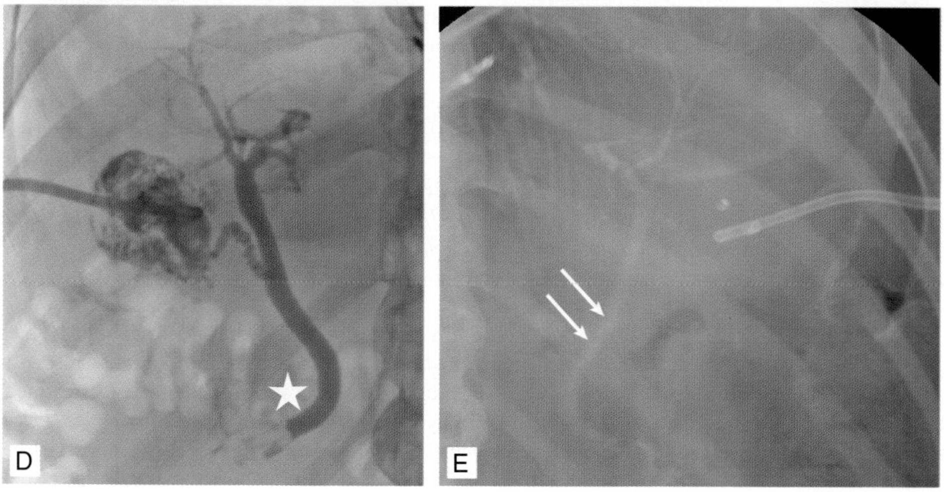

Figure 93.29 Percutaneous cholecystostomy. (A) Axial computed tomography section shows the transhepatic approach (*arrow*) and direct approach (*bold arrow*). (B) Transabdominal ultrasound image with the intercostal approach shows the needle tip in the gallbladder using the transhepatic approach. (C) The catheter tip is seen in the GB (*arrowhead*) (D) Cholecystogram demonstrates a patent cystic duct with distal common bile duct calculus (*star*) causing obstruction. (E) Decompressed common bile duct (*double arrow*) after calculus removal by endoscopic retrograde cholangiopancreatography before cholecystostomy catheter removal.

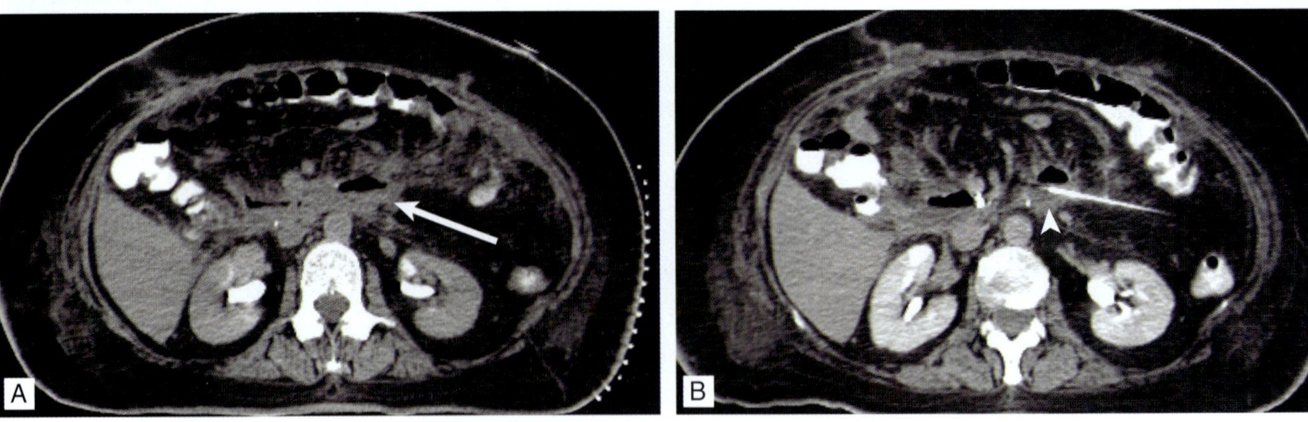

Figure 93.30 Axial computed tomography (CT) images show mesenteric collection (*arrow*) (A) and the percutaneous drainage catheter (*arrowhead*) placed under CT guidance (B).

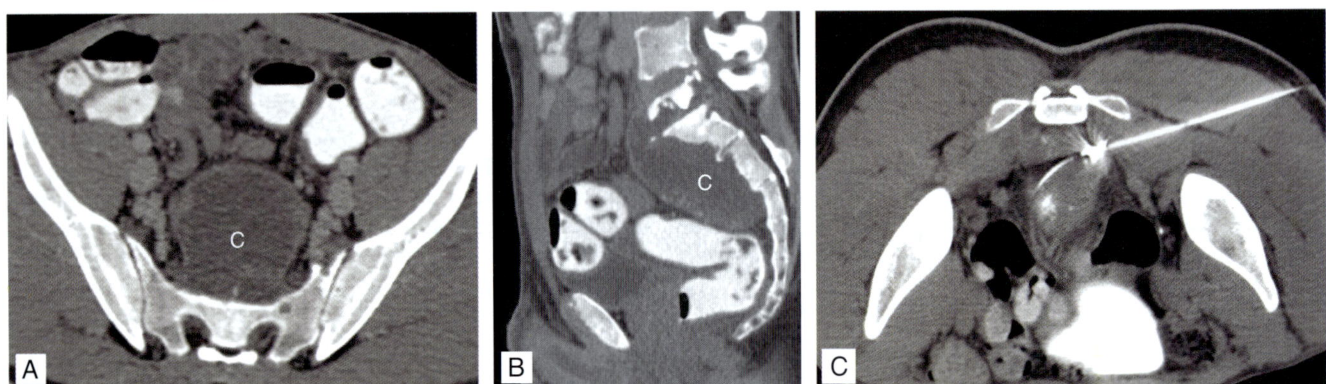

Figure 93.31 Computed tomography (CT) images showing presacral collection. (A) Axial section. (B) Sagittal section. (C) CT-guided drainage using a posterior approach.

and demonstrating free flow of contrast into common bile duct and duodenum (see Fig. 93.29). If the cholecystogram shows calculus obstructing the gallbladder neck or cystic duct and surgery is not feasible because of comorbidities, percutaneous cholecystolithotomy or ablation of the gallbladder can be considered.

Deep Abdominal Collections

Most of the abdominal collections are amenable to catheter drainage under USG guidance, however, deeper collections as seen with appendicular or diverticular perforation may need CT guidance (Fig. 93.30). Loculated pelvic collections may need to be drained using transrectal, transvaginal ultrasound, or CT guidance (Fig. 93.31).

Chylous Ascites and Chylothorax

These are caused by leakage of lipid-rich lymph into the peritoneal or pleural cavity because of disruption of the lymphatic system secondary to traumatic injury or obstruction. The various causes are listed in Table 93.4. The fluid is milky in color and has high triglyceride content (>200 mg/dL) [61,62]. These patients are treated with drainage of fluid along with dietary modification (high-protein and low-fat diets supplemented with medium-chain triglycerides) or total parenteral nutrition and/or somatostatins. Most patients respond well to this treatment.

Resistant cases need percutaneous lymphangiography and embolization. A few cases may require surgical intervention.

Hydatid Cyst

Hydatid cystic disease is a parasitic disease caused by *Echinococcus granulosus*. Hydatid cysts are mostly localized in the liver (50–70%); the next most common site is the lungs (20–30%) [63,64]. Other common sites of involvement in decreasing order of frequency are the peritoneum, kidney, brain, mediastinum, heart, bone, soft tissues, spinal cord, spleen, pleura, adrenal glands, bladder, ovary, scrotum, and thyroid gland [65]. Several classifications exist for liver hydatid cysts, mainly depending on appearance on USG. The classifications by Gharbi et al. and the WHO Informal Working Group on Echinococcosis are the most commonly used [63] (Table 93.5). Patients with hepatic hydatid cysts have been treated surgically for a long time but this is an invasive method with high rates of morbidity, mortality, and recurrence [66]. *PAIR (puncture the cyst, aspirate cyst fluid, inject a scolicidal agent, and reaspirate the cyst content) has been tried with considerable success in type I and II cysts, with encouraging long-term results* [67].

Various randomized studies have shown superiority of PAIR over surgery in terms of shorter hospital stay, complications, and cost-effectiveness [68]. Studies have also shown percutaneous treatment to be safe and effective alternative therapy in treating patients with Gharbi type III hepatic hydatid cysts [69]. For type III cysts, a large-bore sheath (20–24 F) is inserted and stabilized manually in the cyst

TABLE 93.4 Etiology of Chylous Ascites

NONTRAUMATIC			TRAUMATIC
	OTHERS		
Neoplastic	Congenital	Systemic Disease	
▪ Lymphoma	▪ Primary lymphatic hypoplasia	▪ Constrictive pericarditis	▪ Post-surgery: retroperitoneal lymphadenectomy, abdominal aortic aneurysm repair, nephrectomy
▪ Sarcoma	▪ Klippel-Trenaunay syndrome	▪ Celiac sprue	▪ Post-radiotherapy
▪ Lymphangioleiomyomatosis	▪ Lymphangioma	▪ Pancreatitis	

TABLE 93.5 Ultrasonography Classification of Hydatid Cysts

Gharbi Type	WHO Type	Cyst Morphology
I	CE 1	Unilocular anechoic with double line sign
III	CE 2	Multiseptated rosette like honeycomb cyst
II	CE 3A	Cyst with detached membranes (water-lily sign)
III	CE 3B	Cyst with daughter cysts in solid matrix
IV	CE 4	Cyst with heterogenous/hypoechoic contents. No daughter cysts
V	CE 5	Solid plus calcified wall

Adapted from KY Polat, AA Balik, D Oren, Percutaneous drainage of hydatid cyst of the liver: long-term results, HPB (Oxford) 4 (2002) 163–166.

followed by suction of the cyst contents mechanically using a suction apparatus with catheter of 14-Fr size through the sheath (Fig. 93.32).

Role in Pancreatitis

Acute pancreatitis is a common disorder requiring hospitalization and multispecialty care. Most of these patients require catheter-based drainage of multiple collections rather than upfront surgical drainage as per the PANTER trial [70,71]. This is discussed in detail in Chapter 36.

Hematoma and Organized Collections

Most of the hematomas should not be drained percutaneously because of the risk of frequent occlusion of catheter and possibility of introducing infection into the hematoma [72]. These should be drained surgically. If a catheter has been placed in a hematoma or a septated collection instillation of urokinase should be considered to lyse the clot and drain it more effectively [73].

Splenic Abscess

These may need drainage if the patient is septic. The preferred approach for splenic abscess is direct rather than through normal parenchyma unlike hepatic abscess (Fig. 93.33).

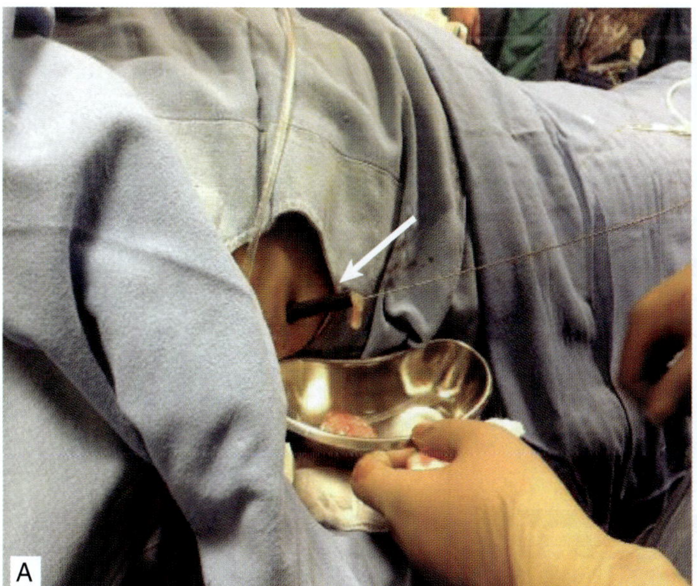

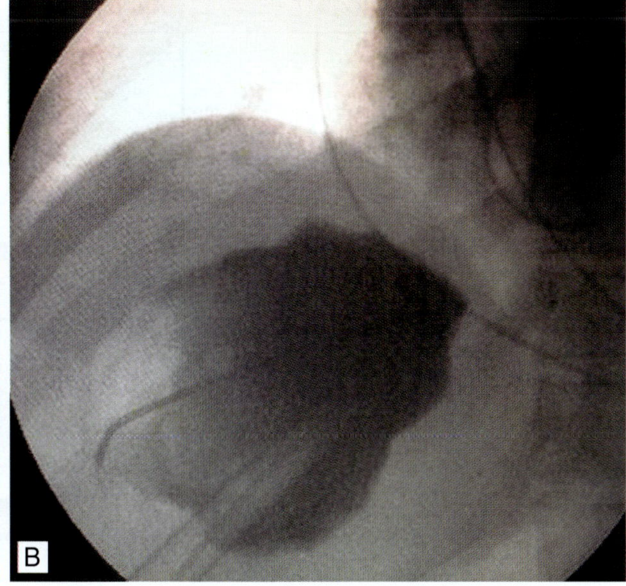

Figure 93.32 (A) A wide-bore sheath (24 Fr) placed percutaneously in a Gharbi type III hepatic hydatid cyst. (B) Cavitogram demonstrates complete aspiration of cyst contents and absence of biliary communication.

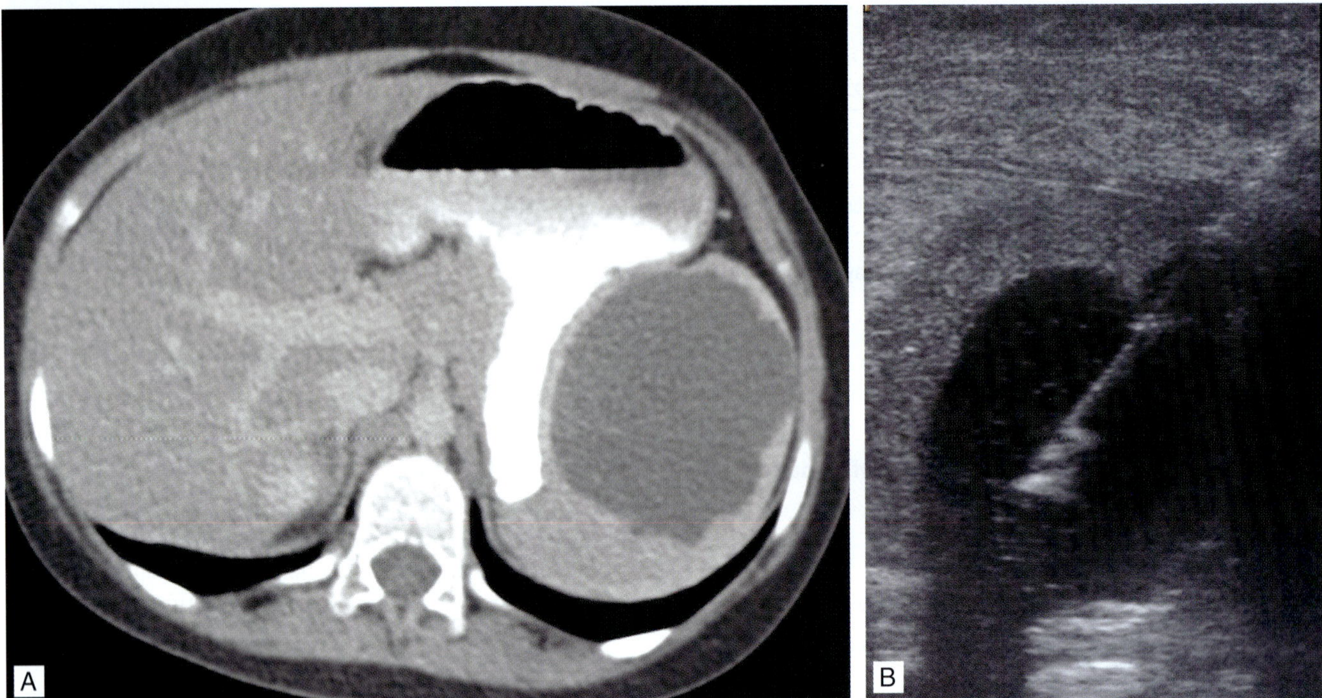

Figure 93.33 Splenic abscess. (A) Axial section computed tomography scan. (B) Needle seen in the abscess through the thinnest parenchyma using a high-frequency linear ultrasound probe.

Basics of Vascular Access

All angiographic procedures start with vascular access. The arterial or venous access route has to be planned according to the planned procedure.

Arterial Access

The femoral artery has been the most common site for arterial access for body angiography, neurointervention, and coronary angiography. There is a recent trend to shift to radial access for diagnostic angiography and therapeutic interventions that can be done through a 6-Fr sheath because larger sheaths are not compatible with the radial artery because of its size.

Femoral or radial access can be done with the palpation method using the Seldinger technique (Fig. 93.34). There are two ways to do this:

1. **Single-wall puncture technique:** After the anterior wall of the artery is punctured as shown by blood flow through the needle, the wire is sent through the needle.

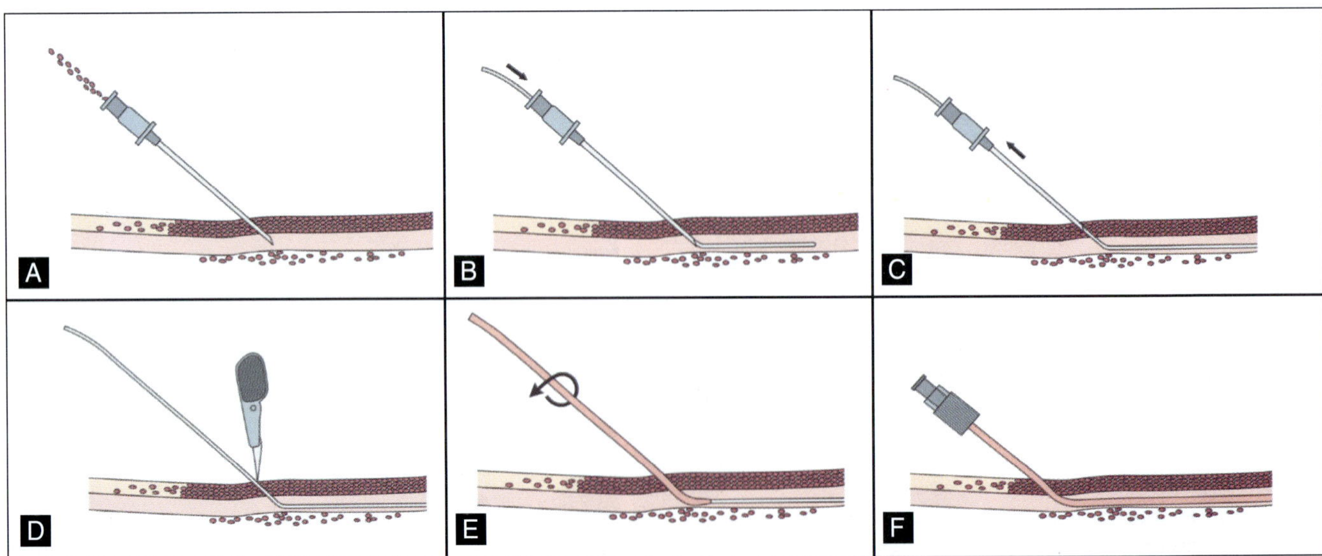

Figure 93.34 Seldinger technique. (A) Needle puncture of the artery. (B) Guidewire passed through the puncture needle. (C) Needle removed over the wire. (D) Skin nick along the wire. (E) Threading of sheath with its dilator over the wire. (F) Wire and dilator removed, leaving the sheath in the artery.

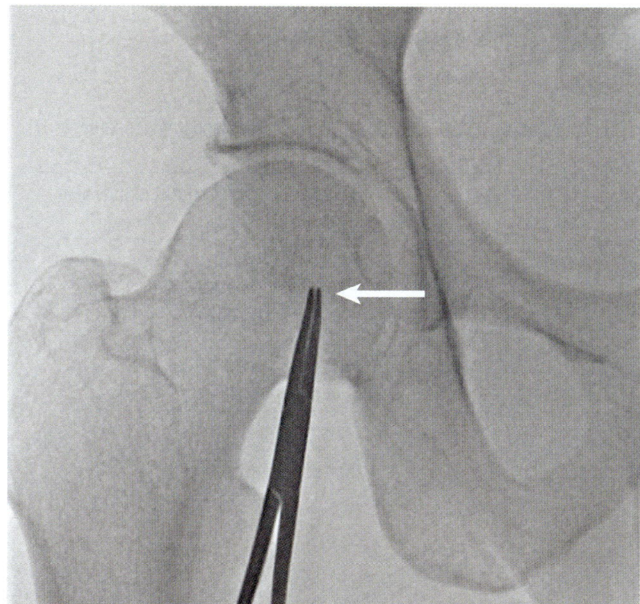

Figure 93.35 Fluoroscopy check before taking femoral access to confirm puncture anterior to the femoral head. A metallic marker is placed over the planned puncture site (*arrow*).

2. **Double-wall puncture technique:** In this technique, after the anterior wall of the artery is punctured, the needle is farther advanced to go through the posterior wall as shown by stoppage of the initial flow of blood through the needle. When the wire is ready to be sent through the needle, the needle is gradually withdrawn until blood flow resumes, and the wire is sent through the needle.

If the pulse is feeble, USG guidance should be taken. This is also helpful in patients who have coagulopathy or who are planned for thrombolysis because the single-wall puncture technique is preferable in such cases. Moreover, ultrasound-guided punctures decrease access site–related complications [74,75].

Femoral Arterial Access

Most of the punctures are done with the palpation method, but it is very important to check on fluoroscopy before taking access. The puncture should be done over the region of femoral head (Fig. 93.35) because after the procedure, it becomes easy to apply compression and achieve hemostasis.

Radial Arterial Access

This is the preferred site in the following circumstances:

1. Patients with aortoiliac occlusive disease
2. Early mobilization is required
3. Ongoing anticoagulation
4. Ease of access because of vascular anatomy (e.g., interventions in the superior mesenteric artery)

A micropuncture needle or radial artery access kit is used for gaining access. It is very important to confirm patency of the palmar arches by the Allen or Barbeau test. If these test results are abnormal, radial access should be avoided. After radial access is taken and a sheath has been placed, a cocktail of calcium channel blocker (e.g., verapamil 2.5 mg), vasodilator (e.g., nitroglycerine 0.25 mg), and heparin (5000 IU) diluted in saline is given through the sheath to prevent vessel spasm and thrombosis [76].

The other arteries that may be accessed are the brachial artery, popliteal artery, and axillary artery.

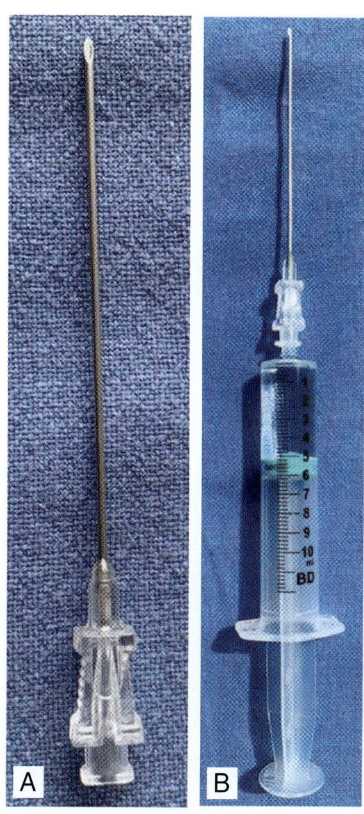

Figure 93.36 (A) Arterial puncture needle. (B) Needle attached with syringe partly filled with saline for venous access.

Venous Access

The femoral vein and internal jugular vein are the most common sites for venous access. These can be accessed by palpation using landmarks or with ultrasound guidance. It is important to attach a syringe (5 or 10 mL) partially filled with heparinized saline to the puncture needle to avoid any embolism unlike the arterial puncture (Fig. 93.36). The Valsalva maneuver during the venous puncture helps to distend the vein and avoid double-wall puncture.

Femoral Venous Puncture

This is most commonly used for

1. Diagnosis and treatment of DVT
2. Inferior vena cava interventions
3. Evaluation and treatment of venous malformations
4. Stenting the superior vena cava in cases of compression by malignant masses

Internal Jugular Vein Puncture

The most common indications for this access are

1. Diagnosis and management of upper limb DVT
2. Central venous access
3. Transjugular liver or kidney biopsy
4. TIPS creation or trans-TIPS variceal embolization
5. Balloon-occluded retrograde transvenous obliteration

Access Sheath

These help in maintaining access of the vessel during the procedure and allow multiple catheter exchanges without any access site injury. Most of the diagnostic angiograms and

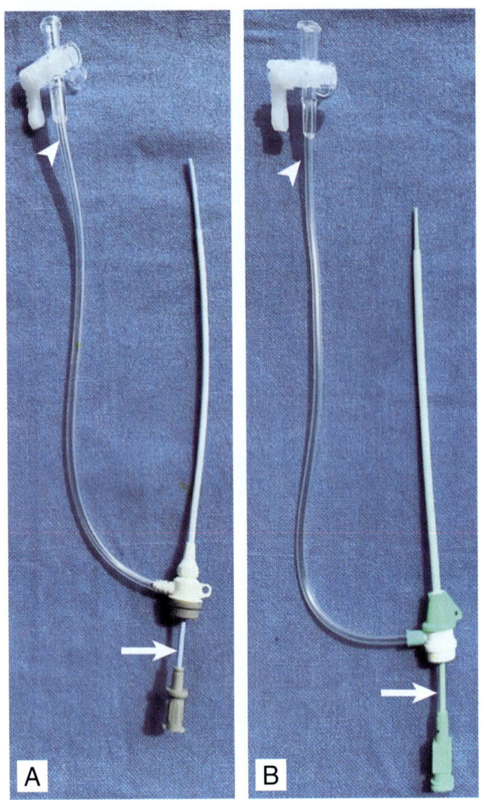

Figure 93.37 Access sheaths. (A) Five Fr (*arrow* showing blue colour of dilator) (B) Six Fr (*arrow* showing green colour of dilator).

venograms can be done using a 4- or 5-Fr sheath. The sheath size represents the inner diameter. However, a larger sized sheath may be required for angioplasty and stenting (e.g., a 10-Fr sheath is used in TIPS).

The sheaths come with an inner dilator, which is removed after placement, and have a side port for flushing and contrast injection (Fig. 93.37). The chances of intrasheath thrombus formation are reduced if the same size catheter is used. If the size of the catheter is smaller than the sheath size, regular flushing should be done to prevent thrombus formation.

TABLE 93.6 Catheters and Their Uses

Catheter	Common Usage
Flush pigtail	Aortograms and venograms in large veins
Cobra 1	Celiac artery, renal artery, adrenal vein sampling
Simmons 1-2	Coeliac artery, SMA, inferior mesenteric artery, cerebral angiography via transradial approach
Multipurpose	TIPS
Headhunter	Cerebral angiography
Picard	Cerebral angiography
Mikaelsson	Bronchial artery

SMA, superior mesenteric artery; *TIPS*, transjugular intrahepatic portosystemic shunt.

Guiding Catheter

These are used for obtaining the angiograms/venograms in the desired vessel. The catheter size represents its outer diameter except in guide catheters where the size represents the inner diameter. Most of these are named after their inventor or the vessel they are meant to engage. Few important guiding catheters are shown in (Fig. 93.38). The important named catheters with their uses are given in Table 93.6.

Microcatheters are used coaxially through the guiding catheter for superselective cannulation of distal branches for angiograms and to deliver embolic material (e.g., polyvinyl alcohol particles of microcoils). These are less than 3 Fr in outer diameter. It is important to pass the microcatheters into the guiding catheter through a Y-connector, which helps in running a continuous flush to avoid thrombus formation in the guiding catheter (Fig. 93.39).

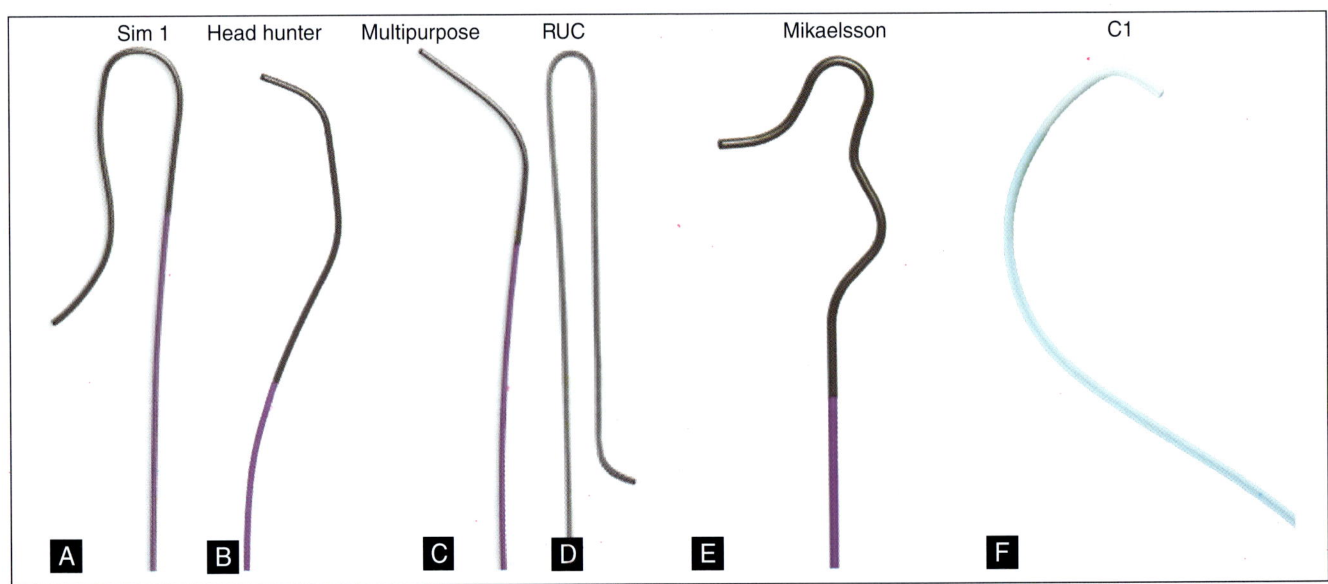

Figure 93.38 (A–F) Angiographic guiding catheters. *RUC,* Robert's uterine catheter.

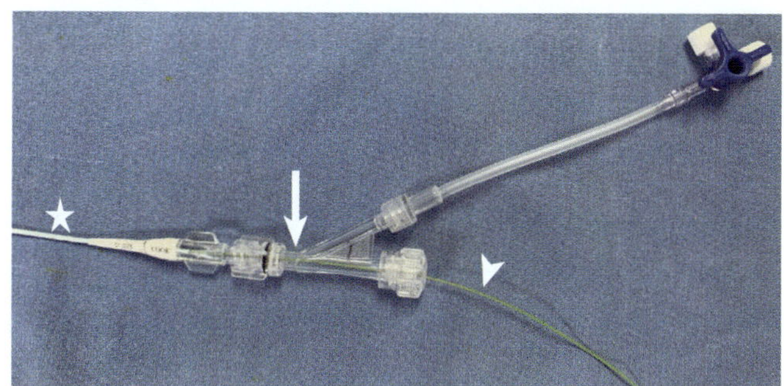

Figure 93.39 Y-connector (*arrow*) for connecting a microcatheter (*arrowhead*) with a guiding catheter (*star*).

Guidewires

Guidewires are used for to gain access, to maneuver into the desired vessel, or to exchange catheters. The most commonly used size are 0.014, 0.018, and 0.035 inch. The most common starting wire is a hydrophilic 0.035-inch wire. Long-length stiff hydrophilic wires are available for catheter exchange in arterial systems, and Amplatz wires are used in the venous system. Microcatheters are advanced using 0.014- or 0.018-inch wires.

Summary

Biopsy and drainage procedures are the backbone of IR over which complicated procedures are based. These are most patient-friendly, minimally invasive techniques with maximum output for optimizing patient treatment. Knowledge of anatomy and hardware is very important before proceeding with any vascular or nonvascular intervention.

Suggested Readings

- S Murphy, The evolution of interventional radiology, Semin Intervent Radiol 22 (1) (2005) 6–9.
- G Guglielmi, History of endovascular endosaccular occlusion of brain aneurysms: 1965–1990. Interv Neuroradiol 13 (2007) 217–224.
- L Pierot, AK Wakhloo, Endovascular treatment of intracranial aneurysms: current status, Stroke 44 (2013) 2046–2054.
- JC Davidson, et al., Society of Interventional Radiology Consensus Guidelines for the Periprocedural Management of Thrombotic and Bleeding Risk in Patients Undergoing Percutaneous Image-Guided Interventions—Part I: Review of Anticoagulation Agents and Clinical Considerations, J Vasc Interv Radiol 30 (2019) 1155–1167.
- IJ Patel, et al., Society of Interventional Radiology Consensus Guidelines for the Periprocedural Management of Thrombotic and Bleeding Risk in Patients Undergoing Percutaneous Image-Guided Interventions—Part II: Recommendations, J Vasc Interv Radiol 30 (2019) 1168–1184.
- Handbook of Interventional Radiologic Procedures, 5th ed. By K Kandarpa, L Machan, JD Durham, Lippincott Williams & Wilkins, 2016.

94 Abdominal Interventions

94.1 Gall Bladder and Liver

Jagadeesh Rampal Singh, Sanjay Baijal

Acute Cholecystitis

Acute cholecystitis can be divided into two groups: acute calculous cholecystitis and acute acalculous cholecystitis.

Percutaneous Cholecystostomy (PC)

Placement of a drainage tube into the gallbladder under imaging control is now a standard treatment option for certain cases of acute cholecystitis where surgery could be high risk, including empyema gall bladder. It carries lower morbidity and equal technical success and patient outcomes, compared to surgery.

The mortality rate from emergency cholecystectomy (13.3%) is 10 times that of elective surgery (1.3%) in patients above 65 years and rises to 25% in case of empyema gallbladder. In such cases, surgery would be a two-stage procedure comprising open cholecystostomy and subsequent cholecystectomy [1].

Indications of percutaneous cholecystostomy:

- To decompress the gallbladder
- To provide access to the biliary tract for therapeutic purposes

Contraindications:

1. Interposed Bowel
2. Coagulopathy (relative contraindication)
3. Malignancy
4. Decompressed gall bladder

Technique: It can be performed under ultrasound (USG), fluoroscopy, or computed tomography (CT) guidance. Catheter placement is performed according to the preference of the radiologist, accessibility of the gallbladder, and coagulation status of the patient by either transhepatic (TH) or transperitoneal (TP) approach.

The technical success of PC is defined as successful placement of the cholecystostomy tube and is reported as high as 95–100% [2]. The clinical success (improvement fever, leukocytosis, pain) is seen within 2–3 days and ranges from 68% to 100% [3]. Procedure-related complications may be seen in 0–26.3% of cases within the first few days which are usually minor, such as catheter displacement and minor bleeding. Catheter dislodgment (6.1–14%) is reported to be the most common late complication [4].

There have been no specific recommendations for the optimal duration of PC drainage. The usual duration ranges from 3 to 6 weeks.

The removal of PC tubes can be considered by performing a cholecystogram via the drain before withdrawal. This ensures the absence of leakage or an obstructed cystic duct and is recommended to reduce the chance of recurrence of cholecystitis [1].

Liver Abscess

Liver abscesses are infectious lesions in the liver. The two most common types of abscesses are pyogenic and amoebic. The severity of pyogenic liver abscess (PLA) depends on the source of the infection and the underlying condition of the patient. Amoebic liver abscesses (ALA) are common in tropical regions mainly where "entamoeba histolytica" is endemic and is more prevalent in individuals with suppressed cell-mediated immunity.

Primary treatment by *percutaneous catheter drainage (PCD)* is performed when:

- The abscess size is greater than 5 cm
- Thick pus
- Thickened walls
- Multiloculated morphology
- Impending rupture (rim <1 cm)

The presence of multiple abscesses necessitates the placement of multiple catheters [5].

ERCP with stent placement or sphincterotomy helps in cases of abscess which have biliary communication.

Incomplete or unsuccessful drainage may result from:

- Improper position of catheter not conducive to adequate drainage
- Premature removal of catheter
- Thick noncollapsible fibrous wall of PLA

Mortality is low with ALA compared with PLA. The risk factors most commonly associated with mortality in PLA include [6]:

- Septic shock
- Clinical jaundice
- Coagulopathy
- Leukocytosis
- Hypoalbuminemia
- Multiple abscesses
- Intraperitoneal rupture
- Malignancy (more in hepatopancreatobiliary malignancy)

Independent risk factors for mortality in ALA are [5]:

- Bilirubin level >3.5 mg/dL
- encephalopathy
- volume of abscess cavity
- hypoalbuminaemia (serum albumin <2.0 g/dL)

Drain removal is considered when the output end-point is <10 mL/day for at least 2–3 consecutive days. Abscesses are slow to resolve. A multidisciplinary approach, including a gastroenterologist, surgeon, and an interventional radiologist are crucial for the successful treatment of these curable infections.

Hydatid Disease of Liver

Hydatid disease is an endemic zoonotic disease caused by tapeworm larvae of the genus echinococcus granulosus. It is a significant public health problem in countries in which it is endemic (Mediterranean, Eastern Europe, South America, and countries in the Far East) [7]. Treatment of liver hydatid cysts is important because it carries the risk of rupture, infection, and anaphylaxis [7].

PAIR (puncture, aspiration, injection, re-aspiration) is a percutaneous radiologic treatment technique for hydatid disease which was proposed in 1986 by the Tunisian team that first used it in a prospective study [8]. The aim of treatment should be to relieve symptoms, inactivate and completely remove viable scolices and germinative membranes, and manage the residual cavity.

Technique—under ultrasonographic guidance, a needle is introduced into the cyst. Cyst fluid is aspirated and analyzed for the presence of scolices. Hypertonic saline or absolute alcohol (95%) is then injected and re-aspirated.

PAIRD (puncture, aspiration, injection, reaspiration, drainage) is similar to PAIR and is often used for large cysts except that a catheter is left in place after completion of the procedure. The safety and efficacy of percutaneous treatment of certain types of hydatid cysts have been well demonstrated with success rate of 97.1–100% [7].

The WHO recommendations for indications for PAIR are [8]:

- Anechoic lesion greater than or equal to 5 cm in diameter
- Cysts with daughter cysts and/or with membrane detachment
- Multiple cysts if amenable for puncture
- Infected cysts
- Patients who refuse surgery
- Cysts that relapse after surgery
- Patients in whom surgery is contraindicated
- Patients who fail to respond to chemotherapy
- Children older than 3 years
- Pregnant women

The WHO recommendations [8] for contraindications for PAIR are:

- Inaccessible or risky location of the liver cyst
- Noncooperative patients
- Cyst in spine, brain, and/or heart
- Cyst communication with the biliary tree
- Inactive or calcified lesion

Liver Trauma

The liver is the second most commonly injured organ in blunt abdominal trauma following the spleen. Injury to the hepatic artery causes significant hemorrhage in the majority of cases. However, venous injury (central hepatic or portal vein) is even more dreadful which requires surgery, irrespective of the hemodynamic status [9].

Until two to three decades ago, most cases of blunt abdominal trauma were managed by exploratory laparotomy [10]. Several innovative multimodal approaches as endovascular routes have allowed to increase the likelihood of nonoperative management (NOM) in selective patients. The majority of patients admitted with liver injuries have minor or moderate injuries (American Association for the Surgery of Trauma-Organ Injury Scale (AAST-OIS I-III)) and are successfully managed by NOM. In contrast, NOM is observed in one-third of severe injuries (AAST-OIS IV, V) [10]. NOM should be considered as the optimal management approach in pediatric patients.

Techniques of Interventional Radiology Management

The main aim of interventional radiology (IR), in trauma, is to save a life by rapidly controlling exsanguinating hemorrhage. The chief mechanism of action of the embolic agents is to reduce perfusion pressure which subsequently reduces or halts the ongoing bleeding. Also, embolization should be done as close as possible to the site of vascular injury. The drawbacks of too proximal embolization include recruitment of collaterals leading to rebleeding whereas distal embolization will result in infarct [9].

Hepatic artery embolization (HAE) is indicated if there is an injury to the hepatic artery or may be done prophylactically in high-grade liver injuries. Surgery is not the preliminary treatment of choice in these cases as during surgery only the main hepatic artery is ligated with potential chances of collateralization leading to rebleeding. In endovascular interventions, site-specific embolization can be performed which prevents collateralization [9]. If superselective catheterization is not feasible or if bleeding is from multiple sites, then nonselective gelfoam embolization can be done. If hemodynamic instability persists, then the patients are taken for rapid "damage control surgery" (DCS) with extensive peri-hepatic packing and temporary abdominal closure [9].

The choice of embolizing material in traumatic injuries is of special concern due to the frequent prevalence of coagulopathy in these patients. Agents like gelfoam or coils need an intact coagulation mechanism to initiate clot formation. On the contrary, the mechanism of clot formation in liquid embolic agents do not depend on coagulation profile. Liquid embolic agents like N-butyl cyanoacrylate or ethylene vinyl alcohol co-polymer (onyx) with a better safety profile may be used in coagulopathy. Some of these are expensive and require expertise for controlled administration at target site so as to limit complications [9].

HAE is an essentially safe procedure with few complications which include delayed hemorrhage, infarction/necrosis, abscess, biloma, or biliary fistula. The risk of complications is more in high-grade liver injuries.

Hepatic artery pseudo-aneurysm (PSA) is a rare complication (1%) [10]. Asymptomatic PSA should be treated at the earliest by endovascular route because of the high risk of rupture and high morbidity [10]. In patients presenting with melena or hematemesis, bleeding from the ampulla of Vater (hemobilia) is highly suggestive of ruptured intrahepatic PSA. Angioembolisation (AE) is the treatment of choice in such cases [10].

Re-bleeding or secondary hemorrhage is the most frequent complication following NOM as in subcapsular hematoma or PSA rupture (1.7–5.9%) with a mortality rate up to 18%. In the majority of cases (69%), "late" bleeding can be managed nonoperatively [10].

Biliary complications include biloma, biliary fistula, bilhemia, and bile peritonitis (2.8–30%) [10]. Most traumatic bilomas resolve spontaneously. Enlarging, symptomatic or infected bilomas can be successfully managed with percutaneous drainage combined with therapeutic endoscopy and eventual endobiliary stent placement. In bile peritonitis, a combination of laparoscopic irrigation/drainage and endoscopic bile duct stent placement may represent a valid alternative [10].

Abscesses are rare after NOM and usually happen in high-grade injury (prevalence 0.6–7%). Percutaneous drainage is the treatment of choice with a high success rate and no reported mortality [10].

A multidisciplinary approach is the best way of managing liver trauma. The best treatment option should be based on clinical condition, anatomical injury grade, and associated injuries.

Biliary Interventions in Obstructive Jaundice

Strategies for the diagnosis and treatment of biliary strictures continue to evolve with advancements in minimally invasive options offered by radiologists and endoscopists.

- For benign strictures, newer techniques, such as large bore catheters, balloon dilatation, and placement of retrievable covered stents, have demonstrated improved results in comparison to previous approaches
- In unresectable malignant strictures, the palliative goal of achieving patency that exceeds survival is possible in some patients with the placement of permanent uncovered, partially covered, or completely covered stents. Palliation that improves patient survival can be achieved with covered stents, drug-coated balloons, and intraductal radiofrequency ablation

Benign biliary strictures (BBSs) have various origins [11]. The most common causes of BBS are iatrogenic like cholecystectomy and orthotopic liver transplantation. Postoperative biliary strictures are further classified as anastomotic or nonanastomotic.

Malignant biliary strictures (MBSs) usually result from local malignancy, most commonly cholangiocarcinoma, pancreatic adenocarcinoma, liver metastases, hepatocellular carcinoma, ampullary carcinoma, or gallbladder adenocarcinoma [11].

Balloon Dilatation

Percutaneous balloon dilation of biliary strictures was first reported in the 1970s and 1980s, with 3-year patency rates of 38–67% [11]. When repeated balloon dilations fail, use of a cutting balloon has been noted with improved results [11].

Another approach to enhance the patency rate of percutaneous management of BBS involves the use of large-bore catheters maintained in place for 6–12 months. This technique is still endorsed by some authors to reduce the restenosis rate. Another strategy is the dual catheter placement technique, where a 8.5-F catheter is advanced into a 14-F catheter and then out of the catheter via a side hole so that the two catheters run parallel at the level of the stricture, reaching a total of 22.5 F.

Biliary Drainage and Stenting

The main indication for endoscopic or percutaneous stenting following percutaneous transhepatic biliary drainage (PTBD) is to relieve jaundice by providing internal biliary drainage

PTBD is an image-guided procedure that is performed under fluoroscopy or combined ultrasound and fluoroscopic guidance.

Indications of PTBD for palliation in obstructive jaundice include:

- Cholangitis
- Pruritus
- To decrease serum bilirubin before chemotherapy
- To access biliary system for further palliative interventions such as stent placement or transhepatic brachytherapy for cholangiocarcinoma
- Rendezvous technique
- Helpful in duct identification during surgery of complex hilar strictures
- Management of biliary fistulas
- Failure of ERCP

Contraindication [12]:

- Absolute
  - Uncorrectable bleeding diathesis
- Relative
  - INR >1.5
  - Platelet counts <50,000
  - Ascites
  - Multiple hepatic cysts or lesions
  - Atrophic lobe

Technique:

Prior to the initiation of the procedure, three-dimensional cross-sectional imaging, i.e., CT or magnetic resonance imaging (MRI) of the patient needs to be reviewed to determine the following (12):

1. Site of obstruction—high or low
2. Selection of appropriate target duct in PTBD—right versus left PTBD

Ultrasound prior to biliary puncture is invaluable for assessing the suitability of puncture as well as any contraindication to the procedure. The preferred site of puncture should be as peripheral as possible as central puncture may cause vascular injury. The procedure can be done under local anaesthesia or conscious sedation. During the procedure, intermittent check cholangiograms with minimal contrast can be done to confirm the level and type of stricture. The site of biliary obstruction is negotiated with a catheter–guidewire combination, and a ring biliary catheter is placed across the stricture into the duodenum. After 48 hours, the ring biliary catheter is capped externally and left solely on internal drainage. Internalization is preferable as it restores the physiological enterohepatic circulation, thus preventing the loss of bile salts and also catheter displacement.

In case of cholangitis, the catheter is placed proximal to the site of obstruction till the cholangitis subsides and later internalised.

Stents

Plastic stents are usually made of Teflon. The use of retrievable covered self-expanding metal stents (CSEMSs) has been proposed predominantly for benign strictures as a treatment strategy on the basis of the higher expansion force and larger diameter of these stents with their sustained dilation effect. These stents are covered by a polytetrafluoroethylene (PTFE) layer and are equipped with a couple of drawstrings attached to the upper margin of the stent for subsequent removal [11]. Stent migration is a significant issue with these stents [13].

The use of biodegradable stents has also been proposed to treat BBS refractory to standard treatment. These stents are made of polydioxanone, which degrades over 3–6 months by a hydrolytic process.

Self-expanding metal stents (SEMSs)—either uncovered (USEMS), partially covered, or completely covered (CSEMS) are the standard palliative options in the management of MBS due to their ease and accuracy of placement, with high technical, clinical success high long-term patency rates. The aim is to drain more than 50% of the liver volume, as this is associated with decreased cholangitis and increased survival [11]. Cholangitis is the most common infectious complication of stent placement, and so the use of periprocedural antibiotics is recommended in all patients [14].

Complications of Biliary Drainage

Potential major complications of both PTBD and Endoscopic biliary drainage (EBD) include bleeding, biliary sepsis, pancreatitis, and cholecystitis. The source of bleeding in PTBD is usually a portal vein branch because of its close proximity to one of the side holes of the catheter. In such cases, it is usually sufficient to adjust the position of the side holes after cholangiography. Arterial injury is uncommon in these patients. The risk of pancreatitis is less than 5%. When a patient is on external catheter drainage short and long-term complications include electrolyte abnormalities and malnutrition which can be reversed by internalizing the catheter [11].

Percutaneous Stone Extraction Through T-Tube Track

Residual gall-stones in the common bile duct occur in up to 4% of patients. These can be extracted along a mature T-tube track, which forms within 4–5 weeks following surgery. Up to 90% of stones can be cleared using a steerable catheter and Dormia basket, by using the track or pushing the fragments across the papilla following stone crushing [14]. Another alternative that can be used is endoscopic extraction.

94.2 Portal Hypertension

Jagadeesh Rampal Singh, Sanjay Baijal

Introduction

Portal hypertension is a hemodynamic abnormality that is commonly seen secondary to cirrhosis and also infrequently as a result of noncirrhotic causes. It can be classified according to its etiology into presinusoidal, sinusoidal and postsinusoidal types [15] (Table 94.1) Portal hypertension arising from cirrhosis causes the serious complications of ascites, variceal hemorrhage, and hepatic encephalopathy. This state of decompensated cirrhosis can further progress to a more severe state of refractory ascites, recurrent variceal hemorrhage, and hepatorenal syndrome which are often life threatening [16].

Increased resistance to portal flow through the liver is the primary cause for portal hypertension which is further aggravated by splanchnic vasodilation, increased portal flow, and hyperdynamic circulation that are seen as part of a hyperkinetic syndrome in cirrhotic patients [17–19]. Portal hypertension can clinically be classified into:

a) Subclinical portal hypertension when hepatic venous pressure gradient (HVPG) is greater than 5 mmHg but lesser than 10 mmHg
b) Clinically significant portal hypertension when HVPG is above 10 mmHg as the risk of varices and decompensation are higher [20]

Hepatic Venous Pressure Gradient

HVPG represents the gradient between pressures in the portal vein and the intra-abdominal portion of the inferior vena cava which is measured by placing a catheter preferably in right hepatic vein (RHV). It is imperative for the procedure to be performed in a standardized manner and for results to be accurate and reproducible [21]. The normal HVPG value lies between 1 mmHg and 5 mmHg. Pressures more than 5 mmHg signifies the presence of portal hypertension, regardless of clinical features [22].

It has been noted that a reduction of the HVPG to <12 mmHg or by ≥20% of the baseline value significantly reduces the risk of recurrent variceal bleeding and mortality [23]. The Baveno VI International Consensus Workshop in 2015 now recommends that "HVPG measurement is the gold standard method to assess the presence of clinically significant portal hypertension" [23].

Technique [22]

HVPG measurement is done after an overnight fast, under conscious sedation, and monitoring for vital signs. Under local anesthesia and aseptic conditions, access is gained into internal jugular vein (IJV), preferably right, by Seldinger technique. With a catheter guidewire combination, RHV is cannulated. Then, a 7-French balloon-tipped catheter (Swan-Ganz) is advanced under fluoroscopic guidance into RHV. Once the tip of the catheter is inside the hepatic vein 3–4 cm from its opening into the IVC, free hepatic venous pressure (FHVP) is measured by keeping the tip of the catheter "free" in the hepatic vein.

WHVP is then measured after inflating the catheter balloon. The wedged pressure should be recorded after the pressure tracing is stable.

TABLE 94.1 Causes of Portal Hypertension

Intrahepatic Presinusoidal PHN	Sinusoidal PHN	Extrahepatic Postsinusoidal PHN
Hepatic schistosomiasis	Cirrhosis	Budd–Chiari syndrome
Congenital hepatic fibrosis	Noncirrhotic alcoholic liver disease	Right heart failure
Noncirrhotic portal fibrosis Nodular regenerative hyperplasia Primary biliary cirrhosis or primary sclerosing cholangitis Extrahepatic Presinusoidal PHN Portal vein thrombosis	Infiltrative disorders: ▪ Amyloidosis ▪ Systemic mastocytosis ▪ Malignancy ▪ Myeloproliferative disorder	Constrictive pericarditis Suprahepatic IVC thrombosis Pulmonary hypertension Tricuspid valve regurgitation Intrahepatic Postsinusoidal PHN Veno-occlusive disease
Superior mesenteric vein thrombosis	Peliosis hepatis	
Splenic vein thrombosis	Hypervitaminosis A	

IVC, inferior vena cava; *PHN*, portal hypertension.
(Adapted from WEA Saad, Portal Hypertension: Imaging, Diagnosis, and Endovascular Management, third ed., Thieme and Society of Interventional Radiology, New York/Stuttgart, 2018.)

WHVP reading should always be preferably taken before injecting the contrast; otherwise falsely high values will be recorded (a) because of the injected contrast, and (b) because the contrast is not a good medium for transmitting the pressure.

Three readings of FHVP and WHVP are taken and their mean value is used. If these readings differ by more than 1 mmHg, all readings need to be obtained again. The total time usually ranges from 10 to 20 minutes. The success of hepatic vein cannulation is greater than 95%.

Free hepatic venous pressure (FHVP): FHVP is usually close to the IVC pressure, the difference being <2 mmHg. Occasionally, the difference is >2 mmHg. In these situations, partial or complete wedging of the catheter, inadequate placement of the catheter, or a hepatic vein obstruction must be ruled out.

Wedged hepatic venous pressure (WHVP): WHVP represents the absolute value of sinusoidal pressure, which is slightly lower than the actual portal vein pressure. In patients with liver cirrhosis, it is closely similar to intravariceal pressure [22].

There are two techniques for measuring WHVP: (a) catheter advancement technique and (b) balloon occlusion technique.

The balloon occlusion technique proposed and validated by Groszmann et al. [22] is preferred because it allows serial measurements of FVHP and WHVP using the same catheter, inflated and deflated repeatedly.

When reporting results of portal hemodynamics, both WHVP and HVPG should be reported since one represents the risk of variceal rupture and the other represents the amount of variceal blood flow.

Applications of HVPG Measurement

1. Diagnosis of portal hypertension: an HVPG value of 6–9 mmHg corresponds to subclinical sinusoidal portal hypertension [24], whereas clinically significant portal hypertension is diagnosed when HVPG is ≥10 mmHg, at which point clinical manifestations such as varices, bleeding, gastropathy, and ascites, might appear.
2. HVPG correlates with the degree of histological liver fibrosis in patients with HBV-related and HCV-related chronic hepatitis [24]. HVPG is over 5 mmHg in the majority of patients with significant fibrosis.
3. Acute alcoholic hepatitis: HVPG (when measured early during hospitalization) provides prognostic information on short-term outcomes; values >22 mmHg were independently associated with a higher risk of death than were valued below this threshold [24].
4. Liver transplantation: HVPG should be the standard measure to assess chronic viral hepatitis recurrence after orthotopic liver transplantation. Diagnosis of portal hypertension at 12 months after orthotopic liver transplantation (value ≥6 mmHg), enables the identification of patients with rapid deterioration of liver function and recurrence of cirrhosis [24].
5. Hepatocellular carcinoma (HCC): HVPG, in addition to albumin levels and viral etiology, is an independent predictor of the risk of developing HCC. This risk is substantially higher in patients with clinically significant portal hypertension (HVPG ≥10 mmHg) than in patients with cirrhosis who have values <10 mmHg. Similarly, in patients with well-compensated cirrhosis and resectable HCC, the presence of clinically significant portal hypertension markedly increases the risk of unresolved hepatic decompensation occurring within 3 months of hepatic resection [24].
6. HVPG is a strong and independent predictor of several outcomes in patients with cirrhosis. In patients who had already developed decompensation, HVPG provides information about the risk of death during follow-up; 16 mmHg was the optimum cut-off value for this correlation [24].
7. Response to therapy for portal hypertension.

Transjugular Intrahepatic Portosystemic Shunt

Along with medical and endoscopic treatments, transjugular intrahepatic portosystemic shunt (TIPS) is considered to be mainstay in the management of portal hypertension and has been widely validated as an effective treatment for the complications of portal hypertension.

TIPS was first described by Josef Rosch in 1969 which began the era of endovascular management of portal hypertension.

With the advent of commercially available expanded polytetrafluoroethylene (ePTFE) grafts in the early 2000s the patency of the TIPS shunt greatly improved and has reduced the number of re-interventions needed to maintain patency. TIPS, when employed with careful patient selection carries low mortality and morbidity. The current era of TIPS use has expanded to novel indications for which the body of evidence is growing. Hepatic encephalopathy remains the main challenge in the management of these patients postprocedure.

Indications: (adapted from The American Association for the Study of Liver Diseases-AASLD guidelines [25])

1. Efficacy determined by controlled trials:
   a) Secondary prevention of variceal bleeding
   b) Refractory ascites
2. Efficacy assessed in uncontrolled series:
   a) Refractory acutely bleeding varices
   b) Portal hypertensive gastropathy (PHG)
   c) Bleeding gastric varices
   d) Gastric antral vascular ectasia (GAVE)
   e) Refractory hepatic hydrothorax
   f) Hepatorenal syndrome (HRS Type 1/Type 2)
   g) Budd–Chiari syndrome
   h) Hepatopulmonary syndrome
3. Emerging indications [26]:
   a) Early management of ascites: consideration after 2–3 large volume paracentesis
   b) Early management of variceal hemorrhage: in patients at high risk of standard therapy failure
   c) Before abdominal surgery: decrease portal hypertension to permit safe abdominal surgery
   d) Recanalization of portal vein thrombosis: chronically occluded portal vein thrombosis with portal hypertensive complications and/or to facilitate liver transplant
   e) Embolization of clinically significant spontaneous portosystemic shunts: refractory hepatic encephalopathy

Contraindications: (AASLD 2009 update) [25]:

1. Absolute:
   a) Congestive heart failure
   b) Severe pulmonary hypertension
   c) Uncontrolled systemic infection or sepsis
   d) Unrelieved Biliary obstruction
   e) Extensive cystic liver disease
2. Relative:
   a) Refractory hepatic encephalopathy
   b) End-stage liver disease (Model for End-stage Liver Disease [MELD] >19, CHILDS C score of 12 or higher)
   c) Volume overloaded state

d) Centrally located liver mass (HCC, metastatic disease)
e) Valvular heart disease
f) Severe coagulopathy (INR >5)
g) Severe thrombocytopenia (platelet count <20,000/cm^3)
h) Moderate pulmonary hypertension
i) Portal vein thrombosis

Factors predicting poor prognosis—(patient selection):

1. Emergency TIPS [27]

Patients undergoing an emergency TIPS procedure who have a Child-Pugh score of 12 or higher along with an APACHE II score of 18 or higher (or patients with a prognostic index of 18 or higher) are expected to have a poor outcome.

2. Elective TIPS

For elective TIPS, MELD >18 is considered high risk and when MELD >25, the mortality ranges from 60% at 3 months to 75% at 6 months [9,10] and total bilirubin >3 mg/dL are the factors.

Preprocedural Imaging

After patient selection, imaging with ultrasound and Doppler needs to be done for assessing the patency of the portal vein, hepatic veins, IJVs and for the presence and quantification of ascites. Triphasic CECT or Triphasic MRI abdomen should be performed to assess the liver parenchyma and vasculature and can act as a roadmap to help determine the appropriate entry site for the portal vein puncture. It also helps in assessing the patency of splenoportal axis for any thrombus and excluding isolated left-sided portal hypertension.

Technique

Standard TIPS involves creating a shunt between the RHV and intrahepatic right portal vein done under general anaesthesia.

- Using USG guidance, right IJV is punctured.
- With a catheter guidewire combination access into RHV is gained.
- The shunt is created between the proximal 2–3 cm of hepatic vein and intrahepatic portion of the right portal vein using ultrasound/fluoroscopic or IVUS guidance [28].
- After balloon dilatation of the TIPS tract, a 10 mm ePTFE graft is deployed with a minimum of at least 5 mm extending into the IVC and uncovered distal 2 cm of the stent in the portal vein (Fig. 94.1).
- Then balloon dilatation of the stent graft is done for incorporation of the graft into the TIPS tract.

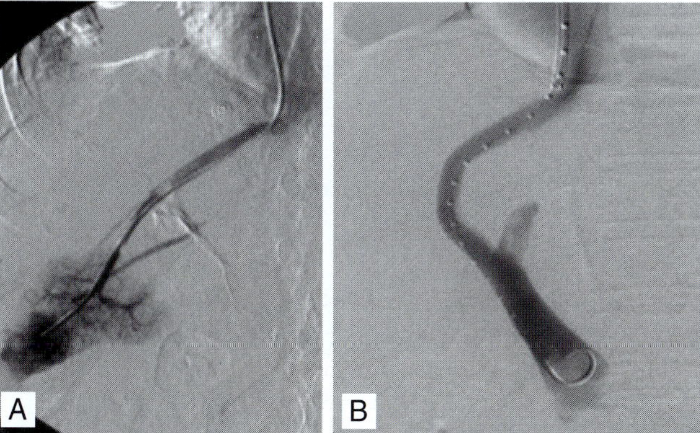

Figure 94.1 (A) Wedged RHV venogram showing parenchymal blush with few portal radicles; (B) Venogram done after placing the PTFE graft extending from RHV ostia into the right portal vein showing the free flow of contrast.

- Post TIPS portosystemic gradient and portovenogram is obtained and if there is persistent contrast filling of the varices or PSG remains >12 mmHg after shunt deployment, the varices are embolized with coils or glue.

Complications [29]

Complications of TIPS and their management are listed in Table 94.2.

Shunt Surveillance

A recommended schedule includes Doppler surveillance at 1, 3, 6, and 12 months after TIPS creation followed by 6–12 monthly thereafter.

Doppler Parameters [30,31]

The sensitivity and specificity of Doppler ultrasound parameters for the detection of shunt dysfunction are 92% and 72% respectively [30]. Findings that could indicate shunt stenosis or occlusion:

- TIPS shunt peak velocities <90 cm/sec or >190 cm/sec
- Main portal vein velocity <30 cm/sec
- Interval change of greater than 25% of peak TIPS velocity
- Intrastent velocity gradient of more than 100 cm/sec
- Reversal of a previously hepatofugal portal vein flow to a hepatopetal flow

Postprocedural Follow-Up [32]

In patients with an initial poor response with nonresolution of symptoms, a TIPS venogram is performed at 3 months (minimum of 3 months required for clinical improvement) along with measurement of portosystemic gradient to rule out other secondary causes for poor clinical response. The creation of a parallel

TABLE 94.2 Complications of TIPS and Their Management

Early Complications	Management
Bile duct injury	Conservative
Intraperitoneal hemorrhage	Blood transfusion when required; Cone beam CT can be done on table to identify source or CECT abdomen done when there is delayed bleeding complications
Extrahepatic puncture	Balloon occlusion of puncture site and deployment of covered stent into the proximal main portal vein
Portal vein dissection	Extension of the TIPS stent across the dissected segment of the portal vein
Hepatic artery injury	Angiography and embolization if needed
Arteriobiliary fistula	Requires embolization/covered stent placement
Acute Hepatic failure	Shunt reduction/occlusion
Hepatic encehalopathy	Medical management and if refractory then shunt reduction
Early shunt occlusion	Thrombolysis/Venoplasty
Liver capsule transgression	Manageable with conservative treatment

TIPS can be considered if symptoms persist or portosystemic gradient continues to remain >12 mmHG after shunt revision.

TIPS revision technique involves angioplasty with or without covered stent placement. Angioplasty alone often leads to recurrence. A few small studies have shown that the use of a covered stent for shunt revision leads to prolonged patency [33].

Hepatic encephalopathy is a frequent complication of TIPS with a reported incidence varying between 22% and 50% [34]. While most episodes of encephalopathy in this setting can be managed medically, approximately 3–7% of these patients can develop TIPS-related refractory encephalopathy (TRHE) and would require shunt reduction [35]. When shunt reduction does not clinically improve hepatic encephalopathy, a spontaneous portosystemic shunt has to be ruled out as the cause and embolized if present.

Balloon-Occluded Retrograde Transvenous Obliteration (BRTO)

Variceal bleeding is a serious complication of portal hypertension. Treatment of esophageal varices is well established with endoscopic methods, but the long-term success is limited in part due to the high flows through the varix and also the location of the varices in the cardia/gastric fundus. Due to their large size, sclerosis of gastric varices usually require large volumes of sclerosant and pose a higher risk of pulmonary system embolization. BRTO has emerged as an alternative treatment method to TIPS, specifically among patients in the United States for whom TIPS is contraindicated [36].

Gastric varices (GV) are classified (Fig. 94.2), as gastroesophageal varices (GOV) and isolated gastric varices (IGV). GOV are further divided as GOV1, which are esophageal varices extending across the gastroesophageal junction along the lesser curve of the stomach, and GOV2, which extend beyond the gastroesophageal junction into the fundus of the stomach. IGV includes IGV1, which are seen in the fundus of the stomach and are also called fundal varices, and IGV2, which refers to ectopic varices present anywhere in the stomach (41).

The portal feeder to the GOV2, IGV1 is usually the posterior or short gastric vein(s), which are closer to the gastrorenal shunt (GRS) (i.e., left side of the portal circulation) whereas the portal feeder to the oesophageal varices/GOV1 (coronary vein/left gastric vein) is to the right side of the portal circulation and is closer to the TIPS (proximity theory). Hence, complex GOV with dominant left gastric veins and poorly supplied by the more distant posterior and short gastric veins respond better to TIPS whereas gastric varices which are predominantly supplied by the posterior or short gastric veins will require BRTO [37].

Management therapies available for gastric varices include:

1. Endoscopic modalities
   a. Gastric variceal sclerotherapy (GVS). For GOV 1
   b. Gastric variceal obturation (GVO) with glue
   c. Gastric variceal band ligation (GVL)
   d. Thrombin injection
   e. Combined endoscopic therapy
2. Endoscopic ultrasound-guided therapy
3. Transjugular intrahepatic portosystemic shunt (TIPS) and BRTO—interventional radiology

The basic portosystemic venous anatomy of gastric varices pertinent to the conventional BRTO procedure is shown in Fig. 94.3.

Indications:

1. Gastric variceal bleeding (impending, prior, or current or active)
2. Clinically recurrent hepatic encephalopathy

Contraindications:

1. Severe uncorrected coagulopathy (which probably in this clinical setting is associated with liver failure)
2. Splenic vein thrombosis (segmental portal hypertension)
3. Portal vein thrombosis
4. Uncontrolled esophageal variceal bleeding

Preprocedural imaging evaluation (upper GI endoscopy, EUS, CECT Fig. 94.4A–F)

1. Splenic and portal vein patency
2. Presence and size of GRSs (for conventional BRTO) or alternative portosystemic shunts and leading systemic veins (for unconventional BRTO)

Procedural steps of the conventional BRTO (Table 94.3) (Fig. 94.4F–J).

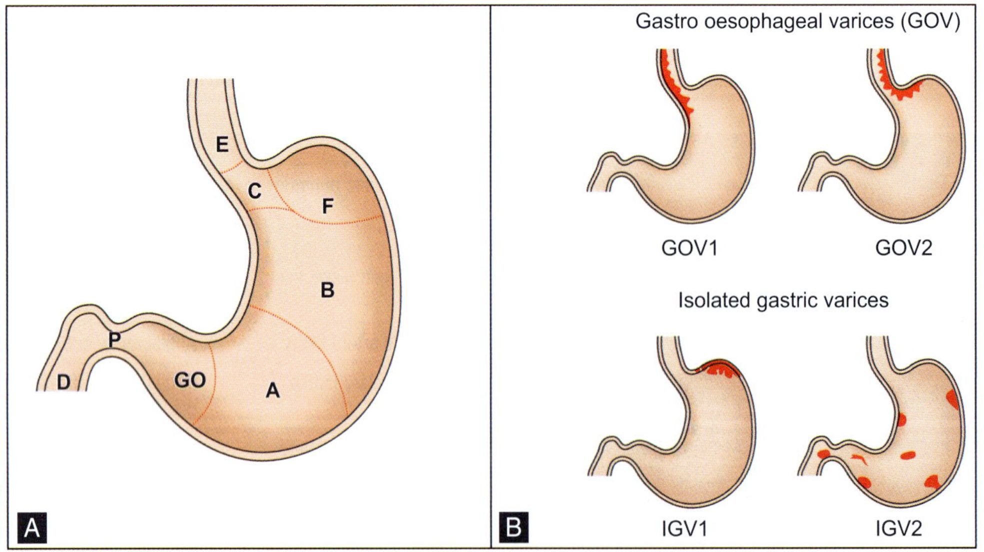

Figure 94.2 Endoscopic classification of gastric and gastroesophageal varices by Sarin et al. 1 (A anatomy of stomach and first part of duodenum. *E*, esophagus; *C*, cardia; *F*, fundus of stomach; *B*, body of stomach; *A*, antrum of stomach; *GO*, gastric outlet which includes the pylorus (P); *D*, first part of duodenum. B) *GOV*, gastroesophageal (esophageal) varices (type-1 and type-2); *IGV*, isolated gastric varices (type-1 and type-2).

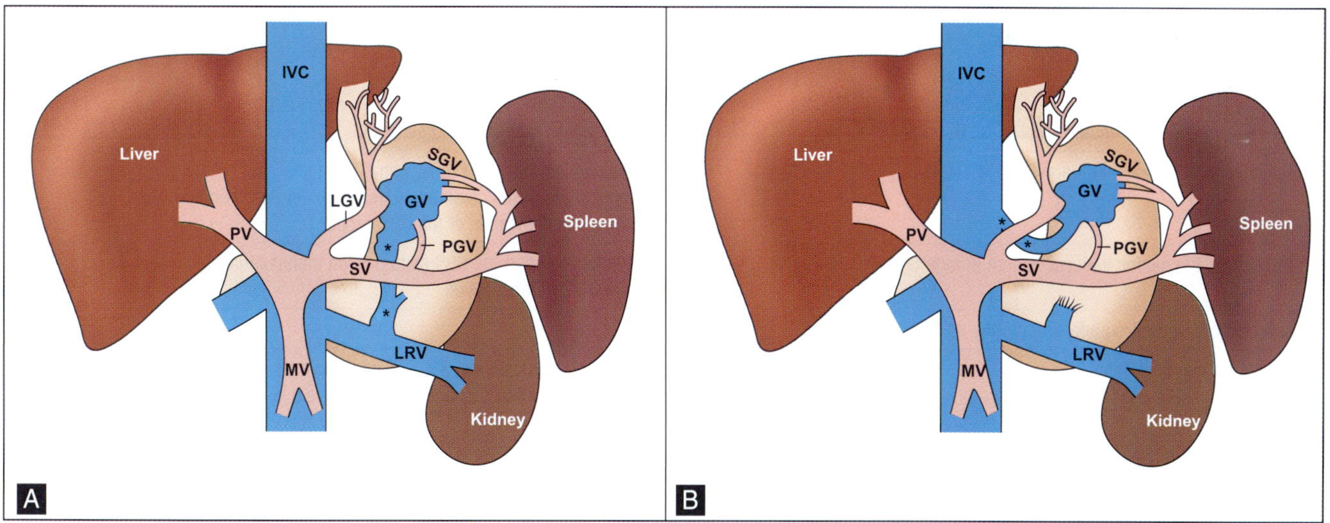

Figure 94.3 The basic portosystemic venous anatomy of gastric varices with gastrorenal shunt (*) in (A) gastrocaval shunt (*) in (B). *GV*, gastric varices; *IVC*, Inferior venecava; *LGV*, Left gastric vein; *LRV*, left renal vein; *MV*, mesenteric veins(s); *PGV*, Posterior gastric vein; *PV*, portal vein; *SGV*, Short gastric vein; *SV*, Splenic vein [38].

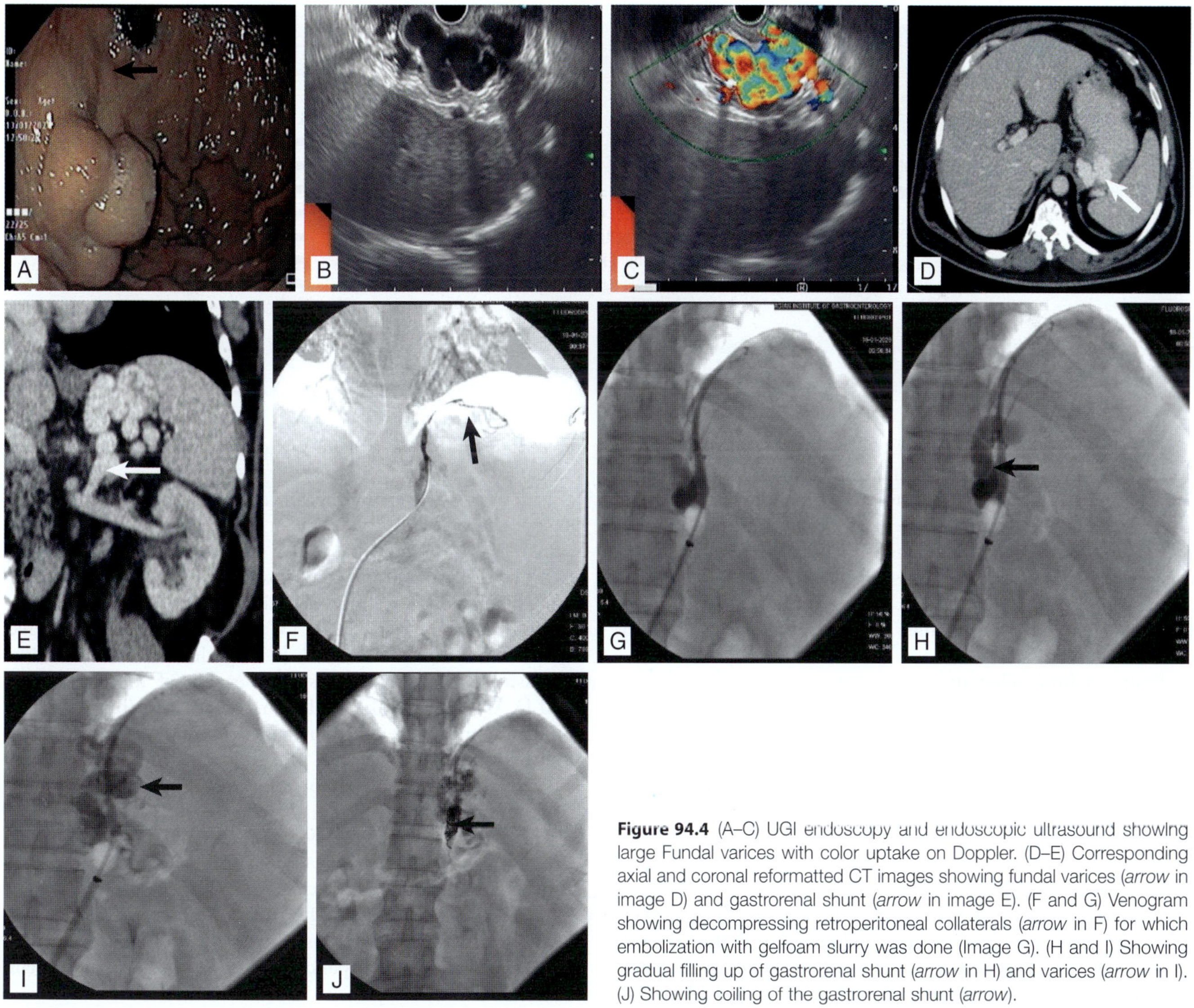

Figure 94.4 (A–C) UGI endoscopy and endoscopic ultrasound showing large Fundal varices with color uptake on Doppler. (D–E) Corresponding axial and coronal reformatted CT images showing fundal varices (*arrow* in image D) and gastrorenal shunt (*arrow* in image E). (F and G) Venogram showing decompressing retroperitoneal collaterals (*arrow* in F) for which embolization with gelfoam slurry was done (Image G). (H and I) Showing gradual filling up of gastrorenal shunt (*arrow* in H) and varices (*arrow* in I). (J) Showing coiling of the gastrorenal shunt (*arrow*).

TABLE 94.3 BRTO Procedure [38]

Broad Procedural Steps	Specific Procedural Steps
Access and approach (Image F in Fig. 94.4)	Venous access (femoral vs jugular)
Selective catheterization (Image F in Fig. 94.4)	Catheterization of the left renal vein Catheterization of the common stump of the adrenal vein and GRS Selective catheterization of the GRS-proper
Trapping of the gastric variceal system (Image G in Fig. 94.4)	Balloon occlusion of the GRS (with balloon manipulation) Collateral vein embolization
Balloon-occluded retrograde venography (BORV)	
Sclerosant administration (Images H and I in Fig. 94.4)	10% Ethanolamine oleate, 3% STS injecting in foam-state by mixing 1 part of lipiodol, 2 part of 3% STS and the 3 part of air, Polidocanol (foam-state sclerosant mixture)
Additional intraprocedural imaging (if any)	Cone-beam dynamic CT
Indwelling sclerosant with indwelling temporary balloon or balloon-occlusion catheter (Image J in Fig. 94.4)	Indwelling balloon catheter can be deflated early by using Coils or Vascular plugs
Deflation of balloon-occlusion catheter	

TABLE 94.4 Complications of BRTO [40,41]

Intraprocedural	Postprocedural	
■ Access site complications ■ Occlusion Balloon Rupture ■ Rupture of the varices or portosystemic shunt ■ Reflux of the sclerosant into the systemic veins	Early ■ Gross hematuria ■ Pulmonary embolism ■ Renal failure ■ Rupture of spleen or mesenteric ischemia (when BRTO performed in the setting of portal vein thrombosis or when portosystemic shunt is the only outflow for splenic and splanchnic venous system)	Long-term ■ Portal hypertensive gastropathy ■ Aggravation of esophageal varices ■ Duodenal varices ■ Ascites ■ Spontaneous bacterial peritonitis ■ Pleural effusion (hydrothorax) ■ Portal vein thrombosis ■ Renal vein thrombosis

Modified BRTO Techniques [39]:

BRTO requires lengthy post-procedural monitoring and has complications (Table 94.4) related to balloon rupture and adverse effects of sclerosing agents. Several modified BRTO techniques have been developed including vascular plug-assisted retrograde transvenous obliteration (PARTO), coil-assisted retrograde transvenous obliteration (CARTO), and balloon-occluded antegrade transvenous obliteration (BATO).

Postprocedural follow-up:

1. Upper GI endoscopy to look for worsening of esophageal varices, recurrence of gastric varices
2. Follow up by imaging
   A. CT Abdomen—noncontrast within 24 hours post procedure to look for completeness of shunt closure
   B. Ultrasound of abdomen to look for worsening or new development of ascites, pleural effusion

Clinical outcomes of BRTO:

Technical efficacy can be defined as the successful injection of sclerosing agent into gastric varices and complete obliteration of gastric varices whereas clinical success can be defined as evidence that the varices have not recurred and absence of evidence of rebleeding from the treated varices on follow-up endoscopic evaluation.

Park et al. [41] reported technical success rate for BRTO was 96.4%; clinical success was 97.3%. The major complication rate was 2.6%.

BRTO diverts portal blood flow toward the liver and thus improves, if not preserving, hepatic function which returns to baseline within 6–9 months [37,42–44]. In a retrospective study conducted by Saad et al. [43], patients with technically successful BRTO procedures were evaluated for changes in MELD, C-P, and MELD/C-P component contribution. They found an improved effect on hepatic reserve from 1.5 to 4 months after BRTO. Serum bilirubin and international normalized ratio were found to improve to significantly below baseline levels.

The clear disadvantage of the increased portal flow in a patient with portal hypertension was worsening of nongastric varices, portal hypertensive gastropathy, ascites, and hepatic hydrothorax.

Conclusion: BRTO is an effective procedure in the management of gastric varices but is associated with worsening of esophageal varices, ascites, and hepatic hydrothorax requiring the patient to be in close follow-up.

94.3 Budd–Chiari Syndrome

Jagadeesh Rampal Singh, Sanjay Baijal

Introduction

It is defined as hepatic venous outflow obstruction which can be located from the small hepatic venules up to the entrance of the inferior vena cava (IVC) into the right atrium [45].

Budd-chiari syndrome (BCS) by causing sinusoidal obstruction leads to liver cell loss and histological changes which are usually seen in the centrilobular region. This can further progress to symptomatic BCS, presenting with ascites and gastrointestinal bleed which can be life threatening. The basic concept of therapeutic radiological intervention is an attempt to decompress the sinusoids to prevent further damage. This can be done by either angioplasty or combined with stents. In some cases where there are no recanalisable hepatic veins, transjugular intrahepatic portosystemic shunts (TIPS) may be required to decompress the system.

The prognosis depends mainly on how rapidly the obstruction has set in, severity of hepatocellular dysfunction and the anatomical location and extent of the block with the presence of associated portal vein thrombosis [45]. Improvements in radiological intervention with early detection of cases have led to improved outcomes in these patients.

While in the West, hepatic vein obstruction is the most common site of block, in Asian population isolated IVC webs are found in 60% of BCS [45]. Majority of Indian studies except one show membranous obstruction of IVC as the most common cause of chronic BCS [45].

Patient workup:

- Laboratory tests should include a complete hemogram, liver function test, prothrombin time, INR, viral serology, auto-immune profile, ceruloplasmin, renal function test, and coagulation profile
- Cardiac evaluation should also be done to rule out mimics of BCS [45]
- Upper GI endoscopy has to be done in all patients to rule out oesophageal and gastric varices. Those who have high-grade oesophageal varices, should undergo prophylactic endoscopic variceal band ligation prior to radiological intervention

Postinterventional therapy, all patients are put on anticoagulants to maintain an INR between 2.0 and 3.

The diagnosis of BCS is established with unequivocal radiological confirmation of hepatic venous outflow obstruction. The site of obstruction is further evaluated using Doppler ultrasound, CT or conventional venography in all patients. The level of obstruction is classified as isolated HV block, isolated IVC block, and combined HV and IVC block. The length of obstruction was sub-classified as short segment (<3 cm) and long segment (>3 cm). Based on clinical presentation it is classified as acute if the duration of the symptoms is less than 1 month, sub-acute if it is between 1 and 6 months, and chronic if more than 6 months [45].

Prognostic Score

Various prognostic scores available are, Child-Turcotte-Pugh (CTP) score, model for end-stage liver disease (MELD), Rotterdam index, BCS-TIPS, original Clichy score [46].

Management Protocol

The following radiological interventions (Table 94.5) are done based on the site of block [47].

TABLE 94.5 Treatment Options Based on the Site of Block in Budd–Chiari Syndrome

Type	Treatment Option
Membranous obstruction of inferior vena cava (MOVC)	IVC balloon Angioplasty with or without SEMS placement
Supra-hepatic IVC block and patent HV	IVC balloon angioplasty with SEMS placement
Juxta-hepatic IVC block and patent HV	IVC balloon angioplasty with SEMS placement
Juxta-hepatic IVC block and short-segment HV block (<3 cm) involving all three HV or two major HV	IVC balloon angioplasty with SEMS placement and HV balloon angioplasty with SEMS placement of any one HV
Juxta-hepatic IVC block and long-segment HV block (>3 cm)	IVC balloon angioplasty with SEMS followed by TIPS placement
Short-segment HV block (<3 cm) involving all three or two major HV	HV balloon angioplasty with SEMS placement of any one HV
Long-segment HV block (>3 cm) involving all three or two major HV	TIPS placement

SEMS, self-expanding metallic stents.

TIPS is now being increasingly used for relieving obstruction in BCS. TIPS has the advantage of avoiding laparotomy and yet achieving adequate outflow through the portal vein in subjects in whom angioplasty and stenting would otherwise be not feasible. It also overcomes the compression effect of the caudate lobe on the stent and has less peri-operative mortality [48]. TIPS is associated with mortality varying between 9% and 30% on follow-up for 4 years [49].

Locoregional Therapies in Hepatocellular Carcinoma

A significant number of patients of hepatocellular carcinoma (HCC) are ineligible for surgical treatment at the time of diagnosis due to an intermediate or advanced stage of disease or severe comorbidities [50]. The prognosis of HCC following systemic chemotherapy, external radiotherapy (RT), or supportive treatments is also poor. Hence, in order to improve outcomes, especially among inoperable patients various percutaneous and image-guided, locoregional therapies, have emerged [50].

Over a period of time, numerous minimal invasive treatment options have been developed in interventional oncology which includes:

- *Curative modalities* such as percutaneous ethanol injection (PEI), radiofrequency ablation (RFA), microwave ablation (MWA), cryoablation (CA), irreversible electroporation (IRE)
- *Palliative therapies* such as bland transarterial embolization (TAE) and conventional mechanisms vary according to the technique [51] transarterial chemoembolization (cTACE) or drug-eluting beads (DEB-TACE) and local endovascular radiotherapy via the trans-arterial delivery of beta-emitting microparticles (selective internal radiation therapy; SIRT)

The Barcelona-clinic liver cancer (BCLC) staging system uses variables related to tumor stage, liver functional status, physical

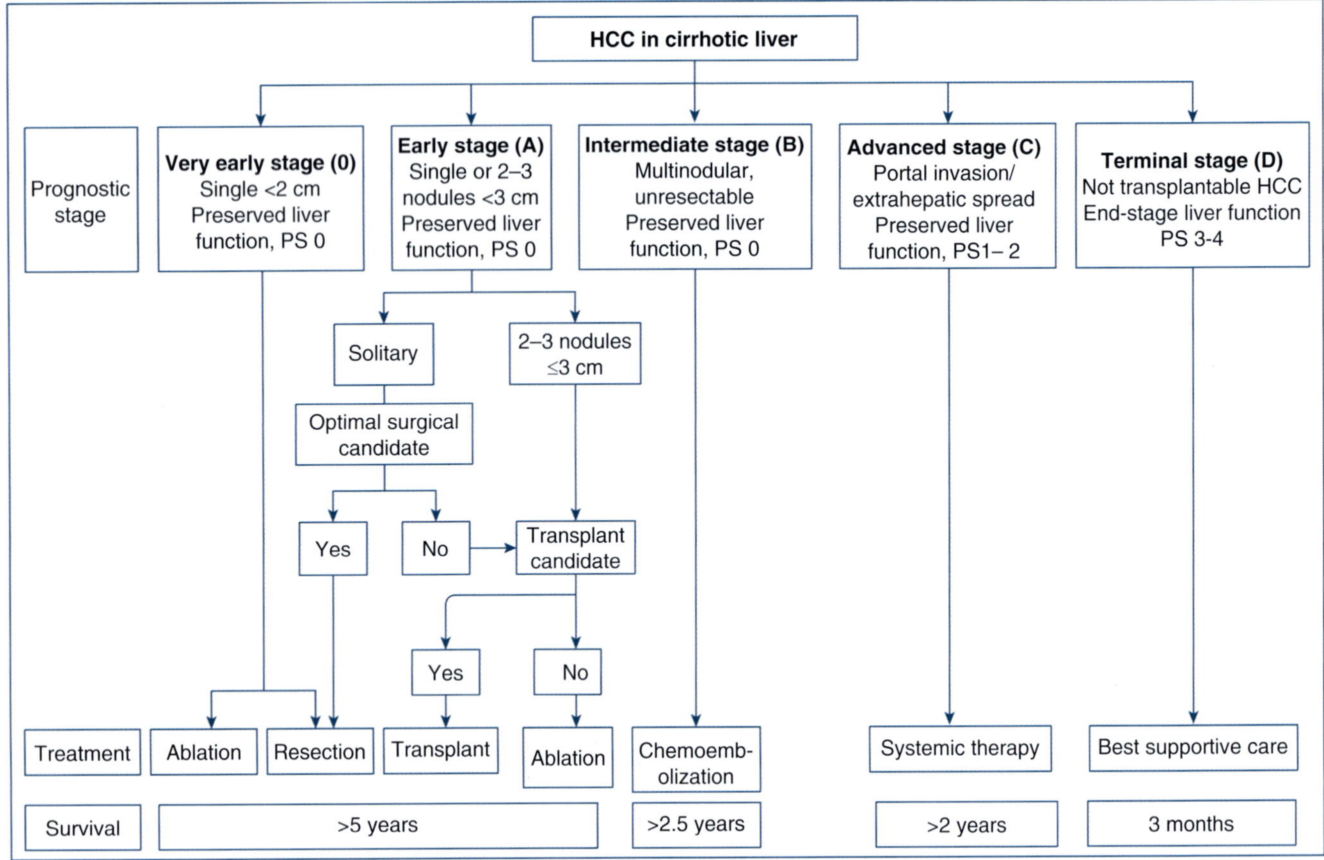

Figure 94.5 Barcelona-clinic liver cancer (BCLC) staging classification and treatment schedule. *BSC*, Best supportive care; *PS*, performance status.

status, and cancer-related symptoms, and links the four stages described with a treatment algorithm (Fig. 94.5) [52,53].

Ablative Therapies

Local ablation along with surgical resection and liver transplantation is considered a potentially curative therapy of small-size HCC [51]. Tumor destruction can be achieved by chemical ablation using PEI, or thermal ablation, which includes RFA, MWA, cryoablation, and laser interstitial thermotherapy (LITT). The mechanisms of each vary according to the technique (Fig. 94.6) [51]. Number (up to three tumors), tumor size (generally <3–4 cm), and location (accessibility to image guidance) limit the use of percutaneous ablation [51].

RFA has been established as the standard ablative therapy for early stages of HCC and has been adopted as first-line primary therapy for single tumors <2 cm, whereas in tumors beyond this size, it remains as an alternative in patients who are not surgically fit [51]. The median overall survival with RFA is 60 months and 5-year recurrence rates range from 50% to 70%. In patients whose waiting period for liver transplantation exceeds 6 months, RFA and TACE have been recommended as bridge therapies. Thermal ablation induces coagulative tumor necrosis and ablate both tumoral and peri-tumoral tissue. Thermal ablation usually aims at inducing a 10 mm margin ring around the tumor edge to remove surrounding small and undetected microsatellites. Fig. 94.7 shows pre and postRFA images on CECT.

Serum α-fetoprotein (AFP) level, tumor size, multinodularity, and Child-Pugh class are seen to be predictors of survival [51].

Micro wave ablation (MWA) has demonstrated similar efficacy to RFA, but increased complication rates in tumors >3 cm. In addition to RFA and MWA, several novel modalities of ablation are entering clinical practice including cryoablation, laser ablation, IRE and high-intensity focused ultrasound (HIFU).

Cryoablation causes tumor necrosis using the Joule-Thomson theory of expanding gases within a needle-like cryoprobe causing cooling at the probe tip [50]. Several probes are usually used with ablation times of up to 25–30 min and the advantage of intraprocedural monitoring of ice ball formation on image guidance (CT/MRI) and the ability to include larger ablative zones.

IRE is a nonthermal ablation technology to induce cell death by pore creation within the cell lipid membrane. The procedure is performed using multiple monopolar 19-gauge probes and, in view of its nonthermal nature, remains a valid alternative to thermal ablation for peri-vascular lesions and those close to large bile ducts [50]. The application of liver IRE for the treatment of HCC requires further investigation and its clinical application remains limited.

Complications and Adverse Effects [51]

Major complications included liver abscess, bleeding, liver failure and tumour seeding. These complications increase with the severity of cirrhosis, extent of ablated zone, use of MWA, and use of multiprobe technology. Liver abscess is the most common major complication and has been usually associated with bilioenteric anastomosis and pre-existing biliary abnormalities.

Transarterial Chemoembolization

Transarterial chemoembolization (TACE), a locoregional therapy (LRT), is widely recommended as first-line treatment for intermediate-stage HCC (BCLC stage B) [4].

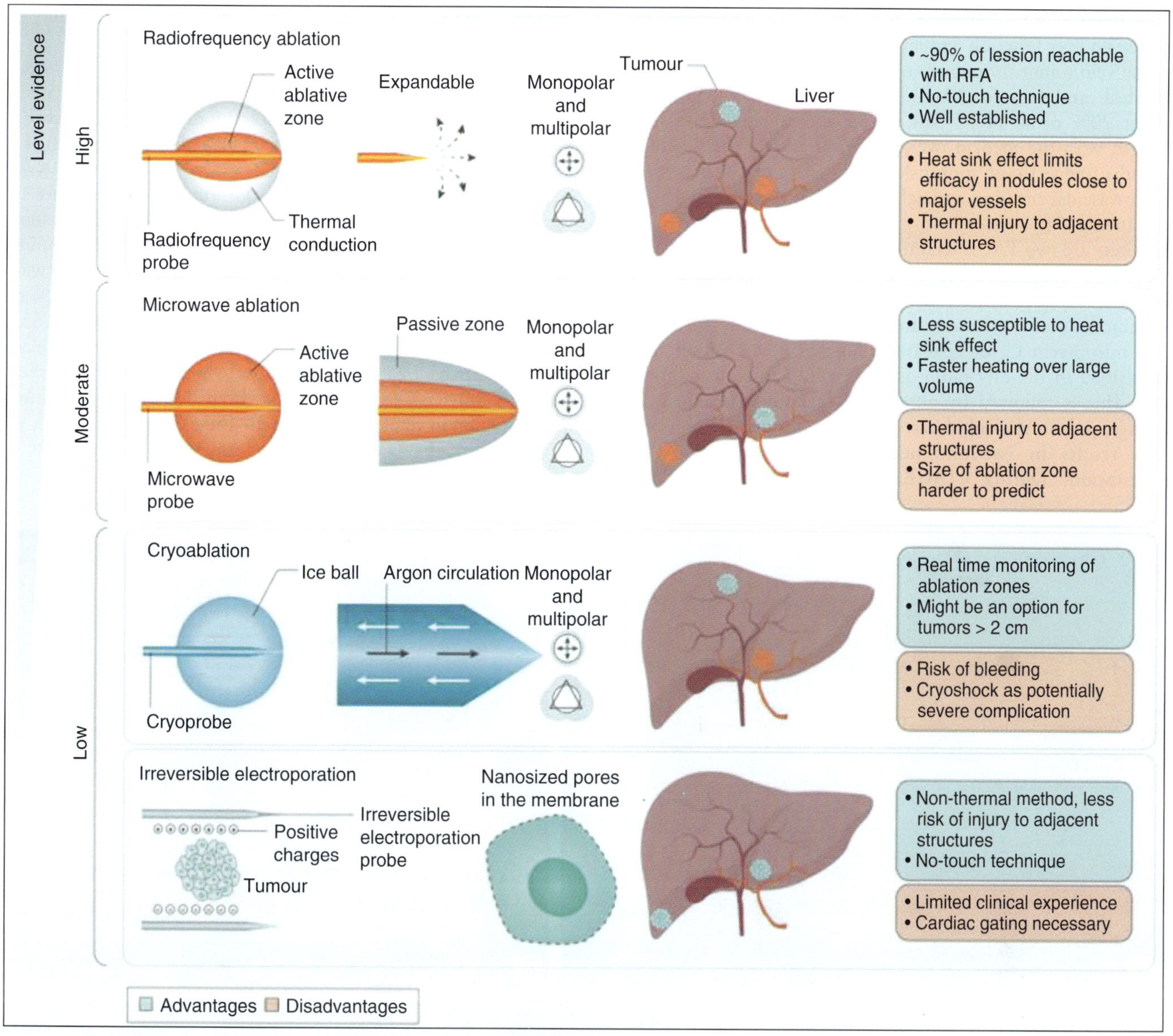

Level evidence

High

Radiofrequency ablation

Active ablative zone
Expandable
Monopolar and multipolar
Tumour
Liver
Thermal conduction
Radiofrequency probe

- ~90% of lession reachable with RFA
- No-touch technique
- Well established

- Heat sink effect limits efficacy in nodules close to major vessels
- Thermal injury to adjacent structures

Moderate

Microwave ablation

Passive zone
Active ablative zone
Monopolar and multipolar
Microwave probe

- Less susceptible to heat sink effect
- Faster heating over large volume

- Thermal injury to adjacent structures
- Size of ablation zone harder to predict

Low

Cryoablation

Ice ball
Argon circulation
Monopolar and multipolar
Cryoprobe

- Real time monitoring of ablation zones
- Might be an option for tumors > 2 cm

- Risk of bleeding
- Cryoshock as potentially severe complication

Irreversible electroporation

Positive charges
Tumour
Irreversible electroporation probe
Nanosized pores in the membrane

- Non-thermal method, less risk of injury to adjacent structures
- No-touch technique

- Limited clinical experience
- Cardiac gating necessary

Advantages Disadvantages

Figure 94.6 Percutaneous local ablative techniques for the treatment of HCC.

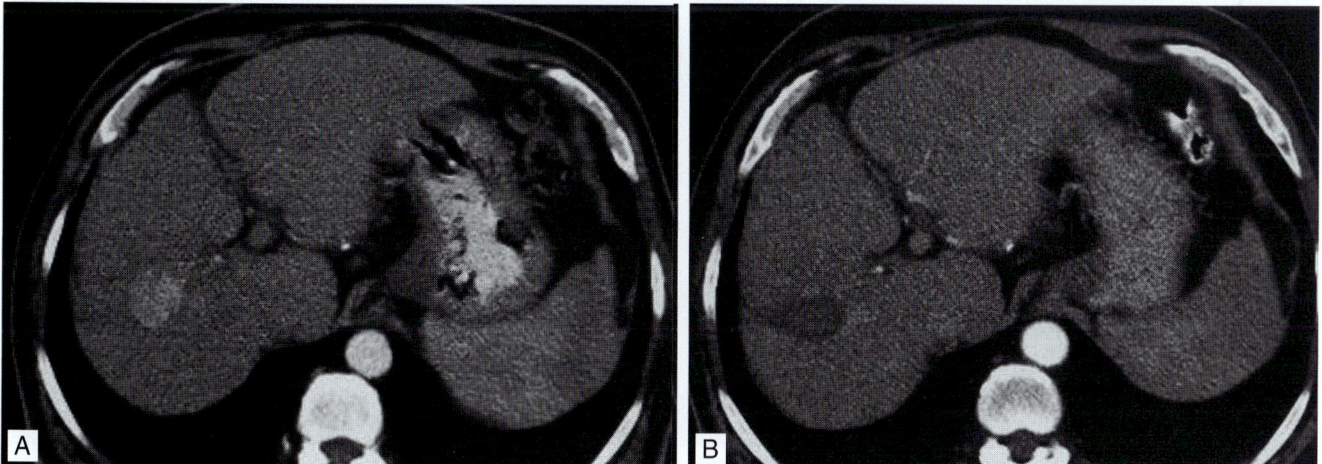

Figure 94.7 (A) A well-defined arterial enhancing lesion on CECT measuring 2.6 cm in segment 8 of the right lobe of the liver and (B) postRFA images after a month showing complete ablation of the lesion.

Patients with intermediate HCC (BCLC stage B) having well-preserved liver function and large or multinodular HCC without portal vein tumor thrombosis or extrahepatic metastasis appear to be ideal candidates for TACE [54]. According to the guidelines, about 20% of all HCC patients are the target population for TACE, with the median overall survival among them being 20 months (range 14–45 months). TACE delays tumor progression, macrovascular invasion and achieves partial response in 15–55% of patients [54].

There are two TACE techniques, namely conventional TACE (cTACE), which uses Lipiodol, and TACE with drug-eluting beads (DEB-TACE).cTACE treatment involves the intra-arterial injection of a cytotoxic drug, such as doxorubicin, epirubicin, mitomycin C, or cisplatin, alone or as a cocktail that is emulsified in the oily radio-opaque agent Lipiodol (ethiodized oil). This is followed by an embolic agent, such as a gelatin sponge, polyvinyl alcohol particles, or microspheres. This occlusion results in ischemic necrosis and slows down tumor progression. During cTACE, Lipiodol carries and delivers chemotherapy to the tumor with subsequent embolization of the tumor microcirculation.

DEBs are nonresorbable embolic microspheres that are loaded with cytotoxic agents with the intent to achieve more sustained drug release and concomitant embolization. 37.5 mg of doxorubicin per mL of microspheres can be loaded in 30 minutes to 2 hours [55].

Systemic complications related to doxorubicin are rare. A recent systematic review of 217 studies have shown that postembolization syndrome (fever, abdominal pain, and ileus) is the most common treatment-related AE, occurring in 47.7% of patients treated with cTACE. A transient increase in liver enzymes was noted in 52% of patients, and the overall postprocedure mortality rate was 0.6% [55].

Ideally, tumor response should differentiate patients who have benefitted from treatment and those who have not. Modified RECIST (m RE-CIST) criteria has been developed to measure the reduction in viable tumor burden. These criteria are predictive for survival if they are measured at least 3 months post cTACE (Fig. 94.8) [55].

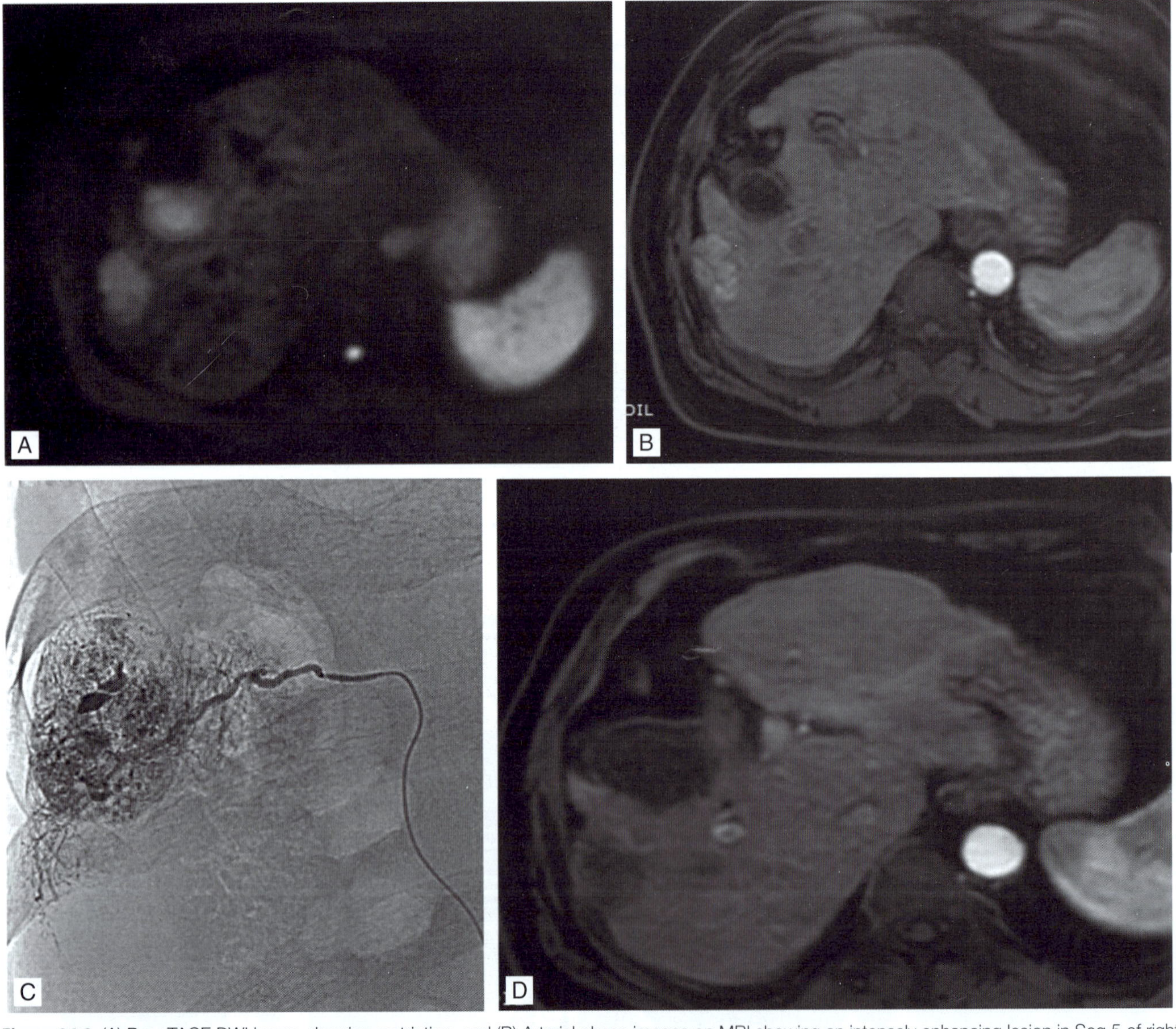

Figure 94.8 (A) Pre cTACE DWI image showing restriction, and (B) Arterial phase images on MRI showing an intensely enhancing lesion in Seg 5 of right lobe liver, (C) cTACE image showing Lipiodol deposition confined predominantly within the tumor, and (D) Postprocedure MRI after 3 months showing no enhancement in the lesion with decrease in size of lesion.

It was recently demonstrated that Lipiodol deposition within the tumor is helpful in survival prognosis for patients with large HCC lesions. Complete Lipiodol tumor deposition is known to indicate tumor necrosis, lack or partial deposition suggests that tumor feeders may have been missed or that Lipiodol uptake in the tumor was low. In such cases, the patient has to be taken up for repeat cTACE without waiting for delayed follow-up imaging. After DEB-TACE, dynamic CT and MRI can be used to assess tumor response.

Tumor burden, radiologic response, BCLC stage at baseline, and Child-Pugh score, are considered the best predictive factors for TACE retreatment and for considering an alternative therapy after two TACE treatments. cTACE should not be repeated when significant necrosis is not achieved after two TACE treatments, deterioration or liver function, worsening of performance status (PS), or the appearance of portal vein tumor thrombosis or extrahepatic metastases [55].

The role of TACE as neoadjuvant therapy has been widely accepted, either as a bridge between treatments while the patient is on the waiting list or to the downstage tumor to within acceptable criteria for transplantation.

It has been observed that in patients who undergo LT after cTACE, recurrence rates are low and tend to have improved post-transplant overall survival, especially when the period on the waiting list exceeds 6–12 months.

Combining TACE with Local Ablation

The superiority of combined treatment (first cTACE and then RFA) over RFA alone was demonstrated in a randomised control trial (2012) of patients with solitary recurrent HCC lesions up to 5 cm in diameter [55]. Combined TACE + RFA can be a good option if there is a surgical risk or if the tumor location makes it difficult to resect (Fig. 94.9).

When considering combination therapies, in lesions greater than 3 cm, RFA plus intravenous systemic lysothermosensitive liposomal doxorubicin (LTLD) treatment has been recently introduced. The doxorubicin-laden liposomes and the RFA-induced target heating, when performed for more than 45 minutes, induce a high target drug concentration, almost 25 times greater than that of free doxorubicin [50].

Transarterial Radioembolization (TARE)/ Selective Internal Radiation Therapy (SIRT)

Transarterial radioembolization/selective internal radiation therapy is selective endovascular intra-arterial administration of microspheres loaded with a radioactive compound such as yttrium-90 (Y90) or Lipiodol labeled with iodine131 or rhenium [56]. It has shown promising results in terms of disease control and is associated with the least side effects depicting it as a very safe procedure.

It consists of the two types of microspheres that are currently available:

- Glass-made microspheres have a diameter of 20–30 µm and activity of 2500 Becquerel (Bq) per sphere at the time of calibration
- Resin microspheres consist of biocompatible resin-based microspheres with a diameter of 20–60 µm and an activity of 50 Bq per sphere [56]

Y90 can be administered via a lobar or segmental injection to patients having a solitary tumor and normal serum bilirubin (Fig. 94.10). For patients with elevated bilirubin but a solitary tumor, TARE/SIRT should only be performed segmentally, which concentrates the Y90 to the tumor and spares the most uninvolved liver. Sequential lobar treatments are performed for patients with multiple tumors and/or bilobar HCC and normal serum bilirubin [57].

Portal Vein Embolization [58]

A significant challenge for a patient to be eligible for a major hepatectomy is the inadequate size of the future liver remnant

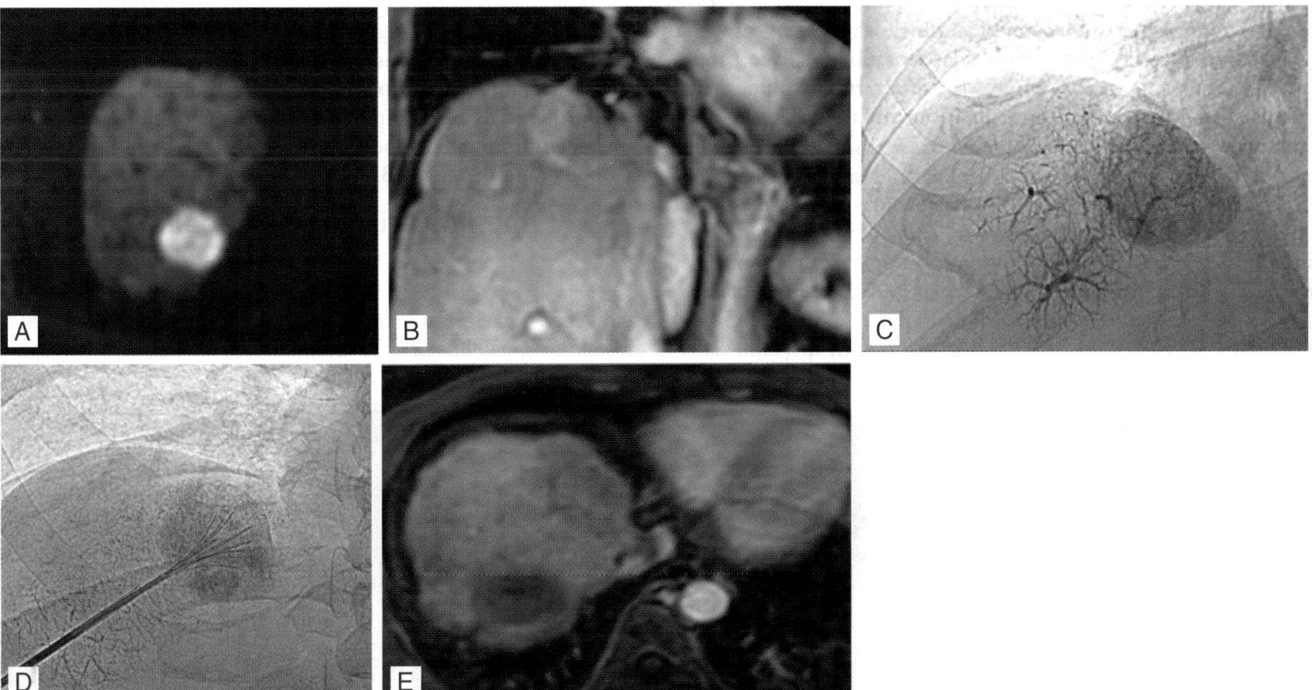

Figure 94.9 Combination of cTACE and RFA. (A) MRI showing a restricted image on DWI in seg 7 of right lobe liver. (B) Portal phase coronal image showing heterogenous enhancement of the lesion. (C) cTACE image showing lipiodol deposition within the tumor. (D) RFA of the segment 7 lesion. (E) Post procedure triphasic MRI after 3 months showing no residual lesion suggesting complete response.

Additionally, during the process of percutaneous necrosectomy, for lesser sac collections with trans-gastric and trans-retroperitoneal drainage, irrigation can be performed via the trans-gastric catheter allowing debris to be aspirated through the larger bore trans-retroperitoneal drain. The percutaneous catheter necrosectomy is usually performed under intravenous conscious sedation especially when patients complain of severe pain.

Other methods of minimal access necrosectomy include; video-assisted retroperitoneal debridement (VARD), laparoscopic debridement, endoscopic necrosectomy when SEMS is in place [67,68].

Follow-up after (repeated) necrosectomy for clinical improvement and radiological resolution of the collection is continued till the drain is less than 10 mL in 48 hours. Nonresolving collections often accompanied by a lack of clinical improvement/deterioration of clinical status and development of life-threatening organ failure is an indication for surgical debridement.

Pancreatic Fistula

Disconnected pancreatic duct syndrome occurs as a result of necrotizing pancreatitis in up to 40% cases wherein the involvement of the central gland causes disruption of the pancreatic duct [60,69,70]. This manifests as persistent drainage of clear fluid from the PCD or as pancreatico-cutaneous fistula when the PCD is prematurely removed. Detection of pancreatic ductal disruption is done by measuring the drain fluid amylase which when more than three times that of the serum amylase value strongly indicates the presence of a ductal disruption. MRCP can further assess the anatomical location of the disrupted segment of the duct.

Traditionally disconnected ducts have been treated endoscopically with an indefinitely placed trans-mural stent allowing drainage of pancreatic fluid into the bowel lumen and this method has been cited in the literature as the main advantage of endoscopic treatment over percutaneous methods.

Surgical options for the treatment of pancreatic fistula include distal pancreatectomy often in combination with splenectomy and pancreatico-jejunostomy [60].

Conclusion

Pancreatitis and associated sequelae, comprising of a varied severity of disease processes and superimposed infection can lead to life-threatening systemic inflammation and subsequent organ failure. It requires a multidisciplinary approach to the treatment of what is often a protracted course of illness. Percutaneous and endoscopic drainage methods following the step-up approach with multiple wide bore catheters with repeated necrosectomy procedures are the mainstay for its management.

94.5 Gastrointestinal Interventions

Harish Bhujade, Naveen Kalra, Sanjay Baijal

Gastrointestinal (GI) interventions are an important subset of visceral interventions. Upper and lower GI bleeding are now being managed by minimally invasive endovascular therapies. The interventional radiologist also plays an important role in the placement of gastrostomy and jejunostomy tubes, which was earlier done by surgical or endoscopic techniques. Moreover, most of these enteral nutrition procedures are carried out under fluoroscopy, which is available in almost all radiology departments.

Percutaneous Gastrostomy

Good supportive nutrition is required to avoid malnutrition in all hospitalized patients [71]. This can be given parenterally in patients who are not able to take oral nutrition. However, parenteral nutrition is costly and has a high risk of complications [72]. Enteral nutrition can be given via nasogastric or nasojejunal tubes for short-term use. For long-term usage, minimally invasive gastrostomy can be performed using fluoroscopic or endoscopic guidance. The advantage of percutaneous gastrostomy (PG) over percutaneous endoscopic gastrostomy (PEG) is that the endoscopy is not required while performing a PG and in patients with an esophageal or pharyngeal obstruction [73].

Percutaneous endoscopic gastrostomy is commonly indicated in the patients with neurologic disorders, impaired swallowing, and esophageal or head and neck masses [74,75]. Other indications include intestinal malabsorption secondary to small bowel pathology such as Crohn's disease, radiation enteritis, and scleroderma; patients with cystic fibrosis or significant burns; and patients with psychologic ailments such as eating disorders [76]. Indications and contraindications for percutaneous gastrostomy are enumerated in Table 94.6.

Technique

Informed and written consent is taken for the procedure. The patient is asked for overnight fasting before the procedure. A nasogastric tube may be placed 1 day before the procedure and is used for stomach insufflation during the procedure (Figs. 94.12 and 94.13). A 4-Fr angiographic catheter may be used in cases in which there is difficulty in placing the nasogastric tube. Oral contrast agents can be given 1 day before to delineate the colonic loops. Generally, the stomach lies directly underneath the anterior abdominal wall with no intervening bowel loops, which can be confirmed using lateral fluoroscopy. Ultrasonography (USG) is used to mark the inferior surface of the left lobe of liver.

Injection of glucagon or n-hyoscine butyl bromide is commonly used to reduce gastric motility. The puncture site should be marked lateral to the rectus sheath to avoid the superior epigastric artery. Computed tomography (CT) guidance can be used in difficult cases for patients who have had prior abdominal surgery.

A gastropexy is performed commonly to fix the stomach wall with the anterior abdominal wall. It also prevents guidewire buckling into the peritoneal cavity and early or late intraperitoneal leakage. It is performed using a T-fastener suture device (Fig. 94.13). The puncture site is marked on the skin midway to the lower third between the superior and inferior margins of the inflated stomach, and the local anesthetic agent is injected at the

TABLE 94.6 Indications and Contraindications for Percutaneous Gastrostomy

Indications	Contraindications
■ Head and neck cancers ■ Esophageal cancers ■ Neurologic disorder causing impaired swallowing ■ Nutritional supplementation for chronic illness or extensive surgery	**Absolute Contraindications** ■ Uncorrectable coagulopathy ■ Life expectancy <1 wk ■ Total gastrectomy ■ Unsatisfactory anatomy **Relative Contraindications** ■ Massive ascites ■ Abdominal varices ■ Prior gastric surgery ■ Inflammatory, neoplastic, or infectious involvement of the gastric wall

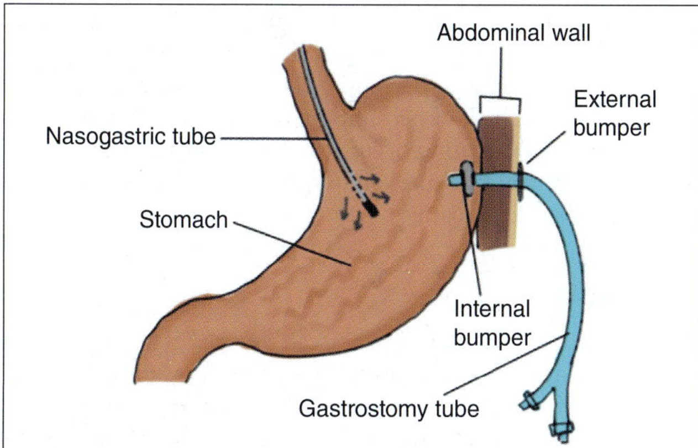

Figure 94.12 Percutaneous gastrostomy.

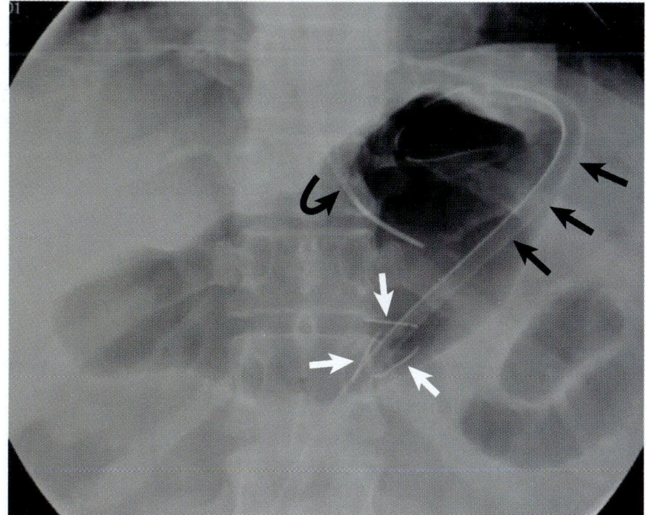

Figure 94.13 Percutaneous gastrostomy. A gastrostomy tube *(black straight arrows)* was placed percutaneously (push technique) after fixing the stomach wall with the anterior abdominal wall using T-fastener (anchor) sutures *(white arrows)*. An angiographic catheter (5 Fr) *(curved arrow)* was used to inflate the stomach.

puncture site and at the three or four corners of a 2-cm square around the puncture site. Using fluoroscopic guidance, puncture of the mid to lower segment of the gastric body is done with each T-fastener–loaded 18-gauge needle. As the needle is advanced, indentation of the anterior gastric wall can often be seen at fluoroscopy. The intraluminal position can be confirmed using contrast injection. The fastener is deployed by pushing it through the needle with a guidewire or by pressing the spring-loaded mechanism on the needle.

The same needle used for the gastropexy can be used to puncture the stomach, and a 0.035-inch stiff guidewire is inserted under fluoroscopic guidance. *The stomach should be kept inflated during gastropexy and gastrostomy tube placement.* Serial fascial dilation of the tract is done using fascial dilators. A peel-away catheter is placed after dilation, through which a 14- to 20-Fr gastrostomy catheter is placed into the stomach (see Fig. 94.13). The intraluminal position of the gastrostomy tube is confirmed by injecting contrast agent. The nasogastric tube is removed after completion of the procedure.

Postprocedure Care

The catheter is placed to gravity drainage for 24 hours to decompress the stomach and monitor for any complications such as bleeding or pain. After 24 hours, tube feeding can start gradually if there are no signs of peritonitis (fever, abdominal pain, tenderness) and there are good bowel sounds. The full nutrition feed is generally achieved within 48 hours. Catheter care instructions are given to the patient or caregivers about tube feedings and catheter maintenance.

Result

The technical success rate for PG is 95% to 100%, and the procedure-related mortality rate is between 0% and 3.2% [73]. A meta-analysis of the literature reported a technical success of 95% for PEG and 100% for surgical gastrostomies [73]. The advantages of percutaneous gastrostomy over other techniques are the capability to place a percutaneous gastrojejunostomy tube at the time of initial PG, replacing existing gastrostomy tubes to gastrojejunostomy tubes, and the capability to perform a gastrostomy in patients with esophageal or pharyngeal strictures.

Complications

The complications related to PG can be major or minor in nature.

- Minor complications are dislodged or leaking tubes and superficial wound infections.
- Major complications include septicemia, aspiration, peritonitis, other GI complications (perforation, bleeding), and dislodgment of the tube, requiring a repeat procedure. Major complication rates of about 3% have been described in different studies [77,78].

Percutaneous Gastrojejunostomy

Some interventional radiologists may prefer to perform percutaneous gastrojejunostomy rather than a percutaneous gastrostomy. The common indication for a percutaneous gastrojejunostomy is a history of reflux or aspiration [76,79]. Jejunal feedings need specially prepared nutrient solutions and must be delivered by a

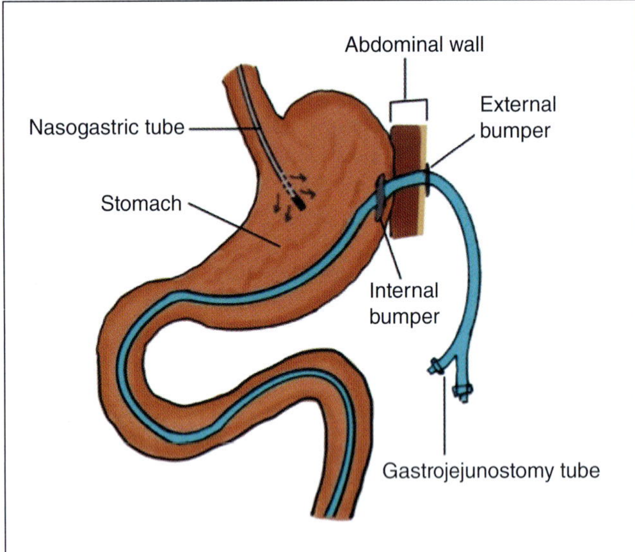

Figure 94.14 Percutaneous gastrojejunostomy.

pump. The gastrojejunostomy catheters are longer and tend to be of narrower calibre than those placed for gastrostomy.

The technique of primary gastrojejunostomy placement is like that of the percutaneous gastrostomy (Fig. 94.14). The puncture is directed toward the pylorus. A 5-Fr angiographic catheter and a 0.035-inch hydrophilic guidewire are used to cannulate the pylorus. The 5-Fr catheter is advanced into the proximal jejunum and the hydrophilic guidewire exchanged for a 0.035-inch superstiff guidewire. After the serial tract dilation, a gastrojejunostomy catheter is placed. At times, the conversion procedures from gastrostomy to gastrojejunostomy can be technically difficult because the initial angle of entry for the gastrostomy is directed toward the fundus of the stomach. The fascial dilators can be used to stabilize the guidewire and aid cannulation.

Success rates for primary gastrojejunostomy placement are high with 95% to 100% successful placement rates [77,80]. Success rates for conversion gastrojejunostomy are also high [81]. The complications of percutaneous gastrojejunostomy are similar to those of PG.

Percutaneous Jejunostomy

Direct percutaneous jejunostomy (PJ) may be indicated when there is failure of gastrojejunostomy tube conversion or when there is abnormal stomach position. In patients with chronic aspirations and gastric outlet obstruction, PJ may be considered [82,83] (Table 94.7). The contraindications for PJ are similar to those of percutaneous gastrostomy.

TABLE 94.7 Indications for Percutaneous Jejunostomy

- Failed gastrojejunostomy
- Chronic aspirations
- Abnormal stomach position
- Gastric outlet obstruction
- Dislodged surgical jejunostomy tube

Technique

The proximal jejunal loop is insufflated through the nasojejunal tube (Fig. 94.15). The puncture can be made under fluoroscopic guidance followed by injection of contrast media to confirm needle position. Alternatively, CT can be used for imaging guidance. After confirmation of intraluminal position of the needle, a 0.035-inch hydrophilic guidewire is inserted followed by a 5-Fr angiographic catheter. Cope sutures or T-fasteners are used to fix the jejunum to the anterior abdominal wall. Dilation of the tract is performed followed by placement of a 14-Fr locking pigtail catheter.

Technical success rates for PJ are between 85% and 95% [84]. Localized pain, infection at the puncture site, and tube blockage are minor complications associated with PJ. Major complications are pericatheter leakage and peritoneal spillage [85].

Percutaneous Cecostomy

Percutaneous cecostomy can be an alternative procedure to surgical cecostomy for patients who are unfit for open surgery [86]. The advantage of percutaneous cecostomy is that it can be done under local anesthesia and sedation unlike surgical cecostomy, which requires general anaesthesia. The main indication for percutaneous cecostomy is decompression of the dilated caecum, which may have a risk of perforation and have a mortality rate as high as 50% if perforation occurs [87]. The contraindications for cecostomy are the presence of bowel ischemia, perforation, or uncorrectable coagulopathy.

Technique

Anterior and posterior approaches can be used for percutaneous cecostomy. The anterior approach is straightforward and can be done under fluoroscopy guidance. The posterior approach is an extraperitoneal approach and is advantageous because there is no

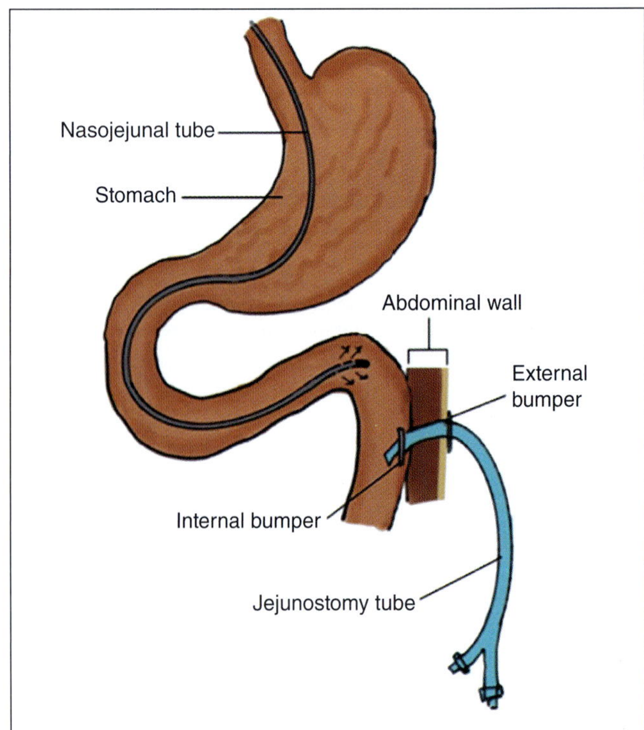

Figure 94.15 Percutaneous jejunostomy.

spillage into the peritoneal cavity. However, peritoneal folds may extend posteriorly in some cases, which is difficult to identify. CT or USG guidance can be used for the posterior approach. The procedure is similar to PG with initial puncture and deployment of T-fasteners to fix the caecal wall to the abdominal wall. The position of the needle is confirmed by injection of contrast media followed by insertion of a super-stiff 0.035-inch guidewire. After serial tract dilation, the cecostomy tube is placed within the lumen.

The catheter may require frequent flushing with 50 to 100 mL of normal saline to prevent blockage caused by the solid components. Close monitoring of cecostomy is needed for any catheter malfunction, pericatheter leakage, or intraperitoneal leak. Technical success rate of percutaneous cecostomy reaches up to 100%. The clinical success rate is up to 89% [88,89].

Complications

Minor complications are pericatheter leak, wound infection, tube blockage, tube dislodgment, and colocutaneous fistula. Catheter blockage can be avoided by frequent flushing. Major complications include peritonitis and sepsis [87].

Balloon Dilation of Gastrointestinal Stricture

Surgical methods have been used for management of GI strictures. Endoscopic and interventional radiologic procedures are rapidly gaining acceptance for management of GI strictures [90]. Balloon dilation is commonly used for esophageal strictures; however, it can also be used for strictures of the stomach, duodenum, or colon.

For esophageal strictures, barium swallow is performed before the procedure to assess the length and location of the stricture. The procedure is performed via the per-oral route with use of a mouthpiece. A topical anesthetic agent can be used to reduce the gag reflux. A 5-Fr angiographic catheter with a hydrophilic guidewire is used to access the esophagus. Contrast injection is done just proximal to the stricture site to confirm the position, and the stricture is then negotiated with the hydrophilic guidewire. After the stricture is crossed, the hydrophilic guidewire is exchanged with a 0.035-inch super-stiff guidewire. The balloon is passed over the exchange-length guidewire and serial dilation is done, starting with 10 to 12 mm up to 20 mm. The patient can be given an analgesic agent to alleviate pain just before dilation. Immediate contrast esophagogram may not be reliable because of acute spasm of the muscular layer during dilation. It is often taken only to rule out esophageal injury during dilation and can be done using a nonionic contrast agent. The technical success rate is between 90% and 95% with appropriate dilation [91].

Colorectal anastomotic stricture can be managed with balloon dilation. The procedure is similar to esophageal stricture dilation and is performed through the anal route. The dilation is done with a 20- or 30-mm balloon. The balloon is inflated until the waist disappears and is left inflated for 2 to 3 minutes. After 4 to 6 hours, contrast enema (iodinated contrast) is performed to evaluate the status of the stricture.

Metallic Stent Placement

There is a limited role for metallic stent placement for a benign GI stricture. Fully covered retrievable metallic stents are used to remodel benign stricture and give long-lasting relief to dysphagia. Metallic stenting is indicated for the palliative management in cases of malignant dysphagia, perforation, or fistula. The placement of a stent at the esophageal sphincter and across the gastroesophageal junction is done with caution because of the risk of aspiration and reflux, respectively [92]. However, dedicated stents are now available for both locations.

The transoral route is used for esophageal stent deployment. The initial procedure is similar to balloon dilation of strictures. Prior dilation is not performed if there is suspicion of a fistula. Proximal and distal stent tips should be kept 1 to 2 cm away from the respective level of obstruction (Fig. 94.16). Technical success rates for esophageal stenting are 97% to 100% [93]. More than 90% of patients will have relief from dysphagia [94]. In 70% to 100% of cases, successful closure of fistula is also possible [95].

Self-expanding stents can be useful for patients with gastroduodenal malignancy, causing obstruction [96] (Fig. 94.17). Both covered and uncovered stents can be used for duodenal obstruction. Currently, the nitinol stents have almost completely replaced other materials because of the marked flexibility and excellent radial force of these stents. Complications related to gastroduodenal self-expanding metallic stents are recurrence of the obstruction caused by stent blockage and stent migration [97].

The indication for colonic stent placement are palliative management of unresectable colonic cancer or for short-term colonic decompression to allow bowel cleansing in preparation for single-stage colonic surgery [98]. The colonic stent is placed through the rectal route or via an existing cecostomy. Fluoroscopic guidance is used for stent placement with the patient in a lateral or oblique position. *Because of the high rates of migration with the covered stents, uncovered stents are preferred.* Dilation is avoided because of a risk of perforation. The technical success rate is between 78% and 100%. Complication rates are between 14% and 42%, which predominantly includes minor complications [99,100].

Gastrointestinal Bleeding

Recent advances in surgical technique, interventions, and imaging tools have led to a reduction in use of conventional angiography for the diagnosis of GI bleeding [101]. However, in small subset of patients, conventional angiography may be useful for evaluation of GI bleeding, which is at times part of important lifesaving interventions [102]. The normal anatomy of mesenteric arteries is depicted in Fig. 94.18.

Acute Gastrointestinal Bleeding

Acute GI bleeding can be upper GI bleeding when the cause of bleed is above the ligament of Treitz or lower GI bleeding when the cause of bleeding lies below the level of ligament of Treitz [103,104]. The various causes for acute GI bleeding are given in Table 94.8.

Catheter Angiography

The first line of management of GI bleeding is to stabilize the patient with intravenous fluid, airway protection, and management of coagulopathy. Blood transfusion should be given in severe cases of GI bleeding.

Catheter angiography is performed based on diagnostic imaging using CT angiography for localization of the bleed. The involved vessel is first evaluated on angiography. In general, for evaluation of upper GI bleeding, celiac arteriogram is taken followed by superior mesenteric arteriogram. If cause of bleed is not identified, selective angiogram of left gastric artery and gastroduodenal artery (GDA) are taken. An inferior mesenteric arteriogram is taken if no cause is identified.

For evaluation of lower GI bleeding, superior mesenteric and inferior mesenteric arteriograms are necessary. Some interventional

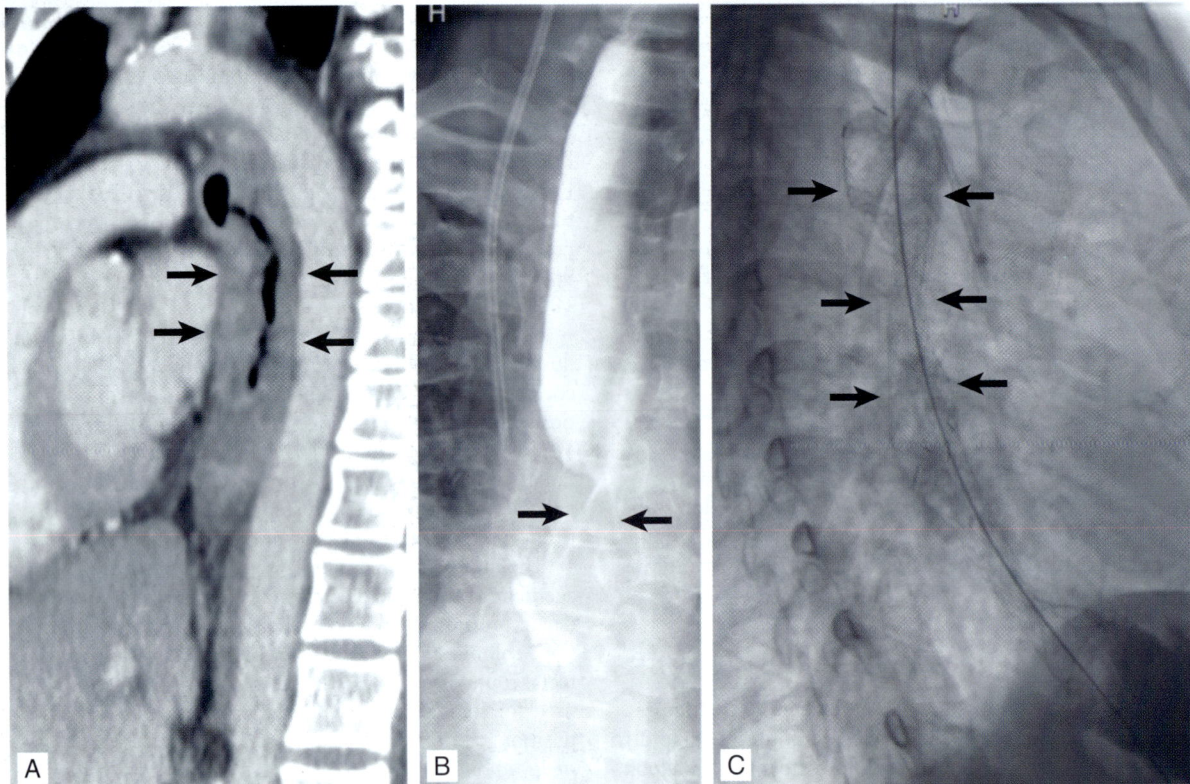

Figure 94.16 Esophageal stenting. (A) Sagittal images of contrast-enhanced computed tomography of a patient with carcinoma esophagus show irregular asymmetric wall thickening with luminal narrowing *(arrows)*. (B) Contrast esophagogram shows a malignant stricture of the esophagus *(arrows)*. (C) A self-expanding metallic stent was placed across the stricture *(arrows)* via a transoral route. (Courtesy of Dr. Abhay Kumar Kapoor.)

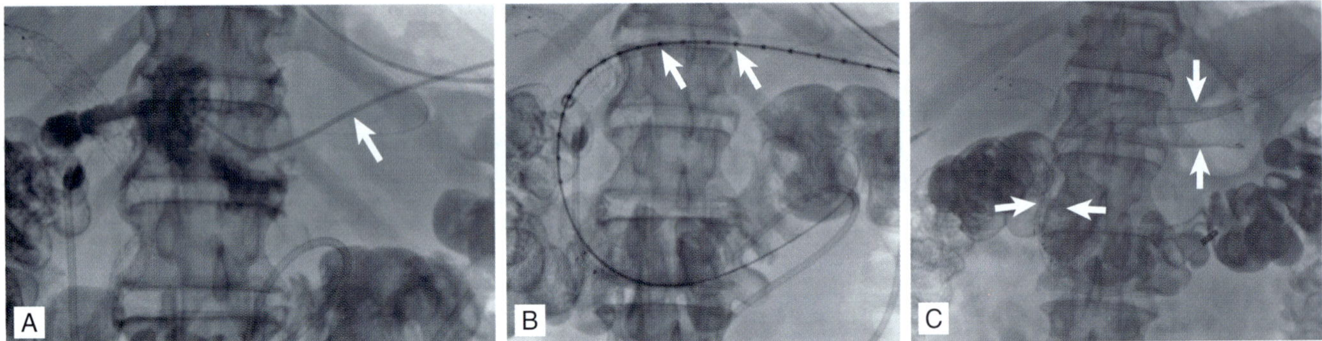

Figure 94.17 Duodenal stenting in malignant duodenal obstruction. (A) The obstruction was negotiated using an angiographic catheter *(arrow)*. (B) Crossing of stricture and placement of the stent over the guidewire *(arrows)*. (C) Fluorographic spot after placement of a self-expanding metallic gastroduodenal stent *(arrows)*. (Courtesy Dr. Abhay Kumar Kapoor.)

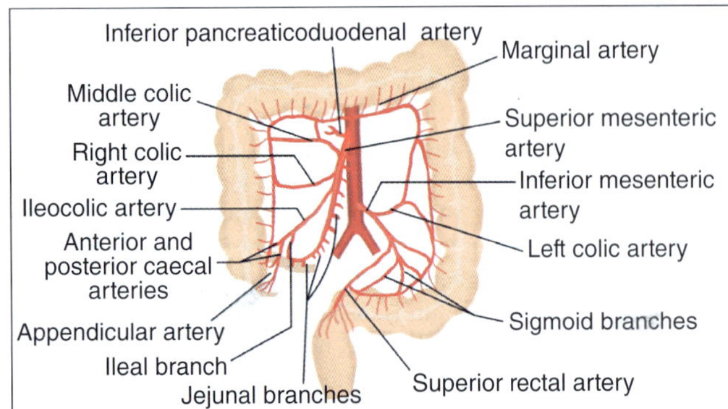

Figure 94.18 Normal anatomy of the superior and inferior mesenteric arteries.

radiologists prefer to cannulate the inferior mesenteric artery first to reduce obscuration by the contrast-filled bladder. If both the angiogram results are negative, then the celiac angiogram is taken.

On angiography, contrast extravasation into the bowel lumen can be identified. *Care should be taken to avoid misinterpretation of bowel artifact, opacified renal pelvis, and hypervascular mucosa as contrast extravasation.*

- Pseudoaneurysm is seen as a contrast-filled outpouching with subsequent washout.
- Early filling of an abnormal cluster of vessels with persistent filling of a draining vein can be seen in cases of angiodysplasia. It may be an incidental finding in an older patient, and other sources of bleeding should also be searched for.
- Congenital arteriovenous malformations also appear similar in characteristics.

TABLE 94.8 Causes of Acute Upper and Lower Gastrointestinal Bleeding

Acute Upper Gastrointestinal Bleeding	Acute Lower Gastrointestinal Bleeding
Peptic ulcer	Diverticulosis
Variceal bleed (portal hypertension)	Hemorrhoids
Malignancies of esophagus or stomach	Malignancies of colon
Mallory-Weiss tear	Postintervention (postsurgery, postbiopsy)
Postintervention (sphincterotomy, postsurgery, postbiopsy)	Ischemic bowel disease
Pseudoaneurysm or aneurysm (GDA, LGA, or splenic artery)	Inflammatory bowel disease
Hemosuccus entericus	Meckel diverticulum
Aortoenteric fisula	Aortoenteric fistula
	Portal hypertension

GDA, gastroduodenal artery; *LGA*, left gastric artery.

Endovascular Therapy

Endovascular embolization is the mainstay of management to occlude the bleeding vessels [105]. The aim of embolization is to prevent bleeding and to maintain bowel perfusion. With the recent advances in interventional tools (microcatheter, coaxial systems, and microcoils), the incidence of bowel necrosis has been decreasing.

Technique

A 5-Fr diagnostic catheter (usually Simmons or Cobra catheter) is used for the main artery. A coaxial system with a microcatheter and microguidewire is used for superselective cannulation of the culprit branch. The microcatheter tip should be kept as close as possible to bleeding point to reduce the risk of bowel gangrene.

The commonly used embolic agents are microcoils, gelfoam, polyvinyl alcohol particles, and cyanoacrylate (glue) [106]. Currently, the role of intraarterial vasopressin injections is very limited and has been replaced by various embolic agents. Most of the pseudoaneurysms require proximal and distal embolization (sandwich technique) to prevent refilling of the sac from the collateral circulation (Fig. 94.19). For example, pseudoaneurysm of the GDA gets filled from the GDA as well as the superior mesenteric artery (SMA). The choice of the embolic agent depends on the location of the bleeding point [107].

Results

The endovascular embolization is successful in about 80% of patients [108]. The common factor for technical failure is an inability to get the proper position of the microcatheter. Patients with inflammatory conditions and vascular malformation may have recurrent bleed. Major adverse effect may occur in fewer than 5% of patients. After embolization, patients should be monitored for signs of ischemia, which may occur in well under 20% of cases [109].

Chronic Gastrointestinal Bleeding

Common causes of chronic GI bleeding are malignancy and vascular malformation. About 5% of patients with GI hemorrhage have persistent, intermittent bleeding that may be difficult to localize (so-called obscure bleeding) [110]. *The common sites for chronic GI bleeding are the small bowel or ascending colon.* The bleeding source can be identified in half of these patients. Some interventionists may prefer provocative angiography with intraarterial injections of a vasodilator or anticoagulation to demonstrate the site of bleed. This should be done carefully because it may increase the risk of bleeding. The site of bleeding is embolized with appropriate embolizing agent depending on the site and underlying pathology.

Acute Mesenteric Ischemia

Many causative factors have been described for acute mesenteric ischemia. The most common cause is thromboembolism of the SMA followed by thrombosis superimposed on SMA stenosis or atherosclerosis [111] (Table 94.9). In fewer than 20% cases, low flow or hypotension leads to nonocclusive mesenteric ischemia [112]. A delay in diagnosis is responsible for the high mortality rate in cases of acute mesenteric ischemia.

The clinical presentation of acute mesenteric ischemia is moderate to severe abdominal pain with or without nausea and vomiting. Symptoms and signs depend on the development of ischemic changes. Imaging tools, especially contrast CT, may tell the status of mesenteric arteries as well as the veins. Doppler USG and magnetic resonance imaging may have a role in diagnosis. On cross-sectional imaging, other findings of bowel ischemia such as wall thickening, enhancement, or intramural gas may be useful to detect the severity of changes.

Catheter Angiography

Catheter angiography is usually performed for endovascular therapy or when there is a high clinical suspicion with equivocal imaging findings, especially in cases of nonocclusive ischemia.

- Surgical management of acute SMA occlusion includes embolectomy, endarterectomy, and bypass grafting along with resection of the infarcted bowel if any [113].

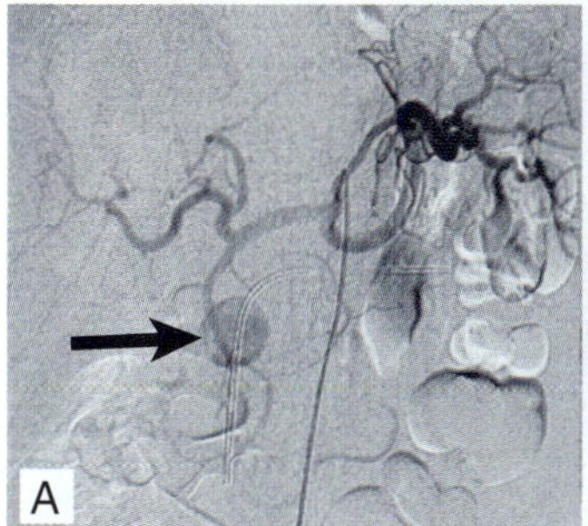

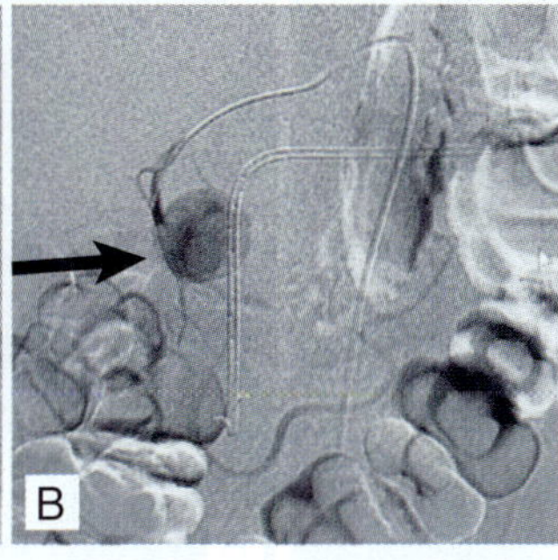

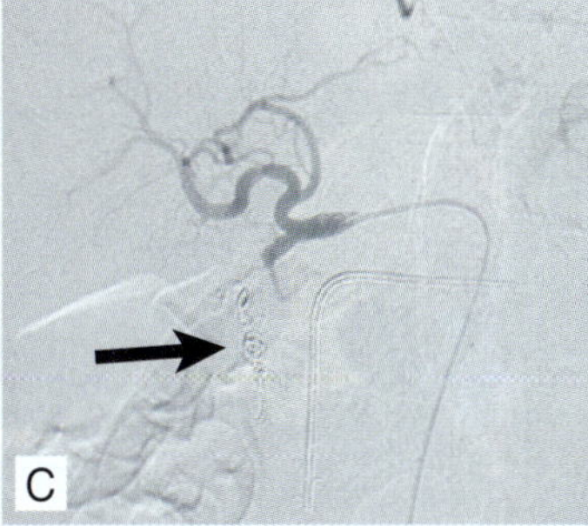

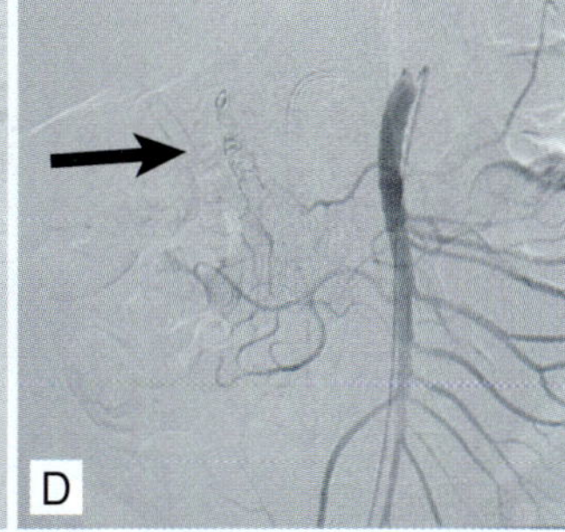

Figure 94.19 Endovascular embolization of a gastroduodenal artery (GDA) pseudoaneurysm in patient with chronic pancreatitis. (A) Celiac angiogram shows contrast outpouching from the GDA *(arrow)*. (B) Superselective angiogram of the GDA shows a large pseudoaneurysm *(arrow)*. Postembolization angiogram through the celiac (C) and superior mesenteric artery (D) shows nonopacification of the pseudoaneurysm. The pseudoaneurysm was embolized using microcoils *(arrows)* (sandwich technique).

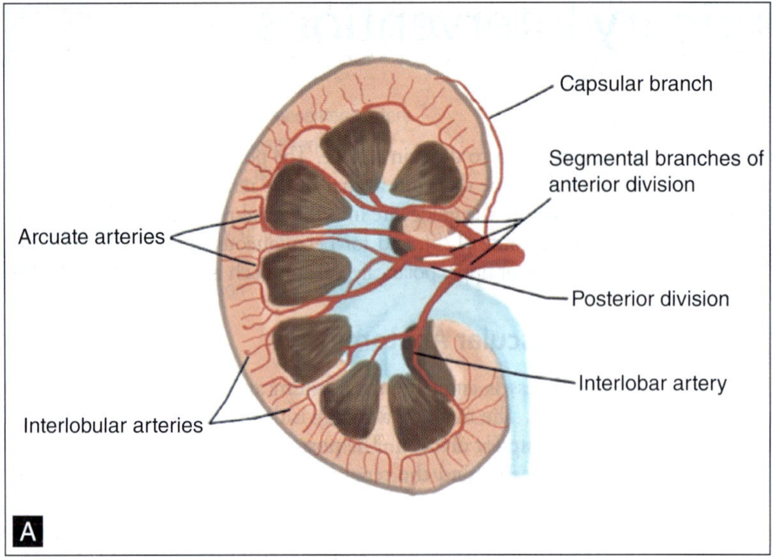

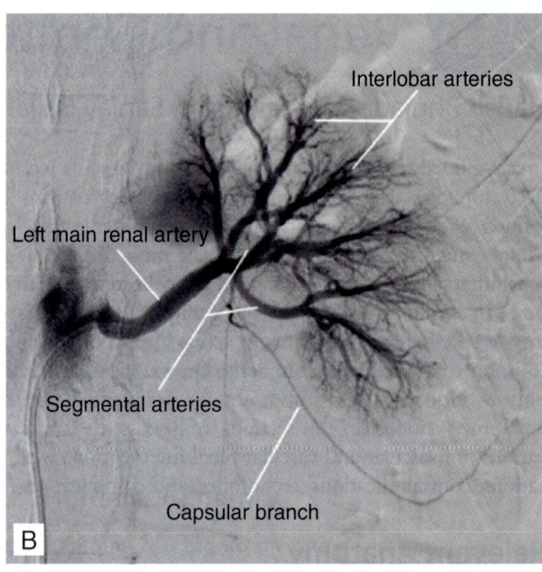

Figure 94.22 Diagram (A) and conventional renal angiography (B) shows the renal arterial anatomy.

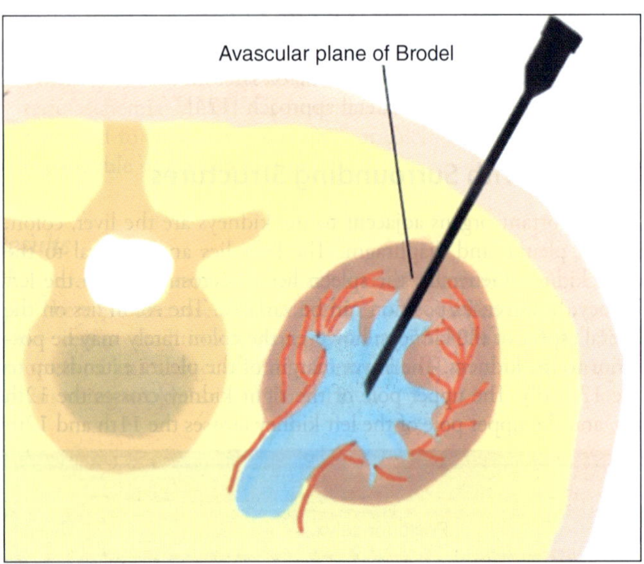

Figure 94.23 Avascular plane of Brodel.

ribs. Therefore, there is more chance of pneumothorax subsequent to percutaneous intervention through the upper pole, particularly on the left side. Because many important organs lie in close relation with the kidneys, assessment of cross-sectional imaging plays an important role before percutaneous renal interventions [126].

Key Points for Relevant Anatomy

- The lower pole is away from the skin surface, and the posterior calyces are near the skin surface.
- The posterior calyces of the lower pole are preferred for renal access.
- The avascular plane of Brodel lies along the posterolateral margin of the kidneys.
- The renal vein, renal artery, and renal pelvis lie from anterior to posterior at the renal hilum. The posterior division of the renal artery courses behind the renal pelvis.
- Knowledge of relation with surrounding structures is important, especially for interventions through the upper polar approach.

TABLE 94.11 Renal and Ureteric Interventions

Intervention	Nonvascular Renal Intervention	Vascular Renal Intervention
Diagnostic	Percutaneous renal biopsy	Transjugular renal biopsy
Therapeutic	Percutaneous nephrostomy Antegrade ureteral stenting Ureteral stricture dilation Perirenal collection drainage	Renal aneurysm or pseudoaneurysm embolization Renal tumor embolization: angiomyolipoma and renal cell carcinoma Renal tumor ablations

The various renal and ureteric interventions can be classified as in Table 94.11.

Patient Preparation

An informed and written consent should be obtained in all cases of renal interventions. The coagulation profile and platelet counts should be checked, and coagulopathies if any, should be corrected before the procedure [127]. The patient should have intravenous (IV) access. Prophylactic antibiotics may be given, especially if there is any evidence of infection. A single dose of a broad-spectrum antibiotic (usually IV 1 g ceftriaxone or 1 g cefazolin) may be given which may be continued depending on the specific course of infection on case-by-case basis [128].

Percutaneous Nephrostomy

Percutaneous nephrostomy (PCN) is the most commonly performed renal intervention. The commonest indication is to relieve renal obstruction [128]. Another common indication is to drain an infected pelvicalyceal system. Urinary obstruction may be acute (caused by calculus or trauma) or chronic (caused by malignancy or retroperitoneal fibrosis).

Emergency PCN may be required to preserve renal function in cases of acute obstruction of bilateral kidneys or of a solitary kidney. The infected calyceal system must be drained as early as

TABLE 94.12 Indications for Percutaneous Nephrostomy

Indication	Specific Causes
To relieve obstruction	Urolithiasis, ureteric stricture, malignancy, external compression by various pathologies, retroperitoneal fibrosis
To drain an infected calyceal system	Pyonephrosis
Diversion of urine	Ureteric injury, urine leak, urinary fistula, hemorrhagic cystitis
Access for percutaneous interventions	Ureteric stenting, ureteric balloon dilation, percutaneous nephrolithotomy, delivery of chemotherapeutic agents or antifungal drugs

possible. In cases of ureteric injury or ureteric fistula, PCN may be necessary for diversion of urine along with placement of the ureteric stent. PCN has also been used for urinary diversion in cases of hemorrhagic cystitis. PCN is often required to perform various therapeutic interventions such as antegrade ureteral stenting, balloon dilation of ureteric strictures, or retrieval of a foreign body. It also provides access for nephroscopy or ureteroscopy [129]. In specific cases of urothelial cancers, intracavitary chemotherapy or immunotherapy and antibiotics can be given through PCN [130,131]. The various indications for percutaneous nephrostomy are given in Table 94.12.

There is no absolute contraindication for PCN [128]. Coagulopathy is a relative contraindication. The decision of whether to perform PCN in cases of coagulopathy depends on the clinical status of the patient and the indications for PCN. A multidisciplinary approach should be followed with the involvement of the referring physicians, urologist, and interventional radiologists.

Image Guidance

Ultrasound guidance is preferred for the initial puncture of the calyx followed by the use of fluoroscopy for the rest of the procedure. Alternatively, the puncture can also be made under fluoroscopy guidance after the opacification of the calyces with the help of an IV contrast agent. CT guidance can also be used to locate the suitable calyx, especially in cases of emphysematous pyelonephritis.

General Technique

The patient is made to lie in a prone position on the fluoroscopy table. If the patient is unable to lie down in a prone position, a supine oblique position can also be used. Analgesia or conscious sedation may be given for pain relief. A suitable site for the puncture is chosen using ultrasound guidance. Then the site is infiltrated with 5 to 10 mL of local anaesthesia (2% lignocaine injection), which is given up to the renal capsule.

The minor calyx is punctured using an 18-gauge needle (Vygon needle). After the needle tip has been confirmed on ultrasonography (USG), the trocar is removed, and a small amount of urine is allowed to flow. The urine sample may be taken in cases of suspected infection. A diluted iodinated contrast is injected to opacify the pelvi-calyceal system (PCS). The rest of the procedure is performed under fluoroscopic guidance.

If the puncture site is acceptable, then a 0.035-inch guidewire (Amplatz stiff guidewire) is inserted and navigated into the ureter. If the initial puncture is not acceptable, then a new puncture is made under fluoroscopy, keeping the previous needle in situ. Alternatively, an 0.035-inch curved tip hydrophilic guidewire (Terumo) may be used to navigate into the ureter or upper pole calyx. A 5-Fr Cobra or Picard catheter can be used in difficult cases for negotiation of the guidewire. The hydrophilic guidewire is then exchanged with a stiff guidewire followed by serial dilation of the tract using a fascial dilator up to the size of the catheter to be inserted. After dilation of the tract, the catheter (usually 8-Fr pigtail catheter) is placed over the guidewire, and the tip is kept in the renal pelvis. The various steps of PCN are depicted in Figs. 94.24 and 94.25.

After the satisfactory placement of the catheter, the catheter is fixed with a skin suture. If the locking pigtail catheter is used for PCN, then the self-retaining suture needs to be pulled to lock the pigtail followed by skin fixation. *Accidental slippage of PCN catheter is very common. Therefore, some interventional radiologists may prefer to fix the catheter with double skin sutures.* Transparent adhesive is placed over the suture site, which allows easy USG assessment of the calyces on follow-up. If the catheter needs to be removed or exchanged, it should be removed or exchanged using fluoroscopic guidance over the guidewire.

Key Points for Percutaneous Nephrostomy

- For future ureteric interventions, the upper or interpolar calyx is preferred.
- Avoid overdistension of the calyces with contrast medium, which may increase the chances of sepsis.
- The beveled edge of the puncture needle should be oriented toward the renal pelvis for easy introduction of the guidewire into the renal pelvis or ureter.
- Use 5-Fr Cobra or Picard catheter for manipulation of the guidewire into the renal pelvis. These catheters can be cut short to make a length of 30 to 40 cm for easy manipulation.
- Minimal manipulation of the guidewire should be done in case of suspected infection.

Complications of Percutaneous Nephrostomy

The complications of PCN are uncommon with an estimated rate of 3% to 4% [128]. The major complications are hemorrhage and sepsis. Hemorrhage can manifest as bloody output from the catheter or as hematuria, which may resolve in 48 to 72 hours. However, major bleeding may require a blood transfusion. The venous bleed may be managed conservatively and may stop spontaneously. The bleeding caused by arterial injury during the procedure requires an angiogram followed by embolization of the culprit arterial branch (Fig. 94.26).

Sepsis may occur because of over distension of the calyces and excessive manipulation of the guidewire [132]. Appropriate antibiotic therapy usually results in a complete resolution of sepsis. Injury to adjacent organs such as the pleura, liver, spleen, or colon is very rare and can be avoided by accurate assessment of preprocedural imaging [133].

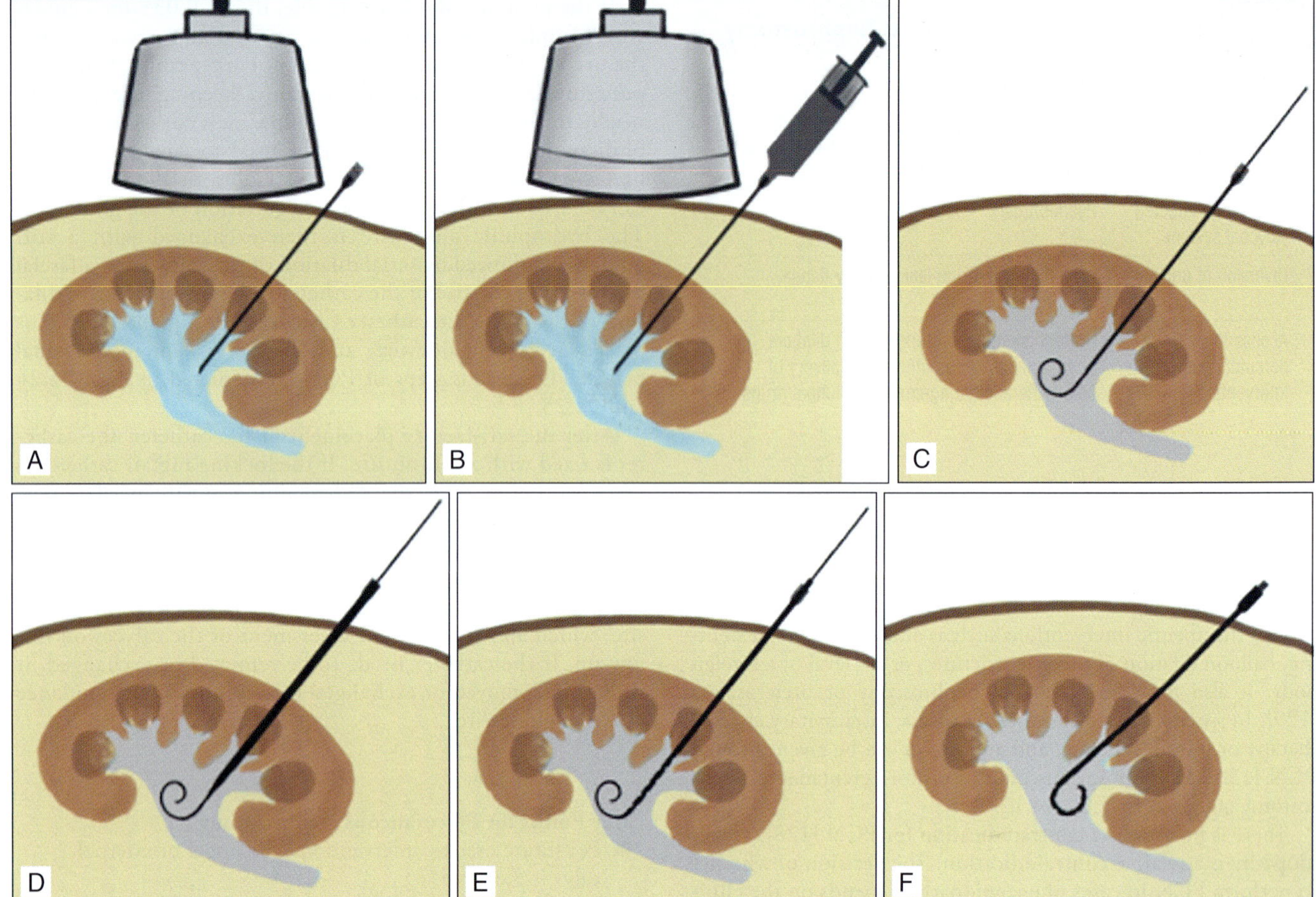

Figure 94.24 General steps of percutaneous nephrostomy. (A) Ultrasound-guided puncture of the calyx. (B) Contrast injection to opacify the pelvicalyceal system. (C) Guidewire insertion through a cannula under fluoroscopy. (D) Dilation of the tract. (E) Pigtail catheter insertion over the guidewire. (F) Removal of the guidewire and final placement of the catheter with the tip in the renal pelvis.

Specific Scenarios

Transplant Kidney

A transplant kidney is very well visualized on USG because of its superficial location [134]. The puncture of the upper pole or interpolar calyx in the supine position is performed to access the calyceal system. The use of a high-frequency linear probe helps to avoid bowel injury or inferior epigastric artery injury. Fibrotic tissue at the operative site may pose difficulty in the dilation of the track. The use of serial dilation with 1- to 2-Fr over-dilation of the track may help in the smooth placement of the catheter (Fig. 94.27).

Horseshoe Kidney

The lower pole of the horseshoe kidney is fused and lies more anterior. The puncture of the lower pole calyx may lead to injury to the anterior division of the renal artery. The upper pole calyx is preferred for calyceal access in a horseshoe kidney.

Nondilated Calyceal System

Percutaneous nephrostomy in nondilated calyces is often challenging because the calyx is difficult to visualize on USG. In this case, a double-puncture technique can be used with the initial puncture of the renal pelvis with a 22-gauge needle under ultrasound guidance and injection of the contrast medium into the collecting system followed by the second puncture of a suitable calyx under fluoroscopy guidance [135]. Alternatively, IV contrast medium may be given, and the calyx is punctured under fluoroscopy during the excretory phase. Also, the use of diuretic agents such as furosemide may help to distend the calyx, which may be identified on USG.

Percutaneous Nephrostomy in Pediatric Patients

Adequate sedation or even general anaesthesia is necessary for PCN in pediatric cases. In children, the pelvicalyceal system is easily visualized on USG. An effort should be made to perform the procedure on only ultrasound guidance to avoid radiation exposure to the children. For pediatric cases, a smaller French catheter (5–7 Fr) is required.

Key Points for Specific Scenarios

- In a transplant kidney, the upper calyx is accessed for PCN, and care should be taken to avoid injury to the bowel and inferior epigastric artery.
- For horseshoe kidney, the upper calyx is preferred for access.
- For nondilated systems, the use of double-puncture, IV contrast medium, or diuretic agents is very helpful.
- In pregnancy, PCN should be done with the patient in the lateral or supine oblique position with minimal use of fluoroscopy.

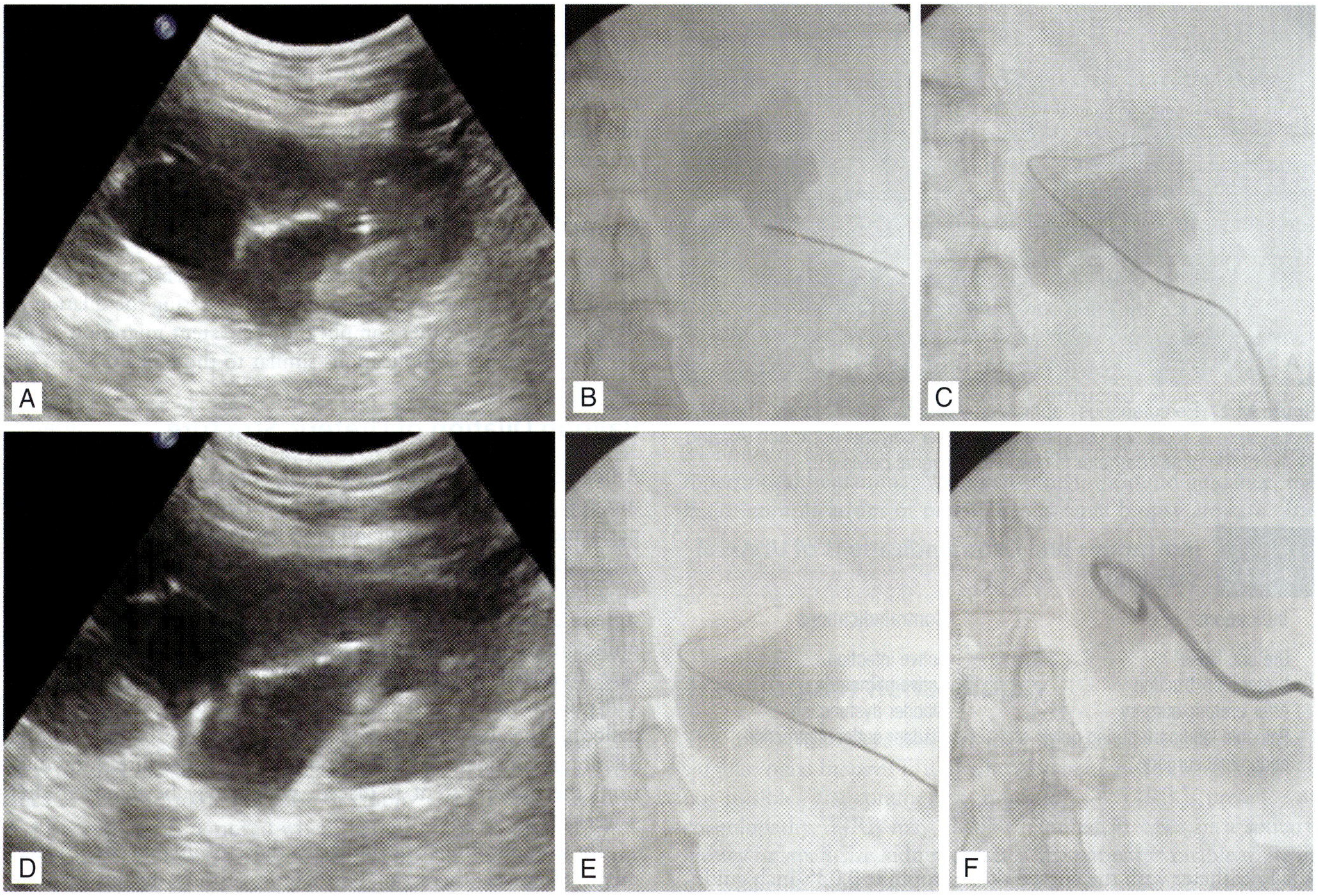

Figure 94.25 Percutaneous nephrostomy. (A) Ultrasound-guided puncture of the lower pole calyx. (B) Injection of contrast medium. (C) Guidewire insertion. (D) Ultrasound confirmation of the guidewire. (E) Dilation of the tract. (F) Insertion of the pigtail catheter.

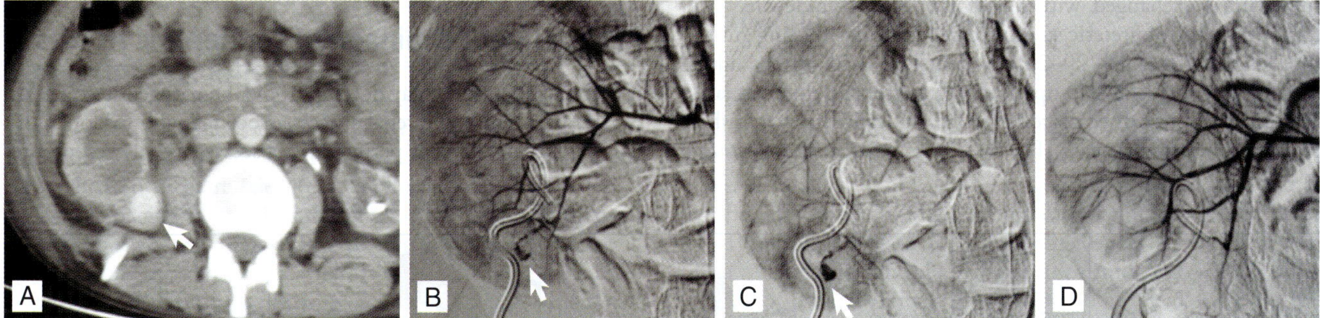

Figure 94.26 Post-percutaneous nephrostomy (PCN) arterial injury. Contrast-enhanced computed tomography (A) shows contrast extravasation *(arrow)* in the right perinephric space in a 22-year-old man after PCN. Right renal angiogram (B and C) shows active leak of contrast *(arrows)* from the lobar branch of the lower pole. Note that there is significant reduction in the caliber of the renal branches suggestive of hypovolemic shock. The culprit branch was embolized using polyvinyl alcohol (D).

Percutaneous Nephrostomy in Pregnant Patients

The interventional radiologist may sometimes be asked to do PCN in a pregnant patient. The procedure should be done with the patient in the lateral or supine oblique position. The use of fluoroscopy should be minimal. Overdistension of calyces and excessive manipulation of the guidewire should be avoided.

Antegrade Ureteral Stenting

Antegrade ureteral stenting can be performed when retrograde ureteral stenting fails [136]. *There are a few advantages of ureteral stenting over PCN such as no external collection bag, no issue of pericatheter leaks or skin irritation, and better patient compliance.* Disadvantages of stenting are stent block and bladder wall irritation. The common indications for antegrade stenting are ureteral leaks, relief of obstruction, and placement after surgery or balloon dilation of ureteric stricture (Table 94.13).

Technique

For antegrade ureteral stenting, the upper or interpolar calyx is punctured for gaining access to the pelvicalyceal system (PCS). The level of obstruction is determined using a nephrostogram.

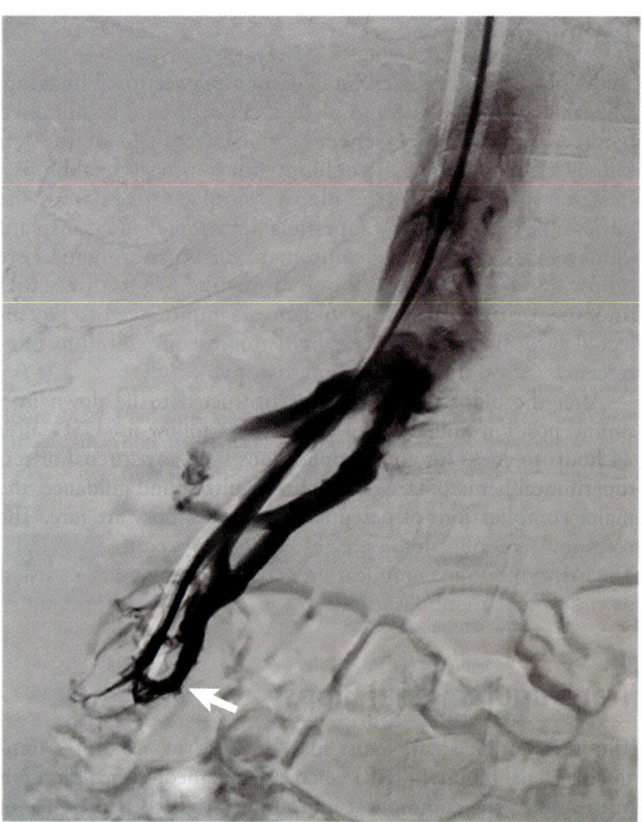

Figure 94.30 Wedge renal venogram *(arrow)*. (Courtesy of Dr. Ujjwal Gorsi, PGIMER, Chd.)

additional safety to avoid a capsular breach. After performing the biopsy, a venogram should be taken from the stiffening cannula to look for any capsular breach.

The complications of TJRB are capsular breach, perirenal hematoma, hematuria, pain, and local hematoma at puncture site and other complications of jugular venous access [145].

Renal Aneurysm and Pseudoaneurysm

The true renal artery aneurysm is rare with an incidence of 0.1% among the general population [146]. The causative factors such as atherosclerosis or fibromuscular dysplasia typically lead to extraparenchymal renal aneurysms, and vasculitis caused by polyarteritis nodosa or infections causes intraparenchymal aneurysms [147]. *The indications for interventions in true renal aneurysms are size more than 2 cm, aneurysms in women of childbearing age, or when associated with symptoms (e.g., renovascular hypertension, hematuria, or rupture) [148].*

Renal pseudoaneurysm usually results because of abdominal trauma or iatrogenic injury. Irrespective of their cause or size, all renal pseudoaneurysms may rupture and must be treated. Computed tomography (CT) angiography is very helpful in the accurate diagnosis of renal pseudoaneurysm and helps in planning the endovascular procedure.

Technique

The endovascular management of true aneurysms is often challenging; however, it is associated with fewer morbidities compared with surgical repair or reconstruction. Emphasis should be given to preserving most of the renal parenchyma with minimal functional renal tissue damage.

The renal arteries usually arise from the aorta at the L2 level. Careful assessment of the initial aortogram is necessary to look for any accessory or aberrant renal artery. A 5-Fr Cobra catheter or a renal double-curve catheter can be used for selective cannulation of the renal artery. A reverse-curve catheter (Simmons) is useful in difficult cases.

- For a true aneurysm, the initial catheter should be exchanged with a long sheath or guiding catheter. Narrow-neck aneurysms can be treated with endovascular detachable coils or endoluminal stent to exclude the neck of the aneurysm in the same way as in the treatment of intracranial aneurysms [149]. A liquid embolizing agent such as Onyx can also be used alone or with concurrent use of an intraluminal balloon to avoid reflux of the liquid agent. Small aneurysms (<2 cm in size) should be followed up annually on imaging.
- The main renal artery pseudoaneurysms are usually treated with a covered stent placed across the neck of the sac. For intrarenal pseudoaneurysms, a coaxial microcatheter is used with mechanical occlusion of the branch supplying the pseudoaneurysm (Fig. 94.31). Because intrarenal arteries are end arteries, only proximal occlusion of the vessel is sufficient for the treatment of intrarenal pseudoaneurysms. Coil embolization is preferred

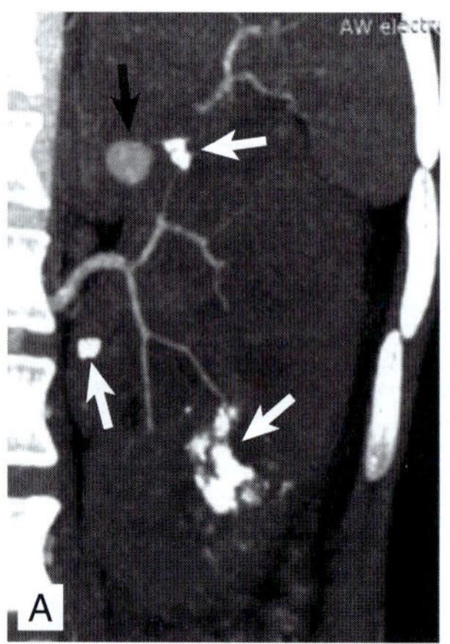

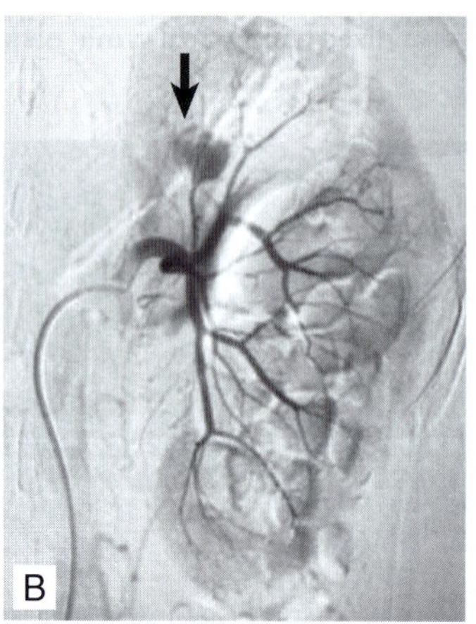

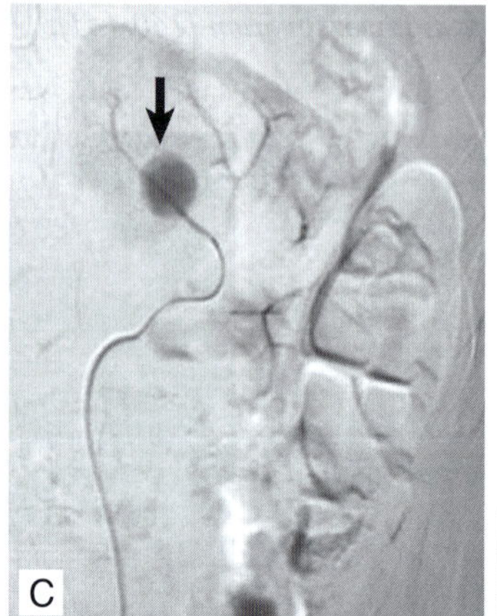

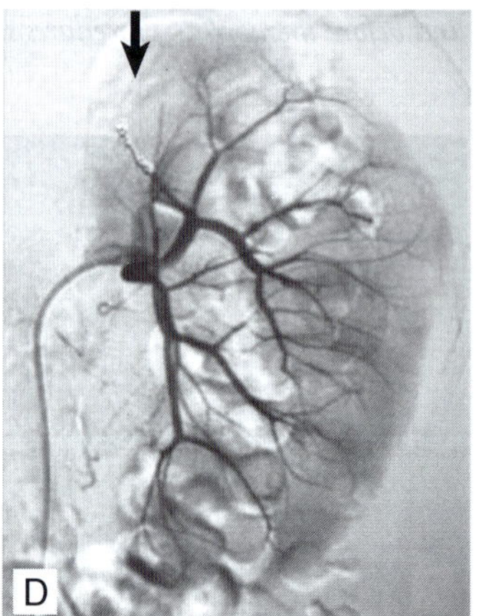

Figure 94.31 Iatrogenic renal pseudoaneurysm (*black arrow*) on computed tomography angiography (A). Note is made of multiple hyperdense calculi (*white arrows* in A). Left renal angiogram (B) and superselective angiogram (C) show a pseudoaneurysm (*black arrow*) arising from the lobar branch at upper pole. (D) Microcoils (*black arrow*) were used to embolize the branch supplying the pseudoaneurysm.

among many available embolizing agents. Liquid embolizing agents such as N-butyl cyanoacrylate (glue) or particulate agents such as polyvinyl alcohol (PVA) may be used for embolization; however, these are more likely to cause nontargeted embolization.

Care must be taken to avoid the reflux of embolizing agents into the aorta, which may cause nontargeted embolization of the spinal artery, leading to paraparesis. The complications of endovascular treatment of renal aneurysms are rare and include nontargeted embolization, incomplete embolization, and rarely postembolization syndrome.

Ultrasound-guided percutaneous embolization can be done using thrombin injection or cyanoacrylate glue with a 22-gauge needle if the sac is peripheral in location and well visualized on USG [150].

Renal Arterio-Venous Shunts

Renal arterio-venous shunts (RAVSs) can be traumatic or congenital. The latter is very uncommon with a prevalence of 0.04% among the general population [151]. Congenital RAVS may have multiple arterial feeders with single or multiple draining veins. At times, it may have a complex network of arterial and venous shunts. Traumatic RAVSs are commonly caused by iatrogenic injury and primarily consist of a single communication between an artery and vein (commonly called a traumatic arteriovenous fistula) with or without a pseudoaneurysm. Color Doppler USG or cross-sectional imaging (CT or magnetic resonance angiography) helps assess the RAVS. The treatment of choice for most RAVSs is endovascular embolization. Surgery may be considered if endovascular management has failed.

Various embolizing agent may be used depending on the number, location, or types of RAVS and include coils, Amplatzer vascular plugs, PVA, absolute alcohol, N-butyl cyanoacrylate, and Onyx. Coil embolization is the preferred mode of treatment in most cases (Fig. 94.32). A combination of embolizing agents may be used in a specific case [152].

Renal Tumor Embolization

The role of endovascular embolization of benign renal tumors is to control hemorrhage, especially in cases of angiomyolipoma (AML). Most AMLs are benign and can be followed up on imaging. The common indications of endovascular treatment of AML include tumor size more than 4 cm in tuberous sclerosis cases or more than 5 cm in sporadic cases, intratumoral aneurysm greater than 5 mm, or symptomatic AML (abdominal pain, ruptured AML, or presence of hematuria) [153,154].

The role of endovascular embolization of renal cell carcinoma (RCC) is not well understood. Embolization can be done before surgery or as palliative treatment for patients with inoperable RCC. The proposed benefits of RCC embolization are reduction in vascularity, ease of surgical resection, reduction in the size of the tumor, and stimulation of immune response. However, there is considerable debate among various authors for preoperative embolization of RCC [155–157].

Technique

The use of particulate embolizing agents is preferred for renal tumors. PVA particles or Embospheres of size 100 to 300 μm should be used for tumor embolization. Additionally, N-butyl cyanoacrylate or coil embolization can be used, especially when there are intratumoral aneurysms. Absolute alcohol with concurrent use of an occluding balloon to avoid reflux can also be used. Chemoembolization with doxorubicin has also been used for patients with RCC.

A coaxial microcatheter should be used for embolization and should be placed as close as possible to the feeding arteries for superselective embolization and to avoid nontargeted embolization. The endpoint of embolization is indicated by the nonvisualization of feeders, stagnation of flow, or reflux of contrast on postembolization angiography (Fig. 94.33).

Postembolization syndrome consisting of pain, fever, and nausea may be seen after the procedure, which usually needs conservative management.

Renal Tumor Ablation

Image-guided ablation of renal tumors has emerged as an alternative to nephron-sparing surgery in select cases of renal cell carcinoma of size 4 cm or smaller (T1a disease), especially when surgical treatment is not possible [158–160]. The indications for ablation are given in Table 94.15 [161]. Many studies have shown the effectiveness of radiofrequency ablation (RFA) and cryoablation in renal tumors. Microwave ablation (MWA) has also shown comparative results in recent data [162]. Recently, the introduction of irreversible electroporation, a nonthermal ablation, has allowed treating the centrally located tumors without damage to the renal collecting system [163]. However, there is no strong

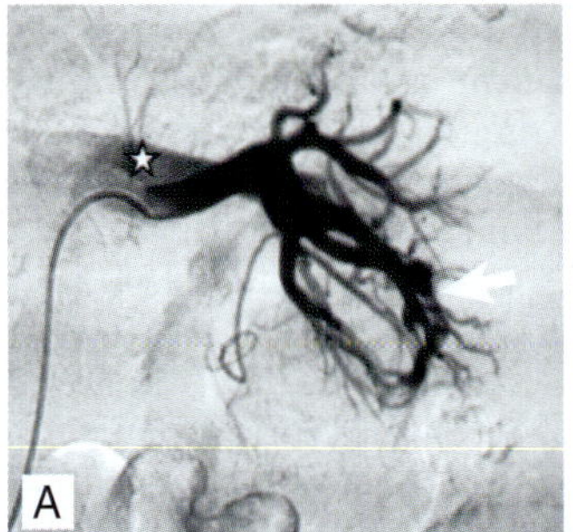

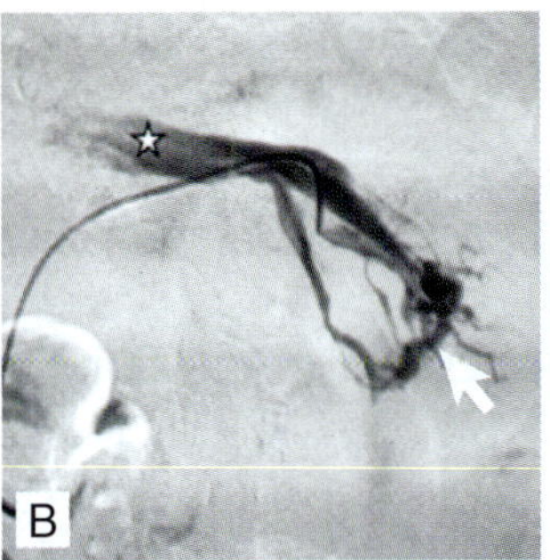

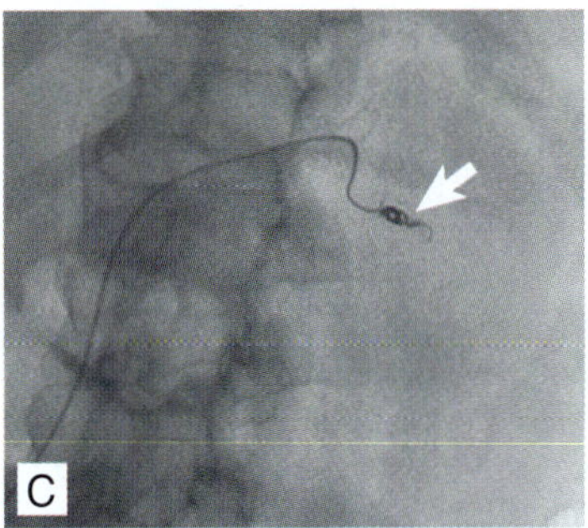

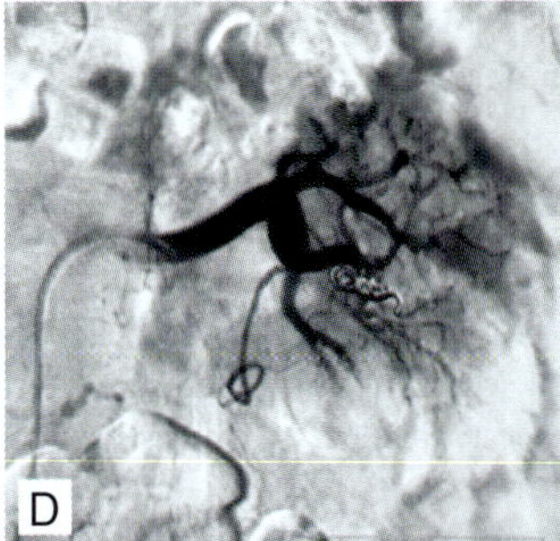

Figure 94.32 Iatrogenic arteriovenous shunt. Left main renal angiogram (A) and superselective angiogram of the segmental branch (B) show arteriovenous shunt *(arrow)* with opacification of the renal vein *(asterisk)*. (C) The segmental branch was embolized using microcoils *(arrow)*. (D) After embolization, there is complete nonopacification of the shunt.

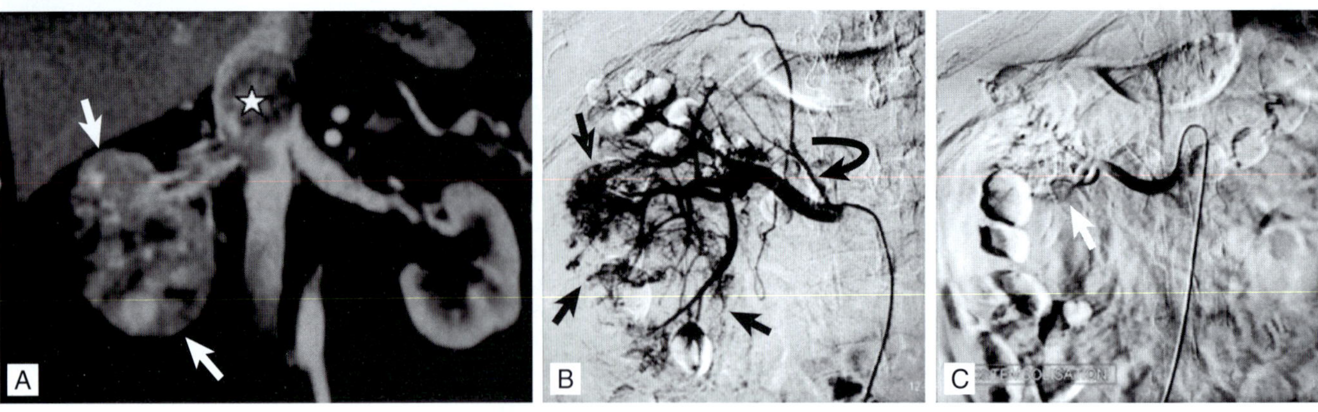

Figure 94.33 Renal cell carcinoma embolization. (A) A contrast computed tomography image shows arterial enhancing heterogenous lesion *(arrows)* of right kidney with extension into right renal vein and IVC *(asterisk)*. (B) A right renal angiogram shows an arterial enhancing lesion *(arrows)* of the right kidney. Note that the capsular branch *(curved arrow)* is also supplying the tumor. (C) The main right renal artery was embolized using Gelfoam and polyvinyl alcohol particles with complete nonvisualization of the renal vascularity *(arrow)* before right radical nephrectomy. Note that the reverse-curve catheter (Simmons 1) helps to cannulate the capsular branch to achieve complete embolization. (*Source:* Department of Radiodiagnosis, PGIMER, Chandigarh).

TABLE 94.15 Indications for Image-Guided Ablation of Renal Tumors

- Unfit for surgery
- Renal insufficiency
- Solitary kidney
- Multiple or bilateral tumors
- Von Hippel–Lindau syndrome
- Transplant kidney
- Palliative in cases of advanced renal cell carcinoma

TABLE 94.16 Ablation Techniques

Chemical	Ethanol or Acetic Acid Injections
Thermal	Radiofrequency ablation Microwave ablation Cryoablation Laser ablation High-intensity focused ultrasound
Nonchemical, nonthermal ablation	Irreversible electroporation

evidence to support the use of one modality over the other. Chemical ablations of renal tumors, though less often done, can be performed using ethanol or acetic acid. The various ablation techniques are listed in Table 94.16.

Technique

The preprocedure blood investigations include coagulation profile, platelet count, complete blood count, renal function test, electrocardiography. Most of the percutaneous ablations are performed under conscious sedation using IV fentanyl and midazolam. Irreversible electroporation (IRE) requires general anaesthesia with proper muscle relaxation.

The total targeted ablation area should include at least a 0.5- to 1-cm "ablative margin" of the normal tissue. USG, CT, magnetic resonance imaging (MRI), and fusion imaging may be used for image guidance as required depending on the visualization of the lesion, ablation procedure, and user preference. Some of the ablations such as RFA, MWA, and cryoablation have been performed by the laparoscopic route. Renal biopsy may be performed just before the ablation. Several renal nephrometry scores may predict outcomes or complications of different ablative modalities.

Radiofrequency Ablation

Radiofrequency ablation is the most commonly used ablation technique for renal tumors (Fig. 94.34). In RFA, the electric energy is converted into heat energy which gets deposited in the surrounding tissue (the Joule effect). Instant coagulative necrosis occurs at 60° to 100°C temperature, which leads to irreversible cell damage [164].

A unipolar radiofrequency (RF) system consists of a generator, electrodes, and grounding pads, and a bipolar system has two interstitial electrodes between which the current oscillates. The diameter of the needle is typically 14 to 18 gauge. The RF system is either a temperature-based or an impedance-based system. The cooled tip RFA electrode has an irrigation system through which ice-cooled saline flows to decrease the temperature at the tip of the electrode, thereby preventing tissue charring [165].

The ablation time for RFA is 7 to 16 minutes for tissue necrosis, which depends on which type of RF system and electrodes are used. *Needle-tract ablation needs to be done during needle removal to avoid tract seeding.*

The advantages of RFA are that it is a minimally invasive procedure, can be done on an outpatient or day-care basis, and has lesser complications compared to surgical resection. Tissue boiling or charring and the heat sink effect (dissipation of heat by flowing blood in an adjacent vessel) may limit the effect of RFA.

Microwave Ablation

Microwave ablation is a thermal-based ablation technique that uses electromagnetic energy to induce tumor cell necrosis using frequencies ranges between 900 and 2450 MHz [166]. The MWA system consists of a microwave generator and a monopolar electrode connected to the generator that is introduced into the lesion through an access needle. No grounding pads are

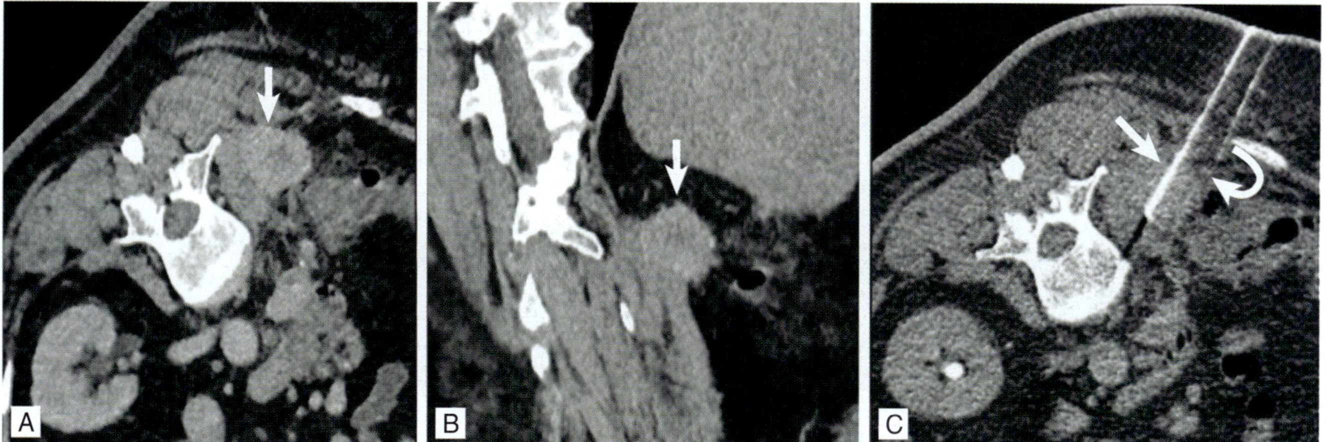

Figure 94.34 Radiofrequency ablation (RFA) in recurrent renal cell carcinoma. A 56-year-old man with an enhancing lesion (*arrow* in A and B) in the renal bed after radical nephrectomy. RFA of the lesion was done under computed tomography guidance (*arrow* in C). Note that the bowel loop has been displaced with 5% dextrose *(curved arrow)*.

required in MWA. The irrigation of fluid or carbon dioxide within the needle is used to prevent skin burn at the site of needle insertion [167].

Microwave ablation has few theoretical benefits over RFA. In MWA, there is a larger zone of active heating, less heat sink effect, and less charring compared with RFA. There is no risk of grounding pad burns in MWA because grounding pads are not used.

Cryoablation

Cryoablation is a thermal-based ablation technique that causes tumor destruction by rapid cell freezing. The inert gases in liquid form (nitrogen or argon) flows through the cryoprobe. The expansion of the gas occurs at the probe tip (the Joule-Thomson effect), which causes the ice-ball formation. The helium is used for active thawing. As helium expands at the probe tip, heat is generated, which causes thawing [168].

The duration of treatment is generally a 10-minute freeze followed by an 8-minute thaw cycle depending on the tumor size. Commonly, two freeze–thaw cycles are used. Temperature monitoring is done by a thermocouple device. The ice ball is visualized directly using USG, CT, or MRI (Fig. 94.35).

Cryoablation has a few advantages over RFA or MWA, including decreased procedure-related pain and better real-time visualization of the ablation zone.

Laser Ablation

Laser ablation or laser photocoagulation is a thermal-based ablation technique that causes coagulation necrosis by heat production. The laser source used in most of the systems is Nd:YAG (neodymium-doped yttrium aluminum garnet), erbium, or holmium, which give accurate wavelength of energy.

High-Intensity Focused Ultrasonography

High-intensity focused ultrasonography (HIFU) is the thermal-based ablation technique in which ultrasonic waves localize at a specific point, which leads to heat deposition in the targeted zone. The important benefit of HIFU is that there is no contact between the applicator and the lesion. MR-guided HIFU also gives real-time monitoring of the ablation. However, because of time constraints, coverage issues, and respiration–movement interference, HIFU is being restricted to treat benign conditions in stationary organs such as the bone, breast, uterus, and prostate.

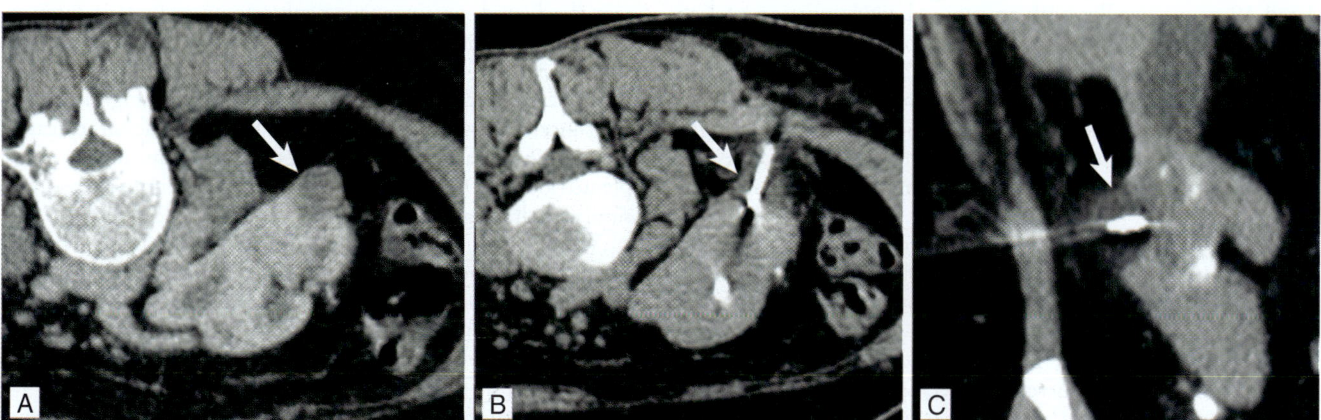

Figure 94.35 Cryoablation of renal cell carcinoma. (A) A 56-year-old woman with an enhancing lesion in the right kidney *(arrow)*. (B) The cryoprobe has been placed within the lesion under computed tomography guidance *(arrow)*. (C) Ice-ball formation *(arrow)* can be seen as the hypoattenuating area around the needle tip.

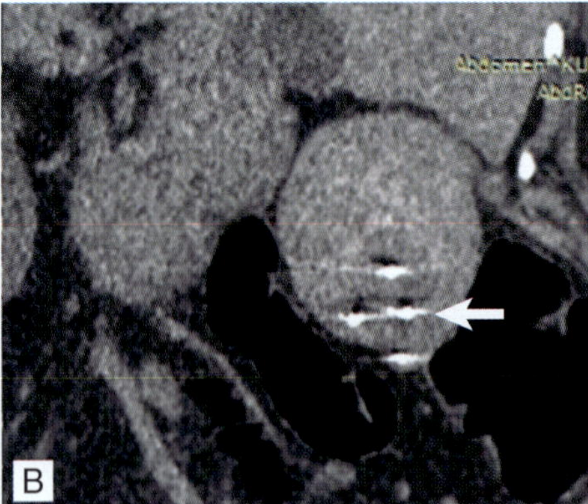

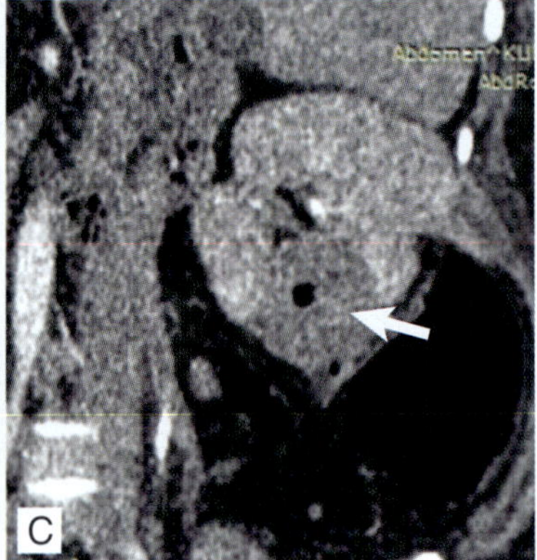

Figure 94.36 Irreversible electroporation (IRE) in solitary functioning kidney in a 44-year-old woman. (A) An enhancing lesion is seen in the right kidney *(arrow)*. Note the nonfunctioning kidney on the left side *(asterisk)*. (B) Placement of four IRE probes, which are parallel to each other *(arrow)*. (C) Air foci *(arrow)* are seen after completion of ablation.

Chemical Ablation

Chemical ablation is the injection of a chemical agent (ethanol or acetic acid) within the tumor under image-guidance. It causes protein denaturation and thrombosis of small vessels. It is performed by inserting a small needle (18–20 gauge) into the tumor. The limitation of chemical ablations includes a lack of control over the injection, a higher rate of recurrence of tumor, and pain during the procedure. Transient hemoglobinuria and direct renal toxicity may occur with acetic acid ablation.

Nonchemical Nonthermal Ablation: Irreversible Electroporation

Percutaneous IRE is a nonchemical, nonthermal ablation method and is a recent advancement in the spectrum of minimally invasive ablation technique. In IRE, high-voltage several-millisecond-long pulses of electric current, up to 3000 V/cm, are applied to the tumor cells, which leads to "irreversible pore formation" within the cell membrane, thereby causing leakage of the intracellular contents and cell death caused by apoptosis [169]. There is no heat sink effect seen with IRE. The renal collecting system, collagenous tissues, and nerves are relatively spared in IRE. Therefore, IRE is useful for lesions close to the renal collecting system.

Irreversible electroporation (NanoKnife) consists of insulated 19-gauge needles with an exposed active portion of 1 to 4 cm. The parallel placement of multiple needles is necessary with an intervening distance of 1.5 to 2 cm to achieve a sufficient electrical field. The procedure needs to be conducted under general anaesthesia with good muscle relaxation as high-voltage pulses are applied to the tumor. CT guidance is preferred for needle placement and assessment of complete ablation (Fig. 94.36).

The major advantage of IRE over thermal ablation techniques is that the tumors adjacent to the renal collecting system or major blood vessels can be treated with IRE because there is no heat production.

The limitations of IRE include the need for general anaesthesia, the long learning curve, the specific contraindications for IRE (pacemaker, cardiac arrhythmias), and the relatively high cost compared with other ablation techniques. Several small study series have already analyzed the safety and feasibility of IRE in the management of patients with solid organ tumors, including those of the liver, kidney, pancreas, and prostate [163,170,171].

Postprocedural Follow-Up After Ablation

For procedures done under conscious sedation, patients are monitored for at least 3 to 4 hours in the recovery or post-operating room and may be discharged on the same day. A few patients may be kept for overnight observation if there is any postprocedure pain or complication. Follow-up imaging (CT, MR, or contrast USG) may be done after 4 to 6 weeks. If the residual or recurrent tumor is suspected at any time on imaging or clinical assessment, reablation or alternative treatment is performed.

Interventions in Transplant Kidneys

A transplant kidney is placed in the right iliac fossa and is superficial in location than native kidneys. The common nonvascular complications after transplantation are perirenal collections, ureteral obstruction, and anastomosis stricture. Biopsy of a transplant kidney is often required to rule out graft dysfunction or rejection. The vascular complications include renal arterial stenosis or thrombosis and renal vein thrombosis. Postbiopsy renal pseudoaneurysm may occur in a transplant kidney.

For access to the collecting system in transplant kidney, typically the upper pole or interpolar calyces are preferred because of their superficial location. After the access to the pelvicalyceal system is achieved, percutaneous nephrostomy or ureteric interventions are performed similar to those in a native kidney (Fig. 94.37). For a percutaneous biopsy, the sample is taken from the upper pole of the transplant kidney. The use of high-frequency transducers helps to avoid bowel injury and inferior epigastric artery injury during percutaneous interventions in the transplanted kidney. Drainage of the perinephric collections is performed similar to drainages of other intraabdominal collections.

Vascular complications can be seen in fewer than 10% of cases of renal transplantation, which include renal artery stenosis, renal arterial or venous thrombosis, pseudoaneurysm, and arteriovenous fistula formation [172].

- Transluminal balloon dilation with or without stent placement is the treatment of choice for renal artery stenosis.
- Mechanical thrombectomy or endovascular thrombolysis may be offered in select cases of graft thrombosis.
- Superselective embolization is the first line of management for pseudoaneurysms and arteriovenous fistulas.

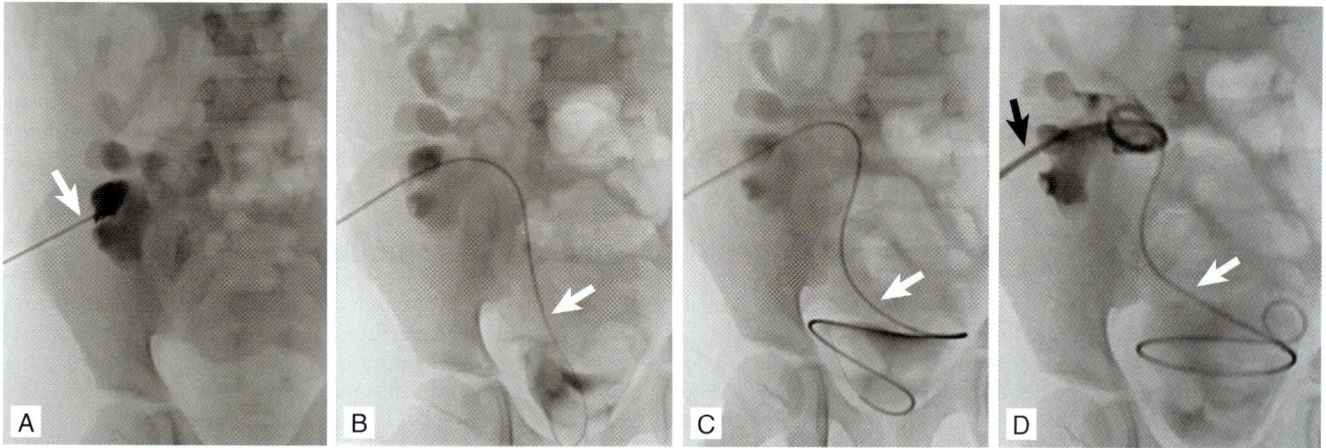

Figure 94.37 Placement of ureteric stent in a transplant kidney. (A) Access of interpolar calyx *(arrow)*. (B) Negotiation of a 5-Fr catheter and guidewire *(arrow)* into the urinary bladder. (C) Placement of a ureteric stent using a pusher. (D) Placement of a nephrostomy tube *(black arrow)* after ureteric stent placement *(white arrow)*. The nephrostomy tube is removed after 24 to 48 hours. (Courtesy Dr Ujjwal Gorsi, PGIMER, Chd.)

94.7 Varicocele

Rohit Khandelwal, Sanjay Baijal

Varicoceles are abnormally dilated veins of the pampiniform plexus, which are typically caused by reflux or less commonly by obstruction. These plexuses primarily drain into the internal spermatic vein (ISV). The right ISV normally drains directly into the inferior vena cava, and the left spermatic vein normally drains into the left renal vein. Varicoceles are more frequent and larger on the left side (Fig. 94.38) [173].

Indications for varicocele treatment are male infertility, testicular hypotrophy in an adolescent, and ipsilateral testicular pain. Varicocele embolization is a safe and durable technique for these patient groups. Percutaneous varicocele embolization is also indicated in postsurgical recurrence of varicocele [174–176].

Varicocele embolization can be done using either right internal jugular or right common femoral venous access. After cannulation of ISV, venography is performed with the patient in a reverse Trendelenburg position or the patient performing the Valsalva maneuver to demonstrate the venous anatomy and retrograde flow in the ISV.

Choice of embolic agent depends on operator preference. Commonly used agents are vascular coils, plugs, sclerosing agents (sodium tetradecyl sulfate), and liquid embolics (N-butyl cyanoacrylate). These embolic agents can also be used in combination [175,177].

At 3 months, follow-up Doppler ultrasonography is performed to see lack of retrograde flow, and at 6 months, semen analysis is done in patients undergoing therapy because of infertility [175].

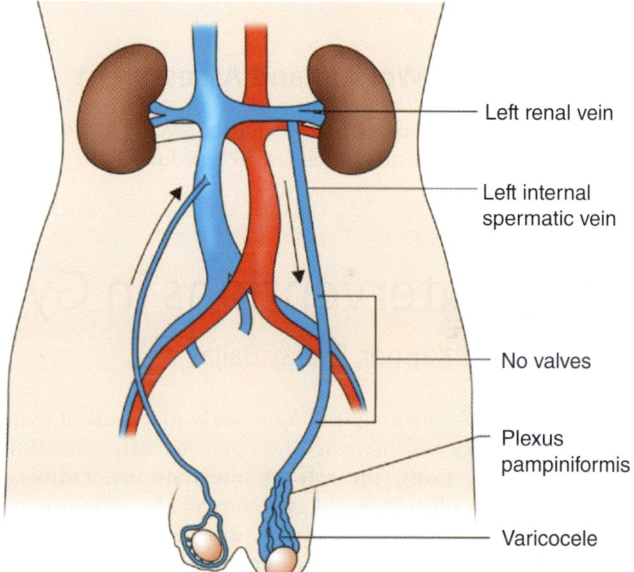

Figure 94.38 Diagram shows reversal of flow in the left internal spermatic vein causing tortuosity in the plexus pampiniformis.

94.8 Prostatic Artery Embolization

Rohit Khandelwal, Sanjay Baijal

Prostatic artery embolization (PAE) is a minimally invasive treatment for lower urinary tract symptoms (LUTS) related to benign prostatic hyperplasia (BPH). PAE leads to alleviation of LUTS by ischemic shrinkage of the prostatic gland. The reduction of α_1-adrenergic receptor density in the embolized prostate also causes relaxation of smooth muscle and potentiates the effect of PAE [178].

Indications

The Society of Interventional Radiology, along with other international societies of interventional radiology, have developed joint positions and recommendations with regard to the use of PAE for LUTS secondary to BPH [179]. These are

- Patients with moderate to severe LUTS and appropriately selected for PAE (having International Prostate Symptom Score [IPSS] >8; quality of life score >3; urine peak flow <15 mL/s; and prostate volume >30–50 mL without upper limit of size)
- Patients with BPH and acute or chronic urinary retention but with preserved bladder function as a method to achieve catheter independence
- Patients with BPH and moderate to severe LUTS who wish to preserve erectile or ejaculatory function
- Patients with hematuria of prostatic origin as a method of achieving cessation of bleeding
- Patients with BPH and moderate to severe LUTS who are not fit to be surgical candidates for any reason, including patients presenting with advanced age, multiple comorbidities, coagulopathy, or inability to stop anticoagulation or antiplatelet therapy

Contraindications

Relative contraindications to PAE are patients with bladder diverticula greater that 2 cm in size, bladder stone, detrusor hyperactivity or hypocontractility, and neurogenic bladder. In case of prostate-specific antigen greater than 4 ng/dL, prostate biopsy should be considered to exclude prostatic carcinoma [180].

Preprocedural Workup and Assessment

The IPSS and urodynamic testing provide the severity of symptoms of BPH. After the treatment, about 30% reduction in IPSS is considered as clinically acceptable for the treatment to be considered effective [181]. Baseline ultrasonography is required to access prostate size and postvoid residual volume. Pre procedure computed tomography angiography is helpful to identify prostatic artery anatomy, arterial course, and tortuosity to access technical complexity and provide a roadmap for the procedure [182].

Procedure Technique

Prostatic artery embolization can be done using either transfemoral or transradial vascular access and performed in local anesthesia. Angiography helps identify the origin of prostatic arteries, anatomic variants, and collateral supply. After the superselective microcatheter cannulation of prostatic arteries is done, embolization is achieved using microspheres (300–500 μm) or polyvinyl alcohol particles (100–300 μm). Embolization of bilateral prostatic arteries is performed; unilateral embolization is done only in the case of a failure to catheterize the other side [180].

Complications

- Perineal pain, dysuria, increased frequency, and other irritative symptoms are part of postembolization syndrome and are frequently seen in the first 3 to 5 days. These symptoms require only symptomatic management [180].
- Minor complications are acute urinary retention requiring catheterization and urinary tract infection requiring antibiotic.
- Major complications are rare and include urinary bladder wall ischemia and glans ischemia [179].

94.9 Interventions in Gynecology

Abhay Kumar Kapoor, Sanjay Baijal

With advances in imaging leading to early diagnosis of gynecologic disorders and increased number of cesarean section-related complications, the role of interventional radiology has increased in obstetrics and gynecology. The various gynecologic interventional procedures can be categorized as follows.

Vascular Procedures

1. **Uterine artery embolization (UAE):** indicated for uterine fibroids, adenomyosis, arteriovenous malformations, and postpartum hemorrhage (PPH)
2. **Venous procedure:** pelvic congestion syndrome (PCS)

Nonvascular Procedures

1. **Biopsy:** percutaneous, transvaginal, or transrectal approach
2. **Drainage:** percutaneous, transvaginal, or transrectal approach for ovarian cyst aspiration and lymphocele obliteration
3. **Fallopian tube recanalization** (FTR)

Obstetric interventions are covered in detail in Chapter 50.

Uterine Artery Embolization

Uterine artery embolization has been in vogue since the 1970s for management of PPH and after gynecologic surgeries [183,184]. It was introduced in 1997 in the United States as a treatment option for patients with fibroids [185]. The safety and efficacy of the procedure have been extensively studied based on long- and short-term outcomes, and UAE is now accepted as a treatment option for patients with fibroids by the American Congress of Obstetricians and Gynecologists [186].

A multicentric study including more than 500 patients treated with UAE reported favorable 3-month outcomes for dominant leiomyoma volume reduction (42%) along with a significant decrease in symptoms such as dysmenorrhea, duration of menses, and urinary frequency [187]. The Uterine Artery Embolization in the Treatment of Symptomatic Uterine Fibroid Tumors (EMMY) randomized trial to compare UAE with total abdominal hysterectomy concluded that patients undergoing UAE had significantly less pain during the first 24 hours postoperatively and returned to work sooner (28.1 vs 63.4 days) than patients who underwent hysterectomy [188]. No statistical difference was found in the rate of major complications in the two wings, though minor complications such as vaginal discharge, leiomyoma expulsion, and hematoma were higher in the UAE group (58% vs 40%) [188].

Magnetic resonance imaging (MRI) can demonstrate the vascularity of fibroids to allow determination of whether embolization will have a good response or not [189]. It also helps in mapping out the total disease burden with regards to number, size, and location of fibroids, which is useful in follow up to objectively look at the response to the procedure.

Indications

- Menorrhagia
- Dysmenorrhea
- Pain
- Pressure
- Urinary symptoms such as urinary frequency and retention related to hydronephrosis
- Infertility

Anatomic Considerations

All fibroid locations (submucosal, intramural, and subserosal) are eligible for embolization, though patients with large uterine fibroids are likely to have less fibroid shrinkage [190] and tend to have less symptom improvement [191]. Patients with intracavitary fibroids have higher chances of expulsion. There is a potential risk of detachment of pedunculated subserosal (PS) fibroids, making them a relative contraindication for UAE per some studies [192]. However, other studies have shown no additional complications in treating patients with PS fibroids with UAE [193,194].

Contraindications

The contraindications of UAE can be absolute or relative as listed in Table 94.17 [195]. The first 10 days after the menstrual cycle are ideal for the procedure. If imaging raises suspicion of malignancy, tissue sampling should be done to exclude this possibility. Any adnexal infection should be treated before UAE. CO_2 angiography should be considered if contrast allergy or renal failure is a concern and cannot be optimized with premedication. Coagulopathy in the form of low platelet count or increased international normalized ratio can be corrected with requisite replacement.

Procedure

Commonly, right common femoral artery access is taken, and embolization is done for bilateral uterine arteries (Figs. 94.39 and 94.40).

TABLE 94.17 Contraindications to Uterine Artery Embolization

Absolute Contraindications
■ Ongoing pregnancy
■ Gynecologic malignancy
■ Pelvic infection
Relative Contraindications
■ Renal failure
■ Contrast allergy
■ Coagulopathy

Adapted from JC Bulman, SM Ascher, JB Spies, Current concepts in uterine fibroid embolization, Radiographics 32 (2012) 1735-1750.

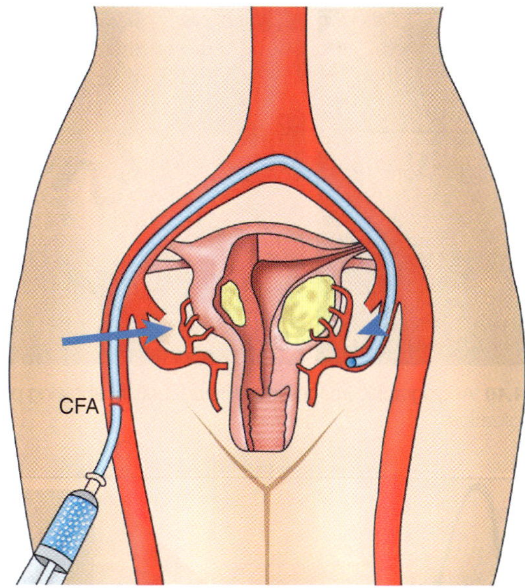

Figure 94.39 Right CFA access. Right uterine artery (*solid arrow*). Left uterine artery (*arrowhead*).

A 5-Fr Roberts uterine catheter (RUC; Cook) (Fig. 94.41) is specially designed for UAE [196]. If this is not available, a cobra-shaped catheter (Fig. 94.41B) can be used. A microcatheter system may or may not be used depending on the anatomy. Embolization is achieved with either polyvinyl alcohol particles (Contour, Boston Scientific or Ivalon, Cook) or trisacryl gelatin microspheres (Embosphere, Merit Medical Systems).

Most of the patients experience moderate pain after the procedure. A hypogastric nerve block (Fig. 94.42) can be given before starting embolization to take care of the pain. Patients can also be given intravenous sedation.

Complications

Apart from puncture site complications, venous thromboembolism is a potential risk because patients undergoing UAE have temporary elevation of procoagulant factors [197]. Ovarian failure is another infrequent potential complication. This was seen in 7.5% of patients in the Fibroid Registry for Outcomes Data (FIBROID) registry [198]. With limited evidence in the literature, it is inferred that UAE should not be the first-line treatment for women who are infertile because of fibroids. But it can be used in patients who have comorbidities and are poor surgical candidates [195,199,200].

Role of Uterine Artery Embolization in Adenomyosis

With extrapolation of the benefits achieved in fibroid management, UAE has also been explored as a treatment option for patients with adenomyosis with favorable results seen in multiple case series [201].

Role of Uterine Artery Embolization in PPH

Uterine artery embolization has a well-established role in treating patients with PPH [202]. Patients with placenta previa and

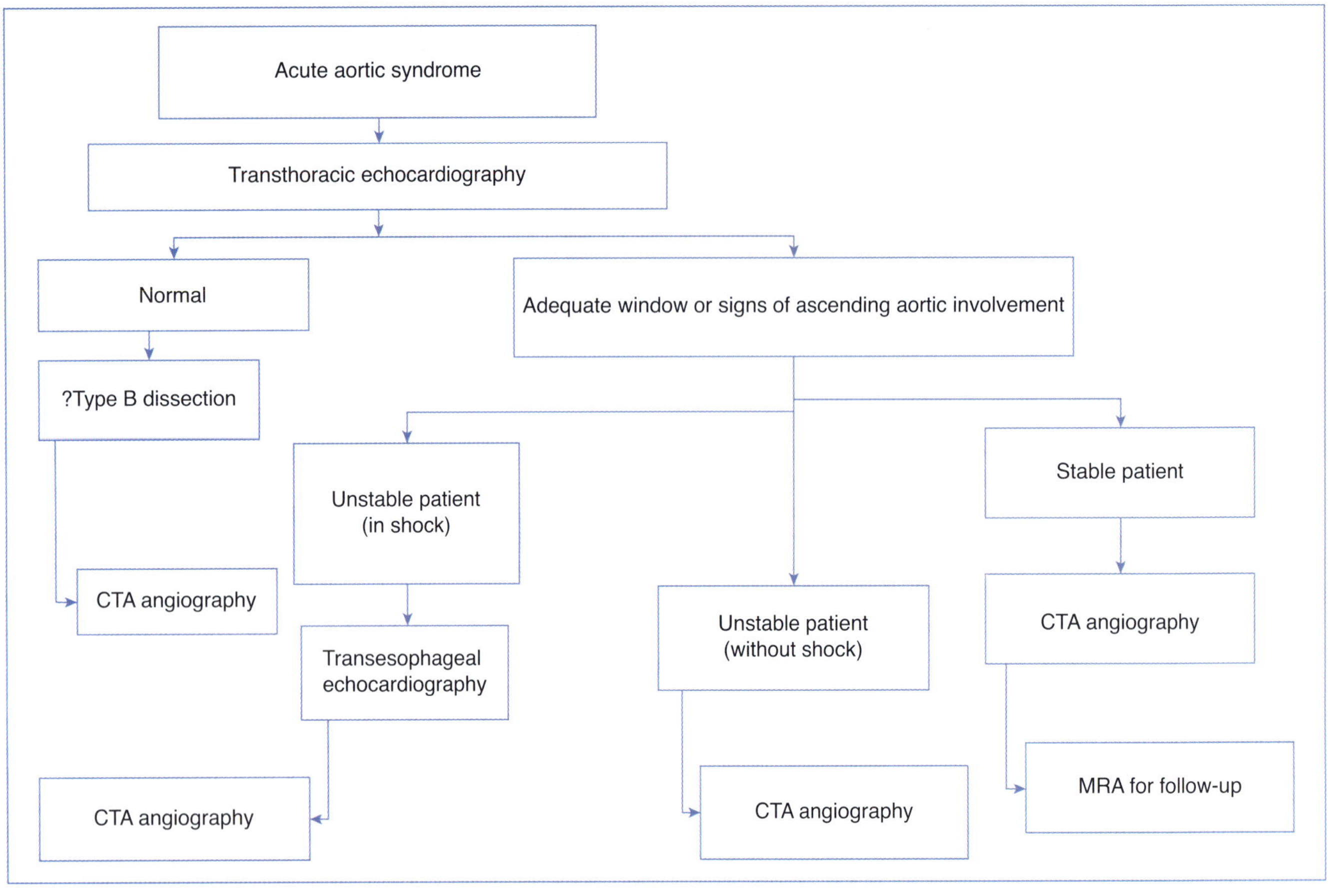

Acute aortic syndrome

Transthoracic echocardiography

Normal

Adequate window or signs of ascending aortic involvement

?Type B dissection

CTA angiography

Unstable patient (in shock)

Transesophageal echocardiography

CTA angiography

Unstable patient (without shock)

CTA angiography

Stable patient

CTA angiography

MRA for follow-up

Figure 95.4 Imaging approach to acute aortic pathologies. *CTA,* computed tomography angiography; *MRA,* magnetic resonance angiography.

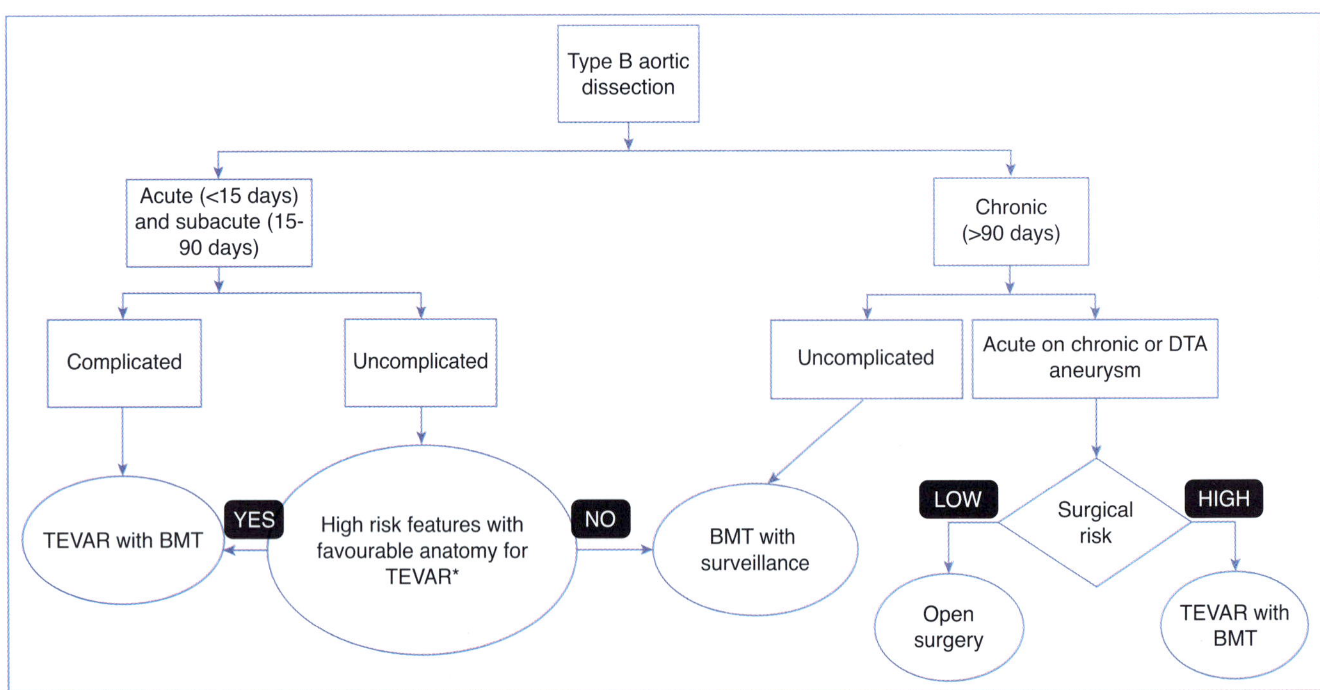

Figure 95.5 An algorithmic approach to management of type B aortic dissection based on the duration of symptoms. *Asterisk* indicates that the high-risk features include total aortic diameter greater than 44 mm, false lumen diameter greater than 22 mm, and false lumen–to–total aortic lumen area greater than 0.7. *BMT,* Best medical therapy; *DTA,* descending thoracic aorta; *TEVAR,* thoracic endovascular aortic repair.

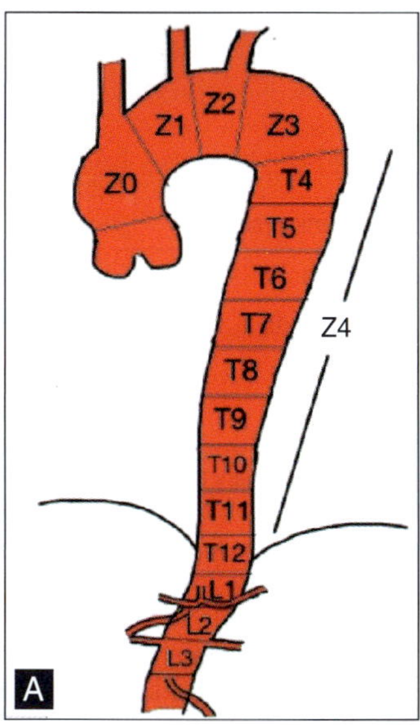

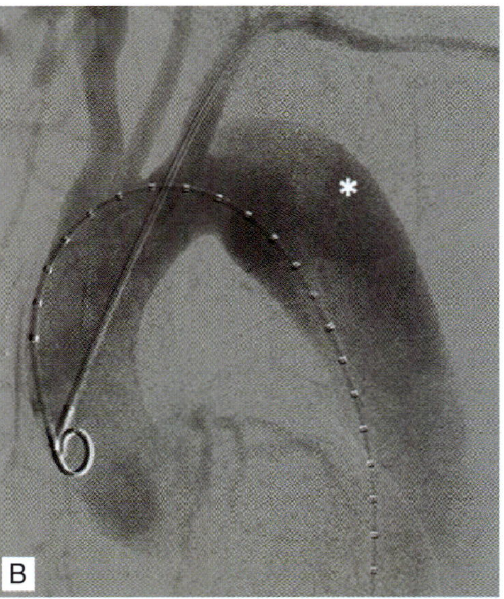

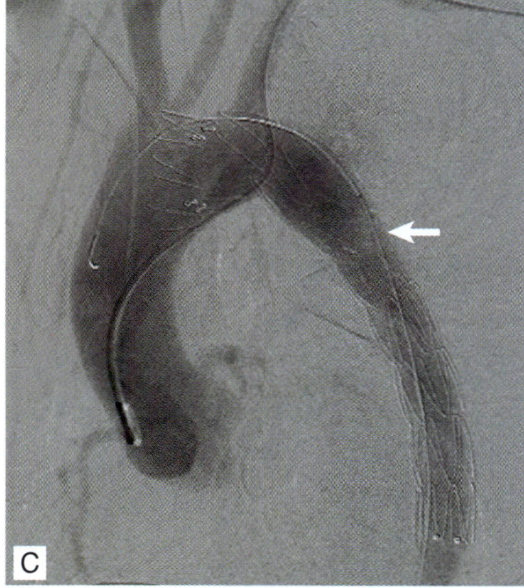

Figure 95.6 (A) Landing zones of the aorta. (B) Thoracic endovascular aortic repair. Baseline angiogram (A) shows a marker pigtail in situ in a patient with complicated type B dissection. *Asterisk* shows the false lumen. (B) Exclusion of the false lumen after stent-graft (*arrow*) placement.

Technique of Thoracic Endovascular Aortic Repair: The aorta can be divided into landing zones ranging from zone 0 in the ascending aorta, zones 1 to 3 in the arch, zones 4 to 12 in the descending thoracic aorta and zones L1 to L4 in the abdominal aorta (see Fig. 95.6A). Endovascular stent grafts can be placed in aortic segments free from any major branches without compromising their patency. When there are major branches arising from an aortic segment where stent graft is intended to be placed, additional techniques may be required to preserve these branches.

The proximal and distal landing zones of the stent are defined as the segment where the proximal and distal ends of the stent graft will land, respectively. *Ideally, the landing zones should be normal segments free from any significant calcification or thrombus and devoid of any major branches.* In case of inadequate landing zone, proximal or distal landing zones can be extended by surgical or endovascular techniques. The surgical techniques include debranching or bypass, and the endovascular techniques include the chimney or snorkel procedure for placing branched and fenestrated devices. The prerequisites for TEVAR are described in Table 95.2.

A stent graft is composed of a woven polyester or expanded polytetrafluoroethylene covering over nitinol or Elgiloy stent frame, which conforms to the wall of the aorta. These devices are usually of large caliber and hence are inserted by a femoral arteriotomy technique. Percutaneous placement is also possible. The goal of treatment of patients with aortic dissection is to seal the primary entry tear. After securing appropriate access, the true lumen is cannulated by a suitable catheter–wire combination. A control aortogram is acquired to adequately profile the arch vessels and the primary entry tear before proceeding with stent-graft deployment (Fig. 95.6B) [7].

TABLE 95.2 Prerequisites for Thoracic Endovascular Repair for Type B Aortic Dissection

Zones	Description
Proximal landing zone of the stent graft	At least 15 mm of normal aorta distal to the LSCA or the left common carotid artery (if the LSCA is being covered). If the landing zones are inadequate, endovascular (use of branched stent graft, chimney, or snorkel technique) or surgical debranching techniques can be used to extend the landing zones. Newer generation devices may be placed even in smaller landing zones.
Distal landing zone	At least 15 mm of normal aorta above the celiac artery
Severe angulation of the proximal or distal aorta	Longer landing zones may be needed, which may necessitate debranching or other hybrid procedure
Access vessels	The minimal common femoral artery diameter required is 7 mm.

LCSA, Left subclavian artery.

Intramural Hematoma

Intramural hematoma is defined as a hemorrhage within the medial layer of the aorta caused by rupture of the vasa vasorum. It constitutes 10% to 20% of acute aortic syndromes. Hypertension is a major risk factor. IMH is classified in a similar way to dissection: type A involving the ascending aorta and type B excluding the ascending aorta. *Imaging findings on CTA include focal crescentic aortic wall thickening in the absence of dissection flap.* The predictors for progression include thickness greater than 10 mm, aneurysm formation, and presence of complications similar to dissection described earlier. The management strategy is similar to dissection—surgery for type A and TEVAR for complicated type B or uncomplicated type B with imaging features predicting progression [4,8].

Penetrating Aortic Ulcer

Penetrating aortic ulcer (PAU) consists of ulceration of atherosclerotic plaque, which disrupts the intima with subsequent extension of the blood into the media. PAU can coexist with IMH or may progress to dissection. *The mid descending aorta is most commonly involved.* CTA is the imaging modality of choice. *Focal ulceration penetrating through the aortic intima into the media is the characteristic finding.* As with dissection and IMH, type A PAU involving the ascending aorta is managed with surgery, and complicated type B PAU is managed with TEVAR. However, ulceration that is 20 mm or greater in diameter or 10 mm in depth should be managed aggressively with TEVAR even if it is not complicated [4,9].

Aortic Aneurysms

Aortic aneurysms are defined as dilatation of an artery more than 50% of the expected normal diameter of the artery. Aneurysms are of two types, true aneurysms and pseudoaneurysms. True aneurysms have all the layers of the arterial wall, whereas there are disruption of the arterial wall in the pseudoaneurysms and extravasation of blood contained by periarterial connective tissue. The locations of aortic aneurysms are

- Thoracic (25.9%)
- Abdominal (62.7%)
- Thoracoabdominal (8.3%) aorta
- Unspecified (3.0%)

Atherosclerosis, infection, trauma, syphilitic aortitis, cystic medial necrosis, and nonspecific aortitis are the most common causes [4].

Surgery is the preferred treatment modality for patients with ascending and thoracoabdominal aneurysm, whereas those with descending thoracic aorta aneurysms are preferably treated via an endovascular approach. The preferred treatment for patients with infrarenal abdominal aneurysm depends on the age. In young patients, a surgical approach is preferred endovascular treatment is preferred in older adults.

The goal of endovascular treatment is deployment of stent graft from normal to normal aorta excluding the aneurysmal sac (Fig. 95.7).

Intervention is indicated in all symptomatic patients irrespective of the size of the aneurysm. In asymptomatic patients, aortic aneurysms are treated if the size is larger than 5 cm in men and larger than 5.5 cm in women (depending on the site of aneurysm and gender) and enlargement in transverse diameter of greater than 5 mm in 6 months. However, the threshold is lower in case of Marfan syndrome and bicuspid aortic valve [10–13].

TABLE 95.3 Types of Aortoarteritis [16]

Type	Involvement
1	Only the aortic arch branches
2a	Ascending aorta and/or at the aortic arch
2b	Only the descending thoracic aorta
3	Descending aorta and abdominal aorta
4	Only the abdominal aorta
5	Entire aorta
	Involvement of the coronary and pulmonary arteries should be indicated as C(+) or P(+), respectively

Nonspecific Aortoarteritis

Nonspecific aortoarteritis (NSAA) is a large-vessel panarteritis of idiopathic cause affecting young women. The types of aortoarteritis are described in Table 95.3. There is idiopathic inflammation of the outer media and adventitia. The most commonly involved vessels worldwide are the arch vessels, especially the left subclavian artery, whereas the abdominal aorta is the most commonly involved vessel in the Indian subcontinent. Clinical presentation in aortic involvement can be in the form of limb claudication or hypertension (aorta or renal artery), stroke (carotid or vertebral artery involvement), or constitutional symptoms.

Imaging of the entire aorta and its branches are critical for diagnosis and preoperative planning. The main imaging modalities are CT, magnetic resonance imaging (MRI), and positron emission tomography/CT/MRI.

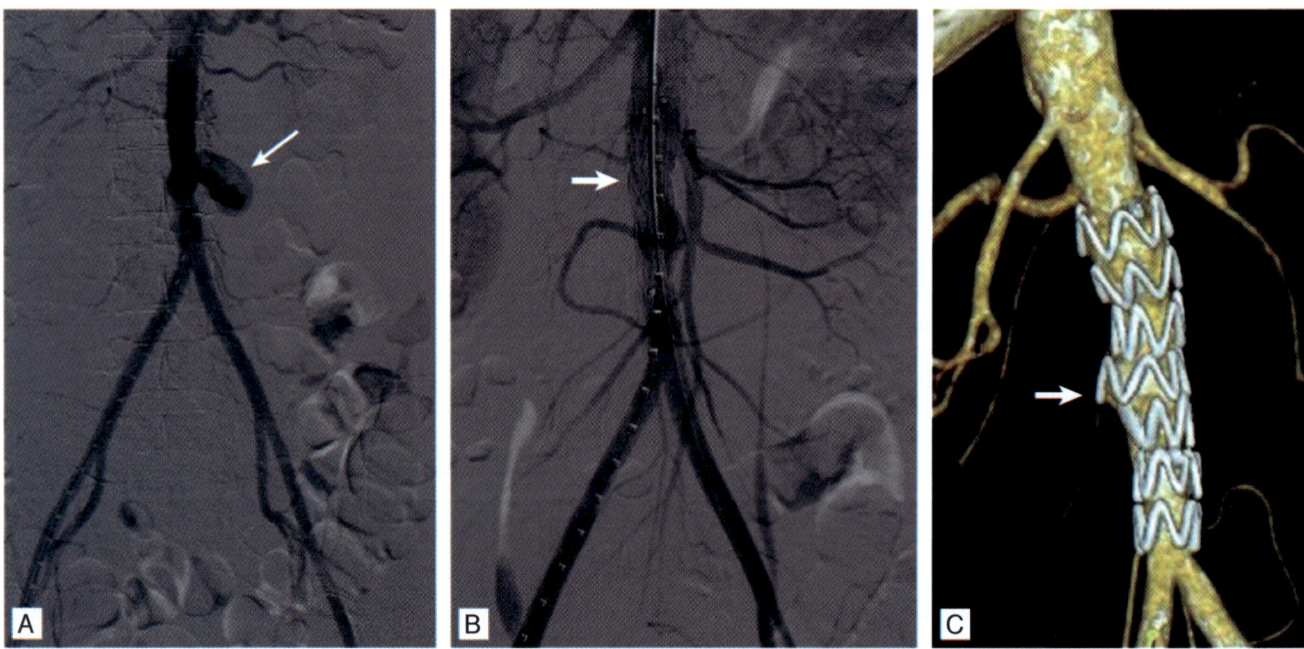

Figure 95.7 Baseline angiogram (A) shows a saccular aneurysm (*thin arrow*) from the infrarenal abdominal aorta. (B and C) The stent graft (*thick arrows*) excluding the aneurysm.

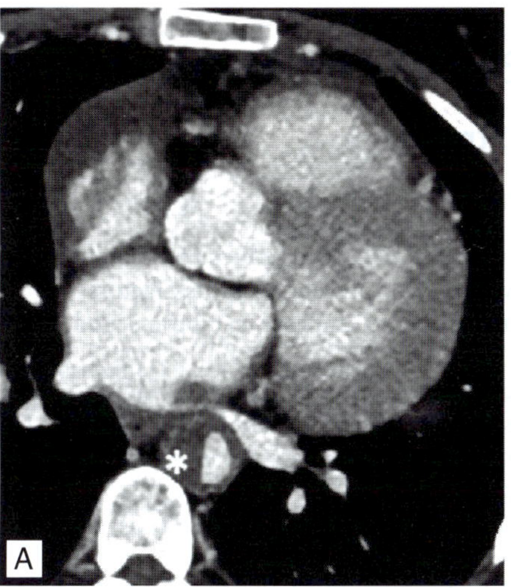

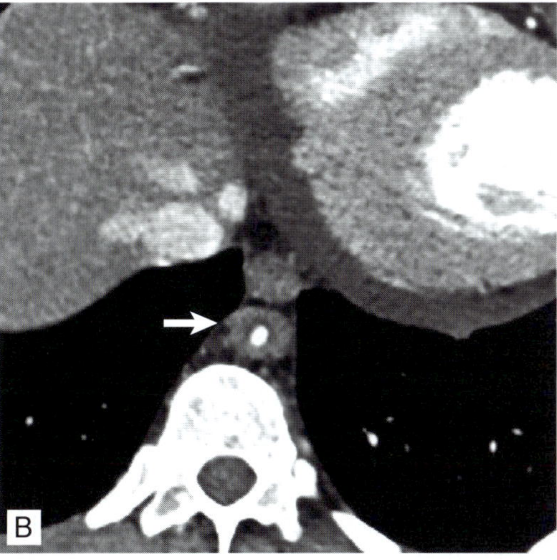

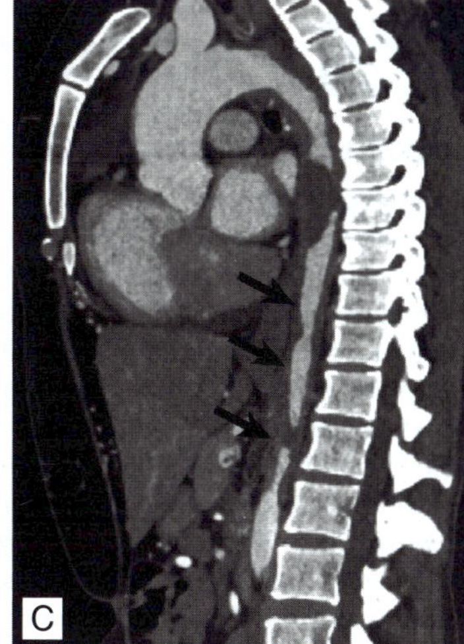

Figure 95.8 Nonspecific aortoarteritis (NSAA). Axial delayed-phase contrast computed tomography image shows a mural thrombus in the descending aorta (*asterisk* in A). Distal to this segment, there is circumferential mural thickening of the aorta with delayed wall enhancement (*arrow* in B) suggesting active disease. Sagittal image (C) shows the diffuse stenotic lesion of aorta (*black arrows*) in this patient with NSAA.

- In the acute stage, there is circumferential mural thickening of the aorta, which can be detected on CT or MRI. T2 weighted MRI shows hyperintense edematous arterial wall, but contrast studies show mural delayed enhancement.
- The chronic stage is characterized by development of stenoses and irregularities in the aortic wall. Long diffuse stenoses with occlusion of the major branches of the aorta at their ostium are common (Fig. 95.8) [14–17].

Management

Patients with active aortoarteritis are treated with steroids and immunosuppressants. *Revascularization is indicated for symptomatic aortoarteritis when the symptoms are not controlled on medical management.* An endovascular approach is preferred in steno-occlusive disease because of its high success rates. Patients with aneurysmal lesions are preferably treated with a surgical approach. It is recommended that intervention be performed in the inactive or chronic phase. However, patients with conditions such as left ventricular dysfunction, flash pulmonary edema, hypertensive encephalopathy, and retinopathy necessitate urgent intervention regardless of disease activity [14,15,18].

Balloon angioplasty is the preferred strategy in patients with chronic symptomatic aortitis with suitable lesion morphology. Balloon length should extend from normal-to-normal segment. The optimum balloon diameter is usually the normal reference vessel diameter measured in the disease-free segment. Elective stenting is usually avoided because the lesions are usually long; there is higher risk of reactivation and in-stent restenosis. Stent placement is indicated only as a bailout strategy when obstructive dissection develops after angioplasty or in patients with recurrent stenosis.

Predictors of poor outcomes of Percutaneous Transluminal Angioplasty (PTA) (high risk of obstructive dissection after balloon angioplasty) are

- Juxtadiaphragmatic stenosis
- Presence of diffuse disease adjacent to the significant stenosis
- Calcific stenosis
- Long disease length (>4 cm)

Image morphology of a combination of these features predicting poor outcome of PTA might be managed by elective stent placement. [14,15,18].

TABLE 95.4 Grades of Aortic Injury [21]

Types	Involvement
I	Intimal tear (10.7%); the tear is typically transverse
II	Intramural hematoma (3.6%)
III	Pseudoaneurysm (78.6%)
IV	Rupture (7.1%)

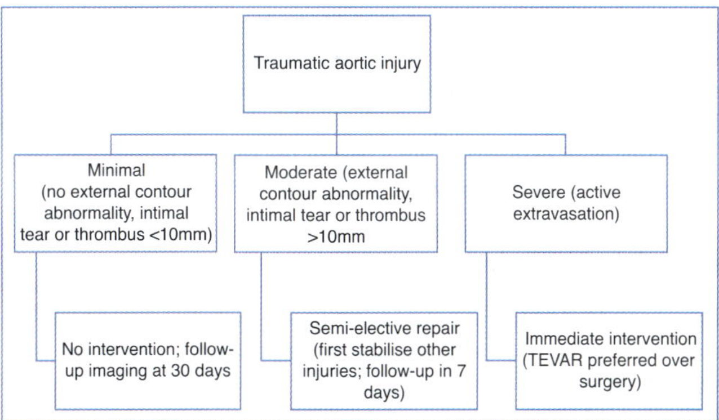

Figure 95.9 Management of traumatic aortic injury according to the University of Washington new Harborview criteria [22]. *TEVAR,* Thoracic endovascular aortic repair.

Traumatic Aortic Injury

Aortic trauma usually results from shearing stress caused by sudden deceleration injuries, most commonly at the isthmus, where the aorta is relatively fixed. The other sites include the aortic arch, brachiocephalic trunk (4.5%), ascending aorta (1%), and descending aorta (2.5%) [19,20]. Grades of aortic injury are described in Table 95.4 [21].

All patients with traumatic aortic injury should receive medical management in the form of beta-blockers, if tolerated, along with antiplatelet therapy. The management strategy is summarized in Fig. 95.9 [22].

TABLE 95.7 Various Types of Balloons Based on Compliance

	Compliant Balloon	Noncompliant Balloon	Semicompliant Balloon
Definition	Increase in inflation pressure → balloon expansion Inequitable distribution of pressure	Do not stretch beyond a predetermined diameter	Inflation in resistant lesion → balloon "hourglasses" or "dog bones" (8–10% growth rate)
Uses	Used for apposition Not used in balloon angioplasty	Stiffer and can deliver high pressure Highly calcified lesions Ideal for focused dilation (4–6% growth rate)	Used in balloon angioplasty Ultra-tight lesions Better trackability: used in difficult-to-reach lesions

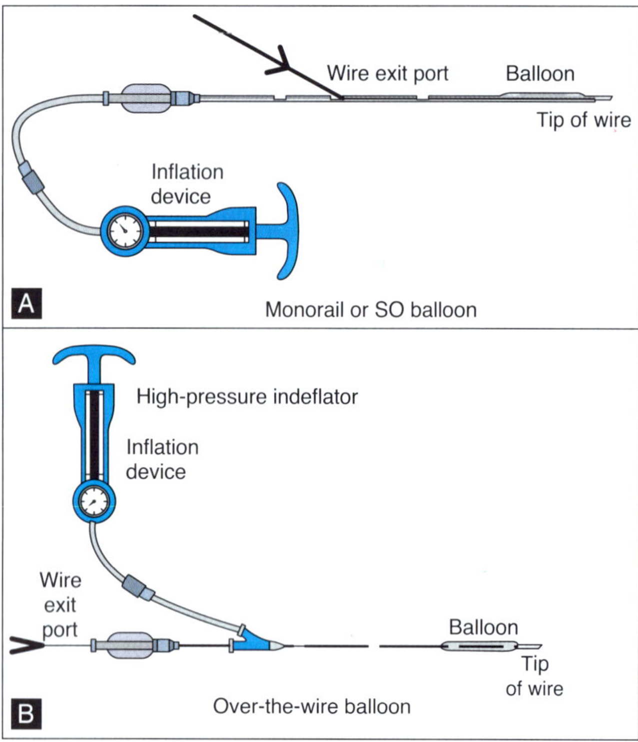

Figure 95.12 Types of balloons based on catheter design. (A) Monorail or Single outlet (SO) balloon. (B) Over-the-wire balloon.

On the basis of catheter design: The balloons can be over the wire or monorail (or rapid exchange). In monorail or rapid exchange catheters, there is a single proximal port for balloon inflation with an exit port for the guidewire (termed the *skive*) approximately 40 cm from the balloon. The advantages of such a balloon include rapid exchange with no need to use exchange-length guidewire. However, there is absence of a port to inject contrast with less trackability through tight or tortuous lesions. In over-the-wire balloons, there are a guidewire port with guidewire tracking along the full length of the catheter and another port for inflation of balloon (Fig. 95.12).

Technique of Angioplasty

The endovascular toolkit includes puncture needles, a variety of guidewires, catheters, balloons, and stents (Fig. 95.13). Any significant inflow disease must be treated first. The ipsilateral approach offers superior purchase, pushability, and trackability,

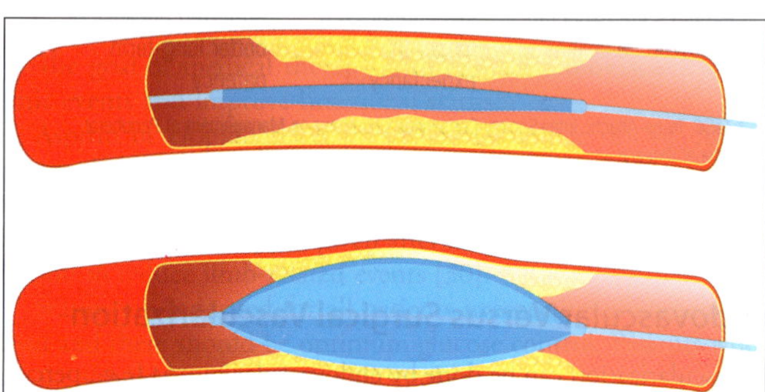

Figure 95.13 Technique of balloon angioplasty.

whereas ipsilateral retrograde access is used in failed antegrade approach or flush SFA occlusion [33].

After crossing the lesion with a suitable catheter–guidewire combination, distal runoff should be assessed. The crossing wire is exchanged with suitable support wire, and balloon angioplasty is performed after confirming intraluminal location. The optimal diameter of the balloon is based on the normal reference diameter, and the length should span from normal-to-normal segment. Angioplasty balloons that approximate the diameter of the normal arterial diameter (90–100%) yield optimal angiographic results [33].

Nominal pressure refers to the pressure at which, when a balloon is inflated, it achieves the listed balloon diameter. Rated burst pressure is the pressure below which 99.9% of the balloons will not burst on single inflation. In balloon angioplasty, prolonged inflation (up to several minutes) is often used at nominal pressures (typically 4–8 atm). Inflation at higher pressures is required in recurrent lesions, residual lesions, and heavily calcified lesions. *Resolution of the waist is an important factor in assessing the adequacy of dilation.*

After deflation and removal of balloon, with wire across the lesion, control angiogram of distal runoff should be taken to determine technical success and exclude complications (distal embolization, dissection) (Figs. 95.14 to 95.17) [34–36].

Endpoints of Angioplasty [14]

- Imaging: less than 30% residual stenosis
- Hemodynamic: reduction of the pressure gradient to less than 5 mm Hg mean or less than 10 mm Hg systolic
- Clinical: restoration of a 2+ Common Femoral Artery (CFA) or Dorsalis Pedis Artery (DPA) pulses

Postintervention ABI (>0.15 improvement) and transcutaneous oximetry ($TcPo_2$) are relevant in below-knee lesions and CLI. *The various*

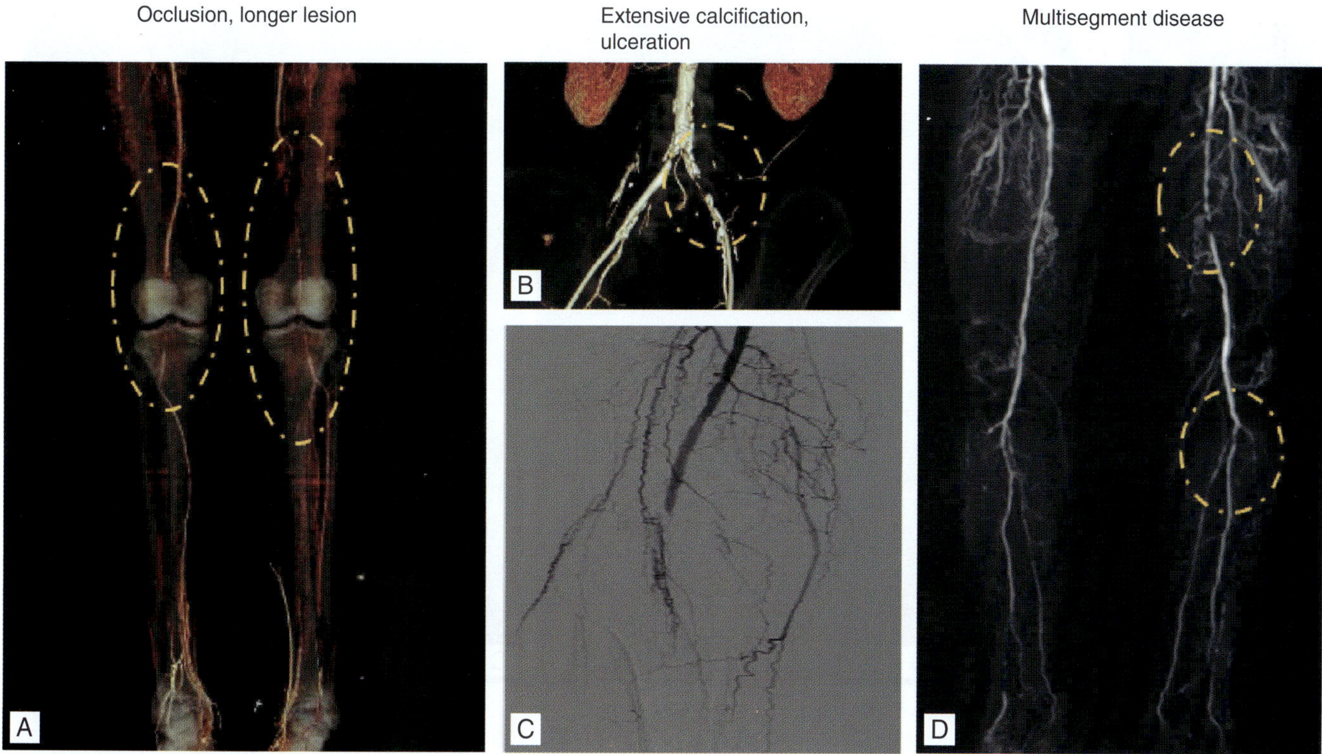

Figure 95.14 Poor prognostic markers of revascularization. (A) Occlusion of the P1 and P2 segments of the right popliteal artery with long-segment stenosis of the left distal superficial femoral artery and popliteal artery. (B) Reconstructed computed tomography image shows left common iliac artery occlusion with extensive calcification and ulceration. (C) Digital subtraction angiography image shows long-segment occlusion of the popliteal artery with poor distal reformation. (D) Reconstructed magnetic resonance angiography image shows multisegment lesions involving the left femoral and tibial artery.

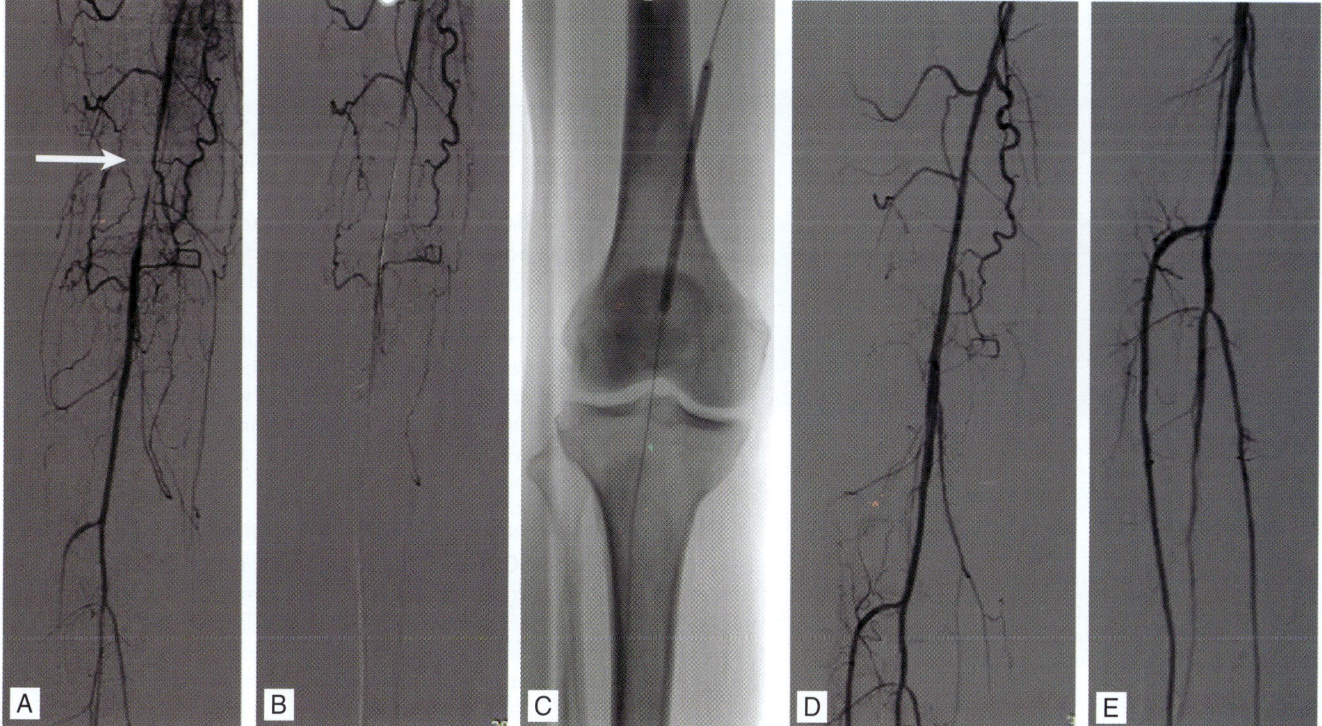

Figure 95.15 Balloon angioplasty for distal right superficial femoral artery (SFA) stenosis in a patient with severe intermittent claudication. (A) Preangioplasty angiogram demonstrates long-segment occlusion of the right distal SFA (*white arrow*). (B) Crossing the lesion with a guidewire. (C) Inflation of the angioplasty balloon across the lesion. (D) Postangioplasty run showing good antegrade flow in the distal SFA with no residual stenosis or dissection. (E) Good distal runoff.

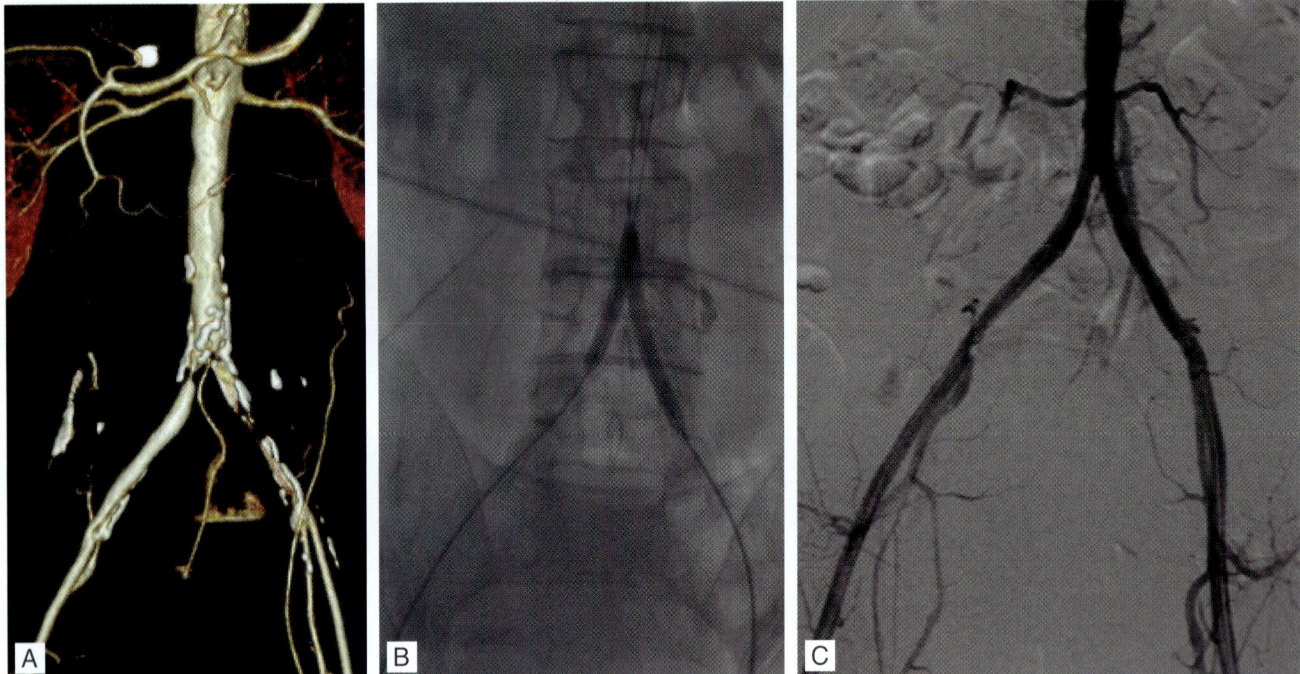

Figure 95.16 (A) Volume-rendered image shows severe stenosis of the right common iliac artery (CIA) with occlusion of the left CIA. Both CIAs show severe calcification. (B) Angiogram shows kissing balloon angioplasty. (C) Postprocedural angiogram after placement of balloon-expandable stents in bilateral CIA shows good antegrade flow with no residual stenosis.

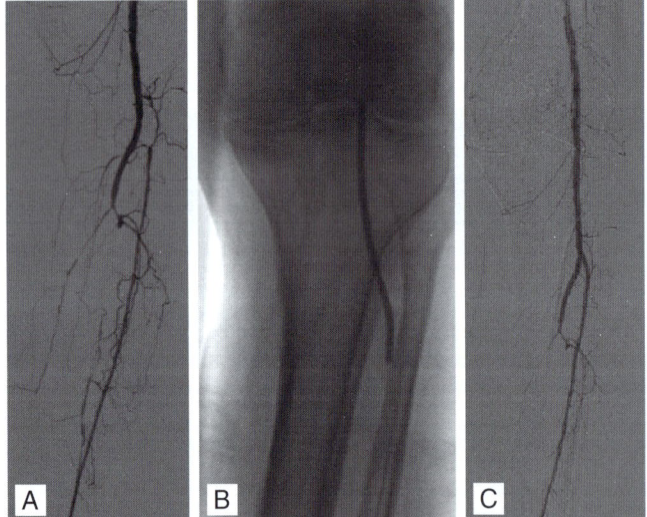

Figure 95.17 Balloon angioplasty for ostioproximal, Anterior tibial artery (ATA) stenosis in a patient with critical limb ischemia. (A) Severe stenosis of the ostioproximal left ATA with mild stenosis of popliteal artery. (B) Balloon angioplasty across the lesion. (C) Postangioplasty angiogram depicts no residual stenosis.

causes of failure of balloon angioplasty include dissection, recoil, residual stenosis, distal atheroembolism, vessel rupture, and restenosis [36].

Role of Stenting

Stent is a metallic scaffold that provides additional support to the lumen to stay patent. The role of stenting can be to supplement the outcome of angioplasty and salvage a complicated angioplasty (provisional stenting) or as an alternative to angioplasty to improve the patency rates in selected lesions such as ostial lesions or chronic total occlusions (primary or elective stenting).

Types of Stents

Stents can be made of nitinol or cobalt and chromium. Nitinol has property of expansion because of thermal shape memory. Cobalt–chromium stents have higher radial strength.

Self-expanding stents have the property of thermal shape memory with the advantage of better conformability and are more crush resistant [37]. Balloon-expandable stents have greater radial force with precise placement and less recoil. However, balloon-expandable balloons are rigid and prone to edge dissections [38]. Self-expanding stents are preferred in treating patients with PAD. Stenting should be avoided across joints because of complex external mechanical stresses.

In selected bailout situations, vasculomimetic stents (closed cell, self-expanding) can be used across the joints (Fig. 95.18) [39]. In cases of primary stenting, predilation with a small-sized balloon creates a profile for the stent. Self-expanding stents may require dilatation with a balloon to fully expand to the intended diameter.

Newer Advances and Works in Progress

Angiosome Concept: The angiosome concept (six angiosomes for the lower extremity) has also been proposed for infrapopliteal lesions, and a metaanalysis has shown improved wound healing and higher limb salvage rates with direct or angiosome-targeted revascularization, but further studies are needed to validate this concept [40].

Advances in Angioplasty Balloons: These advances include cutting balloons, cryotherapy balloons, and laser angioplasty.

- A cutting balloon is a noncompliant balloon with three or four microsurgical blades or atherotomes that "score" the plaque

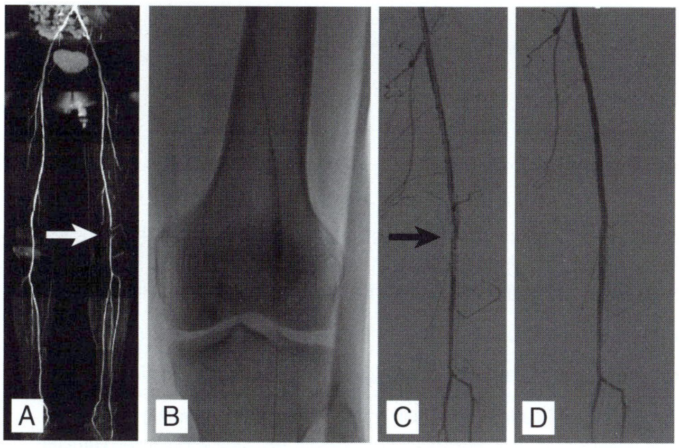

Figure 95.18 Vasculomimetic stent placement for P1 occlusion. (A) Magnetic resonance angiography depicts occlusion of the P1 segment of the left popliteal artery (*white arrow*). (B) Balloon angioplasty across the lesion. (C) Development of a flow-limiting dissection flap (*black arrow*). (D) Post-procedural angiogram after placement of a vasculomimetic stent.

and increase target lesion compliance. They may be considered in severe calcification and recurrent stenosis [41].

- Cryotherapy balloons use the cold caused by nitrous oxide, and a temperature of −10°C has been found to reduce plaque inflammation, and as a result, the elastic recoil and the growth of smooth muscle cells decrease [42].
- Laser angioplasty uses laser radiation to ablate tissue, causing obliteration of occluded or stenosed arteries [43].

Brachytherapy: Brachytherapy is another strategy to treat restenosis after balloon angioplasty. It uses ionizing radiation to inhibit cellular proliferation [38].

Advances in Plaque Removal and Debulking: Atherectomy devices (directional, orbital, and rotational) debulk plaque and modify plaque morphology. They are especially useful in lesions with moderate to severe calcification [38].

Drug-Eluting Technology: Drug-eluting technology, because of its antineoproliferative properties, minimizes neointimal hyperplasia, thus reducing the chance of restenosis and improving long-term patency rates. Currently, the Food and Drug Administration (FDA) recommends informed consent about the risks and benefits of drug-eluting technology with the individual patient and diligent monitoring of patients who have been treated.

Stem Cell Therapy and Therapeutic Angiogenesis: A revascularization strategy may not always be feasible or effective, and hence angiogenic therapies can alleviate the symptoms.

Bone marrow-derived stem and progenitor cells are potential new therapeutic option to induce therapeutic angiogenesis. As these cells grow in hypoxic tissues, they become stimulated to become cells similar to ones they are in contact with [44].

95.3 Pulmonary Artery Interventions

Normal Anatomy

The pulmonary vasculature is constituted by pulmonary arteries and veins, as well as bronchial arteries. Pulmonary arteries and veins, along with the extensive capillary bed, constitute a low-pressure and high-capacitance vascular system. It is involved primarily in gas exchange by providing a large surface area.

The main pulmonary artery (MPA) originates from the right ventricular outflow tract. It goes leftward and posterosuperiorly with respect to the aorta and divides into the right and left pulmonary arteries (RPA, LPA) at the level of the carina. Then the RPA and LPA divide into two lobar branches, each of which divides into segmental and subsegmental branches. The right and left lung are divided into 10 and 8 bronchopulmonary segments, respectively. *The segmental and subsegmental pulmonary arteries run parallel to bronchi. Hence, these are named based on the bronchopulmonary segment being supplied.* These subdivide rapidly and ultimately form a dense web of pulmonary capillaries lining the alveolar wall, providing a larger area for gaseous exchange.

The pulmonary veins carry the blood back to the heart. However, the pulmonary veins do not run parallel to the bronchi but traverse within the interlobular septa. These converge to form bilateral superior and inferior pulmonary veins, which eventually drain into the left atrium.

The bronchial circulation constitutes a low-capacitance and high-pressure circuit, which provides nutrients to the lung and normally does not take part in the oxygenation of blood. It is essential to know about the normal as well as the variant anatomies of the entire pulmonary vasculature, both on cross-sectional imaging and angiography, which is required for making an accurate diagnosis and treatment planning for a subsequent interventional procedure [45,46].

Spectrum of Pathology and Their Management

- Pulmonary embolism
- Pulmonary artery stenosis
- Pulmonary arteriovenous malformations
- Pulmonary artery aneurysms and pseudoaneurysms
- Foreign body retrieval
- Endovascular biopsy
- Intravascular ultrasonography
- Temporary occlusion of the pulmonary artery

Pulmonary Embolism

Pulmonary thromboembolism is one of the leading causes of death from a cardiovascular cause. Massive pulmonary embolism with associated systemic shock has variable mortality rates described in the literature [47,48]. *The established standard treatment strategy for patients with massive, life-threatening pulmonary thromboembolism is medical thrombolysis combined with anticoagulation.* For patients in whom systemic thrombolysis has not been successful, the optimal therapeutic strategy is not known. The various therapeutic strategies

TABLE 95.8 Various Endovascular Interventional Techniques for Pulmonary Thromboembolism

Catheter-Directed Intervention	Description
USG-assisted thrombolysis	■ Use of catheter-directed high frequency USG ■ Advantage: better penetration of the thrombolytic agent into the embolus ■ Without thrombolytics: no proven benefit
Rheolytic embolectomy [49–54]	■ Injection of pressurized saline through the catheter's distal tip followed by aspiration of the macerated thrombus via a catheter port ■ Disadvantage: need for venous cutdown for catheter access and subsequent increased risk of bleeding at insertion site
Rotational embolectomy [55–59]	Rotating the device at the tip of the catheter fragments the thrombus. The fragmented thrombus aspirates continuously.
Suction embolectomy [60–61]	Manual aspiration of thrombus through a large-lumen catheter using an aspiration syringe and a hemostatic valve.
Thrombus fragmentation [62–65]	Using a standard pigtail catheter or balloon angioplasty catheter and manually rotating it into the thrombus can disrupt the thrombus. Small thrombus fragments move distally. This reduces pulmonary vascular resistance. However, catheter fragmentation can lead to increased pulmonary vascular pressures as well (via embolization of larger fragments into distal pulmonary branches). Hence, aspiration of the fragments is simultaneously done to prevent this.

in such cases include repeat systemic thrombolysis, catheter-directed thrombolysis, or catheter or surgical embolectomy. The choice among these options depends on institutional preference, local expertise, and the various resources available.

Endovascular Intervention

The various endovascular techniques are discussed in Table 95.8. The various studies carried out to date have been limited by a small sample size. Moreover, inclusion of heterogeneous patient subsets in the study population (which include hemodynamically stable or unstable patients or patients with or without contraindication to thrombolysis) is another limitation that deserves to be mentioned. Until now, none of the described techniques has shown a definite superiority over the other technique. Hence, currently, the preference of a given intervention is operator or institution dependent.

Surgical Embolectomy

The indications for surgical embolectomy are hemodynamic instability caused by acute pulmonary thromboembolism and

1. Patients with contraindication to thrombolysis (systemic or catheter directed)
2. Failure of thrombolysis
3. Embolus trapped within a patent foramen ovale or present in the right atrium or right ventricle

Although proximal emboli (right ventricle, MPA, RPA, LPA, and extrapulmonary branches of pulmonary arteries) are amenable to surgical removal, distal thrombus (e.g., intrapulmonary branches of pulmonary arteries) is generally not amenable to surgery (Fig. 95.19).

Pulmonary Artery Stenosis

Pulmonary artery stenosis refers to narrowing in the pulmonary artery or its branches. This may be isolated abnormality or may be present in combination with other congenital heart defects (e.g., tetralogy of Fallot, pulmonary atresia, patent ductus arteriosus, truncus arteriosus). In adults, pulmonary artery stenosis is seen mainly in those with pulmonary vasculitis (Behcet disease or Takayasu arteritis) (Fig. 95.20) [71–74]. Therapeutic options include percutaneous transluminal balloon angioplasty and intravascular stent implantation. Balloon angioplasty is performed in children because of the concern of a potential mismatch between the stent and blood vessel size after somatic growth (increase in body size with age, which causes enlargement of pulmonary arteries).

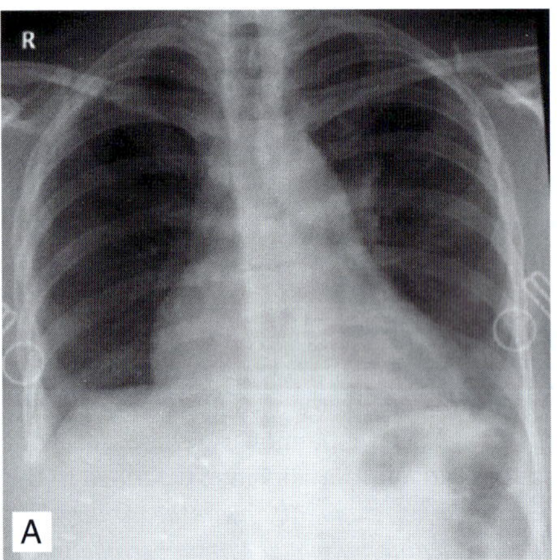

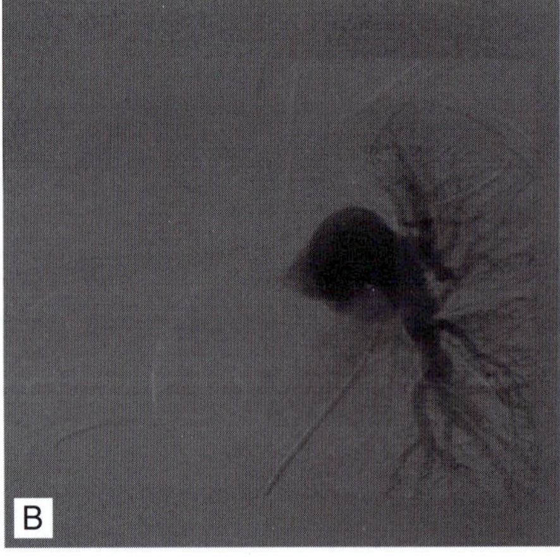

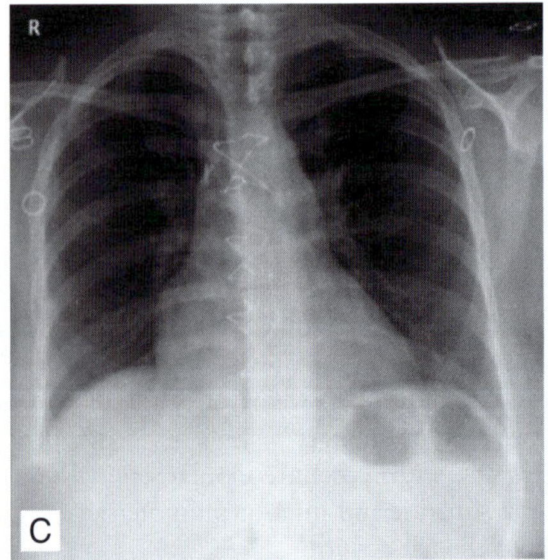

Figure 95.19 Known case of pulmonary thromboembolism involving the right pulmonary artery. Surgical embolectomy was performed. (A) Preoperative chest radiography shows cardiomegaly with differential pulmonary vascularity (mild paucity of vessels on the right side). (B) Catheter angiogram shows complete occlusion of the right pulmonary artery with near-normal vascularity on the left side and patent left pulmonary artery branches. (C) Postoperative chest radiography 6 weeks after surgical embolectomy shows a decrease in cardiac size with equal pulmonary vascularity on both the right and left sides.

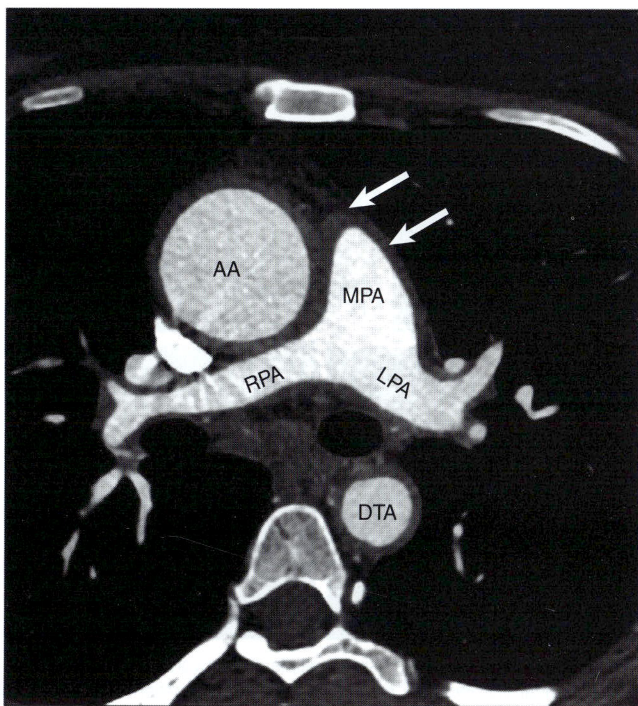

Figure 95.20 Takayasu arteritis. Circumferential mural thickening (marked by *arrows*) seen along the ascending aorta (AA), descending thoracic aorta (DTA) and main pulmonary artery (MPA), and right and left pulmonary arteries (RPA and LPA).

Pulmonary Arteriovenous Malformation

Incidence

Pulmonary arteriovenous malformations (PAVMs) are abnormal communications between pulmonary arteries and veins. These are uncommon in the general population. They are most commonly congenital in origin and associated with Osler-Weber-Rendu syndrome. The various acquired causes include liver cirrhosis, penetrating chest trauma, mitral stenosis, schistosomiasis, Fanconi syndrome, and after surgery for congenital heart disease (Glenn shunt). A female preponderance is seen [75].

Pulmonary arteriovenous malformations are commonly multiple and vary in their number, distribution, and size. Based on previous studies, approximately 36% of patients have multiple lesions, 25% have bilateral disease, and more than half of lesions are seen in lower lung fields [76,77]. PAVMs are typically 1 to 5 cm in size. Their size may occasionally exceed 10 cm. Most PAVMs remain stable over time. However, approximately 25% enlarge slowly, usually at a rate of 0.3 to 2 mm/year. Macroscopic PAVMs (i.e., those seen on computed tomography [CT]) do not spontaneously resolve. Approximately 10% of patients have diffuse microvascular PAVMs that may be seen in combination with radiographically visible PAVMs [78–80].

Classification

PAVMs are classified as either simple or complex as shown in Fig. 95.21.

- Simple PAVMs are perfused by arteries that arise from a single subsegmental artery.
- Complex PAVMs are perfused by more than one subsegmental artery.

Approximately 80% to 95% of PAVMs are of simple type. PAVMs are supplied by pulmonary arteries in approximately 95% of cases with drainage by pulmonary veins. However, they may occasionally be fed by systemic arteries (bronchial artery) or drain directly into the left atrium or inferior vena cava [81,82].

Treatment

Selecting a patient requiring treatment depends on PAVM-related symptoms, feeding artery diameter, and the patient's ability to tolerate the procedure. When indicated, most patients are treated with embolotherapy and angiographic occlusion of the feeding arteries. Patients with asymptomatic PAVMs in whom the feeding artery is smaller than 2 mm can be followed up with yearly clinical observation, and CT every 3 to 5 years. Patients with PAVMs showing progressive enlargement or symptomatic PAVMs during follow up should undergo evaluation for embolotherapy with pulmonary angiography.

For patients who have one or more PAVM, with a feeding artery diameter (FAD) of 2 to 3 mm or greater, endovascular embolization of the PAVM is recommended rather than observation alone. A similar approach is suggested for patients with atypical lesions or PAVMs with FAD smaller than 2 mm who have symptomatic hypoxemia, paradoxical embolism, or hemoptysis. Embolotherapy results in an immediate improvement in the patient's symptom and in oxygenation. Over the long term, there is a reduction in the rate of serious complications (especially neurologic events such as stroke and cerebral abscess) (Figs. 95.22 and 95.23).

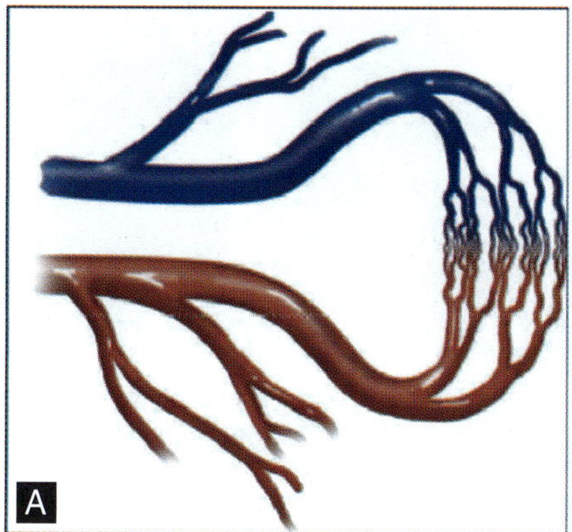

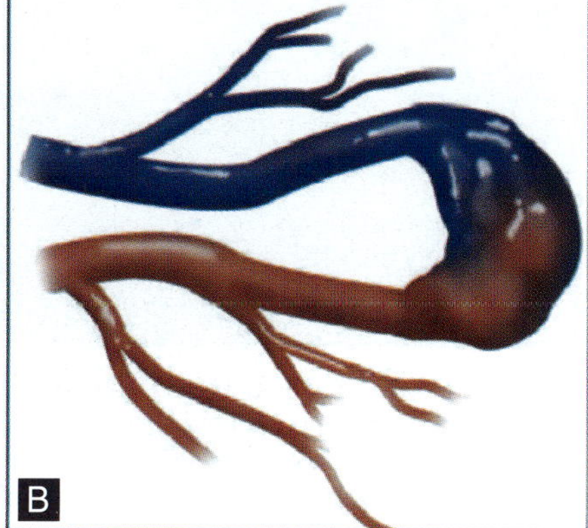

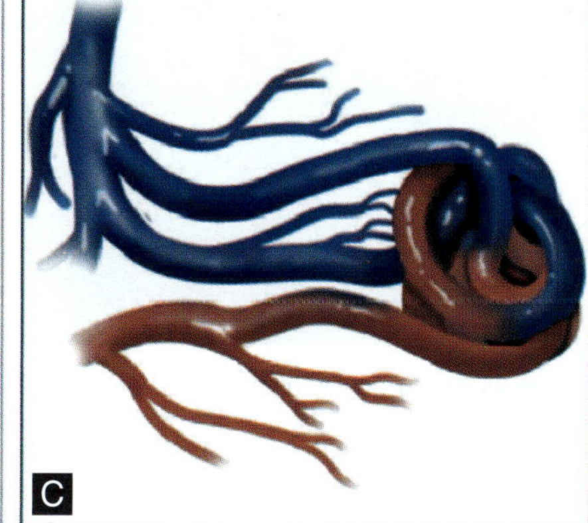

Figure 95.21 (A) Normally capillary bed. (B) Simple pulmonary arteriovenous malformation (PAVM). (C) Complex PAVM.

high incidence of restenosis caused by mucosal trauma, it is usually followed by additional procedures such as stenting (Fig. 95.27). The potential complications include like pneumothorax, pneumomediastinum, and mediastinitis caused by tracheal rupture.

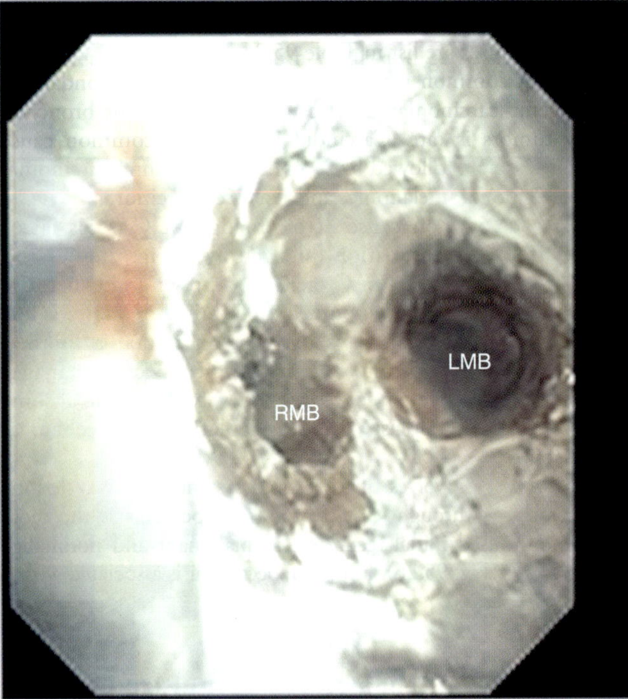

Figure 95.27 Metallic Y-stent deployed in the distal trachea and right and left main bronchi (RMB and LMB) in a case of tracheal bifurcation stenosis.

- Ablation techniques include cryotherapy (nitrous oxide or carbon dioxide at –890°C to rapidly destroy the tissue or tumor) (Fig. 95.28), thermal ablation (electrocautery, laser or argon plasma coagulation), or photodynamic therapy (nonthermal ablation using photosensitizing agents activated by nonthermal lasers). The potential complications include airway fire during thermal ablation, particularly with Nd:YAG (neodymium-doped yttrium aluminum garnet) lasers. This can be avoided by keeping the laser on pulsed mode, maintaining the FiO_2 of 40% or less, and avoiding inflammable anesthetic agents [92]. Cryotherapy and photodynamic therapy do not have this complication. The unique complication of photodynamic therapy is systemic phototoxicity, which can last for several weeks after injection.
- Mechanical debridement is the quickest method for airway debulking and opening up the airway. This is frequently used in conjunction with other ablation modalities. The microdebrider requires a rigid bronchoscope or laryngoscope and is not compatible with a flexible bronchoscope. The potential complications of bleeding and airway perforation are minimal with no risk of airway fire.

Emphysematous Disease

Patients with chronic obstructive pulmonary disease (COPD) have reduced exercise capacity and increased morbidity and mortality rates. COPD is one of the leading causes of death in the world caused by eventual cardiorespiratory failure. The specific

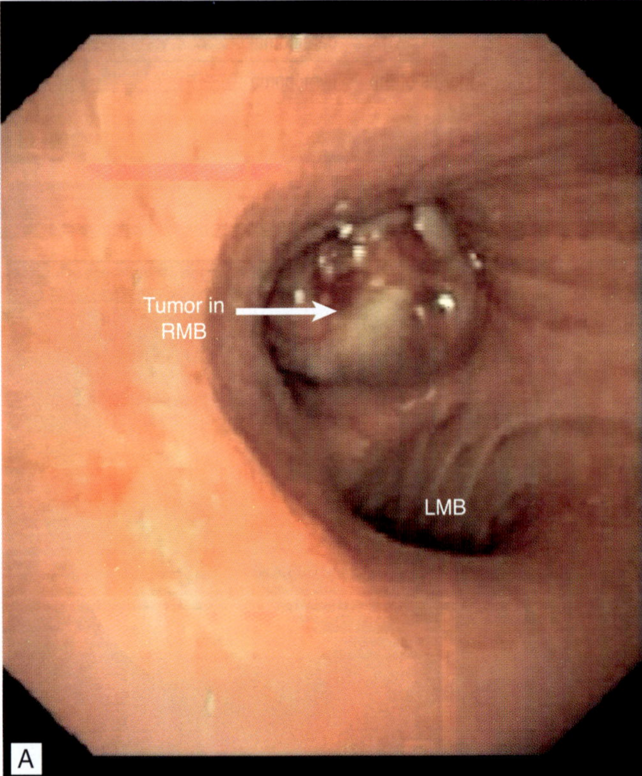

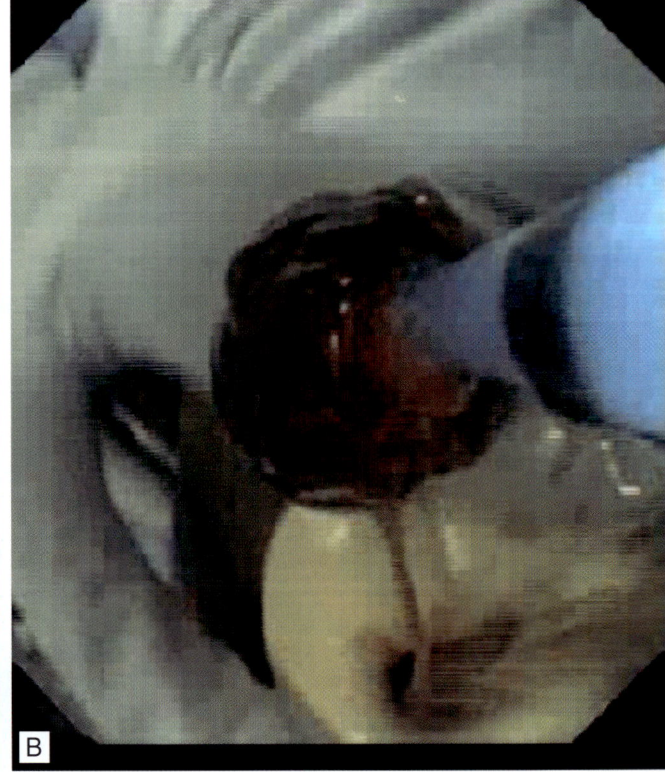

Figure 95.28 (A) Complete occlusion of the right main bronchus (RMB) with tumor. (B) Tumor removed using cryoablation. *LMB,* left man bronchus.

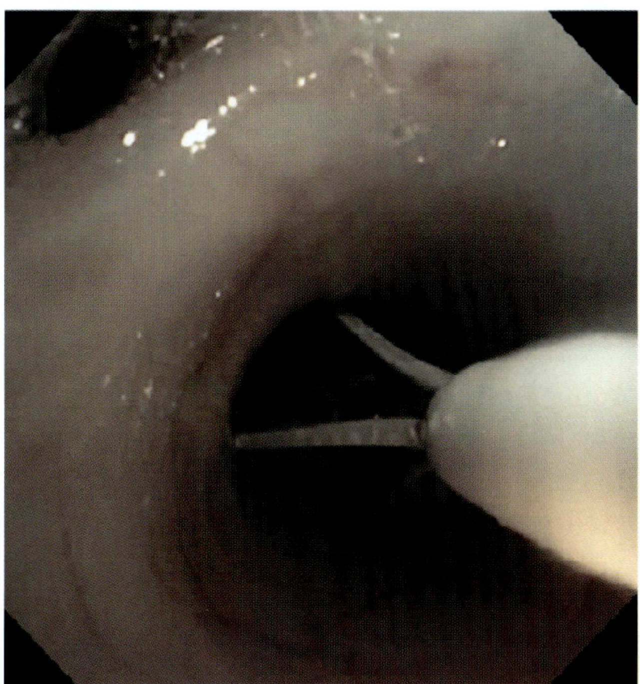

Figure 95.29 Ablation of smooth muscles of airway using bronchial thermoplasty in a case of severe asthma.

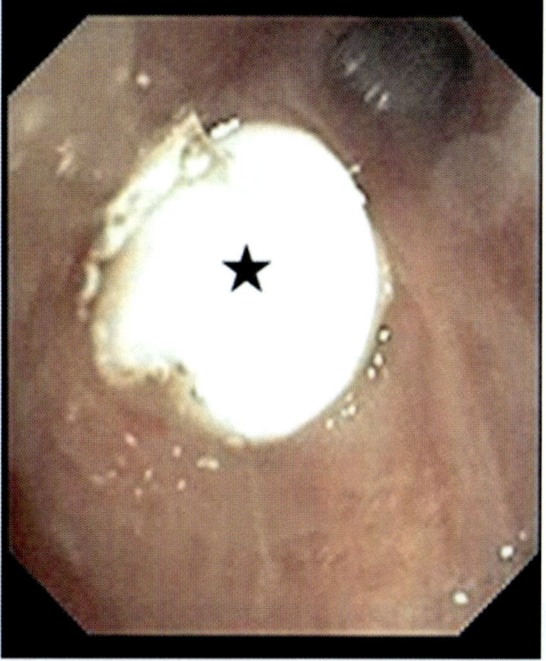

Figure 95.30 Segmental bronchial occlusion for bronchopleural fistula using a plug (endobronchial Watanabe [EWS] spigot) (*star*) in a case of bronchopleural fistula.

subgroup of COPD with emphysematous phenotype has shown a beneficial outcome after the lung reduction surgery as demonstrated first in the National Emphysema Treatment Trial (NETT) trial [93]. Following this, many minimally invasive endobronchial procedures were studied as an alternative to the open surgery.

Bronchoscopic lung volume reduction (BLVR) techniques are minimally invasive methods. They involve placement of an endobronchial coil, one-way valve, or fibrin glue to promote the collapse of the diseased lung parenchyma. The major limiting factor for the success of BLVR is collateral ventilation from the adjacent lung [94–97].

Asthma

Patients with asthma have hyperresponsive airways. *Bronchial thermoplasty (BT)* involves ablation of the smooth muscles of the airways using thermal ablation through a rigid bronchoscope without causing airway scarring or stenosis (Fig. 95.29). The safety and efficacy of BT have been proven with the Research in Severe Asthma (RISA) trial, Asthma Intervention Research (AIR) trial, and AIR-2 trial. The 5-year results of each of these trials showed symptomatic improvement in patients with moderate to severe asthma without major adverse effects [98–100].

Bronchopleural Fistula

This can occur secondary to trauma or secondary to surgical resection of the lung. Endobronchial therapies including glue, coils, or endobronchial one-way valves offer an alternative approach to the traditional surgical management of these patients (Fig. 95.30).

Tracheoesophageal Fistula

Most of these fistulas develop in cases of advanced malignancy and are not candidates for surgical repair. These can be well managed with esophageal or tracheal stenting (Fig 95.31). Injection of chemical glue or laser and argon plasma coagulation have also been used with an endoscopic approach.

Sampling of Peritracheal Tissue

Transbronchial needle aspiration under convex probe endobronchial ultrasonography (EBUS) (Fig. 95.32A) has increased the diagnostic yield in the staging of lung and mediastinal cancers [101]. Radial EBUS-guided sampling (Fig. 95.32B) is an alternative to computed tomography–guided biopsy of the peripheral pulmonary nodules. It has a high diagnostic yield of around 70%, and it is particularly more for nodule of size larger than 2 cm with a very low complication rate [102].

Newer Advances and Works in Progress

The use of bronchial rheoplasty for patients with chronic bronchitis is a promising technique [103,104]. It aims to destroy the mucin-producing goblet cells in the airway while promoting the growth of normal endothelium. A recent study established the safety and feasibility of the procedure, but further studies are required to test the efficacy [105].

Pharmacologic manipulation of the parasympathetic nervous system is the mainstay of COPD management. Targeted lung denervation (TLD) aims to destroy the parasympathetic nerves running along the main bronchi using radiofrequency ablation. The safety and feasibility have been established in previous

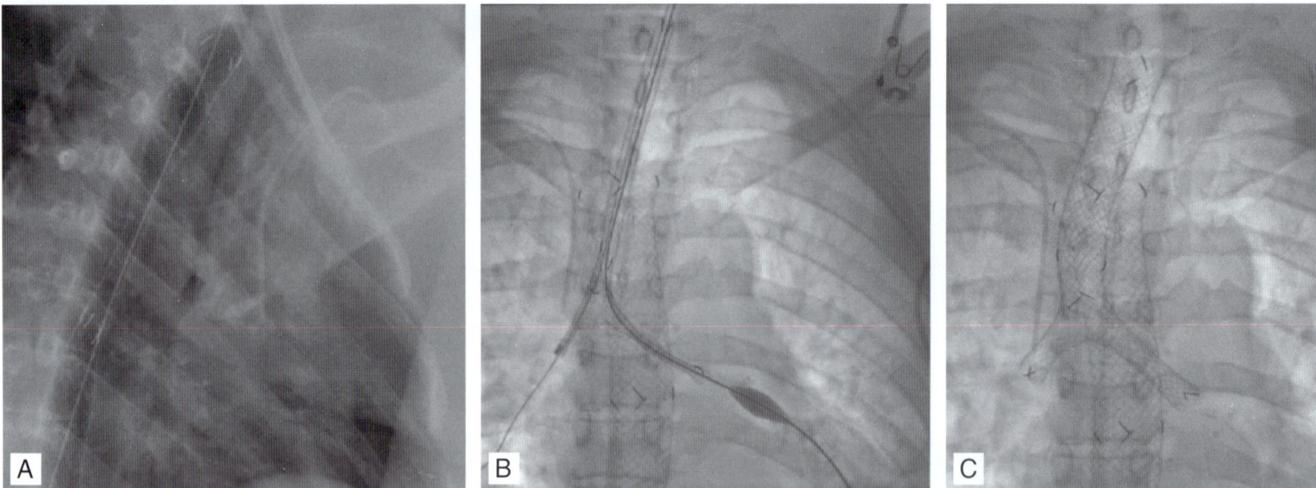

Figure 95.31 (A) Esophageal stent deployment. (B) Tracheal stent being deployed. (C) Postdeployment of esophageal and tracheal stents in a case of tracheoesophageal fistula.

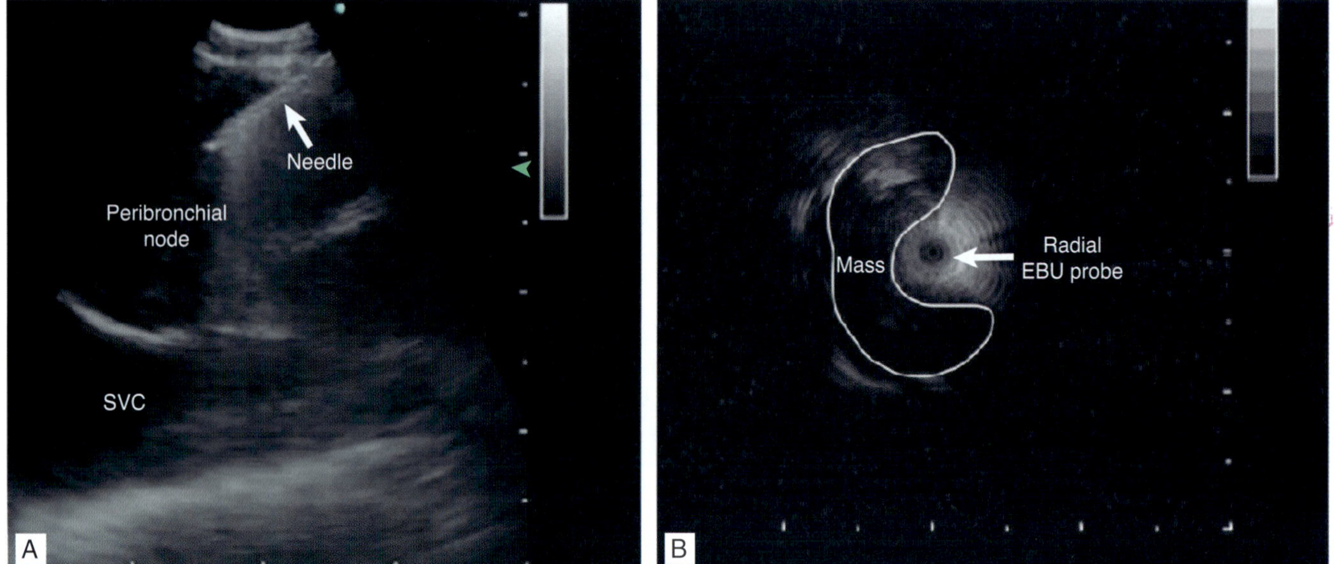

Figure 95.32 (A) Convex endobronchial USG (EBUS)–guided sampling of a peribronchial node in a case of sarcoidosis. (B) Radial EBUS image shows an irregular pulmonary mass lesion. *SVC,* Superior vena cava.

randomized controlled trials (AIRFLOW2 trial). The ongoing AIRFLOW3 trial aims to test the efficacy of TLD [106].

Bronchoscopic thermal vapor ablation is another bronchoscopic lung reduction technique. It has a theoretical advantage of treating the collateral ventilation positive patients. Although the few single-arm studies and a multinational randomized controlled trial have shown positive results, further studies are required to test the efficacy of this procedure [107].

95.5 Bronchial Artery Interventions

Embryology and Anatomy of the Bronchial Arteries

Both lungs are supplied by dual vascular systems composed of pulmonary arteries (PAs) and bronchial arteries (BAs). The PAs supply 99% of blood (deoxygenated) to the lungs at low pressure and essentially participate in gas exchange at the alveolar capillary membrane. The BAs supply 1% of the blood (oxygenated) to the lungs at pressures six times that of the PA. They primarily provide nourishment to the supporting structures of the parenchyma of both lungs, including the PAs, and do not participate in gas exchange [108,109]. Also there exist

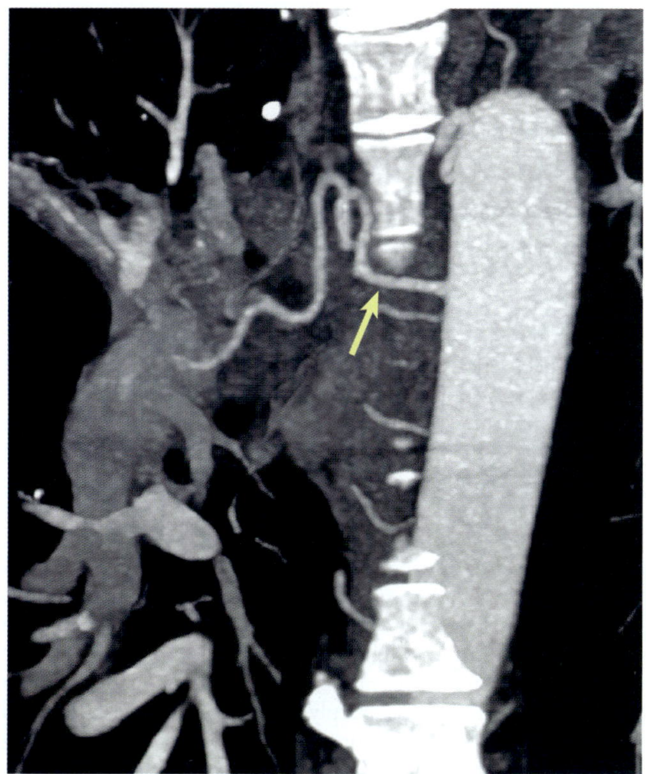

Figure 95.33 Hypertrophied right bronchial artery (*yellow arrow*) from the descending thoracic aorta.

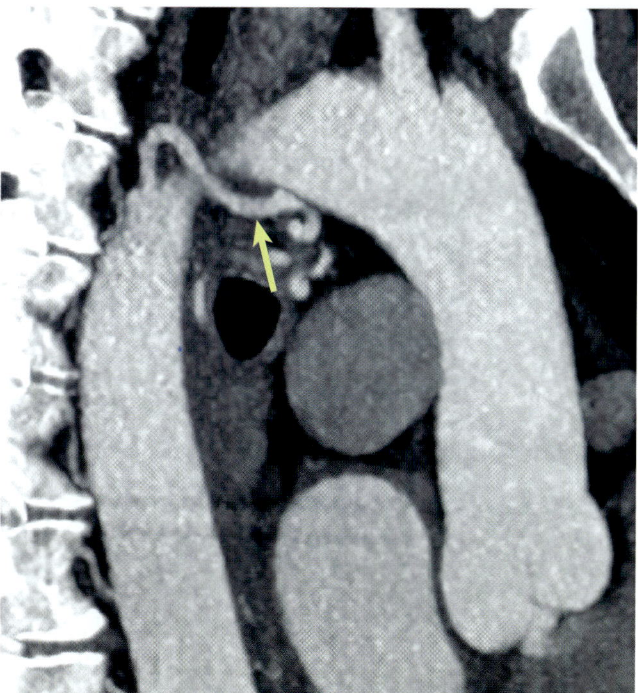

Figure 95.34 Hypertrophied bronchial artery (*yellow arrow*) from under the surface of the aortic arch.

multiple microvascular anastomoses at the level of the alveoli and respiratory bronchioles, through which the BA are connected to the PA [110].

Site of Origin and Variations

Usually, the BAs originate from the proximal descending thoracic aorta (DTA). The BAs are termed orthotopic when the origin is between the superior endplate of the T5 and the inferior endplate of the T6 vertebral bodies and is seen in 64% of patients undergoing computed tomography angiography (CTA) for evaluation of hemoptysis (Fig. 95.33). On angiography, the orthotopic BAs are seen approximately at 1 cm above or below the level of the left main bronchus as it crosses the DTA [111].

The BAs are termed ectopic when they arise elsewhere in the aorta or from branches of the aorta [112–115]. This configuration is seen in 36% (range, 8.3–56% depending on evaluation of the angiography or autopsy) of patients with at least one ectopic BA, commonly originating from the undersurface of the aortic arch (Fig. 95.34) [116–120].

Anatomy

The left BAs arise directly from the DTA. The right BAs most commonly share their origin with the intercostal artery or from a common intercostal bronchial trunk (ICBAT) and is seen in 52% of patients undergoing CTA.

Multiple anatomic variants exist and are described in Table 95.10 [121–126].

Venous return from the bronchial arterial circulation is predominantly via the pulmonary veins. The superior vena cava, azygos, and hemiazygos veins do provide minor contributions. Knowledge of this drainage is important as to determine direct arteriovenous shunting during bronchial angiography.

Cross-Sectional Anatomy of Bronchial Arteries

Normal BAs measure less than 2 mm at their origin and 0.5 mm distally as they enter the bronchopulmonary segment [117].

Bronchial Artery Dilation and Hypertrophy

Abnormal dilated BAs are large (>2 mm in diameter) and often seen to have a tortuous mediastinal course well seen in the multiplanar CT images. The hypertrophied system can accommodate 18% to 30% of cardiac output, especially in chronic pulmonary thromboembolism (Table 95.11). It is important to avoid imaging pitfalls, in which small mediastinal lymph nodes, veins, endobronchial lesions, broncholiths, or enhancement of wall of the esophagus can be mistaken for abnormal BAs [127].

Nonbronchial Systemic Arteries

These are commonly seen in the setting of pleural thickening greater than 3 mm and are seen as tortuous enhancing vessels within hypertrophic extrapleural fat at contrast-enhanced CT. The nonbronchial systemic arteries (NBSAs) can arise commonly from the following arteries:

1. Intercostal artery
2. Branches of the subclavian and axillary arteries
3. Internal mammary artery
4. Inferior phrenic artery

The NBSAs course along the pleura or potentially ascend via the inferior pulmonary ligament, never joining the bronchial tree. NBSAs are common causes of early recurrence of hemoptysis and hemoptysis recalcitrant to optimal bronchial artery embolization (BAE) [128].

Table 95.10 Anatomic Variations of Bronchial Arteries

Types	Incidence (%)	Description
1	40.6	One right bronchial artery arising from a common intercostal bronchial trunk (ICBAT) and two left bronchial arteries
2	21.3	A single bronchial artery on each side, with the right bronchial artery originating from an ICBAT
3	20.6	Two bronchial arteries on each side, with one of the right bronchial arteries originating from an ICBAT
4–9	Unknown	Other variations of bronchial arteries, with up to four arteries on each side

The artery of Adamkiewicz, or greater anterior medullary artery, supplies the lumbar enlargement of the spinal cord. It is a unilateral vessel commonly seen to arise between T9 and T12 in 75% of cases with characteristic "hairpin" configuration at angiography. Although the true prevalence in unknown, in 10% to 15% of cases, the spinal arteries can arise from ICBAT. *Nontarget embolization of the anterior medullary artery leads to transverse myelitis; hence, an optimal technique with a coaxial microcatheter system placed distal to the origin of the anterior medullary artery should be undertaken during BAE.*

The radicular arteries are often visualized during BAE. In our experience, unintentional embolization of radicular arteries does not cause clinical problems such as spinal cord ischemia. It has been stated that the presence of radicular arteries is not considered to be a contraindication for BAE [117,129–132].

Causes of Bronchial Artery Hypertrophy/ Dilatation

BA hypertrophy can be seen in multiple congenital and acquired conditions as described in Table 95.10:

Congenital causes of bronchial artery hypertrophy include

- Major conotruncal anomalies (see Table 95.10) are seen to have systemic supply to pulmonary parenchyma by aortic branches known as major aortopulmonary collateral arteries (MAPCAs) or systemic-pulmonary collateral arteries. MAPCAs are seen in the majority of patients with pulmonary atresia with ventricular septal defect. In these patients, MAPCAs provide for pulmonary perfusion and survival. It has also been seen that MAPCAs likely represent hypertrophied BAs, mimicking the anatomy and branching patterns with absence of native BAs. They cause competing blood flow to the lungs and frequently undergo endovascular embolization at the time of definitive surgery. They are also used to reconstruct the neopulmonary trunk in long-segment pulmonary trunk atresia.

Acquired causes of BA hypertrophy include

- Chronic thromboembolic disease manifests on CT with vascular and parenchymal abnormalities. The vascular abnormalities include partial or complete obstruction of the PAs, which manifests as endoluminal filling defects that are often peripheral, crescentic, calcified, or linear. Complete obstruction manifests with abrupt termination, narrowing, or obliteration of a PA. Secondary signs of pulmonary hypertension include pulmonary trunk dilation (>29 mm), right ventricular or right atrial enlargement or hypertrophy, PA wall calcification, and leftward bowing of the interventricular septum. BA hypertrophy is seen secondary to interruption of the native PA supply. Parenchymal signs include lower lobe subpleural bandlike, linear, or wedge-shaped opacities that represent the sequelae of pulmonary infarction. Mosaic attenuation is often seen and manifests as sharply demarcated regions of normal lung attenuation alternating with regions of decreased lung attenuation, findings caused by differences in vascular perfusion [132–134].
- Fibrosing mediastinitis is a benign but sometimes progressive disorder characterized by infiltrative fibrous tissue in the mediastinum. The two types are nongranulomatous and granulomatous.
  - Nongranulomatous fibrosing mediastinitis usually occurs in association with autoimmune disorders or radiation therapy or as a reaction to drugs such as methysergide.
  - Granulomatous fibrosing mediastinitis can be caused by infections such as tuberculosis, cryptococcosis, and aspergillosis and as an idiosyncratic reaction to histoplasma antigens.

The most common imaging appearance is a focal soft tissue mass that distorts and narrows adjacent structures. There often is dense or stippled calcification within the mass. Ipsilateral BA dilation is seen when fibrous tissue critically encases and narrows a PA as a physiologic response to decreased blood flow to the lung [135–140].

- Chronic or acute inflammation: The bronchial circulation often dilates in patients with inflammatory conditions that affect the lungs and airways. It is thought that vasculitis and thrombosis of pulmonary vessels may occur in response to airway or parenchymal inflammation and infection. Angiogenic growth factors such as vascular endothelial growth factor are postulated to promote collateral supply and neovascularity, with proliferation and expansion of the BAs.

The most common inflammatory lung and airway disorders associated with BA dilation include tuberculosis and nontuberculous mycobacterial infections, cystic fibrosis and other causes of bronchiectasis, mycetoma, and chronic fungal infections. Patients may be asymptomatic or may present with life-threatening hemoptysis resulting from BA hypertrophy, dilation, and eventual rupture. The characteristic CT appearance of mycetoma is a solid round or oval gravity-dependent mass within a cavity. There frequently is a crescent of air separating the mass from the cavity wall, a finding termed the "air crescent" sign. In patients who present with hemoptysis and mycetoma, the radiologist should search for hypertrophied BAs to provide a vascular road map for the interventionalist before BA embolization [141–144].

TABLE 95.11 Causes of Bronchial Artery Hypertrophy

Congenital	Acquired
Pulmonary atresia with ventricular septal defect	Chronic thromboembolic disease
Tetralogy of Fallot	Bronchiectasis, infection, and malignancy
Transposition of great arteries	Fibrosing mediastinitis
Double outlet right ventricle	Pulmonary hypertension
Truncus arteriosus	
Proximal interruption of the pulmonary artery	

Frequently, necrotic squamous cell cancer is the most common cause of massive hemoptysis in adults older than 40 years with neovascularity, destruction of parenchyma by the tumor, and angioinvasion. CT demonstrates abnormal BA or, rarely, active contrast agent extravasation as the source [145,146].

Bronchial Artery Embolization Technique [147–156]

Bronchial artery embolization has become an established procedure in the management of massive and recurrent hemoptysis; its use was first reported in 1973 by Remy et al [147,148].

Angiography: Angiography and intervention are performed under either moderate sedation or general anesthesia, as dictated by the clinical presentation and status of the patient. Standard common femoral arterial access predominates, although brachial artery access may be necessary to address extraordinarily difficult NBSA contributions. All arteriography should be performed with either low-osmolar or iso-osmolar nonionic contrast material because high-osmolar contrast has been implicated in transverse myelitis. Prior multiphasic CTA is used to evaluate the number and site of origin of BAs. It is also useful in the detection of NBSA that supply parenchymal lesions.

Catheterization: The most commonly used catheters to select the BAs are Cobra, Mikaelson, Simmons, or Judkins right catheters. The usefulness of a microcatheter for selective BAE has been emphasized in many recent articles. This superselective catheterization permits stabilization of the catheter position within the BA and safe positioning in the bronchial circulation beyond the origin of spinal cord branches, which prevents severe complications. After catheterization of the BA, bronchial angiography is performed with manual injection of contrast medium.

Angiographic Findings: Angiographic findings in patients with massive hemoptysis include hypertrophic and tortuous BAs (Fig. 95.35), neovascularity, hypervascularity, and parenchymal blush (Fig. 95.36) shunting into the PA or pulmonary vein, extravasation of contrast medium, and BA aneurysm. Although extravasation of contrast medium is considered a specific sign of bronchial bleeding, this finding is rarely seen, and its reported prevalence ranges from 3.6% to 10.7%. Thus, the determination of which arteries are to be embolized should be based on a combination of CT, bronchoscopic, and angiographic findings with clinical correlation. All angiograms, including intercostal arteriograms, must be carefully scrutinized for opacification of spinal arteries to avoid inadvertent embolization.

Embolic Materials: A variety of embolic materials are used for BAE. Therefore, there is no consensus on which embolic material is best; as of now, absorbable gelatin sponge particles or polyvinyl alcohol (PVA) particles are most widely used because they are inexpensive and easy to handle and can be controlled with regard to embolic size.

- **Gelatin sponge:** Absorbable gelatin sponge is widely used because it is inexpensive and easy to handle and has a controllable embolic size. However, disadvantages of absorbable gelatin sponges are their resolvability and lack of radiopacity. Their use may lead to recanalization of the embolized artery and may sometimes be responsible for recurrent bleeding.
- **PVA:** PVA particles are nonabsorbable embolic materials, and particles 350 to 500 μm in diameter are the most frequently used worldwide. Their use may prevent the early recurrence of hemoptysis caused by recanalization of the embolized artery, as might be anticipated with absorbable gelatin sponge. It is essential to avoid the use of embolic materials that can pass through the bronchopulmonary anastomosis. In addition, it is important to

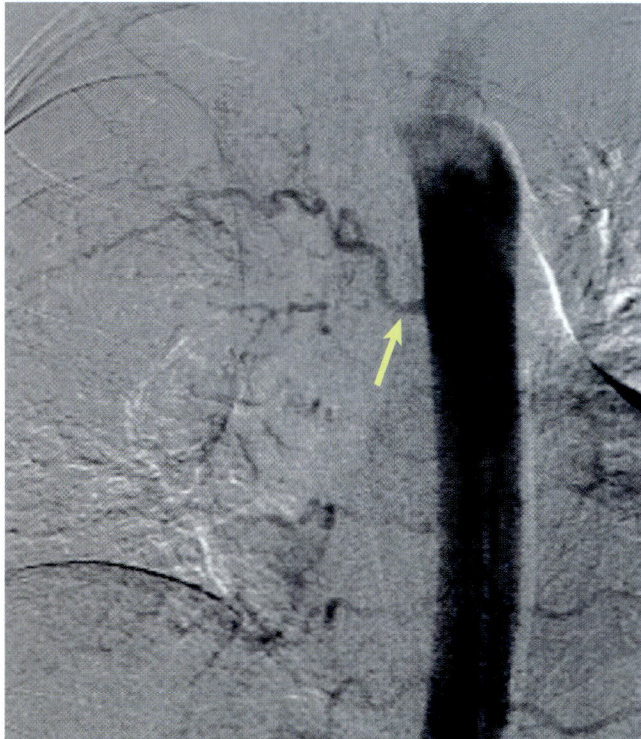

Figure 95.35 Flush aortogram of the descending thoracic aorta showing hypertrophied right bronchial artery (*yellow arrow*).

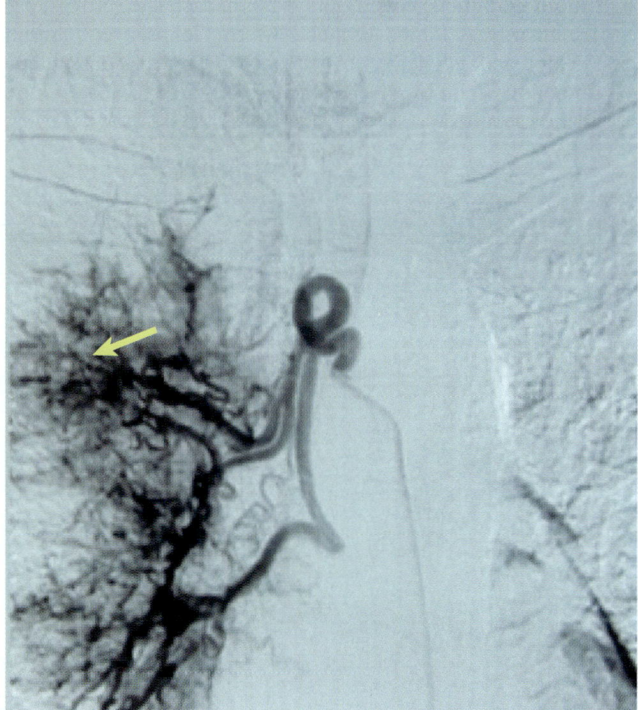

Figure 95.36 Selective angiogram of right bronchial artery showing a hypertrophied and torturous bronchial artery with abnormal parenchymal blush (*yellow arrow*).

avoid using embolic agents that produce distal occlusion to such an extent that normal peripheral branches that supply the bronchi, esophagus, or vasa vasorum of the PA or aorta become occluded, possibly leading to disastrous complications (e.g., bronchial, esophageal, PA, or aortic wall necrosis). To avoid the complications indicated earlier, we recommend the use of polyvinyl alcohol particles with a diameter of 350 to 500 μm for BAE (Fig. 95.37).

- **Microspheres:** Microspheres (e.g., Embosphere Microspheres, BioSphere Medical) are composed of cross-linked gelatin and have been used successfully, in particular for the embolization of uterine fibroids. Because of their smoothly spherical shape and hydrophilic nature, they are less prone to clumping and are more uniform in size than their PVA counterpart. In a recent study, BAE with 500- to 700-μm microspheres achieved short-term clinical success comparable to PVA particles [152,153,157].

In a recent study conducted by Kucukay et al., the technical success rate was 100%. The clinical success rate for preventing massive hemoptysis was 91.9% (160 of 174). There were no procedure-related mortality or morbidities. Minor complications such as chest pain were observed in 9 patients (5.0%). Recurrent hemoptysis (8.1%) was observed within 6 months in 14 patients, 10 of whom were treated with a second embolization session and the remaining 4 with a total of three embolization sessions. The authors concluded that BAE for massive hemoptysis with Embosphere particles 700 to 900 μm in size is a safe and effective method with high technical and clinical success rates [158]. Long-term results are excellent [153,158].

- **Liquid embolic agents:** N-butyl-2-cyanoacrylate (NBCA; e.g., TruFill n-BCA Liquid Embolic System, Johnson & Johnson/DePuy) and ethylene vinyl alcohol polymer (Onyx Liquid Embolic System, eV3 Neurovascular) for BAE have been infrequently reported.

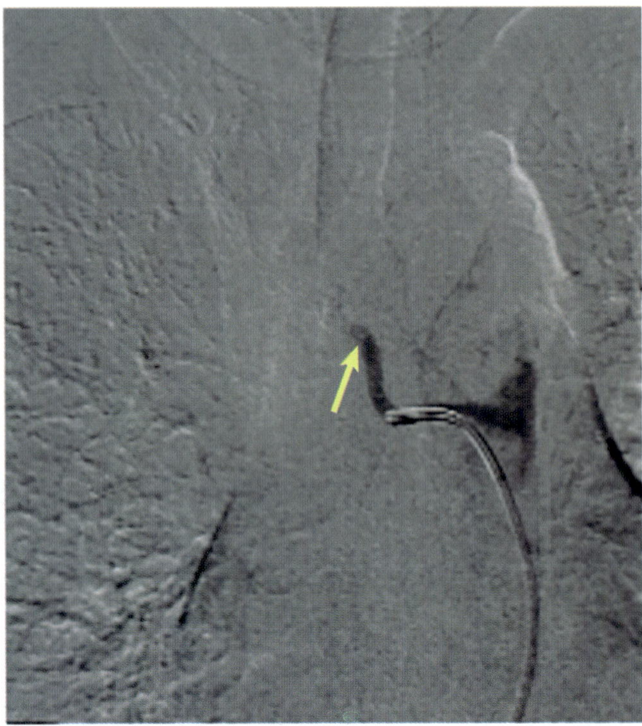

Figure 95.37 Cessation of the flow in the right bronchial artery (*yellow arrow*) *after* polyvinyl alcohol particle embolization.

Neurologic complications, probably caused by nontarget embolization of the spinal artery or vertebral artery, are the most dreaded of BAE-related complications. There has been concern that liquid embolic materials, including NBCA, may increase the risk of nontarget embolization. Another issue regarding liquid embolic agents is the possibility of necrosis of tissues, including of the aorta or bronchi.

Metallic coils: These achieve a relatively proximal occlusion in the vascular bed. In this patient population with a high rate of rebleeding, this position within the vascular tree may jeopardize further embolic attempts. In addition, as with gelatin sponges, proximal occlusion permits collateral flow, resulting in poor control of hemoptysis. Although not first-line therapy for hemoptysis per se, the presence of pseudoaneurysm in the BAs may represent an ideal situation to be managed by application of metallic coils [158,159].

Outcomes

Previous studies have shown that BAE is very effective in controlling acute massive hemoptysis. The initial nonrecurrence rates for BAE have been reported to be 73% to 98%, with a mean follow-up period ranging from 1 day to 1 month. Immediate success rates have increased recently because of the introduction of superselective embolization and the refinement of embolic agents and techniques. However, the long-term success rate of BAE in hemoptysis is unfavorable. Long-term recurrence rates have been reported to be 10% to 52%, with a mean follow-up period ranging from 1 to 46 months. However, the long-term success rate can be improved with repeat BAE.

Hemoptysis may recur after successful BAE if the disease process is not controlled with drug therapy or surgery because embolization does not address the underlying disease but rather treats the symptom. In this sense, BAE is a palliative procedure that prepares the patient for elective surgery for localized disease or continued antimicrobial therapy.

Causes of recurrences include

- Recanalization of embolized vessels
- Incomplete embolization
- Revascularization by the collateral circulation
- Inadequate treatment of the underlying disease
- Progression of basic lung disease or NBSA supply

Depending on the cause, recurrence rates can be highly variable, and in the setting of infectious (e.g., tuberculosis, aspergillus) or neoplastic (e.g., bronchogenic carcinoma) offenders, one can expect nearly all patients to eventually hemorrhage.

Despite technical success, clinical remission is not always achieved. Generally accepted rates of cessation of hemoptysis after technically successful BAE approach 90%. Remobilization is an accepted approach to recurrent hemoptysis; however, surgery remains the definitive treatment for patients with hemoptysis recalcitrant to multiple embolizations and maximum medical therapy [130,159–161].

Complications

Several complications of BAE have been reported in the literature. Chest pain is the most common complication, with a reported prevalence of 24% to 91%. Chest pain is likely related to an ischemic phenomenon caused by embolization and is usually transient. In addition, dysphagia caused by embolization of esophageal branches may be encountered, with a reported prevalence of 0.7% to 18.2%. Dysphagia also regresses spontaneously. Subintimal dissection of the aorta or the BA during BAE is the other minor complication, with a reported prevalence of 1% to 6.3%. There are usually no symptoms or problems related to the subintimal dissection.

The most disastrous complication of BAE is spinal cord ischemia caused by inadvertent occlusion of spinal arteries. The prevalence of spinal cord ischemia after BAE is reported to be 1.4% to 6.5%.

Other rare complications that have been reported in the literature include aortic and bronchial necrosis, bronchoesophageal fistula, nontarget organ embolization (e.g., ischemic colitis), pulmonary infarction, referred pain to the ipsilateral forehead and orbit, and transient cortical blindness. It is hypothesized that cortical blindness develops because of embolism to the occipital cortex, either via a BA–pulmonary vein shunt or via collateral vessels between the bronchial and vertebral arteries. Pain in the orbit or temporal region ipsilateral to the side of embolization may occur but is thought to be referred pain rather than nontarget embolization in these territories [154,162,163].

Conclusion

Optimal management of patients having different pathologies requires a collaboration among interventional radiologists, clinicians, the critical care team, and anesthesiologists in patient management. Nowadays, the endovascular intervention procedures for various pathologies as discussed in this chapter are effective as well as safer substitutes as compared with surgery.

Suggested Readings

- American College of Obstetricians and Gynecologists. ACOG practice bulletin: alternatives to hysterectomy in the management of leiomyomas, Obstet Gynecol 112 (2 pt 1) (2008) 387–400.
- SP Deshmukh, CF Gonsalves, FF Guglielmo, DG Mitchell, Role of MR imaging of uterine leiomyomas before and after embolization, RadioGraphics 32 (6) (2012) E251–E281.
- DD Janette, M Lindsay, Pelvic congestion syndrome, Semin Intervent Radiol 30 (4) (2013 Dec) 372–380.
- ST Amy, Fallopian tube catheterization, Semin Intervent Radiol 25 (4) (2008 Dec) 425–431.

vertebral augmentation, and procedural success is largely dependent on patient selection, duration of the patient's pain, and technique. The consensus opinion supported by a reasonable scientific premise is that severe pain due to osteoporotic fractures of vertebral bodies may be alleviated by vertebroplasty and vertebral augmentation. These results can be sustained by regular physical therapy and reconditioning of paraspinal muscle strength. Alteration of biomechanics by the vertebral augmentation can lead to adjacent level fractures, a risk that is somewhat lower following vertebroplasty without augmentation.

Radiofrequency ablation of vertebral bodies with tumor involvement can also be used before vertebroplasty or vertebral augmentation in pathological vertebral body fractures or collapses. For patients with painful osseous metastases that have failed standard treatments such as systemic chemotherapy and radiation therapy, radiofrequency ablation of the tumor can provide pain relief [91]. This technique was expanded to include painful vertebral body metastases with adjunctive vertebroplasty for stability and aid in analgesia [92,93].

Future Directions

Since its inception in the late 1990s and early 2000s with a good scientific level of evidence for endovascular treatment of ruptured cerebral aneurysms, the specialty of NIR has become more and more established over the past two decades. Currently, the majority of ruptured and unruptured aneurysms are treated endovascularly. Mechanical thrombectomy is a proven treatment for acute ischemic stroke secondary to large vessel occlusion with eligibility criteria that continue to expand. The trajectory of NIR as a specialty over the next two decades holds promise as newer and more robust minimally invasive techniques gain good scientific evidence for improved outcomes in patients with neurovascular and other neurological pathologies.

There is a general anxiety amongst radiologists practicing neurointervention that the field will be taken over by our neurosurgery and neurology colleagues who have established themselves in this practice. However, as diagnostic cerebral angiography is still the gold standard in the diagnosis of many cerebrovascular diseases radiologists play a key role in the field due to the emphasis on the physics of image optimization and the importance of overall radiation dose reduction. As such, most large-volume centers employ all three specialties within the realm of neurointervention. This collaboration is a strength of the field as each specialty brings different perspectives of treatment and overall enhances patient care. Future directions for this field are only limited by the imagination. Devices are constantly improving, and with continued collaboration between radiology, neurosurgery, and neurology, the possibilities are endless.

Suggested Readings

- AY Liu, Update on interventional neuroradiology, Perm J 10 (2006) 42–46.
- OA Berkhemer, PS Fransen, D Beumer, et al., A randomized trial of intraarterial treatment for acute ischemic stroke, N Engl J Med 372 (2015) 11–20.
- TG Brott, RW Hobson, 2nd, G Howard, et al., Stenting versus endarterectomy for treatment of carotid-artery stenosis, N Engl J Med 363 (2010) 11–23.
- TL Rosenberg, JY Suen, GT Richter, Arteriovenous Malformations of the Head and Neck, Otolaryngol Clin North Am 51 (2018) 185–195.
- W Clark, P Bird, P Gonski, et al., Safety and efficacy of vertebroplasty for acute painful osteoporotic fractures (VAPOUR): a multicentre, randomised, double-blind, placebo-controlled trial, Lancet 388 (2016) 1408–1416.

97

Musculoskeletal Interventional Radiology

ROBIN PROCTOR

Introduction

This chapter covers the basic principles and justifications for musculoskeletal interventional procedures with information on methods, indications, contraindications, and the different materials that may be used. More information around the specific application of individual procedures in relation to specific body sites and specific diseases can be found in the relevant chapters covering the relevant area.

Basic Principles of Musculoskeletal Intervention

The basic principle for an interventional procedure is to use imaging guidance to accurately access the relevant area percutaneously, that is, without an open procedure and while avoiding contact with adjacent structures that might be damaged. There is a wide range of procedures that may then be performed under image guidance and broadly they may be diagnostic, therapeutic, or a combination of the two. They may not involve any material being injected or removed (e.g., dry needling or cutting a structure), may involve adding material (e.g., local anesthetic, therapeutic agent, or cement), may involve removing material (e.g., drainage, barbotage, or biopsy), or some combination of the above.

Most national or regional societies offer guidance and peer support for those who are developing an interest in interventional musculoskeletal radiology and there are a number of more specialist reference texts available for those seeking more information [1–6].

Preparation for Musculoskeletal Interventional Procedures

Although an image-guided percutaneous procedure may spare the patient an operation, it remains invasive and the principles of informed consent still apply. Best practice is for the patient to be informed of the range of options available to them, including the likely outcome of doing nothing, as well as the intended benefits and possible complications from the procedure being proposed. If possible they should be given time to consider this information, for instance by receiving written information in advance or being given access to online guidance and afforded an opportunity to ask questions before the procedure is performed. The exact range of complications that should be quoted must be tailored to the patient and this is particularly relevant in musculoskeletal practice where the needs and aspirations of an elite athlete, a child with a suspected sarcoma, and an older patient with osteoarthritis may be very different.

Practical preparation for the procedure is also important. Many potential complications may be avoided by thinking or talking through the procedure in advance ensuring that the necessary staff and equipment are available and that the patient will be appropriately positioned and comfortable enough to remain still for the duration of the procedure.

Routine use of checklists has been shown to reduce medical error in relation to surgery. The degree of parallel with surgical practice depends on the procedure and some jurisdictions will enforce similar procedures before interventional radiology procedures [7]. Even when not required by legislation some adoption of similar techniques, such as skin marking to identify the correct side, level, and location can be advantageous.

Range of Technique and Evidence

Much of the exact technique for individual musculoskeletal procedures varies from one part of the world to another and from one operator to another. The potential variance between what is ostensibly the same procedure performed by different operators together with the modest volume of some procedures makes research more difficult, and in many areas there is a dearth of high-quality evidence [8–10].

There are sometimes strong and politicized opinions and national and regional guidance varies. Understandably, patients with persistent symptoms and their doctors are often willing to try procedures where evidence is weak.

Choice of Technique

Often there are many possible approaches and more than one technique that could reasonably be considered. Other than suitable equipment and an appropriately trained operator being available, the fundamental requirements are that the patient can be positioned in a comfortable enough position that they can remain still for the duration of the procedure and that sterility can be maintained. For some procedures, a full-sterile field may be required and for others it may be more appropriate for a smaller area to be sterilized and an "aseptic no-touch technique" to be adopted.

Just as when radiographic techniques are considered for diagnostic work, the advantages and disadvantages are similar and training, availability, and individual preference may determine which technique is selected.

Understanding the procedure and the potential complications are critical to allow for selection of an appropriate technique. For instance, when performing a guided injection to achieve a cervical nerve root block puncture of the vertebral artery is a potentially very serious complication because it may lead to dissection and more so were any particulate injectate to be administered with potential embolic effects to the posterior circulation. Confident location of the tip of the needle away from structures of concern and aspiration before injection to confirm a nonintravascular position are prudent but depending on training some authors advocate precise location [11], while others prefer fluoroscopy because of its dynamic rather than static nature to detect intravascular spread with a test injection of iodinated contrast [12]. The relative strengths and weaknesses of each technique are considered as they are described below.

Typically ultrasonography (USG), *fluoroscopy, or CT* are used to guide interventional musculoskeletal procedures, although other approaches using x-rays as an adjunct to landmark techniques are described. USG or fluoroscopy are commonly used to access joints for direct MR arthrography but other than in specialist settings use of MRI to guide musculoskeletal interventions is rare [13].

Aseptic technique is required for interventional procedures and the size of the field and exact technique depends on the procedure. In some scenarios, there will be a large field and all of the field will require to remain sterile but in other procedures, for instance if it is possible to puncture some distance from a guiding probe, then a more limited field or no-touch technique sterilizing only the direct path of the needle may be appropriate.

Ultrasonography

USG is very operator dependent but readily available at the bedside and requires more modestly priced equipment than the alternatives. It does not involve radiation and offers real-time guidance but has limited penetration depth and cannot see beyond certain structures, such as the surface of bowel or bone [14].

Because USG requires line of sight to the area of interest, it is generally less useful for osseous procedures, other than accessing the surface of abnormal bone, or for deep procedures. What may be considered deep will vary from one operator to another and it is safer to remain within one's competence and change technique in the acute setting of an individual patient while more slowly upskilling is required than to persevere with an unfamiliar situation.

USG-guided procedures are particularly useful for tendon-related pathology because the diagnostic procedure may be quickly performed at the same time and other than in the largest patients most appendicular tendons are sufficiently close to the surface for extremely good resolution. As for diagnostic procedures *anisotropy* is a key consideration and it may be necessary to "heel-toe" (i.e., to indent one side of the probe further into the overlying soft tissues or to use stand-off gel on the other end of the probe) to maintain an approach perpendicular to the tendon to minimize anisotropy which, if unrecognized, might be mistaken for tendinopathy and lead to unnecessary intervention. Similarly, if neovascularity is being assessed to identify the degree of abnormality before intervention then light pressure with additional gel or a stand-off may necessary to minimize the risk that pressure from the operator would compress the tissues and lead to underassessment of the neovascularity.

Broadly, there are two techniques to insert a needle when using an USG probe:

- *"Out of plane"* where the needle is inserted perpendicular (transverse) to the beam where more vertical penetration following the direction of the beam into the body is usual and where the puncture is adjacent to the probe
- *"In plane"* where the needle is inserted longitudinally along the length of the probe as in Fig. 97.1. In longitudinal guidance, the intention is to see a longer length of the needle, including the tip and to guide it to the intended place. The strongest echo is produced when the beam is perpendicular to an object and having the bevel pointing toward the beam aids visualization of a needle

For longitudinal guidance to be possible, it is necessary to insert the needle at a shallow enough angle to the probe so that it is possible to see the needle. This may necessitate a track starting with a puncture site several centimeters from the edge of the probe and, particularly for deeper interventions, if a puncture is made too close to the probe then the penetration may be too vertical to enable the needle to be adequately visualized. Angling the probe by rocking it "heel-toeing" the probe can help bring it more perpendicular to the track of the needle and most USG machines will allow a degree of beam steering, which can also be useful to angle the beam to be more perpendicular to the needle. Some manufacturers also offer advanced needle visualization software and special needles offering increased passive or actively echogenicity have also been described. Even with those techniques the strongest echo will be generally be produced when the needle is parallel to the probe (i.e., perpendicular to the beam) and the major learning point is to expect progressive loss of visualization as it is angled deeper and more parallel with the beam.

While learning it is necessary to learn to split concentration between the positions of the probe and needle in the operator's hands, which can be directly observed, and also the findings which can be seen on the screen. The aim with longitudinal tracking of the needle is to maintain visualization of the tip and it is important to develop an awareness of whether the needle may be out of the plane of the beam which may often give a similar appearance on screen if it is passing obliquely across the beam.

Larger needles are easier to see and if the bevel can be identified, then it is possible to be sure the tip is in view. Rapidly "bouncing" the needle along the path can help. Keeping the bevel

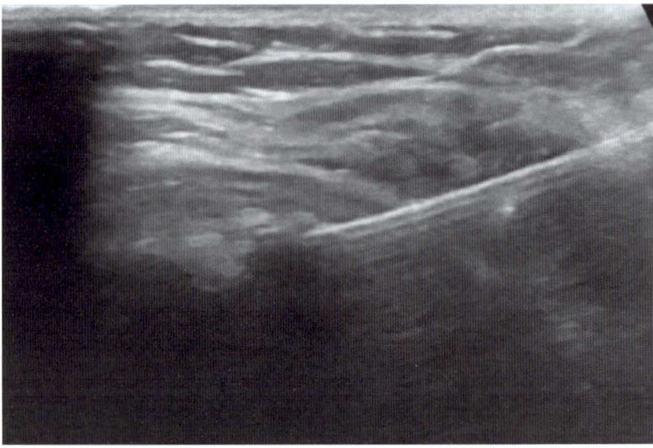

Figure 97.1 USG-guided barbotage of calcific deposit within supraspinatus tendon showing approach of the needle from the right side of the screen. The brightest line near the probe is the needle surface and the multiple parallel lines deep to this within an area of otherwise low signal are reverberation artifact that are strongest when fully in plane with the needle and can aid recognition and tracking of the needle.

up can aid visualization; and awareness of machine settings which may help or hinder visualization (such as steer or harmonics) is also helpful.

Despite these techniques, it can be challenging to maintain the view of the tip of the needle and if it is necessary to adjust the configuration to maintain view or to find the tip of the needle then in general moving either the probe or the needle is more effective than trying to manipulate them both at the same time. If the position of the needle tip is unknown then moving the needle may be hazardous and moving the probe away from the needle, rocking it toward the path and visually aligning the probe with the path before slowly sweeping the probe across this path is effective to find the needle tip.

Needle guides are available for many probes that will hold a needle in the plane of the ultrasound beam and maintain a defined angle of approach. This may be advantageous in some circumstances, but the fixed angle of approach can also become limiting if it is necessary to change angle during the approach, for instance to navigate around a structure on the approach or to avoid an osteophyte or other object near the site of the procedure. Depending on the location, a test injection may be appropriate and when the tip is in view fluid will be seen to flow from the tip. If even a small quantity of air is injected then it creates acoustic shadowing which can hinder further work with USG.

There is no substitute for practice, as well as commercially available phantoms many experts have trained by using their own phantoms constructed from commercially available meat.

Fluoroscopy

Fluoroscopy may also provide real-time guidance and the image, although importantly not the actual tissue, will be less hindered by overlying structures. Typically, the beam may be angled in each plane and by doing this and performing intermittent exposure the progress of the needle can be monitored.

Screening in two planes is one technique to locate the needle tip accurately. An alternative technique is to make an approach along the track of the beam with intermittent exposures after adjusting or advancing the needle. Using this second technique even the longest needle appears as a dot on the screen as the beam is along its length and if it moves out of the line of the beam then the needle will appear to elongate. It then becomes possible to see the hub and tip of the needle separately and for adjustments to be made to return to the intended track as shown in Fig. 97.2.

The need to use radiation and iodinated contrast when confirming position during fluoroscopy may be limiting for some patient populations and locations.

It is possible to increase resolution and magnify the image, but this comes with the penalty of increased radiation dose so resolution should be kept at the minimum required to safely perform the procedure.

To minimize exposure of the operator it is necessary for them to keep their hands out of the primary beam and this can be facilitated by coning the beam to a smaller anatomical area. When working across the beam the tip of the needle can be visualized and moved in real time but intermittent screening between adjustments is required when working along the length of the beam.

Fluoroscopy may be especially effective in navigating a narrow track in a plane that is more oblique than can be delivered with CT or where there are well-defined bony margins or landmarks, for instance traversing a pedicle to access a vertebral body when performing biopsy or augmentation to the vertebral body.

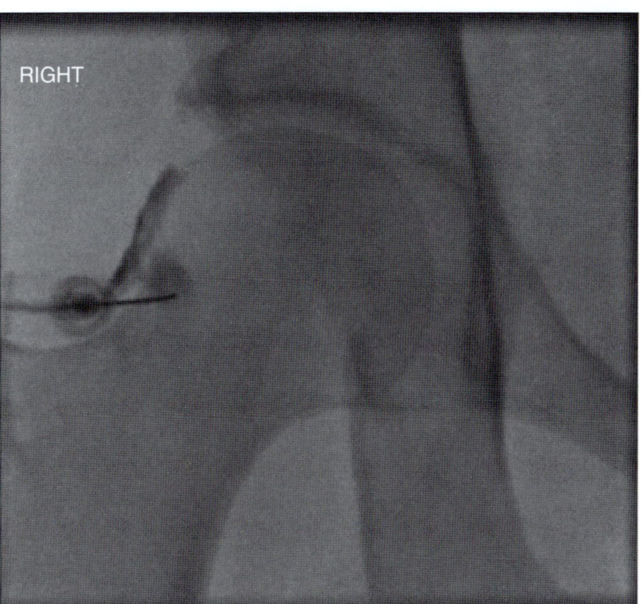

Figure 97.2 Intraarticular injection into right hip to prepare for MR arthrogram. The needle is 9 cm long but because viewed almost along the length it appears much shorter with the hub slightly lateral to the tip and with iodinated contrast having already passed into the joint and visible lateral to the femoral head.

Computed Tomography (CT)

With CT it is possible to see the whole depth of tissue through which an approach is being made and to access deeper structures. CT generally requires a greater amount of radiation than fluoroscopy although with increasingly powerful reconstruction algorithms this dose penalty is diminishing.

Once a needle is inserted a series of images are taken centered on a selected gantry position and the track may then be assessed and modified or the needle advanced before further images are taken. Most CT scanners have a biopsy mode where such slices may be repeated as the approach for a procedure is made.

If an approach can be made in the plane of the scanner gantry and in an orthogonal plane to the room, then it is much easier for most operators to establish and maintain the intended course (Fig. 97.3).

The thickness of the needle should be considered when selecting the thickness and number of the images being acquired and when learning it. Depending on local policy and practice, the operator may wear appropriate personal protective equipment and remain within the room or may wear normal clothing and leave the scan room during each acquisition.

It is possible to utilize CT fluoroscopy where images are obtained in real time and this may provide benefit in certain cases but it can rapidly increase radiation dose and it also becomes harder for the operator to remain out of the primary beam and to minimize their own dose.

Practical Tips

- The more at ease and comfortable the patient can be the more likely they are to stay still and thus the easier the procedure is likely to be. Adequate analgesia is important and because certain tissues are better innervated (skin, periosteum) using adequate local analgesia at the puncture site and going through the subcutaneous tissue quickly is likely to minimize discomfort.

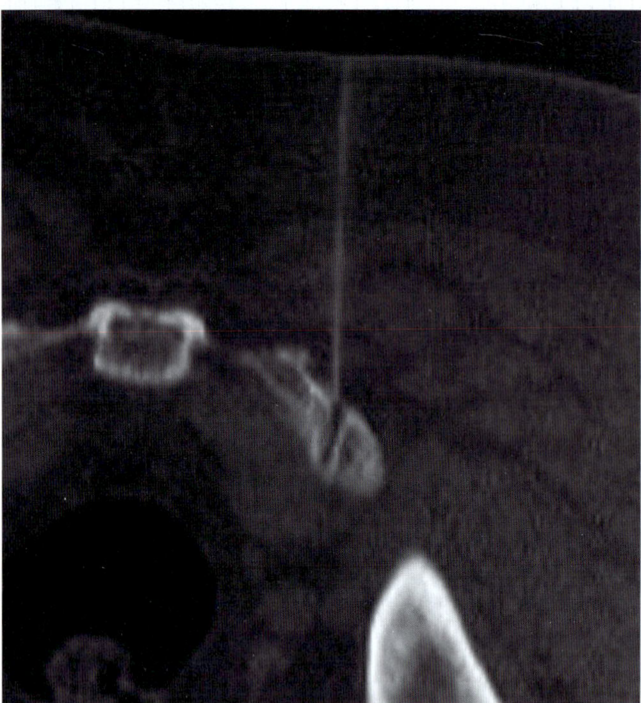

Figure 97.3 CT-guided injection into inferior aspect of left sacroiliac joint. Note the patient is positioned prone for comfort and ease of access and that the needle track is vertical and in the plane of the CT image to make it easier to perform (skin to margin of joint is 9 cm).

- *Syringe exchange:* If it is necessary to exchange the syringe to inject more than one substance, for instance to change to inject a therapeutic agent after first confirming position, then it is important to stabilize the needle to prevent displacement. If the size of the target and volume to be delivered permits, then a connecting tube may be helpful and allow the exchange to be performed distant from the needle to minimize the chance of displacement. Secure attachment of syringe and needle is a requirement but if an exchange is planned then this should not be any more firm than necessary to make a seal as straining to undo a stuck connection can make displacement of the needle more likely.
- *Choice of needles:* The key considerations are the length and diameter of the needle. Some longer needles are only available as spinal needles and compatibility with other available equipment must be considered. Because of safety measures designed to minimize the risk of inadvertent intrathecal administration of intravenous treatments, there is no universal compatibility between needles, connectors, and syringes.
  The wider the needle the easier it will be to make it go in a straight line and to see regardless of the technique but the more difficult it will be to bend and the greater the trauma to tissues it passes through or risk of damage if a structure is contacted unintentionally.
  For aspiration, the radius of the needle is the key feature (flow varies with the fourth power of the radius and inversely with the length); hence, the broadest and shortest needle which will safely access the area being aspirated should be selected.
  Biopsy needles come in a variety of different configurations. Most soft tissue biopsy needles are spring loaded to take a sample and some can be used to selectively take short or longer samples. The key consideration is an awareness of which piece of tissue will be sampled to enable the core to be obtained from the intended area. When the device is "fired" some will sample along the track which has already been traversed and some will sample the material immediately distal to the position of the tip.
- *Steering the needle:* Regardless of the technique used, it is possible to make many needles follow a curved path that may be useful to avoid an obstacle or a hindrance to be minimized if the path to the region of interest is straight.
  The shape of the tip of the needle will influence the direction of travel and with a bevel, the tip will tend to move away from the side of the opening as the needle is advanced, "bevel control". This is more pronounced with thinner needles and some shapes of bevel. The hub of many needles are marked to demonstrate the orientation of the bevel and an operator should become familiar with the orientation of such a marking or make their own mark on the hub so they are confident of the orientation of the needle once it is below the skin surface. The degree of movement in one direction may also be changed by bending the needle, which is also easier with thinner needles but if this is attempted it is imperative that the operator is experienced with the technique and does not apply so much force as to break the needle.
- *Volume of injectate:* The amount injected should be considered both in terms of dose of any drugs administered and the total volume. High-volume techniques (e.g., 50 mL paratenon injection around the Achilles) are advocated by some authors and an appropriate diluent, such as saline with a small amount of local anesthetic must be selected as such volumes of many local anesthetics would be toxic. *Such high-volume techniques are also contentious and not yet supported by strong evidence* [15].

Individual Procedures

Biopsies

Just as in other body systems, a tissue diagnosis may be vital in the diagnosis and treatment of musculoskeletal disease. The basic techniques of fine-needle aspiration for cytology or core biopsy for histopathology are broadly the same as in other techniques; however, certain points should be emphasized as particularly important for musculoskeletal procedures.

Particularly, for suspected bone and soft tissue *sarcomas* and also for other primary bone tumors, the approach for any biopsy may be critical as it may *contaminate the track* and determine the subsequent operative approach. Consequently, the route of a biopsy should be agreed in advance with the relevant surgeon who would perform resection.

Where a lesion is heterogeneous, it may be necessary to agree which element should be biopsied. Broadly, the elements that enhance but which are not vascular structures will be more likely to yield useful tissue rather than necrotic material, although they are often closest to vessels and at greatest risk of bleeding. For some lesions, such as suspected lipomatous tumors, particularly for larger lesions, biopsy may be falsely reassuring as it is not possible to sample the entire lesion and the most relevant component may be missed.

For all these reasons, multidisciplinary team working and centralized treatment of such conditions is the norm in many jurisdictions and familiarity with the arrangements in each center is required.

Although steering needles is possible through soft tissue and some novel devices for steering through bone do exist, it is more

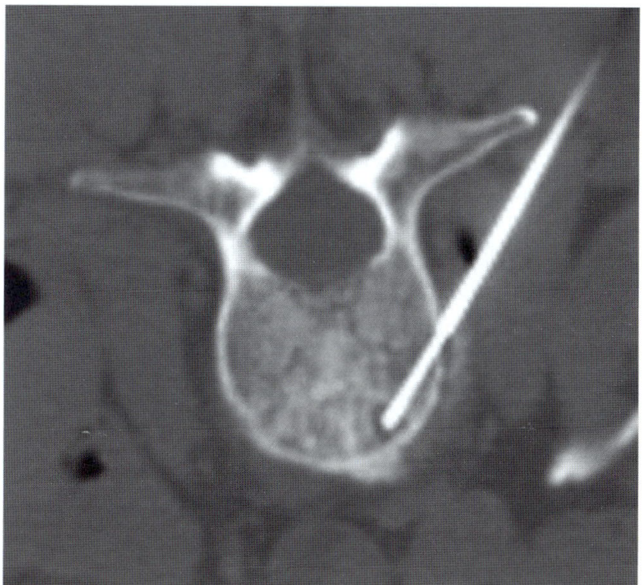

Figure 97.4 Bone biopsy of suspicious lesion within L2 vertebral body in patient with known breast carcinoma. In this case the lesion is distant from the spinal canal with normal intervening bone but more caution would be required if abnormal tissue extended to the dural surface.

usually the case that the site and angle of penetration into a bone will determine the subsequent track so it must be carefully selected, see for example a bone biopsy in Fig. 97.4. The periosteum is well innervated and more local anesthetic will be required there than in the overlying soft tissues.

If a procedure is to pass through a bone and out the other side, then it will be necessary to warn the patient that they will feel the penetration through the deep surface of the bone and further local anesthetic is likely to be required at this location as the deep periosteum is traversed.

Even when the cortex of a bone has been destroyed some mineralized matrix may remain and depending on the extent it may be necessary to use bone biopsy equipment or it may be possible to sample a section without mineralization using a soft tissue biopsy needle taking care to recognize which section of tissue will be taken when a spring-loaded biopsy device is being used when a soft tissue biopsy is performed.

Contraindications to biopsy are similar to those in other body systems

- where it is not safely possible to obtain tissue without damaging adjacent critical structures, or
- where there is a risk of making a situation far worse, for instance the risk of epidural hematoma from a vertebral lesion could alter whether a procedure was performed depending on the integrity of the cortex adjacent to the spinal canal and the amount of space around the cord/cauda equina at that level.

The risks from a biopsy procedure are pain, bleeding, introduction of infection, nondiagnostic sample, and damage to other structures. The precise value of each risk and their relative importance will vary by location, lesion being targeted, and the patient's own values and aspirations.

Aspiration

There are a number of areas where diagnostic or therapeutic aspiration may be performed for musculoskeletal procedures, for instance to drain a collection or to establish if it is infected, to perform arthrocentesis, or to target a ganglion or Baker's cyst. The material being drained should be considered when an appropriate needle is selected: Ganglion contents are typically extremely viscous and aspiration may be difficult if not impossible unless a wide bore (e.g., 16G) needle is used. Similarly, depending on the maturity of hematoma and the viscosity of any collection it may or may not be possible to aspirate to dryness. Where it is not possible to drain material at the initial attempt it may be effective to instill some saline or other fluid to dilute the material of interest and then aspirate the resulting mixture.

Table 97.1 lists the typical characteristics of different types of collection. In practice, it remains necessary to send samples of aspirate for appropriate laboratory testing to confirm the diagnosis although awareness of the likely diagnosis may guide selection of equipment and visual analysis of the material at the time of aspiration may help guide immediate management.

Some collections that are not infected, such as maturing hematoma, offer a very effective growing medium for bacteria and if intervention is considered then asepsis must be maintained to avoid infecting the collection. Following an aspiration some collections may recur and if left untreated others may hydrodissect and enlarge. In some scenarios, for instance when treating Morel–Lavallée lesions a consideration of the balance

TABLE 97.1 Typical Aspirate Findings in Common Conditions

Collection/Joint Aspirate	Appearance of Fluid	Viscosity	White Cell Content	Crystals
Physiological	Translucent, clear, or straw colored	Synovial fluid—thick Serous fluid—not viscous	Low	Absent
Infected	Cloudy, yellow, green, or brown	Thicker than serous fluid but less viscous than normal synovial fluid	Very high, neutrophil predominant	Absent
Hemorrhagic	Bloody/pink Varies with age of hematoma and may yellow with development of xanthochromia	Variable–tends to become less viscous as hematoma matures	Low	Absent
Inflammatory	Cloudy, yellow although often less so than with infection	Reduced viscosity	High	Present in gout, pseudogout (calcium pyrophosphate deposition disease, CPPD), and hydroxyapatite deposition disease

between these factors together with consideration of more conservative measures such as compression is necessary before attempting any aspiration.

Guided Injection

This may be performed alone or in combination with one or more of the other procedures listed and may be diagnostic or therapeutic and the target intraarticular or extraarticular. Typically a joint or other potential space is targeted, such as a tendon sheath, bursa, epineural space, tissue plane adjacent to a retinaculum or other fascia or paratenon space and material is instilled under guidance. The nature and volume of the material depends on the intended treatment. (More information on common procedures is given next and see also Table 97.2).

How to confirm the location is correct:

Under USG it is often possible to directly visualize entry to the target area and to watch injectate passing into the intended location. Under fluoroscopy, it is more usual to inject radiopaque contrast and to assess the spread of the contrast from the tip of the needle to confirm location, for instance as intraarticular, or perineural. In CT, it is possible to directly visualize the tip although some authorities also advocate the use of contrast to demonstrate that the bevel is fully within the intended body cavity.

Volume of Injectate

Whenever making an injection, the volume of the potential space should be carefully considered together with the necessary volume of any therapeutic material. This may dictate that a smaller

TABLE 97.2 Different Substances Commonly Injected During Guided Procedures in Musculoskeletal Radiology

Agent	Indication	Example Agents	Specific Complications
Local anesthetic agents	To facilitate performing procedures or injection of other material Diagnostic block Short-acting therapeutic block	Lidocaine 1% Other agents may have a longer onset and length of action: Bupivacaine Ropivacaine Levobupivacaine See comparison Table 97.3 with dose information	Cardiorespiratory and neurological symptoms with toxic dose or injection into wrong cavity (intravascular, intrathecal) Chondrotoxicity described particularly with bupivacaine
Corticosteroids (also see Table 97.3)	Antiinflammatory agents used to reduce symptoms in inflammatory processes Decreasing frequency of use in treating tendinopathy and chronic injuries but still commonly used	Choice of steroid is contentious and licensing varies by jurisdiction. Awareness of the nature of the preparation, expected duration of action and relative potency is important, for example particulate (prednisolone (depomedrol), triamcinolone (kenalog)) or dissolved (dexamethasone)	*Systemic effects:* immunosuppression, disordered glucose metabolism, *Local effects:* Embolism Post steroid flare Weakening of ligaments and tendons Fat necrosis Chondrotoxicity
Platelet-rich plasma (PRP)	Symptomatic relief and promotion of healing in tendinopathy, chronic tendon, muscle and ligament injuries. Also used in treatment of osteoarthritis and undisplaced labral tears	Prepared by centrifuging the patient's own blood to yield material with increased concentration of growth factors, cytokines, and platelets. This may be acellular or prepared with varying concentrations of leucocytes. See additional information next	Local irritation Flare or reactive effusion particularly with leucocyte-rich PRP (L-PRP)
Dextrose	Hypertonic dextrose as prolotherapy agent and promoting local tissue healing. Lower molarity dextrose may be used for perineural injection to treat allodynia	Hypertonic for prolotherapy (12.5–25%) 5% dextrose for perineural injection therapy	Symptoms usually relate to the injection and procedure rather than the dextrose
Hyaluronic acid	Treatment of osteoarthritis alone or with PRP to increase the concentration of preexisting hyaluronic acid in synovial fluid	Sodium hyaluronate	Generally well-tolerated. Effectiveness not acknowledged by all authorities. May have delayed (several weeks) therapeutic effect
Botulinum toxin	Treatment of spasticity and muscle contracture	Type A botulinum toxin that causes neuromuscular blockade: blocks cholinergic nerve terminals and decreases release of acetylcholine.	Intended to be long acting and cause paralysis which may affect other muscles if injection site or technique is suboptimal.
Chemical ablation agents	Denervation	Neat ethanol Acetic acid Sodium hydroxide	Intended to damage the location in which they are injected and provide irreversible effect so precise targeting is vital

volume of nontherapeutic material or shorter connecting tube must be used or that contrast or local anesthetic be mixed with the therapeutic agent. For instance, if a guided injection to the small joints of the hand was performed with local anesthetic and iodinated contrast it would leave very little intraarticular volume for any further therapeutic substance, such as corticosteroid, because the total potential volume of the joint capsule even when fully distended is small. Full distention of joints is also uncomfortable so patients may better tolerate procedures that do not completely fill a joint, unless this is a requirement such as in hydrodilation of the shoulder joint to treat frozen shoulder when rupture of the capsule is often intended.

Dry Needling (Needle Tenotomy)

Rather than fully cutting through the tendon, the technique is one of repeatedly passing a needle through an area of pathological tissue, such as tendinosis. This is thought to promote increased tissue response and healing. Increasingly, tendinosis has been demonstrated to be a degenerative process and not principally one of inflammation; hence, treatment with antiinflammatory measures such as steroids and nonsteroidal antiinflammatory drugs has become less popular in favor of other techniques. In some body areas, such as tennis elbow (lateral epicondylitis), there is increasing evidence that while steroids may give short-term relief they do not offer a similar improvement longer term and may lead to a worse eventual outcome than other measures [16].

The indications for dry needling are tendinosis and sometimes, and when under the care of a specialist, typical symptoms in the absence of a visible radiological abnormality. The complications are those of any injection, as well as the potential for increased damage to the tendon although it must be made clear that the tendon is already diseased and therefore not of normal strength otherwise the procedure would not be being considered.

True tenotomy and intentionally cutting a tendon or other structure percutaneously is also possible, for instance in performing a full tenotomy of plantaris in selected patients or a release of a finger flexor tendon by cutting an abnormal pulley.

Barbotage

Barbotage is indicated to treat deposits of calcium within a tendon, typically the supraspinatus tendon in the rotator cuff (Fig. 97.1). Depending on the consistency of the calcium, it may be possible to aspirate some or all of the calcium or to puncture it many times to break it up and promote a healing response. Typically, this is accompanied by a steroid injection into the subacromial/subdeltoid bursa at the completion of the barbotage.

With sufficient local anesthetic, it is usually a well-tolerated procedure with risks similar to those of any guided injection going through a tendon. If the calcium has hardened, then it may not be possible to aspirate much material or it may block the needle and some authors describe multiple needle techniques to flush through the region of interest.

Ablation

There are a number of reasons to wish to destroy material, for instance to target a metastasis or primary lesion or to permanently denervate a painful nerve. Several techniques exist that have their own advantages and disadvantages using chemical or thermal agents.

- Chemical ablation may be used for denervation, for instance in the context of chronic pain
- Radiofrequency ablation generates heat and may be used as a primary treatment for selected lesions that would be difficult to access or resect, for example osteoid osteomas
- Cryoablation using cold rather than heat is also available and has been described for the treatment of musculoskeletal lesions

By their very nature all forms of ablation are potentially destructive and should be considered irreversible specialist procedures.

Augmentation Procedures: Cementoplasty, Vertebroplasty, Kyphoplasty

It is possible to percutaneously introduce cement to strengthen bone, relieve pain, and promote fracture healing. This has a range of uses from persistent pain following osteoporotic vertebral fracture, typically after failed conservative management and demonstrating that the fracture is still active on MRI (high signal on fluid sensitive sequences) to treatment of metastatic disease to relieve pain and stabilize the underlying bone.

Choice of Injectate

A very large range of materials have been described as being of potential benefit in guided musculoskeletal procedures. This is a developing and sometimes contentious area where practice and exact protocol varies from jurisdiction to jurisdiction and from institution to institution. Most important is to understand the principles behind the agents being used and to consider their complications.

Prolotherapy is the process of injecting material to promote the patient's own response and achieve healing, for instance using hypertonic dextrose or platelet-rich plasma (PRP).

In any procedure, there is always the potential for no therapeutic response and the risks from any such procedure remain: pain, bleeding, and risk of introduction of infection. In addition, there are some specific complications relating to certain injectates as listed in Table 97.2.

- *Choice of steroids:* Some reports suggest that the risk of fat necrosis varies with choice of steroid and there are a range of claims about efficacy. There has been a move away from using corticosteroids for many pathologies, particularly soft tissue pathologies such as lateral epicondylitis because, although short-term outcomes may be favorable, there is evidence of a worse long-term effect.

  As with any drug there are absolute contraindications (e.g., uncontrolled infection) and relative contraindications (e.g., poorly controlled diabetes, hypertension, or poor preprocedural condition of the joint). Knowledge of local and general side effects of corticosteroids and of relative potency are important, as well as local protocols as has been previously emphasized.

  All steroids give the potential for adrenal suppression and in some patient groups and certain combinations with other drugs this may be markedly potentiated and profound, for example, triamcinolone potentiated by some antiretrovirals (e.g., ritonavir) that can lead to adrenal suppression even after a single dose.

  The solubility of steroids varies and the less-soluble steroids intentionally have particles of the active component within the vials even after shaking. The theory of particulate steroids is

TABLE 97.3 Typical Clinically Useful Concentrations, Dose, Time of Onset and Duration of Selected Local Anesthetics When Used in Soft Tissues [21]

Local Anesthetic	Typical Concentration	Dose	Duration of Onset	Duration of Effect (Soft Tissue)
Lidocaine	1% typical, 2% may be useful in nerve blocks	Adult—max total dose 300 mg	Quick <5 min	2 h
Ropivacaine	0.5%	Up to 200 mg	10–20 min	4–8 h
Bupivacaine	0.25% or 0.5%	Up to 150 mg	10–20 min	5–16 h
Levobupivacaine (S-optical isomer of bupivacaine)	0.25%	Up to 150 mg	10–20 min	5–16 h

they are more likely to be locally active for a long time and will be less systemically circulated and absorbed [17]. Embolic effects are, however, a risk with particulate steroids because they would function as a particulate embolic agent if inadvertently injected intravascularly. Consequently, extreme caution of avoiding them all together is recommended around certain sites, cervical neural foraminal injections, in particular, to avoid causing embolic infarctions.

Methylprednisolone acetate or triamcinolone acetonide are popular choices when a particulate preparation is suitable.

Symptoms may transiently worsen after injection—a "post injection flare." This tends to occur within 1–2 days (sooner than is typical for infection) and typically lasts several days. Such symptoms are common and have been described in up to one-third of patients [18]; hence, appropriate counseling is recommended. The presence of a flare is not associated with either good or bad outcome overall.

Less common but potentially significant local complications of steroids include weakening of the tendons and ligaments and an association with rupture, skin atrophy/depigmentation and fat necrosis. Fat necrosis and skin depigmentation are thought to be less problematic with methylprednisolone than triamcinolone.

There is some evidence of chondrotoxic effect from corticosteroids and they are known to potentiate chondrotoxicity from local anesthetics, at least *in vitro*, see next under local anesthetics.

- *Platelet-rich plasma (PRP) [19]*: PRP is now supported by evidence in a number of areas of the body, such as treatment of lateral epicondylitis, osteoarthritis of the knee, patellar tendinopathy, and plantar fasciitis with mixed evidence in a number of other areas. Its use varies internationally but where established it has taken over from corticosteroid for many of these indications.

  Injection of PRP begins by harvesting the patient's own blood in a tube with anticoagulant and strict asepsis is required. Various proprietary techniques are available which revolve around centrifugation to separate the red blood cells, platelet poor plasma, and the desired PRP. After centrifugation selected layers are harvested to give the intended preparation. This takes between 5 and 20 min and different preparations are possible: those which contain leukocytes are thought to have more pro-inflammatory properties and to be less favored than leukocyte-poor PRP. The optimal concentration is yet to be established but it has been suggested that it is possible for PRP to be too concentrated.

  Some authorities use PRP without prior activation but activation before injection is often thought necessary and may be achieved by physical or chemical methods. The volume depends on the site of injection and is commonly 10 mL for the knee.

  There are many active compounds within PRP and the suggested mechanism of action is that platelets are activated (endogenously or before injection) and release various growth factors, which in turn influence cell migration and the overall effect is to promote tissue repair.

  Because tissue response is important most practitioners encourage patients to stop nonsteroidal antiinflammatory drugs (NSAIDs) for a period before the procedure and post procedure advice is generally to avoid ice, heat, NSAIDs, and other measures that would usually be intended to reduce tissue response, for at least the first 3 days after the procedure.

- *Local anesthetics:* Lidocaine, ropivacaine, bupivacaine, and levobupivacaine have all been demonstrated to be toxic to human chondrocytes *in vitro* which appears to be a dose- and time-dependent effect that is potentiated by the addition of corticosteroids. Ropivacaine may be the least chondrotoxic of these local anesthetics [18].

  These (and many other available local anesthetics) vary by the useful concentrations, dose, speed of onset, and duration. Table 97.3 shows typical clinically useful concentrations, dose, time of onset, and duration of selected local anesthetics when used in soft tissues but there is a wide range of these factors in clinical use and *senior advice should be sought in cases of uncertainty*. The maximum safe dose varies according to the site and relative perfusion of the site, as well as overall patient factors, such as percentage body fat—the maximum dose for some anesthetics should be calculated based on lean body mass (e.g., bupivacaine) and for others an allowance may be made for increasing adiposity (e.g., lidocaine). Their effectiveness depends on the degree of innervation and other tissue factors such as pH and degree of buffering such that areas which are infected may be more difficult to anesthetize.

  Preparations may be made containing epinephrine which induces vasoconstriction to reduce wash out and hence prolong duration of action. This is useful particularly in the most well-vascularized areas of the body (mouth and face) but should not be used in the extremities to avoid a risk of ischaemia.

Post-Procedural Care

The patient should be warned that the presence of local anesthetic may mask any symptoms and in some areas may predispose them to inadvertent pressure injury (e.g., if the sole of their foot is numb). Some authorities advise ice and limited usage for a period of time following therapeutic injection, but there is no general agreement about the degree of reduction in activity required for optimal effect. There is more general agreement that steroids require hours to days to be effective and that there should be a gradual return to activity to prevent a rebound in symptoms. Patients should be counseled about possible complications and be aware of an appropriate contact to use if they develop symptoms of infection or other complication.

The frequency of injections should be determined by previous response, time interval, and consideration of total dose. In general, if joints are so symptomatic as to require percutaneous injections three or more times per year, then alternative treatments should be considered.

Monitoring of response may provide useful feedback for further therapy, particularly if a local anesthetic agent has been injected as a diagnostic test mixed with a therapeutic agent. The patient may usefully be asked to complete some form of scoring or keep a "pain diary" which may vary in complexity from a simple visual analogue scale or quantitative rating scale capturing their experience at certain key times after the procedure to more involved joint- or disease-specific scoring systems.

Suggested Readings

- M Obradov, Jan LMA Gielen, (Eds.), Image-guided Intra- and Extra-articular Musculoskeletal Interventions: An Illustrated Practical Guide, Cham, Switzerland: Springer International Publishing AG, 2018.
- MA Gina, JW David, D Elena, M Mark, Ultrasound Guided Musculoskeletal Injections, Philadelphia, USA: Elsevier, 2017.
- RL Cazzato, J Garnon, G Koch, D Dalili, PP Rao, J Weiss, S Bauones, P Auloge, P de Marini, A Gangi, Musculoskeletal interventional oncology: current and future practices. s.l.: British Institute of Radiology, 2020, British Journal of Radiology.
- JM Morelli, J Fritz, Chapter 15 MR guided interventional radiology of the musculoskeletal system. [book auth.] L Saba (Ed), Magnetic Resonance Imaging Handbook. s.l.: CRC, 2016.
- S Smith, E Scarth, Drugs in anaesthesia and intensive care. s.l.: Oxford University Press.

98 Conventional Nuclear Medicine Imaging

KANHAIYALAL AGRAWAL, GIRISH KUMAR PARIDA, GOPINATH GNANASEGARAN

Introduction

Nuclear medicine is an exciting field of medical practice in which small quantity of unsealed radioactivity is used to diagnose and treat disease. A chemical or pharmaceutical specific to organs is labeled with a radionuclide to form a radiopharmaceutical or radiotracer. *Generally, photons and positron-emitting radionuclides are used in imaging, and alpha and beta particles emitting radionuclides are used for therapeutic applications.* In radiologic procedures such as x-ray and computed tomography (CT), external radiation transmits through the body, which creates an image. In nuclear medicine procedures, radiopharmaceuticals in the human body emit radiation detected externally by sophisticated instruments such as a gamma camera or a positron emission tomography (PET) scanner. Nuclear medicine gamma imaging can be two-dimensional planar or three-dimensional (3D) single-photon emission computed tomography (SPECT) images. SPECT/CT is a hybrid imaging modality that fuses gamma camera functional images with anatomic images acquired on CT, providing morphologic and functional data in a single test. This chapter outlines the current applications of conventional nuclear medicine (excluding PET/CT, which is dealt with in Chapter 99) in routine clinical practice.

A few terms such as *collimator* and *half-life* have been frequently used in this chapter that need little elaboration as explained next.

Collimator

Gamma rays emitted from a point source can be detected anywhere across the field of view. Thus, for the directionality and accurate localization of the source, the emitted gamma rays need to be collimated. Collimators are perforated structures made of lead. They collimate the gamma rays by absorbing and stopping most of the rays except those arriving almost perpendicular to the detector face.

There are two basic types of collimators, which are pinhole and multihole collimators.

- A pinhole collimator operates like that of a box camera. When the gamma rays pass through it, the image is formed on the crystal, which is always magnified and inverted. This type of collimator is usually used for thyroid imaging; cortical scintigraphy of the kidneys; and skeletal imaging, especially for the hip and wrist in children
- The parallel hole collimator is the most commonly used multihole collimator. It has multiple parallel holes perpendicular to the plane of detector. The lead walls between the holes are called *septa*. In-high energy collimators, these septae are thicker than those in low-energy collimators

Half-Life

Radionuclides are unstable forms of their stable nuclide. So, to become stable, they decay to other nuclides by different processes. However, not all radionuclides decay at the same rate. Each radionuclide decays at a particular rate, which is specific to the radionuclide; so is its half-life. In nuclear medicine, *half-life is defined as the time interval during which a given number of radio nuclei (or their radioactivity) decay to half of the original value* [1]. For example, if initially there are N_0 nuclei in a radionuclide and half of them decay in 3 days, then the half-life of this radionuclide is 3 days. Conventionally, the term *half-life* ($t_{1/2}$) represents the *physical half-life* of the radionuclide. Mathematically this can be represented as $N_t = N_0/2$ in which $t = T_{1/2}$, N_0 = initial number of radionuclides, and N_t is the number of radionuclides remaining after time t. *The physical half-lives of a few commonly used radionuclides such as iodine (I-131), technetium-99m (Tc-99m), fluorine-18 (F-18), and gallium-68 (Ga-68) are 8 days, 6 hours, 110 minutes, and 68 minutes, respectively* [1]. Besides physical decay, the radionuclide or radiopharmaceutical disappears from a biologic system with time through metabolism, excretion, simple diffusion, or other ill-defined biomechanism. The interval when a given amount of a radiopharmaceutical or drug reduced to half its original value in a biologic system is called the *biologic half-life* of the same, represented as $t_{1/2\ (Bio)}$. Although in theory we study physical and biological half-life separately, in a biological system, both physical decay and biological elimination (metabolism, diffusion, or excretion) of a radiopharmaceutical occur simultaneously. So, the combined effect of both modes of decay leads to a new term, *effective half-life*, or $t_{1/2(eff)}$. Mathematically, the relationship among these half-lives can be represented as $1/t_{1/2} + 1/t_{1/2(Bio)} = 1/t_{1/2(eff)}$ [1]. So, when the $t_{1/2} >>> t_{1/2(Bio)}$, approximately $t_{1/2\ (eff)} = t_{1/2(Bio)}$, and when $t_{1/2\ (Bio)} >>> t_{1/2}$, approximately $t_{1/2(eff)} = t_{1/2}$.

Musculoskeletal System

The bone scan is one of the most common radionuclide imaging procedures performed in nuclear medicine. In general, it is mostly used for whole-body bone surveys in oncology. However, with the advances in instrumentation, there is an increased use in benign bone diseases.

Radiopharmaceuticals

The radiopharmaceuticals are either phosphates or diphosphonates. The gamma camera agents for bone scintigraphy SPECT are Tc-99m methylene diphosphonate (Tc-99m MDP), Tc-99m hydroxymethylene diphosphonate (Tc-99m HDP or HMDP), Tc-99m hydroxyethylidene diphosphonate (Tc-99m HEDP), and Tc-99m pyrophosphate.

The P-O-P bond present in the phosphate-based bone-seeking tracers (pyrophosphate)is less stable in vivo because of the presence of phosphatase enzyme inside the body, which can easily break down the bond. P-C-P bond, however, is resistant to such phosphatase enzyme and is more stable in vivo. Therefore, diphosphonate containing the P-C-P bond is commonly used radiopharmaceutical in bone imaging [2]. The radiotracer uptake in bone is due to ion exchange phenomena. The diphosphonate-based tracers such as Tc-99m MDP and HEDP binding occurs by chemisorption onto the bone matrix's hydroxyapatite mineral. The radiotracer is primarily excreted through the kidneys.

Radiopharmaceutical Injected Activity [3]

Adults receive intravenous (IV) injection of 740–1110 MBq (20–30 mCi). For obese patients, the dose may be increased to 11–13 MBq/kg (300–350 μCi/kg).

Children receive 9–11 MBq/kg (250–300 μCi/kg), with a minimum of 20 MBq/kg (0.5 mCi).

Imaging Procedure

Patient Preparation

The patient should be well hydrated. After radiotracer administration, the patient should void frequently, and before image acquisition, metallic objects in the area of interest (e.g., pendants, ornaments), should be removed.

Imaging

In whole-body imaging, anterior and posterior views are imaged. Usually, more than 1.5 million total counts are acquired. The energy window is centered at 140 keV. The window width is 15–20%, and the matrix size is 256 × 1024 or higher. If needed, a special spot view (static image) should be acquired with 500,000 to 1,000,000 counts per image.

The three-phase bone scan consists of flow (vascular), blood pool, and a delayed phase. The detector of the gamma camera should be positioned over the area of interest.

- The flow phase is acquired immediately after radiotracer injection for 60 seconds with a frame rate of 1–3 sec/frame and a matrix size 64 × 64 or higher.
- The blood pool phase is acquired immediately after the flow phase within 10–20 minutes of tracer administration. The matrix size should be 256 × 256 and counts 3,00,000 per image or time-based acquisition for 5 minutes.
- The delayed phase is acquired 2–4 hours after tracer injection and approximately 1 million counts.

SPECT acquisition is performed with contoured orbit, 64 × 64 or greater matrix, 3- to 6-degree intervals, and 10–40 sec/stop. Usually, 3D iterative ordered-subsets expectation maximization is ideally 3–5 iterations and 8–10 subsets. CT acquisition parameters in SPECT/CT are 512 × 512 matrix, 80–130 kV; the intensity–time product depends on the body part being imaged and ranges from 10 to 300 mAs.

Common Indications for Bone Scan

- Whole-body survey in oncology to identify bone metastases
- Benign bone tumor (e.g., osteoid osteoma)
- Osteomyelitis, including malignant otitis externa

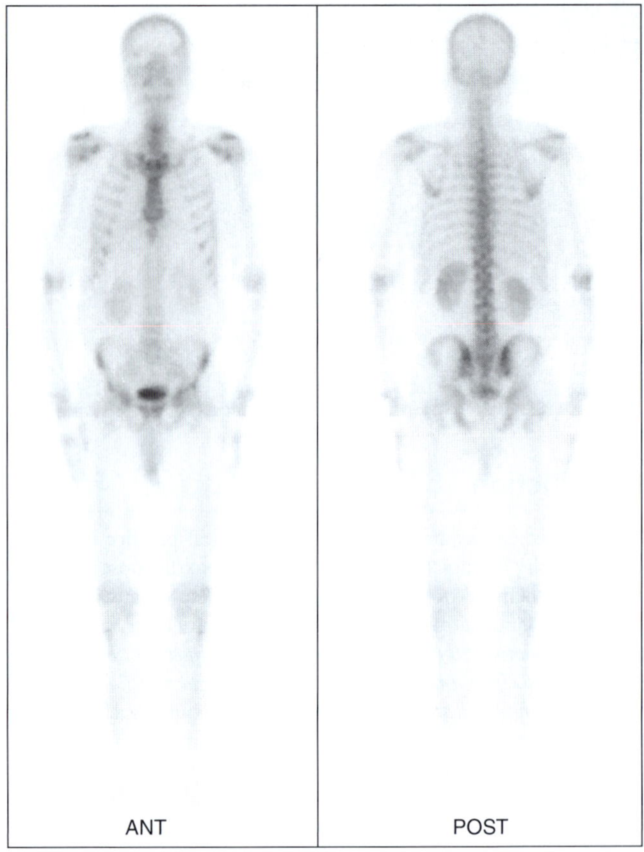

Figure 98.1 Normal bone scan showing homogeneous tracer distribution in the axial and appendicular skeleton. Excretion of tracer is noted through kidneys into the urinary bladder. *ANT*, anterior; *POST*, posterior.

- Stress fracture or shin splint
- Metabolic bone disease
- Osteonecrosis
- Bone dysplasia (e.g., fibrous dysplasia [FD])
- Loosening and infection of hip and knee prostheses
- Unexplained back pain
- Unexplained bone pain in the hip, knee, or foot
- Bone graft viability
- Mandibular condylar hyperplasia
- Complex regional pain syndrome
- Nonunion fracture
- Biodistribution of radiotracer in a bone scan

In general, the normal distribution of radiotracer is homogeneous in the axial and appendicular skeleton (Fig. 98.1). The radiotracer is excreted through the kidneys into the urinary bladder. Some normal variants are commonly seen on the bone scans. For example, "hot skull," or diffuse increase tracer uptake in the skull, is seen mainly in postmenopausal women or after chemotherapy [4]. Focal increased uptake in the ossifying ischiopubic synchondrosis in children between 4 and 12 years is a normal variant [5].

Artifacts and Pitfalls on Bone Scan

Bone scan artifacts are summarized in Table 98.1 and Fig. 98.2 [4]. Several pitfalls should be avoided while reporting a bone scan. Multiple foci of uptake in consecutive ribs in a linear pattern are typical of fractured ribs and should be correlated with the patient clinical history when presented for metastatic workup (Fig. 98.3). The unusual extraosseous tracer accumulation might be misinterpreted as bone uptake (Fig. 98.4). An ectopic or transplant kidney

TABLE 98.1 Bone Scan Artifacts

Instrument Related	Technical	Patient Related	Treatment Related
■ Improper photopeak setting: loss of counts, increase in scatter, and poor image quality ■ Photomultiplier tube defect: photopenic area in the image; usually not missed by expert readers but may be mistaken as a lesion	■ Injection tracer extravasation: poor image quality because a lesser amount of radiotracer reached to the bone; also may lead to lymph node visualization ■ Arterial injection: diffuse intense tracer uptake at the site of injection	■ Patient motion artifact: loss of resolution and blurring of the image ■ Metal artifact (see Fig. 98.2): metal such as jewelry, pacemaker, belt buckle in the region of interest during imaging produces photopenic defect on scan and may be confused as a lytic lesion; therefore, all metallic objects must be removed before scanning if possible and should be documented if they cannot be removed	■ Postsurgical tracer uptake may persist up to months after surgery; hence, treatment history should be recorded during the scan ■ Radiotherapy to a region shows decreased tracer uptake in the bones in the radiation field ■ Recent chemotherapy causes flare (i.e., increased tracer uptake in the existing lesions even if the lesion is healing); the tracer activity reduces after 4–6 months of flare

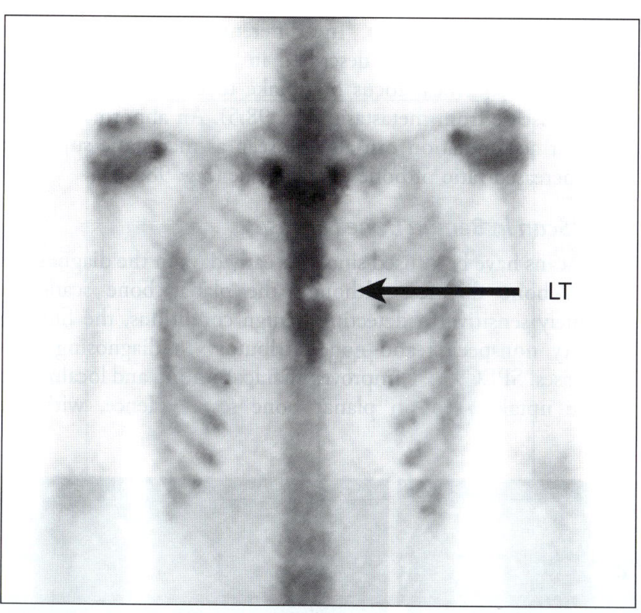

Figure 98.2 A metal artifact showing a photopenic region in the sternum (*arrow*) mimicking a lytic lesion. *LT*, left.

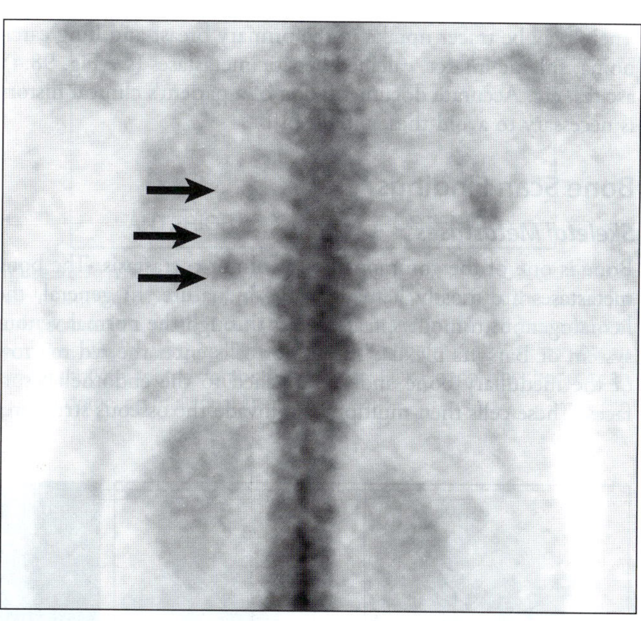

Figure 98.3 Increased tracer uptake in the linear fashion in continuous ribs (*arrows*) typical of fracture.

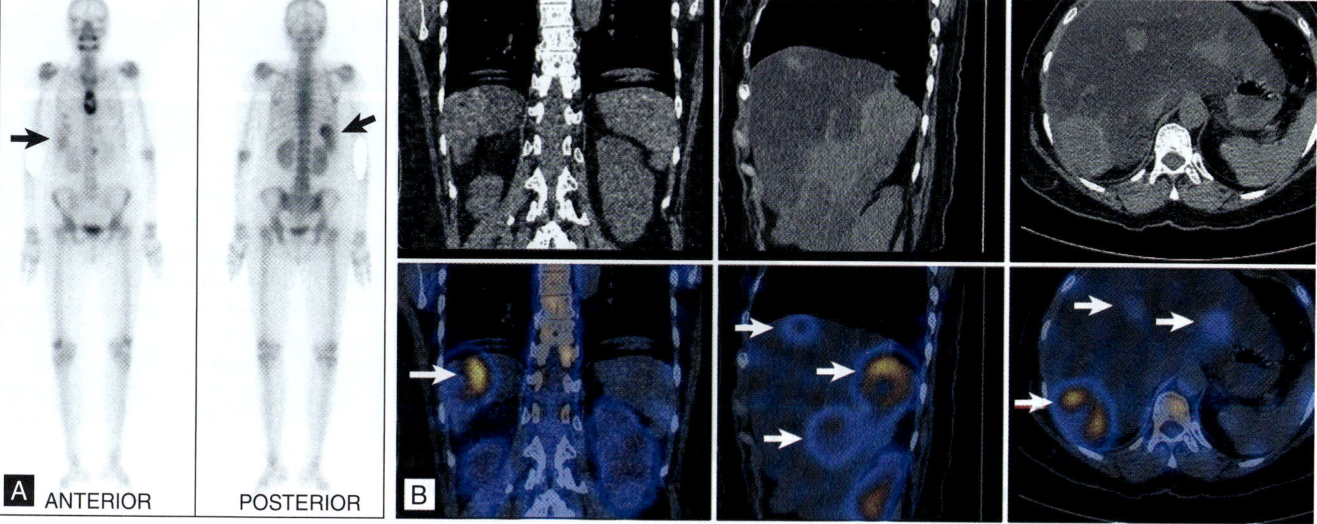

Figure 98.4 Whole-body bone scan in a patient with breast cancer shows increased tracer localization in the sternum with a central photopenic region suggestive of a lytic metastasis. There is abnormal activity in the right lower thorax region (*arrows* in A), which on single-photon emission computed tomography/computed tomography corresponds to multiple hepatic lesions (*arrows* in B) suggestive of soft tissue tracer uptake in the metastatic disease.

disease typically involves the end of the affected bone, whereas FD does not involve the bones' ends.

Osteoid Osteoma: Osteoid osteoma is a benign bone tumor usually present in the adolescent age group, typically as severe night pain that is relieved using salicylate analgesics. It is a cortex-based tumor. In general, results of a three-phase bone scan are positive with focal uptake and double-density sign (i.e., intense tracer accumulation in the central nidus and moderate uptake of tracer in surrounding reactive sclerosis; Fig. 98.9). SPECT/CT is highly sensitive and specific in the identification of osteoid osteoma, particularly in the spine.

Osteomyelitis and Septic Arthritis: Typical pattern on a three phase bone scan is increased tracer accumulation at the infection site in all three phases. Although the bone scan is highly sensitive with more than 95% sensitivity, the specificity is low. Other conditions also show positive three-phase uptake (e.g., malignancy, stress fracture, and osteoid osteoma) [8]. However, in nonviolated bone with clinical suspicion of osteomyelitis, it detects bone infection with good specificity (Fig. 98.10). False-negative findings may be seen in chronic osteomyelitis and vertebral osteomyelitis. Indium-111 labeled white blood cells, along with marrow imaging, is the radionuclide imaging of choice in infection in violated bone. Septic arthritis, such as osteomyelitis, shows increased tracer accumulation in the involved joints in all three phases.

Stress and Insufficiency Fracture: Stress fractures are fractures that occur in normal bone because of repetitive activity or overuse. In contrast, insufficiency fracture is caused by normal stress in a pathological or weak bone. Early diagnosis helps in early recovery and prevention of frank fractures. Bone scan results are positive from the very early or initial phase of stress reaction and are extremely sensitive. Furthermore, because stress reactions may involve multiple sites, the whole-body assessment helps detect additional areas. The uptake is usually focally intense with a shape ranging from oval to fusiform depending on the severity (Fig. 98.11). The first two phases on the bone scan typically

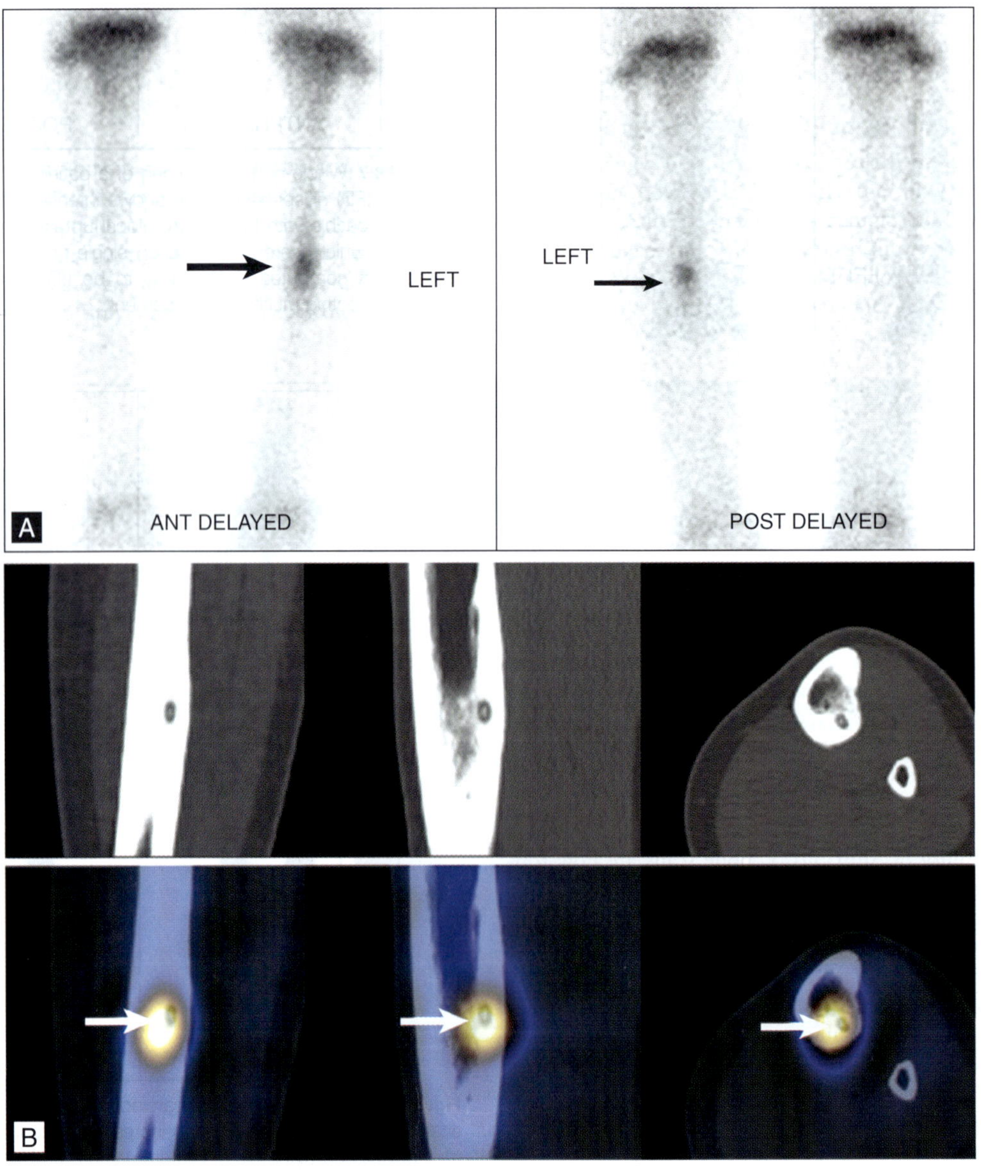

Figure 98.9 A 16-year-old male patient with left leg pain at night. A static planar bone scan of the leg shows focal increased uptake in the left mid tibia (*arrows* in A). This corresponds on single-photon emission computed tomography/computed tomography to a tiny nidus with surrounding reactive sclerosis (*arrows* in B) suggestive of osteoid osteoma.

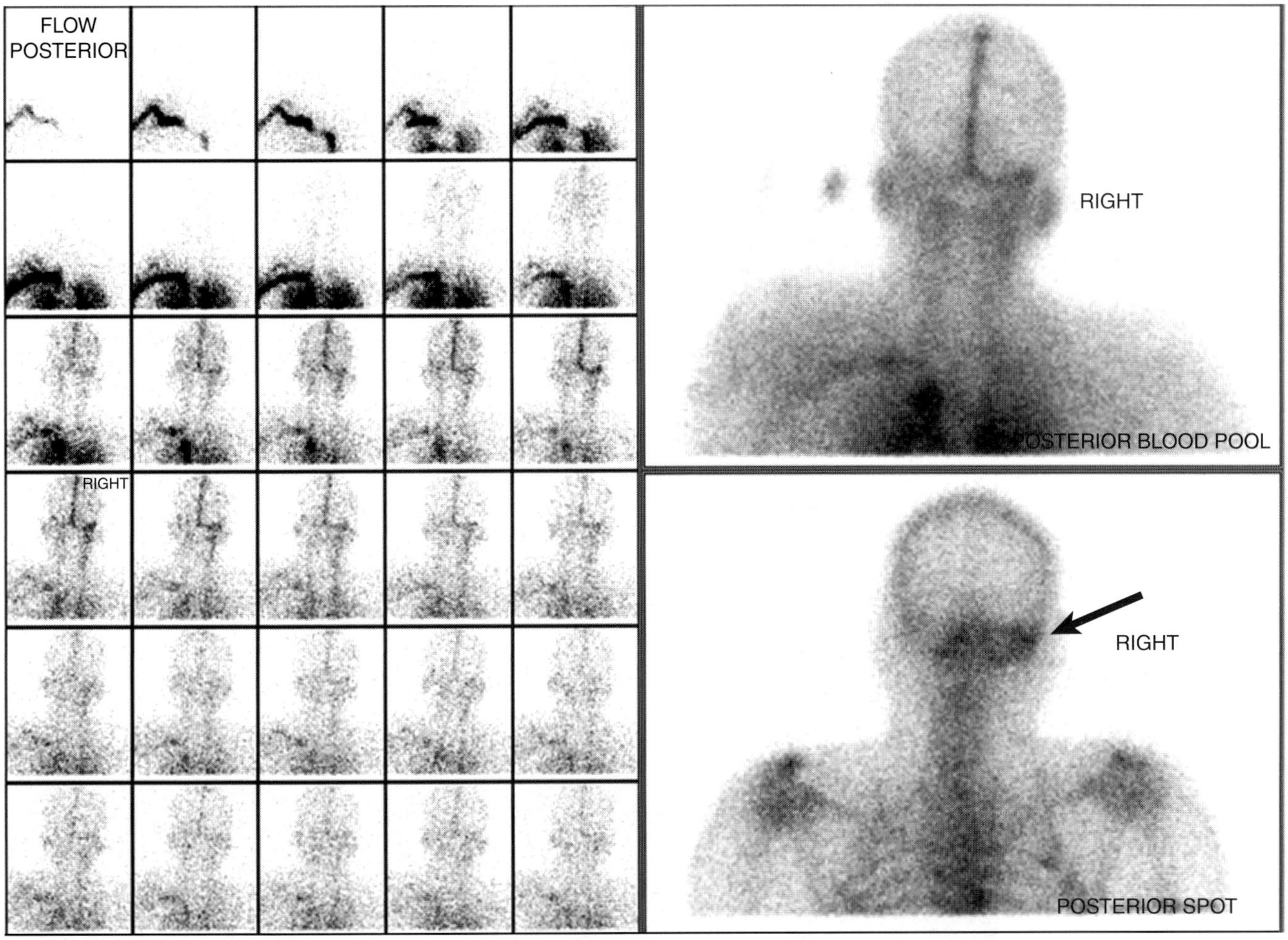

Figure 98.10 Three-phase bone scan in a suspected skull base osteomyelitis shows increased tracer localization at the right-side skull base in the flow and blood pool images with corresponding increased osteoblastic activity (*arrow*) in the delayed image suggestive of acute osteomyelitis.

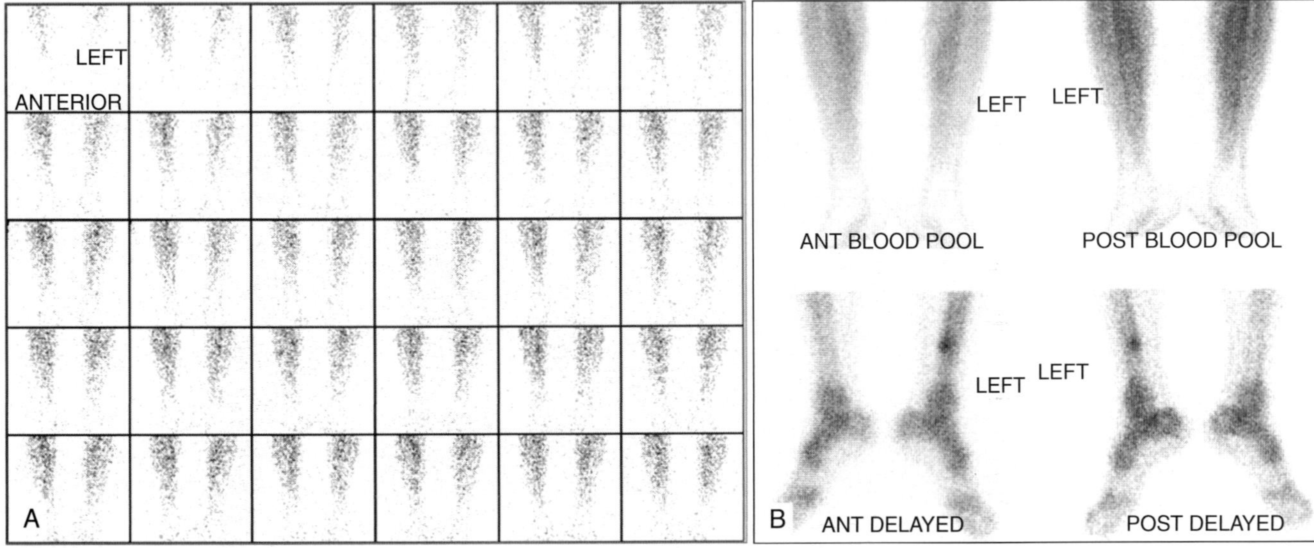

Figure 98.11 A 24-year-old male athlete presented with pain in the left tibia mostly while running. X-ray examination of the left tibia was normal. Three-phase bone scan shows normal flow (A) and blood pool images but increased osteoblastic activity in the left midtibia (B) suggestive of a stress fracture.

show increased hyperemia in a stress fracture. In shin splint or tibial periostitis, there is microavulsion of fibers connecting periosteum to bones. Hence, periostitis is seen as linear tracer uptake, typically in the posteromedial aspect of the tibia involving more than one-third of the tibia. The first two phases of the scan are usually normal.

Metabolic Bone Disease: Metabolic bone disease caused by primary hyperparathyroidism (PHPT) and renal failure produces a metabolic superscan pattern that shows homogenously increased tracer uptake in the axial and appendicular skeleton with faintly visualized kidneys. Sometimes focal increased tracer uptake is seen in the brown tumors in patients with hyperparathyroidism. Because of hypercalcemia, sometimes there is soft tissue uptake in the lungs, stomach, and kidneys.

In patients with rickets, there are changes in endplates of the long bones and beading at costochondral junctions. There may be superscan pattern, increased uptake in the sternum (tie pattern), pseudofractures, or true fractures.

In patients with Paget's disease, abnormal bone remodeling is seen. A bone scan is useful in confirming the diagnosis and assessing the disease extent. However, most often, it is seen incidentally on a bone scan done for other reasons. The typical scintigraphic pattern is intense florid tracer uptake in the involved bones with a blooming uptake appearance (Fig. 98.12).

Osteonecrosis or Avascular Necrosis: The causes of osteonecrosis include trauma, long-term steroid intake, sickle cell disease, and other vascular diseases. During the initial phase, there is a photopenic area in the involved region due to the cut-off of blood supply (Fig. 98.13). Later, there is increased uptake caused by reactive osteoblastic activity. Magnetic resonance imaging (MRI) is usually the gold standard imaging modality in avascular necrosis. However, the bone scan shows changes quite early during the disease process.

Complex Regional Pain Syndrome: Complex regional pain syndrome or reflex sympathetic dystrophy is a response to trauma and immobilization. There is variable presentation; however, typically, there is pain, edema, and muscle wasting. *A three-phase bone scan is helpful, and the most specific finding is the periarticular uptake of tracer.* Classical increased tracer accumulation in all three phases with periarticular uptake in the delayed phase is seen only in early disease. During the later course of the disease, the blood flow phase may be normal (Fig. 98.14).

Miscellaneous Indications

A bone scan is useful in evaluating bone graft viability, and SPECT/CT is usually more specific in such scenarios. (Fig. 98.15). Bone scan is also extremely sensitive in identification of pain generator in unexplained bone pain in the back (Fig. 98.16), pelvis (Fig. 98.17), knee, and foot (Fig. 98.18) [9–12] Often the

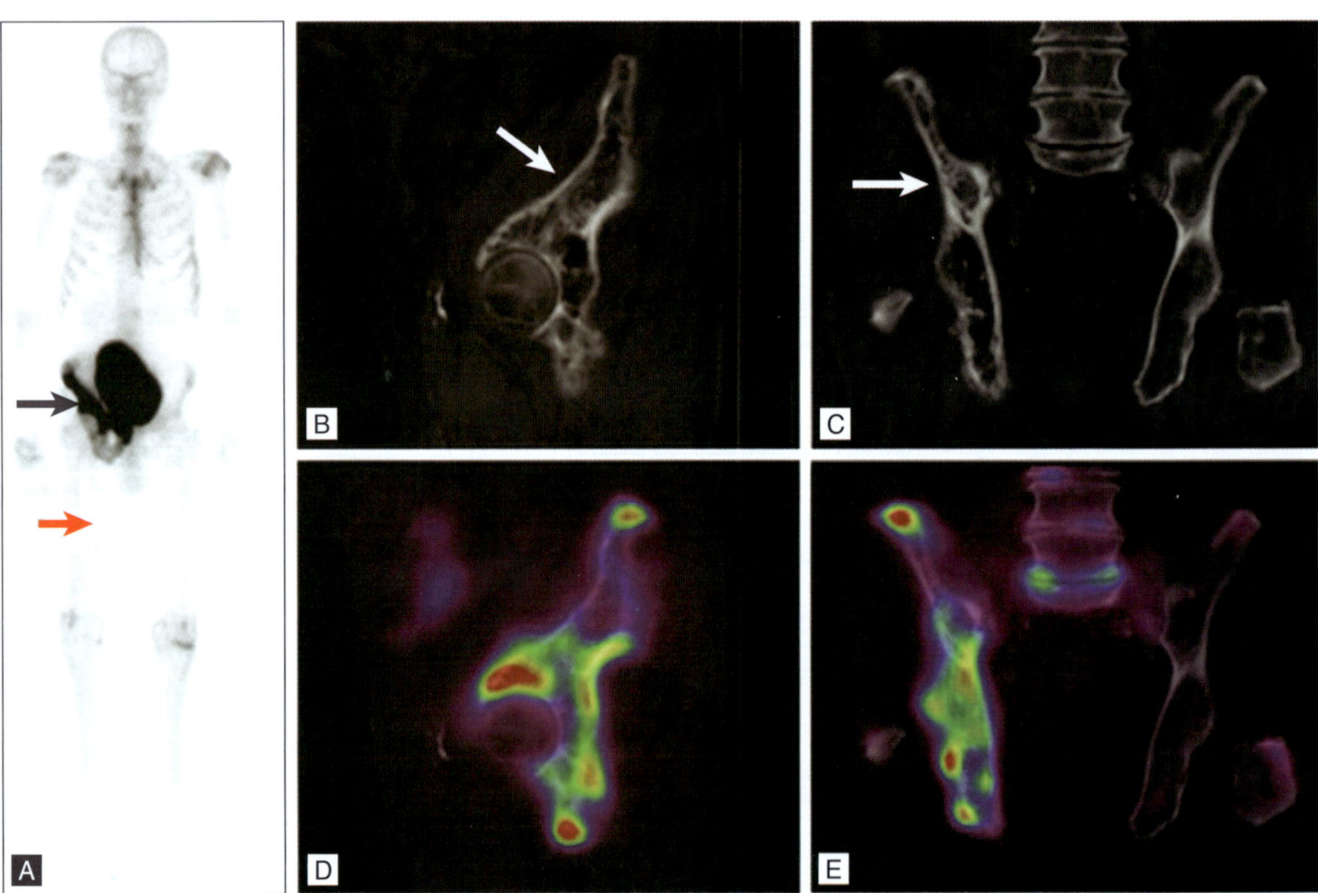

Figure 98.12 The anterior-view whole-body bone scan image (A) of a patient with prostate cancer showed intense tracer uptake in the right hemipelvis (*black arrow* in A), which correlated to cortical thickening and trabecular coarsening on CT component of SPECT/CT study (*arrow* in B and C) suggestive of Paget disease. In addition, on the whole-body study, there is a vertical linear area of increased uptake in the sternum owing to the previous sternotomy (sternal split sign) and uptake in the femoral vessels (*red arrow* in A) likely owing to calcification. (From: K Agrawal, F Marafi, G Gnanasegaran, H Van der Wall, I Fogelman I, Pitfalls and limitations of radionuclide planar and hybrid bone imaging, Semin Nucl Med 45 (5) (2015) 347–372.)

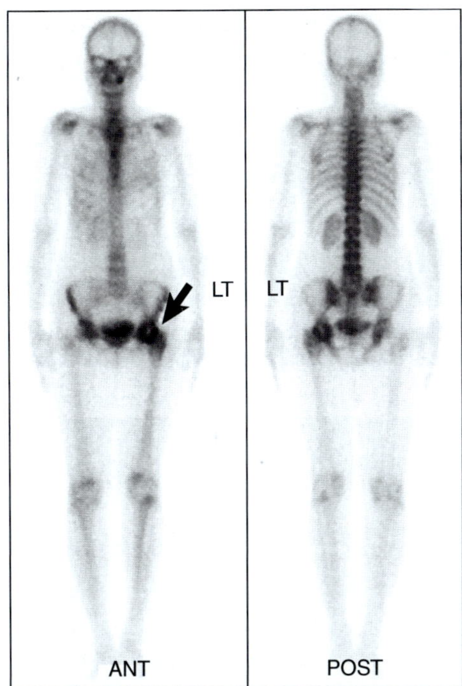

Figure 98.13 In a patient with a left femoral neck fracture, whole-body bone scan shows photopenia in the left femoral head (*arrow*) with increased osteoblastic activity surrounding it suggestive of early avascular necrosis. *ANT*, anterior; *LT*, left; *POST*, posterior.

fractures are seen early in bone scan comparison with conventional radiographs. Aseptic loosening and hip and knee prostheses infection can be differentiated with high sensitivity on a three-phase bone scan.

Endocrine System

Thyroid Imaging

For imaging the thyroid gland, ultrasonography (USG) is the most commonly used modality. However, often functional imaging is needed to either characterize the anatomic abnormality or for confirmation. The nuclear medicine studies in the thyroid gland are mostly based on some hormone synthesis phase in the thyroid gland. Iodine is the most integral part of the thyroid hormone, when taken orally.

Iodine is rapidly reduced to iodide in the small intestine and absorbed into the circulation. It is further trapped in the thyroid gland's follicular cells via sodium iodide symporter. This is usually followed by organification, and iodide is oxidized to iodine by thyroid peroxidase.

This binds to tyrosine present on the thyroglobulin, forming triiodothyronine (T_3) and thyroxine (T_4).

Thyroid-stimulating hormone (TSH) helps in all these trapping processes, organification, and release of thyroid hormones. The thyroid–pituitary feedback mechanism controls the secretion of TSH and thyroid hormones. *Monovalent anions such as*

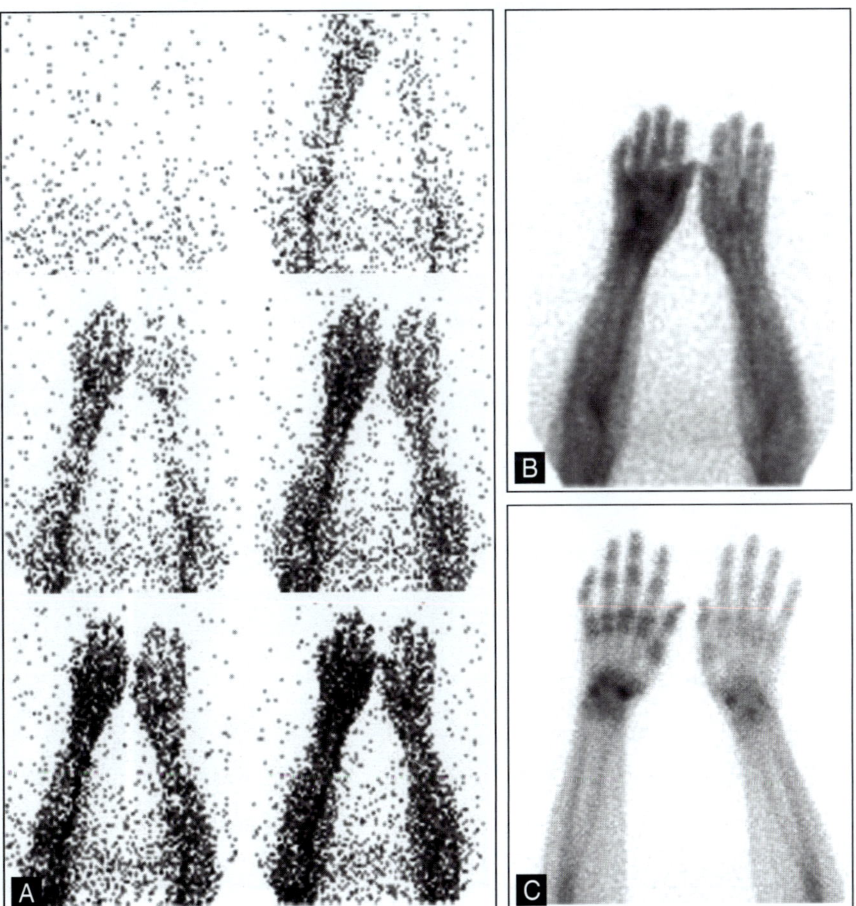

Figure 98.14 Complex regional pain syndrome (A–C). (From: HA Ziessman, JP O'Malley, JH Thrall, FH Fahey (eds.), Nuclear Medicine: The Requisites. fourth ed., Elsevier, Philadelphia, PA, 2014.)

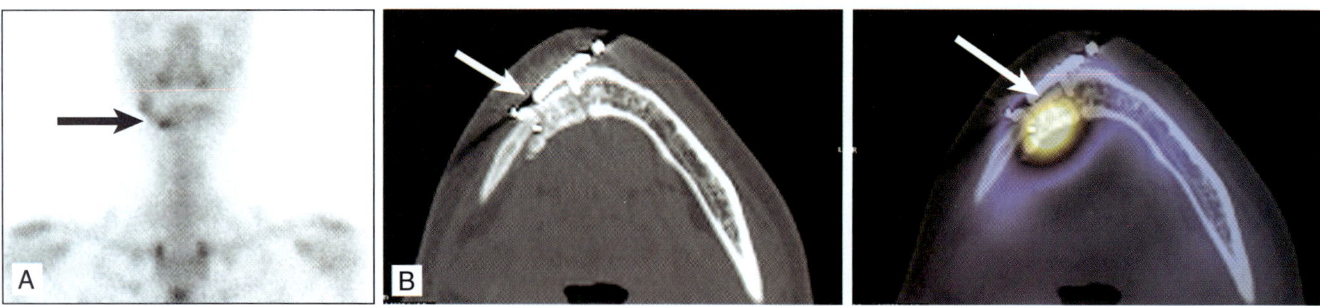

Figure 98.15 Six months after mandibular bone graft following surgery for a mandibular tumour, the planar bone scan shows mild uptake in the graft (*arrows* in A). Single-photon emission computed tomography/computed tomography confirms the uptake in the graft suggestive of the viable graft (*arrows* in B).

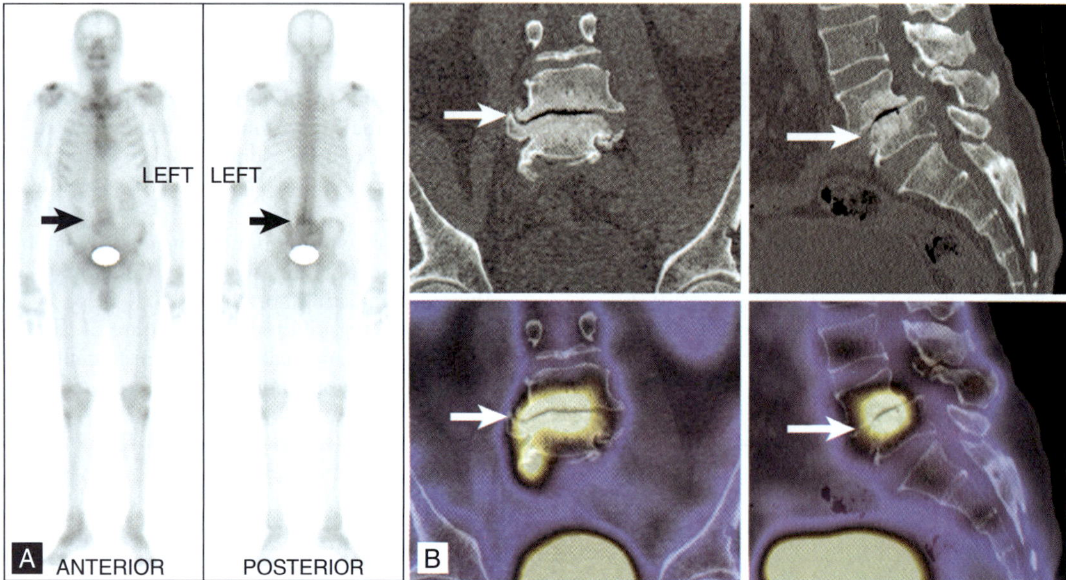

Figure 98.16 A 55-year-old female patient with low back pain shows heterogeneous tracer uptake in the lower lumbar spine (*arrow* in A) on whole-body bone scan. Single-photon emission computed tomography/computed tomography of the lumbar region (B) localizes the uptake to anterior listhesis of L4 over L5 with L4 to L5 endplate degenerative changes (*arrows*) as the cause of pain.

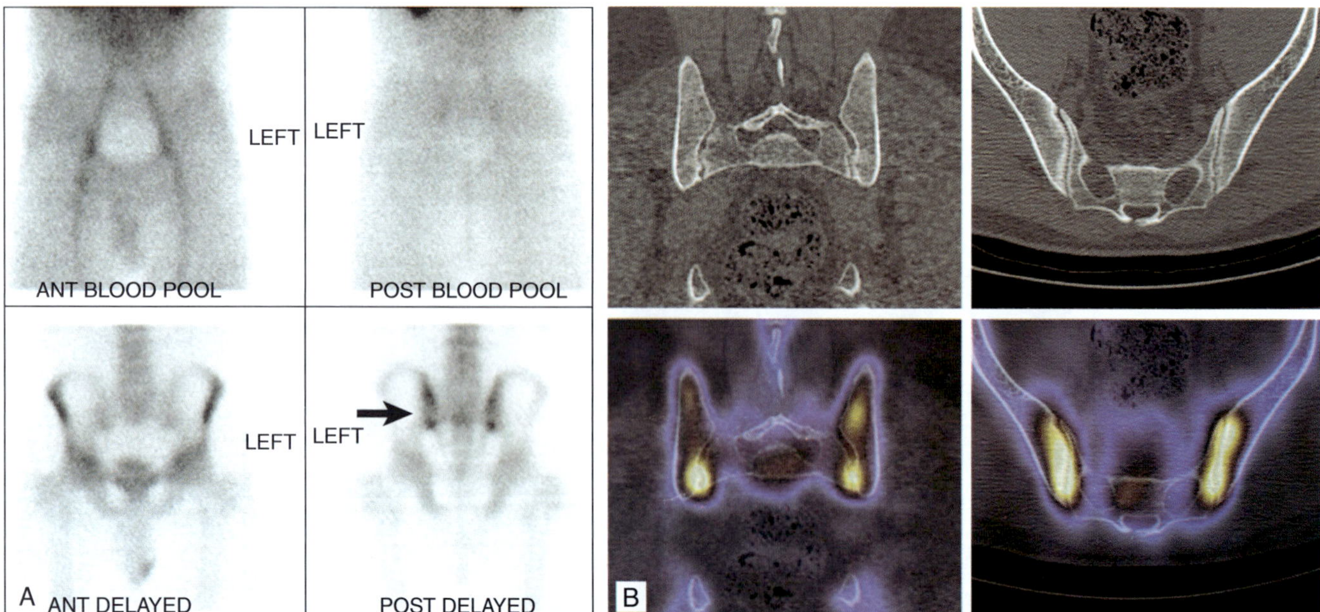

Figure 98.17 A 22-year-old male patient with bilateral hip pain. Three-phase bone scan (A) shows minimal tracer accumulation in the bilateral sacroiliac region on blood pool images with corresponding increased osteoblastic activity in the delayed image (*arrow* in posterior image). Coronal and axial single-photon emission computed tomography/computed tomography image (B) localizes the tracer uptake to irregular endplates with sclerosis suggestive of sacroiliitis.

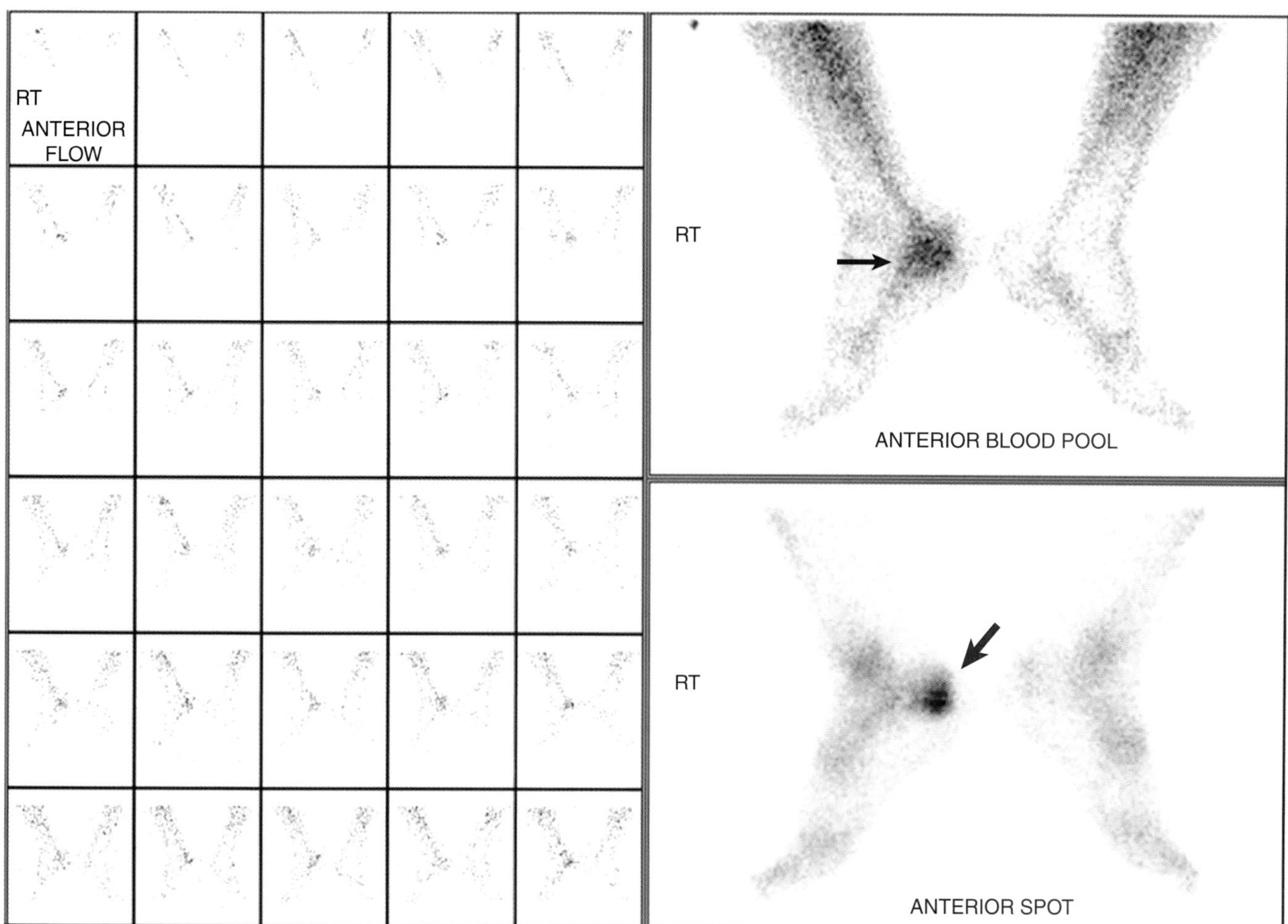

Figure 98.18 A young male patient with right hindfoot pain. Three-phase bone scan shows increased tracer localization at the inferior aspect of right calcaneum in the flow and blood pool images (*thin arrow*) with corresponding increased osteoblastic activity (*thick arrow*) in the delayed image suggestive of plantar fasciitis as the pain generator. *RT*, right.

potassium perchlorate can block the trapping within the thyroid through competitive inhibition. Similarly, organification can be blocked by antithyroid drugs such as carbimazole and methimazole.

Radiopharmaceuticals

Iodine-123 and Iodine-131: Radioactive iodine behaves similar to stable iodine and is the ideal radiotracer in providing information related to the thyroid gland. However, the physical characteristics of radioiodine (RAI) iodine-123 (I-123) and iodine-131 (I-131) allow for the preference of one above the other in clinical practice (Table 98.4). The principal gamma energy of I-131 is 364 keV, which is significantly higher than the ideal imaging energy for a gamma camera, leading to poor counts. Furthermore, it has a half-life of 8.04 days and high beta emission, leading to a higher radiation dose to the thyroid gland when used for imaging. I-123 emits photons with an energy of 159 keV and has a physical half-life of 13 hours. Therefore, this is the ideal choice for thyroid imaging with RAI compared with I-131 [13].

Both tracers get absorbed similar to iodine and are trapped in thyroid follicular cells within minutes of oral ingestion. However, a progressive increase in uptake within the thyroid gland occurs between 24 and 48 hours. *Because the background clearance is slow, usually scanning or uptake is done at 24 to 48 hours after dose administration.* The physiological biodistribution occurs in salivary glands, stomach, choroid plexus, lactating breast tissue, and excretion through kidneys and intestinal route.

Technetium-99m Pertechnetate: Technetium-99m pertechnetate is trapped similar to iodine but is not organified. Hence, imaging must be performed early at 20 minutes after administration because it is not retained in the thyroid. *This tracer's advantages over other tracers are 140-keV photons ideal for imaging, short half-life, no beta particles, and quick imaging. It is also readily available and less expensive than iodine tracers* [13]. The only potential disadvantage is low image quality when uptake is low. Therefore, in characterization of retrosternal mass, RAI is used for better image counts.

Patient Preparation and Precautions for Thyroid Uptake and Imaging

Several drugs and substances interfere with tracer uptake within the thyroid, as mentioned in Table 98.5. The history of these drugs should be taken before the appointment and should be stopped before the thyroid study for the required period if the patient's medical conditions permit. RAI can cross the placenta. Therefore, radiation exposure to fetal thyroid can occur after a higher dose of thyroid tracers, and a pregnancy test must be done before tracer administration. Furthermore, because RAI is excreted in breast milk, lactation should be stopped after I-131 iodide administration in lactating mothers and should not be resumed. For I-123 iodide and Tc-99m pertechnetate, breastfeeding should be stopped for 48 hours and 24 hours, respectively. Iodine-rich foods such as sea fish and dairy products can interfere with the radioiodine uptake (RAIU) and should be restricted before the study.

TABLE 98.4 Characteristics of Radiopharmaceuticals Used in Thyroid Scintigraphy [12]

	Technetium-99m (Tc-99m) Pertechnetate	I-123 Iodide	I-131 Iodide
Use	Imaging the thyroid gland	Imaging the thyroid gland Thyroid uptake	Thyroid uptake Thyroid therapy
Mechanism of uptake	Trapping similar to iodides	Trapping and organification	Trapping and organification
Physical half life	6 hr	13.2 hr	8.04 days
Principal gamma energy	140 keV (ideal for imaging)	159 keV	364 keV
Abundance of principal gamma emission (%)	89	83	81
Beta emission	No	No	Yes (606 keV; can be used in therapy)
Advantages	Low radiation dose Less examination time Easily available Cheaper than radioiodine	Better image quality when count is low Choice for retrosternal goiter or ectopic thyroid in mediastinum	Not ideal for imaging; used as therapeutic agent because of beta particles
Disadvantages	Poor image quality when the tracer uptake is low	Less readily available Higher radiation compared with technetium-99m agents Long examination time	Poor image quality High radiation burden

TABLE 98.5 Drugs and Substances That Interfere With Thyroid Uptake [12]

	Duration of Effects
Increased Uptake	
Lithium	Variable
Decreased Uptake	
Adrenocorticotropic hormone, adrenal steroids	1 wk
Amiodarone (iodinated drug)	3–6 mo
Bromides	1 wk
Cough medicines and vitamin preparations	2–4 wk
Iodine-containing ointments	2–4 wk
Intravenous water-soluble contrast media	3–4 wk
Iodinated (oil-based) contrast agents	In months
Methimazole, carbimazole, propylthiouracil	3 days
Nitrates	1 wk
Perchlorate	Variable
Penicillin	Variable
Propylthiouracil	1 wk
Salicylates (large doses)	1 wk
Sulfonamides	1 wk
Thiocyanate	1 wk
Triiodothyronine (T_3)	2 wk
Thyroxine (T_4)	4–6 wk
Kelp	4 wk

Thyroid Uptake

Although RAI I-123 is preferred, uptake can be performed with I-131 or Tc-99m pertechnetate if thyroid imaging is planned along with it. Essentially, a nonimaging sodium iodide (NaI) crystal–based thyroid uptake probe is required for RAIU. *The most common indication for RAIU is to differentiate different causes of thyrotoxicosis. Generally, RAIU is increased in patients with Graves' disease but is decreased in those with thyroiditis.*

Furthermore, RAIU is used to determine RAI activity (I-131) to be administered to thyrotoxic patients with Graves' disease and toxic nodular goiter. The drugs interfering with the RAIU should be stopped as mentioned earlier.

The patient should be on an empty stomach for approximately 4 hours before RAI intake to ensure good RAI absorption as it is given orally. The RAI dose is 5–10 μCi of I-131 or 50 μCi of I-123 if only RAIU is planned. For scan and uptake, approximately 1–2 mCi of RAI is the preferred dose. The uptake measurement is generally performed 24 hours after administration of RAI; however, some centers measure at 4 hours and others at both 4 and 24 hours [14].

First, the room background activity is measured. Counts are obtained from a known calibrated activity of RAI capsule placed in a neck phantom. This RAI dose is then administered to the patient orally. After 24 hours or the desired time, the patient's neck counts are obtained with 30-cm distance between the crystal's face and the anterior neck of the patient. The patient's body background count is measured as lower thigh counts. Percent RAIU is counted using the following formula:

$$\text{Percent RAIU} = \frac{\text{Neck Counts (counts per minute [CPM])} - \text{Body Background counts (CPM)}}{\text{Administered RAI counts (CPM)} - \text{Room background count (CPM)}} \times 100$$

TABLE 98.6 Causes of Increased or Decreased Radioiodine Uptake

Increased Uptake	Decreased Uptake
▪ Graves' disease ▪ Toxic nodular goiter ▪ Iodine deficiency ▪ Enzyme defect (organification defect) ▪ Pregnancy ▪ Rebound after stopping antithyroid medication	▪ Primary or secondary hypothyroidism ▪ Subacute thyroiditis ▪ Autoimmune thyroiditis ▪ Drug interfering with thyroid uptake ▪ Iodine-containing food or drugs ▪ Congestive heart failure ▪ Renal failure

The uptake can also be measured while a Tc-99m pertechnetate thyroid scan is performed. The advantages are quicker completion of the study within 20–30 minutes. Most of the gamma camera equipment currently available provides software for uptake calculation using Tc-99m pertechnetate. During this, the preinjection and postinjection syringe is imaged, and counts are calculated. The region of interest (ROI) is drawn over the thyroid on the computer, and the uptake is calculated as follows:

$$\text{Percent uptake at 20 minutes} = \frac{\text{Preinjection syringe counts} - \text{Postinjection syringe counts}}{\text{Total administered activity}} \times 100$$

The normal ranges for percent RAIU are approximately 5–15% at 4 hours and 10–30% at 24 hours. The normal range for percent Tc-99m pertechnetate uptake at 20–30 minutes is 0.3–4.5%. The causes of abnormal RAIU is mentioned in Table 98.6 [14].

Thyroid Scintigraphy

Procedure: The patient history is needed as in thyroid uptake, and drugs interfering should be stopped before imaging if possible. The patient's neck should be examined in an upright sitting position to see the nature of swelling, diffuse or nodular. This is required to place a marker during imaging in a supine position. Prior imaging findings and biochemical results should be documented to correlate with image findings. The image is acquired 20 minutes after IV injection of 5 mCi of Tc-99m pertechnetate. Time-based (5 minutes) or count-based (100,000–300,000 counts) images are acquired in the anterior, left, and right anterior oblique views. If I-123 is used, a 200- to 500-μCi dose is given orally, and imaging is done, preferably at 24 hours. Images are acquired for 10 minutes or 50,000 to 100,000 counts [15]. Ideally, a gamma camera with a pinhole collimator is preferred because the thyroid is a small organ. The patient should lie supine with the chin up and the neck extended. If the imaging is for evaluation of nodule, radioactive or radiopaque markers are used to identify palpable nodules' locations. Along with this, anatomic landmarks such as the chin and sternal notch marker image are obtained. The images are obtained with and without a marker in duplicate. Often, the radioactivity in the mouth and esophagus creates confusion, and repeat imaging after asking the patient to rinse the mouth with water and to swallow a glass of water helps.

Interpretation of Thyroid Scan: A thyroid scan should always be interpreted in the context of clinical history and examination and biochemical and radiologic investigation results. In general, a normal thyroid scan shows diffuse homogenous tracer uptake in both lobes of the thyroid (Fig. 98.19). The uptake localization in the isthmus is variable. The pyramidal lobe is not usually seen in a normal thyroid scan. The salivary glands are routinely visualized on Tc-99m pertechnetate scans.

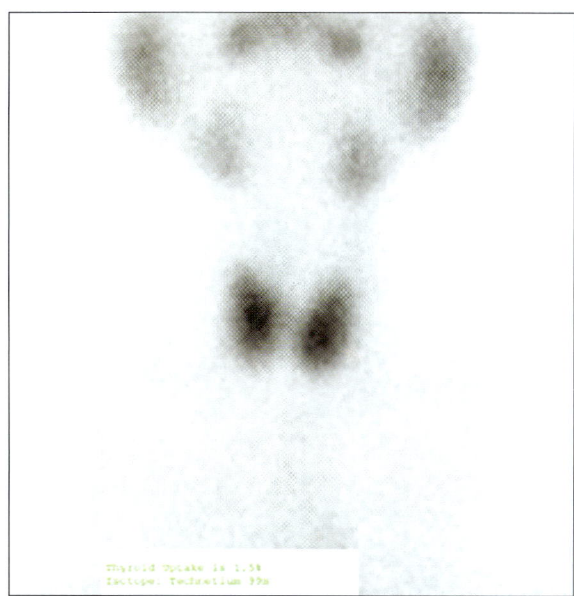

Figure 98.19 Normal thyroid technetium-99m pertechnetate scan shows homogenous tracer uptake in both thyroid lobes and relatively less intense tracer localization in the salivary glands.

Furthermore, Tc-99m pertechnetate scans show higher background uptake than I-123 scans. Sometimes esophageal tracer activity is seen in a normal scan, which is usually just left to the midline. A repeat image of the neck after the patient has swallowed a glass of water helps in differentiating from abnormal uptake. Thyroid enlargement and increased uptake within the gland should be noted. The uptake pattern within the thyroid, whether homogenous or heterogeneous patchy, should be documented. The report should mention any relatively hot or cold regions within the thyroid and any extrathyroidal tracer uptake. In the case of abnormal focal uptake within the gland, the marker image should be taken.

Indications for the Thyroid Scan

- Correlation of thyroid anatomy relative to its function: Mostly it helps in differentiating causes of thyrotoxicosis such as Graves' disease and nodular goiter, which helps in determining the therapy dose and differentiate Graves' disease from thyroiditis
- Evaluation of thyroid nodules
- Evaluation of congenital hypothyroidism
- Evaluation of retrosternal or mediastinal mass to determine whether it is a thyroid tissue
- Evaluation of suspected ectopic thyroid tissue

Clinical Applications

Thyrotoxicosis: Thyroid scans are useful in differentiating the two commonest causes of thyrotoxicosis, Graves' disease and subacute thyroiditis.

Graves' disease is the cause of thyrotoxicosis in approximately 70–75% of patients. It is an autoimmune disorder in which

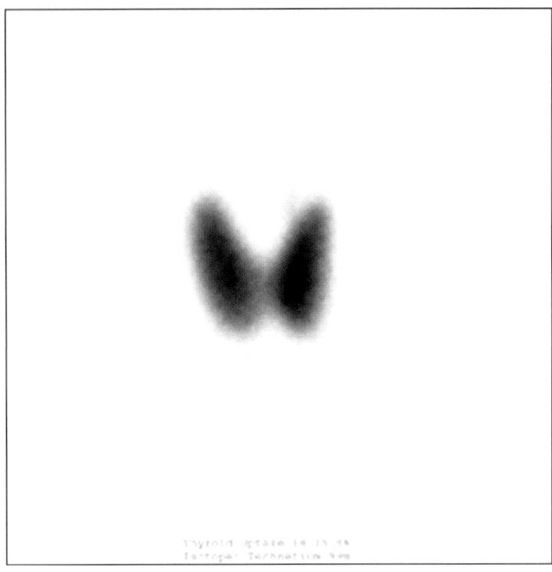

Figure 98.20 In a thyrotoxic patient, technetium-99m pertechnetate thyroid scintigraphy shows enlarged thyroid lobes with homogenously increased tracer uptake in both thyroid lobes (uptake at 20 minutes, 15.8%) suggestive of diffuse toxic goiter. The salivary glands show negligible tracer accumulation.

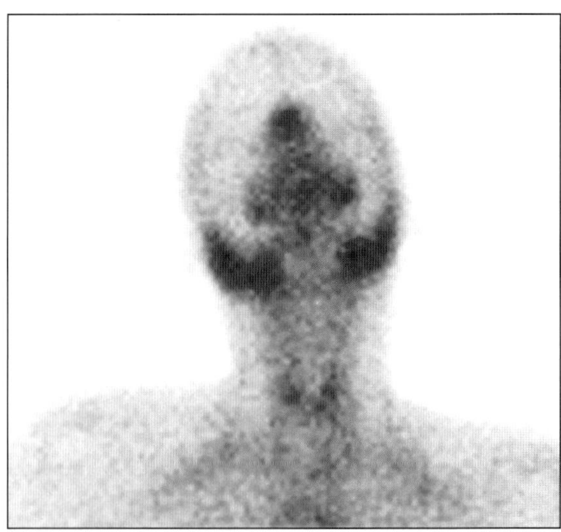

Figure 98.21 In a new-onset thyrotoxic patient with a history of viral fever, technetium-99m pertechnetate thyroid scintigraphy shows negligible tracer uptake in the thyroid gland, increased uptake in the salivary glands, and raised background activity suggestive of subacute thyroiditis.

thyrotropin receptor antibody is produced and has a similar effect to TSH on thyroid follicular cells. Hence, the excessive thyroid hormone is produced independently of thyroid–pituitary feedback. Approximately 30% of patients with Graves' disease show some signs and symptoms of ophthalmopathy. Generally, it is seen in the female gender. The patient usually presents with signs and symptoms of thyrotoxicosis, goiter or proptosis, and is biochemically thyrotoxic.

Subacute thyroiditis could be caused by granulomatous or de Quervain's thyroiditis, silent thyroiditis, or postpartum thyroiditis. During the initial few months of subacute thyroiditis, a patient usually presents with thyrotoxic signs and symptoms with suppressed TSH level similar to Graves' disease. In this period, thyroid scan and uptake are useful to differentiate because management is entirely different in these two entities.

Imaging in Thyrotoxicosis

- Thyroid scan typically shows diffuse homogenous tracer uptake in the enlarged thyroid gland and negligible uptake in the salivary gland in those with Graves' disease (Fig. 98.20). The RAIU is in the range of 40–80%
- In the thyrotoxic phase of thyroiditis, the scan shows significantly reduced or negligible tracer uptake in the thyroid gland (Fig. 98.21) with decreased RAI uptake. In the recovery phase of thyroiditis, the scan pattern is variable and may show patchy tracer accumulation and uptake within the normal range
- Another prominent cause of thyrotoxicosis, toxic multinodular goiter (MNG), shows increased percent RAIU, but the scan pattern is different from that in Graves' disease. In toxic MNG, there is often patchy heterogeneous tracer accumulation with increased tracer accumulation in a hyperfunctioning nodule
- In autonomously functioning thyroid nodule, there is high accumulation within the nodule with near-complete suppression of uptake in the rest of the thyroid gland, but the percent RAI uptake is usually in the normal range
- In iodine-induced thyrotoxicosis or Jod-Basedow phenomenon, which occurs because of iodinated contrast media or very high iodine intake, the percent RAIU is generally decreased. Infrequently, the uptake is increased if iodine activates subclinical Graves' disease or toxic MNG
- Amiodarone-induced thyrotoxicosis (AIT) type 1 usually occurs in a patient with latent Grave's disease or multinodular gland. Amiodarone contains high iodine (i.e., ~37% by weight). In preexisting thyroid disorder, excessive iodine leads to increased thyroid hormone biosynthesis. Vascularity is increased on Doppler USG. Percent RAIU is usually in the low normal range but can be high in iodine-deficient regions
- Contrary to this, AIT type 2 is a destructive process of the thyroid caused by amiodarone's toxic effect, resulting in the release of thyroid hormones. Typically, percent RAIU is negligible in type 2 AIT. AIT type 2 is more common than type 1

Clinically, it is difficult to differentiate between two different types. A small study showed successful use of Tc-99m sestamibi in the differentiation of type 1 and 2 diseases. Tc-99m sestamibi uptake is high in patients with type 1, but uptake is low or absent in those with type 2

- Thyrotoxicosis factitia is a condition caused by the ingestion of exogenous thyroid hormone. The thyroid scan shows reduced tracer accumulation and percent RAIU
- Hashitoxicosis is a cause of thyrotoxicosis that occurs uncommonly in patients with Hashimoto's disease. During this phase of Hashimoto's disease, there is typically diffuse, nontender goiter without nodules. The scan findings and percent RAIU are increased similar to Graves' disease
- Hydatidiform mole, choriocarcinoma, and trophoblastic tumors are rare causes of thyrotoxicosis. In struma ovarii, functioning thyroid tissue is seen in benign ovarian teratomas, and thyrotoxicosis is rarely seen. Percent RAIU in the neck is suppressed; however, on the whole-body thyroid scan, ectopic thyroid tissue is visualized in the pelvis.

Ectopic Thyroid Tissue: Sometimes because of abnormal descent of the primitive thyroid tissue in the embryonic life, thyroid tissue can be seen at places other than normal anatomic location. *The most common site of ectopic thyroid tissue is the lingual area, though it can be*

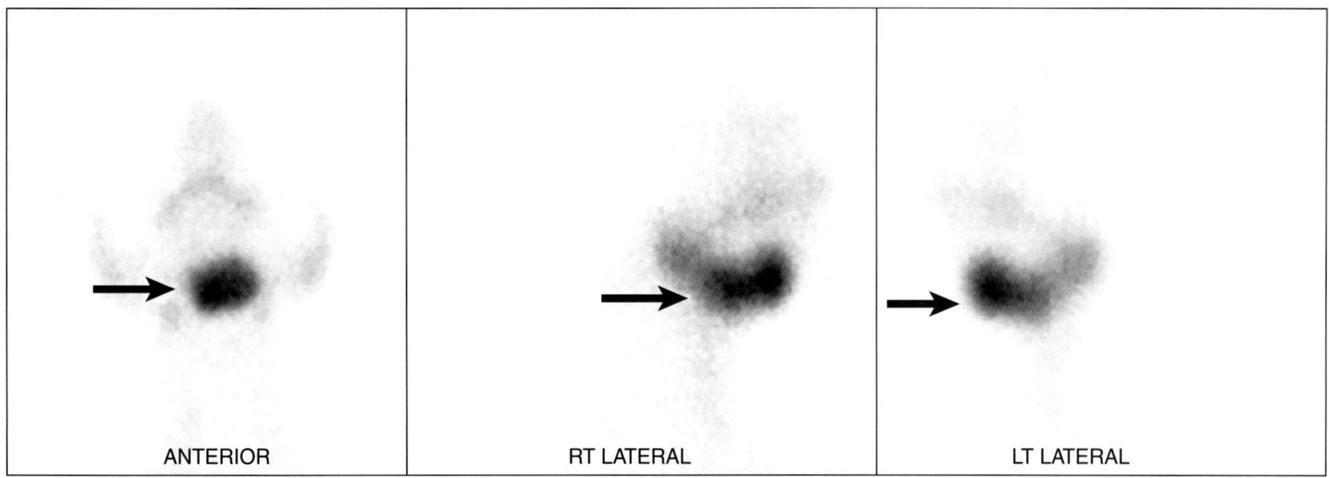

Figure 98.22 Technetium-99m pertechnetate thyroid scintigraphy shows intense abnormal uptake of tracer in the sublingual region (*arrows*) suggestive of ectopic functioning thyroid tissue. There is an absence of tracer uptake in the normal thyroid region in the neck. *LT*, left; *RT*, right.

seen in the mediastinum, ovary, lungs, adrenal gland, pancreas, gallbladder, and heart. Usually, patients present with anterior neck swelling and features of hypothyroidism, although depending on the site and compression of mass, there can be dysphagia, dyspnea, or dysphonia. Thyroid scintigraphy is always considered as the confirmatory imaging modality for the final diagnosis of functioning ectopic thyroid tissue.

Typically, on thyroid scan, there is focal tracer uptake at the base of the tongue in lingual thyroid with the absence of tracer accumulation in usual thyroid location (Fig. 98.22). However, the ectopic thyroid tissue may coexist along with the normal thyroid gland. Sometimes, a thyroid scan detects multiple ectopias that are missed on anatomic imaging. SPECT/CT can help provide both morphologic and functional imaging information, leading to an accurate diagnosis in a location other than the neck.

Thyroid Nodules: Although the prevalence of thyroid nodules is 3–7% by palpation, the prevalence range is very high by high-resolution USG among randomly selected individuals. The typical clinical dilemma is to differentiate between benign and malignant thyroid nodules.

USG is the first-line imaging modality in the thyroid nodules, and fine-needle aspiration (FNA) is the procedure of choice in thyroid nodule assessment. If the thyroid nodule is larger than 1 cm in size, serum TSH is usually performed. If serum TSH is below the normal range, thyroid scintigraphy is indicated. On thyroid scintigraphy, the tracer uptake in the nodule can be (1) greater than the surrounding normal thyroid (hot or hyperfunctioning nodule), (2) equal to the surrounding thyroid (warm or iso-functioning nodule), or (3) less than surrounding thyroid tissue (cold nodule) (Fig. 98.23).

A hot nodule is rarely malignant (<1%), and no cytologic evaluation is necessary (Fig. 98.24) [16]. The risk of malignancy is high in solitary cold nodule (10–15%) than in warm nodules and should be further evaluated by USG and FNA [16]. Similarly, the chance of malignancy is 5% in a dominant cold nodule in multinodular goiter. The differential diagnoses of cold nodules on thyroid scintigraphy include simple cyst, colloid nodules, hemorrhage, abscess, adenoma, focal thyroiditis, hematoma, granuloma, and infiltrative disorders. Although I-123 scintigraphy is preferred because it is both trapped and organified, Tc-99m pertechnetate can also be used. But, rarely, in 5% of patients, nodules are hot on Tc-99m pertechnetate and cold on I-123 scintigraphy. The

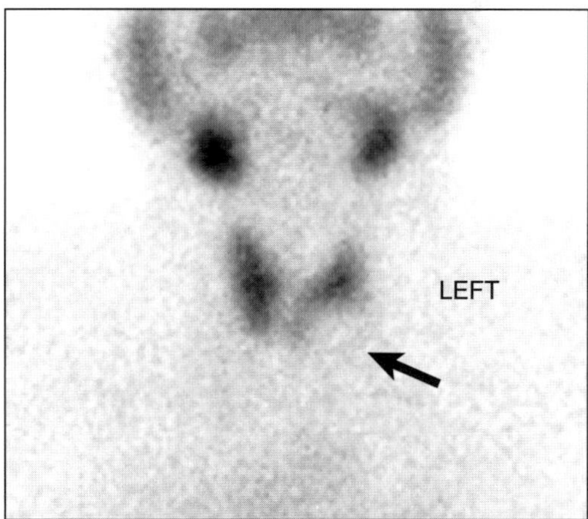

Figure 98.23 A 46-year-old female patient with a large nodule in the neck on the left side. Technetium-99m pertechnetate thyroid scintigraphy shows a large photopenic region (*arrow*) corresponding to the site of a clinically palpable nodule, suggestive of a cold nodule.

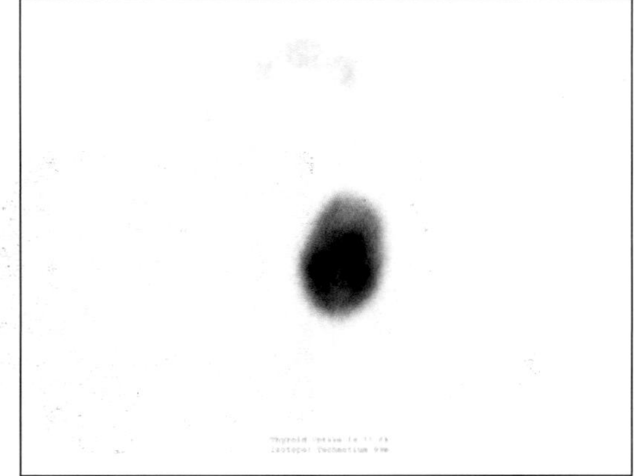

Figure 98.24 Ultrasonography of a thyroid showed a large nodule in the enlarged left thyroid lobe. Technetium-99m pertechnetate thyroid scintigraphy in a thyrotoxic patient shows intense uptake of tracer in the large left thyroid lobe with suppression of tracer uptake in the right thyroid lobe and salivary glands, consistent with autonomously functioning toxic left thyroid lobe nodule.

discrepancy is suggested to be attributable to dissociations of the organic binding of RAI relative to trapping of radioiodide or pertechnetate [17]. *Therefore, a single hot nodule on a Tc-99m pertechnetate scan should be confirmed by I-123 scintigraphy.*

Whole-Body Iodine Scan

Generally, radioiodine whole-body scan (RAI-WBS) is performed in patients with known differentiated thyroid cancer after thyroidectomy. The diagnostic RAI-WBS is performed after thyroidectomy in patients with thyroid cancer to look for the extent of the thyroid remnant or residual disease that cannot be precisely known from the surgical report and neck USG and disease staging (Fig. 98.25).

Patient Preparation: *Diagnostic RAI-WBS is performed 4 to 6 weeks after thyroidectomy. Levothyroxine should be withdrawn for 3 to 4 weeks before RAI-WBS, aiming for serum TSH level greater than 30 mIU/L.* In some patients, levothyroxine withdrawal is not possible because of significant comorbidity such as medical or psychiatric conditions that can worsen because of withdrawal-related hypothyroidism. Sometimes after thyroid hormone withdrawal, an adequate TSH level is not achieved. In such cases, recombinant TSH is recommended to be used; 0.9 mg of recombinant TSH is administered via intramuscular injection on 2 consecutive days in such instances when RAI can be administered on the second day [15]. A low-iodine diet for at least 1–2 weeks before the study should be considered. The RAI activity in diagnostic RAI-WBS is low (i.e., 1–3 mCi I-123 or I-131 to prevent stunning) [18].

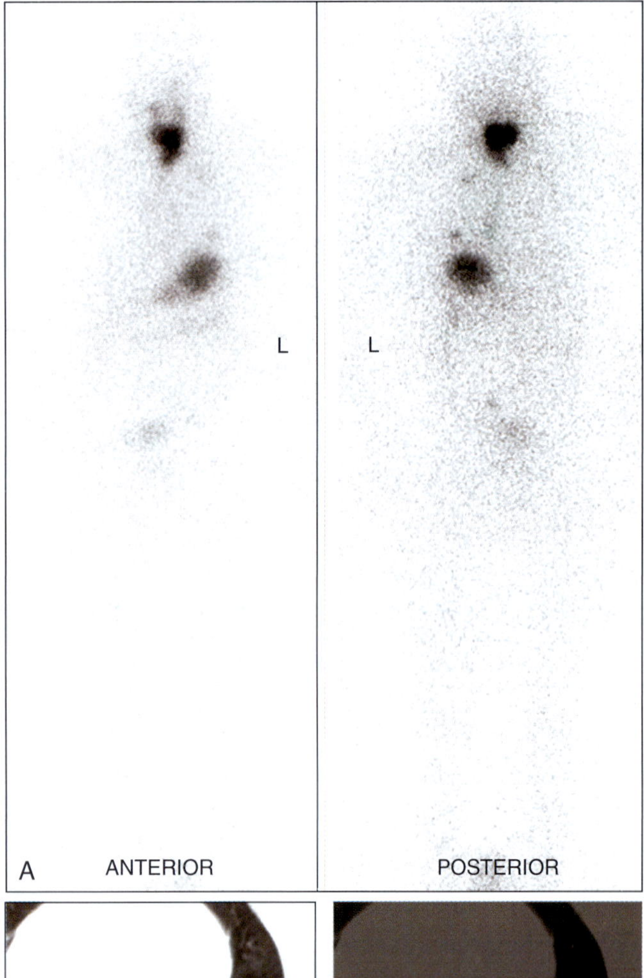

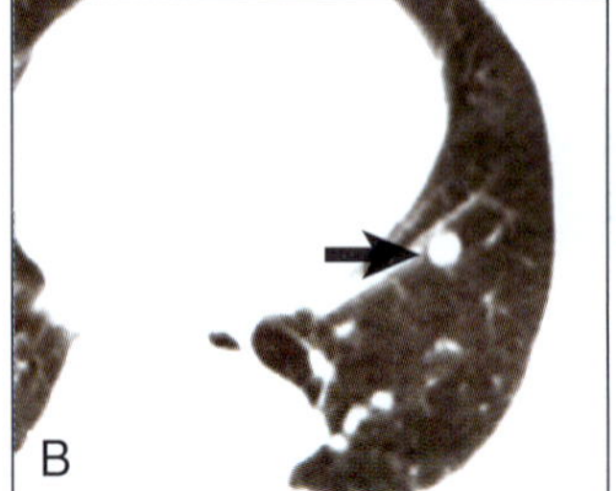

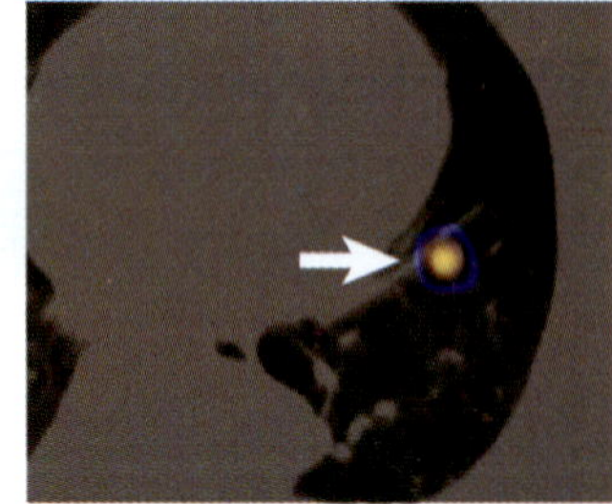

Figure 98.25 Known case of papillary thyroid carcinoma, after thyroidectomy. Whole-body iodine-131 iodine scan (A) shows intense residual disease in the neck and two foci of minimal tracer uptake in the left thorax. Physiological tracer uptake is seen in the stomach and urinary bladder. Single-photon emission computed tomography/computed tomography of the thorax (B) localizes the thoracic uptake to pulmonary nodules (*arrow*), confirming pulmonary metastasis.

Whole-Body Protocol: Whole-body images are acquired 24 hours after I-123 or 48 hours after I-131 administration. For I-123, a medium-energy parallel-hole collimator is preferred because there is concomitant high-energy photons emission from 123I, though a low-energy collimator can be used. But in I-131 imaging, a high-energy parallel-hole collimator with a window centered at 364 keV is used.

Post Radioiodine Therapy Imaging: After high-dose I-131 ablation or treatment, posttherapy WBS is recommended to assess accurate disease staging and document the RAI avidity of any structural disease. It is generally performed 5–7 days after the therapeutic dose of RAI. New lesions not detected on diagnostic RAI-WBS are seen in approximately 10% of patients, which alters patient management [18].

Normal Biodistribution of Tracer: In diagnostic RAI-WBS before treatment, some residual focal thyroid bed uptake is usually seen. The uptake can be seen in the nasal cavity, oropharynx, salivary glands, stomach, and intestine. The posttherapy scan may show liver uptake. The tracer excretion through kidneys into the urinary bladder is visualized. The most common abnormal sites of tracer uptake are the neck, chest, and skeletal sites, which represent metastases from the thyroid cancer.

SPECT/CT Imaging: Because of RAI's poor imaging characteristics, an anatomic landmark is not visualized in the planar imaging. Hence, it is often challenging to differentiate thyroid bed uptake from lymph node uptake; uptake in the thorax region, whether it is within lung or bones; and in other conditions such as surface contamination. SPECT/CT provides anatomic and functional data in one scan and helps in localizing the uptake and characterization of lesions (Fig. 98.26). Furthermore, routine use of neck and chest SPECT/CT after therapy scan alters the postsurgical American Thyroid Association risk of recurrence estimate in approximately 6% of patients. The need for additional cross-sectional imaging is reduced by 20% of patients [18].

Parathyroid Imaging

There usually are four parathyroid glands present in the neck in addition to a fifth one in approximately 10% of the population. These are derived from the third and fourth pharyngeal pouches. The superior parathyroid glands are derived from the endoderm of the fourth pouch and are located posterior to the superior third of both lobes of the thyroid gland. The inferior parathyroid glands, which originate from the third pouch, are usually located posterior to the inferior third of both lobes of the thyroid gland. However, parathyroid glands' location can vary, mostly the inferior glands, because of their embryonic origin and subsequent migration of a more extended pathway. Therefore, the inferior parathyroid glands can be found in the neck in the intrathyroidal location or high in the neck or the thymus, mediastinum, or pericardium or posteriorly in the superior mediastinum in the

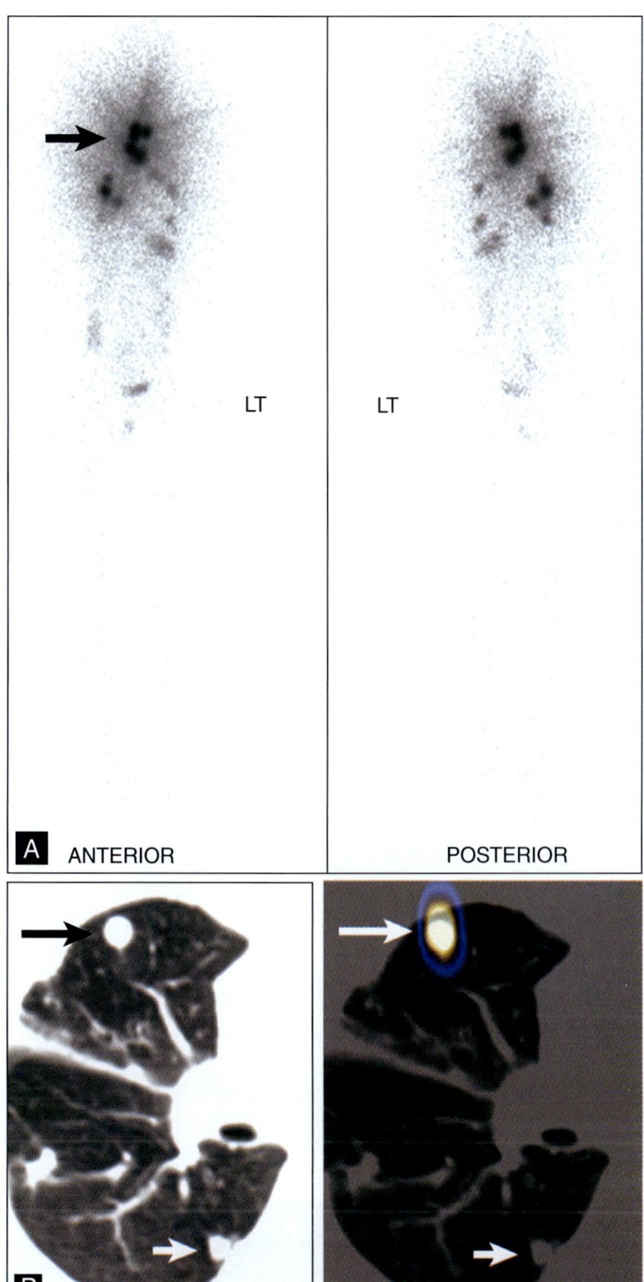

Figure 98.26 In a known case of papillary thyroid carcinoma, after thyroidectomy, whole-body iodine-131 scan (A) shows multiple foci of abnormal uptake in the neck (*arrow*) and the thorax. Single-photon emission computed tomography/computed tomography (SPECT/CT) of the thorax (B) shows tracer uptake in thorax localizes to pulmonary nodules (*black arrow*); however, there were multiple iodine nonavid nodules (*arrow* in the right lower lobe). The overall findings are consistent with neck node and lung metastasis; however, SPECT/CT helped in identifying possible iodine refractory disease. *LT*, left.

tracheoesophageal groove and paraesophageal region. Normal parathyroid glands measure approximately 6 × 3 mm and weigh approximately 20–40 g each. The parathyroid glands contain parenchymal cells (mainly chief cells), oxyphilic and fat cells. The chief cells produce parathyroid hormone (PTH). PTH is a crucial hormone, regulating calcium, phosphorus, and vitamin D homeostasis. There may be pathologically increased production of PTH caused by hyperparathyroidism.

- Primary hyperparathyroidism (PHPT) is caused by autonomous hyperfunction of a parathyroid adenoma, leading to increased serum calcium levels, decreased blood phosphate level, and increased urine calcium and phosphates. Patients usually present with a mass in the neck, bone pain, fractures, and renal colic caused by nephrocalcinosis or urolithiasis. In approximately 85% of patients, the solitary parathyroid adenoma is the cause of PHPT, and adenomas involving more than one gland are seen in around 5%. Parathyroid hyperplasia is seen in approximately 10% of patients of PHPT, and very rarely (in <1% cases of PHPT), parathyroid carcinoma is seen [16]
- Secondary hyperparathyroidism usually occurs in patients with renal failure, gastrointestinal (GI) malabsorption, and regular ingestion of several drugs (e.g., laxatives, phenytoin). Because of chronic low serum calcium levels, continuous compensatory stimulation to produce PTH results in parathyroid hyperplasia
- Tertiary hyperparathyroidism occurs in patients with renal failure. Chronic hypocalcemia leads to parathyroid hyperplasia, which becomes autonomous in function and no longer responsive to serum PTH level and leads to a state of hypercalcemia

Commonly used imaging modalities for the parathyroid gland are radionuclide scan and USG. CT and MRI can be useful in an ectopic parathyroid gland in the mediastinum. USG has the advantages of easy availability and being a nonradiation imaging modality. However, the investigation is highly subjective in nature and operator dependent. Moreover, the sensitivity and specificity of USG are low compared with parathyroid scintigraphy, particularly in the ectopic mediastinal lesion and deeply located neck lesions. USG is complementary in localization of parathyroid adenoma accurately when used with parathyroid scintigraphy and useful to differentiate enlarged parathyroid glands from thyroid nodules in the presence of nodular goiter. Guidelines recommend a combined interpretation of USG imaging and scintigraphy in the same session to confirm the presence of parathyroid adenoma and exclude thyroid nodules.

Parathyroid Scintigraphy

Parathyroid scintigraphy is performed to localize the parathyroid adenoma(s) and to guide minimally invasive surgery. The commonly used radiotracer for parathyroid imaging is Tc-99m sestamibi. Other SPECT tracers are thallium-201 (Tl-201) and Tc-99m tetrofosmin, and PET tracers are C-11 methionine and F-18 fluorodeoxyglucose. Tc-99m sestamibi (2-methoxyisobutyl isonitrile) is a lipophilic cation agent. It localizes and is retained in the mitochondria of the cells. Parathyroid adenoma has high cellularity and vascularity, and oxyphil cells are rich in mitochondria. These two factors lead to high uptake within parathyroid adenoma and slow washout from the mitochondria of the oxyphil cells. The normal functioning glands are not seen on scintigraphy.

Dual-Phase or Washout Parathyroid Scintigraphy

This is used to localize hyperfunctioning parathyroid gland(s) before surgery to guide minimally invasive surgery and recurrent or persistent disease in patients with PHPT. As mentioned before, Tc-99m sestamibi shows differential washout in thyroid and parathyroid tissues with faster clearance from thyroid tissue. Tc-99m sestamibi is the radiotracer of choice for dual-phase scintigraphy.

No patient preparation is usually required. The tracer (15–20 mCi) is injected intravenously [19]. Planar images of the neck and upper thorax in anterior view are acquired using a low-energy, high-resolution, parallel-hole collimator with a matrix size of

128 × 128 or higher. A pinhole collimator has higher sensitivity and should be preferred.

The early images at 10 minutes and delayed images at 1–2 hours are acquired. A further delayed image can be obtained if there is an insufficient washout from the thyroid.

Early images show tracer uptake in the thyroid gland, and parathyroid uptake is a more prominent focal uptake distinct from thyroid uptake. There are washout from the thyroid gland and persistent uptake in the hyperfunctioning parathyroid on the delayed image (Fig. 98.27A). SPECT or SPECT/CT is generally recommended along with planar imaging for more precise localization of the hyperfunctioning parathyroid adenoma. SPECT also has a higher target-to-background ratio than planar images, leading to improved detectability and higher sensitivity in ectopic lesions. It should be performed immediately after an early planar image to avoid false-negative results seen in rapid washout cases. SPECT/CT provides anatomic data and functional imaging, leading to a more accurate interpretation of scintigraphy findings (Fig. 98.27B). It has excellent sensitivity in the detection of parathyroid adenomas of approximately 90% [20]. The adenoma may be missed if the size is too small. Sensitivity in the detection of parathyroid hyperplasia is low, approximately 50–60%. In about 30% of patients, this typical pattern is not seen. In subsets of patients, washout from both the thyroid and parathyroid is seen at the same rate or both washout rapidly and minimal tracer are seen on delayed imaging (Fig. 98.28). False-positive results can be seen in patients with nodular goiter in whom there can be persistent uptake in delayed image in the thyroid nodule. In such cases, dual-tracer subtraction imaging is helpful.

Dual-Tracer Subtraction Parathyroid Scintigraphy

The tracers used in parathyroid imaging are not specific to the parathyroid gland and can be taken up by the thyroid gland. Therefore, a second tracer is used, specific to the thyroid gland in this context, such as Tc-99m pertechnetate or I-123. The thyroid scan is subtracted with computer software from the acquired parathyroid scan using Tc-99m sestamibi or Tl-201 or Tc-99m tetrofosmin images. Tc-99m sestamibi parathyroid scan is preferred because of higher sensitivity and lower radiation than Tl-201. Although I-123 has the advantage of simultaneous imaging with Tc-99m sestamibi scan to avoid image misregistration, it is

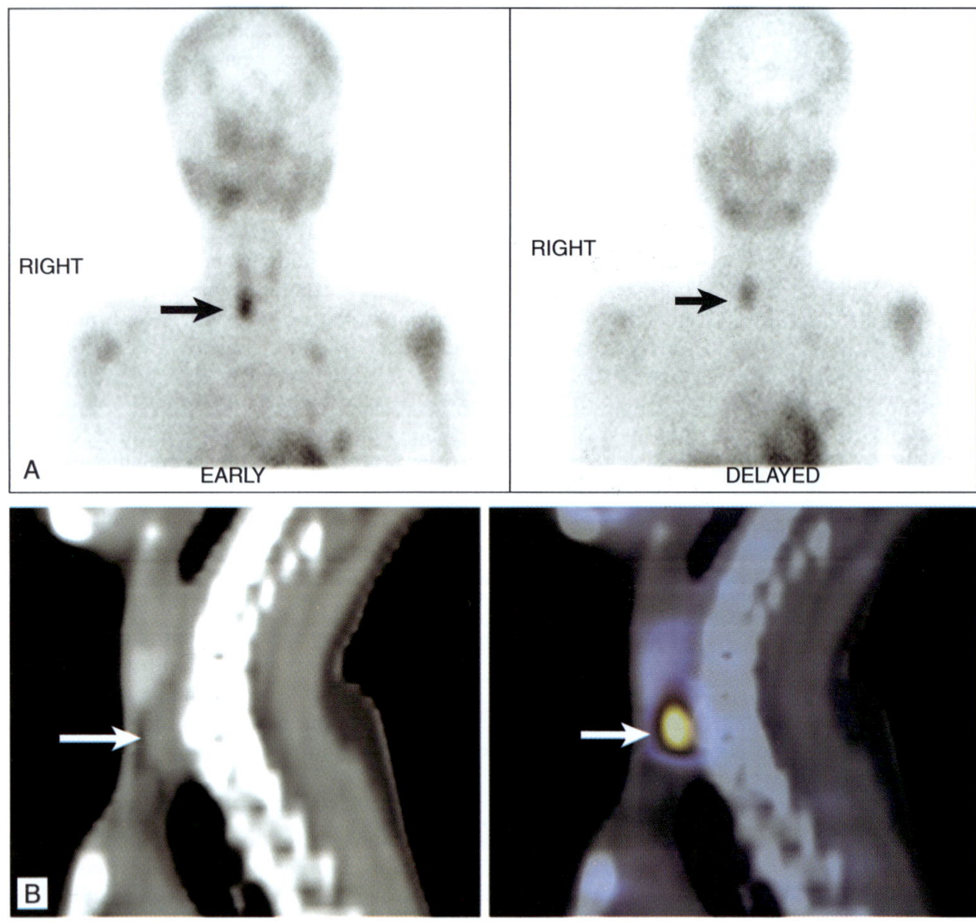

Figure 98.27 A young female patient with pathological fracture of both femora, on evaluation, showed markedly high intact parathyroid hormone level (1803 pg/mL; reference range, 10–65 pg/mL). Dual-phase single tracer technetium-99m sestamibi (A) early image shows homogenous tracer uptake in both thyroid lobes with prominent focal uptake at the inferior pole of the right thyroid lobe (*arrow*). There is complete tracer washout from both thyroid lobes with tracer retention at the inferior pole of the right thyroid lobe (*arrow*) on delayed image suggestive of a parathyroid adenoma. Low-dose single-photon emission computed tomography/computed tomography (SPECT/CT) of the neck (B) localizes the uptake to a soft tissue nodular lesion posteroinferior to right thyroid lobe (*arrow*), thus helping in precise localization of adenoma for minimally invasive surgery. Other abnormal increased uptake in the right maxilla, humeri, and left thorax localizes to lytic lesions on SPECT/CT suggestive of brown tumors (not shown here).

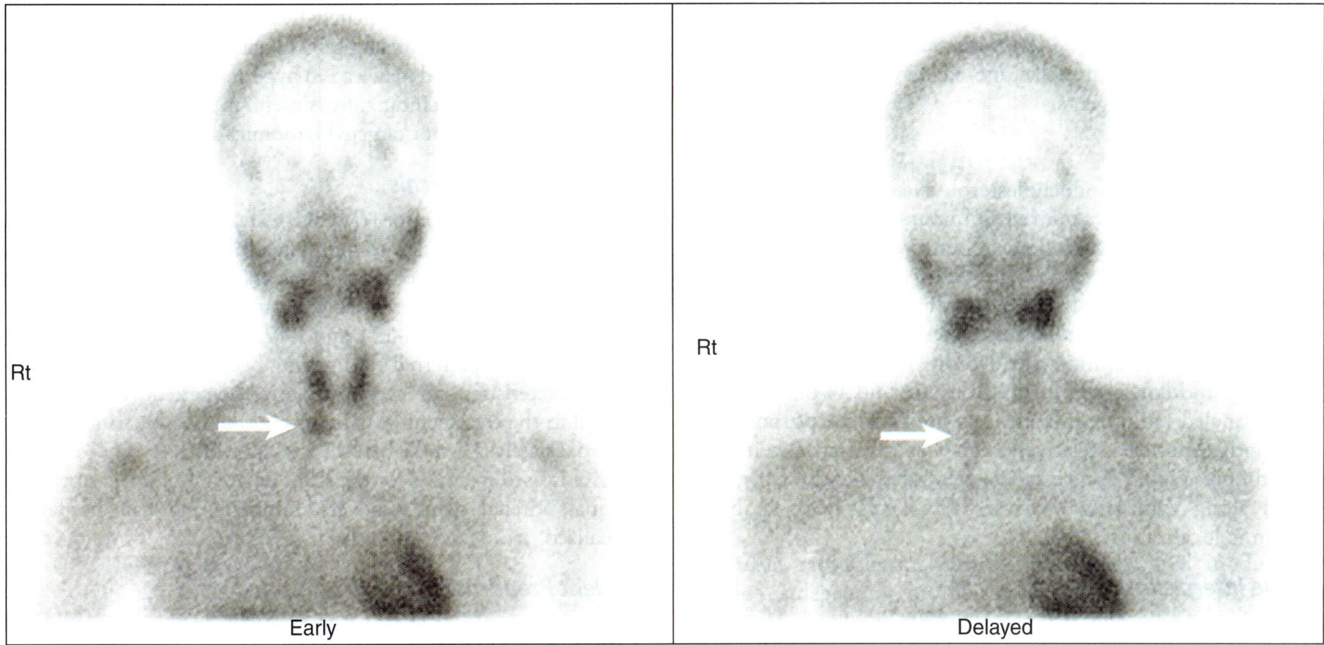

Figure 98.28 Patient with biochemically confirmed primary parathyroidism (1508 pg/mL; reference range, 10–65 pg/mL). Dual-phase single tracer technetium-99m sestamibi early image shows homogenous tracer uptake in both thyroid lobes with focal uptake at the inferior pole of the right thyroid lobe (*arrow*). There is near-complete tracer washout from both thyroid lobes with minimal tracer retention at the inferior pole of the right thyroid lobe (*arrow*) on delayed image suggestive of a parathyroid adenoma. Teaching point: Early washout from the parathyroid adenoma may lead to false-negative findings on dual-phase study. *Rt*, right.

expensive and rarely used. *Tc-99m sestamibi and Tc-99m pertechnetate is commonly used for this purpose.* Subtraction imaging is preferred over dual-phase imaging in some specific situations. In patients with known nodular goiter, subtraction imaging is preferred. Furthermore, it is preferred in patients with recurrent or persistent disease in PHPT and patients suspected of multiple hyperfunctioning parathyroid glands. The patient preparation is similar to that for thyroid scintigraphy. Active vitamin D supplementation should be withheld for 1 week.

The injected activity of Tc-99m sestamibi is approximately 15–20 mCi, and the Tc-99m pertechnetate is 2–4 mCi. There are several sequences in which imaging can be performed in subtraction scintigraphy.

In Tc-99m pertechnetate/Tc-99m sestamibi imaging, the patient is injected with 2 mCi of pertechnetate, and neck images are acquired at 20 minutes. At the end of imaging, 20 mCi of Tc-99m sestamibi is injected, and the neck image is acquired after 15 minutes while keeping the patient in the same position [20]. It has good sensitivity. Some centers prefer using 400 mg of oral potassium perchlorate immediately before thyroid scan acquisition. This helps in the early washout of the pertechnetate from the thyroid gland and fewer counts from the thyroid in the Tc-99m sestamibi image.

Image subtraction of Tc-99m pertechnetate from Tc-99m sestamibi image is performed digitally; however, visual inspection and interpretation help avoid false-negative and false-positive results. Sometimes realignment of images is necessary because there may be patient motion between two-image acquisition.

In general, the focal uptake that persists after subtraction is considered hyperfunctioning parathyroid. Guidelines suggest progressive incremental subtraction with real-time display for optimal subtraction of image (i.e., residual tracer activity in the thyroid should not be lower than surrounding neck tissues after subtraction). This helps to avoid oversubtraction and missing multiple adenomas.

Radionuclide-Guided Minimally Invasive Surgery in Hyperparathyroidism

Intraoperative use of a handheld gamma probe helps to guide the radioactive parathyroid adenoma. It is essential to use a well-collimated probe because the surrounding background thyroid activity could be significantly higher than other radio-guided surgery. Radionuclide-guided minimally invasive surgery helps in less surgery time and shorter hospital stay. Furthermore, on-table verification of excised tissue is possible by measuring counts from the excised specimen. Surgery should be performed 2–3 hours after tracer injection for parathyroid imaging. An in vivo parathyroid-to-thyroid ratio of more than 1.5 and a parathyroid-to-background ratio of more than 2.5 are considered a pathological parathyroid location during surgery.

Adrenal Cortex Imaging

The adrenal cortex consists of the outer glomerulosa zone producing mineralocorticoids, the middle fasciculata zone producing glucocorticoids, and the inner reticulata zone producing sex hormones. The renin–angiotensin–aldosterone axis regulates the outer zone, and the hypothalamic-pituitary–adrenal axis regulates the middle and inner zone.

Radiopharmaceutical

I-131-6β-iodomethyl-19-nor cholesterol (iodocholesterol or NP-59) is the radiotracer of choice for adrenal cortical scintigraphy because of its high avidity to the adrenal cortex. The uptake within the adrenal cortex is related to the precursor status of cholesterol for adrenal steroid synthesis and the transport of iodocholesterol by low-density lipoprotein (LDL). An increase in the cholesterol level downregulates LDL receptors and decreases tracer uptake. Contrary to this, an increase in adrenocorticotrophic hormone (ACTH) level leads to increased tracer uptake.

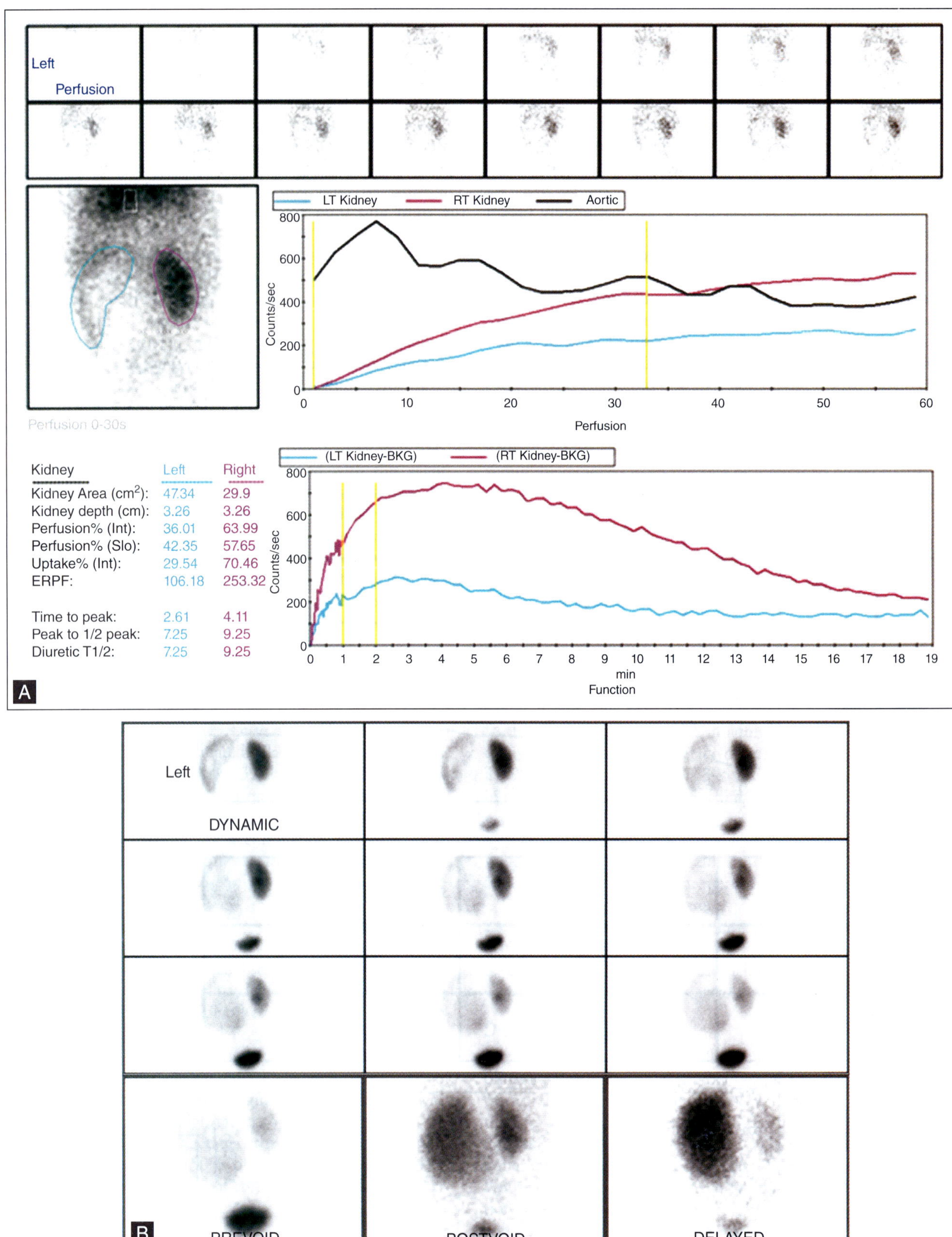

Figure 98.31 Technetium-99m ethylenedicysteine scan in a 4-year-old boy with left hydronephrosis (anteroposterior diameter, 7.5 cm) and recurrent urinary tract infection shows impaired perfusion in the left kidney (top panel images in A). Although the function curve of the left kidney shows a downward trend (lower curve in A) with a diuretic half-life of 7.25 min, the dynamic images show gradual pooling of the tracer in the pelvicalyceal system of the enlarged hydronephrotic left kidney and significant tracer retention until the end of the delayed image at 3 hours (B). The left ureter is not visualized. There is a normal right kidney. Overall findings are suggestive of left pelviureteric junction obstruction. Teaching point: The renal dynamic curve and parameters should be interpreted cautiously; visual analysis gives more accurate information.

Differential Renal Function

Differential or split function is a routinely mentioned parameter in the renography report. The normal range with a 95% confidence interval for Tc-99m MAG3 is 42–58%. It is usually calculated with the ROI placed over the kidney at the peak nephrogram activity between 1 and 3 minutes. *It does not represent the global or absolute renal function.* In early acute obstruction, there may be a relatively equal split function in both kidneys; however, the obstructed kidney may show photopenia in the pelvis with delay in cortical tracer transit. Gradually, there is impairment of function in the affected kidney.

Glomerular Filtration Rate Estimation

Renal dynamic imaging with Tc-99m DTPA can also be used for calculation of GFR. This gamma camera method of GFR estimation is called the Gates' method. In this method, the GFR is obtained by the net counts in the region of the kidneys starting between 1 and 3 minutes from the time point of image acquisition and presyringe and postsyringe counts with the help of software-based formula. Although it is simpler method for obtaining the GFR, it has limited accuracy.

Renovascular Hypertension Evaluation

Renal artery stenosis (RAS) can be an associated incidental finding or cause in patients with hypertension. It is essential to detect if the RAS is the cause of hypertension because early intervention decreases the renal damage and alleviates hypertension. In a significant RAS, there is a decrease in GFR caused by a reduction in afferent arteriolar blood pressure. This in turn leads to activation of the renin–angiotensin axis, releasing renin and subsequently angiotensin II, which acts on efferent arterioles to raise glomerular filtration pressure and GFR. An angiotensin-converting enzyme (ACE) inhibitor (captopril and enalapril) inhibits the production of angiotensin II. *Hence, in patients with RAS and compensated renal function, an ACE inhibitor causes a decrease in GFR, and this decrease in GFR with the ACE inhibitor can be documented with a renography study before and after administration of an ACE inhibitor.* Therefore, ACE inhibitor renography or captopril renography is used in the detection of RVH.

Patient Preparation and Precautions

If the patient is taking ACE inhibitor, short-acting ACE inhibitors such as captopril should be withheld for 3 days, and long-acting should be withheld for 5–7 days before the study if permissible clinically [25]. If it is not possible to stop the drug, it may be continued, and the test will have slightly lower sensitivity. Furthermore, the calcium channel blocker may be discontinued if there is no contraindication. Because an ACE inhibitor administered during the test may cause hypotension, the vital signs should be monitored, and an IV line should be placed before the study.

Radiopharmaceuticals

All three radiopharmaceuticals can be used. However, because of the higher extraction fraction, Tc-99m MAG3 and Tc-99m EC are usually preferred. But GFR can be obtained only in the Tc-99m DTPA study.

Procedure

Captopril recommended dose is 0.5 mg/kg per oral with a maximum dose of 25 mg [25]. The patient should not have taken a solid meal 4 hours before the study, as food decreases GI absorption of this drug. The tracer should be injected 60 minutes after the captopril administration. Injection Enalaprilat can also be used as slow IV injection [25]. The tracer should be injected 15 minutes after the enalaprilat administration. However, Enalaprilat can cause hypotension, and precaution should be taken appropriately.

Two-Day Protocol: ACE inhibitor renography should be performed on the first day. If the ACE inhibitor renogram results are normal, the chance of RVH is low. However, a baseline study should be conducted on another day to increase specificity.

One-Day Protocol: Baseline renography is performed first with a lower activity of radiotracer (~1 mCi). Higher activity of radioactivity is used during the second ACE inhibitor renography (~4–5 mCi). To avoid interference of residual activity from the baseline study, sufficient time interval should occur between the two studies [25].

Study Interpretation

In patients with normal or mildly impaired renal function with a creatinine level of less than 1.7 mg/dL, ACE inhibitor renography has sensitivity and specificity of approximately 90–95% in the diagnosis of RVH [25]. However, impaired renal function decreases sensitivity and specificity. Essentially, with ACE inhibitor, there is a decrease in GFR on renography with improvement in the baseline study. Because of RAS or with a baseline poorly functioning kidney in an already small shrunken kidney, it is difficult to appreciate the decrease in function or GFR caused by the ACE inhibitor.

99mTc-DTPA Study: There is a decrease in GFR in ACE inhibitor renography leading to decreased cortical uptake on the affected side compared with baseline study in those with RVH. There are slower tracer uptake and lower peak on ACE inhibitor renography in patients with RVH. A 10% decrease in differential function or a 10% decrease in estimated GFR compared with the baseline study is considered as having a high probability of RVH. A change in 5–10% is considered an intermediate probability of RVH [25].

99mTc-MAG3 and Tc-99m EC Study: Because renal tubular uptake and secretion are not affected by ACE inhibitors, the critical finding in RVH is cortical tracer retention. However, bilateral cortical retention can be seen because of inadequate hydration, hypotension, or salt depletion.

Renal Transplant Evaluation

Although USG and biopsy are commonly used modalities, renal scintigraphy is an important modality for evaluating renal transplant recipients' medical and surgical complications. In renal transplant evaluation, usually the anterior view centered over the transplanted kidney is acquired. The scintigraphy findings should be interpreted while keeping in mind the time since transplant, clinical history, and type of allograft (cadaveric or living donor transplant). A living donor transplant kidney functions better than a cadaveric allograft. Initially, in a normal transplant kidney, during the perfusion phase, the radiotracer bolus reaches the kidney almost at the same time as the iliac vessels. The normal parenchymal phase is seen at 2–5 minutes. However, there may be a decrease in perfusion and function of the kidney over the years. Clearance of a transplant kidney is slightly slower than that of a normal kidney.

- In both vasomotor nephropathy and acute rejection, there is impaired cortical function and marked cortical retention. However, impaired perfusion is seen in acute rejection
- Furthermore, when initial renal function is normal and deteriorates subsequently, it is more in favor of acute rejection. The initial baseline scan during day 1 or 2 of the transplant is always helpful

- In drug-induced nephrotoxicity, the scan pattern is similar to vasomotor nephropathy. There may be an outflow obstruction in the allograft. Diuretic renography is often helpful in this condition. However, acute rejection may also give an appearance of obstructed clearance
- Postsurgery leaks can occur from the anatomic site. Dynamic renography shows extrarenal tracer accumulation. Sometimes there may be photopenic defect because of the collection of nonradioactive urine
- Scintigraphic pattern in renal artery and vein occlusion is seen as negligible perfusion.

Renal Cortical Imaging

The most common indication for cortical imaging is in the detection of acute pyelonephritis and scarring caused by chronic pyelonephritis. Cortical scintigraphy is twice as sensitive as USG in the detection of cortical defects. Other indications are detection or confirmation of ectopic kidney and horseshoe kidney. Rarely, it is used as differentiation of hypertrophied column of Bertin from the real renal mass. Usually, Tc-99m DMSA is the radiopharmaceutical of choice for cortical imaging.

Procedure

No patient preparation is needed. 4–5 mCi of Tc-99m DMSA is injected intravenously in adults and 50 μCi/kg in children with a minimum of 1 mCi [26]. In general, a low-energy high-resolution parallel-hole collimator is used, and a pinhole collimator gives superior image quality and is preferred. Imaging should start 2–3 hours after radiotracer administration. The patient should void immediately before image acquisition begins. Static images are acquired in anterior, posterior, and oblique views if pinhole imaging not possible.

Interpretation and Pitfalls

A normal scan shows homogeneous tracer accumulation in the renal cortex (Fig. 98.32). There may be some variation in the shape of the kidneys. The sizes, shapes, and positions of the kidneys should be noted. In general, the upper poles show relatively less tracer uptake.

- Scarring or pyelonephritis is seen as a defect in the cortical outline (Fig. 98.33). In the presence of scars, there may be a small, shrunken kidney. It is often challenging to differentiate scar from acute pyelonephritis, and a 3- to 6-month infection-free interval imaging is often necessary. If the defects persist on interval imaging, it is compatible with a scar. The other differential diagnosis of cortical defects is simple cysts, mass, and ischemia. Hence, reading the scan in correlation with USG or other available anatomic imaging is helpful
- In ectopic kidney, both the abdomen and pelvis must be in the field of view, and the bladder should be catheterized (Fig. 98.34)
- In horseshoe kidneys, it is easy to appreciate the fusion of lower poles of both kidneys on DMSA scan, and split function of each moiety can be calculated (Fig. 98.35)
- The feature to differentiate a hypertrophied column of Bertin from a renal mass is that Bertin's column shows tracer accumulation, whereas a renal tumor usually does not accumulate tracer

In renal tubular acidosis or Fanconi syndrome, the uptake of Tc-99m DMSA by proximal tubules is inhibited, and other renal agents such as Tc-99m EC or Tc-99m MAG3 should be used to assess renal function.

Radionuclide Cystography

Vesicoureteral reflux occurs in about 1–2% of the pediatric age group. Approximately 40% pediatric patients with upper urinary tract infections (UTIs) have VUR. If untreated, it may lead to chronic renal failure. Radionuclide cystography (RNC) is useful in the evaluation of VUR with equal sensitivity and significantly less (50–200 times less) gonadal radiation compared with micturating cystourethrography. RNC can detect reflux volume as low as 1 mL [27].

Indications

Indications include valuation of female patients with UTI for VUR, in familial VUR, and to assess treatment response after medical management and antireflux surgery.

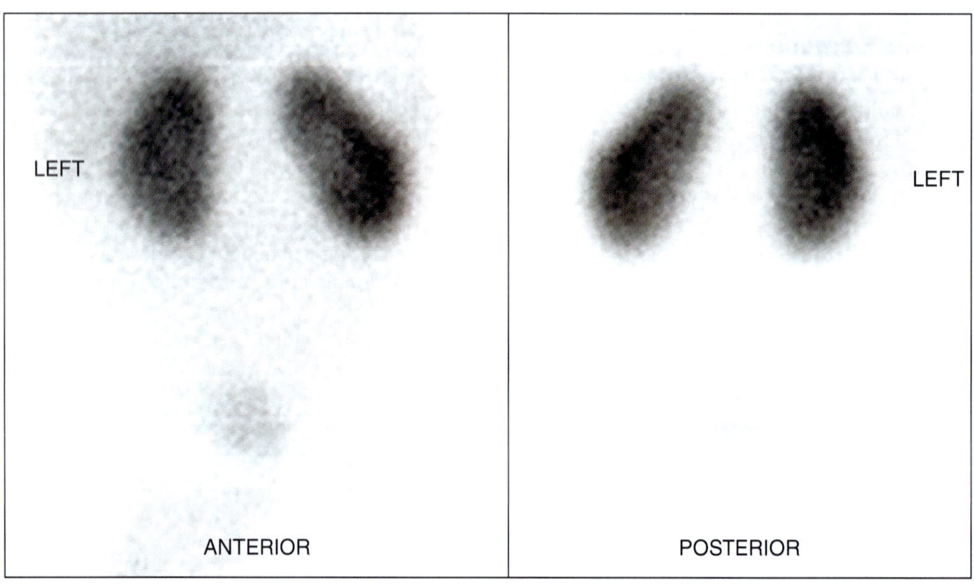

Figure 98.32 Normal dimercaptosuccinic acid scan showing normal size and position of both kidneys with good homogeneous tracer uptake and uniform cortical outline.

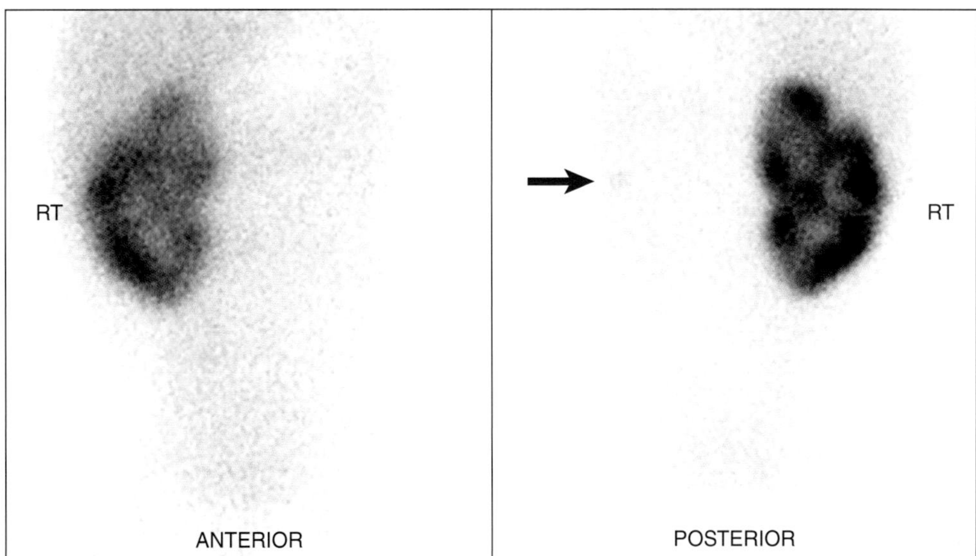

Figure 98.33 Dimercaptosuccinic acid scan of a 4-year-old boy with recurrent urinary tract infection and bilateral hydronephrosis on ultrasonography shows an irregular cortical outline of the right kidney with multiple cortical defects indicative of scarring or acute pyelonephritis. The left kidney is only minimally visualized (*arrow*), suggestive of negligible cortical function. *RT*, right.

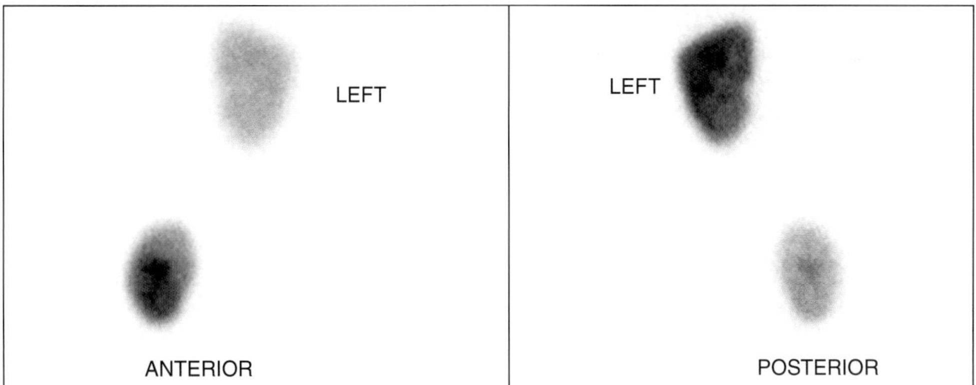

Figure 98.34 This 12-year-old girl was incidentally found to have right ectopic kidney on ultrasonography. Dimercaptosuccinic acid scan shows right pelvic kidney with good cortical function and no evidence of cortical scar.

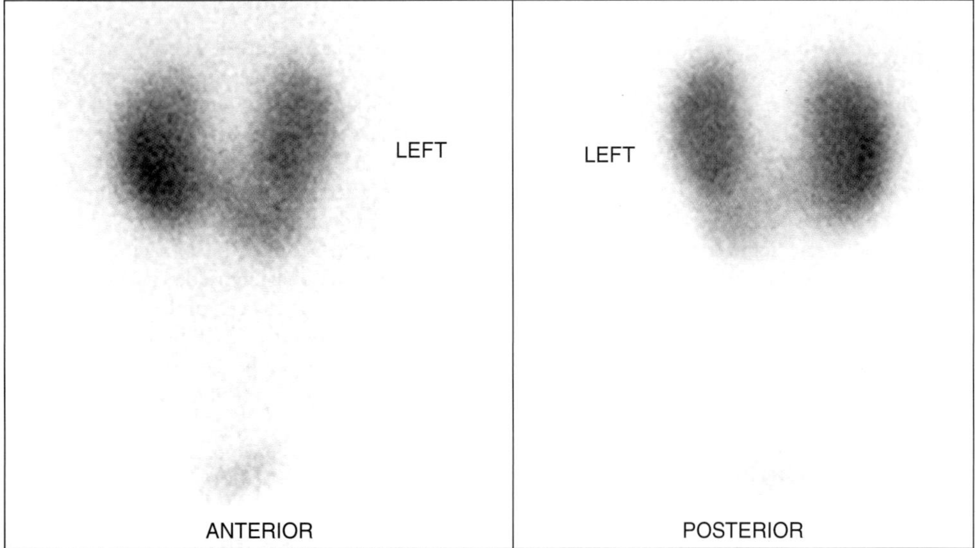

Figure 98.35 A known case of anorectal malformation in a 10-month-old male baby. The dimercaptosuccinic acid scan shows fusion of the lower pole of both kidneys medially, suggestive of horseshoe kidney. Both moieties show good cortical function (split function: left kidney, 45% and right kidney, 55%). There is no evidence of cortical defect to suggest scarring.

Patient Preparation

In general, no specific preparation is necessary. However, in direct radionuclide cystography (DRCG), bladder catheterization under aseptic conditions is needed.

Radiopharmaceutical

Tc-99m sulphur colloid (SC) is the preferred agent. The recommended activity is 0.5–1 mCi.

Procedure

In DRCG, the radiopharmaceutical is mixed with normal saline and instilled into the urinary bladder through a bladder catheter. The fluid should be filled until appropriate bladder volume is achieved. The bladder volume should be calculated as (age in years + 2) × 30 cc [24].

If the patient is cooperative (usually older than 3 years of age), they should sit on a bedpan with a collimator being placed vertically against the back. However, younger children may lie down supine during the filling phase. The catheter balloon is deflated, and the patient should void, if possible, in a sitting position.

The dynamic voiding images are obtained in 2-second time frames until the patient voids. Pre- and postvoid static images are acquired for the calculation of residual bladder volume.

Interpretation

RNC grade I: radiotracer confined to the ureter micturating cystourethrogram (MCU grade I).
RNC grade II: radiotracer reflux to the pelvicalyceal system (MCU II and III).
RNC grade III: radiotracer reflux to the pelvicalyceal system along with a dilated collecting system and dilated tortuous ureter (MCU grades IV and V).

Pitfalls

Small-volume reflux into the lower ureter may be missed because of adjacent bladder activity.

Pulmonary System

Ventilation/perfusion (V/Q) imaging is one of the commonly performed lung imaging studies in nuclear medicine.

Ventilation Imaging

The radiopharmaceuticals used and recommended activity in ventilation imaging are described in Table 98.9.

TABLE 98.9 Radiopharmaceuticals Used and Recommended Activity in Ventilation Imaging

Radiopharmaceutical	Physical Half-Life of Radionuclide	Recommended Dose (mCi)	Gamma Emission Energy (keV)
Aerosols			
Tc-99m DTPA	6 hr	1	140
Technegas	6 hr	1	140
Radioactive Gases			
Xenon-133	5.24 days	15–20	81
Xenon-127	36.4 days	10–20	172, 203, 375
Krypton-81m	13 sec	1–10	190

DTPA, diethylene triamine penta-acetic acid; *Tc-99m*, technetium-99m.

Tc-99m DTPA Aerosols

Tc-99m DTPA aerosols are widely available, inexpensive, and commonly used tracers in nuclear medicine. Tc-99m DTPA aerosols are generated by running oxygen through the aerosol system, which produces particles size in the range of 0.5–0.8 μm in diameter and can reach the alveoli like gases [28]. *Usually, the pulmonary clearance of the tracer has a half-life of approximately 1 hour. Therefore, unlike gases, multiple view of lung images can be obtained.* The disadvantage is that the generated larger particle size is deposited in central airways. Furthermore, there can be excessive deposits in the proximal bronchial tree in obstructed airway disease, which often degrades the image quality.

Tc-99m Technegas (Cyclomedica)

This radiotracer is mainly used in Australia and Europe. The image quality is good because of uniform fine particles; however, its higher cost and limited availability are the disadvantages. An onsite generator is required to produce Technegas.

Xenon-133

There is no central airway deposition and the advantage of having different gamma energy than perfusion agents for imaging. As it clears from the lungs in 2–3 minutes, only the posterior view is possible. Three phases are acquired: wash-in, equilibrium, and washout. Retention of tracer in the lungs beyond 3 minutes is seen in obstructive airway disease.

Xenon-127

This is rarely used because it is cyclotron produced.

Krypton-81m

This is a generator produced radiotracer and produced from a rubidium-81–krypton-81m generator. Because of a very short half-life of 13 seconds, ventilation images are acquired immediately after each perfusion view without moving the patient. Thus, it is the ideal ventilation imaging radiogas. However, it is expensive.

Perfusion Imaging

The radiopharmaceutical Tc-99m macroaggregated albumin (99mTc-MAA) particles are administered intravenously. The particle size usually ranges between 10 and 30 μm. The precapillary arteriole has a diameter of about 0–30 μm. Hence, Tc-99m MAA particles are trapped in the precapillary arterioles. Generally, a typical injected activity in adults contains 500,000 Tc-99m MAA particles, and only about 0.1–0.3% of the precapillary arterioles are occluded. Because the particles are degraded by enzymatic hydrolysis and phagocytized, the arterioles obstruction is only temporary [29]. A lower number of particles (~100,000) should be used in patients with pulmonary arterial hypertension and right-to-left shunts. In neonates, 10,000–50,000 particles are recommended. The critical organ is the lung, which receives 1 rad from a typical 5-mCi injected radiotracer activity. The dose Tc-99m MAA for pediatric patients is 1.11 MBq/kg (0.03 mCi/kg) with a minimum dose of 0.04 mCi.

Pulmonary Embolism

Pulmonary embolism (PE) is a serious condition that can be fatal if not treated. The diagnosis is usually straightforward in the presence of predisposing factors and typical clinical manifestations. CT pulmonary angiography (CTPA) is the most commonly used diagnostic imaging modality because of its easy availability in emergency conditions. CTPA has a high negative predictive value for PE. However, it has significantly higher radiation and has lower accuracy in detecting subsegmental thrombi. CTPA is a contraindication in patients with renal failure and those who are allergic to contrast agents. Although V/Q scans are currently underused, they have an advantage because of lower radiation exposure. Furthermore, with the increased utility of V/Q SPECT/CT, the accuracy is higher than for conventional planar imaging. *V/Q scan is still the imaging modality of choice in pregnant women, patients with compromised renal function, and patients with allergy to contrast media.* A normal scan essentially rules out significant acute PE. A V/Q mismatch is compatible with PE on a V/Q scan (i.e., the normal ventilation region shows a corresponding segmental wedge-shaped area of decreased or absent perfusion).

Image Acquisition

Patient position is supine. The lung images are acquired with a parallel hole, high-resolution collimator using a large field of view camera. Multiple static images in eight standard views (anterior, posterior, right lateral, left lateral, right anterior oblique, left anterior oblique, right posterior oblique, and left posterior oblique) are acquired. In the perfusion phase, each view is acquired for approximately 500,000 counts. In the ventilation phase, each view is acquired for 100,000 counts or 5 minutes. SPECT and SPECT/CT images provide better anatomic and functional information.

Normal Biodistribution and Pitfalls

Normally, the tracers show the homogenous distribution in both lungs without any defect in both perfusion and ventilation studies (Fig. 98.36). However, in an erect posture, a ventilation study shows more tracer localization in the lung base than at the apex and should be interpreted cautiously. Artifacts specific to

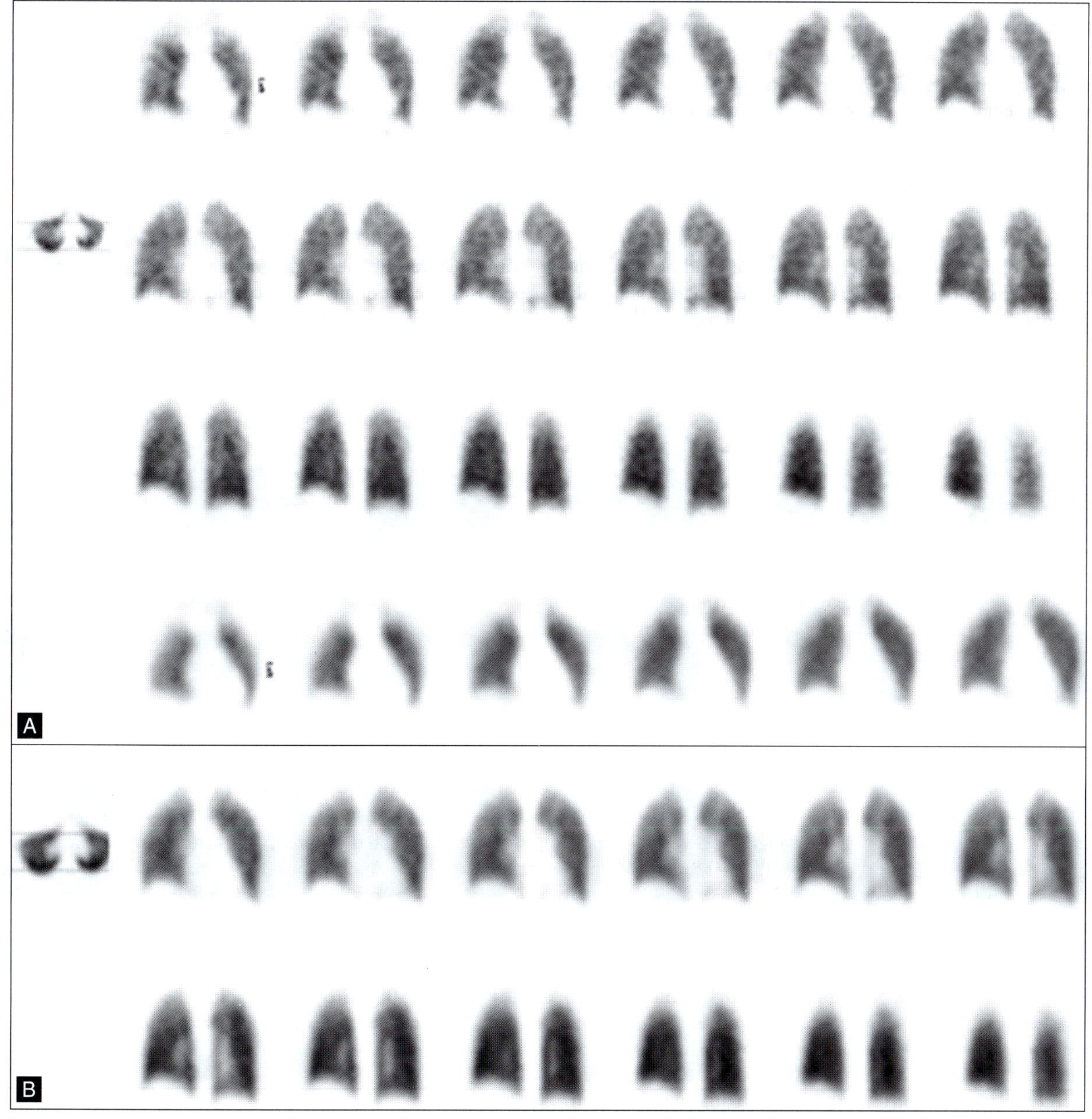

Figure 98.36 Normal Ventilation/perfusion single-photon emission computed tomography coronal ventilation images show normal ventilation with krypton-81m gas (A). Coronal images show normal perfusion. No unmatched perfusion defects were identified (B).

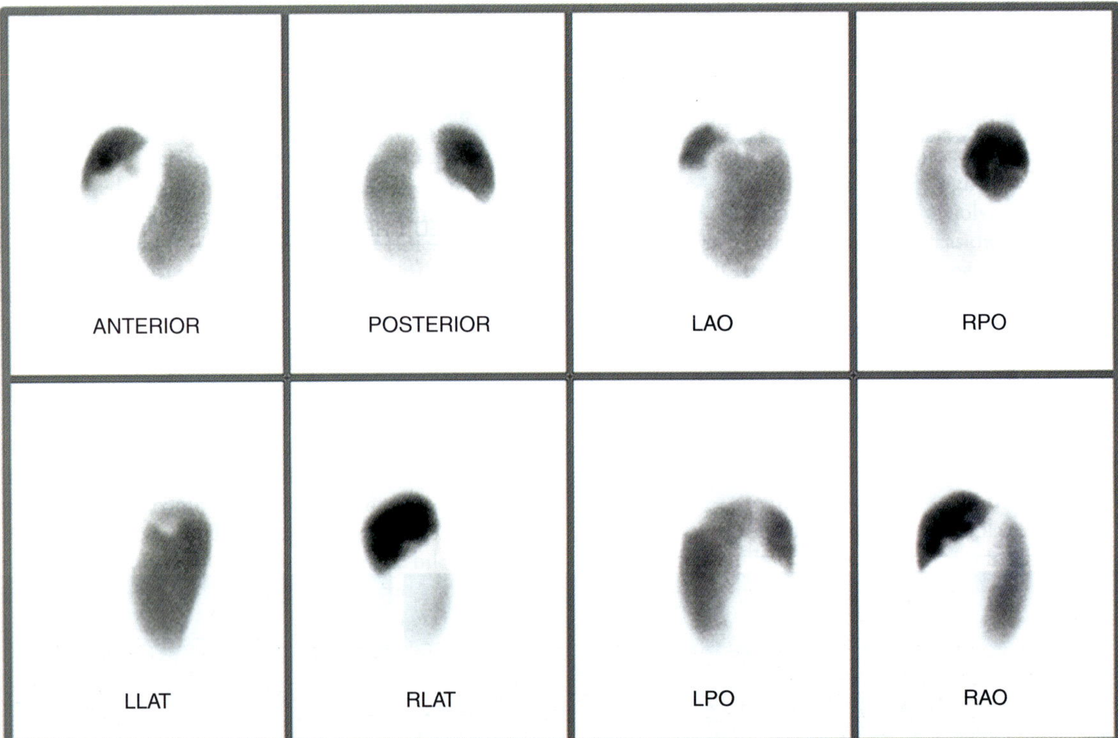

Figure 98.45 A 31-year-old female patient with splenomegaly and features of portal hypertension underwent a liver scan to rule out cirrhosis of the liver. The scan shows preserved trapping function of hepatocyte with no evidence of a colloid shift to the spleen or bone marrow, ruling out cirrhosis. *LAO*, left anterior oblique; *LLAT*, left lateral; *LPO*, left posterior oblique; *RAO*, right anterior oblique; *RLAT*, right lateral oblique; *RPO*, right posterior oblique.

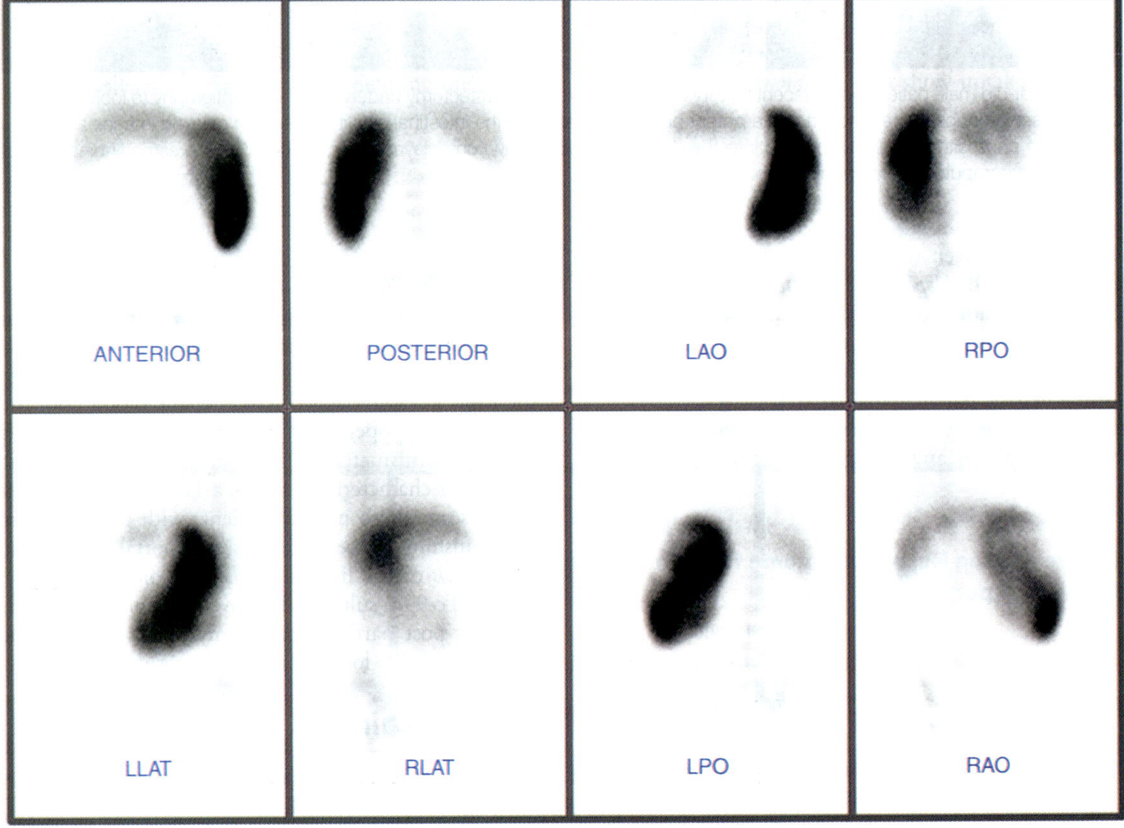

Figure 98.46 A 4-year-old male child with features of portal hypertension and splenomegaly underwent a liver scan. The scan shows impaired hepatocyte extraction of radiotracer with a colloid shift to bone marrow and the spleen, suggestive of liver cirrhosis. *LAO*, left anterior oblique; *LLAT*, left lateral; *LPO*, left posterior oblique; *RAO*, right anterior oblique; *RLAT*, right lateral oblique; *RPO*, right posterior oblique.

1. Seizure focus localization
2. Dementia management
3. Diagnosis of different types of movement disorders
4. Diagnosis of recurrent brain tumors
5. Cerebrovascular diseases management
6. Brain death
7. Normal-pressure hydrocephalus
8. Assessment of ventricular shunt function
9. Detection of cerebrospinal fluid leak

Besides the indications already mentioned, nuclear medicine is also being used in few investigational indications, as in psychiatric diseases, head trauma, and neuroinflammation management. The commonly used radionuclides for the purpose are Tc-99m, I-123, Tl-201, and In-111. These radioisotopes, in combination with different molecules, follow different physiologic functions, which help in the diagnosis of many neurologic disorders.

Seizure Focus Localization

For decades, neuromolecular imaging has been used in noninvasive localization of the epileptic focus in patients planned for epileptic surgery [63,64]. In neuromolecular imaging, ictal and interictal SPECT help in localizing epileptic focus in patients' presurgical evaluation. Two perfusion tracers most commonly used for this purpose are Tc-99m-hexamethyl propylene amine oxime (Tc-99m HMPAO) and Tc-99m ethyl cysteinatediethylester (Tc-99m ECD).

During the ictal state, the seizure focus demonstrates hyperperfusion, and during the interictal and postictal states, it shows hypoperfusion. Both ictal and interictal studies are performed to localize the culprit focus. When subtraction imaging is done by subtracting the interictal image volume from the ictal image volume, the precise location of the ictal-activated hyperperfusion area can be identified. This computer-generated subtraction imaging of ictal and interictal SPECT, superimposed on MRI, is commonly abbreviated as SISCOM/SISCOS. This ictal activation focus strongly corresponds to the epileptogenic zone (Fig. 98.47). The most challenging issue in performing ictal brain SPECT is the prompt injection of radiotracer as soon as the seizure's onset because delayed injection leads to inaccurate localisation of the seizure focus.

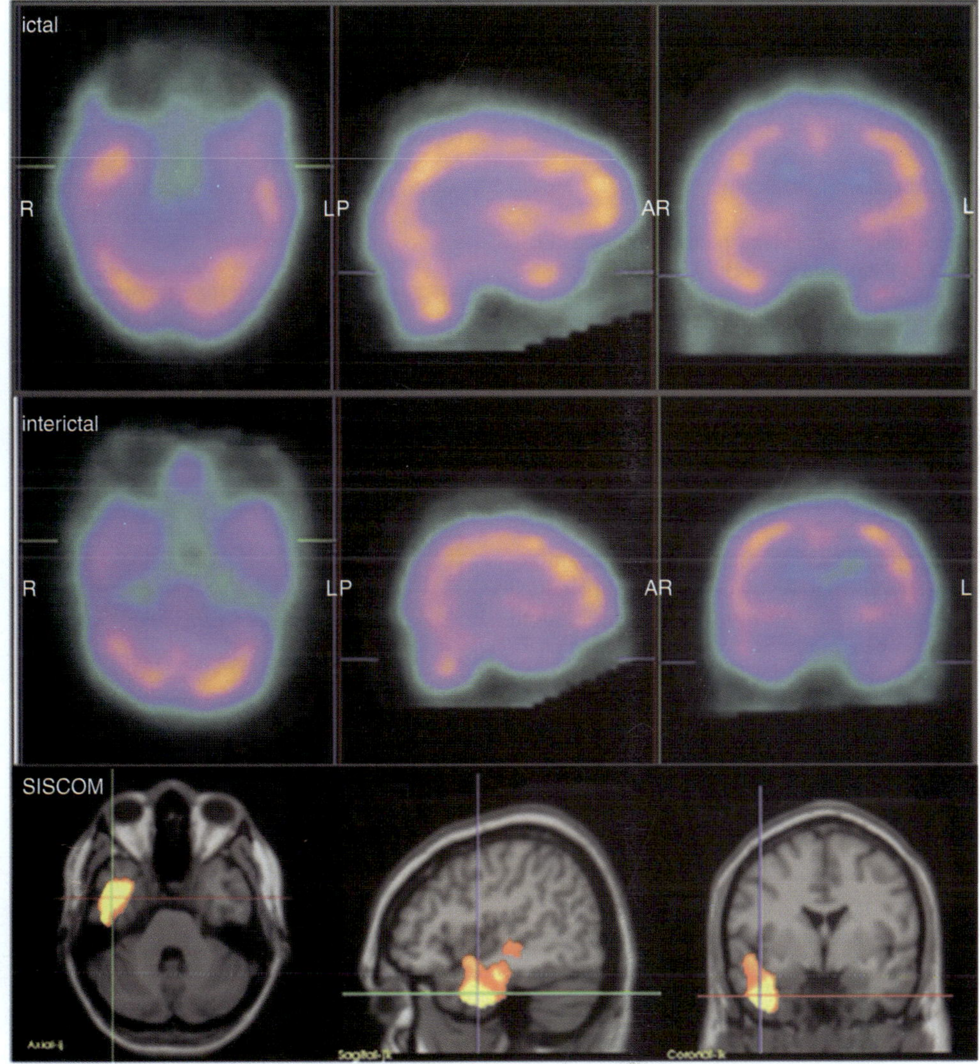

Figure 98.47 A 15-year-old girl with a history of drug-refractory epilepsy underwent ictal and interictal technetium-99m ethyl cysteinatediethylester studies. Ictal images show mildly increased tracer uptake in the right temporoparietal cortex. Interictal images show mild asymmetry in temporoparietal cortex uptake. The same ictal and interictal images were evaluated through subtraction of ictal and interictal SPECT co-registered to MRI (SISCOM), and the subtraction images show focal tracer accumulation in the right temporal cortex, suggestive of the epileptogenic focus.

Dementia Management

There are two primary purposes for neuromolecular imaging in dementia; the first is for early diagnosis, and the other is to differentiate the causes of dementia. The brain function or synaptic activity depends on glucose metabolism, which can be correlated with brain perfusion [65]. Brain perfusion has been studied using SPECT perfusion agents (Tc-99m HMPAO, Tc-99m ECD) for the early diagnosis and management of patients with dementia [65,66].

Many perfusion SPECT studies done to diagnose Alzheimer's disease (AD) have substantiated a definite hypoperfusion pattern. Usually, the posterior cingulate cortex and precuneus are the earliest to show changes, and hypoperfusion in posterior temporoparietal cortices is seen in late stages. The involvement of frontal cortices is seen only in advanced stages. This hypoperfusion is usually bilateral and often asymmetric. As per various metaanalyses, perfusion SPECT's sensitivity and specificity in differentiating AD from healthy individuals are about 80% and 85%, respectively. The sensitivity and specificity in differentiating AD from mild cognitive impairment are 64% and 76%, respectively. The characteristic perfusion pattern in dementia with Lewy bodies is hypoperfusion in the occipital lobe and in progressive supranuclear palsy is frontal hypoperfusion [67]. The typical perfusion pattern is seen in behavioral variant frontotemporal dementia, which includes frontal or anterior temporal hypoperfusion (Table 98.11). Although perfusion SPECT has helped diagnose and differentiate different variants of dementia, PET imaging is currently preferred for this purpose.

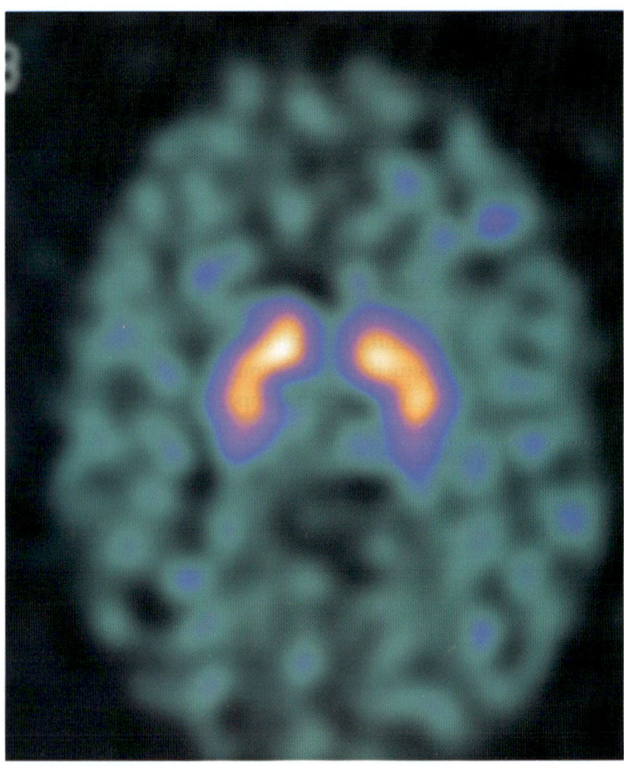

Figure 98.48 Dopamine transporter scan shows normal striatal uptake bilaterally. There is normal background activity. The appearance suggest preservation of the dopaminergic activity within the presynaptic terminals and rules out idiopathic Parkinson's disease or Parkinson's plus syndrome.

Movement Disorders

Several studies have examined the diagnostic performance of SPECT tracers such as I-123-β-carbomethoxy-3β-4-iodophenyltropane (I-123 β-CIT), I-123 fluoropropyl-CIT, Tc-99m TRODAT-1 (Tropane derivative) or I-123 PE21 (cocaine derivative), I-123 Iodobenzamide (IBZM), and I-123 IBF (IBZM analogue) to distinguish degenerative from non-degenerative parkinsonism with preserved nigrostriatal innervation. They show very high sensitivity and specificity of these agents. SPECT imaging can also help in differentiating between idiopathic Parkinson's disease (IPD) and atypical parkinsonism [68]. The integrity of the dopaminergic system can be assessed by dopamine transporter (DaT) imaging.

A normal DaT scan using I-123 ioflupane rules out dopamine-related pathology (Fig. 98.48). However, other differentials such as essential tremor, vascular parkinsonism, and drug-induced parkinsonism should also be considered. It has been seen that in both IPD and multiple system atrophy (MSA), patients show a reduced DaT tracer uptake in putamen than the caudate nucleus (Fig. 98.49). However, the reduced striatal tracer uptake in the

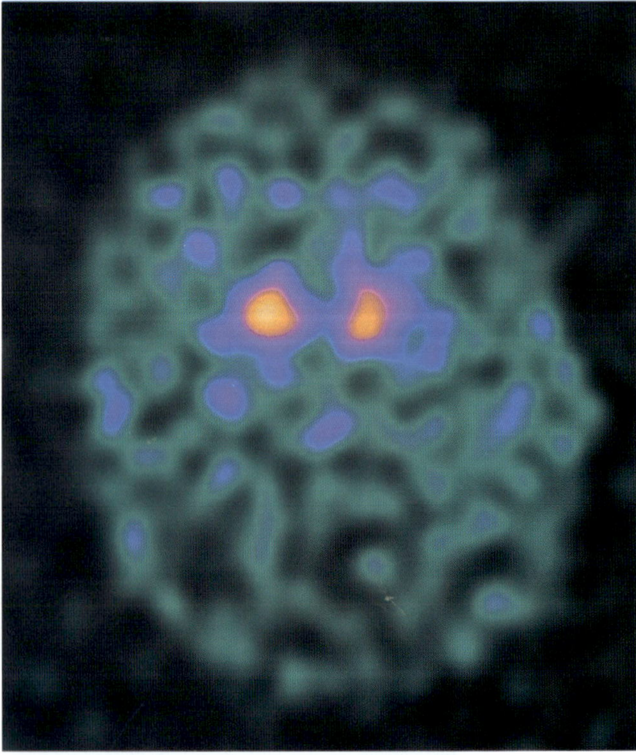

Figure 98.49 Dopamine transporter scan shows markedly reduced tracer uptake in the putamina bilaterally with relatively preserved activity in the caudate nuclei. The appearance suggest the loss of the dopaminergic activity within the presynaptic terminals. Appearance would indicate idiopathic Parkinson's disease or Parkinson's plus syndrome.

TABLE 98.11 Perfusion Pattern in Different Types of Dementia

Dementia Type	Perfusion Pattern
Alzheimer's disease	Hypoperfusion in the posterior cingulate cortex and precuneus with posterior temporoparietal and frontal cortices hypoperfusion in late stages
Dementia with Lewy bodies	Occipital hypoperfusion
Behavioral variant frontotemporal dementia	Frontal and/or anterior temporal hypoperfusion
Progressive supranuclear palsy	Frontal hypoperfusion

DaT scan is more symmetrical in patients with MSA than with IPD. To make the criteria more objective, few researchers have also suggested that patients with a relative asymmetry of more than 15% favor the diagnosis of IPD, whereas patients with an asymmetry between 5% and 15% favor MSA as the diagnosis. Few studies used I-123 IBF (for D2 receptor) along with I-123 β-CIT (DaT scan). It has been found that both IPD and MSA patients show reduced DaT binding, but only those with MSA show reduced tracer uptake in D2 imaging. These results suggest that DAT SPECT may help differentiate IPD from control participants, and D2 receptor imaging can be useful in further differentiating MSA from PD [69]. It is imperative to use multi-tracer imaging to increase the accuracy of diagnosis.

Brain Tumors

Thallium-201 and Tc-99m sestamibi SPECT or SPECT/CT are useful in the evaluation of recurrent brain tumors versus radiation necrosis. However, the factors essential for the uptake of these tracers in the brain tumors are a break in the blood–brain barrier and increased vascularity of the tumors. Besides these, Tc-99m glucoheptonate (GHA) has recently been used in brain tumor management. It is a structural analog of glucose, and a break in the blood–brain barrier is required for its entry. *Whereas the viable tumors show a progressive increase in the GHA uptake, inflammatory cells show rapid clearance.* It has been found that Tc-99m GHA SPECT is a more effective imaging modality compared with other mentioned SPECT tracers in detecting recurrent glioma [70,71]. Nonetheless, PET has mostly replaced brain SPECT for this purpose.

Cerebrovascular Diseases

Brain perfusion studies using radiopharmaceuticals such as Tc-99m HMPAO and Tc-99m ECD can assess the hemodynamic reserve in patients with cerebrovascular disease. The primary role of SPECT in acute stroke is to select patients for thrombolytic therapy. This is assessed by identifying the potentially salvageable brain parenchyma [72]. The cerebrovascular reserved test (CVR test) is also being used for the evaluation of brain perfusion by using vasodilator agents. SPECT perfusion assesses the cerebrovascular activity in response to a vasodilatory challenge. This is usually done by direct administration of acetazolamide, a carbonic anhydrase inhibitor. The acetazolamide challenge can anticipate the possible cerebrovascular event by evaluating the cerebral perfusion reserve. CVR test is also helpful in managing patients with Moyamoya disease who are planned for therapeutic interventions.

A carotid balloon occlusion test is another way of assessing cerebral perfusion reserve, and this evaluates the patency of the collateral circulations in the cerebral vasculature. It can help surgeons to be prepared for any intentional or unintentional sacrifice of the carotid artery during the surgery [73]. Asymmetric perfusion on SPECT imaging may suggest an increased risk of cerebrovascular accidents after internal carotid artery occlusion.

Brain Death Evaluation

The diagnosis of brain death can be confirmed by brain death scintigraphy. The commonly used tracers include Tc-99m HMPAO and Tc-99m ECD. Being lipophilic, they can assess the perfusion to the brain and viability of brain cells. The imaging feature characteristic of brain death is the absence of tracer accumulation in the brain. Currently, brain death scintigraphy is used during organ harvesting.

Diagnosis of Normal-Pressure Hydrocephalus

Cisternography has been used for the functional study of cerebrospinal fluid (CSF) dynamics. In this study, the radiopharmaceutical is administered into the CSF spaces and indirectly assess the CSF flow. The radiopharmaceuticals used are In-111 DTPA and Tc-99m DTPA, though In-111 DTPA is preferred because of its longer half-life. The tracer is administered into the subarachnoid space through a lumbar puncture. It can help in distinguishing communicating from noncommunicating hydrocephalus. The typical cisternographic picture in communicating hydrocephalus or normal-pressure hydrocephalus is the early tracer uptake in the lateral ventricles (by 6 hours of tracer injection) that persists for 1–2 days.

Assessing Shunt Patency

The patency of the shunt can be evaluated by clinical examination of the patient and clinically assessing the subcutaneous CSF reservoir. However, sometimes there may be uncertainty in the diagnosis. In such cases, a radionuclide study with Tc-99m DTPA can add to the diagnosis. The tracer is injected aseptically into the CSF space by a physician who is well aware of the shunt type. Usually, the radiotracer preferred for this purpose is Tc-99m DTPA because of its better image quality and lack of delayed imaging.

Detection of Cerebrospinal Fluid Leak

Radionuclide imaging is one of the most accurate methods used for detecting CSF leak. The radiotracer Tc-99m DTPA is administered into the CSF space through an aseptic lumbar puncture. Then the nasal pledgets are kept in the anterior and posterior part of each nasal cavity. After about 4 hours, the pledgets are collected, and their radioactivity is measured and compared. The radioactivity of nasal pledgets and blood plasma is compared; if the former is more than two times the latter, then a diagnosis of CSF leak is favored. Besides this, gamma camera imaging with an appropriate projection can also help in localizing the source of CSF leak. Usually, for suspected CSF rhinorrhea, the lateral and anterior projection imaging is acquired, whereas posterior projection is helpful for suspected CSF otorrhea. Other views can also be taken if a clear-cut site of leak is not found. Increased tracer accumulation is seen at the site of the leak on the scintigraphic images. Although both methods can be used for localizing CSF leaks, counting the pledgets always has a higher sensitivity.

Nuclear Cardiology

Nuclear medicine procedures are used to evaluate inducible cardiac ischemia, myocardial viability, ventricular function, and cardiac sympathetic innervation.

Myocardial Perfusion Imaging

Myocardial perfusion is evaluated by injecting a radiopharmaceutical that distributes in the myocardium followed by imaging of the heart. The perfusion abnormality is diagnosed as relatively reduced tracer accumulation in the abnormal myocardium compared with that in the adjacent normal myocardium. To increase the sensitivity, different cardiac stress types, such as exercise or pharmacologic stress, are performed during tracer administration. This increases the coronary blood flow compared with resting levels, to render a flow differential between normal and abnormal coronary arteries. These differences can be evaluated visually or quantitatively on myocardial perfusion images.

Radionuclide Ventriculography

Radionuclide ventriculography has long been used for assessment of ventricular function, detection of CAD, and monitoring toxicity of the cardiotoxic drug. There are two ways of doing radionuclide ventriculography, equilibrium radionuclide angiography (ERNA) and first-pass radionuclide angiography (FPRNA) depending on the time of image acquisition [81].

ERNA or MUGA (multigated acquisition) scan requires, an RBC labeling technique, wherein first stannous pyrophosphate or stannous chloride is allowed to create an optimum chemical state inside the RBCs. After 15–20 minutes, Tc-99m pertechnetate is introduced, which enters the RBCs and remains there in the favorable oxidation–reduction environment. The usually administered activity is approximately 800 MBq (20–25 mCi) for adults, and the effective radiation dose received by the patient is approximately 5.6 mSv. There are three methods for RBC labeling, which are in-vivo, modified in vivo–in vitro, and in vitro methods.

- The simplest and fastest method of RBC labeling is in vivo labeling, which gives the lowest labeling efficiency of only 80–90%. In this procedure, the stannous agent is administered intravenously 15–20 minutes before Tc-99m pertechnetate. Tc-99m pertechnetate is injected as a bolus during the imaging for FPRNA. Imaging is performed 15–20 minutes after Tc-99m injection in MUGA scan or ERNA. Because of lower labeling efficiency, the background activity is a little higher in other organs such as the stomach and thyroid in this method
- In the modified in vivo–in vitro method, the reducing agent is administered to the patient. After 20–30 minutes, reduced blood is withdrawn from the patient and kept in a syringe that already contains Tc-99m pertechnetate within it. After the syringe has been gently shaken for 10 minutes, it is administered again to the patient. This method has a labeling efficiency of about 95%
- The in vitro method of labeling, though tedious and the most complicated procedure, provides the highest labeling efficiency. In this procedure, after withdrawing blood from the patient, it is centrifuged and washed to get the RBC pellets. The washed RBC pellets are then incubated in the stannous agent and Tc-99m pertechnetate, respectively. Then the labeled RBCs are reinjected into the patient. The labeling efficiency is more than 97%

For optimum imaging, it is essential to acquire a minimum of 20,000 counts/minute. This provides sufficient count density in the left ventricle to accurately calculate the left ventricular ejection fraction (LVEF). The best septal view or left anterior oblique (LAO) is the most commonly acquired view for estimating LVEF because it provides the optimum images without any ventricular overlap. Additional images in the anterior and lateral view may be acquired if required (Fig. 98.54). The background-corrected

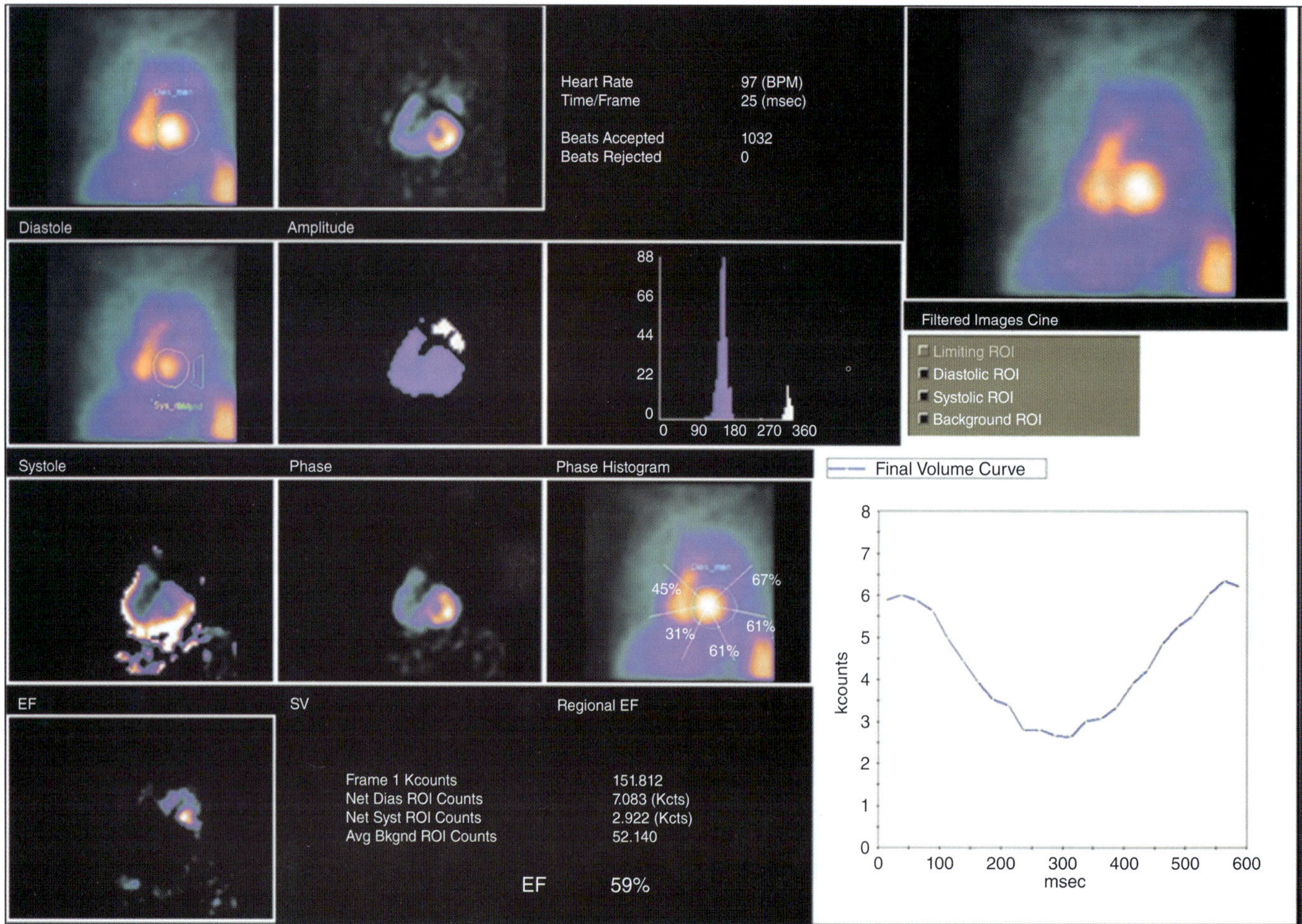

Figure 98.54 A 40-year-old female patient with carcinoma of the breast taking trastuzumab. For baseline evaluation, a multigated acquisition scan was done, which shows left ventricular ejection fraction of 59% and no regional wall motion abnormality. Besides the systolic and diastolic images, it also shows an amplitude image, phase image, and phase histogram, which can be used for dyssynchrony assessment.

counts in the isolated left ventricle are calculated at the ED and ES phases from the LAO view. The following formula is used to estimate the EF:

LVEF = (Background corrected ED counts − Background corrected ES counts)/Background corrected ED counts × 100

Heart Failure Evaluation

Myocardial perfusion study has been an essential part of establishing the etiopathology among newly diagnosed heart failure patients [82]. The literature evidence shows a high negative predictive value of MPI in the detection of CAD among patients with heart failure, and MPI can significantly benefit in better patient management.

Evaluation of Cardiac Dyssynchrony

Left ventricular myocardial dyssynchrony can be evaluated through MPI SPECT as well as MUGA scan by using different commercially available software. These programs usually use the phase histogram to assess the global dyssynchrony. This can also be represented visually. The myocardial dyssynchrony assessment can be done before as well as after the cardiac resynchronization therapy implant [83].

Cardiac Sympathetic Innervation

I-123 MIBG cardiac imaging can localize sympathetic denervated myocardium in post-myocardial injury/ischemia situation. I-123 MIBG imaging can risk-stratify and prognosticate heart failure patients with LV dysfunction. Heart failure patients with cardiac sympathetic denervation in the imaging have higher mortality, dysrhythmia, and more likely to have complications related to heart failure. The ADMIRE-HF study showed the benefits of I-123 MIBG imaging in heart failure patients. I-123 MIBG scanning can be used to prognosticate in ischemic as well as non-ischemic heart failure with the prognosis being directly proportional to the myocardial MIBG uptake [84].

Cardiac Amyloidosis

Heart failure is the usual presentation of cardiac amyloidosis. Pathologically, cardiac amyloidosis can be primary (amyloid transthyretin [ATTR] type) and secondary (amyloid light chain [AL] type) as a part of systemic plasma cell disease. It has been seen that bone-seeking agents such as radiolabeled MDP, 3,3-diphosphono-1,2-pyrophosphate (DPD), and pyrophosphate tracers show myocardial uptake in patients with TTR-type cardiac amyloidosis and not in those with AL-type amyloidosis. Therefore, positive scintigraphy and absence of monoclonal protein in the serum and urine can help in the noninvasive diagnosis of the ATTR type of cardiac amyloidosis [85].

Lymphoscintigraphy

Radionuclide lymphoscintigraphy is a well-established, easy, and commonly performed modality for assessment of the functional status of lymphatics. It is used mostly in two clinical scenarios: for identification of sentinel lymph nodes (SLNs) and for evaluation of lymphedema and lymphatic leaks.

Scintigraphy Evaluation of Sentinel Lymph Nodes

Sentinel lymph node biopsy is used in various malignancies for accurate localization SLNs. The scintigraphic method is one of the most important methods in the identification of the sentinel nodes. The commonly used radiotracers include Tc-99m labeled sulfur colloid, nanocolloid, and phytate. The ideal particle size of the radiopharmaceutical used for this purpose should be approximately 100–200 nm, which does not allow them to enter the capillaries but move along the lymphatic channels and get retained in SLNs. Although various protocols are followed regarding the site of injection, the peritumoral area is the preferred site of tracer injection, especially in breast cancer and malignant melanoma for SLN scintigraphy [86,87]. The usual injection doses are about 500 μCi and 1000 μCi for a single-day and 2-day protocol respectively. After the tracer injection, preoperatively the SLNs can be localized by planar and SPECT/CT imaging. SLNs can also be localized during the surgery through an intraoperative gamma probe. Often, both imaging and probe are used in combination for localizing SLNs in various malignancies.

Scintigraphy Evaluation of Lymphatic Disorders

Lymphedema is caused by chronic obstruction of the lymphatic channels. The common symptom is limb swelling, leading to poor quality of life. Lymphoscintigraphy is a reproducible and easily available method for the assessment of lymphedema. Commonly, Tc-99m–labeled SC and nanocolloid are used for this purpose. The typically administered radiotracer dose is approximately 0.5–1 mCi in divided aliquots for each limb [88]. The injection can be made in epifascial and subfascial planes. Usually, the epifascial injection is preferred, in which tracer is injected in the subcutaneous or intradermal planes along the web spaces. Whole-body imaging is performed. In abnormal lymphatic drainage, the imaging shows dermal backflow of tracer, nonvisualization of inguinal or axillary lymph nodes, asymmetrical tracer uptake in the inguinal or axillary lymph nodes, visualization of the popliteal or epitrochlear nodes, and visualization of lesser number of ilioinguinal nodes (less than three). Any of these findings alone or in combination can help in diagnosing lymphatic abnormality or obstruction (Fig. 98.55). Similarly, lymphoscintigraphy is used for scrotal lymphedema and chylothorax evaluation.

Miscellaneous Investigations

There are a few uncommonly performed but important investigations, including peritoneal scintigraphy, evaluation of protein-losing enteropathy, salivary scintigraphy, and dacryoscintigraphy.

- *Peritoneal scintigraphy* is used to evaluate peritoneal membrane integrity, pleuroperitoneal shunt, and shunt patency. The commonly used radiopharmaceuticals in peritoneal scintigraphy are Tc-99m SC and Tc-99m MAA particles because they do not diffuse through the peritoneum. When injected into the peritoneum, these tracers remain distributed inside the peritoneum, and any uptake in the thorax suggests a communication
- *Protein-losing enteropathy* is associated with massive loss of protein through the GI tract. This can be caused by a variety of diseases such as lymphangiectasia in the intestine, Crohn's disease, Ménétrier disease, etc. The radiopharmaceuticals used for these purposes are Tc-99m HSA, In-111 transferrin, and

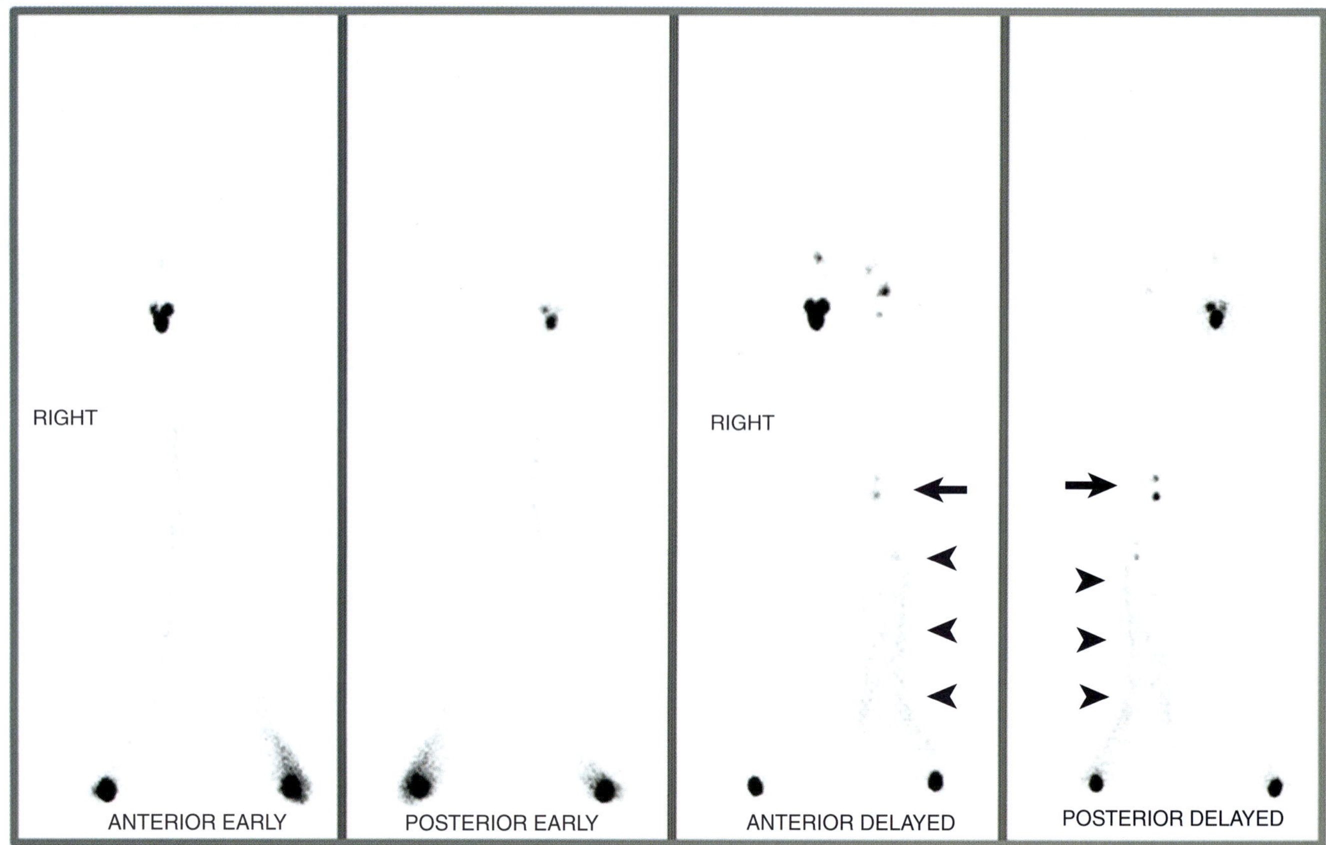

Figure 98.55 A 10-year-old boy with left lower limb swelling for 1 year with normal venous Doppler results. Lymphoscintigraphy shows dermal backflow in the left leg (*arrowheads*), popliteal lymph nodes (*arrow*), and paucity of left ilioinguinal lymph nodes on the left side, suggestive of obstructed lymphatic drainage.

Tc-99m dextran. Tracer accumulation in the abdominal region suggests protein leak from the intestine

- *Salivary scintigraphy* is used to evaluate xerostomia or dry mouth caused by salivary gland hypofunction resulting in reduced saliva production. Causes include radiation therapy, chemotherapy, medications, radioactive iodine therapy, and Sjögren's syndrome. Salivary gland dysfunction can be confirmed by scintigraphy using Tc-99m pertechnetate, which can demonstrate abnormal or normal trapping and poststimulation drainage after administration of lemon juice. Usually 10 mCi of Tc-99m pertechnetate is injected intravenously, and imaging is acquired for 30 minutes with sialagogue is administered orally at 15 minutes
- *Dacryoscintigraphy* is occasionally performed to evaluate the drainage of nasolacrimal ducts, most commonly for epiphora, an overflow of tears that can be caused by obstruction by a variety of anatomic abnormalities. A droplet of normal saline with 100 μCi Tc-99m pertechnetate is instilled into the conjunctiva near the lateral canthus of both the eyes, and serial images are obtained every 15–30 seconds for 15 minutes. It can confirm whether the cause is of obstructive origin
- The *urea breath test* was used for gastric *Helicobacter pylori* infection for a long time. Although it is a simple, noninvasive, and inexpensive investigation modality, currently it is not being used very often. Its overall accuracy is high. Increasingly, the nonradioactive C-13 is more commonly used instead of the C-14 isotope. This test is based on the ability of *H. pylori* to break down urea carbon dioxide, which then is absorbed from the stomach and eliminated in the breath. If the urea breath test is positive and the isotope is detected in the breath, it means that *H. pylori* is present in the stomach

Suggested Readings

- GB Saha, Fundamentals of nuclear pharmacy, fifth ed., Springer, New York, NY, 2004.
- KJ Donohoe, ML Brown, BD Collier, et al., Society of Nuclear Medicine procedure guideline for bone scintigraphy, Society of Nuclear Medicine website (2003). Accepted June 20.
- AT Taylor, DC Brandon, D de Palma, MD Blaufox, E Durand, B Erbas, et al., SNMMI procedure standard/EANM practice guideline for diuretic renal scintigraphy in adults with suspected upper urinary tract obstruction 1.0, Semin Nucl Med 48 (4) (2018) 377–390.
- P Vitali, R Migliaccio, F Agosta, HJ Rosen, MD Geschwind, Neuroimaging in dementia, Semin Neurol 28 (2008) 467–483.
- MJ Henzlova, WL Duvall, AJ Einstein, MI Travin, HJ. Verberne, ASNC imaging guidelines for SPECT nuclear cardiology procedures: Stress, protocols, and tracers, J NuclCardiol 23 (3) (2016 Jun) 606–639.

99

Positron Emission Tomography/ Computed Tomography

KANHAIYALAL AGRAWAL, GIRISH KUMAR PARIDA, GOPINATH GNANASEGARAN

Introduction

Functional imaging with positron emission tomography (PET) has grown manifold both in its technical aspect and its uses in medicine. Being a functional imaging modality, it provides information that is significantly different from what we get from conventional anatomic imaging such as radiography, ultrasonography (USG), computed tomography (CT), and magnetic resonance imaging (MRI). This feature of PET has been exploited in different malignancies for the detection of different pathological changes at an early stage of the disease because functional changes usually precede anatomic changes. With the addition of CT to PET (PET/CT), its usefulness has been further enhanced. Although there are different PET radiopharmaceuticals available, the radiopharmaceutical that revolutionized oncology patient management is *fluorine-18-fluorodeoxyglucose (^{18}F-FDG)*. Currently, however, FDG PET/CT has also been used for different nononcologic indications such as in infection and inflammation imaging, myocardial viability assessment, and neurodegenerative conditions.

The appropriate use criteria (AUC) for FDG PET/CT addresses several clinical scenarios for restaging and response assessment of malignant disease. To improve utilization and guide treatment providers across specialties to use FDG PET, the Society of Nuclear Medicine and Molecular Imaging, the European Association of Nuclear Medicine, and the American Society of Clinical Oncology have collaboratively developed criteria for the appropriate use of this imaging technology. National Comprehensive Cancer Network (NCCN) imaging AUC includes a full complement of imaging AUC in oncology care designed to support clinical decision making based directly on the NCCN guidelines.

Fluorine-18-Fluorodeoxyglucose

Being a glucose analog, FDG enters the cell through the sodium-coupled glucose transporters and glucose transporter facilitators (GLUT) channels [1]. Inside the cells, it gets converted to FDG-6-phosphate by the enzyme hexokinase, but it is not processed further in the metabolic cycle because of the presence of ^{18}F instead of oxygen at the second carbon position. FDG-6-phosphate is not able to move out of the cell unless it gets reconverted to FDG by the enzyme phosphatase as it is not lipophilic. Hence, it gets trapped inside the cells. Therefore, cells that have high glucose affinity or have high GLUT channels on their cell surfaces will have high FDG uptake, and the same can be seen on PET/CT scan.

This visual interpretation of FDG uptake is subjective and may vary depending on technical factors. Therefore, to avoid this technical variation, a quantitative parameter such as the *standardized uptake value (SUV)* is commonly used, which is a semiquantitative indicator of FDG uptake in the tissue. This is calculated as

$$\frac{\text{Mean ROI activity }(\text{MBq/g})}{\text{Injected dose }(\text{MBq})/\text{Bodyweight }(\text{g})}$$

where MBq = mega-Becquerel and g = grams.

Patient Preparation and Image Acquisition

- FDG in the blood can compete with the blood glucose for the GLUT channels because it is a glucose analog. Therefore, blood glucose has to be monitored before FDG injection. A cutoff of 200 mg/dL has been taken as the upper limit for performing FDG PET/CT scan [2]
- The patient should fast for at least 4 hours before the test. Plain unflavored water may be taken without any added sugar. If the patient is on parenteral nutrition, then glucose- and sugar-containing fluids should be discontinued at least 4 hours before FDG injection [2]
- The patient must avoid doing strenuous exercise for 24 hours before the study [2]
- Adequate prehydration is important to ensure optimum background clearance and for radiation safety purposes
- After the injection, the patient has to sit quietly in a room for at least 1 hour for background clearance and to reduce the FDG uptake in the muscles [2]
- The patient should also be kept warm during the whole process to suppress brown fat activity. Sometimes pharmacologic interventions may be required for brown fat activity suppression [2]
- When IV contrast agent is administered as part of the diagnostic CT, the renal function should be assessed beforehand
- The usual adult dose of administered FDG is 5–12 mCi (0.09–0.14 mCi per kilogram of body weight), and the pediatric dose is 0.10 mCi per kilogram of body weight (minimum, 1.0 mCi) [2,3]
- Usually, the patient should be positioned with the arms elevated and alongside the head. However, for head and neck or brain imaging, the arms should be placed down along the torso
- Additional specific imaging protocols are also being used depending on the organs involved for better visualization (e.g., puffed cheeks view for buccal mucosal lesions, a protruded tongue view for tongue lesions, an open mouth view for palate lesions, delayed postdiuretic scan for urinary tract lesions)

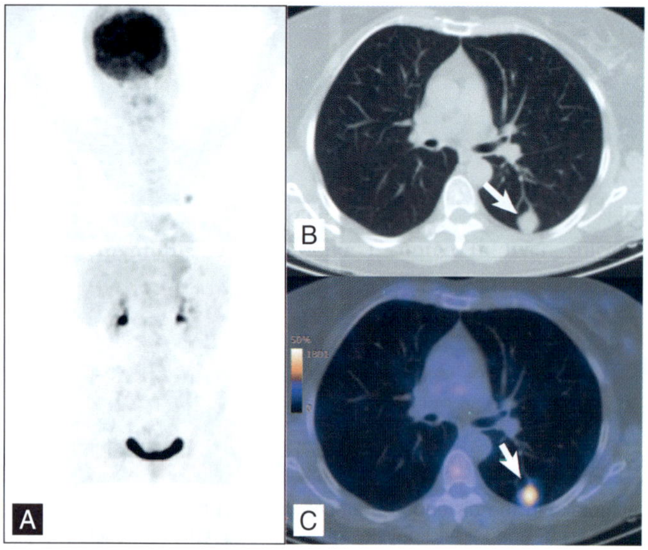

Figure 99.7 FDG PET/CT for solitary pulmonary nodule in the left lung lower lobe shows focal tracer uptake in the left side thorax on the maximum intensity projection image (A). CT (B) and PET/CT (C) images show increased FDG uptake in the left lung nodule suggestive of a malignant cause (*white arrows*).

treatment (colony-stimulating factors), a gap of 3 weeks is essential before doing the FDG PET/CT scan [2].

Positron Emission Tomography/Computed Tomography in Oncology

Many radiopharmaceuticals have been used for the assessment of different malignant diseases; however, in this section, we mainly focus on FDG with mentions of other tumor-specific tracers under specific tumors.

Solitary Pulmonary Nodule (SPN)

Chest radiography and CT scan are the primary imaging modalities for evaluation of a single pulmonary nodule. However, anatomic information from these conventional imaging modalities is often insufficient to differentiate benign nodules from the malignant ones.

Use of PET/CT

FDG PET/CT can help in differentiating benign nodules from malignant ones, by showing the metabolic activity in the SPNs (Fig. 99.7). Usually, a malignant nodule shows a higher degree of FDG uptake than benign nodules on visual interpretation. For a more objective interpretation, quantitative parameters such as SUV can be also used to differentiate benign lesions from malignant ones. Some studies have taken a maximum standard uptake value (SUV_{max}) cutoff of 2.5, and a nodule showing a higher SUV_{max} value than this is usually considered a malignant nodule. Sometimes infective or inflammatory nodules may show high SUV_{max}, leading to false-positive results. However, non-FDG avidity in the nodules most often rules out malignancy, showing a very high negative predictive value of FDG PET/CT [6].

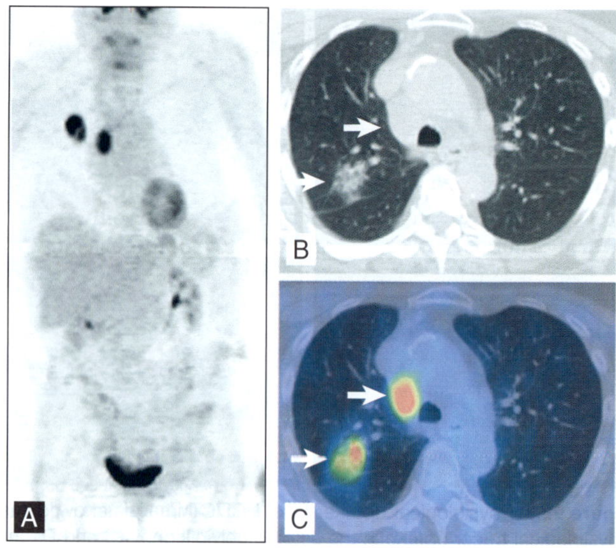

Figure 99.8 Fluorodeoxyglucose (FDG) positron emission tomography/computed tomography (PET/CT) in a patient with a right lung upper lobe cavitating lesion. (A) Increased uptake in the right lung and mediastinum on maximum intensity projection image. (B and C). The uptake in the lung corresponds to a partially cavitating mass lesion in the right lung upper lobe with a maximum standard uptake value (SUV_{max}) of 28.0 and intense uptake in the right paratracheal lymph node with a SUV_{max} of 21.1 (*arrows*) indicative of a solitary pulmonary malignant lesion with mediastinal node metastasis.

Limitations

Falsely increased FDG uptake can be seen in infective or inflammatory pathologies such as tuberculosis (TB) and sarcoidosis. Small nodules (<8–10 mm), however, may show falsely low tracer uptake on PET/CT imaging.

Appropriate Use Criteria

FDG PET/CT should be used for the characterization of indeterminate SPNs of size greater than 8–10 mm. However, it is not very useful for nodules with a high pretest probability of malignancy (>60%) or having a size smaller than 8–10 mm [7].

Lung Cancer

Lung cancer is the leading cause of death among both genders. More than one-third of these patients have metastatic disease at the time of presentation. Histopathologically, lung cancer can be broadly categorized into non–small cell lung cancer and small cell cancer. The primary diagnostic modalities used in the management of patients with lung cancer are chest radiography, CT of the chest and abdomen, and FDG PET/CT; however, tissue diagnosis remains the gold standard.

Use of PET/CT

PET/CT has been seen to have higher accuracy than conventional CT in lymph node staging (Fig. 99.8). But in countries with an endemic infectious granulomatous disease, the specificity of FDG PET/CT for the detection of lymph node metastasis from lung cancer is lower. With respect to distant skeletal metastases, it has also shown higher sensitivity and specificity compared with MRI or whole-body bone scintigraphy (Fig. 99.9).

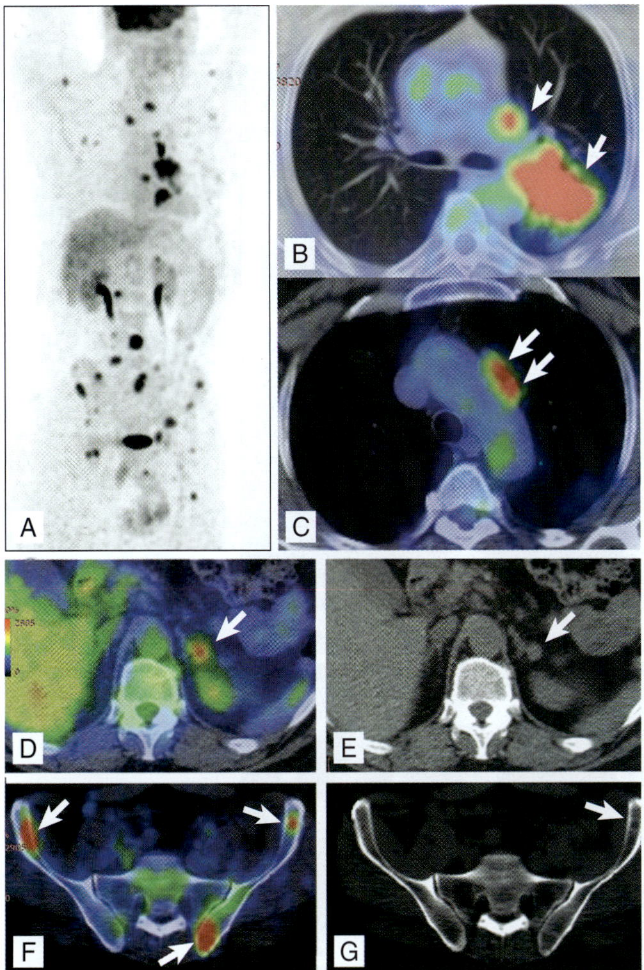

Figure 99.9 Staging fluorodeoxyglucose (FDG) positron emission tomography in a 62-year-old man with a known case of small cell carcinoma of the lung. (A) Multiple foci of abnormal tracer uptake in the body in the maximum intensity projection image. (B) FDG-avid irregular primary soft tissue mass lesion in the left lower lobe lung with a maximum standard uptake value (SUV_{max}) of 11.45 along with uptake in a metastatic mediastinal node (*arrows*) (C) Increased tracer uptake is seen in the mediastinal paraaortic lymph nodes (*arrows*) indicative of metastatic disease. (D and E) FDG-avid soft tissue nodule in the lateral limb of the left adrenal gland (*arrow*) with an SUV_{max} of 6.73 suggestive of metastasis. (F and G) Multiple foci of uptake in the metastatic bones with only a few showing morphologic changes on computed tomography (*arrows*).

Besides staging, FDG PET/CT has shown to be useful in radiotherapy planning and assessment of early response to therapy (Fig. 99.10). In prognostication, quantification parameters such as SUV_{max} and tumor lesion glycolysis have been able to predict tumor invasiveness, survival, and recurrence [8,9] (Table 99.2).

Limitations

Infections such as TB, histoplasmosis, aspergillosis, and cryptococcosis; postsurgical changes; postradiotherapy changes; and flare phenomenon may lead to false-positive results in FDG PET/CT. Low-grade malignancies such as bronchoalveolar carcinoma and carcinoid tumor may not show high FDG uptake, leading to false-negative results.

Breast Cancer

Breast cancer is the most common cancer in women. Mammography and USG of the breast are the initial diagnostic procedures for assessing the local extent of disease. The role of MRI has been described in detail in Chapter 51. For staging workup, contrast-enhanced CT of the thorax and abdomen are commonly recommended; however, FDG PET/CT can also be used in specific cases.

Use of PET/CT

PET/CT is useful in the staging workup in place of conventional imaging modalities such as contrast-enhanced CT of the thorax and abdomen. The sensitivity and specificity of FDG PET/CT for the diagnosis of primary tumor are approximately 90% and 92%, respectively; for axillary lymph node detection, the rates are 80% and 90%, respectively (Fig. 99.11). In approximately 20–30% of patients, FDG PET/CT has been seen to change in management by identifying unsuspected regional nodal disease or distant metastasis in locally advanced breast cancer [11]. Although it is currently recommended for staging workup of inflammatory breast carcinoma, FDG PET/CT has also shown its efficacy in response assessment and prognostication (Fig. 99.12).

Limitations

A few non-neoplastic conditions of the breast can lead to false-positive results, such as abscesses, TB, fungal infections, and postsurgical changes. Similarly, carcinoma in situ, low-grade tumors, and small lesions (<1 cm) usually show significantly lower SUVs and can be misinterpreted as benign, leading to false-negative results.

Head and Neck Cancer

Usually, the malignancies of the paranasal sinuses, nasopharynx, oral cavity, oropharynx, hypopharynx, and larynx constitute the head and neck malignancies. Pathologically, more than 90% of these belong to the squamous cell carcinoma category. The conventional imaging modalities that are commonly used for the staging or restaging of head and neck cancer include USG of the neck, contrast-enhanced CT, and MRI.

Use of PET/CT

PET/CT has been useful in detecting the unknown primary site in patients with metastatic cervical lymph nodes. It also helps in guiding for cytopathologic examination by showing the metabolic activity of the lesions. Although contrast-enhanced CT and MRI are the modalities of choice in staging workup of head and neck cancers, FDG PET/CT can be used in patients with doubtful clinical staging or with stage III or IV disease having a high risk of metastatic disease. It has also been seen that FDG PET/CT has higher sensitivity, as well as specificity, in restaging, response assessment and recurrence detection when compared with conventional imaging modalities. Neck Imaging Reporting & Data System (NI-RADS) is a standardized lexicon for reporting used in posttreatment surveillance imaging of head and neck squamous cell cancers. Besides these, FDG PET/CT can also help in assessing the radiation therapy target volumes during radiation therapy planning by determining the extent of primary as well as regional nodal

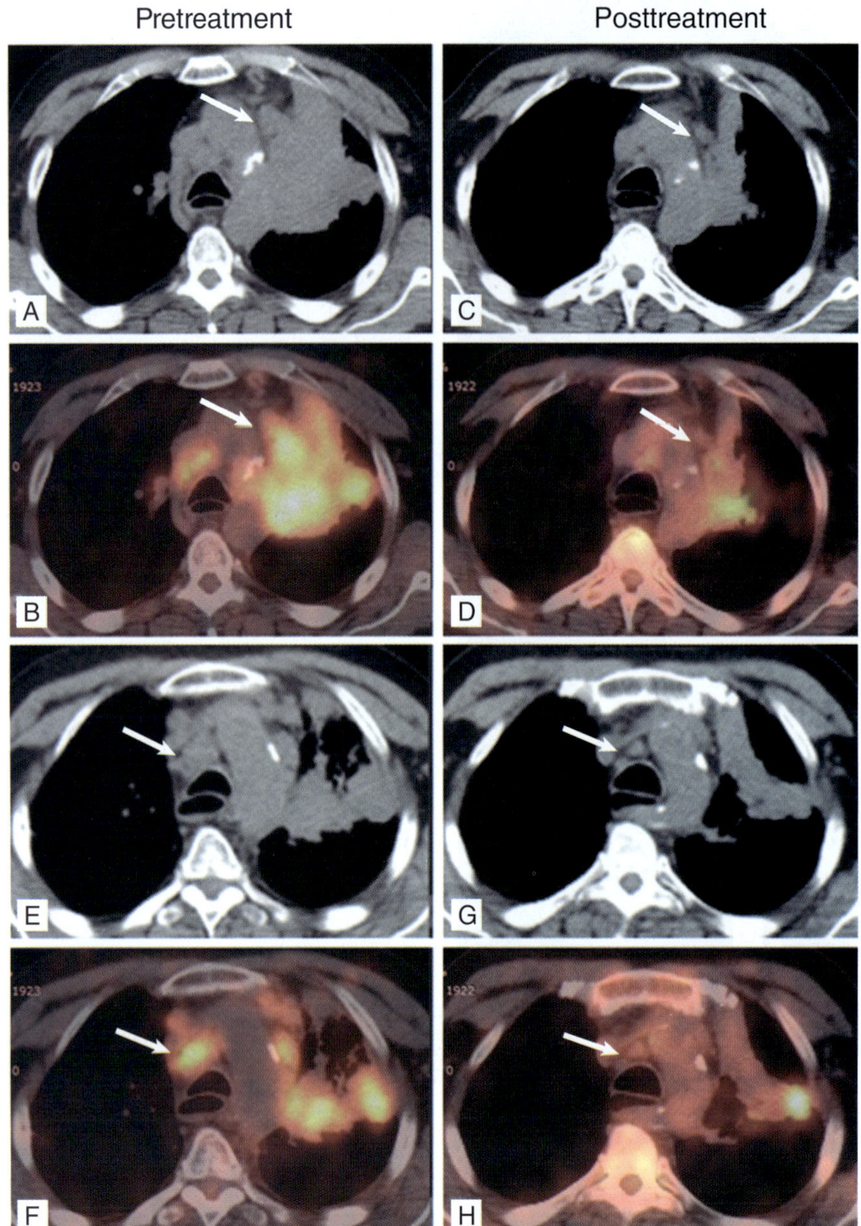

Figure 99.10 Response evaluation after palliative chemotherapy in a 54-year-old man with known bronchogenic carcinoma. Fluorodeoxyglucose positron emission tomography/computed tomography shows significant interval regression in size and metabolic activity of the mass from a maximum standard uptake value (SUV_{max}) of 16.2 in the pretreatment scan (*arrows* in A and B) to an SUV_{max} of 7.6 in the posttreatment study (*arrows* in C and D) mediastinal lymph nodes from an SUV_{max} of 10.5 in the pretreatment scan (*arrows* in E and F) to an SUV_{max} of 4.5 in the posttreatment study (*arrows* in G and H).

TABLE 99.2 Appropriate Use Criteria for Lung Cancer [7,10]

Lung Cancer	Initial Workup	Restaging/Response/Recurrence	Surveillance
Non–small cell lung Cancer	Indicated for initial staging in all cases	To exclude disease progression or interval development of metastatic disease after induction therapy	Not recommended routinely Recommended for RT planning
Small cell lung cancer	If limited stage expected Optional for low or intermediate NET PET/CT has replaced bone scan in NCCN guidelines Recommended for RT planning	Not recommended for routine follow up	Not recommended routinely

CT, computed tomography; *NET*, neuroendocrine tumor; *NCCN*, National Comprehensive Cancer Network; *PET*, positron emission tomography; *RT*, radiotherapy.

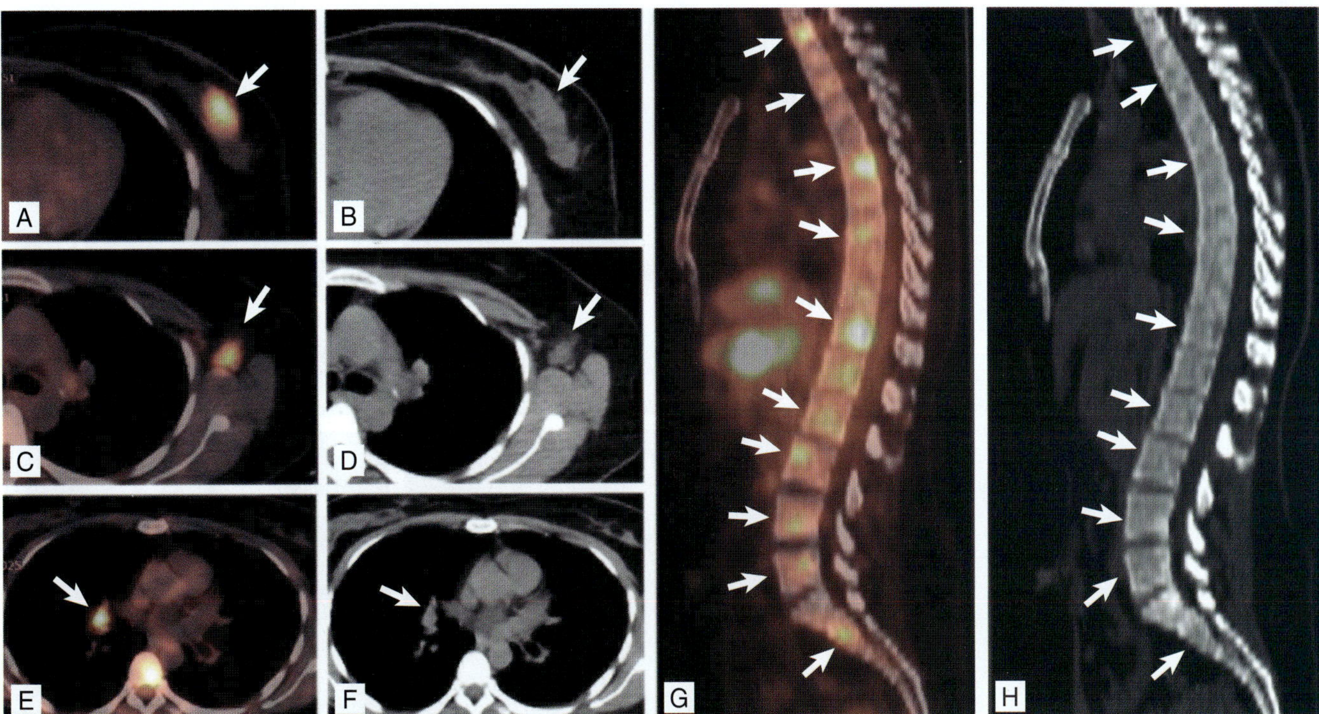

Figure 99.11 A 38-year-old woman with known left breast carcinoma. Staging fluorodeoxyglucose (FDG) positron emission tomography shows an FDG-avid ill-defined soft tissue lesion in the left breast consistent with the primary site (*arrows* in A and B), an FDG-avid left axillary lymph node (metastatic; *arrows* in C and D), and an FDG-avid right hilar lymph node (metastatic; *arrows* in E and F). Furthermore, foci of increased FDG uptake are seen in the bone marrow (*arrows* in G) with no definite morphologic changes on computed tomography (*arrows* in H) indicative of marrow metastatic disease.

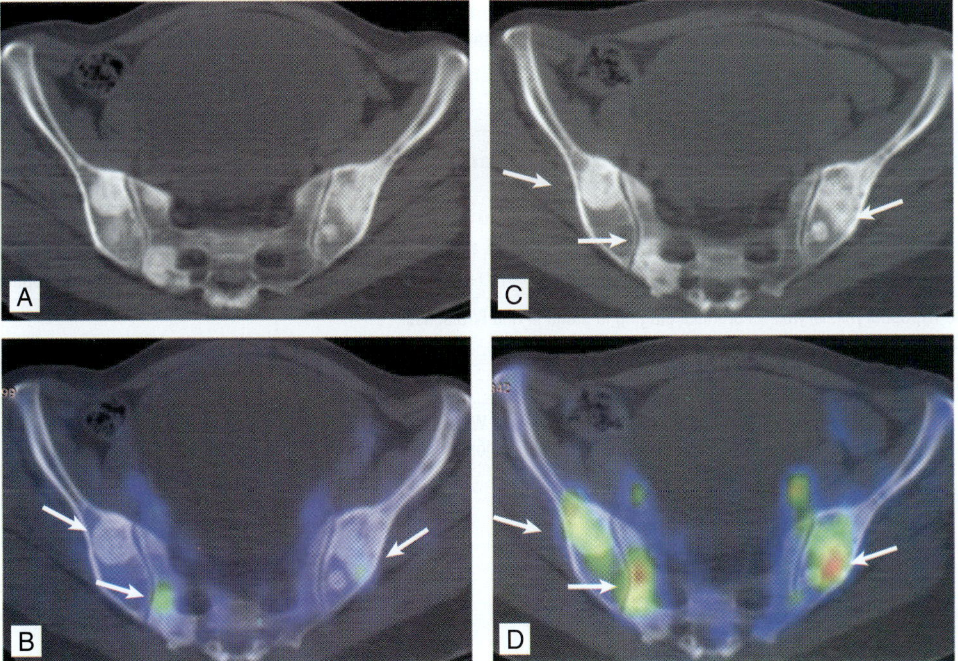

Figure 99.12 A 58-year-old woman with known metastatic left breast carcinoma on hormonal treatment. Pretreatment computed tomography (CT) and fluorodeoxyglucose (FDG) positron emission tomography (PET) (*arrows* in A and B) shows negligible to minimal tracer uptake in the sclerotic bone lesions, whereas posttreatment CT and FDG PET (*arrows* in *arrows* in C and D) show increased tracer uptake suggestive of disease progression. This example shows the importance of FDG PET in response evaluation when there is no significant morphologic change in the lesions on CT.

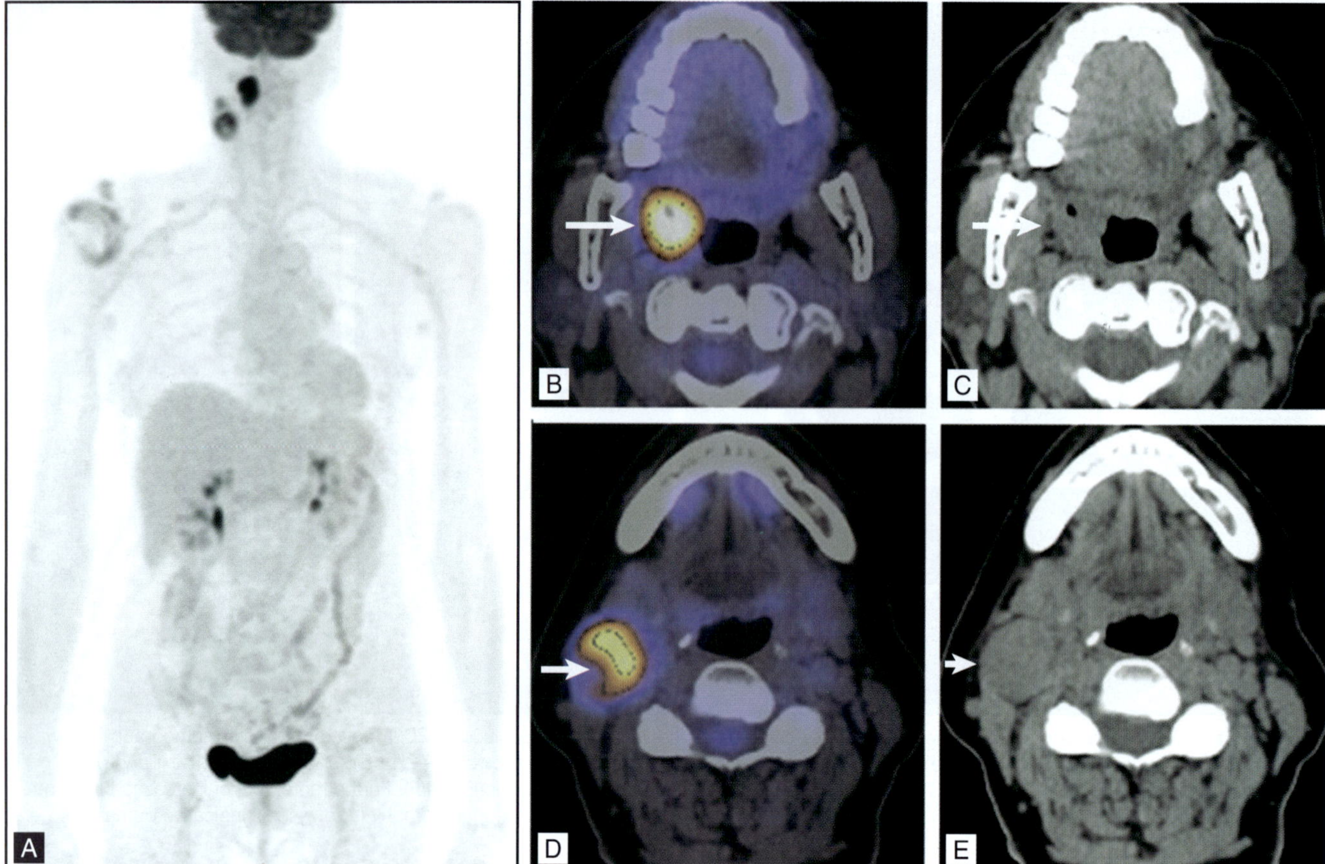

Figure 99.13 A patient with a right level IIB cervical lymph node, which on cytology shows malignant disease. Fluorodeoxyglucose (FDG) positron emission tomography/computed tomography was performed to detect the primary site. Maximum intensity projection (MIP) image shows two abnormal foci of FDG uptake in the neck (A), which localizes to an ill-defined soft tissue lesion on the right side of the oropharynx with maximum standard uptake value (SUV_{max}) of 13.6 suggestive of the primary site (*arrows* in B and C). Further intense tracer uptake with an SUV_{max} of 8.9 is seen in the known ipsilateral metastatic enlarged right level IIB cervical lymph node (*arrows* in D and E). There is uptake at the right shoulder in the MIP image suggestive of capsulitis (A).

TABLE 99.3 Appropriate Use Criteria for Head and Neck Cancer [15]

	Initial Workup	Restaging/Response/Recurrence	Surveillance
Occult primary	Before EUA	PET/CT to be done 12 wk after therapy; if findings are negative, further imaging for restaging is optional	Not indicated
Oral cavity, oro- and hypopharynx, larynx, ethmoid and maxillary sinuses	For initial staging in stage III and IV disease		
Mucosal melanoma	For initial staging		
Nasopharynx	Imaging for distant metastasis in WHO class 2–3/N2–3 disease: PET optional		

CT, computed tomography; *PET*, positron emission tomography; *WHO*, World Health Organization.

metastases, which is more accurate than CT directed radiotherapy planning (Fig. 99.13 and Table 99.3) [13,14].

Limitations

Infective and inflammatory diseases such as tonsillitis and pharyngitis can show falsely increased FDG uptake. Even post-interventional inflammatory changes can show falsely increased FDG uptake. Activated brown adipose tissue is another most important cause that can lead to false-positive results. Lymph nodes with low-grade tumors or with a smaller size (<1 cm) can also cause false-negative results.

Brain Tumors

Primary central nervous system (CNS) tumors are relatively uncommon malignancies. They constitute about 1–2% of all malignancies. The most common CNS malignancy is metastases followed by gliomas. Brain MRI with contrast is the imaging

TABLE 99.4 Appropriate Use Criteria for Brain Tumors [17]

	Initial Workup	Restaging/Response/Recurrence	Surveillance
Glioma/glioblastoma	Radiolabeled amino acid PET may be preferred over FDG PET/CT	To differentiate viable tumor from radiation necrosis	Not recommended
Brain metastasis (If two or more brain lesions and unknown primary)	Recommended (FDG PET/CT)	Not routinely recommended	Not recommended
Primary CNS Lymphoma	Recommended (FDG PET/CT)	Recommended	Not recommended

CT, computed tomography; *CNS*, central nervous system; *FDG*, fluorodeoxyglucose; *PET*, positron emission tomography.

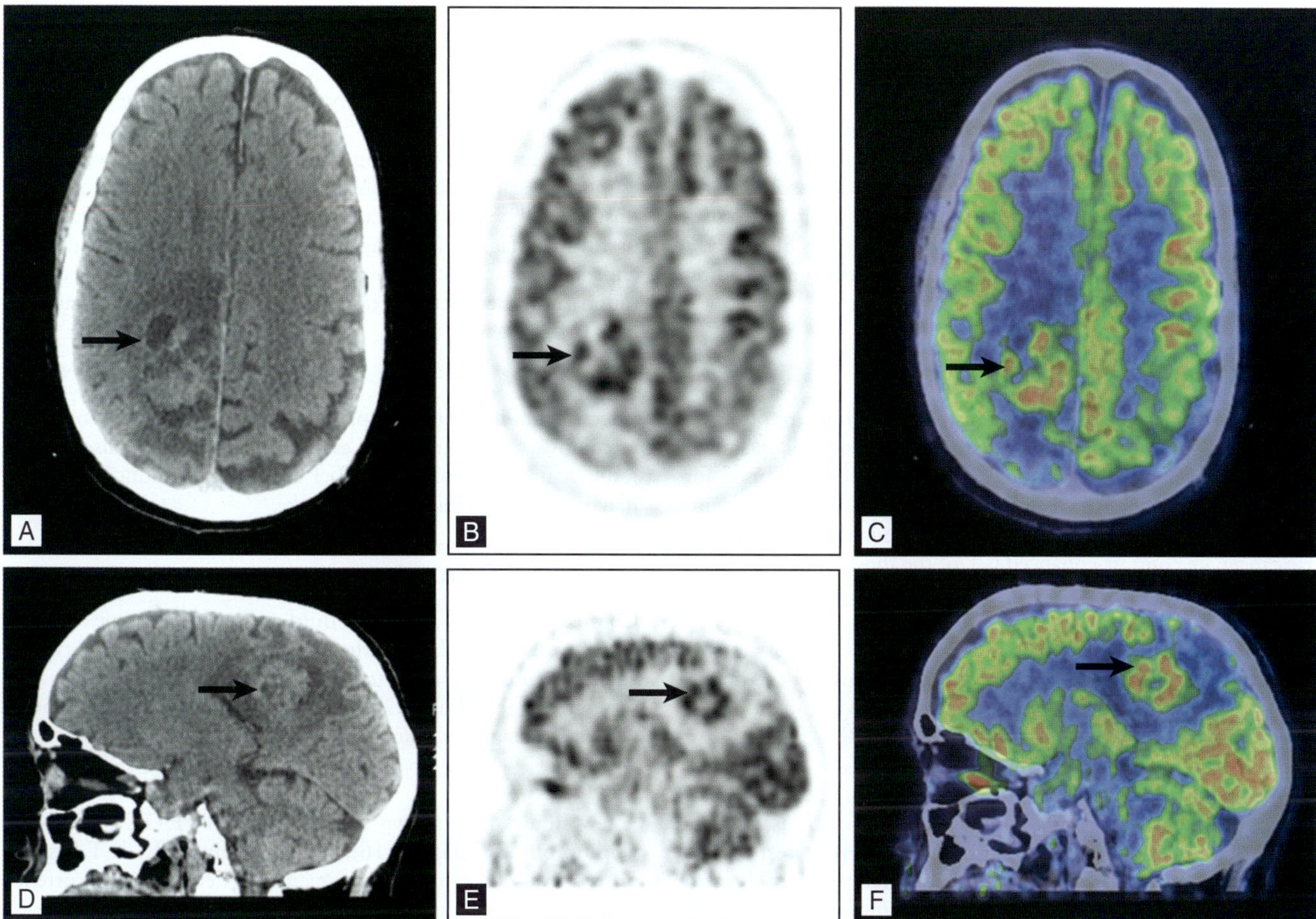

Figure 99.14 A 68-year-old man with diagnosed glioma underwent fluorodeoxyglucose positron emission tomography/computed tomography (PET/CT) as baseline workup. PET/CT shows a metabolically active solid-cystic mass lesion in the right parietal cortex with perilesional edema on CT (*arrows* in A and D), PET (*arrows* in B and E), and fused PET/CT (*arrows* in C and F) images compatible with known high-grade glioma.

modality of choice in the evaluation of brain Space occupying lesions (SOLs) because of its superior soft tissue resolution.

Use of PET/CT

PET/CT measures the glucose metabolism of the tissues, and because it is a functional imaging modality, it has been used in differentiating residual or recurrent disease from postinterventional necrosis or other effects (Table 99.4). However, it has a significant limitation because of its high physiological brain uptake (Fig. 99.14). To overcome this issue, a few amino acid–labeled PET agents have been developed that show lower uptake in normal brain tissue and high uptake in brain tumors. The important beneficial factor of amino acid tracer is their ability to enter the intact blood–brain barrier. The earliest amino acid PET tracer used in brain tumor evaluation was [^{11}C-methyl]-methionine (MET). However, carbon-11 has a very short half-life, so it could not be used on a large scale. Currently, ^{18}F-labelled tracers such as O-(2-[18F]-fluoroethyl)-L-tyrosine (FET) and 3,4-dihydroxy-6-[18F]-fluoro-L-phenylalanine (FDOPA), are being used commonly for this purpose because of their long half-lives. Amino acid PET imaging provides significant additional information regarding the extent and metabolism of the tumor [16]. It has also the ability to accurately differentiate between recurrent lesion and postinterventional

TABLE 99.5 Appropriate Use Criteria for Gastro-esophageal Cancer [20,21]

	Initial Workup	Restaging/Response/Recurrence	Surveillance
Esophageal cancer	Staging if no evidence of M1 For RT planning	5–6 wk after NACT and definitive CTRT for treatment response	Consider for T1b or greater
Gastric cancer	Staging if no evidence of M1 For RT planning	For restaging of unresectable or medically unfit patient after primary treatment	Not recommended routinely

CTRT, Chemotherapy Radiotherapy *NACT*, Neoadjuvant chemotherapy *RT*, radiotherapy.

changes. According to the Response Assessment in Neuro-Oncology (RANO) group, amino acid PET can be useful at all stages of brain tumor management.

Limitations

Recent hematoma and infarct in the brain can show increased amino acid uptake, resulting in false-positive results. Infective and inflammatory pathology of the brain such as abscesses and encephalitis may show increased FDG uptake, leading to false-positive results. Low-grade gliomas may be missed in FDG PET/CT because of the high physiological uptake in the brain, leading to false-negative results.

Gastric Cancer

Adenocarcinoma is the commonest histopathological type of gastric cancers, making up about 95% of all cases. Endoscopy, including endoscopic USG, is the preferred diagnostic procedure used for local disease extent as well as regional lymph node assessment. Other imaging modalities usually used in the management of gastric cancer are contrast-enhanced CT of the thorax and abdomen.

Use of PET/CT

PET/CT has limited utility in T-staging because of its low resolution. However, it has been used efficiently in the detection of lymph nodes and distant metastases in the liver, lungs, and skeleton. Besides staging workup, FDGPET/CT has also been used in response assessment after radiation therapy and chemotherapy, in which it is found to be more accurate than conventional imaging modalities. It can also assess the response at an earlier time, so it can differentiate responders from nonresponders to neoadjuvant therapies. It is also highly useful in the evaluation of recurrence of disease [18] (Table 99.5).

Limitations

It has been a challenging task for FDG PET/CT to detect regional lymph nodes very close to the intensely FDG-avid primary lesion and may cause false-negative results. Besides these, low-grade malignancies or mucinous carcinomas usually show a low-grade FDG uptake that can lead to false-negative results.

Esophageal Cancer

Esophageal cancer is a leading cause of cancer-related death in the world. Metastatic disease is the first presentation in more than one-third of patients with esophageal cancer. The most common histopathological type is squamous cell carcinoma (SCC), making up about 70% of all cases. Endoscopy with or without USG and contrast-enhanced CT of the thorax and abdomen are commonly used diagnostic modalities for the evaluation of esophageal carcinoma.

Use of PET/CT

PET/CT has been successfully used in the staging workup of esophageal cancer (Fig. 99.15). It has been proved to be better than the anatomic imaging modalities in staging workup of esophageal cancer, especially in detection of lymph nodes and unsuspected distant metastases. Besides, FDG PET/CT has been useful in restaging, assessing response after neoadjuvant therapy, and detection of recurrent disease (Table 99.5). It has also been found more beneficial in radiotherapy planning than that with only CT [19].

Limitations

Infective and inflammatory pathologies such as Barrett esophagus, sarcoidosis, and postradiation esophagitis may lead to false-positive results. Similarly, small tumor (<1 cm), mucin-producing tumors, may not show increased FDG uptake.

Colorectal Cancer

Colorectal cancer (CRC) is the third most common type of malignancy worldwide. Histopathologically, the commonest type is adenocarcinoma, making up approximately 90% of all cases. As per current guidelines, CT and MRI are usually being done as part of the staging workup for patients with CRC.

Use of PET/CT

A few studies have shown benefits of FDG PET/CT in staging workup of CRC (Fig. 99.16). Besides staging, PET/CT has also proved its use in response assessment and detection of recurrence in patients with rising serum carcinoembryonic antigen levels [22] (Table 99.6).

Limitations

Inflammatory pathologies such as fistulas, abscesses, diverticulitis, and sometimes adenomas can cause falsely increased FDG uptake. Micrometastases to the lymph nodes and mucinous-secreting tumors can cause false-negative results because of their low-grade FDG uptake.

Hepatobiliary Malignancies

Hepatocellular carcinoma (HCC) is an uncommon malignancy, but it is more common in Asian and African countries and is the most common primary liver cancer. The common diagnostic modalities used in the management of patients with HCC include USG, multiphase CT, and contrast-enhanced multiphase MRI.

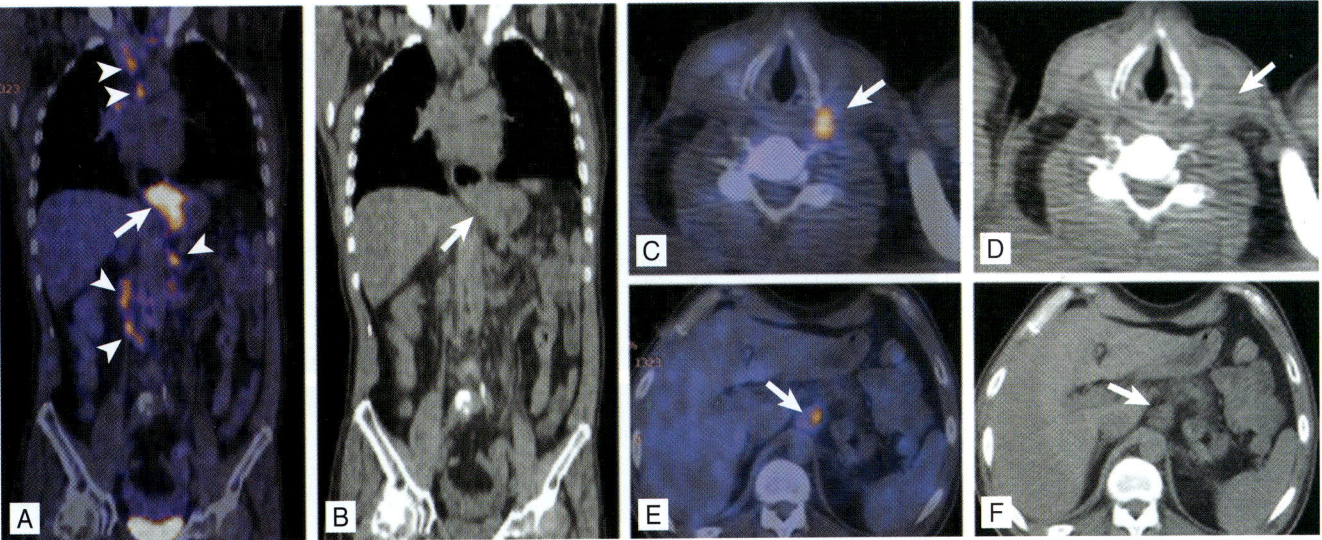

Figure 99.15 In a known case of gastroesophageal carcinoma, staging fluorodeoxyglucose (FDG) positron emission tomography/computed tomography shows intense tracer uptake in the primary site (*arrows* in A and B), along with FDG-avid mediastinal and abdominal lymph nodes suggestive of metastatic disease (*arrowheads* in A). Focal uptake is seen in a subcentimeter left supraclavicular (*arrows* in C and D) and celiac axis lymph nodes (*arrows* in E and F) suggestive of metastases.

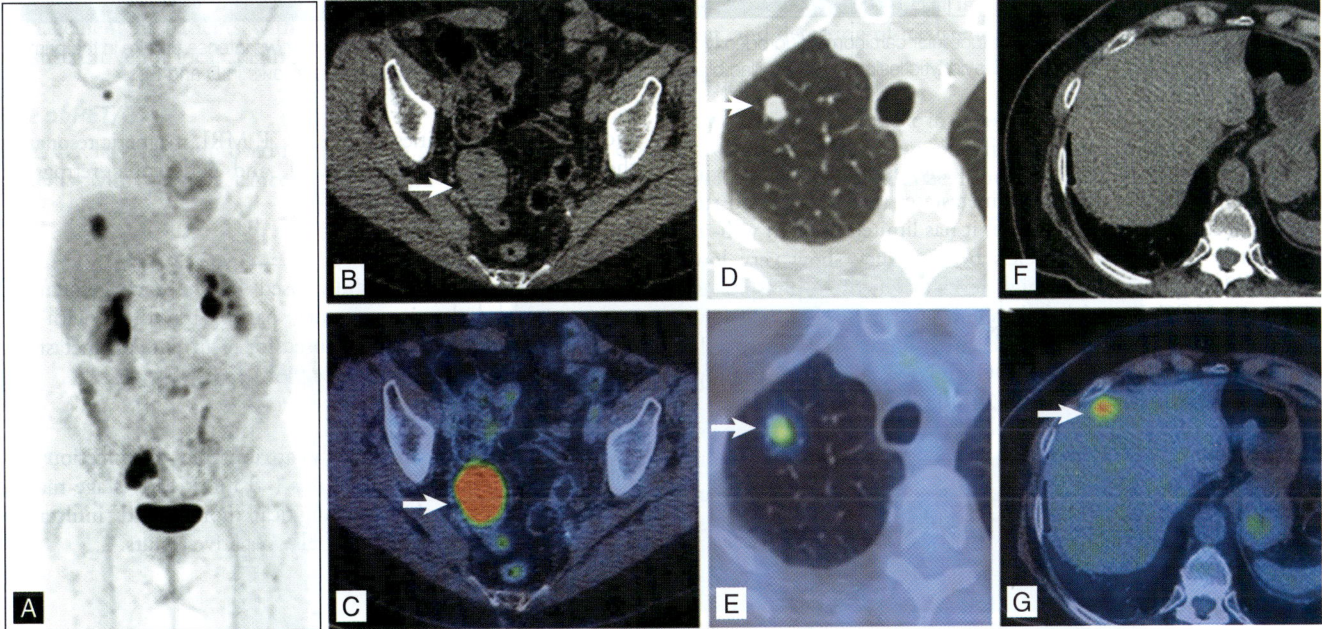

Figure 99.16 In a known case of colon carcinoma, computed tomography showed solitary lesions in the lung and liver. Fluorodeoxyglucose (FDG) positron emission tomography was performed to know the feasibility of the surgical resection of primary. Maximum intensity projection image (A) shows focal uptake in the right thorax, in the liver, and on the right side of the pelvis. There is intense FDG uptake in the primary lesion in the colon (*arrows* in B and C). Furthermore, increased tracer accumulation is seen in the right upper lobe pulmonary nodule measuring 1 cm (*arrows* in D and E) and a small focus in the liver lesion (*arrows* in F and G), confirming the metastatic disease.

TABLE 99.6 Appropriate Use Criteria for Colo-rectal Cancer [23]

	Initial Workup	Restaging/Response/Recurrence	Surveillance
Resectable disease	To be used for staging only if contrast-enhanced CT has an equivocal finding	Not routinely recommended	Not recommended
Metastatic or synchronous adenocarcinoma from large bowel (any T, any N, M1)	For staging to identify other potential disease sites that make it unresectable	Serial CEA elevation to identify other sites of recurrence	Not recommended

CEA, carcinoembryonic antigen; *CT*, computed tomography; *M*, metastasis; *N*, node; *T*, tumor.

TABLE 99.8 Appropriate Use Criteria for Testicular Tumors [36]

Testicular Tumors	Initial Workup	Restaging/Response/Recurrence	Surveillance
Seminomas	Not indicated	Stage IIA, IIB, IIC, and III 6 wk after orchidectomy and chemotherapy, if CT shows residual mass >3 cm and normal tumor markers, PET/CT for restaging; if negative, follow up for recurrence as clinically indicated	Not indicated

CT, computed tomography; *PET*, positron emission tomography.

CT, MRI, bone scan, and ^{18}F sodium fluoride are used in the management. Alternately ^{68}GaPSMA, choline C-11, or ^{18}F fluciclovine PET/CT or PET/MRI can be considered as a one-stop modality and in patients with equivocal results on initial bone scan. ^{68}Ga PSMA, choline C-11, or ^{18}F fluciclovine PET/CT or PET/MRI can also be considered in setting of biochemical failure after prostatectomy or radiation therapy.

Testicular Tumors

Although the overall prognosis for patients with testicular tumors is excellent, accurate staging and surveillance can optimize treatment planning. The primary tumor is usually adequately assessed by USG or, in complex cases, by MRI. CT is the primary imaging modality used for staging because it can visualize adenopathy and lung metastases with reasonable accuracy.

Use of PET/CT

PET has shown its efficacy in the management of patients with seminomatous testicular tumor, but limited data are available with respect to nonseminomatous tumors. FDG PET has been evaluated for its role in testicular tumor recurrence and relapse. It was found that FDG PET may contribute to the management plan of residual seminoma lesions. FDG PET has been used to predict treatment response in patients with testicular cancer [35] (Table 99.8).

Limitations

Physiological uptake in young patients may cause false-positive results. Small lesions (<8 mm) and low-grade tumors may show falsely low grade FDG uptake.

Malignant Melanoma

Malignant melanoma consists of cutaneous and mucosal melanoma. Clinical examination and histopathology of suspicious lesions are the primary diagnostic procedures in the management of patients with cutaneous melanoma. Conventionally CT of the thorax and abdomen is being used for staging purposes.

Use of PET/CT

PET/CT has been already used for metastatic workup in patients with malignant melanoma. It is valuable in patients without metastasis or with limited metastasis in whom radical dissection or distant metastasectomy is planned (Fig. 99.20). So, for the staging of advanced stage III and IV malignant melanoma, FDG PET/CT is found to be promising in detecting lymph node as well as visceral metastatic disease. It can also be used in response assessment. FDG PET/CT has been found to be more specific in detecting metastatic disease for both staging and restaging than CT and MRI [37,38].

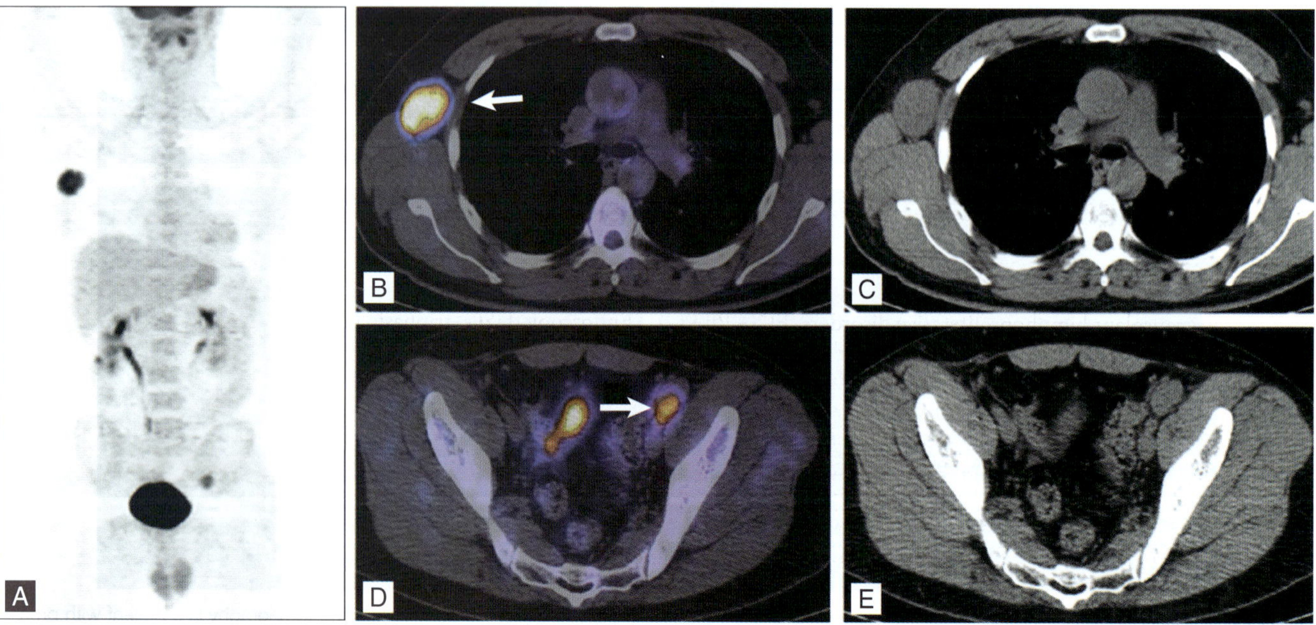

Figure 99.20 Newly diagnosed metastatic melanoma in the right axillary lymph node. Fluorodeoxyglucose positron emission tomography for staging shows Maximum intensity projection image (A), intense metabolic activity within an enlarged right axillary lymph node (*arrow* in B). Further increased metabolic activity in an enlarged left external iliac lymph node (*arrow* in D) is compatible with involvement with malignant melanoma. Images C and E shows corresponding CT sections.

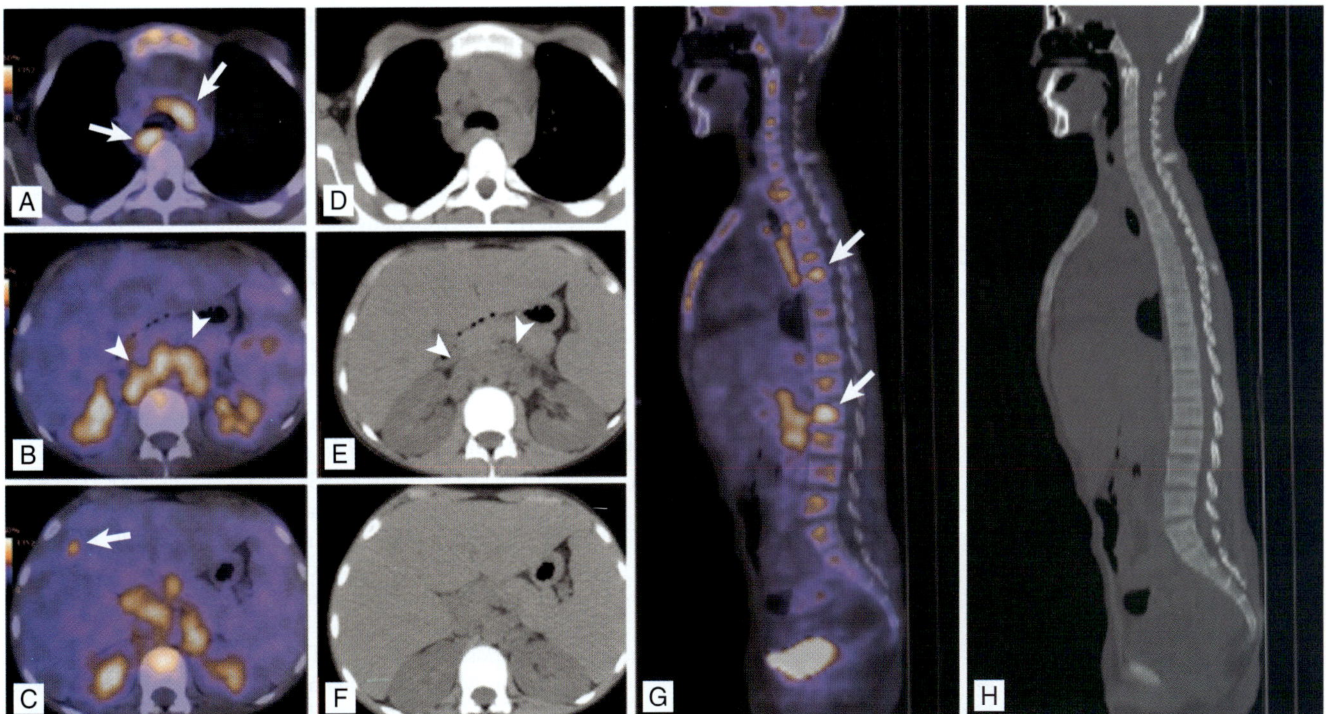

Figure 99.21 An 18-year-old man with Hodgkin lymphoma. Staging fluorodeoxyglucose (FDG) positron emission tomography shows FDG-avid enlarged lymph nodes above and below the diaphragm (*arrows* in A, B) suggestive of lymphomatous involvement. Furthermore, a solitary focus of uptake is seen in a subcentimeter liver lesion indicative of disease involvement (*arrows* in C). Diffuse heterogeneous tracer uptake is noted in the bones (*arrows* in G) suggestive of bone marrow involvement. Images D, E, F, H show corresponding CT sections.

Limitations

Postsurgical inflammatory changes, granulomatous or infectious lesions, and brown fat uptake can lead to false-positive results. High physiological bowel uptake can obscure peritoneal and bowel lesions.

Lymphoma

Lymphoma is one of the most common malignancies worldwide. Broadly, it can be categorized into Hodgkin lymphoma (HL) and non-Hodgkin lymphoma (NHL). NHL, which is more common, is the ninth leading cause of death. History, physical examination, and bone marrow biopsy and aspiration are the primary diagnostic procedures used for the assessment of lymphoma. CT of the thorax, abdomen, and pelvis is the conventional imaging modality.

Use of PET/CT

PET/CT is recommended for staging (Fig. 99.21) and restaging of HL and most NHLs. It has also been used successfully in evaluation of posttransplant lymphoproliferative disorders. FDG PET/CT is found to be more accurate in interim and end-of-therapy response assessment (Figs. 99.22 and 99.23). It can also prognosticate and predict the Richter's transformation. Several studies have observed that FDG PET/CT could be a useful noninvasive method to replace bone marrow biopsy in patients with newly diagnosed HL and in diffuse large B-cell lymphomas (see Table 99.9). For a more objective reporting and interpretation of FDG PET/CT in lymphoma, 5-point scale or Deauville criteria are being used currently [39].

Limitations

Infective and inflammatory lymphadenopathy, lung inflammation (Fig. 99.24), rebound thymic hyperplasia, tonsillitis, and granulocyte-colony stimulating factor–induced bone marrow reactivation are few causes of false-positive results. Low-grade lymphomas such as SLL (Small lymphocytic lymphoma) and FL (Follicular lymphoma) (grades 1 and 2), because of their low-grade uptake, can lead to false-negative results.

Neuroendocrine Tumors

Neuroendocrine neoplasms (NENs) are tumors of neural crest cell origin. The most common site is the gastroenteropancreatic (GEP) system, constituting approximately 70% of NENs. Other locations include the lung, adrenal medulla, pituitary, thyroid, parathyroid, and sympathetic and parasympathetic ganglias. In histopathology, the Ki-67, a tumor proliferative index is a prognostic factor in NENs.

- Ki-67 level of ≤2 for G1 or well-differentiated
- Ki-67 level 3–20 for G2 or moderately differentiated
- Ki-67 level >20 for G3 or poorly differentiated neoplasms

Endoscopic USG, triphasic CT, MRI, MRCP, and ERCP are the primary diagnostic modalities used in the management of patients with NENs.

Use of PET/CT

Fluorodeoxyglucose PET/CT has limited utility in well-differentiated NEN. Several other functional imaging such as ^{68}Ga-DOTA peptides or ^{18}F-dihydroxyphenylalanine (DOPA) PET/CT are being currently used in the evaluation of NENs. ^{68}Ga-SSR (Somatostatin receptor) PET/CT has a very high sensitivity, specificity, and accuracy in GEP neuroendocrine tumors. It is therefore recommended for staging and assessment of suspected recurrence in NENs, especially in G1 tumors (Figs. 99.25 and 99.26).

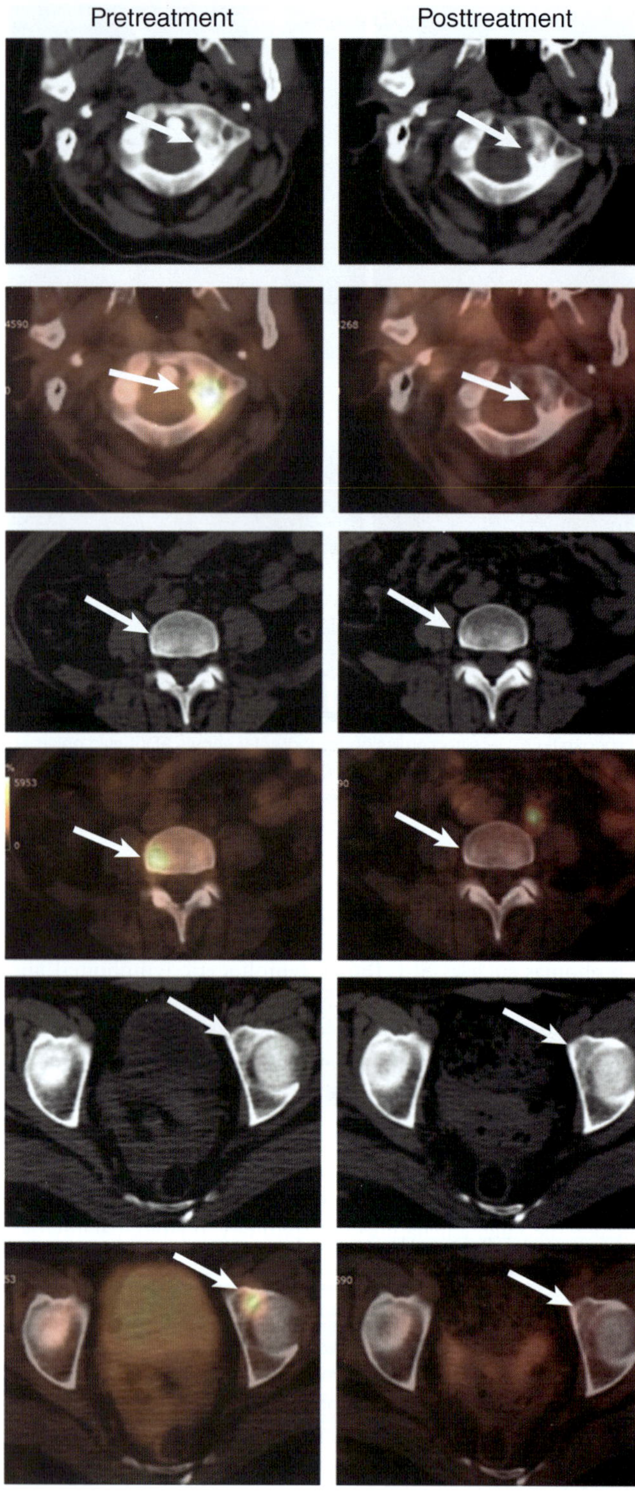

Figure 99.22 In a known case of non-Hodgkin lymphoma after chemotherapy, fluorodeoxyglucose positron emission tomography shows complete resolution of metabolic activity in the posttreatment study (*Arrows* in right side images) compared with the pretreatment study (*Arrows* in left side images) suggestive of complete treatment response with a Deauville score of 1.

^{18}F-DOPA PET/CT has also been used in selected cases of NENs such as insulinoma, neuroblastoma, pheochromocytoma, and paraganglioma. ^{68}Ga-SSR PET/CT has also been used as theragnostic agent for assessing the eligibility of peptide receptor radiolabeled therapy (PRRT) and response assessment after PRRT. The use of FDG PET/CT is usually reserved for patients with poorly differentiated NENs, such as neuroendocrine carcinomas or G3 tumors. It can also be used for prognostication in patients with NENs [42].

Limitations

Uptake in the exocrine pancreas, uncinate process, and adrenal glands; osteoarthritis; recent fracture; vertebral hemangioma; fibrous dysplasia; epiphyseal growth plates; and splenosis may lead to false-positive results. Atypical SSTR (Somatostatin receptor) subtype expression, poorly differentiated tumors, and small-sized lesions (<8 mm) may lead to false-negative results.

Appropriate Use Criteria [43]

- ^{68}Ga-DOTATATE PET/CT (SSR-PET/CT), ^{68}Ga-DOTATATE PET/MRI (SSR-PET/MRI), and SSR scintigraphy (SSR single-photon emission computed tomography [SPECT]/CT) can be used to assess receptor status and disease extent. This is especially important for determining whether a patient may benefit from SSR-directed therapy
- Whenever possible, SSR PET/CT should be performed in combination with contrast-enhanced CT or MRI (dual-phase hepatic CT or MRI is preferred) to minimize the total number of imaging studies
- In selected patients in whom high-grade NET is documented or suspected, FDG PET/ contrast-enhanced CT may be useful to identify high-grade active disease because SSR PET/CT has limited sensitivity in such scenarios

Renal Cell Carcinoma

Renal cell carcinoma (RCC) is one of the most common urological malignancies with clear cell carcinoma being the most common histopathological variety. Contrast-enhanced CT of the abdomen is the primary imaging modality for diagnosis, staging, and treatment planning of RCC.

Uses of PET/CT

PET/CT has significant limitations in local diagnosis of RCC because most of the radiotracers such as ^{18}F-FDG are excreted through kidneys, leading to significant background activity. Even application of diuretics or delayed imaging cannot overcome this limitation so far. However, ^{18}F-FDG-PET has a higher sensitivity in detecting metastatic disease [44].

Limitations

Because FDG is excreted through the kidneys, it has lower sensitivity in detection of primary RCC. Besides this, the clear cell variant of RCC shows lower FDG uptake, so it has limited sensitivity.

Appropriate Use Criteria

Currently, as per NCCN, FDG PET/CT is not indicated in patients with RCC.

Urinary Bladder Cancer

Bladder cancer is the most frequent cancer of the urinary tract. The standard method of diagnosing bladder cancer remains cystoscopy, including biopsy and resection with histopathological evaluation. For local staging, MRI is an accurate technique because of its superior spatial and contrast resolution.

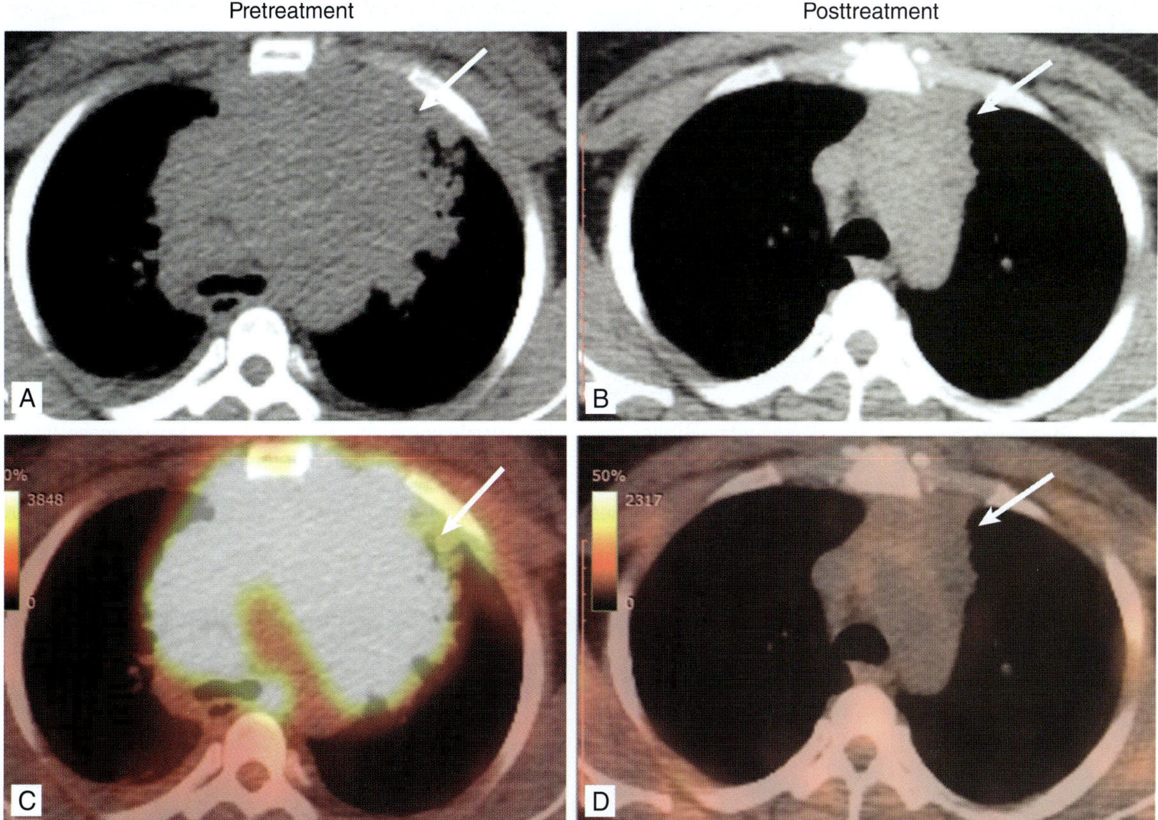

Figure 99.23 A 34-year-old woman with diffuse large B-cell lymphoma after chemotherapy. Interim fluorodeoxyglucose positron emission tomography/computed tomography shows significant regression in the size and metabolic activity of the mediastinal mass (*white arrows* in B and D) with a maximum standard uptake value (SUV_{max}) of 0.9 compared with a pretreatment SUV_{max} of 19.3 (*white arrows* in A and C). Overall, the findings are those of complete metabolic response with a Deauville score of 2, although there is a residual mediastinal mass remaining measuring 4.0 × 2.5 cm.

Uses of PET/CT

PET/CT has limited use in the evaluation in local staging because of its lower spatial resolution of compared with conventional cross-sectional imaging methods, such as MRI. Various mechanisms for improving the diagnostic capabilities of ^{18}F-FDG PET have been investigated, such as delayed pelvic imaging after oral hydration and forced diuresis using furosemide (Fig. 99.27) [45,46]. Currently, FDG PET/CT has been used in metastatic workup, especially in muscle-invasive carcinoma and detection of recurrence (Table 99.10).

Limitations

Physiological tracer activity in the bladder interferes in detection of local and regional nodal diseases. However, postdiuretic imaging has significantly improved the accuracy of FDG PET/CT in this setting.

Multiple Myeloma

Multiple myeloma (MM) is a malignant B-cell and plasma cell disorder that involves the skeleton in more than 80% of patients at diagnosis. Conventionally, skeletal survey radiographs and

TABLE 99.9 Appropriate Use Criteria for Lymphoma [40,41]

Lymphoma	Initial Workup	Restaging/Response/Recurrence	Surveillance
HL	Essential; contrast-enhanced CT may be avoided	1. Early or interim restaging after two to four cycles of standard-dose chemotherapy in patients with advanced or extranodal disease 2. Restaging after chemotherapy or RT completion	Not routinely recommended
NHL (low grade)	Essential if RT planned for Stage I, II	For detection of disease response and to detect high-grade transformation	Not routinely recommended
NHL (high grade)	Essential; contrast-enhanced CT may be avoided	1. Early or interim restaging 2. Restaging after chemotherapy or RT completion	Not routinely recommended
NHL: CLL/SLL	Not indicated unless used to direct nodal biopsy		

CLL, chronic lymphocytic leukemia; *CT*, computed tomography; *HL*, Hodgkin lymphoma; *NHL*, non-Hodgkin lymphoma; *RT*, radiotherapy; *SLL*, small lymphocytic lymphoma.

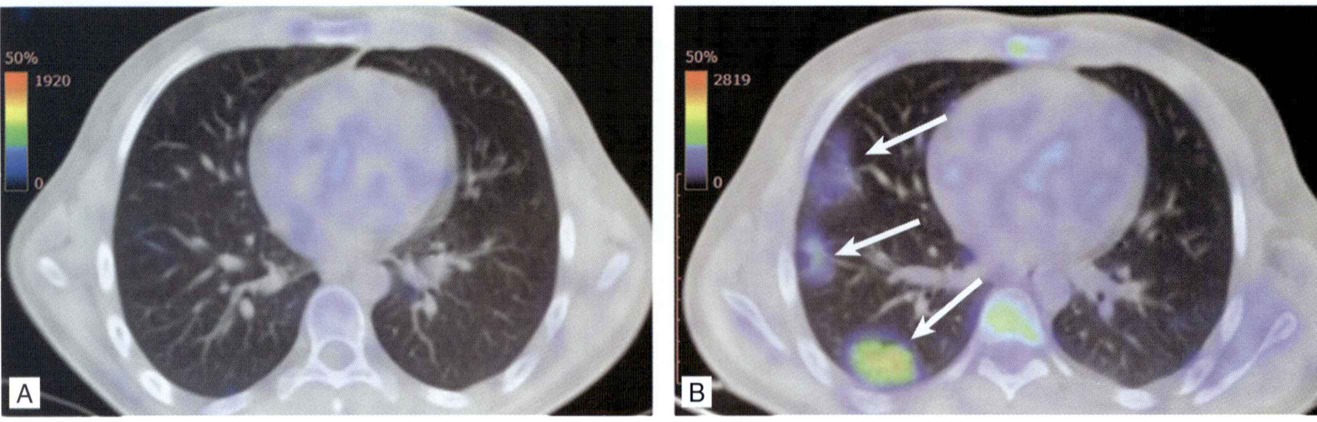

Figure 99.24 A 19-year-old man with Hodgkin lymphoma after completion of chemotherapy. Baseline fluorodeoxyglucose (FDG) positron emission tomography/computed tomography (PET/CT) (A) and post-treatment FDG PET/CT (B) show interval new FDG avid consolidation with ground glass opacities in the lung (*arrows* in B). There is interval resolution of previously seen nodal lesions, and no other hypermetabolic pathological lesions are found in the body. Therefore, the new lung lesions represent inflammatory or infective pathology with a Deauville score of X.

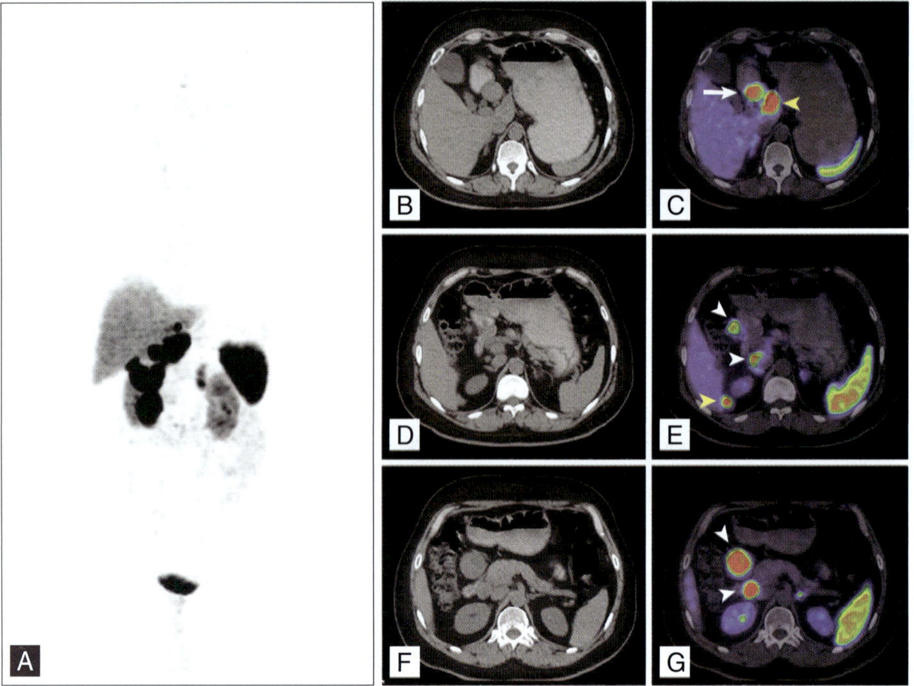

Figure 99.25 A 47-year-old man with known duodenal neuroendocrine tumour (NET) underwent gallium-68 DOTANOC positron emission tomography/computed tomography for staging (A showing maximum intensity projection image). Axial computed tomography and positron emission tomography/computed tomography images (B–G) show somatostatin receptor expressing nodular soft tissue lesion arising from the first part of duodenum (*white arrow* in C), suggesting primary NET with metastases to paraduodenal and precaval lymph nodes (*white arrowheads* in C, E and G) and liver (*yellow arrowhead*).

whole-body MRI are the investigations of choice for these patients for assessment of the skeletal lesions.

Use of PET/CT

^{18}F-FDG PET/CT is commonly used for the detection of myeloma bone disease and extramedullary sites of metabolically active myeloma foci with relatively high sensitivity and specificity. Being a whole-body modality, it helps in evaluation of the patient at one session. Extramedullary disease can also be detected on FDG PET/CT. It helps in response assessment to treatment and imaging findings correlate well with other markers [48].

Limitations

False-positive findings in FDG PET/CT can be caused by metallic implants in situ, fracture sites, infections, postsurgical areas, or recent chemotherapy or radiotherapy. The common causes of false-negative findings are hyperglycemia and the presence of subcentimeter lytic lesions in the skull or close to the brain [48].

Appropriate Use Criteria

^{18}F-FDG PET/CT should be considered as part of the initial investigations in patients with newly diagnosed MM. ^{18}F-FDG

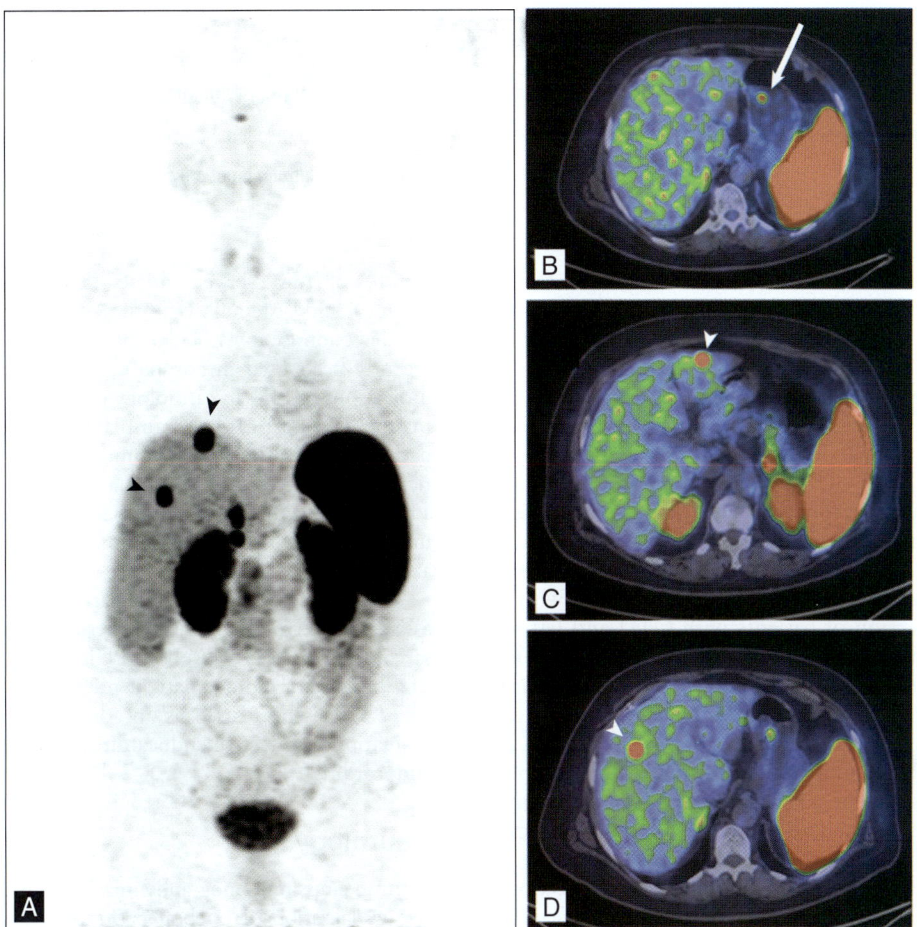

Figure 99.26 A 55-year-old woman with known gastric neuroendocrine tumour staging gallium-68 DOTANOC positron emission tomography/computed tomography shows polypoidal nodular lesion in the body of the stomach along the lesser curvature (*arrow* in B), suggesting primary neuroendocrine tumor with a few somatostatin receptor–expressing lesions in the liver (*arrowheads* in A, C, and D).

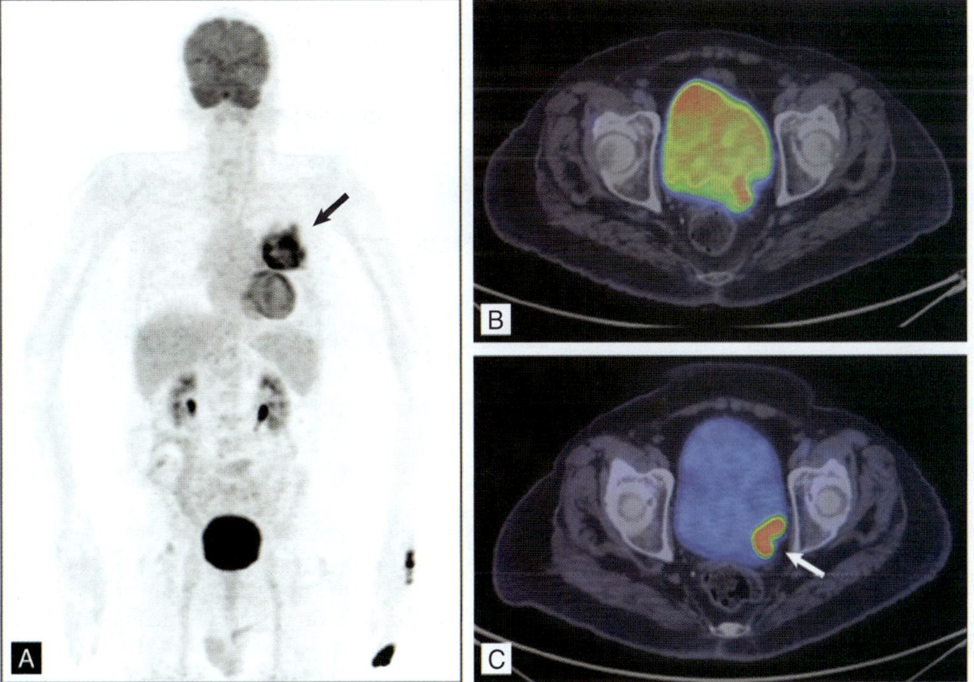

Figure 99.27 A 70-year-old man with known lung cancer. Staging fluorodeoxyglucose positron emission tomography/computed tomography shows a metabolically active mass in left lung upper lobe in the maximum intensity projection (MIP) image (A) compatible with primary malignancy. Additionally, incidental soft tissue lesion is seen along the left posterolateral wall of the urinary bladder, which was not obvious on the MIP as well as transaxial images (A and B) due to intense bladder activity. The delayed postdiuretic study, however, clearly depicts the metabolically active soft tissue lesion along the left posterolateral wall of the urinary bladder (*arrow* in C), suggesting urinary bladder cancer (second primary), which was later confirmed on histopathology.

TABLE 99.10 Appropriate Use Criteria for Urinary Bladder Cancer [47]

Bladder Cancer	Additional Workup	Follow-up With or Without Cystectomy
Muscle-invasive T2 or T3 disease	For staging of selected patients	May be performed if not previously done; if metastasis is suspected
T4 disease	For staging of selected patients	May be performed if not previously done; in high-risk patients

PET/CT is now the preferred technique for evaluating and monitoring response to therapy [48].

Nononcologic Uses of Positron Emission Tomography/Computed Tomography

Cardiology

Positron emission tomography has been used as an imaging tool for the assessment of myocardial perfusion and for the characterization of tissue viability in patients with advanced coronary artery disease (CAD). Viability assessment with ^{18}F FDG is used in selection of patients with CAD and left ventricular dysfunction to determine whether they would benefit from intervention. *FDG-PET imaging shows the glucose metabolism in viable myocardial segments, and it has been seen that most metabolically viable segments on FDG PET recover* (Fig. 99.28).

Ammonia N-13 and rubidium-82 perfusion PET are being used for ischemia assessment as well as for perfusion part of myocardial viability assessment, but they have their limitations because of their short half-lives. Other newer PET tracers such as ^{18}F flurpiridaz have recently shown good results in the detection of myocardial perfusion abnormalities. Another advantage of the PET perfusion tracers is their ability to assess myocardial blood flow, which can provide myocardial flow reserve [49].

Besides CAD, PET/CT has also proved itself useful in the assessment of various types of vasculitis and metabolic diseases. A number of studies have evaluated the value of ^{18}F-FDG in assessing focal and systemic vasculitis. Although not used routinely for the detection of any vascular disease, ^{18}F-FDG PET/CT has also recently been used in coronary plaque assessment. A few other indications of PET in cardiology include the evaluation of cardiomyopathies, post cardiac transplant evaluation, and cardiac sympathetic innervation. The commonly used PET radiopharmaceuticals for imaging presynaptic activity are ^{18}F-fluorodopamine, 11C-hydroxyephedrine, and 11C-ephidrine. Postsynaptic agents include 11C-(4-(3-t-butylamino-2-hydroxypropoxylbenzimidazol-1), and 11C-carazolol.

Currently, ^{18}F-FDG PET is part of the diagnostic criteria and assists in determining treatment response in patients with cardiac sarcoidosis. ^{68}Ga DOTANOC PET is also being tried in this setting because of tedious patient preparation for FDG PET. FDG PET/CT has been used as an adjunctive diagnostic tool in the evaluation of infective endocarditis, especially in prosthetic valve endocarditis.

Neurology

Positron emission tomography imaging of the brain allows noninvasive visualization of cerebral perfusion, metabolism, and receptor binding. Besides oncology, currently, the main indications of PET/CT in neurology are epilepsy, dementias, and movement disorders.

Magnetic resonance imaging is able to identify the source of the seizure in the majority of patients. However, 20–30% of

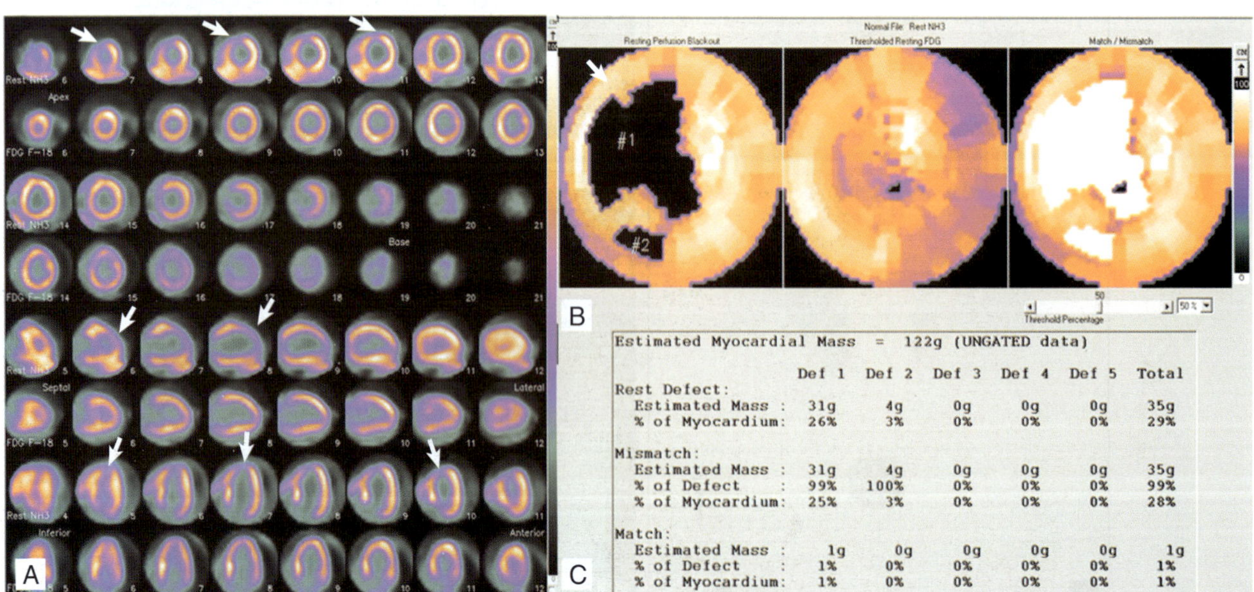

Figure 99.28 A 65-year-old woman with a history of anterior wall myocardial infarction underwent positron emission tomography (PET) for viability assessment that included rest NH_3 perfusion PET and fluorodeoxyglucose metabolic PET. The study shows a mismatched perfusion–metabolic defect (i.e., impaired perfusion with preserved metabolism) involving the mid and distal anteroseptal wall and apex (*arrows* in A and B show mismatched perfusion–metabolic defect in the cardiac slices in three different axes and polar maps, respectively, C shows computer-based quantification), consistent with viable hibernating myocardium.

TABLE 99.11 **The Different Metabolism Patterns and Corresponding Findings on Amyloid PET Imaging**

Dementia	Findings on FDG PET	Findings on Amyloid PET
Alzheimer disease (Fig. 99.29)	Hypometabolism involving the precuneus or posterior cingulate cortex in early phase of disease followed by hypometabolism involving temporoparietal cortices Frontal cortices are involved in late stage of dementia; sensorimotor cortices are usually spared	Increased uptake (positive)
Frontotemporal dementia (Fig. 99.30)	Hypometabolism involving the frontal and temporal cortices with involvement of the parietal cortices in late stages	Usually negative
Dementia with Lewy bodies	Hypometabolism involving the occipital, temporal, and parietal cortices, with sparing of the precuneus and posterior cingulate cortex (posterior cingulate sign)	Could be positive or negative
Vascular dementia	Usually subcortical white matter involved, but hypometabolism is seen in the area of ischemic insult	Negative

FDG, fluorodeoxyglucose, *PET*, positron emission tomography.

potential surgical candidates with focal epilepsy have normal MRI results. In these patients, FDG PET study may provide significant information. *During the ictal phase, it shows an increase in glucose metabolism in the region of the epileptogenic focus, and in the interictal phase, there is decreased glucose metabolism in the epileptogenic focus.* Usually, interictal FDG PET is used for this purpose and sometimes superimposed with ictal SPECT and MRI for better localization of seizure focus.

PET/CT has been a useful tool in the assessment of dementia for a while. The most commonly used tracer is FDG, which demonstrates the regional glucose metabolism of the brain and thereby helps in the diagnosis of different type of dementias. Recently, amyloid PET agents have also been used in this setting. Table 99.11 shows the different metabolism patterns and corresponding findings on amyloid PET imaging [50].

Although FDG PET is also used in movement disorders, more specific receptor-based tracers are being used in this setting. Tracers such as DAT (dopamine transporter) and ^{18}F DOPA (dihydroxy phenyl-alanine) are used in presynaptic dopamine imaging, whereas D2 receptor radioligands are used in postsynaptic dopamine imaging. Table 99.12 depicts different findings of different types of movement disorders [51,52].

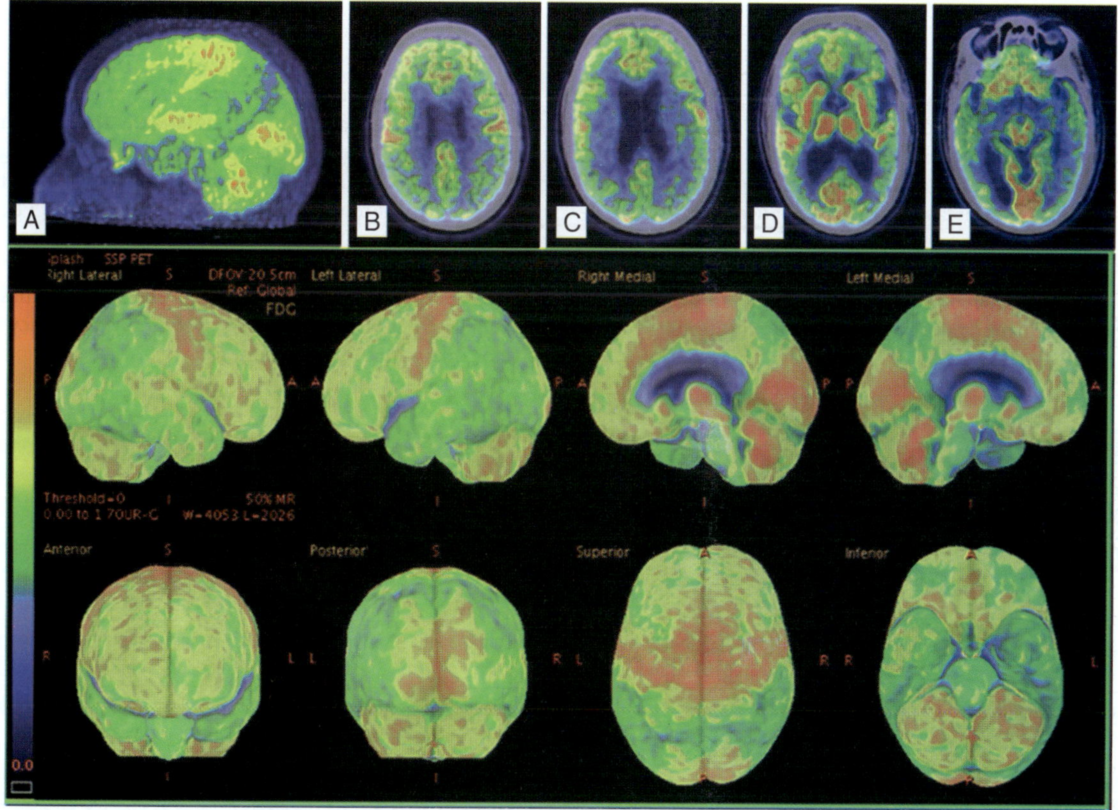

Figure 99.29 A 58-year-old man with a history of dementia and cognitive impairment underwent brain fluorodeoxyglucose positron emission tomography (PET) for evaluation. The study shows hypometabolism involving bilateral parietal, temporal, lateral occipital, and posterior cingulate cortices (A, maximum intensity projection image; B–E, axial fused PET/computed tomography images; *middle* and *lower panels,* three-dimensional SSP images). Overall, the scan findings are suggestive of Alzheimer disease. SSP: Stereotactic surface projection.

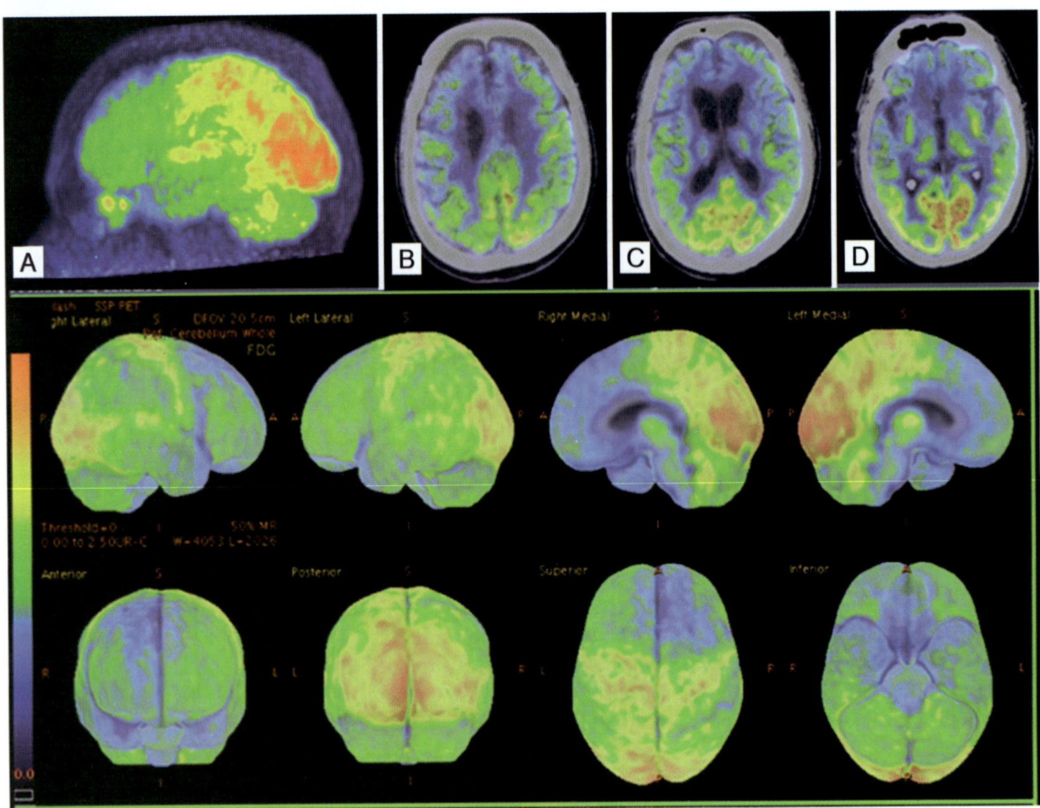

Figure 99.30 A 59-year-old man with history of dementia and aphasia underwent brain fluorodeoxyglucose positron emission tomography (PET) for evaluation. The study shows hypometabolism involving bilateral frontal and temporal cortices (A, maximum intensity projection image; B–D, axial fused PET/computed tomography images; *middle and lower panels,* three-dimensional SSP images). Overall, the scan findings are suggestive of frontotemporal dementia.

Pyrexia of Unknown Origin

The pathophysiology of pyrexia of unknown origin (PUO) can be grouped into four categories: infections, malignancies, noninfectious inflammatory diseases and miscellaneous causes. CT, MRI, and USG are the conventional imaging modalities used in management of patients with PUO. However, inflammatory and infectious lesions can remain undetected because substantial anatomic changes take time to develop and may be absent in the early phase [53].

FDG PET/CT, being a whole-body modality, is a sensitive diagnostic technique for the evaluation of PUO (Fig. 99.32). Being a hybrid anatomic and functional imaging modality, it picks up the pathological lesion before the appearance of anatomic changes. Thus, it guides further diagnostic tests, such as cytopathological tests, to achieve a final diagnosis [54].

Limitations

Although FDG PET/CT has a high sensitivity, it has a limited specificity. It cannot differentiate between malignancy and infective or inflammatory pathology.

TABLE 99.12 Findings in Various Types of Movement Disorders

Movement Disorder	Presynaptic Dopamine Imaging	Postsynaptic Dopamine Imagin	FDG PET Findings
Parkinson disease (Fig. 99.31)	Reduced uptake in the caudate nucleus and putamen with rostrocaudal gradient	Normal or increased uptake in the striatum	Hypometabolism in the frontal, temporal, or parietal cortices; normal or increased metabolism in the basal ganglia and thalamus
Multiple system atrophy	Reduced uptake in the caudate nucleus and putamen with rostrocaudal gradient	Reduced uptake in the striatum	Hypometabolism in both putamen in MSA-P and cerebellum in MSA-C
Corticobasal degeneration	Reduced uptake in the putamen contralateral to the affected side	Reduced uptake in the striatum	Hypometabolism in the basal ganglia and frontoparietal cortices contralateral to the clinically affected side
Progressive supranuclear palsy	Reduced uptake in caudate nucleus and putamen	Reduced uptake in striatum	Hypometabolism involving the anterior cingulate cortex, basal ganglia, and midbrain

FDG, fluorodeoxyglucose; *MSA-C,* Multiple system atrophy – cerebellar subtype; *MSA-P,* Multiple system atrophy – Parkinsonian subtype; *PET,* positron emission tomography.

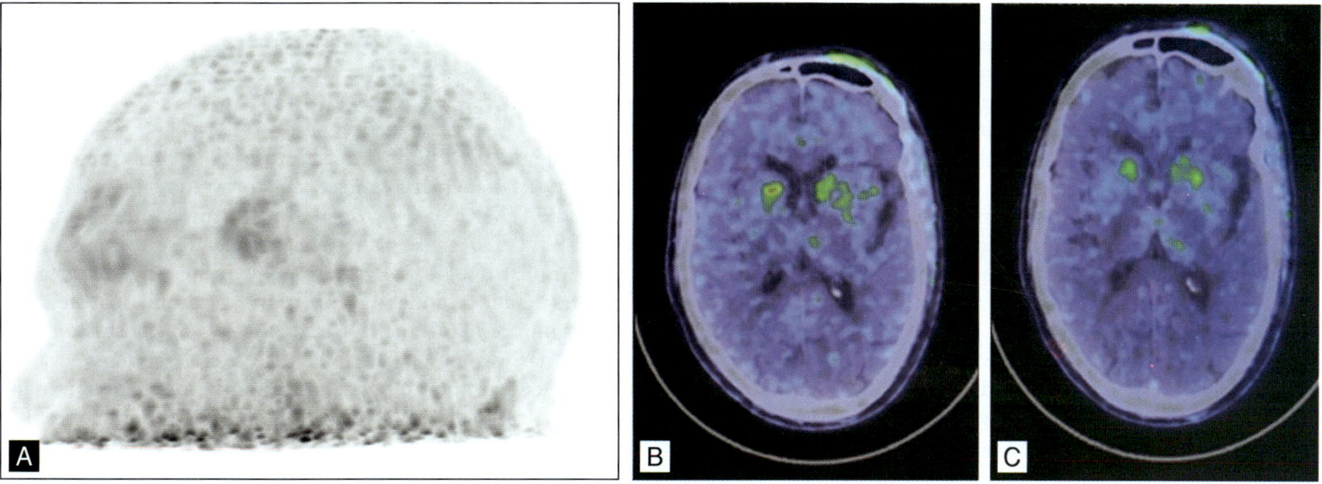

Figure 99.31 A 53-year-old man with a history of tremor and bradykinesia underwent 18-fluorine DOPA positron emission tomography (PET) for evaluation. PET shows reduced tracer uptake in both basal ganglia more severely in the putamen (A, maximum intensity projection image; B and C, fused transaxial PET/computed tomography images), suggesting idiopathic Parkinson disease.

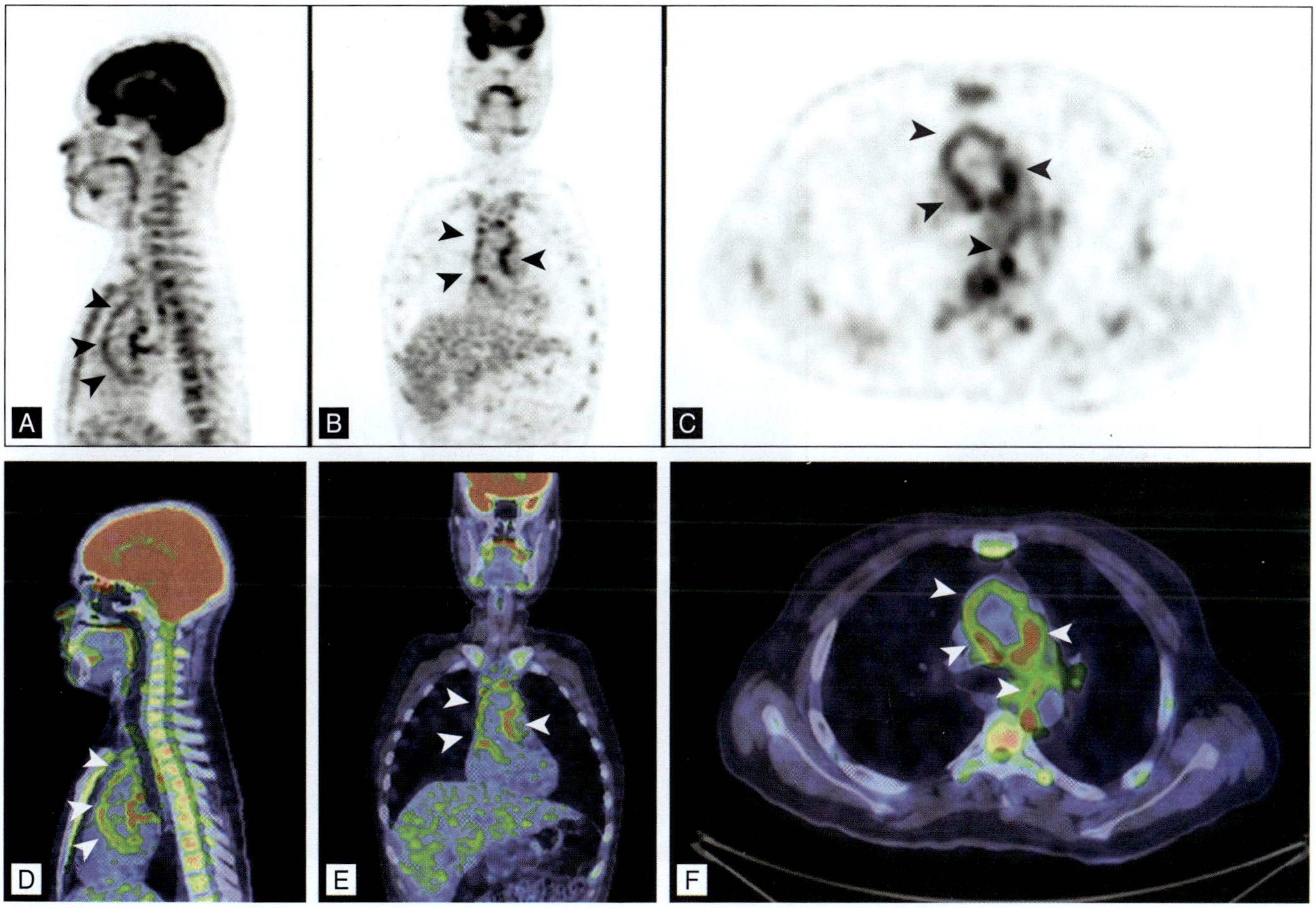

Figure 99.32 A 20-year-old man underwent fluorodeoxyglucose positron emission tomography/computed tomography (PET/CT) for evaluation of pyrexia of unknown origin. PET/CT study shows increased metabolic activity along the walls of the ascending and descending thoracic aorta (*arrowheads* in A–F) and arch of the aorta suggestive of large-vessel vasculitis.

Appropriate Use Criteria

Traditionally, contrast-enhanced CT of the chest, abdomen, and pelvis has been the imaging modality of choice. However, recent evidence suggests that FDG-PET/CT is preferred over the CT for this purpose [55].

Positron Emission Tomography/Magnetic Resonance Imaging

The development of combined PET/CT in the year 2000 marked a milestone in the era of hybrid imaging. With the availability of hybrid PET/CT scanner, PET/CT is currently widely used for oncologic indications mainly because of combined morphologic and functional information obtained in the single study. Recently, another new hybrid imaging technology, PET/MRI, has emerged and has already shown promising potential in different clinical conditions. Although the development of prototype PET/MRI systems began even before the development of combined PET/CT, several technical challenges delayed the development of clinical PET/MRI systems [56]. Information obtained on a true hybrid PET/MRI combines the anatomic and quantitative strengths of MRI with physiologic information obtained from PET [57].

Advantages

Magnetic resonance imaging facilitates obtaining higher anatomic resolution and functional information simultaneously, complementing the functional imaging capabilities of PET, thus opening up new areas of application. Furthermore, there is less radiation exposure on PET/MR than on PET/CT. As hybrid PET/MRI regularly uses respiratory gating, there is improved temporal and spatial co-registration.

Potential Indications

In oncology (Fig. 99.33), head and neck cancers, hepatobiliary cancers, pancreatic cancer, and prostate cancer are areas where PET/MRI has shown its incremental value compared with PET/CT because of better soft tissue resolution. Cardiac applications of PET/MRI are mainly addressing the areas of left ventricular remodeling, infiltrative cardiomyopathies, and gadolinium enhancement–based studies on perfusion and viability assessment. Alzheimer disease and epilepsy evaluation are its main neurologic applications as published in many preclinical and clinical studies [58–62]. Although currently the potential applications of PET/MRI are proposed in oncology, cardiology, and neurology, ever-expanding research interests could never limit the scope of this modality.

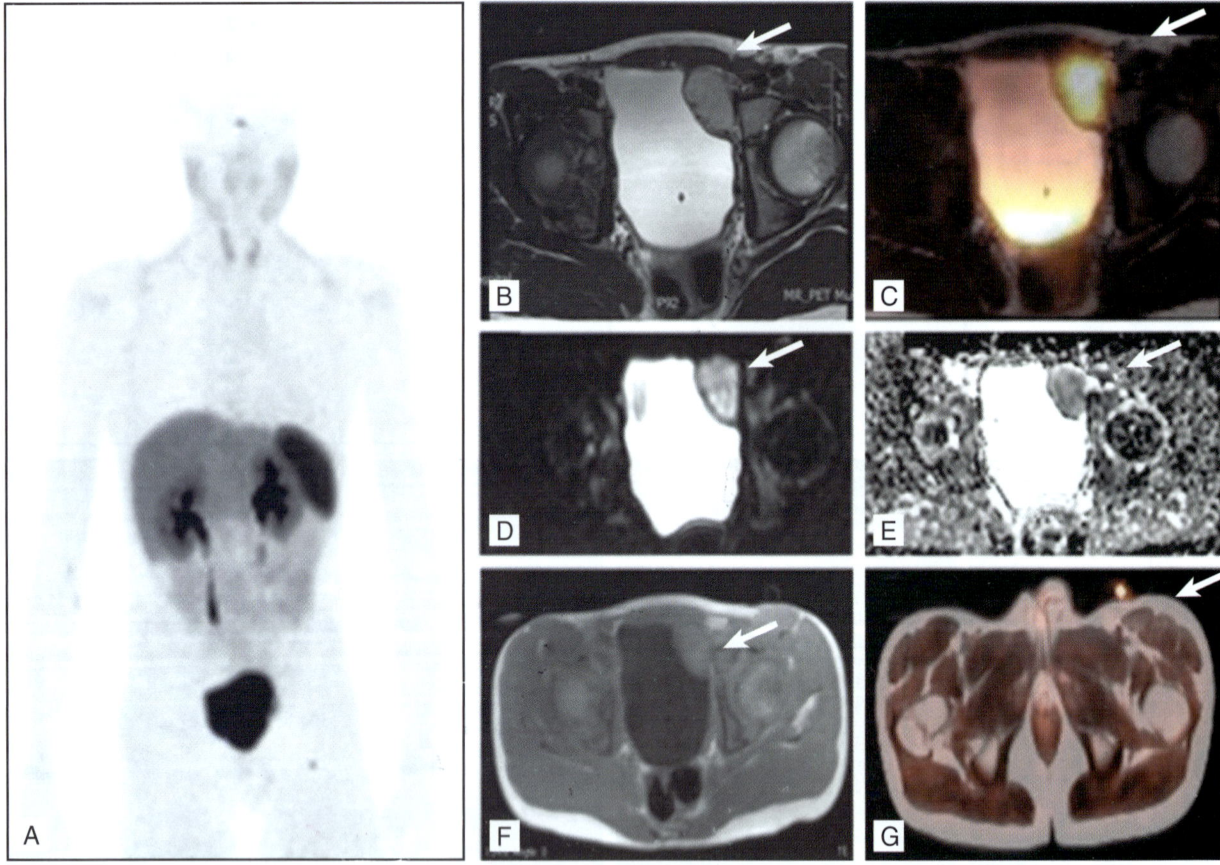

Figure 99.33 Gallium-68 DOTATATE positron emission tomography (PET)/magnetic resonance imaging in urinary bladder paraganglioma. A 13-year-old boy presented with a 1-year history of headache, tachycardia, and pallor every time he passed urine. His urinary and plasma normetadrenaline levels were high. Subsequently, he was referred for PET and scintigraphic studies for further evaluation. (A) Maximum intensity projection (MIP) image shows no evidence of distant metastases. (B) T2-weighted axial images show a lobulated mass of intermediate signal in the left anterolateral portion of the bladder, which appears predominantly extravesicular but closely attached to the bladder wall (*white arrow*). (C) Fused images show intense uptake of tracer in the bladder lesion (*white arrow*). (D) and (E) The diffusion-weighted images show restricted diffusion with increased signal intensity and decreased signal on the corresponding apparent diffusion coefficient image (*white arrows*). (F) T1-weighted fat saturation images show intense contrast enhancement by the mass, indicating the hypervascular nature of the lesion (*white arrow*). (G) Focal uptake in the left groin is activity (*white arrow*) within the urinary catheter, which corresponds to the uptake seen on the MIP.

Conclusion

The addition of combined or hybrid PET/CT modality to the diagnostic toolbox is undoubtedly one of the most significant advancements in oncologic imaging in the past decade. Although currently FDG is the main workhorse in both oncology and non-oncology settings, new tracers are on the rise for more specific results. These tracers are being targeted for detecting certain types and subtypes of malignancies. Besides, to peek further into the future, a potential new field has developed within PET imaging called theranostics, in which in addition to being able to image tumors with PET imaging agents, nuclear medicine physicians are able to use those tracers for treatment as well.

Suggested Readings

- L Gorospe, S Raman, J Echeveste, et al., Whole-body PET/CT: spectrum of physiological variants, artifacts and interpretative pitfalls in cancer patients, Nucl Med Commun 26 (8) (2005 Aug) 671–687.
- W Li, H Pang, Q Liu, J Zhou, The role of ^{18}F-FDG PET or ^{18}F-FDG-PET/CT in the evaluation of solitary pulmonary nodules, Eur J Radiol 84 (10) (2015 Oct) 2032–2037.
- R Goel, W Moore, B Sumer, et al., Clinical practice in PET/CT for the management of head and neck squamous cell cancer, AJR Am J Roentgenol 209 (2) (2017 Aug) 289–303.
- JR García Garzón, M de Arcocha Torres, R Delgado-Bolton, et al., Oncology Task Force of Spanish Society of Nuclear Medicine and Molecular Imaging. 68Ga-PSMA PET/CT in prostate cancer, Rev Esp Med Nucl Imagen Mol 37 (2) (2018 Mar-Apr) 130–138.
- BM Salata, P Singh, Role of cardiac PET in clinical practice, Curr Treat Options Cardiovasc Med 19 (12) (2017 Nov 9) 93.

Appendix

Centres of Ossification

The following illustrations show diagrammatically the dates of appearance of the primary and secondary ossification centres in the various regions of the body. Primary ossification centres are identified by capital letters; secondary ossification centres are identified by small letters.

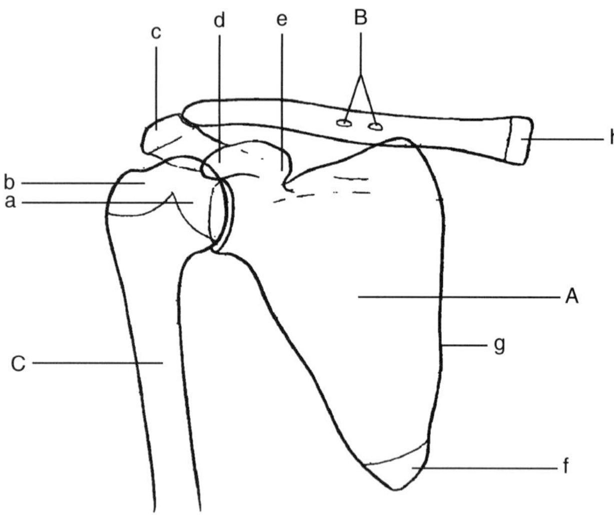

Figure A1 Ossification of bones of the shoulder. *A*, 8th week of fetal life. *B*, 5th and 6th weeks of fetal life, fuse about the 45th day of life. *C*, 8th week of fetal life.

a. Head of humerus 1 year
b. Greater tuberosity 3 years
   Lesser tuberosity 5 years
c. Two epiphyses for acromion 15–18 years, fuse by 25th year
d. Middle of coracoid process 1 year, fuses 15th year
e. Root of coracoid process 17 years, fuses 25th year
f. Inferior angle of scapula 14–20 years, fuses 22–25 years
g. Medial border of scapula 14–20 years, fuses 22–25 years
h. Sternal end of clavicle 18–20 years, fuses 25th year.

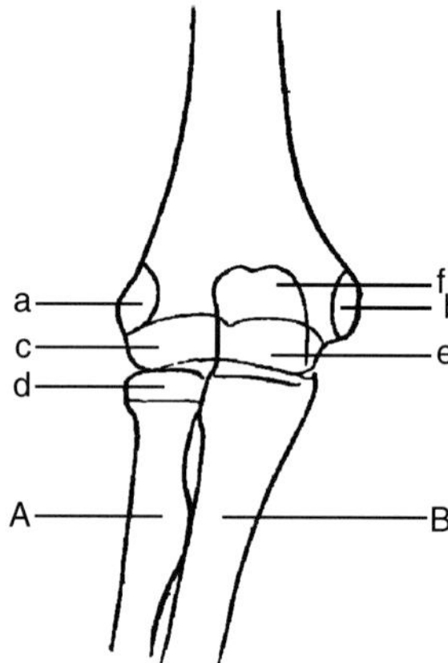

Figure A2 Ossification of bones of the elbow. *A*, 8th week of fetal life. *B*, 8th week of fetal life.

a. Lateral epicondyle 10–12 years, fuses 17–18 years
b. Medial epicondyle 5–8 years, fuses 17–18 years
c. Capitellum 1–3 years, fuses 17–18 years
d. Head of radius 5–6 years, fuses 16–19 years
e. Trochlea 11th year, fuses 18th year
f. Olecranon 10–13 years, fuses 16–20 years.

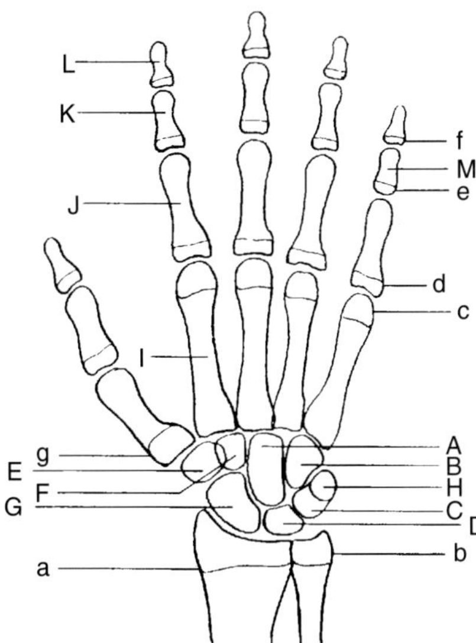

Figure A3 Ossification of the wrist, carpus, and hand. *A*, Capitate 4 months. *B*, Hamate 4 months. *C*, Triquetral 3 years. *D*, Lunate 4–5 years. *E*, Trapezium 6 years. *F*, Trapezoid 6 years. *G*, Scaphoid 6 years. *H*, Pisiform 11 years. *I*, Metacarpals 10th fetal week. *J*, Proximal phalanges 11th fetal week. *K*, Middle phalanges 12th fetal week. *L*, Distal phalanges 9th fetal week. *M*, Middle phalanx of 5th digit 14th fetal week.

a. Lower end of radius 1–2 years, fuses 20th year
b. Lower end of ulna 5–8 years, fuses 20th year
c. Metacarpal heads $2\frac{1}{2}$ years, fuse 20th year
d. Base of proximal phalanges $2\frac{1}{2}$ years, fuse 20th year
e. Base of middle phalanges 3 years, fuse 18–20 years
f. Base of distal phalanges 3 years, fuse 18–20 years
g. Base of 1st metacarpal $2\frac{1}{2}$ years, fuses 20th year.

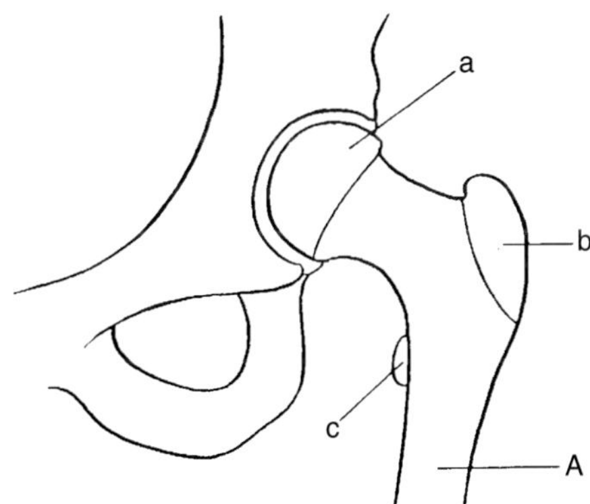

Figure A4 Ossification of bones of the hip. *A*, 7th fetal week.

a. 1st year, fuses 18–20 years
b. 3–5 years, fuses 18–20 years
c. 8–14 years, fuses 18–20 years.

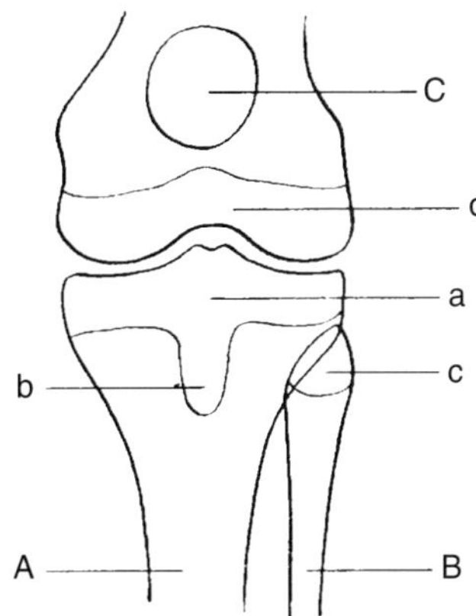

Figure A5 Ossification of bones of the knee. *A*, 7th fetal week. *B*, 8th fetal week. *C*, 5 years.

a. At birth, fuses 20th year
b. Tibial tubercle 5–10 years, fuses 20th year
c. 4th year, fuses 25th year
d. At birth, fuses 20th year.

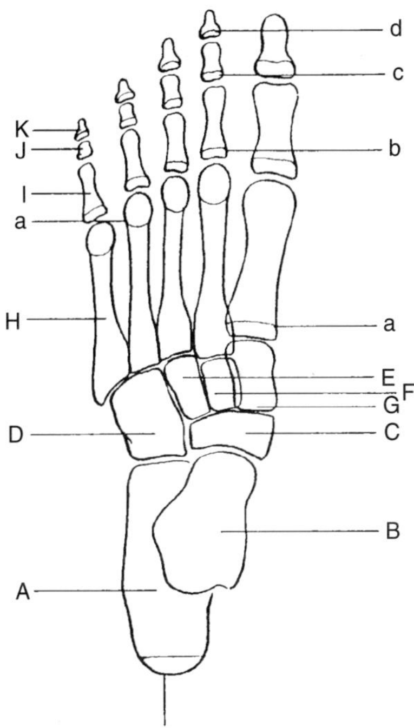

Figure A6 Ossification of bones of the foot. *A*, Calcaneus 6th fetal month. *B*, Talus 6th fetal month. *C*, Navicular 3–4 years. *D*, Cuboid at birth. *E*, Lateral cuneiform 1 year. *F*, Middle cuneiform 3 years. *G*, Medial cuneiform 3 years. *H*, Metatarsal shafts 8–9th fetal week. *I*, *J*, *K*, Phalangeal shafts 10th week.

a. Metatarsal epiphyses 3 years, fuse 17–20 years
b. Proximal phalangeal base 3 years, fuse 17–20 years
c. Middle phalangeal base 3 years, fuse 17–20 years
d. Distal phalangeal base 5 years, fuse 17–20 years
e. Posterior epiphysis of calcaneus 5th year, fuses at puberty.

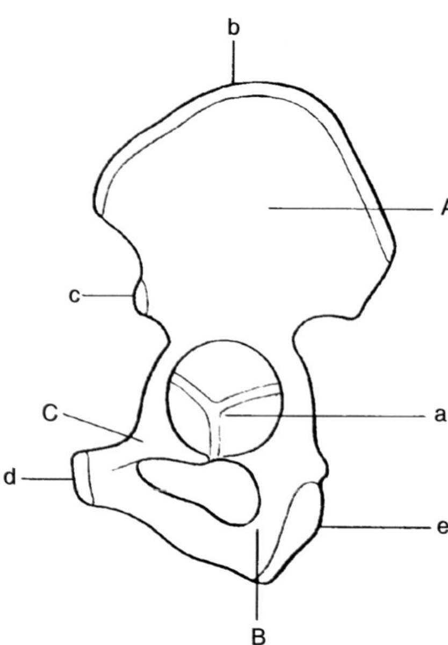

Figure A7 Ossification of bones of the pelvis. *A*, Ilium 3rd fetal month. *B*, Ischium 4th fetal month. *C*, Pubis 5th fetal month. *Note*: ischiopubic ramus fuses at 7th year.

a. Y-shaped cartilage—2 or more centres
b. Iliac crest
c. Anterior inferior iliac spine
d. Pubic symphysis
e. Ischial tuberosity.

} Appear about puberty—fuse 20–25 years.

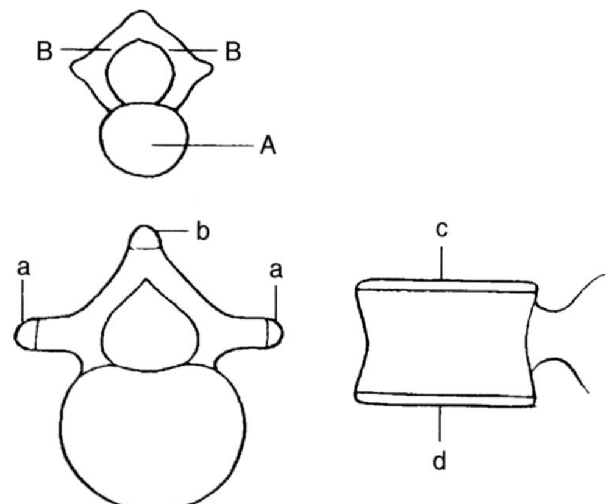

Figure A8 Ossification of vertebrae. *A*, Body 8th fetal week. *B*, Neural arch—one for each side—8th fetal week.

a. Transverse process
b. Spinous process
c. Upper surface of the body
d. Lower surface of the body

All appear at about 16 years and fuse by the 25th year.

Note:
Atlas: 3 centres; one for each lateral mass and one for the anterior arch—unite 6–8 years
Axis: 5 primary centres; one for the body, two for the arch, two for the odontoid process
2 secondary centres; one for the tip of the odontoid, one for the inferior rim of the body
7th Cervical vertebra: extra primary centre for each costal process
Lumbar vertebrae: have two extra secondary centres for the mamillary processes.

Detailed assessment of bone age is discussed in Greulich, W. W., Pyle, S. I. (1959) *Radiographic Atlas of Skeletal Development of the Hand and Wrist.* Stanford University Press.

Index

Note: Page number followed by *f*, *t* and *b* indicates figure, table and box respectively.

Q

R

U

V